D1591411

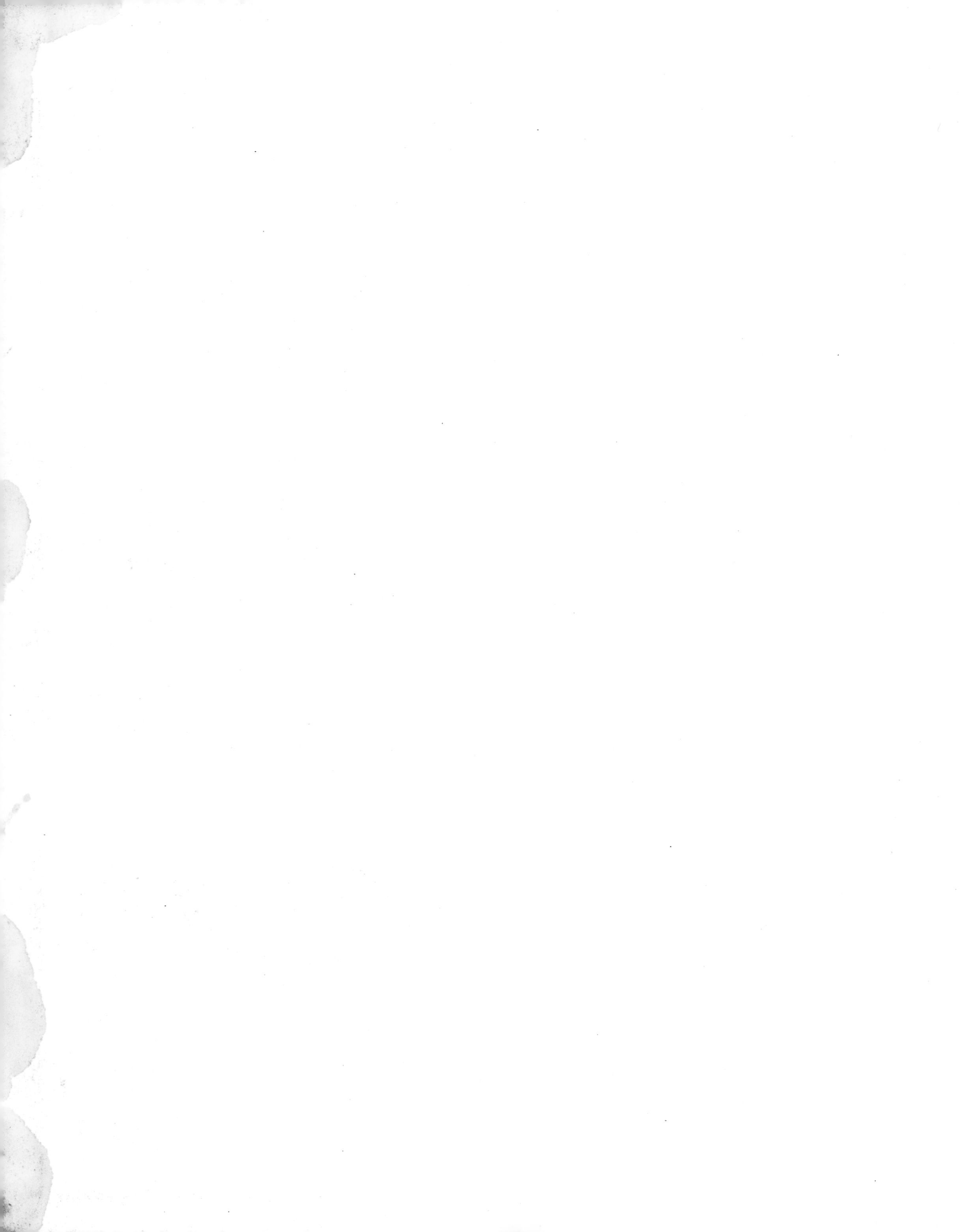

Elaine S. Jaffe, MD
Chief, Hematopathology Section
Laboratory of Pathology
Center for Cancer Research, National Cancer Institute
National Institutes of Health;
Clinical Professor of Pathology
George Washington University School of Medicine;
Series Editor, World Health Organization Classification of Tumours, 4th Edition
International Agency for Research on Cancer
Bethesda, Maryland

Nancy Lee Harris, MD
Editor, Case Records of the Massachusetts General Hospital
New England Journal of Medicine
Austin L. Vickery Professor of Pathology
Harvard Medical School;
Department of Pathology
Massachusetts General Hospital
Boston, Massachusetts

James W. Vardiman, MD
Professor and Director of Hematopathology
Department of Pathology
University of Chicago School of Medicine
Chicago, Illinois

Elias Campo, MD
Chief, Hematopathology Unit
Professor of Anatomic Pathology
Clinical Director, Center for Biomedical Diagnosis
Hospital Clinic, University of Barcelona
Barcelona, Spain

Daniel A. Arber, MD
Professor and Associate Chair of Pathology
Director of Anatomic Pathology and Clinical Laboratory Services
Stanford University
Stanford, California

Hematopathology

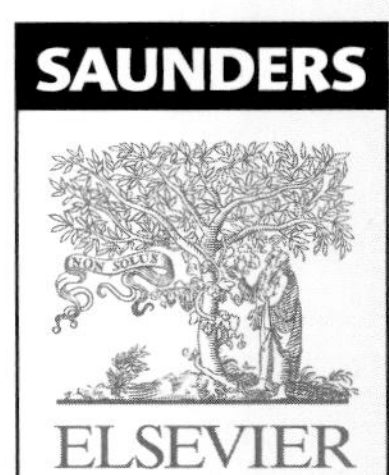

Saunders / Elsevier
Philadelphia, PA

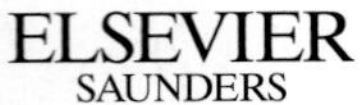

3251 Riverport Lane
St. Louis, Missouri 63043

Hematopathology
ISBN: 978-0-7216-0040-6

Notices

Knowledge and best practice in this field are constantly changing. As new research and experience broaden our understanding, changes in research methods, professional practices, or medical treatment may become necessary.

Practitioners and researchers must always rely on their own experience and knowledge in evaluating and using any information, methods, compounds, or experiments described herein. In using such information or methods they should be mindful of their own safety and the safety of others, including parties for whom they have a professional responsibility.

With respect to any drug or pharmaceutical products identified, readers are advised to check the most current information provided (i) on procedures featured or (ii) by the manufacturer of each product to be administered, to verify the recommended dose or formula, the method and duration of administration, and contraindications. It is the responsibility of practitioners, relying on their own experience and knowledge of their patients, to make diagnoses, to determine dosages and the best treatment for each individual patient, and to take all appropriate safety precautions.

To the fullest extent of the law, neither the Publisher nor the authors, contributors, or editors, assume any liability for any injury and/or damage to persons or property as a matter of products liability, negligence or otherwise, or from any use or operation of any methods, products, instructions, or ideas contained in the material herein.

Library of Congress Cataloging-in-Publication Data
Hematopathology / [edited by] Elaine S. Jaffe ... [et al.].—1st ed.
p. ; cm.
Includes bibliographical references.
ISBN 978-0-7216-0040-6
1. Blood—Pathophysiology. 2. Blood—Diseases—Diagnosis. 3. Hematology. I. Jaffe, Elaine Sarkin.
[DNLM: 1. Hematologic Diseases—pathology. 2. Lymphatic Diseases—pathology. WH 120 H48785 2011]
RB145.H429727 2011
616.1′5—dc22

2009046370

Acquisitions Editor: William Schmitt
Developmental Editor: Andrea Vosburgh
Publishing Services Manager: Debbie Vogel
Senior Project Manager: Jodi Kaye
Project Manager: Bridget Healy
Design Manager: Ellen Zanolle
Illustrations Manager: Mike Carcel

Printed in China

Last digit is the print number: 9 8 7 6 5 4 3 2 1

Contributors

Andrea Abati, MD
Dermatopathologist
Dermpath Diagnostics
Port Chester, New York;
Einstein College of Medicine
Bronx, New York

Daniel A. Arber, MD
Professor and Associate Chair of Pathology
Director of Anatomic Pathology and Clinical Laboratory Services
Stanford University
Stanford, California

Çiğdem Atayar, MD, PhD
Department of Pathology
University Medical Centre Groningen
Groningen, The Netherlands

Adam Bagg, MD
Professor, Director of Hematology
Department of Pathology and Laboratory Medicine
University of Pennsylvania;
Director of Hematology
Director, Minimal Residual Disease Resource Laboratory
Department of Pathology and Laboratory Medicine
Hospital of the University of Pennsylvania
Philadelphia, Pennsylvania

Barbara J. Bain, MBBS, FRACP, FRCPath
Professor, Department of Haematology
Imperial College;
Professor, Department of Haematology
St. Mary's Hospital
London, United Kingdom

Todd S. Barry, MD, PhD
Medical Director
Clarient
Aliso Viejo, California

Michael J. Borowitz, MD, PhD
Professor of Pathology and Oncology
Johns Hopkins Medical Institutions
Baltimore, Maryland

Pierre Brousset, MD
Department of Pathology
CHU Purpan;
Inserm U-563, Department of Oncogenesis and Signaling in Hematopoietic Cells
Centre de Physiopathologie de Toulouse-Purpan
Toulouse, France

Russell K. Brynes, MD
Professor of Pathology, Department of Pathology
University of Southern California Keck School of Medicine;
Director of Hematopathology, Department of Pathology
Los Angeles County-University of Southern California Medical Center
Los Angeles, California

Francisca I. Camacho, MD, PhD
Staff Pathologist, Department of Pathology
Hospital Universitario de Getafe;
Research Associate, Lymphoma Group, Molecular Pathology Program
Spanish National Cancer Research Centre
Madrid, Spain

Elias Campo, MD
Chief, Hematopathology Unit
Professor of Anatomic Pathology
Clinical Director, Center for Biomedical Diagnosis
Hospital Clinic, University of Barcelona
Barcelona, Spain

Ignacio Chacón
Molecular Pathology Program
Centro Nacional de Investigaciones Oncológicas
Madrid, Spain;
Hospital Virgen de la Salud
Toledo, Spain

R. S. K. Chaganti, PhD
Member and Professor, William E. Snee Chair
Medicine and Cell Biology Program
Memorial Sloan-Kettering Cancer Center
New York, New York

Alexander C. L. Chan, MBBS, FRCPA
Consultant Pathologist, Department of Pathology
Queen Elizabeth Hospital
Hong Kong, China

John K. C. Chan, MBBS, FRCPath
Consultant Pathologist, Department of Pathology
Queen Elizabeth Hospital
Hong Kong, China

Wing C. (John) Chan, MD
Amelia and Austin Vickery Professor of Pathology
Co-Director, Center for Lymphoma and Leukemia Research
University of Nebraska Medical Center
Omaha, Nebraska

Karen L. Chang, MD
Director of Clinical Pathology, Department of Pathology
City of Hope National Medical Center
Duarte, California

Wah Cheuk, MBBS, FRCPA
Associate Consultant, Department of Pathology
Queen Elizabeth Hospital
Hong Kong, China

Joseph M. Connors, MD
Clinical Professor and Clinical Director
Centre for Lymphoid Cancer
British Columbia Cancer Agency
University of British Columbia
Vancouver, British Columbia, Canada

Fiona E. Craig, MD
Associate Professor, Department of Pathology
University of Pittsburgh School of Medicine;
Staff Pathologist
Medical Director, Clinical Flow Cytometry Laboratory
Division of Hematopathology, Department of Pathology
University of Pittsburgh Medical Center, Presbyterian Hospital
Pittsburgh, Pennsylvania

Miguel Ángel de la Cruz Mora, MD
Head, Department of Medical Oncology
Hospital Virgen de la Salud
Toledo, Spain

Georges Delsol, MD
Professor of Pathology, Department of Anatomic Pathology
Université de Toulouse III - Paul Sabatier;
Professor of Pathology, Department of Anatomic Pathology
Chu Purpan
Toulouse, France

Miroslav Djokic, MD, MS
Assistant Professor, Department of Pathology
University of Pittsburgh School of Medicine;
Attending Pathologist, Department of Pathology, Hematopathology Division
University of Pittsburgh Medical Center, Presbyterian Hospital
Pittsburgh, Pennsylvania

Lyn McDivitt Duncan, MD
Associate Professor, Department of Pathology
Harvard Medical School;
Chief, Dermatopathology Unit, Pathology Service
Massachusetts General Hospital
Boston, Massachusetts

Kojo S. J. Elenitoba-Johnson, MD
Professor, Department of Pathology
University of Michigan Medical School;
Director, Division of Translational Pathology
Director, Molecular Diagnostics Laboratory and Molecular Genetic Pathology Program
University of Michigan Hospital
Ann Arbor, Michigan

Fabio Facchetti, MD, PhD
Professor of Pathology
Università degli Studi di Brescia;
Chief, Pathology I
Spedali Civili di Brescia
Brescia, Italy

Falko Fend, MD
Professor, Department of Pathology
University of Tuebingen;
Professor, Department of Pathology
University Hospital Tuebingen and Comprehensive Cancer Center Tuebingen
Tuebingen, Germany

Judith A. Ferry, MD
Associate Professor, Department of Pathology
Harvard Medical School;
Associate Pathologist, Department of Pathology
Massachusetts General Hospital
Boston, Massachusetts

Armando C. Filie, MD
Staff Clinician, Laboratory of Pathology
National Cancer Institute
Bethesda, Maryland

Kathryn Foucar, MD
Vice Chair for Clinical Affairs, Department of Pathology
University of New Mexico Health Sciences Center;
Medical Director of Hematopathology
TriCore Reference Laboratory
Albuquerque, New Mexico

Juan F. García, MD, PhD
Head, Department of Pathology
M. D. Anderson International
Madrid, Spain

Randy D. Gascoyne, MD, FRCPC
Clinical Professor of Pathology, Department of Pathology and Laboratory Medicine
University of British Columbia;
Hematopathologist and Senior Scientist, Department of Pathology and Advanced Therapeutics
British Columbia Cancer Agency and the British Columbia Cancer Research Centre
Vancouver, British Columbia, Canada

Philippe Gaulard, MD
Faculté de Médicine
Université Paris;
Département de Pathologie and Inserm U955
Hôpital Henri Mondor
Créteil, France

Timothy C. Greiner, MD
Professor, Hematopathology/Molecular Pathology
Department of Pathology and Microbiology
College of Medicine
University of Nebraska Medical Center;
Medical Director, Molecular Diagnostics Laboratory
Pathology Laboratories
The Nebraska Medical Center
Omaha, Nebraska

Katherine S. Hamilton, MD
Clinical Assistant Professor, Department of Pathology
Vanderbilt University Medical Center;
Staff Pathologist, Department of Pathology
St. Thomas Hospital
Nashville, Tennessee

Nancy Lee Harris, MD
Editor, Case Records of the Massachusetts General Hospital
New England Journal of Medicine;
Austin L. Vickery Professor of Pathology
Harvard Medical School;
Department of Pathology
Massachusetts General Hospital
Boston, Massachusetts

Robert P. Hasserjian, MD
Associate Professor
Harvard Medical School;
Associate Pathologist, Department of Pathology
Massachusetts General Hospital
Boston, Massachusetts

David R. Head, MD
Professor, Department of Pathology
Vanderbilt University Medical Center;
Pathologist, Clinical Laboratories
Vanderbilt University Hospital
Nashville, Tennessee

Amy Heerema-McKenney, MD
Clinical Assistant Professor, Department of Pathology
Stanford University Medical Center
Stanford, California

Hans-Peter Horny, MD
Professor of Pathology
Institute of Pathology
Ansbach, Bavaria, Germany

Jane Houldsworth, PhD
Senior Scientific Officer
Cancer Genetics, Incorporated
Rutherford, New Jersey

Eric D. Hsi, MD
Professor of Pathology
Cleveland Clinic Lerner College of Medicine;
Section Head, Hematopathology, Department of Clinical Pathology
Cleveland Clinic
Cleveland, Ohio

Robert E. Hutchison, MD
Professor, Department of Pathology
Director of Clinical Pathology
State University of New York Upstate Medical University
Syracuse, New York

Elizabeth Hyjek, MD, PhD
Department of Pathology, Hematopathology Section
University of Chicago
Chicago, Illinois

Peter G. Isaacson, FRS
Professor, Department of Pathology
University College London
London, United Kingdom

Elaine S. Jaffe, MD
Chief, Hematopathology Section
Laboratory of Pathology
National Cancer Institute
Bethesda, Maryland

Ronald Jaffe, MB BCh
Professor of Pathology
University of Pittsburgh School of Medicine;
Pathologist, Department of Pediatric Pathology
Childrens Hospital of Pittsburgh of University of Pittsburgh Medical Center
Pittsburgh, Pennsylvania

Pedro Jares, PhD
Specialist, Pathology Department
Hospital Clinic;
Scientific Manager, Genomics Unit
IDIBAPS
Barcelona, Spain

Dan Jones, MD, PhD
Professor, Department of Hematopathology
The University of Texas M. D. Anderson Cancer Center
Houston, Texas

Marshall E. Kadin, MD
Professor, Department of Dermatology
Boston University School of Medicine
Boston, Massachusetts;
Director, Cutaneous Lymphoma Program
Chief, Immunopathology, Department of Dermatology and Skin Surgery
Roger Williams Medical Center
Providence, Rhode Island

Young Hyeh Ko, MD, PhD
Professor, Department of Pathology
Samsung Medical Center, Sungkyunkwan University School of Medicine
Seoul, Republic of Korea

Steven H. Kroft, MD
Professor and Director of Hematopathology, Department of Pathology
Medical College of Wisconsin;
Director of Hematopathology, Department of Pathology
Froedtert Lutheran Memorial Hospital
Milwaukee, Wisconsin

Shimareet Kumar, MD
Quest Diagnostics Nichols Institute
Chantilly, Virginia;
Department of Pathology
Veterans Administration Medical Center
Washington, District of Columbia

Laurence Lamant-Rochaix, MD, PhD
Université Paul-Sabatier;
Laboratoire d'Anatomie Pathologique
CHU Purpan;
Inserm, Oncogenèse et Signalisation dans les Cellules Hematopoïétiques
Centre de Physiopathologie de Toulouse-Purpan
Toulouse, France

Philip E. LeBoit, MD
Professor, Departments of Pathology and Dermatology
University of California, San Francisco
San Francisco, California

Laurence de Leval, MD, PhD
Professor, Department of Pathology
University of Lausanne;
Head of Surgical Pathology, Department of Pathology
Institut Universitaire de Pathologie
Lausanne, Switzerland

Megan S. Lim, MD, PhD
Associate Professor, Department of Pathology
University of Michigan Medical School;
Director, Hematopathology
University of Michigan Hospital
Ann Arbor, Michigan

Robert W. McKenna, MD
Vice Chair for Academic Affairs and Senior Consultant in Hematopathology
Department of Laboratory Medicine and Pathology
Fairview University Hospital
University of Minnesota
Minneapolis, Minnesota

L. Jeffrey Medeiros, MD
Professor, Department of Hematopathology
University of Texas, M.D. Anderson Cancer Center
Houston, Texas

Manuela Mollejo, MD
Department of Pathology
Hospital Virgen de la Salud
Toledo, Spain

Karen Dyer Montgomery, PhD, FACMG
Laboratory Director, Cytogenetics
WiCell Research Institute;
Adjunct Associate Professor, Department of Pathology
University of Wisconsin
Madison, Wisconsin

Gouri Nanjangud, PhD
Senior Research Scientist, Cell Biology Program
Memorial Sloan-Kettering Cancer Center
New York, New York

Yasodha Natkunam, MD, PhD
Associate Professor, Department of Pathology
Stanford University School of Medicine;
Director, Hematopathology
Stanford University Medical Center
Stanford, California

Beverly P. Nelson, MD
Associate Professor, Department of Pathology
Northwestern University Feinberg School of Medicine
Chicago, Illinois

Phuong L. Nguyen, MD
Associate Professor, Department of Laboratory Medicine and Pathology
Mayo Clinic College of Medicine;
Consultant, Department of Laboratory Medicine and Pathology
Mayo Clinic
Rochester, Minnesota

Dennis P. O'Malley, MD
Hematopathologist
Clarient, Inc.
Aliso Viejo, California

Attilio Orazi, MD, FRCPath(Engl)
Professor of Pathology and Laboratory Medicine
Vice-Chair for Hematopathology
Director, Division of Hematopathology, Department of Pathology and Laboratory Medicine
Weill Medical College of Cornell University
New York, New York

German Ott, MD
Professor
Institute of Pathology
Robert-Bosch-Krankenhaus
Stuttgart, Germany

Nallasivam Palanisamy, PhD
Research Assistant Professor
Michigan Center for Translational Pathology
University of Michigan Health System Comprehensive Cancer Center
Ann Arbor, Michigan

LoAnn C. Peterson, MD
Paul E. Steiner Research Professor of Pathology, Department of Pathology
Feinberg Medical School of Northwestern University;
Director of Hematopathology, Department of Pathology
Northwestern Memorial Hospital
Chicago, Illinois

Miguel A. Piris, MD
Director, Molecular Pathology Program
Spanish National Cancer Research Centre
Madrid, Spain

Stefania Pittaluga
Staff Clinican, Laboratory of Pathology, Hematopathology
National Institutes of Health, National Cancer Institute
Bethesda, Maryland

Sibrand Poppema, MD, PhD, FRCPC
President of the Board of the University
University of Groningen;
Professor of Pathology, Department of Pathology
University Medical Center Groningen
Groningen, The Netherlands

Anna Porwit, MD, PhD
Professor, Depatment of Oncology and Pathology
Karolinska Institute;
Chief, Hematopathology Laboratory, Department of Pathology
Karolinska University Hospital, Solna
Stockholm, Sweden

Priv.Doz.Dr. Leticia Quintanilla-Martinez, MD
Associate Professor Institute of Pathology
Eberhard-Karls-University;
Senior Staff, Institute of Pathology
University Hospital and Comprehensive Cancer Center
Tübingen, Germany

Frederick Karl Racke, MD, PhD
Associate Professor, Department of Pathology
The Ohio State University
Columbus, Ohio

Mark Raffeld, MD
Chief, Specialized Diagnostics Unit
Laboratory of Pathology
National Cancer Institute, National Institutes of Health
Bethesda, Maryland

Elisabeth Ralfkiaer, MDSc
Professor, Department of Pathology
Rigshospitalet
University of Copenhagen
Copenhagen, Denmark

Sherif A. Rezk, MD
Assistant Professor of Clinical Pathology
Division of Hematopathology, Department of Pathology
University of California, Irvine Medical Center
Orange, California

Nancy S. Rosenthal, MD
Walter Beirring Professor of Clinical Education, Department of Pathology
University of Iowa Carver College of Medicine;
Director of Hematopathology, Department of Pathology
University of Iowa Hospitals and Clinics
Iowa City, Iowa

Jonathan Said, MD
Professor and Chief of Anatomic Pathology, Department of Pathology and Laboratory Medicine
University of California, Los Angeles David Geffen School of Medicine
Los Angeles, California

Bertram Schnitzer, MD
Professor, Department of Pathology
University of Michigan Health System
Ann Arbor, Michigan

Reiner Siebert, Prof. Dr. med.
Full Professor and Chair of Human Genetics
Institute of Human Genetics
Christian-Albrechts-University Kiel;
Director, Institute of Human Genetics
University Hospital Schleswig Holstein, Campus Kiel
Kiel, Germany

Karl Sotlar, MD
Professor of Pathology
Institute of Pathology
Ludwig Maximilians University Munich
Munich, Germany

Maryalice Stetler-Stevenson, PhD, MD
Director, Flow Cytometry Laboratory
Laboratory of Pathology
National Cancer Institute, National Institutes of Health
Bethesda, Maryland

John L. Sullivan, MD
Professor of Pediatrics and Molecular Medicine
Vice Provost for Research
Department of Molecular Medicine
University of Massachusetts Medical School;
Physician, Department of Pediatrics
University of Massachusetts Memorial Health Care
Worcester, Massachusetts

Steven H. Swerdlow, MD
Professor of Pathology
Director, Division of Hematopathology, Department of Pathology
University of Pittsburgh School of Medicine
University of Pittsburgh Medical Center
Pittsburgh, Pennsylvania

Peter Valent, MD
Professor, Division of Hematology and Hemostaseology, Department of Internal Medicine I
Medical University of Vienna
Vienna, Austria

James W. Vardiman, MD
Professor and Director of Hematopathology, Department of Pathology
University of Chicago School of Medicine
Chicago, Illinois

David S. Viswanatha, MD
Consultant and Associate Professor, Division of Hematopathology
Mayo Clinic
Rochester, Minnesota

Roger A. Warnke, MD
Professor of Pathology, Department of Pathology
Stanford University School of Medicine
Stanford, California

Edward G. Weir, MD
Clinical Pathologist, Division of Hematopathology
Clinical Pathology Laboratories
Austin, Texas

Lawrence M. Weiss, MD
Chairman, Department of Pathology
City of Hope
Duarte, California

Carla S. Wilson, MD, PhD
Professor, Department of Pathology
University of New Mexico Health Sciences Center;
Medical Director, Flow Cytometry Laboratory
Tricore Reference Laboratories
Albuquerque, New Mexico

Bruce A. Woda, MD
Professor and Vice Chairman, Department of Pathology
University of Massachusetts Medical School;
Chief, Anatomic Pathology
University of Massachusetts Memorial Medical Center
Worcester, Massachusetts

Constance M. Yuan, PhD, MD
Staff Clinician, Flow Cytometry Unit
Laboratory of Pathology, National Cancer Institute
National Institutes of Health
Bethesda, Maryland

Fan Zhou, MD, PhD
Staff Pathologist, Department of Pathology and Laboratory Medicine
Southwest Washington Medical Center
Vancouver, Washington

Preface

Hematopathology is a discipline in which the traditional methods of clinical and morphologic analysis are interwoven with newer, biologically based studies to achieve an accurate diagnosis. Studies of hematologic malignancies have been at the forefront in applying the principles of basic research to the understanding of human disease. All cancers are increasingly recognized as genetic diseases, with precise genetic alterations often defining entities. Advances in immunologic and molecular genetic technology have rapidly migrated to the clinical laboratory, where they play a role in routine diagnosis. The authors and editors embrace this new technology. Indeed, it is only possible to understand the histopathologic spectrum of disease if one has an appreciation for the underlying biology and the varied functions of the cells encountered in lymph nodes and bone marrow. The reader will find that the discussion of each disease includes both a description of morphologic features and relevant immunophenotypic, genetic, and clinical features. These data inform our understanding of disease pathogenesis, and provide valuable and often critical adjuncts to diagnosis. The goal is to provide concise, up-to-date, and practical information that is easy for the reader to access.

Pathologic diagnosis cannot occur in a vacuum, and the pathologist must understand the key clinical characteristics of the diseases being considered in the differential. Therefore, discussion of each disease includes a description of expected clinical features at the time of diagnosis, including signs, symptoms, and relevant staging procedures. Chapters dealing with neoplastic disorders incorporate a discussion of patterns of spread, relapse, and prognostic factors.

We hope that this book will be of value to hematologists and oncologists, in addition to pathologists. It is increasingly important that clinicians be aware of basic principles of hematopathology diagnosis; hematologists and hematopathologists must work as a team to achieve the correct diagnosis. Just as the pathologist must use clinical data to make an accurate diagnosis, the clinician should have sufficient knowledge of diagnostic principles to appreciate when the pathological diagnosis just doesn't quite fit.

The use of correct technique is critical in producing a lymph node or bone marrow biopsy specimen that is suitable for accurate diagnosis. Many diagnostic errors stem from poor technique related to fixation, processing, cutting, or staining. The first section of this book deals with technical aspects in the processing of lymph node and bone marrow specimens. While the use of fine needle aspiration for primary diagnosis is controversial, it is critical to be aware of how this diagnostic tool can be used, as well as of its limitations. Thus, a chapter is devoted to this topic. Finally, several chapters deal with the implementation of techniques used in hematopathologic diagnosis, including immunohistochemistry, flow cytometry, molecular genetic techniques in diagnosis, and both classical and interphase cytogenetics.

A discussion of hematologic malignancies derived from myeloid, lymphoid, histiocytic, and dendritic cells represents a major feature of this book. Equally relevant to the diagnostic pathologist is an appreciation of the spectrum of reactive and inflammatory lesions of hematolymphoid tissues occurring in immunocompetent patients as well as those with disimmunity. Thus, the reader will find a discussion of reactive lymphadenopathies and primary and iatrogenic immunodeficiency disorders. Further chapters deal with the bone marrow response to inflammatory, infectious, and metabolic diseases, the findings in a number of inherited and congenital disorders that affect hematopoiesis, and the impact of therapy on bone marrow morphology. Finally, we also include some nonhematopoietic lesions that may be encountered in lymph nodes or bone marrow that are important in differential diagnosis.

The reader will find that most of the chapters deal with a specific disease entity or a group of related diseases. Several key tables have been included in each chapter to facilitate use and access to key facts. These include: major diagnostic features, differential diagnosis, and pearls and pitfalls. The book is generously illustrated, and the consistent use of color photography throughout should make it easy to appreciate key diagnostic features.

The editors appreciate that the reader needs to have access to key source material and that a richly referenced book provides important information for those who wish to delve further into the topic. The scientific literature is voluminous, and we feel it is important to include older historical references as well as the most recent scientific data. Because we increasingly access the medical literature through electronic media, we and the publishers have elected to include the references only on the Expert Consult website for the book. We believe that this minor inconvenience will be outweighed by electronic access to the PubMed links instantaneously, with of course the ability to further research the topic and identify new key references as they appear.

This book has had a long gestation, with the first discussions beginning more than 10 years ago. The editors envisioned a book that would be both practical and accessible but also contain the scientific insights that we feel are critical to understanding pathogenesis and pathophysiology of hematolymphoid disorders. Starts and stops occurred along the way, as both editors and authors were distracted by new scientific developments and the need to create an updated World Health Organization classification of neoplasms of hematopoietic and lymphoid tissues. We believe that the product has met our expectations for an up-to-date and comprehensive text on diagnostic hematopathology, and we hope it meets yours as well. We thank the many authors who both adhered to deadlines and responded to our aims for the book. We hope this book will prove to be a constant and valued resource for pathologists and clinicians dealing with hematologic diseases, and that it will ultimately benefit the patients and their families.

Elaine S. Jaffe, MD

Nancy Lee Harris, MD

James W. Vardiman, MD

Elias Campo, MD

Daniel A. Arber, MD

Contents

PART I
Technical Aspects

PART II
Normal and Reactive Conditions of Hematopoietic Tissues

PART III
Lymphoid Neoplasms

PART VII
Site-Specific Issues in the Diagnosis of Lymphoma and Leukemia

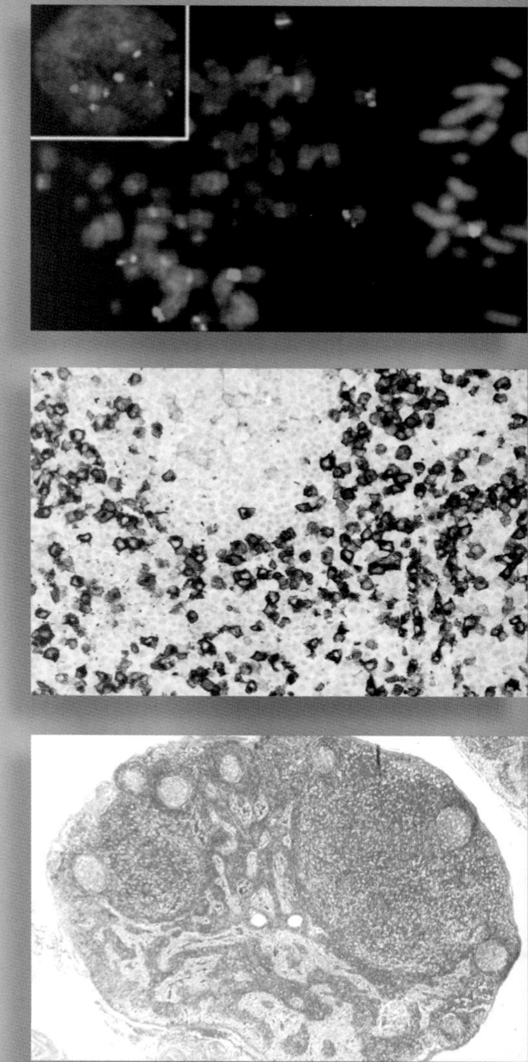

PART I

Technical Aspects

Chapter 1

Processing of the Lymph Node Biopsy Specimen

Yasodha Natkunam and Roger A. Warnke

CHAPTER OUTLINE

In recent years, technical strides in immunophenotyping and molecular genetic testing have revolutionized the diagnosis of hematolymphoid malignancies. Stained sections prepared from paraffin-embedded fixed tissues remain the foundation of histopathologic diagnosis. The accurate classification of lymphoid tumors and the subsequent clinical management of patients rely on the availability of adequate diagnostic tissue. A multiparameter approach to diagnosis is central to the World Health Organization (WHO) and the Revised European American Lymphoma (REAL) classification schemes of hematolymphoid tumors.[1,2] This approach emphasizes the integration of clinical and ancillary data in the formulation of a precise diagnosis. An inadequate lymph node biopsy specimen not only precludes accurate morphologic assessment but also compromises immunophenotypic, cytogenetic, and molecular diagnostic studies. When this first step in making a diagnosis is jeopardized, even the most sophisticated DNA and RNA amplification techniques may not salvage enough information for a definitive diagnosis, and a repeat procedure may be necessary. With the current mandate to provide cost-effective health care, and with mounting pressure to make diagnoses based on needle aspirations and cytologic preparations, repeating an open lymph node biopsy procedure is not trivial. Thus, it is imperative that the pathologist ensure the optimal procurement and processing of lymph node specimens.

The lymph node presents certain unique challenges for the pathologist and the histotechnologist because of its innate organizational structure. The lymph node is composed of millions of small cells held together by fine strands of connective tissue surrounded by a fibrous capsule that is relatively impervious to fixation and processing chemicals. Histologic sections of excellent quality can be obtained only if each step in the processing of a lymph node is handled with care and with knowledge of the underlying factors that result in optimal versus suboptimal preparations. This chapter reviews the essential steps for producing excellent-quality histologic sections of lymph node specimens, discusses the common pitfalls, and suggests how to avoid or correct these errors.

INSTRUCTIONS FOR THE SURGEON

Knowledge of the patient's clinical history and the suspected diagnosis or differential diagnosis facilitates the search for a lymph node sample that best represents the underlying pathologic process. Despite the obvious appeal of convenient access, minimal discomfort, and procedural simplicity of excising a superficial lymph node, these lymph nodes are not always of diagnostic value. The surgeon should be encouraged to examine the patient thoroughly and sample the largest and most abnormal-appearing lymph node whenever possible (Fig. 1-1). This approach avoids the erroneous sampling of enlarged or inflamed nodes adjacent to a previous biopsy site and enables more representative sampling. Imaging studies may help guide the surgeon to the most abnormal lymph node.

Excisional biopsy of an entire lymph node is preferred to an incisional or needle core biopsy because fragments of lymph nodes preclude a proper assessment of architecture, an important feature in establishing a morphologic differential diagnosis. When an infectious cause is suspected, the surgeon should be advised to submit a portion from one pole of the lymph node for appropriate microbiologic studies directly from the sterile environment of the operating room. In all other circumstances, the intact specimen should be submitted fresh to the pathologist in a specimen container and immersed in saline or culture medium to ensure that the specimen does

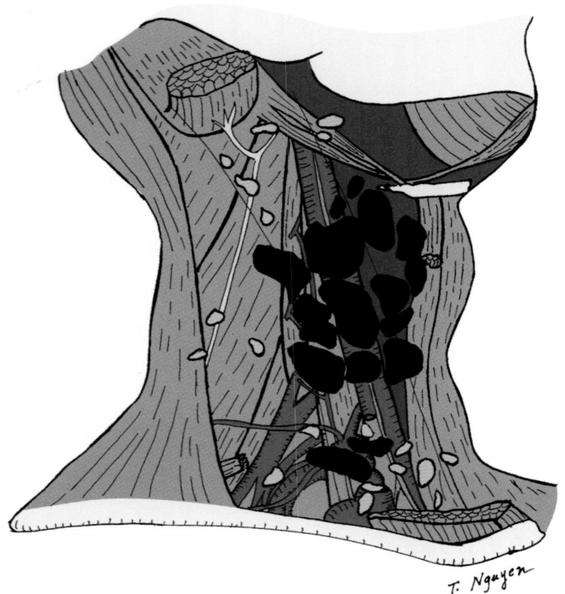

Figure 1-1. Selection of a lymph node for biopsy. Diagram of a neck dissection for Hodgkin's lymphoma, showing the distribution of positive (*black*) and negative (*tan*) lymph nodes. Many of the most superficial and easily biopsied nodes are either benign or only atypical, whereas the diagnostic nodes are deeper, larger, and less accessible. This experience illustrates the need to remove the largest possible lymph node for diagnosis, because it is most likely to contain diagnostic tissue. (Redrawn by Dr. TuDong Nguyen, Stanford University Medical Center, Stanford, CA, from Slaughter DP, Economou SG, Southwick HW. Surgical management of Hodgkin's disease. *Ann Surg.* 1958;148:705-709.)

not dry out during transit. Wrapping the specimen or laying it on gauze, sponges, or towels should be avoided because this leads to desiccation of the lymph node cortex, especially when the specimen is exposed to air. Request for a "lymph node workup" should be clearly indicated on the requisition slip or specimen tag, or both. Ideally, the pathologist should be notified at the time of the biopsy to avoid a delay in the handling of the specimen. When a delay in delivery to the pathologist is anticipated, the specimen should be refrigerated to minimize autolysis. Storage at 4°C for up to 24 hours can yield satisfactory but not optimal morphologic, immunologic, and genetic preservation.[1,3-10] When long delays are expected before the pathologist receives the specimen, the surgeon may be instructed to bisect the lymph node and make air-dried imprints, after which the specimen can be sliced thinly and placed in buffered formalin. Portions should also be set aside for special studies.

GROSS PROCESSING OF THE LYMPH NODE BIOPSY BY THE PATHOLOGIST

Gross Examination

The gross appearance of lymph nodes, including their color, consistency, and changes in contour, may provide useful information about the diagnosis and should be recorded during the gross inspection of the fresh specimen (Fig. 1-2). Preservation of the hilus and the presence or absence of nodularity and fibrosis can offer important diagnostic clues.[1,6,7] Preservation of the hilus is rare in lymphomas, and its presence suggests a reactive process (see Fig. 1-2A and B). Necrosis within the node raises the possibility of an infectious process and may prompt microbiologic studies. Adherence of the node to the surrounding fat may denote extracapsular extension of disease and should be noted in the gross description. Most lymphomas completely efface the nodal architecture, and a nodular appearance or fibrosis can be seen on gross examination (see Fig. 1-2C to E).

Although the gross findings can be helpful in narrowing the differential diagnosis, an accurate pathologic diagnosis is virtually never possible based on the gross findings alone. Thus, these findings must be interpreted in conjunction with microscopic features and immunophenotypic and genetic studies to establish a definitive diagnosis.

Frozen Sections

The diagnosis of lymphoid malignancies can be challenging even on permanent sections. Because of the numerous artifacts generated during the preparation of a frozen section, a diagnosis of lymphoma based on frozen tissue is perilous and best avoided.[1,6-9] Although certain lymphomas can be distinguished on frozen sections, clinical colleagues should be advised of the unreliability of frozen sections for the accurate diagnosis and classification of lymphoma. In the rare event that a rapid interpretation is necessary for patient care, touch imprints or scrape preparations should be examined in conjunction with frozen sections. Imprints yield cytologic details that may not be appreciated on frozen tissue sections; for example, Reed-Sternberg cells may be more readily apparent on imprints than on frozen tissue sections. Even if diagnostic cells are identified on imprints or frozen sections, caution is necessary in the diagnosis of Hodgkin's lymphoma, because atypical cells with Reed-Sternberg cell–like morphology may be present in infectious mononucleosis, posttransplant lymphoproliferative disorders, diffuse large B-cell or anaplastic large cell lymphoma, poorly differentiated carcinoma, sarcoma, melanoma, and fat necrosis.[1,11]

The appropriate use of frozen sections of lymph node biopsy specimens is to estimate the adequacy of the tissue for diagnosis. Frozen sections also offer the pathologist the opportunity to allocate tissue for ancillary studies based on the preliminary differential diagnosis.[1,7-9,12] The frozen portion of the node should always be retained frozen for future immunophenotypic or molecular studies. In addition, microbiologic, cytogenetic, or flow cytometry studies can be initiated rapidly, with optimal preservation of cell viability. If the changes seen on frozen sections suggest a reactive process in a patient in whom there is a strong clinical suspicion of lymphoma, the surgeon can be advised to explore the patient further to find a more abnormal lymph node.

Cytologic Preparations

The utility of imprints in the evaluation of lymphoid lesions should not be underestimated. Cytologic imprint preparations complement tissue diagnosis and are useful both at the time of frozen section and when examining permanent tissue sections. Touch and scrape imprints are encouraged for all intraoperative consultations for lymphoid lesions and should be examined in conjunction with the frozen tissue sections.

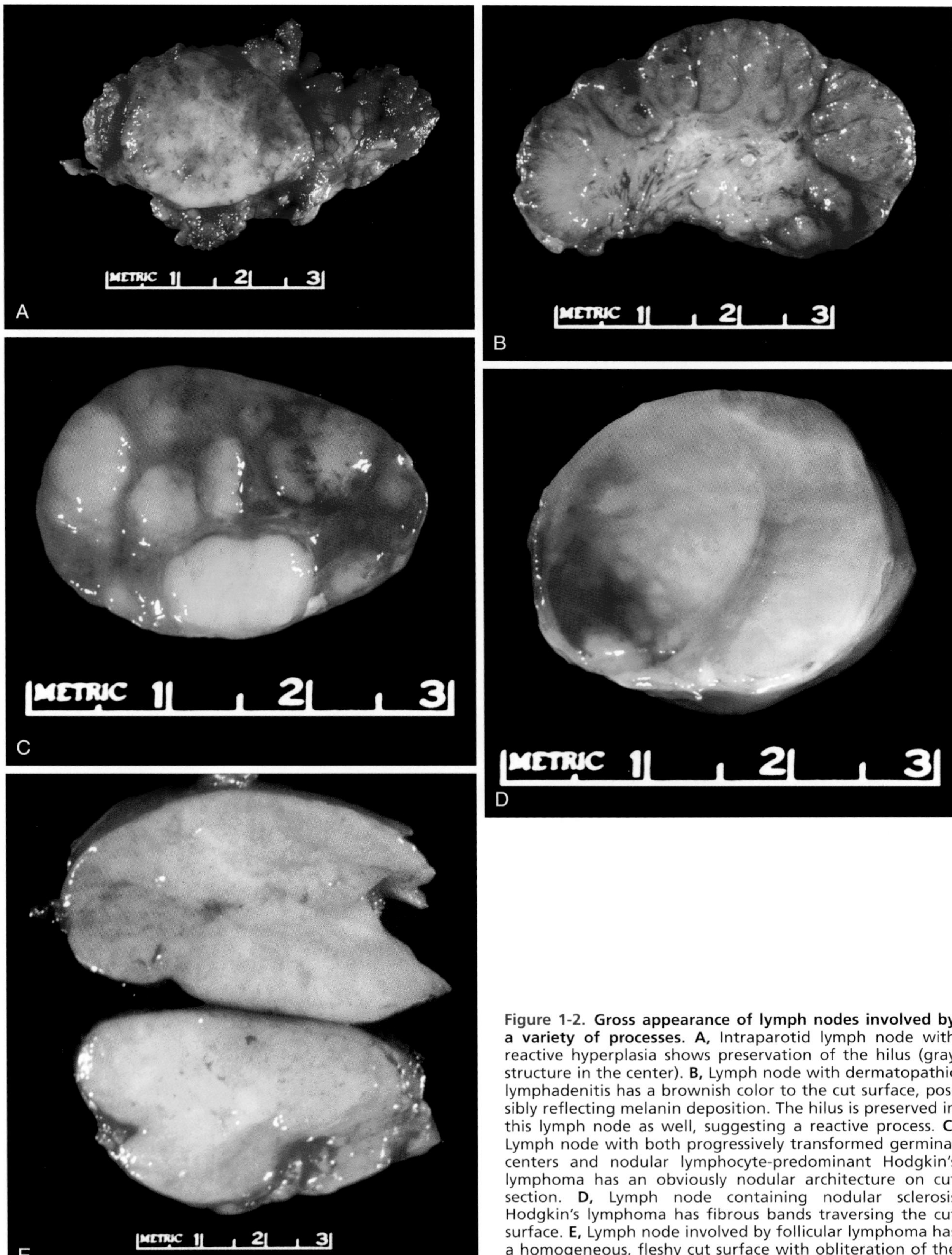

Figure 1-2. **Gross appearance of lymph nodes involved by a variety of processes. A,** Intraparotid lymph node with reactive hyperplasia shows preservation of the hilus (gray structure in the center). **B,** Lymph node with dermatopathic lymphadenitis has a brownish color to the cut surface, possibly reflecting melanin deposition. The hilus is preserved in this lymph node as well, suggesting a reactive process. **C,** Lymph node with both progressively transformed germinal centers and nodular lymphocyte-predominant Hodgkin's lymphoma has an obviously nodular architecture on cut section. **D,** Lymph node containing nodular sclerosis Hodgkin's lymphoma has fibrous bands traversing the cut surface. **E,** Lymph node involved by follicular lymphoma has a homogeneous, fleshy cut surface with obliteration of the hilus, which is typical of lymphomatous involvement.

Most important, imprints can be stored at 4°C for days to weeks or frozen at −70°C indefinitely and used for selected immunophenotypic studies or fluorescence in situ hybridization (FISH) analysis.[6,9,12] Imprints can also facilitate the intraoperative assessment of hematolymphoid lesions of bone when frozen sections cannot be obtained.

When preparing cytologic imprints from lymph node specimens, it is best to prepare and label six to eight slides ahead of time. For touch imprints, the cut surface of the lymph node should be positioned on a flat surface such as a towel. While holding the slide firmly at one end, the slide is gently lowered and brought into contact with the cut surface of the node, avoiding smearing or sideways movement. This process can be repeated three to five times, creating a series of touch imprint slides. The imprint slide should immediately be placed in a Coplin jar with 95% alcohol. Buffered formalin or formaldehyde can also be used as a fixative. A few imprint slides may be air-dried. For scrape preparations, the fresh-cut surface of the lymph node is gently scraped with the edge of a slide or the blunt edge of a scalpel and immediately smeared onto a previously labeled slide. Alcohol- and air-dried slides can be generated as for touch imprints. Although there is almost always enough material available to make touch imprints, scrape preparations are best avoided when dealing with very small samples to prevent inadvertent crushing or distortion of the tissue.

A Wright-Giemsa or Diff-Quik stain is best for identifying and characterizing cells of the hematopoietic system and tumors derived from them. However, the Papanicolaou stain is useful for assessing nuclear details such as membrane irregularity, chromatin configuration, and nucleoli. When necrosis and inflammatory cells are present, a Gram stain can be helpful to highlight bacterial organisms. In general, aspirations of lymph nodes are highly cellular and are characterized by a dispersed cell pattern and lymphoglandular bodies (detached cytoplasmic fragments of lymphoid cells). Indolent lymphomas composed of predominantly small cells or a mixed cellular milieu are much more difficult to diagnose on cytologic preparations than are aggressive lymphomas (Fig. 1-3A).[11] Reactive follicular hyperplasia can be nearly impossible to distinguish from follicular lymphoma on cytologic imprints, although the presence of a limited range of maturation together with the absence of tingible body macrophages favors a malignant diagnosis. In aggressive lymphomas, the presence of monotonous sheets of medium to large cells, especially when associated with karyorrhexis and apoptosis, suggests the differential diagnosis of lymphoblastic, Burkitt's, or large cell lymphoma (see Fig. 1-3B). Similarly, imprints can be helpful in highlighting Reed-Sternberg cells (see Fig. 1-3C) or immunoblastic features in diffuse large B-cell lymphoma (see Fig. 1-3D).[1,11] Cytologic preparations can also be useful in the diagnosis of metastatic melanoma and carcinoma (see Fig. 1-3E and F) and of nonneoplastic lesions in the lymph node such as granulomatous lymphadenitis and Kikuchi's lymphadenitis. Lesions associated with significant sclerosis seldom yield sufficient material for cytologic preparations.[1,9,11]

Sectioning

The two most important initial steps in the processing of a lymph node specimen are sectioning (blocking) and fixation. These steps are entirely the responsibility of the pathologist. Blocking should be performed promptly and should precede fixation because an intact lymph node capsule is impervious to fixation. In addition, touch and scrape imprints are best obtained in the fresh state. The objective of good sectioning of a lymph node is to provide an undisrupted section that maintains the overall architecture of the tissue intact and is thin enough to yield significant cytologic detail. Sections should also preserve the relationship between the capsule and the remainder of the lymphoid compartments (Fig. 1-4). The best cross section of a lymph node results from sectioning perpendicular to the long axis of the node with a sharp knife in one continuous sweep. This technique facilitates excellent preservation of the nodal architecture. For lymph nodes less than 1 cm in diameter, a single cut along the long axis is recommended; such small specimens may be crushed when attempting to perform cross sections perpendicular to the long axis. The entire specimen should be sectioned in 2- to 3-mm slices and then placed promptly in fixative. Portions of lymph nodes should never be left unfixed or fixed without slicing. Because the fibrous tissue in the capsule may contract when exposed to fixatives, scoring of the capsule by introducing small cuts with a sharp scalpel blade may prevent distortion during processing (see Fig. 1-4A). When lymph node specimens are fixed whole or when the central portion of the section is too thick, uneven fixation results (Fig. 1-5). This may lead to autolysis of the central areas or retraction of the tissue, causing erosion or cracking of the sections upon cutting with a microtome blade.[1,7-9,13-16]

Thin slices of 2 to 3 mm should be placed in shallow-profile plastic cassettes (used in most modern surgical pathology laboratories) to allow adequate penetration by fixation and processing reagents. Thorough—if not complete—sampling of the lymph node specimen is essential. This practice prevents sampling errors in disorders that may only partially involve the lymph node, such as nodular lymphocyte–predominant Hodgkin's lymphoma in patients with progressive transformation of germinal centers and in cases of variations in grade or focal progression of a low-grade lymphoma such as follicular lymphoma. Under most circumstances, once portions of the lymph node specimen have been removed for ancillary studies, the specimen is small enough to be submitted entirely in a few cassettes. When multiple lymph nodes are submitted or when a lymph node is so large that 10 or more cassettes are required to submit the entire specimen, knowledge of the clinical differential diagnosis and good gross examination skills are helpful. Multiple sections at 2- to 3-mm intervals should be made throughout the specimen, and sections from various portions should be submitted. It is always preferable to err on the side of submitting too much adequately fixed tissue rather than not having enough to establish a definitive diagnosis or to perform ancillary studies. In any lymph node biopsy in which microscopic examination of the initially submitted sections does not yield a definitive diagnosis, all the remaining tissue should be promptly submitted for microscopic examination.

Fixation

Fixation is the point of no return in the processing of a lymph node specimen. Although subsequent steps, including infiltration, clearing, and dehydration, can be repeated if neces-

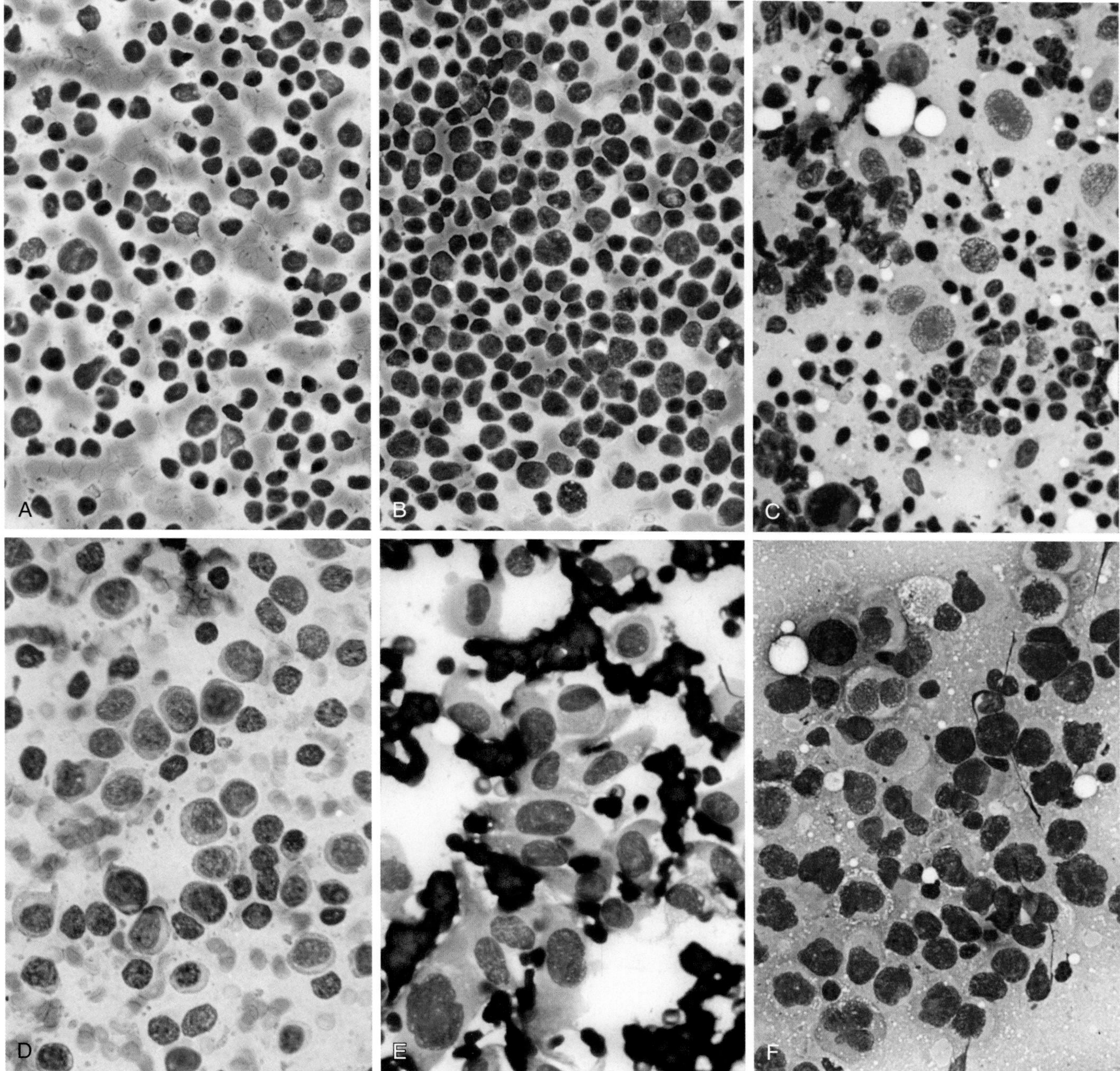

Figure 1-3. Cytologic preparations of low-grade B-cell lymphoma (**A**), lymphoblastic lymphoma (**B**), Hodgkin's lymphoma (**C**), diffuse large B-cell lymphoma with prominent immunoblastic features (**D**), metastatic melanoma (**E**), and metastatic poorly differentiated carcinoma of unknown primary site (**F**).

sary, inadequate fixation cannot be reversed. Poor fixation is the leading cause of uninterpretable lymph node sections.[1,7-9,13-15] Both histotechnologists and pathologists may waste valuable time attempting to reprocess poorly fixed specimens, obtaining special or ancillary studies that may not be necessary, and seeking expert consultation to establish or confirm a diagnosis.

Excellent-quality slides can be prepared from lymph node specimens using a number of different fixatives, as long as the proper volume and strength of fixative are used and, most important, adequate time is allowed for fixation. The advantages and disadvantages of the most commonly used fixatives for lymph node specimens are outlined in Table 1-1. Many laboratories use a combination of neutral buffered formalin and a metal-based fixative; one or two slices are fixed in a metal-based fixative for speed of fixation and optimal morphology, and the remainder are fixed in formalin for preservation of DNA and long-term storage. Although pathologists' preferences for metal fixatives vary, B5 neutral Zenker's solution and zinc sulfate formalin are the most commonly used. Although B5 renders excellent nuclear detail (Fig. 1-6), several factors make its routine use problematic. These include the

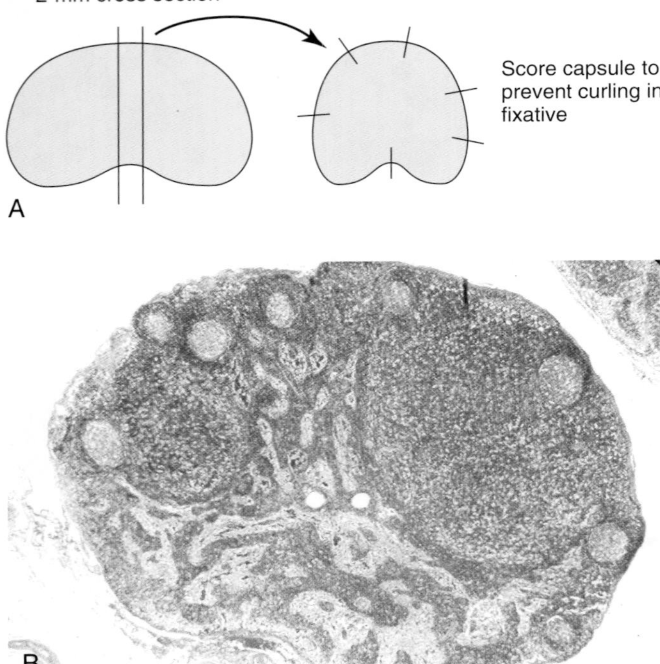

Figure 1-4. Lymph node sectioning. Lymph nodes should be sectioned to provide a complete cross section that allows an appreciation of architecture. **A**, Schematic diagram shows that the lymph node is cut perpendicular to the long axis of the node (best for specimens >1 cm in diameter). The lymph node capsule can be scored, using several small cuts, before placing the section in fixative; this prevents curling as the capsule retracts on exposure to fixative. **B**, Low-power photomicrograph of a properly oriented section of lymph node showing the capsule, cortex, paracortex, and medulla.

relatively high cost, the time-sensitive nature of fixation (2 to 4 hours), and the need to remove mercuric chloride crystals from the sections and dispose of the mercury, an environmental hazard. Zinc sulfate (available commercially as B+ from Biochemicals Corp./BBC, Loveland, OH) is an alternative to B5; it offers good nuclear detail, is less costly, and requires no special procedures for handling and disposal because it contains no mercuric chloride. Fixatives that are highly acidic, such as Zenker's, B5, Bouin's, and Carnoy's, are unsuitable for molecular diagnostic studies because they compromise the efficiency of polymerase chain reaction (PCR) amplification by decreasing the ability of the DNA within tissue to function as a template for the amplification of DNA fragments of desirable length. The best fixatives for molecular diagnostic studies are ethanol, acetone, and Omnifix (FR Chemicals, Albany, NY), although formalin fixation also works well in most instances. Alcohol-based fixatives enhance the preservation of not only DNA and RNA but also certain antigens targeted for immunohistologic studies. Alcohol preserves intermediate filaments better than other fixatives but does not preserve some lymphoid antigens. Alcohol fixation, however, may yield suboptimal morphologic preparations, especially in small biopsies. Several technical modifications are also available to preserve and augment the immunoreactivity of selected antigens. In addition, plastic embedding may be helpful in enhancing cytologic detail.

We find that 10% neutral buffered formalin offers the best overall results by furnishing excellent morphologic preparations with good preservation of immunoreactivity and suitability for molecular diagnostic studies (Table 1-2). In addition, neutral buffered formalin provides the best method for long-term storage of fixed tissue, a particularly important consideration in storing archival material for research purposes. However, for good morphology, fixation in formalin requires at least 12 hours. Thus, when there is sufficient tissue for more than one fixative, a few slices may be fixed in a metal-based fixative, and the remainder in formalin for overnight fixation before additional processing.

Contribution of the Histotechnologist

Once thinly sliced tissue sections are well fixed, the subsequent steps, including dehydration, clearing and infiltration by paraffin, and sectioning, depend on the expertise of the histotechnologist. Although automatic tissue processors are widely used, a processor is only capable of moving the blocks from one compartment to the next. The histotechnologist is

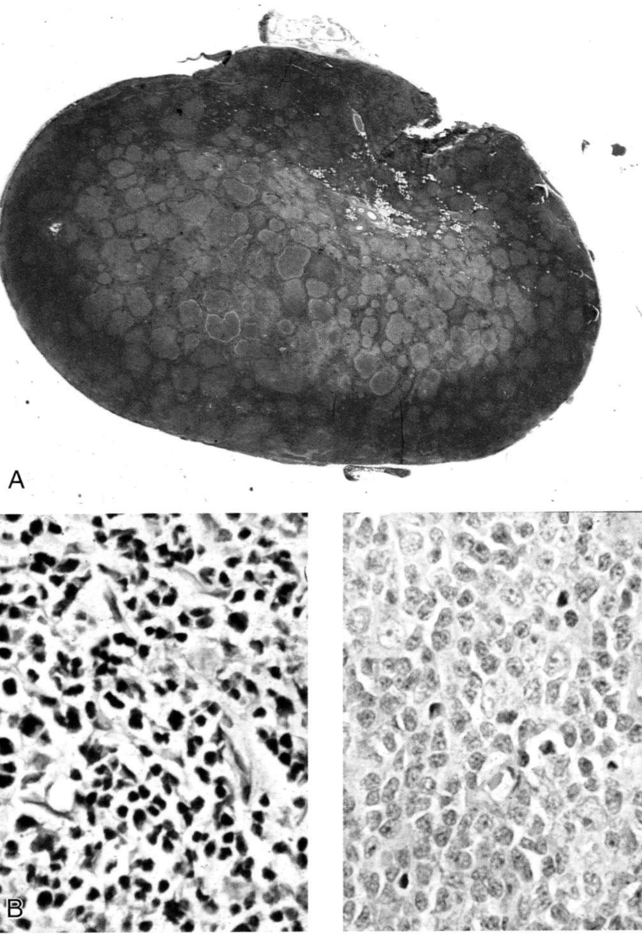

Figure 1-5. Lymph node fixation. This lymph node was placed in fixative without first cutting thin sections. **A**, Only the outer 1.0 mm of this paraffin section stained with hematoxylin-eosin is well fixed and stained; the center shows fainter staining and evidence of cell retraction. **B**, At high magnification, the center of the node (*left*) is autolyzed, with suboptimal cellular detail; the periphery (*right*) shows good cellular detail.

ment minimal residual disease. When ancillary studies are performed in multiple specialized laboratories or sent off site, the issuing of multiple addenda when these results become available may be cumbersome. An accurate and efficient data management system that allows easy access to ancillary test results may be a reasonable alternative to an integrated pathology report. It is imperative that the pathologist ensure that a system is in place to link the results of ancillary studies to the original specimen and to provide an interpretation that relates to the original diagnosis.

Pearls and Pitfalls: Common Errors

Step	Problem	Consequence
Transport	Drying of specimen	Dark, irregular edges on sections Central autolysis if delay is long
Blocking	Thickness >3 mm or encapsulated	Soft, unfixed core may fragment Cells in center show ballooning and pale staining
Fixation	Insufficient time Overfixed in mercury-based fixative	Compromise morphologic and immunopreservation Brittle tissue may shatter Diminished nuclear staining
Dehydration	Insufficient time or aqueous contamination	Sections may crumble, tear, or explode May show small cracks ("dry earth" effect) Faint staining with blurred nuclear detail
Clearing	Excessive time or alcohol contamination	Brittle tissue may shatter Wrinkled sections will not "ribbon"
Infiltration	Paraffin too hot	Brittle tissue may shatter Homogeneous staining, poor nuclear and cytoplasmic detail
Embedding	Delay	Air spaces around tissue in block desist sectioning
Sectioning	Improper knife angle, defective knife edge, section too thick	"Venetian blind" or "shutter" effect Lines across sections Diminished cytologic detail
Floating section	Uneven on bath	Folds or tears
Drying	Temperature too high	Bubbling artifact of nuclei Antigen loss
Staining	Inadequate eosin rinse Inadequate alcohol decolorization	Red hue with obscured cytologic detail Overly blue Giemsa stain with obscured cytologic detail

Data from references 1, 6-9, and 13-15.

References can be found on Expert Consult @ www.expertconsult.com

Chapter 2

Fine-Needle Aspiration of Lymph Nodes

Armando C. Filie and Andrea Abati

CHAPTER OUTLINE

Fine-needle aspiration (FNA) of superficial or deep lymph nodes is a safe, accurate, and sensitive method for assessing lymphadenopathy in adult and pediatric patients.[1-12] The diagnostic sensitivity and specificity of FNA in this role are approximately 94% and 99%, respectively.[13-17] The World Health Organization (WHO) classification system emphasizes the use of ancillary immunophenotypic and genotypic data to define disease entities, and applying these techniques to cells obtained by FNA can enhance diagnostic accuracy beyond that obtained with morphologic evaluation alone.[18-20]

Katz[21] estimates that about 20% of patients with primary or recurrent lymphoma undergo FNA. Using FNA as a first-line procedure has obvious benefits—rapid turnaround time, low cost, and avoidance of surgery. For the assessment of recurrent, progressive, or transforming disease when the tumor characteristics have previously been established, samples should be set aside to confirm ancillary studies (e.g., flow cytometry, molecular diagnostics, fluorescence in situ hybridization [FISH], immunoperoxidase). For the evaluation of primary lymphoma, the differential diagnosis based on cytologic appearance should lead to a cascade of ancillary studies that may yield sufficient information to arrive at a specific diagnostic categorization.[22] The effectiveness of FNA as a diagnostic procedure is dependent on an effective multidisciplinary team to ensure the procurement of an adequate specimen and analysis by appropriate morphologic, immunophenotypic, and genetic techniques. The degree to which FNA can be used to establish a primary diagnosis is controversial.[21,23,24] The prevailing view is that a primary diagnosis of lymphoma by FNA should be confirmed by surgical biopsy, whereas the diagnosis of disease at other sites for staging purposes or at relapse can be made more confidently by FNA alone. However, in rare cases in which excisional biopsy is medically contraindicated, diagnostic decisions must be based on the FNA specimen alone.

For FNA to achieve its true potential as a diagnostic technique for the evaluation of lymphoma, a highly specific approach must be used. Similar to optimal FNA at all organ sites, this approach includes the following:

- A team approach with the cooperation of cytopathologists, hematopathologists, and oncologists
- Competent aspirators
- On-site evaluation for sample adequacy and ancillary studies
- Triage of material for ancillary studies based on a morphologic differential diagnosis
- Cytopathologists experienced in the evaluation of hematopoietic disease processes
- Availability of ancillary diagnostic techniques with committed material for flow cytometry, molecular diagnostics, cell block, and the like

The first step in the cytopathologic diagnosis of the FNA specimen is an on-site, low-tech "eyeballing" for sample adequacy and "triage" for ancillary tests. Katz[21] and Caraway[25] have published the approach taken at MD Anderson, which includes a nonaspiration technique (to minimize bleeding and sample mixing with peripheral blood) and Coulter counters on site for the collection of a minimum of 10 million cells.

FNA has a significant role in the staging of malignant neoplasms as well as the documentation of disease recurrence or transformation in patients with known hematopoietic malignancies.[26,27] As described earlier, however, in certain settings FNA may be the first-line diagnostic procedure for the pathologic diagnosis of lymphadenopathy.[28-41] This chapter provides a guide for the optimal processing and interpretation of a properly obtained cytologic sample.

FINE-NEEDLE ASPIRATION SPECIMEN COLLECTION AND PROCESSING

The initial handling and processing of a lymph node specimen is imperative for maximal diagnostic accuracy. In general, at least three separate needle sticks should be executed.[42] An on-site assessment for specimen adequacy and differential diagnosis should be performed by a pathologist. This is most easily accomplished with a Wright-Giemsa–type stain (usually Diff-Quik [DQ]) carried out on an air-dried smear, which is optimal for the evaluation of hematopoietic processes. The air-drying and Giemsa-type stain provide visual information about the cytoplasm that may be imperative for classification. Although DQ stain offers excellent cytoplasmic and nuclear detail of lymphoid cells and is generally preferable for cytologic evaluation (comparable to the Romanowsky and Giemsa stains used almost exclusively in clinical hematology labs), some authors believe that an alcohol-fixed smear stained with Papanicolaou (Pap) stain should be prepared owing to the enhanced nuclear detail provided. Because of the loss of important cytoplasmic characteristics with Pap stain, we do not support the sole use of alcohol fixation and Pap staining or the use of monolayer technologies that require ethanol or methanol fixation with subsequent Pap staining for the evaluation of hematopoietic processes. If desired, these approaches should be used in addition to air-dried Giemsa-stained material.

Once a differential diagnosis is formulated based on morphology and clinical history, a portion of the sample should be placed in cell culture media such as RPMI (Roswell Park Memorial Institute medium). From this aliquot, cells can be submitted for flow cytometry and molecular diagnostics directly. A cell block or cytospin can also be prepared for immunocytochemistry, FISH, or in situ hybridization for Epstein-Barr virus (EBV) with the EBV-encoded small RNA (EBER) probe. Additionally, an air-dried Giemsa-stained cytospin may be particularly helpful; the cell morphology on the cytospin may be superior to that on the smear owing to the flattening and enlarging effect of cytocentrifugation (Table 2-1; Fig. 2-1).

ANCILLARY STUDIES

Immunocytochemistry

Alcohol fixation of FNA material precludes the performance of some lymphoid markers; thus, it is best to work with a fresh sample that is not prefixed. Cell block sections can be used for immunocytochemistry (ICC) studies with a staining protocol similar to that used for tissue sections.[43,44] ICC can be also performed on air-dried cytospins or smears on charged slides that have been stored desiccated and refrigerated and are postfixed in acetone before staining. The staining protocols used for air-dried cytospins are similar to those used for frozen section material (see Chapter 4). If cellular material is limited, it may be preferable to prepare cytospins rather than attempting a cell block with potentially insufficient material.

ICC on cytospins may be as effective as flow cytometry for the immunophenotyping of cytologic specimens and may be particularly effective for samples with an insufficient number of cells for flow cytometry analysis.[45,46] One distinct benefit of ICC on air-dried cytospins is the detailed visualization of cell size in conjunction with immunophenotypic staining patterns, particularly in mixed populations of cells.

Flow Cytometry

The immunophenotyping of a lymphoid sample may hold the key to the nature of the cells in question, yielding the diagnosis in the vast majority of pathologic lymphoid processes. A recent review highlights the usefulness of flow cytometry (FC) in the diagnosis of lymphoma by FNA.[47] The combination of FC and cytologic morphology can lead to a specific lymphoma classification with a relatively rapid turnaround time (<48 hours) in many cases. The initial cytologic review coupled with the patient's clinical history should yield a differential diagnosis to guide an FC panel of antibodies.[47] FC has the ability to evaluate and quantitate the expression of four or more markers on a single cell and to identify abnormal cells in a mixed population (see Chapter 5).[47] Although it has been suggested that several million cells are required for an adequate FC panel to initially classify a lymphoma, close communication between the cytologist and the other members of the laboratory team can design a limited panel targeting specific diagnostic considerations with as few as 100,000 cells. In particular, when the question is relapse of disease, knowledge of the initial immunophenotype can help select the markers to be analyzed.

FC requires viable cells in suspension. If the FNA sample needs to be stored overnight, it should be placed in RPMI with 10% fetal bovine serum or some other protective medium with protein, such as phosphate buffered saline with 2% bovine serum albumin, and stored at 4°C.

As with any other test, FC may lead to false-negative or false-positive results for FNA material.[47] False-negatives are most commonly due to inadequate sampling, necrosis, and

Table 2-1 Suggested Ancillary Studies Based on Preliminary Diagnosis and Amount of Material Available

Preliminary Diagnosis	Small Amount of Material*	Larger Amount of Material
B-cell lymphoma	Cytospins for immunocytochemistry *IG* gene rearrangement studies	Flow cytometry and/or cell block for immunocytochemistry Cytospins for FISH *IG* gene rearrangement studies
Hodgkin's lymphoma	Cytospins for immunocytochemistry	Cell block for immunocytochemistry
T-cell lymphoma	T-cell gene receptor rearrangement studies	T-cell gene receptor rearrangement and flow cytometry
Lymphoblastic lymphoma	Cytospins for immunocytochemistry	Flow cytometry and/or cell block for immunocytochemistry

*Available material estimated to be sufficient to prepare up to six cytospins.
FISH, fluorescence in situ hybridization; IG, immunoglobulin.

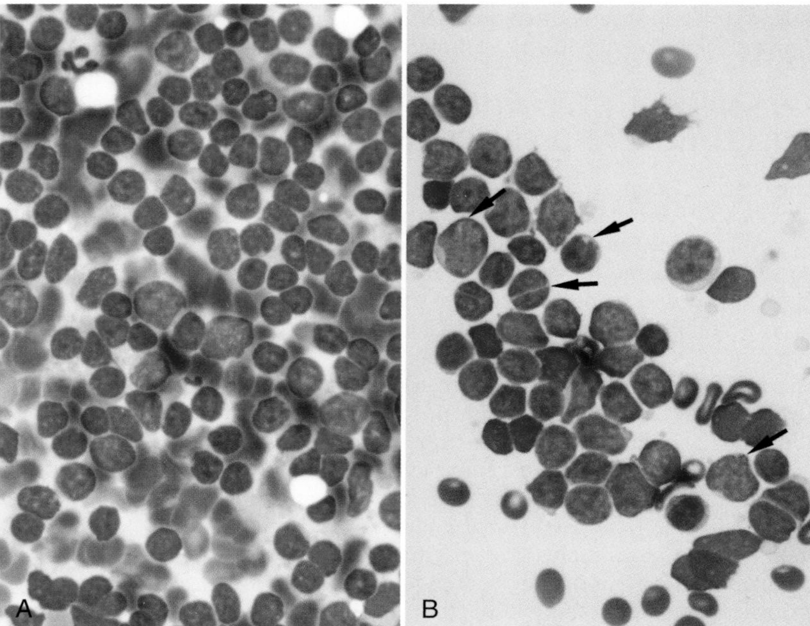

Figure 2-1. **A**, Smear of chronic lymphocytic leukemia–small lymphocytic lymphoma showing mostly small, atypical lymphoid cells with scant cytoplasm and round, slightly irregular nuclei with occasional nuclear clefts. **B**, Cytospin preparation of the same case showing the flattening and enlarging effect on atypical lymphoid cells, accentuating the nuclear irregularity and clefts (*arrows*) (Diff-Quik). Nuclear clefts are an unusual feature for this diagnosis.

fibrosis.[47] False-negatives are most commonly encountered in cases of diffuse large B-cell lymphoma or other aggressive lymphomas due to cell loss or death during FNA and processing. In cases of classical Hodgkin's lymphoma and marginal zone lymphoma, because of the low number of neoplastic cells in a rich reactive background, the malignant clone may not be identifiable by FC, resulting in false-negatives. False-positives may be encountered in reactive lymphoid processes with a skewed light-chain ratio, leading to suspicion of a monoclonal process.[47] These scenarios highlight why FC findings should always be analyzed in conjunction with the morphologic picture. In all these situations, additional studies can be done, such as ICC or polymerase chain reaction (PCR) for *IG* gene clonality, to support or discount the FC outcomes.[47]

When a specific determination cannot be made by FC, additional ancillary tests may be used. PCR may be the key to the diagnosis in a T-cell proliferation that does not show an aberrant clonal immunophenotype via FC yet shows a clonal rearrangement of the T-cell receptor gene at the molecular level. Likewise, FISH may be used for suspected hematopoietic neoplasms with overlapping morphology and an indeterminate flow pattern in which there are specific molecular traits that are easily identifiable by that assay (e.g., mantle cell lymphoma, follicular lymphoma, anaplastic large cell lymphoma).[48-50]

Molecular Studies

PCR studies for B- and T-cell clonality as well as lymphoma-associated viruses, such as EBV and human herpesvirus 8, can easily be performed on fresh or archival FNA samples (via slide scrape lysates). These tests can be used to check and support FC or ICC results, or they can be run on samples with an unexpected morphologic picture when a portion of the sample has not been set aside for ancillary studies. The use of DNA isolated directly from slides containing the cytologic specimen allows the selection of morphologic subpopulations if the specimen is not homogeneous. High-quality PCR products can be readily obtained from both freshly isolated cells and slide scrape lysate material.[51,52]

In the last several years FISH technology has added tremendously to the diagnostic specificity that can be assigned to cytologic specimens of lymphomas using specific genetic alterations identified by commercially available FISH probes.[21,22,25,48-50,52-54] FISH is a particularly useful and highly sensitive technique for the detection of interphase molecular abnormalities. Cytospins of cytologic samples are ideal for FISH because the cells are in a monolayer and are disaggregated, which facilitates the hybridization and scoring of cells.[55] Additionally, performing interphase FISH on cytology monolayer cytospins does not involve the problems inherent in tissue sections, such as scoring of overlapping nuclei and nuclear truncation artifact. For certain translocations, studies have shown that FISH has a higher sensitivity than PCR and Southern blot analysis for the detection of a characteristic translocation.[48]

Recent studies have emphasized the value of FISH studies for the primary diagnosis of lymphoma based on a cytologic sample.[21,22,48-50,53,54] (Where applicable, these are discussed under the particular diagnostic headings in this chapter.) Most centers have used cytospins prepared from fresh samples for FISH, but archival Pap-stained cytologic smears can be examined successfully as well.[54] One such study investigated the *BCL2/IGH@* translocation of follicular lymphoma. Of the 60 archival cases on which FISH was attempted, 9 failed to produce signal sufficient for counting, but there were no false-positives.[54]

In addition to PCR and FISH, gene expression profiling has recently been deemed feasible on FNA material for the discrimination of follicular lymphoma from diffuse large B-cell lymphoma.[56]

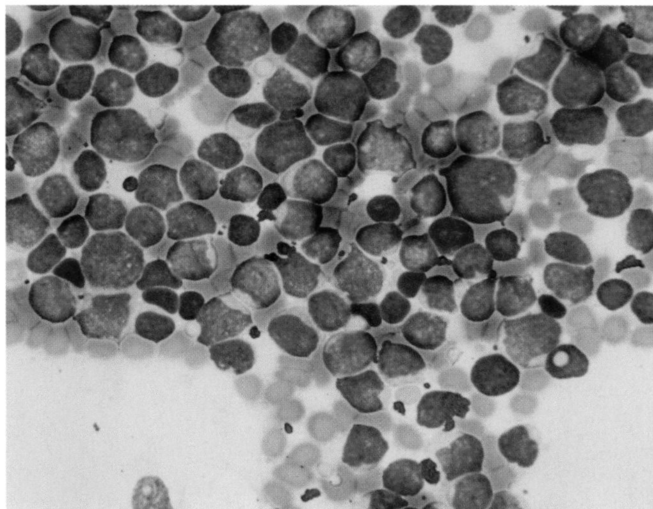

Figure 2-10. Blastoid variant of mantle cell lymphoma. Atypical intermediate-sized to large atypical lymphoid cells with irregular nuclei and small amounts of pale blue cytoplasm (Diff-Quik, smear).

a population of abundant intermediate-sized lymphoid cells with mild atypia (round to slightly irregular nuclei, condensed chromatin, and indistinct nucleoli) (Fig. 2-11).[38,71,72] The background contains small lymphocytes, plasmacytoid lymphocytes, plasma cells, and occasional immunoblasts.[39] These heterogeneous features can make marginal zone lymphoma difficult to distinguish from a reactive process.[72] The neoplastic cells are typically intermediate in size, with moderate to abundant amounts of cytoplasm. They may have a plasmacytoid appearance.[73,74]

Differential Diagnosis. The differential diagnosis includes reactive hyperplasia, follicular lymphoma, mantle cell lymphoma, and small lymphocytic lymphoma.

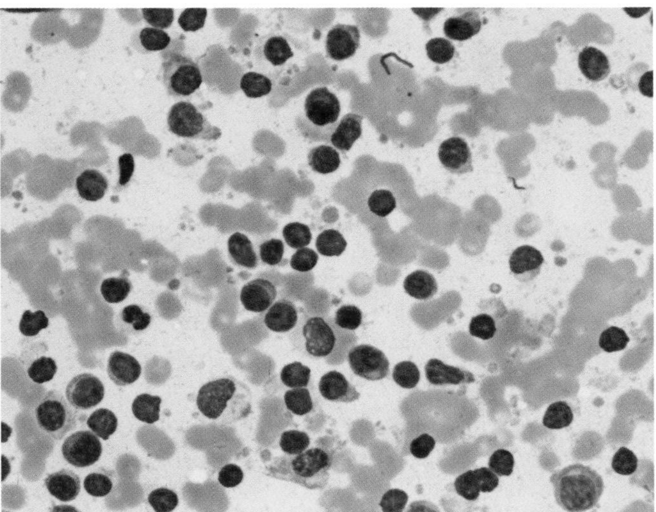

Figure 2-11. Marginal zone lymphoma. Atypical small to intermediate-sized lymphoid cells with slightly enlarged irregular nuclei and variable amounts of basophilic cytoplasm. Isolated benign centrocytes and a mature plasma cell are also identified (Diff-Quik, smear).

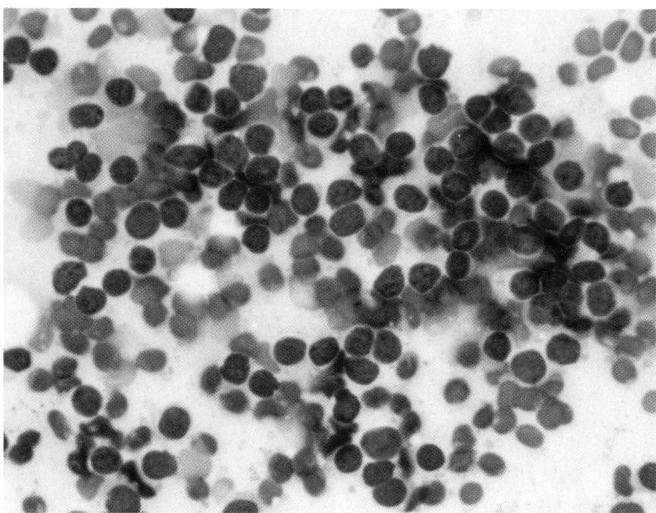

Figure 2-12. Small lymphocytic lymphoma. Numerous small, atypical lymphoid cells with mostly round nuclei, coarsely clumped chromatin, and scant amounts of cytoplasm (Diff-Quik, smear).

Chronic Lymphocytic Leukemia–Small Lymphocytic Lymphoma

Cytomorphology. Aspirates of chronic lymphocytic leukemia–small lymphocytic lymphoma are composed of two cell populations (Fig. 2-12). Most cells are small with round nuclei, coarsely clumped chromatin, occasional nucleoli, and scant cytoplasm. Prolymphocytes are fewer in number and are larger lymphoid cells with round nuclei, a vesicular chromatin pattern, prominent nucleoli, and moderate to abundant amounts of cytoplasm.[38] A uniform population of large transformed cells should suggest Richter transformation.[75-77] Fewer prolymphocytes may imply an accelerated phase and an increased risk for tranformation.[75] Other cytologic features suggestive of progression are an increased number of intermediate-sized or plasmacytoid cells, mitotic figures, the presence of apoptotic bodies and necrosis, and a myxoid and dirty background.[75] The cytologic appearance should be correlated with clinical features indicative of transformation.

Differential Diagnosis. The differential diagnosis includes reactive hyperplasia, follicular lymphoma, mantle cell lymphoma, marginal zone lymphoma, and lymphoplasmacytic lymphoma.

Burkitt's Lymphoma

The lymphoid cells in Burkitt's lymphoma are intermediate in size with round nuclei, a coarse chromatin pattern, several nucleoli, and abundant, deeply basophilic cytoplasm with small cytoplasmic vacuoles (Figs. 2-13 and 2-14). The background shows tingible body macrophages, apoptotic bodies, lymphoglandular bodies, and a watery, basophilic proteinaceous matrix.[38,78] Usually there are very few reactive lymphocytes in the background.

Primary Mediastinal (Thymic) Large B-Cell Lymphoma

Cytomorphology. Aspirates of primary mediastinal large B-cell lymphoma show predominantly single, large lymphoid

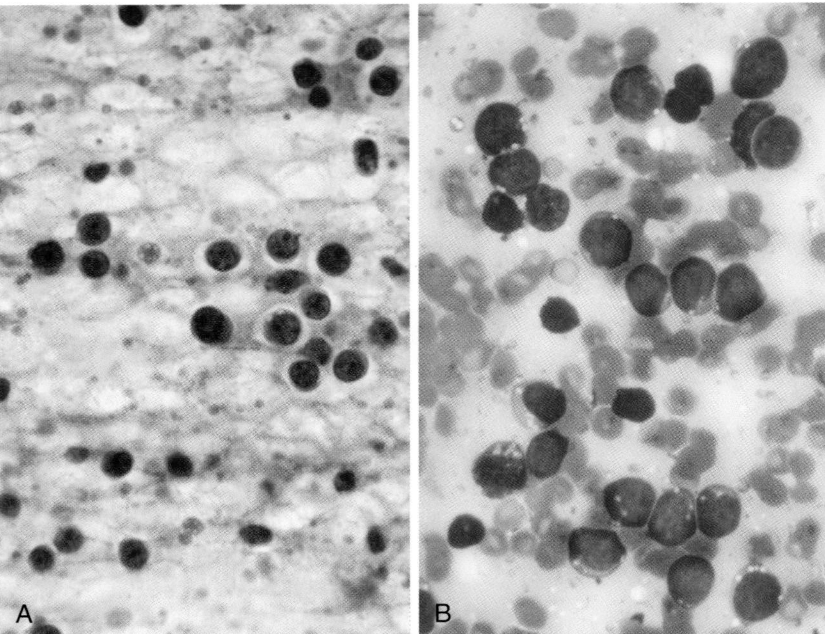

Figure 2-13. Burkitt's lymphoma. Atypical lymphoid cells of intermediate size with enlarged round nuclei, coarse chromatin, prominent nucleoli, and homogeneous well-defined cytoplasm. Some atypical cells display small vacuoles in the cytoplasm. **A**, Pap smear. **B**, Diff-Quik smear.

cells with round to oval nuclei, smooth to irregular nuclear contours, one or more visible nucleoli, and scant to abundant cytoplasm (Fig. 2-15). In some cases the atypical lymphoid cells show markedly lobulated nuclei.[79,80] The cytoplasm is deeply basophilic (DQ-stained slides), and vacuoles may be identified. The background may contain connective tissue fragments with admixed single lymphocytes or groups of lymphocytes. These lymphocytes may have a distorted or elongated morphology due to the fibrosis.[80] It is notable that the majority of primary mediastinal large B-cell lymphomas do not express surface or cytoplasmic immunoglobulin.[79]

Differential Diagnosis. The differential diagnosis includes Hodgkin's lymphoma, lymphoblastic lymphoma, thymoma, and poorly differentiated carcinoma.

Distinctive cytologic features of a mediastinal mass are as follows:

- Hodgkin's lymphoma—presence of classic Reed-Sternberg cells in a background of lymphocytes, plasma cells, and eosinophils
- Lymphoblastic lymphoma—presence of intermediate-sized atypical lymphoid cells with finely dispersed chromatin and inconspicuous, small nucleoli; cytoplasm is

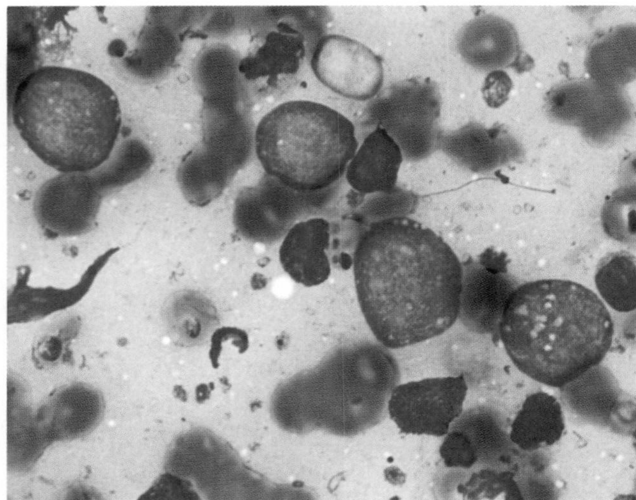

Figure 2-14. Burkitt's lymphoma. The tumor cells are uniform in size and shape, with basophilic cytoplasm and cytoplasmic vacuoles. An inflammatory background is absent, although smudge cells and lymphoglandular bodies are abundant (Diff-Quik, smear).

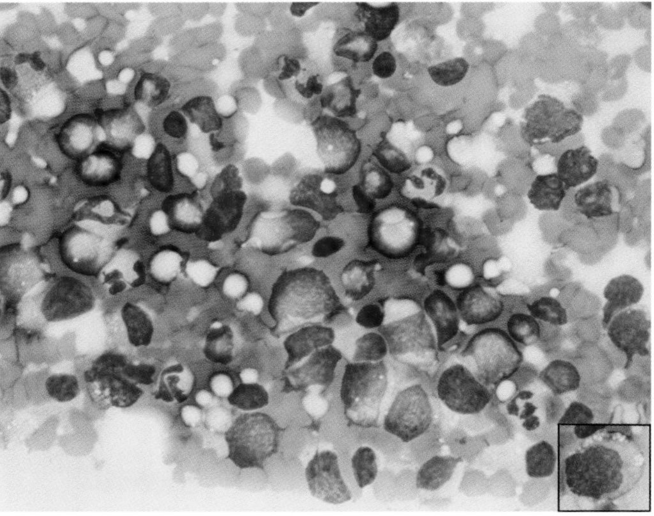

Figure 2-15. Primary mediastinal (thymic) large B-cell lymphoma. Large atypical lymphoid cells with enlarged round to irregular nuclei and variable amounts of cytoplasm in a background of mostly red blood cells. *Inset* shows a large atypical lymphocyte with moderate amounts of basophilic cytoplasm and small vacuoles (Diff-Quik, smear).

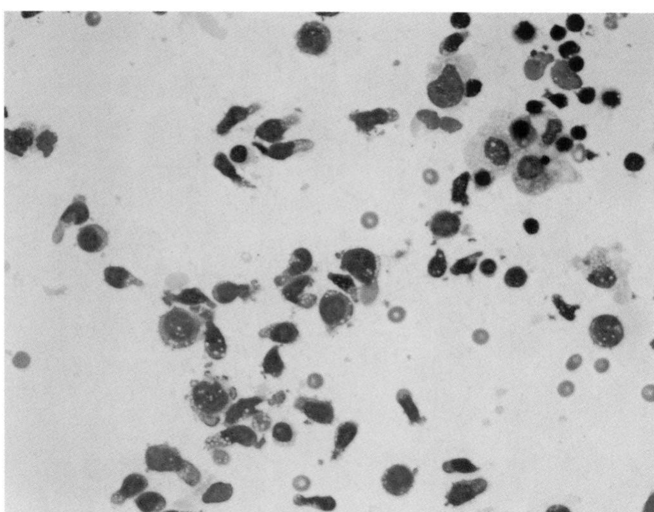

Figure 2-16. Peripheral T-cell lymphoma, not otherwise specified. Small to large atypical lymphocytes in a background containing small mature lymphocytes, histiocytes, and a few red blood cells (Diff-Quik, smear).

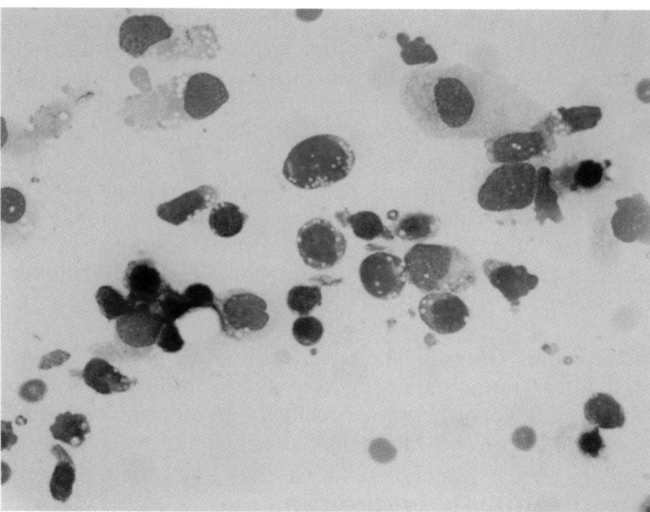

Figure 2-17. Peripheral T-cell lymphoma, not otherwise specified. Small, intermediate, and large atypical lymphoid cells with enlarged, often irregular nuclei, visible to prominent nucleoli, and basophilic cytoplasm. Some cells contain cytoplasmic vacuoles (Diff-Quik, smear).

very sparse (in contrast with primary mediastinal large B-cell lymphoma)

- Thymoma—presence of epithelial cells and lymphocytes; keratinaceous debris may be present if there is cystic degeneration
- Poorly differentiated carcinoma—atypical cells are in clusters, and lymphoglandular bodies are often absent in the background

Mature T-Cell Neoplasms

Peripheral T-Cell Lymphoma, Not Otherwise Specified

Cytomorphology. Aspirates of peripheral T-cell lymphoma show two different patterns (Figs. 2-16 and 2-17). The first pattern consists of a background of a heterogeneous lymphoid cell population (characteristic of T-cell neoplasms) with a combination of epithelioid histiocytes, eosinophils, and plasma cells. Scattered among the background cells are small atypical lymphoid cells that are usually larger than a small, mature lymphocyte and demonstrate nuclear irregularity (protrusions and indentations), clumped chromatin, and scant to moderate amounts of cytoplasm. Also present are large lymphoid cells, which constitute 20% to 50% of the total cell population and often show pale cytoplasm and occasional prominent nucleoli. These large cells may resemble mononuclear variants of Reed-Sternberg cells; however, binucleated or multinucleated forms are uncommon. Aspirates of angioimmunoblastic T-cell lymphoma may display this pattern.[81]

The second pattern has a predominance (>50%) of large, atypical lymphoid cells, with the background displaying variable amounts of small lymphocytes, epithelioid histiocytes, and eosinophils. These large cells may exhibit coarse chromatin, nuclear irregularity, small indistinct nucleoli, and basophilic cytoplasm. Mycosis fungoides involving the lymph node may demonstrate this pattern.[81]

Differential Diagnosis. The differential diagnosis includes reactive hyperplasia; follicular lymphoma; marginal zone lymphoma; diffuse large B-cell lymphoma, not otherwise specified; Hodgkin's lymphoma; poorly differentiated carcinoma; and melanoma.

Anaplastic Large Cell Lymphoma

Cytomorphology. Aspirates of anaplastic large cell lymphoma show numerous aberrant large and medium-sized lymphocytes both singly and in aggregates (Figs. 2-18 and 2-19).[82,83] The atypical cells are large, with variable amounts of dense to pale basophilic cytoplasm; they may be

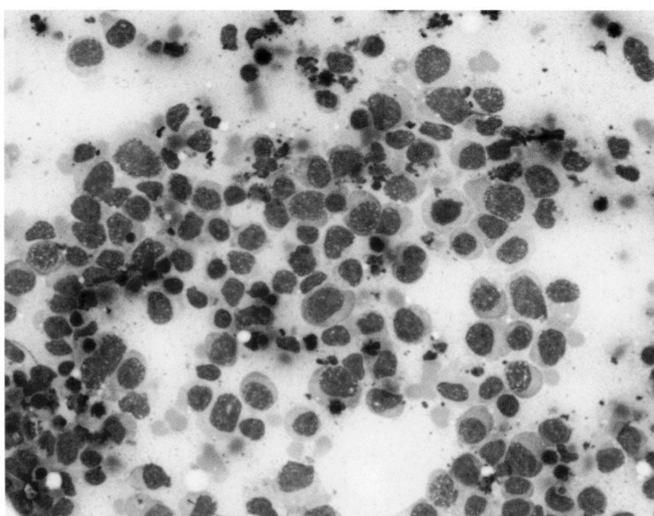

Figure 2-18. Anaplastic large cell lymphoma. Intermediate to large atypical lymphoid cells with enlarged nuclei and pale basophilic cytoplasm. Background shows a few small benign lymphocytes, red blood cells, debris, and absence of lymphoglandular bodies (Diff-Quik, smear).

round to irregularly shaped with infrequent small, fine vacuoles. The nuclei are often hypochromatic with well-defined, irregular nuclear membranes and one to three centrally or eccentrically placed prominent nucleoli. Most of the cells are intermediate sized and mononuclear. Lymphoglandular bodies are usually absent. The background may contain small lymphocytes, histiocytes, necrosis, and a watery, basophilic, proteinaceous matrix material similar to that seen in Burkitt's lymphoma.[82] The presence of abundant neutrophils or eosinophils favors a diagnosis of classical Hodgkin's lymphoma.

Differential Diagnosis. The differential diagnosis includes Hodgkin's lymphoma; histiocytic sarcoma; diffuse large B-cell lymphoma, not otherwise specified; granulocytic sarcoma; poorly differentiated carcinoma; sarcoma; and melanoma.

Lymphoblastic Leukemia and Lymphoma

Cytomorphology. FNA samples of lymphoblastic leukemia or lymphoma of either B- or T-cell origin show similar features (Fig. 2-20). The aspirates often contain a monotonous population of lymphoid cells that are twice the size of a small lymphocyte, with high nuclear-to-cytoplasmic ratios. Nuclei are frequently round, but they may be irregular with nuclear clefts and convolutions. The chromatin is finely granular, and the nucleoli, if present, are small. The cytoplasm is scant and may or may not exhibit small vacuoles. The cells are intermediate in size. The background demonstrates variable amounts of lymphoglandular bodies, tingible body macrophages, and necrosis.[84] There may be frequent mitotic figures and apoptotic bodies.[25]

Differential Diagnosis. The differential diagnosis includes mantle cell lymphoma (blastoid variant), extramedullary myeloid tumor, thymoma, and small cell carcinoma.

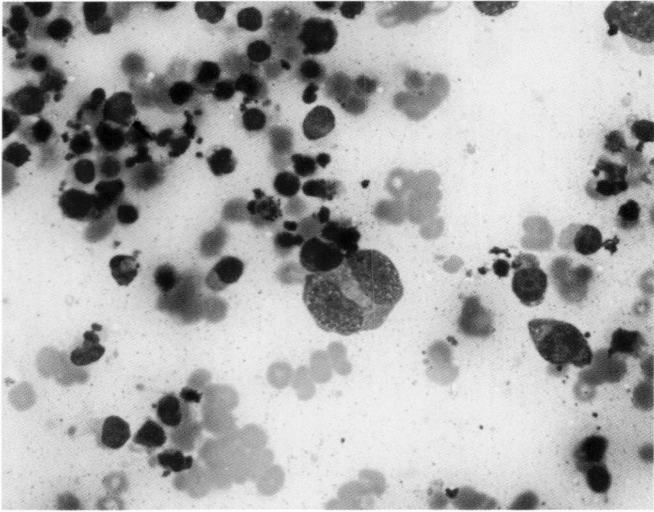

Figure 2-19. **Anaplastic large cell lymphoma.** Large, atypical, binucleated anaplastic large cell lymphoma cell with ample amounts of basophilic cytoplasm and a prominent Golgi region. Background demonstrates smaller atypical lymphoid cells, small benign lymphocytes, red blood cells, and debris (Diff-Quik, smear).

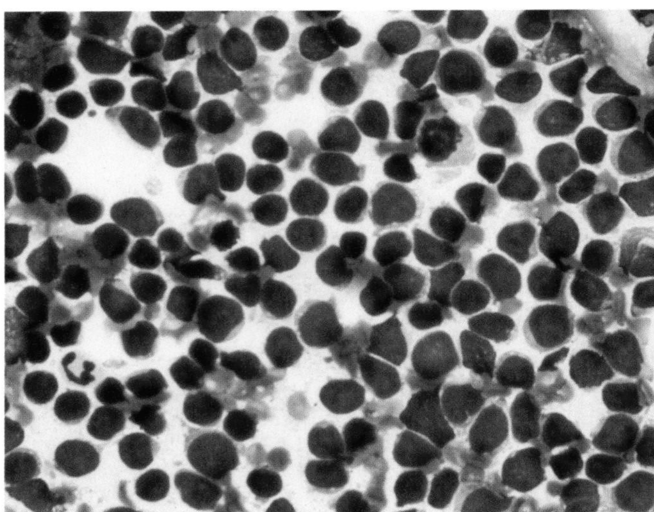

Figure 2-20. **Lymphoblastic lymphoma.** Monotonous population of atypical lymphoid cells (twice the size of small benign lymphocytes) with enlarged, mostly round nuclei, high nuclear-to-cytoplasmic ratios, and scant amounts of pale basophilic cytoplasm (Diff-Quik, smear).

Hodgkin's Lymphoma

Given the morphologic similarities with non-Hodgkin's lymphoma, difficulties in immunophenotyping, and the limitations of FNA, a cytologic diagnosis of primary Hodgkin's lymphoma should be followed by surgical biopsy.[85,86] Some authors claim a high degree of accuracy on FNA alone.[87] Although FNA may suffice for the diagnosis of relapse, excisional biopsy is recommended for the primary diagnosis of Hodgkin's lymphoma.

Classical Hodgkin's Lymphoma

Cytomorphology. Aspirates of classical Hodgkin's lymphoma are characterized by the presence of large atypical mononuclear (Hodgkin [H]) and multinucleated (Reed-Sternberg [RS]) lymphoid cells in a background of reactive inflammatory cells such as benign lymphocytes, histiocytes, eosinophils, and plasma cells (Figs. 2-21 and 2-22).[38,39,85] The number of HRS cells varies according to the histologic type of classical Hodgkin's lymphoma. Classic RS cells display a bilobated or binucleated nucleus, prominent nucleolus (often the size of a red blood cell or larger) in each lobe or nucleus, and variable amounts of cytoplasm.[85] HRS cell variants may be mononucleated, hyperlobated, or multinucleated, with nucleoli ranging from small, single, and inconspicuous to large, multiple, and prominent.

Differential Diagnosis. Because of the wide morphologic spectrum exhibited by RS cells and RS cell variants, the differential diagnosis of classical Hodgkin's lymphoma is quite broad and includes reactive hyperplasia (mononucleosis); granulomatous lymphadenitis; suppurative lymphadenitis; diffuse large B-cell lymphoma, not otherwise specified; peripheral T-cell lymphoma, not otherwise specified; anaplastic large cell lymphoma; T-cell histiocyte-rich large B-cell lymphoma; histiocytic sarcoma; poorly differentiated carcinoma; and melanoma.

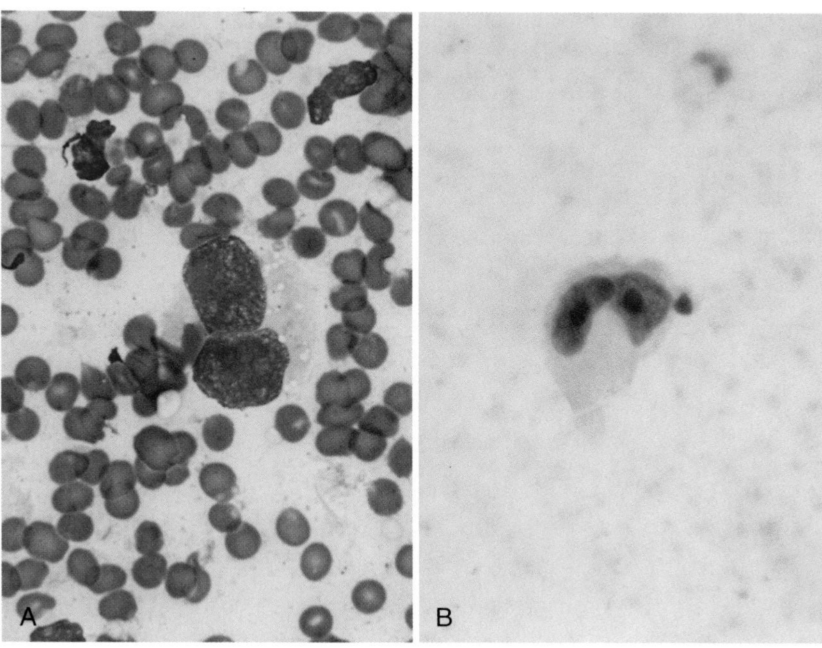

Figure 2-21. **Classical Hodgkin's lymphoma. A,** Classic binucleated Reed-Sternberg cell with enlarged nuclei, visible nucleoli, and moderate amounts of pale basophilic cytoplasm (Diff-Quik, smear). **B,** Classic binucleated Reed-Sternberg cell with enlarged nuclei, finely granular chromatin, prominent eosinophilic nucleoli, and abundant amounts of pale cytoplasm; a small benign lymphocyte is also seen (Pap, filter).

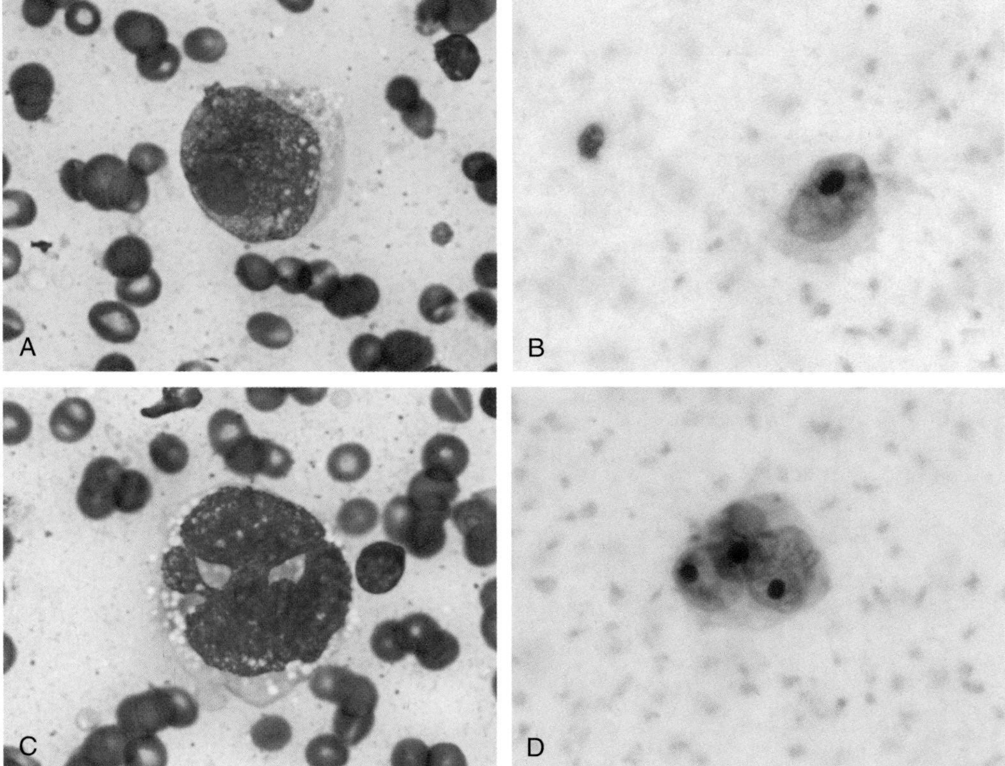

Figure 2-22. **Classical Hodgkin's lymphoma. A,** Mononuclear variant of Reed-Sternberg cell with an enlarged nucleus, visible nucleolus, and pale, ill-defined cytoplasm; a benign lymphocyte is also seen (Diff-Quik stain). **B,** Mononuclear variant of Reed-Sternberg cell with an enlarged nucleus, prominent eosinophilic nucleolus, and moderate amounts of pale cytoplasm; a single small lymphocyte is also present (Pap stain). **C,** Multinucleated variant of Reed-Sternberg cell with enlarged nuclei, large nucleoli, and pale basophilic cytoplasm; a lymphocyte is also present (Diff-Quik stain). **D,** Multinucleated variant of Reed-Sternberg cell with enlarged vesicular nuclei, prominent nucleoli, and moderate amounts of cytoplasm (Pap stain).

Nodular Lymphocyte-Predominant Hodgkin's Lymphoma

To make a cytologic diagnosis of nodular lymphocyte-predominant Hodgkin's lymphoma, one should identify lymphocyte-predominant (LP) cells (formerly lymphocytic and histiocytic [L&H] variants).[19] Morphologically, LP cells often display one large nucleus, usually folded or multilobated; multiple nucleoli; and scant to abundant amounts of cytoplasm.[88] The morphology of LP cells may vary, however, and may include cells more closely mimicking HRS cells and their variants.[74] The background contains lymphocytes and epithelioid histiocytes.[88] Given the rarity of LP cells in the reactive background, the diagnosis is challenging.

LIMITATIONS OF FINE-NEEDLE ASPIRATION

The most common limitations of lymph node aspirates are related to technical issues associated with the procedure, entities that pose diagnostic challenges, and the absence of architectural features. Insufficient sampling of material, inadequate material for ancillary studies, and sampling error are procedure-related problems inherent to FNA in general and are not specific to the aspiration of lymph nodes. Sampling error may be the result of missing the node or lesion, focal involvement of the node by lymphoma, or focal transformation of a lymphoma. Specific entities such as Hodgkin's lymphoma and lymphoma transformation are examples of potential diagnostic challenges. A list of these situations along with suggested solutions is provided in the Pearls and Pitfalls table.[38,39,62]

Another problem limiting the utility of FNA is the lack of expertise in the diagnosis and classification of hematologic neoplasms by many cytologists practicing in the community. To obtain an accurate diagnosis by FNA, clinical and pathologic data must be integrated with ancillary immunophenotypic and genetic techniques. The presence of specific genetic abnormalities in some lymphomas, coupled with characteristic cytologic features in the appropriate clinical setting, may be sufficient for a primary diagnosis in some cases. For example, a primary diagnosis of Burkitt's lymphoma can be based on FNA if supported by suitable genetic testing for a *MYC* translocation. FNA can be used with greater confidence for the diagnosis of relapse or for staging.

Pearls and Pitfalls: Troubleshooting

Problem/Diagnosis	Solution/Recommendation
Unsatisfactory sample	Evaluation of specimen adequacy by a pathologist or cytotechnologist during the procedure If such an evaluation is not possible, make additional passes until the solution is cloudy
Insufficient material for ancillary studies	Evaluation of specimen cellularity by a pathologist or cytotechnologist during the procedure If such an evaluation is not possible, make additional passes until the solution is cloudy Repeat FNA before biopsy (optional)
Sampling error	Make multiple passes (≥3) from different parts of the node or lesion If cytologic findings do not explain clinical features, perform close follow-up with repeat FNA or biopsy
Transformation	Transformed lymphocyte count (TLC) ≥20% highly predictive of large cell lymphoma (in practice, ≥25%) If TLC is ≥25% but <50%, it is important to correlate morphology with clinical and immunophenotypic findings
Immunophenotypically negative lymphoma	Gate on large B cells; absence of immunoglobulin expression supports lymphoma Correlate with clinical and cytomorphologic findings
Hodgkin's lymphoma	Immunocytochemistry on cytocentrifuged samples or cell block preparations Biopsy usually needed for primary diagnosis
T-cell lymphoma	Important to correlate morphology and flow cytometry findings (exclude B-cell lymphoma) Abnormal T-cell phenotype by flow cytometry or T-cell receptor gene rearrangement supports the diagnosis of T-cell lymphoma Biopsy indicated for primary diagnosis (if possible)

References can be found on Expert Consult @ www.expertconsult.com

Chapter 3

Collection, Processing, and Examination of Bone Marrow Specimens

Phuong L. Nguyen

Accurate interpretation of a bone marrow specimen requires an adequate and well-prepared sample. The definition of adequacy depends on the clinical indication for the examination. For example, for staging lymphoma, a bilateral bone marrow core biopsy is superior to a unilateral biopsy[1-3]; thus, for this purpose, a bilateral biopsy defines adequacy. In contrast, for the diagnosis of acute leukemia, a unilateral bone marrow aspiration and core biopsy are usually sufficient, in conjunction with appropriate immunophenotyping and genetic studies. This chapter outlines what constitutes an adequate bone marrow specimen, how to collect such a specimen, and how to process it to ensure optimal interpretation.

MEDICAL INDICATIONS FOR BONE MARROW EXAMINATION

In general, a bone marrow examination is justified if there are hematologic abnormalities that clinical and laboratory data cannot explain. A blood smear should always be carefully evaluated before deciding whether a marrow examination is necessary. For instance, circulating blasts in and of themselves do not necessitate a bone marrow evaluation if the patient has recently been treated with granulocyte colony-stimulating factor and the blood shows a dramatic neutrophilic left shift that manifests as circulating neutrophilic myelocytes and promyelocytes. Should the blasts persist despite the resolution of other neutrophilic precursors, a bone marrow examination should be considered. Aside from the diagnostic purposes outlined in Box 3-1, there are three other broad medical indications for bone marrow evaluation: staging for metastatic disease, monitoring drug therapy that affects hematopoiesis, and evaluating toxicity and antineoplastic effects of antineoplastic regimens. With respect to the last, patients who are treated on study protocols may undergo prescheduled bone marrow examinations. Pathologists should be aware of such ongoing clinical protocols to understand what information is expected from these scheduled examinations.

Several investigators have suggested that if the blood has a sufficient quantity of blasts to meet the definition of acute leukemia and to allow other ancillary studies, such as cytochemical stains, cytogenetics, and flow cytometric immunophenotyping, a bone marrow examination is superfluous.[4] This approach may save time and money, and it may spare the patient discomfort and the risk associated with an invasive procedure. However, this strategy also carries several disadvantages. Weinkauff and associates[4] reported that of 44 cases of acute leukemia in which cytogenetic analysis was performed, the blood yielded an insufficient number of metaphases in 5 of 10 patients with acute lymphoblastic leukemia and in 5 of 29 patients with acute myeloid leukemia. Cytogenetic analysis of the marrow in all these cases was sufficient. Of more immediate concern is the fact that marrow is used to follow patients after the induction of chemotherapy to evaluate tumor burden. Such follow-up requires knowledge of the preinduction marrow blast proportion and the distribution of leukemic cells in the core biopsy in the event leukemic

Box 3-1 *Indications for Bone Marrow Examination*

Diagnostic Purposes
- Unexplained cytopenia or cytosis
- Diagnosis of hematopoietic neoplasms and workup of unexplained blasts or other abnormal cells in the blood suggestive of bone marrow pathology
- Evaluation of mastocytosis, amyloidosis, metabolic storage disorders
- Workup of monoclonal gammopathy
- Workup of fever of unknown origin
- Workup of splenomegaly or other organomegaly

Staging for Malignant Disease
- Staging of malignant lymphoma
- Detection of metastatic tumor

Monitoring
- Follow-up after induction chemotherapy for acute leukemia and, less often, before and during consolidation or maintenance chemotherapy
- Restaging after treatment for lymphoma
- Follow-up after hematopoietic stem cell transplantation
- Follow-up in patients with aplastic anemia, Fanconi's anemia, or paroxysmal nocturnal hemoglobinuria for the development of myelodysplastic syndromes
- Monitoring toxicity and antineoplastic effects of antineoplastic regimens

infiltrates were patchy at diagnosis. Such an assessment is not possible if only the blood is examined at diagnosis.

Comorbid conditions such as coagulopathy, infection in close proximity to the biopsy site, or prior radiation to the posterior iliac crests should be carefully assessed before embarking on a bone marrow biopsy. These factors are not necessarily contraindications to biopsy, and often the procedure can be modified to accommodate these circumstances. Factor replacement or reversal of anticoagulant therapy may be implemented in the case of severe coagulopathy. In the case of infected skin overlying the crests or prior radiation to the posterior iliac crests resulting in persistent marrow hypocellularity in the involved fields, the sternum may be selected for bone marrow aspiration. When the sternum is selected for marrow evaluation, obtaining core biopsies is not feasible. Of note, thrombocytopenia is a relatively common indication for bone marrow examination and a condition that cannot always be easily reversed. Severe thrombocytopenia is usually not a contraindication for bone marrow aspiration and core biopsy as long as pressure is applied to attain hemostasis afterward. Thus, when a marrow examination is truly justified, the aspiration and biopsy procedure can usually be accomplished safely.

COMPONENTS OF A BONE MARROW EVALUATION

Bone Marrow Aspiration or Trephine Biopsy

Once it has been decided that a bone marrow examination is indicated, it is important to determine what specimens to collect. Studies by Brynes[5] and Barekman[3] and their respective colleagues have established that a thorough bone marrow examination includes both marrow aspiration and trephine biopsy. In their review of more than 4000 diagnostic bone marrow specimens over a 10-year period at a single institution, Barekman and colleagues[3] reported that approximately 30% of carcinomas would have been missed if the pathologist had examined only the aspirate. Conversely, in 9% of bone marrow specimens positive for metastatic carcinoma, the diagnosis was made by the aspirate alone. With respect to acute leukemia, in which the presumption may be that bone marrow aspiration alone is sufficient, the same authors reported positive findings in the biopsy but not in the aspirate in 20 of 576 marrow specimens obtained as follow-up for acute leukemia.

The need to examine both the marrow aspirate and core biopsy extends beyond the evaluation of focal processes; it also applies to the workup of pancytopenia. Imbert and coworkers[6] retrospectively examined 213 bone marrow specimens obtained over approximately 4 years at a large tertiary hospital for the evaluation of pancytopenia; "focal" processes such as lymphoma and metastatic tumor accounted for approximately 20% of the final diagnoses. Of the 213 specimens, the authors found that bone marrow aspiration alone was sufficient for diagnosis in 55% of cases; in 27%, a trephine biopsy was necessary for diagnosis. Of note, in this study the bone marrow aspiration was done first, and a supplementary trephine biopsy was performed later in cases of difficult aspiration or hypocellular smears. This sequential approach, and the need to call patients back for another procedure, has obvious disadvantages. Taken together, these data indicate the justification for and expediency of performing both marrow aspiration and core biopsy.

Bilateral or Unilateral Specimen

The issue of bilateral versus unilateral biopsy is an important one. Confirming earlier results by the Brunning[1] and Juneja[2] groups, Barekman and colleagues[3] reported that 32% of carcinomas and 23% of lymphomas examined by them were positive on only one side. The recommendation that bilateral bone marrow biopsy be done in the staging of lymphoma and carcinoma can easily be extrapolated to include other processes that may involve the marrow in a focal manner, such as plasma cell myeloma or mastocytosis in adults and primitive neuroectodermal tumor, rhabdomyosarcoma, and Ewing's sarcoma in children. Ideally, for the initial staging of lymphoma or in other situations in which the documentation of marrow involvement would alter the patient's management, two core specimens should be obtained from each iliac crest, constituting the so-called double-bilateral bone marrow biopsy. Because the aspirate is likewise subject to the artifact of focal sampling, bilateral aspiration may also be considered.

Specimens for Ancillary Studies

In addition to obtaining aspirate and trephine biopsy samples for morphologic examination, consideration should be given to procuring samples for other studies that may be essential for an accurate diagnosis or prognosis. In general, if the differential diagnosis includes malignancy, aspirate samples should be obtained for cytogenetic and molecular genetic analyses. If there is a possibility of acute leukemia or a lymphoid neoplasm, a sample for flow cytometric analysis should also be procured. These suggestions are in accordance with the World Health Organization's recommendation to use "all available information—morphology, immunophenotype, genetic features, and clinical features—to define diseases."[7] Last, samples for bacterial, mycobacterial, fungal, or viral cultures should be collected if an infectious cause is suspected. If the preoperative differential diagnosis is broad, additional anticoagulated aspirates should be obtained in the event special studies become necessary after the morphologic examination.

COLLECTION OF BONE MARROW ASPIRATE AND CORE BIOPSY

Anatomic Sites

In both adults and children, the crest of the posterior superior iliac spine is preferred because of its relative distance from other vital structures and its relatively large surface area, which allows the maneuvering of biopsy and aspiration needles. An alternative site in adults is the sternum, but only marrow aspiration should be performed in this location, and only by an experienced operator; core biopsies are not done at the sternum. The anterior superior iliac spine is rarely used because of its proximity to other vital structures and because the crest is narrow. In very young children, the anterior tibial plateau can be used. Sites within previous fields of radiotherapy should be avoided because irradiation-induced hypocellularity may persist for years.

Collection Procedures

Some authorities recommend that the trephine biopsy be obtained first. Using the same skin incision, a separate needle is then placed through a separate puncture for aspiration. This sequence minimizes the morphologic distortion that can occur from interstitial hemorrhage when the aspirate is obtained first and the trephine needle is advanced through the same puncture site. Other authors suggest that the order of aspiration and trephine biopsy is not important as long as each sample is obtained through a separate puncture and with a separate and appropriate needle.[8]

Detailed instructions on how to perform the bone marrow core biopsy and aspiration are beyond the scope of this chapter. Importantly, the novice should have direct personal supervision. The following discussion focuses on aspects of the procurement procedure that are relevant to the handling of specimens.

General Approach

Because sterile technique minimizes infectious complications, it is worthwhile to work with a trained medical technician or medical technologist who can assist with the handling and disposition of the aspirates, cores, and instruments. Once the procedure begins, it is important to proceed quickly and efficiently to minimize patient discomfort and the clotting of specimens. As mentioned, the types of tissue obtained depend on the preoperative differential diagnosis. It is important to plan in advance the number of core biopsies and aspirate volumes, as well as the types of anticoagulants required. It is also important to plan the sequence in which the various aspirate samples will be obtained, because each successive aspirate is likely to become more hemodiluted. It is helpful to review this sequence with the technical assistant before the procedure. To anticoagulate aspirated marrow, ethylenediaminetetraacetic acid (EDTA) is commonly recommended, but other reagents such as acid citrate dextrose and sodium heparin are also used. However, the best morphology is obtained from aspirated specimens that are not anticoagulated.[9] It is important that the individual performing the aspiration and core biopsy procedure know the requirements of the specialty laboratories so that the correct anticoagulant is used.

Bone Marrow Trephine Biopsy Procedure

Versions of the original Jamshidi biopsy needle for procuring the core biopsy are available in both disposable and reusable forms. Most adult patients require a 4-inch, 11-gauge needle. When patients are osteopenic, a larger bore needle (8-gauge) allows the collection of an intact core biopsy with minimal crush artifact. For pediatric patients, a 2- or 4-inch, 13-gauge biopsy needle is used. Sola and associates[10] described a bone marrow biopsy technique for neonates in which a ½-inch, 19-gauge Osgood needle is used.

With the exception of young pediatric patients, an adequate core biopsy should be at least 2 cm long (exclusive of cortical bone, cartilage, or periosteum) and free of crush artifact or fragmentation (Fig. 3-1).[11,12] Grossly, cores of marrow have a finely mottled, deep red color and a gritty texture; when the marrow is severely hypoplastic, the core may appear pale yellow, but its surface should still be gritty. Marrow that is completely replaced by leukemia, lymphoma, or other neoplasms may appear white. Cortical bone often has an ivory color with a hard, smooth surface. Cartilage is gray-white with a glistening surface—findings that should tell the operator to try again.

To make touch imprints of the core biopsy, the core is gently blotted to remove adherent blood, and several clean glass slides are touched gently to the marrow core. Several touch imprints should be made before placing the cores in fixative. One can also touch the cores to the glass slides, although this approach requires a steady hand to avoid crushing or dropping the specimen. Alternatively, the core is gently rolled between two glass slides; although this method may yield more cells on the imprints, there is also a greater risk of fragmentation of the core.

Bone Marrow Aspiration Procedure

An Illinois aspiration needle or its variant is used to collect the bone marrow aspirate. Although the needle is advanced through the same skin incision used for the biopsy, the point of puncture through the bone should be separate from the puncture site of the trephine biopsy, preferably approximately 1 cm away. Otherwise, the aspirate may consist of only clotted blood or marrow. Because each successive aspiration is likely to become more hemodiluted, a rapid and forceful aspiration of approximately 1 mL of fluid marrow should be obtained first for morphologic examination. Additional aspirate samples can be obtained for flow cytometric analysis, cytogenetics, molecular diagnostic evaluation, and cultures, as needed and in that sequence. (In rare cases in which electron microscopic studies are called for, that sample should be collected after the initial aliquot for morphology but before that obtained for

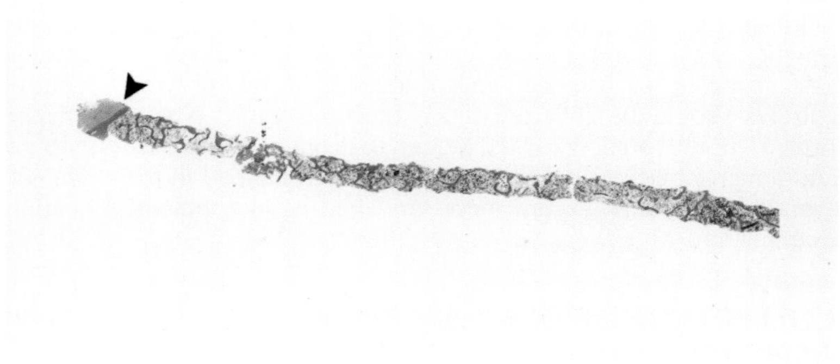

Figure 3-1. Example of an excellent core biopsy (>1 cm long) consisting of mostly marrow, with very little cortical bone or periosteal soft tissue (*arrowhead*) and with minimal crush artifact or hemorrhage. To fit these parameters, one end of this long core biopsy has to be truncated (*right side*).

flow cytometry.) The syringes used for samples obtained for morphologic examination and electron microscopy should be free of anticoagulants; the syringes used for other studies should be coated in advance with the appropriate anticoagulants. Undiluted marrow aspirate is deep red and slightly thicker than blood. Because marrow aspiration can create intense discomfort, patients should be warned in advance, and the aspiration should be done as quickly as possible.

PROCESSING OF MARROW TREPHINE BIOPSY AND ASPIRATE

Trephine Biopsy

The following discussion applies to paraffin embedding. For plastic embedding, the reader is referred to several authoritative reports on the topic.[13-16]

Fixation

Accurate microscopic evaluation of the bone marrow core biopsy can direct the appropriate choice of ancillary immunohistochemical or in situ hybridization techniques or perhaps even obviate their need (Fig. 3-2). However, it is important to recognize the essential role of the immunophenotypic characterization of many myeloid and lymphoid neoplasms and the possibility that when the aspiration yields a dry tap or the aspirate is diluted, the core biopsy may be the only tissue available for ancillary diagnostic studies. For these reasons, factors to consider when choosing the fixative for the core biopsy include not only the preservation of morphologic detail but also the preservation of tissue for subsequent special diagnostic or research studies, as well as whether marrow core biopsies are processed separately from other surgical pathology specimens. In general, mercury-based fixatives such as Zenker's and B5 solutions provide excellent cytologic detail, but they may be incompatible with certain immunohistochemical studies; they are also inconvenient to use because they require special disposal procedures. In laboratories where bone marrow trephine biopsies are processed along with other surgical specimens, neutral buffered formalin is often used. Excellent morphologic detail can be obtained with this fixative, but the laboratory must be very careful to ensure adequate fixation time relative to the thickness or diameter of the core biopsy specimens. Acid zinc formalin has been developed as a compromise that obviates the special disposal requirements for mercury-based fixatives while preserving some of the cytologic detail.

Core biopsies should be placed in 10 to 20 mL of fixative. The recommended fixation time for the various fixatives is as follows: B5, 2 hours; Zenker's fixative, at least 3 to 4 hours, with no adverse effect if fixation is allowed to proceed overnight or over the weekend; neutral buffered formalin, at least 18 to 24 hours; zinc formalin, 3 to 4 hours.

Decalcification

Following fixation, the cores are removed from fixative and rinsed with several changes of water for 3 minutes before being subjected to decalcification, as follows:

1. Place in Decal Stat (Decal Chemical Corp., Tallman, NY) for 1 hour. Other decalcification options include RDO (APB Engineering Products Corp., Plainfield, IL) for 40 to 60 minutes, Surgipath Decalcifier II (Surgipath Medical Industries, Grayslake, IL) for 90 minutes, or hydrochloric acid–formic acid for 2 to 2.5 hours.
2. Wash in several changes of water for 5 minutes.
3. Place in 10% neutral buffered formalin and process in an automatic tissue processor.

Sectioning

Ideally, the paraffin-embedded core biopsies should be sectioned in thicknesses of 3 μm (and preferably no more than 4 μm thick). The importance of adequate sampling cannot be overemphasized, especially when the examination is being performed to determine whether the marrow is involved by a focal process such as metastatic disease. Using a statistical model based on their retrospective review of 46 cases of bilateral bone marrow biopsies with involvement by metastatic carcinoma, sarcoma, or neuroblastoma, Jatoi and coworkers[17] demonstrated that the false-negative rate is inversely proportional to the number of slides examined. For example, when three slides are examined per side, for a total of six slides, the false-negative rate is 5%; when two slides are examined per side, the false-negative rate increases to 11%. In determining the appropriate number of sections to be prepared, individual laboratories also need to consider other factors such as laboratory resources and the types of diseases likely to be encountered. At a minimum, several step sections should be mounted for microscopic examination.

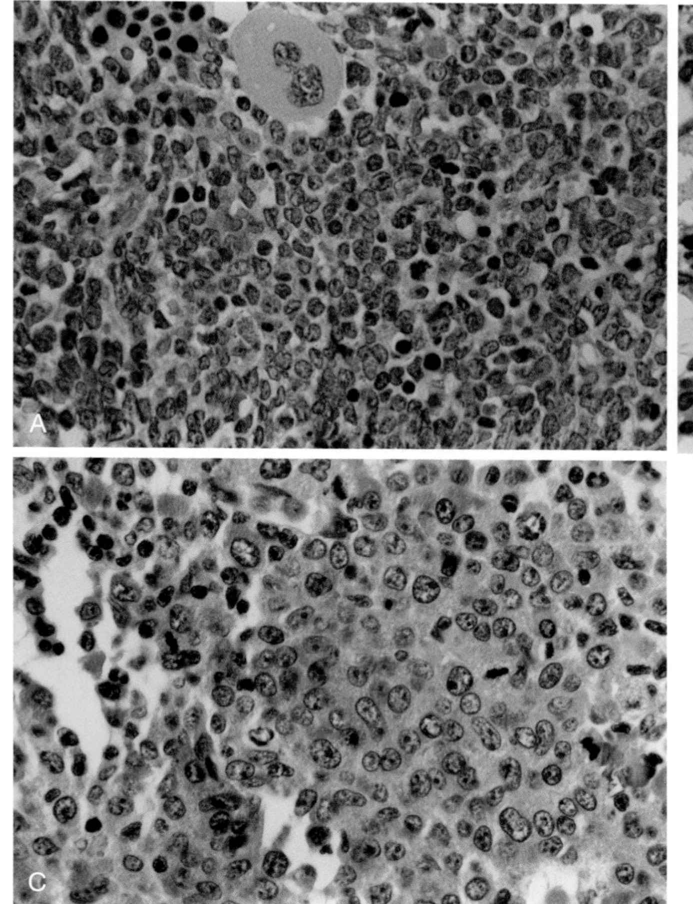

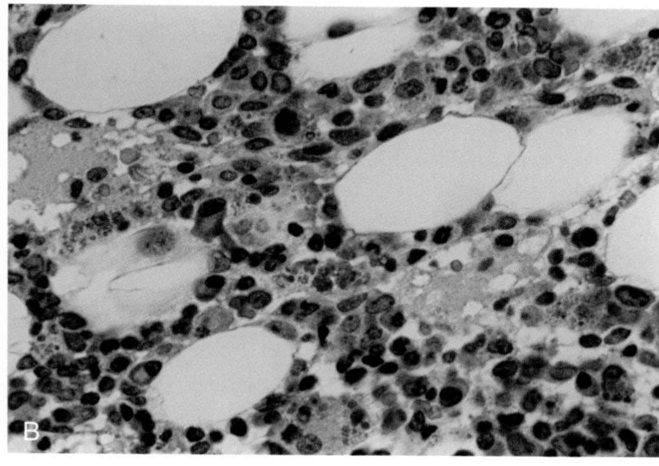

Figure 3-2. Hematoxylin-eosin–stained trephine sections of marrow specimens with leukemia. A, Extensive and diffuse marrow infiltration by precursor T-lymphoblastic leukemia; the upper left corner shows several mature erythroblasts. **B,** Interstitial marrow infiltration by 60% myeloblasts in a patient with underlying Fanconi's anemia. **C,** Focus of left-shifted granulopoiesis with mostly neutrophilic myelocytes in the marrow of a patient with chronic myeloid leukemia in the chronic phase.

Staining

If the core biopsy has been well fixed, decalcified, processed, and sectioned, routine hematoxylin-eosin staining provides excellent histologic detail. Harris hematoxylin stain may be preferred because, as a regressive stain, it allows more flexibility and better control of the intensity of nuclear staining. Zenker's-fixed trephine sections may need a longer staining time in hematoxylin than do B5- or formalin-fixed specimens.

Depending on the individual laboratory and patient population, other stains may be routine. For example, periodic acid–Schiff stains provide an additional means of distinguishing granulocytes and precursors from erythroblasts, highlighting megakaryocytes, and rapidly visualizing fungal organisms; this last feature may be helpful in institutions with large populations of immunosuppressed patients. In cases of myeloproliferative disorders or hairy cell leukemia, assessment of marrow fibrosis is best done with a stain for reticulin; the normal presence of reticulin fibers around arterioles serves as an internal positive control (Fig. 3-3). Collagenous fibrosis is uncommon in the bone marrow and should be looked for on a case-by-case basis. A Giemsa stain can be helpful when looking for mast cells in mastocytosis. There is a high false-negative rate with iron stains of decalcified core sections, caused by the chelation of iron during the decalcification process[18]; therefore, I do not recommend the routine staining of the core biopsy for storage iron. If a satisfactory marrow aspirate was not obtained, iron stains of the clot or biopsy sections are the next best option, keeping in mind the possibility of false-negative results. Staining procedures for hematoxylin-eosin and for reticulin are given in the Appendix.

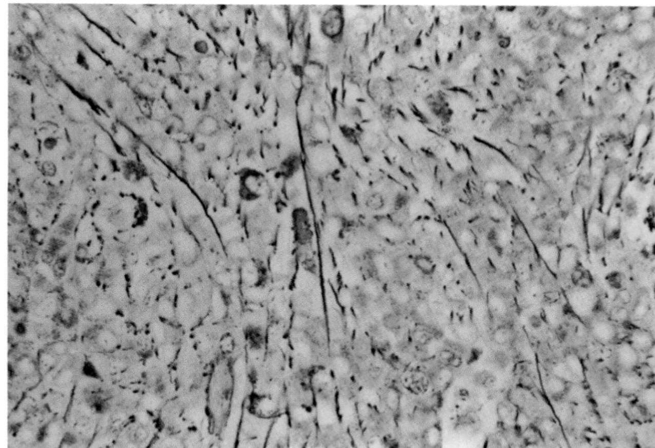

Figure 3-3. Reticulin stain of the marrow core section of a patient with chronic myeloid leukemia showing increased reticulin fibers (*brown-black lines*) within the marrow interstitium, away from the expected normal perivascular location (Wilder reticulin stain).

Bone Marrow Aspirate

From the 1 mL of fluid marrow aspirate obtained for morphologic examination, several preparations are made that allow the maximal use of all components of the sample: direct smears, concentrated or buffy coat smears, particle crush preparation, and particle clot sections. The following procedure is used in my laboratory.

Direct Smears

As quickly as possible after the 1 mL of un-anticoagulated fluid marrow is aspirated, most of it is transferred to a paraffin-coated vial to which disodium EDTA powder has been added (1 mg EDTA for 1 to 2 mL marrow; 0.5 mg EDTA for <1 mL marrow). The paraffin coat prevents the adherence of megakaryocytes to the wall of the vial. The vial is inverted several times to ensure adequate mixing of the marrow and EDTA. This anticoagulated mixture can be brought back to the laboratory for the preparation of additional aspirate smears for morphology or other studies, including iron stains and cytochemistry; it can also be used to prepare the buffy coat smears (see later).

From the remaining un-anticoagulated fluid, individual drops of marrow are quickly placed directly on 6 to 10 glass slides, and a spreader device is used to create aspirate smears. These smears are dried quickly for the preservation of cytologic detail.

Buffy Coat Smears

Based on my own anecdotal experience and that of my colleagues, relative to the amount of preparatory effort required, buffy coat smears of the bone marrow aspirate (also known as concentrated smears) do not add substantially to the information obtained from well-prepared direct smears or particle crush preparations. For the interested reader, the full procedure for preparing buffy coat smears of bone marrow is provided in the Appendix. Briefly, after adequate mixing by inversion of the tube, the EDTA-anticoagulated marrow is placed in a clean Petri dish. The fluid component is collected and transferred to a Wintrobe hematocrit tube, which is then centrifuged. (The marrow spicules are used to prepare the particle crush preparation; see later.) This centrifugation results in the separation of the EDTA-anticoagulated marrow fluid into various distinct layers. One such layer has a tan or "buff" color and is rich in nucleated cells. From this layer, smears are made that are used for routine cytologic examination as well as cytochemical studies. If ultrastructural studies by electron microscopy are planned, the layer is removed for appropriate processing.

Particle Crush Preparation

After the fluid component from the EDTA-anticoagulated marrow in the Petri dish has been collected and placed in the Wintrobe tube for the preparation of buffy coat smears, marrow spicules, if present, should be picked up, placed on three to four clean glass slides, and gently squashed by placing another glass slide on top and pulling the two slides apart in an opposite but parallel direction.

Particle Clot Sections

Any marrow spicules that still remain in the Petri dish are rinsed with 0.015M calcium chloride and pushed close together to form a clot. These particle clots are processed similarly to the core biopsy, but without the decalcification step.

Relative Values of Different Marrow Aspirate Preparations

Not all these aspirate preparations are necessary for every case, and their contribution to the marrow examination sometimes overlaps. Various authors have assessed the relative value of one over another, explored the possibility of substituting one for another, and concluded that the different preparations contribute in different ways in different cases. On the one hand, the direct smears provide excellent cytologic detail with minimal distortion by anticoagulation or centrifugation.[19] On the other hand, examination of a hypocellular specimen can be tedious, and the cell distribution may be uneven because the specimen is not mixed. Buffy coat smears allow a more consistent distribution of cells, and the concentration of erythroblasts facilitates the assessment of sideroblastic iron when a Dacie stain is used. However, the cytologic disadvantages of the buffy coat smears have already been noted, and the preparation is more time-consuming and labor-intensive relative to the amount of diagnostic information gained. In addition, in their examination of 44 pediatric marrow specimens with acute leukemia, Izadi and colleagues[20] reported that buffy coat smears underestimated the proportion of blasts when compared with direct smears (12% to 24% blasts versus 32% to 48% blasts, respectively). In one case of acute promyelocytic leukemia, the authors reported that 9% promyelocytes were seen in the buffy coat preparation, compared with 26% in the direct smear. Neutrophilic precursors were also underestimated in the buffy coat preparation in one case of benign neutropenia. The particle crush preparation bears the closest resemblance to marrow tissue in vivo and allows an approximation of the cells' spatial relationship; however, it also results in more damaged nuclei.

Dry Tap

Approximately 2% to 7% of the time, attempts at aspiration yield no fluid, resulting in the so-called dry tap.[21,22] In his review of more than 1000 bone marrow aspirations and biopsies at a single institution over 6.5 years, Humphries[22] found that faulty technique accounted for only 6.9% of dry taps. Otherwise, the dry tap indicates underlying marrow damage or disease such as aplastic anemia, hairy cell leukemia, advanced-stage myeloproliferative disorder, acute megakaryoblastic leukemia, or mastocytosis. Under these circumstances, one should ensure that sufficient touch imprints are made for cytologic examination and for additional cytochemical studies.[23,24] Because the touch imprints may yield very few cells in cases of severe marrow fibrosis, a bone crush preparation may also be considered; with this technique, the core biopsies are cut into small pieces before being crushed between two glass slides, simulating a particle crush preparation. One should obtain additional cores for most of the special studies, such as cytogenetics, flow cytometric immunophenotyping, molecular genetics, and cultures.[25] The marrow cores can even be minced or subjected to gentle collagenase digestion,[26] although these steps are best left to the discretion of the individual specialty laboratory.

Electron Microscopy

Ultrastructural studies by electron microscopy have become less frequent, partly because of the increasing use of flow cytometric analysis for immunophenotyping. If ultrastructural evaluations are anticipated, an extra 1 mL of fluid marrow should be aspirated. Preferably, this collection should occur after procurement of the sample for morphologic examination but before subsequent aspirates become successively more hemodiluted.[27,28] A summary of the procedure for preparing the marrow aspirate for electron microscopic evaluation is included in the Appendix.

Staining of Marrow Aspirate Smears

Wright-Giemsa Stain

The importance of a well-stained marrow aspirate smear cannot be overemphasized (Figs. 3-4 and 3-5). A poorly stained aspirate smear can mislead and frustrate. For air-dried marrow touch imprints and aspirate preparations, a Romanowsky-type stain is often used. The May-Grünwald-Giemsa stain is also used for staining marrow aspirate preparations. With either staining method, for optimal results, slides should be stained within 24 hours of being prepared. As a "salvage" option, I have found that slides that were previously but poorly stained with Wright-Giemsa can be restained within 1 to 2 months from the time of collection.

Iron Stains

To assess storage iron, a Prussian blue staining method is used on the crush preparation of the fat-perivascular layer (Fig. 3-6A). To evaluate the proportion of sideroblasts and ring sideroblasts, a Dacie method of iron staining is performed on a particle crush preparation, direct marrow aspirate smear, or buffy coat smear. Storage iron can also be assessed in any marrow particles or macrophages present on the buffy coat smear (see Fig. 3-6B). It is important that adequate marrow particles be examined to reliably assess iron stores. Although stainable iron may be found in a single particle, Hughes and associates[29] reported that a minimum of seven particles must be examined to accurately establish the absence of stainable iron. If necessary, an iron stain can be done on the particle clot sections. However, as noted earlier, the interpretation of iron stores on a decalcified trephine section requires caution because the absence of storage iron in such specimens may be due to chelation during decalcification and not true iron depletion.[18] Smears previously stained with Wright stain can be superimposed with Prussian blue reagent to assess sideroblastic iron.[30]

Table 3-1 summarizes the different components of a marrow examination and the various types of stains applicable to the specific preparations. Procedures for Wright-Giemsa staining and for iron stains are provided in the Appendix.

Last, when staining marrow touch imprints and aspirate preparations for routine morphologic examination, the laboratory should save several unstained preparations until the diagnostic evaluation is completed, in case additional studies are necessary.

BONE MARROW EXAMINATION

A complete marrow evaluation entails a review of the relevant clinical and laboratory data as well as examination of the peripheral blood smear, marrow aspirate, and core biopsy. As noted earlier, examining the aspirate alone misses the correct diagnosis of metastatic carcinoma 30% of the time, and examining only the core biopsy misses the diagnosis 9% of the time. Although the reports of the aspiration and core biopsy eventually find their way to the patient's chart, having two seemingly contradictory results on what is really the same sample creates confusion and detracts from efficient patient care. To avoid this pitfall, the final diagnosis should be a unified one. If it is not possible for the same pathologist to examine both the marrow aspirate and the core biopsy, each report must note the existence of the other. Readers of such reports must then collate them for the final interpretation.

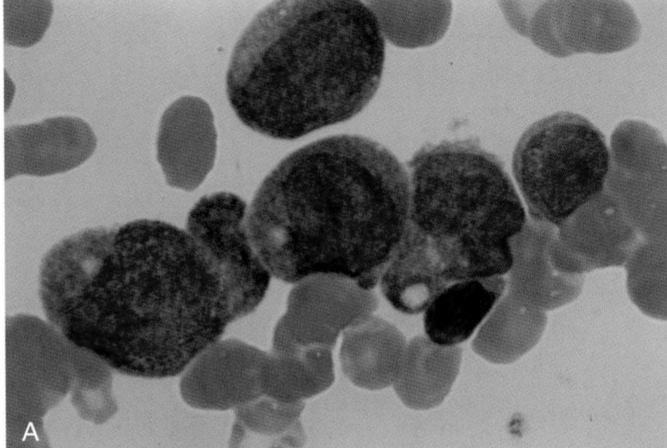

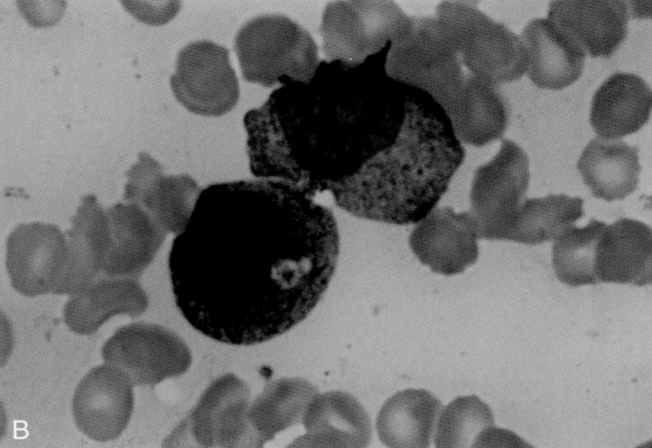

Figure 3-4. Wright-Giemsa–stained marrow aspirate smears of agranulocytosis in a patient who presented with profound neutropenia. **A**, The original stained smear shows a hypocellular specimen with a relative preponderance of early myeloid precursors, raising the differential diagnosis of blasts versus neutrophilic promyelocytes. **B**, Restaining of the smear with Wright-Giemsa shows the presence of azurophilic granules within the precursors, indicative of neutrophilic promyelocytes. Cytogenetic analysis subsequently revealed a normal karyotype. The neutrophil count recovered within a week.

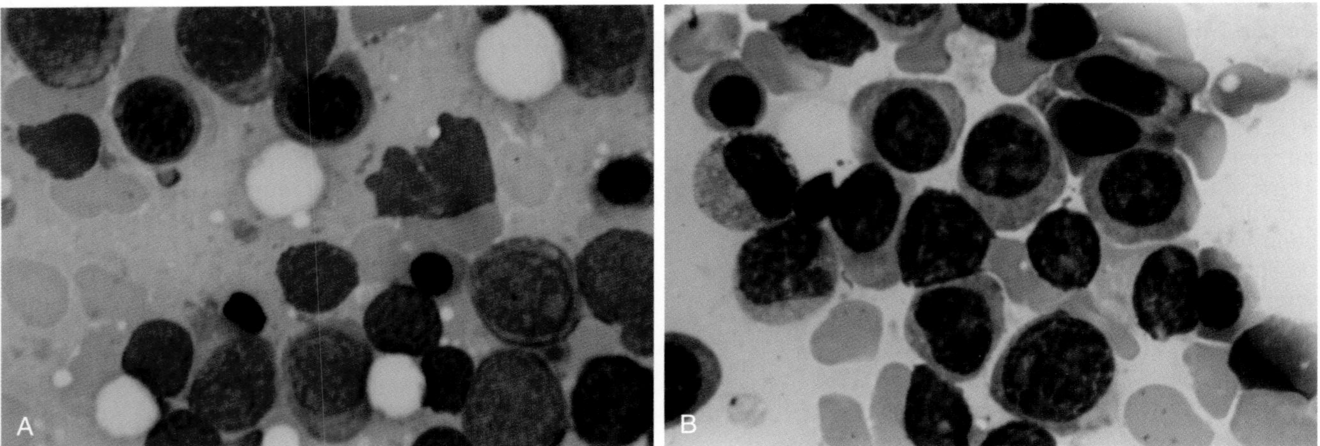

Figure 3-5. Wright-Giemsa–stained marrow aspirate smears of an adult who presented with anemia. A, The original stained smear shows an increased proportion of abnormal cells with overlapping features between plasma cells and basophilic normoblasts. Several polychromatophilic erythroblasts are also present. **B,** Restaining of the smear with Wright-Giemsa confirms the presence of abnormal plasma cells. Subsequent immunohistochemical studies of the core biopsy showed kappa-restricted plasma cell myeloma.

Although I have not specifically discussed the role of the blood smear in the evaluation of marrow specimens, it is clear that the blood is an integral component in any evaluation of a hematologic abnormality.[6] In many cases, the blood first manifests an abnormality that triggers a marrow examination. Occasionally, the blood may show a greater proportion of blasts or a greater degree of differentiation of leukemic cells than the marrow. One may argue that some of these findings are of questionable clinical significance, yet these details may impact one's ability to monitor patients for disease progression or relapse. It is most efficient to obtain blood smears at the time the bone marrow aspiration and biopsy procedure is performed. If a blood smear is not available to the pathologist, at a minimum, hemogram data should be reviewed.

FINAL REPORT

The final report of a bone marrow examination should include the diagnosis, the pathologist's recommendation for further studies if necessary, and supporting data. When multiple laboratories are involved in the analysis and interpretation of a specimen, a concise summary of the salient results from these contributing laboratories should be provided and integrated into the final diagnosis. At the minimum, the hematopathology report should list the specialty laboratories to which aliquots of the specimen were sent.

Inclusion in the report of a detailed differential count of the marrow aspirate or the blood is not always necessary. For example, when the marrow examination is performed to look for metastatic disease but the hemogram and marrow are otherwise normal, or when there is severe pancytopenia and the marrow is markedly hypocellular, differential counts are not required. When a differential count may provide useful information but is not required for determining the diagnosis or subclassification of a process, the International Council for Standardization in Hematology (ICSH) has indicated that a 300-cell count of the nucleated bone marrow cells is sufficient.[9] However, when the disease process involves acute leukemias, myelodysplastic syndromes, or myeloproliferative disorders, and when knowledge of the proportions of

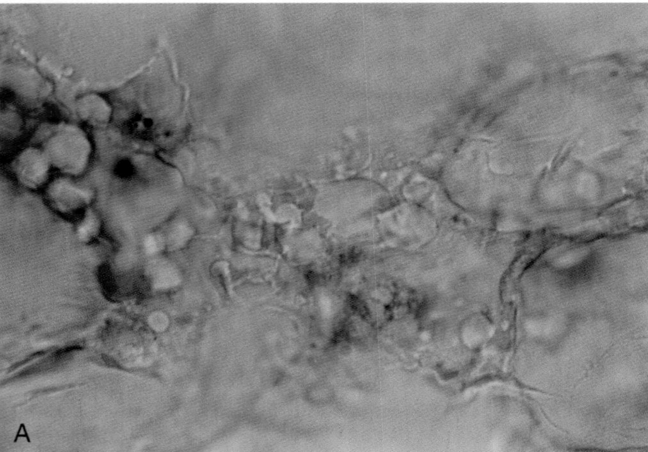

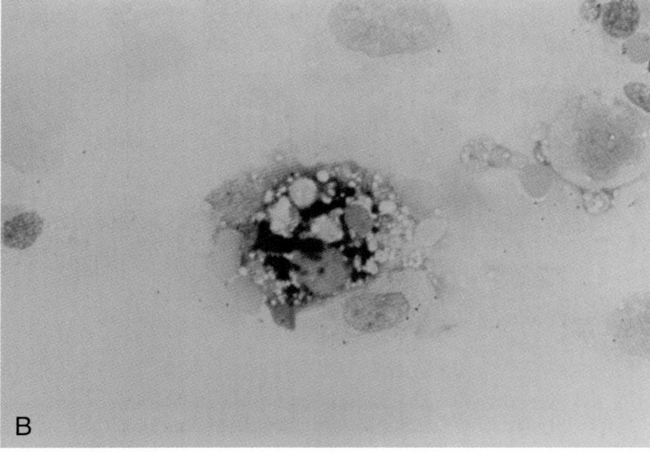

Figure 3-6. Iron stains of marrow aspirate smears. A, Prussian blue reaction of a crush preparation of the fat-perivascular layer showing increased storage iron within macrophages. **B,** Dacie stain of a buffy coat smear showing increased iron within a macrophage.

Table 3-1 Components of a Marrow Examination and Applicable Stains

Examination Component	Stain and Method of Analysis
Bone marrow trephine biopsy	H&E Reticulin PAS Giemsa Immunohistochemistry (can also be used for cytogenetics, flow cytometric analysis, molecular genetics, and cultures if necessary)
Marrow touch imprint and bone crush preparation	Wright-Giemsa Dacie stain Cytochemistry Immunocytochemistry
Bone marrow aspirate	Electron microscopy Flow cytometric analysis Cytogenetics; molecular genetics Cultures
Direct smear	Wright-Giemsa Dacie stain Cytochemistry Immunocytochemistry
Buffy coat smear	Wright-Giemsa Dacie stain Cytochemistry Immunocytochemistry
Particle crush preparation	Wright-Giemsa Dacie stain Cytochemistry Immunocytochemistry
Fat-perivascular layer	Prussian blue stain
Particle clot section	H&E PAS Giemsa Immunohistochemistry Prussian blue stain

H&E, hematoxylin-eosin; PAS, periodic acid–Schiff.

blasts and other abnormal cells is necessary for an accurate diagnosis, classification, or follow-up, detailed differential counts are justified. The World Health Organization recommends that differential counts of 200 leukocytes in the blood and 500 cells in the marrow be performed in determining the percentage of blasts,[31] with additional cells to be counted or additional smears examined if the proportion of abnormal cells is at a "critical threshold for disease stratification" or if there is an uneven distribution of such cells.[9] The ICSH recommends that bone marrow differential counts include blast cells, promyelocytes, myelocytes, metamyelocytes, band forms, segmented neutrophils, eosinophils, basophils, mast cells, promonocytes, monocytes, lymphocytes, plasma cells, and erythroblasts. The nucleated cell count should not include megakaryocytes, macrophages, osteoblasts, osteoclasts, stromal cells, smudged cells, or nonhematopoietic cells such as tumor cells. Lymphoid aggregates, if present, should not be included in the count, but their presence should be commented on.[9]

CONCLUSION

Accurate interpretation of the marrow requires that the marrow specimen be adequate and well prepared. This translates into an examination that includes the blood, the marrow aspirate, and the core biopsy. Rigorous monitoring of the processing and staining procedure ensures optimal morphologic detail for microscopic examination, thus maximizing the likelihood of an accurate diagnosis.

For a detailed analysis of stains and techniques for the effective staining of tissue samples, see the Appendix.

Acknowledgments

The author gratefully acknowledges Dr. A. Jatoi, Department of Oncology, Mayo Clinic, Rochester, Minnesota, for her many helpful suggestions.

Pearls and Pitfalls

Procurement of Bone Marrow Core Biopsy and Aspirate
- Plan ahead: How many cores? Bilateral or unilateral? How many aspirate samples, for what studies, in what types of anticoagulant, in what sequence? Is there any possibility of a sternal aspirate or a dry tap?
- Aspirate quickly and do not exceed 1 mL when aspirating the sample for morphologic examination.
- Obtain additional cores for special studies if the aspiration is hemodiluted or if it yields a dry tap.
- Obtain extra heparinized marrow aspirates (for possible flow cytometry, cytogenetics, or cultures) if the differential diagnosis is broad.
- Use an 8-gauge biopsy needle when experiencing difficulty retaining the marrow cores within the biopsy needle and if the patient is suspected of being osteopenic.

Processing and Staining
- Reactivity for myeloperoxidase fades after a few months; reactivity for Sudan black B does not.
- Dry all smears rapidly. A small tabletop fan can help when the humidity is high.

Examination and Final Report
- Examine and report on both the aspirate and the core biopsy. If this is not possible, indicate that there is another report to be integrated.
- Indicate the status of samples that have been sent to specialty laboratories.

References can be found on Expert Consult @ www.expertconsult.com

Chapter 4

Immunohistochemistry for the Hematopathology Laboratory

Stefania Pittaluga, Todd S. Barry, and Mark Raffeld

CHAPTER OUTLINE

Perhaps in no other subspecialty of pathology does immunohistochemistry (IHC) play as important a role in the accurate diagnosis and definition of disease subtypes as it does in hematopathology. Before the development of this technology, the diagnosis of lymphoproliferative diseases depended on classification systems based solely on morphologic differences. The subjective use of morphology-based classification schemes led to difficulty in defining biologically different entities, and the morphologic categories were often difficult to reproduce even among expert hematopathologists. The advent of IHC allowed the objective identification of specific phenotypic characteristics associated with different lymphoid proliferations. Such phenotypic markers provide information about the cell of lymphoma origin, the production of characteristic oncogenic proteins, and the proliferative characteristics of the lymphoma. By intercalating immunohistochemical studies with morphologic characteristics, more reproducible and biologically relevant classification schemes were developed, reaching their current level of sophistication with the recent publication of the World Health Organization (WHO) classification of lymphoproliferative diseases.[1] The goal of this chapter is to introduce the reader to the practice of IHC and to the wide range of antigenic targets that have proved useful in hematopathology.

BASIC IMMUNOHISTOCHEMISTRY

In theory, IHC is a simple technology that requires only three basic elements: a cellular antigen of interest, a primary antibody targeting the antigen, and a detection system to visualize the location of the antibody-antigen complex. In actual practice, the achievement of good IHC is much more problematic and depends on the condition of the tissue antigen; the type, specificity, and affinity of the primary antibody; and the detection system employed. The interpretation of IHC stains requires knowledge of and control over these elements, as well as an experienced pathologist.

Antigens

At the heart of IHC is the antigen-antibody reaction; therefore, it is crucial that the antigenic epitopes recognized by the cognate diagnostic antibody maintain their reactive conformation. The specific antigenic epitopes present on any given protein or carbohydrate moiety are subject to enzymatic degradation that begins immediately after biopsy or resection and to further conformational changes resulting from fixation. To ensure preservation of the antigen of interest, rapid tissue fixation is important. Some antigenic epitopes, such as those on keratin proteins and other structural proteins of the cell, are relatively resistant to degradation; other antigens, such as phosphoepitopes on signaling proteins, undergo rapid degradation within minutes to hours.[2,3]

Although prompt tissue fixation is essential to preserve antigenicity, the specific fixative and the fixation process itself can interfere with antigenicity by causing conformational changes in antigenic molecules or by actually chemically modifying the antigenic epitopes. Traditionally, tissues have been fixed in neutral buffered formalin (pH 7.0) because it is inexpensive, has sterilizing properties, and preserves morphologic features well. The exact chemical reactions that occur in tissues are not well understood, but it is generally assumed that formalin's ability to cross-link aldehyde groups in proteins is responsible for its fixative properties. This mode of action is potentially deleterious to antigenic structure, and although some antigenic epitopes may not be affected significantly by formaldehyde cross-linking, these chemical modifications clearly have an adverse effect on many antigens. Because formalin penetrates tissues slowly and the chemical reactions are complex, the number of modifications that take place is time dependent. In practice, this means that antigens fall into three basic categories: formalin-resistant epitopes, highly formalin-sensitive epitopes, and epitopes with a time-dependent sensitivity to formalin fixation. Although there have been attempts to generate antibodies specifically to formalin-resistant epitopes,[4] most of the antibodies found to react with formalin-resistant epitopes have been identified through large-scale screenings of available antibody preparations.

Over the years, there has been great interest in identifying methods to overcome or reverse the deleterious effects of formalin fixation. The earliest attempts to retrieve antigenicity used proteolytic enzymes,[5] which presumably act by breaking formaldehyde-induced methylene cross-links in the antigenic molecules, thereby relaxing some of the conformational constraints on the protein epitopes. Such proteolytic methods continue to be used in many IHC laboratories and are particularly useful for recovering the reactivity of the cytokeratins. Nonetheless, proteolytic methods are difficult to control, and careful attention is needed to optimize their retrieval effect and avoid tissue destruction.

Despite some successes with proteolytic methods, the major breakthrough that brought IHC into widespread use was the development of heat-induced epitope retrieval (HIER) procedures.[6] This technique involves heating fixed tissue sections in buffered solutions at or above 100°C for several minutes to more than half an hour. HIER methods vary in terms of the recommended buffer solutions and the mode of heating, but the basic formula of applying wet heat over a period of time is universal.[7,8] The exact mechanism by which HIER reverses the loss of antigenicity in formalin-fixed tissue is unknown. However, hydrolytic cleavage of formaldehyde-related chemical groups and cross-links, the unfolding of inner epitopes, and the extraction of calcium ions from coordination complexes with proteins are among the hypothesized mechanisms.[9,10]

The advent of HIER methods has revolutionized IHC and greatly expanded the number of antibodies that react in formalin-fixed, paraffin-embedded tissue sections.[6,10,11] HIER has also improved the sensitivity of antibodies directed to formalin-resistant epitopes and has enabled the routine assessment of a wide spectrum of antigens in epoxy resin–embedded bone marrow sections.[12] Appropriate retrieval can minimize many of the problems related to overfixation, reducing differences in immunostaining that result from the difficulty of controlling fixation time in the clinical laboratory.[13]

The major disadvantage of HIER is that the high heat can cause considerable tissue damage, particularly when the tissue is underfixed or has a high collagen content, the antigen retrieval time is prolonged, and the buffers contain ethylenediaminetetraacetic acid (EDTA) or have a high pH. Tissue damage can be minimized by ensuring that tissues are optimally fixed, reducing the antigen retrieval time, or changing the retrieval buffer. Despite this potential problem, the ability to detect otherwise nondetectable antigens far outweighs the potential for tissue damage on occasional tissue sections.

Primary Antibodies

There are two major categories of primary antibodies used in diagnostic pathology: monoclonal antibodies and polyclonal antibodies. Polyclonal antibodies are generated by injecting an animal (most commonly a rabbit or goat) with the antigenic preparation of interest and harvesting the animal's serum once an immune response is detected. The serum is subjected to purification and sometimes to differential adsorptions to eliminate unwanted reactivity, but it always comprises a spectrum of antibody molecules originating from multiple unrelated antibody-producing cells (hence the term *polyclonal*). The specificity of a polyclonal antibody preparation is highly dependent on the purity of the initial antigenic preparation and how extensively adsorbed it is. Obtaining highly specific preparations is difficult, and background problems can be troublesome, especially when applied to IHC. Further, because the antibody response is variable over time and from one individual animal to another, complete standardization of antibody composition is not possible. Although developments in recombinant DNA and protein synthesis technology have greatly improved the specificity of polyclonal antibodies by providing tools to generate highly purified protein immunogens or even specific immunogenic peptides, polyclonal antibodies may still contain unwanted specificities.

Monoclonal antibodies, in contrast, are the product of a single immortalized antibody-producing cell, thus avoiding most problems related to antibody heterogeneity and specificity inherent in polyclonal antibody preparations. The hybridoma technology pioneered by Kohler and Milstein[14] in the 1970s allows the immortalization of a single antibody-producing mouse plasma cell by fusing it with a mouse plasmacytoma cell line. Individual hybrid mouse cells can be clonally expanded in tissue culture or in mice as tumors, providing a continuous source of antibody of known composition and reactivity. Because of their high quality and specificity, monoclonal antibodies were rapidly developed as diagnostic reagents in hematopathology, as well as for other clinical applications that require standardized reagents. The specificity advantage of the monoclonal antibody, however, can also be a disadvantage when applied to denatured proteins in tissue sections. Because a polyclonal antibody preparation generally contains a mixture of antibodies reacting to multiple epitopes, it does not matter if some of the epitopes are rendered inactive by the fixation process, as long as one epitope remains in its reactive conformation. However, if the single epitope recognized by a monoclonal antibody is affected by the fixation process, the antibody cannot be used for IHC. A second disadvantage of the mouse monoclonal antibodies is that they generally have weaker affinity constants than do comparable polyclonal rabbit antibody preparations. This led to the development of rabbit plasmacytoma cell lines that could be used as fusion partners to generate high-affinity rabbit monoclonal antibodies.[15,16] Rabbit monoclonal antibodies are now available for many targets of hematopathologic interest, including CD3, CD5, CD8, CD23, CD79a, cyclin D1, and Ki-67.

Table 4-1 Comparison of Detection Systems for Immunohistochemistry

	Avidin-Biotin	Polymer	Tyramide
Sensitivity	Acceptable	High	Very high
Background	Acceptable	Biotin-free	High
Cost	Low	High	High

Regardless of which type of antibody is chosen for an immunohistochemical procedure, careful control over the development and use of the antibody must be maintained. Although antibody specificity is best demonstrated by immunoblotting or immunoprecipitation, this type of biochemical analysis is required only during the initial development of the antibody. However, before placing any antibody into clinical use, extensive validation of its efficacy and staining characteristics on tissue sections in the individual laboratory is necessary. This should include extensive testing of normal and tumor tissues to assess the specificity and sensitivity of tissue staining. The use of tissue microarrays can be extremely helpful during this stage. Once the antibody has been validated and placed in service, the continued use of both negative and positive controls is mandatory with each test sample. Negative controls are best demonstrated by omitting the primary antibody or by substituting the specific primary antibody with an isotype-matched control antibody or immunoglobulin (Ig) preparation.[17,18] Positive controls should include tissues that are known to contain the antigen of interest.[18]

Detection Systems

Detection systems comprise an enzyme, a chromogenic substrate, and a link or bridge reagent that brings the enzyme into proximity with the primary labeling antibody. The choice of a detection system is of great importance, and each method has its own advantages and disadvantages (Table 4-1). Factors influencing the selection of a detection method are related to the type of tissue, the cellular target, its abundance and localization, and laboratory-specific issues (e.g., complexity, time requirements, reagent costs). The most widely used detection systems today are the biotin-based systems—of which the avidin-biotin immunoperoxidase complex (ABC) system developed by Hsu and coworkers[19] may be considered a prototype—and the more recently developed polymer-based systems.[20,21] In the ABC system, a tissue-bound primary unlabeled antibody is reacted with a secondary biotin-conjugated link antibody, and detection is carried out through preformed avidin–biotinylated enzyme (peroxidase) complexes. The peroxidase enzyme in the complex then reacts with a chromogen (e.g., 3,3′-diaminobenzidine [DAB] or 3 amino-9-ethylcarbazole [AEC]) to produce a colored reaction product that is discretely localized to the targeted antigen. More recently, polymer-based detection systems have been developed that do not depend on avidin-biotin links, thereby avoiding the possibility of high backgrounds in tissues rich in endogenous biotin.[20,21] Like in the biotin-based systems, an unlabeled primary antibody is used first, followed in this case by a modified polymer (e.g., dextran) that is linked to a large number of secondary link antibodies and enzyme (peroxidase) molecules. Thus, one reagent contains both a species-specific secondary anti-immunoglobulin linking antibody and the chromogen developing enzyme. Newer detection systems have also been developed to increase the sensitivity for detecting antigens expressed at very low levels or to improve the detection of low-affinity primary antibodies. These systems involve a tyramide-based signal amplification method known as the catalyzed reporter deposition (CARD) or catalyzed system amplification (CSA) method.[22,23]

Interpretive Problems

It is necessary to distinguish specific from nonspecific signals when interpreting IHC. There are many sources of false-positive results, including endogenous biotin or peroxidase, inappropriately high antibody concentrations, poor technique (e.g., excessive antigen retrieval, drying artifacts, prolonged detection), or interpretive errors such as mistaking endogenous pigment for the chromogenic reaction product. Endogenous biotin reactivity can be a serious problem because of its variable occurrence in tumors. This biotin positivity is often amplified by retrieval techniques and displays a granular pattern that can be difficult to distinguish from other granular cytoplasmic staining.[24] Failure to block biotin can lead to problems with interpretation and the reporting of false-positive results.[25,26] Use of one of the newer polymer-based detection systems that avoids the use of a biotin-avidin link can eliminate this problem. False-negative results also have myriad reasons, the most frequent of which are inadequate antigen retrieval, suboptimally fixed tissue, inappropriate primary antibody, or other technical staining issues.

It cannot be overemphasized that the accurate interpretation of IHC stains requires knowledge of the laboratory's methods, the antibodies used, and the expected staining pattern for each antibody. Different antibody preparations to the same antigen may show different patterns and intensities of nonspecific or even specific staining. For instance, the traditional polyclonal carcinoembryonic antigen (CEA) antibodies cross-react with other CEA-like proteins such as CEACAM6 and stain granulocytes, whereas specific monoclonal CEA antibodies do not.[27] Monoclonal antibodies targeting different epitopes of the TREG-associated marker FOXP3 have been shown to stain different subpopulations of cells in comparative studies in paraffin sections.[28] As another example, the anti–Ki-67 monoclonal antibody MIB-1 has been reported to stain the cell membrane of some tumor types, whereas other monoclonal antibodies to the same antigen do not show this type of aberrant staining.[29] Knowledge of the subcellular staining location of the targeted antigen is crucial. There are a number of expected locations for antibody signals, including nuclear, nuclear and cytoplasmic, cytoplasmic, membranous, Golgi, and extracellular (Fig. 4-1). An unexpected staining localization should immediately raise a red flag and should not be considered positive in any situation. For example, in a recent assessment of synaptophysin antibodies by the NordiQC organization, one of several monoclonal antibody preparations was found to produce an unusual dot-like staining reaction in tissues that were known to be negative for synaptophysin. This artifactual staining pattern was believed to be the result of a cross-reaction with a Golgi-associated protein—an artifact that was previously associated with other monoclonal antibodies prepared from mouse ascites,[30] as was the case for this particular antibody. It is also critical that the interpreter be able to distinguish nonspecific background

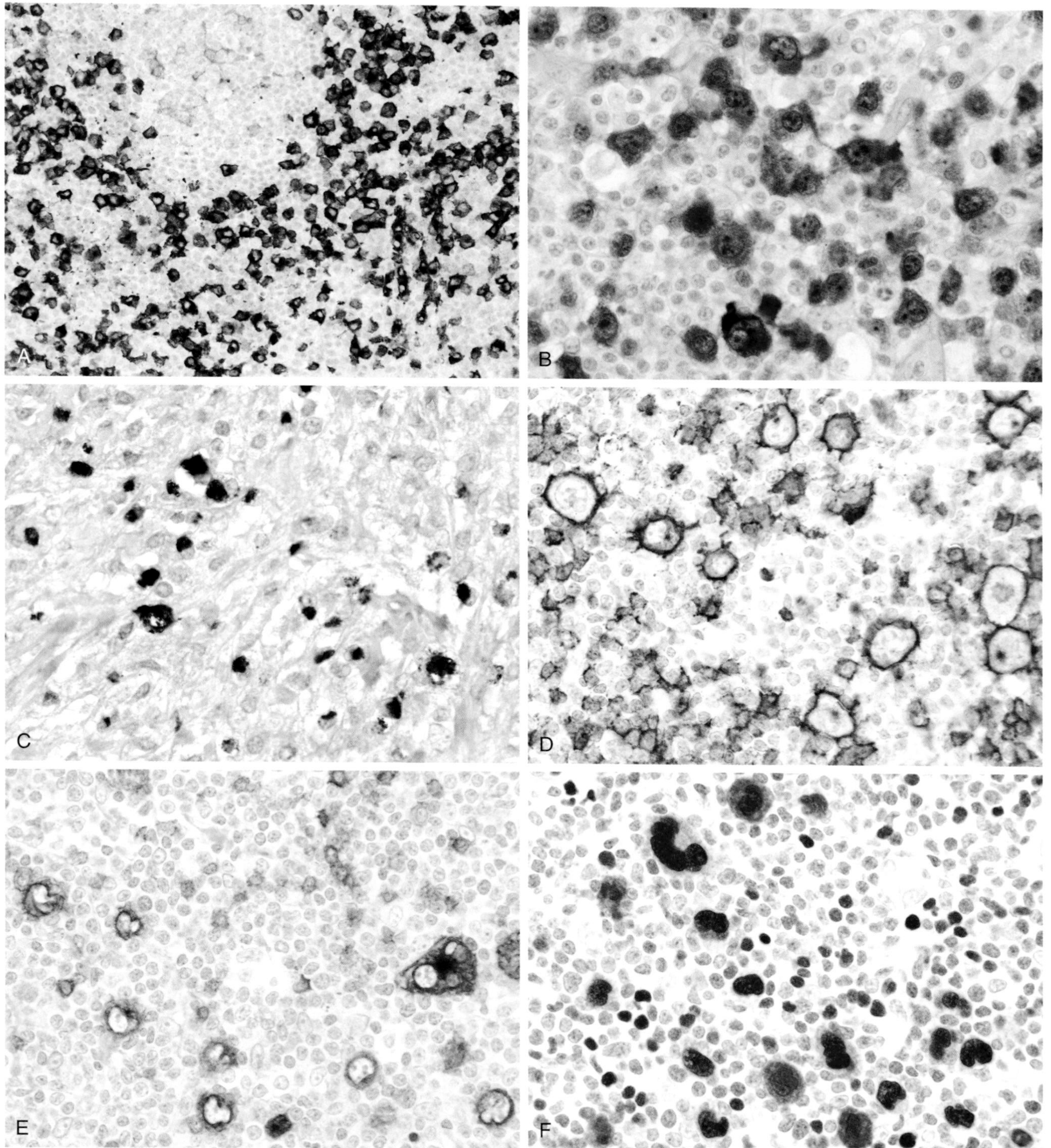

Figure 4-1. Representative patterns of cell-associated immunohistochemical staining (U-view/DAB detection, Ventana, Tucson, AZ; plus hematoxylin counterstain). **A-C,** Examples of immunohistochemical targeting of antigen expression in a case of anaplastic lymphoma kinase (ALK)–positive anaplastic large cell lymphoma. **A,** Membranous and Golgi staining pattern using a monoclonal antibody against CD30. **B,** Nuclear and cytoplasmic staining pattern characteristic of a monoclonal antibody against ALK. **C,** Cytoplasmic granular staining pattern characteristic of a monoclonal antibody against TIA-1. **D,** Membranous staining pattern using a monoclonal antibody against CD20 in nodular lymphocyte-predominant Hodgkin's lymphoma. **E** and **F,** Examples of immunohistochemical targeting of antigen expression in a case of nodular lymphocyte-predominant Hodgkin's lymphoma. **E,** Cytoplasmic staining pattern with membranous and perinuclear accentuation using a polyclonal antibody against immunoglobulin D. **F,** Nuclear and cytoplasmic staining using a monoclonal antibody against OCT-2.

staining or pigment deposits from true staining resulting from the presence of the antigen. It is the ultimate responsibility of the hematopathologist to be familiar with the methods and specific antibodies used by the laboratory, as well as the expected staining patterns of the targeted antigens when using these results to provide diagnoses.

Frozen Sections and Cytospins

Before the development of antigen retrieval and the widespread development of antibodies that react in formalin-fixed, paraffin-embedded tissues, any chapter dealing with IHC would have focused on frozen sections and cytospins. Today, frozen sections are used infrequently, and cytospins are primarily the domain of the cytologist. Although frozen section IHC continues to play a major role in research applications, there are only a few clinically relevant antigens that cannot be assessed in fixed tissues, such as the γδ T-cell receptor. The principles of immunostaining cryostat-sectioned frozen sections and cytospins are essentially identical to those already discussed for formalin-fixed, paraffin-embedded tissues. Nonetheless, there are a few specific differences and considerations that are critical to obtaining optimal results. These differences involve tissue storage, sectioning, fixation, and the immunostaining procedure itself.

Frozen section IHC requires the availability of a properly frozen block of tissue embedded in a mounting medium such as OCT (Sakura Finetek, Torrance, CA). To prepare the frozen block, a thin slice of tissue is covered with the gelatinous OCT compound and quickly frozen by immersing the tissue in a solution of 2-methylbutane and alcohol or in liquid nitrogen. The OCT compound serves the dual purpose of stabilizing the tissue when subjected to cryostat sectioning and preventing desiccation during long-term storage. Rapid freezing is necessary to avoid ice crystal formation and resulting tissue damage. Once the tissue block is prepared, the next challenge is to generate high-quality sections, because poorly cut sections can lead to difficulty interpreting or even misinterpretation of the immunostained tissue. After the block has been cut, it is important to reapply OCT to the cut surface to protect the block from desiccation during storage. The cut tissue sections can be stored refrigerated or at −20°C (with desiccant) for as long as 1 month before staining; however, the correlation between storage time and reactivity should be assessed for each antigen-antibody pair.

The cut frozen sections can be stained directly but are generally gently fixed before immunostaining. The most commonly used fixatives are cold acetone and alcohol-based fixatives. However, terminal deoxynucleotidyl transferase (TdT) and some other nuclear antigens seem to retain better antigenicity following paraformaldehyde fixation. Frozen section immunostaining can be performed using manual procedures or on automated immunostaining platforms. With the latter, a brief secondary fixation in 4% formaldehyde can help prevent tissue detachment during the staining run, generally without compromising staining quality. Pretreatment to block endogenous biotin should be performed, but blocking of endogenous peroxidase should be avoided when not absolutely required. Blocking of peroxidase with hydrogen peroxide–methanol mixtures may lead to a loss of reactivity and can occasionally lead to the detachment of tissue sections if the percentage of peroxide is high. If the preceding advice is adhered to, the success of frozen section IHC will be maximized.

The considerations for immunostaining cytospins are similar to those for staining frozen sections; the differences are related mainly to preparation of the cytospin. The most critical issue in preparing the cytospin is to achieve an optimal cell monolayer with minimal cell overlap. This generally requires running a few pilot cytospins to identify the optimal dilution of cells. The concentration of the cell suspension should be adjusted in 10% fetal calf serum or albumin, which acts as a cushion to preserve the cell morphology during centrifugation. Cells are spun onto slides using a special centrifuge, called a cytocentrifuge, that has been modified to allow the cells to be spun under low centripetal force. Once prepared, the cytospins can be fixed in ethanol or acetone or air-dried before immunostaining. At this point they can be stained in the identical manner described for frozen sections. It may be helpful to wash the cells in an isotonic solution before preparing the final cell concentration. Doing so can reduce nonspecific backgrounds that may occur on the slides following immunostaining as a result of the high and heterogeneous protein content of cellular effusions. In addition, the presence of red blood cells can interfere with staining and immunostain interpretation, so fluids with significant numbers of red blood cells should be subjected to an ammonium chloride or equivalent lysis step before preparation of the cytospins.

Special Considerations for Immunostaining Bone Marrow Biopsies

Examination of bone marrow trephine biopsies is an integral component of the assessment of hematologic disorders and other diseases affecting hematopoiesis. It is particularly useful for the evaluation of marrow cellularity, cell distribution, and the relationship between different cell types. Its role is critical when evaluating patients with a "dry tap"—that is, when examination of the aspirate is unsuccessful owing to fibrosis or other infiltrative processes.

To preserve tissue morphology, the length and type of fixation, tissue processing, sectioning, and quality of staining are crucial. Decalcification procedures represent an additional variable that may influence the staining pattern and affect the preservation of antigenicity in IHC.[31] A variety of fixatives are available, including buffered formalin, mercury-containing solutions such as Zenker's or B5, or a combination based on acetic acid–zinc–formalin (AZF) as proposed by the Hammersmith protocol[32]; the last provides a morphologic quality comparable to B5, but with superior antigen and nucleic acid preservation (if followed by formic acid decalcification). Plastic embedding is still used, despite its technical difficulty and more limited application for downstream procedures such as IHC and molecular techniques. However, newer resin-embedding techniques have resulted in improved performance in both these important ancillary technologies.[12] Subsequent to fixation, the bone marrow trephine needs to undergo decalcification with either calcium-chelating agents such as EDTA or acid-based agents. EDTA decalcification usually lasts 48 to 72 hours; with acid-based solutions the decalcifying time is shorter (1 to 2 hours or up to 6 hours when using 10% formic acid and 5% formaldehyde). Usually each laboratory has a standardized procedure whereby bone

Table 4-2 Immunohistochemistry on Bone Marrow Trephine Biopsies

Cell Type	Antibodies
Precursor	CD34, CD117, TdT, CD10, CD3, CD19
Myeloid	MPO, CD13, CD33, CD10, HLA-DR
Erythroid	Glycophorin A and C, hemoglobin, spectrin
Megakaryocytic	CD42b, CD61, von Willebrand's factor (factor VIIIRA)
Monocytic	CD14, CD68 (KP-1 and PGM-1), CD163

marrow biopsies are monitored during fixation and decalcification to ensure morphologic preservation and the best conditions for IHC and molecular techniques.[33]

Since the introduction of antigen retrieval and improvements in decalcification, the number of antibodies that can be used on bone marrow trephine biopsies has grown dramatically from a few in the early 1990s to more than 100 today.[33] The staining procedures and detection systems are similar to those already described for other formalin-fixed, paraffin-embedded tissue sections. The vast majority of antibodies currently used on lymph node biopsies can also be applied to bone marrow biopsies (Table 4-2).

ANTIGENS OF HEMATOPATHOLOGIC INTEREST

The complexity of hematopathologic neoplasms parallels the complexity of the hematopoietic and immune cells from which they derive, and accurate diagnosis frequently requires the assessment of multiple diverse phenotypic markers. Commonly targeted markers include those related to cell lineage, degree of cellular differentiation, cell function, specific lymphomagenesis, and proliferative activity. The sum of this information allows the hematopathologist to categorize diseases in phenotypic groups that correspond to clinically relevant diagnostic entities. In addition to the characterization of lesional tumor cells, analysis of the microenvironment, which plays an important role during the development and differentiation of hematopoietic and immune cells, can provide diagnostic or prognostic information.

Many antigens that are clinically relevant in hematopathology are designated by a cluster of differentiation (CD) number. The CD nomenclature was established in 1982 at the first International Workshop and Conference on Leukocyte Differentiation Antigens in Paris, France, to organize the increasing number of monoclonal antibodies generated in different laboratories around the world into groups that recognized unique cell surface molecules.[34] Before the establishment of this nomenclature, each laboratory tended to use its own naming system for antibodies that often reacted with identical antigens, causing great confusion. A CD number is assigned when two independent monoclonal antibodies are shown to bind the same molecule, thus cross-validating both the target and the antibody reactivity. CD numbers are not provided for intracellular or nuclear antigens. Over the years the CD nomenclature has been expanded to include surface markers on other cell types, and today it consists of 350 clusters and subclusters. For most if not all CD clusters, the corresponding protein is known, and the CD nomenclature now coexists with the Human Genome Organization (HUGO) gene nomenclature.

Immunohistochemical Characterization of Lymphoid Malignancies

The use of cell lineage and differentiation markers to assist in making a diagnosis is best illustrated with the lymphomas and is predicated on large numbers of studies that have validated the concept that the various lymphoma subtypes arise from or at least appear to reflect different stages of normal lymphocyte development (see Chapters 8 and 13). Coordinated and unique programs of gene expression occur during both B-cell and T-cell differentiation, producing unique combinations of stage-specific protein expression that can be exploited by immunologic techniques, including IHC, to characterize these cell populations; these combinations can also be used to assist in the diagnosis of the corresponding lymphomas (Tables 4-3 to 4-5).

In any given case, the panel of targets assessed by IHC should be based on the differential diagnosis formulated after a review of the hematoxylin-eosin–stained section. Successive panels should be ordered in a stepwise fashion to further refine the diagnosis based on initial results. Although this approach may delay the final diagnosis by a day or two, the process is cost-effective and efficient. One should never order an IHC stain without an understanding of how the result will be used or how it will impact the diagnostic decision process. Table 4-6 outlines some recommended panels for lymph node diagnosis based on common diagnostic questions. The immunophenotypic characteristics of each of the individual entities are discussed in subsequent chapters; therefore, discussion of the immunoprofiles of individual diseases is deferred.

For many hematopoietic tumors, tumor-associated oncogene products provide unique and sometimes specific targets for IHC interrogation. TP53 mutations or deletions have been described in numerous subtypes of mature B- and T-cell lymphomas, and they are usually considered a secondary event associated with a more aggressive clinical course. In follicular lymphomas, p53 mutations were originally described in cases with histologic progression to diffuse large B-cell lymphoma; when detected in the low-grade component, they are associated with a poor prognosis.[35,36] Similarly, the presence of p53 mutations in mucosa-associated lymphoid tissue (MALT) lymphoma,[37] mantle cell lymphoma,[38,39] and chronic

Table 4-3 Immunohistochemical Diagnosis of Mature B-Cell Neoplasms

	CLL/SLL	MCL	FL	MZL	HCL	DLBCL
CD5	+	+	–*	–*	–	–†
CD10	–	–	+	–	–	+†
CD20	+	+	+	+	+	+
BCL6	–	–	+	–	–	+
MUM-1/IRF-4	+‡	–	–	+	–	+†
Cyclin D1	–	+	–	–	–	–
CD23	+	–	+/–	+/–	–	–
CD25	–	–	–	–	+	–

*Some FL and MZL cases can express CD5.
†DLBCL is a heterogeneous group, and different subsets express different antigens such as CD5, CD10, and MUM-1/IRF-4 (see specific chapters).
‡In CLL, proliferation centers express MUM-1/IRF-4.
CLL/SLL, chronic lymphocytic leukemia–small lymphocytic lymphoma; DLBCL, diffuse large B-cell lymphoma; FL, follicular lymphoma; HCL, hairy cell leukemia; MCL, mantle cell lymphoma; MZL, marginal zone lymphoma.

Table 4-4 Immunohistochemical Diagnosis of Mature T-Cell Neoplasms

	T-LBL	PTCL	ALCL	AILT	NK/T Nasal	SPLTCL	HSTCL
TdT	+	–	–	–	–	–	–
CD3	+/–	+	+/–	+	+ cyto	+	+
CD5	+	+/–	+	+/–	–	+/–	–
CD4	+/–	+	+	+	–	–	–
CD8	+/–	+/–	–	–/+	–	+	–
β-F1	–	+			–	+/–	–
TIA-1	–	–	+	–	–	+	+
Gr-B	–	–	+	–	–	+	–
CD10	–	–	–	+	–	–	–
ALK	–	–	+	–	–	–	–
EBER	–	–/+ (B)	–	+ (B)	+	–	–
CD21 (DC)	–	–	–	+	–	–	–

AILT, angioimmunoblastic T-cell lymphoma; ALCL, anaplastic large cell lymphoma; (B), present in background B cells and not in neoplastic cells; cyto, cytoplasmic; (DC), expressed in extrafollicular dendritic cells, not tumor cells; HSTCL, hepatosplenic T-cell lymphoma; NK/T nasal, natural killer/T-cell lymphoma, nasal type; PTCL, peripheral T-cell lymphoma, unspecified; SPLTCL, subcutaneous panniculitis-like T-cell lymphoma; T-LBL, T-cell lymphoblastic leukemia/lymphoma.

lymphocytic leukemia[40] has been associated with aggressive disease. Because the majority of TP53 mutations stabilize the protein and allow it to be detected by IHC, IHC has been used as a surrogate marker for mutation. In B-cell lymphomas, the detection of TP53 protein by IHC correlates relatively well with the presence of mutation; however, in T-cell lymphomas and in classical Hodgkin's lymphoma this correlation is poor.[41,42] With these caveats, assessment of TP53 by IHC remains a useful prognostic marker in some B-cell neoplasms and may also have a role (in conjunction with the assessment of *TP53* target genes) in identifying patients who may benefit from therapies requiring wild-type TP53.[43,44]

Table 4-5 Immunohistochemical Features of Hodgkin's Lymphoma

	LP Cells NLPHL	HRS Cells CHL
Nonlineage Antigens		
CD45	+	–
CD30	–	+
CD15	–	+/–
B-Cell–Associated Antigens		
CD20	+	–/+
CD79a	+	–/+
J chain	+/–	–
IgD	+/–	–
B-Cell–Related Transcription Factors		
BOB.1	+	–/+
OCT-2	+	–/+
PU.1	+/–	–
PAX5	+	+ (weak)
BCL6	+	–
Epstein-Barr Virus Detection		
LMP-1	–	+/–*
EBER	–	+/–*

+, positive in all cases; +/– , positive in a majority of cases; –/+, positive in a minority of cases; –, negative in all cases.
*Often positive in MCCHL and LDCHL; usually negative in NSCHL.
CHL, classical Hodgkin's lymphoma; HRS, Hodgkin Reed-Sternberg; LDCHL, lymphocyte-depleted classical Hodgkin's lymphoma; LP, lymphocyte predominant; MCCHL, mixed cellularity classical Hodgkin's lymphoma; NLPHL, nodular lymphocyte-predominant Hodgkin's lymphoma; NSCHL, nodular sclerosis classical Hodgkin's lymphoma.

Historically, one of the first examples of a tumor-associated oncogene product that proved useful in hematopathologic diagnosis was BCL2. BCL2 was discovered as a result of its involvement in the follicular lymphoma–associated t(14;18)(q32;q21), which juxtaposes the *BCL2* gene to the immunoglobulin heavy-chain locus, resulting in its overexpression.[45] BCL2 resides primarily on the mitochondrial membrane and is the prototypic member of a large family of apoptosis-related proteins.[46] Reactive germinal center B cells do not express

Table 4-6 Recommended Immunohistochemistry Panels for Lymph Nodes and Lymphoma Diagnosis

Diagnostic Panel	Antibodies*
Reactive hyperplasia	CD20, IgD, CD3, CD5, BCL2, kappa, lambda, *CD21, CD123, CD138*
Small B-cell lymphomas	CD20, CD79a, IgD, CD3, CD5, CD10, CD23, CD21, MIB-1, cyclin D_1, BCL2, BCL6, MUM-1/IRF4
Diffuse large B-cell lymphoma, Burkitt's lymphoma	CD20, CD3, CD79a, BCL2, BCL6, CD10, MUM-1/IRF4, p53, MIB-1, EBER
Aggressive B-cell neoplasms	
Plasma cell, plasmablastic neoplasms	CD20, CD79a, CD3, kappa and lambda heavy chains, CD56, CD138, MUM-1/IRF-4, ALK, EMA, EBER
Classical Hodgkin's lymphoma	CD20, CD3, CD30, CD15, PAX5, *OCT-2, BOB.1,* EBER, LMP-1
Nodular lymphocyte-predominant Hodgkin's lymphoma	CD20, CD3, IgD, OCT-2, *BOB.1,* CD21, CD57, PD-1
Peripheral T-cell lymphoma (nodal)	CD20, CD3, CD5, CD4, CD8, *CD2, CD7,* CD10, CD21, CD25, CD30, TIA-1, PD-1, ALK, EBER
Peripheral T-cell lymphoma (extranodal)	CD20, CD3, CD5, CD4, CD8, *CD2, CD7,* CD25, CD30, CD56, TIA-1, granzyme B, β-F1, ALK, EBER
Blastic, blastoid neoplasms	CD20, CD79a, PAX5, CD3, CD4, CD2, *CD34,* CD56, CD68, CD99, CD123, TDT, lysozyme, MPO

*Antibodies shown in italic can be added as needed in selected cases.

BCL2; therefore, detection of this protein is most useful for distinguishing reactive from neoplastic follicles. The pattern of BCL2 expression in follicular lymphomas varies, and interpretation of the stain should be correlated with other markers such as CD10 and BCL6, which are also expressed by germinal center B cells. BCL2 expression as a result of t(14;18) is usually intense and stronger than that of normal B and T cells; however, any amount of BCL2 expression in germinal centers is abnormal and should be carefully evaluated and correlated with other markers (i.e., CD10, BCL6, MIB-1, IgD, CD3). Usually primary follicles, mantle zones of secondary follicles, and intra- and interfollicular T cells stain for BCL2 and can be a useful internal positive control. However, IHC staining for BCL2 has no value in distinguishing follicular lymphomas from other indolent or aggressive B-cell lymphomas or even T-cell lymphomas because they all may express this antiapoptotic protein.

Overexpression of cyclin D1 as a result of t(11;14)(q13;q34) is the hallmark of mantle cell lymphoma involving the immunoglobulin heavy-chain locus and the *CCND1* locus located on 11q13.[47] Cyclin D1 is an important cell cycle regulator in many cell types and controls progression from G_0-G_1 to S phase, but it is usually not expressed in lymphoid cells. As a result of the t(11;14)(q13;q34) translocation, nearly all cases of mantle cell lymphoma accumulate immunohistochemically detectable levels of cyclin D1 in the nucleus.[48] The IHC assessment of cyclin D1 is routinely used in the diagnosis of this lymphoma, and it is particularly helpful in the differential diagnosis of other $CD5^+$ B-cell lymphomas, such as chronic lymphocytic leukemia. Cyclin D1 expression can also be detected in multiple myeloma carrying t(11;14), at low levels in hairy cell leukemia, and in a variety of stromal cells; the last is a useful internal positive control. However, when combined with morphologic features, its nuclear expression is diagnostic of mantle cell lymphoma.

In contrast to the majority of translocations in B-cell lymphomas, the anaplastic large cell lymphoma–associated translocation involving the anaplastic lymphoma kinase (*ALK*) gene located on 2p23 results in a fusion protein with a variety of partner genes on different chromosomes.[49] The most frequent translocation involves the *ALK* gene and the nucleophosmin (*NPM*) gene encoding for a nucleolar phosphoprotein with a chaperone function. This leads to a fusion protein that contains the amino-terminal portion of *NPM* fused to the intracytoplasmic portion, including the catalytic domain of ALK protein. As a result of t(2;5)(p23;q35), ALK protein is expressed in the nucleus and cytoplasm of the malignant anaplastic large cell lymphoma T cells and can be detected by monoclonal antibodies.[50] In cases with variant translocations, the staining pattern of ALK can be cytoplasmic or membranous; the latter staining pattern is usually associated with t(2;X)(p23;q11-12) involving the moesin (*MSN*) gene. The expression of ALK can be also detected in rare cases of diffuse large B-cell lymphoma with immunoblastic or plasmablastic features, but these cases usually show a granular cytoplasmic staining, lack CD30, express B-cell markers, and may be IgA positive. In addition, some nonhematopoietic neoplasms such as rhabdomyosarcoma and inflammatory myofibroblastic tumors express ALK, but they are easily distinguished morphologically from anaplastic large cell lymphoma, and they lack expression of CD30 and epithelial membrane antigen (EMA). The ALK protein is normally expressed only in the brain, so it is a highly specific target for diagnostic application.

Not all translocation targets are diagnostically useful, for a variety of reasons. For some translocations, the expression product is independent of the translocation or gene copy number or the presence of mutations. The best example is BCL6, which is normally expressed in germinal center cells and is necessary for germinal center formation.[51] Similarly, FOXP1 expression, which is usually associated with the non–germinal center B-cell (GCB) phenotype in diffuse large B-cell lymphoma, is independent of translocation or copy number,[52] as are translocation products identified in marginal zone B-cell lymphomas—namely, t(11;18)(q21;q21), t(1;14)(p22;q32), t(14;18)(q32;q21), and t(3;14)(p14.1;q32)—resulting in a chimeric product (*API2-MALT1*) or in transcriptional deregulation of *BCL10, MALT,* and *FOXP1*.

Evaluation of the proliferative rate of the lymphoid populations is also diagnostically useful in many settings. Among the proliferation markers, Ki-67 is by far the most widely targeted antigen in pathology. Ki-67 is a nuclear protein antigen expressed by proliferating cells that are actively dividing and cycling. It is not expressed in G_0.[53] Although it has been shown to have DNA-binding properties and is a major nuclear protein, its function remains unclear. Although the original Ki-67 antibodies were not immunoreactive in formalin-fixed, paraffin-embedded tissue sections, other investigators were successful in generating the now widely used Ki-67 equivalent MIB-1 antibody. The identification of proliferating cells and their distribution within lymphoid tissue are important parameters in the evaluation of reactive and neoplastic disorders. MIB-1 staining can assist in the distinction between follicular hyperplasia and follicular lymphoma; in the former, the reactive germinal centers have a higher proliferative rate, with orderly polarization, compared with low-grade follicular lymphomas.

Within a particular subtype of lymphoma, an increased number of actively proliferating tumor cells is usually associated with a more aggressive clinical course, although the prognostic significance of Ki-67 staining is not always consistent among studies. There are numerous possible explanations for the lack of concordance among different studies, including technical variations and differences in scoring criteria and cutoff values.[54-56] (MIB-1 staining is particularly sensitive to the type of antigen retrieval procedure used.) The poor reproducibility in diffuse large B-cell lymphoma is particularly evident in multicenter studies, where interlaboratory variations play a greater role, whereas the Ki-67 index tends to maintain its significance in defining high-risk groups in series published from single institutions.[56] Furthermore, when Ki-67 immunostaining has been assessed in the context of the "proliferation signatures" generated by gene expression studies in mantle cell lymphoma, transformed follicular lymphoma, and nodal peripheral T-cell lymphoma, it has generally shown excellent correlation.[57-59]

Immunohistochemical Characterization of Myeloid Leukemias, Myelodysplastic Disorders, and Other Myeloproliferative Diseases

In the diagnosis of acute leukemias, immunophenotyping of bone marrow trephine biopsies is usually complementary to flow cytometry, which uses large panels to characterize the

Table 4-7 Recommended Panels for Bone Marrow Immunohistochemistry

Panel	Antibodies
Acute leukemias	CD34, CD117, TdT, CD3, CD19, CD20, CD10, MPO, CD33, CD61 (or CD42b), hemoglobin A, glycophorin A or C, PAX5; also CD123, NPM1, CD68, lysozyme
Myelodysplastic syndromes	CD34, CD117, CD61, MPO, CD33, mast cell tryptase, hemoglobin A
Chronic myeloproliferative neoplasms	CD34, MPO, CD61, CD68 (PGM-1), hemoglobin A
Plasma cell disorders	CD138, kappa, lambda, CD56, CD20
Hemophagocytic syndromes	CD68, EBV in situ, CD20, CD3
Histiocytic and dendritic neoplasms	CD123, CD68, CD163, S-100, CD1a, langerin, lysozyme
Mastocytosis	Mast cell tryptase, CD117, CD25, CD2; also CD34, CD3, CD20

neoplastic populations, identify their lineages, and detect aberrant antigenic expression patterns that can be used to monitor residual or recurrent disease (Table 4-7).

The identification of blasts is critical in the characterization of all potential leukemias and myelodysplastic and myeloproliferative disorders, and this is easily achieved with antibodies against CD34 and CD117. However, it should be pointed out that in about 25% of all cases of acute myeloid leukemia (AML), the blasts do not express CD34. The addition of myeloperoxidase (MPO), glycophorin A or C, hemoglobin, and CD61 is helpful for assessing the distribution and number of different cell types and to identify morphologically abnormal forms such as micromegakaryocytes.

A panel including CD34, TdT, MPO, CD68 (KP-1 and PGM-1), glycophorin A, CD61, CD20, CD79a, PAX5, CD3, and CD1a is useful to distinguish AML from lymphoblastic leukemia. In cases with monocytic differentiation, additional markers include neuron-specific enolase (NSE), CD11c, CD14, CD64, CD163, and lysozyme. In AML, immunophenotyping can be used to identify specific subgroups; typically, AML with t(8;21)(q22;q22) is characterized by the expression of CD13, CD33, MPO, human leukocyte antigen (HLA)-DR, CD34, PAX5, and CD19, whereas AML associated with t(15;17)(q22;q12) lacks expression of HLA-DR and has a more heterogeneous expression of CD13 and CD34 and partial expression of CD2.

Immunohistochemical Characterization of Histiocytic, Dendritic, Mast Cell, and Other Tumor Cell Types

The neoplastic cells of histiocytic sarcoma are positive for CD68, CD163, CD14, and lysozyme, as well as for CD4.[60] S-100, when present, is usually weak and focal. Several markers are useful in the differential diagnosis of Langerhans cell proliferations (CD1a, langerin), follicular dendritic cell tumors (CD21, CD35, clusterin), and proliferations of myeloid origin (CD13, CD33, MPO).[61,62] Histiocytic sarcoma is also negative for keratin, HMB45, EMA, and melanoma markers (except S-100, as described).

All mast cell proliferations can be identified by IHC using an antibody against mast cell tryptase (also effective on bone marrow specimens), irrespective of their degree of maturation.[63] Mast cell tumors also express CD117 (c-Kit) as well as CD68. The mast cells in systemic mastocytosis are usually positive for CD25, and CD2 is positive in about two thirds of cases. In other mast cell syndromes there is more variability in the expression pattern of CD2 and CD25.

The tumor cells of the blastic plasmacytoid dendritic cell neoplasm express CD4, CD43, CD45RA, and CD56, as well CD123 and TCL-1.[64-66] Additional markers include BDCA-2/CD303 and CLA. When CD68 is detectable, it usually has a dot-like staining pattern. TdT is expressed in about one third of cases, and CD34 and c-Kit (CD117) are usually negative.

IN SITU HYBRIDIZATION

Although this is a chapter on IHC, a few words regarding the role of in situ hybridization (ISH) in hematopathology are warranted. These technologies have similarities, in that they both interrogate targets in situ—that is, on frozen or paraffin-embedded tissue sections—and they have similar detection systems. The type of target and the chemistry of its identification are the major differences. ISH is a simple and sensitive technique that permits direct assessment of DNA or RNA targets within tissue sections (both frozen and formalin-fixed), single-cell suspensions, and cytogenetic preparations, whereas IHC targets proteins.

The application of ISH in hematopathology is particularly useful when antibodies are not available, have limited sensitivity, or are associated with high background staining (e.g., kappa and lambda light-chain immunostains).[67] It may also be indicated when proteins are rapidly secreted and are not stored within cells or when nucleic acids are more abundant than proteins. The major technical limitations are related to the abundance and preservation of target sequences within cells; thus, preanalytic factors such as fixation and tissue processing can have a significant impact on target sequence detection by ISH.

Similar to IHC, a primary incubation is performed, substituting DNA or RNA probes instead of a primary antibody. Reactivity (hybridization) is based on complementarity between the sequence of interest and the designed probe, rather than on antigen-antibody recognition. Detection of the annealed products was originally based on the use of radiolabeled probes, which were visualized by slide emulsion autoradiography. Currently, especially in the clinical setting, radioisotopes have been replaced by nonisotopic detection methods. In chromogen-based ISH (CISH), a biotin- or digoxigenin-labeled probe is detected using a secondary antibody and a chromogenic detection system similar to that in IHC. In fluorescence-based ISH (FISH) techniques, signals are detected using a fluorophore in a darkfield setting. These methods offer significant advantages over radioisotope-based ISH, including improved probe stability without waste disposal issues (other than DAB), shortened assay time, excellent sensitivity, superior tissue preservation, and more accurate subcellular localization.

The primary CISH assay used by hematopathologists is for the detection of kappa and lambda immunoglobulin light chains as an assessment of B-cell clonality. Indications for its use are limited to situations in which IHC is not feasible, such as when there is high background in the IHC stain owing to the presence of high levels of interstitial immunoglobulins from serum, and cases that do not express immunoglobulin light-chain proteins, such as some plasma cell dyscrasias. The applicability of CISH for kappa and lambda detection extends to bone marrow sections. ISH should not be used as a replacement test for kappa or lambda IHC because the currently available probes for CISH do not improve the sensitivity of light-chain detection.

CISH is also widely used for the detection of infectious agents, particularly viruses, within cells or tissues. One of the most common clinical CISH tests is the detection of Epstein-Barr virus (EBV) in infected cells.[68-71] In this test, the targets are EBV-encoded RNAs (EBERs), which are short nuclear transcripts that are present early in latent infection and in high copy number (approximately 10^6 to 10^7 copies/cell). Because of these characteristics and their minimal homology to cellular RNA, EBERs are an excellent target for the detection of EBV-infected cells by ISH on formalin-fixed, paraffin-embedded tissue sections and are preferable to the commonly used IHC target, latent membrane protein (LMP).

FISH is commonly used to investigate structural and numerical chromosomal abnormalities and has traditionally been performed on cultured cells in cytogenetics laboratories, but it is increasingly being performed on paraffin sections in histopathology laboratories (see Chapter 7).[72]

CONCLUSION

Immunohistochemistry plays a central role in the practice of hematopathology, and its importance is likely to continue to increase. The rapid growth of genomic and proteomic technologies and their application to normal and neoplastic conditions of the hematopoietic and immune systems have resulted not only in a better understanding of disease but also in the identification of new clinically relevant targets for immunohistochemical interrogation. Further, the recent emphasis on molecularly targeted therapies has focused more attention on the use of IHC to interrogate the presence and activity of therapeutically relevant cellular signaling pathways in archival tissues.

References can be found on Expert Consult @ www.expertconsult.com

Pearls and Pitfalls

- Avoid frequent freezing and thawing of antibodies.
- If the antibody is concentrated (undiluted), it is best to aliquot into small volumes and freeze (−20°C).
- If frozen aliquots are to be used sporadically, retesting and verification are necessary to detect possible changes in reactivity.
- Always use coated or charged slides and bake the slides for 1 hour at 60°C to enhance tissue adhesion.
- Once the primary antibody is applied, do not allow the section to dry, or nonspecific staining will occur.
- Optimization of fixation is required whenever possible, especially if molecular studies might be performed on formalin-fixed, paraffin-embedded tissue.
- Inconsistent results are most frequently due to poor control over preanalytic parameters, especially the antigen retrieval step.
- Antigen retrieval conditions vary, based on the specific antigen.
- The effectiveness of heat-induced epitope retrieval (HIER) is directly proportional to the product of heat × retrieval time in a given solution.
- The cool-down phase following HIER contributes to the overall antigen retrieval time.
- Be aware that overdigestion or excess HIER may result in nonspecific staining or unacceptable morphology.
- HIER can be detrimental for some antigens.
- Positive and negative controls should be run with all test cases, but for some lymphoid specimens, the tissue itself may serve as an internal control owing to the presence of normal hematolymphoid elements.
- Positive control tissues should be low antigen expressers to ensure sensitivity.
- Controls should be handled in the same manner as patient samples in terms of fixation, processing, and so forth.
- Avoid interpreting interstitial staining as membranous.
- The absence of staining may be real, whereas diffuse staining of all tissue elements is likely to be an artifact.

Chapter 5

Flow Cytometry

Maryalice Stetler-Stevenson and Constance M. Yuan

CHAPTER OUTLINE

Flow cytometry (FC) is invaluable in diagnosing and classifying hematolymphoid neoplasms, determining prognosis, and monitoring response to therapy. FC is especially suited for immunophenotypic analysis of blood, fluids (e.g. cerebrospinal fluid [CSF], pleural fluid), and aspirates of bone marrow and lymphoid tissue. FC is also ideal in small samples, where its multiparametric nature allows the concurrent staining of cells with multiple antibodies complexed to different fluorochromes, thus maximizing the amount of data obtained from a few cells. FC can characterize surface as well as cytoplasmic protein expression. Further, FC can accurately quantitate cellular antigens and molecules. With antibody-based therapies (e.g., rituximab, alemtuzumab [Campath]) moving into routine clinical use, the use of FC is likely to increase. Flow cytometric identification of therapeutic targets on the surface of malignant cells impacts the potential utility of these forms of therapy in a given patient. Once a diagnosis is established, FC is highly sensitive in detecting minimal disease (on the order of 1 in 10^4 to 10^6) to monitor disease progression or the impact of prior therapy.

GENERAL PRINCIPLES

In a flow cytometer, cells rapidly pass single file through a finely focused laser at an appropriate wavelength. The cell momentarily breaks the laser beam, scattering light at a low angle (also called forward scatter), much like a small orb casting a shadow. This forward scatter (FSC) can be proportional to cell volume. Laser light is simultaneously scattered at a high angle, called side scatter (SSC), by intracellular and nuclear components. This SSC is proportional to the cell's complexity, which is determined by the type and amount of cytoplasmic granularity and nuclear characteristics. These physical scatter properties accurately identify cell types and are the basis for many commercial hematology analyzers that provide automated differential cell counts.[1]

In addition to FSC and SSC properties, cells are further characterized by staining with multiple fluorescent markers, such as antibodies conjugated to fluorochromes or DNA-binding dyes. If a cell expresses an antigen that binds to a fluorochrome-conjugated antibody, the fluorochrome emits light at a particular wavelength that is measured by detectors. If used in combination with DNA-binding dyes, the DNA content can also be determined, yielding cell cycle data. Multiple fluorochromes (sometimes referred to as "colors"), each emitting uniquely identifiable spectral characteristics, are simultaneously measured with multiple detectors. Most clinical laboratories use four- to eight-color FC, and it is agreed that three-color analysis is the minimal acceptable amount to ensure the reliable discrimination of neoplastic cell populations in a broad range of sample types.[2,3] Ten-color flow cytometric analysis may be available in the clinical laboratory in the near future.[4]

Initially, FC determined the presence or absence of lineage-specific or lineage-associated antigens. However, immunophenotypic interpretation has evolved from a simplistic "positive" or "negative" reaction to a given antigen to an assessment of the degree of expression. This approach is highly reliable in discriminating cell types and identifies flow cytometric features and patterns unique to certain hematolymphoid neoplasias. Because the antigen expression of many hematolymphoid neoplasias overlaps with their normal counterparts, the ability of multiparametric FC to highlight subtle temporal patterns and antigen intensity makes it extremely powerful in the diagnosis of neoplasia.

TECHNICAL CONSIDERATIONS

General

Appropriate samples for FC include blood, bone marrow, lymph node, extranodal tissue biopsy, fine-needle aspirate, and body fluid (e.g., pleural, peritoneal, CSF). International consensus guidelines on the medical indications for FC have been proposed and are based on patient history and presenting symptoms.[5] Timely processing of samples is necessary to maximize cell yield, maintain cell viability and integrity, and prevent loss of abnormal cells of interest.[3] Blood and bone marrow specimens must be collected in an appropriate anticoagulate. Lysis is the preferred approach for removing excess erythrocytes.[3] In patients whose marrow cannot be aspirated or in cases of a "dry tap" (i.e., fibrotic marrow or marrow packed with neoplastic cells), submission of several core biopsies for FC is appropriate. These cores are disaggregated to release cells into fluid suspension before FC.[3] Portions of tissue undergoing FC should represent an area that is also being submitted for histology, to minimize discordance due to sampling. Intact portions of solid tissue (e.g., biopsies of bone marrow, lymph nodes, or other tissue masses) must be made into cell suspensions for FC. Mechanical tissue disaggregation is fairly simple and rapid, and it leaves the cells relatively unaltered; this is achieved by slicing, mincing, and teasing apart the tissue using commercial devices or manual tools.[3] Enzymatic dissociation has been used in processing fibrotic tissue; however, it can alter antigen expression and decrease viability.

Antibody staining protocols differ according to the application and specimen type. Antibody panels are designed for the assessment of lineage, level of differentiation, and subclassification. Their use requires an in-depth understanding of antigen expression patterns in normal and neoplastic cells. The emission spectra of fluorochromes vary, and conjugation should be to appropriate antibodies to maximize detection (e.g., bright fluorochrome with dimly expressed antibody). Multiple antibodies are required for lineage assignment. Most antibodies are not cell lineage specific, and neoplastic cells may lack one or more antigens of a particular lineage. Overall, the number of reagents in a panel should be sufficient to allow the recognition of all abnormal and normal cells in the sample; conversely, limiting the number of antibodies may compromise diagnostic accuracy.[2] In general, the larger the antibody panel, the higher the sensitivity and specificity of detection and characterization. The number of reagents needed to adequately evaluate a specimen for potential hematologic neoplasms depends on the presenting symptoms.[2,6] In addition, surface and intracellular markers may be of prognostic utility and should be studied.

Viability

Decreased viability is noted in solid tissue samples and aggressive lymphomas. Nonviable cells may nonspecifically bind antibodies and interfere with accurate immunophenotyping. A low-viability sample composed entirely of neoplastic cells can yield meaningful results, however. Further, many samples submitted for FC are considered irreplaceable because they are obtained by an invasive procedure with significant trauma or are difficult to impossible to recollect. In this case, every effort must be made to obtain diagnostic information. No specific cutoff exists to dictate specimen rejection for FC, although general guidelines suggest rejecting replaceable samples with less than 75% viability. In an irreplaceable specimen with poor viability, any abnormal populations should be reported. Failure to identify a neoplastic process in a sample of poor viability should not be viewed as a true negative,[3] and subsequent testing may be informative.

Small Specimens

Diagnosis of lymphoma is frequently based on the evaluation of small biopsy specimens, fine-needle aspirates, and body fluids (e.g., CSF, vitreous humor, effusions). Small samples can provide sufficient cells for FC, even when cell numbers are too low to count by conventional methods. FC can be more sensitive than immunohistochemistry, especially when neoplastic cells are admixed with normal counterparts or are associated with a brisk inflammatory response, as in some extranodal marginal zone lymphomas of mucosa-associated lymphoid tissue (MALT lymphoma)[7] or some gastric lymphomas in endoscopic biopsies.[8]

FC provides increased sensitivity for the detection of hematolymphoid neoplasia in fine-needle aspirates.[9-11] Further, because the World Health Organization (WHO) classification incorporates immunophenotypic criteria, flow cytometric evaluation of fine-needle aspirates assists in both the detection and the diagnostic subclassification of lymphoma[9,10,12]; it is particularly robust in the subclassification of B-cell malignancies such as chronic lymphocytic leukemia, mantle cell lymphoma, lymphoplasmacytic lymphoma, Burkitt's lymphoma, and plasmacytoma.[10]

Involvement of the CSF by hematopoietic malignancies may be difficult to document by morphology alone. FC improves the detection sensitivity of non-Hodgkin's lymphoma in CSF.[13-16] In a study assessing FC of CSF in patients at risk of having central nervous system involvement by aggressive B-cell lymphoma, FC was significantly more sensitive than cytology alone in disease detection and prognostication. FC is also useful in identifying central nervous system leukemia and increases the detection rate over cytology alone.[16,17] Thus, FC is useful in the evaluation of CSF for hematolymphoid malignancies.[15]

MATURE B-CELL NEOPLASMS

Flow cytometric detection of malignant B-cell populations requires extensive knowledge of normal B-cell antigen expression and light scatter characteristics. Markers of B-cell neoplasia include light-chain restriction, abnormally large B cells, abnormal levels of antigen expression, absence of normal antigens, and presence of antigens not normally present on mature B cells.[18]

Light-Chain Expression

A B-cell population with monotypic light-chain expression is, with rare exception, considered a B-cell neoplasm.

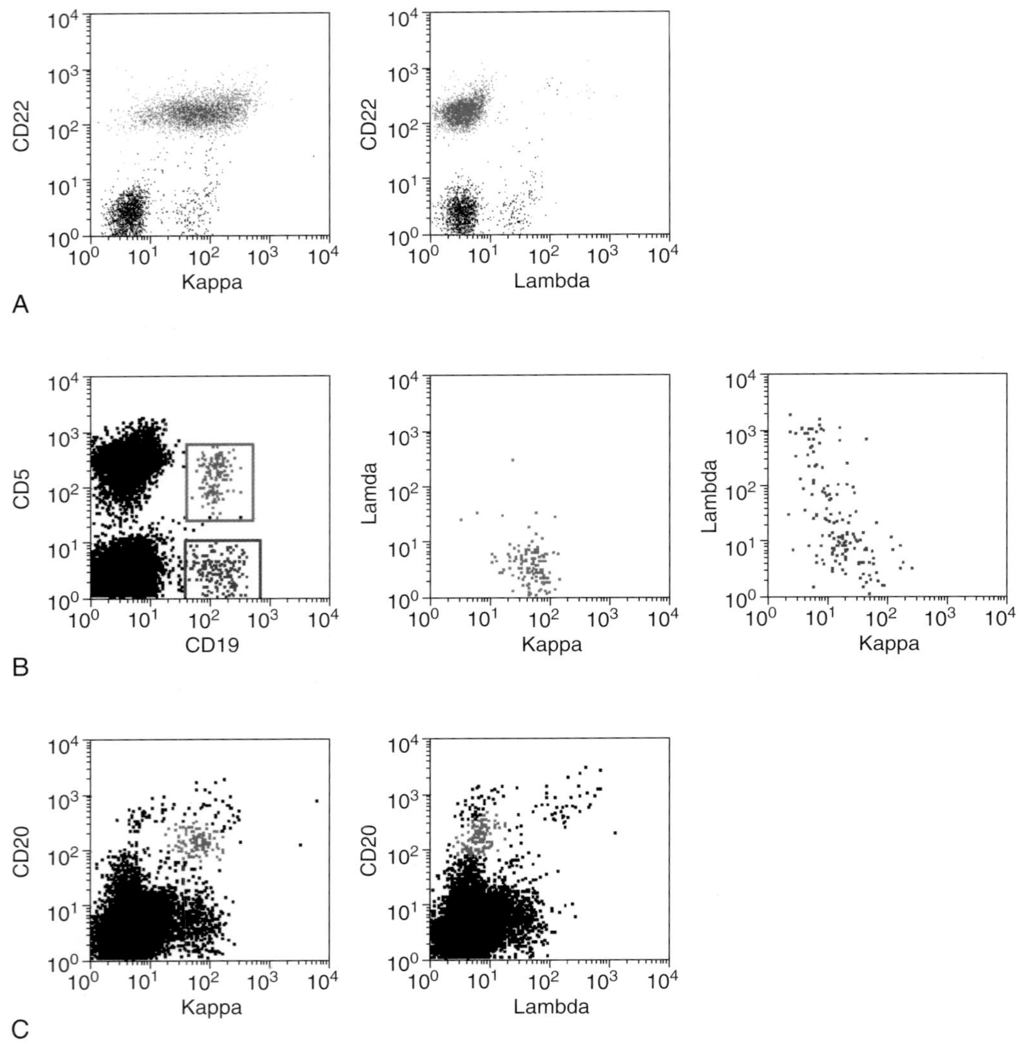

Figure 5-1. Flow cytometric detection of clonal B-cell populations. A, Monoclonal B cells. Y-axis, anti-CD22; X-axis, anti-kappa (*left*) or anti-lambda (*right*) immunoglobulin antibodies. *Red* cells are monoclonal B cells and are CD22⁺, kappa positive, and lambda negative. **B,** Use of a tumor-specific antigen. Y-axis, anti-CD5 (*left*) or anti-lambda (*middle* and *right*); X-axis, anti-CD19 (*left*) or anti-kappa (*middle* and *right*). *Left, Red* cells are CD5⁺ B cells; normal CD5⁻ B cells are *blue. Center, Red* CD5⁺ B cells are monoclonal, kappa positive, and lambda negative. *Right, Blue* CD5⁻ cells are polyclonal. **C,** Abnormal antigen intensity. Y-axis, anti-CD20; X-axis, anti-kappa (*left*) or anti-lambda (*right*). The dim CD20⁺ cells (*red*) are monoclonal, kappa positive, and lambda negative.

Monotypic or monoclonal B-cell populations are infrequently demonstrated in patients with no evidence of lymphoma,[19,20] although this may represent the early, preclinical detection of B-cell malignancy.[21] A monotypic B-cell population is characterized by the expression of a single immunoglobulin light chain,[22] resulting in positive staining with only one light-chain reagent (kappa positive and lambda negative, or vice versa) (Fig. 5-1A). In normal or benign lymphoid tissue, virtually every B cell expresses a single light-chain immunoglobulin, and the ratio of kappa- to lambda-expressing B cells is approximately 60%:40%.[23] Expression of a single light chain is usually but not invariably indicative of a monoclonal population at the molecular level. Restricted expression of lambda light chain has been reported in some B-cell or plasma cell proliferations, without molecular genetic evidence of monoclonality.[24,25] Lack of surface immunoglobulin among mature B cells (see later) or a deviation from this normal ratio suggests a monoclonal B-cell population.

FC is advantageous in that it recognizes monoclonal B cells in B-cell lymphopenia, owing to the rapid analysis of large numbers of acquired B cells, or in a background of polyclonal B cells,[22,23] owing to the detection of aberrant antigens on the neoplastic cells. By examining B-cell subsets with differential CD19, CD20, or CD22 expression, an abnormal monoclonal B-cell population may be discovered (see Fig. 5-1C).[22,26] In fact, detection of a skewed kappa-to-lambda ratio should prompt a diligent search for an underlying monoclonal population that may be discriminated by CD19, CD20, CD22, or other antigens. For example, the CD20 bright (positive) B cells in the peripheral blood specimen from a patient with hairy cell leukemia may be monoclonal, whereas the B cells in total are polyclonal. Antibody panels can be designed to exploit the coexpression of tumor-specific antigens, such as

CD5 in mantle cell lymphoma or CD10 in follicular lymphoma, for the detection of monoclonality.[27] For example, the CD5$^+$ B cells in the peripheral blood specimen from a patient with mantle cell lymphoma may be monoclonal, whereas the CD5$^-$ B cells are polyclonal (see Fig. 5-1B). Clearly, a simplistic, one-dimensional examination of cells staining with kappa, lambda, and CD5 would be ineffective in this case. Multiparametric analysis is essential to detect relevant neoplastic populations.

Absence of surface immunoglobulin may also indicate a mature B-cell neoplasm,[28,29] but caution is imperative when interpreting the significance of such a population. Reactive germinal center cells with dim surface immunoglobulin are increased in follicular hyperplasia and may be mistaken for neoplasm; however, germinal center cells are distinguished by higher levels of CD20, CD10 positivity, and lack of intracellular BCL2.[30,31] Kappa and lambda expression is typically dim but can be detected when compared to immunoglobulin-negative T cells within the sample.[32] In bone marrow aspirates, plasma cells and most normal immature B cells (hematogones, or benign precursor B cells) also lack surface immunoglobulin.

Technical factors, such as antibody choice and cytophilic antibody artifact, can impact a laboratory's ability to assess surface light chain.[22] Cytophilic antibodies may be passively absorbed by Fc receptors present on natural killer cells, activated T cells, monocytes, granulocytes, and some B cells, resulting in apparent surface light-chain expression. Washing a specimen with phosphate-buffered saline before staining and using anti-CD20 or -CD19 for B-cell selection before flow cytometric analysis are sufficient to eliminate this artifact in most cases.[22] Neoplastic B cells may express light-chain epitopes not readily detected by all antibodies. Incorporation of two sets of light-chain reagents results in 100% sensitivity in monoclonal B-cell detection.[22]

Additional Flow Cytometric Abnormalities

Abnormal B-cell antigen expression can identify malignant B cells.[18] Mature, normal B cells express CD19, CD20, and CD22, and failure to express one of these antigens is abnormal, except for plasma cells. An important caveat is a history of monoclonal antibody therapy, because the therapeutic antibody may mask detection of the targeted antigen. For example, CD20 expression cannot be detected on B cells (normal and malignant) after treatment with rituximab, and this feature may persist for 6 months or longer after cessation of rituximab therapy.[33]

The detection of aberrant antigens (not normally expressed on B cells) is also useful in identifying malignant B cells. Aberrant expression of CD2, CD4, CD7, and CD8 occurs in chronic lymphocytic leukemia, hairy cell leukemia, and B-cell non-Hodgkin's lymphomas.[34,35] Demonstration of abnormal levels of expression of various antigens (i.e., abnormally dim or bright staining with antibodies) is also of diagnostic importance and helps in subclassification (see Fig. 5-1C). For example, chronic lymphocytic leukemia is characterized by abnormally dim CD20 and CD22 expression, hairy cell leukemia is characterized by abnormally bright expression of these antigens,[36] and follicular lymphoma frequently exhibits dim expression of CD19.[37] Additionally, light scatter characteristics can help detect malignant B-cell populations, such as the abnormally high FSC observed in diffuse large B-cell lymphoma or the high SSC typically seen in hairy cell leukemia.

PLASMA CELL DISORDERS

FC is useful in characterizing and distinguishing normal from neoplastic plasma cells based on the degree of surface antigen expression, presence of aberrant antigens, and detection of intracytoplasmic immunoglobulin. FC is not routinely used in plasma cell enumeration because cell numbers are usually underrepresented to a significant degree due to hemodilution, sampling artifact, plasma cell fragility, or the nature of the bone marrow aspirate specimen.[38]

In patients with bone marrow plasmacytosis, FC can distinguish normal from neoplastic plasma cells. Normal plasma cells are characterized by intense expression of CD38, coexpression of CD138, low levels of CD45 and CD19, polyclonal intracytoplasmic immunoglobulin light chain, and absence of surface immunoglobulin and common surface B-cell markers (CD20, CD22). Plasma cell neoplasms are characterized by expression of monoclonal cytoplasmic immunoglobulin, aberrant antigens such as CD56 or CD117, diminished CD38 or CD138, and complete absence of CD19 or CD45.[39,40] The simultaneous analysis of CD38, CD56, CD19, and CD117, CD138, or CD45 expression can distinguish normal from malignant plasma cells in the majority of cases, even in the absence of intracytoplasmic immunoglobulin detection.[39-43] Therefore, FC is particularly powerful in characterizing low levels of plasma cells or detecting neoplastic plasma cells obscured by a background of polyclonal plasma cells. For example, FC can be useful in differentiating monoclonal gammopathy of uncertain significance from early plasma cell myeloma because a significant number of normal (polyclonal) residual plasma cells is present in the former but not in the latter.[39] Furthermore, studies suggest a role for flow cytometric monitoring in myeloma after transplantation because the proportion and recovery of normal versus neoplastic plasma cells may predict disease outcome.[44] Assessment of circulating myeloma cells in peripheral blood appears to be prognostically significant.[45] Plasma cell proliferation rate, as determined by flow cytometric measurement of the S-phase fraction, is informative regarding disease status and prognosis in myeloma patients.[46,47]

MATURE T-CELL NEOPLASMS

Flow cytometric immunophenotyping is useful in the diagnosis and may also contribute to the subclassification of mature T-cell neoplasms,[18] although the detection of T-cell neoplasia is more intensive and challenging than that of B-cell malignancies. Typically, subset restriction; absent, diminished, or abnormally increased expression of T-cell antigens; presence of aberrant antigens[48,49]; and expansion of normally rare T-cell populations are indicators of T-cell neoplasia. Therefore, in FC, T cells should be examined for abnormal cell clusters by light scatter or antigen expression compared with normal T cells. Additionally, T-cell clonality can be directly assessed by the flow cytometric analysis of beta chain variants of the T-cell receptor (TCR). Although this requires a larger panel and more extensive analysis, it shares similarities with clonality analysis in B-cell neoplasms.

T cells fall into two main groups based on TCR expression of either the alpha-beta or the gamma-delta chains formed by VDJ segments and a constant region. The vast majority of normal and neoplastic T cells express the alpha-beta chain. Commercial antibodies are available against 70% of the human class-specific sequences among the V segments for the TCR beta chain (Vβ). All T cells in a clonal T-cell population have the same VDJ segment and therefore have identical ("monoclonal") Vβ protein expression. The distribution (proportion) of Vβ classes in normal CD4⁺ or CD8⁺ T cells is well defined.[50] An abnormal expansion of a Vβ population is consistent with a clonal T-cell population, similar to an expansion of light-chain–restricted B cells in a monoclonal B-cell population. Abnormal T-cell populations can be detected using a panel of antibodies; then anti-Vβ antibodies can be used to determine the clonality of the immunophenotypically defined abnormal T cells. This is called Vβ repertoire analysis, and this technique can be used to establish an initial diagnosis and to monitor minimal residual disease.[51,52] Currently, Vβ repertoire analysis is not routinely used in most clinical FC laboratories, but it may have potential utility.

The initial examination of CD4 and CD8 T cells can be informative. Normal reactive lymphoid populations contain a mixture of both CD4⁺ and CD8⁺ cells (with a predominance of CD4⁺ cells), whereas mature clonal T-cell populations are restricted to either CD4 or CD8 expression (usually CD4 > CD8; Fig. 5-2B), coexpression of both CD4 and CD8 (see Fig. 5-2D), or lack of CD4 and CD8 (less frequent; see Fig. 5-2C). Caveats include viral infections, which are characterized by a dramatic increase in CD8⁺ T cells, usually in association with other indications of T-cell activation, such as increased expression of CD2, decreased CD7, and expression of activation markers.[53] Also, a history of human immunodeficiency virus (HIV) infection may diminish or obliterate the number of CD4⁺ T cells.

A significant population of T cells lacking both CD4 and CD8 is abnormal and may be compatible with a T-cell lymphoma; however, some TCR gamma-delta and TCR alpha-beta T cells can be CD4⁻and CD8⁻. A reactive increase in TCR gamma-delta T cells should not be interpreted as a T-cell lymphoproliferative disorder.[54] CD4⁻, CD8⁻ T cells are also present in some abnormal immune states and are a hallmark of autoimmune lymphoproliferative syndrome (ALPS).[55]

Coexpression of CD4 and CD8 (see Fig. 5-2D) is abnormal and is uncommon in mature T-cell neoplasms. Although it can occur, usually in adult T-cell leukemia/lymphoma and T-cell prolymphocytic leukemia, this finding necessitates the exclusion of a T-lymphoblastic leukemia/lymphoma or normal cortical thymocytes, especially if the specimen is from the mediastinum. FC can distinguish a neoplastic T-cell process from normal cortical thymocytes in thymoma or thymic hyperplasia if normal T-cell maturation subsets are examined, as evidenced by the pattern and intensity of CD2, CD3, CD5, CD7, CD4, CD8, CD10, CD34, and CD45.[56,57] Last, apparent coexpression of CD4 and CD8 on T cells may be due to a technical artifact in the staining of unwashed blood[58] and should be interpreted with care.

Because mature T-cell neoplasms frequently fail to express at least one T-cell antigen (i.e., negative for CD2, CD3, CD5, or CD7; see Fig. 5-2E to G), analysis for absence of a T-cell antigen is more useful than subset restriction analysis.[49,59] Thus, it is important to include multiple T-cell antigens (CD2, CD3, CD5, CD7) in a diagnostic panel to ensure sensitivity in detection. Normally, a small percentage of peripheral blood CD3⁺ T cells are CD7⁻, and a subset of normal TCR gamma-delta T cells do not express CD5. However, large numbers of CD7⁻, CD4⁺ T cells (i.e., non–gamma-delta T cells) or CD5⁻ T cells are abnormal. CD2⁻ T cells are rare, and the absence of CD3 is distinctly abnormal.

Neoplastic T cells may be detected as a homogeneous population with an abnormal level of antigen expression (e.g., abnormal CD2, CD3, CD5, CD7, or CD45; see Fig. 5-2H and I).[49,59] For example, CD3 may be expressed at a higher or lower level than normal as measured by staining with anti-CD3 (see Fig. 5-2H and I). Dim CD3 expression is characteristic of Sézary cells and adult T-cell leukemia/lymphoma.[60,61] T-cell large granular lymphocytic leukemias typically have abnormally dim levels of CD5 expression, and CD5 is dimmer in normal CD8⁺ T cells. Abnormal levels of CD2 and CD7 may also be observed in T-cell lymphoproliferative processes. When interpreting data, one must also remember that CD3 is brighter in gamma-delta T cells, and CD2 expression is upregulated in reactive T cells.[18]

A subgroup of clonal T-cell processes is characterized by increased numbers of T-cell subpopulations, normally present in low numbers. In T-cell large granular lymphocytic leukemia, CD8⁺ T cells coexpressing CD57, CD56, or CD16 are increased. Dim CD5 expression and absence of normal T-cell antigens, such as CD7 and CD2, assist in the diagnosis. CD20, considered a B-cell antigen, is expressed by a small subgroup of normal T cells. Detection of a significant population of CD20⁺ T cells is highly abnormal. Also, a high level of gamma-delta T cells is suspicious for malignancy.

In all T-cell neoplasms, correlation with patient history and morphology is essential. When the vast majority of cells are neoplastic by morphology, a corresponding aberrant immunophenotype can be easily interpreted. Caution should be exercised when interpreting single immunophenotypic abnormalities, because these can be found in benign T-cell populations that are highly activated or when subsets are present in higher than normal numbers (e.g., increased gamma-delta T cells, loss of CD7 on T cells in Epstein-Barr virus [EBV] infection). Neoplastic T cells usually have multiple abnormalities that, owing to the multiparametric nature of FC, can be detected in the same cell, differentiating these cells from normal.

MATURE NATURAL KILLER–CELL NEOPLASMS

Mature natural killer (NK)-cell neoplasms are characterized by an increase in malignant CD2⁺, CD16⁺, CD56⁺, CD122⁺ NK cells that are surface CD3⁻ but express the epsilon chain of CD3 (CD3ε) in the cytoplasm.[12,62,63] TCR alpha-beta, TCR gamma-delta, CD4, CD5, CD8, CD16, and CD57 are usually negative. FC is particularly useful in characterizing NK-cell leukemia because it is ideal for immunophenotyping fluids such as blood. FC is also helpful in identifying NK cells in the extranodal, nasal type of NK/T-cell lymphoma, where the tumor often occurs in a background of extensive necrosis and inflammation. Unfortunately, no specific immunophenotypic markers exist that can accurately distinguish between reactive and neoplastic NK cells; however, the number and proportion of NK cells, and the NK cells' FSC properties (presence of large cells), may help confirm the diagnosis.

No truly robust method exists to confirm clonality in NK cells in the clinical setting. Unlike a T-cell neoplasm, a true

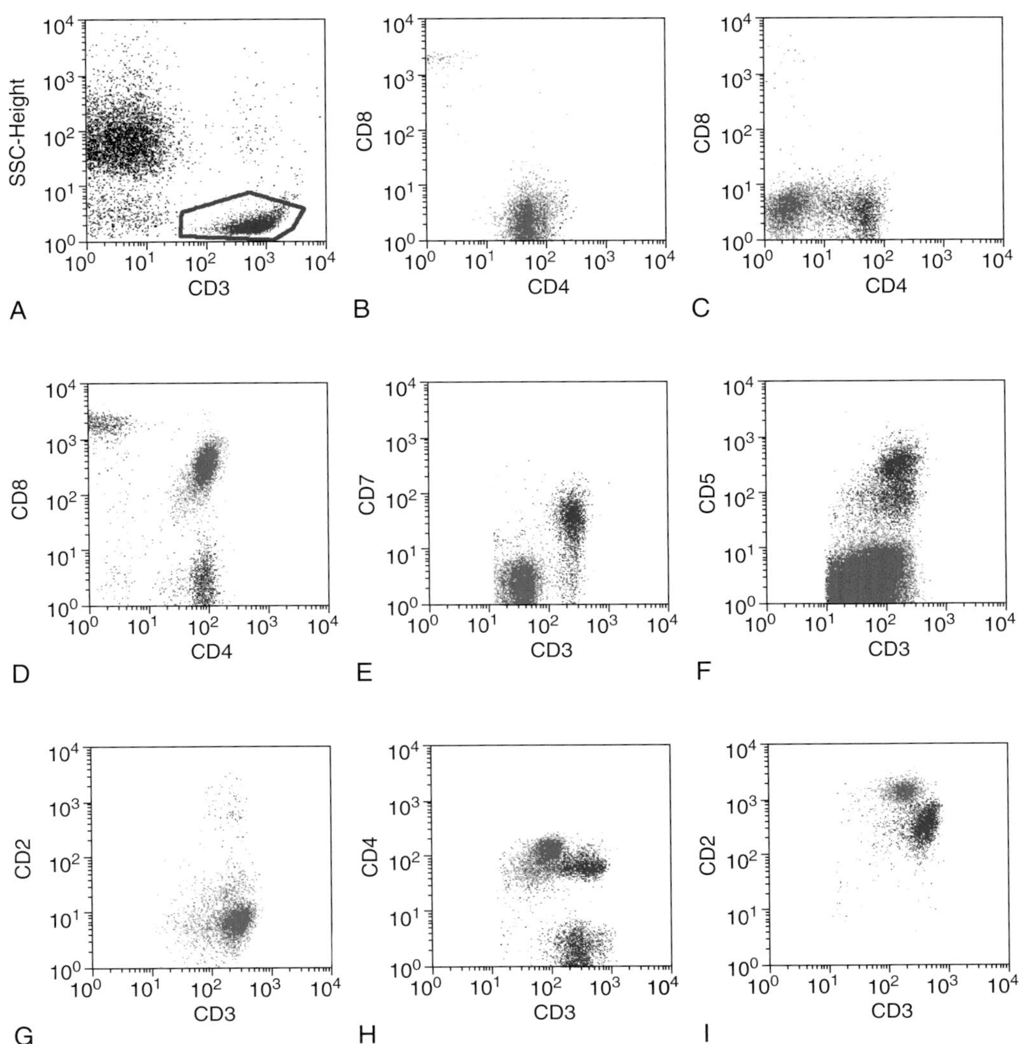

Figure 5-2. Examples of flow cytometric detection of abnormal T-cell populations in mulitiple T-cell lymphomas/leukemias. A, Example of antigen gating. The analysis gate is defined as the CD3$^+$ cells (*blue*). X-axis, anti-CD3; Y-axis, side light scatter (SSC). **B**, T-cell subset restriction. X-axis, anti-CD4; Y-axis, anti-CD8; analysis gate, CD3$^+$ T cells (*blue*). Malignant T cells (*red*) are CD4$^+$, CD8$^-$. **C**, T-cell subset restriction. X-axis, anti-CD4; Y-axis, anti-CD8; analysis gate, CD3$^+$ T cells (*blue*). *Red* cells represent a CD4$^-$, CD8$^-$ T-cell neoplasm. **D**, T-cell subset restriction. X-axis, anti-CD4; Y-axis, anti-CD8; analysis gate, CD3$^+$ T cells (*blue*). *Red* cells represent a CD4$^+$, CD8$^+$ T-cell neoplasm. **E**, Absence of normal T-cell antigen. X-axis, anti-CD3; Y-axis, anti-CD7; analysis gate, CD3$^+$ T cells (*blue*). *Red* cells represent a CD3$^+$, CD7$^-$ T-cell neoplasm. **F**, Absence of normal T-cell antigen. X-axis, anti-CD3; Y-axis, anti-CD5; analysis gate, CD3$^+$ T cells (*blue*). *Red* cells represent a CD3$^+$, CD5$^-$ T-cell neoplasm. **G**, Absence of normal T-cell antigen. X-axis, anti-CD3; Y-axis, anti-CD2; analysis gate, CD3$^+$ T cells (*blue*). *Red* cells represent a CD3$^+$, CD2$^-$ T-cell neoplasm. **H**, Abnormal level of T-cell antigen expression. X-axis, anti-CD3; Y-axis, anti-CD4; analysis gate, CD3$^+$ T cells (*blue*). *Red* cells are CD3$^+$ and CD4$^+$, with abnormally dim CD3. **I**, Abnormal level of T-cell antigen expression. X-axis, anti-CD3; Y-axis, anti-CD2; analysis gate, CD3$^+$ T cells (*blue*). *Red* cells within the oval are CD3$^+$ and CD2$^+$, with abnormally bright CD2 and dim CD3.

NK-cell neoplasm exhibits germline configuration of the TCR gene. Studies have demonstrated the utility of commercial antibodies in assessing the NK-cell killer inhibitory receptor repertoire (CD158-KIR) and the NK-cell expression of CD94-NKG2 heterodimers, an approach similar to Vβ repertoire analysis in T cells. NK cells express a diverse set of KIR surface molecules, and a normal NK cell may express two to eight KIR molecules on its surface.[64] A clonal expansion of an NK-cell population may demonstrate decreased diversity or skewing in the KIR repertoire. Similarly, each NK cell expresses a particular C-type lectin receptor (CD94-NKG2) heterodimer, and a restricted pattern of heterodimer expression may correspond with an NK-cell neoplasm; however, it has also been described in viral processes and EBV-driven lymphoproliferations.[65-67] Currently, these modalities are not routinely used in most clinical FC laboratories, but they may have potential utility.

ACUTE LEUKEMIA

The immunophenotyping of acute leukemia is invaluable in distinguishing myeloid from lymphoid origin. Because true myeloid leukemias can aberrantly express lymphoid markers, and vice versa, the use of a comprehensive panel is vital to prevent misdiagnosis.[2,12,63] The WHO classification has incorporated specific genetic alterations and characteristic translocations that carry prognostic and sometimes therapeutic implications in the diagnosis of leukemia. Associations between specific genetic and immunophenotypic features in acute leukemia have been described, and FC may provide the first clue to the presence of a specific underlying genetic alteration. Last, minimal residual disease detection by FC carries important prognostic implications and may guide further therapeutic options.

Acute Myeloid Leukemia

Flow cytometric immunophenotyping plays an important role in the WHO classification of acute myeloid leukemias. FC is highly sensitive and specific in differentiating acute myeloid leukemia (AML) from lymphoblastic leukemia and in identifying granulocytic, monocytic, erythroid, and megakaryocytic differentiation. Further, FC may provide information to help differentiate between a de novo AML (with a generally favorable prognosis) and one arising from myelodysplasia (with a generally worse prognosis). Generally, blasts in AML exhibit an immature phenotype (dim CD45, CD34, human leukocyte antigen [HLA]-DR, CD117), with some variation, such as lack of CD34 or HLA-DR. Also, AML blasts generally express some combination of myeloid antigens, such as CD13, CD33, CD15, CD11b, and myeloperoxidase. Both the pattern of antigen expression and the intensity and quality of CD45 expression and SSC properties of the blasts help subclassify AML (Fig. 5-3D and E). In the current WHO classification, a few notable subtypes of AML are also described with "recurrent genetic abnormalities" or characteristic genetic features, usually balanced translocations. Many of these AML subtypes respond well to therapy, have a high rate of complete remission, and carry a favorable prognosis. Because many of these AML subtypes often exhibit a characteristic immunophenotype as well, FC is often the first clue that a case of AML may fall into this favorable subgroup, prompting appropriate molecular and cytogenetic studies and correlation.

The immunophenotype of AML with t(8;21)(q22;q22) (*RUNX1/RUNX1T1*) translocation is usually $CD34^+$, with expression of CD13 and CD33. Frequently, the B-lymphoid marker CD19 is coexpressed on a subset of the blasts.[68,69] CD56 is also coexpressed, although less frequently than CD19, and may portend a poor prognosis.[70]

Among the AMLs with characteristic genetic abnormalities, the diagnosis of acute promyelocytic leukemia carries specific clinical, prognostic, and therapeutic implications, setting it apart from the others. These patients have an increased risk of disseminated intravascular coagulation, and the microgranular variant is known for presenting with a high white blood cell count and rapid doubling time. However, acute promyelocytic leukemia with t(15;17)(q22;q12) (*PML/RARA*) is sensitive to treatment with *trans*-retinoic acid and, if identified in a timely fashion, carries a favorable prognosis. The leukemic promyelocytes exhibit a characteristic, although not diagnostic, immunophenotype: CD33 expression is usually homogeneously positive and bright; CD13 positivity is heterogeneous; HLA-DR and CD34 are usually absent or dimly expressed in a minor subset of the leukemic promyelocytes; CD15 is negative, and leukemic promyelocytes frequently coexpress CD2 (typically the microgranular variant).[71,72]

In AML with monocytic features (acute monoblastic and monocytic leukemia), the blasts may exhibit brighter CD45 expression and overlap with the location of normal monocytes on the CD45 versus SSC data plot. In monocytic differentiation, cells initially express HLA-DR and CD36, then develop expression of CD64 and finally CD14 in the mature monocyte. Acute monoblastic and monocytic leukemia can express these antigens to varying degrees. Other characteristic antigens may be expressed, such as CD4, CD11b, CD11c, and lysozyme. Monocytic and myeloid cells share the expression of many common antigens (e.g., CD13, CD33); however, the normal maturation patterns are distinct and exhibit subtle differences in the timing and intensity of expression.[73,74] CD2 coexpression is frequently observed in AML with inv(16)(p13.1q22) (*CBFB-MYH11*). This disease exhibits an abnormal eosinophil component and carries a favorable prognosis.[75,76]

True, pure erythroid leukemia is a rare entity. Immunophenotypically, it can be highlighted by bright expression of CD71 and glycophorin A. Erythroid leukemia blasts with less evidence of maturation may lack glycophorin A. CD36 is also expressed in erythroid progenitors and may be observed in erythroid leukemia.[12,63,76] Interpretation requires care, however, because neither CD36 nor CD71 are lineage specific, and glycophorin-positive red blood cells can cause artifactual results.

Blasts of acute megakaryoblastic leukemia characteristically express CD36 and can exhibit high FSC owing to the larger size and volume of the cell relative to typical myeloblasts. Expression of CD36, the platelet glycoproteins, CD41 and CD61 is also noted. Myeloid antigens CD13 and CD33 may be expressed. Because this entity is uncommon (<5% of all cases of AML), it is important to fully exclude an acute myeloid or acute lymphoblastic leukemia in the immunophenotypic workup.[12,63] Careful examination of lymphoid markers, terminal deoxynucleotidyl transferase (TdT), and myeloperoxidase may be helpful. Also, care should be taken in the interpretation of CD41 and CD61, because platelets adhering to the surface of blasts may mimic the appearance of an acute megakaryoblastic leukemia.[12,63,76] CD42b is expressed by platelets but is absent from megakaryoblasts and assists in determining if staining is due to adherent platelets.

Precursor Lymphoid Neoplasms

Accurate lineage determination by FC in acute lymphoblastic leukemia (ALL) is essential for appropriate treatment. Frequently, ALL coexpresses myeloid antigens (e.g., CD13, CD33), necessitating a thorough immunophenotypic evaluation to fully exclude AML. The appearance of lymphoblasts is typically noted on a CD45 versus SSC plot by the presence of a distinct population of cells with decreased to absent CD45 expression and low SSC. T-cell ALL can exhibit brighter CD45 expression, such that the blast population approaches the population of normal mature lymphocytes on the CD45 versus SSC data plot.[76] Whether the ALL is of B- or T-cell lineage, CD34 is frequently expressed, and in cases in which CD34 expression is equivocal, detection of intracellular TdT is frequently diagnostic.

B-Lymphoblastic Leukemia/Lymphoma

The blasts of B-lymphoblastic leukemia/lymphoma (B-ALL) typically express CD19, CD10, TdT, CD34, and HLA-DR;

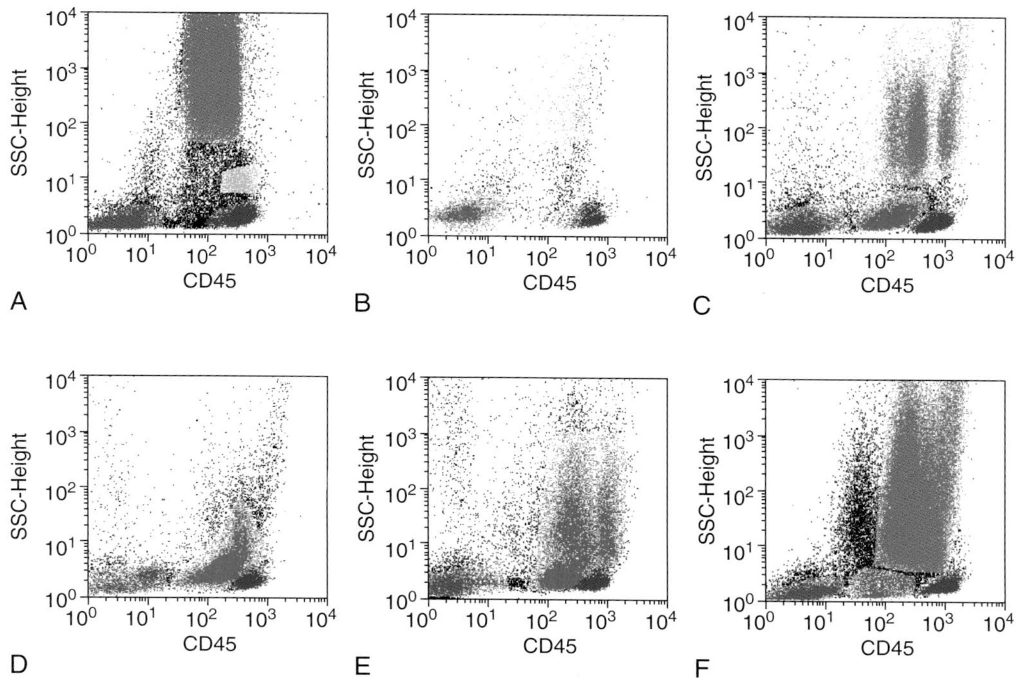

Figure 5-3. CD45 (X-axis) versus side light scatter (SSC; Y-axis) gating in bone marrow. Granulocytes are *gray*, lymphocytes are *blue*, normal monocytes are *aqua*, and erythroid precursors are *green*. **A**,CD45 versus SSC in normal bone marrow. **B**, CD45 versus SSC in acute lymphoblastic leukemia (ALL). The ALL blasts (*red*) are CD45⁻. **C**, CD45 versus SSC in ALL. The ALL blasts (*red*) have dim CD45 expression compared with normal lymphocytes. **D**, CD45 versus SSC in acute myeloid leukemia (AML). Myeloid blasts (*red*) have dim CD45, and SSC is higher than observed in ALL. **E**, CD45 versus SSC in AML with differentiation. Myeloid blasts (*red*) have dim CD45 and a spectrum of SSC that reflects the spectrum of differentiation. **F**, CD45 versus SSC in myelodysplasia. Abnormal hypogranular neutrophils (*gray*) with low side scatter are difficult to separate from monocytes. An increased blast population (*red*) is demonstrated.

have negative to dim expression of CD45 (Fig. 5-3B and C); and lack surface immunoglobulin, consistent with immature B cells. In B-ALL with a more "mature-appearing" immunophenotype, CD45 intensity may increase (see Fig. 5-3C), CD34 expression may diminish, and a cytoplasmic mu chain is present. In rare instances, there is evidence of aberrant surface immunoglobulin expression. Of these, 25% of cases are associated with a t(1;19)(q23;p13.3) translocation fusing the *PBX* and *TCF3* genes, which portends an unfavorable prognosis.[77,78] An association also exists between B-ALL lacking expression of CD10 and CD24 and 11q23 abnormalities involving the *MLL* gene, a poor prognostic feature. Conversely, intense coexpression of CD10 with dim CD9 and dim CD20 is characteristic of the prognostically favorable t(12;21)(p21;q22) (*ETV6/RUNX1*) translocation.[12,63,76] Identifying these immunophenotypic features provides the first clue that cytogenetic studies may yield prognostically important information, prompting appropriate clinicopathologic correlation.

The presence of significant numbers of normal B lymphoblasts (hematogones) in bone marrow makes identifying residual B-ALL a challenge, owing to overlapping morphologic features. In such cases, FC is particularly useful in detecting residual disease. The immunophenotypic patterns observed in normal B-cell maturation are synchronized, regulated, and well defined, based on both the intensity and the temporal patterns of expression of CD19, CD34, CD10, CD45, CD22, CD20, and CD58. In contrast, the immunophenotype of residual B-ALL falls outside this well-defined normal pattern. Examples include unusually bright, homogeneous expression of CD10; persistence of CD34, with evidence of aberrant or arrested CD22 or CD20 expression; or an arrest in the progression of CD45 expression. Additionally, CD58 is extremely useful because it is usually more intensely expressed in residual B-ALL than in hematogone populations. Although interpretation requires extensive knowledge of and familiarity with normal flow cytometric patterns of B-cell maturation, the utility of FC in distinguishing hematogones from B-ALL can prevent a serious misdiagnosis.[79,80]

T-Lymphoblastic Leukemia/Lymphoma

T-lymphoblastic leukemia/lymphoma (T-ALL) blasts have low SSC properties but exhibit CD45 expression that may overlap with the brighter CD45 mature lymphocyte gates.[76] T-ALL can be surface CD3⁻, necessitating the detection of intracytoplasmic CD3 for the diagnosis. T-cell lymphoblasts typically express TdT (detected by intracytoplasmic staining). There is variable expression of the T-cell markers CD1a, CD2, CD3, CD4, CD5, CD7, and CD8. Although CD4 and CD8 may be expressed separately, coexpression is a distinct diagnostic feature, recapitulating the "common thymocyte" stage of T-cell maturation. CD10 is also expressed in a significant subset of these cases. Aberrant myeloid antigen expression of CD13 and CD33 has been observed.[76] Although this finding may prompt the consideration of an AML, use of a comprehensive panel should help resolve lineage discrepancies.

A recognized pitfall is that the CD4⁺, CD8⁺ expression observed in T-ALL is also observed in the common thymocyte seen in a normal thymus, thymic hyperplasia, or a lymphocyte-rich thymoma. However, this pitfall can be avoided by identifying evidence of normal T-cell maturation, which is synchronized and regulated, based on both the intensity and the temporal patterns of expression of CD2, CD3, CD5, CD7, CD4, CD8, CD34, CD10, and CD45. In contrast, the immunophenotype of T-ALL demonstrates maturation arrest and lack of appropriately maturing T-cell subpopulations. Thus, FC can help distinguish neoplastic from nonneoplastic entities with a common thymocyte phenotype.[56,57]

MYELOPROLIFERATIVE AND MYELODYSPLASTIC DISORDERS

The utility of FC has grown to include a potential role in the diagnosis of myelodysplastic syndrome and myeloproliferative neoplasms. The use of four-color (and greater) multiparametric FC has allowed extensive examination and characterization of normal myeloid, monocytic, and immature hematopoietic precursors and their specific, synchronized patterns of antigen expression. Knowledge of these intricate normal patterns allows the detection of multiple abnormalities that aid in the diagnosis and prognosis of myelodysplastic and myeloproliferative processes.

Myeloproliferative Neoplasms

Patients with chronic-phase chronic myelogenous leukemia (CML) are best monitored for residual disease by molecular methods, typically quantitative reverse transcription polymerase chain reaction to detect the BCR-ABL1 transcript. FC has little to no role in patients with chronic-phase CML with stable white blood cell counts. However, FC can provide accurate blast characterization and enumeration in patients with increasing white blood cell counts who may be entering blast crisis, especially if the blasts are not large and are difficult to distinguish by morphology.

Traditionally, FC has not had a role in the diagnosis of non-CML myeloproliferative neoplasms (e.g., polycythemia vera, essential thrombocythemia). Recently, recurring abnormalities in myeloid antigen expression have been well documented in non-CML myeloproliferative disorders with cytogenetic abnormalities. These abnormalities are detected based on a combination of myeloid, monocytic, and hematopoietic precursor markers, many of which are also useful in detecting myelodysplasia. This approach opens the way for FC to become a useful modality in the clinical workup of myeloproliferative neoplasms.[73]

Myelodysplastic Syndrome

Multiple immunophenotypic abnormalities are common in myelodysplastic syndrome (MDS). Although bone marrow biopsy with concurrent cytogenetic study remains the "gold standard" for the diagnosis of MDS, a significant number of patients have blood and bone marrow findings that make diagnosis and classification difficult. For this reason, FC is increasingly being used in potential MDS cases in an attempt to increase the sensitivity and specificity of diagnosis.[73,81,82] This is reflected by the proposed inclusion of flow cytometric immunophenotyping in the minimal diagnostic criteria for MDS developed at a 2006 international working conference[83] and by the WHO classification guidelines. For patients with clinically suspected MDS but inconclusive morphologic findings and no cytogenetic abnormalities, the WHO guidelines recommend that the detection of three or more aberrant features by FC in the erythroid, granulocytic, or monocytic lineage should be considered "very suggestive" of MDS.[12] The utility of FC in the diagnosis of MDS is based on the knowledge that the maturation of hematopoietic lineages is a strictly regulated process that results in a tightly controlled and predictable pattern of normal antigen expression at different stages of differentiation. Because granulocytic, monocytic, and erythroid differentiation is abnormal in MDS, FC identifies dysplasia by detecting deviations from the normal pattern of antigen expression. No single MDS-specific immunophenotype exists. Detection of the multiple characteristic abnormalities depends on the incorporation of large numbers of antibodies in a multiparameter four-color (or greater) panel. The pattern and combination of myeloid abnormalities can distinguish MDS from other disease processes. These include antigenic asynchronous maturation, abnormal intensity of antigen expression, abnormally low SSC in granulocytes (owing to hypogranularity; see Fig. 5-3F), absence of normal antigens, and nonmyeloid (i.e., lymphoid) antigens on myeloid precursors.[73,81,82,84,85] Antigenic asynchronous maturation is often detected by examining the relationship and patterns of CD13, CD33, CD16, CD11b, CD34, CD117, and HLA-DR.[82,85] In MDS, FC can detect abnormal levels of expression of the following antigens: increased expression of CD45, H-ferritin, L-ferritin, and CD105 but decreased expression of CD71 by erythroblasts[81,86]; decreased expression of CD10 and CD45 by granulocytes[84,87-88]; and abnormal levels of CD64, CD13, CD11c, CD34, and CD117 expression in myelocytic series.[81,89,90] Detection of the absence of normal antigens or the presence of abnormal antigens has been useful in the diagnosis of MDS.[81,84,87] Aberrant expression of lymphoid antigens such as CD56, CD19, CD7, and CD5 on myeloid or monocytic cells is also common.[81,84,89] In erythroid precursors, expression of mitochondrial ferritin is associated with ringed sideroblasts in MDS.[86]

Flow cytometric immunophenotypic analysis provides important prognostic information in MDS. Specific immunophenotypic profiles and a variety of immunophenotypic abnormalities are associated with a poor score and risk category by the International Prognosis Scoring System (IPSS).[84,85,89,91-93] Currently, there are several systems available for scoring immunophenotypic abnormalities in MDS and for correlating them with the IPSS score and prognosis.[84,89,91] Moreover, a high number of flow cytometric abnormalities is associated with posttransplantation relapse and poor overall survival, independent of the IPSS prediction of relapse and survival.[84] Further, FC can reportedly identify patients at risk for transfusion dependency and progressive disease.[91] This approach supports the potential utility of FC in the diagnostic and prognostic assessment of MDS.

Acknowledgments

The authors wish to acknowledge Dr. Raul C. Braylan for his pioneering and influential work in the application of flow cytometry to the diagnosis of lymphoproliferative disorders.

Pearls and Pitfalls: Flow Cytometric Immunophenotyping

Pearls	Pitfalls
Mature B-Cell Neoplasia	
• Blood and bone marrow containing excess serum Ig may interfere with binding of anti-kappa and anti-lambda to cells and may bind Fc receptors on cells, masking monoclonality. Washing blood or bone marrow specimens with room-temperature phosphate-buffered saline helps eliminate interference from free serum Ig. • When normal B cells predominate, gating on large cells (cells with increased FSC), cells with abnormal antigen intensity (e.g., dim CD20), or cells expressing specific antigens (e.g., CD10) excludes normal B cells from analysis and allows detection of monoclonality in the abnormal B cells. • Malignant B cells frequently up- or downregulate expression of normal B-cell antigens (e.g., CD19, CD20, CD22), or a normal B-cell antigen may be missing altogether. • In a mature B-cell population, lack of sIg light chain or the appearance of both kappa and lambda light-chain coexpression is abnormal.	• With small samples (e.g., CSF), cell loss during washing with phosphate buffered saline may be considerable. In the absence of significant serum contamination (e.g., no blood), consider reducing or eliminating washing. • Normal germinal center B cells (often increased in follicular hyperplasia) are larger (have increased FSC) and express bright CD20, CD10, and dim sIg. Recognition of this characteristic pattern can avoid misdiagnosis. • Normal plasma cells are usually CD20$^-$. B cells are frequently CD20$^-$ after rituximab (Rituxan) therapy. • Normal plasma cells are sIg$^-$ but have intracellular light-chain expression. Germinal center B cells have dim sIg, and recognition of dim sIg expression may be subtle.
Plasma Cell Dyscrasia	
• Neoplastic plasma cells can be detected and followed based on abnormal patterns of surface antigen expression (e.g., CD38 bright, CD138$^+$, CD19$^-$, CD45$^-$) and expression of aberrant antigens (CD56$^+$, CD117$^+$). • Intracellular light-chain expression can be assessed for monoclonality.	• If a CD45$^-$ population is identified, it is important to consider a nonhematolymphoid malignancy in the differential diagnosis. CD138 and CD56 can be expressed on nonhematolymphoid neoplasms. • Plasma cells are underrepresented in flow cytometry specimens (possibly due to loss during processing). If large numbers of events are not acquired, abnormal plasma cell populations may be missed.
Mature T-Cell Neoplasia	
• Failure to express a T-cell antigen (CD2, CD3, CD5, CD7) is a feature of 75% of T-cell malignancies. • Malignant T cells frequently have abnormal levels of antigen expression; expression may be abnormally up- or downregulated (too bright or too dim). • T-cell clonality can be detected by Vβ repertoire analysis.	• CD7$^-$ T cells are a normal subset and can increase with infection. Normal gamma-delta T cells are frequently CD5$^-$. • Levels of expression of some antigens, such as CD2, are affected by inflammation. • Admixed normal T cells can obscure the presence of clonal subpopulations. Gate on abnormal T cells in such cases.
Acute Leukemia	
• In normally maturing myeloid and lymphoid cells, there is a spectrum of differentiation with an associated spectrum of antigen expression, indicating that cells are not arrested at an immature stage. • A "blast cell" gate that excludes mature cells can be defined based on dim CD45 and low SSC. • Dysynchronous antigen expression (i.e., cell population with coexpression of antigen patterns associated with both early and late stages of differentiation) can be observed in malignancy. • Lineage infidelity can be observed in acute leukemias (e.g., CD13$^+$ or CD33$^+$ ALL or CD7$^+$ AML). • Abnormal antigen intensity is often observed in acute leukemia (e.g., CD10, CD34, CD45, and CD58 in ALL). • CD45 is extremely informative in differentiating a lymphoblastic leukemia (CD45 downregulated) from a mature lymphoid malignancy (CD45 characteristically bright).	• Evaluation of tightly gated populations may examine only a single stage of differentiation, detecting cells that appear to be arrested at an immature stage. By examining all cells in a lineage, the spectrum of differentiation becomes apparent. • Under suboptimal storage conditions (e.g., refrigeration), mature granulocytes can degranulate and lose their normal high SSC characteristics so that they fall into the "blast cell" gate by CD45 versus SSC. The mature immunophenotype allows correct identification. • One must be intimately acquainted with normal patterns of antigen expression, including the normal intensity of cell staining using one's own antibodies and instrumentation, because patterns may appear different from published examples. • CD4$^+$, CD8$^+$ expression observed in T-lymphoblastic leukemia-lymphoma is also seen in the common thymocyte in normal thymus, thymic hyperplasia, and thymoma. • Normal regenerating precursor B cells, when present in large quantities, may initially be confused with ALL. Examination for normal temporal and antigen intensity patterns of B-cell maturation helps distinguish the two and avoid misdiagnosis. • Some lymphoblastic leukemias may exhibit minimal downregulation of CD45 that is difficult to detect. Comparison to CD45 expression of normal lymphoid cells within the sample (as an internal control) may highlight the difference.

ALL, acute lymphoblastic leukemia; AML, acute myeloid leukemia; CSF, cerebrospinal fluid; FSC, forward scatter; Ig, immunoglobulin; sIg, surface immunoglobulin; SSC, side or orthogonal light scatter.

References can be found on Expert Consult @ www.expertconsult.com

Chapter 6

Molecular Diagnosis in Hematopathology

Wing C. (John) Chan, Timothy C. Greiner, and Adam Bagg

CHAPTER OUTLINE

Carcinogenesis is generally initiated by a genetic lesion that results from an error occurring during normal cell function or from unrepaired physical or chemical damage to the genome.[1] Rarely, the abnormal gene is inherited, resulting in an increased susceptibility to cancer for all family members who have inherited the gene.[2] The initial event provides an increased chance for additional genetic lesions to develop, usually over a number of years, resulting in malignancy.

In the past 3 decades, numerous recurrent genetic abnormalities have been discovered, many of which are associated with unique tumor types and play a pivotal role in their pathogenesis.[3] In addition to providing insights into carcinogenesis, these lesions are important diagnostic and prognostic markers and can be used to monitor response to treatment and early relapse in treated patients. Determining the status of a number of these genetic abnormalities is now considered standard practice in cancer diagnosis and management. This chapter summarizes and illustrates the current practice of molecular diagnostics in hematologic malignancies.

Recently, advances in structural genomics and proteomics have been used to obtain a more global understanding of the neoplastic process, with the hope that the molecular mechanisms determining tumor behavior can be understood and a clinically and biologically relevant molecular profile of each tumor can be obtained at diagnosis to individualize therapy.[4-7] A brief discussion of these new investigative efforts using DNA microarrays is also presented.

OVERVIEW OF COMMONLY USED TECHNOLOGIES

Southern Blot

Southern blot hybridization was introduced in 1975[8] and has been widely used in molecular diagnostics since the 1980s. This technique requires high-quality genomic DNA, which is cleaved into defined fragments using appropriate endonucleases (restriction enzymes) that recognize unique sequences for cleavage. These DNA fragments are then size-fractionated using agarose gel electrophoresis. The fragments are transferred ("blotted") from the gel to a membrane (nitrocellulose or nylon) for hybridization with a labeled DNA or RNA probe that is complementary to a genomic sequence of interest. In molecular diagnostics for hematopoietic malignancies, Southern blot analysis has been used mainly for the detection of translocations and clonal T- or B-cell receptor gene rearrangements and occasionally for amplifications or deletions. When a translocation has occurred, the restriction fragment at the chromosomal breakpoint differs in size from the normal fragment because of the introduction or loss of DNA sequences.

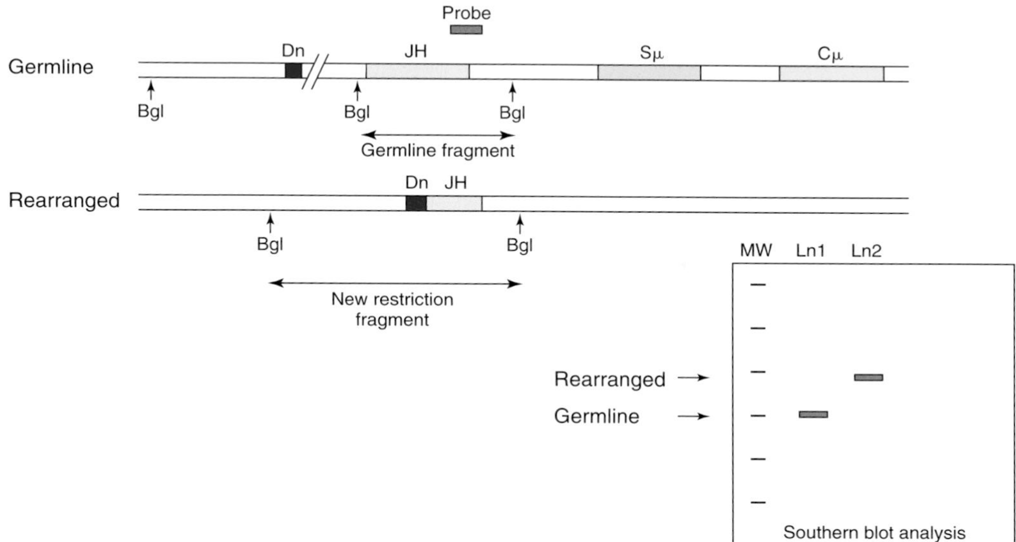

Figure 6-1. Rearrangement of a D segment to one of the J segments, creating a new restriction fragment after BglII digestion. Using a probe to the J_H region, a new fragment (lane 2) different in size from the germline fragment (lane 1) can be detected on Southern blot analysis. Similarly, a complete VDJ rearrangement generates a restriction fragment different in size from the germline fragment.

This new restriction fragment is detectable by a probe specific for the breakpoint region if it is present in a sufficient quantity, typically when the neoplastic cells constitute more than 2% to 3% of the total cellular population (Fig. 6-1). In Southern blot analysis, two or more restriction enzyme digests are examined to ensure that the change in fragment size is not due to an inherited genetic polymorphism that happens to alter a restriction site. Amplifications and deletions are demonstrated by changes in hybridization signal intensity compared with normal controls. Southern blot analysis has been largely supplanted by polymerase chain reaction assays.

Polymerase Chain Reaction

The advent of the polymerase chain reaction (PCR)[9-11] made it possible to perform molecular diagnostic analyses on a small amount of tissue as well as on archival paraffin-embedded material. The high sensitivity of the technique also allows the detection of minimal residual disease (MRD).[12,13] In some instances, it is preferable to perform PCR on complementary DNA (cDNA) rather than genomic DNA, and the starting material is isolated total or messenger RNA (mRNA) followed by reverse transcription of the mRNA to cDNA. This procedure is called reverse transcription PCR (RT-PCR). The primers for DNA PCR may be directed to either exons or introns, whereas the primers used for RT-PCR are exclusively exonic, because introns are removed during mRNA splicing. To reduce the number of reactions that need to be performed or to incorporate an internal standard in a reaction, multiple sets of compatible primers may be used in one reaction to amplify a number of templates—so-called multiplex PCR.

After PCR the products are usually analyzed by gel electrophoresis, and an appropriate gel system with the requisite resolution is essential for correct interpretation. Capillary electrophoresis,[14] which combines high sensitivity, speed, and resolution, has become the most commonly used technique for analyzing PCR products. This method, which uses fluorescent labeled primers, allows fairly precise determinations of product size, which allows comparisons among analyses performed on different tissues and at different time points.

Quantitative Polymerase Chain Reaction

Frequently, PCR is used to indicate the presence or absence of the target DNA sequence, but on occasion, such as the tracking of MRD, quantitative information is important. Real-time PCR is the method of choice for performing quantitative PCR; it provides increased precision, accuracy, and standardization and is amenable to high throughput. There are three major technologies used for real-time PCR. All allow the real-time measurement of amplified products as they accumulate; all are performed in solution, and two are probe based. One of the probe-based methods uses a single (Taqman) probe containing both a fluor and a quencher, with the probe being cleaved by the exonuclease activity of Taq polymerase, so that the fluor is separated from the quencher. As more specific templates are synthesized, more probe hybridizes and is cleaved, and more fluorescence is generated as the label is released from the quencher.[15-17] Another probe-based method uses two probes, with increasing fluorescent resonance energy transfer occurring between the two hybridizing probes as the specific templates are amplified.[18] A third technology does not use probes in the quantification procedure; rather, an intercalating DNA dye (SYBR green) is employed to measure the accumulating double-stranded DNA. In this method, the specificity of the amplified target may be gleaned by melting curve analysis.[19]

Mutational Analysis

Mutations in several genes (e.g., *FLT3, JAK2, NPM1, TP53, ATM*) have clinical, diagnostic, and prognostic significance. In general, segments of a gene that contain "hot spots" of mutation can be amplified by PCR, and the amplicons screened by a gel technique (single-strand conformation polymorphism [SSCP], denaturing gradient gel electrophoresis [DGGE], or temperature gradient gel electrophoresis [TGGE]) for sequence variation from the wild type. The variant product is then sequenced (using either conventional sequencing or pyrosequencing) to determine whether the altered sequence is a genetic polymorphism or will lead to an alteration in protein sequence and function. Alternative methods using denaturing high-performance liquid chromatography (see the section on TP53 mutation), melting curve analysis, and oligonucleotide microarrays have been developed.[20,21]

Methodologies for Detecting Clonality

For hematologic malignancies that lack antigen receptor gene rearrangements or known translocations or mutations (e.g., dendritic cell tumors, myelodysplastic syndromes), assays of X-chromosome inactivation patterns (XCIPs) can be used.[22] These assays, applicable only to females (owing to the requirement for two X chromosomes), have two basic requirements. First, the locus must be sufficiently polymorphic to enable the two alleles thereof to be distinguished from each other, and second, the assay must be able to distinguish an active from an inactive X chromosome. A variety of X chromosome genes have been studied, but perhaps the most informative (because it is highly polymorphic) is the human androgen receptor (*HUMARA*) gene, which has been evaluated fairly extensively in a number of different hematopoietic disorders. The difference in the two alleles is based on size, because the *HUMARA* gene contains between 11 and 31 trinucleotide repeats. The activation-inactivation status of the two alleles is dictated by their methylation status, with this physiologic modification rendering the gene inactive. This distinction has traditionally been made with the use of methylation-sensitive restriction enzymes (e.g., HpaII, HhaI), which are able to digest specific DNA sequences only if they are unmethylated. PCR can then distinguish the two alleles, because no amplification can occur if the target sequence has been digested by the restriction enzyme. A more contemporary approach is to use methylation-specific PCR, in which specific primers can be used to differentially amplify the active and inactive alleles following pre-PCR modification with bisulfite. Interpretation of these XCIP assays may be confounded by skewing phenomena that are either constitutive or age related. Indeed, age-related skewing is a significant issue in hematopoiesis, and it is essential to include appropriate controls for comparison. Recently, however, it was demonstrated that this apparent shortcoming associated with DNA-based assays can be overcome using a transcriptionally based quantitative PCR approach.[23]

In Situ Hybridization

In situ hybridization (ISH) for specific mRNA has the advantage of localizing the positive reaction to particular cells or tissues. In clinical practice, ISH is still largely limited to situations in which the target is present in abundance. This condition is met in the case of latent Epstein-Barr virus (EBV) infection, in which a large quantity of EBV-encoded small RNAs (EBERs) is present in the nuclei of infected cells.[24,25] It is also possible to consistently demonstrate cytoplasmic light-chain mRNA expression in plasma cells.[26] For less abundant messages, ISH is generally not sufficiently robust for clinical assays, even with amplification procedures using tyramine[27] or in situ PCR.[28]

MATURE B-CELL NEOPLASMS

Immunoglobulin Gene Rearrangement

The immunoglobulin heavy-chain (*IGH@*) gene locus[29,30] on chromosome 14q32 contains variable, diverse, joining, and constant regions, stretching over 1.1 megabases. There are approximately 123 variable region genes but only 38 to 46 with open-reading frames. These can be divided into seven families according to their sequence similarity.[31,32] There are 6 joining region segments and about 27 D segments (Fig. 6-2).[33] *IGH@* rearrangement follows a general pattern, starting with joining of the D_H and J_H segments and completed by joining a V_H segment to the rearranged $D_H J_H$ segment. This is followed by κ gene arrangement; if one κ allele is nonproductively rearranged, the other will be rearranged. If both κ rearrangements are nonfunctional, the λ gene will be used, frequently preceded by deletion of both κ genes.[34,35]

Southern blot hybridization was once the standard assay; it can detect more than 95% of clonal rearrangements in the *IGH@* gene using a J_H probe,[30,36] if the neoplastic cells constitute more than about 3% of the total cells in the sample. Typically, three restriction enzymes were used with a com-

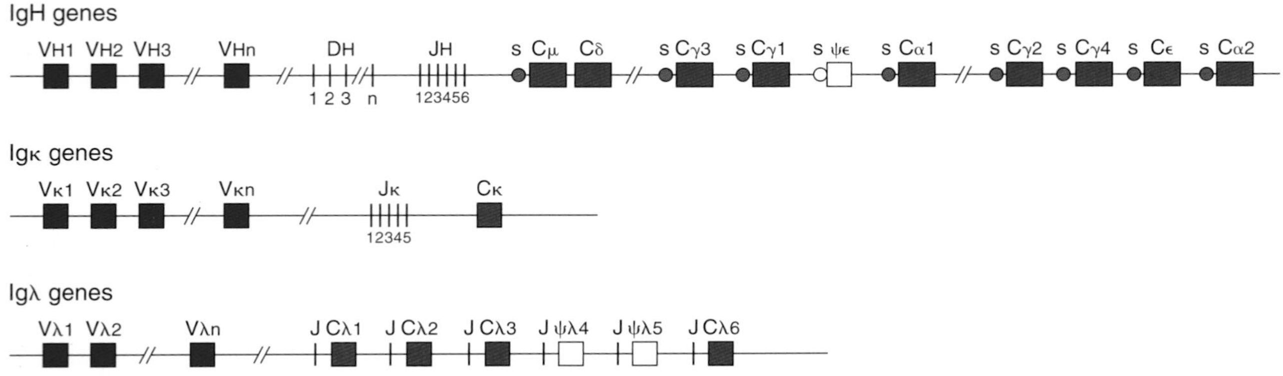

Figure 6-2. Schematic representation of the structure of the immunoglobulin heavy-chain gene.

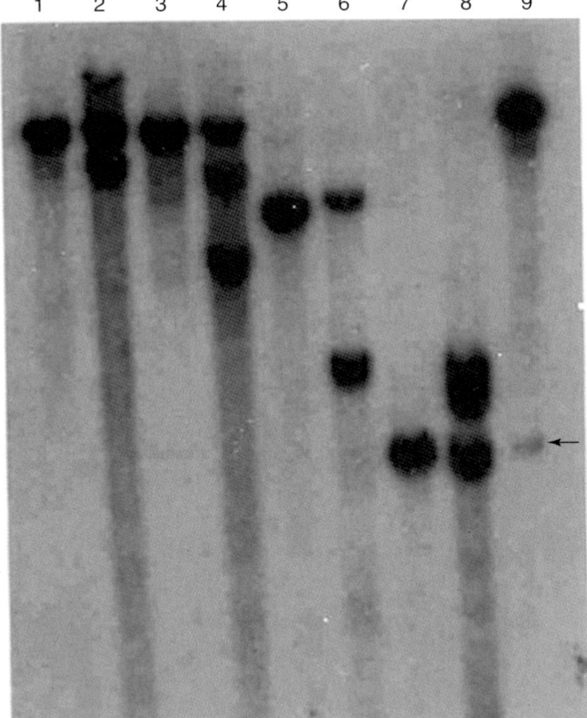

Figure 6-3. **Southern blot hybridization for detecting *IGH@* gene rearrangement.** Lanes 1, 3, 5, and 7, consisting of placental DNA, show germline fragments detected by a JH probe when the DNA is digested with BamH1, EcoR1, Hind III, and BamH1/BglII restriction enzyme, respectively. Lanes 2, 4, 6, and 8 represent tumor sample DNA digested with the same restriction enzymes as the placental sample. Nongermline bands can be observed on each of the lanes. Lane 9 represents a placental sample with a 4% mixture of DNA that gives a nongermline fragment (*arrow*), acting as a control for the sensitivity of the assay.

bined BglII-BamHI digest, which is highly sensitive in detecting nongermline fragments (Fig. 6-3). There is a common polymorphic Hind III site in the J_H region. If the polymorphic site is present in one of the alleles, Hind III digestion will result in two germline bands of equal intensity that could be mistaken for the presence of a clonal rearrangement (Fig. 6-4). For the small percentage of cases with no detectable clonal *IGH@* gene rearrangement, clonal κ gene rearrangement can be examined, generally using a κ constant or joining region probe. Rarely is it necessary to assess lambda light-chain gene rearrangement, and few laboratories offer it as a routine assay.

Southern blot analysis is a labor-intensive assay that usually takes 5 to 7 days to complete. It also requires high-molecular-weight DNA and thus cannot be performed on fixed paraffin-embedded tissue. A moderate amount of DNA is required (about 10 μg/restriction enzyme digest), and for the highest sensitivity, a ^{32}P-labeled probe is still the best choice, although chemiluminescent probes can be used. For these reasons, Southern blot analysis is performed less frequently than PCR (Fig. 6-5). The most frequently employed PCR assays use consensus primers to the J_H and the framework region (FR) III of the V_H gene segments, which amplify complementarity-determining region (CDR) III (Fig. 6-6; see Fig. 6-5). The amplicon is usually less than 150 base pairs long; therefore, the assay is suitable for amplifying short segments of DNA from archival paraffin-embedded tissue.[37-40] The main drawback of PCR for *IGH@* rearrangement is the high false-negative rate, especially for tumors that have a high load of somatic mutations, such as diffuse large B-cell lymphoma and follicular lymphoma[41-43]; the mutations can result in failure of the consensus primers to bind to the target DNA sequence. The false-negative rate can be reduced by the use of additional primers to FR III and the addition of V_H primers to FR II.[40-44] The addition of primers to FR I and leader sequences also improves the detection rate,[41-43] but as the template size increases, the amplificability of DNA from archival tissue becomes progressively poorer. Another very useful approach to increase the detection rate for clonal populations is to add an assay that detects κ gene rearrangements.[45] Although λ gene rearrangement can also be amplified by PCR, it is not generally used in a diagnostic setting.[46] A large European consortium (BIOMED-2) has performed extensive studies on the optimization of PCR procedures for gene rearrangement analysis, leading to significant improvements in the sensitivity and standardization of this approach.[47]

Although PCR is highly sensitive, the primers used amplify rearranged *IGH@* genes from normal B cells in the sample as well as the clonal population. A small clonal population may not be identifiable because of the polyclonal background; thus the sensitivity of the assay is highly dependent on the

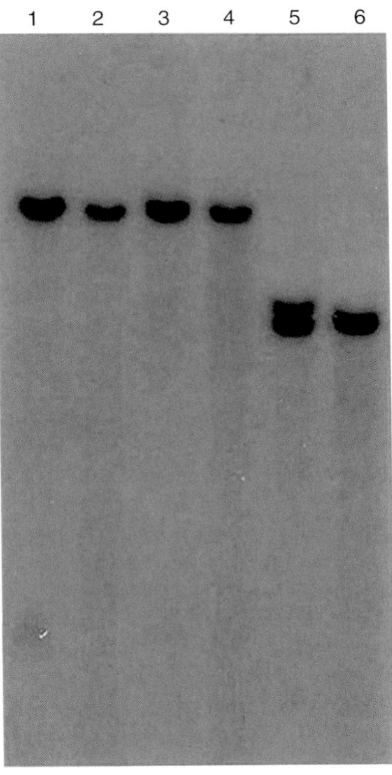

Figure 6-4. Similar to Figure 6-3, lanes 1, 3, and 5 represent the placental control, and lanes 2, 4, and 6 represent a patient specimen. In lanes 1 and 2, the DNA was digested with BamH1; lanes 3 and 4, with EcoR1; and lanes 5 and 6, with Hind III. Only germline bands are observed. Two distinct bands of equal hybridization intensity are seen on lane 5 due to a polymorphism of a Hind III site on one of the alleles of the placental sample used to prepare the control DNA.

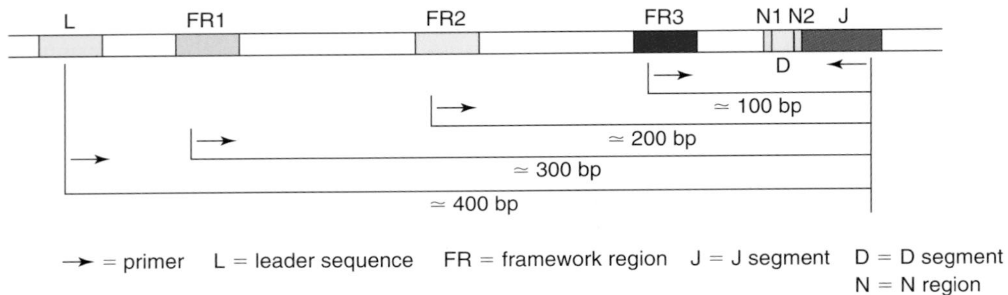

Figure 6-5. Polymerase chain reaction (PCR) for *IGH@* gene rearrangement. This figure illustrates the different strategies that can be used to amplify the VDJ rearrangement. The *arrows* indicate the primers that can be used to amplify different regions of a rearranged VDJ segment. The approximate sizes (base pairs [bp]) of the amplified products are indicated.

proportion of background normal B cells present in the sample (Fig. 6-7). In the detection of MRD, the CDR III sequence in the original tumor should be determined, and then clone-specific primers or probes can be designed to obtain the highest sensitivity.[48]

In samples with highly degraded DNA or those that contain few B cells, especially in small biopsy specimens without a dense B-cell infiltrate, PCR may amplify only a few DNA templates, and one of these may predominate and appear as a distinct band on gel electrophoresis. This may lead to an erroneous interpretation of the presence of a clonal population. However, these pseudoclonal bands are not reproducible, and repeat assays typically show no bands or bands of different sizes (Fig. 6-8). Thus, the results of PCR analysis, particularly on small biopsy specimens lacking a dense B-cell infiltrate, must be interpreted with caution.

BCL2 Translocation

BCL2 translocation occurs in more than 85% of cases of follicular lymphoma and in about 20% of de novo diffuse large B-cell lymphomas (DLBCLs) (Table 6-1).[49-51] In these two tumor types, the *BCL2* breakpoint clusters mainly in three regions (Fig. 6-9): the major breakpoint region (MBR)[52,53] accounts for the majority of cases, and the minor cluster region (MCR) and intermediate cluster region (ICR)[54] account for most of the rest.[55,56] Most of these translocations can be detected by Southern blot hybridization using appropriate probes. Alternatively, fluorescence in situ hybridization (FISH) using appropriate probes can detect practically all *BCL2* rearrangements.[57] Between 50% and 70% of cases of follicular lymphoma[49,58,59] are positive by Southern blot for *BCL2* rearrangement at the MBR and 10% to 20% at the MCR. The MBR and MCR breakpoints can be detected by PCR, but at a lower frequency (see Fig. 6-9). In unselected cases of follicular

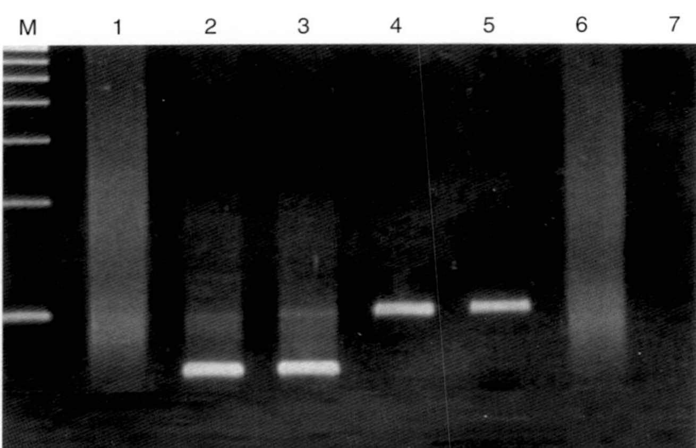

Figure 6-6. Polyacrylamide gel electrophoresis of the amplicons of IgH CDR3 after polymerase chain reaction amplification. Lane M represents a 100–base pair interval molecular weight marker; lane 1, DNA from a bone marrow sample; lanes 2 and 3, DNA from a lymphoma; lanes 4 and 5, different DNA dilutions from a positive control; lane 6, DNA from normal peripheral blood mononuclear cells; lane 7, template containing water only. Lanes 2 and 3 show a monoclonal band similar to the positive control but of a different size. Lanes 1 and 6 do not show any detectable clonal population. Lane 7 shows no amplified products.

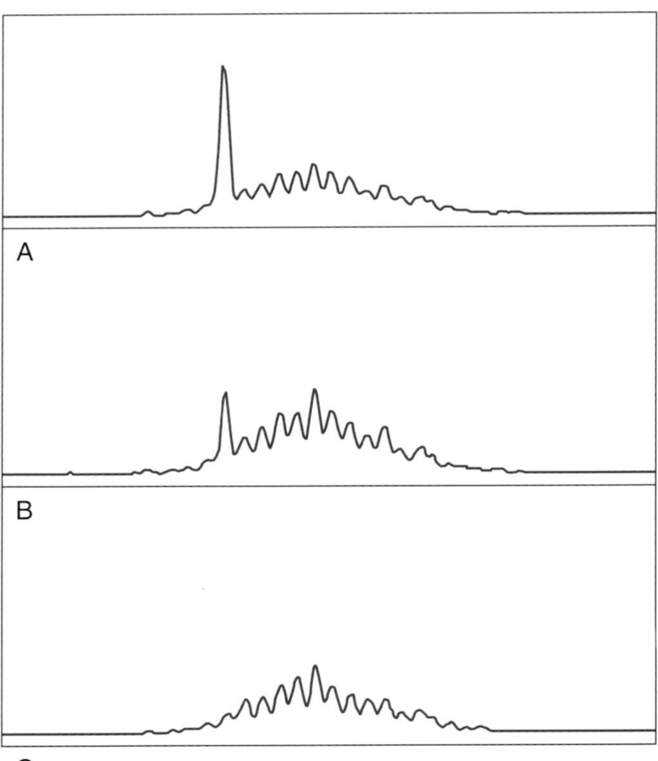

Figure 6-7. DNA from a positive control cell line diluted in DNA from normal peripheral blood mononuclear cells. A-C, The clonal peak becomes less distinct and finally cannot be detected amid the polyclonal background as the ratio of tumor DNA to peripheral blood mononuclear cell DNA is progressively decreased.

Table 6-1 **Recurrent Translocations and the Target Genes Involved in B-Cell Non-Hodgkin's Lymphoma**

Gene Rearrangement	Chromosomal Translocation	Lymphoma Types Commonly Associated*
IGH@	Not characterized	All mature B-cell lymphomas
BCL2	t(14;18)(q32;q21)	Follicular lymphoma Diffuse large B-cell lymphoma
BCL6	t(3;v) (q27;v)	Diffuse large B-cell lymphoma Follicular lymphoma Marginal zone lymphoma
MYC	t(8;14)(q24;q32) and variants	Burkitt's lymphoma Posttransplant and AIDS-associated lymphomas *Diffuse large B-cell lymphoma*
CCND1;IGH@ J region *CCND1;IGH@* S region	t(11;14)(q13;q32)	Mantle cell lymphoma Plasma cell myeloma
MALT1 with *API2/IGH@* and other	t(v;18)(v;q21)	Extranodal marginal zone lymphoma
BCL10	t(1;14)(q22;q32)	*Extranodal marginal zone lymphoma*
ALK	t(2;)(p;q)	ALK-positive large B-cell lymphoma
BCL3	t(14;19)(q32;q13)	Chronic lymphocytic leukemia

*Lymphomas in italic constitute a small percentage (generally <10%) of cases with the translocation.
AIDS, acquired immunodeficiency syndrome; ALK, anaplastic lymphoma kinase; v, variable.

lymphoma, approximately 50% to 60% of cases have *BCL2* translocation detectable by PCR at the MBR and 10% at the MCR[49,60,61] and lower in paraffin-embedded tissues. Additional translocations may be detected by newly designed primer sets targeting other cluster regions,[62,63] including the ICR. Variant translocations involving the light-chain genes or mu switch region[64] cannot be detected using the usual primer sets.

With highly sensitive techniques such as nested PCR, sporadic cells with *BCL2* translocation may be detected in reactive lymphoid tissues and peripheral blood from normal, healthy individuals; the frequency of this finding increases with age.[65,66] In our laboratory, the PCR assay is run in duplicate, and the interpretation of a clonal population with *BCL2* translocation is made only when identically sized products are detected in both assays.

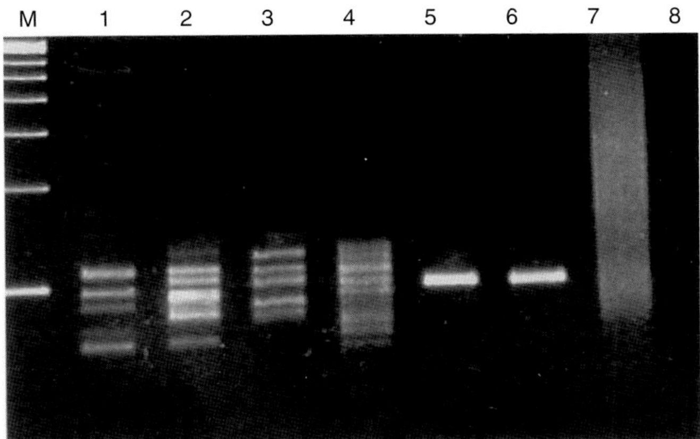

Figure 6-8. False-positive polymerase chain reaction for *IGH@* rearrangement. Lane M represents a molecular weight marker at 100-bp intervals. Lanes 1, 2, 3, and 4 represent amplicons from DNA extracted from a paraffin-embedded section of a small biopsy. Lanes 5 and 6 represent positive control DNA at two different dilutions. Lane 7 represents DNA from normal peripheral blood mononuclear cells, and lane 8 represents a no-DNA template. Lanes 1 to 4 show an increasing concentration of DNA in the template. At lower concentrations, a few distinct bands are observed; at high concentrations, more bands are seen. This illustrates that in small biopsies with highly degraded DNA, pseudoclonal bands may be observed.

BCL2 translocation is a useful diagnostic marker of B-cell lymphomas with germinal center B-cell differentiation (other than Burkitt's lymphoma); it can be used to distinguish benign from malignant follicular proliferations and follicular lymphoma from other tumors such as marginal zone and mantle cell lymphoma, and it is a highly sensitive marker for detecting MRD in patients with follicular lymphoma or DLBCL with the translocation.[48,67,68] In addition, quantitation of *BCL2/IGH@* in the bone marrow at diagnosis may predict treatment response and outcome.[69]

CCND1 (Cyclin D1) Translocation

The t(11;14)(q13; q32) is a hallmark of mantle cell lymphoma (MCL),[70] but it is also present in some cases of plasma cell myeloma (see Table 6-1)[71,72] and B-prolymphocytic leukemia,[73] although the latter is now thought to represent a leukemic presentation of MCL.[74] The translocation leads to upregulation of cyclin D1 mRNA and protein expression. The *CCND1* (formerly known as *BCL1*) breakpoints are scattered over a long stretch of the genomic DNA with clustering in several regions, in particular an area about 120 kb centromeric to the cyclin D1 gene, called the major translocation cluster (Fig. 6-10). However, Southern blot hybridization using probes to the major translocation cluster (see Fig. 6-10B) and up to three additional regions can detect only about 50% of the rearrangements.[75,76] It is possible to design PCR primers to amplify the majority of breakpoints at the major translocation cluster,[77-81] but the detection rate in all MCLs is only in the range of 30% to 40%.

FISH for *CCND1* translocation has an almost 100% sensitivity and is much more useful than Southern blot or PCR as a diagnostic assay for MCL.[82] In most cases, one can confirm the diagnosis by the detection of nuclear cyclin D1 using immunohistochemistry, which also has a higher overall diagnostic yield than Southern blot or PCR assays.[83-85]

Translocations and Mutations of the *BCL6* Gene

The *BCL6* gene, located on chromosome 3q27,[86-88] is one of the most frequent loci involved in translocations in DLBCL,

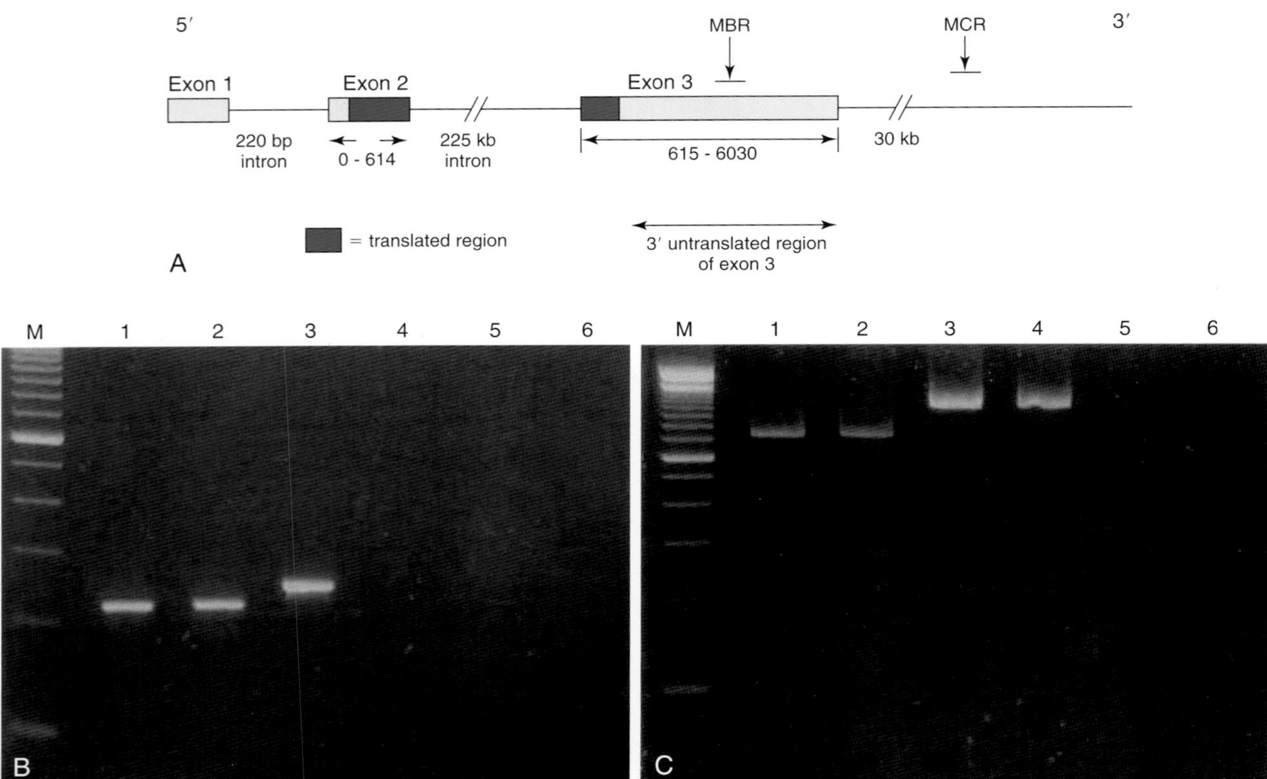

Figure 6-9. Analysis of *BCL2* gene rearrangement in lymphomas. A, Schematic representation of the *BCL2* locus on chromosome 18, with the location of the major breakpoint region (MBR) and minor cluster region (MCR) shown. **B,** Polymerase chain reaction (PCR) amplification of the major breakpoint region. Lane M represents a 100–base pair interval molecular weight marker. Lanes 1 and 2 are duplicate assays of a follicular lymphoma. Lane 3 consists of DNA from a positive control diluted 10,000-fold, and lane 4 represents the control diluted 100,000-fold. Lane 5 represents template DNA from K562, a negative control, and lane 6 represents a no-DNA template. The duplicate patient samples on lanes 1 and 2 show identical size amplification products. The positive cell line control shows an amplicon at 10^{-4} dilution but not at 10^{-5} in this assay. **C,** PCR amplification for the minor cluster region. Lane M represents a 100–base pair interval molecular weight marker; lanes 1 and 2, DNA from a follicular lymphoma; lanes 3 and 4, positive cell line control DNA at 10^{-4} and 10^{-5} dilutions; lane 5, negative DNA control from K562; and lane 6, a template without DNA. The patient samples show amplicons of identical molecular weight on lanes 1 and 2. The DNA from the positive controls at both dilutions are successfully amplified in this assay. The negative controls are appropriately negative.

with a frequency of around 25% (see Table 6-1). Translocations are also found at a lower frequency in other lymphomas. such as follicular lymphoma and marginal zone lymphoma.[89-92] *BCL6* has many translocation partners, including immunoglobulin (Ig) and non-Ig genes. The *BCL6* breakpoints cluster at the 5′ noncoding region and juxtapose heterologous promoters that deregulate its expression.

The BCL6 protein is a POZ/zinc finger transcriptional repressor that is selectively expressed by normal germinal center B cells. The POZ domain is involved in protein-protein interaction such as homo- or heterodimerization, and the zinc finger domain is involved in DNA binding. Many BCL6 target genes have been identified, including genes involved in B-cell differentiation, cell cycle control, growth and survival, and inflammatory response. The repression of BLIMP-1 expression (BLIMP-1 represses numerous genes, including *MYC* and *PAX5*, and promotes terminal differentiation of B cells to plasma cells) may be critical in the oncogenic activity of deregulated BCL6 expression. *CDKN1A* (formerly known as *p21* or *CIP1*), *CDKN1B* (formerly known as *p27* or *KIP1*), and *TP53* have also been identified as BCL6 target genes, and their repression may play a role in lymphomagenesis.[93,94]

BCL6 translocation may be detected by Southern blot hybridization using a probe to the 5′ portion of the gene, including the 5′ flanking sequence, the first noncoding exon, and part of the first intron, where most of the breaks occur (the MBR).[90,95] Because some cases of chromosome 3q27 abnormality do not show a rearrangement by this probe, some of the breakpoints may fall outside of the region,[90] and an alternative breakpoint region 240 to 280 kb 5′ to the MBR has been described and appears to occur more commonly in follicular lymphoma without t(14;18) and follicular lymphoma grade 3B with a diffuse component.[96-99] Because the breakpoint is near the tip of chromosome 3, a significant number of cases may be missed on routine karyotyping.[90] FISH probes for the MBR have been developed.[100,101] Because multiple partners are involved with *BCL6* translocation, a break-apart probe spanning the *BCL6* locus is preferable to *IGH@/BCL6*-specific probes. An additional probe set is required to reliably detect the alternative breakpoint region.[97-99]

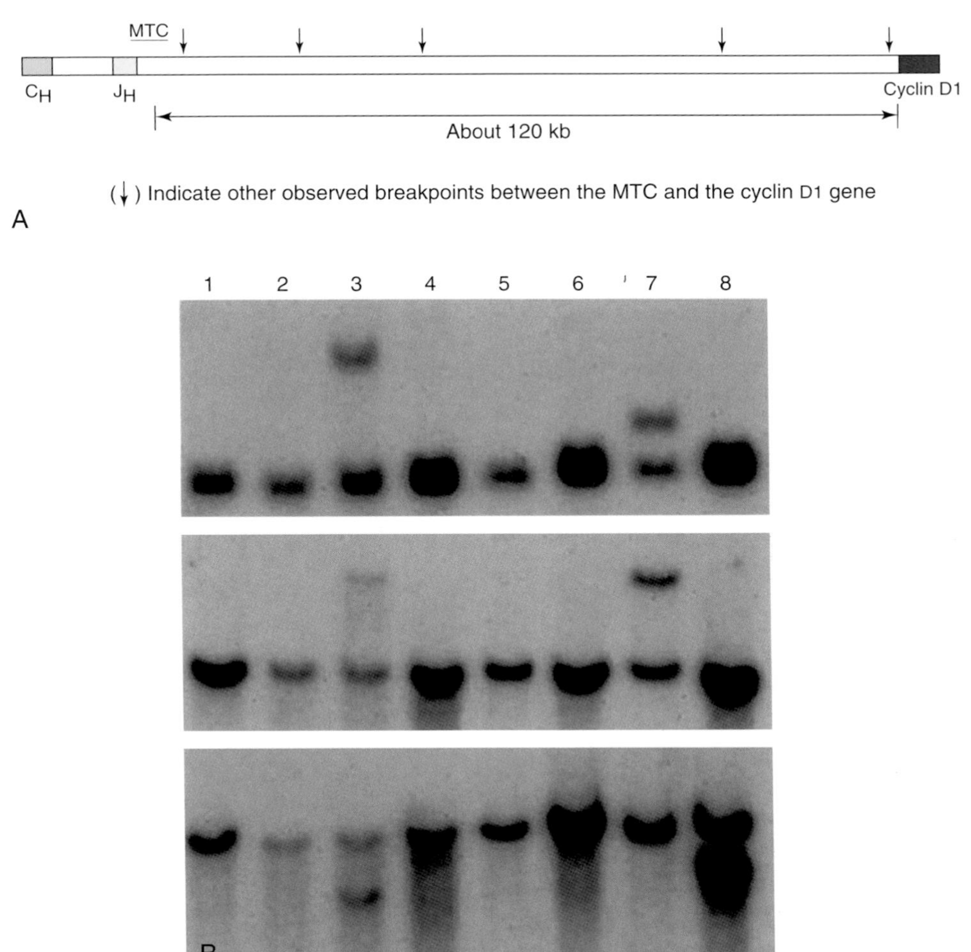

Figure 6-10. ***BCL1*** **(cyclin D1) rearrangement in lymphomas. A,** Diagrammatic representation of a *BCL1* translocation having most of the breakpoint at the major translocation cluster (MTC). The cyclin D1 gene is located about 120 kb from the MTC, and there are many other reported breakpoints scattered within this large region. **B,** Southern blot hybridization assay using a probe to the MTC. Lane 1 shows placental DNA germline control; lanes 2 to 8, DNA samples from seven mantle cell lymphomas. In the *top panel*, DNA has been digested with Sst1; in the *middle panel*, DNA has been digested with EcoR1; and in the *bottom panel*, DNA has been digested with BamH1. Lane 3 shows a nongermline band in all three enzyme digests. Lane 7 shows a nongermline band after Sst1 and EcoR1 digestion. Lane 8 shows a nongermline band only on BamH1 digestion and is therefore not unequivocally positive for a rearrangement at the MTC.

The *BCL6* gene undergoes somatic hypermutation in normal B cells when they transit the germinal center,[102,103] and mutations are also found in the *BCL6* gene in several types of lymphomas. These mutations cluster in the same 5′ regulatory region involved in the translocations. What functional role somatic hypermutation in *BCL6* plays in normal B cells is unclear, as is the role these mutations may play in lymphomagenesis and tumor progression. Mutations affecting the BCL6 binding sites in exon 1 may interfere with negative autoregulation,[104-108] and some of the mutations may disrupt the interferon regulatory factor 4 (IRF-4)-responsive region in the first intron of *BCL6* and block its downregulation by CD40 signaling,[109] thereby deregulating *BCL6* expression in the absence of a translocation.

MYC Translocation

Translocation of the *MYC* gene, located on chromosome 8q24, to the *IGH@* locus and, less frequently, variant translocations involving one of the Ig light-chain loci are characteristically seen in Burkitt's and atypical Burkitt's lymphoma (Fig. 6-11; see Table 6-1).[110] It may also be seen less frequently in posttransplantation lymphoproliferative disorders and myeloma and occasionally in DLBCL and aggressive transformations of indolent lymphomas.[111-113] In endemic Burkitt's lymphoma, *MYC* is translocated to chromosome 14, characteristically near the J_H region, with the break at the *MYC* locus occurring 5′ to exon 1 (see Fig. 6-11). In sporadic Burkitt's lymphoma, the break at the *IGH@* locus occurs at one of the switch regions. The *MYC* breakpoint may be 5′ to exon 1 or within the first intron (see Fig. 6-11). In variant translocations involving the *IGK@* or *IGL@* locus, *MYC* typically remains on chromosome 8, with the breakpoints occurring at various distances 3′ to exon 3. The *IGK@* or *IGL@* locus is translocated to chromosome 8, generally breaking 5′ to the constant region in the V or J segments (see Fig. 6-11). In Southern blot hybridization, probes hybridizing to different *MYC* exons have been used singly or in combination to

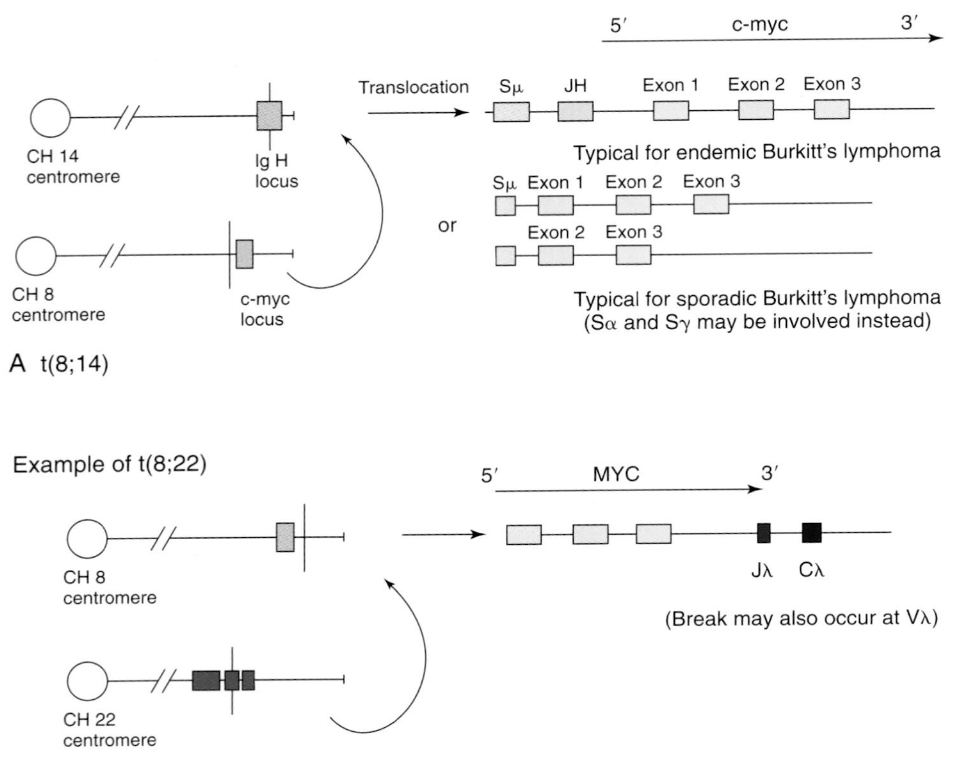

Figure 6-11. Translocations affecting the *MYC* locus. **A,** In t(8;14), the *MYC* locus from chromosome 8 is translocated to chromosome 14 at the IgH locus. **B,** In the variant translocations t(2;8) or t(8;22), the *MYC* locus stays on chromosome 8, and the kappa or lambda light-chain locus telomeric to the break is translocated to chromosome 8, 3′ to the *MYC* locus.

detect most of the translocations that are not too far 5′ or 3′ to the *MYC* gene.[111,114] It is also possible to design PCR primers to amplify many of the translocations involving the switch and J_H region of *IGH@*.[115] Recently, FISH probes have been designed to detect translocations involving the *MYC* locus, including break-apart probes flanking possible *MYC* breakpoints.[116]

Translocations Occurring in Mucosa-Associated Lymphoid Tissue Lymphomas

The most frequent recurrent translocation found in extranodal marginal zone lymphoma of mucosa-associated lymphoid tissue (MALT lymphoma; see Table 6-1) is t(11;18)(q21;q31).[117,118] The translocation involves the *API2* gene on chromosome 11q21 and the *MALT1* gene on chromosome 18q21 (Fig. 6-12).[119] The *API2* gene is a member of a family of genes that encode for proteins that suppress apoptosis, and it has been postulated that the fusion protein resulting from the translocation may retain the antiapoptotic function and promote the survival of the tumor cells. However, there is increasing evidence that the *MALT1* gene is the key component, with activation of the nuclear factor-κB (NF-κB) pathways the major pathogenetic mechanism.[120] Primer sets have been designed that should be able to amplify all known hybrid transcripts by RT-PCR,[121,122] and they can be used to amplify paraffin-embedded specimens. The t(11;18) has been demonstrated in MALT lymphoma from a variety of anatomic sites, with up to a 48% incidence in gastric cases[121] and possibly higher in the lungs.[82,122] Interestingly, this translocation is not detected in aggressive lymphomas in MALT sites or in nodal or splenic marginal zone lymphoma.[82,121-123] The presence of the translocation appears to indicate biologically more advanced MALT lymphomas that do not respond to *Helicobacter pylori* eradication in gastric cases,[124] and it correlates with the nuclear expression of BCL10, albeit not as strongly as with t(1;14).[123] FISH analysis provides an alternative assay for the detection of t(11;18).[125]

The *MALT1* gene can also be translocated to the *IGH@* locus, and this t(14;18)(q32;q21) translocation tends to occur in MALT lymphomas of the liver, skin, and ocular adnexa rather than the stomach and lung, which are common sites for t(11;18).[126-128] This *MALT1/IGH@* translocation can be detected by FISH, and an appropriate break-apart probe spanning the *MALT1* locus should be able to detect both t(11;18) and t(14;18) involving *MALT1*. Different patterns of immunostaining for MALT1 and BCL10 have been described for t(11;18), t(14;18), and t(1;14), and the presence of these translocations may be predictable by immunohistochemistry.[129,130]

The translocation t(1;14)(q22;q32) involves *BCL10* on chromosome 1q22, which is translocated to the *IGH@* locus.[131,132] The *BCL10* gene contains an amino-terminal

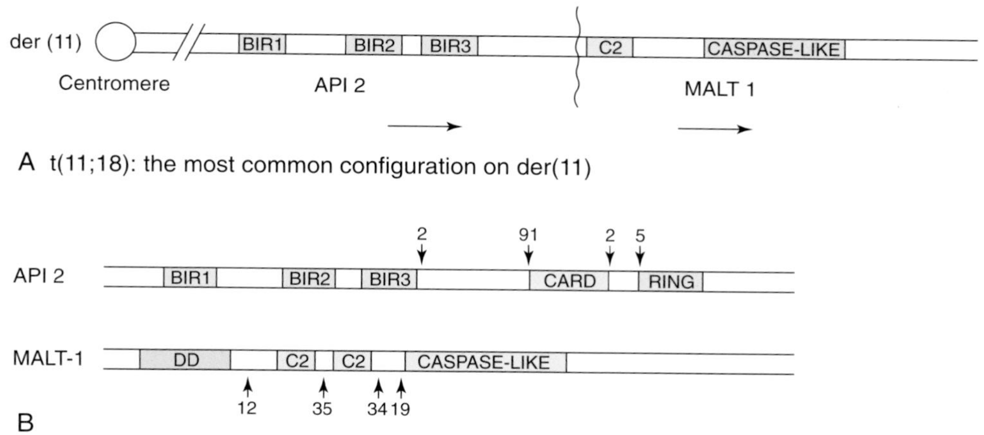

Figure 6-12. **A,** Schematic representation of the most common configuration of der(11) due to t(11;18). The centromere of chromosome 11 is shown, and the *arrows* indicate the transcriptional direction of the two genes. The *vertical wavy line* across the chromosome indicates the point of the break, with the *MALT-1* gene translocated telomeric to the break. **B,** Diagram showing the structure of the *API2* and *MALT-1* genes, with the colored boxes indicating their various domains. The *arrows* indicate the positions of known breakpoints, and the *numbers* above the *arrows* represent the percentage of breaks reported to occur at that site. (Modified from Liu H, Ye H, Dogan A, et al. t[11;18][q21;q21] is associated with advanced mucosa-associated lymphoid tissue lymphoma that expresses nuclear BCL10. *Blood.* 2001;98:1182-1187. Used with permission of the American Society of Hematology; permission conveyed through Copyright Clearance Center, Inc.)

caspase recruitment domain (CARD) that exhibits a variety of mutations giving rise to truncation of the molecule in or distal to the CARD domain.[131,132] *BCL10* mutations are rare and are not confined to any specific type of lymphoma.[133-137] It has been shown that *BCL10* can form a complex with CARD II and MALT1 that activates the I-κB kinase complex and eventually NF-κB.[120] The API2/MALT1 fusion protein may also activate NF-κB by a similar pathway. Abnormal nuclear localization of BCL10 protein has been demonstrated in MALT lymphoma with t(1;14)[138] and also in cases with t(11;18), suggesting that this abnormal localization may play a role in the pathogenesis of MALT lymphoma.[139]

More recently, uncommon novel translocations, including t(3;14)(p14;q32) involving the *FOXP1* gene have been described.[127,140,141] The best diagnostic approach for these translocations has not been established.

MATURE T-CELL NEOPLASMS

T-Cell Receptor Gene Rearrangement Analysis

Since the identification of the various T-cell receptor (TCR) molecules in T lymphocytes, knowledge of the rearrangement process within T cells has been used to support the diagnosis of T-cell lymphomas.[142,143] The TCR is part of the CD3 complex on the surface of T cells. The TCR includes the alpha, beta, gamma, and delta chains (Fig. 6-13). The vast majority (≥90%) of T lymphocytes express the alpha-beta receptor molecule on the cell surface.[144-146] Compared with lymph nodes, there are increased numbers of gamma-delta T cells in the skin, intestine, and spleen. However, regardless of the TCR expressed, T cells more frequently rearrange the gamma

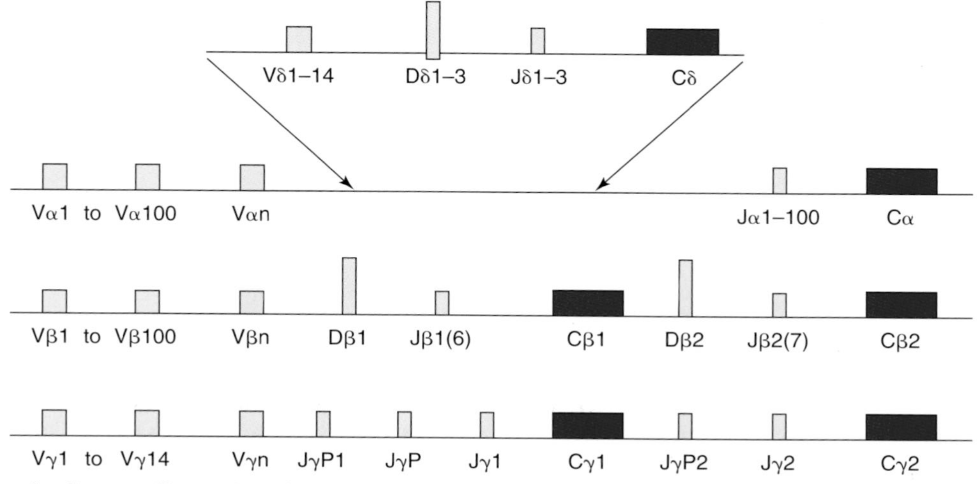

Figure 6-13. Schematic diagram illustrating the gene structure of the T-cell receptor genes. No diversity segment is present in the alpha and gamma genes. The distances are not to scale.

gene than the beta gene.[147] Rearrangements of the *TRG@* or *TRB@* genes do not predict the type of TCR expression on the cell surface.[147] Like Ig genes, each TCR contains variable, joining, and constant region segments. Delta and beta genes also have diversity segments, whereas alpha and gamma genes do not.[148]

In the rearrangement process, a variable region is linked with a downstream joining region segment. The delta gene is the first to rearrange; however, because the delta receptor locus is located within the alpha gene sequence, rearrangement of the alpha gene deletes the delta sequence.[149,150] If delta is deleted, the cell is likely to express the alpha-beta receptor. However, because rearrangements between the alpha variable and joining region genes cover large distances, alpha rearrangements are not amenable to Southern blotting or PCR and are not used in clinical testing. Because the delta gene is often deleted, it is of little utility for diagnostic assays in the vast majority of T-cell lymphomas. However, the *TRD@* gene may be the only TCR gene rearranged in rare cases of T-cell lymphomas.[151] The gamma gene is rearranged before the beta gene. Because the beta and delta genes have a diversity segment with two junctional areas between the variable and joining segments, there is greater variation in these TCR sequences than in the gamma gene. The junctional areas are regions where DNA is lost from the 3′ end of the variable region, the 5′ end of the joining region, and both ends of the diversity gene when it is present. In addition, DNA nucleotides are often inserted or deleted in the junctional or N region by terminal deoxynucleotidyl transferase, as occurs in the Ig genes. This junctional region provides unique identification for the TCR rearrangement of an individual cell.

TRB@ is the most frequent gene used in the detection of TCR rearrangements by Southern blotting.[143,152] Probes to either the constant region or the joining region segments of the beta gene have been used, with greater sensitivity obtained by the use of probes to the two joining region genes. Most laboratories require that a rearrangement be present in two restriction enzyme digests to call a result positive (Fig. 6-14).[143] Because the *TRG@* gene has no diversity gene segment, the junctional region is composed of fewer nucleotides than in *TRB@* rearrangements.[153] In addition, there are a limited number of functional variable and joining region segments.[154,155] Thus, this limited *TRG@* repertoire produces a relatively low number of possible rearrangement combinations, making it difficult to separate rearrangements by Southern blot analysis and identify clonal populations.[156,157]

The simplicity of *TRG@* lends itself to the use of PCR to identify clonal rearrangements.[158-160] A consensus pair of primers, however, cannot be used to cover all the variable region or joining region gene segments.[161,162] Group-specific primers must be used to cover each of the four groups of variable region genes and the three groups of joining region genes. Nonetheless, this set of seven primers is a relatively small number compared with the number of primers necessary to amplify all the gene rearrangement combinations in the *TRB@* family. Complete primer sets are necessary to detect all *TRG@* rearrangements,[161,162] because limited primer sets have an average detection rate of 75%.[163] Group 1 segments, including genes of Vγ2-8, are rearranged most frequently, followed by Vγ9, Vγ10, and Vγ11.[164,165] The Jγ1/Jγ2 pair is rearranged most frequently, followed by JγP2; the least commonly used joining region segment is JγP.[147,165]

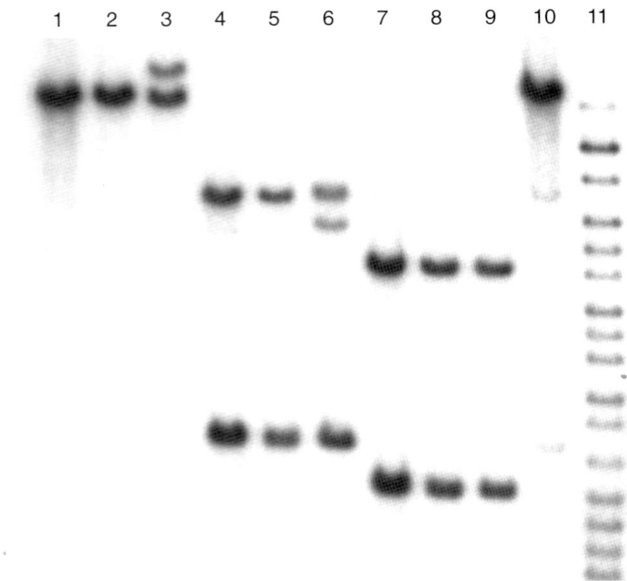

Figure 6-14. Southern blot analysis of T-cell receptor beta. Three cases with three enzymes are illustrated: BamH1 (lanes 1 to 3), EcoR1 (lanes 4 to 6), and Hind III (lanes 7 to 9). One case shows rearrangement in BamH1 (lane 3) and EcoR1 (lane 6), but it is in germline configuration in Hind III (lane 9). The other cases do not show rearrangement of the gene. Lane 10 is the 4% positive control, and lane 11 is the molecular weight marker.

Numerous technologies have been described to analyze TCR beta and gamma gene rearrangements. These include routine agarose or polyacrylamide gel electrophoresis,[159,160,166,167] sequencing gel electrophoresis, DGGE,[164,168-170] SSCP,[171,172] TGGE,[173,174] and heteroduplex analysis.[175] Recently, methods that involve laser scanning of PCR products made with fluorescent labeled primers have been described, with gene scan analysis on a polyacrylamide gel[176-182] and capillary electrophoresis.[14,183-191] Analytical techniques that emphasize biochemical separation of the unique junctional sequences of the neoplastic cells, as opposed to separation by length, include DGGE, SSCP, TGGE, and heteroduplex analysis (Fig. 6-15). MRD can be detected by using junction-specific primers to detect 1 in 10^5 to 10^6 tumor cells.[48,192,193] With this technique, a patient-specific variable or joining region primer is paired with the junction-specific primer to anneal and amplify only the rearrangement of interest.

Capillary electrophoresis represents a flow-through technology as opposed to the gel-based methodologies described in the 1990s. It is a length-based separation method with a single-nucleotide resolution. The use of different fluorochromes on the fluorescent labeled primers allows the identification of variable region genes or joining region genes involved in the rearrangement (Fig. 6-16).[14,174,183,184,186,187,189-191,194] Laboratories find this information valuable because it aids in the follow-up analysis of patient specimens. Polyclonal specimens produce a normal distribution of rearrangements (see Fig. 6-16A). Clonal populations are defined when the suspected peak exceeds the peak height of the polyclonal background by a ratio of 2:1 to 3:1 (see Fig. 6-16B).[187,191] Laboratories need to establish appropriate rules for ratio determination based on the proven sensitivity of their specific assays, which ranges from 1% to 5% of clonal cells. Duplicate analyses are useful to distinguish true positive results from spurious peaks

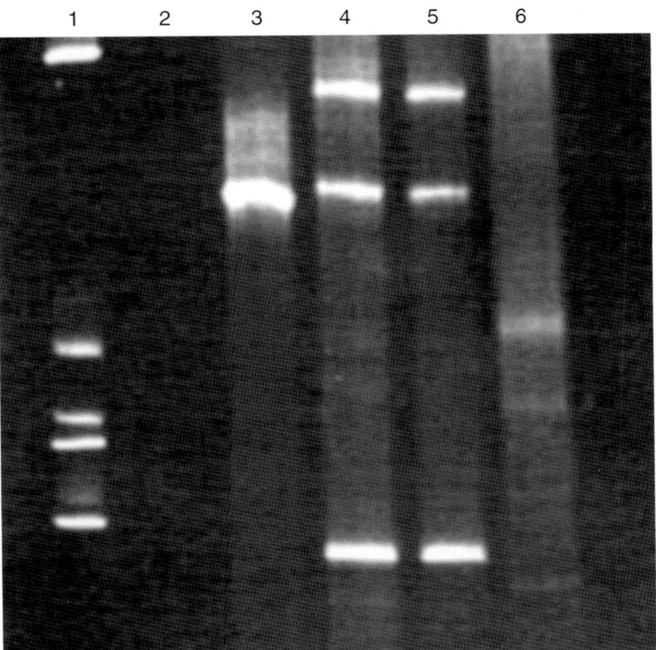

Figure 6-15. Denaturing gradient gel electrophoresis of T-cell receptor gamma rearrangements. There is high-resolution separation of polymerase chain reaction (PCR) products, even though the length of the PCR products has a range of only 50 nucleotides. Lane 1 is a molecular weight marker, lane 2 is a negative control, lane 3 is an HSB2 control, lanes 4 and 5 are paired peripheral T-cell lymphoma, and lane 6 is peripheral blood.

(pseudoclonality) caused by a few T cells in the DNA sample. Assays that have only one fluorochrome and one product size distribution in a single tube are easier to interpret than assays with multiple tubes and multiple product sizes.[191]

TP53 Mutation Analysis

Mutations in the hot-spot coding region of exons 5 to 8 are the most frequent secondary abnormality described in non-Hodgkin's lymphomas and in leukemias.[108,195] Sensitive methods for detecting *TP53* mutations include SSCP,[196] DGGE with guanosine-cytosine (GC)-clamping,[197,198] and denaturing high-performance liquid chromatography (Fig. 6-17).[163,199] Mutations of *TP53* occur in about 15% of non-Hodgkin's lymphomas, with the highest frequency (40%) seen in Burkitt's lymphoma.[109,200] Mutations in *TP53* are associated with transformation of follicular lymphoma and small lymphocytic lymphoma to large B-cell lymphoma[89,201] and a poor prognosis in many types of non-Hodgkin's lymphoma. In MCL they are associated with poor survival and blastic or blastoid morphology.[198,202,203] The poor survival is believed to be due to the absence of functional p53 protein; the other allele is typically deleted, preventing p53-induced apoptosis, and the tumor cells become resistant to chemotherapy.[204-206] This effect is due to the subset of direct DNA-binding mutations.[207] Thus, the type of p53 mutation needs to be identified before enrolling patients in future p53-targeted therapies.

The immunohistochemical analysis of p53 protein expression may result in false-negatives that occur when the mutation causes a stop codon and no protein or a truncated protein is produced.[208] Citrate antigen retrieval and the use of antibodies to epitopes located at the amino terminal end, such as DO-7, are recommended to minimize false-negatives due to truncation of the carboxy end.[209] Also, overexpression of wild-type p53 can occur in some instances from unknown mechanisms.[210-212] To properly evaluate overexpression of p53 in tissue, one needs to simultaneously examine p21 expression, because wild-type p53 is required for p21 expression.[213] If p21 expression is present, p53 expression most likely represents wild-type p53. Owing to these problems, genomic characterization of the mutations is the preferred method.

ACUTE LEUKEMIAS

More than 300 different translocations have been described in acute leukemias, and more than 100 have been cloned, underscoring the remarkable genetic complexity of these diseases. The array of translocations and other genetic abnormalities can be grouped into derangements that affect one of three major pathways (Table 6-2).

There are data that suggest cooperation among some of these dysregulated pathways—for example, enhanced signal transduction via an activated tyrosine kinase conferring proliferative and antiapoptotic activity, whereas disruption of the transcriptional apparatus impairs differentiation. Other pathways affect chromatin modulation and nuclear-to-cytoplasmic shuttling. This rather limited number of deranged pathways may facilitate the development of specific pharmacologic interventions directed at one of them. This section approaches the genetics of leukemia from a disease-based perspective, to highlight the manner in which molecular genetic studies have guided and refined classification, risk stratification, and therapy.

Although many of the genetic lesions are amenable to and have historically been detected by conventional Southern blot analysis, most are now more commonly evaluated by PCR-based technologies. Many of the translocations involve DNA breaks that are quite widely dispersed in introns (albeit usually within a single intron), which would make DNA-based PCR assays somewhat cumbersome. Accordingly, and taking advantage of intronic splicing, most translocation assays are performed by RT-PCR, using exonic primers.

Acute Myeloid Leukemia

Acute myeloid leukemia (AML) is an extremely heterogeneous disease at the genetic level, with at least 160 different recurrent structural cytogenetic abnormalities observed. However, it has now become clear that of all the parameters integrated to yield a final diagnosis and appropriate classification of AML (e.g., clinical features, blood counts, morphology, cytochemistry, immunophenotypic and genetic studies—both classic cytogenetics and molecular genetics), the most relevant feature is the genetic abnormality. This notion has emanated in part from large multicenter cooperative studies that identified three broad prognostic groups (Table 6-3).[214-216] Furthermore, even though AML that develops in the "elderly" (older than 55 years) usually has a poor prognosis, this cytogenetic stratification also holds true for this group of patients.[217]

Translocations

Of the numerous translocations that have been described in AML (Table 6-4), four occur with the greatest frequency:

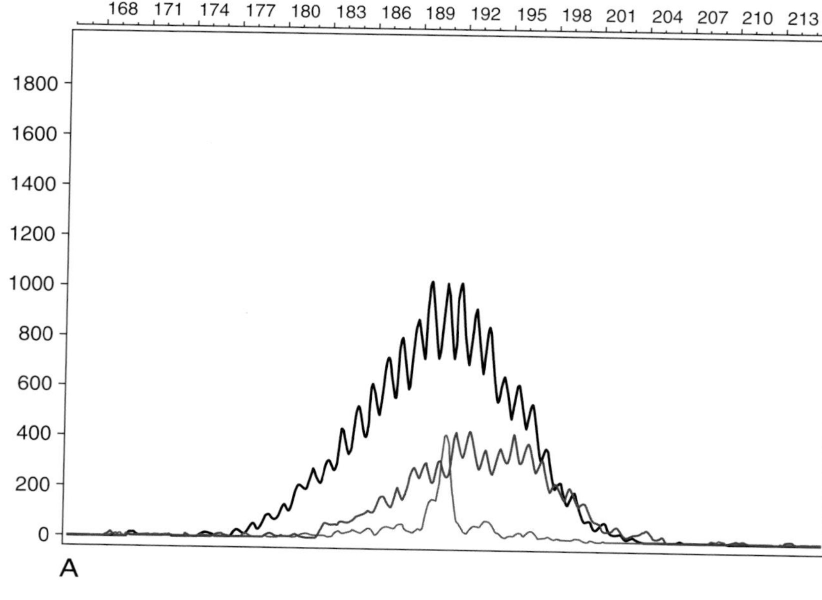

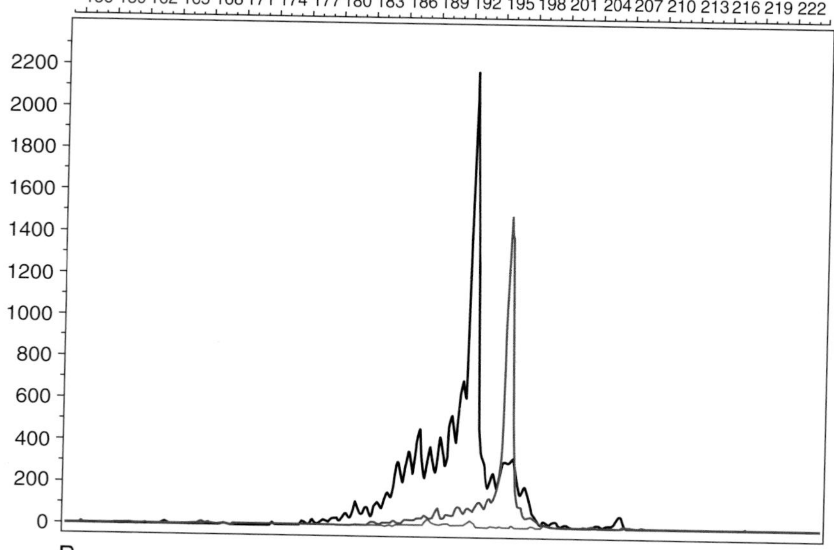

Figure 6-16. Capillary electrophoresis of T-cell receptor gamma rearrangements. A, Polyclonal sample. Note the normal distribution of polymerase chain reaction products spanning 190 nucleotides. **B,** Peripheral T-cell lymphoma. The ratio of the clonal peak to the background exceeds 2.0. Two alleles are rearranged, which occurs in more than 50% of cases.

t(8;21), t(15;17), inv(16), and translocations involving 11q23. The biologic and clinical relevance of these genetic abnormalities is such that each was used to define a specific disease category in the 2001 World Health Organization (WHO) classification of AML.[218] These abnormalities are of prognostic relevance, in that the first three are typically associated with a relatively favorable outcome, whereas most translocations involving 11q23 are predictive of an adverse outcome; however, some reports indicate that t(9;11) is not associated with a poor prognosis.[219] Furthermore, the finding of a t(15;17) or some of the other variant translocations disrupting the *RARA* gene at 17q11 is necessary to justify the use of all-*trans*-retinoic acid (ATRA). Nevertheless, a significant number (up to 50%) of AMLs have a normal karyotype, and it is likely that in many of these cases there are submicroscopic and cryptic genetic lesions that cannot be detected by conventional karyotypic studies. A number of these abnormalities have been discovered and cloned, and it is here that molecular methodologies are likely to have a significant role. In the 2008 WHO classification of AML, three more specific translocations were added—t(1;22), t(6;9), and inv(3)—and the broad 11q23 translocation category was narrowed to include t(9;11) cases only. AMLs defined by t(1;22) involving the *RBM15* (formerly *OTT*) and *MKL1* (formerly *MAL*) genes, t(6;9) involving the *DEK* and *NUP214* (formerly *CAN*) genes, and inv(3) involving the *RPN1* and *EVI1* genes are quite infrequent, each accounting for approximately 1% of AMLs, and they are not discussed here.

t(8;21)(q22;q22). This translocation is believed to be the most common translocation in AML, occurring in approximately 10% of cases, especially in children. It fuses part of the core binding factor (CBF)-A2 encoded by the *RUNX1*

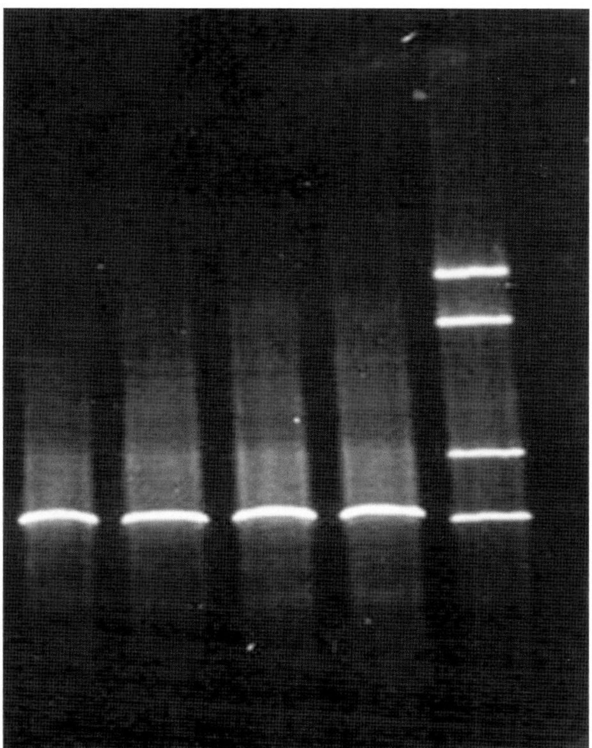

Figure 6-17. Mutations of *p53* detected by denaturing gradient gel electrophoresis. Wild-type samples have a single band. Mutated samples demonstrate a shift in electrophoresis, producing two to four bands (e.g., exon 8 at the right).

(formerly *CBFA2* or *AML1*) gene on 21q22 with part of the *RUNX1T1* (formerly *ETO*) gene on 8q22.[220] The RUNX1 protein is one half of the heterodimer that is a crucial transcription factor in hematopoiesis. This half directly contacts DNA, whereas the CBF-B subunit, which binds to CBF-A2 but not to DNA, facilitates this DNA binding. The genes that encode the two components of the CBF transcriptional factor are common targets of translocations in both AML and acute lymphoblastic leukemia (ALL) and are collectively disrupted in approximately 25% of cases of both these major types of acute leukemia. When *RUNX1* is translocated, the subsequently generated fusion proteins act as dominant inhibitory proteins, inhibiting the transcription of a number of target genes, including myeloperoxidase, *GM-CSF, IL-3*, and *TRB@*. However, a number of studies have indicated that this step alone is unable to induce acute leukemia.

This translocation is most often associated with the subtype of AML historically termed M2 (AML with maturation) in the French-American-British (FAB) classification, and it is found in 40% of M2 cases; more than 90% of t(8;21)-positive cases have M2 morphology. The breakpoints cluster within a single intron of both genes, so that similar *RUNX1/RUNX1T1* chimeric transcripts are generated in every case. Thus, a simple RT-PCR assay, using *RUNX1* and *RUNX1T1* primers, is able to detect this translocation at a molecular level and can be used diagnostically. Leukemias harboring t(8;21) evince particular sensitivity to therapeutic regimens containing high-dose cytosine arabinoside. Although this good prognostic association appears to be well established in adult AML, it is less clear in pediatric AML.

Table 6-2 Major Functional Targets of Genetic Lesions in Leukemias

Group*	Specific Target†	Lesion	Leukemia
Transcription factors	*RUNX1* or *CBFB*	t(8;21)(q22;q22)	AML-M2
		RUNX1 mutation	AML-M0
		inv(16)(p13;q22)	AML-M4Eo
		t(12;21)(p13;q22)	ALL-precursor B
	RARA	t(15;17)(q22;q21)	AML-M3
	TCF3-E2A	t(1;19)(q23;p13)	ALL-precursor B
	MYC	t(8q24)	ALL-B cell‡
	TAL1	t(1p32)	ALL-T cell
	ETV6	t(12p13)	AML, ALL, MPN
	HOX genes	Variable	AML
	CEBPA	*CEBPA* mutation	AML-M2
Signal transduction	Tyrosine kinases	t(9;22)(q34;q11)/*BCR-ABL1*	CML, ALL-precursor B
		FLT3 mutation	AML
		del(4)(q12q12)/*FIP1LI-PDGFRA*	Chronic eosinophilic leukemia
		KIT mutations	Mast cell leukemia, AML
		MPL mutations	Non-CML MPN
		JAK2 mutations	Non-CML MPN
	RAS	*NRAS* mutations	AML, MDS
Chromatin modulation	*MLL*	t(11q23)	AML-M4/5, secondary AML, infantile leukemia
	RBM15-MKL1	t(1;22)(p13;q13)	AML-M7
	MYST3(MOZ)-CBP	t(8;16)(p11;p13)	AML-M5

*A fourth, and currently less common, group of translocations disrupts components of the nuclear pore complex (NUP). For example, *NUP98* on 11p15, which has at least eight different translocation partners, and *NUP214* on 9q34 play a role in transport between the nucleus and cytoplasm. *NPM1*, involved in the t(2;5) translocation associated with anaplastic large cell lymphoma, in a rare variant translocation t(5;17) seen with AML-M3 and t(3;5) in MDS, is also involved in nuclear shuttling. It is also the most commonly mutated gene in AML (see text for details).

†Terms in parentheses are synonyms or accepted abbreviations for the genes.

‡ALL-B cell is now recognized as Burkitt's lymphoma in leukemic phase.

ALL, acute lymphoblastic leukemia; AML, acute myeloid leukemia; CML, chronic myeloid leukemia; MDS, myelodysplastic syndrome; MPN, myeloproliferative neoplasm.

Table 6-3 Cytogenetic Stratification of Acute Myeloid Leukemias

Risk Group	Genetics	Frequency (%)*	CR Rate (%)*	5-Year Survival (%)*
Favorable	t(8;21) t(15;17) inv(16)	25 (5)	85 (70)	60 (35)
Intermediate	Normal +8, +21 11q23	50 (63)	80 (60)	40 (13)
Unfavorable	−5, −7 3q Complex	25 (32)	60 (25)	15 (2)

*Percentages are approximate and are derived from combined data for young patients (<55 or 60 years old) with acute myeloid leukemia (AML) from references 216-218. The percentages in parentheses are for older patients with AML from reference 219; although the distribution of the risk groups is different, the prognostic relevance is still retained, albeit with worse CR and 5-year survival rates.
CR, complete remission.

t(15;17)(q22;q21). Among all the acute leukemias, acute promyelocytic leukemia has the most compelling genotype-phenotype correlation, in that the genetics can frequently be predicted based on the characteristic morphology—either the classic hypergranular form (FAB-M3) or the microgranular variant (FAB-M3v). Although it accounts for about 10% of translocations in AML as a whole, t(15;17)(q22;q21) is seen in approximately 99% of morphologically defined acute promyelocytic leukemias. In the remaining 1% of cases, interesting variant translocations are present. For all of these, the common denominator is disruption of the *RARA* gene at 17q11. In the prototypical t(15;17) translocation, *RARA* is fused to the *PML* gene, the protein product of which is normally located in nuclear bodies or PML oncogenic domains (PODs) within the nucleus. Although the involvement of *RARA* is central to neoplastic transformation, the disruption of *PML* is also thought to play a role.

Wild-type RARA protein acts as a transcriptional activator, but when translocated, it is converted to a transcriptional repressor.[221] Normally, RARA interacts with transcriptional corepressors, and this interaction is abrogated by physiologic concentrations of retinoic acid. However, when RARA is fused to PML, the interaction with the corepressor complex is strengthened, and only pharmacologic doses of retinoic acid (in the form of ATRA) can overcome this repression. At least four variant translocations have been described, as detailed in Table 6-4. The t(11;17)(q23;q11) translocation, fusing *RARA* with *ZBTB16* (formerly *PLZF*), is noteworthy in that it is not

Table 6-4 Recurrent Genetic Abnormalities* in Acute Myeloid Leukemia (AML)

Genetic Lesion	Chromosomal Abnormality	Association	*Frequency (%)*†	
			Subtype	*Overall*
Fusion				
RUNX1-RUNX1T1	t(8;21)(q22;q22)	M2	40	15
PML-RARA	t(15;17)(q22;q21)	M3	99	12
MYH11-CBFB	inv(16)(p13;q22)	M4Eo	85	10
V-MLL	t(V;11)(v;q23)	M4, M5, secondary AML‡	?	5
DEK-NUP214	t(6;9)(p23;q34)	Basophilia	?	2
EVI1-RPN1	t(3;V)(q21;v)	Dysplasia	?	2
ZBTB16-RARA	t(11;17)(q23;q11)	M3	1	<1
NPM1-RARA	t(5;17)(q35;q11)	M3	<1	<1
NUMA-RARA	t(11;17)(q13;q11)	M3	<1	<1
STAT5-RARA	t(17;17)(q11;q11)	M3	<1	<1
NUP98-V	t(11;V)(p15;v)	Secondary AML‡	?	<1
MYST3-V	t(8;V)(p11;v)	M5	?	<1
RBM15-MKL1	t(1;22)(p13;q13)	M7 in infants	?	<1
Numerical Abnormalities				
? *RPS14*	del(5)(q12;q35)/−5	Secondary AML	5	2
Unknown	del (7)(q11;q36)/−7	Secondary AML	5	2
Unknown	+8	Secondary AML	20	10
Unknown	del(20)(q11)	Secondary AML	2	1

*Detectable by both conventional karyotypic cytogenetics and molecular methodologies.
†Frequencies are approximate, have been averaged from a number of multicenter studies, and usually reflect those reported in adults (aged 15 to 55 years). The subtype percentage reflects the frequency in the particular form of AML with which the lesion is typically associated; the overall percentage reflects that of AML as a whole.
‡Previous exposure to topoisomerase II inhibitors.
V or v, variable fusion partners or chromosomal breakpoints.

sensitive to ATRA therapy because the ZBTB16 itself acts as a transcriptional repressor that cannot be abrogated by ATRA. Rather, treatment with histone deacetylase inhibitors is required to induce differentiation in these cases. Thus, from a molecular diagnostic perspective, it is important to identify this rare variant because affected patients will not benefit from ATRA therapy. Interestingly, there may be morphologic correlates with this specific genetic lesion, in that the t(11;17)-positive leukemic cells tend to have regular nuclei, with an increased number of Pelger-Huët–like cells, in contrast to cases with t(15;17), which tend to have irregular (reniform or bilobed) nuclei and typically do not have Pelger-Huët–like cells.[222]

In the common t(15;17) translocation, the breakpoints in *RARA* are well conserved in intron 2, and there are two major breakpoints in the *PML* gene. Thus, a single downstream *RARA* primer and two upstream *PML* primers are required for the detection of most *PML-RARA* fusion transcripts (Fig. 6-18).[223] Interestingly, most cases (about 75%) also express the reciprocal *RARA-PML* transcript; the significance of this is unclear.

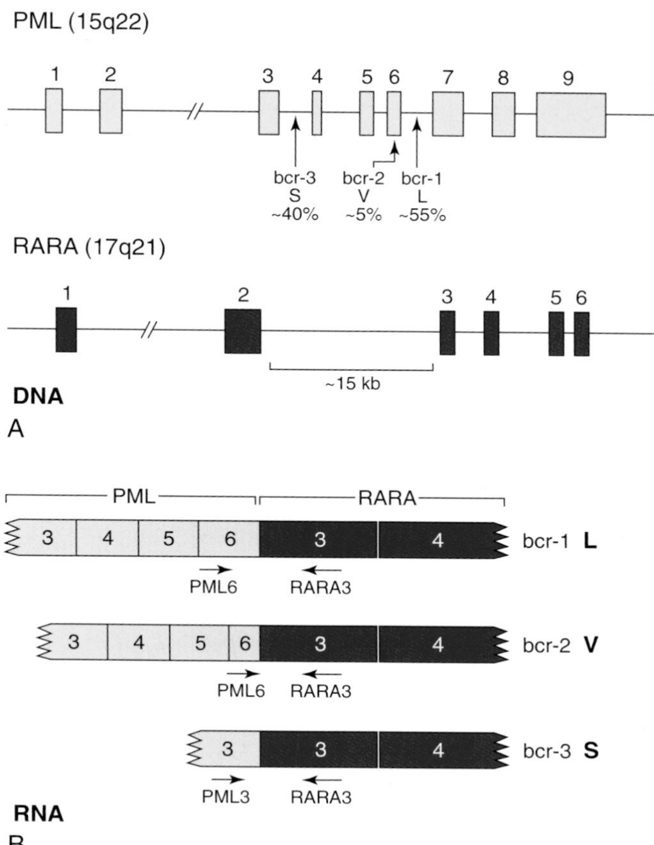

Figure 6-18. Molecular genetics of the t(15;17)(q22;q21) translocation. A, Schematic genomic structure of the *PML* and *RARA* genes, indicating the sites of breakpoint clustering. The breakpoints in the *RARA* gene are confined to intron 2, whereas there are two major breakpoints in *PML:* in intron 3 and intron 6, also referred to as breakpoint cluster region (bcr)-3 and bcr-1, respectively, giving rise to short (S) and long (L) fusion transcripts, respectively (see later). A third, less common breakpoint occurs within exon 6 and is referred to as bcr-2 or variable (V). The approximate frequencies of the different breakpoints are shown. **B,** RNA-cDNA structure of the fused *PML-RARA* genes, showing the three types of transcripts and primers required for reverse transcription polymerase chain reaction amplification. Two *PML* primers, *PML6* and *PML3,* but only a single *RARA* primer, *RARA3,* are required. The *PML6* primer does not clearly amplify bcr-3 breaks, because exon 6 is lost; in contrast, the *PML3* primer—in addition to the *PML6* primer—may amplify bcr-1 breaks, yielding larger than expected products. Even though the bcr-2 break is exonic, it occurs in-frame; it can be detected with appropriate *PML6* primers (those located 5′ of the break, so that the product size is smaller than that seen with bcr-1 breaks), but it may not be discerned with other *PML6* primers (those located 3′ of the break). There are some biologic and clinical correlates with the different breakpoints. There may be decreased all-*trans*-retinoic acid sensitivity with the exonic bcr-2 breakpoints, whereas bcr-3 breaks are associated with a higher presenting leukocyte count, M3v morphology, and CD2 coexpression.[225]

inv(16)(p13;q22). This pericentric inversion, and the molecularly identical t(16;16) translocation, is characteristically seen in acute myelomonoblastic leukemia with abnormal eosinophils (AML-M4Eo). The inversion fuses parts of the *CBFB* (formerly *PEBP2B*) gene with parts of one of the myosin heavy-chain genes, *MYH11* (formerly *SMMHC*). One of the consequences of this is to sequester much of the CBF-B protein in the cytoplasm (where it normally resides), thus precluding its ability to function as part of the CBF transcription factor alluded to earlier.[224] Although this genetic fusion is most often seen in the context of M4Eo, it may also be found in most other subtypes of AML, including M2 and M5.

The inv(16) can sometimes be subtle and may be missed, particularly if the metaphase preparations are suboptimal. Trisomy 22 is the most common secondary abnormality seen in patients with inv(16), but it is uncommon in other situations. Thus, the presence of an apparently isolated +22 should alert one to presence of a possible "cryptic" *CBFB/MYH11* fusion. Molecular studies are important in the detection of this abnormality. The breakpoints in the two genes are heterogeneous, with at least 10 different fusion transcripts. Although 99% of breakpoints in *CBFB* occur in intron 5 of that gene, the breakpoints in the *MYH11* gene are heterogeneous, with seven different exons (7 through 13) variably included in the fusion transcripts. The most common form—designated type A—accounts for approximately 90% of cases, and two other transcripts (types D and E) account for an additional 5%.

11q23 Translocations. The *MLL* (for mixed lineage leukemia, or myeloid lymphoid leukemia) gene on chromosome 11q23 is one of the most promiscuous genes in human leukemias[225] and is involved in at least 80 different translocations; these are seen, as the name indicates, in both AML and ALL, as well as in myelodysplastic syndrome (MDS). This gene has also been termed *ALL1, HTRX,* and *HRX.* Of the numerous translocation partners, the most common are *AFF1* (formerly *MLLT2, FEL,* or *AF4*) on 4q21 in the t(4;11) translocation; *MLLT3* (formerly *AF9*) on 9q21 in the t(9;11) translocation; and *MLLT1* (formerly *ENL*), *ELL,* or *EEN* (three different genes) on 19p13 in the t(11;19) translocation. Together, these account for more than three quarters of the partners, constituting approximately 40%, 27%, and 12%, respectively, of translocations involving *MLL.* However, 99% of cases with the t(4;11) translocation are ALL (see the ALL section later). *MLL* translocations in AML are associated with two scenarios: monoblastic differentiation (both M4 and M5) and prior therapy with topoisomerase II inhibitors (secondary AML).

The breakpoints in *MLL* cluster in a relatively small (8.3-kb) area spanning exons 5 to 11, referred to as a breakpoint cluster region. The breakpoints correlate with some phenotypes: *MLL* translocations in de novo leukemias tend to cluster in the 5′ region of the breakpoint cluster region, whereas those in both infantile and secondary AML occur more often in the 3′ region, where there is a particularly strong DNA topoisomerase II binding site. Although this likely explains the translocations seen in secondary AML, it also suggests that infantile AML may result from exposure to toxic agents in utero.

MLL appears to modulate or maintain the expression of genes—in particular, *HOX* genes—via chromatin remodeling. Many of the fusion partners are putative transcription factors. The mechanisms through which *MLL* translocations lead to leukemogenesis have not been completely unraveled. With the possible exception of the t(9;11) translocation, *MLL* rearrangements are predictive of a poor prognosis.

Rationale for Performing Molecular Genetic Studies for Translocations

Although each of the seven genetically defined AMLs may be readily detectable using conventional karyotypic studies, these analyses have a variable false-negative rate. Some of the translocations are cryptic, in that they are "submicroscopic" (too small to be seen on microscopic analysis of chromosomes); other false-negative results may have a technical basis. There is a variable frequency of false-negative cytogenetics (i.e., leukemia-associated fusion transcript positive, with an apparently normal karyotype) for both *RUNX1/RUNX1T1* t(8;21) and *CBFB/MYH11* inv(16). Although some studies indicated that this false-negative rate was as high as 30%,[226,227] more recent analyses reveal a lower but still sizable frequency of 15%.[228] Up to 15% of acute promyelocytic leukemias may be cytogenetically normal or uninformative. This percentage includes 6% cryptic lesions, due to insertions and complex translocations, and 9% cytogenetic failures. False-negative molecular studies may also occur. Thus, conventional cytogenetics and molecular genetics complement each other, and both have limitations.

Given the importance of detecting these translocations for AML classification and therapy, all newly diagnosed AMLs should be screened for their presence at the molecular genetic level, particularly in cases with an apparently normal karyotype.[229] RT-PCR assays are available for each of the first three translocations. The detection of specific translocations involving *MLL* on 11q23 is confounded by the plethora of translocation partners. There are some well-described individual RT-PCR assays, and a more global approach could be achieved by FISH analysis with *MLL* probes. This assay might be most useful when there is an expectation of a higher frequency of such translocations (e.g., AML following therapy with topoisomerase II inhibitors).

Even in cases with cytogenetically detected translocations at diagnosis, it is reasonable to perform molecular genetic studies to define disease-specific molecular lesions that can be exploited for the subsequent detection of MRD. The following four messages are emerging from studies of MRD testing in AML, as well as in other hematologic malignancies[230]: (1) a single qualitative result is not, in isolation, predictive of subsequent relapse; (2) quantitative results provide more relevant information, with levels on the order of less than 10^{-4} typically associated with long-term remission and higher levels possible harbingers of relapse; (3) stable levels of MRD may not be inconsistent with long-term survival, but rising levels are more predictive of relapse; and (4) the more rapidly MRD is cleared after remission induction therapy, the better the prognosis. In addition to the importance of quantitative PCR in MRD analysis, it has been proposed that high levels of fusion transcript at diagnosis might be of prognostic relevance.[231]

Genetic Lesions Unrelated to Translocations

In addition to cytogenetically detectable translocations, a variety of cryptic genetic lesions have been identified that cannot be discerned by cytogenetics and are likely to be of clinical and prognostic relevance. These include *FLT3* abnormalities, *NPM1* mutations, *CEPBA* mutations, *KIT* mutations, *MLL* partial tandem duplications, *WT1* overexpression, and *BAALC* overexpression (Table 6-5).[232-234]

Table 6-5 Cryptic Genetic Abnormalities* in Acute Myeloid Leukemia (AML)

Gene	Abnormality	Assay	Approximate Frequency (%)†	Prognostic Effect
FLT3	JM-ITD	PCR	23	Negative
	KD-PM	RE-PCR	7	
NPM1	Exon 12 IM	MD	55	Positive
CEBPA	PM	MD	10	Positive
MLL	PTD	PCR	10	Negative
WT1	Increased expression	RT-PCR	100	Negative‡
BAALC	Increased expression	RT-PCR	65	Negative
KIT	PM	MD	45§	Negative
GATA1	PM	MD	100ǀ	Unknown
RUNX1	PM	MD	25¶	Unknown

*That is, there is no cytogenetic correlate.
†In AML with normal cytogenetics, unless otherwise specified.
‡Virtually all AMLs overexpress WT1, but those with a lower level tend to have a superior clinical outcome.[234]
§Frequency in core binding factor AMLs—namely, those with t(8;21) or inv(16).
ǀFrequency in patients with Down syndrome–associated AML, typically megakaryoblastic transient myeloproliferative disorder.[232]
¶Frequency in minimally differentiated AML.[233]
IM, insertion mutation; ITD, internal tandem duplication; JM, juxtamembrane domain; KD, kinase domain; MD, mutation detection (variable methodologies); PCR, polymerase chain reaction; PM, point mutation; PTD, partial tandem duplication; RE-PCR, PCR with restriction enzyme digestion; RT-PCR, reverse transcription PCR.

***FLT3* Abnormalities.** FLT3 is a class III receptor tyrosine kinase and Ig receptor superfamily member that is expressed by hematopoietic progenitor cells and downregulated during differentiation. Once physiologically activated through FLT3 ligand binding, phosphorylation of regions in the juxtamembranous (JM) domain leads to growth induction and apoptosis inhibition via STAT5 and MAPK signaling. Two major types of abnormalities of the *FLT3* gene have been described: internal tandem duplication of the JM domain, and a missense mutation at Asp835.[235] Internal tandem duplication is more common, occurring in approximately 23% of all cases; the point mutation is seen in about 7% of cases. Thus, together they are seen in about 30% of all AMLs, making *FLT3* one of the most common identified genetic targets in AML. These mutations are even more common in AMLs with normal cytogenetics (occurring in up to 50%). Functionally, these lesions result in the constitutive activation of the tyrosine kinase domains via autophosphorylation, leading to a persistent on-signal in the transformed leukemic cell. Importantly, from a clinical perspective, this dysregulation of FLT3 has been shown by some to be the single most important prognosticator for overall survival in AML patients younger than 60 years, and this correlation with poor prognosis is independent of the powerfully prognostic karyotypic groups alluded to previously. The greater the amount of mutant FLT3 compared with wild type, the worse the prognosis; thus, it is important to measure the mutant–to–wild-type ratio. The tandem repeats are easily detected by standard fluorescent-labeled PCR (both DNA and RT) with capillary electrophoresis, and the point mutations are detected by systems such as conformational sensitive gel electrophoresis or restriction enzyme-based analysis. Capillary electrophoresis is best suited for detecting internal tandem duplications, whereas resistance to ECoRV digestion is useful for detecting the common missense mutation. As with most molecular lesions, mutations of *FLT3* provide a useful marker for MRD testing, although there are concerns about their stability in relapsed specimens.[236]

***NPM1* Mutations.** NPM1 (nucleophosmin) is a molecular chaperone that shuttles ribosomal proteins between the nucleus and the cytoplasm, with the *NPM1* gene sometimes affected by translocation in a subset of hematologic neoplasms (commonly in anaplastic lymphoma kinase–positive anaplastic large cell lymphoma; rarely in AML). More recently, insertion (typically 4–base pair) mutations affecting *NPM1* have been described, occurring quite commonly in all AMLs (about 35%) but even more frequently in those AMLs with normal cytogenetics (up to 60% of cases).[237-239] As a consequence of this mutation, the nucleolar localization signal is disrupted, and the protein accumulates in the cytoplasm (providing a potentially useful immunophenotypic surrogate). Functionally, this is believed to contribute to leukemogenesis by destabilizing the *p19/ARF* tumor suppressor.[240] The presence of these mutations is associated with increasing patient age, higher white cell counts, monocytic differentiation, CD34 and CD133 negativity, *FLT3* mutations, and an increased response to therapy and improved survival, particularly in those who lack *FLT3* mutations.

***CEBPA* Mutations.** The *CEBPA* gene encodes a transcription factor (CCAAT enhancer binding protein alpha) that plays a central role in granulocytic differentiation and has antiproliferative effects. Mutations are found in approximately 10% of AMLs and are dispersed throughout the gene, albeit with some clustering.[241] Most AMLs with *CEBPA* mutations have normal cytogenetics; are likely to be of the FAB M1, M2, or M4 subtype; and have a favorable outcome

***KIT* Mutations.** *KIT* encodes the class III receptor tyrosine kinase (CD117), which is the receptor for stem cell factor. Mutations affecting this gene are traditionally associated with mast cell neoplasms; however, more recently they have been described in AMLs as well, particularly those with *CBF* translocations t(8;21) and inv(16).[242] There are various sites of mutation, with *D816* mutations (the typical mutation in mast cell neoplasms) associated with t(8;21) and exon 8 mutations associated with inv(16). The former, in particular, portends an adverse outcome. There appear to be fairly consistent associations between the specific "second hit" (affecting proliferation) in the three prototypic, cytogenetically good-prognosis AMLs: *FLT3* mutations with t(15;17), *KIT* mutations with t(8;21), and *RAS* mutations with inv(16). The first two may have a negative prognostic impact, but the last appears to be neutral.[243]

Partial Tandem Duplication of *MLL*. Partial tandem duplication of the *MLL* gene is another example of a cryptic abnormality that appears to have biologic relevance.[244] Although there are usually cytogenetic pointers to the presence of *MLL* partial tandem duplication, in that approximately 90% of cases with trisomy 11 are associated with this abnormality, it is also present in about 10% of AMLs with normal cytogenetics. *MLL* partial tandem duplication is readily detected by RT-PCR by amplifying exons 2 to 6 or 2 to 8; it is prognostically important, being associated with an unfavorable outcome.

***WT1* Overexpression.** *WT1* has the somewhat perplexing ability to function as either a proto-oncogene or a tumor suppressor gene, with these divergent actions largely dictated by cellular milieu and protein interactions. The transcription of *WT1* is upregulated in acute leukemias, in which context it is presumed to act as a bona fide oncogene.[245] There are data indicating that higher levels of *WT1* expression are associated with an adverse prognosis, that expression increases at relapse, and that it is a good target for MRD testing.[246] Accordingly, molecular evaluation of *WT1* might have a number of potential applications.

***BAALC* Overexpression.** The brain and acute leukemia, cytoplasmic (*BAALC*) gene encodes a protein that is a marker of the mesodermal lineage, especially muscle, and is upregulated in $CD34^+$ hematopoietic precursors. Overexpression of *BAALC* is seen in the majority of AMLs, particularly those with a normal karyotype, and it appears to be an important adverse prognostic factor.[247]

Acute Lymphoblastic Leukemia

A major change in the 2008 WHO classification was the incorporation of a number of genetically defined ALLs (similar to AMLs in 2001). Some of the major types are detailed here. In addition to the study of these pathologic genetic abnormalities, the study of physiologic gene rearrangements (antigen receptor genes) is valuable in a number of contexts.

Immunoglobulin and T-Cell Receptor Gene Rearrangements

Although assays of antigen receptor gene rearrangements are usually not required for diagnostic purposes—because most cases of ALL can be assigned lineage using flow cytometry—the study of antigen receptor gene rearrangements has a role in monitoring MRD. In particular, the rate at which molecular remission is attained is one of the most prognostically relevant assays, especially in pediatric ALL.[248,249] Antigen receptor gene rearrangements in ALL may undergo changes over time, so a clonal rearrangement evident at diagnosis may no longer be evident at the time of disease recurrence. Accordingly, it is recommended that more than one antigen receptor gene rearrangement be used to track the disease. This is usually not a problem because many lymphoblastic leukemias contain "cross-lineage" or illegitimate rearrangements. For example, up to 70% of precursor B-cell ALLs harbor monoclonal TCR gene rearrangements. Another context in which such studies might be helpful is to resolve the clonal nature of increased numbers of precursor B cells in the bone marrow following chemotherapy for precursor B-cell ALL (physiologic hematogones versus pathologic blasts).[250]

Translocations

Unlike in AML, where specific translocations often confer a good prognosis, the opposite is generally (but not universally) observed in ALL. In AML, translocations generally result in in-frame fusion of transcription factors, and translocations that result in the increased expression of intact, structurally normal genes are unusual. In contrast, both types of translocation are seen in ALL. The increased expression of intact, structurally normal genes is often seen in the context of translocations that involve one of the antigen receptor genes (Ig and TCR genes), with the promoters or enhancers of these physiologically active genes driving the expression of the translocated proto-oncogene.

t(9;22)(q34;q11). In addition to being the hallmark of chronic myeloid leukemia (CML), this translocation is quite common in ALL. It is the most common translocation in adult ALL, occurring in approximately 25% of cases; it is seen almost exclusively in precursor B-cell ALL (as defined by CD10 expression), and quite often in the context of the coexpression of the myeloid antigens CD13 and CD33. It is also seen in approximately 5% of pediatric ALL cases. Importantly, this abnormality is associated with a uniformly poor prognosis, with some data suggesting that it is the most important predictor of poor long-term survival, despite intensified chemotherapy.[251] At a molecular level, the breakpoints in the *ABL1* gene are usually consistent in both CML and ALL—typically 5′ of *ABL1* exon 2, but occasionally 5′ of exon 3; they vary in the *BCR* gene (Fig. 6-19). To optimally detect the presence of a *BCR-ABL1* chimeric transcript in ALL, it is necessary to perform two separate RT-PCRs using two different upstream *BCR* primers—one complementary to exon 1 and the other to exon 13. Each reaction contains a single downstream *ABL1* primer, typically one complementary to exon 2 (or 3). In vivo, those breakpoints in the minor breakpoint cluster region yield a p190 fusion protein, whereas those in the major breakpoint cluster region yield a p210 fusion protein. This oncoprotein has heightened tyrosine kinase activity that is now cytoplasmic (as opposed to the usual nuclear localization of ABL1) and is key to the neoplastic transformation of the cells. Not unexpectedly, the p190 protein is more potent at transformation than is p210, and this correlates with the respective biologies of ALL and CML. Some data indicate that this might be true in ALL as well, with p190-positive ALL possibly having a more aggressive clinical course than p210-positive ALL.[252]

This is a crucial molecular fusion in terms of prognostication and therapeutic decision making. Conventional cytogenetic analysis underestimates the prevalence of this translocation, with RT-PCR detecting a *BCR-ABL1* fusion in up to 10% of ALL cases that are karyotypically normal.[253] Thus, it is reasonable to screen all adult precursor B-cell ALLs at the molecular level, particularly in the context of CD13 and CD33 coexpression. Given the advent of targeted therapy (imatinib mesylate [Gleevec]), there is even more reason to be certain that the molecular lesion is present at diagnosis.

It has recently been demonstrated that *BCR-ABL1*–positive ALLs, whether de novo cases or those evolving from CML, are frequently accompanied by deletions of *IKZF1*, which encodes the ikaros protein, a transcription factor that is central to early lymphoid development.[254]

t(12;21)(p13;q22). This is the most common translocation in pediatric ALL, particularly in children between 2 and 5 years of age, and it is generally (but not uniformly) associated with a favorable prognosis.[255] Typically, such patients have a relatively low leukocyte count ($<50 \times 10^9$/L), nonhyperdiploidy (DNA index = 1), and coexpression of myeloid antigens on precursor B lymphoblasts. Despite the relatively good outcome in such patients, they are potentially at increased risk for late relapse. Most important from a diagnostic perspective, the translocation cannot be identified by conventional karyotypic analysis, requiring molecular genetic studies (RT-PCR or FISH) for its documentation. It is thus a prototypic example of a cryptic translocation. This translocation results in an in-frame fusion of a portion of the *ETV6* (formerly *TEL*) gene on chromosome 12p13 with the *RUNX1* gene from chromosome 21q22. Typically, the breakpoint occurs in intron 5 of the *ETV6* gene and intron 1 of the *RUNX1* gene, with the chimera driven by the promoter of the *ETV6* gene. The translocation is present in 25% of pediatric but only 3% of adult B-lineage ALLs. In most cases of ALL with this translocation, the other *ETV6* allele is deleted, suggesting that the fusion may function in a recessive manner, requiring the loss of the normal *ETV6* allele. Interestingly, both the *ETV6* and *RUNX1* genes are quite promiscuous, in that both can be translocated to a variety of different partners in a number of different hematologic malignancies, including AML and MDS.

t(1;19)(q23;p13). The TCF3 (formerly E2A)-PBX1 chimeric oncoprotein is generated as a consequence of this translocation. Of note, this translocation is more often unbalanced (75% of cases) than balanced (25%), resulting in –19, der(19) t(1;19). Each partner gene is physiologically involved in transcription; *TCF3* encodes a number of basic helix-loop-helix transcription factors (including E12 and E47) that are crucial for B-cell development, whereas *PBX1* encodes a DNA-binding homeodomain protein that is not normally expressed in B cells. This genetic fusion is characteristically associated with a

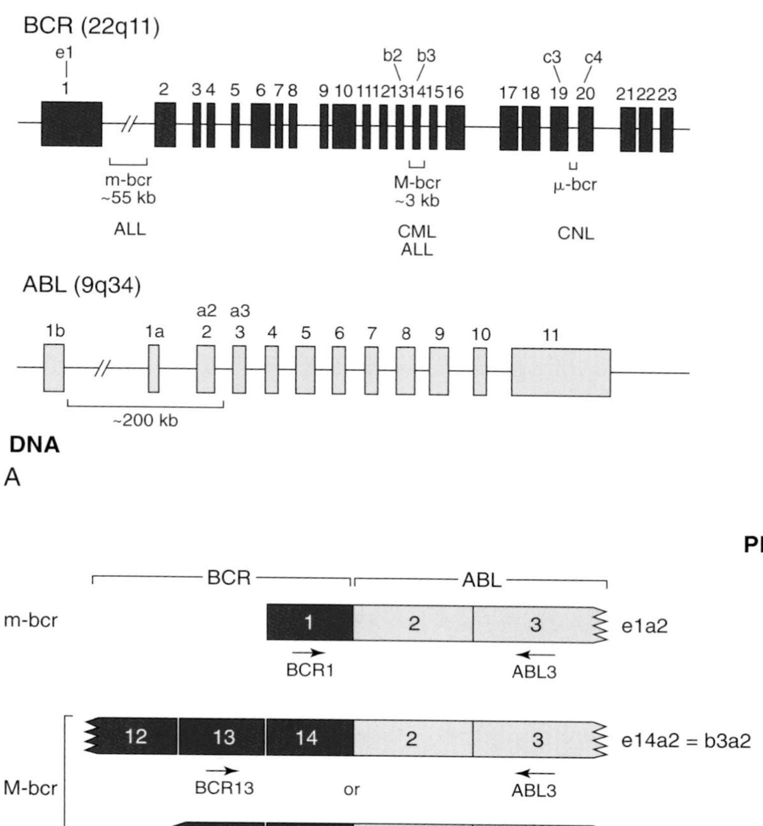

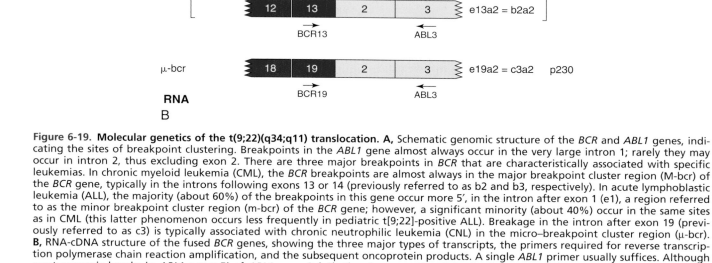

Figure 6-19. Molecular genetics of the t(9;22)(q34;q11) translocation. A, Schematic genomic structure of the *BCR* and *ABL1* genes, indicating the sites of breakpoint clustering. Breakpoints in the *ABL1* gene almost always occur in the very large intron 1; rarely they may occur in intron 2, thus excluding exon 2. There are three major breakpoints in *BCR* that are characteristically associated with specific leukemias. In chronic myeloid leukemia (CML), the *BCR* breakpoints are almost always in the major breakpoint cluster region (M-bcr) of the *BCR* gene, typically in the introns following exons 13 or 14 (previously referred to as b2 and b3, respectively). In acute lymphoblastic leukemia (ALL), the majority (about 60%) of the breakpoints in this gene occur more 5′, in the intron after exon 1 (e1), a region referred to as the minor breakpoint cluster region (m-bcr) of the *BCR* gene; however, a significant minority (about 40%) occur in the same sites as in CML (this latter phenomenon occurs less frequently in pediatric t[9;22]-positive ALL). Breakage in the intron after exon 19 (previously referred to as c3) is typically associated with chronic neutrophilic leukemia (CNL) in the micro–breakpoint cluster region (μ-bcr). **B,** RNA-cDNA structure of the fused *BCR* genes, showing the three major types of transcripts, the primers required for reverse transcription polymerase chain reaction amplification, and the subsequent oncoprotein products. A single *ABL1* primer usually suffices. Although most genomic breaks in *ABL1* occur 5′ of *ABL1* exon 2 (a2), thus incorporating it in the fusion transcript, an *ABL1-3* primer may be required to avoid missing the rare intron 2 breakpoint. The fusion transcripts illustrated, however, reflect the more common a2 breaks, as designated on the right side. Transcripts generated by the m-bcr breakpoint require a downstream *BCR1* (e1) primer. Either of the M-bcr breakpoints can be detected with a single *BCR13* (e13/b2) primer; if the break is after exon 14, the subsequent product will be 75 base pairs longer than if the breakpoint is after exon 13. Transcripts from the μ-bcr require a *BCR19* (e19/c2) primer. *BCR1* and *BCR13* primers are always required for routine diagnosis. A *BCR19* primer is not commonly used unless CNL is strongly suspected. Fusion transcripts generated from genomic breaks in the M-bcr might be detected with the *BCR1* primer, as a consequence of alternative splicing.

specific subtype of B-lineage ALL—namely, pre-B-ALL—that is immunophenotypically defined by the presence of cytoplasmic mu heavy chains and often by the absence of CD34. Pre-B-ALL is seen more commonly in pediatric than adult patients, and t(1;19) can be seen in approximately 20% of pre-B-ALL cases. By contrast, at least 90% of t(1;19)-positive ALLs have this pre-B-cell immunophenotype. The genomic breaks in these two genes are quite consistent, in that they almost invariably involve the same introns (between exons 13 and 14 of *TCF3*, and between exons 1 and 2 of *PBX1*). Accordingly, a simple RT-PCR assay, using a single pair of primers, is able to detect more than 90% of t(1;19)-positive cases. In some cases, a variant transcript with an additional 27 nucleotides, likely due to differential splicing, is seen.

This genetic lesion has traditionally been associated with an adverse prognosis. However, its recognition at the time of diagnosis, leading to the use of more intensive therapy, represents one of the triumphs of genetics-based diagnosis and risk-adapted therapy, and these patients no longer have an adverse outcome.[256] Importantly, a significant number of cases have uninformative cytogenetics,[257] once again underscoring the need for molecular genetic studies at the time of diagnosis.

t(4;11)(q11;q23). The t(4;11) translocation, fusing *MLL* and *AFF1*, is fairly common in both adult and pediatric ALL (about 5% of cases), but it is extremely common in infantile ALL, occurring in approximately 70% of cases. This translocation is particularly associated with the pro-B-cell (early precursor B cell) immunophenotypic profile (lacking CD10) and with the coexpression of myeloid antigens CD15 and CD65.

RT-PCR analyses for this translocation are relatively simple in design but can be complex in their interpretation. A single exon 8 *MLL* primer and a single exon 7 *AFF1* primer should suffice in detecting all known fusion transcripts. However, more than 10 different fusion transcripts can be generated by two mechanisms: differential breakpoints in different introns, and alternative splicing. Clinically, the presence of this fusion is associated with an adverse prognosis in both infants and adults. As has become thematic, there are also reports of this fusion being detected in situations in which conventional cytogenetic analysis was negative.[258]

Genetics of T-Cell Acute Lymphoblastic Leukemia

Precursor T-cell ALL is less common than B-cell ALL, accounting for approximately 15% to 25% of cases. Translocations in ALL typically result in the increased expression of intact, structurally normal genes more commonly in T-cell ALL than in B-cell ALL. The *TCRA@/TCRD@* locus is more often involved than the *TRB@* and *TRG@* loci. The more common genetic abnormalities associated with T-cell ALL are detailed in Table 6-6.[259] T-cell ALL is almost always an aggressive disease, and unlike B-cell ALL, the various genetic lesions apparently do not impart any significant prognostic information and are not routinely evaluated in the diagnostic context. Molecular genetic studies in such patients are appropriate primarily to discern a tumor-specific fingerprint—either a monoclonal *TCR@* gene rearrangement or a submicroscopic lesion that can be used for posttherapeutic monitoring.

More recently, a number of key discoveries have begun to shed light on the molecular pathogenesis of T-cell ALL and provide possible prognostic and therapeutic insights. Gene expression profiling has revealed at least three subsets, which can be delineated based on the overexpression of single genes previously shown to be involved in translocations. These are *LYL1*, *TLX1* (formerly *HOX11*), and *TAL1*, which are associated with distinct stages of thymocyte maturation—namely, double-negative, early cortical, and late cortical, respectively. The *LYL1* and *TAL1* profiles are associated with a bad prognosis, and the *TLX1* cases are associated with a better prognosis.[260,261] These expression profiles can occur independent of (known) translocation events. *NOTCH1*, which encodes a transmembrane receptor and is converted into a transcription factor upon ligation, is central to the development of T cells; although rarely involved in translocations, activating mutations have been described in greater than 50% of cases of T-cell ALL, and some may be amenable to targeted therapy with gamma-secretase inhibitors.[262,263] Finally, *ABL1* is dysregulated by the generation of *NUP214-ABL1* episomal amplifications in about 6% of T-cell ALLs, and this phenomenon may be associated with a response to target therapy with imatinib mesylate (Gleevec).[264]

Rationale for Performing Molecular Genetic Studies for Translocations

There are several situations in which molecular genetic studies can facilitate diagnosis and prognosis in ALL. Conventional

Table 6-6 Recurrent Genetic Abnormalities in T-Lineage Acute Lymphoblastic Leukemia

Genetic Lesion	Chromosomal Abnormality	Approximate Frequency (%)	Function of Dysregulated Protein
Mutation			
NOTCH1	9q34*	55	Aberrant transcription
Fusion†			
TAL1	1p32	10-25	bHLH transcription factor
TRA@/TRD@-TLX3	t(10;14)(q24;q11)	5-10	Homeobox
TRA@/TRD@-LMO2	t(11;14)(p13;q11)	5-10	LIM domain
TRA@/TRD@-TAL1	t(1;14)(p32;q11)	2	bHLH transcription factor
TRA@/TRD@-MYC	t(8;14)(q24;q11)	2	bHLH transcription factor
TRA@/TRD@-LMO1	t(11;14)(p15;q11)	1	LIM domain
TRB@-NOTCH1	t(7;9)(q34;q34)	1	Aberrant transcription
TRB@-TAL2	t(7;9)(q34;q32)	<1	bHLH transcription factor
TRA@/TRD@-TCL1‡	inv(14)(q11;q32)	<1	? Prosurvival pathway
Loss of Function (Deletion, Transcriptional Silencing)			
CDKN2A/CDKN2B	del(9)(p21)	>50	CDKI
Amplification			
NUP214-ABL1	Episomal	6	Increased tyrosine kinase activity

*This is a submicroscopic lesion and is not evident cytogenetically (see text for details).
†For translocations involving the T-cell receptor genes, these most commonly involve the *TRA@/TRD@* locus; however, variant translocations involving *TRB@* on 7q35 and *TRG@* on 7p15 may also occur.
‡This translocation is prototypically associated with T-cell PLL but may occur in T-cell acute lymphoblastic leukemia as well.
bHLH, basic helix loop helix; CDKI, cyclin-dependent kinase inhibitor; LIM, Lin11, Isl 1, Mec-3.

cytogenetic analysis may fail to detect a biologically and prognostically relevant translocation typified by t(12;21). Detection of clonal antigen receptor gene rearrangements that cannot be discerned cytogenetically may aid in diagnosis and classification. Molecular genetic studies may also provide a specific molecular fingerprint of the neoplastic clone that can be used to detect MRD. Other molecular lesions, unrelated to translocations, are also common, some of which can be discerned only by molecular genetic techniques.

Genetic Lesions Unrelated to Translocations

Alterations of Cyclin-Dependent Kinase Inhibitors. Inactivation of cyclin-dependent kinase inhibitors (CDKIs) appears to play an important role in ALLs. CDKIs regulate passage through the cell cycle, acting primarily at the G_1 phase of the cell cycle via the inhibition of cyclin-dependent kinases (CDKs). CDKIs may function as tumor-suppressor genes, and decreased expression has been implicated in neoplastic transformation.[265] There are two major CDKI families, based on their structure and targets, although there is some overlap with regard to the pathways they affect. One family contains the INK4 proteins (so named because their activity is somewhat specifically restricted to inhibiting CDK4 as well as CDK6), with members including $p16^{INK4a}$, $p15^{INK4b}$, $p18^{INK4c}$, and $p19^{INK4d}$. The other family, the CIP/KIP family, contains more broadly acting CDKIs, including $p21^{CIP1/WAF1}$, $p27^{KIP1}$, and $p57^{KIP2}$. Alterations of the former group of CDKIs have long been recognized in ALL, especially in T-cell ALL (>50%). In contrast to the mechanism of inactivation of tumor suppressor genes noted in other tumors via point mutation, they are usually inactivated by either deletion (in particular, del[9][p21]) or transcriptional silencing via hypermethylation of 5′ CpG islands. Southern blot analysis, real-time PCR, methylation-sensitive PCR, and RT-PCR can be employed to assess this phenomenon. However, the prognostic significance of these alterations is controversial

Microdeletion 1p32. The *TAL1* gene (formerly known as *SCL* or *TCL5*) at this locus was identified by cloning the relatively uncommon t(1;14)(p32;q11) translocation, which occurs in about 2% of T-cell ALL and in which *TAL1* is fused to the *TRA@* or *TRD@* gene. An intrachromosomal, submicroscopic fusion of *TAL1* with a gene termed *SIL* (for SCL interrupting locus), normally located about 90 kb upstream, is seen in up to 25% of T-cell ALLs, making this the most common known genetic fusion in T-cell ALL.[266] This fusion cannot be detected on conventional karyotypic studies and requires either Southern blot or PCR. A PCR assay using a single upstream *SIL* primer, together with three downstream *TAL1* primers, can detect most fusion transcripts. The fusion, which is mediated by illegitimate V(D)J rearrangement mechanisms, places *TAL1* under the transcriptional control of the *SIL* promoter. Although this event appears to lack prognostic relevance, it may be a useful marker for tracking MRD.

MYELOPROLIFERATIVE NEOPLASMS

Chronic Myelogenous Leukemia

Identification of the Philadelphia chromosome in 1960 heralded the era of cancer cytogenetics that culminated, more than 40 years later, in the use of rational, targeted therapy (imatinib mesylate) directed against the molecular consequences (chimeric BCR-ABL1 oncoprotein) of the associated t(9;22)(q34;q11) translocation. This drug inhibits the enhanced tyrosine kinase activity that arises as a consequence of this fusion. The exact mechanism through which this oncoprotein transforms cells is complex, in that multiple pathways are dysregulated. These include the JAK/STAT, RAS/RAF, JUN, MYC, and P13K/AKT pathways, which likely lead to a variety of biologic consequences such as increased proliferation, resistance to apoptosis, and adhesion defects.

CML is now essentially defined by the presence of a *BCR-ABL1* fusion that is usually, but not always, accompanied by the classic karyotypically determined translocation.[267] Even when the cytogenetic data are unequivocal, it is prudent to document the presence of the fusion mRNA transcript. This is important not only to indicate that the target of the planned therapy is present (if imatinib mesylate is to be used) but also to discern the molecular fingerprint that is likely to become most important for the subsequent tracking of MRD.

The breakpoints in the *BCR* gene in CML are quite homogeneous, mostly occurring after exon 13 or exon 14, in the major breakpoint cluster region of the gene (see Fig. 6-19). Thus, a simple RT-PCR assay using a single upstream *BCR* exon 13 (b2) primer and a single downstream *ABL1* exon 2 (a2) primer suffices for the molecular detection of this event in virtually all cases of CML. An exon 3 (a3) primer can also be used to avoid a false-negative result in the event of a rare intron 3 break. There appears to be no definitive clinical or biologic significance associated with the site of the major breakpoint cluster region breakpoint; however, due to alternative splicing, an intron 14 break may yield both e13 and e14 (equivalent to b2 and b3) transcripts. The e1a2 transcripts can be identified in the context of bona fide CML, unrelated to an e1 breakpoint; rather, this is a manifestation of alternative splicing and might have some clinical significance. There are reports of breakpoints other than those occurring in the regions noted here, and these can lead to alternative product sizes or false-negative molecular results; however, these are rare.

In addition to the value of RT-PCR testing at diagnosis, monitoring MRD is mandatory in most therapeutic contexts. Although stem cell transplantation (SCT) is the only therapeutic modality that can definitely cure CML, extensive data support the role of molecular genetic–based MRD testing in patients treated with imatinib mesylate, which has become the preferred first-line therapy. Based on current knowledge, the following key points emerge[268-270]: (1) there are two scenarios in which MRD testing is appropriate in CML—following SCT to allow the early detection of relapse, and following imatinib to gauge response; (2) there is usually a high concordance between peripheral blood and bone marrow testing, indicating that the less invasive former procedure may suffice for monitoring MRD; (3) a single qualitative (and probably also quantitative) positive RT-PCR result is not predictive of relapse in an individual patient; (4) most patients are qualitatively RT-PCR positive in the first 6 months after SCT, and this is not of consequence; (5) patients who are RT-PCR positive more than 6 months post-SCT are at high risk of relapse; (6) in a relapsing patient, RT-PCR positivity precedes cytogenetic and hematologic relapse by several months; (7) using quantitative RT-PCR, low or falling levels correlate with continued remission, whereas high or rising levels predict relapse; (8) molecular relapse can reasonably be defined as a 10-fold or greater increase in the expression of *BCR-ABL1*, determined by a minimum of three consecutive quantitative PCR analyses; (9) notwithstanding the different technologies and therapeutic contexts, it appears that the critical level above or below which outcome differs is about 0.02%, which is on the order of 10^{-4} and, interestingly, is similar to that for other targets in other leukemias and lymphomas; (10) in patients treated with imatinib, the attainment of a "major molecular response," defined as a 3-log or greater reduction in *BCR-ABL1* transcript level compared with the pretreatment level, after 12 months is highly predictive of sustained cytogenetic remission and improved survival; and (11) for patients treated with SCT, molecular testing should probably be performed once every 3 to 6 months initially, then annually thereafter, whereas patients treated with imatinib should be monitored at intervals not exceeding 3 months.

RT-PCR is not helpful in the detection of transformation to either accelerated or blast phase; conventional karyotypic analysis is more appropriate in the identification of clonal evolution. Molecular-only monitoring also misses the emergence of t(9;22)-negative clones, which have been reported in patients treated with imatinib.[271] Thus, it is important to appreciate the potential pitfalls of any molecular assay and to realize that other genetic studies (conventional cytogenetics, FISH, or newer technologies such as spectral karyotyping) may be required to complement one another.

Although the advent of imatinib has dramatically altered the therapeutic landscape of CML, resistance to this form of targeted therapy occurs in a subset of patients. The major mechanism for this resistance is the expansion of cells with *ABL1* point mutations.[272] More than 100 different mutations have been described; however, those occurring in the region encoding the P-loop of the molecule and *T315I* mutations are most often associated with imatinib resistance, requiring a change in therapy. In contrast, some mutations in other sites may benefit from dose escalation. A rise in BCR-ABL1 levels typically prompts screening for mutations, which can be performed using a variety of techniques.

Other Myeloproliferative Neoplasms

Unlike CML, which is essentially defined by a specific genetic lesion, other myeloproliferative neoplasms (MPNs) lacked such specific lesions until recently, and the *absence* of a *BCR-ABL1* fusion was used as a diagnostic criterion. The identification in 2005 of V617F mutations in the *JAK2* gene in large subsets of MPNs has provided an important diagnostic tool, in addition to helping to unravel the biology of these disorders.[273-275] JAK2 is a nonreceptor tyrosine kinase downstream of surface receptors (including those for some hematopoietic growth factors) and is involved in intracellular signaling following the binding of ligand (growth factor) to the receptor. The point mutation leads to activation in the absence of ligand. This mutation is seen in more than 90% of cases of polycythemia vera and in about 50% of cases of essential thrombocythemia and primary myelofibrosis. A number of mutation detection assays can be used to identify this key event.[276] A minor subset of polycythemia vera patients who lack the V617F mutation (which occurs in exon 14) have alternative exon 12 mutations. Similarly, minor subsets of primary myelofibrosis and essential thrombocythemia patients have mutations in the *MPL* gene, which encodes the thrombopoietic receptor. Before the discovery of *JAK2* mutations, the detection of PRV1 overexpression appeared to have diagnostic utility in the evaluation of the MPNs, especially polycythemia vera[234]; however, the value of this assay may now be diminished.

Chronic neutrophilic leukemia is an extremely rare MPN characterized by sustained mature neutrophilia, hepatosplenomegaly, and a high LAP score. Data indicate that some cases might be associated with the variant *BCR-ABL1* fusion in which the breakpoint in the breakpoint cluster region occurs following exon 19, yielding an e19/a2 fusion transcript, which results in a p230 oncoprotein (see Fig. 6-2). Others suggest that this is reflective of neutrophilic CML and that bona fide chronic neutrophilic leukemia is not associated with t(9;22).[277] The *FIP1L1-PDGFRA* fusion gene is generated by a cryptic interstitial chromosomal deletion, del(4)(q12q12), in about half of patients with another rare MPN, chronic eosinophilic leukemia, as well as in some patients with a diagnosis of systemic mast cell disease associated with eosinophilia; this abnormality is readily detected by RT-PCR or FISH.[278] The discovery of this fusion in cases diagnosed as systemic mast cell disease (protoypically associated with *CKIT* mutations) may result in these cases being redefined as chronic eosinophilic leukemia. There are additional hematologic malignancies associated with eosinophilia that are amenable to molecular diagnostic testing.[279] These include the 8p11 myeloproliferative disorders (associated with T-lymphoblastic lymphoma), in which the *FGFR1* gene is translocated to one of a number of different partners, and chronic myelomonocytic leukemia with eosinophilia, often associated with 5q33 translocations that affect the *PDGFRB* gene. When there is no neoplasm-associated molecular genetic defect, XCIP-based assays such as *HUMARA* may be of value in determining the presence of monoclonality (discussed earlier); this approach is not restricted to MPNs and is theoretically applicable to any female patient with an atypical cellular proliferation, including dendritic cell disorders such as Langerhans cell histiocytosis and MDS.

MYELODYSPLASTIC SYNDROMES

This heterogeneous group of hematologic malignancies is associated with a variety of well-recognized cytogenetic abnormalities. These abnormalities are found in approximately 50% of de novo cases but much more commonly (80%) in secondary cases, arising in the context of prior cytotoxic chemotherapy. In contrast to many of the cytogenetic abnormalities described in the other hematologic malignancies, there is a predominance of unbalanced, numerical chromosomal abnormalities in MDS.[280] This predilection toward the loss of genetic material is the hallmark of tumor suppressor genes and suggests that this is an important step in the neoplastic transformation of MDS cells either in a recessive fashion (akin to the Knudson two-hit model) or via haploinsufficiency. A list of candidate genes has been proposed, based on the commonly deleted chromosomal segments involved; however, other than the recent indication that *RPS14* is the targeted gene in 5q− syndrome,[281] nothing has been definitively established to date.[282,283] Thus, the role of molecular techniques in the diagnosis and prognosis of MDS is limited.

A variety of other genetic lesions not detectable by routine cytogenetics have been identified in MDS. Many of these are not specific for MDS, although they are both frequent and of prognostic relevance and thus may have a role in routine diagnostic testing. These include point mutations of the *RAS* (especially affecting *NRAS*) and *TP53* genes, each of which is significantly associated with a poor prognosis.[284,285] *RAS* mutations occur in 10% to 30% of MDS patients, but the timing of such events (early or late) is unclear. Mutations in the *NF1* (neurofibromin) gene, incriminated in neurofibromatosis, are also seen in a subset of patients, including about 30% of those with juvenile myelomonocytic leukemia, a disease with features of both MDS and MPN. Interestingly, inactivation of *NF1* leads to *RAS* activation, because NF1 has GTPase activity that dampens RAS signaling. A third component of the RAS signaling pathway, *PTPN11*, is often targeted in juvenile myelomonocytic leukemia. Thus, it appears that the RAS pathway may be deranged quite frequently in MDS and, in particular, in juvenile myelomonocytic leukemia.[286]

Although the cytogenetic lesions identified in MDS are largely numerical and unbalanced, some recurrent balanced translocations have been reported, including t(5;12)(q33;p12), t(11;16)(q23;p13), t(3;5)(q25;q34), and t(3;21)(q26;q22). Although these events are uncommon, they could potentially be exploited for molecular genetic testing by RT-PCR analysis, given the knowledge of which genes are fused. Other molecular genetic abnormalities have been described in MDS with variable frequency, such as transcriptional silencing via methylation of *CDKN2B* ($p15^{INK4b}$), mutation of the *FMS* gene that encodes the macrophage colony-stimulating factor (M-CSF) receptor, and the quite common (up to 80% in one series) mutations of the mitochondrial cytochrome-*c* oxidase gene in MDS patients.[287] Microarray analysis of expression profiles of MDS blasts suggests that the *DLK* gene may be a candidate that distinguishes MDS blasts from AML blasts.[288]

Another group of genetic lesions is related to the role of chemical agents in the pathogenesis of MDS, with polymorphism in certain detoxification enzymes associated with a predisposition toward the development of MDS. For example, glutathione *S*-transferase genotypes may be associated with a higher incidence of MDS, and individuals with genetic polymorphisms leading to both a high level of activity of the *CYP2E1* gene and low activity of the *NQO1* genes (involved in the detoxification of benzene) are at increased risk for the development of MDS following benzene exposure.

As in the MPNs, XCIP analysis has been used in the molecular genetic evaluation of MDS. Although this technology has been applied to the documentation of monoclonality, some issues exist. Specifically, the interpretation of XCIP studies in MDS patients may be confounded by age-related skewing, as discussed earlier.

In summary, although no consistent and specific molecular genetic abnormalities have been described in MDS, a panel of molecular genetic assays may play a role in the diagnosis of this group of diseases and can facilitate the diagnosis when classic morphologic and cytogenetic features are lacking. Such a panel might include assays for *RAS* mutations, cytochrome-*c* oxidase mutations, and XCIP analysis.

DNA MICROARRAY AND MOLECULAR DIAGNOSTICS

There is a growing realization that molecular diagnostics should not be limited to providing an accurate diagnosis or serving as an assay for an abnormal parameter to aid in diagnosis. Ideally, molecular diagnostics should provide additional information that is useful in treatment decisions and in prognostication. With the development of genome-scale investigations, the pace of discovery is markedly accelerated, and the goal of defining and eventually measuring the key molecular mechanisms that determine the behavior of a tumor may be achieved in the not too distant future. One major research thrust in this direction is the gene expression profiling of large series of hematologic malignancies, most commonly by using DNA microarray technology.

A DNA microarray is, in principle, a reverse Northern blot, with thousands of DNA probes immobilized on a nonporous solid support.[289,290] The sample to be studied is then labeled and hybridized to the array, and the concentration of mRNA species corresponding to each of the immobilized probes is determined. A profile of gene expression, as specified by the composition of the microarray, is thus obtained. There are two major platforms of DNA microarray. In cDNA microarrays, cDNA clones are spotted on a solid support, usually a glass slide,[291,292] whereas in oligonucleotide arrays, oligonucleotides are spotted or synthesized in situ on the solid matrix.[293,294]

Because an enormous number of measurements are taken in each experiment, data management and analysis are crucial components of these assays.[295-297] Data management starts with the construction of the microarray, including the database of the genes on the array and their thorough annotation. The construction of the microarray must be carefully controlled to ensure good spot quality and uniformity. Many of these issues have been discussed in detail elsewhere.[291,292] In prefabricated arrays, many of the informatics and technical issues should have been addressed by the manufacturer. Image processing after hybridization includes algorithms for measuring fluorescence from each of the spots, background subtraction, and data normalization. However, the main challenge is interpretation of the data.

Several major constraints in the evaluation of clinical samples can significantly impact data analysis in microarray studies. Samples may not be collected and processed in a uniform fashion, and this variability can introduce variations in gene expression patterns that are unrelated to real biologic differences. Although thousands of parameters are measured in each sample, the number of samples studied is often in the range of tens to low hundreds, making statistical analysis challenging. Furthermore, in most instances, samples are being assayed only once because of limited materials or cost constraints. This decreases the statistical confidence of the measurements obtained. Validation of data accuracy, analysis, and conclusions drawn is essential in microarray studies. Obviously it is not possible to validate each measurement obtained, but for the expression of selected genes or pathways that appear to be important based on data analysis, the accuracy of the microarray data can be verified by independent assays such as RT-PCR or expression of the corresponding protein. Many analytical tools have been designed and employed in microarray data analysis.[296] Data can be examined using different tools and statistical manipulations to test the robustness of the derived conclusions. One way of validating the conclusions is to perform the analysis first on one set of cases (the test set) and then repeat the analysis on a separate set of cases (the validation set) to see whether the conclusions are confirmed. Variations of this approach include leaving out cross-validation.[298] Finally, the conclusions can be examined for correlations with clinical, pathologic, genetic, and independent biologic observations.

Many microarray studies on lymphomas and leukemias have been reported, and they have demonstrated that many of the entities in the current classification scheme have distinct gene expression profiles (class prediction).[5,299] There is also evidence that gene expression profiling can discover new entities (class discovery) that appear to have distinct biologic and clinical characteristics. Thus, DLBCL can be divided into at least two distinct subtypes, with one showing the gene expression signature of germinal center B cells and the other the expression signature of activated blood B lymphocytes.[300,301] In addition, primary mediastinal B-cell lymphoma has a gene expression profile that is distinct from the aforementioned subtypes, indicating that it is indeed a unique entity.[302,303] Interestingly, the gene expression profile of primary mediastinal B-cell lymphoma bears significant similarity to Hodgkin's lymphoma, suggesting some shared biologic characteristics. In MCL there appear to be uncommon cyclin D1–negative cases that share the gene expression profile of typical cases.[304] The spectrum of MCL may thus be expanded to include these unusual cases that have been difficult to classify.[305] The study of peripheral T-cell lymphoma and natural killer cell lymphoma has lagged behind that of their B-cell counterparts because they are uncommon and it is difficult to obtain a sufficient number of cases for analysis. Nevertheless, a number of studies have been performed,[306-313] and one of the most interesting findings is the possible derivation of angioimmunoblastic lymphoma from T-follicular helper cells.[310,312] Studies of ALL and AML have demonstrated that gene expression profiling can accurately predict cytogenetic subgroups.[314,315] Novel subgroups have also been defined,[315-317] and interestingly, gene expression profile signatures associated with unique genetic abnormalites may allow the identification of related cases without the characteristic abnormalities.[318]

Measuring the expression of certain genes or groups of genes in DLBCL, MCL, and follicular lymphoma has prognostic value independent of the International Prognostic Index.[6,300,302,315,319] Attempts have also been made to find predictors of response to specific therapies, such as rituximab in follicular lymphoma[320] and the addition of rituximab to the treatment of DLBCL.[321] In acute leukemias, cytogenetic subgroups, some unique mutations (e.g., *FLT3*, *CEBPA*), and abnormal expression of specific transcripts (*HOX11*, *TAL1*, *LMO2*) are powerful predictors of prognosis. Additional independent predictors of prognosis or response to treatment have been sought.[316,322,323] These studies need to be validated in the future by large, well-defined patient groups. In chronic lymphocytic leukemia, gene expression profiling has identified a set of genes that can predict the Ig mutational status of the tumor cells.[324,325] One of these genes, *ZAP-70*, is an excellent discriminator of the two prognostic subtypes of chronic lymphocytic leukemia, and measurement of the expressed protein is being incorporated into clinical practice.[326,327] Some of the genes that show highly significant differential expression between entities with distinct gene expression profiles are not yet characterized expression sequence tags, which could be fruitful targets for future study (gene discovery).[328] A number of genes represented by these expression sequence tags have been cloned and studied in more detail both biologically and in the clinical setting.[329-332] Other global investigations such as micro-RNA profiling,[333,334] array comparative genomic hybridization,[335-339] methylation studies,[340] and mutation analysis[341-343] are being pursued, and all this information can be integrated to achieve a better understanding of the pathogenesis and evolution of hematologic malignancies.

In conclusion, early studies using microarrays have been promising, and it is anticipated that gene expression profiling and other genome-wide studies will provide information that will have enormous impacts on molecular diagnostics. It is uncertain how this information will be used in the clinical setting. Useful information from gene expression profiling can be condensed and represented by a much smaller number of transcripts than the probe sets on the microarrays used for discovery. A diagnostic array with several hundred probes may be adequate for hematologic malignancies. Alternative platforms using quantitative RT-PCR[344] or immunohistochemistry[345] may also be developed, especially if we want to apply the knowledge gained to the study of paraffin-embedded materials. It is also not clear whether a single diagnostic platform can be designed that incorporates important findings from multiple sources (e.g., gene expression profiling, array comparative genomic hybridization, methylation, mutation) or whether several assays will have to be used to capture all relevant information. However, it is likely that some form of diagnostic assay for hematologic malignancies based on these global analyses will emerge in the next few years to provide additional relevant molecular information for clinical use.[346]

Pearls and Pitfalls

- Molecular testing has significantly enhanced our ability to make rational and specific hematopathologic diagnoses and has identified numerous nascent biologically and therapeutically relevant subtypes.
- Essentially no molecular test is 100% sensitive or specific, and it is crucial to be aware of the limitations of each assay including false-positives and false-negatives.
- Clonality testing for antigen receptor gene rearrangements is fraught with caveats; for example, it is essential to perform such assays in duplicate to exclude the possibility of pseudoclonality due to the paucity of lymphocytes in small biopsies.
- A subset of cytogenetically defined entities (e.g., CML, subtypes of AML and ALL) is missed by conventional cytogenetics, which highlights the need for judicious molecular testing when such entities are suspected.

References can be found on Expert Consult @ www.expertconsult.com

Chapter 7

Cytogenetic Analysis and Related Techniques in Hematopathology

Gouri Nanjangud, Nallasivam Palanisamy, Jane Houldsworth, and R. S. K. Chaganti

CHAPTER OUTLINE

Cytogenetic analysis of leukemias and lymphomas has been instrumental in identifying recurring translocations and establishing the principle that translocations cause deregulation of genes at the breakpoints, leading to aberrant cell function and initiation of neoplastic proliferation. They have also shown, especially in acute leukemias, that certain chromosome changes are associated with favorable outcomes and others with unfavorable outcomes, thereby enabling therapeutic decisions based on the results of chromosome analysis. In contrast to leukemias, detailed cytogenetic information on non-Hodgkin's lymphomas (NHLs) was unavailable until recently.

Genetic analysis is a powerful approach to resolve the biologic complexity of tumors and gain insights into their clinical behavior. This approach involves conventional cytogenetic analysis by G-banding and molecular cytogenetic analysis by methods such as fluorescence in situ hybridization (FISH), spectral karyotyping (SKY), multicolor FISH (M-FISH), and comparative genomic hybridization (CGH) with both low and high resolving power (chromosomal CGH and array CGH). With this combination of conventional and molecular-based methods of cytogenetic analysis, an array of novel recurring chromosome abnormalities has been identified, and the application of cytogenetic analysis has been expanded in both clinical and basic research.

CONVENTIONAL CYTOGENETIC METHODS

Since Tjio and Levan[1] and Ford and Hamerton[2] discovered in 1956 that the human chromosomal complement comprises 46 chromosomes (22 pairs of autosomes and the X and Y sex chromosomes), the development of human cytogenetics has been one of continuous discovery and impressive advances in methodology. The first of these was the observation by Hsu[3] that hyposmotic treatment swells cells and leads to the dispersion of chromatin and chromosomes. Hyposmotic treatment, in combination with the metaphase-arresting drug colchicine, scatters chromosomes, thereby enabling their counting and identification.[3] Shortly thereafter, Nowell and Hungerford[4] discovered that treatment of peripheral blood lymphocytes with phytohemagglutinin stimulates them to undergo mitosis, thus providing a ready source of dividing cells for chromosome analysis. These initial discoveries led to the early demonstration that constitutional chromosome abnormalities contribute significantly to the causes of infertility, reproductive loss, birth defects, and mental retardation. The first successful application of cytogenetics to neoplastic disease was the discovery by Nowell and Hungerford[4] that in chronic myeloid leukemia (CML) one of the small acrocentric (G-group) chromosomes is replaced by a much smaller acrocentric chromosome that appeared to be diagnostic of this disorder and was termed the Philadelphia (Ph) chromosome. During the 1970s special stains or chemical treatments were used to reveal structural variation along the length of the chromosome to aid in the identification of individual chromosomes and their regions. This effort led to the development of several so-called banding methods that provided the basis for detailed subregional mapping of the human chromosome complement as well as the development of a system of nomenclature for the description of normal and abnormal chromosome complements. The International System for Human Chromosome Nomenclature is updated from time to time based on new information and continues to be the currently accepted standard for chromosome description.[5] The development of banding techniques also had a significant effect on efforts under way to unravel the molecular organization of chromatin and chromosomes.

The main banding techniques are those that produce the so-called quinacrine (Q), Giemsa (G), centromeric (C), and reverse (R) banding methods. In Q-banding, the chromosomes on a metaphase preparation, stained with quinacrine dihydrochloride, exhibit brighter fluorescence of A-T–rich regions compared with G-C–rich regions. This pattern of bright and dull fluorescence is consistent and yields a reproducible banding pattern.[6] Q-banding is the most efficient and economic method to identify the Y chromosome in both metaphase and interphase nuclei. In G-banding, the chromosome preparation is subjected to treatment with sodium salt citrate at a warm temperature or to a mild, brief treatment with an enzyme such as trypsin, followed by staining with a weak solution of Giemsa. This procedure also leads to linear differentiation of the chromosome into darkly stained and lightly stained regions, or bands, that correspond to the brightly fluorescent and dully fluorescent regions revealed by Q-banding.[6,7] Currently, G-banding is the method of choice for most cytogenetic analysis (Fig. 7-1).

R-banding is produced by incubation of the chromosome preparation in very hot phosphate buffer, followed by staining with Giemsa.[8] R-banding yields a banding pattern that is the reverse of G-banding; thus, bands staining dark with G-banding stain light with R-banding, and vice versa. R-banding is useful for identifying deletions or translocations that involve the telomeric regions of chromosomes and the late-replicating, inactive X chromosome. C-banding involves treating the chromosomes on a metaphase preparation with a weak solution of alkali, such as barium hydroxide, for a few seconds, followed by staining with Giemsa as in the case of G-banding.[9] C-banding suppresses staining all along the chromosome except at the centromeric heterochromatin regions. C-banding was instrumental in discovering constitutional polymorphisms in the heterochromatin segments around the centromeric regions of human chromosomes.[10] C-banding can also be applied to polymorphism analysis of donor and recipient cells to evaluate the outcome of bone marrow transplantation, but it is limited to metaphase chromosomes only.

Together, these banding techniques are collectively referred to as conventional cytogenetics or banding methods. These techniques have been responsible for delineating a large number of dysmorphic syndromes and are routinely used in the pre- and postnatal diagnosis of birth defects and infertility.

Rowley[11] made the discovery, using Q-banding, that the Ph chromosome is the result of a reciprocal translocation between chromosomes 9 and 22, with breaks at 9q34 and 22q11. Since then, more than 31,000 hematopoietic tumors have been karyotyped, and several recurring chromosome abnormalities have been identified, including approximately 360 reciprocal translocations.[12] In leukemias, many of the recurring chromosome abnormalities are associated with characteristic morphologic and clinical features, and their detection has become essential for accurate diagnosis and classification. These aberrations and their molecular counterparts were included in the World Health Organization (WHO) classification of hematologic malignancies and, together with morphology, immunophenotype, and clinical features, are used to define distinct clinical entities with unique patterns of responses to treatment.[13] In lymphomas, the recurring abnormalities are associated mainly with histologic subsets and are useful in the differential diagnosis. Owing to the complexity of the disease and the karyotype, only a few recurring abnormalities have been found to be clinically relevant.[14] Given the importance of cytogenetic analysis, efforts are constantly being made to obtain good chromosome preparations. Table 7-1 provides an overview of specimen requirements and culture techniques routinely used in the analysis of hematologic malignancies. Additional technical details can be obtained from *The AGT Cytogenetics Laboratory Manual,*[15] which is the standard reference.

Although conventional cytogenetic analysis is a powerful tool for characterizing tumor karyotypes, it has some

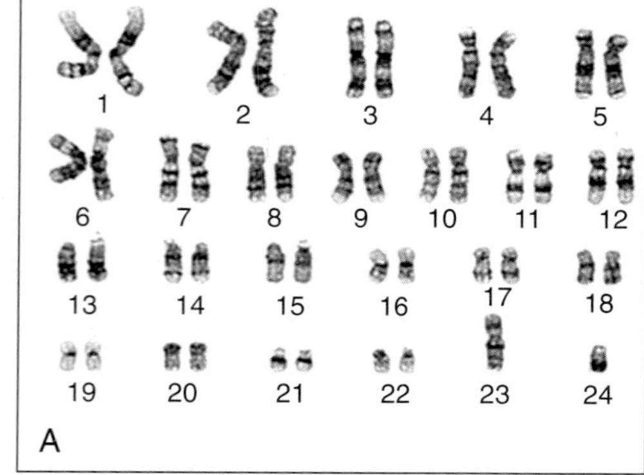

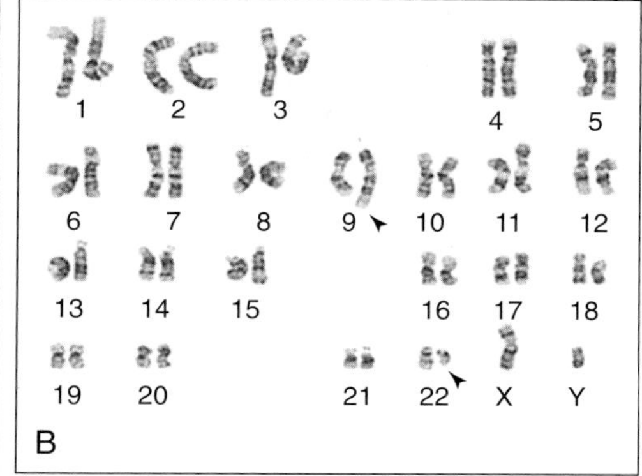

Figure 7-1. G-banded karyotype. A, G-banded karyotype of a normal male (46, XY). **B,** G-banded karyotype showing 46, XY, t(9;22)(q34;q11) (*arrowheads*).

Table 7-1 Specimen and Culture Techniques Routinely Used in Hematologic Malignancies

Technique	Malignancy	Comments
Specimen*		
Bone marrow (0.5-2 mL)	Myeloid neoplasms, precursor lymphoid neoplasms, some chronic myeloproliferative neoplasms	Cell density is critical (optimal cell density: $10^{5\text{-}6}$cells/mL) Hypercellularity is common in B- and T-cell ALL and CML
Peripheral blood (1-5 mL)	Chronic lymphoproliferative disorders	>25% blasts must be present when used in B- and T-cell ALL
Lymphoid tissue (at least 1 cm^3)	Most mature B- and T-cell lymphoid neoplasms	Cultures must be set up on the same day; surrounding nonlymphoid tissue and fat must be removed before culture
Culture Methods[†]		
Direct (1-6 hr)	Precursor B- and T-cell ALL, neoplasms with high mitotic index	Not suitable for AML
Overnight colcemid[‡]	Most neoplasms	Can produce short chromosomes
Short-term culture (18-24 hr)		
Unsynchronized	Most neoplasms	
Synchronized	Most neoplasms; used when a higher banding resolution[§] is required or when the mitotic index is low	
Mitogen-stimulated cultures (3 days)	B- or T-cell chronic lymphoproliferative disorders; check constitutional karyotype	Most B-cell mitogens also stimulate T cells, and vice versa; can stimulate normal cells to divide

*EDTA is not a suitable anticoagulant for cytogenetic studies and should be avoided.
[†]Multiple cultures should be set up to maximize the chance of obtaining abnormal metaphases.
[‡]Colcemid is a mitotic inhibitor and arrests the cells at metaphase.
[§]The typical resolution in the haploid set of 23 chromosomes is about 400 bands. Dividing cells are synchronized with amethopterin or fluorodeoxyuridine and arrested in prometaphase or prophase to obtain a banding resolution of about 550 or 800 bands, respectively.
ALL, acute lymphoblastic leukemia; AML, acute myeloid leukemia; CML, chronic myeloid leukemia.

limitations. Karyotype analysis can be performed only on dividing cells. In many hematologic malignancies, particularly lymphomas, the mitotic index is often low and the quality of metaphases is poor. In addition, the karyotypes of many advanced lymphoid tumors are highly complex and cannot be completely resolved by conventional cytogenetic analysis. Another critical limitation of conventional cytogenetic analysis is its inability to distinguish molecularly distinct rearrangements that appear to be cytogenetically identical. For example, the t(14;18)(q32;q21) translocation is observed in both follicular lymphoma and extranodal marginal zone B-cell lymphoma of the mucosa-associated lymphoid tissue (MALT) type, but the genes at 18q21 deregulated by the translocation are different. The fusion product in follicular lymphoma is *IGH-BCL2,* whereas in extranodal marginal zone B-cell lymphoma of the MALT type it is *IGH-MALT1*. It is important to distinguish between the two translocations because each is associated with a distinct histologic subtype.

MOLECULAR CYTOGENETIC METHODS

The limitations of cytogenetic analysis led investigators to seek alternative molecular methods that would enable the analysis of nondividing cells as well as offer better resolution. FISH was the first such molecular method developed, and several others followed rapidly.[16,17] All molecular methods are based on the principle of in situ hybridization, in which single-stranded complementary sequences of DNA or RNA (probe) are hybridized to target DNA or RNA under appropriate conditions to form stable hybrid complexes. These complexes are then visualized by a direct or indirect detection system in morphologically preserved chromosomes, cells, or tissues or in high-resolution adaptations to microarrays containing thousands of arrayed spots of DNA of known genomic localization and representative of the genome complement.

The sensitivity, specificity, and resolution of the technique depend on the length of the probe, method of labeling, accessibility of target DNA, and stringency of posthybridization washing. The three most widely used molecular cytogenetic methods in the study of hematologic malignancies are FISH, SKY or M-FISH, and CGH (chromosomal and array). The applications, advantages, and disadvantages of these three methods in comparison to conventional G-banding are summarized in Table 7-2.

Fluorescence in Situ Hybridization

In FISH, fluorescently labeled DNA probes are hybridized to metaphase spreads or interphase nuclei. FISH is usually performed on samples prepared for standard cytogenetic analysis but can also be applied to a wide range of cellular preparations such as G-banded slides, air-dried bone marrow or blood smears, fresh tumor touch prints, frozen or paraffin-embedded tissue sections, or nuclear isolates from fresh or fixed tissues. FISH can also be combined with immunophenotyping, which is particularly useful in identifying the cell lineage of a cytogenetically aberrant neoplastic clone. A variety of FISH probes, each targeting a specific region or the entire chromosome, are available. Probes routinely used in the analysis of hematologic malignancies include chromosome-specific centromeric probes, gene- or locus-specific probes, whole chromosome painting probes, arm-specific sequence probes, and telomeric probes.

Chromosome-specific centromeric probes are derived from the highly repetitive alpha-satellite DNA sequences located within the centromeres. Because the target size is several hundred kilobases in length, the probes exhibit bright,

Table 7-2 Comparison of Conventional and Molecular Cytogenetic Techniques

Feature	G-Banding	SKY/M-FISH	FISH	CGH
Resolution	>5 Mb	>2 Mb	0.5 kb	3-10 Mb
Identification				
Balanced translocations	Yes	Yes	Yes	No
Unbalanced translocations	Sometimes	Yes	Yes	No
Structural rearrangements within a single chromosome	Sometimes	No	Yes*	No
Origin of marker chromosome	No	Yes	No	No
Copy number changes†	Yes	Yes	Yes	Yes
Deletions <10 Mbp	No	No	Yes	No
Allelic loss	No	No	Yes	No
High-level amplification	Sometimes‡	Sometimes‡	Yes	Yes
Subtelomeric rearrangements	No	No	Yes	No
Resolves complex and cryptic chromosomal alterations	No	Yes	Yes	No
Requires specifically labeled probes	No	Yes	Yes	Yes
Requires prior knowledge of DNA sequences of the aberration	—	No	Yes	No
Scans the entire genome	Yes	Yes	No	Yes
Identifies tumor heterogeneity	Yes	Yes	No	No
Requires viable cells	Yes	Yes	No	No
Requires tumor metaphase spreads	Yes	Yes	No	No
Applicable to interphase nuclei and nondividing cells	No	No	Yes	No
Applicable to DNA extracted from archived tissue	No	No	No	Yes
Labor intensive	Yes	Yes	No	No
Interpretation highly dependent on experience and knowledge	Yes	Yes	Yes	Yes
Expensive for small diagnostic laboratories	No	Yes	No	Yes
Applicable and cost-effective as a routine screening method	Yes	No	Yes	No
Turnaround time (days)	3-10	2-7	2-7	5-7

*Only with appropriately designed probes.
†None of the methods can detect uniparental disomy.
‡When present in the form of a homogeneous staining region.
CGH, comparative genomic hybridization; FISH, fluorescence in situ hybridization; M-FISH, multicolor FISH; SKY, spectral karyotyping.

discrete signals and are easy to evaluate in both metaphase and interphase nuclei of various tissue preparations. Centromeric probes are useful in identifying numerical abnormalities (aneuploidy), dicentric chromosomes, and the origin of marker chromosomes. Currently, centromeric probes are available for all chromosomes except chromosomes 13, 14, 21, and 22. Sequence similarities in the pericentromere region between chromosomes 13 and 21 and between chromosomes 14 and 22 preclude their unique identification. Clinically important aberrations such as +12 in chronic lymphocytic leukemia (CLL), −7 in acute myeloid leukemia (AML), and high hyperploidy in acute lymphoblastic leukemia (ALL)—all of which are detected at a lower incidence by conventional cytogenetics owing to low mitotic index or poor morphology —are now routinely evaluated by FISH in many clinical laboratories. Another common example is the use of differentially labeled probes specific for chromosomes X and Y in monitoring engraftment in sex-mismatched allogeneic bone marrow transplants.

Gene- or locus-specific probes are derived from unique DNA sequences or loci within the chromosome. Using banding techniques on highly extended chromosomes, the smallest detectable chromosome abnormality is 2000 to 3000 kb; in contrast, gene- or locus-specific probes can detect regions as small as 0.5 kb.[17] As such, these probes have wide application in both basic and clinical research. Gene or locus probes have proved to be extremely useful in gene mapping and in defining structural rearrangements, chromosomal amplification, and origin of marker chromosomes in both metaphase chromosomes and interphase nuclei. Rearrangements in leukemias and lymphomas are often multiple or complex; hence, the strategy employed for their detection is critical and has evolved over the years from the conventional dual-color fusion signal methods to multicolor signal detection systems. In one approach, two sets of probes are derived from regions outside the involved gene (including all the breakpoints) on each of the translocating chromosomes and labeled with either one color, to yield a dual-color dual-fusion signal, or two colors, to yield a four-color signal in nuclei with the translocation; the latter is called F-FISH.[18] Dual-color dual-fusion and F-FISH analysis of the Ph chromosome translocation using these new approaches is illustrated in Figure 7-2, which demonstrates the ease and precision with which variant translocations, region-specific deletions, and amplifications can be identified in a single hybridization. Such probes are thus highly efficient and economical. Another variation of this approach is the use of one probe set to detect two translocations that involve both homologues of one chromosome common to the two translocations, such as chromosome 14 in B-cell lymphomas. Thus, as shown in Figure 7-3, the same probe set can detect two different translocations in the same or different nuclei. In addition to being economical, these probes are valuable in assaying for translocation combinations in given tumors, such as t(14;18)(q32;q21) and t(8;14)(q24;q32) or t(14;18)(q32;q21) and t(11;14)(q13;q32). Such combinations are helpful in establishing a correct diagnosis or predicting the clinical outcome. In lymphoid malignancies, locus- or gene-specific probes have also been effective

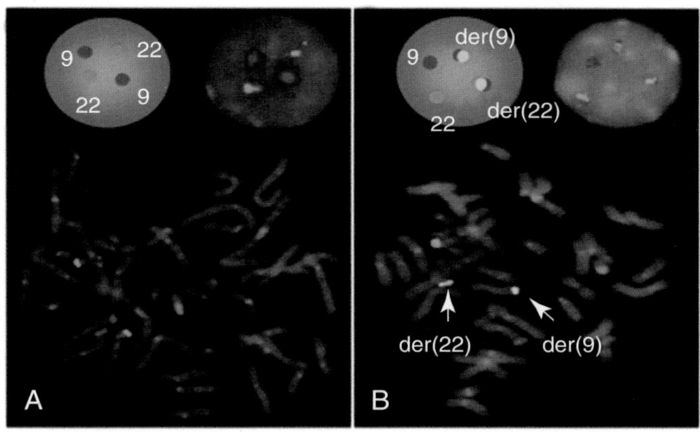

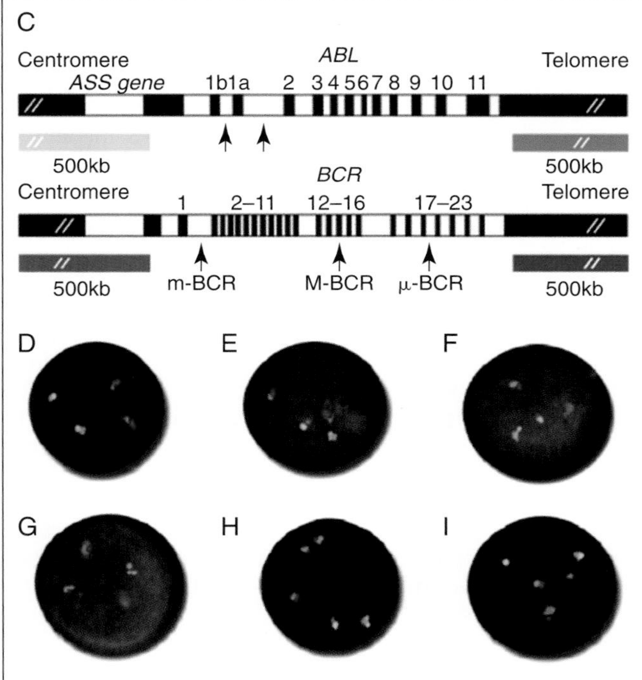

Figure 7-2. Fluorescence in situ hybridization (FISH) analysis of t(9;22)(q34;q11) with BCR/ABL probes. A, *Top,* Schematic representation and an interphase nucleus showing the normal signal patterns for chromosomes 9 (red) and 22 (green). *Bottom,* Normal metaphase showing the red and green signals on chromosomes 9 and 22. **B,** *Top,* Schematic representation and an interphase nucleus showing the dual-fusion signal pattern of the t(9;22)(q34;q22) translocation—one red, one green, and two fusion signals. *Bottom,* Metaphase with t(9;22)(q34;q22) showing appropriate signals. The fusion signals on der(9) and der(22) are indicated by *arrows.* **C,** Illustration of the F-FISH method. Schematic diagram of the genomic organization of *ABL* and *BCR* genes, with *arrows* indicating the breakpoint regions. The yellow, green, red, and blue bars indicate the positions of probes labeled with ULS-Dy-630, ULS-dGreen, ULS-Rhodamine, and ULS-DEAC, respectively. Probes cover a region of 500 kilobase pairs (kbp) on either side of the *ABL* and *BCR* gene without overlapping the breakpoints. **D,** Normal interphase with two yellow-green (*ABL*) and two red-blue (*BCR*) signals, **E,** Tumor interphase nucleus with one yellow-green (*ABL*), one red-blue (*BCR*), one yellow-blue (der[9], *ABL/BCR*), and one red-green (der[22], *BCR/ABL*) signal. **F,** Interphase nucleus with deletion of the BCR region on der(9). **G,** Interphase nucleus with deletion of ABL on der(9). **H,** Interphase nucleus with two Ph chromosomes. **I,** Interphase nucleus with a variant translocation. (Courtesy of Cancer Genetics Inc., Milford, MA.)

in delineating minimal regions of deletion on chromosomes 6q,[19] 11q,[20] and 13q[21] and in demonstrating monoallelic losses of *RB1* and *TP53* genes.

Whole chromosome painting probes or arm-specific sequence probes use mixtures of fluorescently labeled DNA sequences derived from the entire length or arm of the specific chromosome, usually obtained by flow-sorting of individual chromosomes, followed by DNA amplification by polymerase chain reaction and fluorescent labeling.[16,22] They are helpful in characterizing complex rearrangements and marker chromosomes. Cryptic rearrangements affecting terminal regions may remain undetected, however, owing to suppression of the repetitive DNA sequences within these regions. The application of chromosome painting probes is limited to metaphase analysis because the signals are often large and diffuse in interphase. Chromosome-specific telomeric or subtelomeric probes are derived from DNA sequences located at or adjacent to the telomeres and are effective in detecting terminal, interstitial, and cryptic translocations that are below the resolution of conventional cytogenetics or are undetected by whole chromosome painting probes.

By using a combination of these probes, virtually every karyotype can be comprehensively characterized. Probe sets are now available commercially for the detection of most rearrangements associated with specific subtypes of leukemia or lymphoma and are routinely used in cytogenetic laboratories to establish a diagnosis, select and monitor the effects of therapy, and detect minimal residual disease (Table 7-3). Although the probe sets can be easily applied to and analyzed on cytogenetic or other preparations, paraffin-embedded sections can be difficult to work with and require additional standardization techniques. Loss of signal due to low hybridization efficiency and high nonspecific background autofluorescence can lead to atypical signal patterns, making signal interpretation difficult. Nevertheless, probe sets for the detection of t(14;18)(q32;q21), t(11;14)(q11;q32), t(11;18)(q21;q21), t(3q27), t(11q13), and *TP53* deletion have been used successfully in paraffin and frozen sections or nuclei isolated from them and other cytologic preparations.

Spectral Karyotyping and Multicolor Fluorescence in Situ Hybridization

SKY and M-FISH enable the simultaneous visualization of all 24 human chromosomes, each in a different color, at the same time. Flow-sorted chromosomes are labeled with one to five fluorochromes to create a unique color for each chromosome pair. In SKY, image acquisition is based on a combination of epifluorescence microscopy, charge-coupled device imaging, and Fourier spectroscopy.[23] In M-FISH, separate images are captured for each of five fluorochromes using narrow band-pass microscope filters; these images are then combined by dedicated software.[16] Both these methods have the ability to characterize complex rearrangements, define marker chromosomes, and identify cryptic translocations (Fig. 7-4).[23,24] The resolution of SKY for the detection of interchromosomal rearrangements is between 500 and 2000 kbp and depends significantly on the quality of the metaphases and the resolution of the chromosomes involved in the rearrangement. Additional FISH experiments are often required to clarify or confirm ambiguous results. Subtelomeric translocations and high-level amplifications cannot be

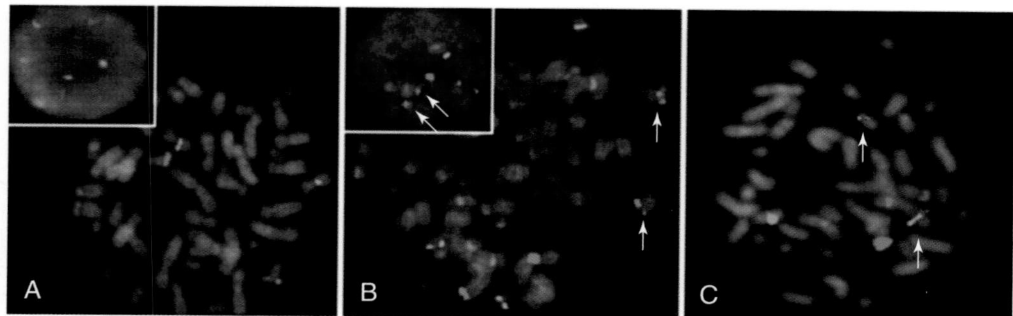

Figure 7-3. Fluorescence in situ hybridization analysis of 14q32 (*IGH*)-associated translocations in B-cell lymphomas with the tricolor probe. A, Normal metaphase and an interphase nucleus (*inset*) showing two each of blue (chromosome 11), red (chromosome 14), and green (chromosome 18) signals. **B,** Metaphase and interphase nuclei (*inset*) showing two red-green fusion signals representing the t(14;18)(q32;q21) translocation. **C,** Metaphase showing two red-blue fusion signals representing the t(11;14)(q13;q32) translocation. The fusion signals are indicated by *arrows.* (Courtesy of Cancer Genetics Inc., Milford, MA.)

detected by SKY. Without banding information, intrachromosomal aberrations such as duplication, deletion, and inversion cannot be identified, and specific breakpoints cannot be assigned to the abnormalities by SKY. Therefore, SKY or M-FISH is most useful as an adjunct to conventional G-banding analysis.

Comparative Genomic Hybridization

CGH is designed to scan the entire genome for gains, losses, and amplification.[25] In this method, tumor and reference (normal) DNAs are differentially labeled and cohybridized to normal metaphase spreads (chromosomal CGH) or to microarrays (array CGH). CGH has the advantage of requiring only tumor DNA extracted from either fresh or archived material. The reference DNA does not need to be from the same patient. For chromosomal CGH, the tumor DNA is usually labeled with a green fluorochrome (FITC), and the reference DNA is labeled with a red fluorochrome (TRITC/spectrum-RED). For array CGH, the DNAs are directly labeled with Cy3 and Cy5 fluorescent dyes, with tumor DNA pseudocolored red and reference DNA green. For chromosomal CGH, the differences in copy number between the tumor and normal DNA are reflected by differences in green and red fluorescence along the length of the chromosome (Fig. 7-5). A number of hematologic malignancies have been analyzed by chromosomal CGH to identify genomic imbalances. One valuable finding has been the identification of high-level amplification of genes such as *REL, MYC,* and *BCL2* in B-cell lymphoma.[26-29] The importance of gene amplification as a genetic mechanism in the biology of NHL had remained unrecognized by G-banding analyses.[26-29] A caveat related to this assay is its inability to detect rearrangements. Moreover, to be reliably detected, a gain or loss must be present in at least 35% of the tumor cells, and the altered regions must be at least 10 Mb. For detection of high-level amplification, the size of a given amplicon must amount to at least 2 Mb.[30] Several of these limitations have been markedly reduced with the higher resolution afforded by array CGH, where differences in copy number between the tumor and normal DNA are reflected by differences in green and red fluorescence at each spot. The spots are either DNA isolated from clones such as bacterial artificial chromosomes (BACs) containing human genomic DNA or oligonucleotides synthesized directly on the glass slide. Extensive statistical analyses are required to analyze each spot with respect to signal-to-noise ratio, Cy3-to-Cy5 ratio, regional placement along the chromosome, and regional copy number alteration (CNA) or genomic imbalance. High-density oligonucleotide arrays have improved the ability to detect gains and losses of fewer than 5000 bp, thus permitting the identification of smaller amplicons and microdeletions that were previously undetectable.[31]

Application of this technology and the related oligonucleotide array platform, which uses only single indirectly labeled tumor DNA for hybridization, has revealed that many normal copy number variations occur throughout the genome complement within the general population.[32] With the ability to define the genomic regions spotted on the arrays, and the

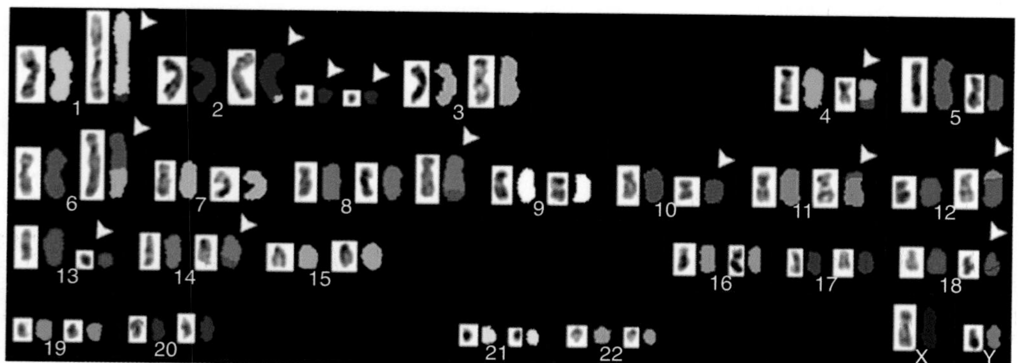

Figure 7-4. Spectral karyotype of a follicular grade 3 lymphoma with t(14;18)(q32;q21) and additional subtle translocations, such as t(1;2)(q32;q33), t(11;12)(p13;p11), and der(18)t(10;18)(q24;q21). Aberrations are indicated by *arrowheads.*

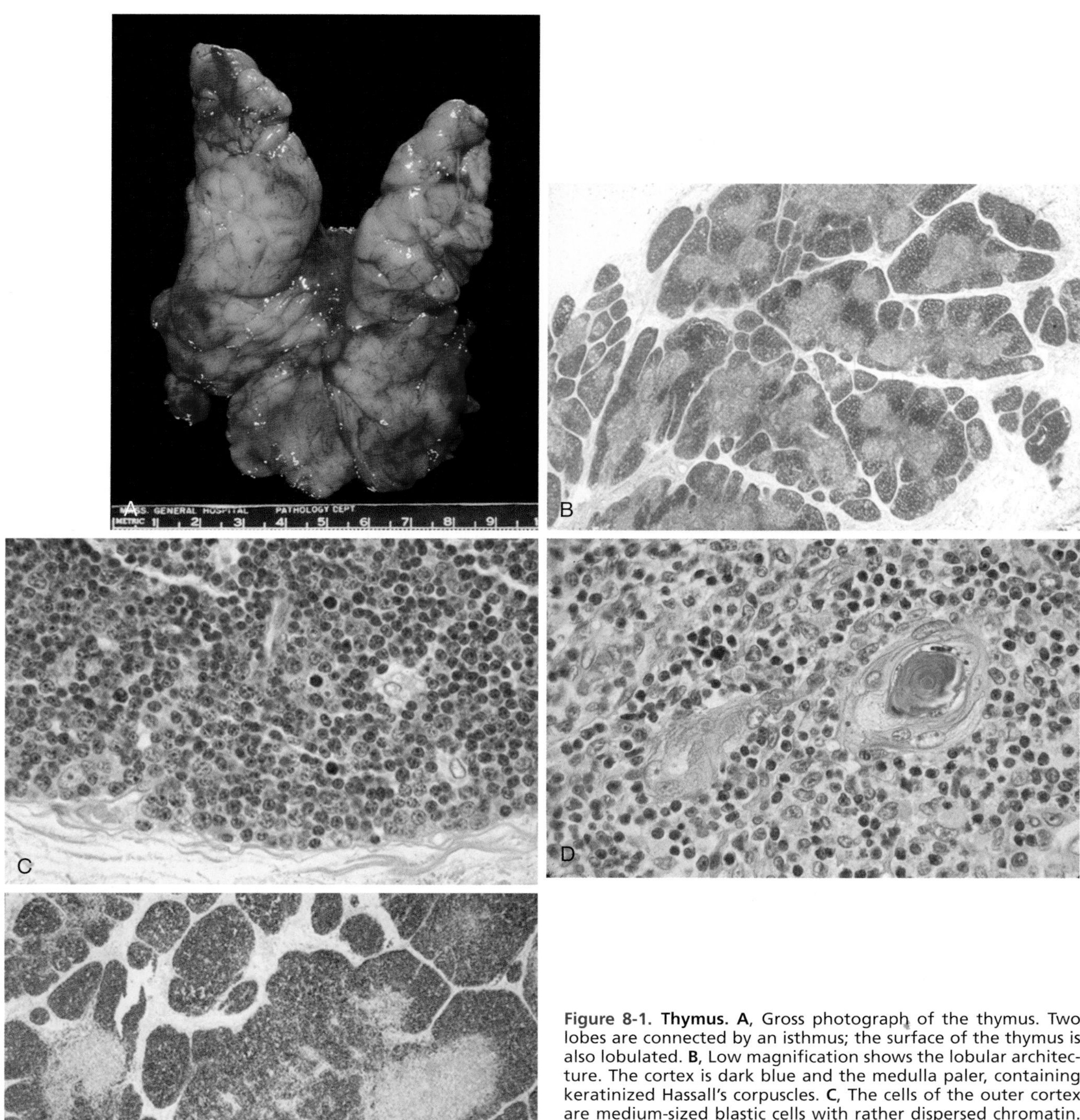

Figure 8-1. Thymus. A, Gross photograph of the thymus. Two lobes are connected by an isthmus; the surface of the thymus is also lobulated. **B**, Low magnification shows the lobular architecture. The cortex is dark blue and the medulla paler, containing keratinized Hassall's corpuscles. **C**, The cells of the outer cortex are medium-sized blastic cells with rather dispersed chromatin. Large oval cortical epithelial cells are visible, with distinct nucleoli and indistinct cytoplasm. **D**, The cells of the medulla are mature-appearing lymphocytes, associated with more spindle-shaped epithelial cells. **E**, With immunostaining for terminal deoxynucleotidyl transferase, the cortical thymocytes are stained, and the medullary thymocytes are negative.

perivascular spaces resemble those in the medulla.[7] Both have the immunophenotype of mature T cells (TdT$^-$, CD1a$^-$, CD3$^+$, CD4$^+$ or CD8$^+$).

The thymic medulla also contains a particular population of B cells with dendritic morphology that expresses mature B-cell markers CD23, CD37, CD72, CD76, immunoglobulin (Ig) M, and IgD. These cells form rosettes with non–B cells and have been called *asteroid cells*. The close relationship with T cells and epithelial thymic cells suggests that they may play a functional role in the T-cell differentiation process.[9-11] It has been suggested that they may be the cell of origin for primary mediastinal large B-cell lymphoma.

The thymic epithelial space begins to atrophy at age 1 year; it shrinks by about 3% per year through middle age and then 1% per year thereafter[7]; concomitantly, the perivascular space increases. The "fatty infiltration" noted in the adult thymus occurs in the perivascular space.[12-17]

Secondary (Peripheral) Lymphoid Tissues

Lymph Nodes

Lymph nodes are strategically located at branches of the lymphatic system throughout the body to maximize the capture of antigens and chemokines present in lymph drained from most organs via the afferent lymphatics (Fig. 8-2). The lymph nodes are protected by an external fibrotic capsule with internal prolongations that form trabeculae, providing the basic framework for the organization of the different cellular, vascular, and specialized stromal components.

The cellular compartments are distributed among three discrete but not rigid regions: cortex, paracortex, and medullary cords. The cortex or cortical area is the B-cell zone and contains the lymphoid follicles; the paracortex contains mainly T cells and T-cell antigen-presenting cells. The medullary cords in the inner area of the lymph node contain B cells, T cells, plasma cells, macrophages, and dendritic cells.

Cortical Area. The initial cortical structure is the primary lymphoid follicle, composed of aggregates of naïve B cells with a small network of follicular dendritic cells (FDCs) (see Fig. 8-2B). The lymphoid cells are small and have round nuclei with dense chromatin and scant cytoplasm. These cells express mature B-cell markers as well as IgM, IgD, CD21, and

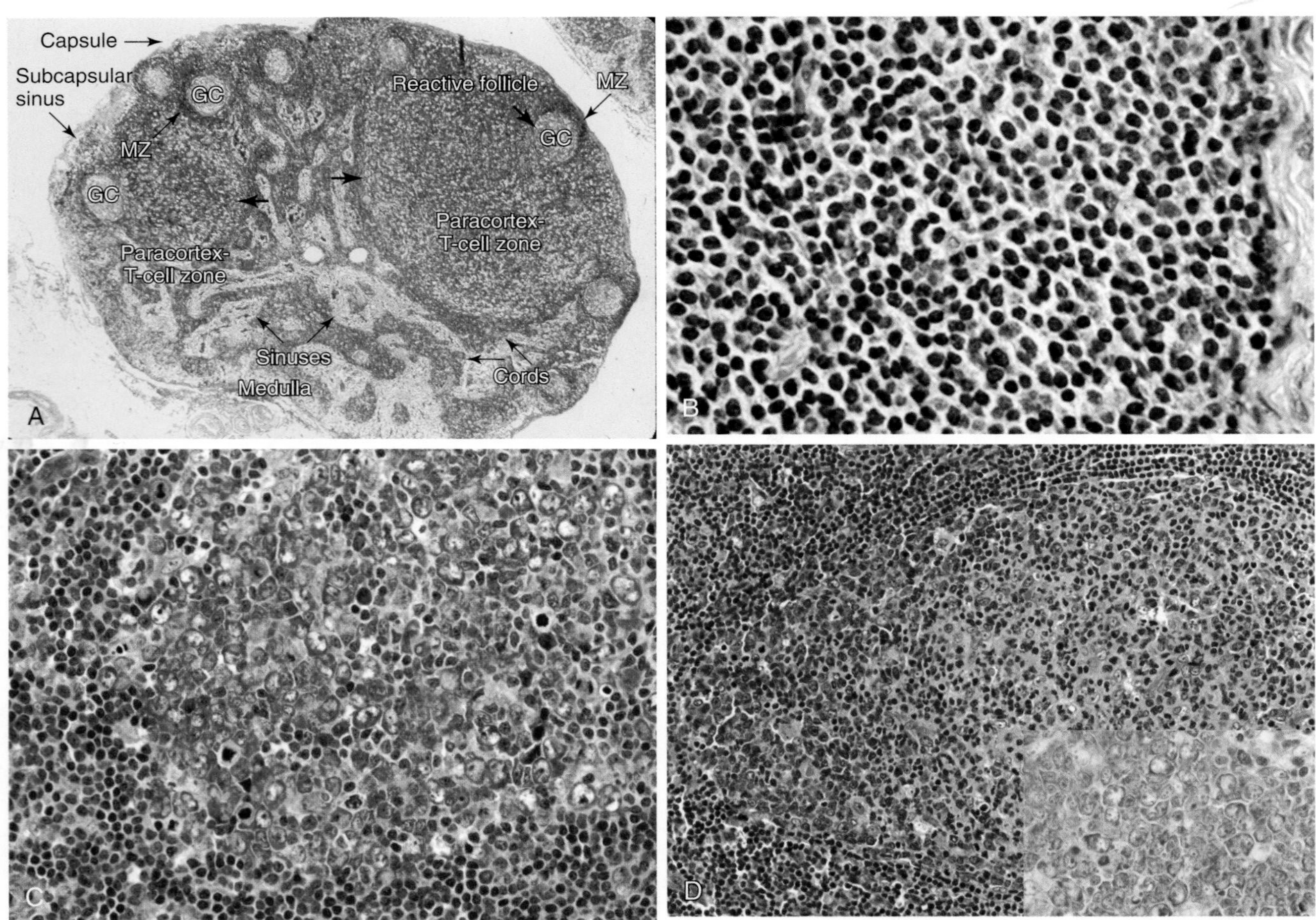

Figure 8-2. Lymph node. A, Low magnification illustrates the architecture of a reactive lymph node. Lymph nodes have a capsule, a cortex, a medulla, and sinuses (subcapsular, cortical, and medullary). The sinuses contain histiocytes (macrophages), which take up and process antigen, which is then presented to lymphocytes. The cortex is divided into follicular (*long, thin arrows*) and paracortical (*short, thick arrows*) regions, and the medulla is divided into medullary cords and sinuses. Both T-cell and early B-cell reactions to antigen occur in the paracortex, and the germinal center (GC) reaction occurs in the follicular cortex. Plasma cells and effector T cells generated by immune reactions accumulate in the medullary cords and exit via the medullary sinuses. MZ, mantle zone. **B,** Primary follicle composed of small, predominantly round lymphocytes arranged in a cluster that appears somewhat three-dimensional. These cells express IgM, IgD, and CD23. **C,** Secondary follicle with an early germinal center contains predominantly centroblasts—large blast cells with vesicular chromatin, one to three peripherally located nucleoli, and basophilic cytoplasm. Occasional centrocytes are present—medium-sized cells with dispersed chromatin, inconspicuous nucleoli, and scant cytoplasm that is not basophilic (Giemsa stain). **D,** The germinal center has polarized into a light zone and a dark zone, surrounded by a mantle zone of small lymphocytes. The dark zone contains mostly centroblasts, with admixed closely packed centrocytes (*inset*) (Giemsa).

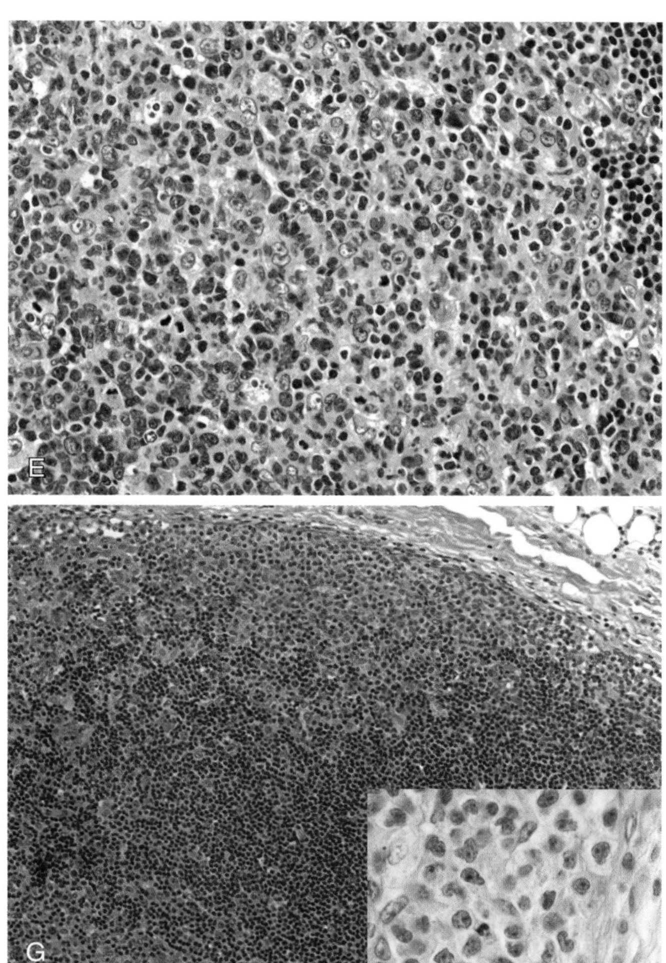

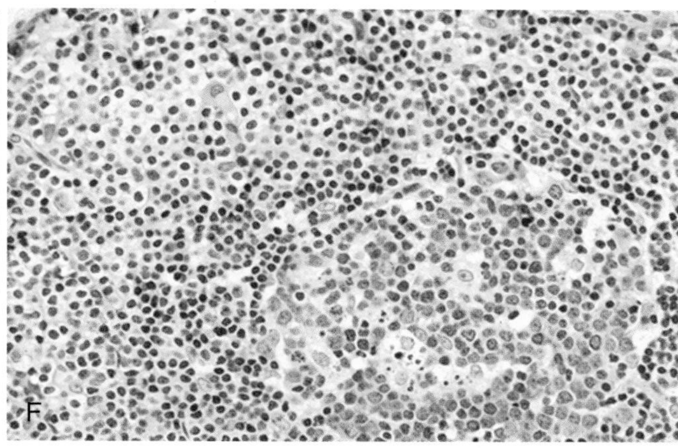

Figure 8-2, cont'd. E, The light zone contains centrocytes, numerous T cells, and many follicular dendritic cells with oval, vesicular nuclei that are often bilobed or binucleate. **F,** Follicle from a mesenteric lymph node has an expanded marginal zone composed of cells with centrocyte-like nuclei and pale cytoplasm. **G,** Lymph node with a monocytoid B-cell aggregate forming a pale band beneath the subcapsular sinus. *Inset* shows the cells at higher magnification; they have folded, monocyte-like nuclei and abundant pale to eosinophilic cytoplasm.

CD23. Antigen stimulation of these cells generates the expanded and highly organized secondary lymphoid follicle with a mantle cell corona, a germinal center, and a dense meshwork of FDCs (Fig. 8-3; see also Fig. 8-2C to F).

The mantle zone is composed mainly of the small B cells of the primary lymphoid follicle that are pushed aside by expansion of the germinal center. Like primary follicle B cells, mantle zone B cells express IgM, IgD, CD21, and CD23. Occasional B cells coexpressing CD5 are also located in this area but are difficult to identify in routine histologic sections. The mantle corona also contains memory B cells when the outer marginal zone is not developed.

The germinal center is a specialized lymphoid compartment in which the T-cell–dependent immune response occurs. This structure sustains the proliferative expansion of antigen-activated B-cell clones and the generation of high-affinity antibodies by the induction of antigen-driven somatic hypermutation of the immunoglobulin genes. Immunoglobulin genes also undergo the class or isotype switch from IgM or IgD to IgG, IgA, or IgE. This process is not exclusive to the germinal centers; it also occurs in other sites, to a lesser degree, in the T-cell–independent response. The germinal center also provides a microenvironment that selects the antigen-stimulated clones that produce high-affinity antibody, whereas B cells that do not produce high-affinity antibody to the specific antigen undergo apoptosis. Antigen-selected cells then exit the germinal center, becoming memory B cells or long-lived plasma cells.

Morphologically, the early germinal center contains predominantly small and large centroblasts (large, noncleaved follicular center cells). These cells are medium-sized to large B cells with an oval to round vesicular nucleus containing one to three small nucleoli close to the nuclear membrane, as well as a narrow rim of basophilic cytoplasm; these features are best seen on Giemsa staining (see Fig. 8-2C). After several hours or days, the germinal center becomes polarized into two distinctive areas: the dark zone and the light zone (see Fig. 8-2D). The dark zone is composed predominantly of centroblasts. Mitotic figures are common in this area. Closely packed centrocytes (cleaved follicular center cells) are also present in the dark zone (see Fig. 8-2D, *inset*). These are small to large B cells with irregular, sometimes deeply cleaved nuclei, dense chromatin, inconspicuous nucleoli, and scant cytoplasm that is not basophilic on Giemsa staining. Macrophages phagocytizing apoptotic nuclear debris are also present (tingible body macrophages). The light zone contains predominantly quiescent centrocytes.

The light zone also contains a high concentration of FDCs, and their vesicular and often double nuclei with small nucleoli are easily seen in this area (see Fig. 8-2E). Contrary to

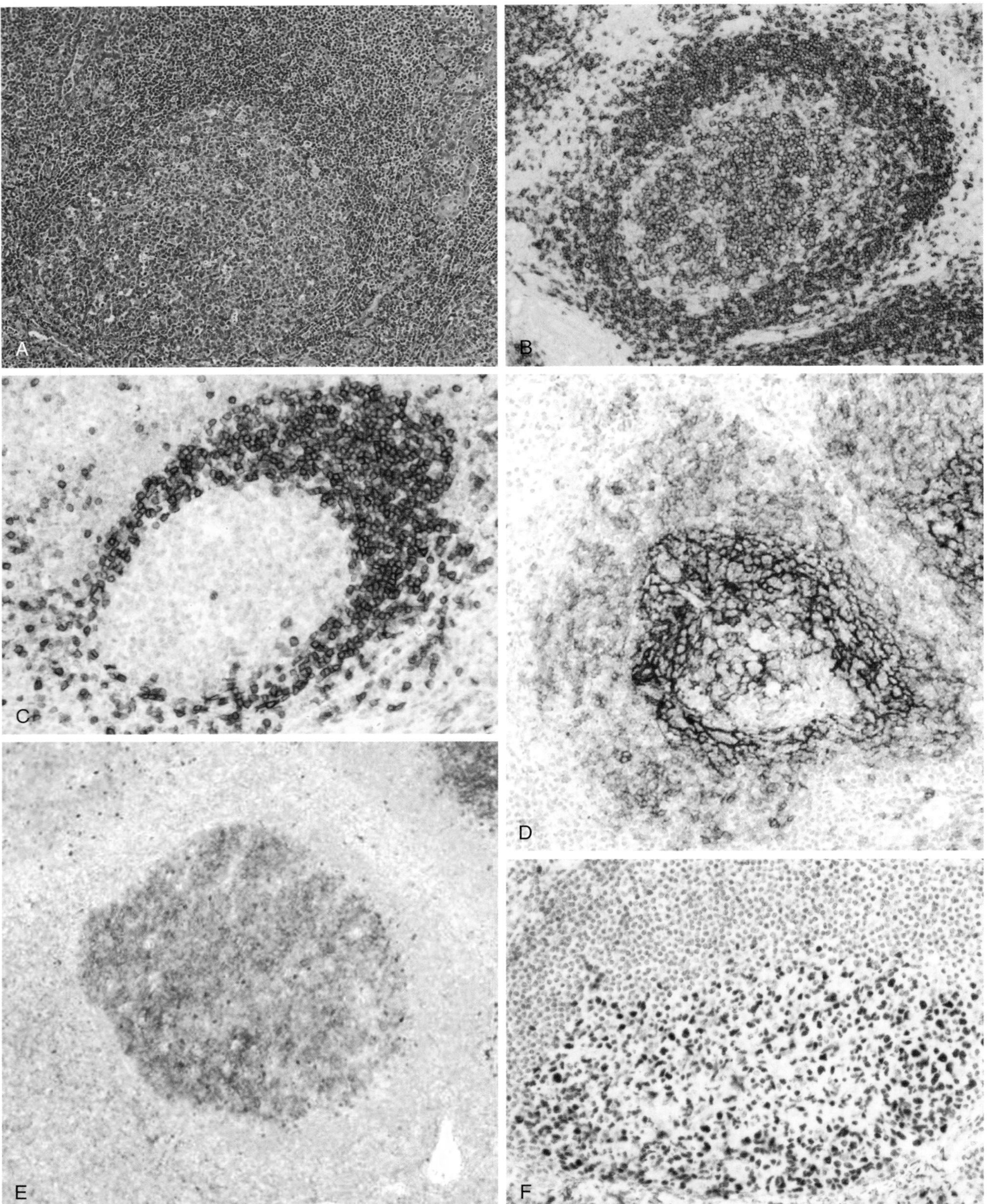

Figure 8-3. Secondary follicle. A, Reactive follicle with a polarized germinal center (dark zone to the left and light zone to the right) and a mantle zone area more developed near the light zone of the germinal center. **B**, Immunostain for CD20 shows staining of both the mantle zone and the germinal center. **C**, Immunostain for IgD shows staining of the mantle zone lymphocytes. **D**, CD23 stains follicular dendritic cells predominantly in the light zone, as well as mantle zone B cells. **E**, CD10 highlights the germinal center. **F**, BCL6 shows nuclear staining of most germinal center cells.

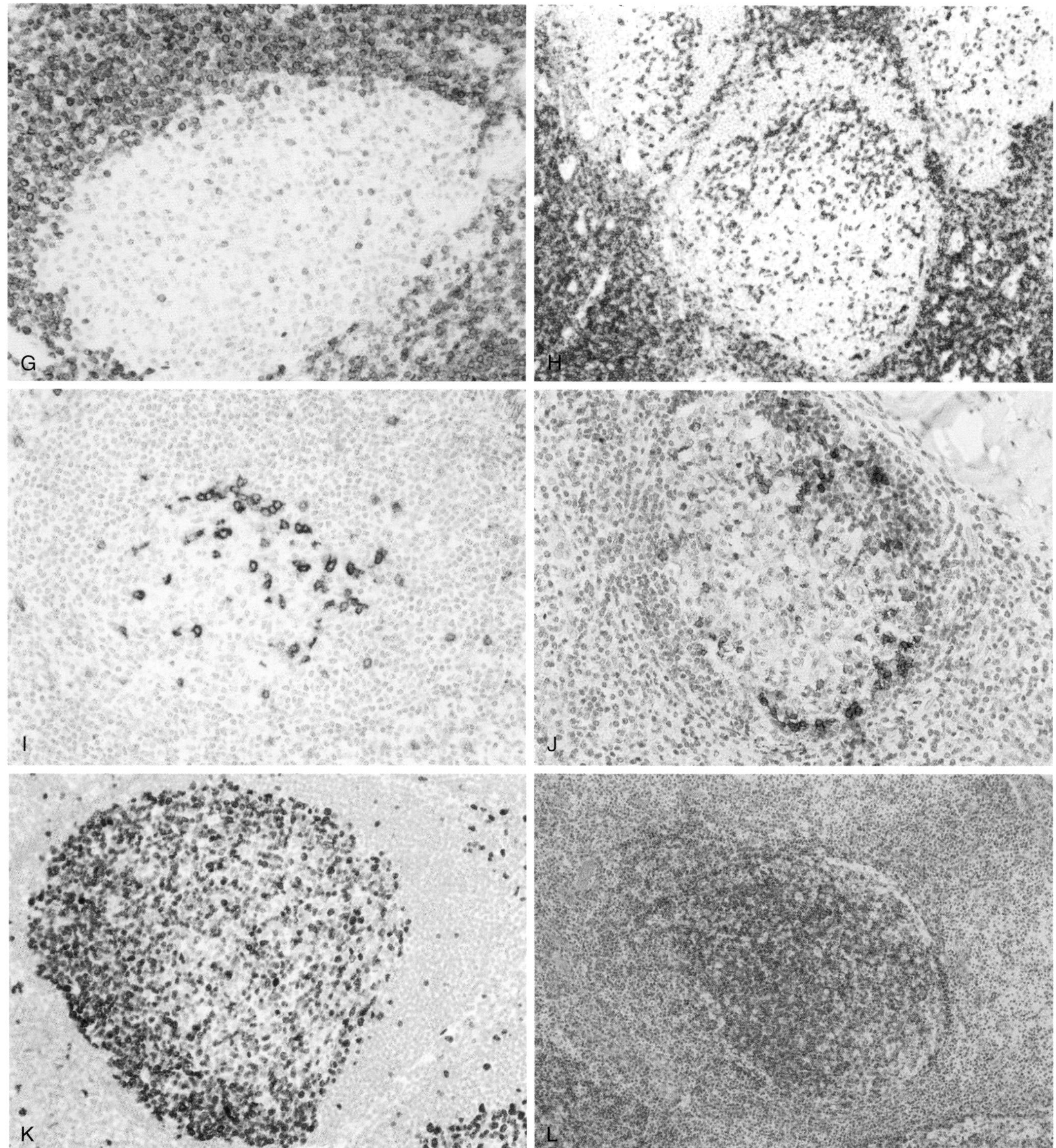

Figure 8-3, cont'd. **G**, BCL2 is expressed by mantle zone B cells and some intrafollicular T cells, but germinal center B cells are negative. **H**, CD3 stains the T cells in the paracortex, as well as numerous T cells within the germinal center. They are more numerous in the light zone than in the dark zone and form a crescent at the junction of the germinal center and the mantle zone. **I**, CD57 is expressed by a subset of germinal center T cells. **J**, CD279 (PD1) is expressed by germinal center T cells of the follicular helper subset. **K**, The majority of cells in the dark zone are in cycle, staining for Ki-67, whereas fewer cells in the light zone are proliferating. **L**, CD21 stains FDC predominantly in the light zone as well as mantle zone B cells.

other dendritic cells, FDCs are derived from mesenchymal cells and are important organizers of the germinal centers and the T-cell–dependent immune response. These cells express a profile of molecules that attract B and T cells and facilitate the antigen-presenting process. Thus, FDCs secrete CXCL13, a chemokine that recruits B and T cells expressing CXCR5 (see Table 8-1). They also express CD23, the adhesion molecules ICAM-1 and VCAM-1, and complement receptors (CD21, CD35) that fix immunocomplexes (see Fig. 8-3).

Phenotypically, both centroblasts and centrocytes express mature B-cell antigens (CD19, CD20, CD22, CD79) and the germinal center markers BCL6 and CD10 (see Fig. 8-3). Centroblasts lack surface immunoglobulin or express it at low levels because the immunoglobulin gene undergoes somatic hypermutation and class switch in these cells.[12-17] Surface immunoglobulin is reexpressed by centrocytes that have a higher affinity for the driving antigen. BCL6 is an essential nuclear zinc-finger transcription factor required for germinal center formation and the T-cell–dependent immune response. It is expressed in germinal center B cells but not in naïve B cells, mantle zone B cells, memory B cells, or plasma cells.[12-17] CD10 is a membrane-associated molecule (also known as *common acute lymphoblastic leukemia antigen* [CALLA]) that is normally expressed in early pro-B cells in the bone marrow but is lost in naïve cells and reexpressed in germinal center cells. Its function is not well known, but it seems to be indispensable for germinal center formation. CD10$^+$ mature lymphoid cells are restricted to germinal centers, and their identification outside this compartment should suggest the presence of a follicular lymphoid neoplasm. An important functional phenotypic change in germinal center cells is the downregulation of the antiapoptotic molecule BCL2, constitutively expressed in naïve and memory lymphoid cells.[12-17] Thus, these cells are susceptible to death through apoptosis, and only the clones encountering the specific antigens will be rescued and survive in this microenvironment. Germinal center B cells also express surface molecules involved in cell interactions with FDCs and T cells. In particular, CD40, CD86, and CD71 facilitate the association with T cells,[12-17] whereas CD11a/18 and CD29/49d recognize the FDC ligands CD44, ICAM-1, and VCAM-1. Similarly, germinal center lymphoid cells express receptors for the FDC molecules CD86D and interleukin (IL)-15, providing proliferative signals and B-cell activating factor (BAFF), which triggers survival signals that facilitate the rescue of BCL2$^-$ cells from apoptosis.[18-22]

Germinal centers contain specialized subpopulations of T cells that play an important role in the regulation of the B-cell differentiation process and T-cell–mediated immune response (see Fig. 8-3). One recently recognized subset is the follicular T-helper (T_{FH}) cell, which is mainly localized in the light zone and in the mantle zone area.[23] These cells express CD4, CD57, ICOS, PD-1 (programmed death-1, or CD279), and CXCR5, the receptor for the CXCL13 chemokine secreted by FDCs. T_{FH} cells promote B-cell differentiation through activation-induced cytidine deaminase (AID), immunoglobulin class switch, and immunoglobulin production. Germinal centers also contain a subset of T regulatory (T-reg) cells that express CD4, CD25, and FOXP3 and play a role in preventing autoimmunity and limiting T-cell–dependent B-cell stimulation. These cells also seem to directly suppress B-cell immunoglobulin production and class switch.[24] T-reg cells are also found in interfollicular areas.

Marginal zones are sometimes seen around follicles in lymph nodes, although these are usually not as prominent as those in the spleen; they are often more conspicuous in mesenteric lymph nodes (see Fig. 8-2F). Marginal zone B cells have nuclei that resemble those of centrocytes, but with more abundant pale cytoplasm; they appear to be a mixture of naïve and memory B cells. In some reactive conditions, slightly larger B cells with even more abundant pale to eosinophilic cytoplasm appear in aggregates between the mantle zone and cortical sinuses; these are known as *monocytoid B cells* (see Fig. 8-2G). Like marginal zone B cells, they appear to be a mixture of naïve and memory B cells.

Paracortex. The paracortex is the interfollicular T-cell zone (see Fig. 8-2A). This compartment contains mainly mature T cells and dendritic cells of the interdigitating cell subtype that specialize in presenting antigens to T cells (Fig. 8-4A). This area is organized by the production of the chemokines CCL19 and CCL21 by stromal cells of the paracortex and endothelial cells of the high endothelial venules (HEVs) present in this area. These chemokines recruit the T cells and dendritic cells expressing their receptor CCR7. The T cells in these areas are heterogeneous, with a predominance of CD4$^+$ cells; some CD8$^+$ and T-reg cells are also found. The interdigitating cells are positive for S-100, class II major histocompatibility complex (MHC), CD80, CD86, and CD40 but negative for CD1a, CD21, and CD35; they have complex interdigitating cellular junctions, seen on electron microscopy. In some reactive conditions, particularly those associated with rashes, the paracortical areas contain Langerhans cells that have migrated from the skin.

Interfollicular areas also contain isolated large B cells with immunoblastic morphology; these cells may be numerous in some reactive conditions. Immunoblasts are large cells similar in size to centroblasts but with prominent single nucleoli and more abundant basophilic cytoplasm (Fig. 8-4B). These cells express mature B-cell markers and abundant cytoplasmic immunoglobulins and are considered intermediate steps toward plasma cells. A less frequent subset of large B cells with a dendritic morphology was recently identified in nodal T-cell areas.[25] These cells carry immunoglobulin gene somatic mutations and express mature B-cell markers and CD40 but are negative for germinal center markers (BCL6 and CD10), CD30, and CD27. The functional role of these cells is not known, but they resemble the thymic asteroid cell.

The paracortex contains high endothelial venules (HEVs), postcapillary venules through which both T and B lymphocytes enter the lymph node from the blood (Fig. 8-4C). HEVs have large, plump endothelial cells whose nuclei often appear to virtually occlude the lumen. These endothelial cells express adhesion molecules that anchor circulating lymphocytes and also act as tissue-specific recognition molecules (called *addressins*) that bind to specific molecules on the lymphocytes (called *homing receptors*). These include E-selectin, P-selectin, VCAM-1, ICAM-1, ICAM-2, peripheral node addressin (peripheral lymph nodes), and mucosal addressin (mesenteric lymph nodes) cell adhesion molecules (MAdCAMs). The addressins bind to L-selectin and $\alpha_4\beta_7$-integrins on the lymphocytes. Postcapillary venules in other tissues do not express lymphocyte adhesion molecules unless they are stimulated by inflammatory mediators; however, those in the lymph nodes express them constitutively and thus recruit lymphocytes

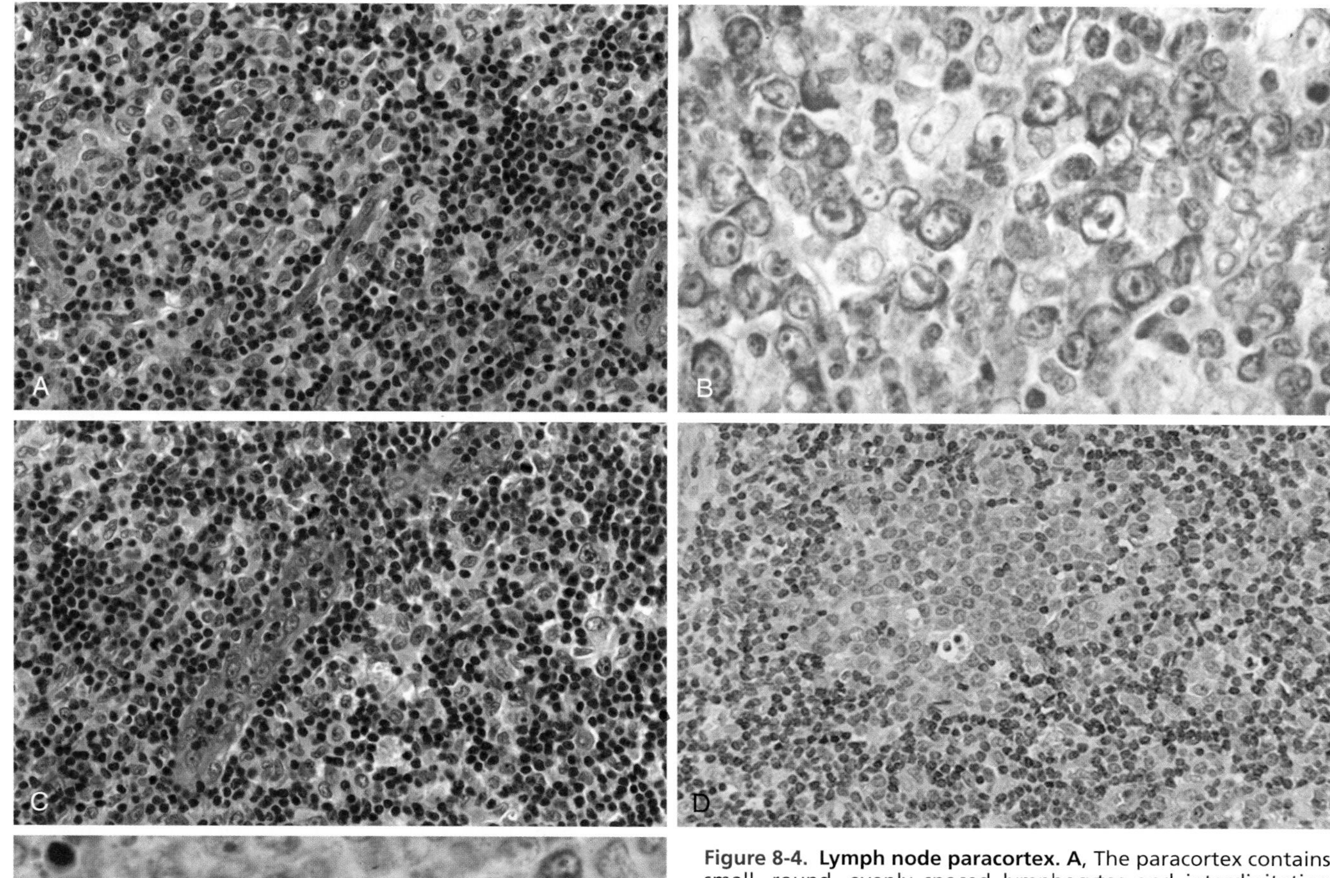

Figure 8-4. Lymph node paracortex. **A**, The paracortex contains small, round, evenly spaced lymphocytes and interdigitating dendritic cells with pale, grooved or irregular nuclei and indistinct cytoplasm; these cells present antigen to T cells and also to B cells that may migrate through the paracortex. **B**, In early reactions to antigen, an immunoblastic reaction occurs, and numerous B immunoblasts are present in the paracortex. Immunoblasts are two to three times the size of small lymphocytes and have vesicular chromatin, single central nucleoli, and abundant basophilic cytoplasm (Giemsa stain). **C**, High endothelial venules (HEVs) are prominent in the paracortex. HEVs have plump endothelial cells, and lymphocytes are typically seen migrating between them. Lymphocytes migrate into the lymph node via the HEVs, which have receptors for lymphocytes on the endothelial cells. **D**, At the junction of the paracortex and the medulla, an aggregate of plasmacytoid dendritic cells is seen. The cells have dispersed chromatin and amphophilic cytoplasm; apoptosis and nuclear dust may be seen. **E**, On Giemsa staining, the cytoplasm is faintly basophilic and eccentric, resembling a plasma cell.

continuously.[26] The HEVs usually contain lymphocytes both within the lumen and infiltrating between the endothelial cells and the basement membrane.

Under some circumstances, collections of plasmacytoid dendritic cells may be found in the paracortex, usually at its junction with the medullary cords. These are medium-sized cells with dispersed chromatin, small nucleoli, and eccentric, amphophilic cytoplasm; they typically occur in small clusters, sometimes with apoptotic debris and histiocytes, mimicking a small germinal center (Fig. 8-4D). Vollenweider and Lennert[27] noted that these cells have abundant rough endoplasmic reticulum on electron microscopy, resembling plasma cells; they named them *T-associated plasma cells*. Other names over the years have been *plasmacytoid T cells* and *plasmacytoid monocytes*. In vitro studies on these cells have shown that they produce high amounts of interferon-α and function in the regulation of T-cell responses. They express CD68, CD123, TCL1, and BDCA2 and lack specific markers of T-cell, B-cell, or myeloid differentiation.[28,29]

Lymph Node Vasculature and Conduit System. The interaction among lymph, blood, and the different cell components of the lymph node is facilitated by a highly organized vascular system. Arteries arrive at the hilus and branch to reach the subcapsular area and paracortex, where the capillaries form loops and specialize into postcapillary HEVs.

Lymph arrives through the afferent lymphatic vessels at the opposite pole of the node, which open to the subcapsular sinus, and flows through the trabecular and medullary sinuses toward the efferent lymph vessels at the hilus. Macrophages in the subcapsular sinuses capture large antigens, immune complexes, and viruses and may present them to nearby B cells in the cortical areas. Small soluble antigens may diffuse through the sinus wall and reach the cortical areas.[30]

The nodal conduit system is a specialized structure that connects the lymphatic sinuses with the walls of the blood vessels, particularly the HEVs in the paracortex, allowing the rapid movement of small antigenic particles (around 5.5 nm and 70 kDa) and cytokines from the afferent lymph deep into the portal of entry of lymphocytes to the nodal parenchyma.[31] This structure consists of small conduits composed of a core of type I and III collagen fibers associated with cross-linked microfibrils of fibromodulin and decorin, all of them surrounded by a basal membrane of laminin and type IV collagen. This entire conduit system is wrapped by the cytoplasm of fibroblastic reticular cells. At certain places not totally covered by fibroblastic reticular cells, the dendritic cells contact the basal membrane and reach inside the conduit to capture antigens.

Spleen

The spleen has two major compartments—red pulp and white pulp—related to its two major functions as a blood filter for damaged formed elements of the blood and a defense against blood-borne pathogens, respectively. The white pulp organization is similar to that of the lymphoid tissue of lymph nodes (Fig. 8-5A to F). Follicles and germinal centers are found in the malpighian corpuscles, and T cells and interdigitating cells are found in the adjacent periarteriolar lymphoid sheath. The red pulp also contains antigen-presenting cells; lymphocytes, particularly a subset of gamma-delta T lymphocytes; and plasma cells. A distinctive feature of the spleen is the presence of a prominent marginal zone, composed of lymphoid cells with abundant pale cytoplasm and macrophages, which surrounds both the B- and T-cell zones (see Fig. 8-5D).[32,33]

White Pulp. The B-cell and T-cell areas in the spleen are organized around the branching arterial vessels (see Fig. 8-5A to F). Similar to the lymph nodes, the T- and B-cell compartments are recruited and maintained by specific chemokines. CCL19 and CCL21 are produced mainly by stromal cells in the T-cell areas, and the FDCs secrete CXCL13; these chemokines recruit cells expressing the receptors CCR7 and CXCR5, respectively (see Table 8-1). T cells surround the arterioles in a discontinuous manner, whereas B-cell follicles may be found adjacent to the T-cell sheaths or directly attached to the arteriole without a T-cell layer (see Fig. 8-5F).[34] A distinctive area of the splenic white pulp is the marginal zone, which is more evident in follicles with an expanded germinal center. B cells in this area have slightly irregular nuclei, resembling those of centrocytes but with more abundant pale cytoplasm (see Fig. 8-5D). These cells express CD21 and IgM, but contrary to mantle cells, IgD expression is negative or weak. These cells predominantly surround the follicles but are almost absent from the surface of the T-cell regions. Some studies in human spleen distinguish between an inner and outer marginal zone separated by a shell-like accumulation of $CD4^+$ T cells and a layer of peculiar fibroblasts that extend to the T-cell areas as a meshwork. These cells express smooth muscle α-actin and myosin, MAdCAM-1, VCAM-1, and VAP-1.[34] In contrast to murine white pulp, human spleen lacks the marginal zone sinus, where the arterial blood opens into the sinusoidal system. Instead, the human marginal zone is surrounded by a perifollicular area with more widely separated fibers and capillaries sheathed by abundant macrophages that are positive for sialoadhesin. A large amount of the splenic blood passes through this area, where the flow seems to be retarded. This anatomic relationship between an open blood area and the marginal zone seems to facilitate direct contact between blood-borne antigens and B cells.[32,33]

Red Pulp. The red pulp is composed of sinuses and cords. The sinuses form an interconnected meshwork covered by a layer of sinusoidal endothelial cells and surrounded by annular fibers of extracellular matrix; these annular fibers may be seen on periodic acid–Schiff staining (see Fig. 8-5G). The cells have cytoplasmic stress fibers that regulate the passage of blood cells. The capillaries open into the cords, and the blood cells that cannot pass through the sinusoidal cells are destroyed by the abundant macrophages resident in the cords. Sinusoidal blood flows into the venous system. The sinusoidal cells express endothelial markers such as factor VIII, but they are also positive for CD8 (see Fig. 8-5H). The red pulp cords also contain plasmablasts and plasma cells. Upregulation of CXCR4 in these cells may play a role in this movement because it binds to the CXCL12 expressed in the red pulp; on the contrary, CXCR5 and CCR7, which bind to the white pulp chemokines CXCL13, CCL19, and CCL21, are down regulated in these cells (see Table 8-1).[33]

Mucosa-Associated Lymphoid Tissue

Specialized lymphoid tissue is found in association with certain epithelia, in particular, the gastrointestinal tract (gut-associated lymphoid tissue—Peyer's patches of the distal ileum, mucosal lymphoid aggregates in the colon and rectum), the naso- and oropharynx (Waldeyer's ring—adenoids, tonsils), and, in some species, the lung (bronchus-associated lymphoid tissue). Collectively, this is known as *mucosa-associated lymphoid tissue* (MALT). In each territory MALT comprises four lymphoid compartments: organized mucosal lymphoid tissue, lamina propria, intraepithelial lymphocytes, and regional (mesenteric) lymph nodes (Fig. 8-6).[35] The organized lymphoid tissue is exemplified by Peyer's patches of the terminal ileum and is also found in Waldeyer's ring. The lymphoid follicles are structurally and immunophenotypi-

Figure 8-5. Spleen. A, At low magnification, the white pulp contains a reactive follicle with a germinal center (*left*) and a T-cell zone (*right*); both are surrounded by a pale-staining marginal zone. **B,** CD20 staining highlights the B-cell nodules. **C,** Splenic follicle contains a germinal center, a marginal zone, and a pale-staining marginal zone composed of medium-sized cells with abundant pale cytoplasm. **D,** Marginal zone area of the B-cell follicle. The cells have pale cytoplasm. **E,** T-cell zone has an appearance similar to that of nodal paracortex, with interdigitating dendritic cells present in a background of small lymphocytes. **F,** CD3 stains the periarteriolar T cells. **G,** Periodic acid–Schiff stain highlights the basement membrane of the sinuses, which are fenestrated, allowing nucleated red blood cells to be trapped in the cords. **H,** CD8 stains the red pulp sinusoidal cells strongly.

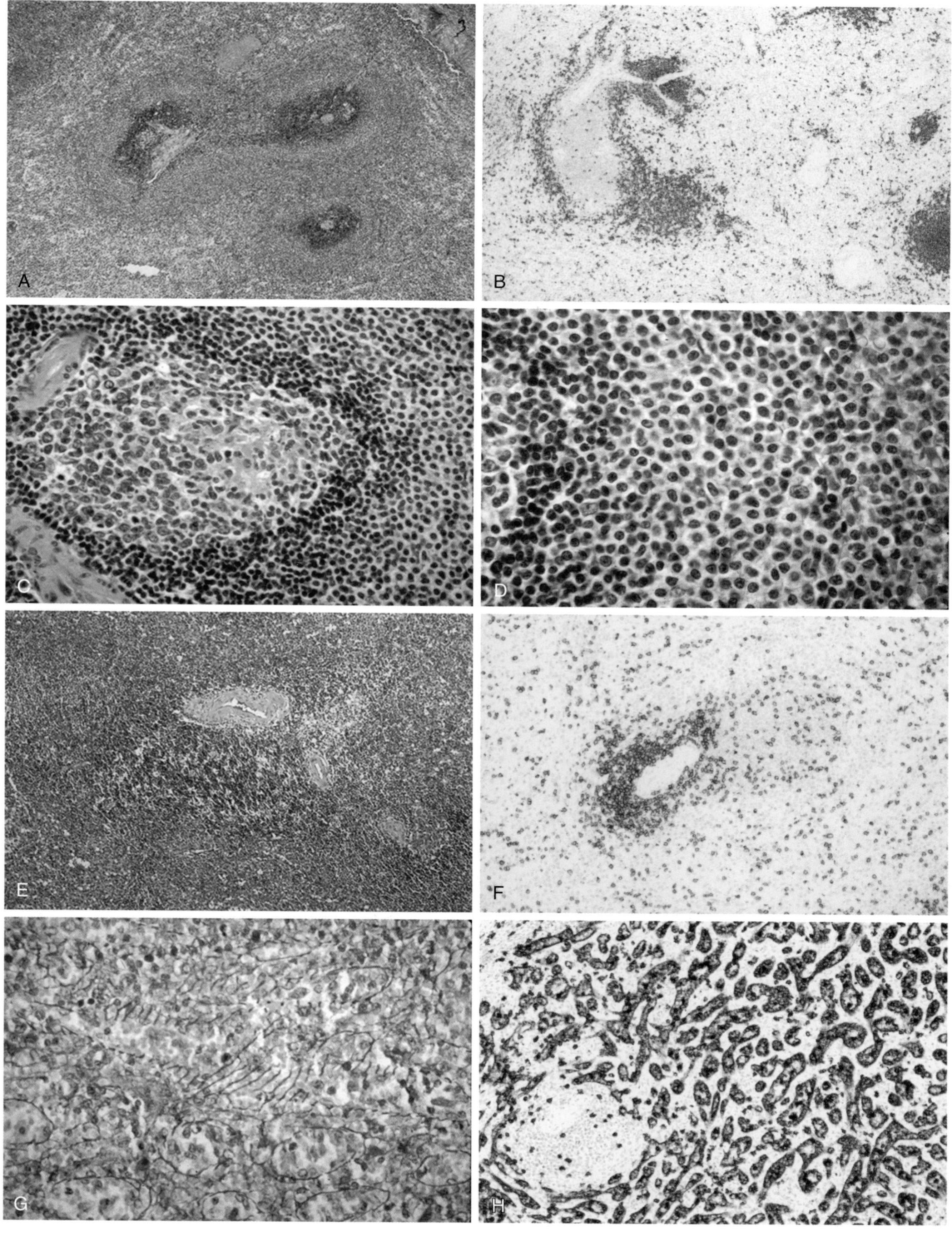
A
B
C
D
E
F
G
H

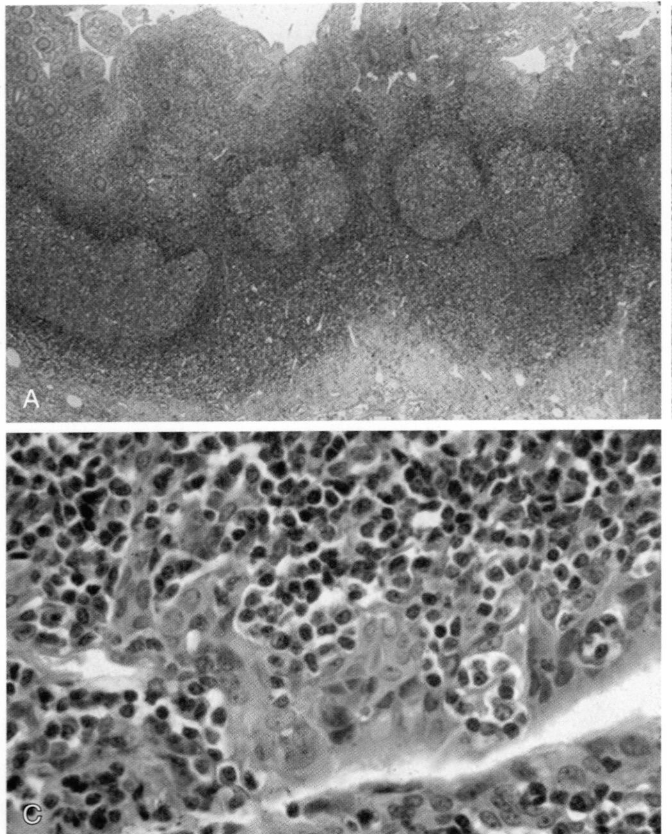

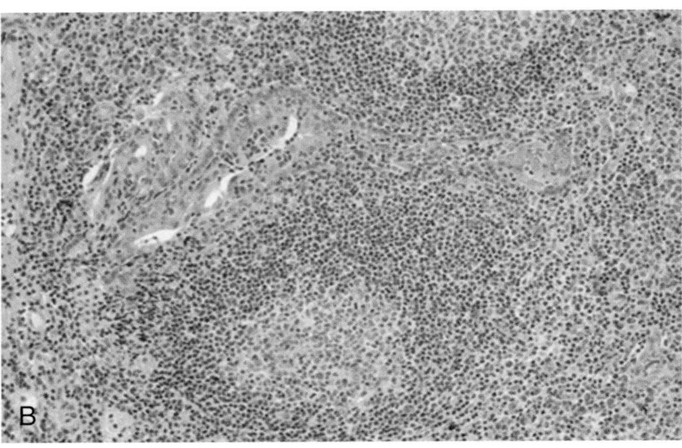

Figure 8-6. Mucosa-associated lymphoid tissue (MALT). A, Low magnification of Peyer's patches of the terminal ileum shows lymphoid follicles with reactive germinal centers and mantle zones; a pale area of marginal zone cells extends upward into the lamina propria. The overlying mucosa is somewhat flattened and eosinophilic. **B,** Adenoid showing a reactive follicle with pale-staining marginal zone cells extending toward a crypt. **C,** Adenoid showing marginal zone cells within the epithelium (lymphoepithelium).

cally similar to those found in lymph nodes. The only difference here is the expanded marginal zone, which tends to reach the superficial epithelium. MALT marginal zone cells are morphologically similar to those found in the spleen. The interfollicular areas are occupied by T cells and interdigitating dendritic cells. The mucosal lamina propria contains mature plasma cells and macrophages and occasional B and T lymphocytes. These plasma cells secrete mainly dimeric IgA, but small populations producing IgM, IgG, and IgE are also present. The dimeric IgA and pentameric IgM are secreted into the intestinal lumen bound to the secretory component, a glycoprotein produced by the enterocytes. The T lymphocytes in the lamina propria are a mixed population of $CD4^+$ and $CD8^+$ cells, with a slight predominance (2:1 to 3:1) of the former. Intraepithelial lymphocytes are observed between the epithelial cells and are composed of a heterogeneous population of T cells. The predominant cells are $CD3^+$, $CD5^+$, and $CD8^+$, whereas 10% to 15% are $CD3^+$ and double negative for CD4 and CD8. $CD3^+$, $CD4^+$ cells are a minority, and only rare cells are $CD56^+$.[36] Most of the T cells express the alpha-beta form of the T-cell receptor (TCR), and around 10% of the cells are TCR gamma-delta. The epithelium above the Peyer's patches contains clusters of B cells and specialized epithelial cells called *membranous* or *microfold cells* (M cells). These cells are also found more dispersed in other parts of the gastrointestinal tract and other mucosal sites, particularly in the epithelium over lymphoid follicles.[37] M cells play a sentinel role for the mucosal immune system by capturing luminal antigens and delivering them to the underlying immune cells. The basic structure of mesenteric lymph nodes is similar to that of other lymph nodes, but the marginal zone surrounding the follicles is usually expanded and visible.

The organization of the immune system in mucosal sites is orchestrated by the coordinated action of several adhesion molecules, chemokines, and their respective receptors. Lymphoid cells that respond to antigen in the MALT acquire homing properties that enable them to return to these tissues.[38,39] This homing is mediated in part by expression of high levels of $\alpha_4\beta_7$-integrin, which binds to MAdCAM-1 on HEVs in gut-associated lymphoid tissue.[26] In addition, the MALT immune cells express $\alpha_E\beta_7$-integrin (CD103), whose ligand E-cadherin is expressed on the basolateral surface of the epithelial cells. Epithelial cells also secrete CCL25, which recruits immune cells expressing its receptor CCR9 (see Table 8-1).[40]

B-CELL AND T-CELL DIFFERENTIATION

In both the T-cell and B-cell systems, there are two major phases of differentiation: foreign antigen independent and foreign antigen dependent (Figs. 8-7 and 8-8). Foreign antigen–independent differentiation occurs in the primary lymphoid organs—bursa equivalent (bone marrow) and thymus—without exposure to foreign antigen. This produces a pool of lymphocytes that are capable of responding to foreign antigens (naïve or virgin T and B cells) and in general do not respond to self- or autoantigens. The early stages of

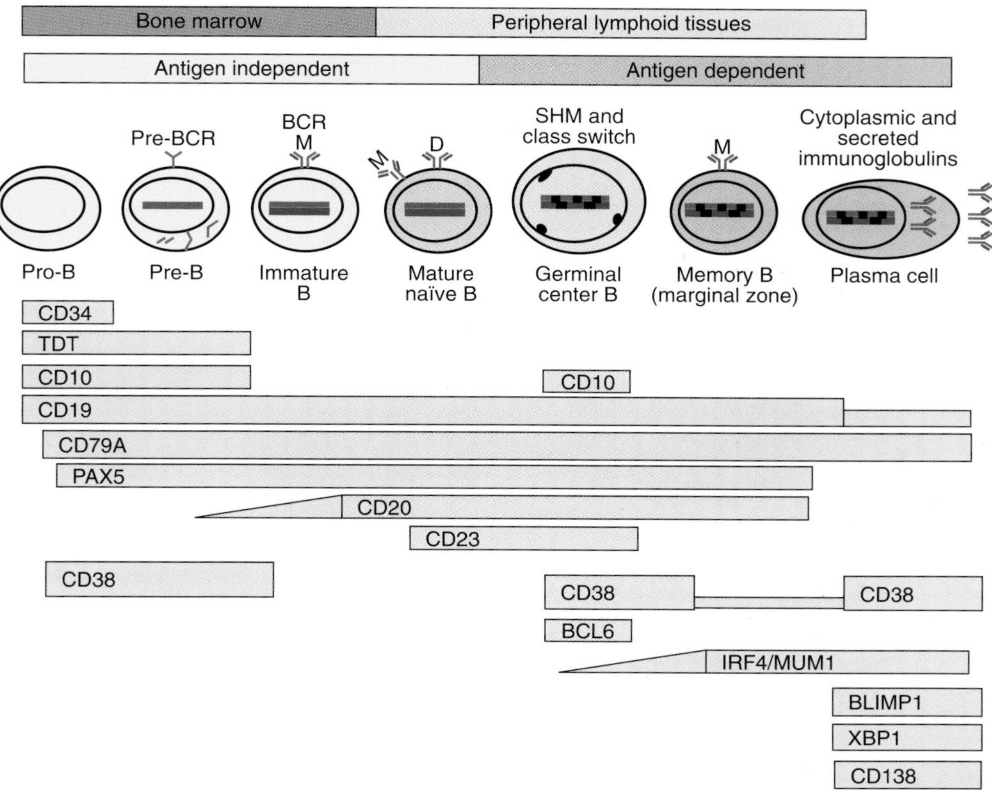

Figure 8-7. Schematic diagram of B-cell differentiation. Early B-cell precursors express CD34, terminal deoxynucleotidyl transferase (TDT), and CD10. CD19 is an early B-cell differentiation antigen that is maintained during the entire B-cell differentiation program, and its expression is attenuated in plasma cells. CD79A and PAX5 appear at nearly the same time as heavy-chain gene rearrangement. CD20 is not expressed until the stage of light-chain rearrangement. Germinal center cells are positive for BCL6 and reexpress CD10 and CD38. The plasma cell differentiation program is characterized by the downregulation of PAX5 and the expression of CD138, BLIMP1, and XBP1. BCR, B-cell receptor of mature B cells; pre-BCR, pre–B-cell receptor consisting of a heavy chain and the surrogate light chain (which is composed of two linked small peptides, VpreB and λ5, represented in *green*); SHM, somatic hypermutation; *red bar, IGH* gene rearrangement; *blue bar, IGL* gene rearrangement; *red bar and blue bar with black insertions,* rearranged *IGH* and *IGL* genes with somatic hypermutations.

foreign antigen–independent differentiation are stem cells and lymphoblasts (blast or progenitor cells of the entire lymphoid line), which are self-renewing; the later stages are resting cells with a finite life span ranging from weeks to years. Naïve B cells and T cells carry surface molecules that are receptors for antigens (the T-cell antigen receptor and surface immunoglobulin). On exposure to antigens that fit their surface receptors, naïve lymphocytes transform into large, proliferating blast cells (immunoblasts for progenitor cells of immune effector cells, or centroblasts for blast cells of the germinal center). These blasts give rise to progeny that are capable of direct activity against the inciting antigen: antigen-specific effector cells. The early stages of both antigen-independent and antigen-dependent differentiation are proliferating cells; the fully differentiated effector cells do not divide unless they are stimulated by antigen. B cells and most T cells belong to the adaptive immune response system—that is, they have surface receptors that are specific for certain antigens and, on encountering antigen, undergo proliferation and affinity maturation, giving rise to a large population of antigen-specific effector cells and memory cells. In contrast, NK cells and gamma-delta T cells belong to the innate immune response.

Differentiation of Cells of the Adaptive Immune Response

B cells and most T cells described earlier represent mediators of the adaptive immune system, which can recognize a virtually unlimited number of antigens using specific receptors generated by the somatic recombination of the receptor genes. Memory cells are also generated, which help respond faster during subsequent contact with the antigen.

B-Cell Differentiation

Antigen-Independent B-Cell Differentiation

Precursor B Cells. Precursor B cells develop from hematopoietic stem cells and differentiate in the bone marrow before they migrate to the peripheral lymphoid tissues as naïve mature B lymphocytes. Fetal early B-cell development occurs in the liver, bone marrow, and spleen, whereas in adults it is restricted to the bone marrow. B-cell differentiation produces a broad repertoire of B-cell antigen receptors by the recombination of the variable (V), diversity (D), and join (J) segments of the immunoglobulin genes. In this process, the gene

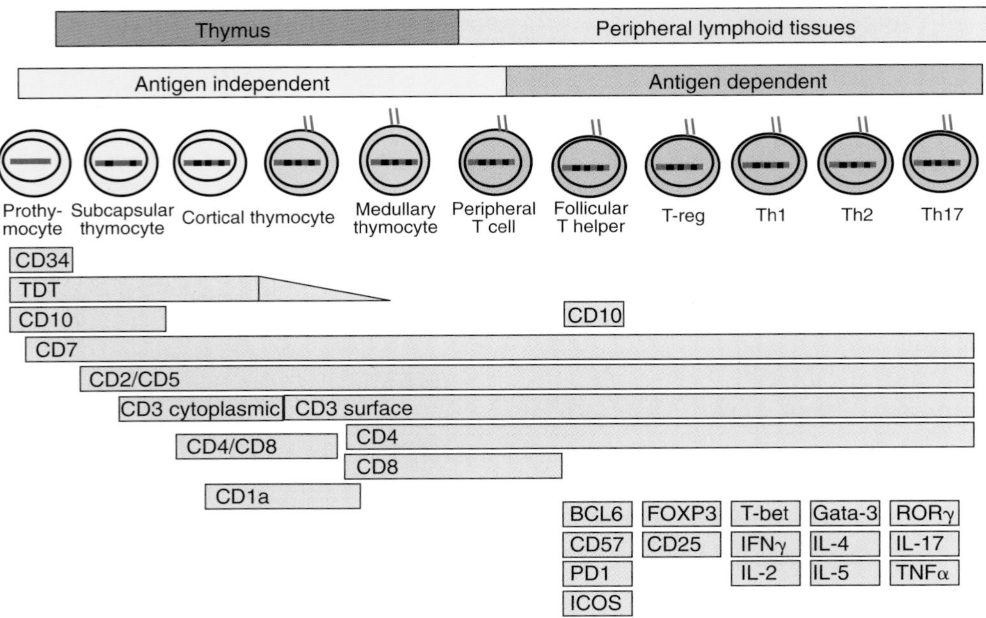

Figure 8-8. Schematic diagram of T-cell differentiation. Early T-cell precursors express CD34, terminal deoxynucleotidyl transferase (TDT), and CD10. CD7 is the first T-cell–specific antigen expressed, followed by CD2/CD5 and cytoplasmic CD3. Cortical thymocytes are double positive for CD4 and CD5 and express CD1a. Medullary thymocytes are already either CD4 or CD8 and express surface CD3. Different subpopulations of mature T cells have been recognized. This simplified diagram illustrates follicular T-helper (Th) cells that express CD10, BCL6, CD57, PD1, and ICOS. T-regulatory cells, Th1, Th2, and Th17 CD4^{+} cells are characterized by expression of the transcription factors FOXP3, T-bet, Gata-3, and RORγ, respectively. Germline T-cell receptor (TCR) genes are represented schematically with a *solid red bar*. Additional *blue segments* represent gene rearrangements. The *TRG@* gene is the first one rearranged, followed by *TRB@* and *TRD@*. Alpha-beta T cells delete the *TRD@* gene during the *TRA@* rearrangement as delta segments are included in the *TRA@* locus. Gamma-delta T cells may have *TRB@* gene rearrangements without assembly of a complete alpha-beta TCR. These gene rearrangements generate two main populations of T cells—alpha-beta and gamma-delta—with expression of the TCR complex in the cell membrane (represented here as *double solid bars*).

segments V, D, and J are joined to encode the heavy-chain (H) variable region that is then fused to the constant region.

The earliest stages lack surface immunoglobulin and are called *progenitor B cells* (pro-B cells).[41] These cells first carry out DH-JH rearrangements, followed by the VH rearrangement to the DH-JH element. Some of the common chromosomal translocations in B-cell lymphomas occur at this stage of differentiation, when the cell is initiating the immunoglobulin gene rearrangement with the recombination of the VDJ segments. In the next steps the precursor B cells (pre-B cells) acquire cytoplasmic mu heavy chain and later express surface mu heavy chain with a surrogate light chain composed of two linked small peptides consisting of a variable region ($V_{pre\text{-}B}$) and a constant region (λ5). The physiologic *IGK/IGL* gene rearrangements start later. When light-chain rearrangement is complete, a complete surface IgM molecule is expressed (immature B cell). Finally, the mature cells that leave the bone marrow express both IgM and IgD.

At early stages of B-cell differentiation, the cells contain the intranuclear enzyme TdT and express CD34, a glycoprotein present on immature cells of both lymphoid and myeloid lineage; human leukocyte antigen (HLA)-DR (class II MHC antigens); and CALLA (CD10).[42-45] CD34 is lost in pre-B cells. PAX5, a crucial transcription factor determining and maintaining the B-cell differentiation pathway, is expressed early in this process, as is CD19, a target of PAX5.[46] Pre-B cells express CD79a, a molecule associated with surface immunoglobulin and involved in signal transduction after engagement of surface immunoglobulin with antigen,[47,48] analogous to CD3 and the TCR molecule. Expression of class II MHC antigens persists throughout the life of the B cell and is important in interactions with T cells; in contrast, CD10 and TdT are lost before the cells leave the bone marrow. The mature B-cell antigen CD20 is expressed weakly in pre-B cells and increases in the immature B cells. The leukocyte common antigen (CD45) does not appear until surface CD20 is expressed.

Naïve B Cells. The product of antigen-independent B-cell differentiation is the mature, naïve (virgin) B cell, which expresses both complete surface IgM and IgD molecules; lacks TdT, CD10, and CD34; and is capable of responding to antigen. Naïve B cells have rearranged but unmutated immunoglobulin genes.[49] Each individual B cell is committed to a single light chain, either kappa or lambda, and all its progeny express the same light chain.[50] In addition to surface immunoglobulin, naïve B cells express pan–B-cell antigens (CD19, CD20, CD22, CD40, CD79a), HLA class II molecules, complement receptors (CD21, CD35), CD44, Leu-8 (L-selectin), and CD23; some also express the pan–T-cell antigen CD5.[51] Many of the surface antigens expressed by mature B cells are involved in "homing" or adhesion to vascular endothelium, interaction with antigen-presenting cells, and signal transduction. Surface immunoglobulin, CD79a, CD19, and CD20 appear to be involved in signal transduction[52]; CD22 is involved in signaling[53]; and CD40 is involved in interaction with T cells[12] and in further differentiation of B cells. Resting B cells also express the BCL2 protein, which promotes survival in the resting state.[54] CD5^{+} B cells produce immunoglobulin that often has broad specificity (cross-reactive idiotypes) and reactivity with self-antigens (autoantibodies).[51]

Morphologically, naïve B cells are small resting lymphocytes. In fetal tissues, they are the predominant lymphoid cell in the spleen; in children and adults, they circulate in the blood and also constitute a majority of the B cells in primary lymphoid follicles and follicle mantle zones (so-called recirculating B cells).[51,55] There are thought to be at least three subsets of naïve B cells: (1) a recirculating subset expressing CD23 and non–autoantigen-reactive immunoglobulin receptors, (2) a recirculating subset expressing CD23 and low-affinity autoreactive immunoglobulin receptors (also known as *B1 cells)*, and (3) a subset of sessile naïve B cells lacking CD23 and expressing non–autoantigen-reactive immunoglobulin receptors. Studies of single cells picked from the mantle zones of reactive follicles show that they are clonally diverse and contain unmutated immunoglobulin genes, consistent with naïve B cells.[56]

Chronic lymphocytic leukemia (CLL) and mantle cell lymphoma were traditionally considered neoplasms of naïve B cells (Table 8-2). However, the identification of immunoglobulin somatic mutations in subsets of these lymphomas and the recognition of a clear bias in the use of family genes and stereotyped amino acid sequences by the immunoglobulin genes in CLL has changed that view, suggesting that CLL is derived from CD5^{+} memory B cells that have experienced antigen, possibly having passed through the germinal center, or matured through an extrafollicular pathway.[57,58] Whether unmutated mantle cell lymphoma is also related to antigen-experienced cells is not yet clear, but the identification of some bias in the use of certain immunoglobulin family genes suggests that this may be the case. The gene expression profiles of both mutated and unmutated CLL cells have more similarities to memory B cells than to either naïve or germinal center B cells.[59]

Antigen-Dependent B-Cell Differentiation

T-Cell–Independent B-Cell Reaction. Some antigens, particularly those with repeat structures, are able to trigger a B-cell immune reaction without T-cell cooperation. These antigens may activate the B cells directly or may be presented by antigen-presenting cells. When naïve B cells encounter antigen, they transform into proliferating blast cells; some of the daughter cells mature into short-lived plasma cells, producing the IgM antibody of the primary immune response, but no memory cells are generated.[50,60-62] These antibodies have a lower affinity for antigen than the antibodies generated in the T-cell–dependent immune reaction because somatic hypermutation in the immunoglobulin genes is not induced or occurs at a low level. Studies of the T-cell–independent immune response in the spleen have shown that naïve B cells from the marginal zone are activated and rapidly transform into plasmablasts that localize in the sinuses. These cells are supported in part by dendritic cells to survive through signals mediated by BAFF and APRIL (a proliferation-inducing ligand), that stimulate the nuclear factor-κB (NF-κB) pathway in the activated B cells.[63-65] These signals likely have an effect similar to CD40L-CD40 interactions in the germinal center.

T-Cell–Dependent Germinal Center Reaction. Later in the primary response (within 3 to 7 days of antigen challenge in experimental animals) and in secondary responses, the T-cell–dependent germinal center reaction occurs. The mechanisms triggering this response are not fully understood, but it seems that the type of antigen is an essential element. Each germinal center is formed from 3 to 10 naïve B cells and ultimately contains approximately 10,000 to 15,000 B cells; thus, more than 10 generations are required to form a germinal center.[56,61] Proliferating IgM^{+} B blasts formed from naïve B cells that have encountered antigen in the T-cell zone (paracortex) migrate into the center of the primary follicle and fill the FDC meshwork by about 3 days after antigen stimulation, forming a germinal center.[61,66]

The movement from the T cell to the follicular area is determined by the upregulation of CXCR5 in the primed B and T cells. This receptor binds to the CXCL13 ligand produced by the FDCs and adjacent stromal cells (see Table 8-1).[67] The germinal center reaction is an efficient mechanism to generate expanded B-cell clones with a highly selected antigen receptor and two types of effector cells—memory B cells and long-lived plasma cells. This process includes four major steps: proliferation, induction of immunoglobulin somatic hypermutation and class switch, selection, and differentiation.

An important event in germinal center development is the expression of BCL6 protein, a nuclear zinc-finger transcription factor expressed by both centroblasts and centrocytes and germinal center T cells, but not by naïve or memory B cells, mantle cells, or plasma cells.[68,69] The upregulation of this gene is necessary for germinal center formation, and its transcription program targets a series of genes directly involved in the basic mechanisms of the germinal center reaction.[70] BCL6 downregulates genes involved in negative cell cycle regulations and the genotoxic response. One of the major targets is *p53*. Its inhibition in the germinal center leads to the downregulation of the cell cycle inhibitor p21 and consequently facilitates proliferation. In addition, the downregulation of *p53* as well as *ATM* and *ATR*, genes involved in the cell response to DNA damage, facilitates the germinal center cells' tolerance to the DNA breaks and rearrangements that occur during the somatic hypermutation and class switch process. Finally, BCL6 represses the differentiation of centrocytes to plasma cells and memory cells, particularly by inhibiting the plasma cell differentiation transcription factor BLIMP1, among others.[70]

Proliferation. The antigen-stimulated B blasts differentiate into centroblasts, which appear at about 4 days and accumulate at the dark zone of the germinal center.[54,61,71,72] These cells have a rapid cell cycle that is completed in 6 to 12 hours. This high proliferation is associated with the inactivation of cell cycle inhibitors and the expression of cell cycle activators. However, the expression program of these cells also differs from that of proliferative cells in other tissues. Thus, centroblasts activate telomerase to prevent the shortening of telomeres in each cell cycle. In addition, centroblasts downregulate antiapoptotic genes, such as *BCL2* and other members of the family, and they upregulate proapoptotic molecules such as CD95 (Fas). The effect of this proapoptotic default program is to facilitate the survival of only those cells that will be rescued by the generation of highly selected receptors to the specific antigen present in the germinal center.[70]

Somatic Hypermutation. Centroblasts undergo somatic hypermutation of the immunoglobulin V region genes, which

Table 8-2 Immunohistologic and Genetic Features and Postulated Normal Counterpart of Common B-Cell Neoplasms

Neoplasm	Postulated Normal Counterpart	sIg; cIg	CD20	CD5	CD10	CD23	CD43	CD103	Cyclin D1	CD38/ CD138	Genetic Abnormality	Immunoglobulin Genes
Chronic lymphocytic leukemia	Antigen-experienced B cell	+; –/+	+ (weak)	+	–	+	+	–	–	–	Trisomy 21; del(13q); del(11q); del(17p)	R, U (50%); M (50%)
Lymphoplasmacytic lymphoma	Post-follicular B cell that differentiates to plasma cell?	+; +	+	–	–	–	+/–	–	–	+	del 6(q23)	R, M
Hairy cell leukemia	Memory B cell?	+; –	+	–	–	–	+	++	+/–	–	None known	R, M
Splenic marginal zone lymphoma	Marginal zone cells	+; –/+	+	–	–	–	–	+	–	–	del 7(q31-32)	R, M
Follicular lymphoma	Germinal center cell	+; –	+	–	+/–	–/+	–	–	–	–	t(14;18); BCL2	R, M, O
Mantle cell lymphoma	Mantle zone cell Antigen-experienced cell?	+; –	+	+	–	–	+	–	+	–	t(11;14); cyclin D1	R, U (70%), M (30%)
MALT lymphoma	Marginal zone cell	+; +/–	+	–	–	–/+	–/+	–	–	–	Trisomy 3 t(11;18); t(14;18) *MALT1*; t(1;14) *BCL10*; t(3;14) *FOXP1*	R, M, O
Diffuse large B-cell lymphoma	Germinal center cell Activated B cell	+/–; –/+	+	–	–/+	NA	–/+	NA	–	–	t(14;18), t(8;14), t(3q27); *BCL2, MYC, BCL6, BLIMP1* mutation, NF-κB pathway mutation	R, M (O in germinal center B-cell type)
Burkitt's lymphoma	Germinal center cell	+; –	+	–	+	–	–	NA	–	–	t(8;14), t(2;8), t(8;22), *MYC*, EBV$^{-/+}$	R, M
Plasmablastic lymphoma	Plasmablast	+	–	–	–/+	–	–	–	–	+	?, EBV^{+}	R, M, U
Plasma cell myeloma	Bone marrow plasma cell	+	–/+	–	+/–	–	–/+	–	–/+	+	Hyperdiploidy del(13q14) t(11;14), t(14;16), t(4;14), t(6;14), t(14;20)	

+, >90% positive; +/–, >50% positive; –/+, <50% positive; –, <10% positive.

cIg, cytoplasmic immunoglobulin; EBV, Epstein-Barr virus; M, immunoglobulin gene hypermutated; MALT, mucosa-associated lymphoid tissue; NA, not available; NF-κB, nuclear factor-κB; O, ongoing immunoglobulin gene mutations; R, immunoglobulin gene rearranged; sIg, surface immunoglobulin; U, immunoglobulin gene unmutated.

alters the antigen affinity of the antibody produced by the cell.[73,74] This process requires the activity of AID, which is induced in these cells. Somatic hypermutation results in marked intraclonal diversity of antibody-combining sites in a population of cells derived from only a few precursors. Studies of single centroblasts picked from the dark zone of germinal centers suggest that in the early stages, a germinal center may contain about 5 to 10 clones of centroblasts, which show only a moderate amount of immunoglobulin V region gene mutation; later, the number of clones diminishes to as few as three, and the degree of somatic mutation increases.[56] This process introduces somatic mutations in other genes expressed in the germinal center, such as *BCL6* and *PAX5*, although at a lower frequency than is seen in the immunoglobulin genes.[75-77]

Selection. Centroblasts mature to nonproliferating centrocytes, which accumulate in the opposite pole of the germinal center—the light zone. Centrocytes reexpress surface immunoglobulin, which has the same VDJ rearrangement as the parent naïve B cell and the centroblast of the dark zone. Cells in the light zone also undergo heavy-chain class switch, which changes the IgM constant region to IgG, IgA, or, less commonly, IgE. This process also requires the enzyme AID. The somatic hypermutation alters the antigen binding site of the antibody.[56] Centrocytes whose immunoglobulin gene mutations have resulted in *decreased* affinity for antigen rapidly die by apoptosis (programmed cell death); the prominent "starry sky" pattern of phagocytic macrophages seen in germinal centers at this stage is a result of the apoptosis of centrocytes. In contrast, centrocytes whose immunoglobulin gene mutations have resulted in *increased* affinity are able to bind to native, unprocessed antigen trapped in antigen-antibody complexes by the complement receptors on the processes of FDCs. The centrocytes are able to process the antigen and present it to T cells in the light zone of the germinal center. The activated T cells express CD40 ligand (CD40L), which can engage CD40 on the B cell. Both ligation of the antigen receptor by antigen and ligation of CD40 on the surfaces of germinal center B cells "rescues" them from apoptosis.[50,66,71,72,78]

Differentiation. Termination of the germinal center program and post–germinal center differentiation of selected centrocytes into plasma cells or memory B cells require inactivation of the master regulator BCL6. This inactivation probably involves several mechanisms. The increasing signaling activity from the selected high-affinity B-cell receptor induces the ubiquitination of BCL6 and subsequent degradation. Similarly, the CD40-CD40L activation of B cells induces the expression of the transcription factor IRF4, which represses BCL6.[70] The stimulus to direct the rescued centrocytes into memory B cells is not clear, but interaction with the numerous T cells present in the light zone, through CD40-CD40L, appears to be important in the generation of these cells.[61,66] The plasma cell differentiation pathway involves the upregulation of IRF4 and BLIMP1 and the inactivation of PAX5. IRF4 and BLIMP1 seem to cooperate as potent inductors of plasma cell differentiation, whereas PAX5, which has maintained the B-cell program from the early stages of B-cell differentiation, needs to be shut off to allow plasma cells to develop. The transcription of BLIMP1 is negatively regulated by BCL6, and this inhibition is released by the downregulation of BCL6 at the end of the germinal center program. BLIMP1, in turn, represses PAX5, opening the pathway to plasma cell differentiation. BLIMP1 also stimulates the transcription of XBP1, which is required to maintain and tolerate the reticulum stress signals that appear during the secretory phenotype of the plasma cells.[70,79]

Most B-cell lymphomas originate in cells derived from the germinal center (see Table 8-2). The paradigm is follicular lymphoma, which recapitulates the whole organization of the secondary follicle. The basic oncogenic mechanism is the t(14;18) translocation, which constitutively upregulates BCL2 in a tissue compartment that physiologically represses its expression. Burkitt's lymphoma has the phenotype and expression profile of a germinal center cell and carries the t(8;14) translocation that activates *MYC*. Gene expression array profiling has identified two major molecular subtypes of diffuse large B-cell lymphoma (DLBCL): a germinal center B-cell (GCB) type and an activated B-cell (ABC) type. The GCB type of DLBCL is probably related to the centroblastic compartment of the germinal center, whereas the ABC type has features of a B cell committed to secretory differentiation.[80] DLBCL has frequent translocations involving *BCL6*, and interestingly, some ABC-type DLBCLs, but not GCB types, carry inactivating *BLIMP1* mutations. These alterations may interfere with the normal differentiation process of the cells, facilitating malignant transformation.[81] In addition, DLBCL carries multiple gene mutations that constitutively activate survival of the NF-κB pathway.[82,83]

Memory B Cells. Antigen-specific memory B cells generated in the germinal center reaction leave the follicle and are detectable in the peripheral blood and different tissue compartments, mainly in the marginal zones. The memory B cells seem to be composed of different subsets of cells. The initial idea of memory cells was represented by the class-switched B cells expressing IgG, IgA, or IgE with somatic mutations. However, a large subpopulation of memory cells expresses only IgM, without having undergone the immunoglobulin class switch.[84,85] These cells are detected in the peripheral blood and represent 10% of all B cells, whereas the class-switched cells account for 15% and the naïve cells for about 75%. Similar IgM memory cells are present in tissues, particularly in splenic and MALT marginal zones, tonsils, and lymph nodes.

On rechallenge with antigen, splenic marginal zone B cells migrate first into the germinal center and then quickly appear in the T-cell zone as immunoglobulin-positive blast cells, which give rise to antigen-specific plasma cells; thus, they are thought to be memory B cells.[61] Studies on single marginal zone B cells from the spleen and Peyer's patches show that they have mutated V region genes, may be oligoclonal, and are not clonally related to the adjacent germinal center.[86-88]

Intriguingly, a population of IgM^+, IgD^+, $CD27^+$ B cells has been detected in the human peripheral blood and splenic marginal zone; these cells have low levels of somatic mutations, suggesting antigen exposure, but a high clonal diversity that resembles that observed in naïve B cells. These cells are similar to the low mutated B cells generated in patients with hyper-IgM syndrome owing to a CD40-CD40L genetic deficiency, in whom the germinal center reaction is not generated. These patients have a subset of IgM^+, IgD^+, $CD27^+$ B cells with a low frequency of somatic mutations that have been generated in a T-cell–independent pathway. Such observations suggest that the B cells populating the marginal zone are heterogeneous and include IgM-only memory cells and some cells with low levels of somatic mutations generated in a T-cell–independent pathway.[67,89]

Monocytoid B lymphocytes are cells that resemble marginal zone B cells but have even more nuclear indentation and abundant cytoplasm. These cells occur in clusters adjacent to subcapsular and cortical sinuses of some reactive lymph nodes,[90] peripheral to and often continuous with the follicle marginal zone. In contrast to marginal zone B cells, the monocytoid B cells found in reactive lymph nodes appear to have either unmutated immunoglobulin V region genes or only a small number of randomly distributed mutations that do not suggest selection by antigen.[88]

Nodal and splenic tumors resembling normal marginal zone and monocytoid B cells have been described (see Table 8-2).[91-94] Analysis of immunoglobulin V region genes suggest that most of these have mutations consistent with germinal center exposure and antigen selection.[95,96] In addition, about 50% of B-cell CLLs or small lymphocytic lymphomas have mutated immunoglobulin V region genes and appear to correspond to a CD5$^+$ memory B-cell subset.[97]

Plasma Cells. Plasma cells are heterogeneous. The precursor of a mature, antibody-secreting plasma cell is a cell that retains proliferating activity, known as a *plasmablast*. Mature plasma cells are divided into short- and long-lived subsets.[79] Plasmablasts express MHC but lose mature B-cell markers such as CD20 and PAX5 and the CXCR5 and CCR7 receptors that maintain the lymphoid cells in the B and T compartments in response to CXCL13, CCL19, and CCL21. They acquire CXCR4, which attracts the cells to the CXCL12-secreting tissues in the bone marrow and other plasma cell niches, such as the lymph node medullary cords and splenic red pulp cords.[79]

Short-lived IgM-secreting plasma cells are generated in the T-cell–independent immune response, whereas long-lived IgM$^+$, class-switched plasma cells are effector cells of the T-cell–dependent immune response. IgG-producing plasma cells accumulate in the lymph node medulla and splenic cords, but it appears that the immediate precursor of the bone marrow plasma cell leaves the node and migrates to the bone marrow.

Plasma cells lose surface immunoglobulin, pan–B-cell antigens, HLA-DR, CD40, and CD45, and cytoplasmic IgM, IgG, or IgA accumulates. Plasma cells also express CD38 and CD138 (syndecan). PAX5 is lost at the plasma cell stage, whereas BLIMP1, XBP1, and IRF4/MUM1 are expressed. These cells have rearranged and mutated immunoglobulin genes, but they do not have the ongoing mutations seen in follicle center cells.

Tumors of bone marrow–homing plasma cells correspond to osseous plasmacytoma and plasma cell myeloma (see Table 8-2). Some aggressive lymphomas have the morphology and cell proliferation activity of centroblasts or immunoblasts but the immunophenotype of plasma cells (lack of mature B-cell markers and expression of CD38 and CD138) and may correspond to the malignant counterpart of plasmablasts (see Table 8-2). These lymphomas include plasmablastic lymphoma, primary effusion lymphoma, and large B-cell lymphomas associated with multicentric Castleman's disease.[98]

Mucosa-Associated Lymphoid Tissue. A subset of B cells, including all the differentiation stages listed earlier, are programmed for gut-associated rather than nodal lymphoid tissue. In these tissues (Waldeyer's ring, Peyer's patches, mesenteric nodes), similar responses to antigen occur, but both the intermediate and end-stage B cells that originate in the gut or mesenteric lymph nodes preferentially return there rather than to the peripheral lymph nodes or bone marrow. Thus, the plasma cells generated in gut-associated lymphoid tissue home preferentially to the lamina propria rather than to the bone marrow.[38,39] The mechanisms facilitating this tissue-specific traffic of effector cells include chemokines and their receptors and different adhesion molecules (see earlier).

Many extranodal low-grade B-cell lymphomas are thought to arise from MALT (see Table 8-2).[99] Because most MALT lymphomas contain prominent marginal zone–type B cells, in addition to small B lymphocytes and plasma cells, and because similar lymphomas occur in non-MALT sites, the term *extranodal marginal zone lymphoma of MALT type* has been proposed for these tumors.[100] MALT-type lymphomas have somatically mutated V region genes, consistent with an antigen-selected post–germinal center B-cell stage.[101]

T-Cell Differentiation

Antigen-Independent T-Cell Differentiation

Cortical Thymocytes. The earliest antigen-independent stages of T-cell differentiation occur in the bone marrow; later stages occur in the thymic cortex. The exact site at which precursor cells become committed to the T lineage is not known because the thymus contains cells that can differentiate into either T cells or NK cells, but not B cells.[102] The earliest thymic precursors are able to generate T and NK cells. Cortical thymocytes are lymphoblasts that contain the intranuclear enzyme TdT. The earliest committed T-cell precursors are CD34$^+$ and CD45RA$^+$; express the CD13 and CD33 antigens usually associated with myeloid cells; and lack CD3, CD4, and CD8 ("triple negative" cells). Within the thymus they sequentially acquire CD1a, CD2, CD5, and cytoplasmic CD3, and first the CD4 "helper" and then the CD8 "suppressor" antigen ("double positive"). In the thymus, rearrangement of the TCR genes is initiated, beginning with the gamma and delta chains, followed by the beta and then the alpha chain genes; these proteins are then expressed on the cell surface. Surface CD3 expression appears at the same time as expression of the T-cell antigen receptor beta chain, with which it is closely associated, and participates in signal transduction. Cortical thymocytes express the CD45RO epitope of the leukocyte common antigen instead of CD45RA[103] and lack the antiapoptosis protein BCL2.[54]

In addition to providing a pool of mature T cells through the proliferation of precursor cells, the thymus plays a major role in the selection of T cells so that the resulting pool of mature T cells recognizes self-HLA molecules, in which antigen is presented to T cells, and does not react to self-antigens. Both positive and negative selection occurs in the thymus at the double-positive (CD4$^+$, CD8$^+$) stage. Thymocytes that have anti-self specificity bind strongly via their TCR alpha-beta complex to self-antigens presented by MHC molecules on thymic dendritic cells, and they die by apoptosis. Those that lack anti-self reactivity are positively selected for strong reactivity with self-HLA molecules on thymic epithelial cells. These selected cells then express increased levels of surface CD3, acquire CD27 and CD69, switch their CD45 isotype from RO back to RA, lose CD1a, express BCL2, and lose either CD4 or CD8 to become mature, naïve T cells.[102]

The tumor that corresponds to the stages of T-cell differentiation in the thymic cortex is T-lymphoblastic lymphoma/leukemia; the varieties of immunophenotypes and antigen receptor gene rearrangements found in precursor T-cell neoplasia correspond to the stages of intrathymic T-cell differentiation.

Naïve T Cells. Mature, naïve (virgin) T cells have the morphologic appearance of small lymphocytes, have a low proliferation fraction, lack TdT and CD1, and express either CD4 or CD8 (but not both), as well as surface CD3 and CD5,[104] CD45RA, and BCL2.[54,103] These cells leave the thymus and can be found in the circulation, in the paracortex of lymph nodes, and in the thymic medulla.

These are migratory cells with a surveillance function. They arrive at the secondary lymphoid tissues via the bloodstream and exit the circulation through the HEVs in the nodes and MALT and through the sinusoids in the spleen. Naïve T cells express CCR7 and CD62L (L-selectin), which are instrumental at these sites, by recognizing the CCL21 and vascular addressins, respectively, expressed by the HEVs.

Some cases of T-cell prolymphocytic leukemia and peripheral T-cell lymphoma, unspecified, may correspond to naïve T cells (Table 8-3).

Antigen-Dependent T-Cell Differentiation

A complex interaction of T-cell surface molecules with molecules on the surface of antigen-presenting cells is required for T-cell activation in response to antigen.[12] On the T cell, the CD4 or CD8 molecules bind to MHC class II or class I molecules, respectively, on the antigen-presenting cell. A complex of CD3 and the T-cell antigen receptor (which may be either gamma-delta or alpha-beta and has a combining site that "fits" the specific peptide antigen) binds to the antigen-MHC complex on the antigen-presenting cell. The adhesion molecule LFA-1 on the T cell binds to ICAM-1 on the antigen-presenting cell; the activation-associated molecule CD40L on the T cell binds to CD40; and CD28 and CTLA4 on the T cell bind to B7-1 (CD80) and B7-2 (CD86) on the antigen-presenting cell.[16] The binding of CD40-CD40L provides an activation stimulus for both the T cell and the antigen-presenting cell, and binding of CD28 or CTLA4 to B7 provides a crucial second stimulus for the T cell, without which anergy develops.[105] In addition, both the T cell and the antigen-presenting cell release stimulatory molecules, such as interferon-γ and interleukins, which provide further mutual activation stimuli.[12]

T Immunoblasts. On encountering antigen, mature T cells transform into immunoblasts, which are large cells with prominent nucleoli and basophilic cytoplasm that may be indistinguishable from B immunoblasts. T immunoblasts, in contrast to T lymphoblasts (thymocytes), are TdT$^-$ and CD1$^-$, strongly express pan–T-cell antigens, and continue to express either CD4 or CD8 (not both). Activated or proliferating T cells express HLA-DR, as well as CD25 (IL-2 receptor) and both CD71 and CD38. Antigen-dependent T-cell reactions occur in the paracortex of lymph nodes and the periarteriolar lymphoid sheath of the spleen, as well as at extranodal sites of immunologic reactions.

Effector T Cells. From the T-immunoblastic reaction come antigen-specific effector T cells of either CD4 or CD8 type, as well as memory T cells. Antigen-stimulated T cells switch their CD45 isotype from CD45RA to CD45RO. Effector T cells of the CD4 type typically act as helper cells, and those of the CD8 type as suppressor cells in vitro. However, both types can be cytotoxic.[106] CD4 cells are cytotoxic to cells that display antigen complexed with MHC class II antigen, and CD8 cells are cytotoxic to cells that display it complexed with MHC class I antigen. Activated CD8$^+$ cells produce interferon-γ and have cytoplasmic cytotoxic granules containing granzyme-B, perforin, and TIA-1, which permit their recognition in tissue sections.

Different subsets of specialized CD4$^+$ effector cells are now recognized. Three subsets, T-helper 1 (Th1), Th2, and Th17, are involved mainly in cytokine production. Thus, Th1 cells secrete interferon-γ and are important activators of macrophages, NK cells, and CD8$^+$ cells. These cells seem to be involved mainly in systemic immunity. Th2 cells secrete IL-4, IL-5, IL-6, IL-13, and IL-25. These cells mobilize eosinophils, basophils, mast cells, and alternatively activated macrophages. Th17 cells produce IL-17 and tumor necrosis factor-α and regulate acute inflammation. T-bet, Gata-3, and RORγ are critical transcription factors in the commitment of these CD4 subsets, respectively. CD4 cells involved in the B-cell response seem to constitute a specific subset of T_{FH} cells. These cells express CXCR5 and are recruited by the CXCL13 produced in the germinal centers. They also express the costimulatory molecule ICOS and the receptor PD1 (CD276), and a subset is CD57$^+$. A subpopulation of CD4$^+$ T-reg cells is increasingly recognized as an important element to limit the expansion of the immune responses. These cells express CD25 and secrete IL-10 and are generated by the activity of the transcription factor FOXP3.

After the clearance of the pathogens, most T cells undergo apoptosis. However, a small subset of memory T cells persists for a long time, often for the life of the host.

Most cases of peripheral T-cell lymphoma are thought to correspond to stages of antigen-dependent T-cell differentiation (see Table 8-3). Angioimmunoblastic T-cell lymphoma seems to be a malignant counterpart of T_{FH} cells.[107] Mycosis fungoides corresponds to a mature effector CD4$^+$ cell, and T-cell large granular lymphocytic leukemia corresponds to a mature effector CD8$^+$ cell—however, the relationship between neoplastic and normal T cells is not nearly as well understood as in the B-cell system. The systemic symptoms such as fever, rashes, and hemophagocytic syndromes associated with some peripheral T-cell lymphomas may be a consequence of cytokine production by the neoplastic T cells.

Differentiation of Cells of the Innate Immune Response

The innate immune system is conserved through evolution and constitutes a first line of defense based on relatively nonspecific germline-encoded receptors. The cells involved in the innate immune response are localized mainly in barriers such as mucosa and skin and do not require antigen-presenting

Table 8-3 Immunohistologic and Genetic Features and Postulated Normal Counterpart of Common T-Cell Neoplasms

Neoplasm	Postulated Normal Counterpart	CD3 (S;C)	CD5	CD7	CD4	CD8	CD30	CXCL13	TCR	NK (16, 56)	Cytotoxic Granule†	EBV	Genetic Abnormality	T-Receptor Genes
T-PLL	? Immature/ naïve T lymphocyte	+	–	+, +	+/–	–/+	–	–	αβ	–	–	–	inv14 Trisomy 8q	R
T-LGLL	?/Naïve T lymphocyte	+	–	+, +	–	+	–	–	αβ	+, –	+	–	None known	R
NK-LGLL	NK cell	–	–	+, –	–	+/–	–	–	–	–, +	+	+	None known	G
Extranodal NK/T-cell lymphoma	NK cell	–; +	–	–/+	–	–	–	–	–	NA, +	+	++	None known	G
Hepatosplenic T-cell lymphoma	Gamma-delta T cell	+	–	+	–	–	–	–	γδ > αβ	+, –/+	+	–	Iso 7q	R
Enteropathy-type T-cell lymphoma	Intraepithelial T lymphocyte	+	+	+	–	+/–	+/–	–	αβ >> γδ	–	+	–	None known	R
Mycosis fungoides	Mature skin-homing CD4+ T cell	+	+	–/+	+	–	–	–	αβ	–	–	–	None known	R
Subcutaneous panniculitis-like T-cell lymphoma	Mature cytotoxic alpha-beta T cell	+	+/–	+/–	+/–	–	++	–	αβ	–	–/+	–	None known	R
Primary cutaneous gamma-delta T-cell lymphoma	Gamma-delta T cell	+	+	+	–	+	–/+	–	γδ	–, +/–	+	–	None known	R
PTCL, NOS	Mature T cell	+/–	+/–	+/–	+/–	–/+	–/+	–	αβ > γδ	–/+	–/+	–/+	inv 14, complex	R
Angioimmunoblastic T-cell lymphoma	Follicular T-helper cell	+	+	+	+/–	–/+	–	+	αβ	–	NA	+/–	None known	R
ALK+ ALCL	?	+/–	+/–	NA	–/+	–/+	++	–	αβ	–	+	–	t(2;5); *NPM/ALK*	R

+, >90% positive; +/–, >50% positive; –/+, <50% positive; –, <10% positive.

ALCL, anaplastic large cell lymphoma; ALK, anaplastic lymphoid kinase; C, cytoplasmic; EBV, Epstein-Barr virus; G, ; Ig, immunoglobulin; M, mutated; NA, not available; NK, natural killer; NK-LGLL, NK-cell large granular lymphocytic leukemia; PTCL, NOS, peripheral T-cell lymphoma, not otherwise specified; R, rearranged; S, surface; TCR, T-cell receptor gene; T-LGLL, T-cell large granular lymphocytic leukemia; T-PLL, T-cell prolymphocytic leukemia.

†Cytotoxic granule = TIA-1, perforin, and/or granzyme.

cells or the association of antigens with the MHC. The main lymphoid cells involved in innate immune responses are NK cells and gamma-delta T cells. Phagocytes, mast cells, eosinophils, and basophils are also involved in innate responses.

Gamma-Delta T Cells

Mature gamma-delta T cells express these two chains of the TCR. Gamma-delta TCR binds directly to the antigens and does not require specialized antigen processing and presentation, as alpha-beta T cells do. These cells do not seem to have a thymic differentiation phase and are derived directly from bone marrow precursors. They are positive for CD3, CD2, and CD7 but negative for CD4 and CD8, and they express cytotoxic granules in the cytoplasm. Gamma-delta T cells are present in mucosa, skin, and splenic red pulp. The number of these cells is low, and their function is not completely clear. They participate in innate immune responses and also in tissue repair by expressing epithelial growth factors.[108-110]

Hepatosplenic gamma-delta T-cell lymphoma and primary cutaneous gamma-delta T-cell lymphoma are considered to be neoplasms derived from these cells (see Table 8-3).

Natural Killer Cells

A third line of lymphoid cells, called *NK cells* because they can kill certain targets without sensitization and without MHC restriction, appears to derive from a common progenitor with T cells.[102] NK cells recognize self–class I MHC molecules on the surfaces of cells through killer cell immunoglobulin-like receptors, and they kill cells that lack these antigens.[111] Activated NK cells express the epsilon and zeta chains of CD3 in the cytoplasm, but these cells do not rearrange their TCR genes or express TCRs or surface CD3. They are characterized by certain NK-cell–associated antigens (CD16, CD56, CD57), which can also be expressed on some T cells; they also express some T-cell–associated antigens (CD2, CD28, CD8). Similar to gamma-delta T cells, these cells have cytotoxic granules that specifically contain granzyme-M. NK cells appear in the peripheral blood as a small proportion of circulating lymphocytes; they are usually slightly larger than most normal T and B cells, with abundant pale cytoplasm containing azurophilic granules—so-called large granular lymphocytes. Nasal NK/T-cell lymphoma and aggressive NK-cell leukemia, and possibly NK-cell large granular lymphocytic leukemia, are thought to be neoplasms of NK cells (see Table 8-3).

Pearls and Pitfalls

- The immune system has two differentiated arms—the innate and the adaptive immune system. The innate system is a first line of defense mediated by cells that express germline-coded receptors, recognize a wide but relatively nonspecific number of antigens, and do not generate immunologic memory. The adaptive system reacts specifically against antigens presented to lymphocytes associated with the MHC. The immune cells express specific receptors encoded by somatically rearranged genes that may recognize a virtually universal spectrum of antigens and generate cells with immunologic memory.
- Lymphoid tissues are highly organized microenvironments in which different cell populations, vascular structures, and stromal components facilitate the selective interactions between lymphocytes and antigens for the initiation and expansion of immune responses.
- The follicular lymphoid germinal center is a complex structure where cells of the adaptive immune system expand clonally and the immunoglobulin gene is somatically mutated to select high-affinity receptors. The immunoglobulin gene also undergoes idiotype switch, and the cell commits to memory or plasma cells.
- The high proliferation and DNA breaks that occur in germinal center cells are mechanisms that facilitate the development of lymphoid neoplasms. Most B-cell lymphomas carry somatically mutated immunoglobulin genes, indicating that they derive from cells with germinal center experience.
- Most lymphoid neoplasms are related to a normal cell counterpart of the immune system. Some lymphomas, however, do not correspond to a known normal stage of differentiation, and others display aberrant phenotypes, lineage heterogeneity, or changes in cell lineage that may represent the malignant counterpart or the physiologic plasticity of the immune cells.

References can be found on Expert Consult @ www.expertconsult.com

Chapter 9

The Reactive Lymphadenopathies

Eric D. Hsi and Bertram Schnitzer

CHAPTER OUTLINE

The major question that confronts the surgical pathologist when examining a lymph node biopsy is whether the process is benign or malignant.[1] Familiarity with the histologic changes of a diverse group of nonneoplastic disorders is necessary to differentiate them from both Hodgkin's and non-Hodgkin's lymphomas as well as to render a specific diagnosis or differential diagnosis on morphologic grounds. A specific diagnosis often requires correlation among the morphologic features, the clinical history, and the results of additional studies such as immunohistochemistry, stains for microorganisms, cultures, serologic studies, and molecular analysis for microbial genetic material.

We group the reactive lymphadenopathies into four major categories according to their predominant architectural histologic pattern: follicular-nodular, sinus, interfollicular or mixed, and diffuse. Although this approach is convenient, multiple nodal compartments may be involved in a single process, and variation exists from case to case. Furthermore, reactive conditions of the lymph node are dynamic processes, and the predominant pattern may differ depending on when during the course of the disease the biopsy is performed.

Box 9-1 lists the major reactive conditions that cause lymph node enlargement and may result in lymph node biopsy. Several benign disorders and borderline lesions such as immune deficiency–related lymphadenopathy, sinus histiocytosis with massive lymphadenopathy, and the plasma cell variant of Castleman's disease are covered in other chapters.

FOLLICULAR AND NODULAR PATTERNS

Follicular Hyperplasia

Follicular hyperplasia is defined as an increase in the number and usually the size and shape of secondary lymphoid follicles (Fig. 9-1). It is among the most common reactive patterns encountered by the surgical pathologist. The antigens responsible are usually not known. Hyperplastic follicles contain germinal centers with a mixture of centroblasts (noncleaved cells) and centrocytes (cleaved cells) that vary in proportion depending on the duration of the immune response. Tingible body macrophages containing apoptotic cellular debris are common and impart a "starry sky" pattern to the germinal center (see Fig. 9-1A and B). The prominence of the "starry sky" pattern correlates with the proliferative index in the germinal center. Typically, some follicles show polarization of the germinal center, with a proliferative dark zone, composed mostly of centroblasts, located toward the medullary side of the germinal center, and with an apical light zone, containing a predominance of centrocytes, located on the capsular side of the follicle (Fig. 9-2A; see Fig. 9-1C). Early in a hyperplastic reaction, germinal centers may consist almost exclusively of centroblasts (Fig. 9-3). The high proliferative index is highlighted by staining with MIB-1 (Ki-67) (see Figs. 9-1D and 9-3B). Centrocytes, plasma cells, and varying numbers of T cells ($CD4^+$) and follicular dendritic cells (FDCs) are present in the light zone. FDCs have intermediate-sized, bilobed pale

Box 9-1 *The Reactive Lymphadenopathies*

Follicular and Nodular Patterns
- Follicular hyperplasia
- Autoimmune disorders (rheumatoid arthritis)
- Luetic lymphadenitis
- Castleman's disease, hyaline vascular type
- Progressive transformation of germinal centers
- Mantle zone hyperplasia
- Mycobacterial spindle cell pseudotumor

Predominantly Sinus Pattern
- Sinus histiocytosis
- Specific causes: lymphangiogram, storage disease, prosthesis, Whipple's disease
- Vascular transformation of sinuses
- Hemophagocytic syndrome

Interfollicular or Mixed Pattern
- Paracortical hyperplasia and dermatopathic reaction
- Granulomatous lymphadenitis
  - Nonnecrotizing granuloma
  - Necrotizing granuloma
  - Tuberculosis
  - Fungal infection
  - Cat-scratch disease
- Kimura's disease
- Toxoplasmic lymphadenitis
- Systemic lupus erythematosus
- Kikuchi's lymphadenitis
- Kawasaki's disease
- Inflammatory pseudotumor
- Bacillary angiomatosis

Diffuse Pattern
- Infectious mononucleosis
- Cytomegalovirus infection
- Herpes simplex lymphadenitis
- Dilantin lymphadenopathy

nuclei that contain small central nucleoli; many are binucleated, with opposing nuclear membranes appearing flattened (see Fig. 9-2B). A variably prominent mantle zone composed of small lymphocytes surrounds the germinal center. In a polarized germinal center, the mantle zone is expanded around the light zone (see Fig. 9-1C). Other features of follicular hyperplasia include large, irregular germinal centers with oddly shaped geographic outlines (see Fig. 9-1B) and, occasionally, follicular lysis (Fig. 9-4). The latter is characterized by disrupted germinal centers due to infiltration by mantle zone lymphocytes. The interfollicular area may show variable expansion with scattered transformed cells, small lymphocytes, plasma cells, and high endothelial venules.

Germinal centers are composed predominantly of $CD20^+$ B cells, with varying numbers of $CD4^+$ T cells and $CD57^+$ cells as well as $PD\text{-}1^+$ cells.[1a] BCL2 is not expressed by reactive germinal center B cells, whereas BCL6 and CD10 are expressed in both benign and neoplastic germinal center B cells. A subset of inter- and intrafollicular T cells coexpresses CD4 and BCL6.[2]

Differential Diagnosis

The main differential diagnosis in follicular hyperplasia is follicular lymphoma. Features that favor a benign process include polarization, tingible body macrophages with a "starry sky" pattern, the presence of plasma cells within follicles, and a well-defined mantle zone. Immunostains show a lack of BCL2 protein in B cells.[3,4] Because T cells express BCL2, this stain should always be interpreted in conjunction with B- and T-cell markers so that relative percentages of each type of cell can be determined, allowing appropriate interpretation of the BCL2 stain. Although the t(14;18)(q32;q21) transformation, characteristic of follicular lymphoma, may be detected in hyperplastic lymph nodes by polymerase chain reaction (PCR),[5] this finding does not appear to be a significant problem with assays that have a sensitivity of 1 in 10^4 or less.[6]

Monocytoid B-Cell Proliferation

Follicular hyperplasia may be associated with the proliferation of monocytoid B cells in and around cortical sinuses, around venules, or in a parafollicular location.[7-9] Although this proliferation may be associated with nonspecific follicular hyperplasia (Fig. 9-5), it is characteristic of *Toxoplasma* lymphadenitis, human immundeficiency virus (HIV)–associated lymphadenopathy, cytomegalovirus (CMV) lymphadenitis, and disorders associated with suppurative granulomas, especially cat-scratch disease. Monocytoid B cells are medium-sized cells with abundant pale to clear cytoplasm and round to slightly indented nuclei with moderately dispersed chromatin. Neutrophils and immunoblasts are usually scattered among the monocytoid cells (see Fig. 9-5). The differential diagnosis when the monocytoid B-cell proliferation is prominent includes marginal zone (monocytoid B-cell) lymphoma. Although this differentiation may be difficult in some cases, evidence of light-chain restriction is diagnostic of lymphoma and can be established in paraffin sections if plasmacytoid differentiation is present. Morphologic features favoring lymphoma include partial effacement of the architecture and increased numbers of large cells with an increased mitotic index. Molecular genetic analysis for immunoglobulin (Ig) gene rearrangement by PCR may be helpful.

Autoimmune Disorders: Rheumatoid Arthritis

Patients with autoimmune disorders such as rheumatoid arthritis (RA), juvenile rheumatoid arthritis, and Sjögren's syndrome often develop lymphadenopathy characterized by follicular hyperplasia.[10-13] Although biopsies are not ordinarily performed in these patients, they may be done if there is clinical suspicion of lymphoma. The features of RA-associated lymphadenopthy are well characterized, and RA is the focus of this secton.

The lymph node histologic changes seen in RA are follicular hyperplasia, inter- and intrafollicular plasmacytosis, and neutrophils within sinuses (Fig. 9-6).[10,13] The lymph node capsule may be thickened but is not infiltrated by plasma cells. The lymphoid reaction may expand into perinodal tissue but does not necessarily denote malignancy. Compared with nonspecific follicular hyperplasia, the reactive germinal centers of RA are smaller and more regularly spaced, with a predominance of centrocytes exhibiting less mitotic activity.[13] Immunohistochemical studies have shown that $CD4^+$ T cells predominate in the interfollicular areas, with $CD8^+$ T cells within germinal centers.[10,13] Increased numbers of polytypic $CD5^+$ B cells, which may be expanded in autoimmune disor-

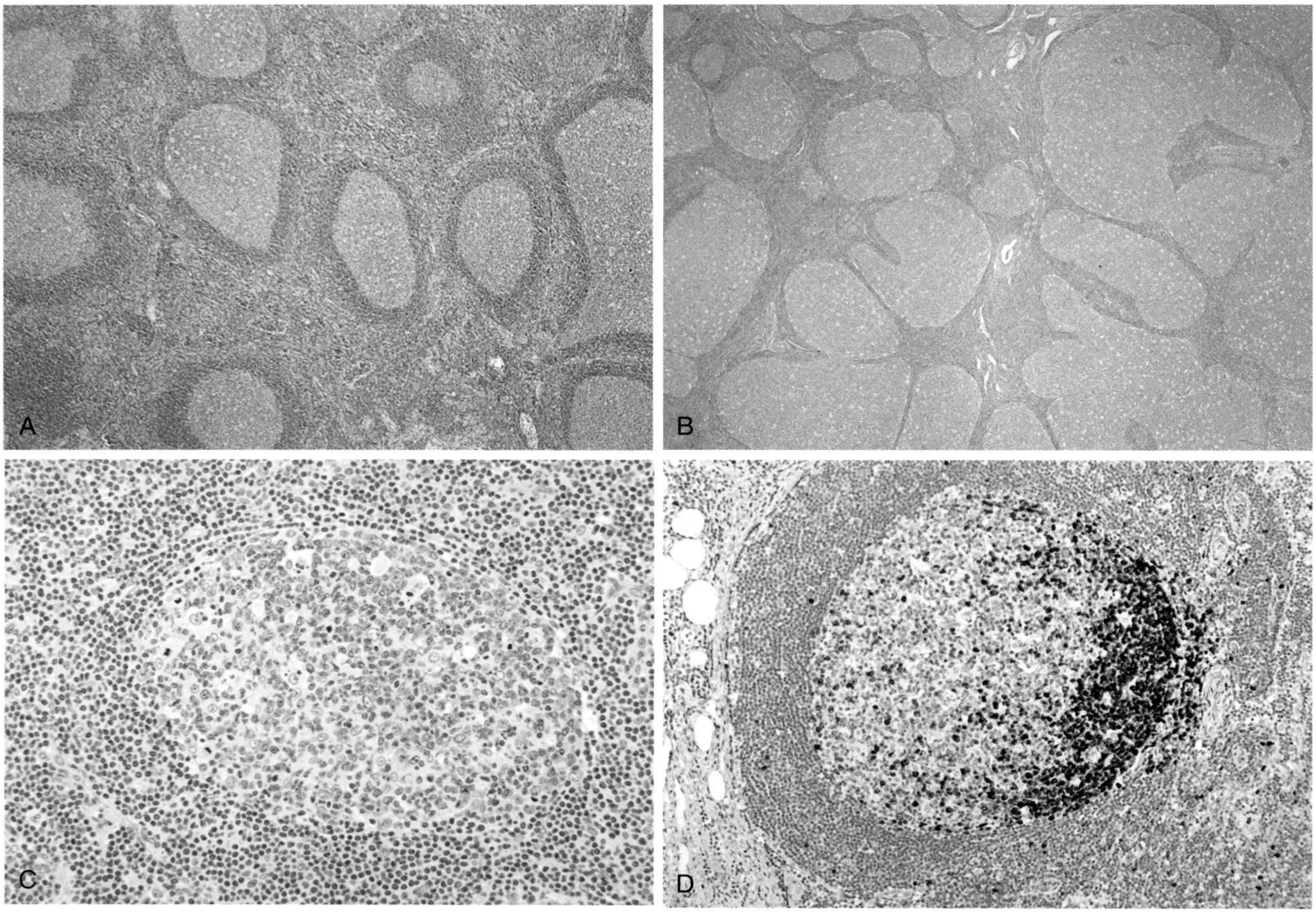

Figure 9-1. Follicular hyperplasia. A, Increased numbers of follicles with large, irregular germinal centers; preserved mantle zones; and ample interfollicular areas. **B**, Germinal centers may be large and irregular, forming large, bizarre structures. **C**, Polarization of the germinal center with a dark zone composed of centroblasts and tingible body macrophages and a light zone with a predominance of centrocytes. **D**, MIB-1 stain showing that almost all cells in the dark zone are positive. The mantle zone is expanded adjacent to the light zone.

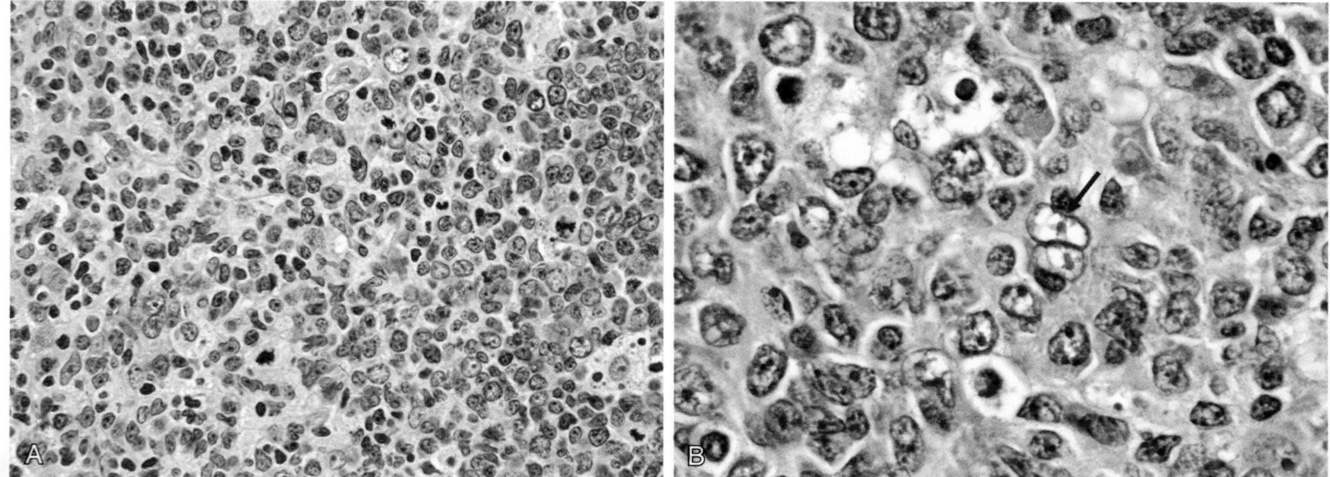

Figure 9-2. A, Higher magnification of a germinal center. The light zone (*left*) shows a predominance of centrocytes, whreas the dark zone (*right*) contains mostly centroblasts interspersed with tingible body macrophages. **B**, Follicular dendritic cell (*arrow*). These cells have cleared chromatin with a small central nucleolus; they often appear bilobed, with flattening of the nuclear membranes.

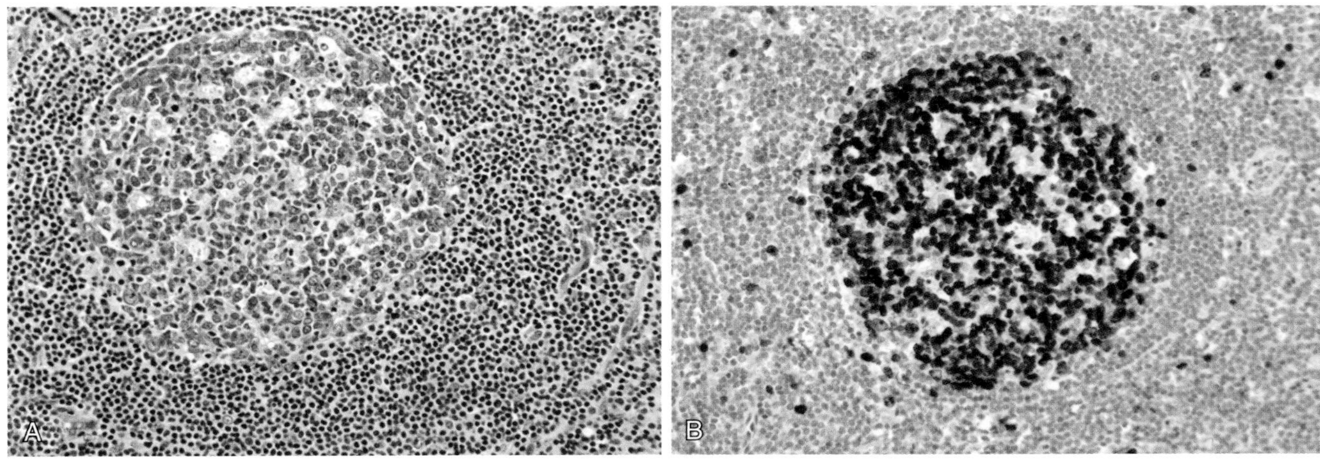

Figure 9-3. A, Germinal center consisting almost exclusively of centroblasts. Tingible body macrophages are scattered throughout. **B,** MIB-1 staining of the germinal center in **A** showing positivity in all centroblasts, indicating that these cells are proliferating.

ders, may be seen.[10] These features are also seen in other disorders such as Sjögren's syndrome. Monocytoid B-cell hyperplasia is more frequent in the latter.

The differential diagnosis of follicular hyperplasia associated with RA includes follicular hyperplasia due to other causes. The presence of plasma cells within germinal centers should raise the suspicion of RA or another autoimmune disorder. Appropriate clinical history and laboratory findings should help confirm the diagnosis of RA-associated lymphadenopathy.

Syphilis may show histologic features similar to those in RA (see later). However, granulomas, infiltration of the thickened capsule by plasma cells and lymphocytes, and endarteritis or venulitis are typically present. Special stains for spirochetes may be diagnostic. HIV infection, particularly early in the course of the disease, may show histologic changes similar to those in RA. Follicular lymphoma might also be considered in the differential diagnosis. Demonstration of BCL2 protein–positive germinal center B cells or the presence of t(14;18)(q32;q21) confirms the diagnosis of follicular lymphoma, although their absence does not exclude a diagnosis of follicular lymphoma.[14]

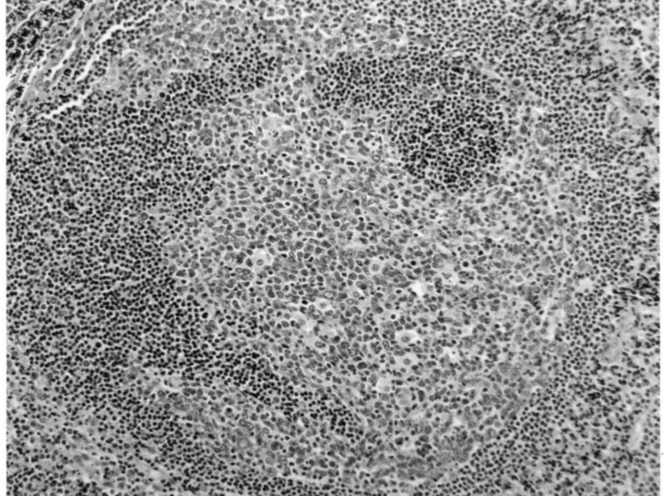

Figure 9-4. Follicular lysis of a germinal center. Mantle cell lymphocytes infiltrating and disrupting the germinal center.

In follicular hyperplasia associated with Sjögren's syndrome, marginal zone lymphoma should be excluded. Features suggesting lymphoma include large confluent areas of monocytoid B cells. Demonstration of monoclonality may be necessary to confirm the diagnosis in cases of follicular hyperplasia with extensive monocytoid B-cell proliferation.[15]

Luetic Lymphadenitis

Although lymph node biopsy does not play a significant role in the diagnosis of syphilis, the localized or generalized lymphadenopathy of primary and secondary syphilis may be clinically suspicious for lymphoma, and biopsies may be performed.[16] The typical histologic picture is follicular hyperplasia with interfollicular plasmacytosis, similar to that seen in RA-associated lymphadenopathy.[16,17] Features that point to luetic lymphadenitis include capsular and trabecular fibrosis with infiltration by plasma cells and lymphocytes (Fig. 9-7). Sarcoid-type or, rarely, suppurative granulomas in the paracortex, clusters of epithelioid histiocytes, and endarteritis or venulitits may be present.[18] Rarely, a suppurative form of syphilitic lymphadenitis produces a necrotizing lymphadenitis. Warthin-Starry or Steiner stains may demonstrate spirochetes anywhere in the lymph node, but they are most consistently found within the walls of blood vessels and epithelioid histiocytes.[16] Spirochetes may be difficult to identify, but serologic studies should be positive.[19] Immunohistochemistry may aid in detecting the organisms.[20]

The differential diagnosis includes other causes of follicular hyperplasia and, because of the increased number of plasma cells, autoimmune disorders such as RA (see earlier).

Hyaline Vascular Castleman's Disease

Castleman's disease may be localized or multicentric. Localized Castleman's disease is typically of the hyaline vascular type (HVCD), but the plasma cell variant may also be localized. HVCD (also called *angiofollicular lymphoid hyperplasia* or *giant lymph node hyerplasia*) is typically a disease of young adults, although it can affect patients of any age. Clinically it

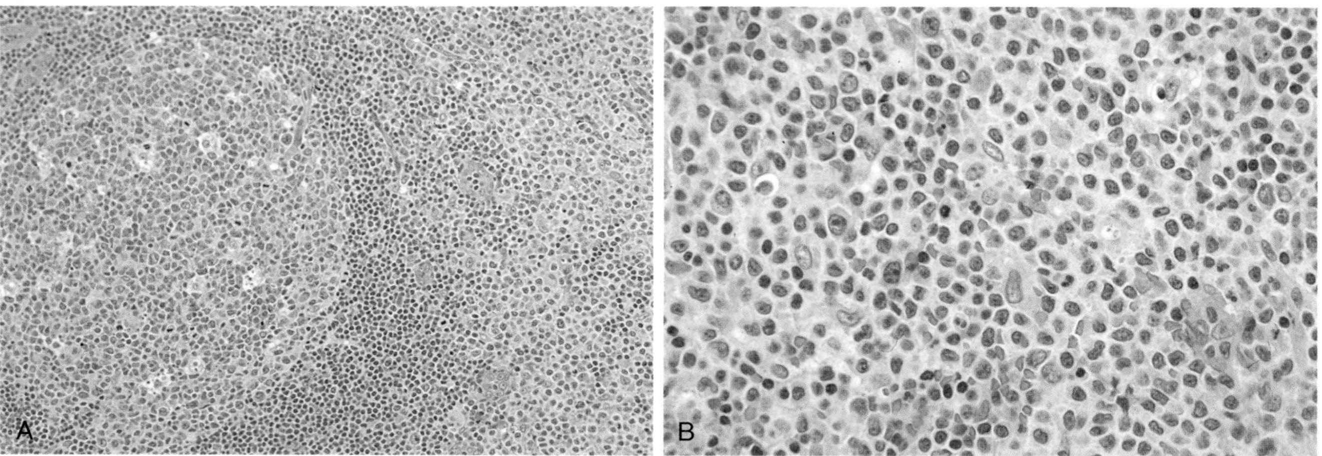

Figure 9-5. **A,** Reactive follicle with adjacent monocytoid B-cell proliferation. **B,** The monocytoid cells are medium-sized, with slightly indented nuclei and ample cytoplasm. Neutrophils are scattered among the monocytoid cells.

presents as a localized mass, with the mediastinal and cervical lymph nodes the most common sites involved. Patients with HVCD are usually asymptomatic, unlike those with the plasma cell type, and are not infected with HIV.[21] In general, localized Castleman's disease can be successfully treated with surgical resection, whereas multicentric forms require systemic therapy.[22]

Histology

The histologic features of HVCD include numerous small, regressively transformed germinal centers surrounded by expanded mantle zones, and a hypervascular interfollicular region (Fig. 9-8A and B).[23] The cells within the regressively transformed germinal centers are predominantly FDCs and endothelial cells. Relatively few follicle center B cells remain. The mantle cells tend to form concentric rings, lined up along FDC processes, imparting an "onionskin" pattern. Blood vessels from the interfollicular area may penetrate at right angles into the germinal center to form a "lollipop" follicle (see Fig. 9-8C). The interfollicular area contains increased numbers of high endothelial venules and varying numbers of small lymphocytes. A useful diagnostic feature is the presence of more than one germinal center within a single mantle (see Fig. 9-8D). Occasional clusters of plasmacytoid dendritic cells (formerly plasmacytoid monocytes) are found (see Fig. 9-8F).[23a] The relative numbers of follicular and interfollicular components may vary from case to case. Sclerosis in the form of perinodal fibrosis and fibrous bands, often perivascular, within the lesion is common.

A stroma-rich variant of HVCD has been described, with stromal cells consisting of an angiomyoid component expressing actins. This variant is also clinically benign.[24,25] In some cases there may be atypical FDCs with enlarged, irregular nuclei, which some investigators regard as dysplastic.[26] These cells may be precursors to FDC sarcoma; a case of FDC tumor has been reported in a patient with HVCD, and a karyotypic

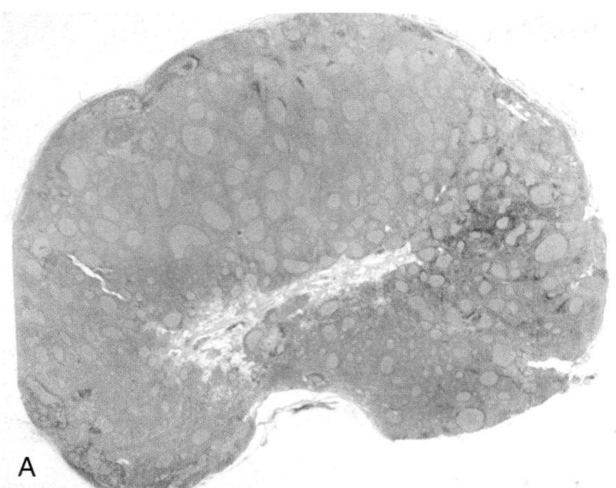

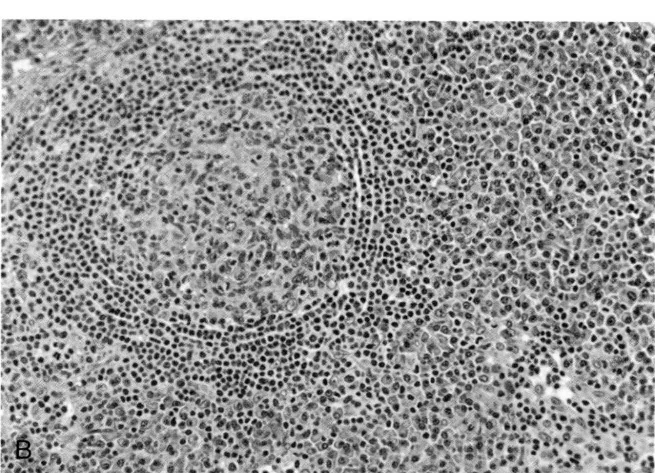

Figure 9-6. Follicular hyperplasia in a lymph node from a patient with rheumatoid arthritis. A, Follicles with enlarged germinal centers varying in size and shape are present throughout the cortex and medulla. **B,** Follicle surrounded by sheets of plasma cells. (**A** and **B** from Schnitzer B. Pathology of lymphoid tissue in rheumatoid arthritis and allied diseases. In: Glynn LE, Schlumberger HD, eds. *Bayer Symposium VI, Experimental Models of Chronic Inflammatory Diseases.* New York: Springer-Verlag; 1977:331-348; and Schnitzer B. Reactive lymphoid hyperplasia. In: Jaffe ES, ed. *Surgical Pathology of the Lymph Nodes and Related Organs.* Philadelphia: Saunders; 1985:22-56.)

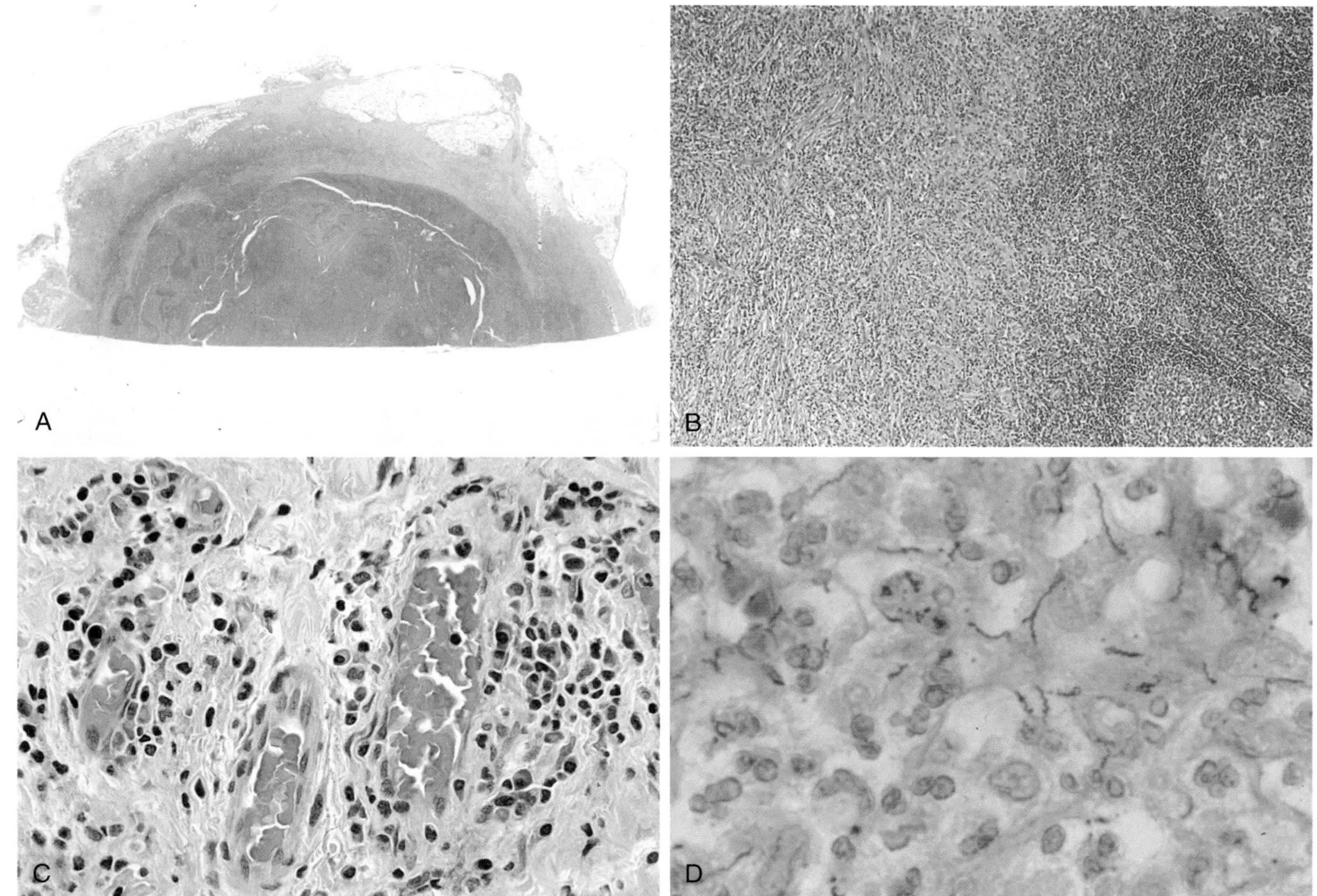

Figure 9-7. Syphilitic lymphadenitis. A, The thickened, fibrotic capsule is infiltrated by chronic inflammatory cells. Follicular hyperplasia and interfollicular plasmacytosis are present. **B,** Higher magnification of heavily inflamed fibrotic capsule and two large reactive follicles. **C,** The vessels in the capsule are surrounded by plasma cells, along with lymphocytes. **D,** Steiner stain shows numerous spirochetes in a case of necrotizing syphilitc lymphadenitis. (**D,** Courtesy of Dr. Judith A. Ferry, Massachusetts General Hospital.)

abnormality has been reported in a patient with HVCD lacking evidence of lymphoid monoclonality.[24,27,28]

Plasma cell Castleman's disease (PCCD) may be localized (approximately 10% of localized cases). It may be associated with constitutional symptoms that resolve with resection. The predominant features of PCCD are follicular hyperplasia with intense interfollicular plasmacytosis. Hyalinized vessels may also be seen in the interfollicular areas. The plasma cells are not cytologically atypical. These features are not entirely specific, and occasional hyaline vascular follicles are present, assisting in the diagnosis.

Immunophenotype

The immunophenotype of the follicles in HVCD is similar to that of reactive follicles. Expanded, concentric meshworks of FDCs stain with antibodies to CD21 (Fig. 9-8E); multiple germinal centers may be found within a single expanded FDC meshwork.[29] Patches of plasmacytoid dendritic cells are highlighted by stains for CD123, CD68, and CD43.[30] Staining for human herpesvirus 8 is typically negative in HVCD. Plasma cells in localized PCCD are generally polytypic; however, as with multicentric PCCD, monotypic plasma cells (usually λ-light chain restricted) may be present.

Differential Diagnosis

The morphologic features of HVCD are not entirely specific, and the differential diagnosis includes late-stage HIV-associated lymphadenopathy, early stages of angioimmunoblastic T-cell lymphoma, follicular or mantle cell lymphoma, and nonspecific reactive lymphadenopathy. Clinical history and serologic testing can exclude HIV infection. Angioimmunoblastic T-cell lymphoma is typically a diffuse process containing expanded meshworks of FDCs outside of B-cell follicles, highlighted by CD21 staining. However, atrophic germinal centers may occasionally be present. In early stages, the atypical infiltrate of angioimmunoblastic T-cell lymphoma may be interfollicular, and the proliferation of high endothelial venules may resemble the hypervascular interfollicular region of HVCD. Atypia of the lymphoid cells, including characteristic clear cells, is usually seen, and $CD10^+$ T cells and PD-1^+ cells[1a] outside of germinal centers have been described in some cases.[31] In situ hybridization for Epstein-Barr virus (EBV)–encoded RNA (EBER) may reveal EBV^+ B immunoblasts in the interfollicular region in early angioimmunoblastic T-cell lymphoma; these should not be present in HVCD.

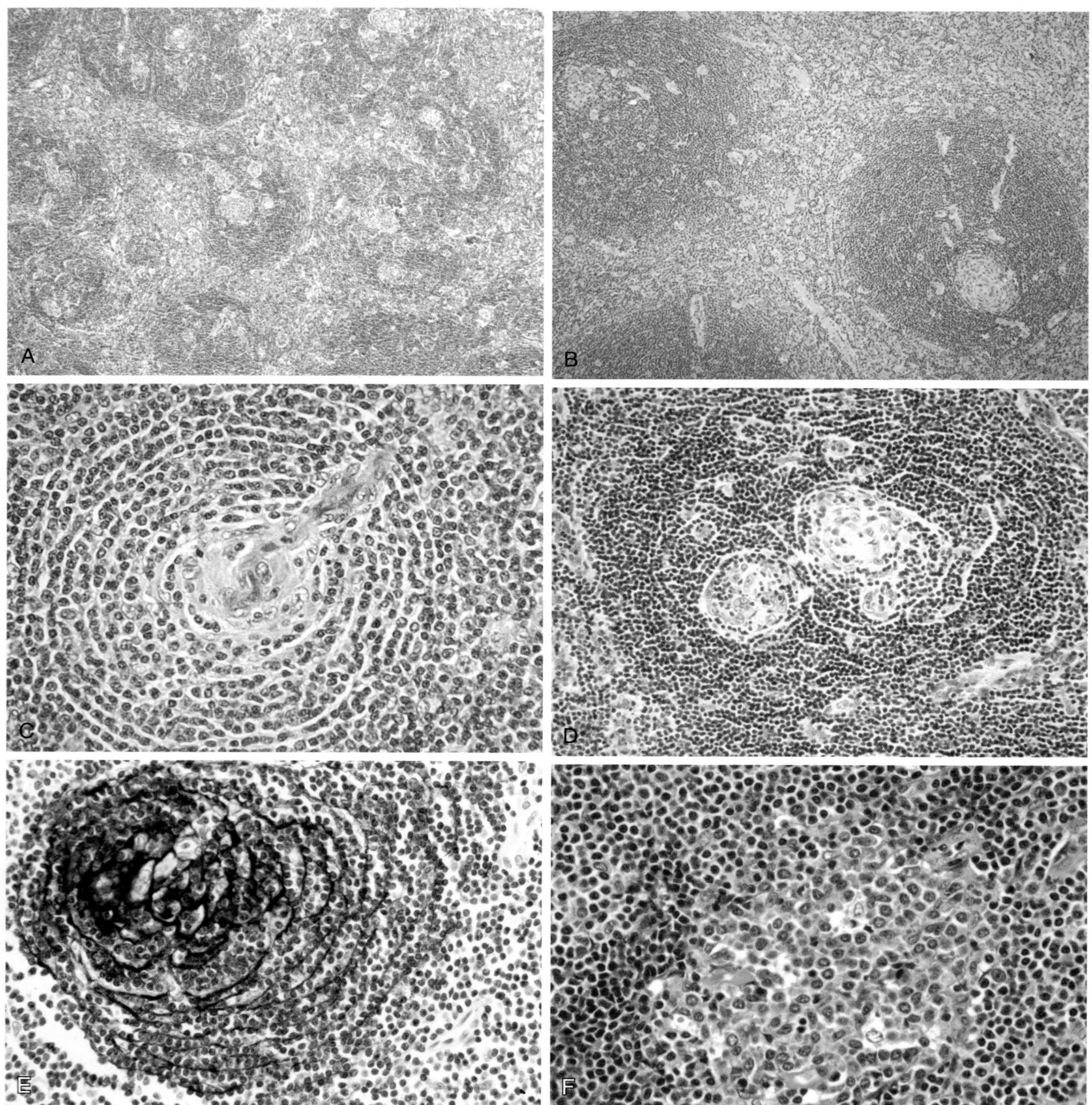

Figure 9-8. Hyaline vascular Castleman's disease. A, Follicles with expanded mantle zones containing regressively transformed germinal centers. Interfollicular vascular proliferation is prominent. **B,** Higher magnification of expanded mantle zones penetrated by vessels from the interfollicular areas and atrophic germinal centers. **C,** Residual germinal center penetrated at a right angle by a hyalinized vessel, giving the follicle a "lollipop" appearance. Small lymphocytes palisade around the germinal centers ("onionskin" appearance). **D,** Two atrophic germinal centers within a single mantle zone. **E,** CD21 staining shows the tight follicular dendritic meshwork within the atrophic germinal center extending in a loosely arranged pattern into the mantle zone. **F,** Plasmacytoid dendritic cells are characteristically seen in hyaline vascular Castleman's disease.

The mantle zone pattern of mantle cell lymphoma may mimic HVCD. However, the lymphoid component in mantle cell lymphoma is atypical, monotypic, and $CD5^+$ and expresses cyclin D_1. The characteristic interfollicular vascularity of HVCD is absent. Small follicles of follicular lymphoma can be mistaken for the regressively transformed germinal centers of HVCD. However, immunostains demonstrate the typical phenotype of follicular lymphoma ($CD20^+$, $CD10^+$, $BCL2^+$).

Exclusion of autoimmune processes such as RA or HIV infection is important when considering a diagnosis of PCCD.

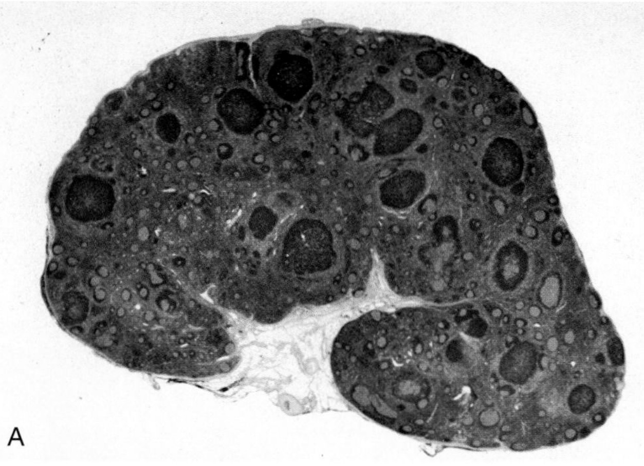

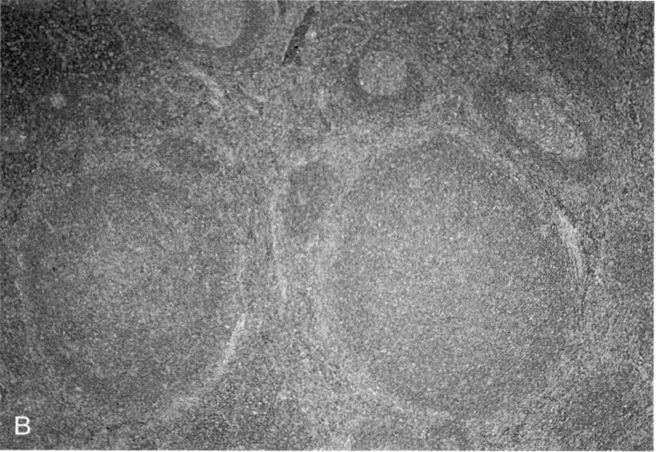

Figure 9-9. Progressive transformation of germinal centers. A, Follicular hyperplasia characterized by increased numbers of reactive follicles among progressively transformed germinal centers, recognized by their large size (CD20 stain). **B,** Reactive follicles and two large, progressively transformed germinal centers composed predominantly of small lymphocytes.

Progressive Transformation of Germinal Centers

Progressive transformation of germinal centers (PTGC) usually occurs in a background of follicular hyperplasia. It presents most commonly as a single enlarged lymph node in an asymptomatic young adult (peak incidence in the second decade and predominantly in males), although it is also seen in children. Cervical and axillary lymph nodes are most commonly involved.[32-34]

PTGC occurs as macronodules scattered in the background of typical follicular hyperplasia (Fig. 9-9). The nodules are usually at least twice as large as the hyperplastic follicles (and often much larger) and are composed predominantly of small lymphocytes with scattered follicle center cells present singly or in small clusters. In most cases, single or a few transformed germinal centers are present in a lymph node. However, in florid PTGC, numerous transformed germinal centers are present, especially in young males.[35] Even in these cases, typical reactive follicles are always present between the transformed germinal centers. Epithelioid histiocytes may occasionally be seen surrounding the follicles.[32,35] Immunophenotypically, the small cells are predominantly IgM$^+$, IgD$^+$ mantle zone B cells.[36] Concentric, smooth meshworks of CD21$^+$, CD23$^+$ FDCs outline the follicles.

The main differential diagnostic consideration is nodular lymphocyte-predominant Hodgkin's lymphoma (NLPHL). NLPHL and PTGC resemble each other, and both may occur in the same lymph node. NLPHL may be present focally in cases of florid PTGC, making it imperative that the entire lymph node be submitted for histologic examination. Like PTGC, NLPHL contains macronodules, but in contrast to those in PTGC, they efface the nodal architecture and lack interspersed reactive follicles. As in PTGC, the nodules also consist predominantly of small B cells with scattered large cells. However, the large cells in NLPHL are Reed-Sternberg cell variants also known as "popcorn" cells or LP cells. The Reed-Sternberg variants, unlike the centroblasts in nodules of PTGC, have large, lobulated nuclei and variably sized nucleoli. T cells and CD57$^+$ cells are often present in small clusters in NLPHL, whereas they are more uniformly scattered in PTGC. A feature useful in the differential diagnosis is the rosetting of T cells and PD-1$^+$ cells[1a] around the neoplastic CD20$^+$ cells in NLPHL,[37] a finding typically absent in PTGC. Popcorn cells are epithelial membrane antigen–positive in some cases of NLPHL, whereas residual centroblasts in PTGC are negative.[37] In addition, the nodules in PTGC usually have sharply defined borders, whereas in NLPHL the nodules have ragged, "moth-eaten" edges.[38] These features are accentuated in sections stained with CD20 or CD79a. Epithelioid histiocytes are also commonly seen not only around but also within the nodules in NLPHL; thus the presence of epithelioid histiocytes within nodules should raise suspicion for NLPHL rather than PTGC. Morphologic and immunophenotypic features should be carefully evaluated in areas where the nodules are closely packed, to rule out NLPHL.

Surgical excision is often curative, but PTGC may recur in the same site. Some investigators suggest a histogenetic relationship between PTGC and NLPHL because PTGC can precede, present simultaneously with, or occur after a diagnosis of NLPHL.[33,39] Most studies show that the risk of developing NLPHL in a patient with PTGC is quite low, but the magnitude of risk is not known.[35] Thus, patients with florid or recurrent PTGC should be followed closely, and suspicious lymph nodes should be biopsied to rule out the development of NLPHL.[32]

Mantle Zone Hyperplasia

Mantle zone hyperplasia rarely causes lymph node enlargement.[40] Mantle zones may be expanded around either hyperplastic or atrophic germinal centers. Mantle zone hyperplasia may arouse suspicion for HVCD, mantle cell lymphoma, or marginal zone lymphoma. The interfollicular vascularity seen in Castleman's disease is lacking. Mantle cell lymphoma usually involves the entire node, whereas mantle cell hyperplasia is most often limited to the cortex or involves only selected follicles (Fig. 9-10). Fusion of adjacent mantle zones may be present in mantle cell lymphoma. Stains for

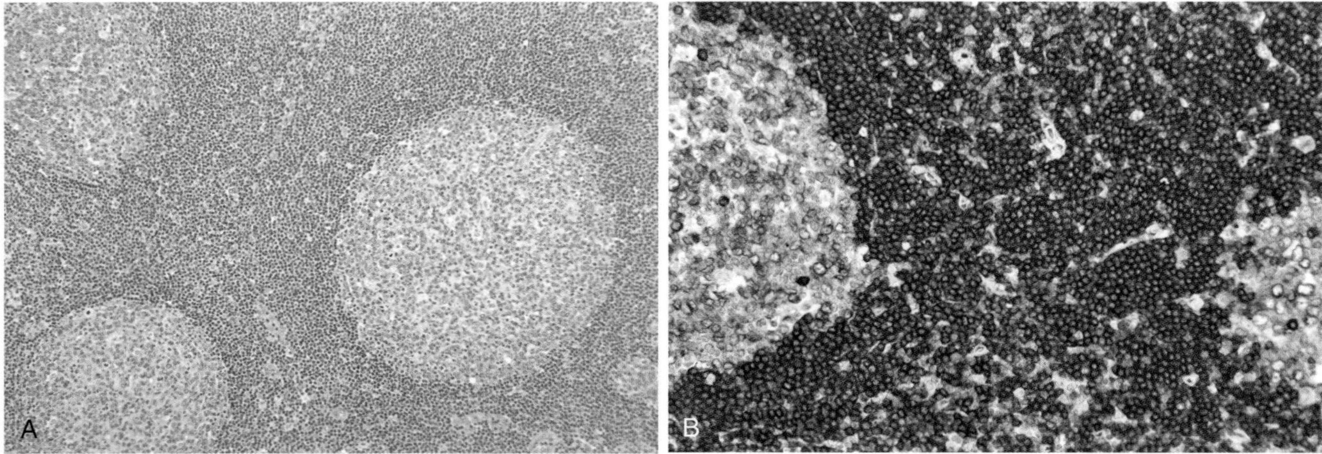

Figure 9-10. Mantle zone hyperplasia. A, Three follicles with expanded mantle zones that have virtually replaced the interfollicular area. **B**, CD79a stain shows positive mantle zone B cells, with an absence of interfollicular areas and parts of two germinal centers.

CD5, CD43, cyclin D_1, and Ig light chains can be useful in excluding mantle cell or marginal zone lymphoma; rarely, gene rearrangement analysis may be required to exclude lymphoma.[40]

PREDOMINANTLY SINUS PATTERN

Sinus Histiocytosis

Sinus histiocytosis (SH) is a common, nonspecific reaction characterized by the expansion of sinuses by histiocytes. It is often seen in lymph nodes draining a tumor. Its prognostic significance (a marker of immune response) in this setting is debated, with some studies suggesting better survival when SH is present.[41-43] SH may also be a reaction to recent surgery for malignancy such as breast cancer.[44]

SH is a nonspecific and benign finding in a clinically enlarged lymph node.[42,45-48] The degree of histiocytic reaction is variable. Cytologically, the histiocytes are bland (Fig. 9-11), without mitoses, a key distinguishing feature between this entity and sinusoidal involvement by malignancies such as melanoma, mesothelioma, and anaplastic large cell lymphoma. All these malignancies may preferentially involve the sinuses with an infiltrate of noncohesive cells, but in contrast to SH, they are composed of cytologically atypical cells. Uncommonly, SH may take on a "signet ring" appearance and mimic metastatic adenocarcinoma.[48] Immunohistochemistry for markers specific for these tumors and for histiocytes (CD68) can be used to sort out rare problematic cases.

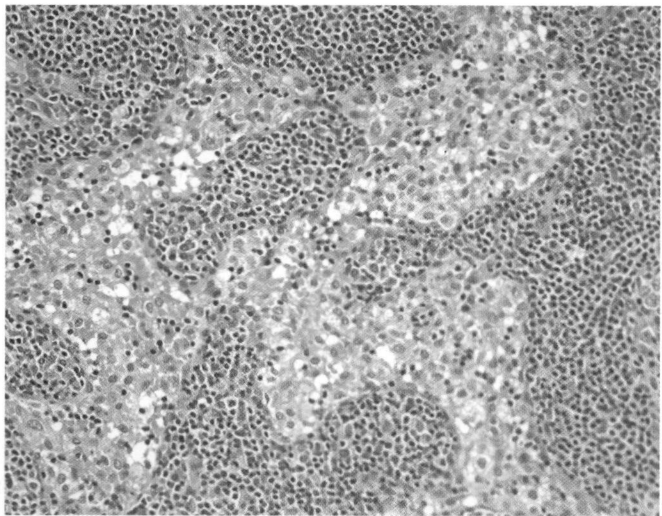

Figure 9-11. Sinus histiocytosis. The sinus is distended with histiocytes that have ample cytoplasm and bland-appearing nuclei without nucleoli.

Histiocytic Expansion with a Specific Cause

Histiocytic reactions involving lymph nodes are sometimes attributable to specific causes, which are briefly described here. However, they may not manifest primarily as a sinusoidal histiocytosis.

Lymphangiograms, Prostheses, and Storage Diseases

Lymphangiograms, performed in the past for the staging of lymphomas, produce large vacuoles formed by lipid-rich contrast material and may result in the formation of lipogranulomas and foamy histiocytes in sinuses (Fig. 9-12).[49]

Histiocytic reactions may also result from the release of foreign material from deteriorating joint or silicone prostheses, causing regional lymphadenopathy.[50-54] Foreign material may be present in sinuses in the regional lymph node, with extension into the paracortex and granuloma formation. Metal fragments and refractile prosthetic material can be demonstrated in the histiocytes. Polarized light examination can be helpful in demonstrating certain types of material, such as polyethylene.[55] Silastic prostheses reportedly produce granulomas with multinucleated giant cells containing yellow, refractile, nonbirefringent silicone.[56] Breast implants can also result in lymphadenopathy, with diffuse infiltrates of vacuolated and foamy histiocytes and large cystic spaces containing silicone.[54]

Hereditary storage diseases such as Gaucher's and Niemann-Pick diseases may also be associated with nodal infiltrates of storage product–laden macrophages. The histiocytes retain

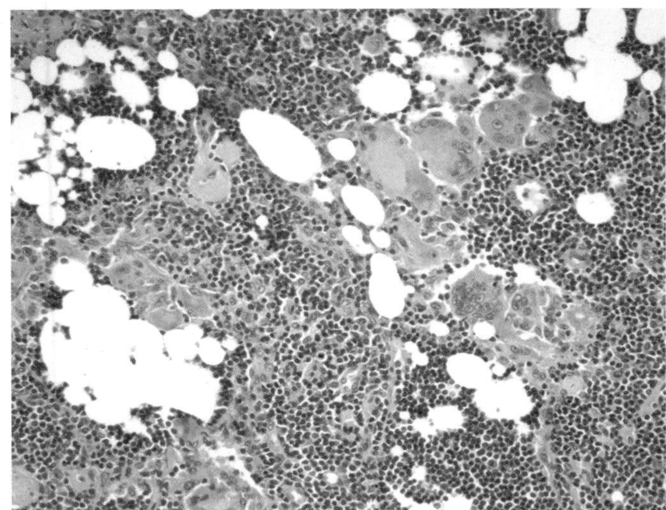

Figure 9-12. Abdominal lymph node following a lymphangiogram. The sinuses are distended by large vacuoles surrounded by sinus histiocytes and foreign body–type giant cells.

the characteristics of the particular disease seen in other sites (e.g., a "tissue paper" appearance in Gaucher's disease).[34,57]

Whipple's Disease

Whipple's disease, first described by George Whipple in 1907,[58] is an infection caused by the bacterium *Tropheryma whippelii*.[59] It occurs most commonly in middle-aged men with symptoms of weight loss, diarrhea, abdominal pain, and often arthralgia. Abdominal lymphadenopathy is usually present, with peripheral or mediastinal lymphadenopathy in about 50% of cases. Although Whipple's disease is often diagnosed by small bowel biopsy, a lymph node may be the first tissue biopsied, especially in patients without abdominal complaints.

Lymph node sinuses contain large, pale-staining, finely vacuolated histiocytes that harbor diastase-resistant, periodic acid–Schiff (PAS)–positive sickle-form structures as well as large cystic vacuoles (Fig. 9-13). Electron microscopy confirms the presence of bacteria.[58,60,61] Not all cases have the characteristic findings; some patients have nonnecrotizing granulomas resembling sarcoidosis.[62,63] The PAS stain may be only focally positive when few organisms are present.[59] A high index of suspicion is required not to miss this diagnosis.

The differential diagnosis of Whipple's disease includes lymphangiogram effect; mycobacterial infection, such as with *Mycobacterium avium-intracellulare*; sarcoidosis; and leprosy.[64] The last can show diffuse infiltrates of histiocytes with abundant vacuolated cytoplasm; cystic spaces, however, are absent. In *M. avium-intracellulare* infection, the organisms are both PAS and acid-fast positive, whereas in leprosy the organisms are acid-fast positive but PAS negative. The presence of *T. whippeli* in fixed tissues can be confirmed by PCR.[58]

Vascular Transformation of Sinuses

Vascular transformation of sinuses (stasis lymphadenopathy, nodal angiomatosis, or hemangiomatoid plexiform vascularization) is an uncommon vasoproliferative lesion that occurs in patients of all ages and is usually an incidental finding in a lymph node removed for other reasons. Histologically, subcapsular sinuses and, less frequently, other sinuses are expanded by thin-walled blood vessels lined by flat endothelial cells. The vascular spaces are more cellular in the intermediate sinuses and become ectatic and less cellular in the subcapsular sinuses (Fig. 9-14).[65] Arborizing slit-like spaces may also be formed. The histologic appearance varies; some cases have a more solid appearance owing to plump endothelial cells and smaller vascular spaces. A plexiform variant consists of dilated and anastomosing spaces with flat lining cells. Extensive vascular transformation of sinuses may form spindle cell nodules.[65-68]

The pathogenesis is thought to be lymphatic or vascular obstruction.[66-69] The differential diagnosis includes Kaposi's sarcoma (KS), hemangioma, and bacillary angiomatosis. KS involves subcapsular sinuses in its early stages and is composed of slit-like vascular spaces. The nodal capsule, which is often involved in KS, is never infiltrated in vascular transformation of sinuses. Sclerosis is minimal in KS, and there are long spindle cell fascicles, whereas bacillary angiomatosis forms nodules and contains granular eosinophilic material and neutrophilic debris not seen in vascular transformation of sinuses. Hemangiomas have well-developed vascular spaces and form nodules.[70,71]

Hemophagocytic Syndrome

Hemophagocytic syndrome (HPS) can be subdivided into three types: infection associated, malignancy associated, and familial (see Chapter 51). Histologically, they are all characterized by a systemic proliferation of benign histiocytes. Although the histiocytes are not neoplastic, the disease is often fatal. Patients have constitutional symptoms, fever, anemia, hepatosplenomegaly, abnormal liver function tests, and often coagulopathies. Infection-associated HPS most commonly occurs in patients who are iatrogenically immunocompromised. It was originally described in association with herpes group viral infections such as CMV or EBV.[72] Subsequently it has been associated with infection by other viruses, bacteria, mycobacteria, rickettsia, and fungi.[73-76] Patients not obviously immunocompromised may have subclinical immunodeficiencies.[77,78]

T-cell/natural killer cell lymphomas may be complicated by HPS. Subcutaneous panniculitis-like T-cell lymphoma is particularly associated with this disorder.[79]

Familial HPS is a rare autosomal recessive syndrome that usually occurs in infants or young children, often younger than 2 years old, with multiorgan involvement. About 40% of the cases have been traced to perforin deficiency. Other abnormalities include mutations in MUNC13-4 and Syntaxin 11 (see Chapter 54).[80-83] Patients are constitutionally ill and have organomegaly, fever, and rash. Common laboratory findings include hyperlipidemia, cytopenia, and liver dysfunction.[84,85]

In infection-associated HPS there is generalized lymphadenopathy, and early in the disease there may be an immunoblastic proliferation with partial effacement of the lymph node. As the disease progresses, the lymph node becomes depleted of lymphocytes, and the sinuses become filled with bland-appearing phagocytic histiocytes. These cells may be stuffed with erythrocytes, but other hematopoietic cells may also be phagocytosed (Fig. 9-15). The latter appearance

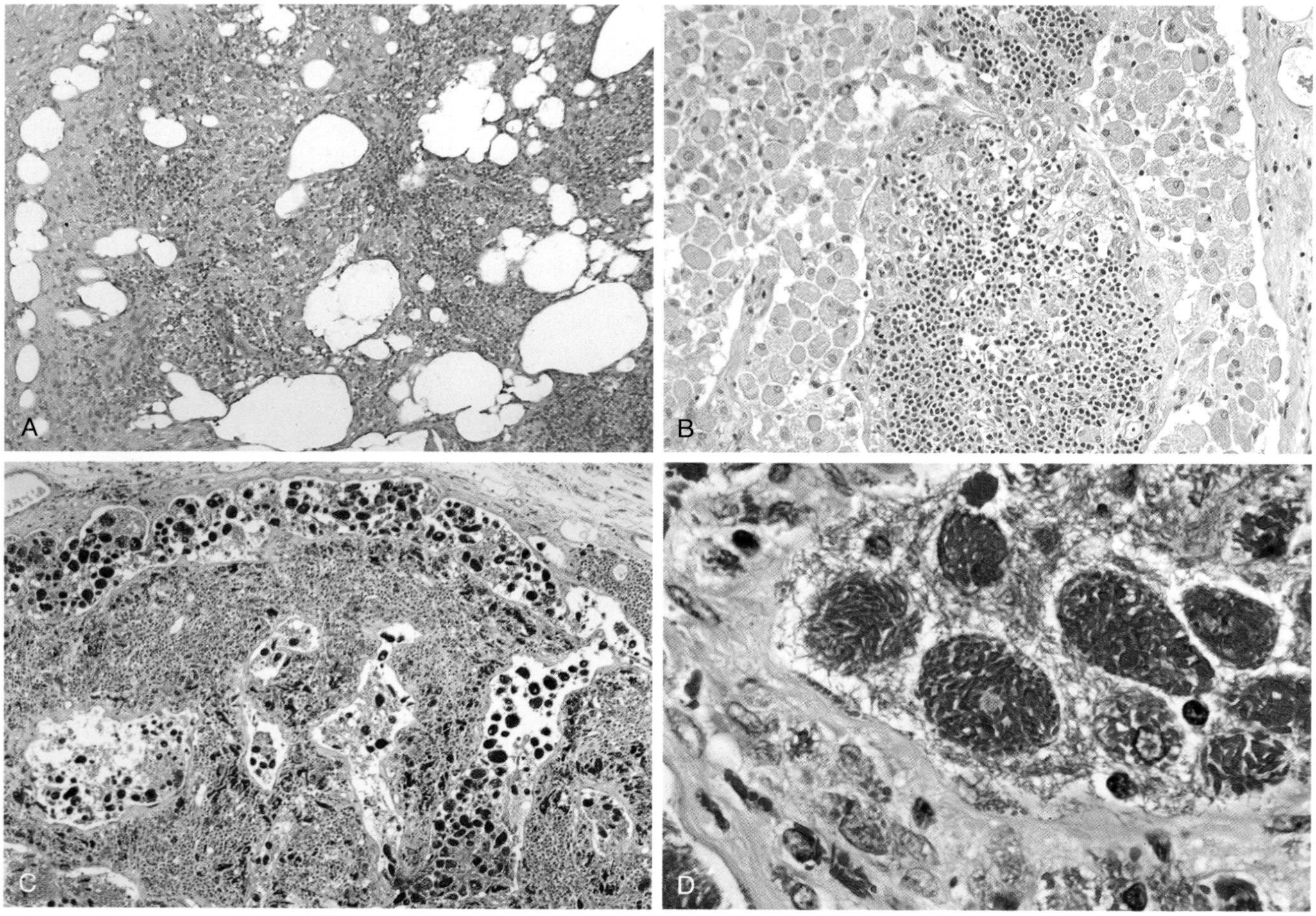

Figure 9-13. Whipple's disease involving a lymph node. A, Sinuses contain vacuoles of varying sizes and few histiocytes. **B**, Sinuses filled with large, pale-staining histiocytes. **C**, Periodic acid–Schiff (PAS)–positive histiocytes fill the sinuses. **D**, High magnification of histiocytes filled with PAS-positive sickle-form particles.

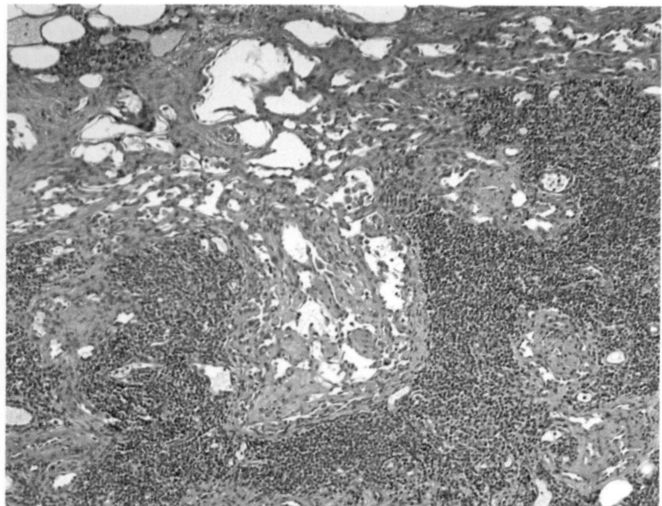

Figure 9-14. Vascular transformation of sinuses. The subcapsular and intermediate sinuses are replaced by vascular structures ranging from slit-like spaces, especially in the intermediate sinus, to ectatic vessels in the subcapsular sinus, as well as associated fibrosis.

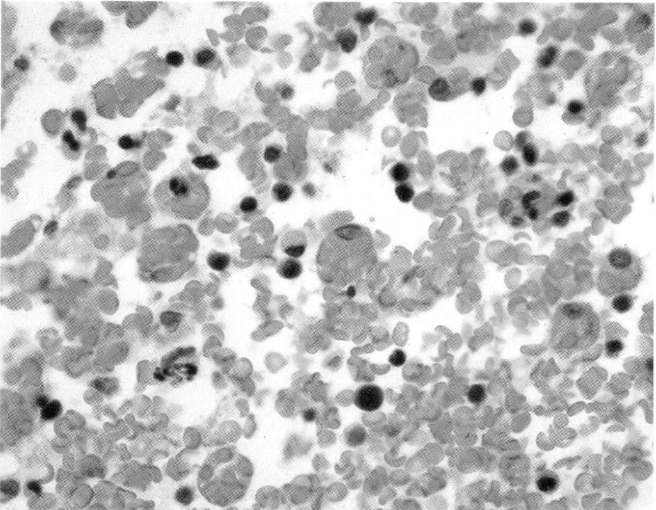

Figure 9-15. Lymph node from a patient with hemophagocytic syndrome. The distended sinus contains histiocytes engorged with phagocytosed red blood cells.

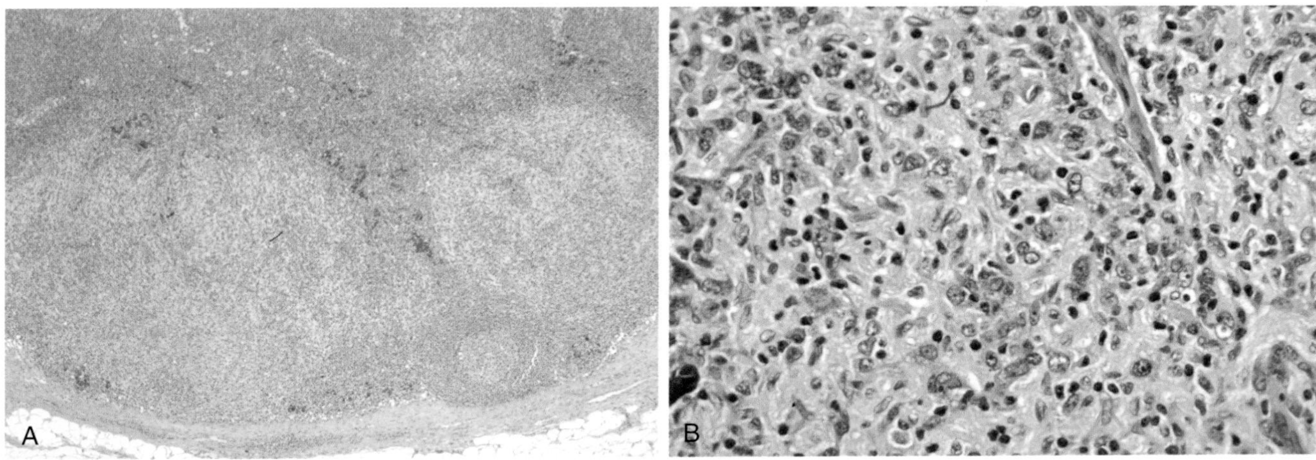

Figure 9-16. Dermatopathic lymphadenitis. A, Two pale-staining nodules in the expanded paracortex composed of Langerhans cells and histiocytes, some containing melanin. A follicle is compressed adjacent to the capsule. **B,** Higher magnification showing mixtures of pigment-containing macrophages and Langerhans cells.

is seen especially well in smears of bone marrow aspirates.[77,86] In lymphoma-associated HPS, the lymph node may or may not be involved by neoplasia. Lack of evidence of malignancy in the lymph node does not exclude the possibility of a lymphoma-associated HPS. Familial HPS, or familial hemophagocytic lymphohistiocytosis, also involves lymph nodes, which usually appear to be lymphoid depleted, with cytophagocytosis seen in sinusoidal histiocytes.[84,85]

The differential diagnosis includes SH with massive lymphadenopathy (Rosai-Dorfman disease). This disorder is characterized by a sinusoidal infiltrate of large histiocytic cells with prominent nucleoli demonstrating emperipolesis of lymphocytes and occasionally plasma cells rather than true cytophagocytosis.[87] The histiocytes are strongly S-100$^+$, whereas the histiocytes in HPS or SH are S-100$^-$ or variably weakly positive.

Cells of Langerhans cell histiocytosis also involve sinuses, but they are CD1a$^+$ in addition to being S-100$^+$. Furthermore, the nuclei have a characteristic nuclear groove or crease and are accompanied by an inflammatory infiltrate that often includes eosinophils. Electron microscopy demonstrates diagnostic Birbeck granules.[88,89]

INTERFOLLICULAR OR MIXED PATTERNS

Paracortical Hyperplasia and Dermatopathic Reaction

Paracortical hyperplasia—expansion of the paracortical (T-zone) region of the lymph node—may be a cause of lymphadenopathy. It can represent a response to a viral infection or a reaction to a nearby malignancy, or it can be part of an autoimmune process.[90-92] Histologically, there is a mixed population of small lymphocytes, variable numbers of immunoblasts, prominent vascularity (high endothelial venules), and interdigitating dendritic cells.[90,93,94]

Dermatopathic lymphadenitis is a specific type of paracortical hyperplasia that typically manifests in lymph nodes draining areas of chronic skin irritation. Histologically, there are paracortical lymphoid nodules with increased numbers of interdigitating dendritic cells and Langerhans cells and histiocytes containing melanin or, less commonly, iron (Fig. 9-16). The histiocytes and interdigitating dendritic cells and Langerhans cells impart a mottled appearance at low magnification. Studies have shown that dermatopathic changes can often occur in the absence of dermatitis.[95]

The major differential diagnosis is mycosis fungoides, in which dermatopathic change is common. Lymph node involvement by mycosis fungoides may take several forms, ranging from the presence of atypical cells in clusters without obvious effacement of the lymph node architecture to diffuse involvement by lymphoma. Scoring systems to grade this involvement and predict behavior have been suggested,[96] but multivariate survival analysis calls into question their utility.[97] Gene rearrangement studies may be helpful in evaluating histologically equivocal cases and predicting outcome.[98,99]

Granulomatous Lymphadenitis

Granulomatous lymphadenitis can be divided into nonnecrotizing, necrotizing, and suppurative forms. Often a specific cause cannot be determined.

Nonnecrotizing Granuloma

Nonnecrotizing epithelioid granulomas are often seen as nonspecific reactions to malignancy such as Hodgkin's lymphoma, non-Hodgkin's lymphoma, or carcinoma. The lymph node may or may not be involved with the malignancy.[100-102] Types of lymphoma particularly associated with granulomas include classical Hodgkin's lymphoma, NLPHL, lymphoplasmacytic lymphoma, and some peripheral T-cell lymphomas (Lennert's lymphoma), although clusters of histiocytes smaller than granulomas are characteristic of the last. Metastatic nasopharyngeal carcinoma may be associated with a florid granulomatous reaction that obscures the tumor.

Sarcoidosis involving the lymph node results in discrete, well-formed epithelioid granulomas with or without multinucleated giant cells and scattered lymphocytes. The granulomas first involve the paracortical regions but often become confluent and can eventually replace the entire lymph node (Fig. 9-17). Schaumann's, asteroid, and Hamazaki-Wesenberg bodies may be seen but are not specific for

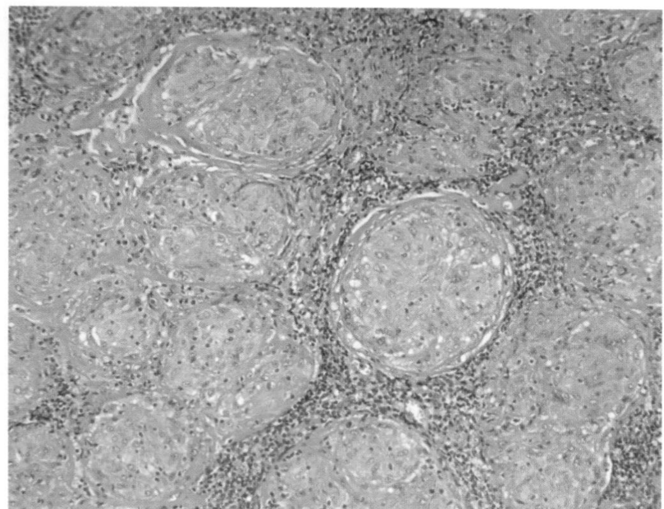

Figure 9-17. Sarcoidosis. Sarcoidosis in a lymph node characterized by epithelioid granulomas, some surrounded by delicate fibrous bands.

sarcoidosis.[103-106] PAS-positive and acid-fast Hamazaki-Wesenberg bodies (1- to 15-μm ovoid to spindle-shaped intracellular and extracellular structures) should not be mistaken for microorganisms.[106] The granulomas may be surrounded and replaced by fibrous tissue. Immunophenotyping shows a predominance of $CD4^+$ T cells.[107] Although almost any tissue can be involved, lung and mediastinal lymph nodes are most commonly affected. Cultures and special stains for microorganisms should be done to exclude infectious causes, particularly looking for fungi and acid-fast organisms.[108]

Necrotizing Granuloma

Necrotizing granulomas are caused by a variety of infectious organisms, including mycobacteria, fungi, and bacteria. Some show characteristic histologic features.

Tuberculosis. Mycobacterial infections, particularly *Mycobacterium tuberculosis*, are common throughout the world.[109] After increasing in the 1980s and 1990s, the incidence in the United States has stabilized at 6.8/100,000 per year.[109,110] In tuberculosis patients who present with peripheral lymphadenopathy, cervical lymph nodes are most commonly involved.[111] Cervical lymphadenopathy may also be the presenting feature in atypical mycobacterial infection with organisms such as *Mycobacterium scrofulaceum*, particularly in children.[112,113] Epitrochlear, axillary lymph, or inguinal nodes may be infected with *Mycobacterium marinum* from cutaneous lesions (swimming pool granuloma).

Histologically, lymph nodes infected by mycobacteria of any kind contain multiple well-formed, sarcoid-like granulomas consisting of epithelioid histiocytes and multinucleated Langerhans giant cells. Caseating necrosis may be seen. In immunocompromised patients, the granulomas may not be well formed and may contain neutrophils. Mycobacterial organisms may be demonstrated in the granulomas with acid-fast stains. Culture is usually required to definitively identify species, although PCR has also been used.[114,115] Brucellosis may cause a granulomatous lymphadenitis similar to that seen in tuberculosis; organisms are difficult to demonstrate in tissue sections.

Fungal Infection. Fungal infections of lymph nodes typically cause granulomatous lymphadenitis that may be necrotizing and indistinguishable from mycobacterial infection. Fibrosis and calcification may occur in older lesions. Generally the lymphadenitis occurs as part of pulmonary-based disease or a disseminated infection. Disseminated infections usually occur in immunocompromised patients, in the setting of HIV infection, malignancy, or iatrogenic immunosuppression.[108,116,117] In immunocompromised patients the granulomas may not be well formed. In a large series of cases, *Histoplasma capsulatum* was the most common cause of fungal infection in immunocompetent patients.[108] Gomori methenamine silver or PAS stains aid in the identification of organisms, although organisms are often absent in older lesions. The differential diagnosis includes necrotizing granulomas due to other infectious causes such as mycobacteria.

Suppurative Granuloma

Cat-Scratch Disease. Cat-scratch disease, caused by *Bartonella henselae*, is characterized histologically by suppurative granulomas.[118,119] It is likely underrecognized and may be one of the more common causes of chronic lymph node enlargement in children.[120] Patients usually present with axillary or cervical lymphadenopathy and mild fever of 1 to 2 weeks' duration.[120,121] Because cats are the reservoir of the causative organism, there is often (but not always) a history of exposure to cats, particularly kittens, which have higher levels of bacteremia and are more likely to scratch than are adult cats.[120] The disease usually resolves spontaneously in several months.

The histologic features of cat-scratch disease are characteristic but not entirely specific. Well-developed lesions are characterized by follicular hyperplasia, monocytoid B-cell reaction, and suppurative granulomas (Fig. 9-18). Suppurative granulomas consist of a central necrotic focus containing neutrophils surrounded by palisaded macrophages forming the classic stellate granuloma.[118] Various stages in the development of the characteristic suppurative lesion are often seen in the same node. Early lesions show small foci of necrosis within clusters of monocytoid B cells containing small clusters of neutrophils. Later lesions are surrounded by histiocytes. Very old lesions may contain central areas of caseation, similar to that seen in mycobacterial infection. The bacillus can be identified within the granulomas or walls of vessels with a Warthin-Starry stain.[119] Organisms are most readily identified in early lesions, where they tend to cluster in the walls of blood vessels (see Fig. 9-18). Cultures are rarely successful, but PCR tests in fixed tissue have been successful in detecting the organism.[122] Confirmation of the diagnosis can be obtained by acute and convalescent serologic testing.

The differential diagnosis of suppurative granulomas includes other infectious agents such as *Chlamydia trachomatis* (lymphogranuloma venereum), *Francisella tularemia* (tularemia), *Yersinia pseudotuberculosis* (mesenteric lymphadentitis), *Listeria monocytogenes* (listeriosis), *Burkholderia mallei* (glanders), and *Burkholderia pseudomallei* (melioidosis). Many of these disorders are rare but have a specific clinical picture or history of exposure to animals that aids in the clinical diagnosis when combined with appropriate microbiologic studies.[123-127] The potential use of some of these agents in

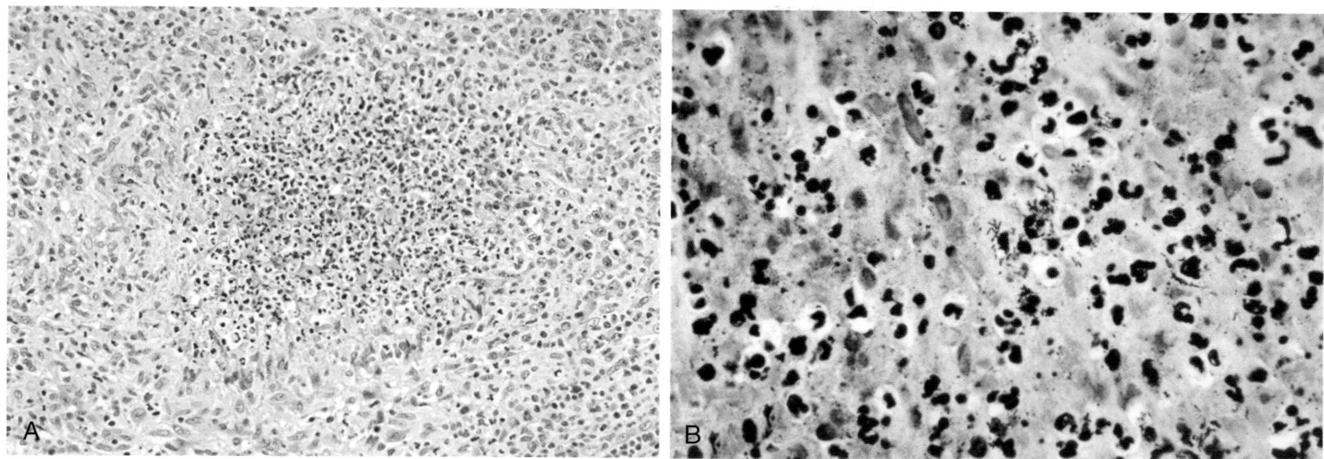

Figure 9-18. Lymph node from a patient with cat-scratch disease. A, Suppurative granuloma with a central area composed predominantly of neutrophils surrounded by palisading histiocytes and fibroblasts. **B,** Warthin-Starry stain showing the causative *Bartonella henselae* organisms.

bioterrorism has led to an increased awareness of their virulence and manifestations.[128,129]

Kimura's Disease

Kimura's disease is a chronic inflammatory condition of unknown cause that affects young to middle-aged patients, most often males of Asian descent.[130] Patients usually present with a mass in the head and neck region with involvement of subcutaneous tissue, soft tissue, salivary glands, and single or multiple regional lymph nodes. Peripheral blood examination shows eosinophilia and increased serum IgE levels. The disease is self-limited, although recurrences can occur over a period of years.[130]

Key histologic features include florid follicular hyperplasia that may contain a proteinaceous precipitate (IgE in a follicular dendritic network pattern) and vascularization of the germinal centers (Fig. 9-19). The interfollicular areas show prominent high endothelial venules with a mixture of lymphocytes, plasma cells, eosinophils, and mast cells. Follicle lysis is often present, and eosinophilic abscesses are characteristic within germinal centers as well as in the paracortex. Polykaryocytes are usually seen in the germinal centers and paracortex. A varying degree of fibrosis is seen.

In lymph nodes, the differential diagnosis includes other entities associated with eosinophilia, including allergic and hypersensitivity reactions and parasitic infestation. However, none of these disorders is associated with follicular hyperplasia, vascularization, and eosinophilic abscesses of follicles and paracortex.

The entity most likely to be confused with Kimura's disease is angiolymphoid hyperplasia with eosinophilia, which also involves the head and neck region. Long thought to be synonymous with Kimura's disease, angiolymphoid hyperplasia with eosinophilia is a vascular neoplasm characterized by the proliferation of blood vessels lined by plump endothelial cells with abundant eosinophilic cytoplasm, imparting a hobnail appearance. This lesion is part of the spectrum of histiocytoid or epithelioid hemangiomas, and it is a low-grade vascular tumor. There is a dense, mixed inflammatory cell infiltrate consisting of lymphocytes, plasma cells, and eosinophils. The prominent histiocytoid endothelial cells seen in angiolymphoid hyperplasia with eosinophilia are not seen in Kimura's disease, making this feature the most reliable means of distinguishing the two entities.[131-134]

Toxoplasmic Lymphadenitis

Infection by *Toxoplasma gondii* in immunocompetent patients most commonly results in solitary cervical lymphadenopathy. The organism has a worldwide distribution, with 30% to 40% of adults in the United States having been exposed to it.[135] Patients with an acute infection may be asymptomatic or, less frequently, may have nonspecific symptoms such as malaise, sore throat, and fever, a constellation of symptoms similar to those seen in infectious mononucleosis. In addition, reactive lymphocytes may be found in peripheral blood smears, thus clinically resembling the features of infectious mononucleosis.[135-137] The disease is self-limited, but immunodeficient patients may develop severe complications such as encephalitis. Infection during pregnancy may result in birth defect or fetal loss.

Histologically, lymph nodes show prominent follicular hyperplasia with expansion of monocytoid B cells in a sinusoidal and parasinusoidal pattern. Small clusters of epithelioid histiocytes in the paracortex encroach on and are present in germinal centers (Fig. 9-20). The germinal centers have ragged, "moth-eaten" margins and contain numerous tingible body macrophages. Granulomas and multinucleated giant cells are absent. Parasitic cysts are seen only rarely, and earlier attempts to detect the organisms by PCR were mostly unsuccessful.[138,139] Serodiagnosis is the primary means of confirming the diagnosis.[137] However, one study showed a PCR detection rate of 83% in cases with the histologic triad of florid reactive follicular hyperplasia, clusters of epithelioid histiocytes, and focal sinusoidal distention by monocytoid B cells.[140]

Although the histologic features are characteristic of toxoplasmic lymphadenitis, the differential diagnosis includes leishmanial lymphadenitis, which can result in a histologic picture similar to toxoplasmosis. In leishmaniasis, organisms may be seen in the granulomas. Ultrastructurally, *Leishmania*

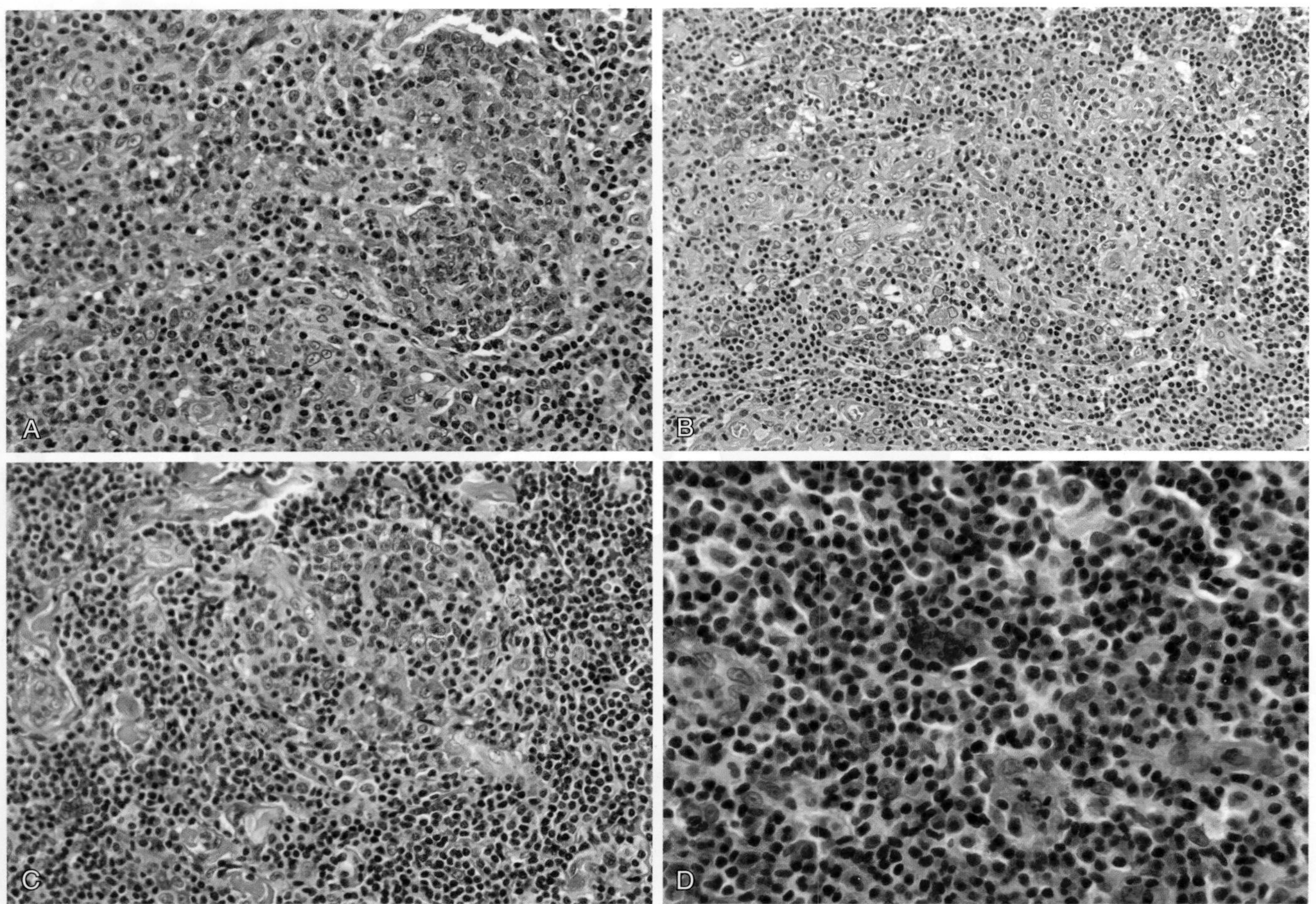

Figure 9-19. Kimura's disease in a lymph node biopsy from a young man with a mass in the parotid gland region. A, Follicular lysis with eosinophils in a hyperplastic germinal center. **B,** Eosinophilic abscess in a germinal center. Residual clusters of large germinal center cells are present. **C,** Vascularization of a germinal center and high endothelial venules in the paracortex. **D,** Numerous eosinophils in the paracortex, along with a polykaryocyte.

can be distinguished from *Toxoplasma* by the presence of kinetoplasts and basal bodies in the former.[141] Early stages of cat-scratch disease, infectious mononucleosis, and CMV lymphadentis may also have morphologic features similar to that of *Toxoplasma* lymphadenitis.

Systemic Lupus Erythematosus

Patients who have systemic lupus erythematosus (SLE) are at increased risk for the development of lymphoma, and lymphadenopathy is present in up to 60% of patients, most commonly involving cervical and mesenteric nodes.[142,143] The histologic features of lymph nodes in SLE include nonspecific follicular hyperplasia, with or without an interfollicular expansion of lymphocytes and immunoblasts, often with numerous plasma cells both within germinal centers and in the medullary cords. A characteristic feature of lupus lymphadenitis is coagulative necrosis, often involving large areas of the lymph node (Fig. 9-21).[142,144-146] The necrotic areas contain ghosts of lymphoid cells, often abundant karyorrhectic debris, and histiocytes; segmented neutrophils are scant but may be present, in contrast to Kikuchi's lymphadenitis (see later). The presence of hematoxylin bodies—extracellular amorphous hematoxyphilic structures probably composed of degenerated nuclei that have reacted with antinuclear antibodies—is specific for SLE. The hematoxylin bodies are found in areas of necrosis as well as in sinuses. Hematoxylin bodies are absent in Kikuchi's disease.

Kikuchi's Lymphadenitis

Histiocytic necrotizing lymphadenitis, also known as Kikuchi's or Kikuchi-Fujimoto lymphadenitis, was described in Japan in 1972.[147,148] It has a worldwide distribution and affects predominantly young adults, especially young women of Asian descent. In most cases the disease resolves spontaneously within several months. Patients most often present with cervical lymphadenopathy, sometimes associated with fever and leukopenia. Three histologic subtypes, probably representing various stages in the evolution of the disease, have been described.[149]

The early-stage, proliferative type is characterized by the presence of numerous immunoblasts with prominent nucleoli and basophilic cytoplasm in the paracortex, raising the differential diagnosis of large cell lymphoma. The immunoblasts are admixed with large mononuclear cells, including histiocytes, some with curved nuclei (crescentic histiocytes) and some with twisted nuclei; aggregates of plasmacytoid

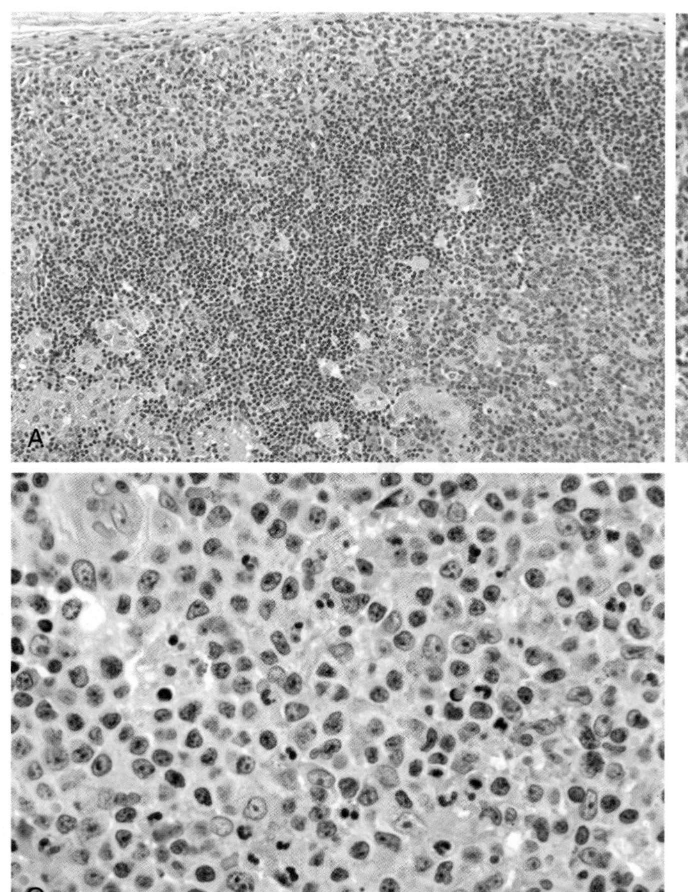

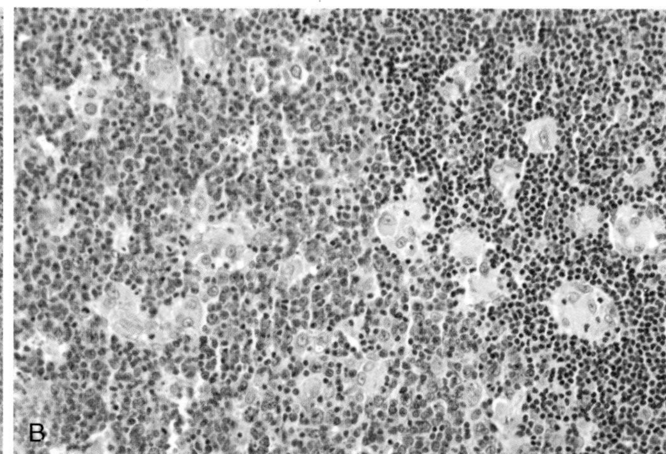

Figure 9-20. Toxoplasmic lymphadenitis. A, Reactive follicle and epithelioid histiocytes, some in clusters, in the paracortex, encroaching on and within the germinal center. The subcapsular sinus is dilated and filled with monocytoid B cells. **B,** Higher magnification showing histiocytes close to and within the germinal center. **C,** Higher magnification of the monocytoid B cells, which have ample cytoplasm, indented nuclei, and slightly condensed chromatin. Intermingled neutrophils are present.

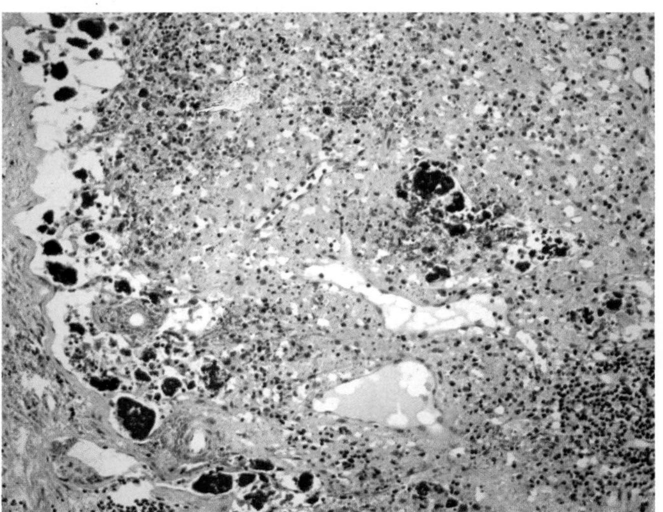

Figure 9-21. Lymph node from a patient with systemic lupus erythematosus. Extensive necrosis with apoptotic debris and hematoxylin bodies found predominantly within sinuses. Neutrophils are absent.

dendritic cells may be prominent. The latter cells are intermediate-sized with round to oval nuclei and granular chromatin placed eccentrically within an amphophilic cytoplasm. As the name implies, plasmacytoid dendritic cells resemble plasma cells but lack a clear Golgi area. They are often difficult to identify within the mixture of cells. Karyorrhectic bodies are often interspersed among the plasmacytoid dendritic cells, and the necrosis seen in Kikuchi's disease often appears to begin in nests of these cells.

The necrotizing type, which is most common, is characterized by patchy areas of necrosis within the paracortex (Fig. 9-22). The necrosis contains no neutrophils, has abundant karyorrhectic nuclear debris, and is surrounded by a mixture of mononuclear cells identical to those found in the proliferative type. The karyorrhectic debris is extracellular as well as phagocytosed by histiocytes.

The xanthomatous type is the least common and most likely represents the healing phase of this entity. It contains many foamy histiocytes and fewer immunoblasts than the other types. Necrosis may or may not be present in the xanthomatous type.

The minimal criteria for the diagnosis of Kikuchi's lymphadenitis include paracortical clusters of plasmacytoid dendritic cells admixed with karyorrhectic bodies and crescentic histiocytes.[150] The noninvolved part of the node has a mottled appearance owing to the presence of immunoblasts scattered

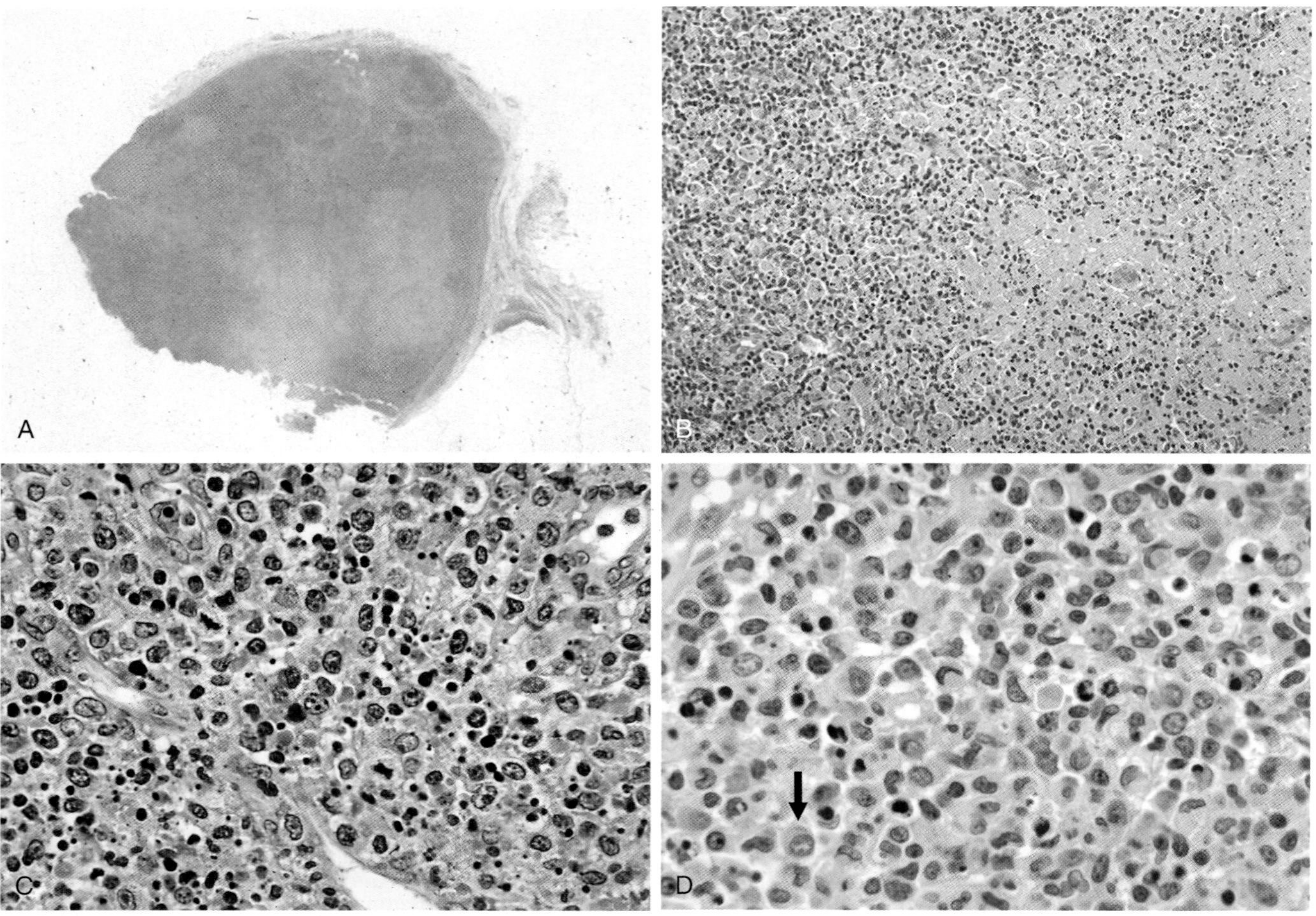

Figure 9-22. Lymph node from a young woman with Kikuchi's disease. A, Confluent foci of necrosis in the paracortex surrounded by large mononuclear cells. **B**, Higher magnification showing necrosis with karyorrhectic debris, histiocytes, and immunoblasts. **C**, Predominance of immunoblasts, histiocytes, necrosis, and apoptotic debris. **D**, Mononuclear cells—most of which are histiocytes, some of which have crescentic nuclei—as well as a few plasmacytoid monocytes (*arrow*) and immunoblasts.

among small lymphocytes. Reactive lymphoid follicles may be seen. There is also a proliferation of high endothelial venules.[150] This histologic picture resembles that seen in viral-associated lymphadenopathy.

Immunophenotypically, the infiltrate is composed of T cells, with $CD8^+$ cells outnumbering $CD4^+$ cells; $CD68^+$ histiocytes; and $CD68^+$, $CD4^+$, $CD43^+$, CD123 plasmacytoid dendritic cells. B cells are rare.

The differential diagnosis includes lupus lymphadenitis and non-Hodgkin's lymphoma. The findings in Kikuchi's lymphadenitis may be indistinguishable from those in lupus lymphadenitis, and some investigators have raised the possibility of a relationship between the two; however, cases reported as Kikuchi's lymphadenitis in association with SLE are almost certainly lupus lymphadenitis misdiagnosed as Kikuchi's.[144,151] Extensive necrosis, the presence of hematoxylin bodies, and plasma cells or neutrophils favor SLE.[144] Most patients with Kikuchi's lymphadenitis lack antinuclear antibodies.[150] Because of the difficulty in distinguishing histologically between the two, whenever a diagnosis of Kikuchi's lymphadentis is made, serologic testing for SLE is advisable; if tests are positive, the diagnosis is lupus lymphadenitis.

Cases with abundant immunoblasts may be mistaken for lymphoma. Patchy involvement of the lymph node, abundant karyorrhectic debris, a mixed cell population that includes the crescentic histiocytes described earlier, absence of B-cell markers on immunoblasts, and lack of a B- or T-cell receptor gene rearrangement favor Kikuchi's lymphadenitis.[144]

Kawasaki's Disease

Kawasaki's disease (mucocutaneous lymph node syndrome) is an acute exanthematous childhood disease of unknown cause.[152] The male-to-female ratio is 1.5:1, and there is a peak incidence at age 3 to 4 years.[153] Diagnosis rests on the presence of five of the six following features that cannot be attributable to other causes: fever unresponsive to antibiotics, bilateral conjunctivitis, oral mucositis, distal extremity cutaneous lesions, polymorphous skin exanthems, and cervical lymphadenopathy.[154] The disease appears to be a systemic vasculitis, and the term *juvenile polyarteritis nodosa* has been proposed. Although most children recover, patients are at high risk for coronary artery aneurysm. Sudden death occurs in approximately 1% of patients.[155,156] Histologically, the lymph nodes show nongranulomatous foci of necrosis, with or without neutrophils, associated with vasculitis and thrombosis of small vessels. Scattered lymphocytes, plasma cells, and immunoblasts are seen in the background. The overall nodal architecture is often effaced. The differential diagnosis is extensive and includes other entities with necrosis such as SLE and Kikuchi's lymphadenitis.[144,157] Observation of fibrin thrombi in nodal vessels with the appropriate clinical history strongly favors Kawasaki's lymphadenitis.

Inflammatory Pseudotumor

Inflammatory pseudotumor is an idiopathic reactive condition of lymph nodes affecting young adults (median age, 33 years) without a gender predilection.[158] Patients have constitutional symptoms and often laboratory abnormalities such as hypergammaglobulinemia, elevated erythrocyte sedimentation rate, and anemia. Single peripheral or central lymph nodes or multiple lymph node groups and the spleen may be involved.[158,159] Inflammatory pseudotumor can spontaneously resolve; surgical excision or anti-inflammatory agents can relieve symptoms.[160]

The key histologic feature is a fibroinflammatory reaction of the connective tissue framework of the lymph node, with extension into the perinodal soft tissue. The capsule, trabeculae, and hilum are involved by a proliferation of small vessels, histiocytes, and myofibroblastic cells with admixed lymphocytes, plasma cells, eosinophils, and neutrophils. The myofibroblastic cells are spindly to polygonal, with bland nuclei and abundant cytoplasm. They can form ill-defined fascicles or appear in a storiform pattern. Fibrinoid vascular necrosis, karyorrhexis, and focal parenchymal infarction may be seen. Medium-sized vessels may be invaded and destroyed. Lymphoid follicles are uncommon.[158,159,161,162] Immunophenotyping shows that the lymphoid cells are predominantly T cells. CD68⁺ histiocytes and vimentin-posistive, actin-positive spindle cells are present, supporting the fibrohistiocytic nature of the proliferation.[159,161,162] As the lesions age, the node becomes replaced by fibrotic tissue with a scant inflammatory infiltrate.[159]

The differential diagnosis includes KS and FDC tumors. Early involvement by KS shows capsular, subcapsular, and trabecular spindle cell areas that may suggest the connective tissue framework pattern of inflammatory pseudotumor. Vascular structures are poorly formed in KS, in contrast to their appearance in inflammatory pseudotumor. The PAS-positive hyaline globules of KS are not present. The bland cytologic features of inflammatory pseudotumor, the lack of a mass-forming nodule, and the absence of FDC markers such as CD21 and CD35 aid in making the distinction from FDC tumors.[163,164] Hypocellular anaplastic large cell lymphoma has an edematous fibromyxoid background with scattered myofibroblastic cells that may form fascicles, mimicking inflammatory pseudotumor. CD30 and anaplastic lymphoma kinase expression in atypical cells that tend to cluster around vessels confirms lymphoma and excludes inflammatory pseudotumor.[165]

Bacillary Angiomatosis

Bacillary angiomatosis due to infection with *B. henselae* or, less commonly, *Bartonella quintana*[166-170] may cause lymphadenopathy in immunocompromised patients, particularly those infected with HIV. Patients present with skin lesions, lymphadenopathy, and occasionally hepatosplenomegaly.

The lymph nodes demonstrate single or confluent nodules composed of small blood vessels lined by plump endothelial cells, interstitial granular eosinophilic material, and varying numbers of neutrophils with leukocytoclasis. Warthin-Starry staining demonstrates tangles of bacilli in the eosinophilic material[171,172] (Fig. 9-23), and organisms may be detected by immunohistochemistry and PCR.[173-176]

The differential diagnosis includes other vasoproliferative disorders.[70] In immunocompromised patients, KS must be considered. In KS, the vascular structures are less well formed, and the fascicular pattern and hyaline globules of KS are not seen in bacillary angiomatosis. The endothelial cells of bacillary angiomatosis are positive for *Ulex europaeus* and factor VIIIRA, whereas they are negative in KS. Detection of bacteria in bacillary angiomatosis and human herpesvirus 8 in KS are helpful in establishing a diagnosis.

DIFFUSE PATTERN

Diffuse paracortical proliferations are the most difficult benign lymphadenopathies to differentiate from lymphomas because there is often subtotal effacement of the nodal architecture and immunoblasts with atypical cytologic features, occasionally mimicking large cell or Hodgkin's lymphomas. Clinical history, results of laboratory studies, immunophenotyping, and molecular analysis are crucial in distinguishing benign from malignant proliferations.

Infectious Mononucleosis

Infectious mononucleosis caused by EBV infection commonly produces lymphadenopathy and enlargement of tonsils in adolescents and young adults, although older adults may also be affected. Clinical features including pharyngitis, fever, cervical lymphadenopathy of short duration, and splenomegaly, along with laboratory features such as reactive peripheral blood lymphocytes and the presence of heterophile antibody, usually lead to a diagnosis without a lymph node biopsy. However, lymph nodes may be biopsied to exclude lymphoma, and tonsils may be removed for relief of airway obstruction.

The histologic features vary during the course of the disease.[8,177-180] Early in the disorder, there is follicular hyperplasia, often with monocytoid B-cell aggregates and epithelioid histiocytes, resembling Toxoplasmic lymphadenitis. Later, expansion of the paracortex predominates. Although the architecture of the lymph node or tonsil may be distorted, it is not effaced. There is a polymorphous paracortical infiltrate with a mottled pattern caused by the presence of large immunoblasts in a background of medium-sized and small lymphocytes and plasma cells (Fig. 9-24). The immunoblasts are occasionally binucleate and resemble classic Reed-Sternberg cells. In some areas there may be a diffuse proliferation of immunoblasts, resembling large cell lymphoma. However, in contrast to large cell lymphoma, intermediate-sized lymphocytes, plasma cells, and plasmacytoid cells are present among the immunoblasts, high endothelial venules are often prominent, and single-cell necrosis is common. The sinuses are often distended and filled with monocytoid B cells, small lymphocytes, and immunoblasts.

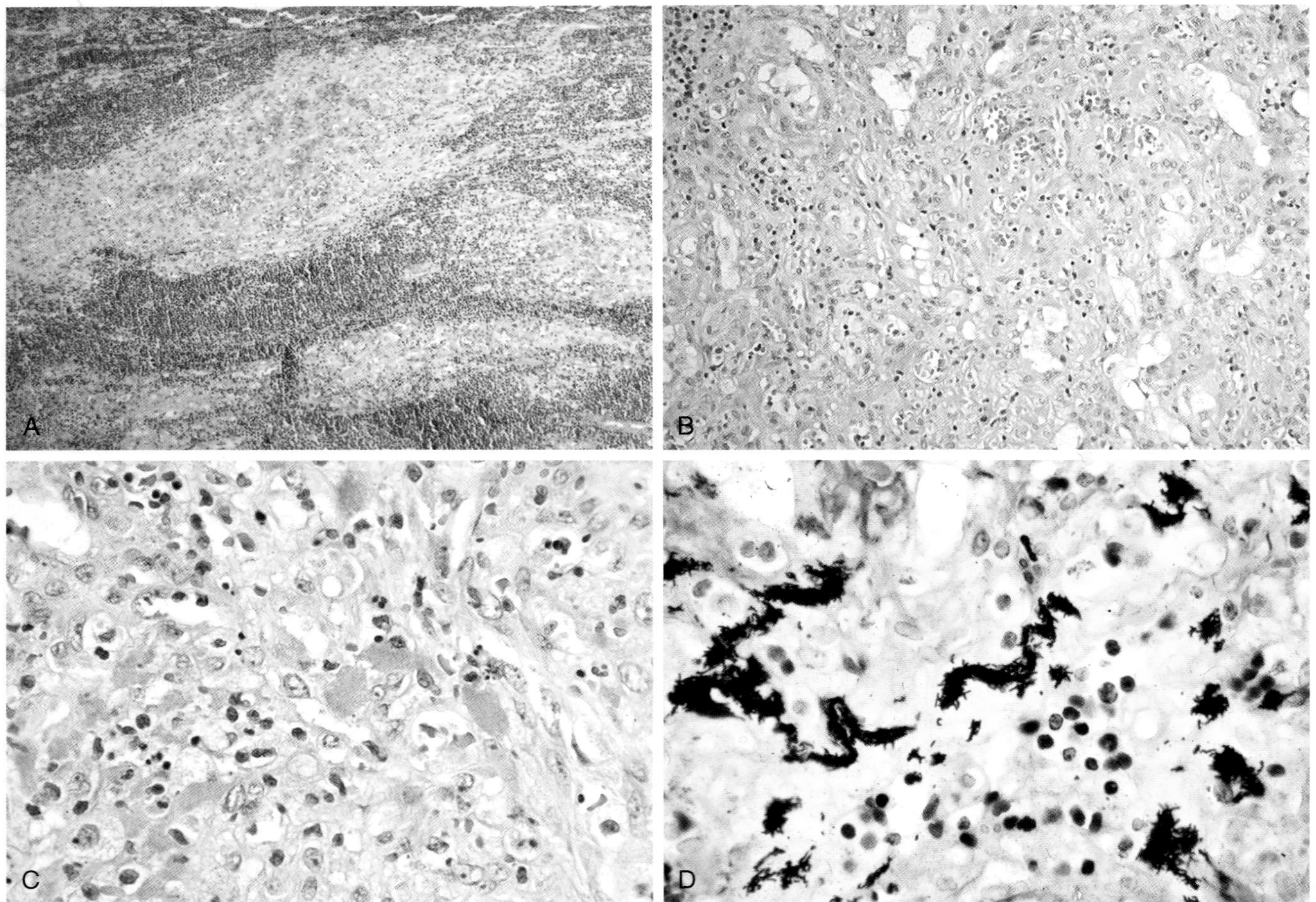

Figure 9-23. Bacillary angiomatosis involving a lymph node. A, Multiple coalescent nodules of proliferated blood vessels. **B,** Blood vessels, some barely canalized, lined by plump endothelial cells with pale cytoplasm. **C,** Amphophilic material representing tangles of bacteria among endothelial cells. **D,** Tangles of *Bartonella henselae* (Warthin-Starry).

Immunophenotyping shows both T and B immunoblasts, with B immunoblasts usually predominating.[181] The immunoblasts, including Reed-Sternberg–like cells, often express CD30, but they are CD15⁻ (see Fig. 9-24).[182] CD8⁺ T cells outnumber CD4⁺ cells. In situ hybridization for EBER shows numerous positive immunoblasts in the paracortex but not in the germinal centers; monocytoid B cells may also contain EBV RNA.[183,184]

LMP-1 protein is also expressed and may be related to the accumulation of p53 within the cells, as the two proteins appear to colocalize.[185,186]

The most important differential diagnoses are high-grade non-Hodgkin's lymphoma and classical Hodgkin's lymphoma. When paracortical immunoblasts are numerous, large cell (immunoblastic) lymphoma of B- or T-cell type may be considered. Morphologic features favoring a benign process include incomplete architectural effacement, mixed cellular infiltrate, patent sinuses, and presence of high endothelial venules among the large cells. Immunohistochemical features include the presence of both B- and T-cell immunoblasts and a predominance of CD8⁺ T cells. The presence of classic Reed-Sternberg–like cells may suggest Hodgkin's lymphoma, but these cells lack expression of CD15, mark with either B- or T-cell antibodies, and are usually CD45⁺. In addition, they are not in the cellular environment of the subtypes of Hodgkin's lymphoma. Tonsillar location and young patient age should prompt a conservative approach and testing for EBV.

Other viral infections such as CMV and herpes simplex may resemble infectious mononucleosis. The presence of characteristic viral inclusions or the demonstration of viral proteins by immunohistochemistry aids in their distinction from infectious mononucleosis.

Cytomegalovirus Infection

CMV infection may cause the clinical picture of infectious mononucleosis, but the heterophile antibody test is negative.[187] Lymph nodes show follicular or paracortical hyperplasia with scattered immunoblasts, which may resemble Reed-Sternberg cells.[188] A monocytoid B-cell reaction in sinuses is usually prominent, and epithelioid histiocytes may be present within the clusters. Intranuclear and intracytoplasmic viral inclusions typical of CMV infection may be found within epithelioid histiocytes or, less often, vascular endothelial cells, although in immunocompetent individuals they may be sparse (Fig. 9-25). They should be diligently searched for in a lymph node biopsy with an unexplained prominent monocytoid B-cell proliferation.

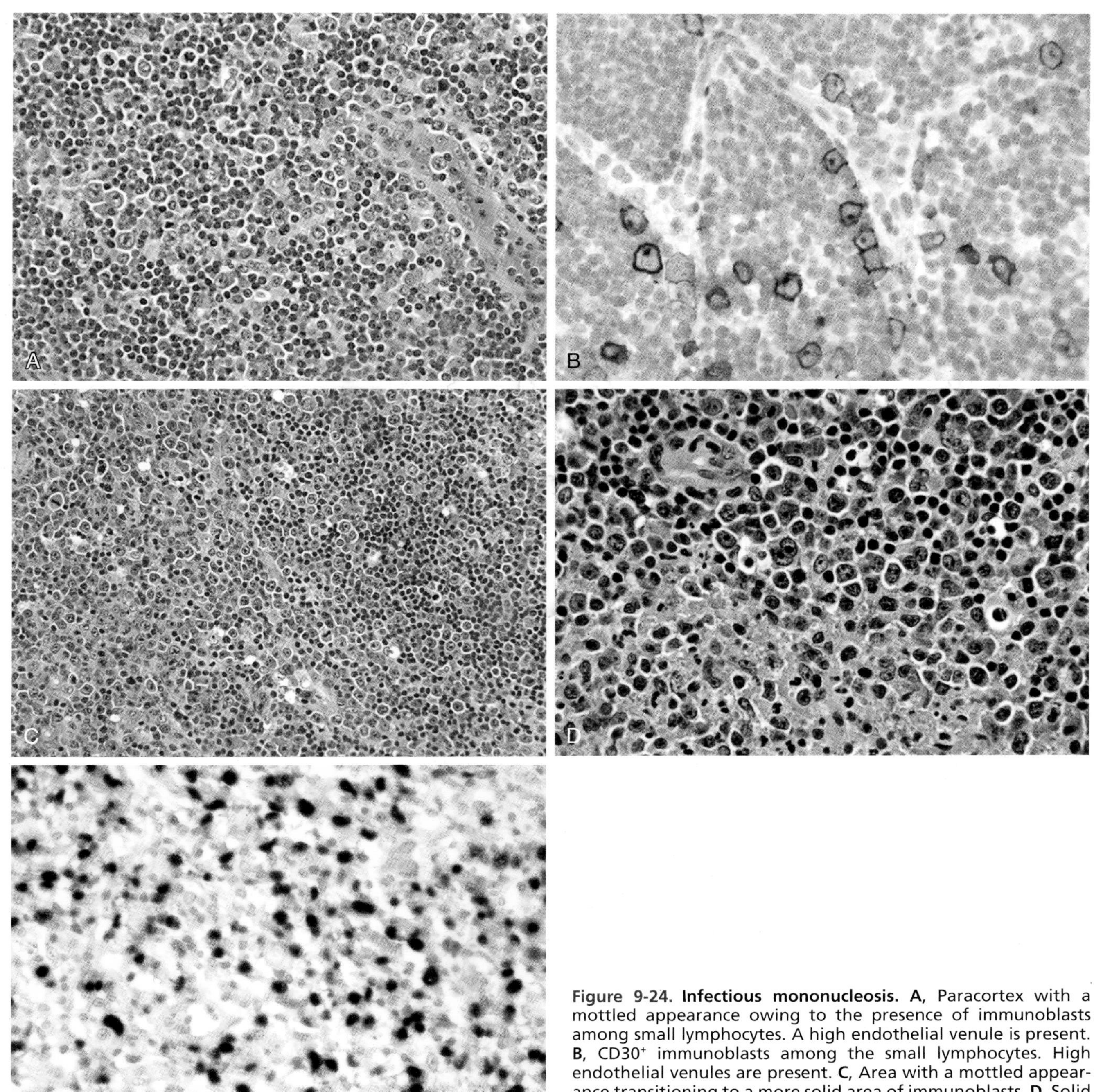

Figure 9-24. Infectious mononucleosis. A, Paracortex with a mottled appearance owing to the presence of immunoblasts among small lymphocytes. A high endothelial venule is present. **B,** CD30⁺ immunoblasts among the small lymphocytes. High endothelial venules are present. **C,** Area with a mottled appearance transitioning to a more solid area of immunoblasts. **D,** Solid focus of immunoblasts with necrosis. A Reed-Sternberg–like cell is present. **E,** Epstein-Barr virus (EBV)–encoded RNA (EBER) in situ hybridization showing numerous EBV-infected cells.

Immunophenotyping shows paracortical T cells and immunoblasts that may express CD30. Infected histiocytes may express cytoplasmic, but not membrane, CD15. This phenotype and the presence of cytomegalic cells may cause confusion with Hodgkin's lymphoma.[189] Lack of classic Reed-Sternberg cells and the absence of the typical background of classical Hodgkin's lymphoma favor CMV lymphadenitis. CMV antigens can be demonstrated by immunohistochemistry, which is useful in cases without well-developed inclusions.[190]

Herpes Simplex Lymphadenitis

Herpes simplex (type I or II) produces a lymphadenitis that is most often localized to inguinal lymph nodes but may be disseminated. It is seen predominantly, but not exclusively, in immunocompromised hosts.

The histologic picture varies. There may be follicular hyperplasia with expansion of the paracortex by a proliferation of immunoblasts, resembling other viral infections. Monocytoid B cells may be prominent and mimic marginal

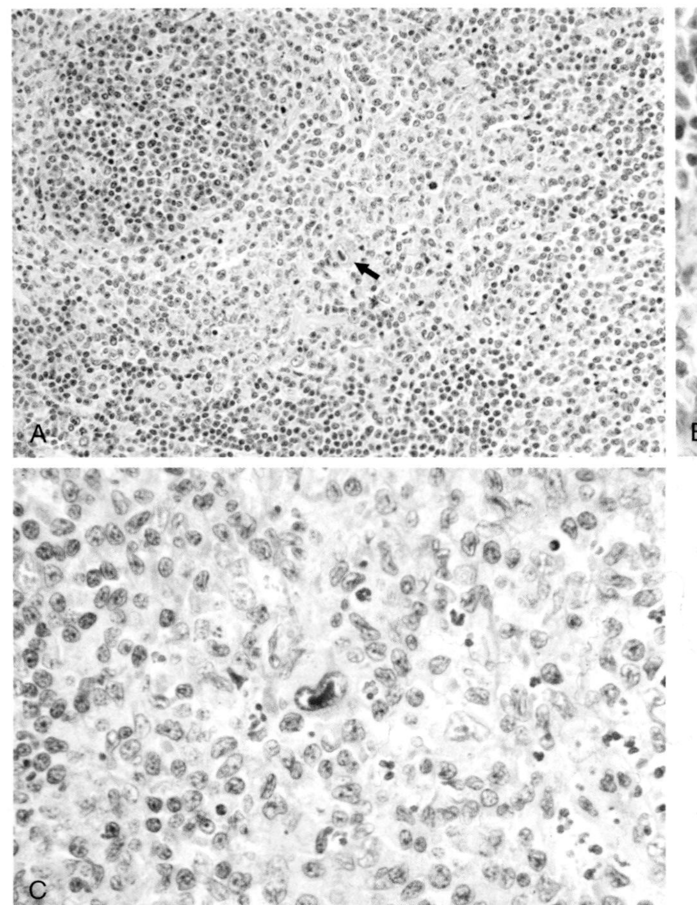

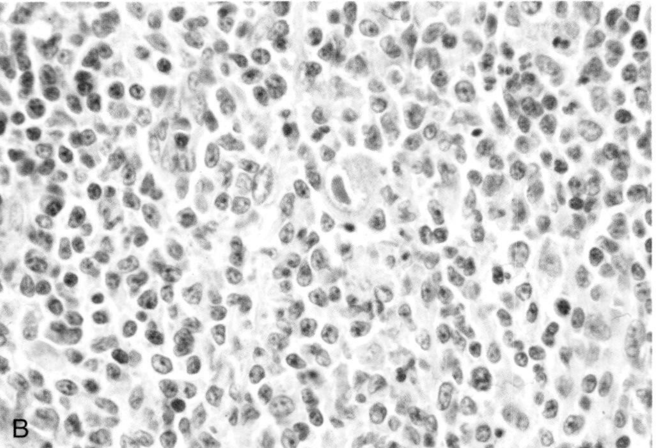

Figure 9-25. Lymph node from an immunocompetent patient with cytomegalovirus (CMV) infection. A, Among the parafollicular monocytoid B cells is a large cell (*arrow*) with a prominent intranuclear inclusion. **B**, Higher magnification of the intranuclear inclusion. **C**, Anti-CMV antibody–positive intranuclear inclusion (immunoperoxidase [anti-CMV]).

zone lymphoma.[191] Usually, foci of necrosis are present, containing neutrophils and varying numbers of large cells with margination of nuclear chromatin and prominent nuclear inclusions, resulting in a "ground glass" appearance (Fig. 9-26). Intranuclear eosinophilic inclusions with clear halos have also been reported. Histiocytes often surround necrotic foci, but granulomas are absent.[191] The diagnosis can be confirmed by immunostaining, serology, or in situ hybridization.[192,193]

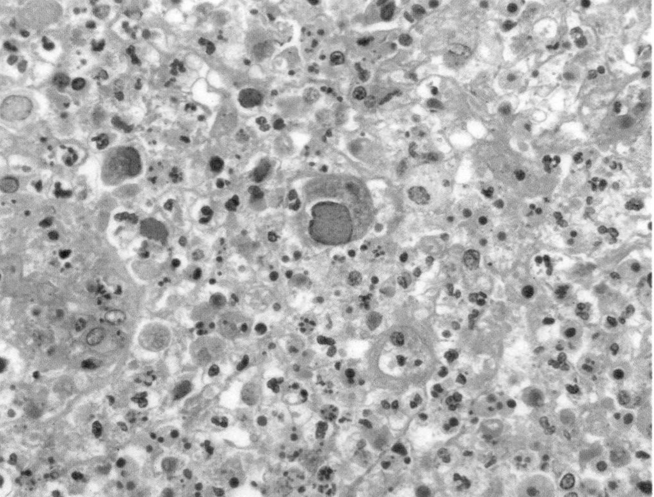

Figure 9-26. Lymph node from a patient with chronic lymphocytic leukemia shows a focus of necrosis containing large cells, with margination of nuclear chromatin and a "ground glass" nucleus, characteristic of herpes simplex infection.

Dilantin-Associated Lymphadenopathy

Lymphadenopathy associated with anticonvulsant therapy (most commonly phenytoin [Dilantin]; less often carbamazepine)[194,195] has been the subject of numerous case reports and a few larger series. Rare cases of lymphoma have developed in patients using phenytoin,[196] but a causal role in the development of lymphoma has not been demonstrated.[197] Most patients undergoing lymph node biopsy have been on therapy for prolonged periods (median, 2 years), although some have been treated for less than 6 months. Common symptoms include fever, rash, weight loss, fatigue, organomegaly, and eosinophilia. Lymphadenopathy may be localized or generalized.[197]

The histologic appearance is variable. The most common feature is paracortical expansion by a polymorphous popula-

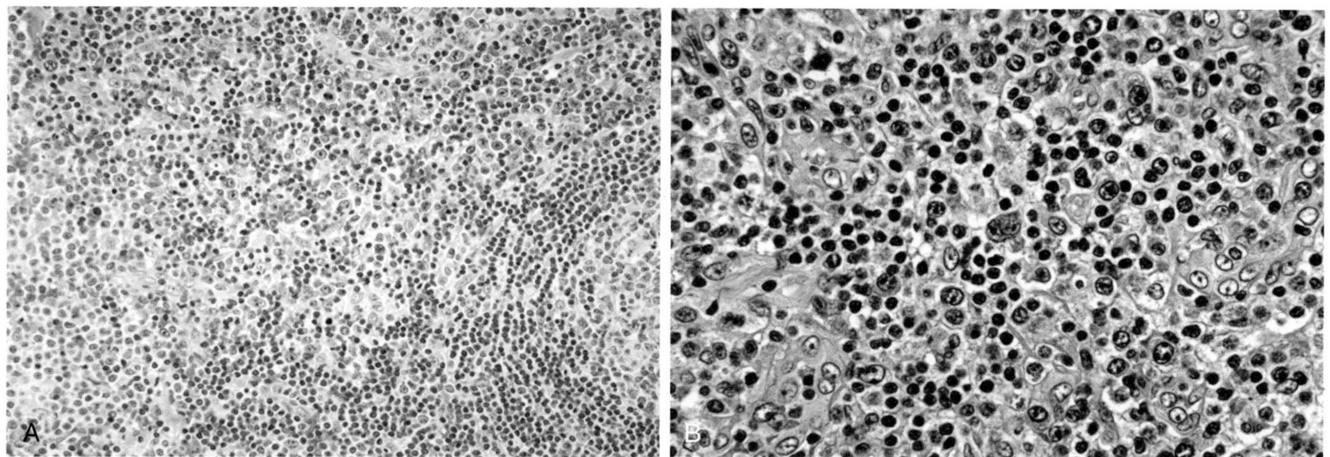

Figure 9-27. Lymph node from a patient taking phenytoin (Dilantin) for epilepsy. A, The interfollicular area is expanded by a polymorphous infiltrate. A portion of a follicle is present on the right. **B,** Interfollicular area containing lymphocytes, immunoblasts, histiocytes, eosinophils, and high endothelial venules. A Reed-Sternberg–like cell is present.

tion of immunoblasts, plasma cells, histiocytes, and eosinophils, with high endothelial venules; Reed-Sternberg–like cells may be found (Fig. 9-27).[18,34] There is variable follicular hyperplasia, and some cases show regressed germinal centers.[197] Immunophenotyping usually shows an intact immunoarchitecture, and many of the immunoblasts are B cells.[197]

The differential diagnosis includes both classical Hodgkin's lymphoma and non-Hodgkin's lymphomas, as well as viral lymphadenitis. The absence of CD15$^+$, CD30$^+$, B- and T-antigen–negative Reed-Sternberg cells helps exclude Hodgkin's lymphoma. When immunoblasts predominate, gene rearrangement studies can be useful to assess clonality[198,199]; however, rare cases of anticonvulsant-related lymphadenopathy can be monoclonal. The bone marrow may also be involved, making the diagnosis of a benign condition even more problematic.

The clinical history is essential to making this diagnosis. Cessation of the drug should result in resolution of the lymphadenopathy within several weeks.[198,200]

Pearls and Pitfalls

- Knowledge of normal lymph node structure and function is essential for accurate diagnosis.
- Immunohistochemical stains are valuable for highlighting architectural and ctyologic components.
- Immunohistochemical stains should be performed as a panel, with pertinent stains selected based on the histologic appearance in routine hematoxylin-eosin sections.
- Atypical cells should be evaluated in the company they keep; cells mimicking Reed-Sternberg cells can be seen in reactive conditions, particularly infectious mononucleosis.
- Limited clonal B-cell and T-cell populations can sometimes be identified by PCR in reactive hyperplasia; interpret all data in the context of clinical and histologic features.

References can be found on Expert Consult @ www.expertconsult.com

Chapter 10

The Normal Bone Marrow

Barbara J. Bain

CHAPTER OUTLINE

Although hematopoietic stem cells circulate in small numbers, hematopoiesis, in steady-state conditions in adult life, is largely confined to the bone marrow. All lymphopoietic and hematopoietic cells are ultimately derived from pluripotent hematopoietic stem cells—slowly cycling cells with a capacity for self-renewal.[1] Pluripotent stem cells give rise to common lymphoid stem cells and multipotent myeloid stem cells. The multipotent myeloid stem cells give rise to lineage-committed progenitors. None of the stem cells and progenitor cells is morphologically recognizable. Such cells can be identified in vitro by their capacity for self-renewal and their ability to differentiate to produce cells of specific lineages. Some of them can also be putatively identified by flow cytometry, immunocytochemistry, and immunohistochemistry, detecting the expression of antigens characteristic of stem cells such as CD34, with or without CD38. Stem cells in the marrow are located in stem cell "niches" adjacent to either bone or blood vessels, where they have a close relationship with stromal cells. Cells beyond the stage of a lineage-committed progenitor can be recognized from cytologic as well as functional and immunophenotypic characteristics. Some platelets are produced from megakaryocytes that have entered the circulation and lodged in the lungs. With this exception, all mature blood cells in healthy adults are produced in the bone marrow by a process involving repeated cell division and cellular maturation (Fig. 10-1).

Hematopoiesis occurs in a specific bone marrow microenvironment, in cavities surrounded and traversed by bony spicules. The intertrabecular spaces are occupied by stroma and hematopoietic cells, with the two elements having a dynamic interrelationship. The stroma is composed of stromal cells and a matrix of proteins such as laminin, thrombospondin, and fibronectin. Recognizable stromal elements include blood vessels, nerves, fat cells, other mesenchymal cells (e.g., reticular cells, macrophages, fibroblasts), and a delicate fiber network. The fiber network is detectable on a reticulin stain; if graded 0 to 4,[2] most normal subjects have grade 0 to 1 reticulin, but some have grade 2. Reticulin is deposited preferentially around arterioles and adjacent to bony spicules. In normal bone marrow, collagen is not detectable on a hematoxylin-eosin (H&E) stain or a trichrome stain. The earliest recognizable granulocyte precursors—myeloblasts and promyelocytes—are located against the periosteum and in a band around arterioles. Myelocytes, metamyelocytes, and neutrophils are found progressively farther from the endosteum. Recognizable cells of eosinophil lineage do not show the same distribution; eosinophil myelocytes and eosinophils are more randomly distributed. The distribution of basophils is not known. Maturing erythroid cells and megakaryocytes are found more centrally in the intertrabecular space. Erythroblasts are clustered, forming erythroid islands in which erythroid cells of varying degrees of maturity surround a central macrophage. Megakaryocytes are found preferentially in relation to sinusoids, and serial sections of bone marrow show that part of the megakaryocyte cytoplasm abuts a sinusoid. They may form small clusters, but these comprise no more than two or, occasionally, three cells. Other cellular components of the bone marrow include mast cells, lymphocytes, plasma cells, monocytes, and macrophages. Normal bone marrow architecture is shown diagrammatically in Figure 10-2.

The regulation of hematopoiesis is highly complex. It involves the interaction of adhesion molecules on hematopoietic cells with their ligands on stromal cells and the action of hematopoietic growth factors such as stem cell factor, inter-

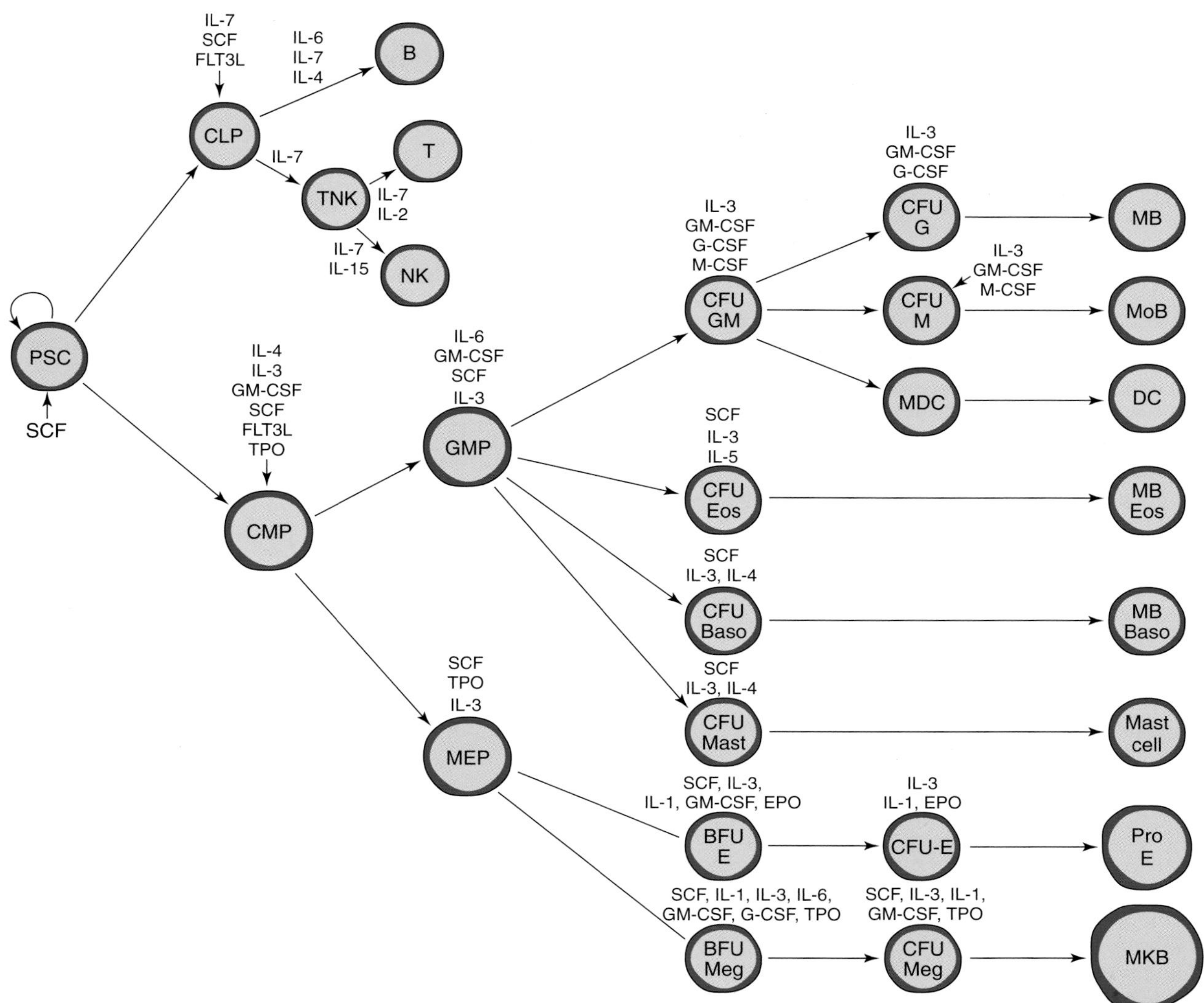

Figure 10-1. Diagrammatic representation of one proposed scheme of the stem cell hierarchy,[1] showing the growth factors believed to operate at each stage. Alternative models of hematopoiesis have been proposed,[18,19] including one in which the common erythroid and megakaryocytic progenitor arises directly from the pluripotent lymphoid-myeloid stem cell (PSC; also known as the *common lymphoid-myeloid progenitor)* rather than from the common myeloid progenitor (CMP; also known as *multipotent myeloid stem cells*). B, B lymphocyte; Baso, basophil; BFU, burst-forming unit; CFU, colony-forming unit; CLP, common lymphoid progenitor; DC, dendritic cell; E, erythroid; Eos, eosinophil; EPO, erythropoietin; FLT3L, ligand of FLT3; G, granulocyte (neutrophil); G-CSF, granulocyte colony-stimulating factor; GM, granulocyte-macrophage; GM-CSF, granulocyte-macrophage colony-stimulating factor; GMP, granulocyte-monocyte progenitor; IL, interleukin; M, macrophage; Mast, mast cell; MB, myeloblast; M-CSF, monocyte colony-stimulating factor; MDC, myeloid dendritic cell; Meg, megakaryocyte; MEP, myeloid erythroid progenitor; MKB, megakaryoblast; MoB, monoblast; NK, natural killer; ProE, proerythroblast; SCF, stem cell factor; T, T lymphocyte; TNK, T/NK cell progenitor; TPO, thrombopoietin.

leukin (IL)-3, IL-4, IL-5, IL-6, granulocyte-macrophage colony-stimulating factor, granulocyte colony-stimulating factor, monocyte colony-stimulating factor, erythropoietin, and thrombopoietin.[3] Growth factors may be secreted locally by bone marrow stromal cells (e.g., granulocyte-macrophage colony-stimulating factor), or they may be secreted at distant sites (e.g., erythropoietin). The ultimate effects of growth factors on hematopoiesis are mediated by transcription factors. Through their regulation of gene expression, these proteins coordinate the many proliferation and differentiation signals that reach the cell and are important for establishing the ultimate characteristics and phenotype of the mature blood cell. Although most diagrams of hematopoiesis suggest that cellular differentiation is unidirectional along one lineage, recent evidence suggests that it may be possible to reprogram cells of one lineage to differentiate into another lineage by altering the expression of various transcription factors.[1] Whether this takes place only under experimental conditions, in certain pathologic situations, or perhaps even occasionally in normal hematopoiesis, is not clear. The stages at which various growth factors are believed to operate are shown in Figure 10-1.

The proportions of different hematopoietic cells normally present in the bone marrow are best determined by examining bone marrow from healthy volunteers, but it is also possible to examine marrow obtained from volunteer patients who are apparently hematologically normal. Patients with normal blood counts who require surgery for conditions that are unlikely to have any influence of bone marrow activity are

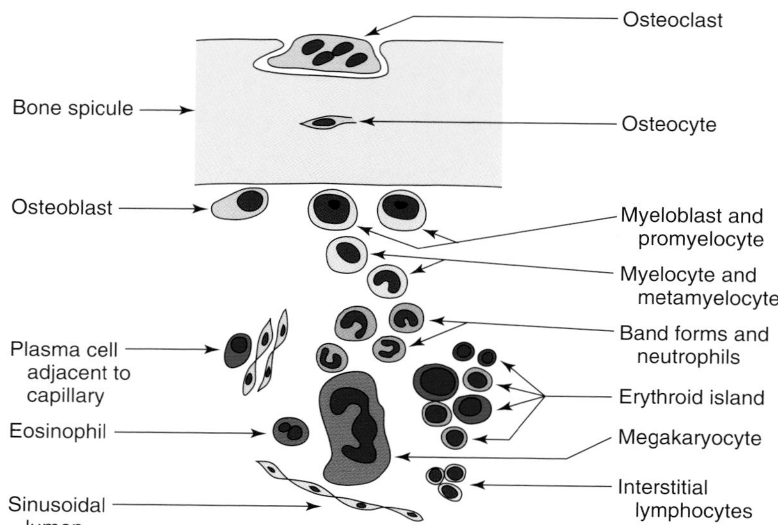

Figure 10-2. Diagrammatic representation of the topography of normal bone marrow. Osteoclasts, osteoblasts, myeloblasts, and promyelocytes are adjacent to the spicule of bone. Deeper in the intertrabecular space are maturing cells of neutrophil lineage, erythroid islands with a central macrophage, and interstitial lymphocytes. Eosinophils and their precursors are apparently randomly scattered, plasma cells are interstitial or form a sheath around capillaries, and megakaryocytes abut a sinusoid at one extremity of the cell.

suitable. Differential counts can be performed on wedge-spread films prepared directly from the bone marrow aspirate, on buffy coat preparations, or on films of crushed marrow particles. For wedge-spread films, the first 0.1 to 0.2 mL of the aspirate should be used so that there is minimal dilution by peripheral blood. The effects of dilution should be further minimized by counting the trails behind individual particles. For films of crushed particles, dilution is less of a problem; however, the films may be thicker, so identification of individual cells is more difficult. Whether wedge-spread films, buffy coat preparations, or films of crushed particles are used, a large number of cells must be counted because some of the cells of interest are present in a low proportion, and the count would otherwise be very imprecise. The International Council for Standardization in Hematology recommends that at least 500 cells be analyzed whenever the cell percentages will be used for diagnostic purposes[4]; following this guidance is particularly important when the percentage will be used to assign a diagnostic category (e.g., acute myeloid leukemia versus myelodysplastic syndrome). Results of studies using these methods are summarized in Table 10-1.[5-12] In one study the myeloid-to-erythroid ratio was found to be higher in women than in men,[10] but this was not confirmed in two other studies.[11,13]

Bone marrow cellularity in health is dependent on the age of the subject. The proportion of the marrow cavity occupied by hematopoietic and lymphoid cells rather than adipose cells varies from 100% at birth to between 30% and 65% after age 80 years. Between age 30 and 70 years, cellularity is of the order of 40% to 70%. Figure 10-3 shows a bone marrow biopsy section with normal cellularity in comparison with hypocellular and hypercellular bone marrow specimens.

HEMATOPOIESIS

Erythropoiesis

The morphologic features of erythroid precursors in bone marrow films and sections are summarized in Table 10-2 and illustrated in Figures 10-4 to 10-8. In normal bone marrow, cells of each successive stage of maturation are more numerous than those of the preceding stage. Erythroid islands may be noted in bone marrow aspirates (Fig. 10-9) but are more readily appreciated in trephine biopsy sections, where they are located in the intertrabecular space away from the surface of the bone (Fig. 10-10). In normal subjects, a low proportion of erythroblasts may show binuclearity, cytoplasmic bridging, detached nuclear fragments, and irregular hemoglobinization (see later).

Assessment of erythropoiesis in aspirate films requires not only a Romanowsky stain (e.g., Wright-Giemsa or May-Grünwald-Giemsa stain) but also a Perls Prussian blue stain; the latter both assesses storage iron and determines the presence, number, and distribution of erythroblast siderotic granules. A Perls stain identifies hemosiderin but not ferritin. Normal late erythroblasts have a small number of scattered fine hemosiderin granules (Fig. 10-11). Occasional intermediate erythroblasts may also contain siderotic granules. A Perls stain on trephine biopsy sections is informative if specimens have been plastic embedded; storage iron can be assessed, and abnormal sideroblasts can be detected. A Perls stain on sections from a paraffin-embedded, decalcified biopsy specimen is much less reliable because storage iron may have been removed in whole or in part by the process of decalcification, and regardless of whether storage iron is present, siderotic granules cannot be assessed.

Granulopoiesis

The morphologic features of granulocytic (specifically neutrophil) precursors in bone marrow films and sections are summarized in Table 10-3 and illustrated in Figures 10-12 to 10-15. Maturating cells of eosinophil and basophil lineage can be recognized morphologically from the myelocyte stage onward. When there is reactive eosinophilia, it is often possible to recognize eosinophil promyelocytes, cells with a persistent nucleolus and a paranuclear Golgi zone that have brightly staining primary granules and a few eosinophilic granules.

Text continued on page 147

Table 10-1 Mean Values and 95% Ranges for Bone Marrow Cells in Sternal or Iliac Crest Aspirates of Healthy White Adults

	Jacobsen[6]	Segerdahl[7]		Vaughan and Brockmyr[8]	Wintrobe et al[9]	Bain[10]	den Ottonlander[11]	Girodon et al[12]
Age (yr)	20-29	20-30		17-45	Not stated	21-56	Not stated	60-82
Number and gender	28 males and females	52 males	40 females	42 males, 8 females	12 males	30 males, 20 females	53 males, 14 females	40 males, 14 females
Site	Sternum	Sternum	Sternum	Sternum	Sternum	Iliac crest	Not stated	Sternum
Myeloid-to-erythroid ratio	3.34	—	—	6.9	2.3 (1.1-3.5)*	2.4 (1.4-3.6)	2.2 (0.8-3.6)	1.8-4.4
Myeloblasts	1.21 (0.75-1.67)	1.32 (0.2-2.5)	1.2 (0.1-2.3)	1.3 (0-3)	0.9 (0.1-1.7)	1.4 (0-3)	0.4 (0-1.3)	0-2.4
Promyelocytes	2.49 (0.99-3.99)	1.35 (0-2.9)	1.65 (0.5-2.8)	—†	3.3 (1.9-4.7)	7.8 (3.2-12.4)	13.7 (8-19.4)	3.6-10
Myelocytes	17.36 (11.54-23.18)	15.00 (7.5-22.5)	16.6 (11.4-21.8)	8.9 (3-15)	12.7 (8.5-16.9)	7.6 (3.7-10)**		6-13
Metamyelocytes	16.92 (11.4-22.44)	15.7 (9.2-22)	15.8 (11.0-20.6)	8.8 (4-15)	15.9 (7.1-24.7)	4.1 (2.3-5.9)	35.5 (22.2-48.8)	28-45
Band cells	8.7 (3.58-13.82)	10.5 (3-17.9)	8.3 (4-12.4)	23.9 (12.5-33.5)	12.4 (9.4-15.4)			
Neutrophils	13.42 (4.32-22.52)	20.9 (9.9-31.8)	21.7 (11.3-32)	18.5 (9-31.5)	7.4 (3.8-11)	34.2 (23.4-45)		
Eosinophils	2.93 (0.28-5.69)‡	2.8 (0.1-5.6)‡	3 (0-7.2)‡	1.9 (0-5.5)	3.1 (1.1-5.2)‡ 2.2 (0.3-4.2)	2.2 (0.3-4.2)	1.7 (0.2-3.3)	1.6-5.4
Basophils	0.28 (0-0.69)‡	0.14 (0-0.38)	0.16 (0-0.46)	0.2 (0-1)	<0.1 (0-0.2)§	0.1 (0-0.4)	0.2 (0-0.6)	0-1
Monocytes	1.04 (0.36-1.72)	2.3 (0.5-4)	1.61 (0.2-3)	2.4 (0-6)	0.3 (0-0.6)	1.3 (0-2.6)	2.5 (0.5-4.6)	2-5
Erythroblasts	19.26 (9.12-29.4)‖	12.9 (4.1-21.7)	11.5 (5.1-17.9)	9.5 (2.5-17.5)	25.6 (15-36.2)	25.9 (13.6-38.2)	23.6 (14.7-32.6)	16-31.4
Lymphocytes	14.6 (6.66-22.54)	16.8 (7.2-26.3)	18.1 (10.5-25.7)	16.2 (7.5-26.5)		13.1 (6-20)	16.1 (6.0-26.2)	6-18.8
Plasma cells	0.46 (0-0.96)	0.39 (0-1.1)	0.42 (0-0.9)	0.3 (0-1.5)	1.3 (0-3.5) 16.2 (7.5-26.5)	0.6 (0-1.2)	1.9 (0-3.8)	1-4.4

*Neutrophils plus precursors: erythroblasts.
†Promyelocytes were categorized with either myeloblasts or myelocytes.
‡Including eosinophil and basophil myelocytes and metamyelocytes.
§Including basophil precursors and mast cells.
‖Approximate (sum of ranges for different categories of erythroblast).
**Neutrophil plus eosinophil myelocytes: mean, 8.9 (range, 2.14-15.3); macrophages: mean, 0.4 (range, 0-1.3).
Modified from Bain BJ, Clark DM, Wilkins BS. *Bone Marrow Pathology*, 4th ed. Oxford: Wiley-Blackwell; 2009.

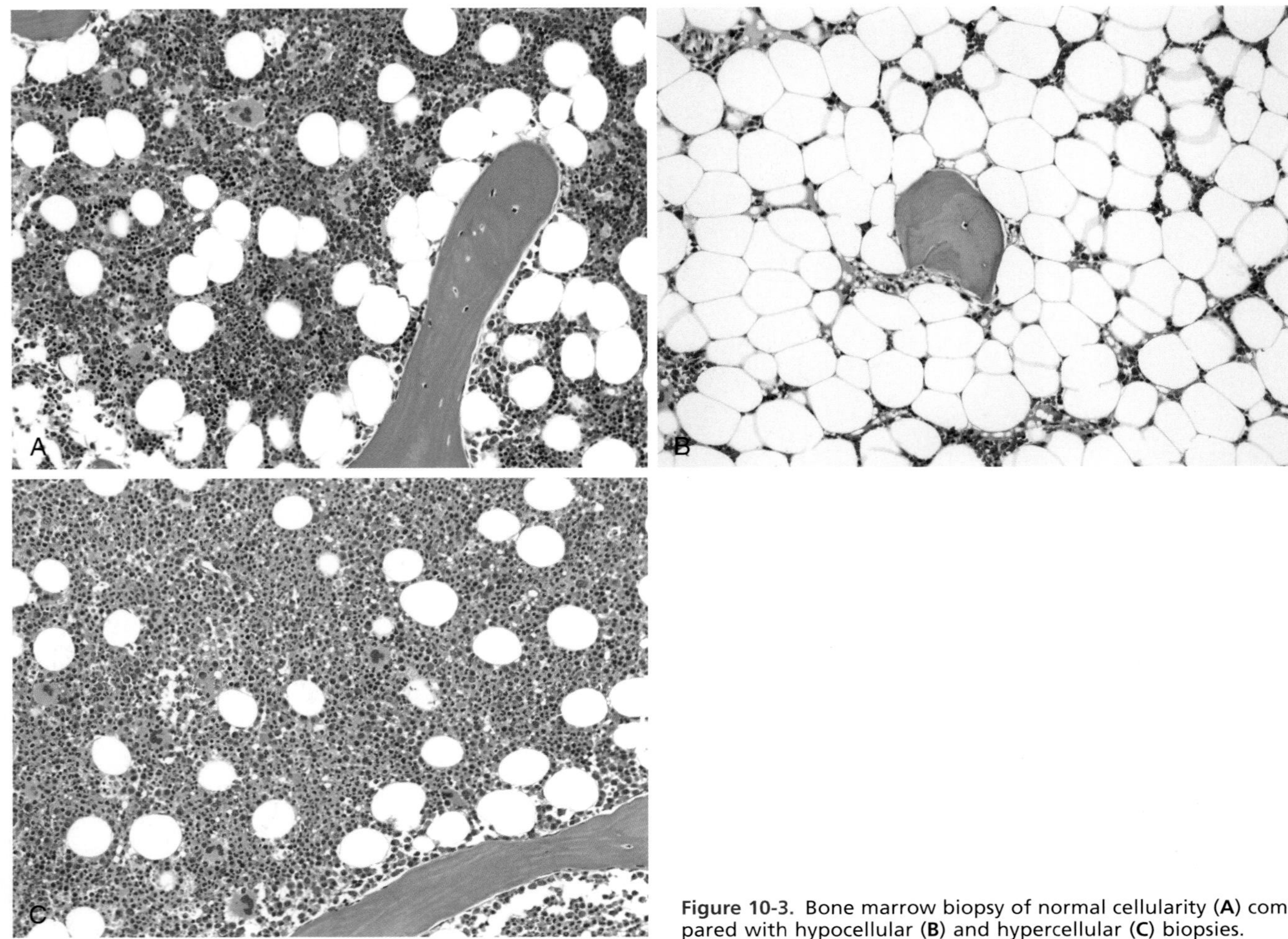

Figure 10-3. Bone marrow biopsy of normal cellularity (**A**) compared with hypocellular (**B**) and hypercellular (**C**) biopsies.

Table 10-2 Cytologic Features of Erythroid Precursors in Bone Marrow Aspirates and Trephine Biopsy Sections

Cell	Bone Marrow Aspirate	Bone Marrow Trephine Biopsy Section*
Proerythroblast	Large round cell, 12-20 μm in diameter, with finely stippled or reticular chromatin pattern and strongly basophilic (deep blue) cytoplasm; one or more nucleoli, which may be indistinct; there may be a perinuclear clear Golgi zone	Large round cell with round or slightly oval nucleus and one or more visible nucleoli, which are often linear or irregular and may abut the nuclear membrane; cytoplasmic basophilia is marked and is most readily detected on a Giemsa stain
Early erythroblast (basophilic erythroblast)	Similar to proerythroblast but smaller, and some chromatin clumping is now apparent; hemoglobin synthesis starts at this stage, but cytoplasm still appears deeply basophilic; perinuclear Golgi zone may be apparent	Somewhat smaller than proerythroblast, but otherwise with similar features
Intermediate erythroblast (polychromatic erythroblast)	Intermediate-sized cell with less basophilic cytoplasm than early erythroblast and lower nuclear-to-cytoplasmic ratio; moderate chromatin condensation into coarse clumps; paranuclear, often partly perinuclear Golgi zone may be apparent; if Golgi zone is paranuclear, nucleus may be somewhat eccentric	Intermediate-sized cell with less cytoplasmic basophilia than early erythroblast; moderate chromatin clumping; sections of paraffin-embedded biopsy specimens may exhibit artifactual perinuclear halo owing to cytoplasmic shrinking
Late erythroblast (sometimes called orthochromatic erythroblast)	Small cell, not much larger than erythrocyte, with lower nuclear-to-cytoplasmic ratio and less cytoplasmic basophilia than intermediate erythroblast; chromatin clumping is marked, and cytoplasm is acquiring a pink tinge owing to increasing amounts of hemoglobin; however, when erythropoiesis is normoblastic, there is still some cytoplasmic basophilia, so this cell is not truly orthochromatic	Small cell with condensed chromatin, pink (eosinophilic) cytoplasm on hematoxylin-eosin stain, little basophilia on Giemsa stain, and prominent perinuclear halo; nucleus is more round and regular than that of lymphocyte

*Erythroblasts of various stages of maturation are found clustered around a macrophage to form an erythroid island.

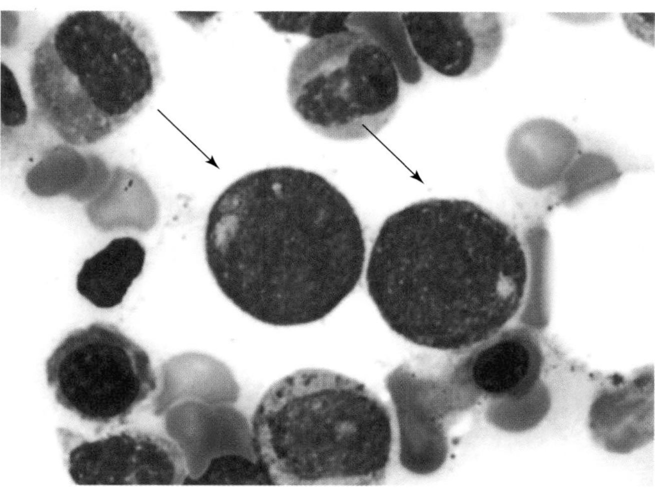

Figure 10-4. Two proerythroblasts (*arrows*) in a bone marrow aspirate from a hematologically normal man.

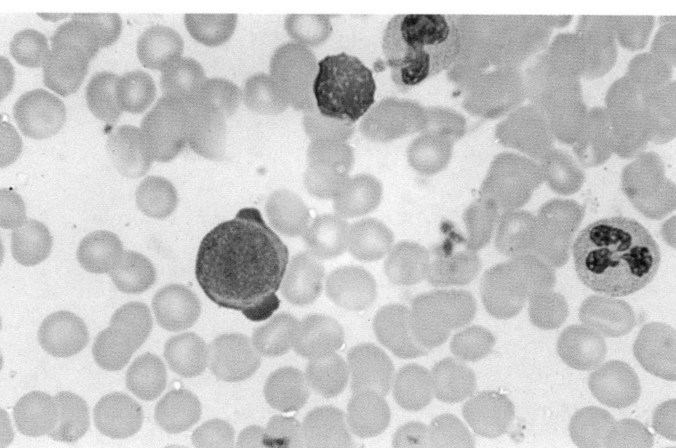

Figure 10-5. Early erythroblast and neutrophil in a bone marrow aspirate from a healthy volunteer; note the perinuclear Golgi zone in the early erythroblast.

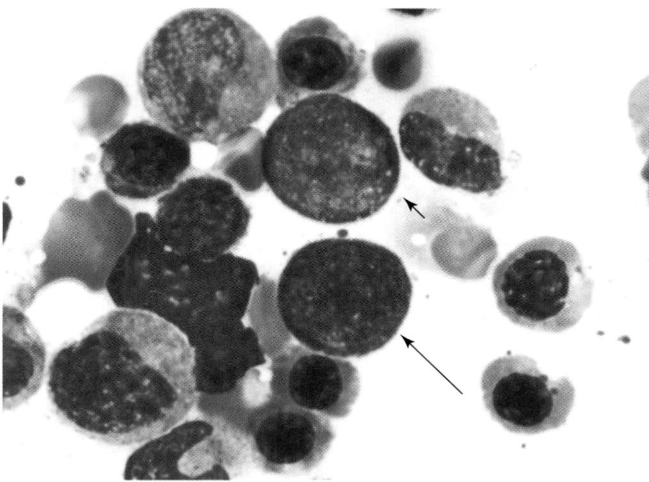

Figure 10-6. Compared with the two proerythroblasts in Figure 10-4, the erythroid precursor (*short arrow*) in this figure is intermediate between a proerythroblast and an early erythroblast (*long arrow*). Intermediate and late erythroblasts, two myelocytes, and a metamyelocyte are also present.

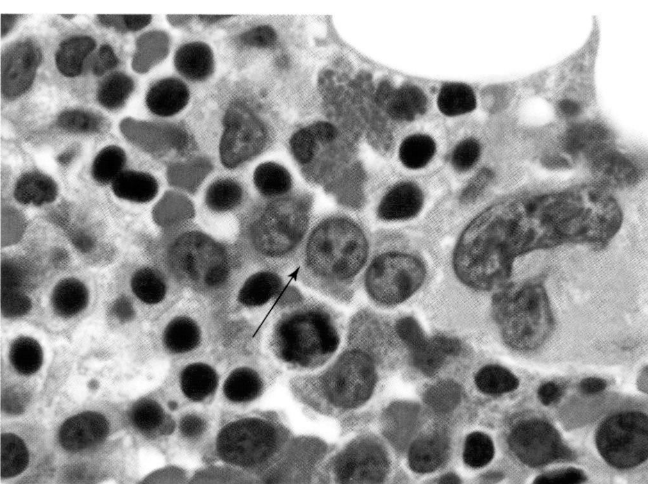

Figure 10-7. Four proerythroblasts (*arrow*) surrounded by erythroid precursors in later stages of maturation, a megakaryocyte, and some immature granulocytes in a trephine biopsy from a hematologically normal man. Note the strong amphophilic cytoplasm of the proerythroblasts and their linear or comma-shaped nucleoli, which often abut the nuclear membrane.

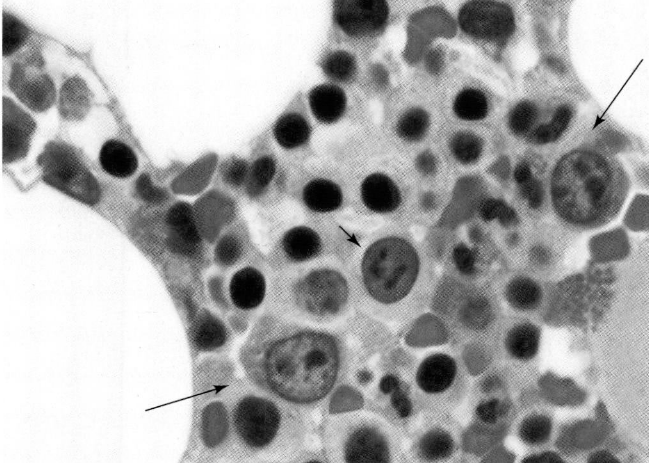

Figure 10-8. Two proerythroblasts (*long arrows*) and a late pronormoblast to early erythroblast (*short arrow*) surrounded by late erythroid precursors.

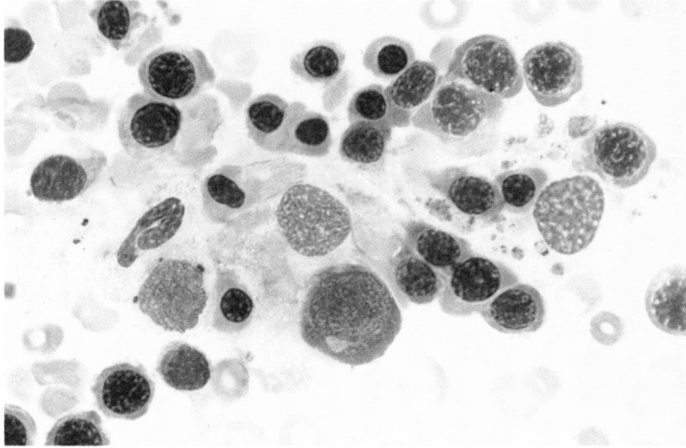

Figure 10-9. Disrupted erythroid island showing early, intermediate, and late erythroblasts in a bone marrow aspirate from a healthy volunteer.

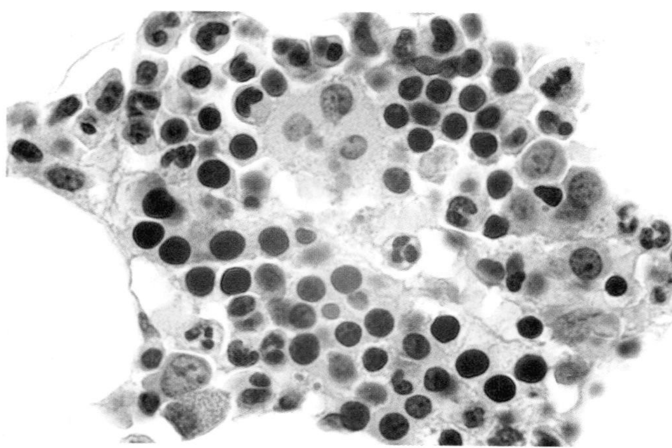

Figure 10-10. Erythroid island composed mainly of intermediate and late erythroblasts in a section of a trephine biopsy specimen from a hematologically normal patient. A megakaryocyte, eosinophil myelocyte, and several neutrophils are also apparent.

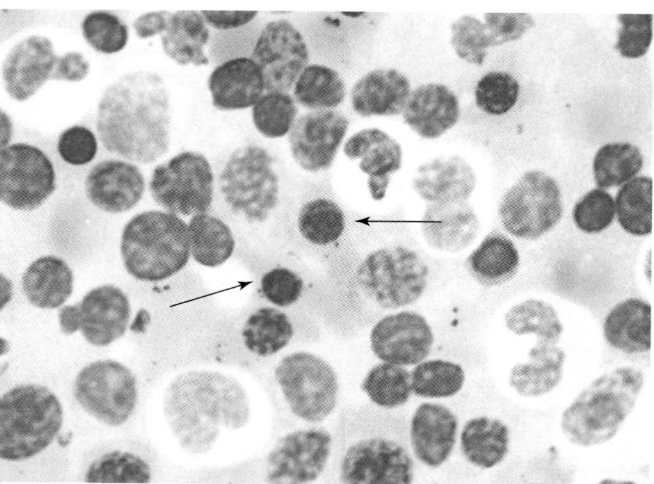

Figure 10-11. Late erythroblasts containing siderotic granules (*arrows*) in a bone marrow aspirate stained with Perls stain.

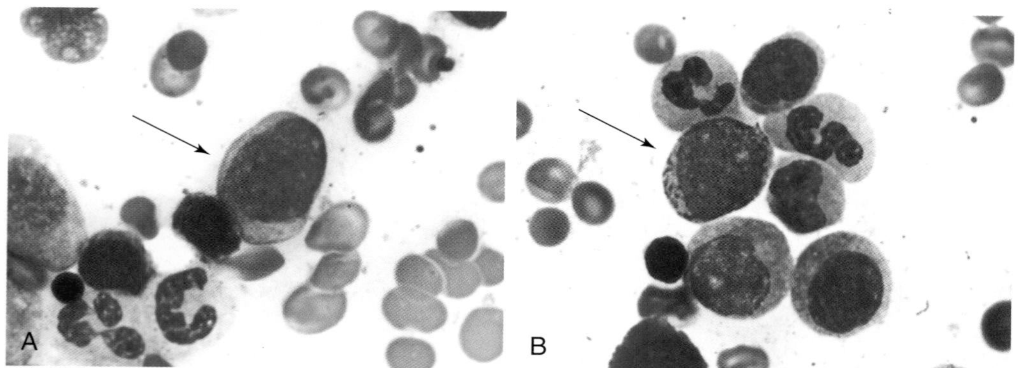

Figure 10-12. Myeloblast (**A**, *arrow*) and promyelocyte (**B**, *arrow*) in a bone marrow aspirate from a healthy volunteer. The promyelocyte is surrounded by maturing granulocytic (neutrophilic) precursors.

Table 10-3 Cytologic Features of Granulocyte (Neutrophil) Precursors in Bone Marrow Aspirates and Trephine Biopsy Sections

Cell	Bone Marrow Aspirate	Bone Marrow Trephine Biopsy Section
Myeloblast	Large cell, 12-20 μm in diameter, with high nuclear-to-cytoplasmic ratio, moderate cytoplasmic basophilia, and diffuse chromatin pattern, often with one or more round or oval nucleoli; myeloblast is more irregular in shape than proerythroblast, and its cytoplasm is less basophilic; there may be small numbers of azurophilic (reddish purple) granules	Large cell with high nuclear-to-cytoplasmic ratio, located near surface of bony spicule or near arteriole; nucleolus is more round than that of proerythroblast and does not touch nuclear membrane; on Giemsa stain, cytoplasmic basophilia is less than that of proerythroblast
Promyelocyte	Larger cell than myeloblast, 15-25 μm in diameter, with more plentiful basophilic cytoplasm and more abundant reddish purple azurophilic or primary granules; paranuclear Golgi zone; eccentric nucleus containing a nucleolus	Larger cell than myeloblast, with similar nucleus but more abundant granular cytoplasm, similarly located near bony spicules or arterioles
Myelocyte	Medium-sized to large cell, 10-20 μm in diameter; nucleus lacks a nucleolus and shows some chromatin condensation; cytoplasm is more acidophilic (pinker) than that of promyelocyte and contains azurophilic granules (which now stain less strongly) and finer, lilac-colored neutrophilic granules; Golgi zone is not conspicuous, but its presence may lead to slight nuclear indentation	Smaller cell than promyelocyte, located farther away from bone surface; cytoplasm is granular, and oval nucleus has no apparent nucleolus
Metamyelocyte	Medium-sized cell, 10-12 μm in diameter; resembles myelocyte, with granular acidophilic cytoplasm but indented or U-shaped nucleus	Medium-sized cell resembling myelocyte and similarly situated, but with indented or U-shaped nucleus
Band form and neutrophil	Medium-sized cells with granular pink cytoplasm and band-shaped or segmented nucleus, respectively; chromatin is coarsely clumped, particularly in mature neutrophil	Medium-sized cells located some distance from bony spicule or arteriole, with granular cytoplasm and coarsely clumped chromatin in band-shaped or lobulated nuclei

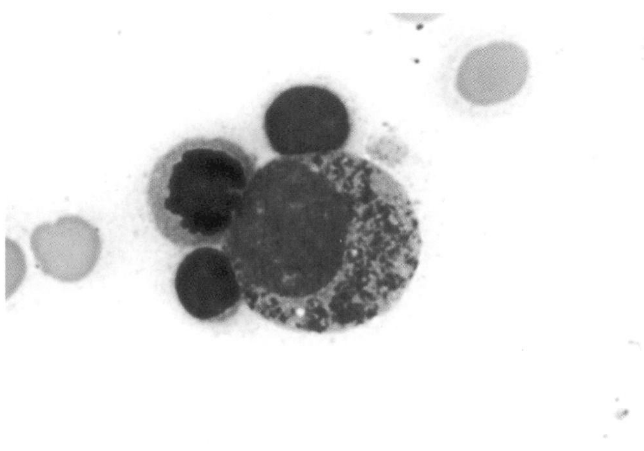

Figure 10-13. Promyelocyte, together with two lymphocytes and a mitotic figure, in a bone marrow aspirate from a hematologically normal patient.

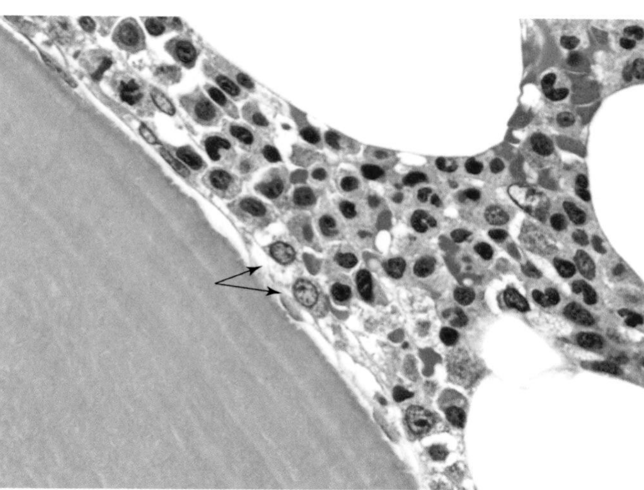

Figure 10-15. Immature granulocytes along a bony trabecula. The most immature cells are next to the bone, including blasts (*arrows*), with more mature granulocytes deeper in the intertrabecular space.

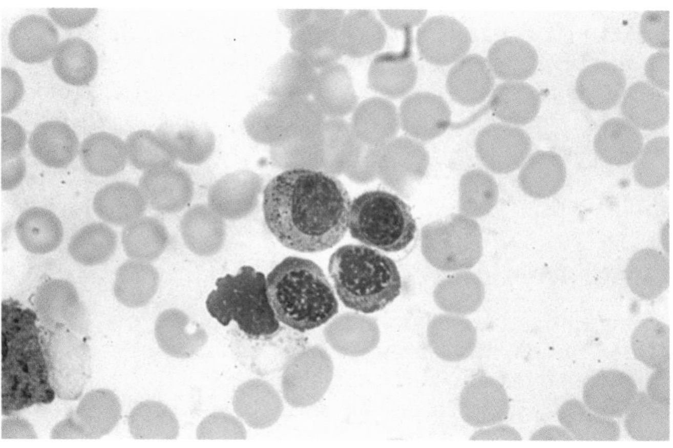

Figure 10-14. Myelocyte and three intermediate erythroblasts in a bone marrow aspirate from a healthy volunteer (May-Grünwald-Giemsa stain).

Megakaryocytes and Thrombopoiesis

Three stages of megakaryocyte maturation can be recognized in normal bone marrow. All recognizable normal megakaryocytes are large polyploid cells. The smallest immature megakaryocytes measure 30 μm or more in diameter and have a high nuclear-to-cytoplasmic ratio and basophilic, often "blebbed" cytoplasm. Mature megakaryocytes are large cells, up to 160 μm in diameter, generally with a lobulated nucleus and pink or lilac granular cytoplasm (Fig. 10-16); sometimes platelets are apparent, budding from the surface. A late megakaryocyte (Fig. 10-17) is similar in size to an immature megakaryocyte because virtually all cytoplasm has been shed as platelets, leaving only a rather pyknotic nucleus with a thin rim of cytoplasm. Caution should be exercised in interpreting cytologic features of megakaryocytes because these large cells are very prone to crushing during the spreading of a bone marrow film; this may fragment a nucleus or cause some parts of the nucleus to be partly extruded from the cell. The

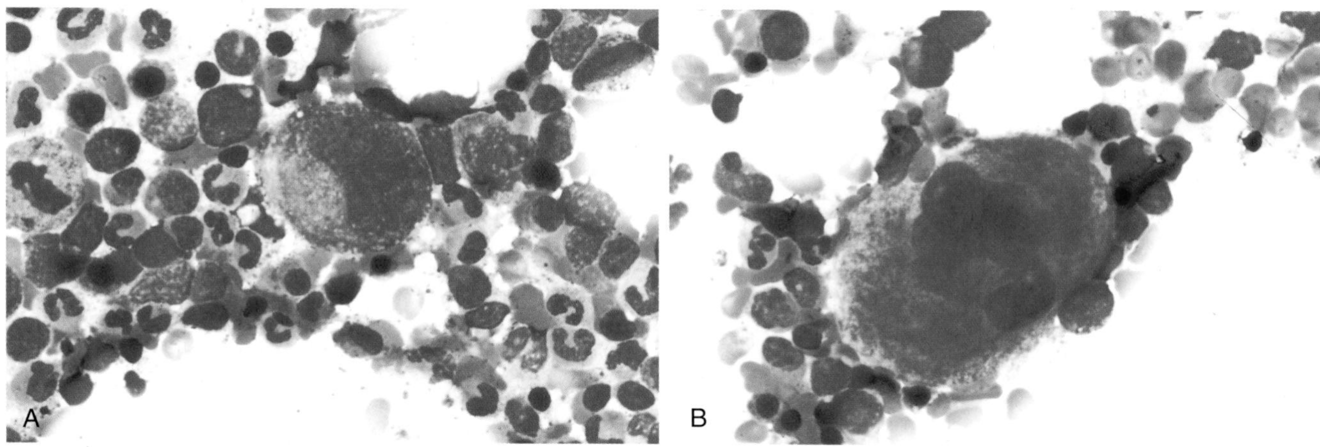

Figure 10-16. Immature (**A**) and mature (**B**) megakaryocyte in a bone marrow aspirate from a hematologically normal individual.

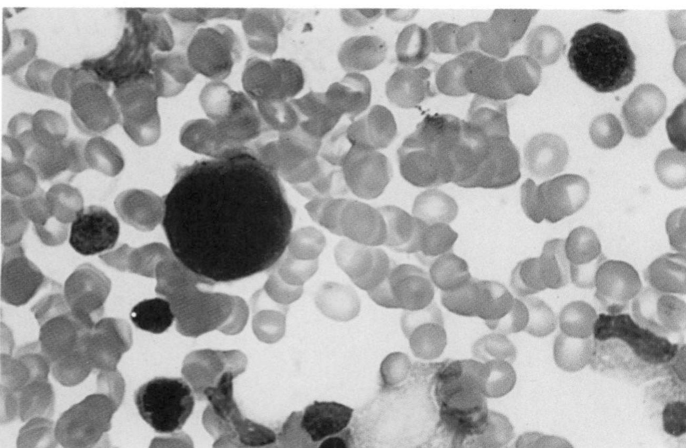

Figure 10-17. Late megakaryocyte, which has shed almost all its cytoplasm as platelets and appears as an almost bare nucleus, in a bone marrow film (May-Grünwald-Giemsa stain).

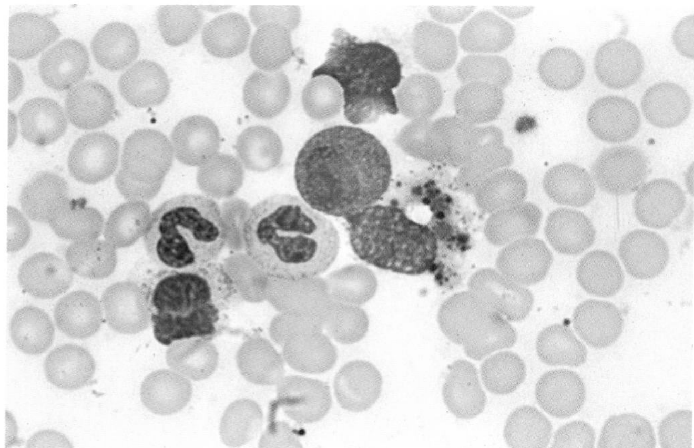

Figure 10-19. Debris-laden macrophage, eosinophil myelocyte, and two neutrophil band forms in a bone marrow aspirate from a healthy volunteer.

cytoplasm of megakaryocytes may appear to contain intact cells of other lineages; these are actually within the surface-connected canalicular system. This phenomenon, known as *emperipolesis,* is physiologic but may be exaggerated in various pathologic states.

In histologic sections, mature megakaryocytes are easily recognized by their large size, plentiful cytoplasm, and lobulated nuclei (Fig. 10-18). They can be highlighted by a Giemsa stain, which also demonstrates platelet demarcation zones in the cytoplasm, or by a periodic acid–Schiff (PAS) stain, which shows glycogen-rich pink cytoplasm. Late megakaryocytes are readily recognized as apparently bare megakaryocyte nuclei, which are larger than the nuclei of bone marrow cells of any other lineage and are more pyknotic than other nuclei of comparable size. Early megakaryocytes can be more difficult to recognize because they are not much larger than other bone marrow cells, and their features are not very distinctive. They are more readily appreciated by immunohistochemistry with a monoclonal antibody directed at platelet antigens such as

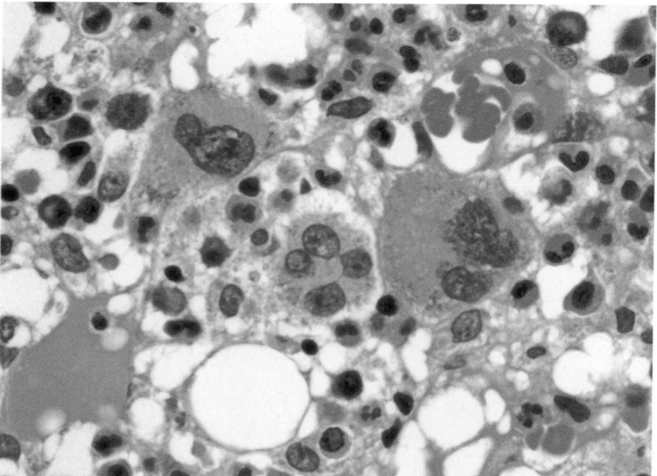

Figure 10-18. Three megakaryocytes in a section of a trephine biopsy specimen from a hematologically normal patient. The variation in size and the nuclear lobulation are due to sectioning across a large, three-dimensional megakaryocyte in the biopsy.

CD61 for platelet glycoprotein IIIa or CD41 for platelet glycoprotein IIb.

Megakaryocytes are irregularly distributed in the bone marrow, and determining whether the number of megakaryocytes in a bone marrow aspirate is normal is difficult and necessarily subjective; it often relies on the quality of the film as well as the experience of the observer. In bone core biopsy sections from hematologically normal subjects, there are usually three to six megakaryocytes in each intertrabecular space; clusters of three or more megakaryocytes are not normally seen.

Other Myeloid Cells

Monocytes, macrophages, mast cells, and osteoclasts are all of myeloid origin. Low but variable numbers are recognized in the bone marrow in healthy subjects.

Monocytes and macrophages are a minor population in normal bone marrow aspirates. Macrophages may be seen as isolated cells or in relation to erythroblasts in an erythroid island. Macrophages may contain cellular debris or hemosiderin (Fig. 10-19).

Normal mast cells, although infrequent, are readily recognizable in bone marrow aspirate films because of their distinctive cytologic features. They generally have central, round or oval nuclei, and their cytoplasm is packed with brightly staining purple granules (Fig. 10-20); a minority may be more fusiform. In H&E-stained sections, the scattered mast cells present in normal bone marrow are not readily recognizable. However, they are easily demonstrated on a Giemsa stain, which stains their granules purple; they are preferentially located adjacent to bone and around arterioles but are also scattered in small numbers throughout the marrow. Mast cells can also be demonstrated by immunohistochemical stains such as mast cell tryptase.

Osteoclasts are large, generally multinucleated cells with quite heavily granulated cytoplasm (Fig. 10-21). Their multiple nuclei are oval and very uniform in appearance; each has a single lilac nucleolus. Only small numbers are seen in aspirates from healthy adults, but they are more numerous in aspirates from children. In histologic sections, osteoclasts are apparent as multinucleated cells adjacent to bone (Fig. 10-22).

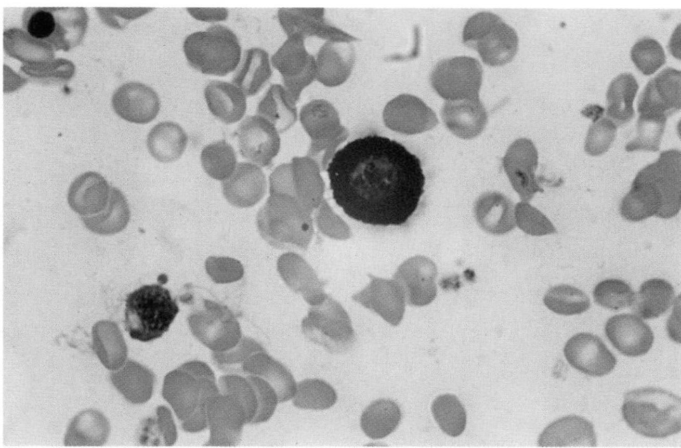

Figure 10-20. Mast cell in a bone marrow aspirate from a healthy volunteer.

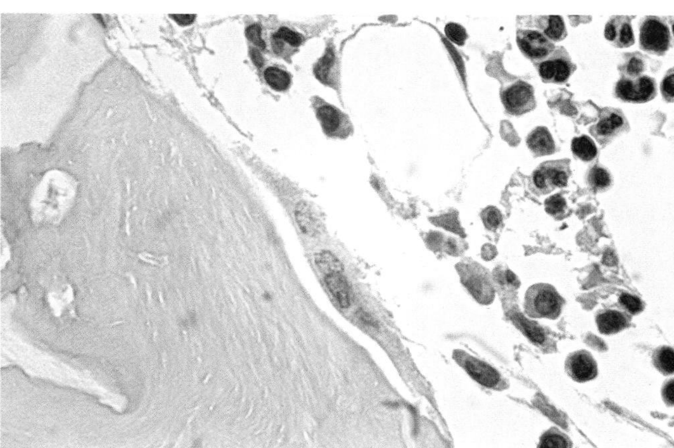

Figure 10-22. Osteoclast adjacent to a bony spicule in a section of a trephine biopsy specimen from a child.

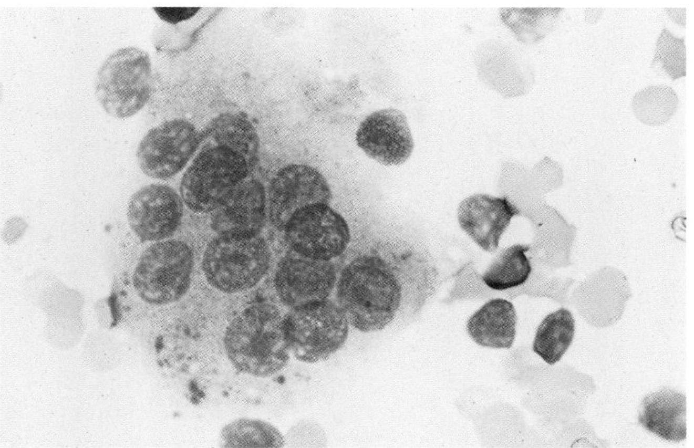

Figure 10-21. Normal osteoclast in a bone marrow aspirate.

Occasionally, apparently mononuclear osteoclasts can be recognized from their position and cytologic features.

Cytologic Abnormalities in Myeloid Cells in Hematologically Normal Subjects

It should be noted that the bone marrow aspirate of healthy volunteers may show some features that could be interpreted as indicative of dysplasia, such as dyserythropoietic features or the presence of nonlobulated or multinucleated megakaryocytes (Table 10-4).[10] Studies of apparently hematologically normal surgical patients indicate that dysplastic changes in erythroid,[14] granulocyte,[14] and megakaryocyte[12] lineages increase with age. Certain dysplastic features are not seen or are rarely seen in healthy subjects and thus likely indicate bone marrow damage or disease; these include agranular

Table 10-4 Frequency of Dyserythropoietic Features and Dysmegakaryopoiesis in 50 Young Healthy Volunteers and 54 Elderly, Apparently Hematologically Normal Patients*

	Healthy Young Volunteers[10]		Apparently Hematologically Normal Elderly Patients[12]	
Abnormality	Number of People in Whom Observed	Percentage of Cells in Which Observed	Number of People in Whom Observed	Percentage of Cells in Which Observed
Binuclearity	12/42	1-2		
Nuclear lobulation	3/42	1		
Detached nuclear fragments (Howell-Jolly bodies)	3/42	1	3/30	<10
Nuclear bridging	0/42			
Irregular nuclear membrane	5/42	1-2		
Cytoplasmic bridging	21/42	1-6		
Vacuolated, irregular, or poorly hemoglobinized cytoplasm	31/42	1-7	3/30	<10
Basophilic stippling	8/42	1-3	19/30	<10
Macronormoblastic maturation	—	—	18/30	<10
Hypolobated megakaryocytes	15/50	1-2	45/54	1-5
Multinucleated megakaryocytes	4/50	1-2	25/54	1-3
Giant megakaryocytes	—	—	5/54	1-4
Mononuclear micromegakaryocytes	—	—	5/54	1-2

*Storage iron was present either in all individuals[10] or in the subset of individuals in whom erythropoiesis was assessed.[12]

neutrophils, the acquired Pelger-Huët anomaly, and ring sideroblasts.[10] Micromegakaryocytes (defined as megakaryocytes <30 μm in diameter) are not seen in healthy young subjects[10,12] but have been reported in elderly subjects without any apparent hematologic disease.[12]

BONE MARROW LYMPHOID CELLS

Bone marrow lymphocytes in healthy adults are small and mature, resembling those in the peripheral blood. To assess their number accurately, it is important to make films from the first few drops of aspirated marrow, thus minimizing dilution by peripheral blood. Aspirates of children not only have more lymphocytes than those of adults[5] but also are likely to contain immature lymphocytes. These range from cells somewhat larger than a mature lymphocyte, with the nucleolus sometimes being apparent, to larger cells that are cytologically indistinguishable from leukemic lymphoblasts, with a high nuclear-to-cytoplasmic ratio, a diffuse chromatin pattern, and nucleoli. These immature lymphoid cells, often designated *hematogones*, can be seen even in the marrow of healthy children, such as those acting as bone marrow donors. They can be distinguished from leukemic cells by the fact that there is a spectrum of cells from lymphoblasts to mature lymphocytes, and even though they may constitute a high percentage of bone marrow cells (e.g., 20% to 30%), normal hematopoiesis is not ablated.

In histologic sections, lymphocytes are mainly interstitial, and there are fewer lymphocytes than in bone marrow aspirates, even small-volume aspirates, which should have minimal dilution by sinusoidal blood. In one study, around 10% of nucleated cells in trephine bone marrow sections were lymphocytes, with the ratio of T/B cells being 6:1 as determined by immunohistochemical stains.[15] In another study with a small number of subjects, the T/B ratio was 4:1 to 5:1.[16] In a third investigation, median numbers were on the order of 2%, representing approximately equal numbers of B and T cells; the range of B cells was 0% to 5.97%, and the range of T cells was 0% to 6.7%.[17] With increasing age, lymphoid aggregates are found in an increasing proportion of individuals. Girodon and colleagues,[12] for example, observed lymphoid aggregates, with associated increased mast cells, in 7 of 54 elderly subjects without apparent relevant disease. Although lymphoid aggregates are most readily observed in sections of trephine biopsy specimens, they are occasionally detected if films are made by crushing aspirated bone marrow fragments. Wedge-spread films of aspirates from individuals with increased lymphoid aggregates do not usually show any increase in lymphocytes.

Plasma cells (Figs. 10-23 and 10-24) are quite infrequent in aspirates and trephine biopsy specimens from healthy subjects. They are preferentially localized adjacent to capillaries (Figs. 10-25 and 10-26). Occasional binucleate forms may be present.

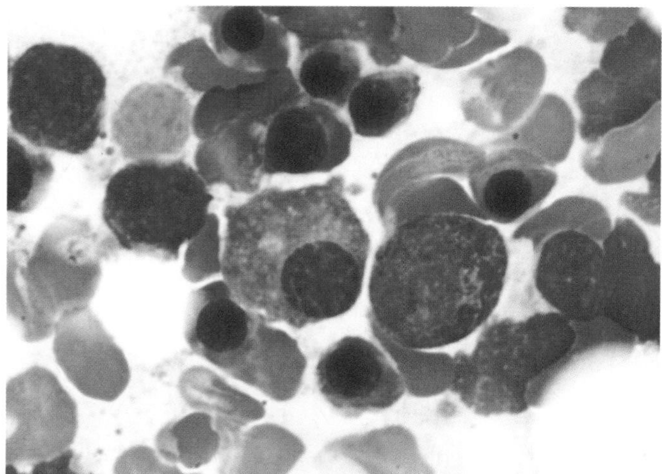

Figure 10-23. Plasma cell, promyelocyte, and several erythroid precursors in a bone marrow aspirate from a healthy individual.

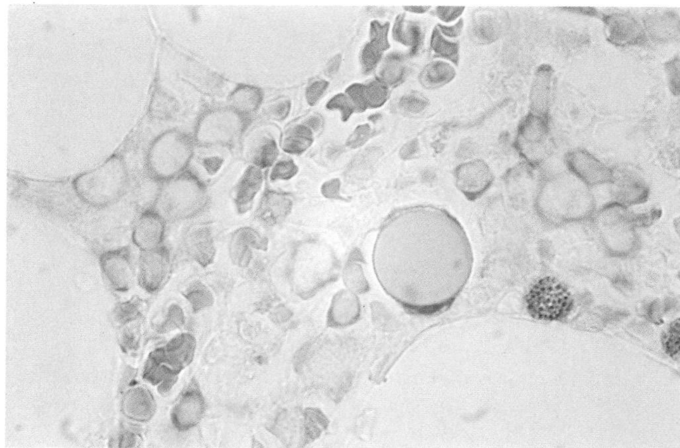

Figure 10-24. Plasma cell containing a Russell body—a large, homogeneous, rounded immunoglobulin inclusion—in a section of a trephine biopsy specimen from a healthy volunteer (Giemsa).

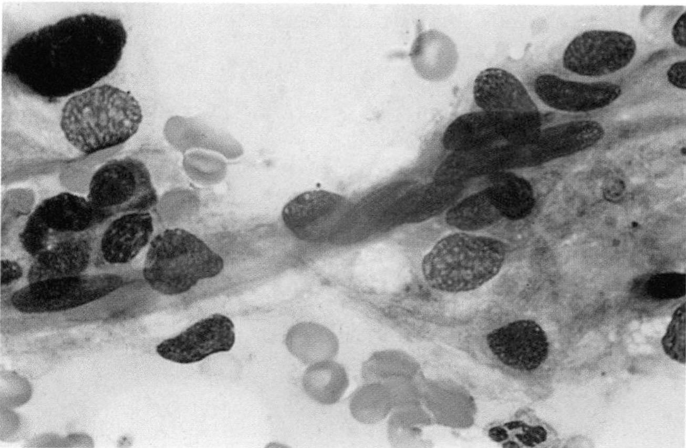

Figure 10-25. Two pericapillary plasma cells adjacent to a capillary in a bone marrow aspirate from a healthy volunteer.

OTHER CELLS PRESENT IN NORMAL BONE MARROW

Normal Bone Marrow Components

Small numbers of osteoblasts are present in normal aspirates (Fig. 10-27). Larger numbers are seen in aspirates from chil-

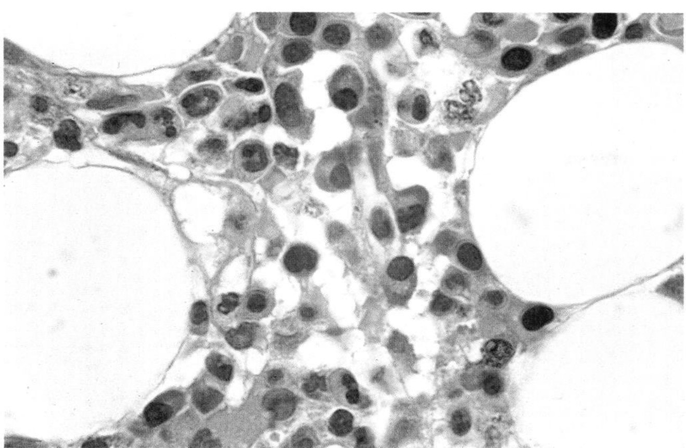

Figure 10-26. Pericapillary plasma cells in a section of a trephine biopsy specimen.

dren. They are readily distinguished from plasma cells by their slightly larger size, more voluminous cytoplasm, and the fact that the readily apparent Golgi zone is not immediately adjacent to the nucleus. Stromal cells that may be recognized in aspirates include fat cells and reticulum cells. Capillaries may be aspirated, being recognized as parallel sequences of fusiform cells (see Fig. 10-25).

Osteoblasts are readily recognized in trephine biopsy sections on the basis of both their position and their cytologic features (Fig. 10-28). Fat cells, capillaries, and sinusoids are readily recognizable.

Extraneous Cells and Tissues

It is important to recognize extraneous cells that are normal but have been introduced into the bone marrow during the biopsy procedure. In aspirates these include epithelial and endothelial cells. In trephine biopsy sections, they include epidermis, sweat glands, and sebaceous glands. The reader is referred to Bain and associates[5] for a detailed discussion of the appearance of extraneous material and artifacts that may complicate the interpretation of bone marrow biopsies.

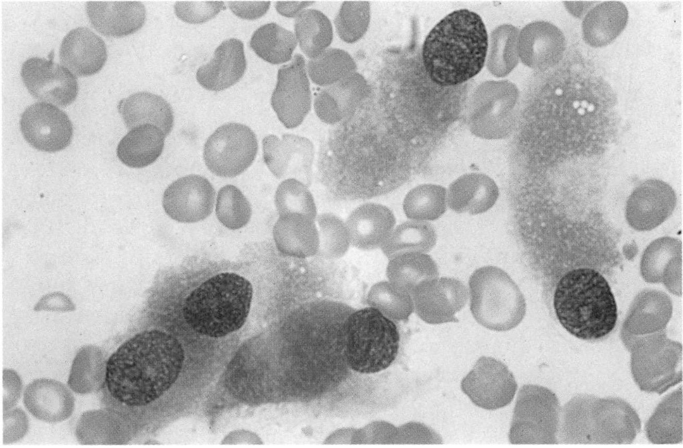

Figure 10-27. Cluster of osteoblasts in a bone marrow aspirate from a child.

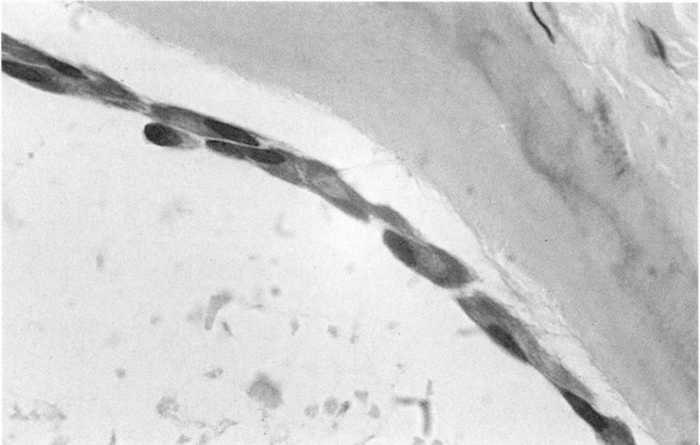

Figure 10-28. Osteoblasts lining bone in a section of a trephine biopsy specimen.

CYTOCHEMISTRY AND HISTOCHEMISTRY

All the stains routinely performed on bone marrow aspirate films and trephine biopsy sections are cytochemical or histochemical in nature. However, by convention, this term is usually not applied to those that are routinely performed, such as a Romanowsky-type stain on an aspirate or an H&E, Giemsa, or reticulin stain on a section.

Cytochemical and histochemical stains, other than Perls stain, are mainly of value in the investigation of suspected hematologic or lymphoid malignancies and for the detection of microorganisms. With advances in immunophenotyping techniques, cytochemical stains are losing importance. However, if immunophenotyping is not readily available, cytochemistry should not be neglected, because it still yields valuable information. Histochemical stains, other than those for iron, reticulin fibers, collagen, amyloid, and microorganisms, are now of little importance in diagnosis.

Cytochemistry

The Perls stain for hemosiderin is diagnostically important and should be performed on the initial bone marrow aspirate in all patients. Other cytochemical reactions remain important in the diagnosis of acute leukemia, but their usefulness has diminished as immunophenotyping has become widely available. For this reason, the PAS stain and acid phosphatase reaction are now largely redundant. The tartrate-resistant acid phosphatase (TRAP) reaction continues to be useful in the diagnosis of hairy cell leukemia, particularly if the specific antibody panel necessary for an immunophenotypic diagnosis is not available; however, TRAP can also be readily detected by immunohistochemistry performed on trephine biopsy sections. It should be noted that normal osteoclasts also show TRAP activity. The most useful cytochemical stains are shown in Table 10-5.

Histochemistry

If H&E, Giemsa, and reticulin stains (Fig. 10-29) are performed routinely, the only other stain needed with any frequency is a Perls stain. The normal findings with this and

Table 10-5 Cytochemical Stains in Bone Marrow Aspirate

Stain	Reactivity in Normal Bone Marrow	Comments
Perls Prussian blue	Hemosiderin in macrophages and developing erythroid cells	Diagnostically important
Myeloperoxidase	Primary granules of promyelocytes and all later cells of neutrophil lineage (myeloblasts may have scattered fine granules); primary and secondary granules of cells of eosinophil lineage, from promyelocyte stage onward; granules of basophil myelocytes but not normal mature basophils; granules of monocytes—finer and less numerous than granules of neutrophils; erythroblasts and erythrocytes show diffuse cytoplasmic positivity	Immunophenotyping with antimyeloperoxidase antibodies is more sensitive than a cytochemical reaction dependent on enzyme activity; uncommonly, there is a congenital peroxidase deficiency in hematologically normal subjects
Sudan black B	As for myeloperoxidase; eosinophil granules appear hollow	Immunophenotyping is more sensitive for detecting granulocytic differentiation; Sudan black B staining is negative in individuals with a congenital peroxidase deficiency
Naphthol AS-D chloroacetate esterase (specific [neutrophil] esterase)	Granules of neutrophils and their precursors from promyelocyte stage onward (normal eosinophils are negative); mast cell granules	Less sensitive than myeloperoxidase or Sudan black B for detecting granulocytic differentiation; immunophenotyping is also more sensitive
Alpha naphthyl acetate esterase (nonspecific esterase)	Granules of monocyte precursors, monocytes, and macrophages; granules of megakaryocytes and platelets; many T lymphocytes are positive; normal neutrophils and erythroblasts are negative	Immunophenotyping is an alternative means of demonstrating monocytic differentiation (e.g., with CD14 and CD64 monoclonal antibodies) and megakaryocytic differentiation (e.g., with CD42 and CD61 monoclonal antibodies)
Alpha naphthyl butyrate esterase (nonspecific esterase)	Granules of monocyte precursors, monocytes, and macrophages; some T lymphocytes are positive	More specific for monocyte lineage than alpha naphthyl acetate esterase
Toluidine blue	Granules of mast cells and basophils	
Periodic acid–Schiff (PAS)	Neutrophil lineage, strongest in mature cells; eosinophil cytoplasm is positive, but granules of normal eosinophils are negative; basophil cytoplasm may show large, irregular positive blocks, but granules are negative; monocytes show variable diffuse plus granular positivity; megakaryocytes and platelets usually show strong diffuse plus granular or block positivity; plasma cells have strong diffuse positivity; some lymphocytes show granular positivity	Normal erythroblasts are PAS negative; PAS is redundant in diagnosis of acute lymphoblastic leukemia if immunophenotyping is available
Acid phosphatase	Positive in most bone marrow cells: neutrophils, macrophages, megakaryocytes, and plasma cells are strongly positive; reactivity of eosinophils, monocytes, and platelets is more variable	Redundant in diagnosis of acute leukemia if immunophenotyping is available
Tartrate-resistant acid phosphatase	Osteoclasts	Still useful in diagnosis of hairy cell leukemia

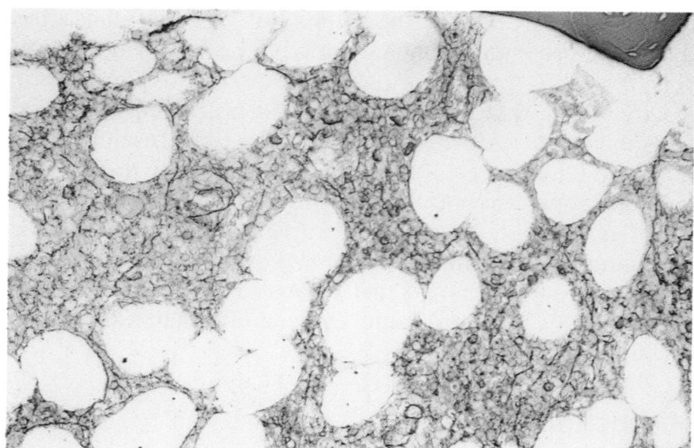

Figure 10-29. Reticulin stain of a section of a trephine biopsy specimen from a healthy volunteer shows Bauermeister[2] grade 2 reticulin deposition.

other histochemical stains are summarized in Table 10-6. If a bone marrow aspirate containing fragments is available, the Perls stain on histologic sections is unlikely to provide additional useful information. It is also important to note that if a biopsy specimen has been paraffin embedded and decalcified, some or all of the hemosiderin originally present will have been removed; it may therefore be possible to report that iron is present in such sections, but it is not possible to report that iron is reduced or absent. Collagen deposition can be detected on an H&E-stained section, but a collagen stain, such as a Martius scarlet stain, can be useful for confirmation and to assess the severity of fibrosis. A Leder stain can be useful for the detection of mast cells and for highlighting cells of neutrophil lineage. However, it should be noted that only plastic-embedded specimens or paraffin-embedded specimens decalcified with a chelating agent rather than with acid are suitable for this cytochemical stain. A PAS stain does not provide any useful information on sections of normal bone

Table 10-6 Histochemical Stains in Bone Marrow Trephine Biopsy

Stain	Reactivity in Normal Marrow	Comments
Perls stain	Hemosiderin in macrophages; hemosiderin in erythroblasts is detectable only if plastic embedding is used	More useful in aspirate, as long as it contains bone marrow fragments. Decalcification procedure may remove iron from bone marrow trephine biopsy.
Naphthol AS-D chloroacetate esterase (Leder stain)	Neutrophil lineage; mast cells	
Gomori or Gordon-Sweet stain for reticulin	See text	Important for highlighting abnormal areas of bone marrow and in the diagnosis of myeloproliferative neoplasms
Martius scarlet blue	None	Collagen and fibrin or fibrinoid
Periodic acid–Schiff (with or without diastase)	Highlights plasma cells, megakaryocytes, mature neutrophils	
Congo red	None	Positive staining with apple-green birefringence on polarized light

marrow, but the pathologist needs to be aware of the usual pattern of staining of normal bone marrow cells.

Immunophenotyping

Immunophenotyping on bone marrow specimens is now usually done by flow cytometry on aspirates or by immunohistochemistry on bone marrow trephine biopsy sections. The former permits the simultaneous labeling of cells with multiple antibodies and is more quantitative, but the latter permits assessment of the expression of specific antigens in relation to histologic features.

CONCLUSION

The important principles in interpreting a normal bone marrow aspirate or trephine biopsy section are (1) to have high-quality material, (2) to know the range of normality so that normal features are not misinterpreted as pathologic, and (3) to be aware of artifacts that can be misinterpreted as evidence of a pathologic process.

The interpretation of a bone marrow aspirate and trephine biopsy must be based on a thorough knowledge of the cytologic and histologic features of the bone marrow in healthy subjects of similar age to the patient.

Pearls and Pitfalls

Pearls	Pitfalls
Bone Marrow Aspirate Films	
• The pathologist must be totally familiar with the appearance of all normal cells that might be found in the bone marrow. • Interpretation must be done in light of the clinical history and with knowledge of the blood count and appearance of the blood film. • Aspirates must be particulate for a valid interpretation. • Differential counts greatly enhance detection of a minor abnormal population of cells.	• A wrong opinion may be rendered because of failure to interpret the aspirate in light of the clinical and hematologic features and age of the patient. • A wrong opinion may be rendered because of a lack of familiarity with the full range of normal appearances (e.g., hematogones may be misinterpreted as leukemic lymphoblasts). • Normal cells may be interpreted as pathologic (e.g., osteoclasts may be mistaken for dysplastic megakaryocytes, osteoblasts may be misinterpreted as abnormal plasma cells, crushed erythroid cells or clumps of osteoblasts may be mistaken for tumor cells). • Extraneous cells and tissues may not be recognized and may therefore be misinterpreted (e.g., sweat glands may be mistaken for clumps of tumor cells). • Artifacts may be misinterpreted as evidence of a pathologic process (e.g., poorly fixed erythroblasts may show apparent leakage of nuclear contents into the cytoplasm, wrongly suggesting dyserythropoiesis); if anticoagulated marrow is stored before films are made, features such as nuclear lobulation may develop.
Trephine Biopsy Sections	
• The pathologist must be totally familiar with the histologic features of normal bone and bone marrow and with the artifacts that may complicate interpretation. • Specimens must be sufficiently large. • Specimens must be adequately fixed before further processing. • Sections must be sufficiently thin to permit the recognition of individual cells.	• A wrong opinion may be rendered because of failure to interpret the sections in light of the clinical and hematologic features, age of the patient, and bone marrow aspirate findings. • A wrong opinion may be rendered because of lack of familiarity with the full range of normal appearances (e.g., reactive lymphoid aggregates may be misinterpreted as infiltration by lymphoma). • Extraneous material may be misinterpreted as evidence of a pathologic process (e.g., components of the dermis may be driven into the biopsy specimen or, if correct technical procedures are not followed, dysplastic or neoplastic tissue from another patient may become attached to a biopsy specimen). • An inadequate, damaged, or badly processed specimen may be misinterpreted as abnormal (e.g., a biopsy specimen obtained at the wrong angle and that contains only subcortical bone marrow may be misinterpreted as hypoplastic, or twisting artifact may be mistaken for fibrosis).

References can be found on Expert Consult @ www.expertconsult.com

Chapter 11

Evaluation of Anemia, Leukopenia, and Thrombocytopenia

Carla S. Wilson and Russell K. Brynes

CHAPTER OUTLINE

Quantitative and qualitative abnormalities of the peripheral blood are routinely detected with an automated complete blood count (CBC) and examination of a peripheral blood smear. The peripheral blood evaluation serves as a screening test for potential bone marrow abnormalities and diseases that affect bone marrow function. When peripheral blood abnormalities are identified, the decision to further assess hematopoiesis by performing an invasive bone marrow procedure is influenced by a moderate number of quantitative findings from the CBC and a greater number of qualitative abnormalities found on inspection of the peripheral blood smear. The decision also relies on a carefully obtained history, thorough physical examination, and evaluation of current and historical laboratory values. The utility of a thorough history in the evaluation of bone marrow specimens cannot be overemphasized. The history should include information about the present and past illnesses, including how and when the cytopenia or cytosis presented and how it was discovered (Fig. 11-1). Occupational history and a history of exposure to therapeutic or recreational drugs, alcohol, and toxins should be sought. Finally, physical examination often provides the critical clue to the responsible mechanism or disease process. Without this essential integrated information, reliable interpretation of bone marrow findings is often incomplete or misleading. This chapter focuses on anemia, leukopenia, and thrombocytopenia. The differential diagnosis of increased numbers of red blood cells, leukocytes, and platelets is discussed elsewhere in this book.

EVALUATION OF ANEMIA

The World Health Organization (WHO) defines anemia as a hemoglobin concentration of less than 12 g/dL in women and less than 13 g/dL in men.[1] The initial evaluation of anemia begins with a careful evaluation of the CBC data and a comprehensive examination of a well-prepared peripheral blood smear. The blood smear should initially be evaluated at scanning power to detect abnormalities such as rouleau formation and red blood cell (RBC) agglutination, followed by careful examination of individual RBCs with a high-powered lens. Review of pertinent history and physical findings can help determine what additional laboratory tests are needed and whether a bone marrow examination is required to further define the process.

Anemias can be divided into those due to production problems, with insufficient or ineffective erythropoiesis, and those caused by either blood loss or decreased RBC survival. The reticulocyte count is the best test to differentiate between abnormalities of production and survival, and it is often the first test considered in algorithms for the evaluation of anemia. Because the reticulocyte count may not be high during the initial stages of hemolysis and blood loss, anemia may be better stratified first by the CBC data, using size (mean cell volume [MCV]), hemoglobinization (mean cell hemoglobin concentration [MCHC]), RBC count, and degree of anisocytosis (red cell distribution width [RDW]) (Fig. 11-2). This approach can then be extended with an algorithm that adds

Clinical Diagnosis/Suspicion (check all appropriate categories):

☐ Anemia
☐ Thrombocytopenia
☐ Neutropenia
☐ Myelodysplastic syndrome
☐ Non-Hodgkin's lymphoma
☐ Hodgkin's lymphoma
☐ Acute myeloid leukemia
☐ Precursor lymphoid neoplasm
☐ Chronic myelogenous leukemia
☐ Other myeloproliferative neoplasm
☐ Chronic lymphocytic leukemia
☐ Other B-cell lymphoproliferative disorder
☐ T-cell lymphoproliferative disorder
☐ Plasma cell neoplasm
☐ Systemic infection
☐ HIV infection
☐ Other

Reason for Bone Marrow Study (include a brief history, past and current): ____________________

Pertinent Physical Findings/Presenting Symptoms:

☐ Lymphadenopathy (location:_______________)
☐ Splenomegaly
☐ Ecchymoses
☐ Petechiae
☐ Fever
☐ Night sweats
☐ Weight loss
☐ Other:____________________

Occupational History/Exposure: ☐ Radiation ☐ Organic chemicals ☐ Heavy metals

Current Drug/Chemotherapy (type and dates of administration): ____________________

Cytokine therapy: ☐ G-CSF ☐ EPO

Other Tests Requested:

☐ Flow cytometry
☐ Cytogenetics
☐ Fluorescence in situ hybridization
☐ Molecular genetics:_______________
☐ Bacterial culture
☐ AFB culture
☐ Fungal culture
☐ Other:____________________

PATIENT NAME: ____________________
CHART NUMBER: ____________________
BIRTHDATE: ____________________
SEX: ☐ Male ☐ Female
ETHNICITY: ☐ White ☐ Black ☐ Asian ☐ Hispanic ☐ Other:__________

Figure 11-1. Example of a requisition form for bone marrow evaluation.

reticulocyte count, serum iron studies, and vitamin B_{12} and folate values as needed. Using this algorithm, bone marrow examination is required most frequently for normocytic or macrocytic anemias with low reticulocyte counts that cannot be explained by vitamin B_{12} or folate deficiency, liver disease, drug or alcohol effects, or other clearly defined causes. Bone marrow examination is essential in the diagnosis of aplastic anemia, myelodysplastic syndromes, and myelophthisic anemia. Of course, anemia is quite common in patients undergoing bone marrow examination for other indications, such as tumor staging.

Microcytic Anemia

In microcytic anemia, the MCV is less than the normal laboratory reference range, generally less than 80 fL for adults and dependent on age for children. The small RBCs result from defective or ineffective production of hemoglobin. Heme, the iron-containing porphyrin ring component of hemoglobin, is synthesized from succinyl coenzyme A (CoA) and glycine through a series of enzymatic steps that occur in the mitochondria (Fig. 11-3). Disorders affecting heme synthesis, the globin genes, or iron availability prevent adequate hemoglobinization and maturation of RBC cytoplasm, resulting in hypochromic microcytic cells. Table 11-1 lists additional findings for the hypochromic microcytic anemias.

Iron Deficiency

Iron deficiency occurs when iron utilization or loss exceeds iron absorption and results in depletion of body stores. Early in iron deficiency, iron stores are decreased, but the red cells are morphologically unaffected. Serum ferritin (normally 12 to 300 ng/mL) is in equilibrium with tissue stores and serves as an indirect measure of storage iron in uncomplicated cases. However, ferritin is an acute phase protein, and patients with chronic inflammation or liver disease may have elevated

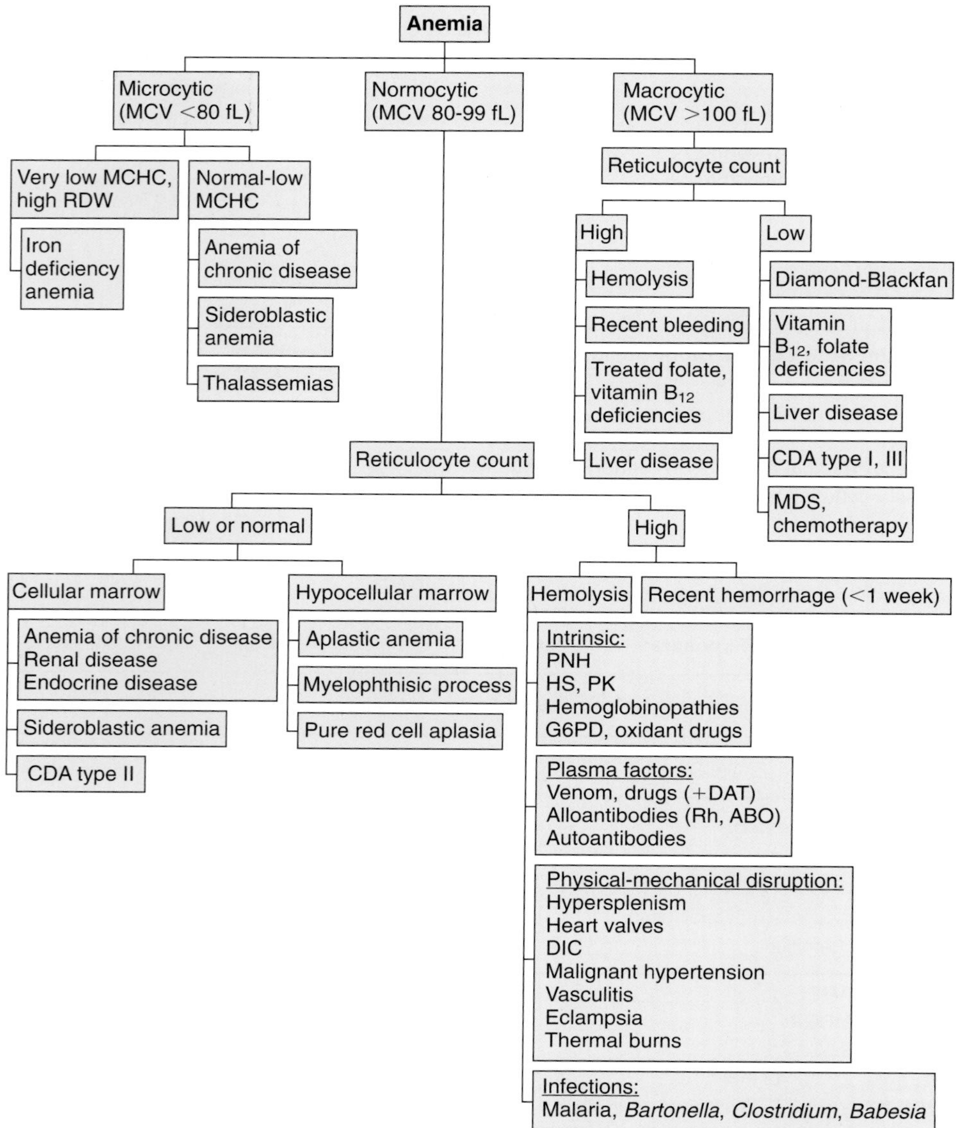

Figure 11-2. Anemia algorithm. Mean cell volume (MCV) is based on adult values; reference ranges must be considered for pediatric patients. CDA, congenital dyserythropoietic anemia; DAT, direct antiglobulin test; DIC, disseminated intravascular coagulation; G6PD, glucose-6-phosphate dehydrogenase; HS, hereditary spherocytosis; MCHC, mean cell hemoglobin concentration; MDS, myelodysplastic syndrome; PK, pyruvate kinase deficiency; PNH, paroxysmal nocturnal hemoglobinuria; RDW, red cell distribution width.

values even in the presence of iron deficiency. After iron stores are depleted, serum iron drops and the iron transport protein, transferrin, increases, so that the total iron binding capacity is increased. The red cells become microcytic and normochromic, and finally microcytic and hypochromic (Figs. 11-4 and 11-5).[2] Transferrin saturation (serum iron/total iron binding capacity) of less than 15% is virtually diagnostic of iron deficiency. Iron homeostasis, including iron uptake from the intestine and release from stores, is regulated by the liver-secreted protein hepcidin.[3] Serum iron concentration has diurnal variation and should be measured in the morning, when it is at its highest level. The sensitivity and specificity of the CBC, transferrin saturation, and ferritin values are usually sufficient to make the diagnosis of iron deficiency without the need to perform a bone marrow study. Additionally, serum-soluble transferrin receptor (sTfR) levels, which are elevated in iron deficiency but usually unaffected by inflammation, and the sTfR-ferritin index (sTfR/log ferritin) may be helpful in interpreting iron status in patients with inflammatory disease.[4,5] Bioactive forms of serum hepcidin are also being investigated as markers of iron status and erythropoietin resistance in states of inflammation.[6] In ambiguous cases, such as patients with elevated acute phase proteins or hepatic disorders, a bone marrow evaluation for iron assessment is indicated. Bone marrow iron stores and sideroblast iron should be evaluated on an aspirate smear (Fig. 11-6), because iron is chelated by acidic decalcifying agents and is generally underestimated in clot or trephine biopsy sections (Table 11-2). In iron deficiency, the Prussian blue reaction demonstrates loss of reticuloendothelial marrow stores and iron incorporation into normoblasts (Fig. 11-7). In normal bone marrow, one or two small siderotic granules are

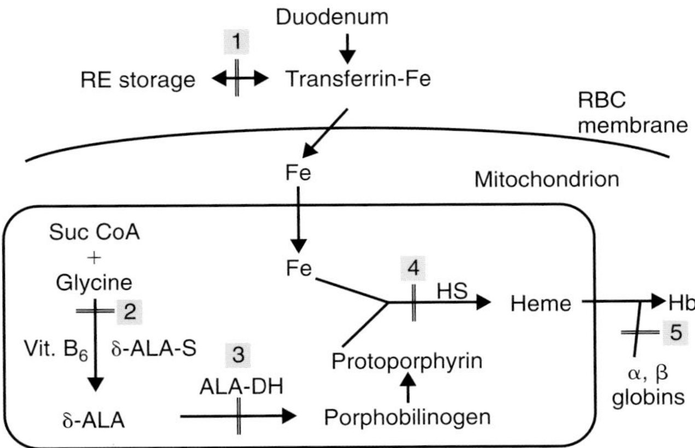

Figure 11-3. Defects causing microcytic anemias. Ferric iron is absorbed by the duodenum and transported via ferroportin receptors to serum transferrin (measured as total iron binding capacity). Hepcidin, produced by the liver, regulates iron (Fe) uptake and transport through ferroportin in response to iron stores, inflammation, erythropoiesis, and hypoxia. Most serum iron is delivered to the bone marrow for red blood cell (RBC) production. Erythroid precursors have classic transferrin receptors that selectively bind and internalize diferric transferrin. When transferrin saturation exceeds 60%, iron is shunted into histiocyte storage in the bone marrow, spleen, and liver. Blockade of this pathway and inability to mobilize iron back into the serum through ferroportin receptors on macrophage surfaces (1) is characteristic of *anemias of chronic disease*. Deficiency or blockade of key steps in heme synthesis by heavy metals and various drugs (e.g., isoniazid) causes iron to accumulate within mitochondria, producing *sideroblastic anemias*. Congenital deficiency of δ-aminolevulinic acid synthase (δ-ALA-S), or lack of vitamin B_6 (pyridoxine) (2), prevents the formation of δ-aminolevulinic acid (δ-ALA) from succinyl coenzyme A (Suc CoA) and glycine. Congenital deficiency and heavy metal (lead) inhibition of aminolevulinic acid dehydratase (ALA-DH) (3) or heme synthetase (HS) (4) produce a similar effect. Decreased synthesis of globin chains (5) contributes to the microcytosis of *thalassemia syndromes*. Blood loss or dietary deficiency of iron ultimately produces *iron deficiency anemia*. Hb, hemoglobin; RE, reticuloendothelial.

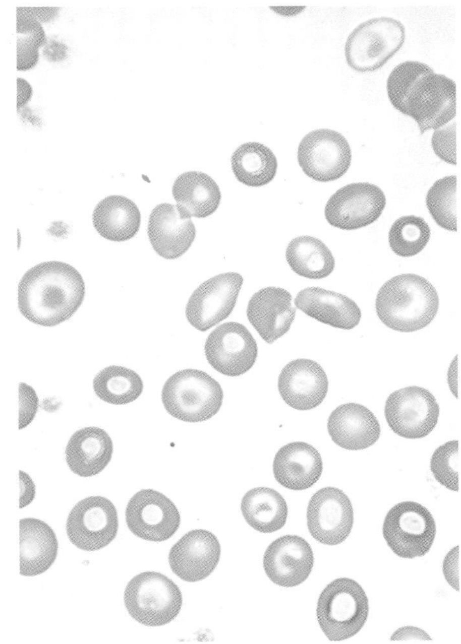

Figure 11-4. Iron deficiency anemia in a child. The red cells are hypochromic and microcytic. Note the many target cells, a feature reported in long-standing iron deficiency.

normally identifiable in at least 10% of the normoblasts (see Fig. 11-6). The absence of iron stores differentiates iron deficiency from advanced anemia of chronic disease, which may mimic an iron deficiency state. However, some authors suggest the evaluation of multiple marrow spicules before declaring the marrow as iron deficient because the iron may be irregularly distributed.[7] If recent parenteral iron or RBC transfusion has been given to an iron-deficient individual, these findings may be misleading because the bone marrow iron stores may appear adequate. Bone marrow morphology

Table 11-1 Classification of Hypochromic Microcytic Anemia

Disorder	Peripheral Blood	Comments
Iron deficiency	CBC: ↓ RBCs, ↓↓ MCHC, ↓ MCV, ↑↑ RDW, ↑-normal-↓ platelets, ↓ reticulocytes PBS: anisopoikilocytosis, especially elliptocytes ("cigar" or "pencil" cells), prekeratocytes, occasional target cells	Iron required for rate-limiting step in heme synthesis Deficiency caused by chronic blood loss (especially menstrual), GI dietary deficiency (breastfed children aged 6 mo to 2 yr at risk), postgastrectomy (gastric acid required for iron absorption), upper GI malabsorption, *Helicobacter pylori* infection
β-Thalassemia	CBC: normal-↑ RBCs, ↓↓MCV, ↓-normal MCHC, normal-↑ RDW PBS: target cells, coarse basophilic stippling	Absent or ↓ synthesis of beta globin chains due to gene mutations Frequent in Mediterranean populations ↑ HbF has heterogeneous distribution in RBCs
α-Thalassemia	Similar to β-thalassemia	Absent or ↓ synthesis of alpha globin chains due to gene deletions Frequent in Southeast Asian and African populations
Anemia of chronic disease	CBC: ↓ RBCs, normal-↓ MCV, normal-↓ MCHC, normal RDW PBS: possible hypochromic cells even if normocytic	More often presents as a normochromic normocytic anemia, caused by ↑ hepcidin secondary to cytokines (IL-6) Normal-↓ serum iron, normal transferrin saturation
Sideroblastic anemia	Dimorphic RBCs, moderate poikilocytosis, hypochromic teardrop forms, coarse basophilic stippling, Pappenheimer bodies	See Box 11-1 ↓ Reticulocyte count Variable anisocytosis, but may be marked

CBC, complete blood count; GI, gastrointestinal; Hb, hemoglobin; IL, interleukin; MCHC, mean corpuscular hemoglobin concentration; MCV, mean cell volume; PBS, peripheral blood smear; RBC, red blood cell; RDW, red cell distribution width.

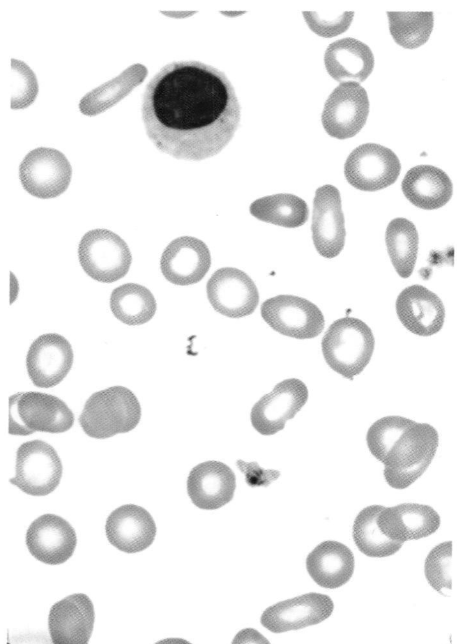

Figure 11-5. Severe iron deficiency anemia. The red cells are hypochromic and microcytic. Their small size is apparent when compared to the nucleus of the lymphocyte. Hypochromic elliptocytes are common in iron deficiency anemia.

is otherwise nonspecific in iron deficiency. In severe anemia, the erythroid precursors may appear smaller, with only a narrow rim of cytoplasm. Rare individuals have iron-refractory iron deficiency anemia that is congenital. Some cases are due to gene mutations involving the transferrin gene or iron transport genes (*DMT1*, *GLRX*); other individuals may have cellular iron export abnormalities.[8,9] Exclusion of *Helicobacter pylori* infection as a cause of unexplained iron deficiency anemia is important, because eradication of the organisms leads to amelioration of the anemia.[10]

Thalassemias

Thalassemias are a common cause of hypochromic microcytic anemia in which adult hemoglobin (HbA [$\alpha_2\beta_2$]) synthesis is quantitatively affected by decreased alpha or beta globin chain synthesis (Table 11-3; see Fig. 11-3). Thalassemia is common in Mediterranean regions, tropical Africa, and Asia; β-thalassemia is also seen in the Middle East and India. It is caused by nearly 200 different mutations that affect one or both of the beta globin chain genes on chromosome 11. These are primarily point mutations affecting transcription, splicing, or translocation of beta globin messenger RNA. The diagnosis is best made by high-performance liquid chromatography or hemoglobin electrophoresis. In its most benign form (β-thalassemia minor), only one of the two genes is mutated, causing either decreased (β^+) or absent (β°) beta globin protein synthesis by the affected allele. The normally produced alpha chains have insufficient beta chains with which to pair, and the excess combines with delta chains to produce HbA_2 ($\alpha_2\delta_2$). A mild elevation in HbF ($\alpha_2\gamma_2$) is also found in about one third of patients. If both beta chain genes are mutated, scant ($\beta^+\beta^+$ or $\beta^\circ\beta^+$) or no beta chains ($\beta^\circ\beta^\circ$) are made, causing a serious childhood anemia, β-thalassemia major (Cooley's anemia). This is usually diagnosed in the first year of life as hemoglobin switches from HbF to HbA; it is associated with severe microcytic anemia, marked hemolysis, marked erythroid hyperplasia, hepatosplenomegaly, and failure to thrive (Figs. 11-8 and 11-9). Leukopenia and thrombocytopenia may occur with progressive splenomegaly. Patients who are not transfusion dependent or are diagnosed later in life are classified clinically as having β-thalassemia intermedia. Methyl

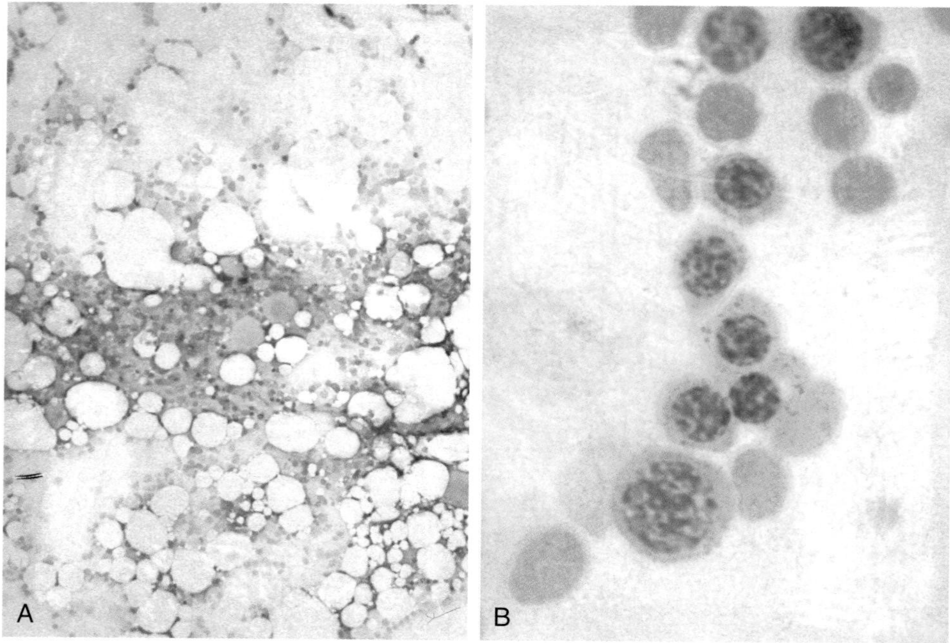

Figure 11-6. Bone marrow particle smear with normal iron stores and incorporation. Storage iron in stromal histiocytes stains blue with the Prussian blue reaction (**A**). Sideroblast (incorporated) iron granules are seen in 10% to 20% of normoblasts (**B**).

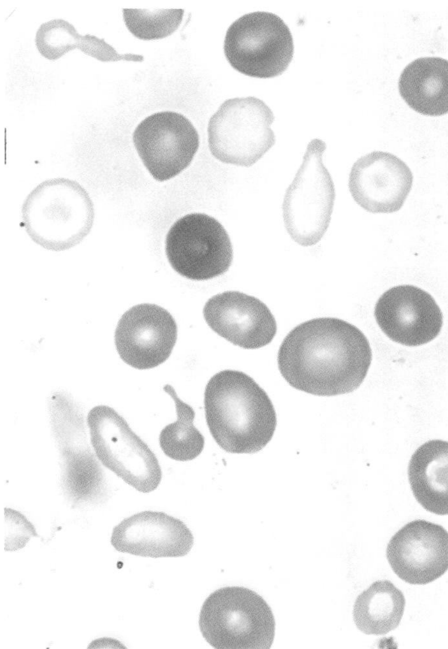

Figure 11-15. Pyridoxine-responsive sideroblastic anemia showing a dimorphic population of normochromic normocytic red cells and hypochromic microcytes. Hypochromic teardrop forms are common in sideroblastic anemia.

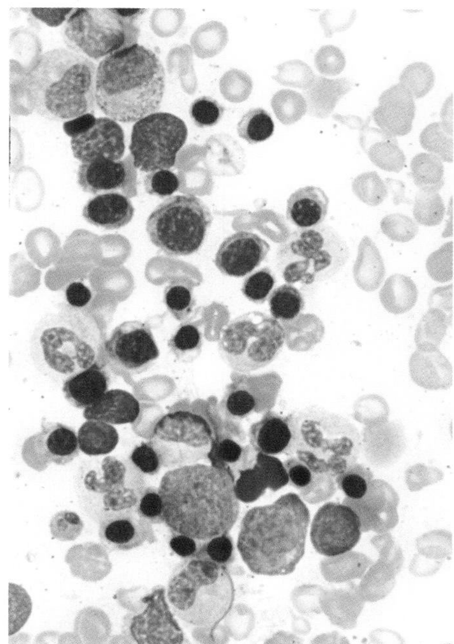

Figure 11-17. Ineffective erythropoiesis produces erythroid hyperplasia in most cases of sideroblastic anemia.

in patients with primary acquired sideroblastic anemia, but their significance in the pathophysiology of the disease process is not yet clear.[22]

The secondary and less common forms of acquired sideroblastic anemia are the result of drugs and exposure to toxins, many of which have been characterized. For example, the drug isoniazid inhibits pyridoxine metabolism; lead inhibits δ-ALA dehydratase and heme synthetase; and alcohol produces a direct toxic effect on erythroid precursors (found in 30% of hospitalized alcoholics). The anemia can be reversed by administration of pyridoxal phosphate and discontinuation of the offending drug. Copper deficiency anemia, often secondary to zinc overload, is discussed in more detail in the neutropenia section of this chapter; the red cells may be microcytic, normocytic, or macrocytic. A number of cases of

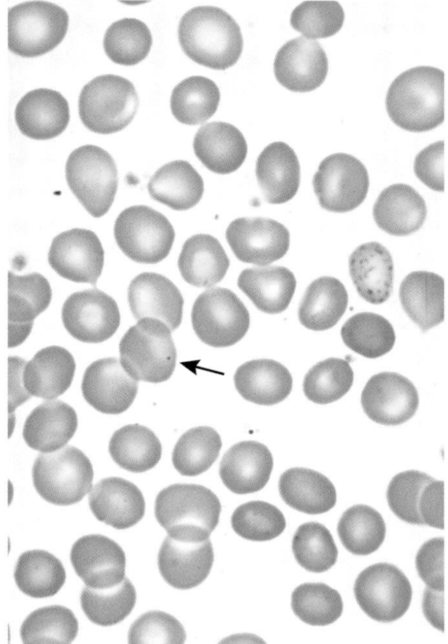

Figure 11-16. Coarse basophilic stippling and Pappenheimer granules (*arrow*) are seen in this case of sideroblastic anemia associated with lead poisoning.

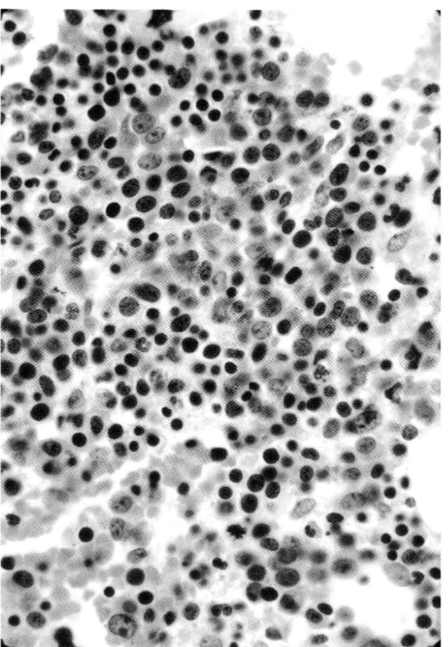

Figure 11-18. Markedly hypercellular bone marrow with erythroid hyperplasia in pyridoxine-responsive sideroblastic anemia.

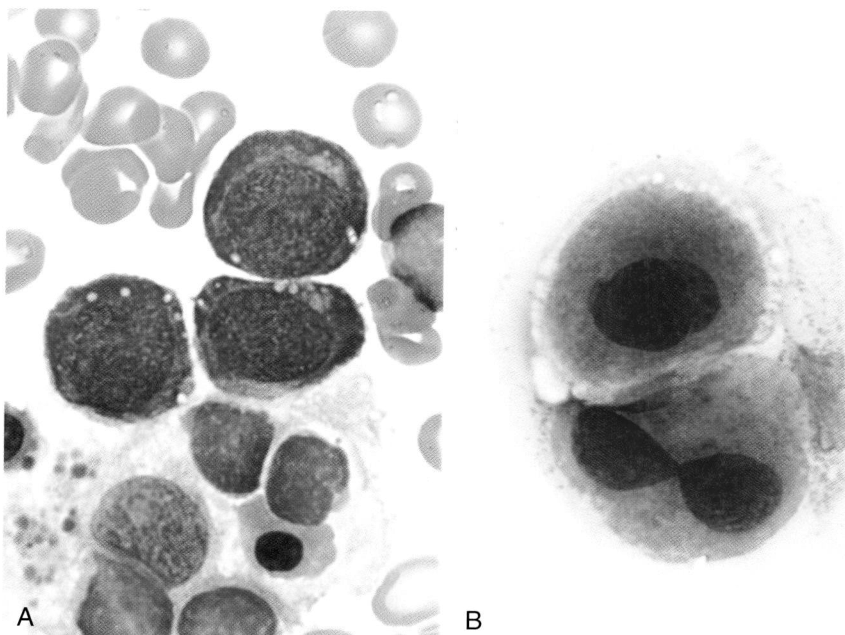

Figure 11-19. Cytoplasmic vacuoles in pronormoblasts (**A**) and megakaryocytes (**B**) are often found in Pearson's syndrome. This rare form of sideroblastic anemia is associated with exocrine pancreas failure and is caused by a mutation in mitochondrial DNA.

sideroblastic anemia have been found to be due to mtDNA mutations.[23] Perhaps the best example is Pearson's marrow-pancreas syndrome, a congenital disorder that occurs sporadically and is characterized by lactic acidosis, exocrine pancreatic insufficiency, sideroblastic anemia, and large deletions or duplications in mtDNA.[24,25]

Normochromic Normocytic Anemia, Underproduction

The normochromic normocytic anemias are characterized by red cells of normal size and hemoglobin content. They are most easily divided by reticulocyte count into disorders of underproduction (low or normal reticulocyte count), discussed in this section, and increased production (high reticulocyte count), discussed in the next section (see Fig. 11-2).

Pure Red Cell Aplasia

Pure red cell aplasia is an isolated failure of erythropoiesis that results in anemia with reticulocytopenia and normal neutrophil and platelet counts. The marrow shows absent or diminished erythroid precursors, often with a left shift in erythroid maturation (Fig. 11-21). The anemia may be acute and transient or chronic, depending on the cause (Box 11-2). The

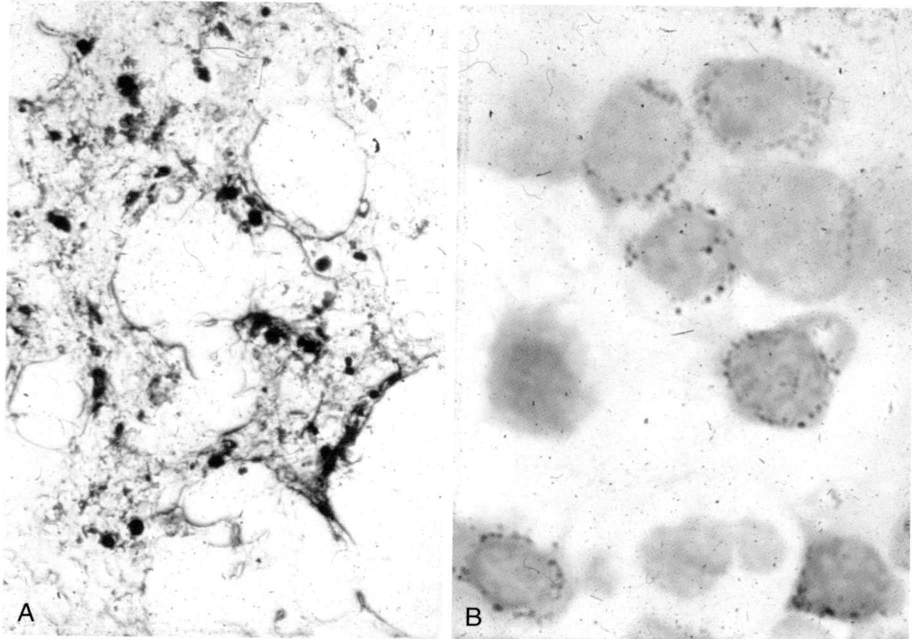

Figure 11-20. Increased iron stores (**A**) and numerous ring sideroblasts (**B**) are the diagnostic hallmarks of all forms of sideroblastic anemia.

Box 11-1 *Classification of Sideroblastic Anemias*

Hereditary
- X-linked
- Autosomal recessive

Acquired, Clonal
- Myelodysplastic syndromes (e.g., refractory anemia with ring sideroblasts)
- Therapy-related myeloid neoplasms

Acquired, Nonclonal
- Drugs*: isoniazid, chloramphenicol, cycloserine, penicillamine, azathioprine
- Alcohol
- Lead poisoning, arsenic
- Copper deficiency

Acquired, with Mitochondrial DNA Mutations or Deletions
- Pearson's marrow-pancreas syndrome
- Some nonclonal refractory sideroblastic anemias

*Drug list is not all-inclusive.

Box 11-2 *Classification of Pure Red Cell Aplasia*

Acute Transient Anemia
- Idiopathic: transient erythroblastopenia of childhood
- Viral infection: parvovirus B19, hepatitis, Epstein-Barr virus
- Drugs*: azathioprine, cephalothin, chloramphenicol, dapsone, diphenylhydantoin, isoniazid, procainamide

Chronic Anemia
- Constitutional: Diamond-Blackfan anemia
- T-cell mediated: thymoma, T-cell large granular lymphocytic leukemia, chronic lymphocytic leukemia, myelodysplastic syndrome
- Immunoglobulin G autoantibody mediated: systemic autoimmune disorders (rheumatoid arthritis, systemic lupus erythematosus, Sjögren's syndrome, myasthenia gravis)
- Insufficient antibody production: AIDS with parvovirus, pregnancy, organ transplantation
- ABO-incompatible stem cell transplants

*Drug list is not all-inclusive.
AIDS, acquired immunodeficiency syndrome.

congenital form, Diamond-Blackfan syndrome, is described under the macrocytic anemias. The acquired forms of pure red cell aplasia more frequently present with normochromic normocytic anemia. Parvovirus B19 is the most common identifiable cause of red cell aplasia in children and immunocompromised adults.[26] The virus selectively invades and replicates in erythroid progenitor cells, causing direct cytotoxic effects with interruption of erythrocyte production. In children, it is associated with erythema infectiosum (fifth disease), a transient, asymptomatic drop in hemoglobin of about 1 g/dL, with recovery in 10 to 19 days. Children with a hemolytic disorder that shortens the RBC life span, such as red cell enzyme deficiencies, membrane abnormalities, hemoglobinopathies, or malaria infection, often have a more profound anemia and "aplastic crisis" (Fig. 11-22). Parvovirus B19 may persist in immunocompromised individuals who fail to produce neutralizing antibodies to eradicate the virus. Infection manifests as a chronic instead of acute pure red cell aplasia unless patients are treated with intravenous immunoglobulin therapy.[26] Bone marrow findings depend on the timing of the evaluation. Initial RBC depletion may be followed by a wave of early progenitors without maturation. Giant proerythroblasts with intranuclear viral inclusions are transient but may be occasionally identified, particularly in immunocompromised individuals. Viral-associated suppression of myelopoiesis and megakaryopoiesis occurs with rare cases of marrow necrosis. Serum polymerase chain reaction studies for parvovirus B19 DNA, elevated immunoglobulin (Ig) M antibody titers, and immunohistochemistry or in situ

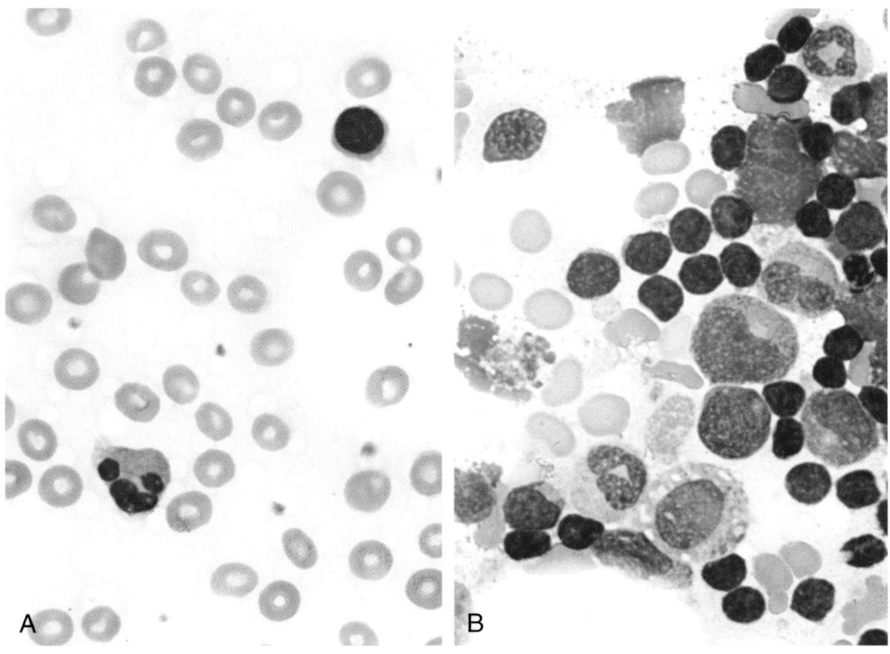

Figure 11-21. A, Severe anemia with reticulocytopenia was the presenting feature in this child with pure red cell aplasia. **B,** The bone marrow aspirate shows an absence of erythroid precursors. Granulocytic maturation is normal. Increased numbers of hematogones are present.

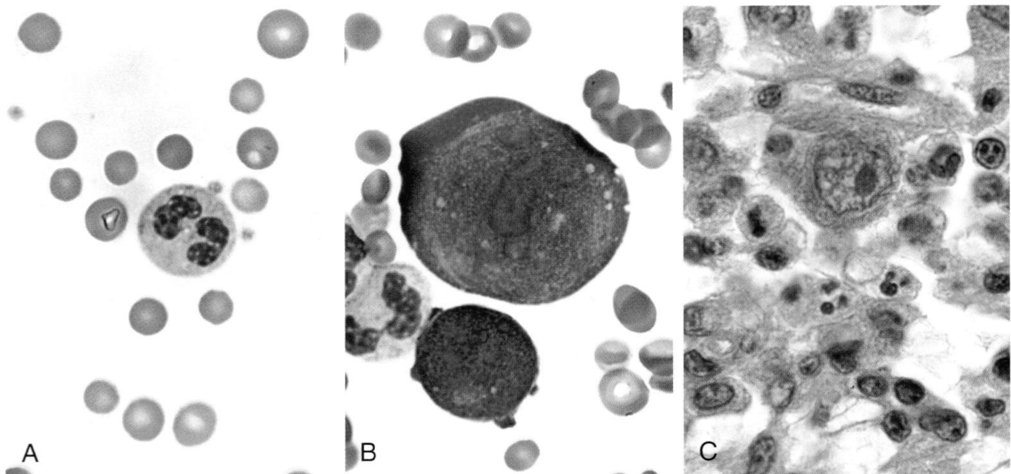

Figure 11-22. Peripheral blood smear from a patient with hereditary spherocytosis who developed severe anemia due to a parvovirus B19–associated "aplastic crisis" (**A**). The bone marrow aspirate (**B**) and trephine biopsy (**C**) contained giant pronormoblasts with large, nucleoli-like parvovirus inclusions.

hybridization for parvovirus on marrow biopsy sections are diagnostic.

The sudden onset of pure red cell aplasia is often associated with a history of a recent respiratory or gastrointestinal viral infection or the use of drugs administered for infectious or inflammatory conditions. Box 11-2 provides a partial list of drugs that may be responsible, with resolution of the aplasia typically occurring with drug cessation. The rare formation of antierythropoietin antibodies secondary to erythropoietin treatment, particularly in patients with renal failure, is more of a problem. Red cell aplasia persists despite stopping erythropoietin treatment, and immunosuppressive therapy is required.[27] Transient erythroblastopenia of childhood is a common finding in children undergoing bone marrow examination for anemia.[28] The cause of this acute, transient disorder remains elusive. Most chronic, acquired pure red cell aplasias have an autoimmune basis, with impairment or suppression of erythropoiesis by humoral or cellular immune mechanisms.[29] Classic causes include thymoma, hematologic malignancies, and systemic autoimmune disorders. Despite the clearly established association between red cell aplasia and thymoma, less than 10% of individuals with aplasia are found to have thymomas on radiographic evaluation. Clonal proliferations of T cells or altered Th1/Th2 ratios have been implicated in many cases of chronic pure red cell aplasia. Additionally, a significant proportion of idiopathic cases are likely secondary to the frequently underdiagnosed T-cell large granular lymphocytic leukemia.[30] Antibody-mediated processes may affect cells directly or indirectly through complement-mediated processes. Alternatively, erythropoietin may be targeted, as previously described.[31] In refractory patients without a clear underlying cause and normal cytogenetic studies, bone marrow cultures examining erythroid burst-forming units are reportedly helpful in excluding MDS.[32] If erythroid maturation is present after serum antibody is removed, the patient is unlikely to have MDS, and additional therapy with immunologic agents is warranted. Patients with MDS may have aberrant expression of antigens on their erythroid precursors, such as CD71 and CD105, which may be useful in distinguishing MDS from other causes of persistent anemia.[33]

Aplastic Anemia

Aplastic anemia usually presents with pancytopenia and is discussed under bone marrow failure syndromes.

Myelophthisic Anemias

Myelophthisic anemias are caused by replacement of normal marrow cells by tumor, granuloma, histiocytes in storage disease, or fibrosis and usually exhibit bicytopenia or pancytopenia. Although the anemia is typically normochromic and normocytic, red cell fragmentation, spherocytes, and teardrop forms are frequently encountered. Normoblasts and left-shifted granulocyte precursors produce a "leukoerythroblastic" blood picture in most cases associated with metastatic tumor or fibrosis (Figs. 11-23 and 11-24). Bone marrow evaluation is essential to identify the underlying disorder.

Anemia of Chronic Renal Failure

Anemia of chronic renal failure often has a multifactorial cause, including the effect of certain still ill-defined plasma factors. However, a primary cause is erythropoietin underproduction by the damaged kidneys (see Chapter 12).

Normochromic Normocytic Anemias, High Output

The remaining normochromic normocytic anemias, which include acute posthemorrhagic anemia and the hemolytic anemias, show increased erythropoiesis with elevated reticulocyte counts.

Posthemorrhagic Anemia

Posthemorrhagic anemia due to recent blood loss is normochromic and normocytic and is accompanied by a reticulocytosis that first manifests 3 to 5 days after blood loss. By 7 to 10 days, the reticulocytes may be so numerous that they increase the MCV up to 100 to 110 fL. Shortly after the hemorrhage, the first notable change in the blood is thrombocytosis, followed by demargination of neutrophils from the release of adrenergic hormones. Finally, the hemoglobin falls as extravascular fluids enter the vascular space.

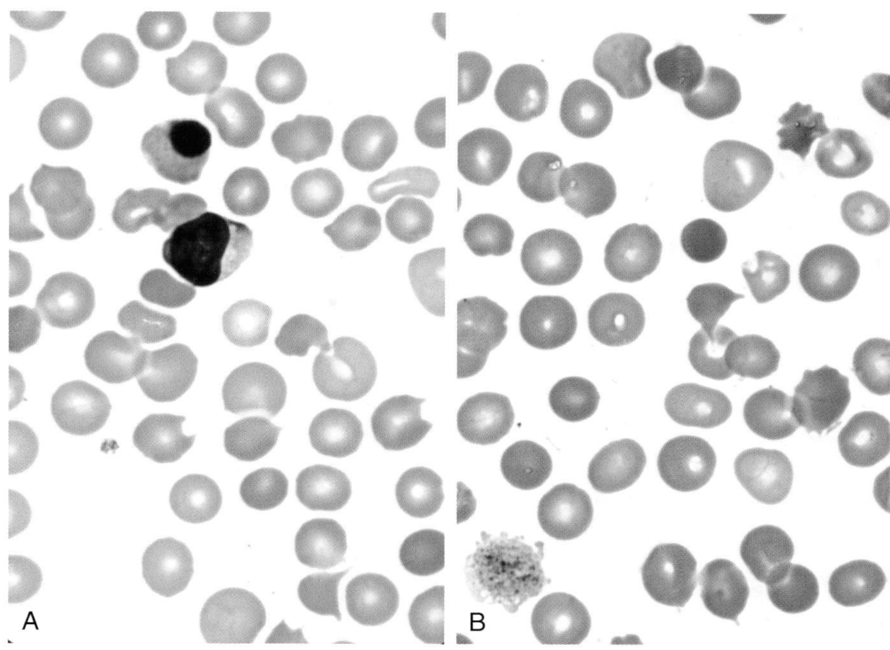

Figure 11-23. Myelophthisic anemia typically shows circulating normoblasts and red cell fragmentation (**A**). A left shift in all cell lines is common. Note the giant platelet (**B**).

Hemolytic Anemias

Hemolytic anemias are usually normochromic normocytic anemias in which an elevated reticulocyte count reflects compensation for increased RBC destruction. The process may be episodic or persistent. Hemolysis is caused by four basic abnormalities: intrinsic red cell defects, plasma factors, disruption of the cells by mechanical or thermal damage, and infectious agents (Table 11-4; see Fig. 11-2). Patients with hemolytic anemia often have similar clinical and laboratory findings: normochromic normocytic anemia, reticulocytosis, shortened red cell life span, elevated erythropoietin level, increased indirect bilirubin, increased lactate dehydrogenase, and jaundice. Those with extravascular hemolysis also develop splenomegaly and gallstones. Bone marrow evaluation invariably shows erythroid hyperplasia, even in patients with only mild compensated hemolysis. Circulating red cells with characteristic shape changes (i.e., sickle cells or spherocytes) are helpful in the diagnosis, whereas the erythroid precursors in the marrow usually have an unremarkable appearance. Identifying or confirming the cause of a hemolytic anemia relies on the patient's history (including the family history) and on definitive laboratory studies, as summarized in Table 11-4.

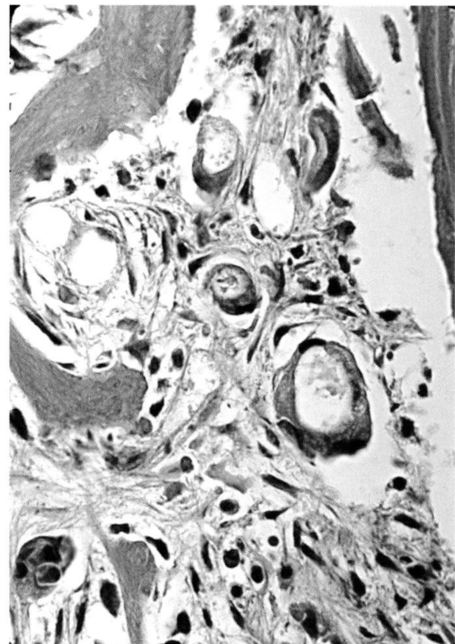

Figure 11-24. Metastatic adenocarcinoma of the small intestine involving bone marrow produced the myelophthisic picture illustrated in Figure 11-23.

Hemolysis Due to Intrinsic Red Cell Disorders. Because these anemias are inherited, a history of lifelong anemia or a family history of anemia, cholelithiasis, jaundice, or mild splenomegaly is helpful. A notable exception is paroxysmal nocturnal hemoglobinuria (PNH), an acquired defect described later with the bone marrow failure syndromes.

Red Blood Cell Membrane Disorders. The molecular basis of a number of RBC membrane disorders has been elucidated in the past few years (Table 11-5).[34,35] The red cell membrane is composed of a lipid bilayer, a network of "horizontally" positioned proteins on the inner surface called the *skeletal proteins,* and transmembrane proteins that "vertically" traverse the lipid bilayer. The skeletal proteins maintain shape and deformability, and the transmembrane proteins provide membrane cohesiveness. Among the more than 50 transmembrane proteins are transport proteins, receptors, and antigens. Mutations in genes encoding key membrane proteins, particularly spectrin, ankyrin, protein 4.1R, protein 4.2, and band 3, lead to inherited red cell membrane disorders.

Hereditary Spherocytosis. Hereditary spherocytosis (HS) is a common cause of nonimmune hemolytic anemia due to abnormalities in the RBC transmembrane proteins.[36] The

Table 11-4 Hemolytic Anemias

Cause	Disorder	Diagnostic Test
Intrinsic RBC Defects		
RBC membrane defects	Hereditary spherocytosis Hereditary elliptocytosis Hereditary pyropoikilocytosis Hereditary stomatocytosis	Incubated osmotic fragility Negative direct antiglobulin test Flow cytometric analysis of eosin-5′-maleimide–labeled RBCs Membrane protein analysis or quantification Genomic DNA analysis
RBC enzyme defects		
HMPS	Glucose-6-phosphate dehydrogenase Rare: GSH synthetase, γ-glutamylcysteine synthetase, glutathione reductase	Quantitative enzyme assays Fluorescent screening tests Polymerase chain reaction Genomic DNA analysis
Glycolytic pathway*	Pyruvate kinase Rare: hexokinase, aldolase, glucose phosphate isomerase, phosphofructokinase, triose phosphate isomerase, phosphoglycerate kinase	
Abnormal Hemoglobin		
Altered solubility	Hemoglobin SS, SC, S/D, S/O-Arab, DD, EE, S/β-thalassemia	Hemoglobin electrophoresis
Oxidative susceptibility	Unstable hemoglobins (100 variants)	High-performance liquid chromatography Isopropanol stability test
Abnormal structure	Thalassemias	
Plasma Factors		
Immune mediated		
AIHA	Idiopathic, infection, autoimmune disorders, malignancy	Direct antiglobulin test
Alloimmune	Hemolytic disease of the newborn	ABO and Rh testing
Drug induced		
Direct toxic effect	Spider bites, bee, snake (cobra) venom	Coagulation tests
Mechanical or Thermal Damage	Burns, heart valves, vasculitis, eclampsia, malignant hypertension, TTP, DIC, HUS	PT, PTT, D-dimer, fibrinogen, BUN, creatinine
Infection	Malaria, *Babesia, Bartonella, Clostridium perfringens*	Peripheral smears, cultures
Splenic Sequestration	Hypersplenism—usually distribution abnormality	Physical exam, radiographic studies

AIHA, autoimmune hemolytic anemia; BUN, blood urea nitrogen; DIC, disseminated intravascular coagulation; GSH, reduced glutathione; HMPS, hexose monophosphate shunt; HUS, hemolytic uremic syndrome; PT, prothrombin time; PTT, partial thromboblastin time; RBC, red blood cell; TTP, thrombotic thrombocytopenic purpura.
*Embden-Meyerhof.

Table 11-5 Red Blood Cell Membrane Disorders

Disorder	Defect (Inheritance)	RBC Morphology	Comments
Hereditary spherocytosis	β spectrin (D); *SPTB* gene α spectrin (R); *SPTA1* gene Ankyrin (D, R); *ANK-1* gene Protein 4.2 (R); *EPB42* gene Band 3 (D); *SLC4A1* gene	Spherocytes + acanthocytes (5%-10%) Spherocytes, microspherocytes, poikilocytes Spherocytes Few spherocytes, ovalocytes, stomatocytes Spherocytes + "pincered" cells (<5%)	All ethnic groups, ↑ in those of northern European ancestry (1 : 200 incidence), North American, Japanese 75% autosomal dominant; 25% autosomal recessive or sporadic 50%—ankyrin or combined ankyrin-spectrin protein deficiency
Hereditary elliptocytosis	α spectrin (D) β spectrin (D) Protein 4.1 (D) Glycoprotein C	Elliptocytes—usually >25% of RBCs If moderate to severe anemia: schistocytes, budding RBCs	Heterogeneous clinical, genetic disorder ↑ in those of African and Mediterranean ancestry Majority—partial α and β spectrin deficiencies 10% isolated spectrin deficiency
Southeast Asian ovalocytosis	Band 3 (D)	Ovalocytes (20%-50%) with transverse bars or single longitudinal slit	Very rigid red cell membrane but mechanically stable Little hemolysis
Hereditary pyropoikilocytosis	Spectrin (D)	Fragile cells fragment into bizarre shapes in circulation, including budding, fragments, spherocytes, triangulocytes	Subset of hereditary elliptocytosis ↑ in those of African ancestry Infant and children present with severe hemolytic anemia and develop associated complications (e.g., growth retardation, bone abnormalities) Cells have ↑ thermal sensitivity
Hereditary stomatocytosis	Stomatin? (regulates sodium and potassium transport) (D)	Macrocytosis common; stomatocytes, target cells, schistocytes, spiculated cells	Molecular basis not defined

D, dominant; R, recessive; RBC, red blood cell.

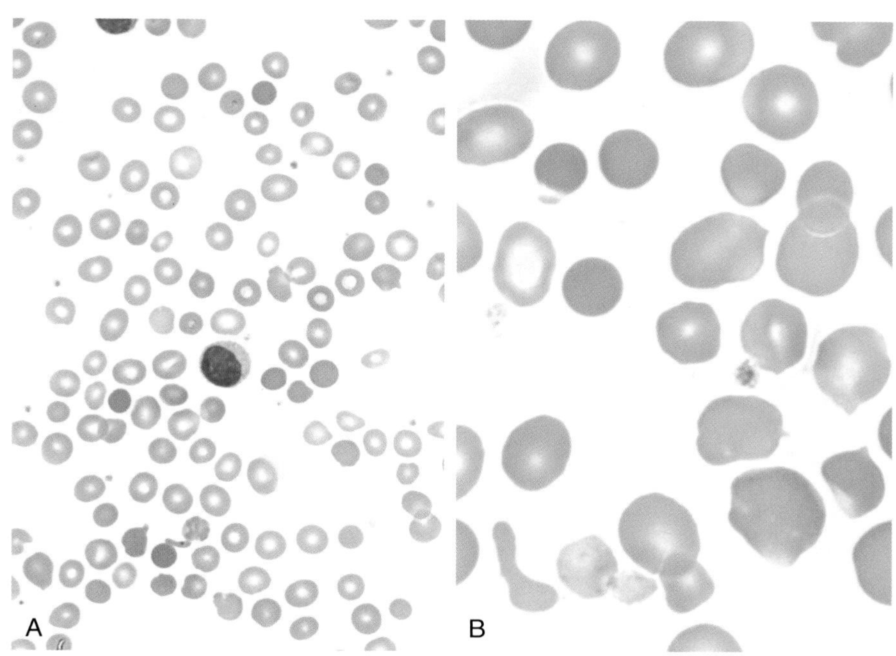

Figure 11-25. In this case of hereditary spherocytosis, the number of red cells is moderately decreased, and spherocytes are readily apparent **(A)**. Spherocytes are smaller and stain more darkly than the surrounding normocytes and large polychromatophilic red cells **(B)**.

defect leads to local dyscohesion of the membrane skeleton from the lipid bilayer, which creates a microvesicle with subsequent loss of membrane and formation of a spherocyte. Spherocytosis is the hallmark of HS and should be suspected if the red cell indices include a normal or low MCV and the MCHC after warming remains 36 g/dL or greater (Fig. 11-25). The less deformable spherocytes are selectively trapped in the spleen and are vulnerable to further surface membrane loss and destruction. Genetic defects vary among different racial groups, with heterogeneous molecular abnormalities that are often family specific. Gene mutations typically shift the normal reading frames or introduce premature stop codons that result in mutant alleles that fail to produce protein. The specific gene involved (i.e., the molecular phenotype) may not strictly relate to the biochemical phenotype (i.e., the abnormal protein produced).[37] For example, an ankyrin gene defect may manifest as spectrin protein deficiency. It is usually the spectrin content of the red cell that best correlates with the degree of anemia, percentage of circulating spherocytes, reticulocyte count, and increased osmotic fragility.

Clinically, anemia is the presenting complaint in nearly half of patients, although disease severity varies widely among individuals. Mild compensated hemolysis is observed in about 20% of individuals, with the majority of affected people (60%) having moderate hemolysis with a hemoglobin of 8 to 11 g/dL and reticulocyte percentage generally higher than 8%. At birth, HS patients usually have a normal hemoglobin value that may sharply and transiently decrease during the first 20 days of life to a level that requires blood transfusions.[38] The more asymptomatic forms of HS may not be identified until a hemolytic crisis develops during childhood, often triggered by a viral infection. Less commonly, an aplastic crisis develops secondary to parvovirus B19 infection (see Fig. 11-22). Although a family history of HS is often elicited in individuals suspected of having HS, the most severe forms of the disease are recessive and associated with α-spectrin and some ankyrin defects.[39] Sporadic mutations are particularly common in the autosomal recessive forms of HS. The most widely used diagnostic test is an incubated osmotic fragility study coupled with examination of the peripheral blood smear. More recently, flow cytometric analysis of eosin-5′-maleimide (EMA)–labeled red blood cells was reported to have greater than 95% specificity and sensitivity for HS.[40] Although EMA binds specifically with band 3 protein, membrane protein abnormalities in HS other than band 3 deficiency affect binding and therefore the fluorescent intensity of the dye measured by flow cytometry.[33] Splenectomy has been the primary mode of therapy.

Hereditary Elliptocytosis and Hereditary Pyropoikilocytosis. Hereditary elliptocytosis (HE) and hereditary pyropoikilocytosis (HPP) were originally described as distinct entities, but recent molecular studies have established that HPP is a subset of HE (see Tables 11-4 and 11-5).[34] They are caused by defects in the horizontal protein interactions that hold the membrane skeleton together. The abnormality that best correlates with disease severity is a failure of spectrin homodimers to self-associate into heterodimers, the basic building blocks of the membrane skeleton. Differences in the clinical severity of HE cannot always be explained by a specific genetic defect. The most prevalent form of the disease is a single gene defect (heterozygous) that causes the red cells to elongate and form elliptocytes in circulation, without anemia or significant splenomegaly. The more severe form of the disease, HPP, is due to a combination of two defective membrane protein genes that result in marked spectrin deficiency in addition to functionally abnormal proteins. The MCV may be very low because of marked RBC fragmentation, rendering the clinical presentation atypical for a hemolytic anemia, with possible microcytic rather than normocytic RBC indices (Fig. 11-26). A disorder related to HE, called *Southeast Asian ovalocytosis*, is found in people from Malaysia, Indonesia, the Philippines, and Papua New Guinea. Only a subset of affected individuals has hemolytic anemia, with distinctive oval stomatocytes.

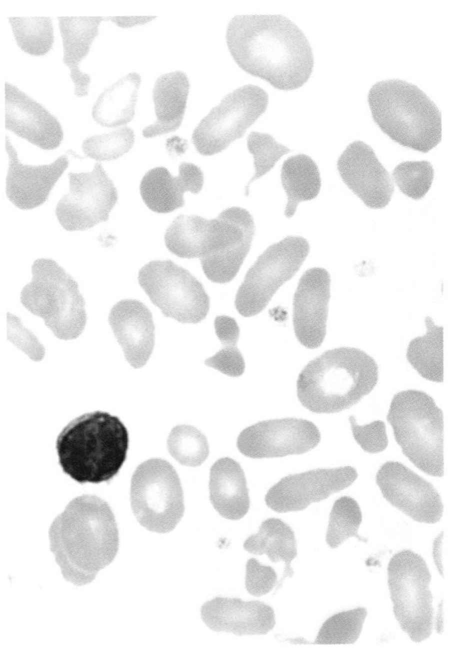

Figure 11-26. Hereditary pyropoikilocytosis. Numerous elliptocytes, fragmented red cells, and teardrop forms were found in this child's blood. The mother's blood looked similar. The father's blood was normal.

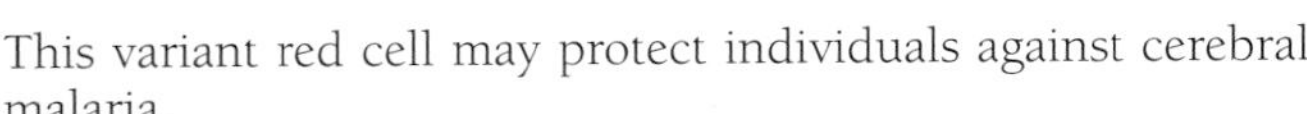

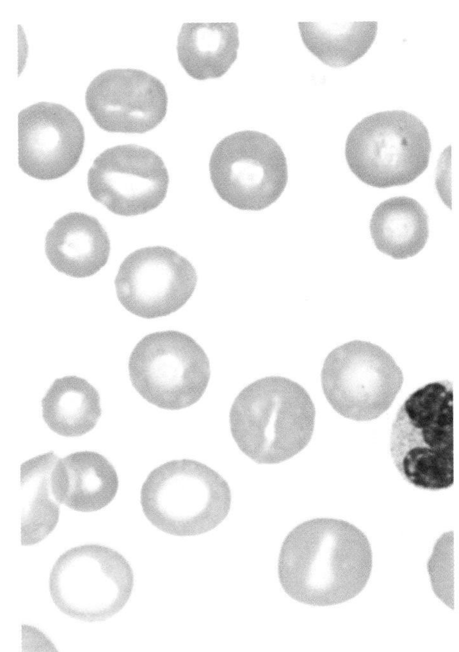

Figure 11-27. Hereditary stomatocytosis. Stomatocytes are often darker than surrounding red cells and have a slit-like central pallor due to the loss of intracellular fluid.

This variant red cell may protect individuals against cerebral malaria.

Hereditary Stomatocytosis Syndromes. Hereditary stomatocytosis syndromes are a group of disorders of the RBC membrane characterized by a mouth-shaped central area of pallor and abnormal permeability to sodium and potassium (Fig. 11-27).[41] Loss of potassium leads to RBC dehydration and a mild to moderately severe hemolytic anemia. Automated counts show an increased MCHC and normal MCV (falsely elevated on some automated counters). A misdiagnosis of atypical HS is often made. Patients with hereditary stomatocytosis have severe thrombotic complications after splenectomy, and avoidance of this procedure is important.

Red Blood Cell Enzyme Defects. RBC energy requirements are met primarily through the metabolism of glucose by the glycolytic pathway. Alternatively, approximately 10% of glucose is metabolized by the hexose monophosphate shunt. Erythrocyte disorders due to enzyme deficiencies of the glycolytic pathway are extremely rare, and approximately 90% of these are deficiencies of pyruvate kinase caused primarily by *PK-LR* gene mutations on chromosome 1q21 (see Table 11-4).[42] The majority are inherited as autosomal recessive traits and first detected in infancy or childhood with the clinical presentation of chronic hemolysis. The direct antiglobulin test (Coombs test), hemoglobin electrophoresis, and osmotic fragility are normal. The peripheral blood film shows normochromic normocytic RBCs without spherocytes. The remaining morphologic findings are nonspecific but include reticulocytosis and erythroid hyperplasia.

Hereditary disorders of the hexose monophosphate shunt enzymes are also rare, except glucose-6-phosphate dehydrogenase (G6PD) deficiency. G6PD deficiency is one of the most prevalent inborn errors of metabolism.[43] More than 400 variants of G6PD and at least 30 mutations (missense point mutations) have been described (Table 11-6). It is particularly prevalent in populations from geographic areas with endemic malaria, suggesting that evolutionary polymorphisms were formed to counteract the effects of this parasite. The *G6PD* gene is carried on the X chromosome, and full expression of G6PD deficiency is found only in males; female carriers may have partial deficiency. Clinical manifestations of G6PD deficiency include neonatal jaundice and hereditary nonspherocytic hemolytic anemia. The most serious consequence of G6PD deficiency is neonatal jaundice leading to kernicterus, which is worsened by associated Gilbert's disease.[44] Although a few patients have chronic hemolytic anemia, the majority

Table 11-6 Common Glucose-6-Phosphate Dehydrogenase (G6PD) Variants

Isoform	Ethnic Group	Comments
G6PD B	All	Most common, normal variant
G6PD A	Blacks (20%)	Normal variant, no hemolysis
G6PD A^-	Blacks (11%)	Group of variants with same mutation as G6PD A, but with one additional mutation Moderate hemolysis Unstable enzyme, ↑ decay
G6PD^{MED}	Greeks, Arabs, Sicilians, Sephardic Jews	Severe hemolysis Protects against *Plasmodium falciparum*
G6PD^{CANTON}	Asians	Moderate hemolysis

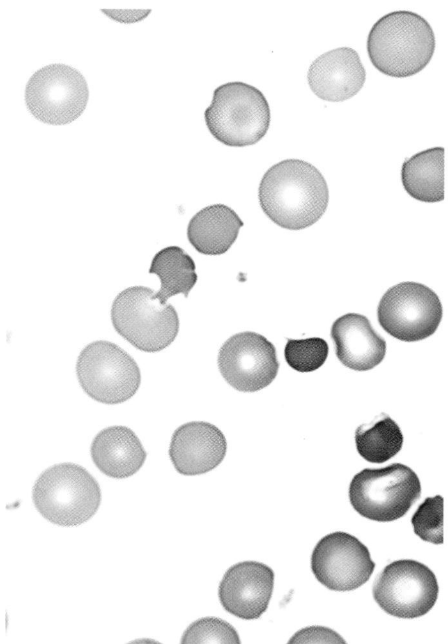

Figure 11-28. Oxidant hemolysis causes hemoglobin to precipitate at the cell membrane. The spleen removes the aggregates of hemoglobin and associated membrane, producing "bite" cells and spherocytes.

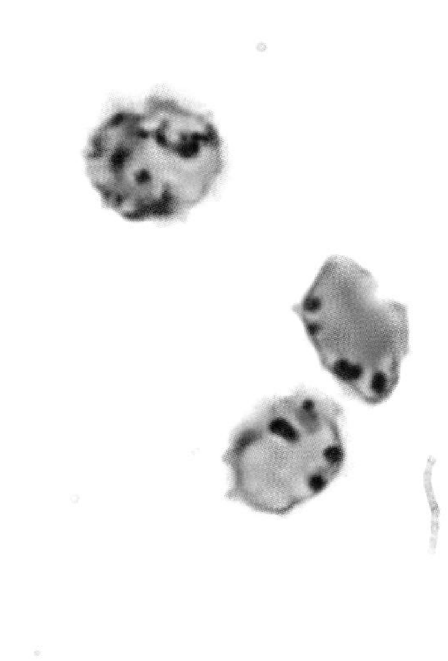

Figure 11-29. This wet mount illustrates membrane-associated Heinz bodies in oxidant hemolysis.

have episodic anemia induced by increased oxidative stress in erythrocytes from certain foods (fava beans), a number of drugs (sulfonamides, nitrofurans, quinine derivatives, aspirin), and chemicals (naphthalene, toluidine blue).[45] Erythrocytes deficient in G6PD are unable to maintain sufficient reduced glutathione for the generation of NADH, a cofactor that maintains hemoglobin integrity. The WHO has classified G6PD variants based on their degree of enzyme deficiency and severity of hemolysis: class I, less than 10% enzyme activity with severe chronic (nonspherocytic) hemolytic anemia, to class V, increased enzyme level with no hemolysis or clinical sequelae. Oxidant damage is reflected by marked anisopoikilocytosis with "bite" cells and increased polychromatophilia on the peripheral blood film (Fig. 11-28). Supravital staining demonstrates denatured hemoglobin precipitates (Heinz bodies) (Fig. 11-29). The bone marrow most commonly demonstrates erythroid hyperplasia.

Hemoglobinopathies. Hemoglobinopathies are abnormalities of hemoglobin structure due to abnormal amino acid sequences in either the alpha or beta globin chains. The most prevalent abnormal hemoglobin is HbS, produced by the substitution of glutamate for valine at the sixth position of the beta globin chain. The gene for HbS has autosomal dominant inheritance and is found in areas of the world where malaria is common. Approximately 8% to 10% of the African American population carries at least one HbS gene.[46] Sickle cell disease occurs in individuals with homozygous sickle mutations (termed *HbSS* or *sickle cell anemia*) or compound heterozygous mutations, most commonly sickle cell β-thalassemia or hemoglobin SC disease. RBC sickling is induced under conditions of deoxygenation, vasoconstriction, acidosis, increased HbS concentration, and infection. The clinical symptoms of the sickle cell disorders vary greatly in severity among individuals,[47,48] but they are often due to the increased tendency of sickle cells to adhere to vascular endothelium and to the ensuing vaso-occlusive complications.[49] Cells become irreversibly sickled and are removed by the reticuloendothelial system. The hallmark of these disorders is morphologically altered red cells (Fig. 11-30). In addition to the sickle cells, irregularly shaped cells, targets, spherocytes, and polychromatophilic cells may be found on the blood film. Howell-Jolly bodies are usually identified in older individuals as a

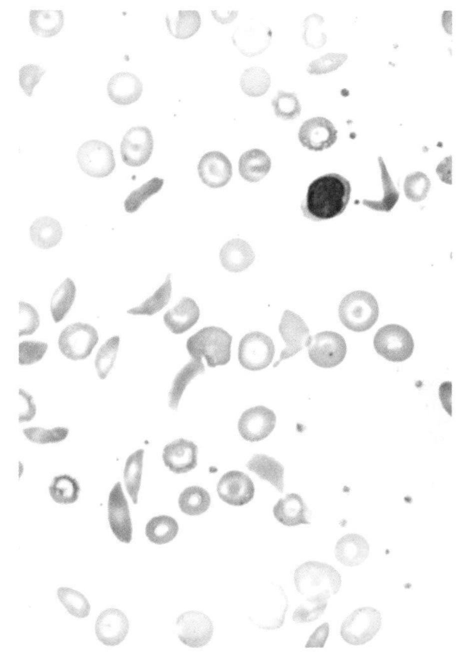

Figure 11-30. Numerous sickled red cells and target cells are seen in this patient with sickle cell anemia.

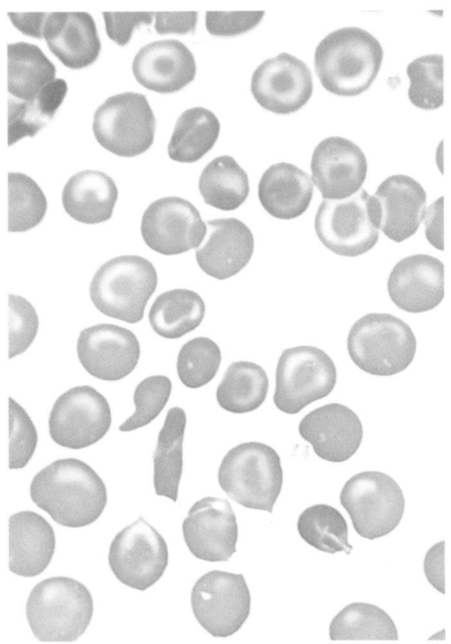

Figure 11-31. Target cells predominate, and plump angulated sickle cells are found in hemoglobin SC disease.

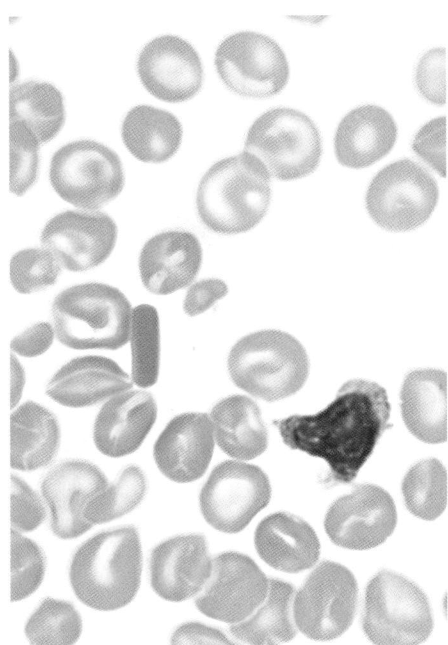

Figure 11-32. In hemoglobin C disease, target cells are numerous. Note the rod-shaped crystal in the "boxcar" cell at the *top center* of the figure.

result of autosplenectomy. A left-shifted neutrophilia with toxic features and thrombocytosis are common during an acute crisis. Heterozygous disorders may additionally show microcytosis (Sβ-thalassemia) and intracellular crystals (HbSC) (Fig. 11-31). Patients with sickle cell anemia may also develop acute splenic sequestration, parvovirus-related red cell aplasia, and bone marrow necrosis. In addition to erythroid hyperplasia, bone marrow biopsies frequently show increased arterial fibrosis.[50]

Among the numerous other known hemoglobinopathies, HbC and HbE are the next most common causes of chronic hemolysis. The HbC gene mutation is most prevalent in West Africans; the HbE gene is found primarily in Southeast Asians. Homozygous HbE is unusual in its presentation as a mild to moderate, hypochromic microcytic anemia (MCV 50 to 65 fL). HbC is recognized morphologically by the unique intracellular crystalline structures in erythrocytes on the blood film (Fig. 11-32).

Immune-Mediated Hemolytic Anemia

Autoimmune Hemolytic Anemias. Autoimmune hemolytic anemias (AIHAs) are categorized by the temperature at which the autoantibody has the greatest avidity for the target red cell antigen, and they are detected by a positive direct antiglobulin test. Warm AIHA is most common (70% of AIHAs) and is clinically significant because it occurs at body temperature. IgG antibody– or occasionally IgA antibody–coated RBCs act to bind Fc receptors on splenic macrophages and, with or without subsequent complement fixation, are removed from circulation. Partial phagocytosis of the RBC membrane produces spherocytes (Fig. 11-33). Cold AIHA is due to IgM coating of red cells at low temperatures, leading to RBC agglutination and complement fixation. The antibody is most often directed at the I antigen on the red cell membrane. Some hemolysis occurs secondary to intravascular destruction of the agglutinated cells. However, if the antibody is active at temperatures approaching 37°C, complement becomes activated, and clinically significant intravascular and sometimes extravascular complement-mediated hemolysis occurs in the liver (80% of time).[51] Smears typically show agglutinated cells unless the blood tube was previously warmed; spherocytes are less frequent (Fig. 11-34). Autoantibody formation in both warm- and cold-type AIHA most likely represents a derange-

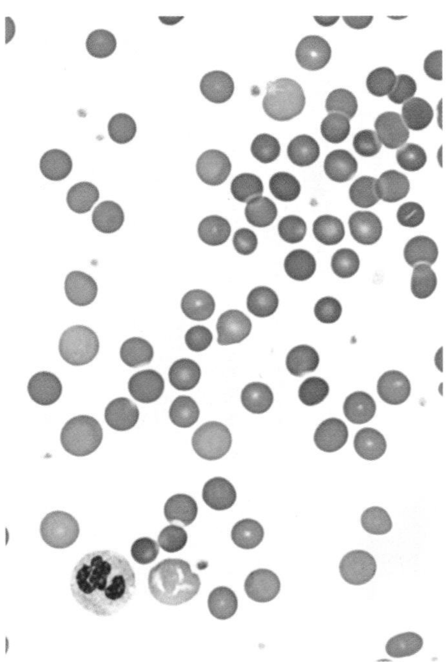

Figure 11-33. In warm antibody hemolytic anemia, numerous spherocytes are seen.

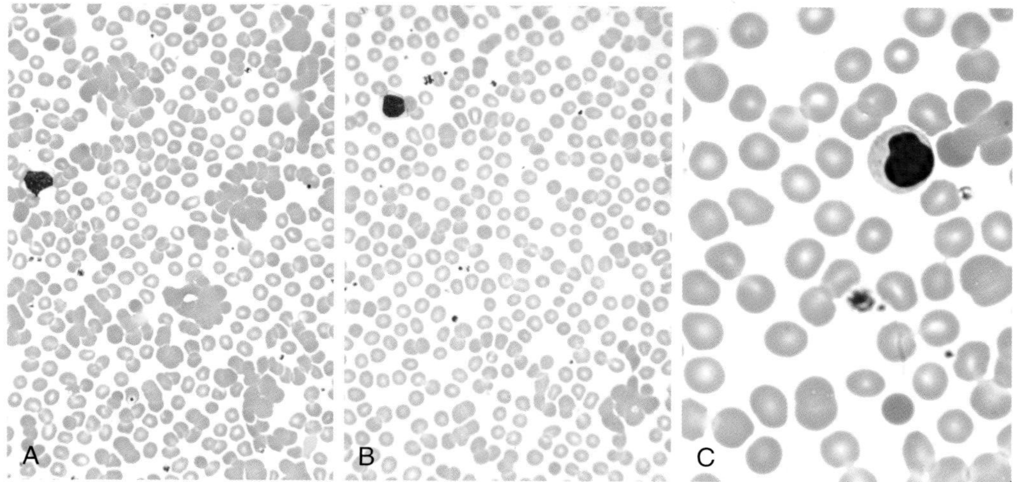

Figure 11-34. In cold agglutinin disease, numerous aggregates are seen in blood smears made from blood at room temperature (**A**). When the blood is warmed to 37°C (**B**), the agglutination phenomenon is reversed. Red cell morphology is essentially normal in cold agglutinin disease. Only a rare spherocyte is seen (**C**).

ment of normal immune function. Approximately 50% of AIHA is idiopathic (primary) and observed in older patients.[52] In contrast, secondary AIHA develops in patients with underlying disease, predominantly lymphoproliferative disorders but also carcinoma, autoimmune disorders, and infections. Young patients, in particular, develop a self-limited cold-type AIHA after *Mycoplasma pneumoniae* infection or infectious mononucleosis.

Drug-Induced Immune Hemolysis. Drug-induced immune hemolysis occurs through three main mechanisms: autoantibody formation (warm-type AIHA), often directed at the Rh locus of the red cell; hapten formation with IgG antibody to drug that is adsorbed on the red cell surface; and drug-antibody complex that attaches to the RBC surface and activates complement.[53] Examples of drugs that typify these mechanisms are α-methyldopa; penicillin and cephalosporins; and quinine, isoniazid, and insulin, respectively. Certain drugs, such as the cephalosporins and methyldopa (Aldomet), can alter RBC membranes, causing nonspecific binding of IgG or IgM. RBCs are lost through splenic sequestration and destruction. The direct antiglobulin test is positive, and bone marrow evaluation is not required.

Hemolysis Due to Physicomechanical Disruption. Hemolysis due to physicomechanical disruption develops when red cells are exposed to mechanical trauma or to heat above body temperature. Mechanical trauma occurs through a variety of mechanisms, including disruption by fibrin strands in disseminated intravascular coagulation, vasculitis, and possibly thrombotic thrombocytopenic purpura, and the effects of vortexing in aortic insufficiency, malignant hypertension, and eclampsia (see Fig. 11-2). The blood smear typically contains numerous schistocytes and small numbers of spherocytes (Fig. 11-35). These anemias are commonly referred to as *microangiopathic hemolytic anemia*, even though red cell destruction may occur in the left ventricle, aorta, or other large vessels. When blood is heated to greater than 50°C, red cells fragment into microspherocytes (Fig. 11-36). This phenomenon is typical of patients suffering severe thermal burns of the skin.

Infection-Associated Hemolytic Anemia. Infection-associated hemolytic anemia is due to organisms that parasitize or otherwise disrupt the RBCs, such as malaria, babesiosis, and bartonellosis (Figs. 11-37 and 11-38).

Macrocytic Anemia

Macrocytic anemia is defined as an MCV greater than 99 fL in adults and is dependent on age for infants and children. Because reticulocytes are larger than normal red cells, a mild degree of macrocytosis (MCV rarely >110 fL) may be seen following recent hemorrhage (>1 week), hemolytic anemia, or treated anemia with a brisk reticulocyte response. A

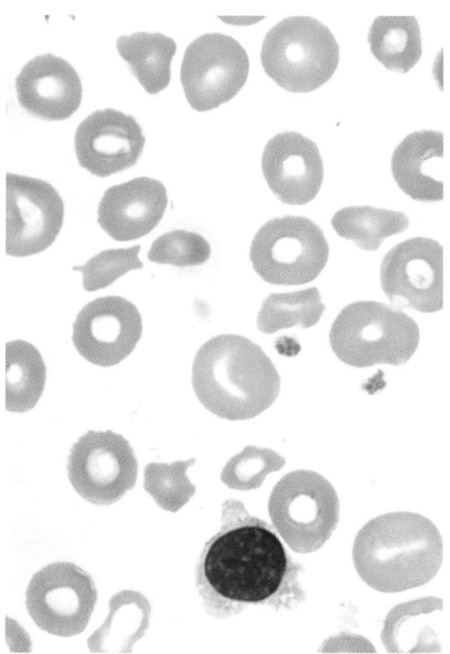

Figure 11-35. Fragmentation syndrome produced by a defective prosthetic aortic valve.

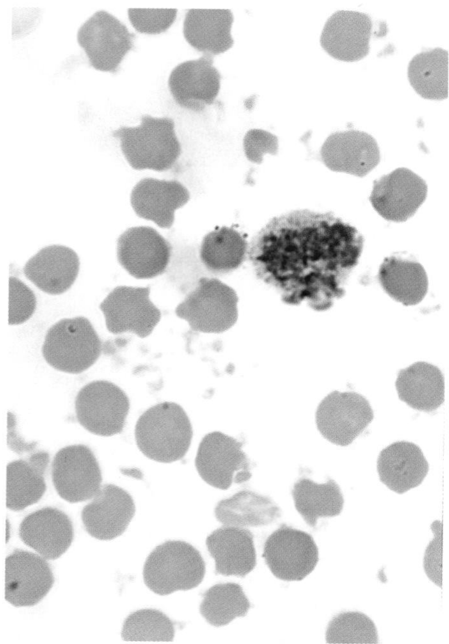

Figure 11-36. This blood smear was made from a specimen inadvertently exposed to high temperatures in a defective pneumatic tube system adjacent to a steam line. Numerous spherocytes, cytoplasmic red cell fragments, and a degenerating white cell are present.

secondary reticulocytosis is observed in a subset of patients with liver disease; the RBCs have increased cholesterol and lecithin incorporation, producing thin macrocytes and target cells that have a shortened life span.[54] The increase in reticulocytes in all these processes is reflected by a high RDW. The remaining macrocytic anemias (Table 11-7) exhibit decreased or ineffective hematopoiesis, with low reticulocyte numbers and a frequently normal RDW.

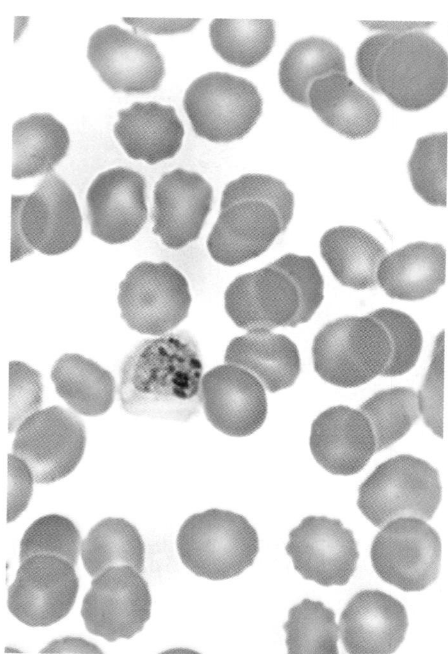

Figure 11-37. Mature schizont of *Plasmodium vivax*.

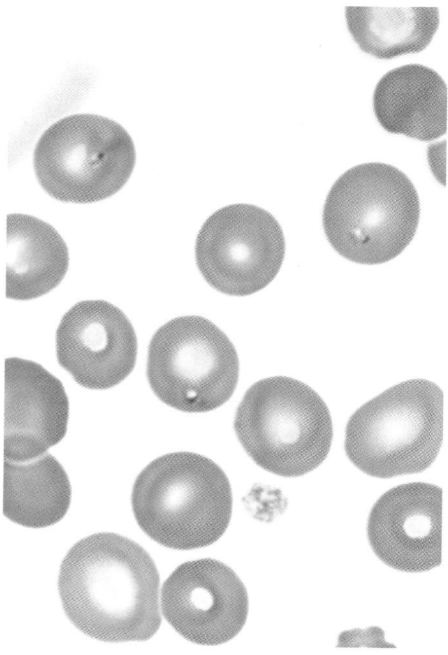

Figure 11-38. Small microgametocytes of *Babesia microti* are present in multiple RBCs.

Megaloblastic Anemias

Megaloblastic anemias are the most common macrocytic anemias, particularly those due to vitamin B_{12} (cobalamin) or folate deficiency (see Table 11-7). Megaloblastic anemias are the consequence of ineffective erythropoiesis due to defects in DNA synthesis.[55] The coenzyme form of folate is an important cofactor in the rate-limiting step and many additional steps of DNA (pyrimidine) synthesis; cobalamin plays an interdependent role involving methionine synthesis and the conversion of methylmalonyl CoA to succinyl CoA. Enlargement or "gigantism" of hematopoietic precursors is seen because cytoplasmic maturation proceeds while cell division is delayed by the lack of sufficient DNA to undergo mitosis. Increased intramedullary cell death ensues, with compensatory hyperplasias and the development of anemia characterized by oval macrocytes. Anemia is often a late event in folate or vitamin B_{12} deficiency; hypersegmentation of neutrophils usually appears earlier (Figs. 11-39 to 11-42). The hematologic findings in patients with megaloblastic anemia are readily identified (see Table 11-7). Bone marrow examination is usually not required but may be performed for the evaluation of pancytopenias or when the typical peripheral blood findings are masked by concurrent iron deficiency anemia or a constitutional microcytic anemia. It is extremely important to recognize that severe megaloblastic anemia may have sufficiently bizarre cells and increased pronormoblasts to be mistaken for MDS or erythroleukemia. Recognizing the absence of trilineage dysplasia and the absence of an increase in myeloblasts is essential to making a morphologic distinction. Serum and red cell folate and serum vitamin B_{12} levels simplify this task.

Folate deficiency is most commonly nutritional in origin and is most prevalent in alcoholics, indigents, and the elderly. Mood disorders, particularly in elderly patients, may be attributed to undiagnosed folate deficiency. A normal diet contains a large excess of vitamin B_{12}; thus, total body stores of cobal-

Table 11-7 **Causes of Macrocytic Anemia**

Disorder	Bone Marrow Morphology	Comments
Congenital Disorders		
Diamond-Blackfan syndrome	Isolated profound ↓ in erythroid elements, defective erythroid maturation, ↑ hematogones	Familial with autosomal dominance (40%-45%) Sporadic or familial with different inheritance types Familial cases associated with anomalies (e.g., short stature, abnormalities of head and upper limbs)
CDA I	Megaloblastic maturation, 1%-3% erythroid precursors have intranuclear chromatin bridges, binucleation, or nuclear budding	Autosomal recessive, *CDAN1* mutations (15q15.1-q15.3) Mild to moderate anemia
CDA II (HEMPAS)	Normoblastic or megaloblastic, 10%-40% erythroid precursors have bi- or multinucleation, karyorrhexis	Autosomal recessive, genetic heterogeneity (*CDNA2* on chromosome 20q11.2) Mild to severe anemia
CDA III	Megaloblastic maturation, 10%-40% erythroid precursors are multinucleated, including giant erythroblasts (up to 12 nuclei); karyorrhexis	Autosomal dominant, *CDAN3* mutations (15q21-25) Mild to moderate anemia
Megaloblastic Disorders		
Cobalamin (vitamin B_{12}) deficiency	Dyssynchronous nuclear-cytoplasmic maturation Erythroid and often myeloid hyperplasia—↓ myeloid-erythroid ratio	Caused by inadequate intake (strict vegan diet) or impaired absorption (pernicious anemia, gastrectomy, fish tapeworm [*Diphyllobothrium latum*], ileal resection or disease, pancreatic insufficiency, blind loop syndrome)
Folate deficiency	Erythroid lineage—larger cells with immature nucleus (open chromatin) compared to cytoplasmic maturation, possible multinucleation, abnormal nuclear configurations, Howell-Jolly bodies, basophilic stippling, Cabot rings	Caused by inadequate intake (poor diet, premature infant, hemodialysis), impaired absorption in small intestine (celiac sprue, enteritis, resection), increased utilization (chronic hemolysis, pregnancy, chronic infections)
Drugs	Myeloid lineage—giant serpentine bands and metamyelocytes, hypersegmented neutrophils (6 lobes)	Inhibitors of DNA metabolism (deoxynucleotide synthesis inhibitors, antimetabolites, dihydrofolate reductase inhibitors), anticonvulsants, oral contraceptives
Inborn errors	Megakaryocytes—large with multiple lobes, large platelets	Congenital deficiencies (intrinsic factor, transcobalamin II), errors of metabolism, hereditary orotic aciduria, Lesch-Nyhan syndrome
Other		Liver disease, thyroid disease, toxins, alcohol, aplastic anemia

CDA, congenital dyserythropoietic anemia; HEMPAS, hereditary erythroblastic multinuclearity with positive acidified serum.

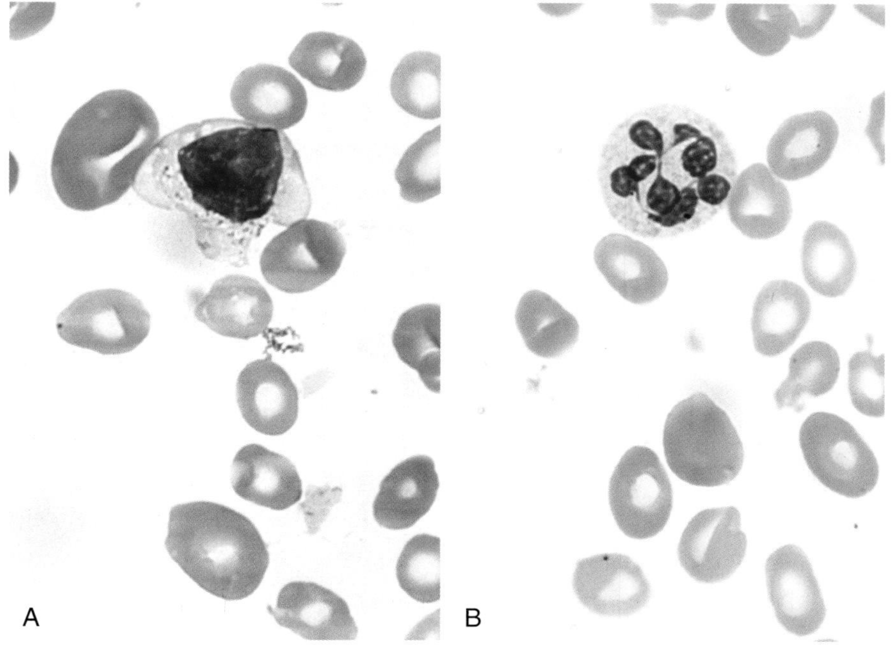

Figure 11-39. Macro-ovalocytes (**A**) and hypersegmented neutrophils (**B**) are typical features of megaloblastic anemia.

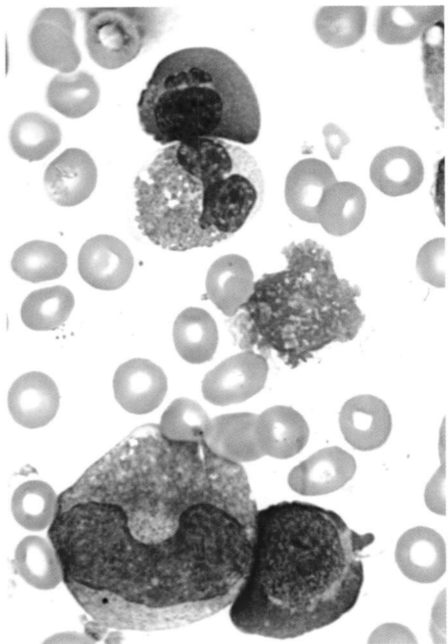

Figure 11-40. Bone marrow aspirate from a patient with cobalamin deficiency illustrates a giant C-shaped neutrophil band and megaloblastic normoblasts.

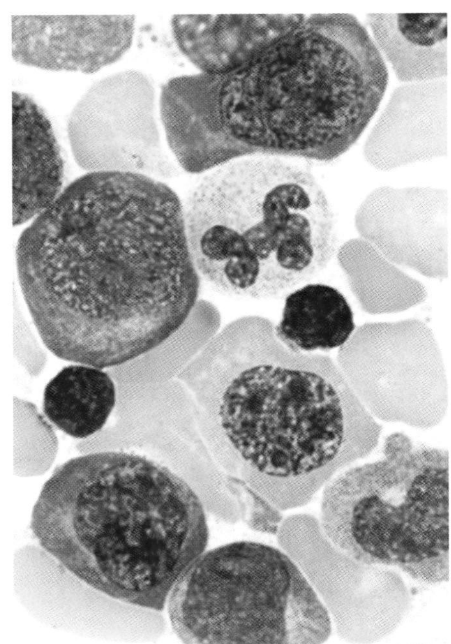

Figure 11-41. Bone marrow aspirate from a patient with pernicious anemia shows dissociation of nuclear and cytoplasmic maturation in megaloblasts. Band neutrophils often have serpentine nuclear contours.

amin are abundant. The most common cause of cobalamin deficiency in the Western world is pernicious anemia. Under normal conditions, cobalamin complexes with intrinsic factor, a product of gastric parietal cells, and binds to intrinsic factor receptors in the terminal ileum. In pernicious anemia, parietal cells are destroyed through autoimmune mechanisms, and little or no cobalamin is absorbed. In contrast to folate deficiency, cobalamin deficiency also causes a demyelinating disorder with numerous neurologic manifestations. Controversy exists regarding the best diagnostic approach to identifying these vitamin deficiencies. The most commonly used indicators of deficiency are the red cell folate level and serum cobalamin; however, these tests are not entirely specific or sensitive. Serum cobalamin levels may be normal or only slightly reduced in some patients with vitamin B_{12} deficiency. Additional tests currently used include serum or plasma methylmalonic acid and plasma homocysteine levels, which better detect low tissue cobalamin stores among individuals

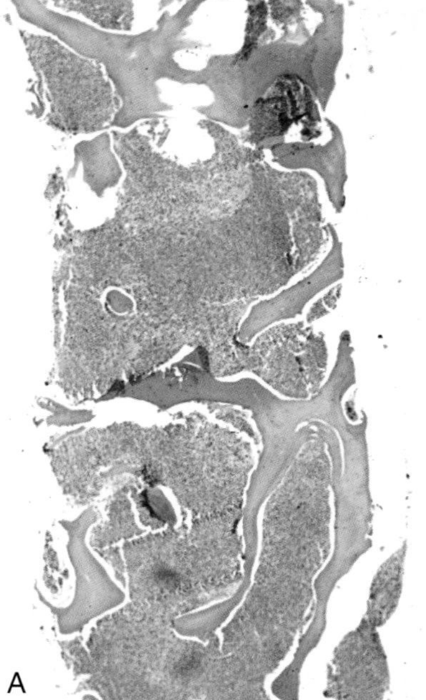

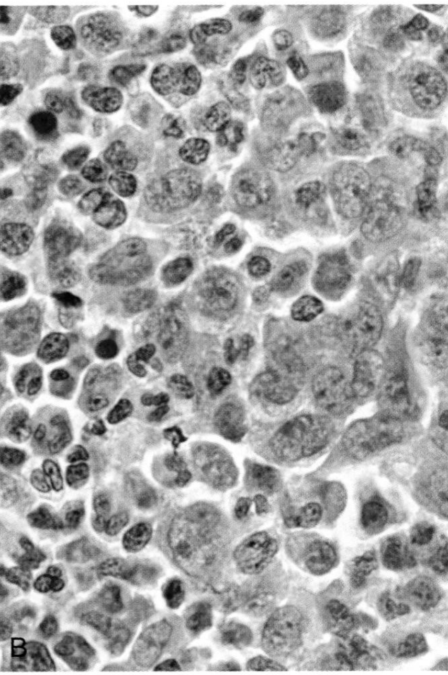

Figure 11-42. The trephine biopsy section of pernicious anemia is often markedly hypercellular (**A**) and contains clusters of large pronormoblasts (**B**). It is important to distinguish this picture from myelodysplastic syndromes and acute erythroleukemia.

with early deficiencies.[56] Hyperhomocysteinemia may be seen in folate deficiency. The measurement of serum holotranscobalamin II, a subfraction of cobalamin, is also a good marker of early vitamin B_{12} deficiency in patients with normal renal function.[57] Pernicious anemia is associated with several autoantibodies; measurement of parietal cell and intrinsic factor antibodies is diagnostically helpful.[58]

Drugs that cause megaloblastic anemia are those that act primarily on DNA synthesis and include antifolates (e.g., methotrexate), purine analogues, pyrimidine analogues (zidovudine), and ribonucleotide reductase inhibitors (e.g., hydroxyurea). Additionally, the metabolism of a number of anticonvulsant and antidepressant drugs is dependent on adequate folic acid for appropriate drug response.[59]

Constitutional Causes

Constitutional causes of macrocytic anemia are much less common. Diamond-Blackfan syndrome is a heterogeneous genetic disorder that usually presents within the first few months of life and by 1 year of age in 90% of cases (see Table 11-7).[60] It is the first human disease found to be caused by mutations in a ribosomal structural protein (*RPS19* gene on chromosome 19q13.2). Mutations of this gene are found in 25% of sporadic and familial cases. Additional genes have been implicated (e.g., *RPS24*), all of which encode ribosomal proteins; approximately 50% of patients studied have a gene mutation.[61] The failure of erythroid production is hypothesized to be caused by faulty ribosome production leading to apoptosis of erythroid precursors.[62] Not surprisingly, the clinical manifestations of the disorder are heterogeneous. Affected family members may have dramatically different degrees of anemia, responses to therapy, and presence of congenital anomalies. Most commonly, the disease presents as a nonresolving severe macrocytic anemia with reticulocytopenia. Bone marrow specimens demonstrate few or no erythroid precursors. Some cases exhibit increased numbers of hematogones. Circulating red cells contain increased HbF (heterogeneous distribution) and have a fetal distribution of intracellular enzymes. In addition to the blood and marrow findings, increased erythropoietin, elevated red cell adenosine deaminase levels, and i antigen expression help to support the diagnosis.

Congenital Dyserythropoietic Anemias

Congenital dyserythropoietic anemias (CDAs) are rare hereditary disorders characterized by abnormalities of erythropoiesis.[63] The three originally described forms, CDA I, II, and III, are defined by distinctive morphologic abnormalities of erythroblasts (see Table 11-7). Additional rare, unique types and variant forms (CDA IV) are also recognized. The morphologic hallmark of CDA is prominent erythroid hyperplasia and striking dyserythropoiesis, with normal myeloid and megakaryocytic lineages (Figs. 11-43 to 11-45). Erythropoiesis is ineffective, as manifested by reticulocytopenia and usually a mild to moderate macrocytic anemia in CDA I and III or moderate normocytic anemia in CDA II. Anisopoikilocytosis is common to all types. Circulating RBCs occasionally have basophilic stippling, cytoplasmic vacuolization, or Cabot rings. CDA II patients have strong expression of protein antigens i and I on their RBCs. Generally, the clinical findings are those associated with a chronic hemolytic anemia, including increased lactate dehydrogenase and bilirubin levels, jaundice, splenomegaly, tendency to form gallstones, and iron overload. CDA II is the most common CDA and may be the most frequently misdiagnosed; the correct diagnosis is often not made until patients are teenagers or even adults, despite the identification of a chronic hemolytic anemia earlier in life.[64] Unlike the other CDAs, CDA II may have associated microspherocytes and a positive osmotic fragility test, suggesting a diagnosis of HS, or a positive Ham acidified serum lysis test, suggesting PNH.[65] Treatment with interferon-α has been effective in a few patients with CDA I.

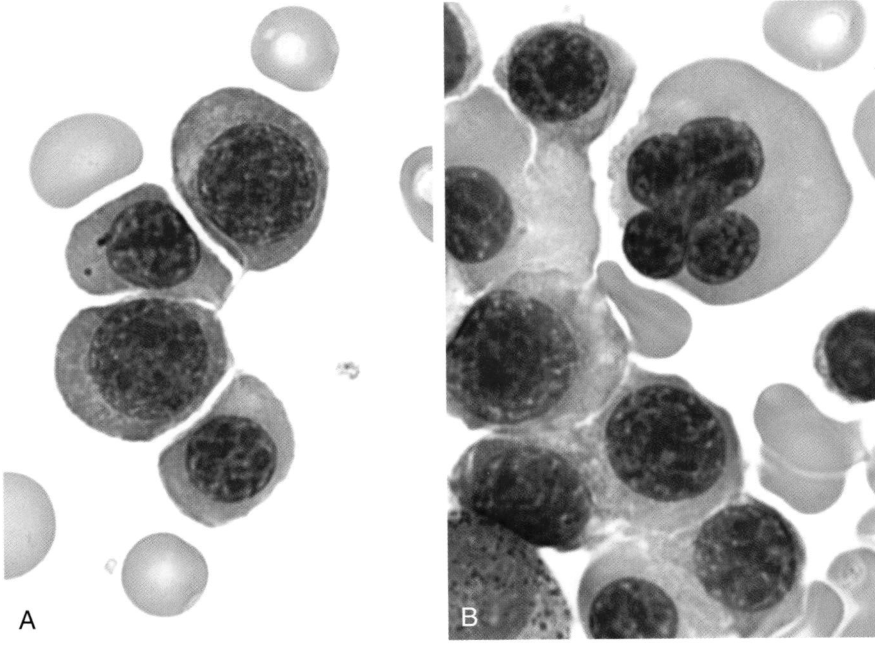

Figure 11-43. Bone marrow aspirate of congenital dyserythropoietic anemia type I shows megaloblastic maturation, intranuclear bridging by chromatin filaments (**A**), and multinucleation (**B**).

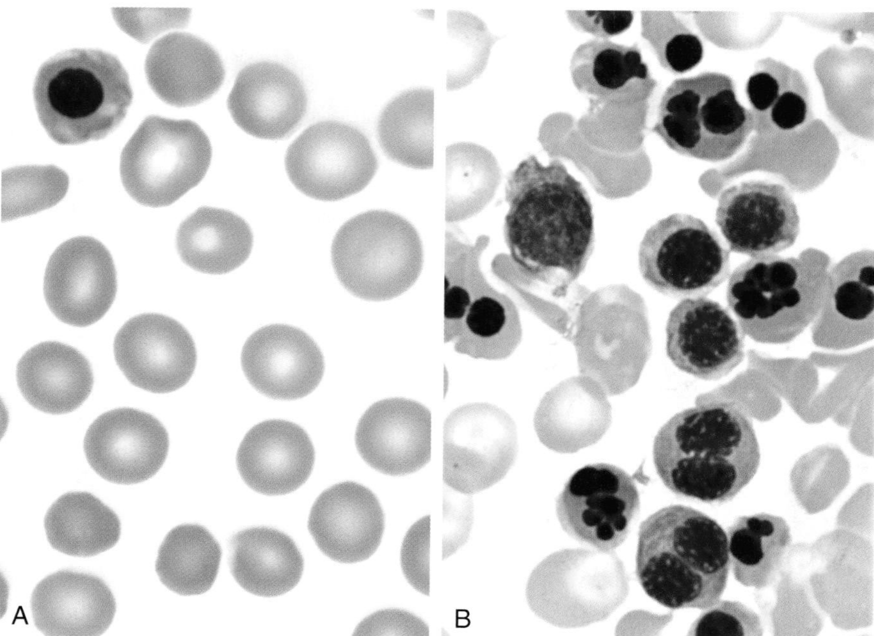

Figure 11-44. Peripheral blood smear from a 16-year-old girl with congenital dyserythropoietic anemia type II (hereditary erythroblastic multinuclearity with positive acidified serum [HEMPAS]) shows mild normochromic normocytic anemia and a normoblast (**A**). The patient underwent a bone marrow study for unrelated tumor staging. Numerous binucleated and multinucleated normoblasts were found (**B**). Her younger brother had similar changes. Both had a positive acidified serum test.

EVALUATION OF LEUKOPENIA

Neutropenia

Neutrophils are the most prevalent leukocyte in circulation before 1 week and after approximately 5 years of age. Neutropenia is therefore the most common cause for a decreased white blood cell count. Age, sex, and ethnic background affect neutrophil counts, and appropriate reference ranges must be considered. Without taking into account sex and ethnic biases, neutropenia is usually present if absolute neutrophil counts (ANCs) are less than 0.7×10^9/L in newborns, less than 2.5×10^9/L in infants, and less than 1.5×10^9/L in children and adults. Compared with whites, Latinos have slightly higher neutrophil counts, and persons of African origin, Sephardic and Falasha Jews, and black Bedouin Arabs have slightly lower neutrophil counts, owing to differences in myeloid production or the inability to modulate white cell trafficking.[66,67] One quarter of healthy individuals of African ancestry have ANCs of 1.0 to 1.5×10^9/L. Their lower neutrophil counts are linked to Duffy antigen receptor chemokine gene polymorphisms, which may play a role in *Plasmodium vivax* malaria resistance, and to C-reactive protein levels.[68] Individuals are at significantly greater risk for life-threatening infection, particularly from endogenous bacteria, if severe neutropenia ($<0.5 \times 10^9$/L) persists for more than a few days. Neonates are particularly vulnerable because they have qualitative neutrophil defects, a limited bone marrow neutrophil storage pool, and an inability to rapidly increase neutrophil production. Up to 38% of septic neonates become neutropenic.[69]

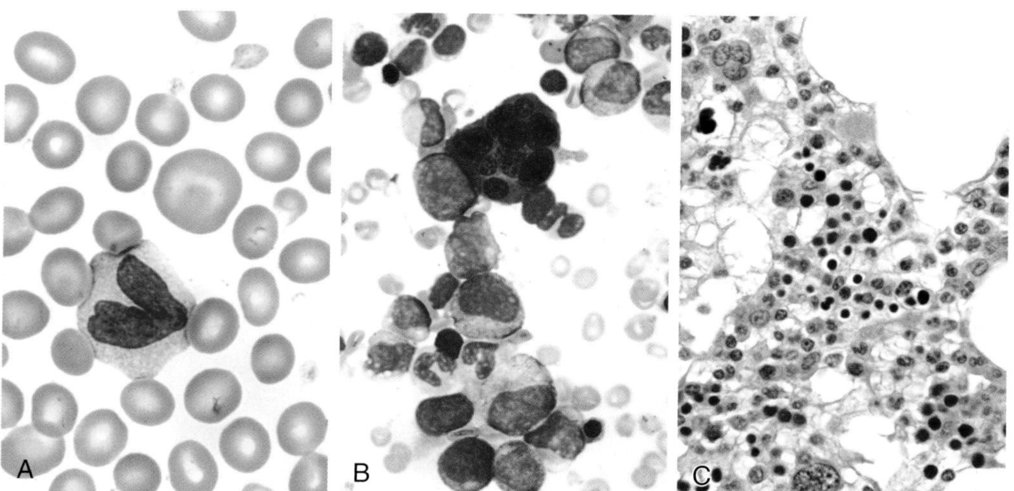

Figure 11-45. Peripheral blood smear of congenital dyserythropoietic anemia type III shows macrocytic red cells and a megaloblastic neutrophil band (**A**). The bone marrow smear (**B**) contains a gigantoblast with eight nuclei. Occasional multinucleated erythroid precursors are seen in the trephine biopsy section (**C**).

Acquired Neutropenia in Infancy and Childhood

Acquired neutropenia in infancy and childhood is much more common than constitutional disorders. It is often transient or chronic and self-resolving; causes are typically infectious or immunologic in nature (Box 11-3).

Neonatal Alloimmune Neutropenia. Neonatal alloimmune neutropenia is caused by transplacental passage of maternal IgG antibodies that are sensitized to paternally inherited antigens on fetal neutrophils (HNAs).[70] The number of postpartum women having HNAs is significantly higher than the incidence of neutropenia, suggesting that many of the antibodies are clinically irrelevant. Neutropenia varies from relatively mild to severe; thus, an affected infant may be either asymptomatic or septic in extremely severe cases. The neutropenia is transient, lasting 2 to 4 months (average, 11 weeks) and is ameliorated by the administration of granulocyte colony-stimulating factor (G-CSF).[71] Granulocyte agglutination or immunofluorescent tests are usually sufficient for diagnosis. A bone marrow examination, although not normally required, shows normal to increased cellularity with a decrease in mature neutrophils.

Box 11-3 *Causes of Acquired Neutropenia*

Drug Induced*
- Antibiotics
- Anticonvulsants
- Anti-inflammatories
- Antithyroid agents
- Antidepressants
- Sedatives
- Cardiovascular drugs
- Diuretics

Primary Immune Mediated
- Neonatal alloimmune neutropenia
- Autoimmune neutropenia of childhood
- Transfusion reaction

Secondary Immune Mediated
- Autoimmune disorders: rheumatoid arthritis, systemic lupus erythematosus, primary biliary cirrhosis, polyarteritis nodosa, scleroderma, Castleman's disease, Sjögren's syndrome
- Infection: *Helicobacter pylori*, HIV, parvovirus B19
- Neurologic diseases: multiple sclerosis
- Malignancy: Hodgkin's lymphoma, T-cell large granular lymphocytic leukemia, Wilms' tumor
- Drug induced: rituximab, fludarabine, propylthiouracil
- Transplantation: stem cell, bone marrow, kidney
- Bone marrow injury: aplastic anemia, paroxysmal nocturnal hemoglobinuria

Other
- Chronic idiopathic neutropenia†
- Infection*
  - Viral: HIV, respiratory syncytial virus, cytomegalovirus, Epstein-Barr virus, hepatitis A or B, influenza, measles, mumps, rubella
  - Bacterial: rickettsia, typhoid, miliary tuberculosis, typhus
  - Protozoan: malaria, kala-azar, trypanosomiasis
  - Fungal: histoplasmosis
- Nutritional deficiencies: vitamin B_{12} (cobalamin), folic acid, copper
- Bone marrow infiltration*: carcinoma, leukemia, lymphoma, myeloma, granulomatous diseases, fibrotic processes
- Endocrine or metabolic disorders*: Addison's disease, hyperthyroidism, hypopituitarism, hyperglycemia, acidemia, tyrosinenima, glycogen storage disease type 1B
- Hypersplenism
- Radiation
- Toxins, alcohol
- Hemodialysis
- Maternal hypertension

This list is not inclusive, but instead represents major types of causes.
*Causes that overlap with secondary immune-mediated mechanisms.
†Etiology is unclear but may be immune mediated.
HIV, human immunodeficiency virus.

Primary Autoimmune Neutropenia. Primary autoimmune neutropenia, or autoimmune neutropenia of childhood, is the most common cause of chronic neutropenia in infants and children and shows no association with other pathology (e.g., secondary neutropenia). This condition afflicts newborns and children younger than 38 months, with spontaneous resolution in 95% of cases by 2 to 3 years of age.[72] Infectious complications are usually less severe than expected for the degree of neutropenia. The majority of patients have antineutrophil antibodies directed against HNA-1a or HNA-1b. The bone marrow is normocellular to hypercellular, often with left-shifted myelopoiesis and a decrease in mature neutrophils. An arrest in myeloid maturation at the metamyelocyte-myelocyte stage has been reported in severe cases.[73] A bone marrow examination is usually not required unless additional hematopathologic abnormalities are identified on the blood film or the child is older than typical for this disorder. Administration of G-CSF is helpful in severe cases.

A transient neutropenia of unknown mechanism can be seen in small-for-gestational-age newborns or neonates of hypertensive women.[74] Three days after birth, neutropenia is more commonly associated with necrotizing enterocolitis or nosocomial infection. Vertical transmission of human immunodeficiency virus (HIV) infection must always be considered in newborns with unexplained neutropenia. Acute isolated neutropenia in children is most often the consequence of a recent viral infection.[75] Neutropenia develops within 48 hours of infection and may persist up to 6 days. In addition to primary loss by extensive neutrophil infiltration into infected tissue, splenic sequestration or antineutrophil antibody formation (with Epstein-Barr virus infection) may accelerate neutrophil destruction. Monitoring blood counts for evidence of recovery is usually all that is required.

Acquired Neutropenia in Adults

Acquired neutropenia in adults has a large number of causes (see Box 11-3). These can be broadly categorized into drug-induced neutropenia, primary and secondary immune neutropenia, and nonimmune-mediated neutropenia.[76] A bone marrow examination is often required when the clinical history and physical examination do not elicit a likely cause for the neutropenia, and particularly when other cell lineages are affected. Neutropenia may be caused by myeloid production problems secondary to direct toxic effects by free radicals or metabolites, immune-mediated destruction, defective myeloid proliferation or maturation, and increased apoptosis. Alternative mechanisms include decreased neutrophil survival, increased utilization of neutrophils, and neutrophil redistribution. The cause of neutropenia in a given individual is often multifactorial.

Drug-Induced Neutropenia. Drug-induced neutropenia is the most common cause of neutropenia in adults. The neutropenia is often secondary to chemotherapy or radiotherapy and shows a dose-dependent relationship, with possible multilineage involvement. An idiosyncratic drug reaction is the most common cause for an unexpected isolated neutropenia in an outpatient setting. Idiosyncratic drug-induced agranulocytosis (ANC <0.5 × 10^9/L) is defined as an adverse reaction in an abnormally susceptible individual with previously normal neutrophil counts.[77] Individuals with mild to moderate neutropenia (ANC 0.5 to 1.5 × 10^9/L) are alternatively referred to as having *drug-induced neutropenia.* The onset of neutropenia is unpredictable in these processes but usually occurs 1 to 2 weeks after initial drug exposure or immediately after drug reexposure. The most common offending drugs are antithyroid medications and sulfonamides; however, almost any drug can be involved.[75] Causative mechanisms are difficult to pinpoint and differ, depending on the drug involved. Roles for immune-mediated (immune complex, hapten, or autoimmune) or nonimmune-mediated mechanisms, such as active drug metabolite toxicity to neutrophils or marrow stroma, have been described. Why only rare patients are susceptible to this phenomenon is unclear; increased myeloid precursor sensitivity to a normal drug concentration or gene polymorphisms that alter drug metabolism or drug pharmacokinetics are hypothesized. If a drug-related neutropenia is suspected and the cause is unknown, all nonessential drugs and over-the-counter medications must be discontinued, with substitution of essential medications.

Secondary Autoimmune Neutropenia. Secondary autoimmune neutropenia is associated with many disorders in adults (and children), including systemic autoimmune disorders, infectious diseases, neoplasms, neurologic disorders, transplants, and certain medications.[72] Concurrent thrombocytopenia or hemolytic anemia may be seen. Diagnosis is based on the identification of antineutrophil antibodies, but unlike primary autoimmune neutropenia of childhood, the autoantibody specificity is often unknown, and the mechanism for neutropenia is commonly multifactorial. Chronic autoimmune neutropenia is most commonly seen in systemic autoimmune disorders, particularly rheumatoid arthritis (Felty's syndrome) and systemic lupus erythematosus (SLE). Felty's syndrome closely resembles and likely represents a spectrum of disease with T-cell large granular lymphocytic leukemia, whereby expansions of large granular lymphocytes in blood and bone marrow become clonal. In addition to rheumatoid arthritis, this type of leukemia is seen in a number of other autoimmune conditions and may present with isolated neutropenia, anemia, thrombocytopenia, or pancytopenia.[78] Neutropenia associated with Felty's syndrome or T-cell large granular lymphocytic leukemia is of multifactorial origin, with a role for antineutrophil autoantibodies, myelopoiesis inhibition by cytokines, soluble Fas ligand–mediated apoptosis (shed from large granular lymphocytic cells), and splenic sequestration. In addition to peripheral blood and possibly bone marrow morphology, flow cytometric or immunohistochemical evaluation to identify large granular lymphocytes, in conjunction with a *TCR* gene rearrangement, confirms the diagnosis. A bone marrow evaluation is usually not required for chronic autoimune neutropenia unless the cause of the neutropenia is unclear. For example, neutropenia in patients with SLE is often due to factors other than antineutrophil autoantibodies.

Nonimmune Chronic Idiopathic Neutropenia. Nonimmune chronic idiopathic neutropenia is defined as a persistent (>3 months), nonoscillating, and unexplained reduction in neutrophils for age and ethnic group (ANC <1.8 × 10^9/L for whites; <1.5 × 10^9/L for those of African ancestry).[79] This is essentially a diagnosis of exclusion after extensive evaluation for other causes, including repeat negative antineutrophil antibody testing and normal bone marrow cytogenetic analysis.[80] It is seen more frequently in females, particularly those with an HLA-DRB1*1302 genetic predisposition, who may have concurrent mild anemia or thrombocytopenia and osteopenia. Spontaneous remissions occur rarely among adults, unlike in infants or children. The bone marrow is typically normocellular, with a left shift in myelopoiesis and a slight decrease in the myeloid-to-erythroid ratio. The cause is unclear, but the disease likely represents a mild form of T-cell and cytokine-mediated suppression of hematopoiesis. G-CSF is the preferred treatment when necessary.

Infection-Related Neutropenia. Infection-related neutropenia may be significant and may be due to a number of infectious agents. Mechanisms for the neutropenia are multiple and ill defined. Some cases may involve infection of progenitor cells or immunologically mediated bone marrow suppression (particularly viral infections), whereas others cause excessive destruction (especially bacteremia with endotoxemia).

Nutritional Deficiency–Related Neutropenia. The myeloid cells in the bone marrow generally show normal morphology in the majority of acquired neutropenias. Notable exceptions include megaloblastic anemia (see Table 11-7) and copper deficiency. Copper deficiency should be considered when cytoplasmic vacuoles are present in myeloid (particularly promyelocytes and myelocytes) and erythroid precursors. Ring sideroblasts are frequently present, and hemosiderin-containing plasma cells may be seen as well.[81,82] The bone marrow may be hypocellular, normocellular, or hypercellular, with variable myeloid and erythroid dysplasia. Patients have concurrent normocytic, macrocytic, or microcytic anemia, neurologic disorders, and rarely thrombocytopenia. Copper deficiency is being seen more frequently owing to excess zinc intake (through supplements, medications, or dietary means). It can also be associated with total parenteral nutrition and gastrointestinal disorders (e.g., partial gastric resection).

Congenital Neutropenia

Congenital neutropenia refers to neutropenias with genetic mutations and not simply those that are present at birth. Many of these disorders have intrinsic defects that cause premature apoptosis of cells, ineffective neutrophil production, and recurrent infections. These are discussed in the following paragraphs and summarized in Table 11-8.

Severe Congenital Neutropenia. Severe congenital neutropenia (SCN) represents a heterogenous group of disorders characterized by severe, persistent neutropenia and a maturation arrest in neutrophilic myeloid production.[83,84] Kostmann originally described a recessive form of the disease that is now considered a separate syndrome (see Kostmann's

Table 11-8 Causes of Constitutional Neutropenia with Associated Peripheral Blood and Bone Marrow Findings

Disorder	Peripheral Blood Findings	Bone Marrow Findings	Comments
Severe congenital neutropenia	Chronic, marked neutropenia (<0.5 × 10^9/L) Often monocytosis, eosinophilia	Normocellular with marked myeloid hypoplasia, maturation arrest with rare myeloblasts and promyelocytes, occasional multinucleation, promyelocytes with cytoplasmic vacuolation Increased monocytes, eosinophils, macrophages, plasma cells	Sporadic or autosomal dominant Rare X-linked or autosomal recessive forms with *ELA2* gene mutations *CSF3R* gene mutations: Acquired: ↑ MDS, AML transformation Constitutive: ↓ G-CSF responsiveness
Kostmann's neutropenia	Chronic, marked neutropenia (<0.2 × 10^9/L)	Similar to above	Autosomal recessive, familial disorder *HAX1* mutations
Cyclic neutropenia	Cyclic, marked neutropenia at nadir of cycle (<0.2 × 10^9/L) Oscillations in monocyte, reticulocyte, and platelet counts (normal to ↑)	Myeloid aplasia or hypoplasia with marked left shift prior to periods of marked neutropenia	25% autosomal dominant, sporadic *ELA2* gene mutations 10% fatal infections Leukemic transformation is rare G-CSF shortens cycle length and increases neutrophil counts
Shwachman-Diamond syndrome	Neutropenia (88%-100% of patients) ⅓ chronic, ⅔ intermittent Anemia (42%-82%) Thrombocytopenia (24%-88%)	Variable cellularity Myeloid hypoplasia with possible left shift Decreased $CD34^+$ cells	Autosomal recessive, increased hemoglobin F *SBDS* gene mutation Exocrine pancreatic dysfunction, short stature, skeletal abnormalities, bone marrow stromal defects, hepatic and cardiac disorders
Chédiak-Higashi syndrome	Chronic neutropenia, large cytoplasmic inclusion bodies in granulocytes and other granule-producing cells	Cytoplasmic azurophilic granules or inclusion bodies in granulated cells are myeloperoxidase and CD63 positive	Autosomal recessive *CHS1/LYST* gene mutations; protein likely regulates lysosome-related organelle size and movement
Myelokathexis (WHIM syndrome)	Chronic, severe neutropenia Hypersegmented neutrophils with cytoplasmic vacuoles and degenerative changes	Hyperplasia, hypersegmented granulocytes with apoptotic features, fine interlobar bridging, and cytoplasmic vacuolation	Autosomal dominant ↑ CXCR4 activity, often mutation in *CXCR4* gene (gain of function) Retention, senescence, and apoptosis of mature neutrophils in marrow Improved neutrophil release with G-CSF or GM-CSF therapy

AML, acute myeloid leukemia; G-CSF, granulocyte colony-stimulating factor; GM-CSF, granulocyte-macrophage colony-stimulating factor; MDS, myelodysplastic syndrome; WHIM, warts, hypogammaglobulinemia, infections, and myelokathexis.

Neutropenia). SCN occurs most commonly as a sporadic or autosomal dominant disorder. Patients present with life-threatening pyogenic infections in early infancy and, unless treated with G-CSF or hematopoietic stem cell transplantation, often die by 3 years of age (Fig. 11-46).[85] Approximately 50% to 60% of patients have heterozygous *ELA2* mutations, with at least 50 distinct mutations described in SCN and cyclic neutropenia (see later). *ELA2* encodes for a serine protease called *neutrophil elastase,* which is produced in promyelocytes and stored in primary granules of neutrophils. Recent studies show that *ELA2* mutations produce misfolded neutrophil elastase protein.[86] This abnormal protein activates the unfolded protein response mechanism (similar to cystic fibrosis and osteogenesis imperfecta) and ultimately leads to neutrophil apoptosis. Genetic testing for disease-specific *ELA2* mutations confirms SCN; its presence may correlate with more severe disease.[87] Rare mutations found in SCN patients include those of *GFI-1*, *AP3B1*, *WAS*, *TAZ1*, and *MAPBPIP*. Some of these mutations are known to increase granulocytic apoptosis. SCN is considered a preleukemic condition, with one study showing a 21% cumulative incidence of transformation to MDS or acute myeloid leukemia after 10 years.[88] Acquired G-CSF receptor truncating mutations predict transformation but are not required for it (see Fig. 11-46).[89] Whether chronic G-CSF therapy plays a role in leukemic transformation is unclear, but it is suggestive. The effect of G-CSF in ameliorating neutropenia in more than 90% of SCN patients may be accomplished through increased neutrophil survival.

Kostmann's Neutropenia. Kostmann's neutropenia is an autosomal recessive neutropenia that was first described by Kostmann in 1956 among a consanguineous cohort in Sweden. The clinical and morphologic features are similar to SCN; therefore, some investigators consider this an autosomal recessive subtype of SCN with lower neutrophil counts.[84] A majority of patients have homozygous *HAX1* gene mutations that encode for a mitochondrial protein with apoptosis-regulating functions, similar to BCL2.[90] A subset of these individuals develop neurologic symptoms (epilepsy, cognitive defects, mental retardation) and have been found to have a *HAX1* transcript variant that is expressed in brain tissue.

Cyclic Neutropenia. Cyclic neutropenia is characterized by episodes of severe neutropenia recurring at about 21-day intervals (intervals vary from 14 to 36 days). The marrow exhibits a myeloid maturation arrest before the period of severe peripheral neutropenia. Accelerated apoptosis of bone marrow progenitor cells is found in all stages of the cycle, with insufficient myeloid output.[91] Most individuals have

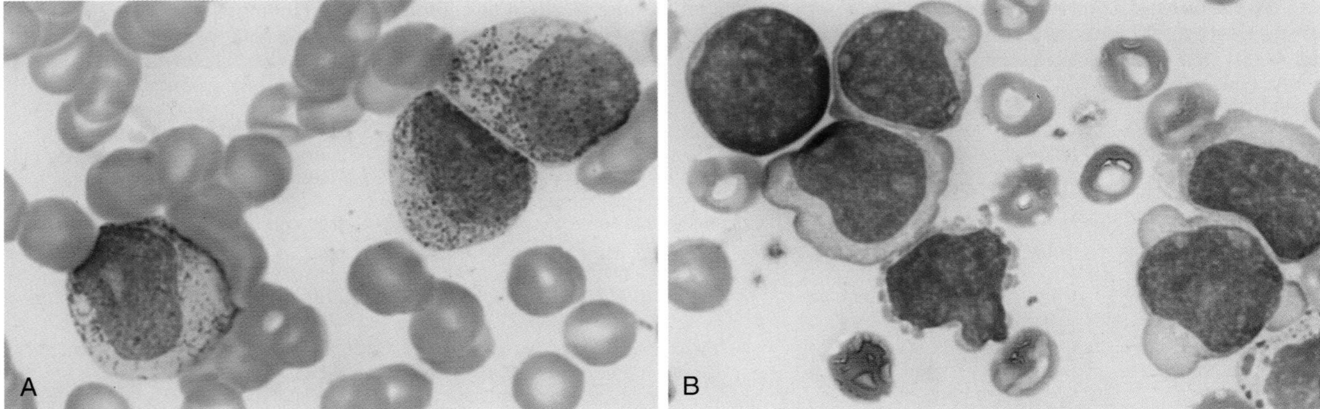

Figure 11-46. Bone marrow smear of severe congenital neutropenia in a 3-year-old boy illustrates a maturation arrest at the promyelocyte stage of development **(A)**. Ten years later, following therapy with granulocyte colony-stimulating factor (G-CSF), he developed acute myeloid leukemia **(B)**. Point mutations in the G-CSF receptor gene were detected.

ELA2 gene mutations that likely play a role in apoptosis, similar to SCN, but the pathomechanisms responsible are not yet understood.[92] The diagnosis is most easily established by monitoring serial neutrophil counts over a 6- to 8-week period. G-CSF provides effective therapy, and symptoms often improve as individuals grow older.[93]

Shwachman-Diamond Syndrome. Shwachman-Diamond syndrome (SDS) is a rare multisystem disorder of diverse symptoms, with pancreatic exocrine and bone marrow dysfunction being the central features.[94] It is the second most common cause of congenital pancreatic insufficiency after cystic fibrosis. Affected infants invariably have malabsorption, steatorrhea, and failure to thrive, with ultimate growth retardation. Increased infections are due to decreased neutrophils with impaired neutrophil chemotaxis and, commonly, T-cell and B-cell abnormalities. Approximately 90% of patients have biallelic mutations of the Shwachman-Bodian-Diamond syndrome gene (*SBDS*).[95] The SBDS protein is involved in ribosome biogenesis, mitotic spindle stabilization, and chromosome segregation. SBDS-deficient cells have increased Fas-mediated apoptosis.[96] How the mutated gene relates to the report of clonal cytogenetic abnormalities that may wax and wane and occasionally disappear is unclear.[97] The possible role of defective mitotic spindle stabilization is intriguing. The most commonly reported cytogenetic abnormalities are of chromosome 7 and del(20)q. These are also seen in MDS and may represent a very early form of this disorder; children with SDS have an increased propensity to develop MDS or acute myeloid leukemia. The clinical course is variable. Although most patients present with neutropenia, SDS is considered a bone marrow failure disorder owing to the development of progressive cytopenias and aplastic anemia.

Chédiak-Higashi Syndrome. Chédiak-Higashi syndrome is a rare disorder (<500 cases in the past 15 years) with diverse clinical manifestations related to abnormally enlarged lysozymes or lysosome-related organelles in all cells of the body.[98,99] The disorder is characterized by severe immunodeficiency, mild coagulation defects, variable oculocutaneous albinism, progressive neurologic dysfunction, and possible defective plasma membrane repair. Defective neutrophil chemotaxis and function lead to the frequent and severe pyogenic infections that characterize this disorder, whereas a deficiency in platelet dense bodies contributes to the tendency for easy bleeding. Accelerated disease is associated with a multiorgan lymphohistiocytic infiltrate that may result in organ failure and death. Without bone marrow transplantation, the disease is usually fatal in the first decade of life.[100]

Myelokathexis. Myelokathexis is a histologic pattern of increased myeloid cells with excessive neutrophil apoptosis in the bone marrow. It is associated with the immunodeficiency disorder WHIM (warts, hypogammaglobulinemia, infections, and myelokathexis) syndrome.[101] Patients with WHIM have recurrent infections secondary to neutropenia, B-cell lymphopenia, and hypogammaglobulinemia. They are particularly susceptible to human papillomavirus infection and require careful surveillance of related lesions. This was the first example of a disease mediated by a chemokine receptor dysfunction. Most but not all patients have heterozygous C-terminus deletion mutations of the chemokine receptor CXCR4.

Dyskeratosis Congenita. Dyskeratosis congenita is a multisystem disorder that affects tissues with a high turnover rate, such as skin, mucous membranes, and blood. Although neutropenia is often the presenting hematologic manifestation, approximately 80% to 90% of patients develop bone marrow failure. Therefore, this disorder is more fully described under the bone marrow failure syndromes. Additionally, patients with Fanconi's anemia, inherited immunodeficiency disorders such as reticular dysgenesis and cartilage-hair hypoplasia, and metabolic disorders such as Barth's syndrome and glycogen storage disease type IB may present with neutropenia.

Lymphopenia

Lymphopenia or lymphocytopenia is defined as an absolute lymphocyte count of less than 1.5×10^9/L in adults and less than 2.0×10^9/L in young children. It may occur in isolation or as part of pancytopenia. Lymphopenia can be further categorized as decreased B cells, T cells, natural killer (NK) cells, or their subsets. The causes of lymphopenia are extensive and include a variety of infectious, drug-related, autoimmune, and congenital causes (Box 11-4).

Box 11-4 *Causes of Lymphopenia*

Infections
- HIV
- SARS coronavirus
- Influenza
- Respiratory syncytial virus
- Ebola
- Anaplasmosis (ehrlichiosis)
- *Legionella pneumophila*
- Tuberculosis
- Bacterial sepsis

Therapy
- Steroids
- Rituximab
- Chemotherapy, especially purine analogues and alkylating agents
- Antibiotics
- Antithymocyte globulin
- Immunosuppressive therapy
- Radiation therapy

Autoimmune
- Systemic lupus erythematosus
- Rheumatoid arthritis
- Crohn's disease
- Vasculitis

Malignancy
- Carcinoma
- Hodgkin's lymphoma
- Non-Hodgkin's lymphoma

Hematologic Disorders
- Aplastic anemia

Congenital
- Severe combined immunodeficiency
- DiGeorge syndrome (thymic aplasia)
- Wiskott-Aldrich syndrome

Other
- Physiologic stress
- Idiopathic CD4 lymphocytopenia

HIV, human immunodeficiency virus; SARS, severe acute respiratory syndrome.

Lymphopenia may also be seen in a variety of viral, fungal, bacterial, mycobacterial, and parasitic infections. Reactive lymphocyte morphology in these disorders provides a clue to the underlying infection. A decreased lymphocyte count is the hematologic hallmark of HIV infection. The destruction of $CD4^+$ memory T cells, followed by increased memory T-cell turnover and damage to the thymus and other lymphoid tissues, results in profound lymphopenia.[102]

Therapeutic Agents

Therapeutic agents are sometimes associated with decreased lymphocyte counts. Within hours of administration, corticosteroids initiate lymphopenia, primarily of T cells, through a glucocorticoid receptor–associated apoptotic mechanism.[103] Chemotherapeutic agents, particularly alkylating agents and purine analogues, induce lymphocyte depletion through several different apoptotic mechanisms. The CD4 cells are especially sensitive, and lymphopenia following therapy may be prolonged.[104] The anti-CD20 monoclonal antibody rituximab binds to B cells and produces cell death by complement-mediated lysis and apoptosis.[105]

Congenital Disorders

Congenital disorders are classified as producing humoral, cellular, or combined immunodeficiency. Several types of severe combined immunodeficiencies also involve the loss of NK cells. These rare severe deficiency states usually present in infancy or early childhood and manifest as severe infections. Nearly half are X-linked. Although B-cell numbers may be normal, their activity is diminished by T-cell hypofunction, thymic and paracortical lymphoid depletion, and T lymphopenia. Most cases are due to mutations in the cytokine receptor common gamma chain of IL-2, -4, -7, -9, -15, and -21 or absence of the purine salvage pathway enzymes adenosine deaminase and purine nucleoside phosphorylase.[106]

Reactive Disorders

Decreased lymphocyte counts are a criterion for the diagnosis of SLE and are encountered in other autoimmune diseases as well, particularly rheumatoid arthritis, Crohn's disease, and vasculitis. Lymphocytotoxic antibodies have been implicated in SLE, but the mechanisms remain unclear.[107,108]

Autoimmune Disorders

Stress lymphopenia is seen in the setting of myocardial infarction, major surgery, sickle cell crisis, acute stroke, and intense exercise. Release of cortisol with subsequent apoptosis results in decreased lymphocyte numbers.[109,110] Idiopathic CD4 lymphopenia is a rare disease associated with persistent lymphopenia ($CD4^+$ cells $<0.3 \times 10^9$/L). It manifests clinically with severe opportunistic infections in the absence of HIV infection or other recognized causes of low CD4 cell counts. The pathogenesis is not clear but may be due to increased apoptosis via the Fas pathway, decreased T-cell production, or defective tumor necrosis factor-α or interferon-γ production.[111]

EVALUATION OF THROMBOCYTOPENIA

Thrombocytopenia is a decrease in the circulating platelet count to less than 150×10^9/L. It is encountered frequently in clinical practice, and when severe, it is a common cause of hemorrhage. Thrombocytopenia is the result of decreased production, increased destruction, increased utilization, or abnormal distribution of platelets. Evaluation of megakaryocytes in patients with unexplained thrombocytopenia is one of the most common indications for a bone marrow examination in clinical practice. An important caveat before bone marrow evaluation is to confirm that the platelet count is not spuriously low as a result of platelet clumping in vitro. This phenomenon is most commonly caused by naturally occurring antibodies directed against a normally hidden platelet epitope (glycoprotein IIb/IIIa complex) that becomes exposed in the presence of EDTA.[112] Blood collection in citrate or heparin usually alleviates this problem. Review of the peripheral blood film before bone marrow evaluation is essential to exclude this possibility and to evaluate for platelet rosetting around white blood cells (satellitism) and platelet–white blood cell aggregates.

Evaluation of bone marrow megakaryocytes is an important initial step in the workup for unexplained thrombocytopenia. Decreased megakaryocytes are indicative of decreased platelet production, whereas normal or increased megakaryocytes point toward ineffective megakaryopoiesis (intramedullary cell death or excessive apoptosis) or loss of platelets from the circulation.

Table 11-9 lists the differential diagnosis for thrombocytopenia when megakaryocytes are absent or decreased. Age is an important consideration; an isolated loss of megakaryocytes (amegakaryopoiesis) suggests a congenital or, rarely, an autoimmune process with antimegakaryocyte or antithrombopoietin antibodies. Constitutional disorders are more likely to present in infancy and to be associated with other hematopoietic and nonhematopoietic abnormalities as part of a syndrome.[113,114] Identifying the cause of the underlying disorder (e.g., Fanconi's anemia, acute leukemia) may be a challenge when isolated thrombocytopenia is the presenting finding. Evaluation for subtle dysplasia, viral effects, or abnormal cellular infiltrates is required; cytogenetic evaluation, chromosome breakage studies (Fanconi's anemia), and molecular analysis (e.g., *c-MPL* gene mutation) are warranted as clinically indicated. Chemotherapy, toxin exposure, or prolonged use of certain drugs can selectively affect the megakaryocytes in some patients. Chronic platelet destruction or consumption may rarely induce amegakaryopoiesis.

Causes of thrombocytopenia when the bone marrow megakaryocytes are normal to increased in number are listed in Tables 11-10 and 11-11. A compensatory increase in megakaryocytes with a shift toward more immature forms is customarily present during times of increased platelet destruction or utilization (Fig. 11-47). Megakaryocytes are smaller and exhibit less nuclear lobation. Platelets produced from these cells are larger than the normal platelet diameter of 4 to 7 μm. In this setting, platelet accumulation in bone marrow sinuses also suggests increased platelet consumption when bone marrow artifacts or a myeloproliferative neoplasm is excluded.

Immune-Mediated Thrombocytopenic Purpura

Immune-mediated thrombocytopenia is the most frequent cause of platelet destruction. There are primary and secondary forms.

Primary Immune Thrombocytopenia

Primary immune idiopathic thrombocytopenic purpura (ITP), is defined as an acquired isolated thrombocytopenia of no definitive cause.[115] It is classified as acute or chronic in duration and by age of onset (adult or childhood). The pathogenesis of ITP is similar in children and adults. The primary mechanism is antibody-mediated destruction, with IgG autoantibodies binding to platelet glycoproteins (glycoproteins IIb/IIIa and Ib/IX).[116] Additional mechanisms include T-cell–mediated platelet destruction, autoantibody-mediated interference with megakaryocyte maturation, and immune tolerance defects consistent with an autoimmune syndrome.[117] An insufficient thrombopoietin response is seen in chronic ITP patients. Although a number of causes have been ascribed to primary ITP, none has a strong association once an

Table 11-9 Thrombocytopenias with Decreased Bone Marrow Megakaryocytes

Disorder	Comments
Constitutional	
Isolated Thrombocytopenia	
Thrombocyopenia with absent radii	Variable inheritance, chromosome 1q microdeletions, clinical syndrome of unknown genetic basis, infants (<1 mo), small megakaryocytes if present Usually recover platelet counts by 1 yr, possible mild intermittent thrombocytopenia in adults Bilateral radial aplasia; other skeletal, renal, and cardiac anomalies
Congenital viral infection	Rubella, rubeola, CMV
Thrombocytopenia ± other Lineage Abnormalities	
Congenital amegakaryocytic thrombocytopenia	Autosomal recessive; *c-MPL* gene mutations; risk of MDS, AML Isolated marked thrombocytopenia at birth Development of trilineage bone marrow failure: type 1 mutations—early onset (2 yr); type 2 mutations—later onset (5 yr)
Bone marrow failure syndromes* (dyskeratosis congenita, Fanconi's anemia, Shwachman-Diamond syndrome)	May present initially with isolated thrombocytopenia
Acquired	
Infection	Viral (measles, varicella, EBV, CMV, hantavirus, HIV-1, parvovirus, dengue) Mycoplasma, mycobacteria, ehrlichiosis, malaria
Immunoregulatory defects	Autoimmune disease, T-cell large granular lymphocytic disorders, some cases of chronic ITP
Toxins/drugs	Alcohol; chemotherapy; drugs, especially after prolonged use (thiazide diuretics, chloramphenicol, estrogen, prednisone, progesterone)
Nutritional deficiency	Vitamin B_{12} or folate deficiency
Bone marrow replacement	Leukemia, metastatic carcinoma, myeloma, granuloma, fibrosis
Paroxysmal nocturnal hemoglobinuria*	
Myelodysplastic syndrome	May initially present with isolated thrombocytopenia, dysplastic megakaryocytes
Aplastic anemia*	

*See Table 11-2 for additional information.
AML, acute myeloid leukemia; CMV, cytomegalovirus; EBV, Epstein-Barr virus; HIV, human immunodeficiency virus; ITP, idiopathic thrombocytopenic purpura; MDS, myelodysplastic syndrome.

Table 11-10 Acquired Thrombocytopenia with Normal to Increased Megakaryocytes

Mechanism	Disease/Cause	Comments
Increased Destruction or Utilization		
Immunologic	Childhood immune thrombocytopenic purpura	Acute onset, often occurs 2-3 wk after viral infection or immunization (especially MMR); about 80% resolve within 6-12 mo; slight platelet enlargement
	Adult immune thrombocytopenic purpura	Similar to childhood, except insidious onset; need to exclude secondary cause; chronic course; increased in females younger than 40 yr, especially during first trimester of pregnancy; usually responds to glucocorticoids, but may relapse
	Diseases	Autoimmune collagen vascular disorders (e.g., SLE), rheumatoid disorders, lymphoproliferative disorders (e.g., CLL, lymphoma, T-LGL leukemia), antiphospholipid syndrome, thyroid disease, solid tumors, common variable immunodeficiency disorder, ALPS, autoimmune hemolysis/Evans syndrome
	Drugs	A number of drugs involved; variety of mechanisms, including hapten-dependent antibody formation, drug-glycoprotein complex antibody formation, autoantibody formation, ligand-induced binding site creation, drug-specific antibody formation, and immune complex–mediated antibody formation; circulating antibodies to PF4-heparin complexes
	Heparin	Type I: immediate onset with minimal sequelae; may resolve during continued therapy Type II: direct platelet aggregation effect with significant thromobembolic complications; develops 5-14 days after exposure with 30%-40% drop in platelet count
	Infection	HIV, *H. pylori*, HCV, VZV; generates antibodies that cross-react with platelet antigens or immune complexes that bind platelet Fc receptors
	Neonatal alloimmune thrombocytopenia	IgG alloantibodies transferred from maternal circulation to baby, formed against incompatible paternal platelet antigens, most often HPA-1a
	Platelet transfusion	Alloantibodies to host platelets
Thrombotic microangiopathies	Thrombotic thrombocytopenic purpura (TTP)	Increase in woman in third to fourth decades of life Pentad of findings: thrombocytopenia, microangiopathic hemolytic anemia, fever (25%), neurologic abnormalities (70%-80%), and renal dysfunction (40%) Antibody or inhibitor of ADAMTS 13 is causative Idiopathic (80%); secondary to infection, drugs, pregnancy, other (10%-15%); congenital (<5%) Congenital disorder caused by mutated *ADAMTS 13* gene; no inhibitor; chronic relapsing disease
	Hemolytic uremic syndrome (HUS)	Similar clinical symptoms to TTP but less extensive and predominantly involves the kidneys; common cause of acute renal failure in children Normal ADAMTS 13 levels Triggered by infection with Shiga toxin–producing bacteria (e.g., *Escherichia coli* O157:H7); has a favorable outcome Atypical HUS (10% of cases) associated with mutations in genes that regulate the complement system; has a poor prognosis
	Disseminated intravascular coagulation (DIC)	Syndrome seen in a variety of diseases or with marked tissue damage; thrombohemorrhagic disorder secondary to intravascular activation of coagulation (with fibrin thrombi deposition) and simultaneous consumption of coagulation factors and platelets
Other	HELLP syndrome	Develops in pregnant, often white, multiparous women older than 25 yr
	Mechanical injury	Prosthetic heart valves, burns, malignant hypertension, vasculitis, transplantation-associated microangiopathy
Ineffective Megakaryopoiesis	Infection	HIV, CMV, other
Abnormal Distribution	Splenomegaly	Increased splenic sequestration—up to 80%-90% of circulating platelets (normal, 30%-35%); chronic liver disease, pediatric sickle cell disease, hemoglobinopathies, chronic infection, myeloproliferative disorders, lymphomas, storage diseases
	Hypothermia	Pooling of platelets in splenic sinusoids, especially at body temperature <25°C
	Massive transfusion	Hemodilution
	Gestational thrombocytopenia	Platelet count >70,000/μL in healthy pregnant woman; pathogenesis is unclear but probably related to hemodilution or increased platelet clearance

ALPS, autoimmune lymphoproliferative syndrome; CLL, chronic lymphocytic leukemia; CMV, cytomegalovirus; HCV, hepatitis C virus; HELLP, hemolysis, elevated liver enzymes, low platelet count; HIV, human immunodeficiency virus; MMR, measles-mumps-rubella; PF, platelet factor; SLE, systemic lupus erythematosus; T-LGL, T-cell large granular lymphocytic; VZV, varicella-zoster virus.

Table 11-11 Constitutional Thrombocytopenia with Normal to Increased Megakaryocytes

Disease	Inheritance/Defect	Morphology	Comments
Platelet Adhesion Defect			
Bernard-Soulier syndrome	Autosomal recessive; mutations of *GP1BA, GP1BB, GP9*; reduced or absent GP Ib-IX-V receptor complex	Large platelets, large megakaryocytes with increased ploidy, mild (heterozygous) or marked (homozygous) thrombocytopenia	Extremely rare; reduced GP Ib-IX-V (CD42a-d) on platelets, abnormal megakaryocyte membrane maturation Early childhood mucocutanous tissue bleeding, severe bleeding during surgery or trauma Defective ristocetin-induced platelet aggregation (homozygous)
von Willebrand's disease type 2B	Autosomal dominant; *VWF* gene mutation	Large platelets, sometimes circulating platelet aggregates, variable thrombocytopenia	Spontaneous binding of mutated vWF to platelet GP Ibα enhances ADAMTS 13 cleavage of large vWF multimers; defective vWF-dependent platelet function; defective ristocetin-induced platelet aggregation
Montreal platelet syndrome	Autosomal dominant; *VWF* mutation (V1316M)	Enlarged platelets, moderate thrombocytopenia, platelet clumps	Best considered a variant of von Willebrand's disease type 2B
Pseudo–von Willebrand's disease	Autosomal dominant; *GP Ib* gene mutation	Normal platelet morphology	Intermittent thrombocytopenia; GP Ib has increased affinity for vWF, accelerates removal of vWF multimers from circulation
Secretion Defect			
Gray platelet syndrome	Autosomal recessive; genetic defect unknown; deficiency or abnormal function of platelet α-granules and α-granule proteins	Large "gray" platelets without granules, mild to moderate thrombocytopenia, possible bone marrow reticulin fibrosis, emperipoiesis	Bleeding disorder with a number of platelet aggregation defects; empty α-granules on electron microscopy
Wiskott-Aldrich syndrome	X-linked recessive; *WAS* gene mutations; decreased WAS protein	Small platelets, usually marked thrombocytopenia	Underlying immunodeficiency, mild thrombocytopenia at birth, usually diagnosed at 6-12 mo Eczema; recurrent infections; increased phosphatidylserine on platelets leads to splenic engulfment; T-cell defects; propensity to develop lymphomas
X-linked thrombocytopenia	X-linked recessive; *GATA-1* or *WAS* gene mutations	Small platelets, hypercellular bone marrow, large megakaryocytes with nuclear abnormalities	Mild form of Wiskott-Aldrich syndrome; possible mild immunodeficiency; RBC abnormalities; nonsyndromic
Hermansky-Pudlak syndrome (7 types)	Autosomal recessive; gene mutations involving *HPS* complex, *APDB1*, or gene coding for dysbinden protein	Reticuloendothelial	Disorders involving oculocutaneous albinism with vision problems; variably severe bleeding due to few or no dense bodies in platelets (diagnosed by electron microscopy); ceroid deposits leading to lung, intestine, kidney, or heart dysfunction; major complication of all types is pulmonary fibrosis
Chédiak-Higashi syndrome	Autosomal recessive; *CHS1/LYST* gene mutations	Giant inclusion bodies in granule-containing cells	Often chronic neutropenia (see Table 11-8)
MYH9-Related Disorders			
May-Hegglin anomaly	Autosomal dominant; mutations in myosin heavy-chain 9 (*MYH9*) gene	Large platelets, leukocytes with Döhle-like bodies, variable thrombocytopenia	Often asymptomatic; defect in megakaryocyte maturation or fragmentation, abnormal organization of platelet microtubules
Epstein's syndrome	Alterations of the protein nonmuscle myosin IIA lead to formation of giant platelets	Large platelets, no leukocyte inclusions	Abnormal organization of platelet microtubules; hearing loss, nephritis
Fechtner's syndrome		Large platelets; leukocytes with small, round inclusions	Resembles Alport's syndrome; interstitial nephritis, deafness, cataracts
Sebastian platelet syndrome		Large platelets; leukocytes with small, round inclusions	Similar platelet and neutrophil morphology to Fechtner's syndrome, but milder disease and may not have additional anomalies
Other			
Kasabach-Merritt syndrome	Vascular lesion causes platelet trapping and activation, with consumption of coagulation factors; platelet activation promotes further growth of vascular tissue	Normal platelets	Localized intravascular coagulation within a congenital vascular tumor; visible cutaneous giant hemangioma or multiple smaller hemangiomas are often the presenting feature but regress with age

GP, glycoprotein; RBC, red blood cell; vWF, von Willebrand factor.

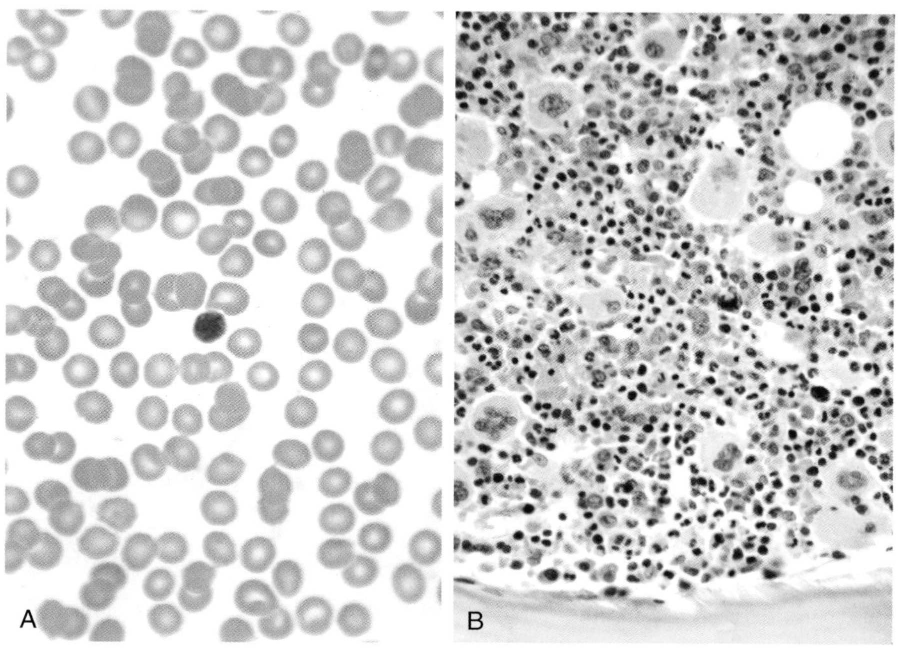

Figure 11-47. **A,** Peripheral blood smear of immune thrombocytopenic purpura. A single large platelet is seen at the *center*. Large platelets reflect early release from the bone marrow. **B,** The bone marrow trephine biopsy section contains increased numbers of megakaryocytes.

infectious process is excluded.[118] The majority of cases of acute ITP of childhood are attributed to recent infection or immunization. Approximately 20% of children with ITP relapse or have a chronic form more similar to adult ITP. Constitutional platelet disorders need to be excluded in these individuals, who usually present without a viral prodrome.

Secondary Immune Thrombocytopenia

Secondary immune thrombocytopenia is most often secondary to medication, concurrent disease, or chronic infection.[119] These thrombocytopenias may be clinically indistinguishable from the classic (primary) type until an underlying disorder is identified. Drug-induced thrombocytopenia is becoming increasingly common, and the list of implicated drugs is extensive.[120] Historically, vancomycin, quinine, and quinidine were well-known culprits. Despite the numerous drugs known to be involved, the diagnosis is frequently difficult and often becomes one of exclusion. The immune mechanisms involved are also varied and drug dependent, but they act primarily to increase peripheral platelet clearance, with some drugs also causing marrow suppression.

Heparin-Induced Thrombocytopenia

Heparin-induced thrombocytopenia is a clinicopathologic syndrome in which platelet counts at the nadir are typically less severe (60×10^9/L) than those seen in classic drug-induced thrombocytopenia (10×10^9/L). Heparin-induced thrombocytopenia occurs in approximately 5% of individuals receiving heparin, and there are two types at clinical presentation (see Table 11-10).[121] The clinical features of the more severe type II are thrombocytopenia, venous and arterial thrombosis, and platelet activation triggered by platelet factor-4–heparin-containing immune complexes.[122] Diagnosis is made by sensitive enzyme-linked immunoassays for heparin-induced thrombocytopenia antibodies. Bone marrow examination is required only when platelet counts are not ameliorated with discontinuation of heparin.

Infection-Associated Thrombocytopenia

Infection, especially viral infection, is a frequent cause of thrombocytopenia. HIV-associated thrombocytopenia was reported in 5% to 30% of infected individuals before the advent of highly active antiretroviral therapy (HAART).[118] HIV-associated thrombocytopenia involves multiple mechanisms: HIV directly infects megakaryocytes through CD4 and CXCR4 receptors and coreceptors; megakaryocytes are normal to increased in number but are ineffective in producing platelets; and accelerated platelet clearance occurs through immune-mediated destruction, with either specific or nonspecific binding of anti-HIV antibodies or immune complexes to platelets (e.g., glycoprotein IIb/III). Megakaryocytes undergo increased intramedullary apoptosis and appear pyknotic, with near-naked hyperchromatic nuclei that have scant associated cytoplasm (Fig. 11-48).[123]

The recently identified relationship between *Helicobacter pylori* infection and thrombocytopenia may involve cross-reactivity between platelet-associated immunoglobulins and *H. pylori* CagA protein.[124] The prevalence of *H. pylori* in patients with thrombocytopenia is similar to that in healthy adults matched for age and geographic area. Platelet counts improve after *H. pylori* eradication in about 50% of adult thrombocytopenia patients, but the response is dependent on geographic area; high responses are seen in studies from Italy and Japan, with poor responses among populations from other countries. The variable responses may be related to differences in *H. pylori* strains in different locations.[118]

In newborns, thrombocytopenia caused by perinatal complications such as infection or asphyxia rarely requires bone marrow evaluation before platelet counts resolve. Severe platelet reductions in the first month of life are usually due to alloimmunization with platelet-specific antigens that are incompatible between mother and child. This diagnosis of neonatal alloimmune thrombocytopenia is best made by examination of maternal, paternal, and sometimes fetal blood specimens rather than bone marrow examination.[125]

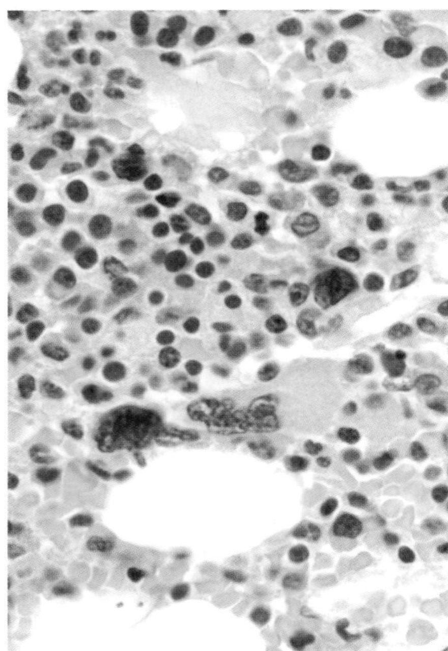

Figure 11-48. Several small hypolobated megakaryocytes are seen in this bone marrow biopsy section from a patient with HIV-associated thrombocytopenia.

Microangiopathic Processes

Microangiopathic processes are associated with thrombocytopenia, but the anemia and red cell fragmentation (i.e., schistocytes) may not be evident until a few days after the initial clinical presentation (Figs. 11-49 and 11-50). Mechanical fragmentation of erythrocytes occurs during flow through partially occluded high-shear microvessels. The partial arteriolar and capillary occlusion results from excessive platelet deposition or the formation of thrombi in disorders such as thrombotic thrombocytopenic purpura, hemolytic uremic syndrome, and disseminated intravascular coagulation.[126,127] Thrombotic thrombocytopenic purpura is caused by a deficiency of functionally active metalloproteinase (ADAMTS 13) that is responsible for cleaving ultralarge von Willebrand's factor multimers released by endothelium.[128] These multimers directly induce vessel wall platelet aggregation unless degraded by ADAMTS 13. Assays for ADAMTS 13 activity and associated antibodies help in the diagnosis. A bone marrow evaluation is indicated for questionable diagnoses or for the evaluation of an underlying immune disorder such as SLE.

Splenic Sequestration

Splenic pooling of platelets causes their displacement from the peripheral circulation; the platelets are not destroyed and remain exchangeable with the peripheral pool. Therefore, megakaryocytes may not be increased in number. This condition is most often seen in patients with chronic liver disease with portal hypertension and splenomegaly, and it may explain in part the loss of circulating platelets in some patients with Wiskott-Aldrich syndrome.[129]

Constitutional Thrombocytopenia

Mild forms of hereditary thrombocytopenia may not be obvious and are picked up incidentally in patients who have no record of a normal platelet count. Platelet survival studies may be required to confirm a hereditary process when minimal signs of bleeding cannot be elicited in patients or their relatives. Among patients with hereditary disorders, the medical history and physical examination provide important information regarding whether the thrombocytopenia is part of a syndrome. Megakaryocytes are produced in the bone marrow of patients with the inherited disorders listed in Table 11-11.[130-132] Megakaryopoiesis is ineffectual, and platelet survival may be decreased. Evaluation of platelet size is helpful. The presence of small platelets is typical of Wiscott-Aldrich syndrome and X-linked thrombocytopenia; only the

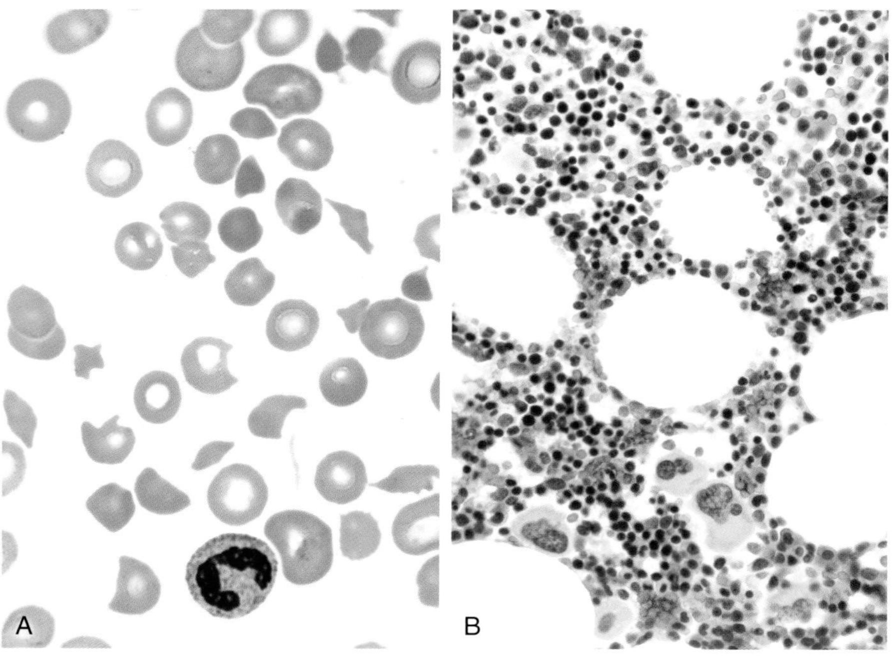

Figure 11-49. A, Peripheral blood smear of thrombotic thrombocytopenic purpura. Numerous red cell fragments (schistocytes) are present. No platelets are seen in this field. **B,** The bone marrow trephine biopsy section demonstrates increased numbers of megakaryocytes.

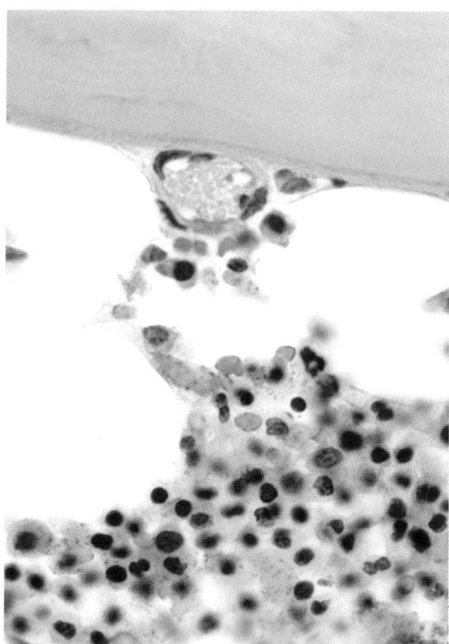

Figure 11-50. A platelet thrombus is seen in a small vein of the trephine biopsy section of the patient shown in Figure 11-49.

latter is nonsyndromic. Large or giant platelets (larger than normal RBCs) are seen in a majority of patients with constitutional thrombocytopenia. Platelet counts and mean platelet volume may be inaccurate in these individuals if platelets are gated erroneously by automated counters. Concurrent neutrophil inclusions indicate *MYH9*-related diseases. Platelets are usually normally granulated, except in the rare gray platelet syndrome (Fig. 11-51). Familial thrombocytopenia is relatively common in the Mediterranean countries, particularly Bernard-Soulier and Wiskott-Aldrich syndromes, which can be diagnosed by flow cytometric analysis (Fig. 11-52).[133] Flow

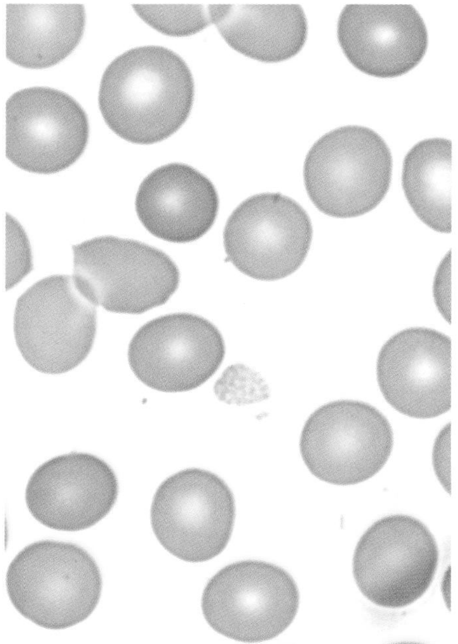

Figure 11-51. Peripheral blood smear of gray platelet syndrome. The large platelet is agranular due to the absence of alpha granules.

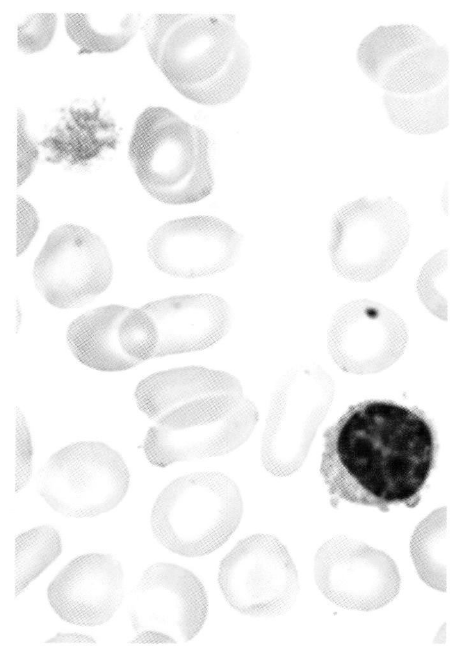

Figure 11-52. Peripheral blood smear of Bernard-Soulier syndrome. The large platelets in this disorder have absent or dysfunctional glycoprotein Ib-IX-V receptors. The patient also has β-thalassemia minor.

cytometric analysis is also diagnostic for X-linked thrombocytopenia. Other parameters can help diagnose macrothrombocytopenia in DiGeorge, gray platelet, Montreal, and Paris-Trousseau syndromes. Normal-sized platelets are more commonly seen in syndromes that have decreased bone marrow megakaryocytes (see Table 11-9).

A number of congenital platelet disorders are due to qualitative defects in platelets in the absence of thrombocytopenia.[132] These patients generally have hemostasis complications and the finding of abnormal platelet sizes on blood films. Included in this category are Glanzmann's thrombasthenia, disorders of agonist receptor and signaling pathways (collagen receptors, adenosine diphosphate receptors, G proteins, phospholipase C), enzyme deficiencies (cyclooxygenase, thromboxane synthetase), Scott's syndrome, and type I von Willebrand's disease.[133]

EVALUATION OF SPECIFIC BONE MARROW FAILURE SYNDROMES

Bone marrow hypoplasia involving more than one lineage, also termed *bone marrow failure*, is discussed in this section and includes congenital disorders and acquired aplastic anemia and PNH (Table 11-12). Acquired multilineage cytopenias may also be caused by nutritional deficiencies (copper, vitamin B_{12}, folate), drug reactions, toxic effects (alcohol), and infections (especially viral); these are discussed in other sections of this chapter.

Paroxysmal Nocturnal Hemoglobinuria

PNH is caused by a clonal expansion of hematopoietic stem cells that acquire a mutant *PIG-A* gene (see Table 11-12). These PNH stem cells are present in normal bone marrow and appear to have a growth or survival advantage over normal

Table 11-12 Acquired and Constitutional Bone Marrow Failure Syndromes

Disorder	Inheritance/Defect	Morphology	Clinical Features	Comments
Paroxysmal nocturnal hemoglobinuria (PNH)	Acquired: somatic X chromosome *PIGA* gene mutation; loss of GPI-APs on RBCs, neutrophils, monocytes platelets	Normochromic normocytic anemia, increased polychromasia Normocellular or hypercellular bone marrow Erythroid hyperplasia, normal morphology	Florid intravascular hemolysis (hemoglobinuria), thrombosis (40%), smooth muscle dystonias, abdominal pain	All ages and ethnic groups, less common in children; thrombosis main cause of death Complement-mediated lysis of GPI-AP–deficient cells Flow cytometry: often >50% of PMNs are GPI-AP deficient Neutrophils may have short telomeres
	In setting of other bone marrow failure syndrome	Evidence of concomitant syndrome (often aplastic anemia or low-grade MDS)	Intermittant hemolysis or no hemolysis (subclinical)	Usually <30% of PMNs are GPI-AP deficient, or <1% of PMNs are GPI-AP deficient
Aplastic anemia	Acquired: cytotoxic T-cell–induced apoptosis of CD34$^+$ stem cells ⅓ of cases have short telomeres Mutations in *TERC* (4%), *TERT* (4%), *SBDS* (5%), *TERF1/2* (1%)	Cytopenias—slowly progressive (idiopathic) or abrupt (secondary) Bone marrow hypoplasia (often <10%), lymphocytes, plasma cells, hematogones (children), ± mast cells Possible dyserythropoiesis, but no significant dysplasia in myeloid or megakaryocytic lineages, No increase in CD34$^+$ cells	Development of infections, bleeding, cardiac output failure Evolution to PNH, MDS, or AML possible	Majority (60%) idiopathic; may arise after injury from chemotherapy, idiosyncratic drug or chemical reactions, infections (especially seronegative hepatitis), radiation, immune disorders Increased frequency in developing countries, especially Southeast Asia and Far East in patients with HLA-DR2 or cytokine gene polymorphisms
Fanconi's anemia	Autosomal or X-linked recessive: biallelic mutations of *FANC-A* to *FANC-N* 13 known genes are involved in the Fanconi's anemia pathway	Neutropenia and thrombocytopenia may precede anemia; possible macrocytosis; gradual development of pancytopenia and aplasia (90% by fifth decade); MDS or AML may develop Aplastic anemia or, rarely, AML may be the presenting feature	25% lack clinical anomalies Skin discoloration (55%), skeletal anomalies (51%), abnormal reproductive organs (35%), facial dysmorphic features (26%), short stature, gastrointestinal anomalies, renal malformations, abnormal thumbs	Median age at diagnosis is 7 yr (range, 0-49 yr); 85% cumulative probability of cancer by age 40-50 yr, especially squamous cell carcinoma of head, neck, esophagus Increased chromosome breakage with mitomycin C or diepoxybutane is diagnostic; carriers cannot be detected
Dyskeratosis congenita	X-linked: *DKC1* (≈36%) Autosomal recessive: *TERC* (≈6%), *TINF2* Autosomal dominant: *NOP10*, *TERT* (1%) Mutated genes are involved in telomere maintenance	Progressive neutropenia and/or thrombocytopenia followed by pancytopenia; initial compensatory hypercellularity, megaloblastic changes, with progressive loss of cellularity Aplastic anemia in 33% of X-linked, 60% of autosomal recessive cases before adulthood; may be the presenting feature	Reticular pigmentation, dysplastic nails, oral leukoplakia, pulmonary fibrosis, liver fibrosis, osteoporosis, microcephaly	Median age at diagnosis is 15 yr (range, 0-74 yr); 50% are older than 15 yr at time of diagnosis Diagnosis: gene mutation tests or screening for short telomeres in all leukocyte subsets; diagnostic if <1% length for age 35% cumulative probability of cancer by 40-50 yr, especially squamous cell carcinoma

AML, acute myeloid leukemia; GPI-AP, glycosylphosphatidylinositol-anchored protein; MDS, myelodysplastic syndrome; PMN, polymorphonuclear neutrophil; RBC, red blood cell.

hematopoietic stem cells in the setting of immune-mediated bone marrow injury.[134] Further genetic or epigenetic events enhance their clonal proliferation. The progeny of PNH stem cells have reduced or absent glycosylphosphatidylinositol (GPI)-anchored proteins. These include important complement regulatory proteins, such as CD55 and CD59, on erythrocytes, granulocytes, monocytes, and platelets (Figs. 11-53 to 11-56). Flow cytometric analysis to detect the loss of GPI proteins or a fluorescein-labeled proaerolysin variant (FLAER) that binds to the GPI anchor (best on neutrophils) is diagnostic.[135] The natural history of PNH is variable, with some patients having well-tolerated minor cytopenias and others progressing to aplastic anemia.

Aplastic Anemia

Aplastic anemia (AA) may be of variable severity. Severe AA is characterized by a markedly hypocellular bone marrow

Box 12-1 *Causes of Reactive Neutrophilia*

- Infection
- Autoimmune disorders
- Collagen vascular disease
- Malignancy
- Exogenous growth factor therapy (granulocyte-macrophage colony-stimulating factor, granulocyte colony-stimulating factor)
- Acute stress
- Epinephrine administration
- Corticosteroid therapy

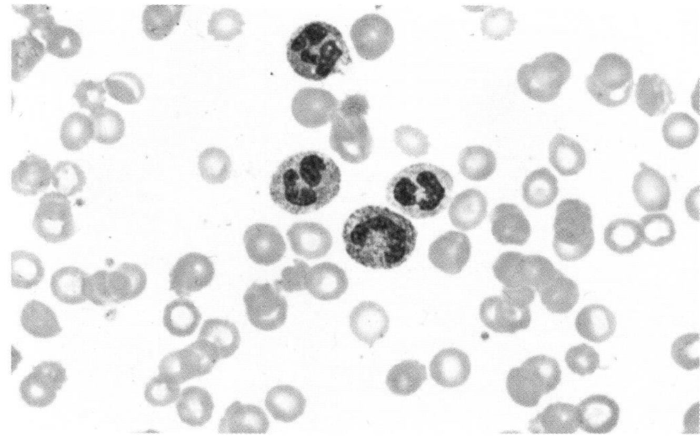

Figure 12-1. Toxic granulation and vacuolization in peripheral blood neutrophils due to infection.

monly related to viral infections (Epstein-Barr virus [EBV], cytomegalovirus [CMV], hepatitis, human herpesvirus 6, human immunodeficiency virus [HIV]) or drug reactions (particularly phenytoin),[4] but it may also be seen in "stress" conditions.[5,6] The latter conditions may be related to endogenous epinephrine release.[7] Rare cases of polyclonal T-cell lymphocytosis have been described in patients with thymomas.[8] The peripheral lymphocytosis secondary to infection is predominantly a T-cell reaction.[9]

Reactive marrow lymphocytosis is characterized by an increase in benign-appearing lymphocytes. The increase may or may not be associated with a peripheral lymphocytosis and may be due to either an interstitial increase in lymphoid cells or an increase in lymphoid aggregates. Increased precursor B-lymphoid cells (hematogones) may be seen in variety of conditions, especially in children, but they are common after chemotherapy in both adults and children (Fig. 12-3). These cells are often difficult to distinguish from lymphoblasts in acute lymphoblastic leukemia (see Chapter 41). The patient's age is important in determining whether lymphoid cells are increased because children normally have more lymphocytes (up to 35%) in the marrow.[10] In adults, the normal value for lymphocytes on the aspirate smear is approximately 6% to 25%.[11]

Persistent polyclonal B-cell lymphocytosis is a rare disorder seen primarily in young women who are often cigarette smokers (Box 12-2).[12] Patients are typically asymptomatic and rarely have lymphadenopathy or splenomegaly.[13] There is an association with human leukocyte antigen (HLA)-DR7.[14] EBV has been found in the peripheral blood cells of some patients, and the cells appear to have a defective CD40 activation pathway.[15,16] Increased polyclonal immunoglobulin (Ig) M is found in the serum.

The peripheral blood shows increased lymphocytes with moderate amounts of cytoplasm and bilobed nuclei (Fig. 12-4). These cells may be seen in the bone marrow aspirate smear and biopsy, typically in an intrasinusoidal or intravascular pattern.[17] Immunophenotypic evaluation shows a polyclonal proliferation of B cells that are often IgD$^+$ and CD27$^+$; multiple *BCL2/Ig* rearrangements have been detected.[12,18] Isochromosome i(3q) and trisomy 3 are present in some cases.[19-21] The lymphoid proliferation may persist for many years without any clinical evidence of the development of malignancy.

REACTIVE EOSINOPHILIA

Reactive eosinophilia is caused by a wide variety of underlying conditions (Box 12-3).[22-43] Mild elevations in the eosinophil count are usually due to allergic conditions; moderate eosinophilia is more common in lymphomas, rheumatoid arthritis, and nonhematologic malignancies; and severe elevations are seen in parasitic infections, pulmonary eosinophilia, and clonal eosinophilic disorders.[44,45] Rarely, reactive eosinophilia

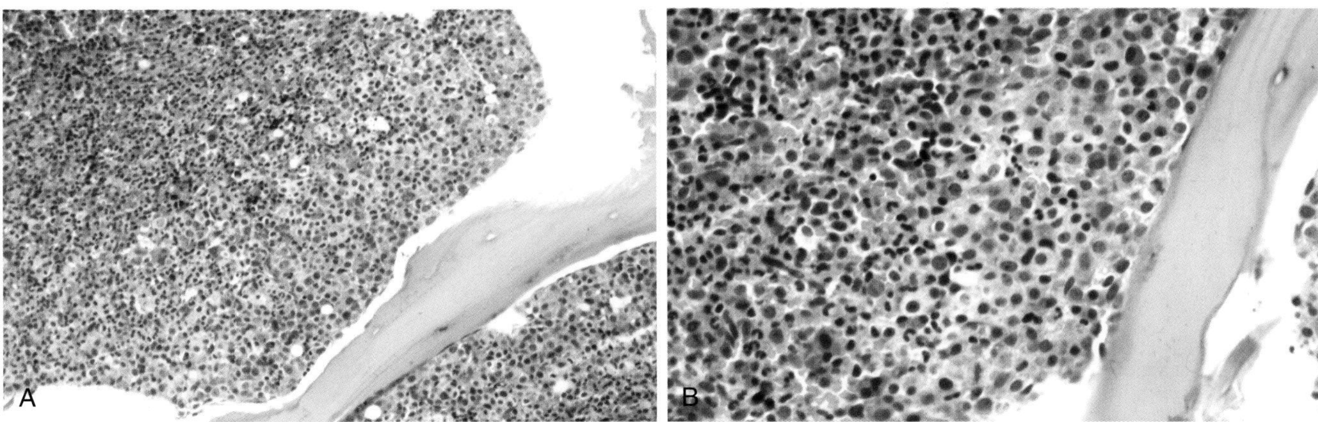

Figure 12-2. Peritrabecular myeloid precursors in bone marrow biopsy at low (**A**) and high (**B**) power, resembling metastatic carcinoma.

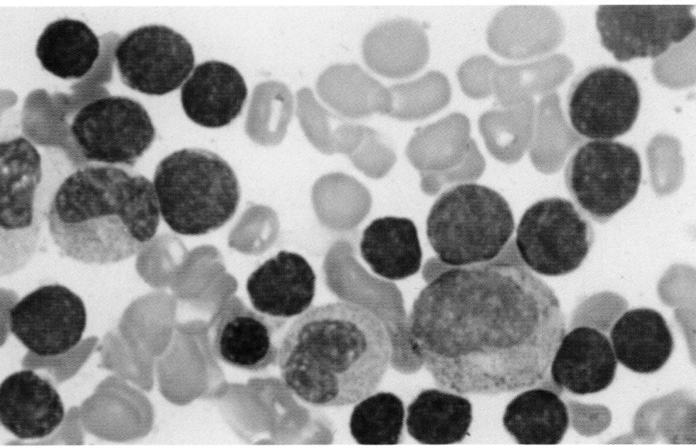

Figure 12-3. Precursor B cells (hematogones) in the bone marrow aspirate from a child with neutropenia. The cells have a high nuclear-to-cytoplasmic ratio, with condensed chromatin and no nucleoli.

Box 12-3 *Causes of Reactive Eosinophilia*

- Atopic disorders: allergy, asthma, eczema[22-24]
- Parasitic infections: *Toxacara canis* most common in the United States[25]
- Connective tissue disease[26]
- Drug reactions[27,28]
- Hematopoietic growth factor and interleukin-3 therapy[29,30]
- Inflammatory skin disorders[31]
- Carcinoma[32]
- T-cell malignancies
  - Acute lymphoblastic leukemia with t(5;14)(q31;q32)[33]
  - Mycosis fungoides[34]
  - Peripheral T-cell lymphoma[35,36]
- B-cell lymphomas[37]
- Hodgkin's lymphoma[38]
- Pulmonary eosinophilic syndromes[39]
- Transplant rejection[40]
- Vasculitis[41,42]
- Constitutional abnormality[43]

Box 12-2 *Characteristics of Persistent Polyclonal B-Cell Lymphocytosis*

Clinical Findings

- Female predominance
- Age 20 to 40 years
- Asymptomatic
- Cigarette smoker

Laboratory Findings

- Peripheral lymphocytosis
- Bilobed lymphocytes
- Increase in polyclonal serum immunoglobulin M
- Multiple *BCL2/IgH* gene rearrangements
- Epstein-Barr virus in peripheral blood
- Polyclonal immunophenotype—memory B cells
- Increased frequency of HLA-DR7
- Isochromosome i(3q)

has been reported as a constitutional abnormality; two of the reported patients had a chromosomal abnormality—a pericentric inversion of chromosome 10.[43]

In cases of reactive eosinophilia, the marrow aspirate smears show increased eosinophils and precursors, usually greater than 5% of the bone marrow nucleated cells.[46] Eosinophilic myelocytes frequently show small basophilic granules. Such myelocytes represent a normal stage of eosinophil development, and the basophilic granules likely represent eosinophil primary granules.[47] In tissue sections of the bone marrow, there is often a diffuse increase in eosinophils and precursors, but focal eosinophilia may be seen surrounding the lesions of marrow involvement by Hodgkin's disease, malignant lymphoma, benign lymphoid aggregates, systemic mast cell disease, and Langerhans histiocytosis (Fig. 12-5).[48,49] In these cases increased eosinophils may not be seen in the peripheral blood or in the aspirate smear.

A more detailed discussion of the evaluation of patients with nonneoplastic and neoplastic eosinophilia can be found in Chapter 49.

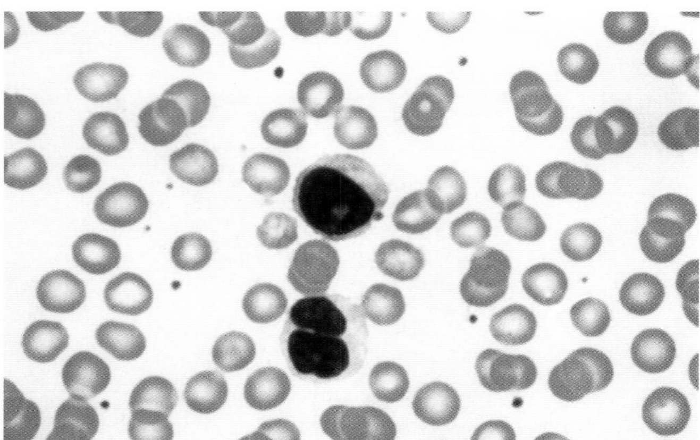

Figure 12-4. Polyclonal B-cell lymphocytosis in the peripheral blood smear. Atypical bilobed lymphocytes are seen. (Courtesy of Linda Sandhaus, MD.)

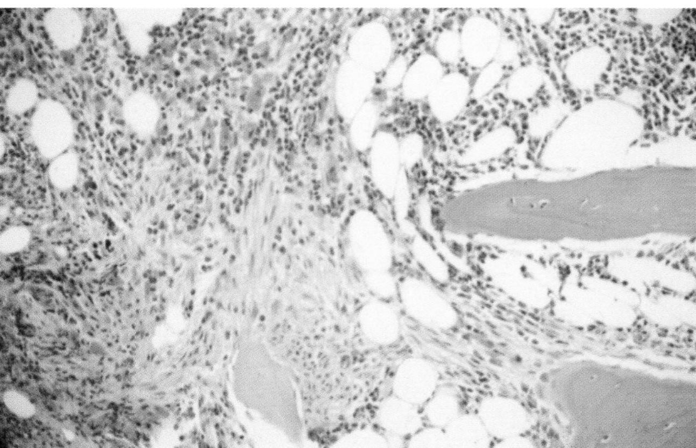

Figure 12-5. Increased eosinophils are seen surrounding a bone marrow lesion of mast cell disease.

Box 12-4 *Causes of Reactive Monocytosis*

- Acute and chronic inflammation
- Acute myocardial infarction
- Carcinoma
- Hodgkin's lymphoma
- Hypothyroidism
- Neutropenia
- Splenectomy

REACTIVE BASOPHILIA

Reactive basophilia is not a common finding. In some cases it may be seen with a reactive eosinophil proliferation. Peripheral blood findings show an absolute basophil count greater than 0.2×10^9/L. Marrow aspirate smears show an increase in basophils and precursors, accounting for more than 2% of cells.

Commonly associated conditions are allergies, carcinoma, inflammation, malignant lymphoma, multiple myeloma, radiation, and renal failure.[50,51]

REACTIVE MONOCYTOSIS

A peripheral blood monocytosis is defined as greater than 1×10^9/L monocytes; an increased monocyte level in the bone marrow aspirate smear is often defined as greater than 3% of the differential count.[11] Associated conditions include acute and chronic inflammation, collagen vascular disorders, acute myocardial infarction,[52] carcinoma,[53] hypothyroidism,[54] and splenectomy[55] (Box 12-4). Monocytes are also commonly increased in the presence of neutropenia after chemotherapy or due to a congenital deficiency.[56]

BONE MARROW IN INFECTIOUS DISORDERS

Bacterial Infection

Bacterial infections often cause an increase in neutrophils in the peripheral blood, with an increase in immature myeloid cells, or a left shift. Exceptions are seen in neonates and in elderly or debilitated patients who cannot mount a neutrophilic response. Morphologic changes associated with bacterial infection include toxic granulation, Döhle bodies, and cytoplasmic vacuolization. In rare cases bacteria may be seen within neutrophils and monocytes. An increase in circulating neutrophils results in a subsequent increase in myeloid precursors in the bone marrow.

Rare bacterial infections such as pertussis may cause a lymphocytosis in the peripheral blood, which consists of predominantly $CD4^+$ cells (Fig. 12-6).[57] In children, these lymphocytes often have clefted, irregular nuclei, similar to the cells seen in peripheralization of follicular lymphoma. Neutropenia may be seen with *Salmonella* or *Brucella* infections. Uncomplicated tuberculosis infection does not typically cause a change in the neutrophil count.

Red cell abnormalities are rarely seen in bacterial infections. *Mycoplasma* pneumonia can lead to the development of a cold agglutinin. Severe hemolysis can be seen in *Clostridium* infection owing to the presence of a hemolysin, phospholipase C.[58]

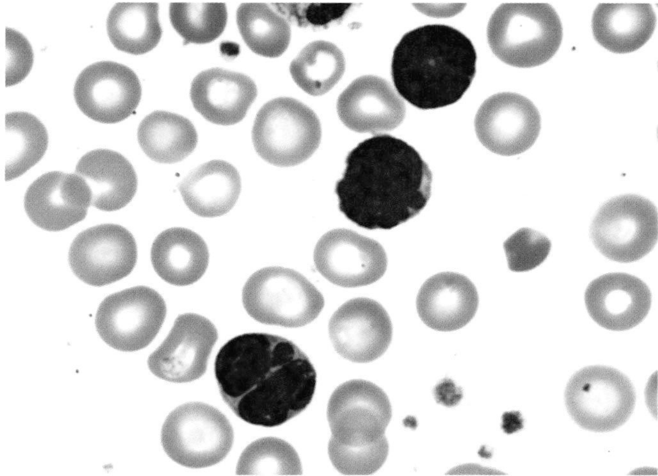

Figure 12-6. Small clefted lymphocytes in the peripheral blood smear from a child with pertussis infection.

The only bacterial infections diagnosed with any frequency within the bone marrow are those due to mycobacteria (see later). Rare cases of infection with *Tropheryma whippelii*, the causative agent of Whipple's disease, have been described.[59] Periodic acid–Schiff–positive organisms are seen within marrow macrophages. Confirmation can be accomplished by polymerase chain reaction or electron microscopy. *Salmonella typhi* infection has been associated with pancytopenia due to hemophagocytosis,[60,61] granulomas, ring granulomas, or bone marrow necrosis.[62] *Salmonella* organisms may be seen within neutrophils and monocytes. Bone marrow involvement by lepromatous leprosy is characterized by a proliferation of foamy histiocytes that contain the bacilli or by the presence of bacilli lying free in the marrow interstitium.[63] Brucellosis can cause marrow granulomas, hemophagocytosis, and a peripheral pancytopenia (Fig. 12-7).[64]

Mycobacterial infection of the bone marrow is most commonly caused by *Mycobacterium tuberculosis* or *Mycobacterium*

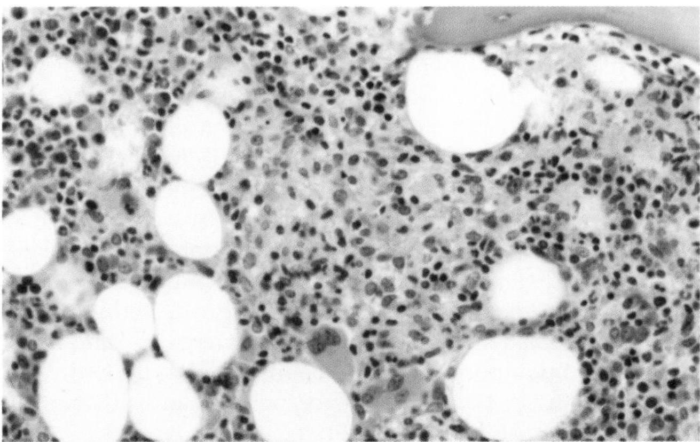

Figure 12-7. Noncaseating granuloma in a bone marrow core biopsy from a patient with brucellosis.

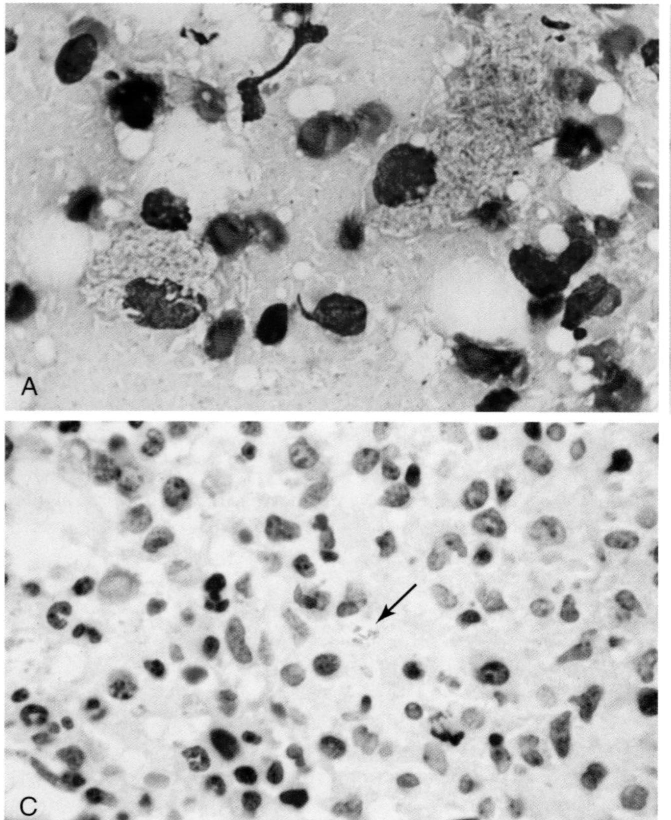

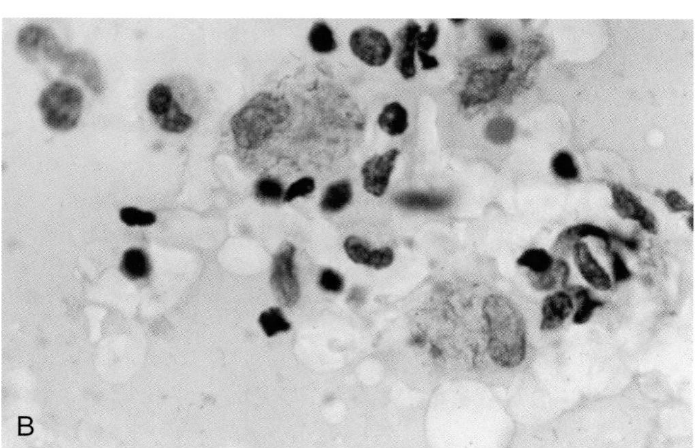

Figure 12-8. **A,** Touch preparation of bone marrow from an HIV patient with *Mycobacterium avium-intracellulare* infection. The histiocytes show linear, negatively stained inclusions on the Wright-Giemsa stain. **B,** The inclusions in **A** are seen to be mycobacteria on the acid-fast stain. **C,** Rare *Mycobacterium tuberculosis* organisms are identified on this acid-fast stain in a granuloma from a different patient.

avium-intracellulare. Rare cases of infection with other mycobacteria have been described.[65] Patients with pulmonary tuberculosis may have thrombocytosis, leukocytosis, or monocytosis.[66] Peripheral blood abnormalities in miliary tuberculosis include the anemia of chronic inflammation, leukopenia, thrombocytopenia, and pancytopenia. Peripheral lymphopenia or thrombocytopenia suggests marrow involvement by granulomas in *M. tuberculosis*.[67,68] Patients with *M. avium-intracellulare* infection often have peripheral blood abnormalities associated with an underlying HIV infection. Negatively stained linear inclusions may be seen within histiocytes on Wright-stained preparations in *M. avium-intracellulare* infection (Fig. 12-8A and B).[69] Granulomas can rarely be found on an aspirate smear but are typically detected on the clot section or core biopsy. Caseation within marrow granulomas is rare, but when present it is highly suggestive of infection with *M. tuberculosis*. In *M. avium-intracellulare* infection, the granulomas may not be well formed, or there may be diffuse infiltration by histiocytes. Special stains for acid-fast bacilli show rare organisms in *M. tuberculosis* (see Fig. 12-8C); the bacilli are more easily found in cases of *M. avium-intracellulare* infection and may be numerous. Blood cultures are a more sensitive technique for detecting mycobacteria, especially in the setting of HIV infection,[70] and it has been argued that bone marrow examination has limited value in this setting.[71] Detecting the organism with an acid-fast bacilli stain can significantly shorten the time it takes to make a diagnosis, which may have a positive clinical impact.[72] Rarely, granulomas and organisms can be found in culture-negative patients.[73]

Rickettsial Infection

Rickettsial infections, including Q fever and ehrlichiosis, have been diagnosed in the bone marrow and blood. Infection with *Coxiella burnetii* causes Q fever, which leads to a characteristic donut or ring granuloma in marrow clot sections or core biopsies. The granuloma consists of a ring of epithelioid histiocytes and neutrophils surrounding a central vacuole with an outer fibrin ring (Fig. 12-9).[74,75] These granulomas are not specific for Q fever and have been seen in CMV infections as well as Hodgkin's lymphoma, infectious mononucleosis, and typhoid fever.[76]

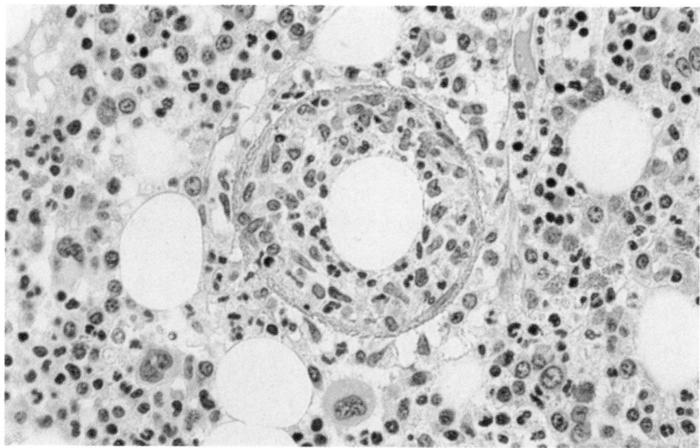

Figure 12-9. Fibrin ring granuloma on a core biopsy from a patient with Q fever.

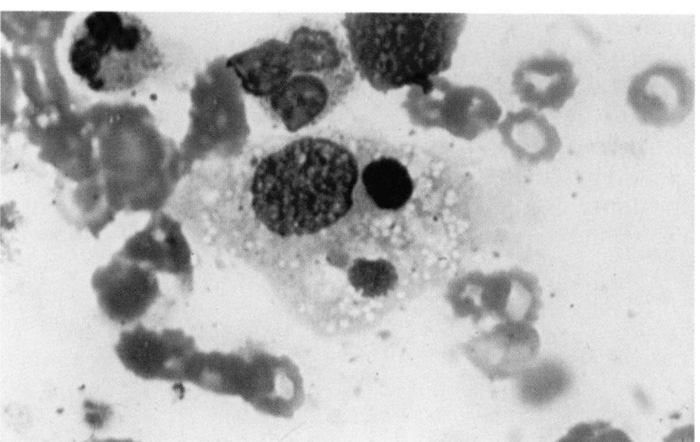

Figure 12-10. Bone marrow aspirate smear showing ehrlichiosis. The organisms are contained within histiocytes.

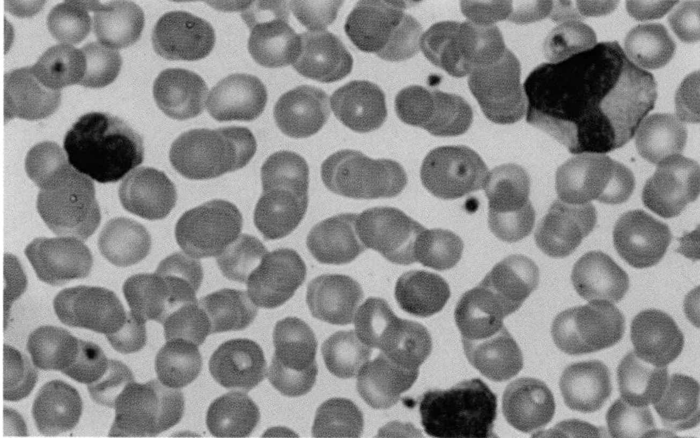

Figure 12-11. Peripheral blood smear showing reactive lymphocytes from a patient with cytomegalovirus infection.

Human ehrlichiosis is caused by infection with *Ehrlichia chaffeensis*, *Anaplasma phagocytophilum*, or, less commonly, *Ehrlichia ewingii*.[77] The first organism infects monocytes, and the other two infect granulocytes. Any of these infections can cause leukopenia, with a left shift, and thrombocytopenia.[78-80] Fever and elevated hepatic transaminases may also be seen. The organisms can be identified in the peripheral blood smear, in which small clusters of darkly stained bacteria may be found in circulating monocytes or neutrophils. Bone marrow pathology has been better studied in monocytic ehrlichiosis. Granulocytic hyperplasia is common; organisms may be seen within histiocytes in the aspirate, and 67% of patients have granulomas on biopsy sections (Fig. 12-10).[81] The bone marrow in patients infected with *Anaplasma* is either normocellular or hypercellular, with rare infected cells present.[82] Lymphoid aggregates, plasmacytosis, and erythrophagocytosis may be seen.[83] Polymerase chain reaction testing of peripheral blood can confirm the diagnosis.[84]

Parasitic Infection

Infections with tissue-invasive parasites result in an increased eosinophil count in the peripheral blood and bone marrow. *Toxoplasma gondii* pseudocysts have been seen in association with bone marrow necrosis in patients with acquired immunodeficiency syndrome (AIDS).[85] Leishman-Donovan bodies can be seen with macrophages in patients with leishmaniasis. Leishmaniasis is a severe disease caused by *Leishmania* species found in endemic areas, but it is also an opportunistic infection in immunocompromised individuals, including those with HIV infection or bone marrow transplantation.[86,87] Clinical findings include fever, hepatosplenomegaly, and pancytopenia. A reactive increase in plasma cells is seen on the aspirate smear. Granulomas may be seen on the core biopsy or clot section. The amastigotes are typically visible within histiocytes. The cytoplasm of the amastigote stains blue, with a red nucleus and a rod-shaped kinetoplast.[88]

Viral Infection

Cytomegalovirus

CMV is a DNA virus that is a member of the herpes family. Acute CMV infection may be associated with a proliferation of reactive lymphocytes in the peripheral blood, similar to those seen with infectious mononucleosis due to EBV infection (Fig. 12-11).[89] In rare cases, CMV-infected cells with abundant cytoplasm and nuclear inclusions may be seen in the peripheral blood.[90] These cells are most easily seen in the feathered edge of the blood smear. Other peripheral blood findings include hemolysis, neutropenia, and thrombocytopenia.[91-93]

Bone marrow biopsy abnormalities include granulomas or ring granulomas.[94] Rarely, large intranuclear inclusions can be seen in endothelial cells (Fig. 12-12). A myeloid maturation arrest leading to neutropenia can also be seen on the aspirate smear. CMV is one of the causes of hemophagocytic syndrome.

In infants, either congenital or acquired CMV infection can mimic the features of juvenile myelomonocytic leukemia.[95] Genetic evaluation and studies to determine hypersensitivity to granulocyte-macrophage colony-stimulating factor, which is typical for juvenile myelomonocytic leukemia, may be required for the final diagnosis.[96] CMV infection has also been reported to mimic myelodysplasia in adults who present with thrombocytopenia.[97] CMV infections are commonly seen in patients infected with HIV. Rare intranuclear inclusions may be present, but no other specific findings can be attributed to CMV infection. CMV infection after stem cell transplantation

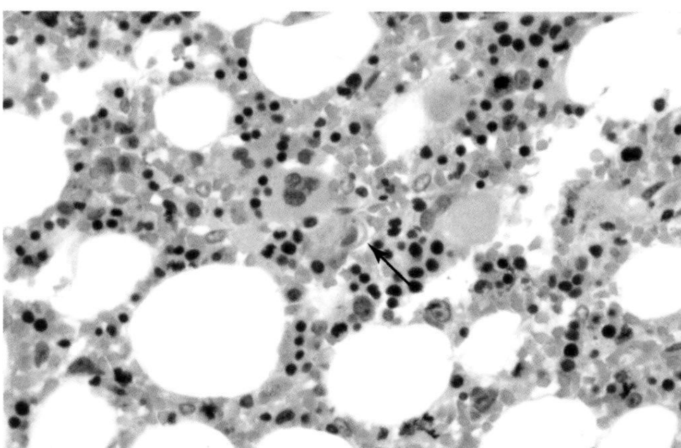

Figure 12-12. Bone marrow core biopsy showing a large eosinophilic cytomegalovirus inclusion (*arrow*).

can lead to delayed engraftment, especially with respect to recovery of platelet counts.[98] Similar bone marrow suppression can be seen with human herpesvirus 6 infection.[99]

Epstein-Barr Virus

EBV infection causes peripheral blood and bone marrow abnormalities. The most characteristic finding in the peripheral blood in patients with infectious mononucleosis is an absolute lymphocytosis with many reactive lymphocytes. Older patients often have fewer reactive lymphocytes in the peripheral blood.[100] These circulating lymphoid cells are predominantly CD8$^+$ T cells.[101] Apoptosis of lymphoid cells is also a frequent finding (Fig. 12-13A to C).[102] In addition to exhibiting lymphocytosis, patients may be anemic or thrombocytopenic. In rare patients with EBV infection, hemolytic anemia develops due to a cold agglutinin. If the patient devel-

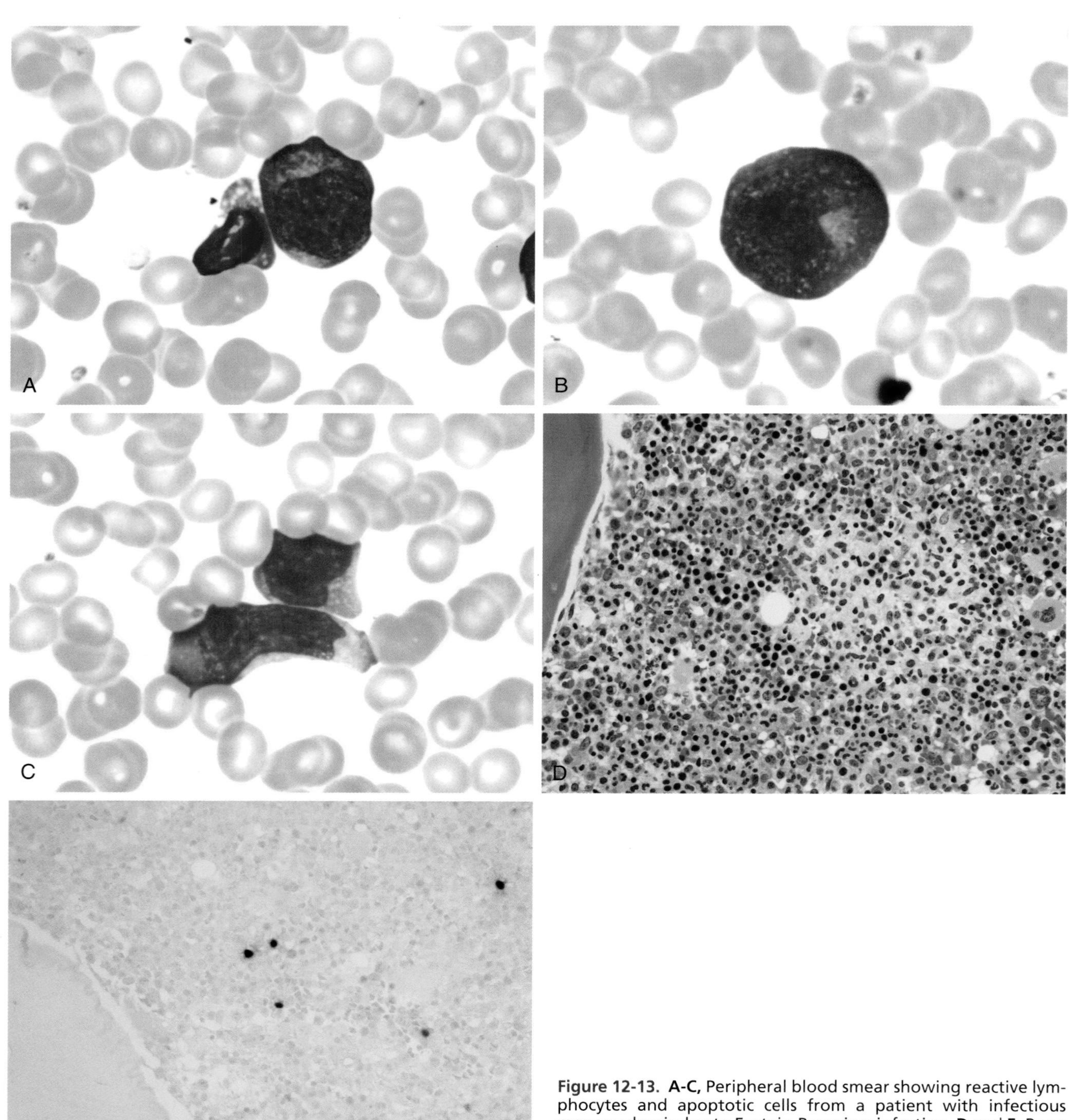

Figure 12-13. A-C, Peripheral blood smear showing reactive lymphocytes and apoptotic cells from a patient with infectious mononucleosis due to Epstein-Barr virus infection. **D** and **E,** Bone marrow from the same patient shows small, ill-defined histiocytic-lymphocytic aggregates. In situ hybridization for EBER1 shows several scattered hybridization signals.

ops hemophagocytic syndrome or marrow suppression secondary to EBV, pancytopenia may be present. Rare cases of atypical myelomonocytic proliferations have been seen secondary to EBV infection; this disorder resembles juvenile myelomonocytic leukemia.[103] Aplastic anemia has also been described as a sequela of EBV infection.[104,105]

EBV is associated with malignant lymphoid proliferations, including Burkitt's lymphoma, lymphomatoid granulomatosis, and immunodeficiency lymphoproliferative disorders, which are discussed in other chapters.

Studies to determine whether a patient has EBV infection should be performed on the peripheral blood. A monospot test for the detection of heterophil antibodies confirms the diagnosis. This test is more likely to be negative in young children and the elderly, owing to the limited production of heterophil antibodies. If the monospot test is negative and the clinical picture is consistent with mononucleosis, additional tests for specific viral antibodies directed against viral capsid antigen, early antigen, and Epstein-Barr nuclear antigen should be performed.

Bone marrow examinations are generally not done in patients with infectious mononucleosis; however, when marrow biopsies have been performed, benign lymphoid aggregates and noncaseating granulomas without giant cells have been described.[106] In situ hybridization studies for EBV-encoded RNA (EBER1) may be performed on biopsy tissue to substantiate the diagnosis (see Fig. 12-13D and E). Marrow aplasia and hemophagocytic histiocytes are seen if aplastic anemia or hemophagocytic syndrome complicates acute EBV infection.

Hepatitis

Acute viral hepatitis may be associated with a reactive lymphocytosis in the peripheral blood. Hepatitis A, B, and C have been associated with the development of aplastic anemia. Patients with hepatitis C develop a variety of hematologic complications, including monoclonal gammopathies and cryoglobulinemia; they also have an increased risk of low-grade lymphoproliferative disorders.[107] Type II mixed cryoglobulinemia has been associated with atypical lymphoid aggregates in the bone marrow. These aggregates often consist of monomorphic small lymphocytes and may be paratrabecular in location (Fig. 12-14).[108] Immunophenotyping reveals the cells to be B cells that express BCL2, and they may show light-chain restriction. Molecular analysis shows an oligoclonal expansion of B cells in many cases. Care should be taken in diagnosing lymphomatous involvement in the marrow in the absence of other clinical or molecular evidence of lymphoma.[109]

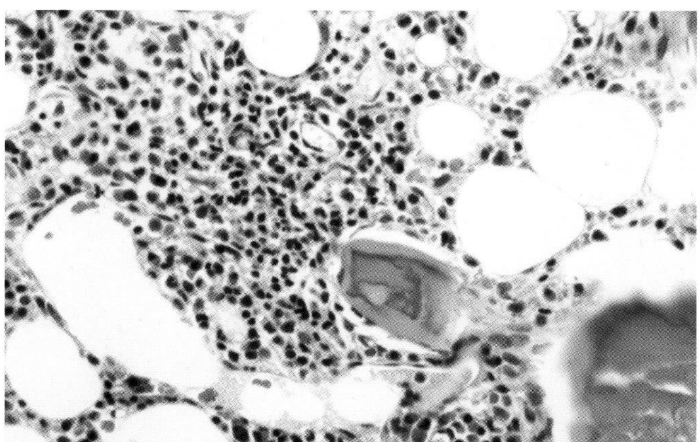

Figure 12-14. Bone marrow core biopsy showing atypical lymphoid aggregates from a patient with hepatitis C infection.

Hantavirus

Hantavirus pulmonary syndrome was first described in 1993 in the southwestern United States. The infection is caused by Sin Nombre virus.[110] In the prodromal phase, thrombocytopenia is the only finding.[111] The peripheral blood findings that accompany the pulmonary leak syndrome are thrombocytopenia, hemoconcentration, leukocytosis with a left shift, and lymphopenia with more than 10% immunoblasts. Immunoblasts may also be seen in the bone marrow.[112,113]

Parvovirus B19 and Human Immunodeficiency Virus

The bone marrow findings associated with parvovirus B19 and HIV infection are found in Chapters 11 and 56, respectively.

Fungal Infection

Fungal infections of the bone marrow are most often due to *Histoplasma* or *Cryptococcus*[114-116] and are most common in patients with underlying immunodeficiencies.[117,118] Other fungal infections such as coccidioidomycosis, blastomycosis, and aspergillus have rarely been described. In patients with histoplasmosis, peripheral blood findings may include anemia, thrombocytopenia, and leukopenia. In disseminated infection, fungemia may be present, and *Histoplasma* organisms can be seen in circulating monocytes or neutrophils (Fig. 12-15A). Hemophagocytic syndrome has been described in HIV patients with disseminated histoplasmosis[119] and in rare patients with crytoptococcal meningitis.[120]

Bone marrow examination is often useful for the evaluation of disseminated histoplasmosis, particularly in the setting of HIV infection, in which case the marrow is involved in up to 80% of patients.[114] Wright stain can identify organisms in the aspirate smear in many cases (see Fig. 12-15B).[121] Rarely the organisms are confined to the megakaryocytes owing to emperipolesis.[122] Granulomas may be seen on the clot section or core biopsy. *Histoplasma* organisms are positive for both periodic acid–Schiff and Gomori's methenamine silver. Cryptococcal organisms can also be recognized on Wright-stained aspirate smear material as variably sized budding yeasts (Fig. 12-16). Granulomas can be seen on histologic sections, and a Gomori's methenamine silver or mucin stain can be used to stain the organism. Confirmation by antigen testing can be done on a urine specimen for histoplasmosis or on serum for *Cryptococcus*. Coccidioidomyocosis is also a rare cause of granulomas within the marrow.

Bone Marrow Necrosis

Bone marrow necrosis is defined as necrosis of hematopoietic tissue and marrow stroma without necrosis of the adjacent bone. It can be seen in severe infections and in disseminated intravascular coagulation, although it is more commonly associated with malignancies.[123] The most common malignancies

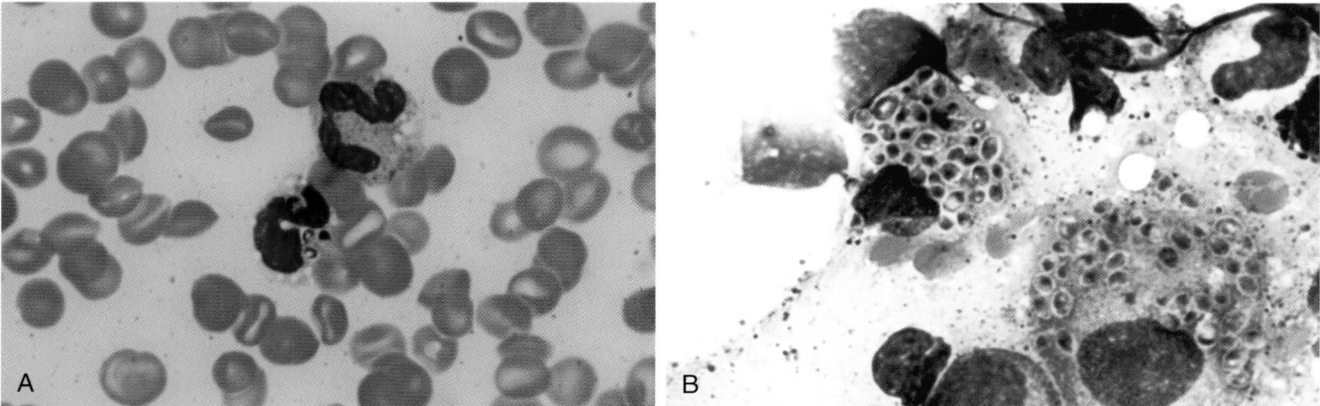

Figure 12-15. Peripheral blood neutrophils that have phagocytized *Histoplasma* organisms (**A**) and histiocytes in the bone marrow stuffed with the same organism (**B**).

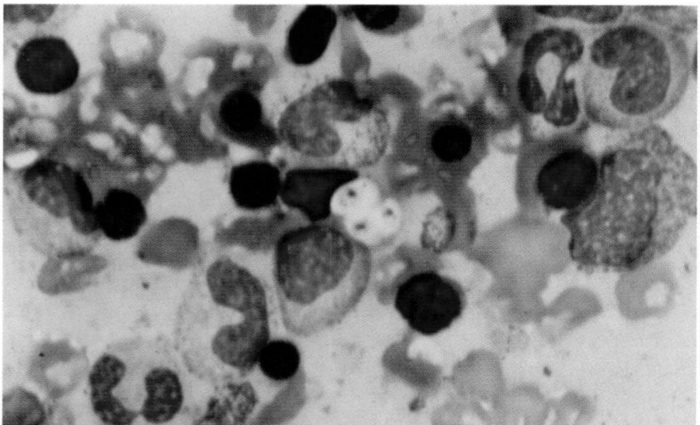

Figure 12-16. Bone marrow touch preparation from a patient with underlying chronic lymphocytic leukemia and *Cryptococcus* infection. Several encapsulated yeasts are seen.

are hematologic, including acute lymphoblastic leukemia, acute myeloid leukemia, and lymphoma. Necrosis due to carcinoma is less common but has been described with lung, stomach, breast, and prostate carcinomas. In many cases the site of the primary tumor is not identified.[124] Severe bone pain is the most common symptom. Other findings associated with the patient's underlying disease, such as fever, weight loss, malaise, and night sweats, are also common. Bone tenderness may be evident on physical examination. The prognosis depends on the underlying disorder.

The most common peripheral blood findings are anemia, thrombocytopenia, and a leukoerythroblastic reaction.[123] However, the findings depend on the underlying disease and the extent of the necrosis. Elevated lactate dehydrogenase levels and hypercalcemia are often present.

On gross examination the bone marrow aspirate may appear brown, with poorly defined particles. The Wright-stained aspirate shows eosinophilic, necrotic cells in a granular background (Fig. 12-17A). The clot section and core biopsy show necrotic smudgy cells with nuclear pyknosis (see Fig. 12-17B). The necrosis may be extensive or focal, with viable normal marrow present in the remainder of the biopsy.

The underlying abnormality in bone marrow necrosis is thought to be occlusion of small blood vessels, leading to disruption of blood supply to the marrow.

Fever of Unknown Origin

It is controversial whether bone marrow examination and culture should be performed in the evaluation of a fever of unknown origin. Some studies show no increased yield

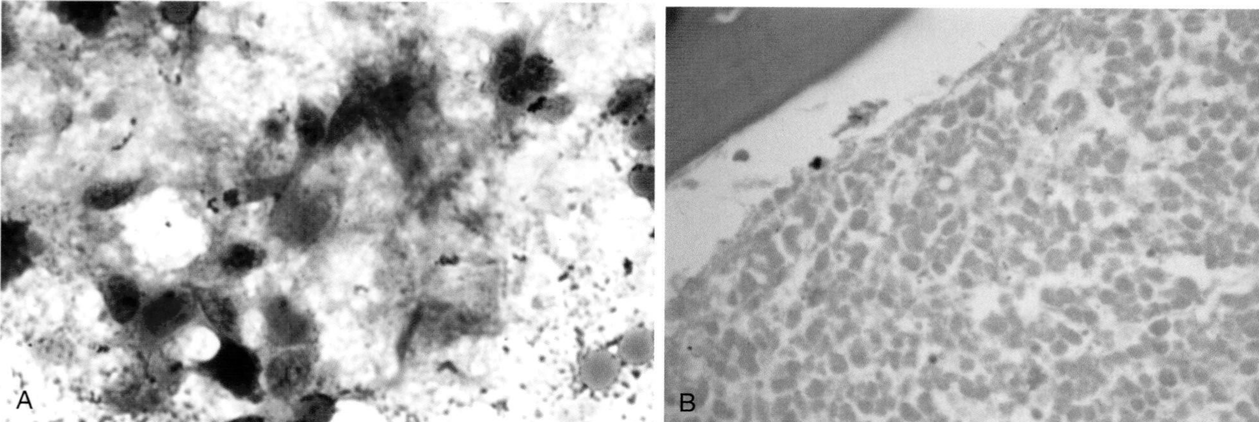

Figure 12-17. Bone marrow aspirate smear (**A**) and core biopsy (**B**) showing severe marrow necrosis. Only degenerated cellular material is seen.

compared with blood culture,[125] whereas others show a higher yield with bone marrow culture.[121] It is clear that the usefulness of special stains in the absence of granulomas is minimal.[125]

BONE MARROW IN NONINFECTIOUS SYSTEMIC AND INFLAMMATORY DISORDERS

Noninfectious Granuloma

Granulomas in the bone marrow have a variety of noninfectious causes, including Hodgkin's lymphoma, non-Hodgkin's lymphoma, nonhematopoietic malignancies, sarcoidosis, drug reactions, and a variety of connective tissue diseases.[126] Five percent of patients with Hodgkin's lymphoma have granulomas,[127] as do 2% to 3% of those with non-Hodgkin's lymphoma,[128,129] regardless of whether the marrow is involved by lymphoma. Granulomas have been described with numerous other malignancies, including acute lymphoblastic leukemia, acute myeloid leukemia, multiple myeloma, and lung, colon, ovarian, and breast carcinoma[130-132]; as in lymphomas, granulomas may be seen regardless of whether the marrow is involved by disease. Drugs most often implicated are procainamide and sulfonamide, although many others, including penicillamine, chlorpropamide, tolmetin, and amiodarone, are associated with granuloma formation.[133-136] A wide variety of connective tissue diseases have been associated with granulomas, although most reports are of isolated cases. Patients with granulomatous hepatitis may have noncaseating granulomas within the marrow.[137] Small noncaseating granulomas, which are likely nonspecific in nature, are often seen in marrow after transplantation.[138] In up to 13% of patients with granulomas, no apparent cause is identified.[126]

Noncaseating granulomas are seen primarily on clot and core biopsy sections, although in rare cases aspirate smears contain granulomas (Fig. 12-18). No characteristic morphologic findings have been associated with any of the aforementioned underlying causes. Special stains for acid-fast bacilli and fungi should be performed on these specimens to eliminate the possibility of an underlying infectious disease. Repeat biopsy with culture may be needed if an infectious cause is suspected.

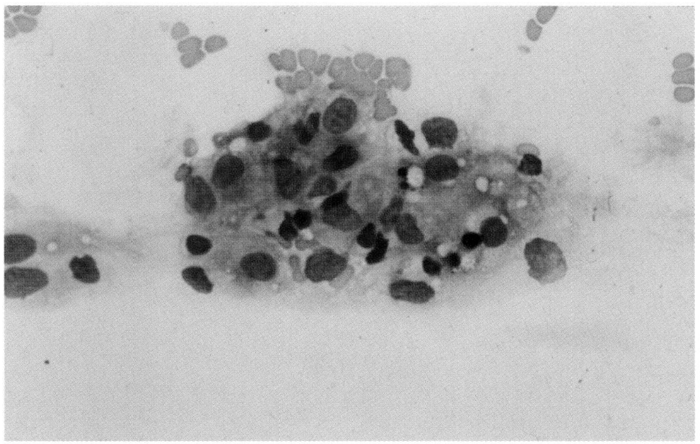

Figure 12-18. Bone marrow aspirate smear with a small granuloma.

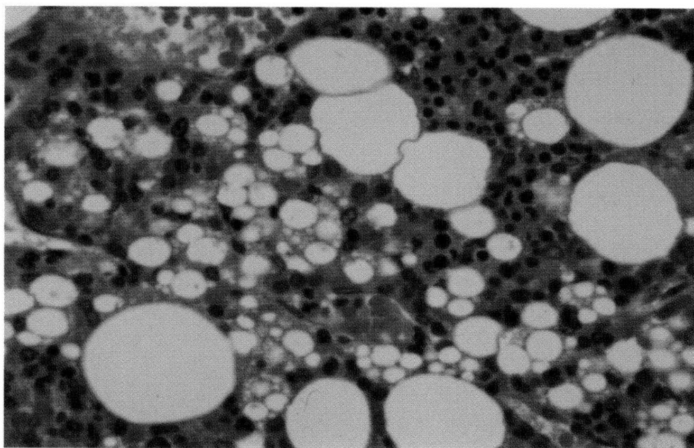

Figure 12-19. Bone marrow core biopsy showing a typical lipogranuloma consisting of histiocytes, lymphocytes, and small fat cells.

Lipogranulomas may be seen in up to 4% of marrow biopsies.[139] These collections of microvesicular fat, lymphocytes, and histiocytes are often associated with benign lymphoid aggregates (Fig. 12-19). These granulomas have no clinical significance, and no further evaluation is required.

The differential diagnosis of granulomatous lesions within the bone marrow includes the lesions of systemic mast cell disease, marrow involvement by Hodgkin's lymphoma, non-Hodgkin's lymphoma (particularly T-cell and T-cell–rich B-cell lymphomas), and focal involvement by hairy cell leukemia.

Connective Tissue Disease

Peripheral blood and bone marrow abnormalities have been associated with a variety of connective tissue diseases, including systemic lupus erythematosus (SLE), rheumatoid arthritis, mixed connective tissue disease, scleroderma, Sjögren's syndrome, and polymyositis.[140] These patients have a variety of abnormalities in the peripheral blood and bone marrow that may be related to their underlying disease or its treatment (Box 12-5).

Cytopenias are common in patients with connective tissue disease. In SLE there may be a variety of underlying causes (Box 12-6).[141] Anemia may be due to chronic inflammation, renal insufficiency, immune hemolysis, and, in rare cases, pure red cell aplasia.[142] Neutropenia and thrombocytopenia may also be caused by an immune mechanism.[143] A microangiopathic hemolytic anemia and thrombocytopenia may be seen in thrombotic thrombocytopenic purpura, which has been reported in association with SLE.[144] Thrombocytopenia may also be a complication of vasculitis with peripheral consumption of platelets.[145] Rare cases of amegakaryocytic thrombocytopenia have also been described.[146] Small platelets are typically seen on the peripheral blood smear owing to decreased production within the marrow.

In rheumatoid arthritis the most common cause of anemia is anemia of chronic disease, and the severity parallels the disease activity. Neutropenia is seen in Felty's syndrome, which consists of neutropenia, splenomegaly, and rheumatoid arthritis. Neutrophil counts range from 0.5 to 2.5 × 10^9/L. The bone marrow is typically hypercellular, with a maturation

Box 12-5 *Connective Tissue Disorders and the Bone Marrow*

Laboratory Findings
- Anemia
  - Anemia of chronic inflammation
  - Hemolytic anemia
  - Red cell aplasia
- Immune-mediated neutropenia
- Steroid-induced neutrophilia
- Eosinophilia
- Thrombocytopenia
  - Immune mediated
  - Amegakaryocytic thrombocytopenia
- Thrombocytosis

Morphologic Findings
- Variable cellularity
- Lymphoid aggregates
- Plasmacytosis
- Increased iron stores
- Granulomas
- Marrow fibrosis

arrest at the myelocyte stage of development (Fig. 12-20). A proliferation of large granular lymphocytes with a T-cell phenotype may be found in patients with Felty's syndrome, and there seems to be clinical and immunologic overlap between Felty's syndrome and large granular lymphocytic leukemia.[147]

Thrombocytosis may be seen in patients with chronic inflammatory conditions. Typically, platelet counts are less than 1 million, and thrombocytosis is not associated with an increased risk of either thrombosis or hemorrhage.

Leukocytosis is frequently present in patients with polymyalgia rheumatica, Still's disease, and Behçet's disease, which may be due to increased cytokine (granulocyte colony-stimulating factor) activity.[148]

Marrow specimens from patients with any of the connective tissue disorders may contain benign lymphoid aggregates and increased reactive plasma cells (Fig. 12-21). Granulomas are rarely seen and are typically noninfectious; however, care must be taken to exclude an infectious cause, because these patients are often immunosuppressed. Rheumatoid nodules can rarely be seen within the marrow space.

Other marrow findings include serous fat atrophy, necrosis, and hemophagocytosis.[149] Macrophage activation syndrome,

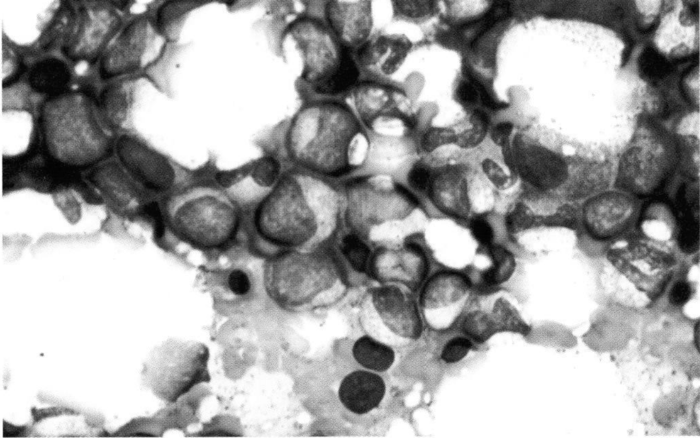

Figure 12-20. Bone marrow touch preparation showing a maturation arrest of the myeloid cell line in a patient with Felty's syndrome.

which is similar to hemophagocytic lymphohistiocytosis, has been described in juvenile arthritis.[150] Necrosis has been documented as a complication of antiphospholipid antibody syndrome.[151,152]

Rare patients have been described with autoimmune myelofibrosis.[153] These patients may have SLE or progressive systemic sclerosis, but they may also have nonspecific immune symptoms such as hemolytic anemia or synovitis. The marrow is variably cellular. In some cases the marrow may be depleted (Fig. 12-22), whereas in others the marrow is cellular and even has prominent megakaryocytic hyperplasia, which raises the possibility of a myeloproliferative neoplasm. In the latter case, however, the megakaryocytes are not clustered, as is commonly observed in myeloproliferative neoplasms, and no basophilia is seen. Marrow fibrosis is present; this responds to corticosteroid therapy.[154] Benign lymphoid aggregates and plasmacytosis, particularly in perivascular locations, may accompany the fibrosis.

Therapy for a connective tissue disorder may also cause peripheral blood and bone marrow abnormalities. Corticosteroid therapy is associated with a peripheral neutrophilia due to increased release from bone marrow stores. Lymphopenia is caused by apoptosis of lymphocytes. Eosinophils may also

Box 12-6 *Hematologic Findings in Systemic Lupus Erythematosus*

- Anemia
  - Anemia of chronic disease
  - Autoimmune hemolytic anemia
  - Renal-insufficiency anemia
  - Pure red cell aplasia
  - Microangiopathic hemolytic anemia
- Neutropenia
- Thrombocytopenia
- Myelofibrosis
- Hemophagocytic syndrome
- Necrosis

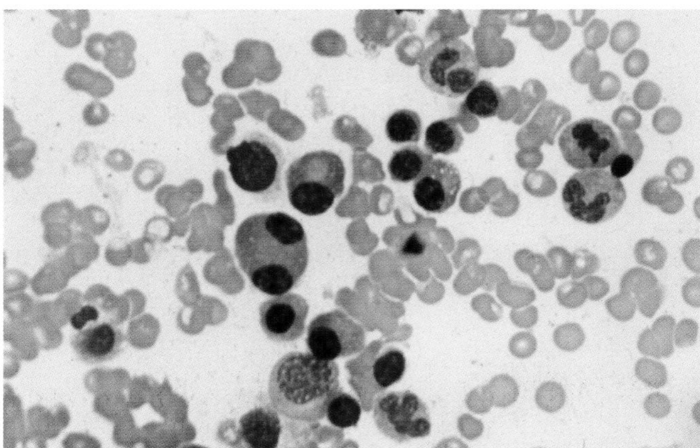

Figure 12-21. Increased reactive plasma cells are seen in the aspirate smear from a patient with rheumatoid arthritis.

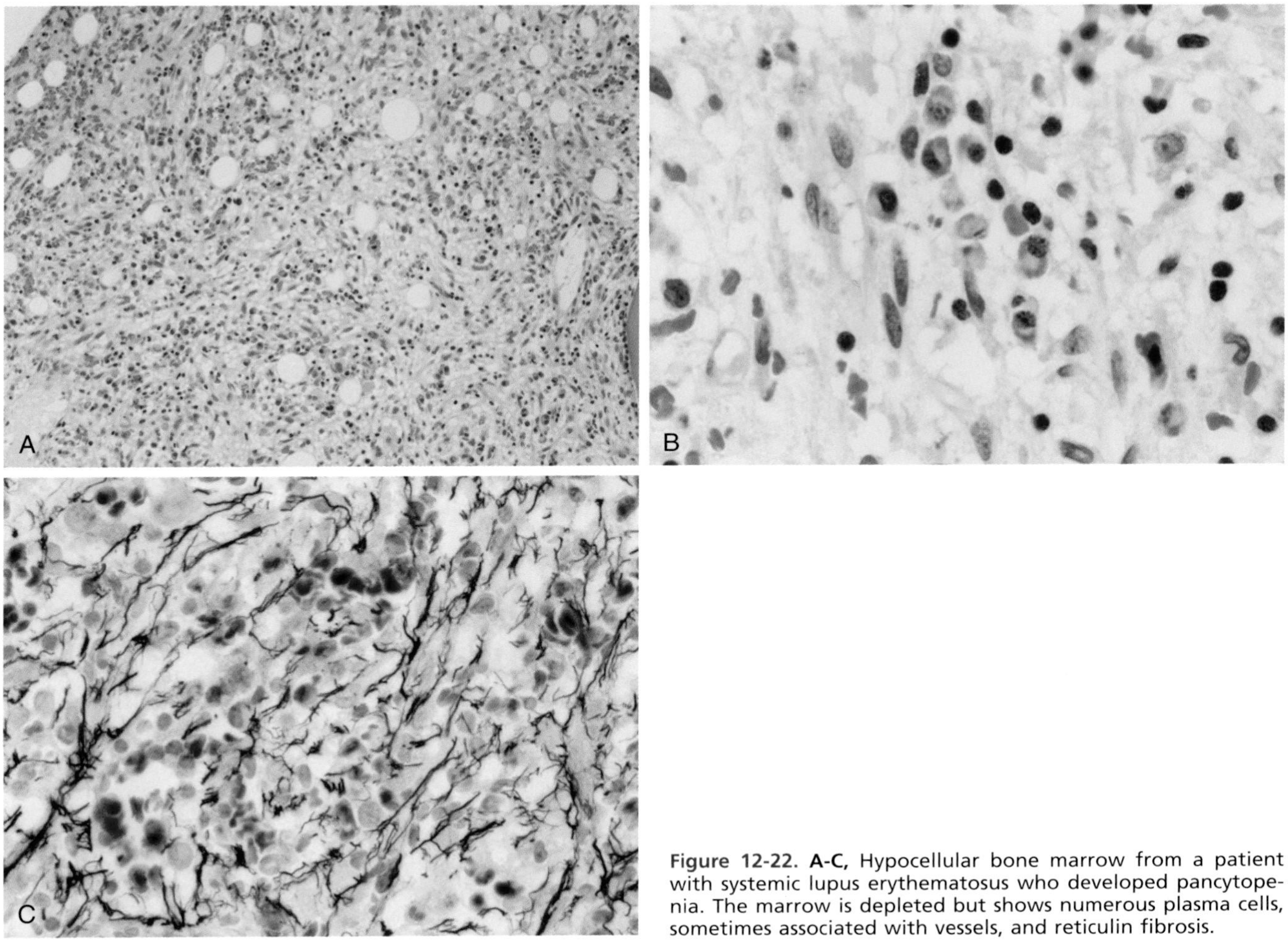

Figure 12-22. A-C, Hypocellular bone marrow from a patient with systemic lupus erythematosus who developed pancytopenia. The marrow is depleted but shows numerous plasma cells, sometimes associated with vessels, and reticulin fibrosis.

be decreased. Gastrointestinal blood loss due to nonsteroidal anti-inflammatory medications may cause iron deficiency anemia. Azathiaprine can cause leukopenia, thrombocytopenia, or pancytopenia and can give the marrow a dysplastic appearance.[155] Methotrexate causes an increase in the mean corpuscular volume in 50% of patients treated with this drug. Leukopenia and thrombocytopenia may also occur. On rare occasions, methotrexate therapy has been associated with pancytopenia, megaloblastic change, and hypocellular marrow.[156] Development of myelodysplasia has also rarely been linked to methotrexate therapy.[157] Alkylating agent chemotherapy is associated with myelodysplastic syndrome and acute myeoloid leukemia due to DNA damage by these drugs.[158,159]

Sarcoidosis

Patients with sarcoidosis may have anemia and leukopenia.[160] Increased eosinophils are common but rarely constitute more than 10% of the peripheral white cell count.[161] Peripheral blood eosinophilia does not correlate with tissue eosinophilia in sarcoidosis.

Bone marrow biopsies contain granulomas in up to 53% of patients.[162] Granulomas can be singular, multiple, or confluent within the marrow biopsy (Fig. 12-23). The granulomas are typically noncaseating and composed of epithelioid histiocytes. Asteroid bodies, Schaumann's bodies, and calcium oxylate crystals may be seen. Stains for acid-fast bacilli and fungi are negative. Hemophagocytosis has been described in rare patients.[163]

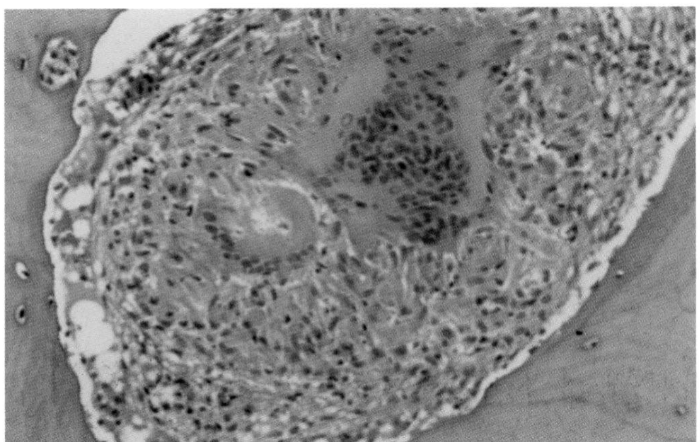

Figure 12-23. Bone marrow core biopsy showing a noncaseating granuloma with a multinucleated giant cell from a patient with sarcoidosis.

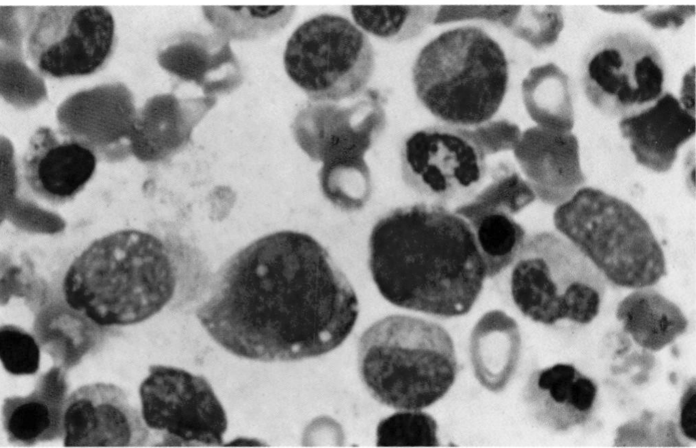

Figure 12-24. Bone marrow aspirate smear showing vacuolated erythroid precursors due to alcohol abuse.

Alcohol Abuse

Ethanol abuse causes numerous hematologic effects that often overlap with the findings in liver disease. Laboratory studies show anemia with macrocytosis due to the direct toxic effect of ethanol, liver disease, or concomitant folate deficiency[164]; stomatocytes may also be seen. Thrombocytopenia is due to the direct toxic effect of ethanol on megakaryocytes or increased splenic sequestration. Leukopenia can be a result of splenic sequestration or a maturation arrest at the promyelocyte stage. Leukoerythroblastosis may be found if alcoholic hepatitis is present.[165,166]

Marrow aspirate smears show a decreased myeloid-to-erythroid ratio, vacuolated erythroid and myeloid precursors,[167,168] megaloblastic change, and multinucleated erythroid precursors (Fig. 12-24).[169] Megakaryocytes may be decreased or absent. Ring sideroblasts are often seen.[170,171] Plasma cells are often increased and stain for cytoplasmic iron, a finding almost exclusively found in chronic alcoholism. Iron stores are often increased. If bleeding leads to iron deficiency, storage iron is absent.

Marrow sections may show decreased cellularity, a rare finding,[172] in addition to those described earlier. Precursor vacuolization, ring sideroblasts, and hypoplasia may resolve with abstinence from alcohol.[173,174] Ring sideroblasts have been reported to persist in patients taking disulfiram.[175]

Hepatic Disease

Numerous peripheral blood and bone marrow findings have been described in patients with liver disease (Box 12-7). Some of these findings overlap with the hematologic effects of alcohol. Macrocytic anemia is often present, with target cells seen. Severe liver disease may lead to hemolytic anemia, in which numerous acanthocytes or spur cells may be seen on the peripheral blood smear (Fig. 12-25). The development of hemolysis is associated with a poor prognosis.[176] Hypersplenism due to portal hypertension leads to pancytopenia.

Hypersplenism is often associated with a hypercellular bone marrow in which all three hematopoietic cell lines are increased. Aplastic anemia has been described in patients with viral hepatitis and after orthotopic liver transplantation.[177,178]

Box 12-7 *Hepatic Disease and the Bone Marrow*

- Macrocytic anemia
- Thrombocytopenia
- Pancytopenia
- Aplastic anemia
- Hypersplenism
- Hemolytic anemia

Renal Disease

Peripheral blood and bone marrow abnormalities in patients with both acute and chronic renal insufficiency have been described. Patients with chronic renal failure are anemic primarily due to erythropoietin deficiency. Other causes include iron and folate deficiency, aluminum overload, hemolysis, and secondary hyperparathyroidism with osteitis fibrosa.[179] Patients also may have a bleeding diathesis due to abnormalities of platelet function. Treatment with recombinant erythropoietin therapy has lessened transfusion dependency in these patients.

Acute renal failure can also lead to impaired erythropoietin production, but anemia is typically related to the disorder causing the renal impairment. For example, hemolytic uremic syndrome, thrombotic thrombocytopenic purpura, and systemic vasculitis cause hemolysis, and red cell fragmentation can be seen on the peripheral blood smear.

The anemia of chronic renal insufficiency is normochromic and normocytic, with burr cells or echinocytes seen on the peripheral blood smear. The white blood cells and platelets are normal in number and morphologically unremarkable.

The erythroid precursors may be slightly decreased on the aspirate smear but are morphologically normal. Biopsy sections may reveal bony abnormalities due to secondary hyperparathyroidism. Bone changes that have been described include peritrabecular fibrosis, widened osteoid seams, and increased bony remodeling (Fig. 12-26). The amount of fibrosis can be extensive and lead to pancytopenia in some cases. The myeloid-to-erythroid ratio is often slightly high, and there is an increase in storage iron. Exogenous erythropoietin decreases the myeloid-to-erythroid ratio owing to an increase in erythroid precursors and an increase in overall marrow

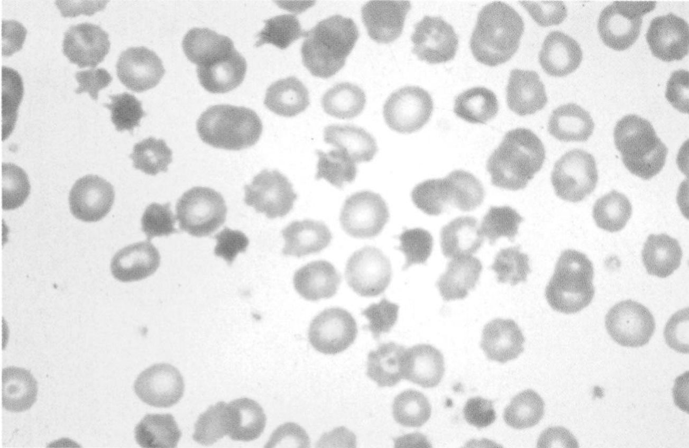

Figure 12-25. Peripheral blood smear with numerous acanthocytes due to severe liver disease.

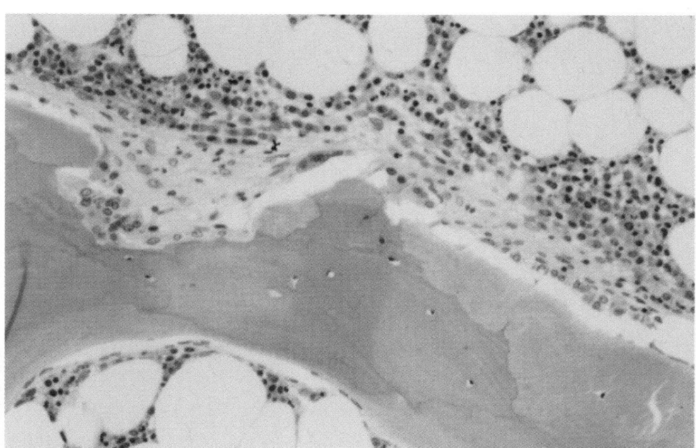

Figure 12-26. Bone marrow core biopsy showing widened osteoid seams and peritrabecular fibrosis in a patient with chronic renal failure.

cellularity.[180,181] Pure red cell aplasia is rarely seen in patients on erythropoietin owing to antierythropoietin antibodies.[182] Patients with extensive marrow fibrosis due to hyperparathyroidism may be resistant to treatment with erythropoietin.[183] Storage iron in the marrow may be completely or relatively depleted after treatment with recombinant erythropoietin, and iron replacement therapy may be needed.[184]

Hypothyroidism

Hematologic findings in hypothyroidism include pancytopenia, reduced red blood cell mass and plasma volume, macrocytosis with or without anemia, decreased reticulocytes, and decreased plasma levels of erythropoietin. Bone marrow biopsy may reveal hypoplasia.[185,186] In myxedema, findings similar to gelatinous transformation of the marrow may be seen.[187]

Hyperthyroidism

The hyperthyroid state causes anemia and neutropenia that reverses with treatment. Microcytosis is common, with or without anemia. Graves' disease may lead to an autoimmune hemolytic anemia. Treatment with propylthiouracil and methimazole can cause agranulocytosis. Exposure to radioactive iodine (I^{131}) has not been shown to increase the risk of leukemia or myelodysplastic syndromes.[188]

CONCLUSION

In this chapter a wide variety of findings in inflammatory, infectious, and metabolic conditions have been discussed. In many cases the findings are nonspecific, but often the marrow findings are indicative of a specific cause. Clinicopathologic correlation is essential to an accurate diagnosis of these disorders.

Pearls and Pitfalls

- Atypical lymphoid aggregates morphologically suggestive of lymphoma are seen in patients with viral infections such as Epstein-Barr virus or hepatitis C virus.
- Marrow dyspoiesis suggestive of a myelodysplastic syndrome can be seen with cytomegalovirus infection or treatment with immunosuppressive agents such as azathiaprine or methotrexate.
- Small clefted lymphocytes, suggestive of follicular lymphoma, may be seen in peripheral blood in *Bordetella pertussis* infection.
- Reactive lymphocytosis is almost always composed predominantly of T cells.
- Persistent polyclonal B-cell lymphocytosis is often characterized by lymphocytes with moderate amounts of cytoplasm and bilobed nuclei; in the bone marrow they may occur in an intrasinusoidal or intravascular pattern.

References can be found on Expert Consult @ www.expertconsult.com

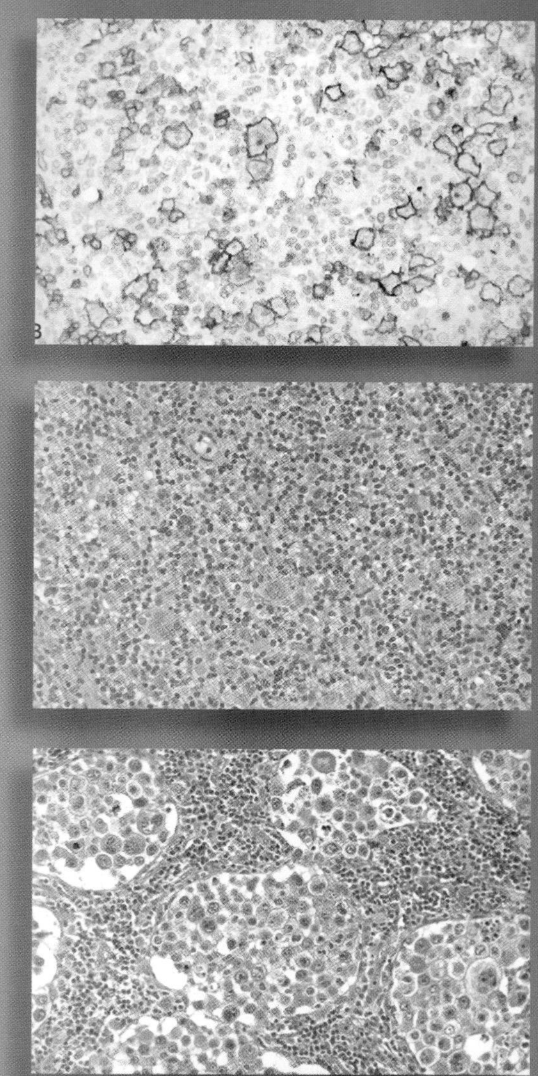

PART III

Lymphoid Neoplasms

Chapter 13

Principles of Classification of Lymphoid Neoplasms

Elaine S. Jaffe, Nancy Lee Harris, and Elias Campo

CHAPTER OUTLINE

HISTORICAL BACKGROUND

The classification of lymphoid neoplasms used in this book is the one published by the World Health Organization (WHO) in *WHO Classification of Tumours of Haematopoietic and Lymphoid Tissues*.[1] Published in 2008, WHO's fourth edition builds on the success of the third edition (2001),[2] defining new entities and proposing solutions for problematic categories. However, the basic principles underlying this classification are essentially unchanged from those of the Revised European American Lymphoma (REAL) classification of lymphoid neoplasms published by the International Lymphoma Study Group (ILSG) in 1994.[3] The REAL classification represented a new paradigm in the classification of lymphoid neoplasms (Fig. 13-1), focusing on the identification of "real" diseases rather than a global theoretical framework such as survival, as had been used in the working formulation,[4] or cellular differentiation, as had been applied in the Kiel[5,6] and Lukes-Collins[7] classification systems. Key events in the evolution of the classification of lymphoid malignancies are summarized in Table 13-1.

The REAL classification defined distinct entities using a constellation of features: morphology, immunophenotype, genetic features, and clinical presentation and course. Each of these elements plays a part, and no one feature takes precedence over the others consistently. For some diseases, morphology alone is highly characteristic, allowing one to confidently make the diagnosis without additional ancillary studies. Most cases of chronic lymphocytic leukemia (CLL) or follicular lymphoma (FL) presenting in lymph nodes fall into this category. For other diseases, knowledge of the underlying genetics may be essential, such as in the diagnosis of anaplastic lymphoma kinase (ALK)–positive anaplastic large cell lymphoma (ALCL) (Fig. 13-2). The relative importance of each of these features varies among diseases, depending on the state of current knowledge, and there is no one "gold standard" by which all diseases are defined. Still, lineage is a defining feature and forms the basis for the classification system's structure, recognizing B-cell, T-cell, and natural killer (NK)–cell neoplasms. Additionally, a basic premise is the distinction between precursor lymphoid neoplasms and those derived from mature lymphoid cells.

In the 20th century the field of immunology shed light on the functional and immunophenotypic complexity of the immune system.[8] Traditional morphologic approaches were recognized as insufficient to decipher the many benign and malignant cellular components of lymphoid malignancies. Monoclonal antibody technology provided a seemingly endless array of immunophenotypic markers that could delineate the various cells types,[9] and technologic advances soon permitted the immunohistochemical detection of most relevant antigens in routinely processed formalin-fixed, paraffin-embedded sections.[10] Many lymphoid malignancies have characteristic immunophenotypic profiles, but even among some very homogeneous entities, immunophenotypic variation may be seen. For instance, not all cases of CLL are $CD5^+$ and $CD23^+$; not all FLs are $BCL2^+$ or $CD10^+$. CD5 may be expressed in otherwise classic FL. Expression of ALK is essential for the diagnosis of ALK^+ ALCL, but it is also expressed in ALK^+ large B-cell lymphoma and some myofibroblastic

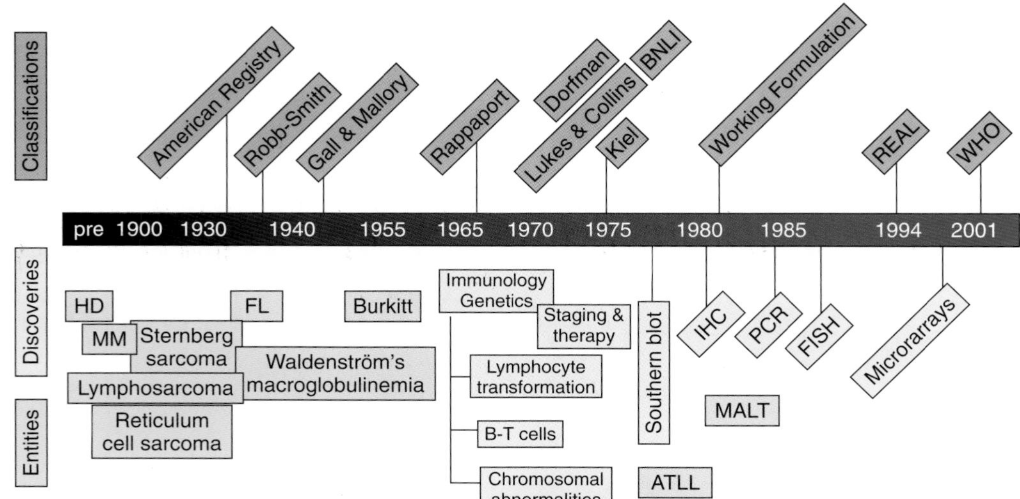

Figure 13-1. Diagram illustrating advances in the classification of lymphoid malignancies (*above the time line*) and corresponding events (*below the time line*) related to insights into the biology of lymphoid cells, the recognition of significant clinicopathologic entities, and advances in treatment and clinical evaluation. Technologic advances identifying the heterogeneity of lymphoid cells in the 1960s and 1970s precipitated a flurry of new classification systems that related lymphoid malignancies to the normal cells of the immune system. Improvements in the treatment and clinical evaluation of patients with lymphoid malignancies facilitated the recognition of clinical correlations and made accurate classification essential for patient management. The Revised European American Lymphoma (REAL) and World Health Organization (WHO) classifications represented a new perspective, emphasizing the recognition of disease entities and integrating morphologic, immunophenotypic, molecular, and clinical data. This multiparameter approach provides objective criteria for diagnosis, facilitating reproducibility and consensus. BNLI, British National Lymphoma Investigation; FISH, fluorescence in situ hybridization; FL, follicular lymphoma; HD, Hodgkin's disease; IHC, immunohistochemistry in frozen and, later, paraffin-embedded sections; MALT, marginal zone lymphoma of mucosa-associated lymphoid tissue; MM, multiple myeloma; PCR, polymerase chain reaction studies for rearrangements of immunoglobulin and T-cell receptor genes.

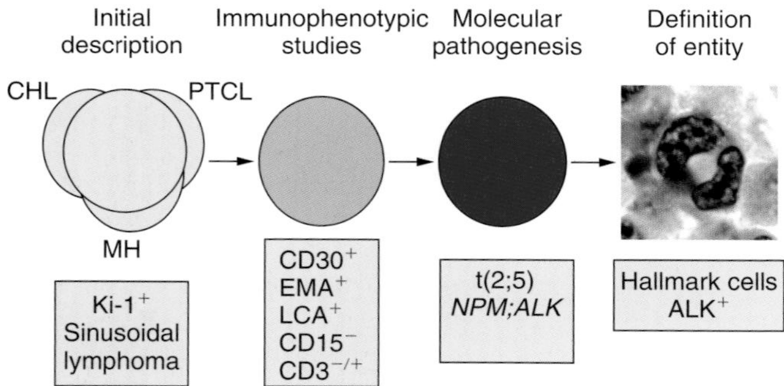

Figure 13-2. The recognition of anaplastic lymphoma kinase (ALK)–positive anaplastic large cell lymphoma (ALCL) is emblematic of the stepwise advances in the identification of new disease entities. ALCL was first recognized by distinctive morphologic features. The identification of a characteristic immunophenotype, with strong expression of CD30, led to better recognition of the entity and facilitated studies to determine its molecular pathogenesis. Identification of the *NPM/ALK* translocation, with high levels of ALK expression, led to the development of polyclonal and, later, monoclonal antibodies to identify ALK in formalin-fixed, paraffin-embedded sections. These tools, when incorporated into daily practice, both broadened and narrowed the original concept of ALCL as a morphologic entity. Small cell variants were included, whereas highly anaplastic and Hodgkin's-like forms were largely excluded from the disease spectrum. CHL, classical Hodgkin's lymphoma; MH, malignant histiocytosis; PTCL, peripheral T-cell lymphoma.

tumors in children. Thus, knowledge of the immunophenotype is a highly effective tool, but one that must be used in context.

There has been equally dramatic progress in understanding the genetics of lymphoid malignancies. Recurrent cytogenetic abnormalities have been identified for many lymphoma subtypes. The first to be recognized were the t(14;18)(q32;q21) of FL and the t(8;14)(q24;q32) of Burkitt's lymphoma (BL).[11-13] Subsequent studies led to the cloning of the genes involved in these translocations. The laboratories of Leder and Croce in 1982 both identified *MYC* as the gene that was translocated into the immunoglobulin genes in human BL[14,15]; other similar discoveries soon followed, such as *BCL2/IGH@* in FL[16] and *CCND1/IGH@* in mantle cell lymphoma.[17,18] The most common paradigm for translocations involving the immunoglobulin heavy-chain gene, *IGH@* at 14q24, is that a cellular proto-oncogene comes under the influence of the *IGH@* promoter. There are also less frequent but parallel alterations involving the T-cell receptor genes in T-cell malignancies.

The REAL classification recognized the importance of genetic abnormalities in defining disease entities. However, it has become clear that a purely genetic approach to defining diseases is not feasible. Although the *MYC* translocation is universally present in BLs, *MYC* translocations involving the immunoglobulin genes are found as either secondary or, less commonly, primary genetic abnormalities in other lymphoid malignancies, including some diffuse large B-cell lymphomas (DLBCLs), plasmablastic malignancies, and some cases of B-lymphoblastic lymphoma/leukemia. Similarly, *BCL2/IGH@* is found in only 85% to 90% of FLs and is present in up to 25% to 30% of de novo DLBCLs with no prior evidence of FL.

Table 13-1 Milestones in the Evolution of the Classification of Lymphoid Neoplasms

Year	Reference	Principal Contributors	Event
1806	73	Alibert	Clinical description of mycosis fungoides
1828	113	Carswell	"Cancer cerebriformis of the lymphatic glands and spleen"—first case of what was later recognized as Hodgkin's disease
1832	113	Hodgkin	"On some morbid appearances of the absorbent glands and spleen"—clinical report of what would later be known as *Hodgkin's disease*
1845 1863	114	Virchow	Description of both leukemia and lymphosarcoma
1865	113	Wilks	Proposal of eponym "Hodgkin's disease"
1898 1902	113	Sternberg Reed	Definition of microscopic features of neoplastic cell of Hodgkin's disease, establishing an accurate microscopic description of the disease—the first lymphoma to be defined histologically
1914 1928 1930	114	Ewing Oberling Roulet	Description of "reticulosarcomas" (reticular cell sarcomas) of bone and lymphoid organs
1916	114	Sternberg	Description of "leukosarkomatose," a process with characteristic features of precursor T-lymphoblastic lymphoma
1925 1927	115-117	Brill Symmers	Description of "giant follicle hyperplasia" and "follicular lymphadenopathy"—processes with features of follicular lymphoma and florid follicular hyperplasia
1934	114	Callender	American Registry of Pathology (AFIP) classification
1938	114	Robb-Smith	Robb-Smith classification of reticulosis and reticulosarcoma
1941 1942	118, 119	Gall Mallory	Accurate description of follicular lymphoma and proposal of first modern lymphoma classification system
1947	114	Jackson Parker	Proposal of classification of Hodgkin's disease
1958	120	Burkitt	Description of clinical syndrome of Burkitt's lymphoma in African children
1960	121	Nowell	Phytohemagglutinin used to "transform" lymphocytes in vitro
1961	122	O'Conor	Histopathologic description of Burkitt's lymphoma
1964	123	Epstein	Description of viral particles (Epstein-Barr virus) in cultured cells from Burkitt's lymphoma
1956 1966	124, 125	Rappaport	Proposal of alternative classification for "non-Hodgkin's" lymphoma
1966	126	Lukes, Butler	Proposal of modern classification of Hodgkin's lymphoma
1972	127	Stein	Identification of high levels of IgM in "histiocytic" lymphomas
1973	114	Lennert	Lennert and colleagues meet to form European Lymphoma Club, predecessor of European Association for Haematopathology
1974	128	Lennert	Proposal of Kiel classification of lymphoma
1974	129	Taylor, Mason	Immunohistochemical detection of immunoglobulin in cells in formalin-fixed, paraffin-embedded sections
1974	130	Jaffe	Identification of complement receptors on cells of "nodular lymphoma," linking them to lymphoid follicle
1975	4	NCI	Failed consensus meeting of proponents of lymphoma classification systems, leading to working formulation study by NCI
1975	131	Southern	Development of Southern blot technique to separate and analyze DNA fragments
1976	11	Klein	Identification of t(8;14)(q24;q32) as recurrent translocation in Burkitt's lymphoma
1979	12	Fukuhara, Rowley	Identification of t(14;18)(q32;q21) as recurrent translocation in "lymphocytic lymphoma" (follicular lymphoma)
1979	132	McMichael	Discovery of first monoclonal antibody to human leukocyte differentiation antigen, later defined as CD1a
1980-1982	133-136	Stein, Poppema, Warnke, Mason	Characterization of lymphoid cells by immunohistochemistry on frozen and paraffin sections
1982	137	Bernard, Boumsell	First international workshop on human leukocyte differentiation antigens
1982	14, 15	Leder, Dalla-Favera, Croce	Cloning of *MYC* gene; identification of *MYC* and *IGH@* as reciprocal partners in t(8;14)
1982	13	Yunis	Identification of recurrent translocations in follicular lymphoma, Burkitt's lymphoma, and chronic lymphocytic leukemia
1982	4	Berard, Dorfman, DeVita, Rosenberg	Publication of NCI-sponsored working formulation for clinical classification of non-Hodgkin's lymphomas
1985	138	Mullis	Development of polymerase chain reaction technique for amplification of specific DNA sequences
1986	139	Cremer	Development of in situ hybridization techniques for analysis of chromosome aberrations in interphase nuclei
1991-1992	140	Isaacson, Stein	Founding of ILSG and publication of consensus report on mantle cell lymphoma

Continued on following page

Table 13-1 Milestones in the Evolution of the Classification of Lymphoid Neoplasms (Continued)

Year	Reference	Principal Contributors	Event
1994	141	Kuppers, Rajewsky	Identification of IgH@ gene rearrangements in Reed-Sternberg cells picked from tissue sections of classical Hodgkin's lymphoma
1994	3	Harris, ILSG	Publication of REAL classification of lymphoid neoplasms
1997	142	Armitage	Validation of REAL classification by International Lymphoma Classification Project study
2000	143	Staudt	Application of gene expression profiling to human lymphomas
2001	2	EAHP & SH	Publication of WHO monograph: *Pathology and Genetics: Tumours of Hematopoietic and Lymphoid Tissues* (3rd ed.)
2008	1	EAHP & SH	Publication of *WHO Classification of Tumours of Haematopoietic and Lymphoid Tissues* (4th ed.)

AFIP, Armed Forces Institute of Pathology; EAHP & SH, European Association for Haematopathology and the Society for Haematopathology; ILSG, International Lymphoma Study Group; NCI, National Cancer Institute; REAL, Revised European American Lymphoma; WHO, World Health Organization.

Finally, the inclusion of clinical criteria was one of the novel aspects of the ILSG approach.[19] The REAL classification recognized that the site of presentation is often a signpost for underlying biologic distinctions, such as in extranodal lymphomas of mucosa-associated lymphoid tissue (MALT),[20] primary mediastinal large B-cell lymphoma, and many types of T/NK-cell lymphomas. The ILSG appreciated that accurate diagnosis cannot take place in a vacuum and requires knowledge of the clinical history, because biologically distinct entities may appear cytologically similar. Integration of clinical features is an essential aspect in the definition of disease entities and in accurate diagnosis in daily practice. The pathologist must be provided with relevant clinical details to arrive at a correct diagnosis, and it is the pathologist's responsibility to insist on sufficient clinical data if it is not provided. The subsequent chapters in this part emphasize the pertinent clinical features of each disease entity discussed.

It is also evident that clinical features are important prognostic indicators, and in many instances, the treatment approach chosen is based on the clinical setting in conjunction with the pathologic diagnosis. For instance, some patients with FL can be followed with a watch-and-wait approach, whereas in others a heavy tumor burden at diagnosis mandates immediate therapy. Response to therapy is influenced not only by underlying clinical features but also by biologic and prognostic factors. Cytologic grade varies in many disease entities and is discussed in the chapters that follow. Other prognostic factors are based on tumor cell biology, such as ZAP-70 expression in CLL,[21,22] or host factors, such as the tumor microenvironment.[23] For this reason, it is not possible to stratify lymphoma subtypes in a linear fashion according to their clinical aggressiveness. The pathologist and clinician are part of a management team that determines the therapeutic approach in each case.

The REAL classification was based on the building of consensus, and it recognized that a comprehensive classification system was beyond the experience of any one individual. The 19 members of the ILSG contributed their diverse perspectives to achieve a unified point of view. In addition, the ILSG made the decision to base its classification exclusively on published data; thus, for an entity to be included in the REAL classification, it had to be validated in more than one publication.

Recognition that the development of classification systems should be a cooperative effort was expanded with the third edition of the WHO classification.[2] It represented the first true worldwide consensus classification of hematologic malignancies and was the culmination of the efforts of a 7-member steering committee, 11 pathology committee chairs, 75 author contributors, and 44 clinician participants in a clinical advisory committee meeting. In 2008 the fourth edition of the WHO classification involved the efforts of 138 authors and two clinical advisory committees comprising 62 clinical specialists with expertise in lymphoid and myeloid disorders. The clinical advisory committee meetings were organized around a series of issues, including disease definitions, nomenclature, grading, and clinical relevance. As with the third edition, the effort was coordinated by the European Association for Haematopathology and the Society for Hematopathology, led by the eight editors who served as a steering committee.

Disease definitions are not static, and new disease entities or variants continue to be recognized. Some of these new entities were incorporated into the fourth edition of the WHO classification and are discussed in this chapter. For example, recent studies have drawn attention to the biologic overlap between classical Hodgkin's lymphoma (CHL) and DLBCLs. Similarly, there is a greater appreciation of the borders between BL and DLBCL. Strategies for the management of these borderline lesions are proposed. Additionally, age-specific and site-specific factors play an important role in the definition of several new entities, which also have biologic underpinnings. The 2008 WHO classification draws attention to early events in lymphomagenesis. These lesions help delineate the earliest steps in neoplastic transformation and generally mandate a conservative therapeutic approach. The 2001 classification was rapidly adopted for clinical trials and successfully served as a common language for scientists comparing genetic and functional data. The modifications made in the 2008 classification are the result of this successful partnership among pathologists, clinicians, and biologists, but they are only a steppingstone to the future.

EMERGING CONCEPTS: 2008 WORLD HEALTH ORGANIZATION CLASSIFICATION

Changes in the classification of lymphoid malignancies have largely resulted from new insights derived from clinical and laboratory research to better define heterogeneous or ambiguous categories of disease. The areas of modification relate to several discrete topics: (1) a greater appreciation of early or in situ lesions that challenge us to define the earliest steps in neoplastic transformation; (2) the recognition of age as a defining feature of some diseases in both the young and the elderly; (3) a further appreciation and recognition of the site-specific impact on disease definitions; and (4) a recognition of borderline categories in which current morphologic, immunophenotypic, and genetic criteria do not permit sharp delineations into existing disease categories. Finally, the fourth edition incorporates some provisional entities for which sufficient data are lacking, either clinically or biologically, leading to uncertainty in definitional criteria.

Continued challenges remain in the stratification and subclassification of major disease groups, including FL and DLBCL. Genomic and genetic studies have led to significant new insights with the identification of biologic and clinical subgroups. Nevertheless the authors concluded that the application of this research to clinical practice on a daily basis was premature, because many of the relevant techniques are not yet available in the clinical laboratory. The thematic approach to peripheral T-cell lymphoma (PTCL) is unchanged. Some diseases are defined based on clinical, pathologic, immunophenotypic, or genetic parameters, whereas others are provisionally defined as PTCL, not otherwise specified (NOS).

The 2008 classification incorporated minor changes in terminology, reflecting our better understanding of disease entities and their relationship to the immune system. For example, the authors concluded that the modifier *B-cell* was no longer required for nodal, extranodal, or splenic marginal zone lymphomas (MZLs) because there are no T-cell marginal zone neoplasms (Box 13-1). The modifier *B-cell* had previously been eliminated from CLL. In addition, the names for the precursor lymphoid neoplasms were simplified to eliminate redundancy; thus, the modifier *precursor* is no longer required for either B- or T-lymphoblastic leukemia/lymphoma because the term *lymphoblastic* carries this meaning.

Box 13-1 *WHO 2008: Mature B-Cell Neoplasms*

- Chronic lymphocytic leukemia–small lymphocytic lymphoma
- B-cell prolymphocytic leukemia
- Splenic marginal zone lymphoma
- Hairy cell leukemia
  - *Splenic lymphoma/leukemia, unclassifiable*
  - *Splenic diffuse red pulp small B-cell lymphoma**
- *Hairy cell leukemia variant**
- Lymphoplasmacytic lymphoma
  - Waldenström's macroglobulinemia
- Heavy-chain diseases
  - Alpha heavy-chain disease
  - Gamma heavy-chain disease
  - Mu heavy-chain disease
- Plasma cell myeloma
- Solitary plasmacytoma of bone
- Extraosseous plasmacytoma
- Extranodal marginal zone lymphoma of mucosa-associated lymphoid tissue (MALT lymphoma)
- Nodal marginal zone lymphoma
  - *Pediatric-type nodal marginal zone lymphoma*
- Follicular lymphoma
  - *Pediatric-type follicular lymphoma*
- Primary cutaneous follicle center lymphoma
- Mantle cell lymphoma
- Diffuse large B-cell lymphoma (DLBCL), not otherwise specified
- T-cell/histiocyte-rich large B-cell lymphoma
- *DLBCL associated with chronic inflammation*
- *Epstein-Barr virus–positive DLBCL of the elderly*
- Lymphomatoid granulomatosis
- Primary mediastinal (thymic) large B-cell lymphoma
- Intravascular large B-cell lymphoma
- *Primary cutaneous DLBCL, leg type*
- ALK^+ large B-cell lymphoma
- Plasmablastic lymphoma
- Primary effusion lymphoma
- *Large B-cell lymphoma arising in human herpesvirus 8–associated multicentric Castleman's disease*
- Burkitt's lymphoma
- *B-cell lymphoma, unclassifiable, with features intermediate between DLBCL and Burkitt's lymphoma*
- *B-cell lymphoma, unclassifiable, with features intermediate between DLBCL and classical Hodgkin's lymphoma*
- Hodgkin's lymphoma
  - Nodular lymphocyte-predominant Hodgkin's lymphoma
  - Classical Hodgkin's lymphoma
  - Nodular sclerosis classical Hodgkin's lymphoma
  - Lymphocyte-rich classical Hodgkin's lymphoma
  - Mixed cellularity classical Hodgkin's lymphoma
  - Lymphocyte-depleted classical Hodgkin's lymphoma

*Provisional entities or provisional subtypes of other neoplasms.
Diseases in italic are newly included in the 2008 World Health Organization (WHO) classification.
Adapted from Swerdlow SH, Campo E, Harris NL, et al, eds. *WHO Classification of Tumours of Haematopoietic and Lymphoid Tissues.* Lyon, France: IARC; 2008.

Early Events in Lymphoid Neoplasia: Borders of Malignancy

The multistep pathway of tumorigenesis has parallels in most organ systems and is best documented in the evolution of colonic adenocarcinoma.[24] Histologic progression is a well-recognized feature of many lymphoid neoplasms, but the earliest events in lymphoid neoplasia are difficult to recognize. In fact, the lymphoid system historically has had no recognized "benign neoplasms," a fact that may be related to the propensity of lymphoid cells to circulate and not remain confined to a single anatomic site.[25] The 2008 WHO classification addresses the problem of clonal expansions of B cells or, less often, T cells that appear to have limited potential for histologic or clinical progression.

The use of flow cytometry on a routine basis led to the recognition that populations of monoclonal $CD5^+$ B cells could be identified in the healthy, unaffected first-degree relatives of patients with CLL and in 3% of healthy adults older than 40 years.[26,27] Many of these clones have genetic abnormalities associated with CLL, including 13q14 deletion and trisomy 12, similar to sporadic CLL.[28] Nevertheless, only a small percentage of these patients progress to clinically significant CLL, at a rate of less than 2% per year. This condition has been termed *monoclonal B-cell lymphocytosis* (MBL) and should be distinguished from CLL. The minimal diagnostic criteria for CLL have been modified to require at least 5×10^9/L of monoclonal B cells in the peripheral blood or evidence of extramedullary tissue involvement. A level below this threshold is considered MBL. One group suggested that the cutoff point between MBL and CLL should be increased to a B-cell count of 11×10^9 L.[29] The data suggest that most patients ultimately diagnosed with CLL go through a prolonged prodromal phase, with evidence of the circulating clone found many years before diagnosis.[30] Thus, at present the distinction between MBL and CLL is largely one of practice guidelines. There are no proven biologic parameters that can distinguish MBL from CLL or identify which patients will progress to clinically significant disease more rapidly. However, a recent study identified differences in the immunoglobulin gene repertoire in cases of MBL as compared with both mutated and nonmutated CLL, suggesting that such biologic differences may exist and that not all MBL cases are destined to progress.[31]

Another area that challenges us to define *lymphoma* involves early events in FL. Up to 70% of normal, healthy adults have circulating clonal memory B cells with the t(14;18)(q32;q21) translocation; however, these cells presumably lack other genetic alterations necessary for the development of malignant behavior.[32,33] The tissue equivalent of this process is thought to be in situ FL, also termed *intrafollicular neoplasia* in the WHO classification.[34] These lesions are often discovered incidentally and are composed of isolated, scattered follicles colonized by monoclonal t(14;18) B cells overexpressing both BCL2 and CD10 within an otherwise uninvolved lymph node. Rarely the in situ FL lesion is discovered in lymph nodes involved by a clonally unrelated process.[35] Further evaluation reveals evidence of FL at another site in about half the patients, but in approximately 50% of cases, progression to FL does not occur, at least with current follow-up. The challenge is to distinguish true in situ FL from lymph nodes with partial involvement by FL due to the naturally occurring dissemination of the disease. In cases of partial involvement by FL, many or most of the follicles are involved, but definitive criteria for this distinction are lacking.

A possibly related condition is localized FL presenting as small polyps in the duodenum; these duodenal FLs rarely if ever progress to nodal or systemic disease.[36,37] Duodenal FL cells express intestinal homing receptors that may retain the clonal B cells within the intestinal mucosa.[38] An in situ form of mantle cell lymphoma, with cyclin D1$^+$ cells restricted to mantle zones of reactive follicles in lymph nodes with preserved architecture, has been described in a few isolated cases, although little is known about the clinical outcome of this lesion.[39,40] Other instances of clonal proliferations with limited potential for clinical aggressiveness may be encountered. This phenomenon is exemplified by Epstein-Barr virus (EBV)–driven B-cell proliferations arising in the setting of altered immunity, but it also pertains to early gastric extranodal marginal zone (MALT) lymphomas lacking secondary genetic alterations. These lymphomas appear to be dependent on continued antigen activation from *Helicobacter pylori* and may regress with only antibiotic therapy.[41] In the T-cell system, lymphomatoid papulosis, part of the spectrum of primary cutaneous CD30$^+$ T-cell lymphoproliferative disorders, is a clonal T-cell proliferation that also has limited malignant potential.[42-44]

The third edition of the WHO classification included a category of B-cell or T-cell proliferations of uncertain malignant potential. This category encompassed conditions such as lymphomatoid papulosis or lymphomatoid granulomatosis, in which spontaneous regression may occur. However, the decision was made to eliminate this designation because a broader view of lymphoid malignancies indicates that proliferations of uncertain malignant potential are encountered within many well-recognized disease entities. This is especially true of some pediatric lymphomas (discussed later). It is incumbent on the pathologist and clinician to be aware of the spectrum of disease and to manage each case appropriately, taking into consideration biologic and clinical factors. These early events of lymphomagenesis can also provide instructive models of lymphocyte homing and migration.

Age as a Feature of Disease Definition

The 2008 WHO classification uses patient age as a defining feature in a number of newly incorporated disease entities. For example, within the categories of FL and nodal MZLs there are distinctive variants that present almost exclusively in the pediatric age group and differ from their adult counterparts clinically and biologically. The pediatric variant of FL usually presents with localized disease and is of high histologic grade. These lymphomas lack *BCL2/IGH@* translocations and do not express BCL2 protein. They may present at nodal or extranodal sites (testis, gastrointestinal tract, Waldeyer's ring).[45] Pediatric FLs have a good prognosis, although the optimal management has not yet been determined.[45-47] A challenging area of diagnosis involves rare cases of florid reactive follicular hyperplasia in children that have been reported to contain clonal populations of CD10$^+$ germinal center B cells yet do not progress to overt lymphoma.[48]

Nodal MZLs in children, although monoclonal at the immunophenotypic and genetic levels, also appear to have a low risk of progression.[49] Most patients present with stage I disease and have a low risk of recurrence following conservative therapy. Pediatric nodal MZLs are often associated with marked follicular hyperplasia and changes resembling progressive transformation of germinal centers, and the distinction from pediatric FL is sometimes problematic. Because there is no molecular hallmark for adult nodal MZLs, knowledge of the biologic underpinnings of this diagnosis is lacking. Interestingly, pediatric nodal MZLs are relatively more common in males, in contrast to the female predominance in adult nodal MZLs.

The 2008 classification also recognizes two rare EBV-associated T-cell diseases: systemic EBV$^+$ T-cell lymphoproliferative disease of childhood and hydroa vacciniforme–like lymphoma (Box 13-2). These diseases occur almost entirely in children and primarily in those of Asian origin, although they are also seen in ethnic populations from Mexico and Central and South America. Both types of lesions have been included under the broad heading of "chronic active EBV infection" in the Japanese literature[50] and are derived from EBV$^+$ clonal T cells.[51] Hydroa vacciniforme–like lymphoma has a chronic and protracted clinical course, with remissions often occurring during the winter months. It may resolve spontaneously in adult life or progress to more systemic and aggressive disease. Systemic EBV$^+$ T-cell lymphoproliferative disease is highly aggressive, with survival measured in weeks to months, and is usually associated with a hemophagocytic syndrome.[52]

By contrast, some diseases occur most often in those of advanced age, such as EBV$^+$ DLBCL of the elderly, which likely arises because of decreased immune surveillance.[53] These lymphomas are clinically aggressive and occur more often in extranodal than nodal sites. The neoplastic cells may

Box 13-2 *WHO 2008: Mature T-Cell and NK-Cell Neoplasms*

- T-cell prolymphocytic leukemia
- T-cell large granular lymphocytic leukemia
- Chronic lymphoproliferative disorder of NK cells*
- Aggressive NK-cell leukemia
- *Systemic EBV⁺ T-cell lymphoproliferative disease of childhood (associated with chronic active EBV infection)*
- *Hydroa vacciniforme–like lymphoma*
- Adult T-cell leukemia/lymphoma
- Extranodal NK/T-cell lymphoma, nasal type
- *Enteropathy-associated T-cell lymphoma*
- Hepatosplenic T-cell lymphoma
- Subcutaneous panniculitis-like T-cell lymphoma
- Mycosis fungoides
- Sézary syndrome
- Primary cutaneous $CD30^+$ T-cell lymphoproliferative disorder
  - Lymphomatoid papulosis
  - Primary cutaneous anaplastic large cell lymphoma
- *Primary cutaneous aggressive epidermotropic $CD8^+$ cytotoxic T-cell lymphoma**
- *Primary cutaneous gamma-delta T-cell lymphoma*
- *Primary cutaneous small/medium $CD4^+$ T-cell lymphoma**
- Peripheral T-cell lymphoma, not otherwise specified
- Angioimmunoblastic T-cell lymphoma
- Anaplastic large cell lymphoma, ALK^+
- *Anaplastic large cell lymphoma, ALK^-**

*Provisional entities or provisional subtypes of other neoplasms.
Diseases in italic are newly included in the 2008 World Health Organization (WHO) classification.
ALK, anaplastic lymphoma kinase; EBV, Epstein-Barr virus; NK, natural killer.
Adapted from Swerdlow SH, Campo E, Harris NL, et al, eds. *WHO Classification of Tumours of Haematopoietic and Lymphoid Tissues.* Lyon, France: IARC Press; 2008.

mimic Hodgkin/Reed-Sternberg cells and exhibit marked pleomorphism, with a broader range of morphology than typically seen in CHL. Necrosis and an inflammatory background are common. EBV^+ DLBCL of the elderly should be distinguished from reactive hyperplasia associated with EBV, also encountered in the elderly, which usually has a benign outcome and spontaneous regression in most patients.[54,55]

Although the lesions mentioned in this section cluster in particular age groups—either the very young or the very old—it is unlikely that these entities are entirely age restricted. Some cases of pediatric-type FL may be seen in adults, and EBV^+ DLBCL is sometimes seen in individuals younger than 60 years. However, age has been useful in identifying these relatively uncommon forms of lymphoma.

AGGRESSIVE B-CELL LYMPHOMAS AND BORDERLINE MALIGNANCIES

In the past 20 years there has been a greater appreciation of morphologic and immunophenotypic overlap between CHL and some large B-cell lymphomas—usually primary mediastinal large B-cell lymphoma (PMBL) and mediastinal nodular sclerosis CHL.[56,57] The use of gene expression profiling further confirmed a biologic relationship.[58,59] Prior case reports had identified cases of primary mediastinal large B-cell lymphoma followed by CHL or vice versa, or other cases in which both lymphomas were composite in the same tumor mass.[60] Notably, both neoplasms occur in young adults and involve the mediastinum. In most biopsies one or the other diagnosis can be made, but in some cases the lymphoma exhibits transitional features that defy traditional diagnostic categories; these tumors have been termed *gray zone lymphomas.* The 2008 WHO classification recognizes a provisional category of B-cell neoplasms with features intermediate between DLBCL and CHL.[60,61] These tumors occur predominantly in young men and appear to be more aggressive than either primary mediastinal large B-cell lymphoma or nodular sclerosis CHL.[62] There are other settings in which the distinction between DLBCL and CHL is challenging. For example, some EBV-associated B-cell lymphomas may exhibit features that closely resemble or mimic CHL.[63] The borderline category should be used sparingly but is appropriate when a distinction between CHL and DLBCL is not possible.

The 2008 WHO classification recognizes a group of high-grade B-cell lymphomas that are not readily classified as either BL or DLBCL. This provisional category is termed *B-cell lymphoma, unclassifiable, with features intermediate between DLBCL and BL.* These rare lymphomas, which occur predominantly in adults, have a germinal center phenotype that resembles BL, but they exhibit atypical cytologic features for BL.[64] Also included are cases with translocations of both *MYC* and *BCL2* ("double hit"). Although gene expression profiling may show similarities with classic BL,[65,66] other data, including a very aggressive clinical course, support segregation from BL.[67]

The 2008 WHO classification eliminated the variant category of *atypical BL*, which had been included in the 2001 classification.[2] Thus, a case with the typical BL phenotype ($CD20^+$, $BCL6^+$, $CD10^+$, $BCL2^-$) and genotype (so-called *MYC*-simple or *MYC/IG* in the absence of other major cytogenetic anomalies) may be classified as BL even if there is some cytologic variability in the morphology of the neoplastic cells. Likewise, cases of otherwise typical DLBCL with a very high growth fraction should not be included in this "intermediate" group.[68] It should be noted that a *MYC* translocation does not mandate a diagnosis of either BL or the borderline category, and *MYC* translocations may be found in cases of otherwise typical DLBCL.[65,66] Thus, the final diagnosis rests on the integration of morphologic, immunophenotypic, and molecular data.

Other changes in the classification of aggressive B-cell lymphomas recognize the importance of site or clinical factors in defining variants of DLBCL. The age-associated subtype EBV^+ DLBCL of the elderly has already been mentioned.[69] DLBCL associated with chronic inflammation is another EBV^+ DLBCL arising in a specialized clinical setting; it is most often associated with long-standing pyothorax,[70] but it can also occur in cases of prolonged chronic inflammation, such as chronic osteomyelitis, or reaction to metallic implants in a joint or bone.[71] Other site-specific categories are primary DLBCL of the central nervous system[72] and primary cutaneous DLBCL, leg type.[73] Interestingly, the leg type of primary cutaneous DLBCL exhibits an activated B-cell (ABC) gene expression profile in most cases.[74] Both primary central nervous system DLBCL and other DLBCLs arising in privileged sites, such as the testis, may exhibit distinctive biologic features, such as loss of human leukocyte antigen (HLA) class I and II expression.[75-77] One might expect that in the future, biologic and genetic parameters will drive the subclassification of DLBCL rather than clinical features. However, clinical features remain important in clinical management.[72] In addition, primary central nervous system DLBCL has a distinctive gene expression signature that may continue to justify it as a separate entity.[78,79]

Despite the identification of new subtypes of DLBCL, we are still left with a large group of DLBCLs lacking pathologic features that can stratify them in terms of predicting prognosis or response to therapy. These are designated *DLBCL, NOS* in the WHO classification. Stratification according to gene expression profiling as germinal center B-cell (GCB) versus activated B-cell (ABC) types has proven prognostic value.[80] However, the GCB and ABC subtypes were not formally incorporated into the classification owing to the lack of availability of gene expression profiling as a routine diagnostic test and the imperfect correlation of immunohistochemical surrogate markers with genomic studies. Moreover, these designations do not direct therapy, although recent studies suggest that ABC versus GCB lymphomas exhibit differential sensitivity to certain drugs.[81] Further development of targeted therapies and recognition of additional markers of clinical behavior will likely result in modifications to this category in the future.[82,83]

Several aggressive B-cell lymphomas have an immunoprofile resembling the plasma cell stage of differentiation. These include plasmablastic lymphoma, ALK^+ large B-cell lymphoma, human herpesvirus 8–associated malignancies, primary effusion lymphoma, and large B-cell lymphoma associated with multicentric Castleman's disease. Most cases of plasmablastic lymphoma are EBV associated and arise in the setting of immunodeficiency, usually secondary to human immunodeficiency virus (HIV) infection but also in those of advanced age.[84]

FOLLICULAR LYMPHOMA: GRADING AND GENETIC HETEROGENEITY

The grading of FL was the subject of spirited discussion among both the authors and the participants on the Clinical Advisory Committee. FL has traditionally been graded according to the proportion of centroblasts and stratified into three grades. However, most studies have shown poor interobserver and intraobserver reproducibility. Moreover, the clinical significance of separating grades 1 and 2 has been questioned, with minimal differences seen in long-term outcome. Thus, the 2008 WHO classification combines cases with few centroblasts as *FL grade 1-2 (low grade)* and does not require or recommend further separation.

FL grade 3 is divided into grades 3A and 3B, based on the absence of centrocytes in the latter category. Several studies have identified biologic differences between these two subtypes, with most cases of FL grade 3B being more closely related to DLBCL at the genetic level.[85-88] However, in clinical practice, the separation of grades 3A and 3B can be challenging and thus imperfect. Diffuse areas in any grade 3 FL should be designated DLBCL (with FL); these areas are more commonly observed in grade 3B.[87] Further studies are likely to lead to more precise delineation of the grade 3 cases that truly belong within the FL category and those representing an intrafollicular variant of the GCB type of DLBCL.

Pediatric and intestinal FL have already been mentioned as distinctive variants, with pediatric FL lacking an association with t(14;18). Primary cutaneous follicle center lymphoma is now a distinct disease entity, whereas it was considered a variant of FL in the 2001 edition. Notably, primary cutaneous follicle center lymphoma may contain a high proportion of large B cells, including large centrocytes and centroblasts.[73] Evidence of the t(14;18) translocation is uncommon, and most cases are $BCL2^-$. Dissemination beyond the skin is rare, and the prognosis is usually excellent.

PERIPHERAL T-CELL LYMPHOMAS

PTCL, NOS remains a "wastebasket" category, analogous to DLBCL, NOS. Most cases lack distinct genetic or biologic alterations, and prognostic models have largely relied on clinical features or generic factors such as proliferation.[89,90] Nevertheless, progress has been made in the understanding of a number of PTCL entities. Angioimmunoblastic T-cell lymphoma bears a close relationship to the T_{FH} cell of the germinal center, and the follicular variant of PTCL, NOS shares a similar phenotype, although, interestingly, it differs genetically and clinically.[91-93] The majority of nodal PTCLs appear to be related to effector T cells.

The 2008 WHO classification applied more stringent criteria to the diagnosis of *enteropathy-associated T-cell lymphoma*, and the change in the diagnostic term from *enteropathy-type T-cell lymphoma* reflects these changes. It is appreciated that a variety of PTCLs can present with intestinal disease, and not all these cases are associated with celiac disease. For example, intestinal involvement can be seen at presentation, or with progression, in extranodal NK/T-cell lymphoma and some gamma-delta T-cell lymphomas. To make the diagnosis of enteropathy-associated T-cell lymphoma, one should have evidence of celiac disease either at the genetic level, with the appropriate HLA phenotype, or histologically, in the adjacent uninvolved small bowel mucosa. A new variant, termed the *monomorphic variant of enteropathy-associated T-cell lymphoma*, or *type II*, was introduced into the classification. These cases have some distinctive immunophenotypic and genotypic features. The tumor cells are $CD8^+$ and $CD56^+$, and *MYC* amplifications have been shown in a subset of cases.[94,95] The monomorphic variant occurs in the setting of celiac disease but also occurs sporadically.

ALK^+ ALCL is considered a distinct disease that must be distinguished from the provisional entity of ALK^- ALCL. This distinction is supported by clinical as well as biologic differences.[96-98] More serious debate revolved around the decision to segregate ALK^- ALCL cases from PTCL, NOS. Recent clinical studies appear to support this resolution, because the former has a better prognosis and evidence of a plateau, at least in a proportion of patients.[99] Stringent morphologic and immunophenotypic criteria are required for the diagnosis of ALK^- ALCL because CD30 may be expressed in a variety of PTCL subtypes, and CD15 may be negative in CHL.

Three new variants of primary cutaneous PTCL were introduced: primary cutaneous gamma-delta T-cell lymphoma, and the provisional entities of primary cutaneous $CD4^+$ small/medium T-cell lymphoma and primary cutaneous aggressive epidermotropic $CD8^+$ cytotoxic T-cell lymphoma. Cutaneous gamma-delta T-cell lymphomas have a diverse histologic and clinical spectrum and may display a panniculitis-like pattern.[100] However, this disease has a much poorer prognosis than subcutaneous panniculitis-like T-cell lymphoma,[101] which is defined as a lymphoma exclusively of alpha-beta phenotype in the 2008 WHO classification.[102]

PRECURSOR LYMPHOID NEOPLASMS

A basic premise of the classification system is the distinction between neoplasms derived from precursor cells or blasts and those derived from fully differentiated cells. Most precursor B- and T-cell neoplasms present as leukemia, but some cases present first as a mass lesion involving a lymph node or other site outside the bone marrow. Thus, the classification retains the convention that precursor neoplasms are designated *leukemia/lymphoma*, and regardless of the mode of presentation, the diagnosis is the same. For some clinical protocols, the distinction between leukemia and lymphoma may be requested for eligibility criteria. In that event, for patients presenting with a mass lesion and increased blasts in the bone marrow, a threshold of 25% blasts is used as the defining feature of leukemia.[103]

The terminology of the precursor lymphoid neoplasms has been simplified to reduce redundancy. In the 2001 classification, the terms *precursor B-lymphoblastic* and *precursor T-lymphoblastic leukemia/lymphoma* were used. Because a lymphoblast is recognized as an immature or precursor cell by definition, the terminology was simplified to *B-lymphoblastic leukemia/lymphoma* and *T-lymphoblastic leukemia/lymphoma*, omitting the unnecessary modifier.

The 2008 classification places a greater emphasis on genetic features in the definition of some forms of B-lymphoblastic malignancies.[103] Several categories with recurrent genetic abnormalities are now delineated (Box 13-3). These were selected because they are associated with distinctive clinical and immunophenotypic features, and their recognition has prognostic implications. One such example is Philadelphia chromosome–positive (Ph^+) B-lymphoblastic leukemia, associated with *BCR-ABL1*. This disease is more common in adults than in children and is very high risk, regardless of other factors.[104] Another variant with distinctive clinical features at presentation is B-lymphoblastic leukemia/lymphoma with t(5;15)(q31;q32) (*IL3-IGH*). These patients present with a marked increase in eosinophils, which may mask a relatively small number of blasts in the bone marrow—a diagnostic pitfall worthy of note.

T-lymphoblastic leukemia/lymphoma is also associated with considerable genetic variability. The most commonly involved genes include the HOX transcription factors. However, although genotyping is recommended in the workup of the disease, it is not used as a criterion to define distinct entities at this time.

Box 13-3 *Precursor Lymphoid Neoplasms*

- B-lymphoblastic leukemia/lymphoma, not otherwise specified
- B-lymphoblastic leukemia/lymphoma with recurrent genetic abnormalities
  - B-lymphoblastic leukemia/lymphoma with t(9;22)(q34;q11.2); *BCR-ABL1*
  - B-lymphoblastic leukemia/lymphoma with t(v;11q23); *MLL* rearranged
  - B-lymphoblastic leukemia/lymphoma with t(12;21)(p13;q22); *TEL-AML1* (*ETV6-RUNX1*)
  - B-lymphoblastic leukemia/lymphoma with hyperdiploidy
  - B-lymphoblastic leukemia/lymphoma with hypodiploidy (hypodiploid acute lymphocytic leukemia)
  - B-lymphoblastic leukemia/lymphoma with t(5;14)(q31;q32); *IL3-IGH*
  - B-lymphoblastic leukemia/lymphoma with t(1;19)(q23;p13.3); *E2A-PBX1* (*TCF3-PBX1*)
- T-lymphoblastic leukemia/lymphoma

Adapted from Swerdlow SH, Campo E, Harris NL, et al, eds. *WHO Classification of Tumours of Haematopoietic and Lymphoid Tissues.* Lyon, France: IARC Press; 2008.

Box 13-4 *Histiocytic and Dendritic Cell Neoplasms*

- Histiocytic sarcoma
- Langerhans cell histiocytosis
- Langerhans cell sarcoma
- Interdigitating dendritic cell sarcoma
- Follicular dendritic cell sarcoma
- Fibroblastic reticular cell tumor
- Indeterminate dendritic cell tumor
- Disseminated juvenile xanthogranuloma

Adapted from Swerdlow SH, Campo E, Harris NL, et al, eds. *WHO Classification of Tumours of Haematopoietic and Lymphoid Tissues.* Lyon, France: IARC Press; 2008.

HISTIOCYTIC AND DENDRITIC CELL NEOPLASMS

The histiocytic and dendritic cell neoplasms are mentioned here briefly, although technically, these tumors are not of lymphoid origin and, in terms of ontogeny, are probably more closely related to the myeloid lineage. Nevertheless, the diagnosis of a histiocytic or dendritic cell tumor often falls to the anatomic pathologist, and these tumors come to mind in the differential diagnosis of many aggressive lymphomas. The classification has retained the traditional approach of separating these neoplasms into histiocytic and dendritic cell lineages (Box 13-4). Histiocytic tumors are considered functional macrophages, whereas dendritic cells serve as antigen-presenting cells. However, particularly when it comes to neoplasms, there may be considerable overlap in immunophenotype.[105]

Historically, many lymphomas composed of large lymphoid cells were thought to be of histiocytic or reticulum cell derivation. The advent of modern immunology provided evidence that most such tumors were of lymphoid, rather than histiocytic or macrophage, derivation. However, recently it has become apparent that hematolymphoid cells are capable of considerable lineage plasticity, even in a fully differentiated form. Thus, downregulation of the transcription factor PAX5 can lead to reprogramming of mature B cells into macrophages and even T cells.[106] Moreover, histiocytic sarcomas have been reported as secondary tumors in a variety of B-cell lymphomas, but at least in some cases, they were shown to be clonally related to the initial B-cell process.[107] Thus, histiocytic or dendritic cell neoplasms may be seen following FL, MZL, and CLL.[107-110] Even more common is the occurrence of a histiocytic or dendritic cell neoplasm following precursor lymphoid neoplasms.[111,112] Greater lineage plasticity in immature cells is an expected phenomenon.

CONCLUSION

The 2008 WHO classification is a continuation of the successful international collaboration among pathologists, biologists, and clinicians interested in the hematologic malignancies. The 2001 classification was rapidly adopted for clinical trials and successfully served as a common language for scientists comparing genetic and functional data. The modifications made in the 2008 version are the result of this successful partnership, but it is evident that many areas are still the subject of intense investigation, including the admittedly heterogeneous groups of DLBCL, NOS and PTCL, NOS. The inclusion of borderline categories is an intermediate step, and further modifications in these areas are expected.

References can be found on Expert Consult @ www.expertconsult.com

Chapter 14

Mature B-Cell Neoplasms: Chronic Lymphocytic Leukemia–Small Lymphocytic Lymphoma, B-Cell Prolymphocytic Leukemia, and Lymphoplasmacytic Lymphoma

David S. Viswanatha, Karen Dyer Montgomery, and Kathryn Foucar

CHAPTER OUTLINE

B-CELL CHRONIC LYMPHOCYTIC LEUKEMIA–SMALL LYMPHOCYTIC LYMPHOMA

Definition of Disease

Among the mature B-cell neoplasms reviewed in this chapter, B-cell chronic lymphocytic leukemia–small lymphocytic lymphoma (CLL/SLL) is by far the most common (Table 14-1). This clonal disorder is derived from mature B lymphocytes characterized by small, round nuclei; inconspicuous nucleoli; and generally scant cytoplasm. Within lymph nodes, larger clonal B cells termed *prolymphocytes* or *paraimmunoblasts* often form pale foci called *proliferation centers*. The diagnostic distinction between CLL and SLL is based primarily on disease distribution and the number of circulating leukemic cells. Disorders with a predominant extramedullary disease distribution and few, if any, leukemic cells in blood ($<5.0 \times 10^9$/L) are termed SLL, whereas CLL, by definition, exhibits a leukemic blood picture (Box 14-1).[1,2]

Diagnostic criteria for CLL include an absolute mature lymphocytosis that is sustained for at least 3 months and

Table 14-1 Primary Entities and Variants

Primary Entity	Variants
CLL/SLL	Atypical CLL (morphology) Atypical CLL (immunophenotype) CLL with plasmacytoid differentiation CLL with Reed-Sternberg cells Mu heavy-chain disease
B-cell prolymphocytic leukemia	No variants described, but overlap with leukemic MCL is problematic
Waldenström's macroglobulinemia–lymphoplasmacytic lymphoma	Gamma heavy-chain disease Other B-cell lymphomas with IgM paraprotein (e.g., MZLs)

CLL, chronic lymphocytic leukemia; CLL/SLL, chronic lymphocytic leukemia–small lymphocytic lymphoma; IgM, immunoglobulin M; MCL, mantle cell lymphoma; MZL, marginal zone lymphoma.

clinically unexplained.[1,2] The degree of absolute lymphocytosis required for diagnosis varies somewhat among investigators, but in general, the minimal absolute lymphocyte count required is 5.0×10^9/L for patients without significant extramedullary disease.[1,3] Although a bone marrow lymphocytosis is also present, bone marrow examination is often not required for the diagnosis of CLL. Many cases of CLL can be successfully diagnosed by morphologic review of blood smears, but immunophenotypic confirmation is advised. In addition to confirming the prototypic immunophenotyping profile of CLL (see Box 14-1), the use of immunophenotyping to delineate prognostic features has assumed greater importance in recent years. Furthermore, immunophenotyping may be required to establish a diagnosis of CLL when the absolute lymphocyte count is only modestly higher than normal. The term *monoclonal B lymphocytosis* may be applied to these cases, especially if there is neither significant lymphocytosis nor any cytopenia (see Differential Diagnosis).[1,2]

Epidemiology and Incidence

CLL is by far the most common mature B-cell leukemia in Western countries, where it accounts for up to 30% of all leukemias; CLL is also the most common familial leukemia.[4-6] In Western countries, incidence rates increase dramatically in the elderly, with more than 20 cases per 100,000 in this population. In contrast, a substantially lower incidence rate of CLL has been documented in Asian patients.[7,8]

SLL accounts for about 7% of all non-Hodgkin's lymphoma.[1] Both CLL and SLL exhibit a male predominance and affect largely middle-aged to elderly patients, with a median age of about 65 years. The rare cases of CLL-like disorders that occur in young patients appear to be biologically distinct from prototypic CLL in the elderly and are not covered in this chapter.

Box 14-1 *Major Diagnostic Features of Chronic Lymphocytic Leukemia (CLL) and Small Lymphocytic Lymphoma (SLL)*

CLL
- Absolute mature lymphocytosis of $\geq 5 \times 10^9$/L sustained for at least 3 months
- Monoclonal B cell with mature phenotype, CD5 coexpression, weak CD20, weak surface immunoglobulin, CD23, weak CD22, weak CD11c
- Antigens typically *not* expressed include CD10, FMC7, and CD79b

SLL
- Extramedullary sites of disease predominate
- Diffuse infiltrate of small lymphocytes, proliferation foci
- Monoclonal B cell with mature phenotype similar to CLL

See references 1 and 2.

Clinical Features

At presentation, many elderly patients with CLL are either asymptomatic (70% of cases) or only mildly symptomatic, and this disease is often detected as an incidental finding on complete blood cell counts.[8] Many CLL patients have preserved hematopoietic lineages, and the absolute lymphocyte count varies from mildly to markedly increased. Some CLL patients manifest clinically apparent anemia that is secondary to immune-mediated erythrocyte destruction, a distinctive and relatively common complication that reflects the high incidence of autoimmune aberrations in these patients.[8,9] Other types of anemia that can affect CLL patients include anemia of chronic disease and, very rarely, acquired pure red cell aplasia.[8] However, in most cases, cytopenias are the consequence of bone marrow infiltration. Serum studies may reveal monoclonal gammopathy in some patients, which does not seem to affect disease outcome.[10] Hypogammaglobulinemia is much more common, occurring in more than half of CLL patients.[8]

Other CLL/SLL patients present with manifestations of extramedullary disease, primarily lymphadenopathy, but also splenomegaly in a subset of patients. Like their leukemic counterparts, these patients with SLL are often asymptomatic.[11] Infiltrates of CLL/SLL can be detected infrequently in a wide variety of other sites, but except for in the liver and skin, these are not commonly encountered in clinical practice.[12-14]

In individuals younger than 55 years, CLL may be less indolent, and these patients may present with fatigue or symptomatic organomegaly.[15] Likewise, the incidence of transformation of CLL/SLL to large cell lymphoma (Richter's syndrome) seems to be more common in patients who develop CLL at a younger age.[15] It is likely that these differences in older versus younger patients are attributable to molecular, genetic, or epigenetic differences in the neoplastic clones (see later sections).

Morphology

Lymph Node

Lymph node involvement in CLL/SLL is generally characterized by diffuse effacement of the architecture with variably preserved sinuses.[1,16] The infiltrate consists of small, round lymphocytes with condensed chromatin and scanty amounts of cytoplasm, imparting a dark color on low magnification. Mitotic activity is virtually absent in these areas. Interspersed among these diffuse sheets of small, round lymphocytes are proliferation foci that produce a vague, pale nodular pattern (Fig. 14-1A). On high magnification, proliferation foci are composed of larger lymphoid cells with more

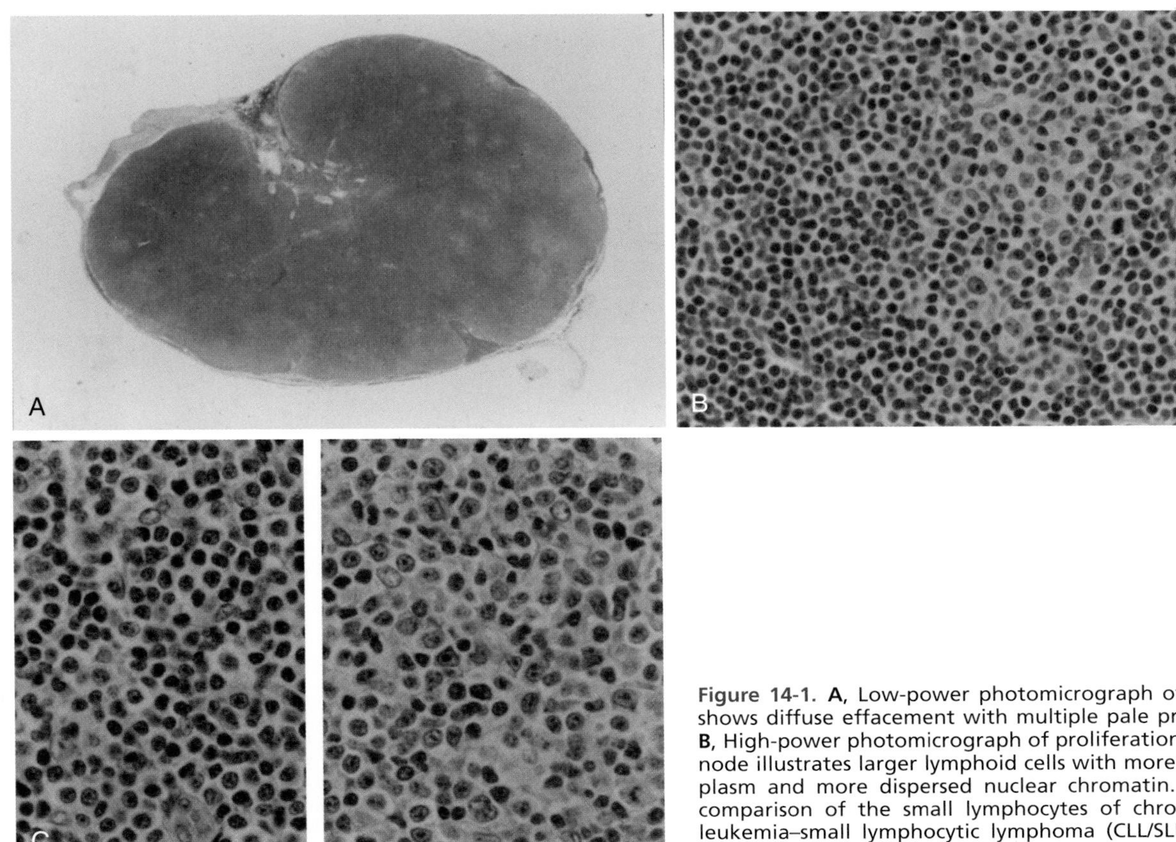

Figure 14-1. **A,** Low-power photomicrograph of a lymph node shows diffuse effacement with multiple pale proliferation foci. **B,** High-power photomicrograph of proliferation foci in a lymph node illustrates larger lymphoid cells with more abundant cytoplasm and more dispersed nuclear chromatin. **C,** Side-by-side comparison of the small lymphocytes of chronic lymphocytic leukemia–small lymphocytic lymphoma (CLL/SLL; *left*) and the larger lymphoid cells constituting proliferation foci (*right*).

abundant cytoplasm and more conspicuous nucleoli (see Fig. 14-1B and C). By the assessment of DNA synthesis, such as Ki-67 staining, these proliferation foci are shown to represent the mitotically active portion of the neoplastic clone. Occasionally, proliferation foci may be very large and confluent, raising concerns of transformation to large cell lymphoma (Fig. 14-2).

In a minority of CLL/SLL cases, the pattern of lymph node infiltration is interfollicular or exhibits a perifollicular or marginal zone–type pattern, resulting in potential confusion with mantle cell lymphoma, marginal zone lymphoma (MZL), or other B-cell neoplasms.[17] Likewise, some cases exhibit greater nuclear irregularity of the small lymphocytes, reminiscent of mantle cell lymphoma or even follicular center cell lymphoma. However, the presence of proliferation foci, the distinctive immunophenotypic profile, and the absence of cyclin D1 expression support a diagnosis of CLL/SLL.[18-20]

Spleen

The degree of splenomegaly is highly variable in CLL patients, with some patients exhibiting significant and symptomatic splenic involvement.[21] Splenic involvement by CLL/SLL is characterized by white pulp expansion that produces a miliary micronodular appearance grossly.[21] The white pulp infiltrates consist of small, round lymphocytes with scant cytoplasm, similar to those seen in lymph nodes (Fig. 14-3).[22] Although occasional prolymphocytes and paraimmunoblasts may be present, typical proliferation foci generally are not readily apparent. Extension of the lymphoid infiltrate into the periarteriolar lymphoid sheath, along splenic trabeculae, and into both the red pulp cords and sinuses is common.[21,22]

Blood

A mature lymphocytosis is a diagnostic requirement for CLL, with 5.0×10^9/L the generally accepted minimum absolute lymphocyte count (see Box 14-1).[1,2] These lymphocytes are typically monotonous with relatively homogeneous features, including small, round nuclei with highly condensed nuclear chromatin and inconspicuous nucleoli (Fig. 14-4). The exaggerated chromatin clumping may impart a “cracked mud” appearance to these nuclei. These leukemic lymphocytes are easily disrupted during smear preparation, creating smudge cells that may be numerous (Fig. 14-5). Larger lymphoid cells or lymphocytes with irregular nuclear contours may be evident, but these cells usually constitute less than 2% of the leukemic population (Fig. 14-6).[1] When these “atypical” forms are conspicuous, a diagnosis of atypical CLL may be preferred to convey to the clinician these aberrant morphologic features (see the section on morphologic variants). Cytogenetic assessment is recommended in these atypical cases because an association between adverse karyotype and nuclear morphology has been proposed (see the section on genetics). In general, the agranular cytoplasm is scant, but some cases of CLL demonstrate moderate amounts of cytoplasm. Distinctive cytoplasmic vacuoles or crystals are noted occasionally.

The number of prolymphocytes and clonal cells with a larger nuclear size and a single, distinct nucleolus should be assessed (see Fig. 14-6). When prolymphocytes predominate

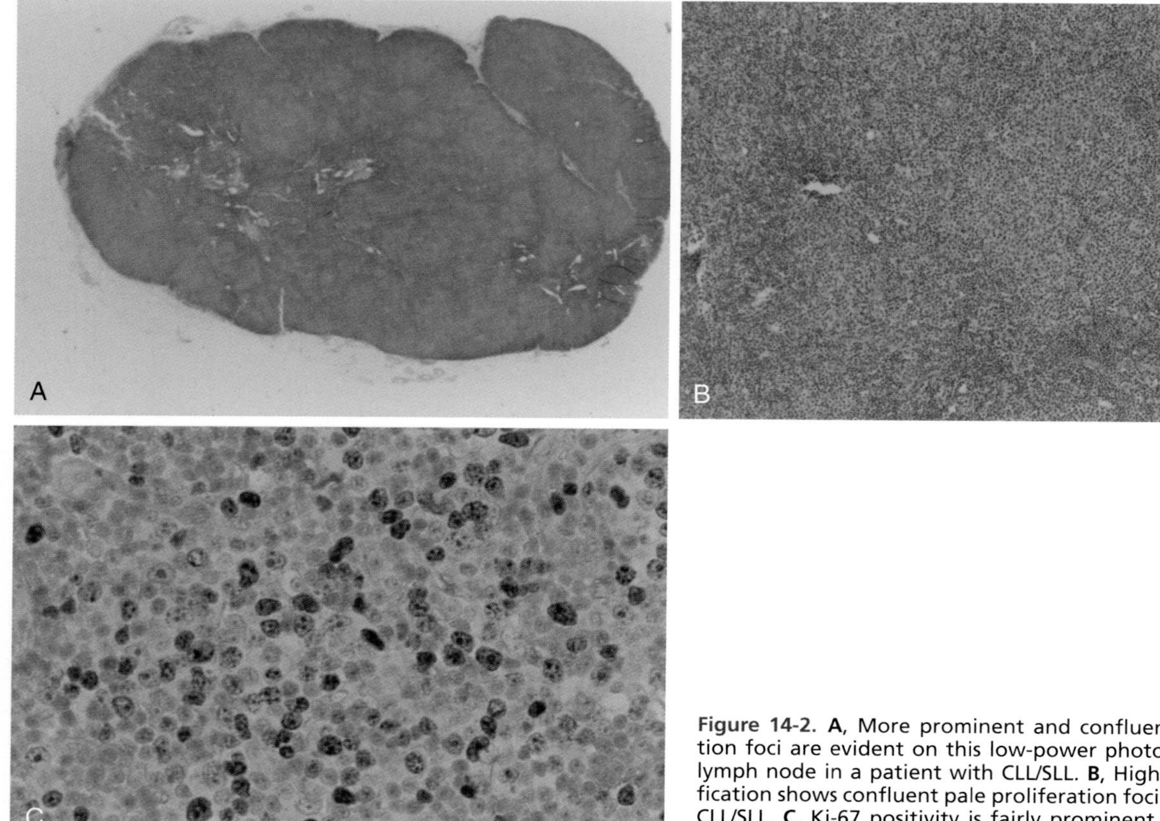

Figure 14-2. **A**, More prominent and confluent pale proliferation foci are evident on this low-power photomicrograph of a lymph node in a patient with CLL/SLL. **B**, Higher-power magnification shows confluent pale proliferation foci in a patient with CLL/SLL. **C**, Ki-67 positivity is fairly prominent in the confluent proliferation foci in this case of CLL/SLL.

at presentation, a diagnosis of B-cell prolymphocytic leukemia should be strongly considered (see later). In some patients, an increasing proportion of prolymphocytes may be a harbinger of clonal transformation, whereas other cases of stable CLL demonstrate consistently high numbers of prolymphocytes.[16] Any significant change in the blood picture should prompt a reevaluation of the patient's disease status as well as specialized testing for the assessment of prognostic factors (e.g., flow cytometry, genetic testing).

Bone Marrow

Although not necessary for diagnosis, bone marrow examination in CLL patients may be useful in assessing residual hematopoiesis and in determining the pattern and extent of bone marrow effacement. On aspirate smears, CLL cells exhibit similar cytologic features to circulating clonal cells (Box 14-2).[1,16,23,24] These small mature lymphocytes are generally abundant on aspirate smears, although variability is expected

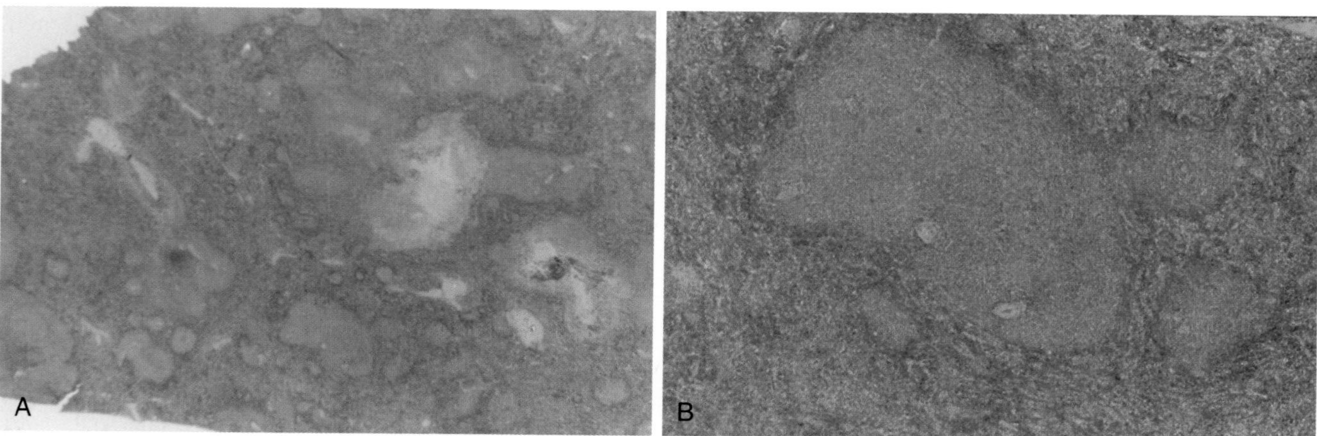

Figure 14-3. Expanded, dark-staining white pulp infiltrates of CLL/SLL are evident at low (**A**) and intermediate (**B**) magnification in this spleen.

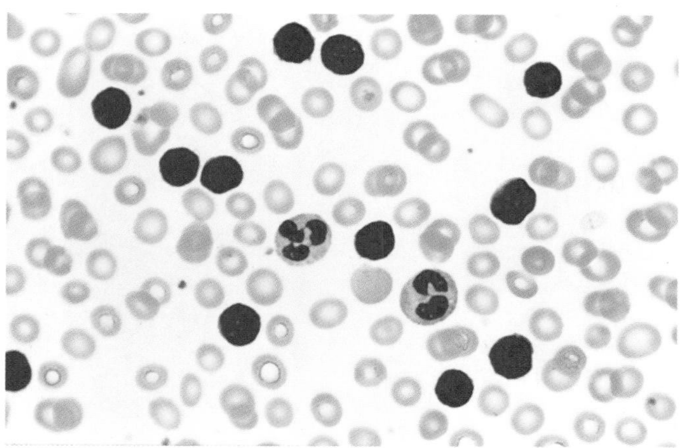

Figure 14-4. A marked mature lymphocytosis characterized by round nuclei with highly condensed chromatin and scant cytoplasm is evident in the blood of this patient with chronic lymphocytic leukemia (CLL).

Box 14-2 *Bone Marrow Findings in Chronic Lymphocytic Leukemia*

Morphology

- Small lymphoid cells with round nuclear contours, condensed chromatin, and inconspicuous nucleoli, analogous to the appearance in blood
- Lymphocytes usually constitute at least 30% of total nucleated cells

Core Biopsy

- Nonparatrabecular lymphoid nodules with closely packed round nuclei, scant cytoplasm, and minimal mitotic activity
- No predilection for paratrabecular localization
- Possible diffuse increase in interstitial lymphocytes admixed with hematopoietic elements
- Diffuse, solid bone marrow effacement is relatively uncommon
- Proliferation foci are rare, and true germinal centers are even rarer (two cases)

See references 1, 16, 23, and 24.

owing to the multifocal nature of neoplastic infiltration of the bone marrow. However, in most cases lymphocytes constitute more than 30% of total cells.[1] The extent of bone marrow replacement by CLL generally parallels the proportion of lymphocytes on differential cell counts, although the extent of disease is best assessed on core biopsy specimens. There is some evidence that the lymphocyte percentage on differential cell counts provides additional prognostic information.[24]

On core biopsy sections, the pattern of bone marrow infiltration may be useful for both distinguishing CLL from other diagnostic possibilities and providing prognostic information.[25] In CLL, the bone marrow core biopsy may exhibit a range of infiltration patterns, including focal, nonparatrabecular nodules; an interstitial infiltrate in which CLL cells are admixed with hematopoietic elements; and diffuse, solid lesions (Figs. 14-7 and 14-8). Multiple patterns may be evident in a single core biopsy specimen. The typical nodular infiltrates of CLL are readily apparent on low magnification, and their dark appearance is quite distinct from that of normal hematopoietic cells. This dark appearance is due to closely packed nuclei with scant cytoplasm, which typify this disorder (see Box 14-2). On high magnification the densely packed nuclei exhibit round contours and minimal, if any, mitotic activity. The borders of these nonparatrabecular nodules may show infiltrative margins with diffusion of lymphocytes into adjacent hematopoietic tissues. Likewise, diffuse interstitial infiltrates of CLL may be evident throughout the bone marrow, widely separated from discrete nodular lesions. In these areas adipose cells and hematopoietic elements are at least partially preserved, although on low magnification the CLL infiltrates impart a darker appearance than uninvolved bone marrow (see Fig. 14-7). The most extensively effaced bone marrow core biopsy sections are characterized by solid areas of complete replacement of both hematopoietic and fat cells, with CLL filling the entire hematopoietic cavity between bony trabeculae. The presence of extensive diffuse, solid infiltrates would predict cytopenias and, consequently, a higher clinical stage. Recent studies suggest an association between diffuse bone marrow infiltration and 70-kDa zeta-associated protein (ZAP-70) expression by immunophenotyping studies (see

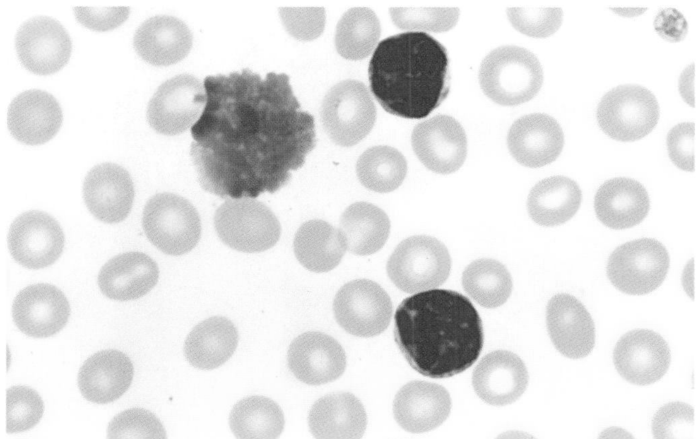

Figure 14-5. Broken CLL cells (so-called smudge cells) are evident on this peripheral blood smear from a patient with CLL. Smudge cells consist largely of nuclear material.

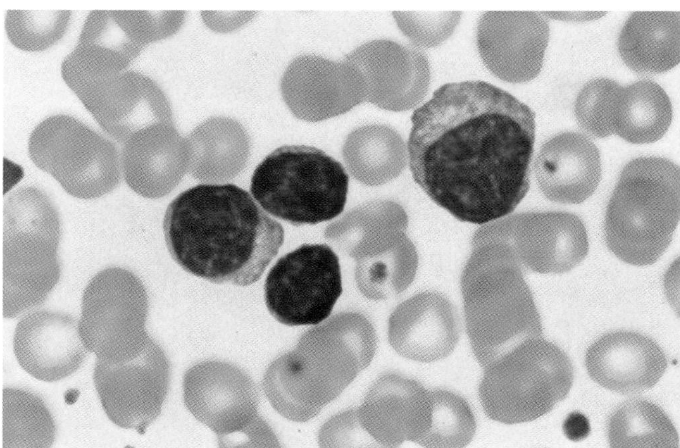

Figure 14-6. Larger lymphoid cells with more dispersed chromatin and a distinct nucleolus (so-called prolymphocytes) can usually be identified in the peripheral blood of patients with CLL.

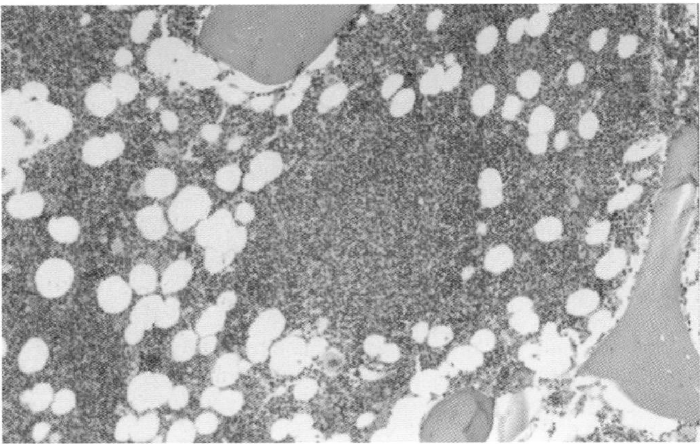

Figure 14-7. This bone marrow core biopsy section from a patient with CLL illustrates a focal, nonparatrabecular infiltrate of leukemia. Note the dark blue color of this infiltrate due to the back-to-back nuclei that typify CLL infiltrates.

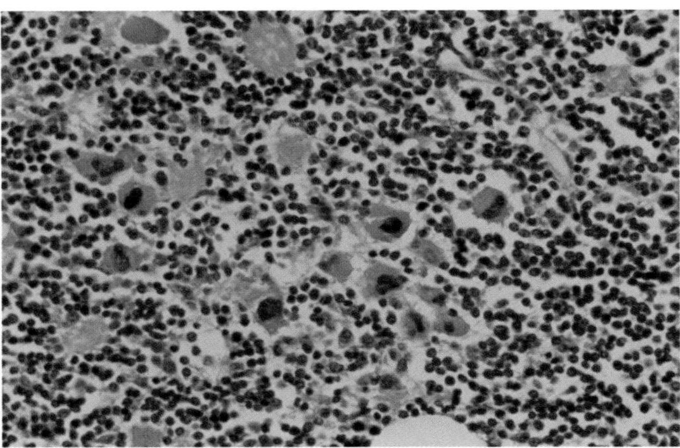

Figure 14-8. This bone marrow biopsy section from a CLL patient illustrates the diffuse, interstitial infiltration that can occur. Abundant preserved megakaryocytes are evident.

later).[26,27] The extent of bone marrow effacement in CLL is best estimated from technically optimal core biopsy specimens at least 10 mm long that do not consist of large portions of hypocellular subcortical regions.

Although proliferation foci are a typical feature of nodal infiltrates of CLL/SLL, these foci of larger, transformed prolymphocytoid cells are generally not conspicuous in bone marrow sections, possibly reflecting the relatively limited sample size of core biopsies (Fig. 14-9). Only very rarely are true germinal centers evident in bone marrow specimens from CLL patients; the presence of germinal centers should prompt the systematic exclusion of other B-cell chronic lymphoproliferative disorders.[23] In rare CLL patients, foci of large cell lymphoma transformation are first appreciated in bone marrow specimens. Owing to the large overall cell size and the presence of moderate amounts of cytoplasm, these large cell lymphoma infiltrates are quite distinct even on low magnification, where they are a pale pinkish color (see the later section on transformation).

Increased angiogenesis may be involved in the pathogenesis of CLL.[28,29] Based on the measurement of vascular endothelial growth factor in serum, Western blot analysis of clonal cells for vascular endothelial growth factor, or the assessment of small vessel density on actual core biopsy sections, studies have documented that an increase in angiogenesis may be involved in CLL.[28,29]

Other Organs

Liver involvement is common in CLL, but clinically significant hepatic dysfunction is encountered in only a small subset of patients (Fig. 14-10).[12,30] Portal infiltrates of neoplastic cells predominate, and fibrosis may also be noted. Likewise, a small subset of CLL patients presents with cutaneous manifestations of disease, including generalized papules or isolated plaques, nodules, and discrete masses.[14] The dermal infiltrates of CLL range from patchy perivascular or periadnexal infiltrates to solid dermal masses. In some patients the cutaneous lesions are a manifestation of large cell lymphoma transforma-

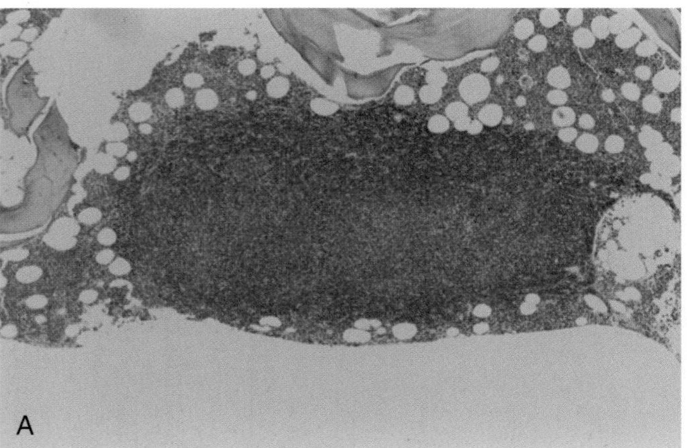

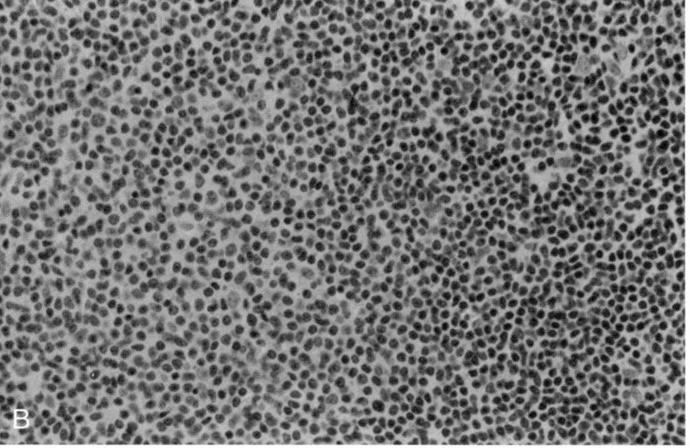

Figure 14-9. **A,** Low-power photomicrograph of a bone marrow core biopsy in a patient with CLL illustrates a large focal infiltrate with pale central proliferation foci—an unusual finding in bone marrow specimens. **B,** High-power photomicrograph shows the larger prolymphocyte-like cells (*left*) composing the proliferation foci, compared to the small, dark typical CLL cells with scanty cytoplasm and highly condensed chromatin (*right*).

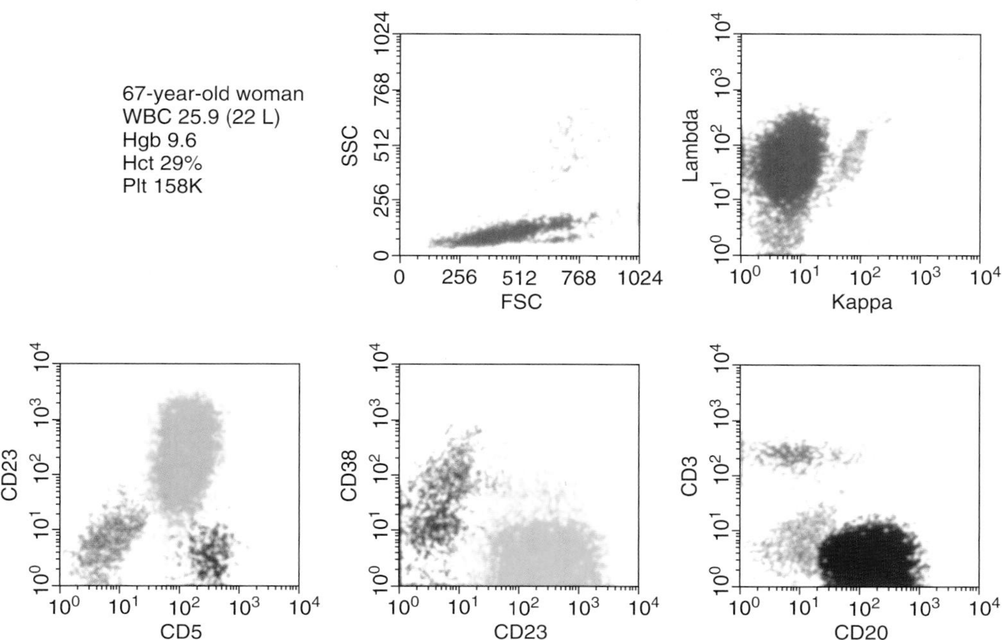

Figure 14-15. The classic immunophenotypic profile of CLL/SLL is illustrated in this flow cytometric histogram. FSC, forward scatter; SSC, side scatter.

cells showed distinct differences.[99] The dissimilarity was further expanded by using a micro-RNA microchip to develop a micro-RNA signature, leading to significant prognostic associations among specific micro-RNAs, *IGH@* V mutational status, and ZAP-70 expression.[103] Specific micro-RNA genes (*miR15* and *miR16*), mapped to 13q14, are downregulated or deleted in the majority of CLL cases.[98]

Using FISH, *IGH@* V mutation assessment, and other molecular techniques, specific prognostic categories of CLL can be established related to accompanying morphology. Appropriate therapy can then be chosen, based on underlying biology.[96,104-107]

The most frequent cytogenetic abnormalities associated with CLL are described in the following sections, in order of increasing pathogenicity.

Deletion of 13q14

Deletion of 13q14 is the most common cytogenetic abnormality associated with CLL, detected in more than 50% of cases with abnormal FISH results (see Fig. 14-17).[89] The deletion

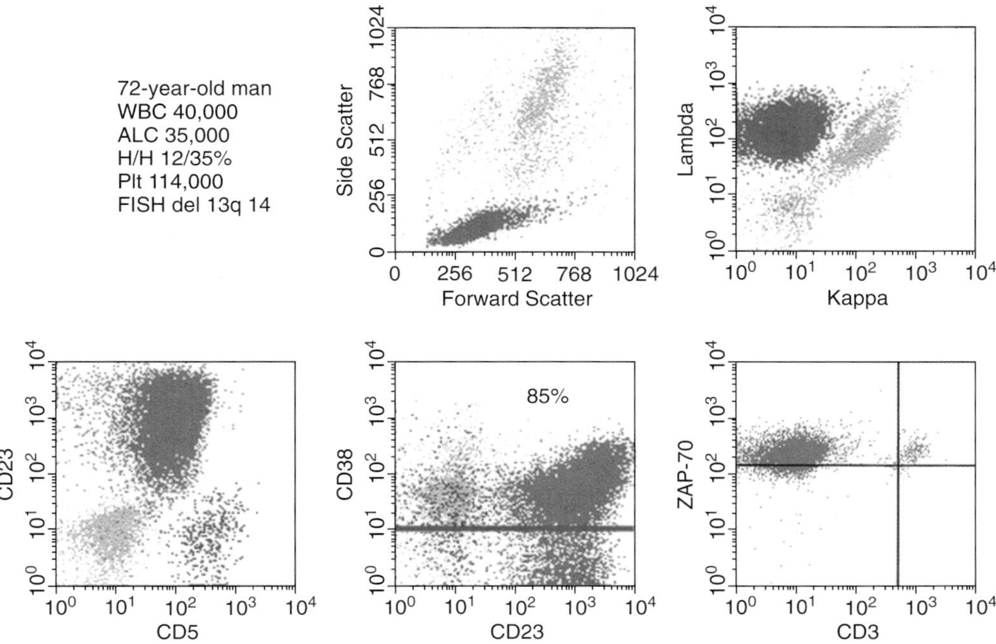

Figure 14-16. Both CD38 and ZAP-70 expression are evident in this flow cytometric phenotyping profile in a patient with CLL.

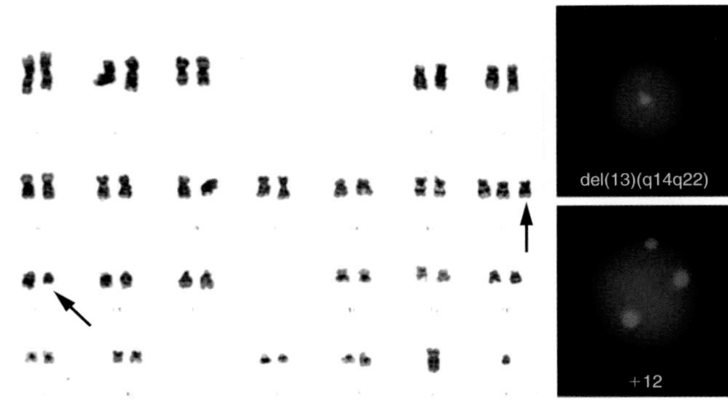

Figure 14-17. Deletion of 13q14 and trisomy 12 are identified by fluorescence in situ hybridization in this case of CLL.

is monoallelic 80% of the time and biallelic in the remainder.[108] Loss of sequences at this locus is also reported in other B-cell neoplasms (including mantle cell lymphoma and myeloma) and solid tumors, suggestive of a common tumor suppressor gene. A number of genes have been identified in the minimally deleted region of 13q14, including *CAR*, which encodes a putative RING-finger–containing protein, and two noncoding genes, *DLEU2* (1B4/Leu2) and *DLEU1* (EST70/Leu1).[108,109] Detailed mutational, loss of heterozygosity, and expression studies have not supported the involvement of these genes. The deleted region contains two micro-RNA genes, *MIR15A* and *MIR16-1*. Both of these genes are deleted or downregulated in the majority of cases of CLL, and this loss of gene function is directly correlated with allelic loss at 13q14.[99] A minimal 26-kb region of deletion overlap in 13q14 was detected by ROMA that spans the two micro-RNAs; however, multiple genetic lesions were found in 13q14, indicative of complex pathobiology.[93]

Deletion of 13q14 occurs in patients with both unmutated and mutated *IGH@* V, although it is better represented in the latter group.[110] Survival of patients with deletion 13q14 is better than that of those whose tumors have apparently normal karyotypes, other chromosomal changes, or cytogenetic abnormalities in addition to loss of 13q14.[89]

Trisomy 12

Trisomy 12 occurs in less than 20% of cases with abnormal karyotypes analyzed by FISH (see Fig. 14-17).[89] The molecular basis for the association of trisomy 12 and CLL is unknown, although overexpression of multiple candidate genes has been detected by protein expression analysis.[111] This anomaly is often associated with atypical morphology, but it occurs in only a subset of tumor cells.[112] Minimal levels of *IGH@* V mutations are reported.[112] Trisomy 12 as a sole anomaly appears to have limited prognostic implications.[89]

Deletion of 11q22-q23

Deletions of the distal long arm of chromosome 11 occur in about 20% of CLL patients with abnormal FISH patterns.[89] The loss of a putative tumor suppressor gene in this area is reported to be related to decreased expression of specific adhesion molecules.[82] CCG-trinucleotide repeats have also been implicated in this deletion, possibly associated with instability of this chromosome segment.[113] Gene expression profiling of CLL patients with 11q23 deletions has identified a cluster of associated expressed genes.[114,115] Deletions involving the ataxia-telangiectasia mutated (*ATM*) locus at 11q22.3 appear to be associated with CLL disease progression and with the development of significant lymphadenopathy.[116,117]

Deletion of 17p13

Deletions of the short arm of chromosome 17 occur in about 5% to 10% of CLL patients and are related to allelic loss accompanied by mutation of the *TP53* gene.[89] This tumor suppressor gene is a transcription factor active in cell cycle control.[118] Deletion of 17p is a significant independent adverse prognostic factor, related to the shortest survival time of any subset of CLL associated with a cytogenetic abnormality.[69,89,119] This deletion is a recurring secondary aberration associated with disease progression.[69] Micro-RNAs may also play a role in the tumorigenicity of *TP53* abnormalities. Transcriptional activity of *MIR34* requires binding with *TP53*; loss of *TP53* may then have significant effects on the silencing of genes implicated in cancer.[120]

Postulated Cell of Origin and Normal Counterpart Cell

Although cases of CLL segregate into two distinct biologic entities, both are derived from antigen-experienced B cells that differ in the level of immunoglobulin V gene mutations.[59] The distribution of cases of CLL into either unmutated or mutated categories varies in the literature; recent evidence suggests that the majority of cases exhibit somatic hypermutation.[1]

Clinical Course, Prognostic Factors, and Transformation

CLL is generally an indolent disease characterized by gradual leukemia cell accumulation rather than rapid cell proliferation. However, the disease course of CLL covers a broad spectrum, with median survival times ranging from less than 10 years to more than 25 years.[121] In general, the disease course is best predicted by combining stage of disease as determined by either the Rai or Binet staging system with assessment of CD38 and ZAP-70 expression by flow cytometry, cytogenetics, and mutation status of immunoglobulin variable-chain genes by sequence analysis studies.[1,61,62,69,83,122] Prognostic factors such as CD38, ZAP-70 expression, and mutation analysis are especially predictive when concordant. For example, the shortest interval to therapy and shortest overall survival time occur in patients whose CLL cells are $CD38^+$ and $ZAP\text{-}70^+$ and show unmutated *IGH@* V genes.[62,64,121] Similarly, survival time is best for patients whose CLL cells exhibit concordant favorable features, with an intermediate prognosis for discordant cases.[62,63,121] The literature is less clear-cut in delineating the dominant prognostic factor that independently predicts prognosis in discordant cases. Some investigators describe ZAP-70 as the strongest risk factor, but others conclude that cytogenetics is most predictive of outcome.[63,64,95,121,123] Some authors have reported that ZAP-70 is a better predictor of need for therapy than is the mutational status of *IGH@* V genes[63,64]; however, some laboratories no longer offer ZAP-70 testing by flow cytometry because of technical concerns and immediately resort to mutation analysis.

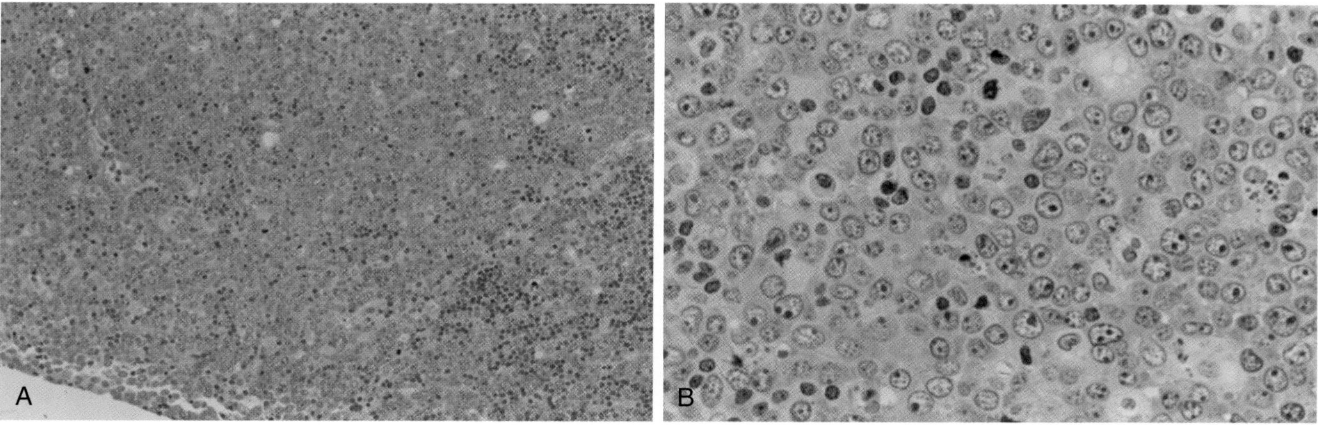

Figure 14-18. **A**, Low-power photomicrograph of a lymph node shows an area of large cell lymphomatous transformation (Richter's syndrome). **B**, Cytologic features of large cell lymphoma arising in CLL are illustrated on high-power magnification in this lymph node section from a patient who developed Richter's syndrome.

Other reportedly independent prognostic factors in CLL include lymphocyte doubling time, serum lactate dehydrogenase, bone marrow pattern of infiltration, and laboratory parameters such as serum thymidine kinase, soluble CD23 doubling time, and β_2-microglobulin levels.[15,68,122,124,125] Some of these prognostic factos are more useful in patients with low-stage disease by standard assessment.[125] Finally, age may be a factor, in that younger CLL patients (younger than 55 years) have a higher rate of transformation to large cell lymphoma and are more likely to die of direct consequences of CLL than are elderly patients.[15]

Transformation of CLL into a biologically more aggressive neoplasm is a well-known phenomenon that occurs in 2% to 12% of patients.[1,126-128] The two most frequently encountered types of clonal transformation in CLL are prolymphocytoid transformation, characterized by a progressive increase in the proportion of prolymphocytes in blood and bone marrow, and Richter's syndrome, the development of overt clinically aggressive large cell lymphoma.[129] All other types of transformation of CLL, including Hodgkin's lymphoma and proposed blastic, plasmacytoid, and paraimmunoblastic transformations, are exceedingly rare and not generally encountered in clinical practice.[128]

Although definitions vary somewhat, prolymphocytoid transformation of CLL is associated with abundant prolymphocytes, gradually progressive cytopenias, and refractoriness to therapy.[16,130-132] The increasing proportion of leukemic cells with prominent nucleoli may be linked to clonal progression by cytogenetic studies and changes, often minor, in the immunophenotypic profile of the neoplasm.[16,133]

The clonal association between overt large cell lymphoma and antecedent CLL has been established for most, but not all, cases of Richter's syndrome.[126,127] Factors linked to the development of large cell lymphoma in CLL patients include CD38 polymorphisms, lack of 13q14 deletion, and lymph node size.[127,134] The large cell lymphoma generally exhibits pleomorphic, immunoblastic features, yet some cases may fulfill morphologic criteria for Hodgkin's lymphoma (Fig. 14-18).[46,126,128] Although transformations generally predominate in extramedullary sites, large cell lymphoma can sometimes be detected initially in bone marrow, where it produces discrete large cell infiltrates (Fig. 14-19). An increased incidence of Richter's syndrome has been reported in patients receiving fludarabine therapy for CLL, with the transformation occurring within the first year of therapy. Not uncommonly, these cases are related to Epstein-Barr virus.[135,136]

Differential Diagnosis

The differential diagnosis of CLL ranges from nonneoplastic reactive lymphocytosis at one end of the spectrum to the diverse family of other leukemias and lymphomas that constitute the B-cell chronic lymphoproliferative disorders (Tables 14-2 to 14-4). The distinction of CLL from these neoplastic and nonneoplastic "look-alikes" can generally be achieved by a systematic assessment of cells; this begins with a morphologic review followed by multicolor flow cytometry when appropriate. In blood samples, cell uniformity is characteristic of CLL, whereas cytologic heterogeneity is more typical of either reactive processes or other B-cell chronic lymphoproliferative disorders, especially peripheralizing lymphomas. The morphologic spectrum of lymphoid cells in acute viral infections is generally readily distinguishable from clonal disorders; immunophenotyping is not necessary, especially in

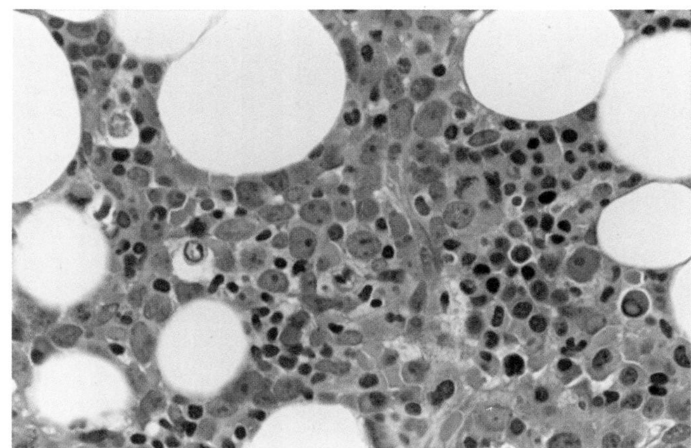

Figure 14-19. Large cell lymphomatous transformation was initially detected in this bone marrow biopsy specimen from a patient with long-standing CLL.

Table 14-2 **Comparison of Morphologic Features of B-Cell Chronic Lymphoproliferative Disorders in Lymph Node and Spleen**

Feature	CLL/SLL	B-PLL	MCL	FCC	LPL/WM	SMZL	HCL
Nuclei	Small, round	Medium, round	Small, irregular	Small to medium; clefted, with variable large centroblasts	Small, round; subset of transformed cells is large	Small, round to reniform	Small, reniform
Cytoplasm	Scant	Scant to moderate	Scant	Scant	Scant to moderate	Moderate to abundant	Moderate to abundant
Mitotic activity	Minimal	Variable	Variable	Minimal	Minimal	Minimal	Minimal
Pattern of LN infiltration	Diffuse with proliferation foci	Diffuse or vaguely nodular; no proliferation foci	Nodular or diffuse with spared germinal centers	Follicular	Diffuse or vaguely nodular; subtotal involvement can be seen; amyloid present in some cases	Variable, usually nodular; may show marginal zone pattern with spared germinal centers and mantle zones or sinusoidal pattern; follicle colonization often present	Diffuse
Pattern of splenic infiltration	Primarily white pulp with secondary involvement of red pulp	Both diffuse red pulp and prominent white pulp involvement	Primarily white pulp with spared germinal centers	Primarily white pulp	Mainly white pulp with numerous patchy red pulp infiltrates	Primarily white pulp with variable pattern, often including marginal zone pattern with compartmentalization or zoning of white pulp	Red pulp with erythrocyte lakes and attenuated white pulp

B-PLL, B-cell prolymphocytic leukemia; CLL/SLL, chronic lymphocytic leukemia–small lymphocytic lymphoma; FCC, small cleaved follicular center cell lymphoma; HCL, hairy cell leukemia; LN, lymph node; LPL/WM, lymphoplasmacytic lymphoma–Waldenström's macroglobulinemia; MCL, mantle cell lymphoma; SMZL, splenic B-cell marginal zone lymphoma.
See references 143-149.

Table 14-3 Pattern and Morphology of Bone Marrow Involvement in B-Cell Chronic Lymphoproliferative Disorders

Disorder	Aspirate Morphology	Core Biopsy Features
CLL/SLL	Monotonous small, round lymphocytes with scant cytoplasm	Focal nonparatrabecular infiltrates predominate, but either diffuse interstitial or diffuse solid infiltrates may be seen
B-PLL	Intermediate-sized lymphocytes exhibiting round nuclei with relatively condensed nuclear chromatin and prominent central nucleoli	Usually diffuse
MCL	Small to intermediate-sized lymphocytes with variably condensed chromatin and irregular nuclear contours; variable number of cells may exhibit either prolymphocytic or blastic features	Usually focal nonparatrabecular and paratrabecular infiltrates evident, although interstitial and diffuse lesions also described
FCC	Variable, but small cleaved lymphoid cells typically predominate	Focal paratrabecular lesions predominate
MZL (including splenic MZL)	Variable with admixture of plasmacytoid forms; some cells may exhibit shaggy cytoplasmic contours that tend to be bipolar	Variable; sinusoidal infiltrates common, but usually in association with discrete lesions; "naked" germinal centers may be seen
LPL/WM	Spectrum of lymphoplasmacytoid cells and plasma cells; Dutcher bodies; abundant mast cells may be seen	Focal, interstitial, or diffuse lesions may be noted; amyloid deposition may be seen
HCL	Distinctive cell with oblong to reniform nuclei, spongy "checkerboard" nuclear chromatin, and moderate to abundant amounts of slightly basophilic cytoplasm exhibiting shaggy contours	Diffuse interstitial and sinusoidal infiltrates characteristic; can be very subtle and best appreciated by immunophenotypic assessment

B-PLL, B-cell prolymphocytic leukemia; CLL/SLL, chronic lymphocytic leukemia–small lymphocytic lymphoma; FCC, small cleaved follicular center cell lymphoma; HCL, hairy cell leukemia; LPL, lymphoplasmacytic lymphoma; MCL, mantle cell lymphoma; MZL, marginal zone lymphoma; WM, Waldenström's macroglobulinemia.
See references 1, 16, 130, and 150-155.

young patients who exhibit the typical clinical manifestations of acute viral infections, notably infectious mononucleosis. However, a rare condition termed *benign polyclonal lymphocytosis* exhibits more overlap with CLL, and flow cytometric immunophenotyping is generally required to identify this disorder, which is characterized by a sustained, unexplained mature B lymphocytosis.[137,138] Although binucleate and activated lymphocytes may be present, the majority of circulating cells are small, with scant cytoplasm and round, condensed nuclei.[137,138] Patients with polyclonal B lymphocytosis tend to be young to middle-aged women, usually smokers. A link to a specific paternal human leukocyte antigen haplotype has been established, suggesting an underlying genetic disorder in familial cases.[137]

During the past 10 years, the application of multicolor flow cytometric immunophenotyping on blood samples from various normal, healthy subjects has revealed occult B-cell clones in a small percentage (1% to 5%) of healthy individuals.[139-142] The incidence of monoclonal B lymphocytosis increases with both patient age (>5% in subjects older than 60 years) and the presence of a mild absolute lymphocytosis (>14% in individuals with absolute lymphocyte counts of 4 to 4.9×10^9/L).[141] Although monoclonal B lymphocytosis is a precursor to overt CLL, progression rates to overt CLL are only 1% per year, and the majority of individuals with these occult clones never manifest CLL.[4,18,139,141] In fact, the incidence of monoclonal B lymphocytosis is at least 100 times that of overt CLL.[18] However, in healthy adults enrolled in a nationwide cancer screening clinical trial, virtually all patients who developed overt CLL had an occult B-cell clone that was detected retrospectively in cryopreserved banked specimens that had been obtained up to 6.4 years earlier.[142]

In lymph node sections, nodular lymphocyte-predominant Hodgkin's lymphoma may exhibit some morphologic overlap with SLL, although both assessment for large lymphocyte-predominant L & H- (lymphocytic and histiocytic)-type

Table 14-4 Classic Immunophenotypic Profile of B-Cell Chronic Lymphoproliferative Neoplasms

Disorder	sIg	CD19	CD20	CD22	CD23	CD25	CD5	FMC7	CD11c	CD10	CD79a	CD79b	CD103	Cyclin D1
CLL/SLL	w	+	w	w	+	–	+	–	w	–	w	–	–	–
B-PLL	+	+	+	+	–	+ (s)	v	+	+ (s)	–	+	+	–	–
MCL	+	+	+	+	– (w)	–	+	+	–	–	+	+	–	+
FL	+	+	+	+	v	–	–	+	–	+	+	+	–	–
SMZL	+	+	+	+	v	–	–/+ (s)	+	v	–	+	+	–	–
HCL	+	+	+	+	–	+	–	+	+	+ (s)	+	–	+	+ (s)
LPL/WM	sIg/cIg+	+	+	+	–	–	–	–	–	–	+	+	–	–

B-PLL, B-cell prolymphocytic leukemia; cIg, cytoplasmic immunoglobulin; CLL/SLL, chronic lymphocytic leukemia–small lymphocytic lymphoma; FL, follicular lymphoma; HCL, hairy cell leukemia; LPL/WM, lymphoplasmacytic lymphoma–Waldentröm's macroglobulinemia; MCL, mantle cell lymphoma; s, subset of cases; sIg, surface immunoglobulin; SMZL, splenic B-cell marginal zone lymphoma with villous lymphocytes; v, variable expression; w, weakly expressed.
See references 1, 9, 16, 19, 130, 149, 150, 153, 156-165.

Reed-Sternberg cells and immunoperoxidase staining generally facilitate the distinction betweeen these two disorders. However, the more common and potentially problematic situation in clinical practice involves the distinction of CLL/SLL from other mature clonal B-cell disorders. This differential diagnosis can be a challenge in blood, bone marrow, and solid tissue such as lymph node or spleen (see Table 14-2).[143-149] In solid tissues, features that should be assessed include nuclear size and contour (round versus irregular); amount of cytoplasm, as reflected by the amount of space between nuclei; mitotic activity; and monotony versus heterogeneity of the infiltrate. On low magnification it is important to determine the pattern of infiltration and the specific anatomic region of the lymph node or spleen that shows selective involvement by the neoplasm. The presence of proliferation foci in the setting of diffuse nodal effacement is highly characteristic of CLL/SLL, even if some nuclear irregularity is present.[1,19,150] In the spleen, infiltrates should first be separated into white pulp and red pulp lesions; white pulp lesions are further subdivided by pattern of infiltration (germinal center, mantle, or marginal zone) when feasible.

In bone marrow, the pattern of infiltration is useful in both the differential diagnosis and the prognosis in cases of bona fide CLL (see Table 14-3).[1,16,130,150-155] The assessment of nuclear and cytoplasmic features is similar to that described in solid organs. Attention should be paid to identifying the pattern of infiltration as focal paratrabecular, focal nonparatrabecular, interstitial, diffuse, or sinusoidal, recognizing that more than one pattern may be evident in an individual case. Sinusoidal infiltrates can be very inconspicuous on hematoxylin-eosin stained sections and are best appreciated by immunoperoxidase staining for CD20 or CD79a.

Immunophenotypic assessment is essential in the accurate subclassification of B-cell chronic lymphoproliferative disorders, and a panel of antibodies evaluated by flow cytometric techniques is optimal, although immunoperoxidase stains can also provide significant information about the neoplastic clone. With multicolor flow cytometric immunophenotyping, both the profile and the intensity of antigen coexpression can be determined (see Table 14-4).[1,9,16,19,130,149,150,153,156-165] Although detailed immunophenotypic profiles provide critical information for the subclassification of chronic lymphoproliferative disorders, variations from classic profiles are commonly encountered in practice. Consequently, the integration of hematologic, morphologic, clinical, and genetic features is required for accurate classification. One particularly challenging area is the distinction between atypical CLL and mantle cell lymphoma (Figs. 14-20 and 14-21). Assessment for cyclin D1 expression by immunoperoxidase staining or cytogenetic or molecular studies for *CCND1(BCL1)* gene rearrangement or translocation is required to make this distinction.[45] Cyclin D1 positivity, although a highly sensitive marker for mantle cell lymphoma, has also been noted in cases of hairy cell leukemia and other disorders.[153] However, cyclin D1 positivity excludes CLL/SLL from consideration.

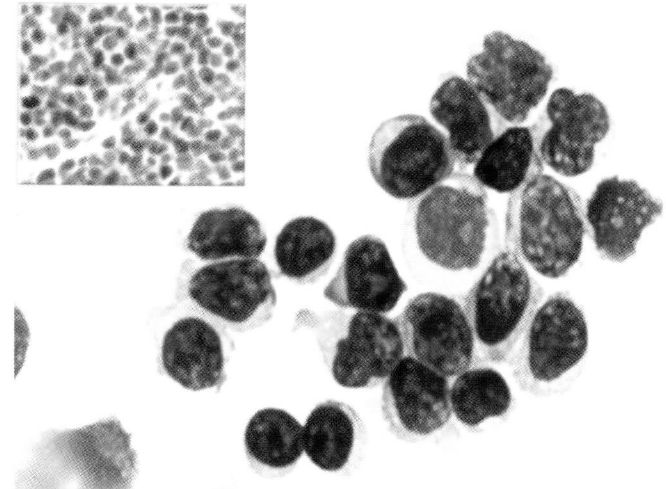

Figure 14-20. Composite illustrates the cytologic features of mantle cell lymphoma in blood (cytospin) in conjunction with nodal cyclin D1 nuclear expression (*inset*).

B-CELL PROLYMPHOCYTIC LEUKEMIA

Definition of Disease

B-cell prolymphocytic leukemia (B-PLL) is a rare malignant lymphoid tumor characterized by predominant blood, bone

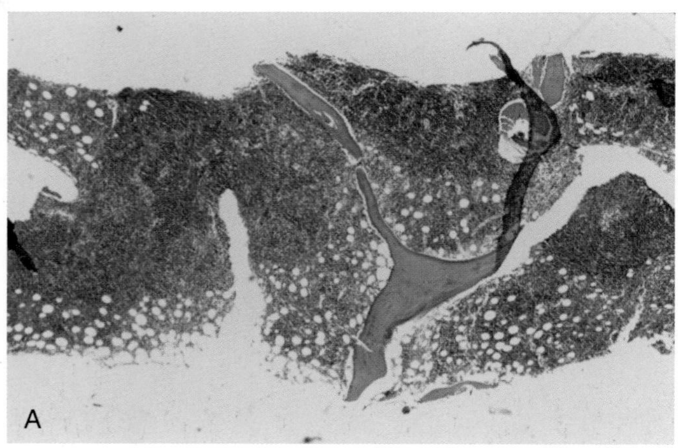

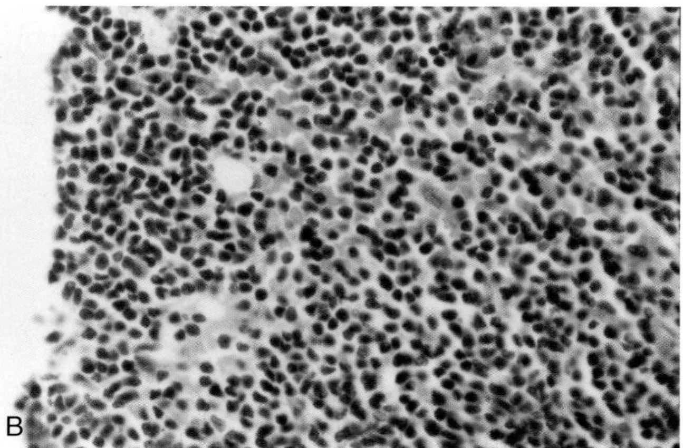

Figure 14-21. **A**, Low-power photomicrograph of a patient with prominent bone marrow involvement by mantle cell lymphoma illustrates focal paratrabecular and nonparatrabecular infiltrates. **B**, On high-power magnification, the nuclear irregularity that characterizes most cases of mantle cell lymphoma is evident.

marrow, and splenic involvement by a clonal proliferation of prolymphocytes.[16,25,166,167] More specifically, B-PLL constitutes a de novo chronic B-cell leukemic presentation with greater than 55% circulating peripheral blood prolymphocytes.[145,156,168,169] Patients with transformed CLL or preexisting CLL with increased prolymphocytes are thus excluded. Although the cytologic features of B-PLL are considered to be relatively distinctive, exclusion of potential disease mimickers (such as unusual presentations of mantle cell lymphoma) is required before a definitive diagnosis of B-PLL can be made. The application of ancillary immunophenotypic and molecular cytogenetic techniques is of great value in this regard.

Epidemiology and Incidence

B-PLL is a relatively rare tumor, accounting for 1% or less of lymphoid leukemias.[145] Consequently, few large studies have been described, and much of our knowledge of the epidemiologic variables in this disorder is derived from earlier reports.[166,169] Males are affected slightly more commonly than females, and the median age at diagnosis is 65 to 70 years.

Clinical Features

Patients with B-PLL exhibit marked leukocytosis (frequently >100 × 10^9/L), with absolute lymphocytosis and splenomegaly.[166,169] Extensive bone marrow involvement by the neoplastic prolymphocytes produces anemia and thrombocytopenia in approximately half of patients, although the absolute neutrophil count is often within the normal range. Splenic enlargement can be massive, with associated clinical symptoms.[166,169] Involvement of the liver may also occur, although to a lesser degree and less frequently. Characteristically, lymphadenopathy is absent or relatively minimal; the presence of bulky peripheral adenopathy in addition to an abnormal peripheral blood lymphocytosis should raise the differential diagnosis of a non-Hodgkin's lymphoma with a leukemic component. A modest serum monoclonal gammopathy, usually of IgG or IgM type, can be detected in some patients with B-PLL.

Morphology

See Tables 14-2 and 14-3.

Peripheral Blood and Bone Marrow

In the peripheral blood, the vast majority of circulating leukocytes are prolymphocytes, characterized by medium nuclear size, moderately condensed chromatin, and a single prominent nucleolus (Fig. 14-22). Cells with finely dispersed or "blastoid" chromatin are not present in B-PLL. Nuclear contours are rounded, without significant nuclear membrane irregularity, and there is generally minimal cell-to-cell variability. The cell cytoplasm is minimally to moderately abundant, with well-defined borders in Wright-Giemsa preparations. The bone marrow aspirate typically shows marked hematopoietic replacement by neoplastic prolymphocytes. In fixed bone marrow core biopsy sections, there is extensive diffuse or interstitial involvement of the marrow space, although a focal nodular, nonparatrabecular pattern can also be observed.[25] The abnormal prolymphocytes are relatively uniform and display a small to medium nuclear size, with prominent small, central nucleoli and a rim of amphophilic cytoplasm. Although the appearance and cytologic features of B-PLL in the bone marrow are somewhat characteristic, other B-cell lymphomas or chronic leukemias can display partially overlapping morphologic findings; thus, comprehensive immunophenotypic and often molecular cytogenetic evaluation is generally required for diagnosis.[130]

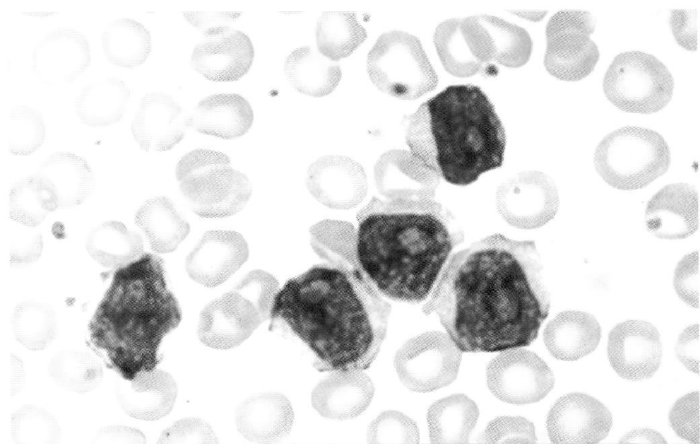

Figure 14-22. Peripheral blood smear illustrates a striking lymphocytosis with a monotonous population of lymphoid cells exhibiting prominent nucleoli in this elderly patient with B-cell prolymphocytic leukemia.

Spleen

Splenic infiltration by B-PLL involves both red and white pulp regions.[16,145,156,166,170] The red pulp sinusoids are variably expanded by neoplastic lymphocytes demonstrating medium-sized nuclei with central prominent nucleoli. The white pulp is usually greatly expanded, with a multinodular appearance; particularly large foci may result in coalescence of adjacent involved white pulp nodules.

Lymph Node

Although clinical lymphadenopathy is not common in this B-cell neoplasm, the morphologic features of involved lymph nodes demonstrate diffuse or vaguely nodular effacing infiltrates composed of cells similar in appearance to those described in spleen or marrow tissue sections (Fig. 14-23). A pattern of distinct proliferation centers or "pseudofollicles" characteristic of CLL/SLL is not identified in B-PLL. Nevertheless, the nodal histology of B-PLL may be similar to some cases of CLL/SLL with particularly prominent or confluent proliferation centers. A subset of mantle cell lymphomas, B-cell marginal zone lymphomas (MZLs), and occasional presentations of diffuse large B-cell lymphoma can also overlap with B-PLL morphologically.

Other Tissue Sites

Hepatic involvement in B-PLL is less pronounced than in the spleen. Liver infiltration by B-PLL appears as sinusoidal hepatic infiltrates, in keeping with the predominantly leukemic nature of the disease. Other tissue sites involved in B-PLL have been reported, such as rare cases of cutaneous and central nervous system disease.[171,172]

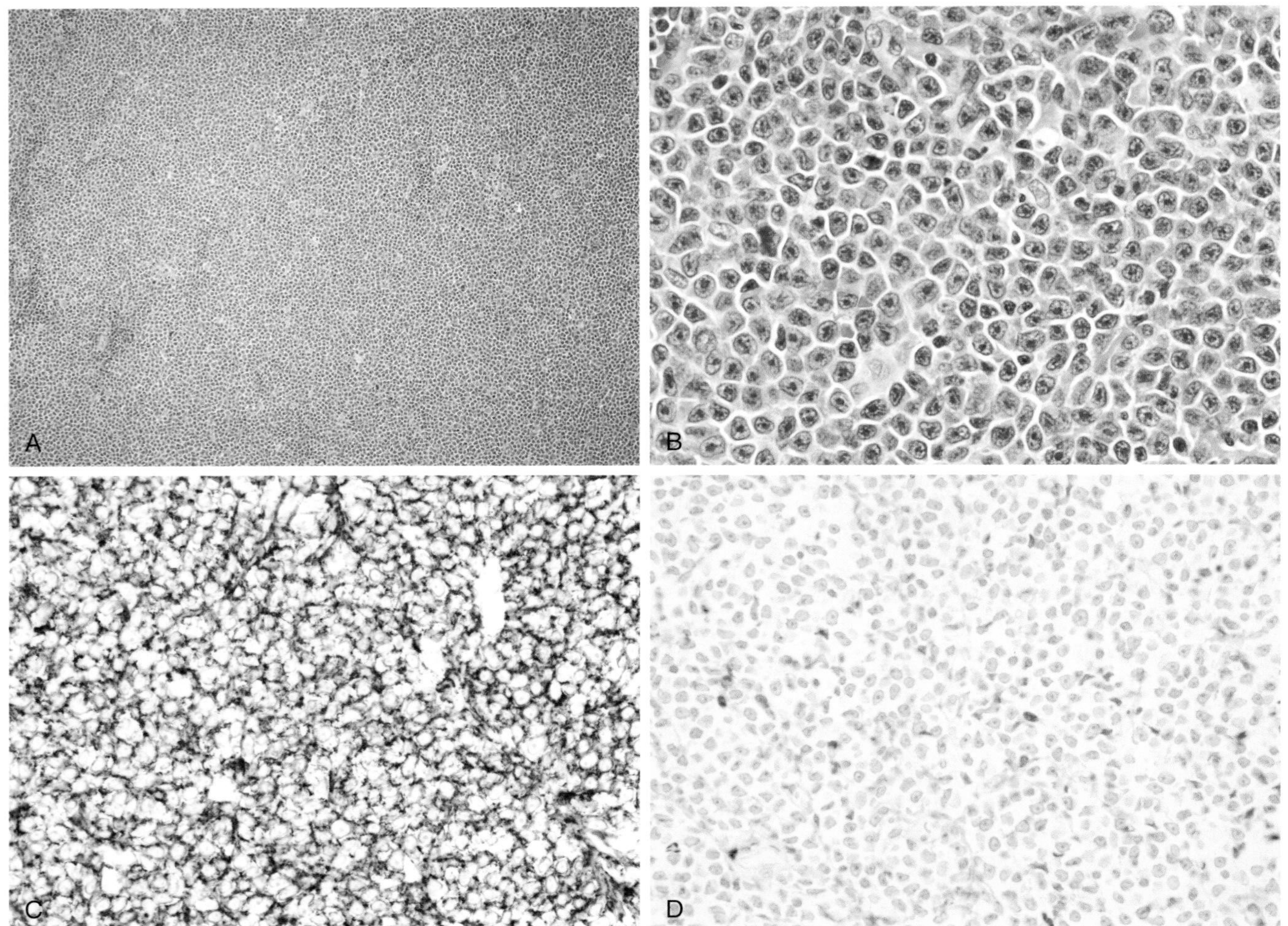

Figure 14-23. This patient presented with a neck mass and sinus infiltration by B-cell prolymphocytic leukemia (**A** and **B**). Cells are CD20+ (**C**) and lack cyclin D1 (**D**). At presentation, the peripheral white blood cell count was 80×10^9/L, with 80% classic prolymphocytes showing a B-cell immunophenotype with partial CD5 expression by flow cytometry (not shown). (Courtesy of Dr. Burton Kim, Austell, CA.)

Immunophenotype

Flow cytometric evaluation of B-PLL constitutes an important aspect of the diagnostic evaluation (Fig. 14-24). Cell surface markers expressed by B-PLL cells include B-cell antigens CD19, CD20, CD22, CD79a, monotypic surface light-chain immunoglobulin, and the CD20-associated antigen FMC7 (see Table 14-4).[145,173] Aberrant CD5 antigen expression is present in less than 50% of cases. CD23 antigen expression is infrequently seen in B-PLL,[157] although some investigators have reported positive cases.[130] The intensity of surface light-chain immunoglobulin is moderately bright. CD38 expression is variably observed in B-PLL. Expression of the ZAP-70 protein kinase (>20% of cells) has been noted in nearly 60% of cases.[174]

Cytogenetic and Molecular Genetic Features

The genetic features characterizing B-PLL remain incompletely understood owing to the relative rarity of the disease and the occurrence of other entities that previously may have been considered B-PLL. Tumor cells of B-PLL demonstrate clonal rearrangements of the immunoglobulin heavy-chain gene (*IGH@*), with the preferential VH3 and VH4 family gene segment usage.[174,175] Specific genetic locus abnormalities have been described in B-PLL, including a high frequency (approximately 50%) of 17p deletions involving the *TP53* gene, as well as rearrangements of the *MYC* oncogene at 8q24.[176-178] Cytogenetic or FISH studies of B-PLL have also revealed abnormalities involving chromosomes 7, 11q23, and 13q14, as well as more complex karyotypes, although none of these represent tumor-specific markers.[179] Most significantly, the t(11;14)(q13;q32) *CCND1/IGH@* genetic lesion was previously reported to occur in nearly 20% of cases described as B-PLL.[180] Evaluation of such cases in the current era, however, indicates that these "prolymphocytoid" B-cell leukemias represent leukemic manifestations of mantle cell lymphoma.[130,181-187]

Cell of Origin

The normal mature B-cell counterpart for B-PLL remains elusive. Molecular genetic studies of somatic hypermutation status have shown that B-PLL cases are divided nearly equally into those with unmutated (<2%) and mutated (>2%) *IGH@*

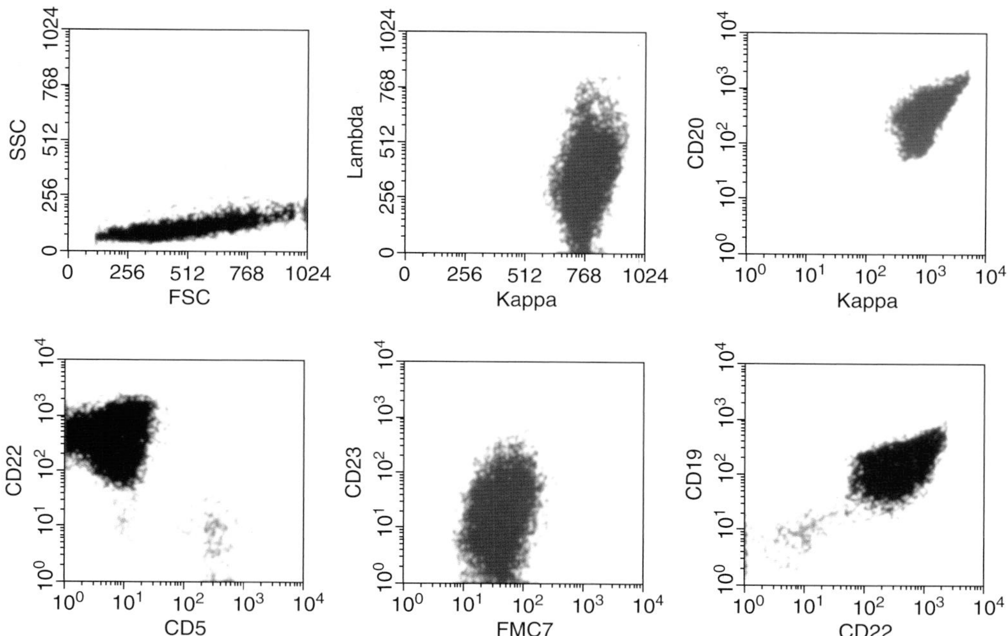

Figure 14-24. Composite flow cytometric histogram illustrates the immunophenotye in a case of B-cell prolymphocytic leukemia. Note expression of CD19, CD20, FMC7, CD22, and monoclonal kappa light chain. There is weak to minimal expression of CD23; CD5 is absent. FSC, forward scatter; SSC, side scatter.

V regions, compared with germline sequences.[174] This apparent heterogeneity in mutation status is strikingly similar to the situation for CLL, suggesting the possibility of different pre– and post–germinal center pathways in the pathogenesis of the disease. A more precise definition of the lymphoid ontogeny of B-PLL requires additional study.

Clinical Course

Earlier clinicopathologic studies documented a rapid clinical course with poor outcome for B-PLL patients, with median survival times ranging from 4 months to 3 years.[166,188] One series of 35 B-PLL patients documented a more heterogeneous population, with correspondingly nonuniform clinical and biologic behavior.[189] These investigators were able to identify three nearly equally sized groups of patients, with the main differences being the degree of spleen enlargement and the level and progression of peripheral lymphocytosis. Adverse clinical and laboratory prognostic factors in B-PLL include advanced patient age, marked splenomegaly, high absolute prolymphocyte count, and anemia (hemoglobin <11 g/dL).[173,188,189] Clearly, a potential drawback to early studies of B-PLL is the possibility that other B-cell lymphoproliferative diseases with prolymphocytoid morphologic features were included, owing to less precise disease definitions. A more recent analysis of 19 B-PLL patients did not identify *IGH@* mutation status, CD38, or 17p deletion as prognostic factors[174]; paradoxically, this study suggested that ZAP-70 positivity was associated with better overall survival than ZAP-70$^-$ status. Other small case studies have suggested that 17p and 8q24 genomic deletions are associated with a poor outcome in B-PLL.

Therapeutic options for B-PLL are not standardized. Typical alkylating agent chemotherapy is relatively ineffective. Multiagent regimens (e.g., CHOP chemotherapy) have shown improved response rates.[189] The use of purine nucleoside analogues, particularly in conjunction with therapeutic antibodies (e.g., rituximab, anti-CD20) may be more promising in this regard.[189-193]

Differential Diagnosis

As indicated, the diagnosis of B-PLL requires the exclusion of several other lymphoid neoplasms by the use of appropriate immunophenotypic and molecular cytogenetic investigations, in addition to histopathologic observations (see Tables 14-2 to 14-4). From a morphologic perspective, prolymphocytoid cytologic features can be observed in CLL with increased prolymphocytes, the leukemic phase of mantle cell lymphoma, splenic marginal zone lymphoma (SMZL), large B-cell lymphoma, rare cases of so-called hairy cell leukemia variant (HCLv), and T-cell prolymphocytic leukemia. (Note that HCLv is currently designated "splenic B-cell lymphoma/leukemia" by the World Health Organization's 2008 criteria.)[194] CLL in prolymphocytic transformation is readily distinguished by the presence of a substantial population of small lymphocytes with condensed, classic CLL-like features and less than 55% prolymphocytes. Large B-cell lymphoma involving the peripheral blood is seldom associated with a marked lymphocytosis; moreover, the abnormal lymphoma cells generally appear larger and more pleomorphic than those of B-PLL. T-cell prolymphocytic leukemia generally presents with bulky lymph node disease and is readily identified by its mature CD4 T-cell immunophenotype and the presence of *TCL1A* gene translocations in 80% of cases.

The remaining considerations, including mantle cell lymphoma, SMZL and HCLv, can each resemble cases of true B-PLL and thus pose a more substantial challenge. It is now recognized that B-cell neoplasms with prolymphocytic features and the t(11;14) translocation are in fact leukemic presentations of mantle cell lymphoma, often with prominent splenomegalic disease.[130,182,183,187] Thus, evaluation for the t(11;14) *CCND1/IGH@* abnormality by karyotyping or FISH techniques, or cyclin D1 overexpression by immunohistochemistry, is required to exclude mantle cell lymphoma. SMZL is an uncommon mature B-cell leukemia/lymphoma characterized by circulating atypical lymphocytes, splenomegaly, and bone marrow involvement. SMZL may contain a proportion of PLL-like cells; however cytologic variability is often present, and some cases show more distinct findings such as plasmacytoid differentiation, or "villous" circulating lymphocytes. In the bone marrow, SMZL demonstrates either nodular aggregates of monocytoid cells or a subtle intrasinusoidal infiltration, in contrast to the more leukemic interstitial pattern of B-PLL.[195] Clinically, SMZL is associated with relatively indolent behavior. The entity HCLv is controversial and describes a B-cell neoplasm with features overlapping with those of classic HCL, B-PLL, and SMZL.[196,197] This tumor is currently included in the category of "splenic B-cell lymphoma/leukemia, unclassifiable."[194] Patients with HCLv present with marked splenomegaly and high peripheral white blood cell counts. Cytologically, HCLv cells show some similarity to B-PLL cells, including the presence of a single prominent nucleolus (Fig. 14-25). In most cases, the cells of HCLv retain delicate fibrillary cytoplasmic membrane borders and may have a sponge-like chromatin pattern similar to that of typical HCL or a more unusual blastoid or convoluted nuclear cytology. Distinction of HCLv from B-PLL can be achieved morphologically in the spleen, with HCLv showing a pure red pulp pattern of splenic involvement. In bone marrow trephine biopsies, HCLv also produces an interstitial or sometimes diffuse pattern, but it usually has the characteristic appearance of HCL (i.e., "fried egg" cell morphology). HCLv can also be readily distinguished from B-PLL by immunophenotyping studies, which reveal positivity for CD103 and bright coexpression of CD11c and CD22 (Fig. 14-26).[197]

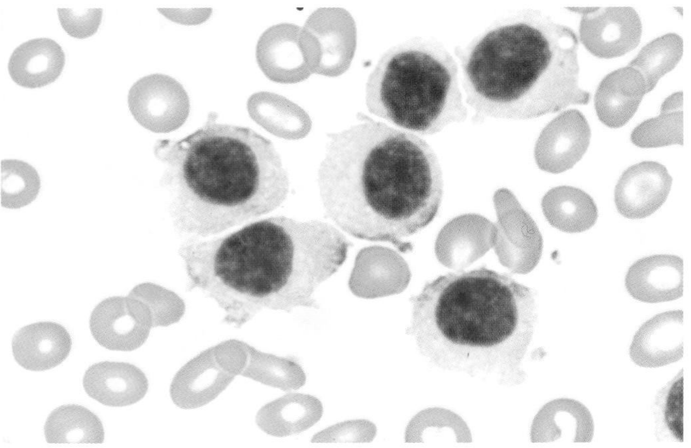

Figure 14-25. Peripheral blood composite illustrates the cytologic features in a patient with so-called hairy cell leukemia variant (splenic B-cell lymphoma/leukemia, unclassifiable).

LYMPHOPLASMACYTIC LYMPHOMA AND WALDENSTRÖM'S MACROGLOBULINEMIA

Definition of Disease

Lymphoplasmacytic lymphoma (LPL) is a disseminated B-cell lymphoproliferative disorder characterized by a spectrum of small B cells, plasmacytoid lymphocytes, and plasma cells. This neoplasm mainly involves the bone marrow, although splenic and nodal disease can be seen, as well as involvement

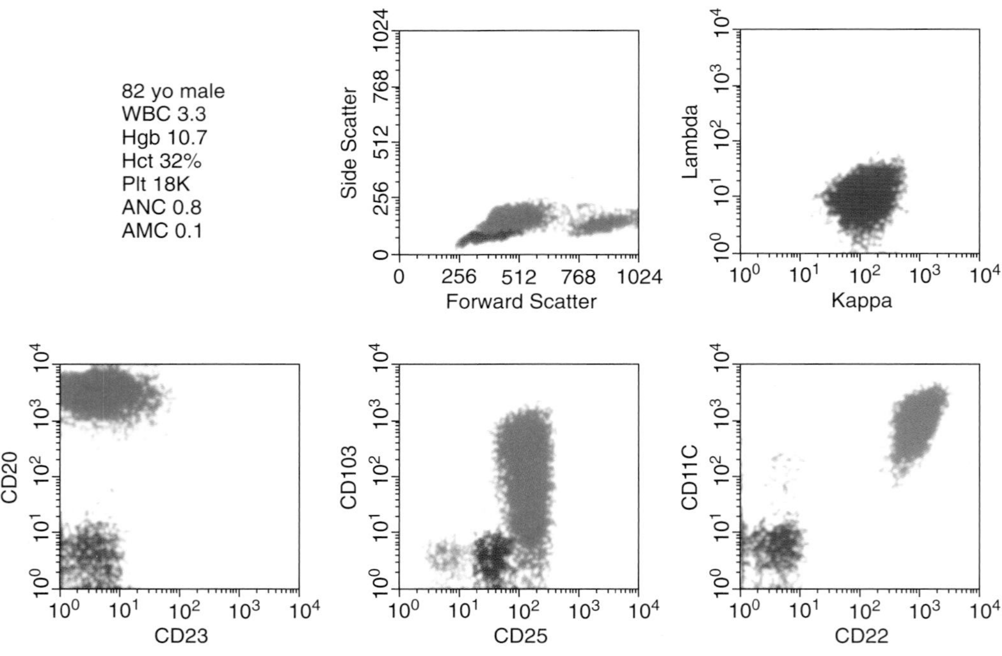

Figure 14-26. Flow cytometric immunophenotyping composite illustrates the typical immunophenotypic profile of hairy cell leukemia. Note strong expression of CD22 in addition to other B-cell markers, as well as strong coexpression of CD103, CD25, and CD11c.

of other tissue sites. LPL is typically but not always associated with an IgM gammopathy. The clinical syndrome of Waldenström's macroglobulinemia (WM) is currently defined as LPL with an associated monoclonal IgM protein of any level.[160,198-200] LPL/WM is a major entity in the spectrum of IgM gammopathies, which includes IgM monoclonal gammopathy of uncertain significance (MGUS) and very rare presentations of IgM myeloma (see Differential Diagnosis). It is also important to note that other B-cell neoplasms, often with features of plasmacytic differentiation (e.g., MZLs), are occasionally associated with IgM paraprotein production, reflecting the still imprecise nosologic aspects of this disorder.[50] Conversely, rare patients with B-cell lymphoproliferations and symptomatic WM-like features have been described in association with non-IgM (i.e., IgG or IgA) gammopathy. Rarely, a primarily node-based presentation of LPL is encountered in hematopathology practice; however, this entity is incompletely understood, is not necessarily associated with symptomatic WM, and exhibits clinical behavior intermediate between other indolent and aggressive nodal B-cell lymphomas.

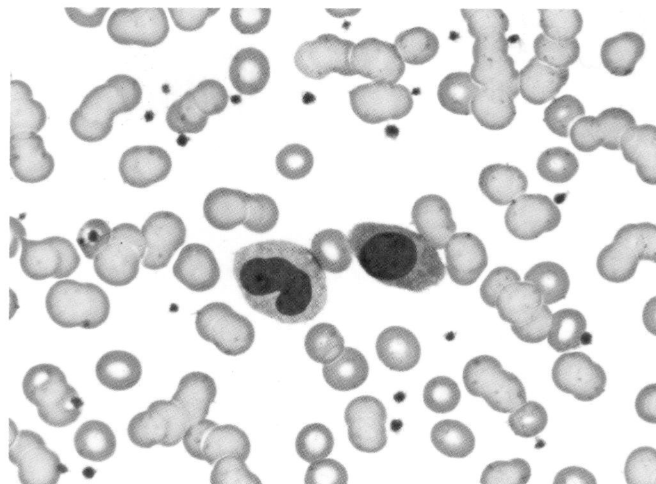

Figure 14-27. Peripheral blood smear from a patient with Waldenström's macroglobulinemia shows prominent rouleau formation in addition to circulating lymphoplasmacytoid cells.

Epidemiology and Incidence

LPL is an uncommon lymphoid neoplasm, accounting for approximately 5% of B-cell lymphoproliferative disorders. The disease has a slight male predominance and occurs at a median age of 60 to 65 years. Analysis of familial risk in LPL/WM suggests a genetic predisposition in some cases.[201-204] Autoimmune and infectious diseases are additional risk factors identified by population-based studies.[205,206] The role of hepatitis C virus (HCV) in LPL remains controversial. At least in some geographic areas, a link among HCV infection, the development of type II (mixed) cryoglobulinemia, and LPL has been noted, although other studies have shown no significant correlation (see Cell of Origin).

Clinical Features

The clinical manifestations of LPL/WM can be divided into two major types: hematologic and gammopathy-related abnormalities.[160,198,207-209] A spectrum of disease severity is present, encompassing relatively asymptomatic individuals as well as patients with variably relapsing-remitting or progressive disease. The bone marrow is consistently involved, and extensive replacement of normal hematopoietic cells by LPL can result in peripheral cytopenias. Accompanying lymph node disease may be present, although bulky adenopathy is uncommon. Splenomegaly of mild to moderate degree is present in some individuals. Involvement of the liver, as well as multiple additional tissue sites (e.g., skin, gastrointestinal tract, lung), can be seen in more advanced disease. Osteolytic bone lesions are not observed, and hypercalcemia is rare. The majority of patients with LPL/WM have an IgM paraproteinemia, although rare occurrences of IgG or mixed IgM-IgG production can be encountered. Higher IgM levels (>3.0 g/dL) are associated with greater risk of hyperviscosity symptoms, including fatigue, mental status changes, and visual disturbances.[210] Abnormal IgM proteins can also contribute to hemostatic dysfunction, with bleeding, hemolytic anemia (cold agglutinin or autoimmune mediated), and cryoglobulinemia.[211] In addition, deposition of IgM paraprotein may cause peripheral neuropathies and renal impairment.[212,213] In rare patients, amyloidosis can become a serious complication during the course of the disease.[214,215]

Morphology

Peripheral Blood and Bone Marrow

Lymphocytosis may be present, but many patients with LPL do not have significantly elevated lymphocyte counts. Circulating lymphocytes are small, with condensed nuclei and inconspicuous nucleoli. A subset of lymphocytes can demonstrate plasmacytoid cytoplasmic features characterized by eccentric nuclei and slightly more abundant basophilic cytoplasm (Fig. 14-27). Rare plasma cells may be seen. Red blood cell rouleau formation is typically noted owing to the abnormal serum IgM paraprotein. On bone marrow aspirate smears, the neoplastic lymphocytes show a spectrum of morphology, including small, round lymphocytes, plasmacytoid lymphocytes, and plasma cells (Fig. 14-28). Plasma cells show

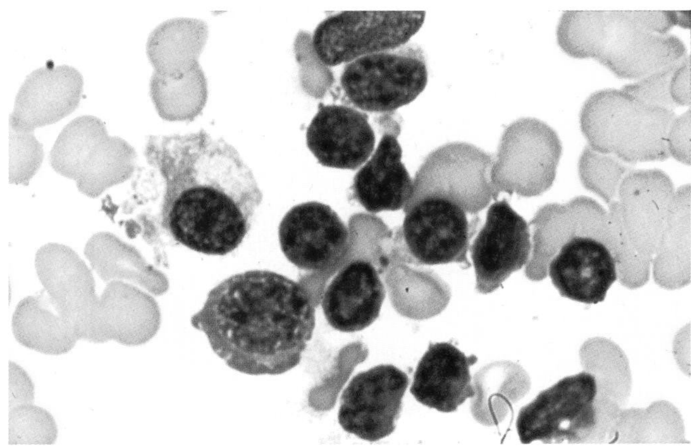

Figure 14-28. Bone marrow aspirate smear from a patient with Waldenström's macroglobulinemia highlights the spectrum of plasma cells, plasmacytoid lymphocytes, and lymphocytes that characterizes this lymphoplasmacytic disorder.

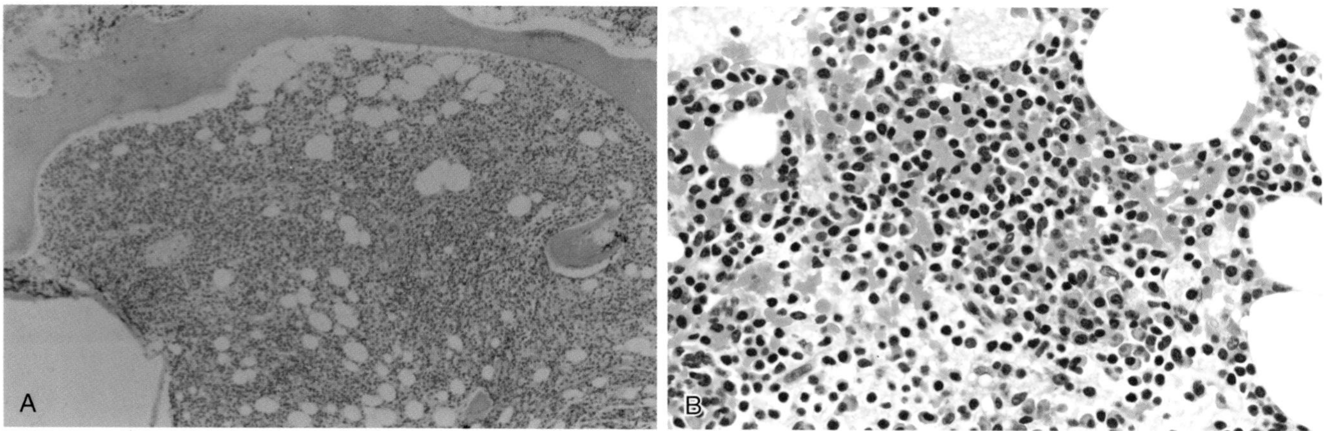

Figure 14-29. Morphologic features of Waldenström's macroglobulinemia in bone marrow core biopsy sections on low (**A**) and high (**B**) magnification. Note the Dutcher bodies in **B**.

minimal to mild cytologic atypia. Trephine biopsy samples can exhibit several patterns of infiltration by mainly small lymphocytes and plasma cells. Scattered large centroblastic or immunoblastic cells may also be present. The variable composition of small lymphocytes, plasmacytoid lymphocytes, plasma cells, and large lymphocytes in tissue biopsies of LPL has led to historical descriptions of lymphoplasmacytoid, lymphoplasmacytic, and polymorphous morphologic subtypes. Polymorphous cytology is distinguished by the presence of noticeable admixed centroblasts or immunoblasts (e.g., 5% to 10%), whereas the other subtypes have rare to absent large cells. The tumor may form ill-defined, patchy interstitial collections, nodular aggregates, or loose paratrabecular foci (Fig. 14-29).[25,161,216] In some cases, pronounced interstitial or even diffuse, sheet-like replacement of the hematopoietic marrow is observed. Dutcher bodies (intranuclear pseudoinclusions of immunoglobulin) are frequently found in plasma cells and lymphocytes but may be sparsely distributed (see Fig. 14-29B). A frequently associated feature of LPL is the presence of increased mast cells in the marrow; these can be readily identified lying within or surrounding marrow particles on Wright-Giemsa aspirate preparations or by immunohistochemistry for tryptase or CD117 (c-Kit) in trephine biopsy sections (Fig. 14-30).[151] Immunoglobulin or amyloid deposition may be observed in rare cases; the latter finding is confirmed by staining with Congo red (Fig. 14-31). Other useful markers in LPL/WM include CD20, CD138, and MUM-1 (Fig. 14-32). Biopsies should also be carefully evaluated for focal transformation to diffuse large B-cell lymphoma.[217]

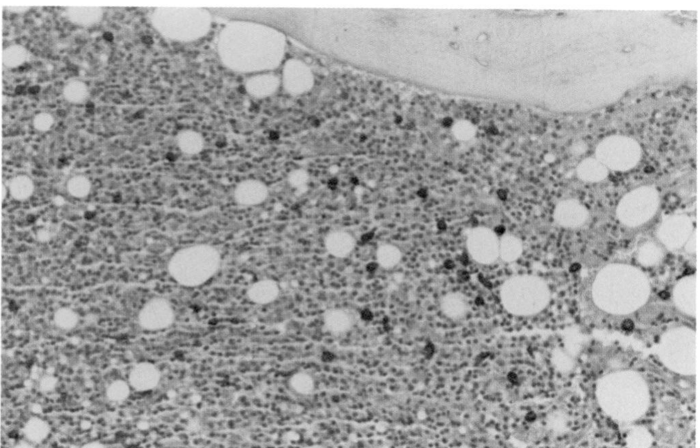

Figure 14-30. Increased mast cells in lymphoplasmacytic lymphoma are highlighted by immunoperoxidase for tryptase.

Lymph Nodes

LPL often involves lymph nodes in a spotty or subtle distribution within the paracortex and perisinusoidal regions, sparing the overall nodal architecture and the patency of trabecular sinuses. In other cases, the lymph nodes may be replaced by a vaguely nodular or more diffuse effacing pattern. "Pseudofollicles" or proliferation center foci classically associated with CLL/SLL are not noted in LPL. Cytologically, the neoplastic cells comprise small lymphocytes and varying numbers of plasma cells. Plasma cells may be distributed in small, distinct clusters or admixed with small lymphocytes. Dutcher bodies are often readily found. Importantly, "monocytoid" or marginal zone cytologic features are absent, and other related findings of MZL (e.g., follicle colonization) are not observed. Intermixed mast cells are common, and in rare instances, epithelioid histiocytes may be abundant, imparting a non-necrotizing granulomatous appearance.[218] Hemosiderin deposition is typically noted. Rarely, extracellular immunoglobulin or amyloid deposition is found. The mitotic rate is generally low in nodal biopsies of LPL. Centroblastic or immunoblastic large lymphocytes generally constitute a minor subset of the neoplastic cells and are admixed with the ubiquitous small lymphoid and plasma cell populations in most cases. However, in some tumors, large cells are more predominant (5% to 10% of cells), representing a polymorphous morphology. A more substantial presence of large lymphocytes in LPL should prompt a careful evaluation for discrete foci or aggregates suggesting the possibility of transformation to large B-cell lymphoma.

Spleen, Liver, and Other Tissue Sites

The spleen in LPL is infiltrated mainly in a white pulp manner, although patchy red pulp lymphoid aggregates are often

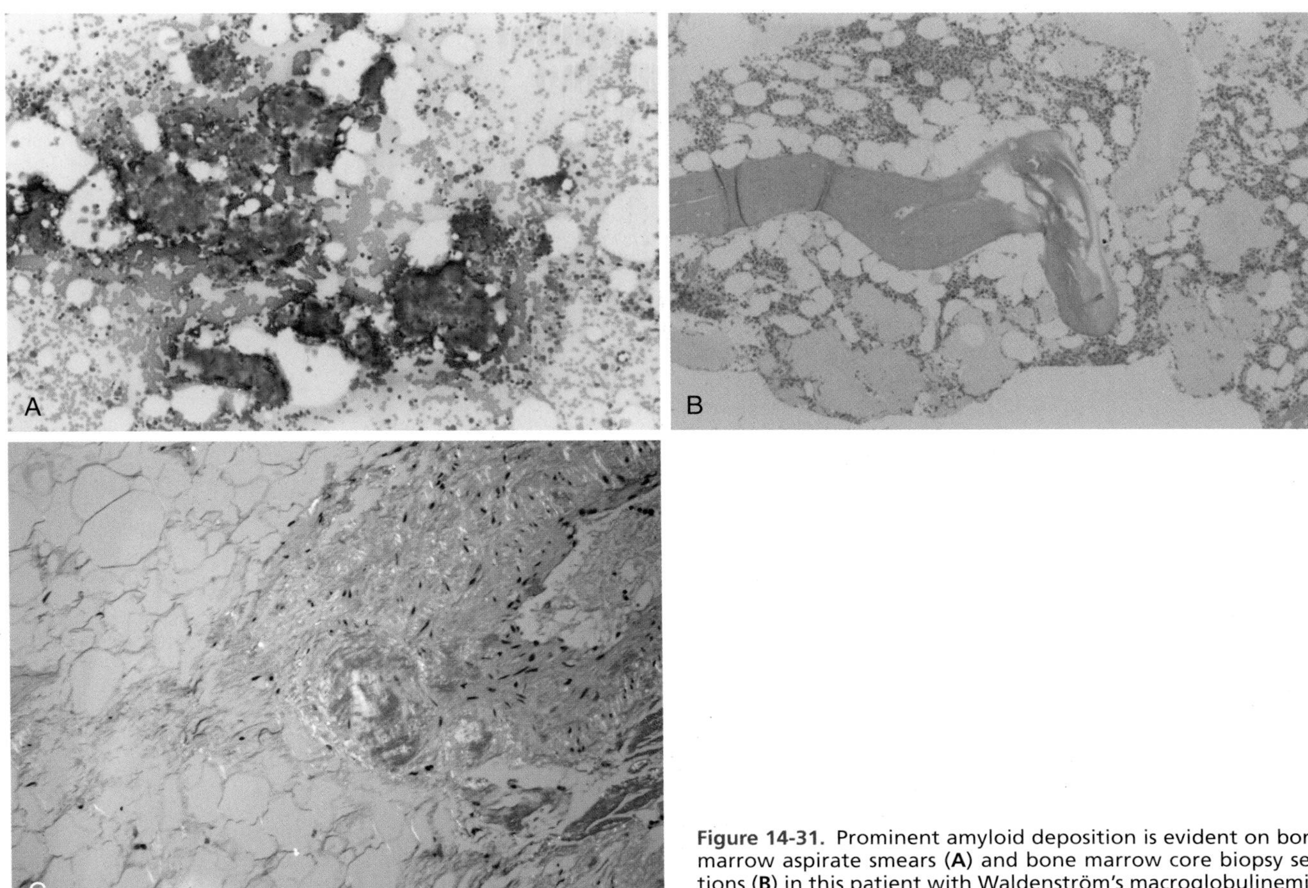

Figure 14-31. Prominent amyloid deposition is evident on bone marrow aspirate smears **(A)** and bone marrow core biopsy sections **(B)** in this patient with Waldenström's macroglobulinemia. Birefringence is noted by polarization of Congo red stain **(C)**.

present as well. The neoplastic cells show a cytologic spectrum similar to that of lymph node and bone marrow. The distribution and cytologic appearance may create difficulty in differentiating LPL from SMZL, particularly if tissue fixation is suboptimal. Again, the presence of distinctive monocytoid features and a marginal zone growth pattern should raise the possibility of SMZL. LPL probably should not be diagnosed from splenic pathology alone; those findings should be integrated with bone marrow or lymph node biopsy findings, serum protein electrophoresis results, and the clinical scenario. Liver biopsies are seldom obtained in LPL, but when the liver is involved, there is an abnormal lymphoplasmacytic population predominantly in portal areas. Sporadic reports of skin involvement by LPL have been documented.[219,220] Cutaneous disease may manifest as plaque-like lesions due to diffuse reticular dermis infiltration by LPL cells or, less commonly, as papular lesions of eosinophilic proteinaceous material containing IgM paraprotein. Additional sites of extramedullary tissue involvement have been described in WM patients, most often characterized by infiltrates of morphologically typical LPL, although some cases are difficult to distinguish from B-cell MZL.[221]

Immunophenotype

The small B lymphocytes in LPL demonstrate expression of pan–B-cell antigens (CD19, CD20, CD22, CD79a, PAX5) with monotypic surface light-chain restriction. In many cases there is no additional phenotypically distinct marker profile, unlike in other subtypes of B-cell lymphoma (see Table 14-4).[160-162,222] A significant subset of cases can coexpress CD5 or CD23, or both, although with a pattern distinct from that of classic CLL/SLL. The diagnosis of LPL should therefore not be dismissed in the immunophenotypic setting of CD5 or CD23 copositivity.[223] Rare examples of LPL with CD10 coexpression are also recognized.[224] In tissue sections, light-chain restriction is usually easily demonstrated in both small lymphocytes and associated plasma cells by immunohistochemistry. The plasma cell component can also be highlighted using antibodies recognizing CD138 or MUM-1 (IRF4) proteins (see Fig. 14-32B and C). Heavy-chain immunoperoxidase is infrequently employed for diagnosis, but the vast majority of LPLs are clearly IgM$^+$. Recent flow cytometric studies have noted that LPL-associated plasma cells are CD19$^+$, in contradistinction to the plasma cells of multiple myeloma.[225]

Cytogenetic and Molecular Genetic Features

Early genetic associations attributed the presence of a t(9;14)(p13;q32) abnormality to 50% of low-grade B-cell lymphomas characterized by plasmacytoid differentiation.[226] Subsequent cloning of the breakpoints revealed fusion of

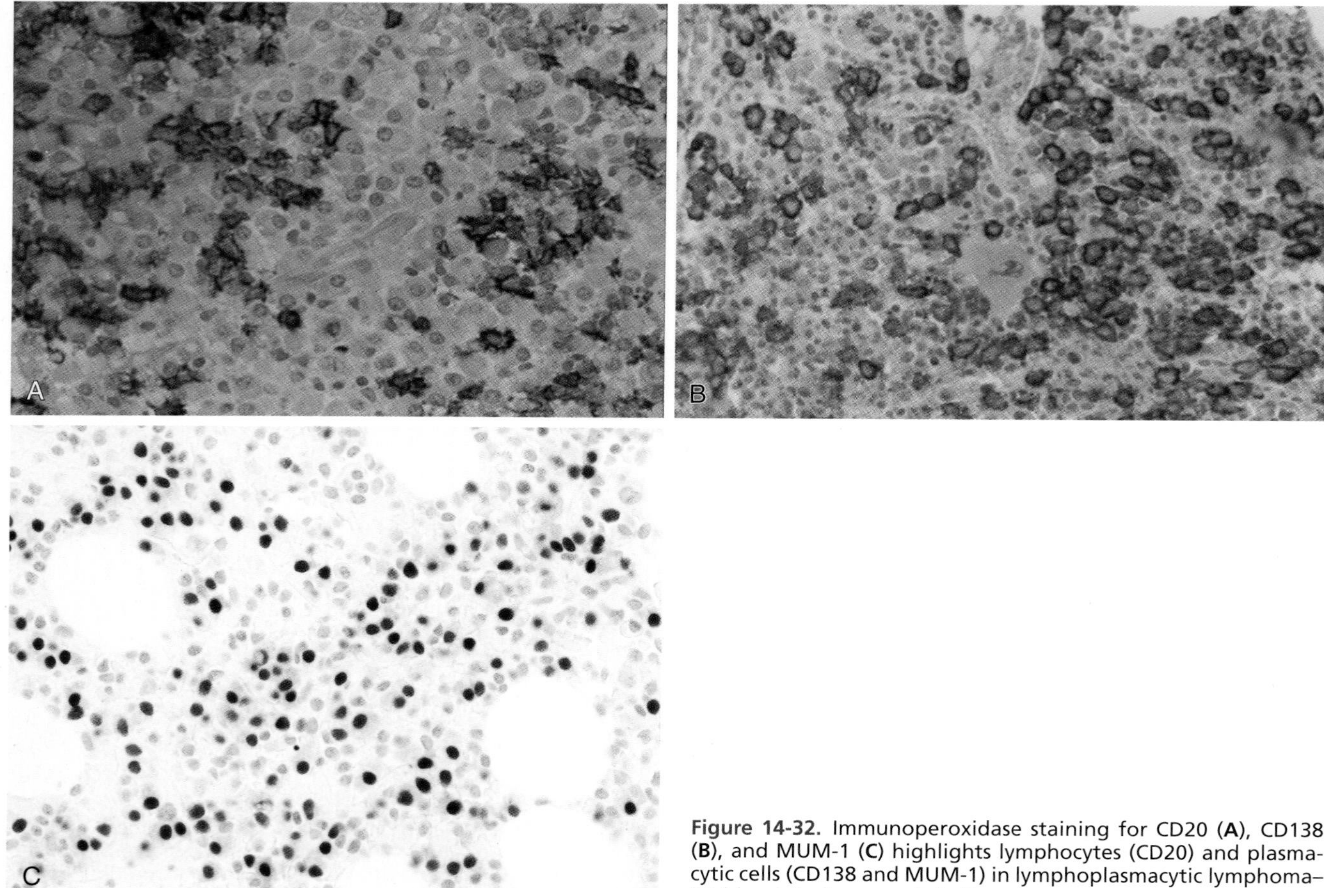

Figure 14-32. Immunoperoxidase staining for CD20 (**A**), CD138 (**B**), and MUM-1 (**C**) highlights lymphocytes (CD20) and plasmacytic cells (CD138 and MUM-1) in lymphoplasmacytic lymphoma–Waldenström's macroglobulinemia.

the *PAX5* gene on 9(p13) to the *IGH@* locus.[227] More recent studies have not shown t(9;14) in cases of LPL, and some have suggested an association with large B-cell lymphoma instead.[228-234] This discrepancy most likely reflects the more precise current definition of LPL and the use of more comprehensive laboratory methods for the evaluation of genetic anomalies. In fact, using FISH techniques, rearrangements of the *IGH@* locus are very infrequent in LPL.[235] Deletion of the long arm of chromosome 6 (6q−) has emerged as the most common abnormality in LPL (40% to 60% of cases), even though this finding is relatively nonspecific as a tumor marker.[231,233,234,236] Trisomy of chromosome 4 has also been reported in a subset of LPL patients.[237] In one study, LPL cases with increased large cells (i.e., polymorphous cytology) were more strongly associated with complex or aneuploid karyotypes.[231] Notably, cytogenetic abnormalities often associated with CLL, such as +12 or 13q−, are infrequently identified in LPL.[231,238-240] New approaches, perhaps employing array-based genomic analysis, may be able to better define the genetic features of LPL.[241] Of note, a case series specifically investigating node-based LPL revealed the absence of the 6q− and *PAX5* gene rearrangements, as well as the lack of many typical genetic changes associated with MZLs; this study emphasizes our incomplete understanding of rare lymph node–predominant presentations of LPL.[242]

Cell of Origin

The lymphocytes of LPL are mature B cells capable of differentiating to plasma cells.[50,222,243] Mutational analysis of the *IGH@* gene in LPL has shown the presence of extensive somatic hypermutation, in keeping with a post–germinal center cell origin[244]; however, these cells have failed to undergo heavy-chain class switching and may be physiologically impaired in this ability.[245-247] Most reports in this regard have not found evidence of substantial intraclonal variation.[248-251] Recent insights from gene expression profiling and proteomics approaches have further demonstrated the role of gene deregulation in pathways governing late B-cell transition and plasma cell differentiation in the pathogenesis of LPL.[252-257]

Several studies have described an intriguing association between HCV infection and the rare development of non-Hodgkin's lymphomas, mainly in Italian patients.[258-260] HCV infection is strongly associated with type II or mixed cryoglobulinemia and, in this setting, is thought to lead to excess B-cell lymphoproliferation and subsequent clonal outgrowth.[261] Some epidemiologic surveys have found that MZL and LPL are overrepresented in HCV-positive patients,[262] whereas other series suggest an increased risk for mature B-cell neoplasms overall.[263] The apparent link between HCV infection and the occurrence of low-grade B-cell LPL or MZL implicates chronic antigenic stimulation in the genesis of the neoplastic clone; this hypothesis is supported to some extent by the finding of partial regression of splenic lymphomas in HCV-positive patients treated with interferon-α.[264] Nonetheless, the association between HCV infection and LPL/WM remains uncertain because similar findings have not been observed in other geographic populations.[265]

Increasing attention has been directed toward the cellular and stromal background accompanying LPL. Mast cells, long considered a bystander cell population, have become the focus of investigation as a result of the potent inflammatory and immune cytokine effects these cells can generate in the microenvironment. Some investigators have postulated a permissive role of mast cells and other nontumor components in supporting the growth of LPL.[266,267] Although not strictly related to the cytologic origin of LPL, the lymphoma microenvironment is likely important to the pathogenesis of LPL and possibly as a novel therapeutic target.

Clinical Course

Patients with LPL/WM exhibit the general features of most low-grade B-cell lymphomas—that is, a waxing and waning disease course that eventuates in progressive disease and treatment refractoriness. The disease can be asymptomatic, with a relatively prolonged survival; however, many patients have more advanced symptomatic disease at presentation, and their median overall survival is approximately 5 years. Supervening complications of cytopenia, hyperviscosity, and bleeding increase the morbidity in LPL/WM patients and may have an adverse impact on survival. Plasmapheresis can be performed for patients with symptomatic hyperviscosity manifestations. Treatment options for LPL range from expectant management (for patients with no or minimal symptoms) to immunochemotherapeutic regimens and stem cell transplantation.[198,207,268-275] Therapy with alkylating agents or purine nucleoside analogues, often with rituximab (anti-CD20 therapeutic antibody), is frequently considered first-line management.[276-281] These combinations have demonstrated good activity against LPL, although complete, durable remissions are not the rule. Furthermore, use of these agents is associated with a variety of early and late complications, including hypersensitivity reactions (to rituximab), profound marrow suppression, and the risk of developing secondary hematopoietic cancers (e.g., aggressive lymphoma, acute myeloid leukemia, myelodysplasia).[282] Large B-cell lymphomas arising in a background of LPL are associated with a poor outcome, likely reflecting the more complex tumor genetics of underlying transformation.[217,231,283,284]

A number of prognostic factors encompassing clinical symptoms, laboratory markers, and histopathologic findings have been described in LPL/WM.[208,209,285-294] Advanced age, poor performance status, hyperviscosity, cryoglobulinemia, progressive neuropathy, amyloidosis, bulky organ or nodal disease, and the presence of "B" symptoms have all been associated with inferior outcome. Some studies have described particular laboratory findings in more aggressive LPL/WM, including high serum β_2-microglobulin levels, peripheral blood cytopenias, and decreased serum albumin.[208,209,285,287-296] These clinical and laboratory findings have led some investigators to propose a "simplified" prognostic scoring system to guide the timing and nature of therapeutic interventions. An International Prognostic Scoring System for WM has recently been advanced for the evaluation of symptomatic and previously untreated patients. It defines five high-risk variables: age (older than 65 years), hemoglobin (<11.5 g/dL), platelet count (<100×10^9/L), serum β_2-microglobulin level (>3 mg/L), and serum IgM paraprotein (>7 g/dL).[297] These five parameters have been used to establish low-, intermediate-, and high-risk categories for determining initial therapeutic interventions.[298,299] Some reports have suggested an adverse outcome for LPL with the 6q− cytogenetic abnormality[300]; however, other investigators have not shown this relationship.[236,301] Serum free light-chain levels in LPL/WM have been correlated with clinical outcome.[302,303] Polymorphous morphology with increased large transformed cells in LPL has been associated with complex karyotypic abnormalities and a poorer clinical outcome.[231] Novel micro-RNA profiling studies in LPL/WM have revealed specific expression patterns in neoplastic B cells of patients that correlate with prognosis and International Prognostic Scoring System status.[257]

Differential Diagnosis

In light of the cellular composition of LPL, tissue biopsy findings may overlap with those of reactive conditions (see Tables 14-2 to 14-4). Autoimmune diseases or infectious processes can result in significant plasmacytosis in both lymph nodes and bone marrow, but these conditions are readily distinguished by clinical history and the lack of monoclonal B-cell and plasma cell populations. The unusual entity of IgG4-associated sclerosing disease generally involves exocrine glands, often typified by conditions such as autoimmune pancreatitis.[304] Recent descriptions of lymph node involvement by this disorder have emerged, including some features that can resemble LPL infiltrates.[305] The lack of a clonal B-cell and plasma cell population, the presence of increased serum IgG4, and an increased IgG4-to-IgG plasma cell ratio by immunohistochemistry help establish this diagnosis. Castleman's disease, especially the plasma cell type, can also demonstrate some features reminiscent of LPL in lymph nodes, especially given the presence of a marked interfollicular plasmacytosis. Castleman's disease can be associated with monoclonal plasma cells, almost always of the IgG- or IgA-lambda type. The clinical presentation and the lack of a monoclonal B-cell component help differentiate Castleman's disease from LPL.

Other low-grade B-cell lymphomas are frequently considered in the differential diagnosis of LPL. The MZLs are perhaps the most challenging to distinguish from LPL, particularly in small tissue biopsy samples. MZL often exhibits plasmacytic differentiation and shares a relatively nonspecific B-cell immunophenotype with LPL. However, MZL is seldom associated with the clinical features of WM and IgM paraprotein production. Furthermore, the tissue site distribution of MZL (i.e., splenic, extranodal, or extensively nodal) is frequently informative. The "monocytoid" features of MZL are also quite distinctive, even in the presence of plasmacytic differentiation. In lymph node or extranodal sites, follicular colonization and lymphoepithelial lesions are helpful histologic findings. Bone marrow biopsies tend to show either nodular nonparatrabecular foci of monocytoid-type cells or, in some cases of SMZL, a discrete intrasinusoidal pattern. Molecular genetic studies for *BIRC3* (*API2*), *BCL10*, and *MALT1* translocations can be useful to identify a subset of extranodal MZL cases occurring in the stomach and lungs.[306,307] CLL/SLL is occasionally included in the morphologic differential diagnosis with LPL. The presence of proliferation centers in tissue biopsies and the characteristic CLL immunophenotype help resolve this uncommon situation. Nonetheless, it has been recognized that IgM gammopathy can accompany other types of low-grade B-cell lymphoma.[50,308,309] Although the diagnostic criteria for WM are defined primarily by the presence of a bone marrow lymphoplasmacytic neoplasm and IgM paraproteinemia, it is occasionally difficult to classify some tumors with variant or overlapping pathologic features. In these cases, the designation of "low-grade B-cell lymphoma with plasmacytic differentiation" is acceptable, given that the precise morphologic distinction between LPL and MZL is probably of minimal significance in the clinical setting of symptomatic WM.[222]

Gamma heavy-chain disease (GHCD) is a very rare hematopoietic tumor characterized by LPL-like infiltrates involving lymph nodes, spleen, liver, bone marrow, and blood, with resultant lymphadenopathy and hepatosplenomegaly.[41,310] Autoimmune cytopenias are common, and peripheral eosinophilia can occur. The tumor cells in GHCD secrete gamma immunoglobulin heavy chains without light chains, owing to deletions in the gamma heavy-chain gene that abrogate the assembly of light-chain immunoglobulin. Lymph nodes and bone marrow show infiltration by a variable population of small lymphocytes, centroblasts, plasma cells, and eosinophils, which also raises the consideration of classical Hodgkin's lymphoma or peripheral T-cell lymphoma. GHCD is considered more aggressive than typical LPL/WM, although recent data suggest a more indolent course with improved therapy. GHCD is distinguished from LPL by the absence of surface and cytoplasmic light chain on neoplastic B cells, but it has been considered a variant of LPL because of the overlapping histopathologic features and clinical presentation.

The differential diagnosis of LPL must also include diseases in the spectrum of IgM gammopathy.[243] The IgM subtype accounts for only a small proportion of patients who develop MGUS. IgM MGUS has been defined as follows: IgM monoclonal protein less than 3 g/dL, absence of histopathologic bone marrow involvement (<10%) by a lymphoid or plasmacytic neoplasm, and absence of WM symptoms. (Nevertheless, some patients with IgM MGUS may suffer clinically from IgM paraprotein effects. These individuals are considered to have so-called IgM-related disorders, given that morphologic and immunophenotypic evidence for LPL is not present.) Long-term evaluation indicates that IgM MGUS patients have a significantly elevated risk of developing B-cell malignancies over time, particularly LPL/WM and, to a lesser extent, CLL/SLL.[311-315] Any patient with apparent IgM MGUS must therefore be thoroughly evaluated to exclude LPL and should be closely followed in light of the natural history of this process. Multiple myeloma of the IgM type is extremely rare, accounting for 1% of de novo cases. Although this diagnosis should always be considered very carefully by the hematopathologist, IgM multiple myeloma presents in a similar manner to non-IgM plasma cell tumors, with osteolytic lesions and hypercalcemia.[316] No features of lymphoid marrow infiltration, concurrent monoclonal B-cell population, peripheral lymphadenopathy, or splenomegaly should be present in cases of true IgM multiple myeloma. Of note, very rare presentations of primary AL-type amyloidosis associated with IgM monoclonal protein production have been identified, and these patients appear to have relatively distinctive clinicopathologic features.[317]

Finally, patients treated for LPL may have morphologic changes in follow-up bone marrow specimens that can cause confusion in the absence of complete clinical information. Examples of marked terminal plasmacytic differentiation can be encountered, resembling foci of myeloma in the bone marrow.[318,319] Knowledge of serum protein electrophoresis studies, flow cytometry to detect monoclonal B cells, and pertinent history can help resolve this situation. Similarly, rare presentations of LPL/WM with residual extracellular light-chain or amyloid deposits can be problematic if these occur or are persistent after therapeutic intervention for LPL/WM. As an adjunct to immunohistochemistry, novel methods such as mass spectroscopic analysis of protein deposits in fixed tissue biopsies can be helpful to assess the nature of extracellular material in these instances.[320]

Pearls and Pitfalls: CLL/SLL

Pearls
- Successful diagnosis of CLL/SLL requires the integration of morphologic and immunophenotypic properties (especially multicolor flow cytometric immunophenotyping)
- Cyclin D1 expression has high sensitivity and reasonable high specificity for mantle cell lymphoma; cyclin D1 positivity excludes a diagnosis of CLL/SLL
- Proliferation foci in lymph node sections are a reasonably specific feature of CLL/SLL, even if some nuclear irregularity is noted; proliferation foci are generally not encountered in bone marrow specimens
- The comprehensive evaluation of CLL/SLL requires the integration of both diagnostic and prognostic information
- Prognostic factors in CLL/SLL include standard clinical staging, CD38 and ZAP-70 expression by flow cytometry, cytogenetic assessment, and *IGH@* V mutation status determination
- Potential new prognostic factors such as micro-RNA profiles may become clinically relevant

Pitfalls
- In blood, bone marrow, and lymph node, it is critical to distinguish $CD5^+$ CLL/SLL from $CD5^+$ mantle cell lymphoma
- In clinical practice, CD23 expression is found in a substantial proportion of non-CLL B-cell lymphoproliferative disorders
- Only a small proportion of bona fide cases of CLL lack CD5 expression
- Rare cases of CLL with admixed Reed-Sternberg cells must be distinguished from overt Hodgkin's lymphoma

References can be found on Expert Consult @ www.expertconsult.com

Chapter 15

Hairy Cell Leukemia

Robert P. Hasserjian

CHAPTER OUTLINE

DEFINITION OF DISEASE AND NOMENCLATURE

Hairy cell leukemia (HCL) is a mature B-cell neoplasm that involves primarily the blood, bone marrow, and splenic red pulp. The neoplastic lymphocytes have surface "hairy" projections and express the B-cell–associated antigens CD19, CD20, and CD22; characteristically, they are also positive for CD103, CD25, and CD11c. The disease was originally described in 1958 and termed *leukemic reticuloendotheliosis*.[1] The long, slender cell surface projections identified initially on smear preparations and subsequently by scanning and electron microscopy gave the disease its vivid descriptive name.[2,3]

EPIDEMIOLOGY

HCL is rare, with only about 600 cases per year diagnosed in the United States and accounting for only 2% of all leukemias.[4] It affects predominantly middle-aged men and does not occur in children. In the largest published series of HCL patients, the mean age was 54 years (range, 23 to 85 years) and the male-to-female ratio was 4:1.[5]

ETIOLOGY

HCL is not associated with Epstein-Barr virus or other infectious pathogens.[6] Several reports of HCL occurring in family members have raised the possibility of a genetic predisposition for the disease.[7-9] In many families the cases were linked with an A1, B7 haplotype, and association with other haplotypes has been reported.[8,9] Nevertheless, the vast majority of HCL cases appear to be sporadic.

CLINICAL FEATURES

Symptoms and Signs

Patients with HCL present most often with symptoms related to cytopenia. In one large series, infections (29%) and weakness or fatigue (27%) were the most common initial symptoms. Not uncommonly (26% of patients), HCL is diagnosed incidentally as a result of routine hematologic screening in patients lacking symptoms attributable to HCL.[10]

Abnormalities found on physical examination and in laboratory studies in HCL patients at presentation are summarized in Table 15-1.[5,11-13] HCL is characterized by a leukopenic or pancytopenic presentation rather than a leukemic presentation. An elevated white blood cell count ($>10,000 \times 10^9/L$) is present in only 10% to 15% of cases[5]; marked leukocytosis with numerous circulating neoplastic cells is rare in HCL and, if present, raises the possibility of the so-called HCL variant (see later) or another disease. Notably, monocytopenia is seen in almost all cases of HCL and is considered one of the most sensitive markers of disease. Leukoerythroblastosis is usually not present, in spite of the common presence of bone marrow reticulin fibrosis.[14] Palpable splenomegaly is present in 72% to 90% of patients, and peripheral lymphadenopathy is uncommon.[5,10,15] Polyclonal hypergammaglobulinemia is present in 22% of patients at presentation, but a monoclonal paraprotein is present in less than 2% of patients.[10]

Imaging Studies

Retroperitoneal lymphadenopathy is detected by computed tomography (CT) in about 15% of patients at presentation and in up to 56% of patients later during the course of the disease.[12,16] Massive abdominal lymphadenopathy has been associated with a poorer response to therapy, leading some to suggest that abdominal CT scans be used to stage HCL; however, CT imaging to stage HCL is not common practice, and its usefulness is controversial.[16,17]

Diagnostic Procedures

Although a diagnosis of HCL can be based on peripheral blood morphology and immunophenotype, examination of bone marrow is recommended in all newly diagnosed cases to assess the extent of marrow involvement and provide a baseline for assessing response to treatment. The key diagnostic features of HCL are summarized in Table 15-2. A good bone marrow core biopsy is essential because the bone marrow aspirate is often poorly cellular or unobtainable.[18] If an aspirate cannot be obtained, the diagnostic HCL immunophenotype can usually be demonstrated in the peripheral blood; circulating neoplastic cells are present in almost all patients, even when they are difficult to identify on smears.[19] Rarely, HCL presents with splenomegaly without bone marrow or peripheral blood involvement,[20,21] requiring splenectomy for diagnosis.

Table 15-1 Clinical and Laboratory Findings of Hairy Cell Leukemia at Presentation

Finding	% of Patients with Finding	Comments
Splenomegly	86	Massive in 25% of patients
Hepatomegaly	73	If biopsied at presentation, the liver is nearly always involved[11]
Lymphadenopathy	13	Mostly abdominal and retroperitoneal; peripheral lymphadenopathy is uncommon[12,13]
Anemia (hemoglobin ≤12.0 g/dL)	77	
Neutropenia (≤1500 × 10^9/L)	79	
Monocytopenia (<500 × 10^9/L)	98	Marked monocytopenia (<150 × 10^9/L) is present in 90% of patients
Thrombocytopenia (<100,000 × 10^9/L)	73	
Hairy cells detected on peripheral smear examination	85	Often few in number; identification may require careful examination by an experienced observer

Table 15-2 Major Diagnostic Features of Hairy Cell Leukemia

Study	Findings
Morphology of hairy cells	Oval or indented nuclei and abundant pale blue cytoplasm Absent or inconspicuous nucleoli Circumferential cell surface "ruffled" projections
Bone marrow biopsy morphology	Diffuse or interstitial bone marrow infiltration, without discrete nodular aggregates Clear cells with "fried egg" or spindled appearance Reticulin fibrosis
Flow cytometry	Clonal B cells expressing CD103, CD25, and CD11c and lacking CD5 expression
Immunohistochemistry	Positive for DBA.44, TRAP, and ANXA1

Staging

A clinical staging system, proposed by Jansen and Hermans[22] in 1982, measured hemoglobin level and spleen size to define stages of disease and predict outcome and benefit of splenectomy; the current infrequent use of splenectomy to treat this disease has reduced the utility of this system. The "hairy cell index," representing the proportion of bone marrow space occupied by hairy cells, has been shown to correlate with platelet response to splenectomy[23] and is still useful in comparing bone marrow samples before and after treatment.

MORPHOLOGY

Cell Morphology on Smear Preparations

HCL morphology is ideally represented on well-prepared peripheral blood smears. Hairy cells are 1.5 to 2 times the size of small lymphocytes and are characterized by oval to bean-shaped nuclei, dispersed chromatin with features intermediate between a mature lymphocyte and a blast, and absent or inconspicuous small nucleoli. Hairy cell cytoplasm is moderately abundant, pale blue, and often flocculent, with ill-defined or ruffled borders with "wispy" projections (Fig. 15-1A-C).[24,25] Occasional cytoplasmic granules or small rod-shaped structures may be evident. These correspond to the ribosome-lamellar complexes frequently seen in hairy cells by electron microscopy.[26] Hairy projections are best seen in thin areas of the smears and, when well demonstrated, are present all around the cell membrane. Poorly prepared or thick smears (particularly from bone marrow aspirations) may cause artifactual hairy-like projections or cytoplasmic ruffling in other cell types, mimicking hairy cells. Moreover, the cell trauma associated with preparing the bone marrow aspirate renders the characteristic hairy cell cytomorphology more difficult to appreciate in aspirate smears or even touch preparations than in peripheral smears.[14]

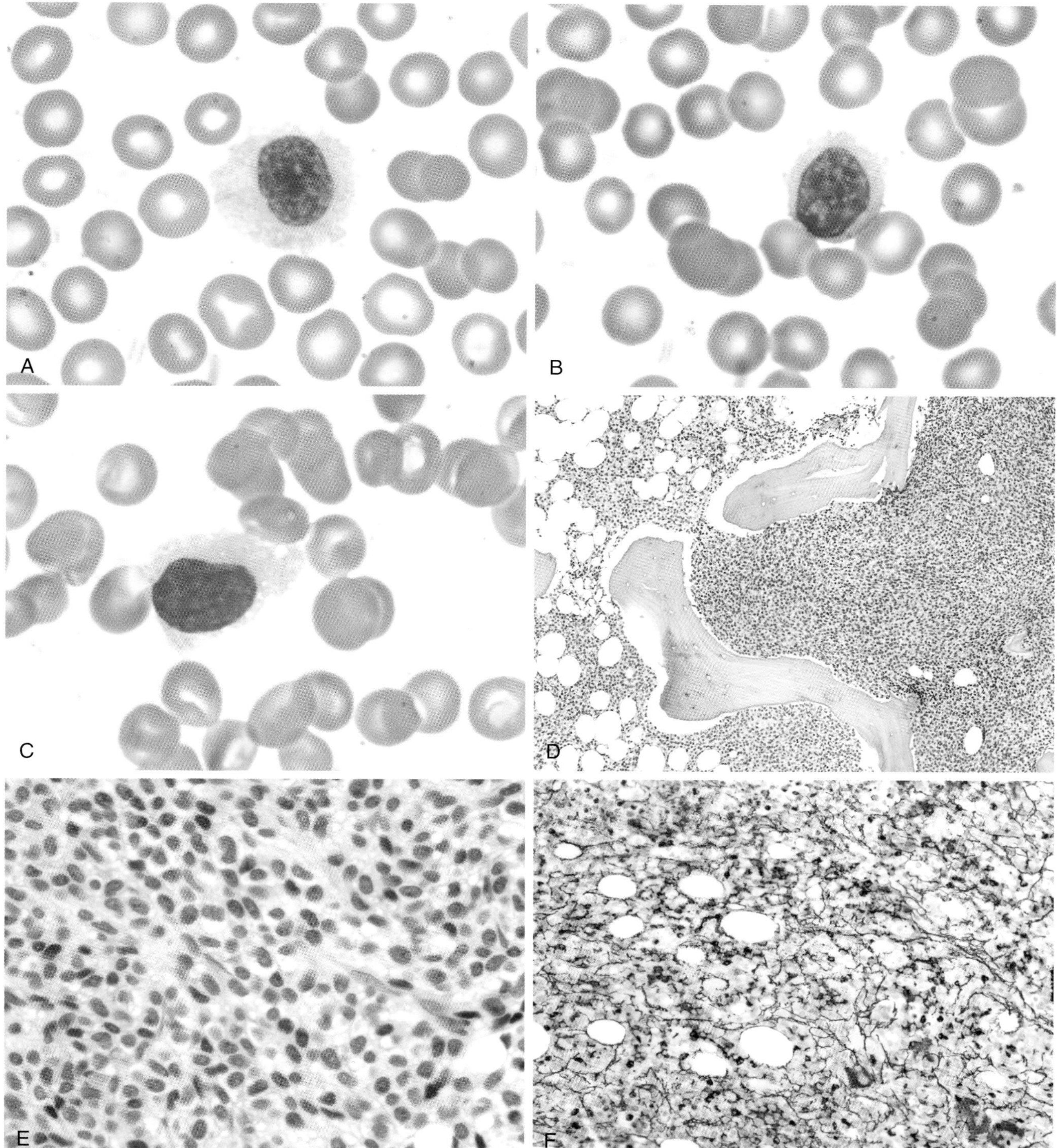

Figure 15-1. **A,** Hairy cell on peripheral blood smear. The nucleus is oval, with slightly dispersed chromatin, and the cytoplasm is pale blue with an ill-defined, ruffled border. **B,** Hairy cell on peripheral blood smear. In thicker areas of the smear or in bone marrow aspirates, the cytoplasm may appear more scant. Small nucleoli may be present in some hairy cells. **C,** Hairy cell on bone marrow aspirate. Hairy cells are often poorly preserved in aspirate smears, with stripped or ragged-appearing cytoplasm. **D,** Hairy cell leukemia (HCL) in bone marrow biopsy section (low power), illustrating the characteristic diffuse and interstitial infiltration patterns. **E,** HCL in bone marrow biopsy section (high power), illustrating wide spacing of the folded and bean-shaped nuclei. Depending on the fixation and processing method, the cytoplasm may appear clear or pale pink. **F,** HCL in bone marrow biopsy (reticulin silver stain). Reticulin is increased in almost all HCL cases, often resulting in a poor or failed aspirate.

Cell Morphology in Bone Marrow Sections

At low power, the bone marrow infiltrate in HCL is mainly interstitial or diffuse and does not form the well-defined aggregates that characterize most other small B-cell lymphomas (see Fig. 15-1D). At diagnosis, the bone marrow is hypercellular in most cases, with diffuse sheets of hairy cells.[25] However, in early stages of the disease the bone marrow may be hypocellular or may have a subtle interstitial infiltrate that is not readily apparent on routine stains.[27] At higher power, the hairy cells appear round and monotonous, with oval to indented to occasionally convoluted nuclei set in an abundant clear cytoplasm that holds the nuclei equidistant and imparts the characteristic "fried egg" appearance; large cells are virtually absent.[14,28] Depending on the fixation and processing method, the cytoplasm may appear clear, uniformly pale pink, or flocculent on hematoxylin-eosin stain (see Fig. 15-1E). Hairy projections are usually not evident on routine stains, although these may be visualized with DBA.44 immunohistochemistry.[29] Immunohistochemical stains for CD20 or DBA.44 may also reveal an intrasinusoidal component to the infiltrate that is observed in up to 70% of cases.[30,31] In some cases, particularly when there is extensive involvement, the neoplastic cell infiltrate may appear spindled.[28]

The amount of residual hematopoiesis is variable, but there is often a reduction in normal hematopoietic cells, particularly of the myeloid lineage.[32,33] Hematopoietic elements may manifest morphologic dysplasia, mimicking a myelodysplastic syndrome[32,34]; in some cases the marrow may appear hypoplastic, mimicking aplastic anemia.[27] These observations suggest that HCL influences and suppresses hematopoiesis beyond a mere space-occupying effect, presumably by disruption of the bone marrow microenvironment and by the abnormal release of cytokines such as transforming growth factor-β.[35,36] Not infrequently, there is a modest increase in the number of plasma cells and mast cells.[37]

Significant reticulin fibrosis due to the deposition of pericellular fibronectin is found in almost all cases of HCL at diagnosis, and this is the presumed cause of poor aspirate smears or the inability to aspirate marrow (see Fig. 15-1F).[38] Collagen fibrosis is uncommon.[39] The bone marrow fibrosis resolves following effective therapy for HCL.[40]

Spleen and Other Organs

HCL almost always involves the spleen. In contrast to most other B-cell lymphomas (including splenic marginal zone lymphoma [SMZL]), HCL preferentially involves the splenic red pulp rather than the white pulp. On gross examination, the spleen is massively enlarged (median weight, 1300 g) and exhibits inconspicuous white pulp (Fig. 15-2A).[23] Microscopically, the hairy cells in the spleen appear similar to those in involved bone marrow sections.[28,41] Microscopic areas of hemorrhage (so-called pseudosinuses or blood lakes) are characteristic but not specific for HCL and result from hairy cell adhesion and damage to sinus endothelial cells.[28,42] Extramedullary hematopoiesis is infrequent.[14] Owing to recent advances in HCL diagnosis and therapy, pathologists now rarely encounter splenectomy specimens from HCL patients.

HCL almost always involves the liver at presentation and commonly causes modest hepatomegaly, although the liver is usually not biopsied. In liver biopsies, the hairy cells are located in small clusters in the sinuses and portal tracts. As in the spleen, there may be associated hemorrhage, which in the liver may mimic peliosis.[11]

HCL involves lymph nodes in a paracortical distribution and may surround germinal centers in a pattern mimicking nodal marginal zone lymphoma (see Fig. 15-2B).[41] Examination of the peripheral blood and bone marrow (including immunophenotyping) is helpful in accurately separating marginal zone lymphoma from HCL involving lymph nodes. HCL not uncommonly involves abdominal and retroperitoneal lymph nodes, particularly after splenectomy or in patients with long-standing disease. In such cases the HCL cells may appear larger, and the disease may be refractory to therapy, suggesting transformation to a higher-grade disease biology.[17,43] However, transformation to bona fide diffuse large B-cell lymphoma is rare.[41]

VARIANTS

About 10% of cases of HCL are reported to display morphologic, immunophenotypic, and clinical features that deviate significantly from typical HCL and are encompassed in an ill-defined and poorly understood provisional lymphoma entity in the 2008 World Health Organization classification: hairy cell leukemia variant (HCL-v).[44] HCL-v patients tend to be older than typical HCL patients (median age, 71 years). At presentation, splenomegaly is often massive and, in contrast to classic HCL, there is usually marked leukocytosis (median white blood cell count 116×10^9/L) with numerous circulating neoplastic cells.[45,46] The leukemic cells resemble hairy cells but have prominent central nucleoli that are not typically seen in classic HCL (see Fig. 15-2C).[46] Unlike in classic HCL, monocytopenia is not seen, and there is usually no or minimal myelosuppression and relatively little marrow fibrosis.[46] The pattern of bone marrow and splenic red pulp infiltration is similar to that in typical HCL. Immunophenotypically, HCL-v has a similar profile to HCL but is usually $CD25^-$; tartrate-resistant acid phosphatase (TRAP), CD123, and annexin A_1 are also negative.[45] More than half of cases express immunoglobulin (Ig) G heavy chain, often in combination with other heavy chains—an unusual feature shared with typical HCL.[46] The clinical course is somewhat more aggressive than that of typical HCL, and about 50% of patients are resistant to purine analogues.[45,46] Some authorities believe that HCL-v is not merely a variant of HCL but represents a distinct B-cell lymphoproliferative disorder, perhaps arising from a lymphoid cell in the red pulp of the spleen.[30,47]

About 75% of Japanese patients with HCL manifest features distinct from those of classic HCL; these cases have been termed *Japanese variant HCL*.[48] This variant exhibits clinicopathologic features intermediate between HCL and HCL-v.[48] A blastic form of HCL has been described both as a de novo disease and as a transformation of classic HCL.[49,50] Because of the small number of cases, it is uncertain if this represents a true HCL variant with distinctive clinicopathologic features.

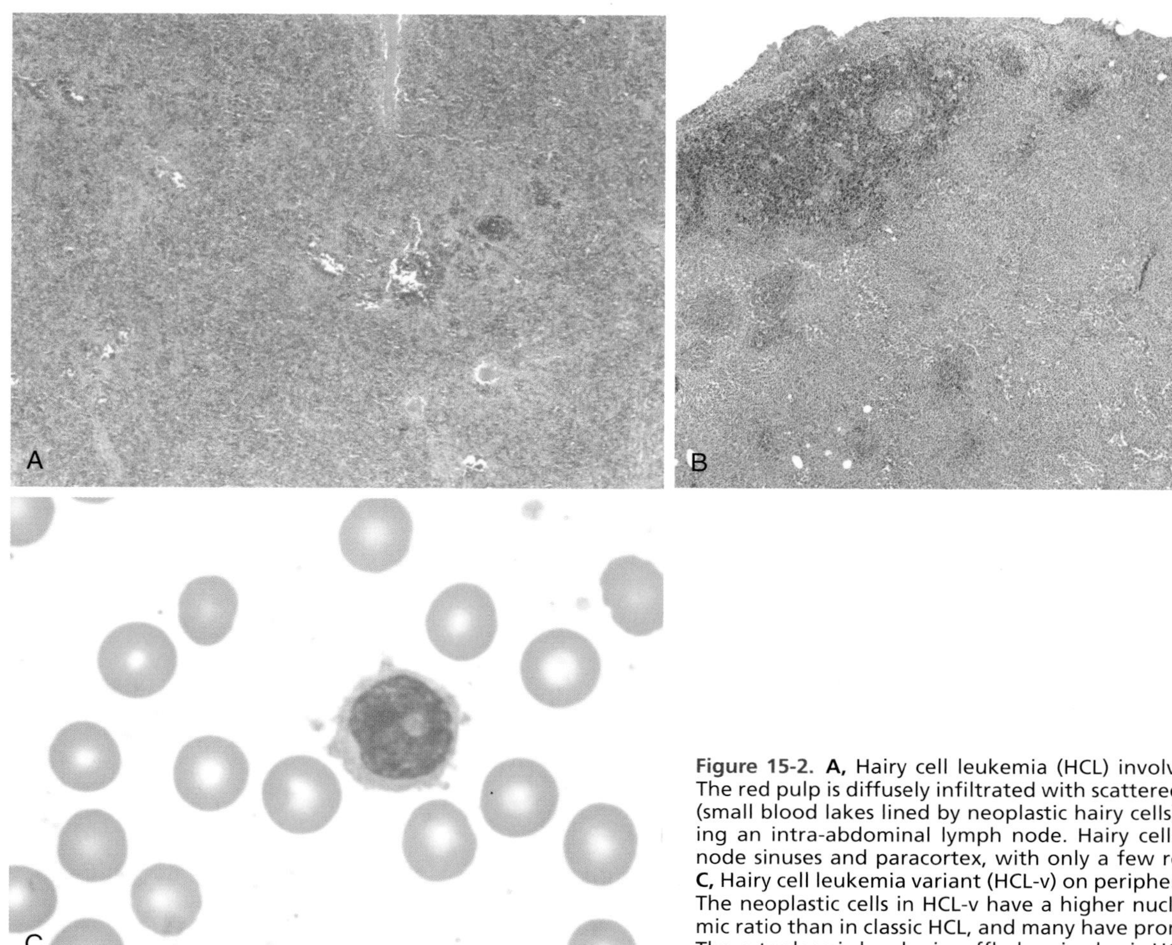

Figure 15-2. A, Hairy cell leukemia (HCL) involving the spleen. The red pulp is diffusely infiltrated with scattered pseudosinuses (small blood lakes lined by neoplastic hairy cells). **B,** HCL involving an intra-abdominal lymph node. Hairy cells fill the lymph node sinuses and paracortex, with only a few residual follicles. **C,** Hairy cell leukemia variant (HCL-v) on peripheral blood smear. The neoplastic cells in HCL-v have a higher nuclear-to-cytoplasmic ratio than in classic HCL, and many have prominent nucleoli. The cytoplasmic border is ruffled, as in classic HCL and unlike in prolymphocytic leukemia.

PHENOTYPE

Flow Cytometry

Flow cytometric demonstration of the characteristic hairy cell immunophenotype, in combination with morphology, is the cornerstone of HCL diagnosis. HCL expresses CD45 (at bright intensity) and the B-cell markers CD19, CD20 (at bright intensity), FMC-7, CD22, and CD79a and is negative for CD5, CD10, and CD79b.[51,52] Although CD10 is typically negative, it can be positive in 10% to 26% of otherwise classic HCL cases, and CD23 is positive in up to 17% of cases; CD5 is positive in less than 5% of cases.[51,53-55] HCL expresses monotypic surface immunoglobulin at high intensity. Bright expression of CD11c, CD25, and CD103 is characteristic of HCL,[51] and these markers should be added to the immunophenotyping panels in all cases of possible HCL subjected to flow cytometry. In addition, an antibody that identifies the alpha chain of the interleukin-3 receptor, CD123, is reportedly expressed in 95% of cases of HCL but not in HCL-v, SMZL, or other B-cell lymphomas[56]; thus, it may be helpful in distinguishing other diseases with "hairy" or "villous" morphology from HCL. If the characteristic but often elusive hairy cells are not recognized on the peripheral smear, the characteristically high forward and side light scatter qualities of hairy cells on flow cytometry may be helpful clues (Fig. 15-3A). Care must be taken when performing flow cytometry to recognize that hairy cells often fall outside of the usual lymphocyte region within the monocyte gate.[57]

There is no absolutely specific immunophenotypic marker for HCL; the pathologist should evaluate the overall immunophenotype in the context of the morphologic and clinical findings. The vast majority of HCL cases—and only very rare cases of other B-cell lymphoproliferative disorders—express at least three of the four characteristic HCL markers (CD11c, CD103, CD25, and CD123, or the less commonly used HC2).[56,58-60] Cases with some atypical immunophenotypic features, such as CD10 or CD5 expression or lack of CD103 or CD25 expression, may still be diagnosed as HCL if the clinical features, marrow infiltration pattern, and cytomorphology are otherwise typical.[55]

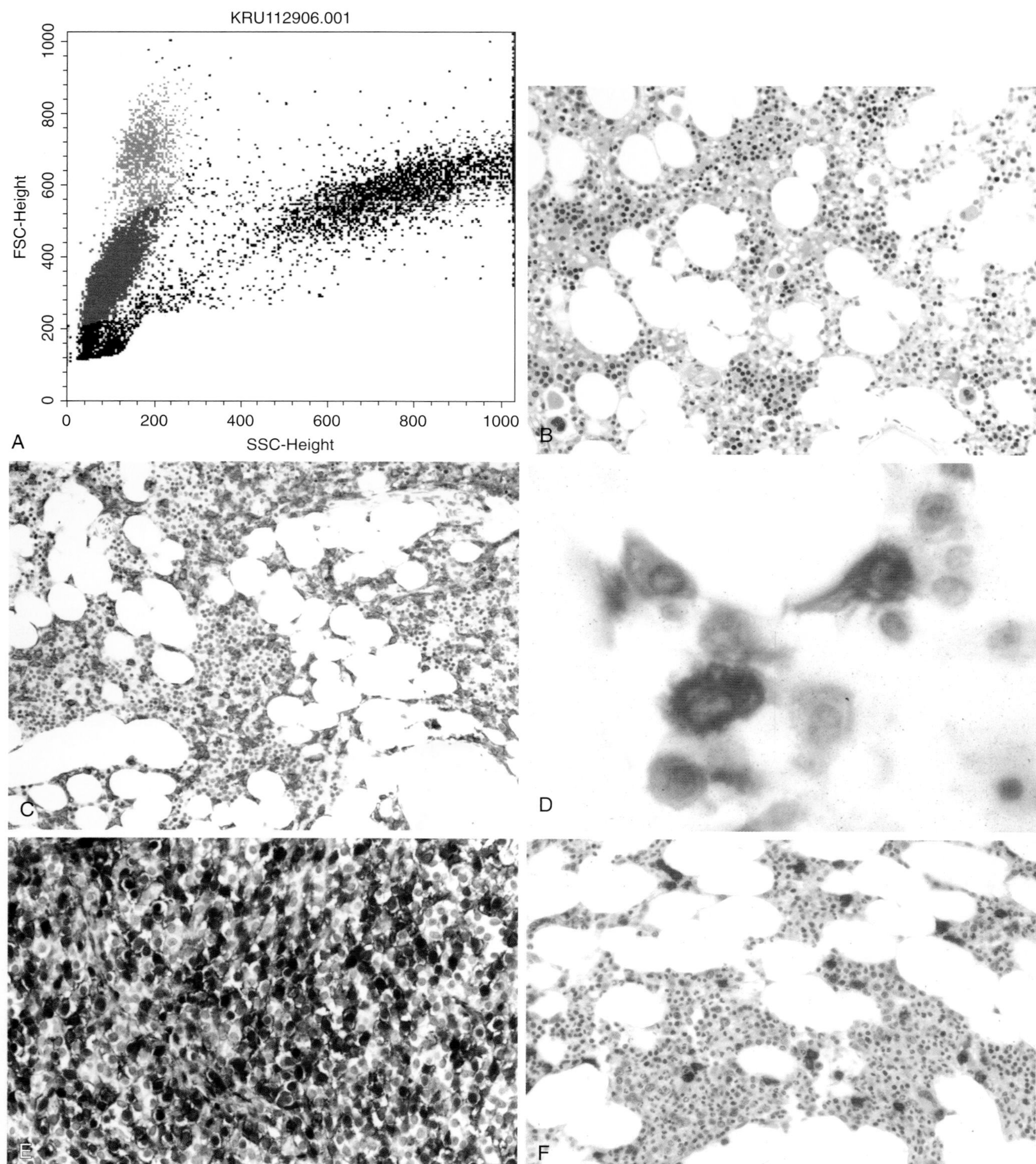

Figure 15-3. A, Light scatter characteristics of hairy cell leukemia (HCL) in peripheral blood (flow cytometry). The hairy cells (*green*) have higher forward light scatter (FSC, vertical axis) and slightly higher side light scatter (SSC, horizontal axis) than the normal lymphocytes (*red*). Also note the absence of monocytes, which would be located between the *red* lymphocytes and the *black* granulocytes. **B,** Subtle case of HCL in the bone marrow of a 57-year-old man presenting with leukopenia and anemia on screening. Hairy cells are not obvious on a hematoxylin-eosin (H&E) stain of the bone marrow biopsy. **C,** CD20 immunohistochemical study of the case in **B** discloses a heavy interstitial infiltrate of cells with characteristic features of HCL. **D,** DBA.44 immunohistochemical study on hairy cells in an involved bone marrow biopsy reveals the ruffled, irregular cytoplasmic border, not evident on H&E stain. **E,** Annexin 1 staining of HCL involving a lymph node. **F,** Minimal residual HCL following therapy, as evidenced by scattered DBA.44$^+$ cells with the typical irregular cytoplasmic borders of hairy cells. (E, Courtesy of Dr. Laurence de Leval, Liege, Belgium.)

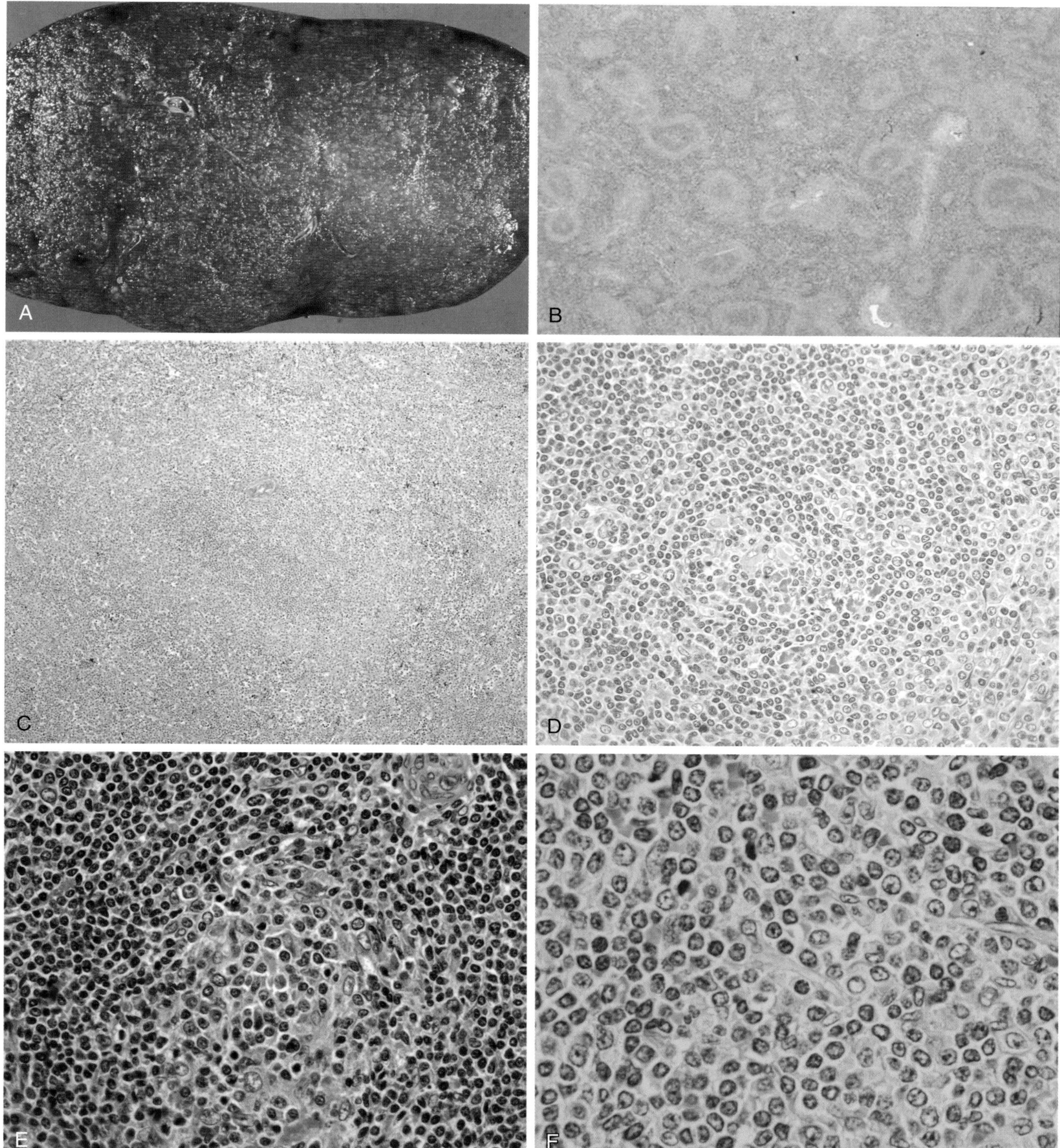

Figure 16-1. **Splenic marginal zone lymphoma morphology in the spleen. A**, Gross photograph shows a micronodular homogeneous pattern. **B**, Low magnification shows marginal zone differentiation and biphasic cytology, with pale-staining cells in the marginal zone, darker cells in the interior of the follicle, and occasional pale central areas, indicating residual reactive germinal centers. **C** and **D**, Replacement of lymphoid follicles by neoplastic cells (Giemsa stain). **E**, Germinal center infiltration by neoplastic cells at a higher magnification; this case shows plasmacytic differentiation within the germinal center. **F**, Cytologic features. Cells in the marginal zone component have slightly enlarged nuclei and abundant pale cytoplasm in contrast to the neoplastic small cell component in the center of the nodules (Giemsa stain).

the similarities between SMZL and so-called hyperreactive malarial splenomegaly.[12]

CLINICAL FEATURES

The most frequently reported symptoms at diagnosis are fever, weight loss, or night sweats, present in 25% to 58% of cases. Splenomegaly is the most common sign, observed in 75% of patients; anemia, thrombocytopenia, or leukocytosis is reported in 25%. Autoimmune hemolytic anemia is found in 10% to 15% of patients, and infection in 10%.[7,9] SMZL is infrequently diagnosed incidentally on routine examination.

Almost without exception, SMZL involves the bone marrow at diagnosis, and roughly a third of patients have liver involvement. Tumor involvement of peripheral blood (defined as the presence of absolute lymphocytosis or >5% tumor lymphocytes in peripheral blood) was detected in 68% of cases by Chacon's group[7] and in 57% by Berger's.[9] Abdominal lymphadenopathy was observed in 25%; peripheral lymphadenopathy was observed more rarely (17%). Because of the high frequency of bone marrow or liver involvement, most patients are at Ann Arbor stage IV at diagnosis. Serum paraproteinemia (usually IgM) is observed in 10% to 28% of cases.[7,9]

Although the diagnostic criteria were initially based on splenic morphology, the conjunction of clinical features, immunophenotype, and morphology usually allows a diagnosis with a reasonably high level of confidence on bone marrow biopsy specimens.

MORPHOLOGY

Splenic involvement in SMZL is characterized by a micronodular lymphoid infiltrate in which white pulp follicles are increased in both size and number, with a variable degree of red pulp involvement always present (Fig. 16-1). The follicles typically have a biphasic appearance, with the presence of both a small cell and a marginal cell component. The cells in the center of the follicles are small lymphocytes with generally round nuclei and scant cytoplasm; the cells in the marginal zones have irregular nuclear contours and moderately abundant pale cytoplasm. In addition, most cases contain scattered large B cells resembling centroblasts or immunoblasts; in the spleen, these appear in the marginal zone and red pulp, but they can also be seen in the bone marrow and lymph node.[13] A reactive or regressed germinal center may be seen in the centers of some nodules, but these are often absent. Neoplastic plasma cells may be present within the germinal centers, forming clusters in rare cases, and in the splenic red pulp. The cellular composition of the tumor follicles may reflect the capacity of marginal zone B cells to induce germinal center development through the transport of immune complexes to the follicular dendritic cells.[14]

In contrast with the organoid pattern of involvement of the white pulp, mimicking the architecture of normal splenic lymphoid follicles, the red pulp more frequently shows a diffuse pattern of involvement, with infiltration of both the cords and the sinuses. Aggregates of lymphoid cells can also be seen in the red pulp. The cells in the red pulp include both small lymphocytes and large centroblasts or immunoblasts. Epithelioid histiocytes may be present in some cases.

Splenic hilar lymph nodes are commonly involved in SMZL (Fig. 16-2), but lymph node involvement is infrequent in other localizations. In lymph nodes, a marginal zone pattern is only rarely observed. The pattern is typically micronodular, and the cells are predominantly small; sinuses may be dilated.[15] The variability of the cellular composition of the tumor in various sites suggests that the microenvironment is relevant to the pattern of tumor growth.[1,2]

Bone marrow infiltration is the rule in SMZL, although it may be difficult to recognize on routine morphologic sections (Fig. 16-3). CD20 staining helps reveal the presence of intertrabecular lymphoid aggregates and intrasinusoidal small tumor cells. The intertrabecular nodules mimic the architecture and cell composition of tumor nodules in the spleen, with occasional reactive germinal centers surrounded by tumor cells. Characteristically, CD20 staining reveals the presence of linear aggregates of intrasinusoidal B cells.[16,17] None of these findings is restricted to SMZL, but their combination is quite characteristic.

Peripheral blood involvement is less frequent than bone marrow infiltration. However, it is relatively common to find a small number of neoplastic B cells in the blood, some of which may have a villous morphology. This usually takes the form of small cytoplasmic projections at one pole of the rather abundant cytoplasm (Fig. 16-4).

Cases characterized by massive splenomegaly and a morphologic picture of increased large lymphocytes have been described.[13,18,19] Unlike in classic SMZL, these cases had a conspicuous component of larger lymphocytes distributed in the marginal zone, occasionally overrunning it, with the isolated presence of the same cells within the central small cell component and in the red pulp. The bone marrow and peripheral lymph nodes showed similar histologic findings to those described for SMZL in these locations. The genetic and molecular features of these cases showed no alterations specific to other lymphoma types, such as t(14;18) and t(11;14). Instead, there was 7q loss in three of five cases, p53 inactivation in two of six cases, scattered cyclin D_1^+ cells in two of six cases, and the presence of translocations involving the 1q32 region in two of four cases.

IMMUNOPHENOTYPE

Immunophenotypic features are summarized in Box 16-1 and shown in Figure 16-5. The most common profile is $CD20^+$, $CD3^-$, $CD23^-$, $CD43^-$, $CD38^-$, $CD5^-$, $CD10^-$, $BCL6^-$, $BCL2^+$, cyclin D_1^-, IgD^+, $p27^+$, annexin A_1^-. DBA:44 expression has been described in a small fraction of cases.[20] MIB-1 staining shows a distinctive annular pattern, indicating the presence of an increased growth fraction in both the germinal centers and the marginal zones.

Low expression of p53 is the most common finding, although a small proportion of cases may show increased p53 expression that is commonly associated with *p53* mutations.

GENETICS

Genetic Abnormalities

Until recently, no characteristic genetic alterations had been described for this entity, rendering the diagnosis of SMZL

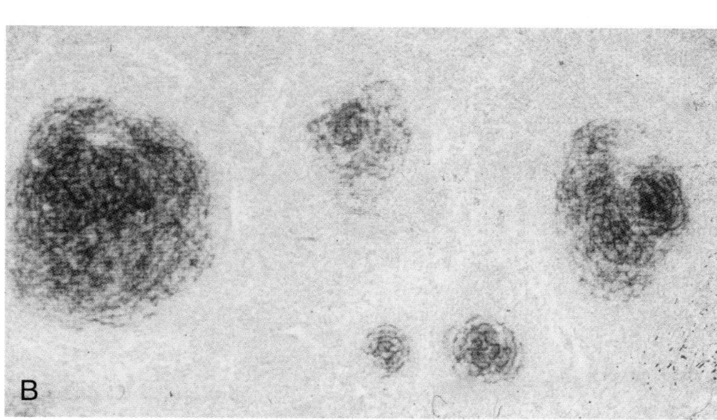

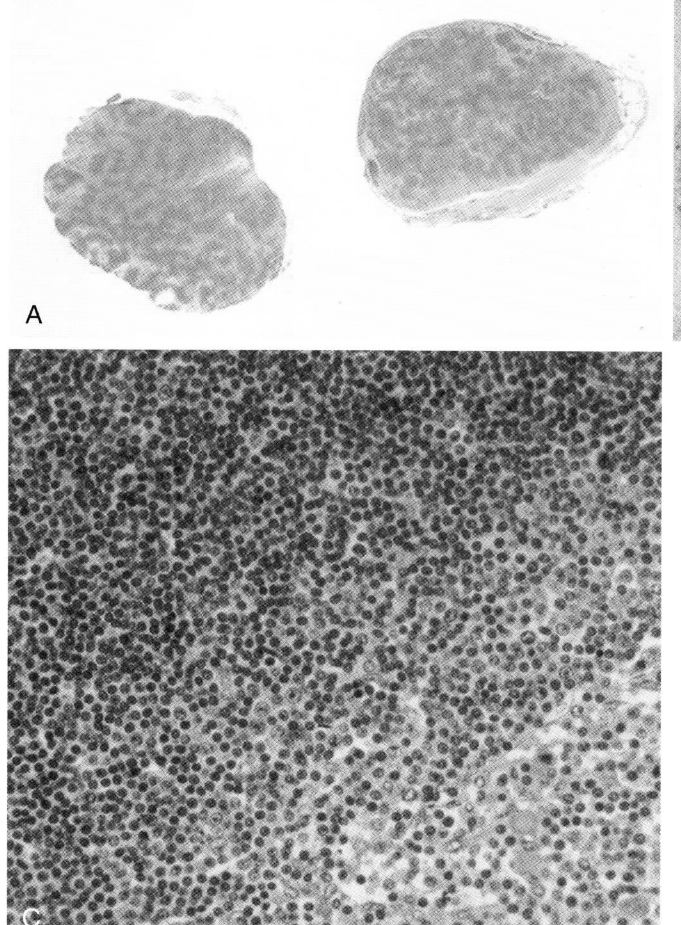

Figure 16-2. Lymph node involvement by splenic marginal zone lymphoma. A, Low magnification of a splenic hilar lymph node with a micronodular pattern and prominent sinusoidal dilation. **B,** Tumor is centered in lymphoid follicles, highlighted by staining for follicular dendritic cells (immunoperoxidase stain for CD23). **C,** Higher magnification shows small tumor cells in lymph node, with scant cytoplasm and clumped chromatin and lacking marginal zone differentiation.

difficult in some cases. The analysis of chromosome region 7q22-36 for loss of heterozygosity and karyotyping demonstrated allelic loss in 40% of cases, a frequency higher than that observed in other B-cell neoplasms (8%).[21-23] The most frequently deleted microsatellite was D7S487. Surrounding this microsatellite, a small, commonly deleted region of 5cM has been identified, defined between D7S685 and D7S514. These results provide a cytogenetic marker for this neoplasm, which may be used in conjunction with other morphologic, phenotypic, and clinical features. SMZL with 7q loss tends to behave more aggressively, with more frequent tumor progression. This region has been demonstrated to contain a cluster of micro-RNA, including MiR29a1 and MiR29b, with the potential capacity to regulate TCL1a.[24]

Other clonal chromosome abnormalities detected in SMZL are gain of 3q (10% to 20%) and involvement of chromosomes 1, 8, and 14. No t(11;14)(q13;q32) or t(14;18)(q21;q32) translocations are seen. Occasional cytogenetic abnormalities involving 14q32, such as t(6;14)(p12;q32) and t(10;14) (q24;q32),[25] or 7q21 (with deregulation of cyclin-dependent kinase 6) have been reported.[26] Deletion of 17p13 (*p53*) has been observed in 3% to 17% of cases.[20,25,27]

Antigen Receptor Genes

The frequency of immunoglobulin heavy-chain variable region (IgVH) somatic mutations has also been investigated in SMZL. Analysis of 35 cases demonstrated molecular heterogeneity, with 49% of cases having unmutated variable region genes (<2% somatic mutations); these patients had a higher frequency of 7q31 deletions and shorter overall survival than those with IgVH mutations. Additionally, a high percentage of cases showed selective use of the V(H)1-2 segment, suggesting that this tumor is derived from a highly selected B-cell population.[10,28] Cases with IgVH mutations also display somatic mutations in the 5´ noncoding region of the *BCL6* gene, although at a lower frequency than that of IgVH mutations.[29]

Gene Expression Profiling

Gene expression profiling studies reveal potential diagnostic markers and pathogenetic pathways involved in tumor cell survival. Thus, the signature obtained in different studies coincides with the upregulation of different families of genes:

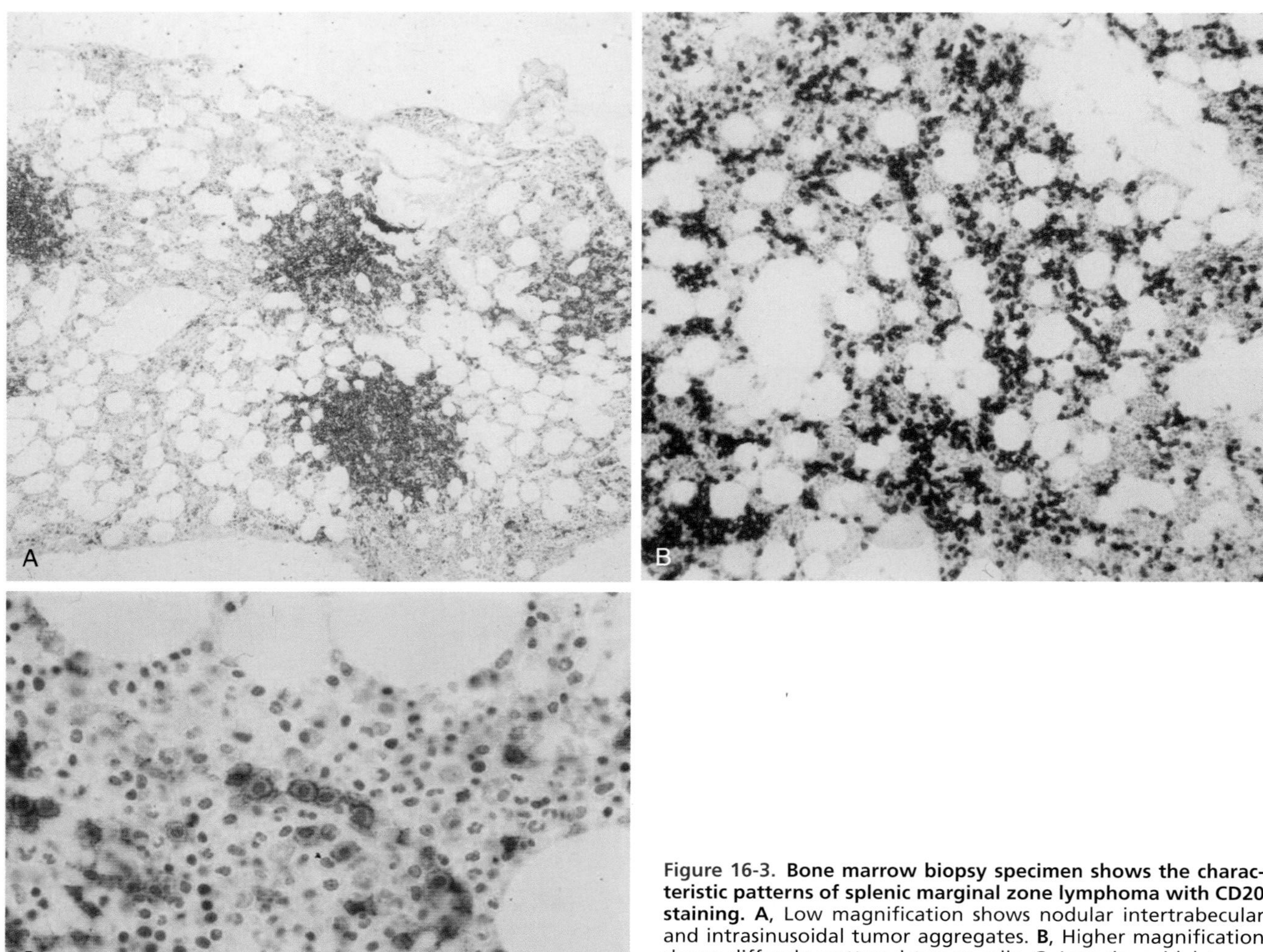

Figure 16-3. Bone marrow biopsy specimen shows the characteristic patterns of splenic marginal zone lymphoma with CD20 staining. **A**, Low magnification shows nodular intertrabecular and intrasinusoidal tumor aggregates. **B**, Higher magnification shows diffusely scattered tumor cells. **C**, Intrasinusoidal tumor cells.

Figure 16-4. **A** and **B**, Peripheral blood morphology shows villous lymphocytes. Villi are typically short and are described as polar—that is, they are concentrated at one pole of the cytoplasm, in contrast to the longer, circumferential villi typically seen in hairy cell leukemia. Villi are usually seen in only a subset of cells.

Box 16-1 *Major Diagnostic Features of Splenic Marginal Zone Lymphoma*

Clinical Features
- Splenomegaly
- Bone marrow involvement
- Lymphocytosis with or without villous cells

Morphologic Features
- Spleen: micronodular pattern; biphasic cytology; follicular replacement; marginal zone differentiation; diffuse, micronodular infiltration of red pulp
- Peripheral blood: villous cells, small lymphocytes
- Bone marrow: intrasinusoidal involvement; intertrabecular nodules, occasionally with a marginal zone pattern
- Lymph nodes: micronodular pattern, small lymphocytes, scattered blasts, rare marginal zone differentiation

Immunophenotypic Features
- $CD20^+$, IgD^+, $BCL2^+$, $CD3^-$, $CD23^-$, $CD43^-$, $CD5^-$, $CD10^-$, cyclin D_1^-, $BCL6^-$, annexinA_1^-
- Ki-67 (MIB-1) low (target pattern with higher proliferation in germinal center and marginal zone); residual germinal centers may be $BCL2^-$, $CD10^+$, $BCL6^+$

Genetic Features
- del 7q: 40%
- *p53* gene alterations: 0 to 20%[20,45]
- *p16* gene alterations: rare
- *BCL6* gene somatic mutations: 13%[29]
- *IgVH* gene somatic mutations: 51%[10]

- Genes involved in apoptosis regulation, BCR and TNF signaling, and nuclear factor-κB activation, such as *SYK*, *BTK*, *BIRC3*, *TRAF3*, *TRAF5*, *CD40*, and *LTB*.
- Genes associated with the splenic microenvironment, such as *SELL* and *LPXN*.
- Lymphoma oncogenes such as *ARHH* and *TCL1*.[30] The increased expression of TCL1 is linked with the AKT1 activation in SMZL, as proposed by Thieblemont and colleagues.[31]
- AP-1 and Notch 2 transcription factors.[32]

Consistent with previous cytogenetic studies, genes located in the 7q31-7q32 region, such as *CAV1*, *CAV2*, and *GNG11*,[30] are downregulated.

CELL OF ORIGIN

The debate over the cellular origin of SMZL has been fueled by conflicting morphologic and molecular findings. A large proportion of tumor cells in SMZL are IgD^+ small lymphocytes, in which marginal zone differentiation is produced only in the microenvironment provided by the splenic marginal zone. The absence of somatic mutation in *IgVH* genes in half the cases of SMZL does not help establish a close relationship with normal marginal zone B cells, which typically have somatic mutations, indicating passage through the germinal center.[33] One hypothesis to explain this paradox is the existence of an as yet undescribed subpopulation of small B cells in the primary lymphoid follicles of the spleen with the potential capacity to differentiate into marginal zone B cells in the appropriate environment and to acquire somatic mutations after exposure to antigens present in the germinal center.

CLINICAL COURSE

SMZL is a low-grade tumor with a survival probability at 5 years that varies from 65% (for patients diagnosed with SMZL after splenectomy) to 78% (for patients diagnosed with splenic lymphoma with villous lymphocytes (SLVL) in peripheral blood).

The few studies performed on relatively large series show that adverse clinical prognostic factors are related to high tumor burden and poor performance status. The biologic parameters associated with adverse outcome are p53 mutation or overexpression, 7q deletion, and the absence of somatic mutation in *IgVH* genes. SMZL therefore seems to behave similarly to chronic lymphocytic leukemia (CLL), in which an unfavorable clinical course is associated with p53 inactivation and unmutated (naïve) *IgVH* genes.

Although very little information about SMZL is available from clinical trials, some clear points are emerging. These include the lack of efficacy of 2-chlorodeoxyadenoside,[34] the relatively favorable course of patients treated with splenectomy,[7] and the potential efficacy of fludarabine in patients who relapse after splenectomy or are resistant to chlorambucil.[35] Hepatitis C–positive patients seem to benefit from antiviral therapy.[11] Specific recommendations for staging and therapy have recently been published.[6]

Patients with SMZL appear to have a greater frequency of transformation to large B-cell lymphoma (13% of cases with adequate follow-up) compared with CLL (1% to 10%), although the incidence of large cell transformation in SMZL is lower than in follicular lymphoma (25% to 60%). In the few cases studied to date, it seems that progression in SMZL is mainly independent of p53 or $p16^{INK4a}$ inactivation, and it is preceded by a higher growth fraction and more frequent 7q deletion.[27]

DIFFERENTIAL DIAGNOSIS

The differential diagnosis of SMZL and other small B-cell lymphomas requires the integration of clinical, morphologic, immunophenotypic, and genetic information (Table 16-1). A micronodular pattern of splenic involvement with villous cells in the peripheral blood can be observed in other conditions, such as follicular and mantle cell lymphomas (Fig. 16-6). Immunophenotyping and genetic features are usually diagnostic; follicular lymphoma is typically $CD10^+$, and mantle cell lymphoma expresses CD5 and cyclin D_1. The absence of t(11;14) and t(14;18) is also helpful in ruling out these entities.[36-39] Particularly helpful features are the intrasinusoidal pattern of involvement in the bone marrow[16,17] and IgD expression by tumor cells.[1,2]

Distinguishing lymphoplasmacytic lymphoma may be problematic, because SMZL shows a gradient of plasmacytic differentiation with serum monoclonal paraproteinemia in up to 28% of cases in some series.[2,7,9] There are no specific immunophenotypic features that distinguish these disorders; however, detection of the characteristic 7q abnormalities favors SMZL. Patients with SMZL rarely have a sufficient serum IgM concentration to result in hyperviscosity syndromes. Bone marrow trephine examination may be useful because lymphoplasmacytic lymphoma typically produces a subtle, diffuse lymphoplasmacytic infiltrate; if lymphoid aggregates with a marginal zone pattern or intrasinusoidal involvement are recognized, a diagnosis of SMZL should be

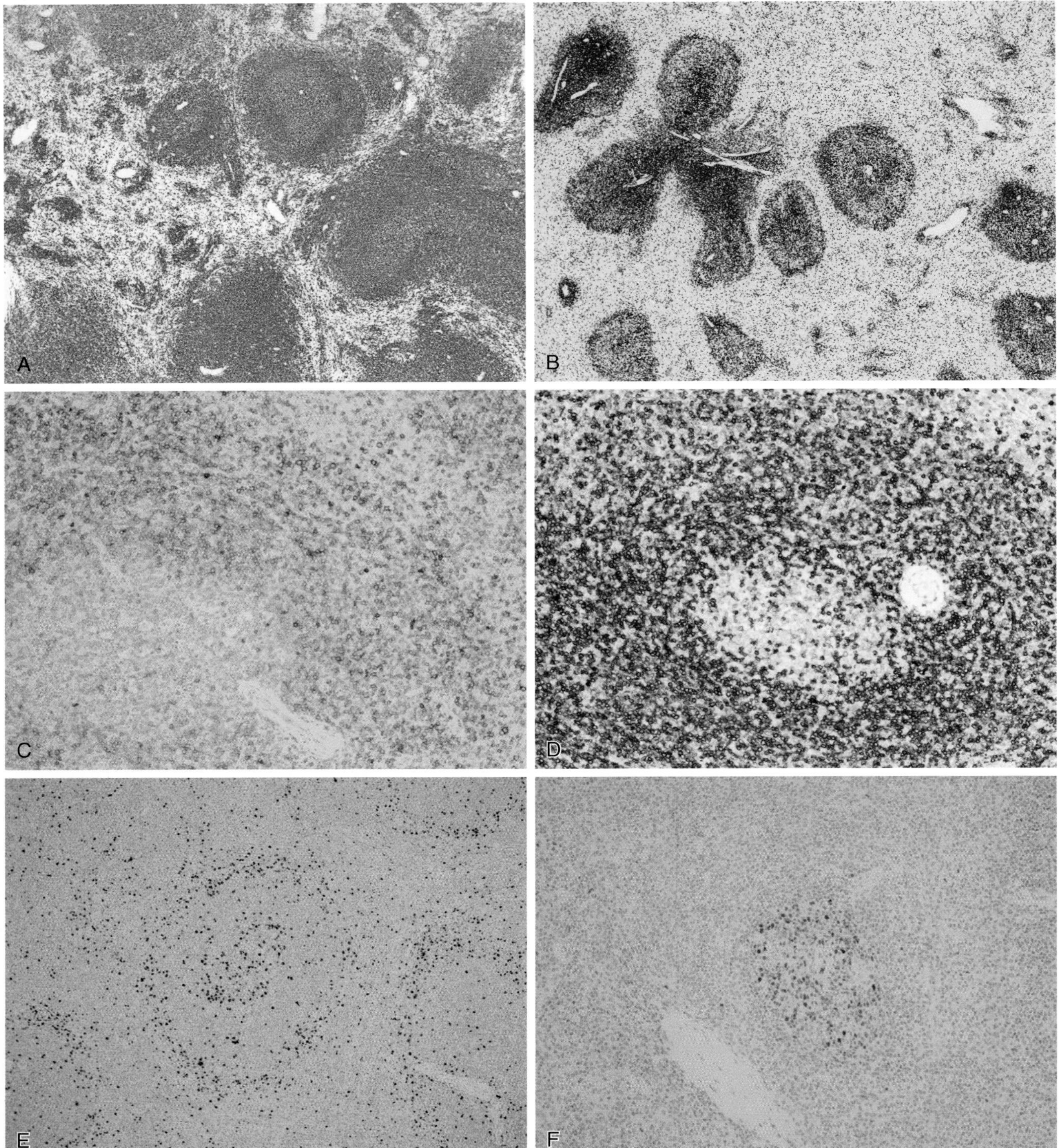

Figure 16-5. Immunophenotypic features of splenic marginal zone lymphoma (SMZL) involving the spleen. A, CD20 reveals prominent red pulp infiltration. **B**, $CD3^+$ T cells in the follicle centers and red pulp, highlighting the micronodular pattern. **C**, IgD staining in the tumor cells. **D**, BCL2 staining shows a $BCL2^-$ germinal center surrounded and partially replaced by tumor cells. **E**, Target pattern with MIB-1 (Ki-67) staining; there are proliferating cells in the germinal center and in the peripheral marginal zone. **F**, BCL6 staining outlines the reactive germinal center cells.

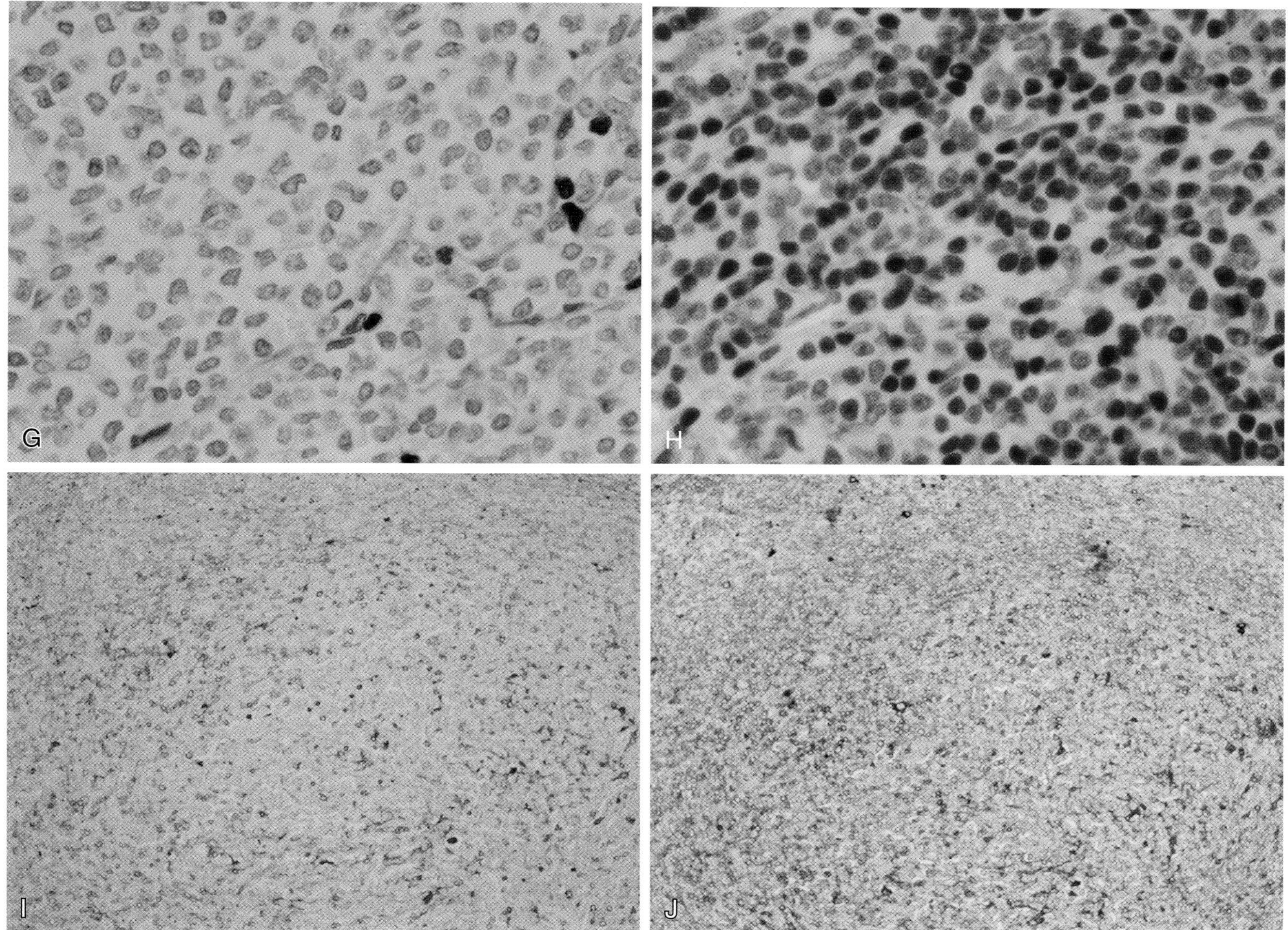

Figure 16-5, cont'd. G, Cyclin D_1 negativity. **H**, Rarely, SMZL shows strong p53 staining. **I** and **J**, Light-chain restriction revealed by cytoplasmic staining for kappa (**I**) and absence of lambda staining (**J**).

suspected. Finally, on splenectomy specimens, the pattern of infiltration in lymphoplasmacytic lymphoma is typically diffuse red pulp involvement, in contrast to the nodular involvement of both white and red pulp in SMZL.[40]

Rarely, MALT-type MZL may infiltrate the spleen with a micronodular pattern, characteristically involving the splenic marginal zone and thus causing diagnostic problems. Useful distinguishing features are the absence of t(11;18) in SMZL,[41] the presence of 7q abnormalities in SMZL, and the characteristic IgD expression in SMZL, which is only rarely observed in MALT-type MZL. Additionally, the typical translocations of MALT lymphoma have not been described in SMZL.

OTHER SPLENIC B-CELL LYMPHOMAS

Splenic Diffuse Red Pulp Small B-Cell Lymphoma

Cases of splenic B-cell lymphoma have been described, with predominantly red pulp involvement, absence of follicular replacement, and a monomorphous population of tumor cells resembling marginal zone B cells, with scattered nucleolated blast cells.[42,43] Some cases have reactive hyperplastic follicles in the white pulp isolated in the middle of a diffuse infiltrate of neoplastic cells. Within the spleen and bone marrow, these cases have a characteristic intrasinusoidal pattern of involvement. More frequent expression of IgG and DBA.44 has been found in these cases compared with SMZL.

Hairy Cell Leukemia Variant

Despite its name, this very unusual low-grade B-cell lymphoma bears no relation to hairy cell leukemia in terms of morphology, immunophenotype, or response to therapy. Cases are characterized by large, prolymphocyte-like cells with prominent nucleoli; absence of annexin A_1, CD25, and CD123; and resistance to conventional hairy cell leukemia therapy.[44]

Table 16-1 **Differential Diagnosis of Splenic Marginal Zone Lymphoma**

Feature	SMZL	CLL	MCL	FL	LPL	MALT MZL
Morphology						
Cytologic composition	Small lymphocytes Large B cells Marginal zone cells	Small lymphocytes Prolymphocytes Paraimmunoblasts	Monomorphous (centrocytes)	Centrocytes Centroblasts	Small cells Plasmacytoid cells Plasma cells	Small lymphocytes Blast cells Marginal zone cells
Marginal zone pattern in spleen	+ (not in LN)	–	±	±	–	+ in all sites
Immunophenotype						
IgD	+	+	+	–	±	–
CD43	–	+	+	–	±	±
CD5	–	+	+	–	–	–
CD23	–	+	–	–	–	–
CD10	–	–	–	+	–	–
Cyclin D_1	–	–	+	–	–	–
BCL6	–	–	–	+	–	–
MIB-1	Target pattern	Low	Low-medium	Low	Low	Low
Genetic Features						
Trisomy 3 (%)	17	3	—	—	—	50-85
Trisomy 12 (%)	10-50	20	5-15	—	—	5-15
7q– (%)	40	—	—	—	—	—
t(11;14) (%)	—	—	100	—	—	—
t(14;18) (%)	—	—	—	90	—	—
t(11;18) (%)	—	—	—	—	—	40-60
IgVH somatic mutations (%)	51	54	25	90	100	100
Clinical Findings						
Splenomegaly	+	+	+	+	+	–
BM involvement	+	+	25%	+	+	20%
PB involvement	+	+	20-58%	9%	+	–
M-component	10-30%	–	–	–	+	Rare
Peripheral LN	Rare	Rare	+	+	+	Rare
Nonhematopoietic extranodal sites	Rare	—	GI Waldeyer's ring	GI	Rare	+

BM, bone marrow; CLL, chronic lymphocytic leukemia; FL, follicular lymphoma; GI, gastrointestinal; LN, lymph node; LPL, lymphoplasmacytic lymphoma; MCL, mantle cell lymphoma; MALT MZL, mucosa-associated lymphoid tissue marginal zone lymphoma; PB, peripheral blood; SMZL, splenic marginal zone lymphoma.

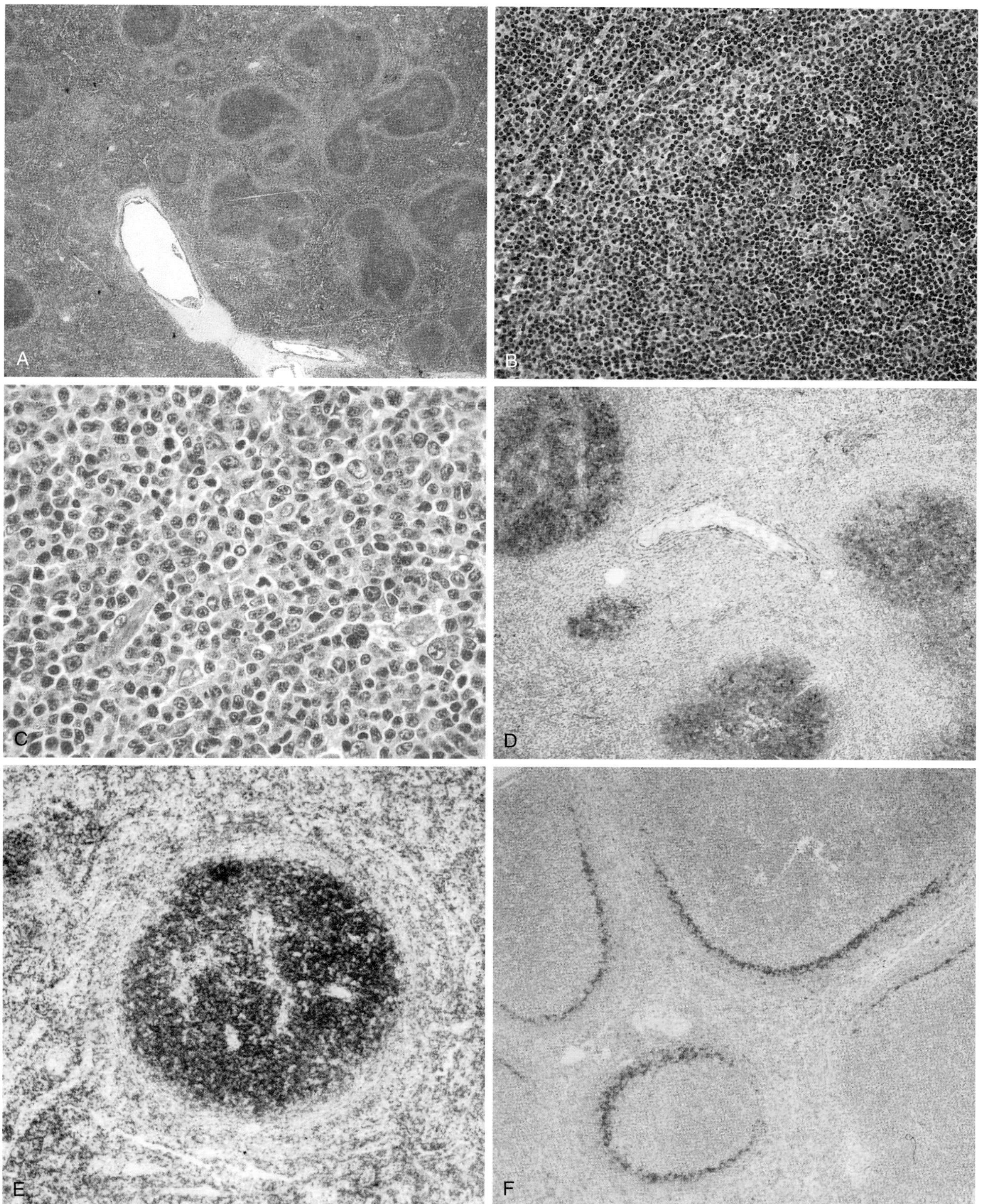

Figure 16-6. Follicular lymphoma with splenic infiltration, mimicking splenic marginal zone lymphoma (SMZL). A and **B,** Micronodular pattern with marginal zone differentiation. **C,** On higher magnification, the cells in the follicles are a mixture of centrocytes and centroblasts, typical of germinal center cells (Giemsa stain). **D,** CD10 staining highlights the entire follicle rather than just a residual germinal center, as would be seen in SMZL. **E,** Homogeneous BCL2 expression within the follicle. **F,** Characteristic IgD staining of residual mantle cells; the neoplastic cells are negative.

Pearls and Pitfalls

Feature	Comments
Follicular replacement (MIB-1 and BCL2 staining)	MIB-1 shows a target pattern, and $BCL2^+$ tumor cells mixed with residual $BCL2^-$ germinal center cells highlight follicular replacement. This contrasts with neoplastic follicles with homogeneous BCL2 staining and proliferating cells evenly distributed throughout the follicles in follicular lymphoma.
IgD staining	IgD is expressed in most cases of SMZL. Residual mantle cells are absent from this lymphoma. In follicular lymphoma and MALT-type MZL, preserved IgD^+ mantle cells may be observed.
Bone marrow infiltration	Bone marrow biopsy shows intertrabecular nodules of small lymphocytes and scattered blasts overrunning residual germinal centers. Intrasinusoidal involvement (demonstrated by CD20 staining) is quite characteristic of this entity.
Splenic hilar lymph node morphology	Lymph node involvement by SMZL displays characteristic histologic and immunohistochemical features, with frequent loss of marginal zone differentiation.
7q deletion	7q31-32 loss is a relatively specific genetic marker of SMZL, present in 40% of cases.
IgVH somatic mutations	Analysis of somatic mutations in the *IgVH* gene reveals 49% of unmutated cases. This group is associated with shorter overall survival and 7q loss.
Marginal zone pattern	A marginal zone pattern can be observed in other small B-cell lymphomas involving the spleen. Marginal zone differentiation in bone marrow and lymph node involvement by SMZL are usually absent.
Villous cells in peripheral blood	Although SMZL and SLVL mostly overlap, not all SMZLs show villous cells in peripheral blood; villous lymphocytes may appear in mantle cell lymphoma, follicular lymphoma, LLC-B, and lymphoplasmacytic lymphoma.
Cyclin D_1^+ cells	Scattered cyclin D_1^+ cells independent of t(11;14) translocation can be found in a few cases of SMZL.

LLC, chronic lymphocytic leukemia; SLVL, splenic lymphoma with villous lymphocytes.

References can be found on Expert Consult @ www.expertconsult.com

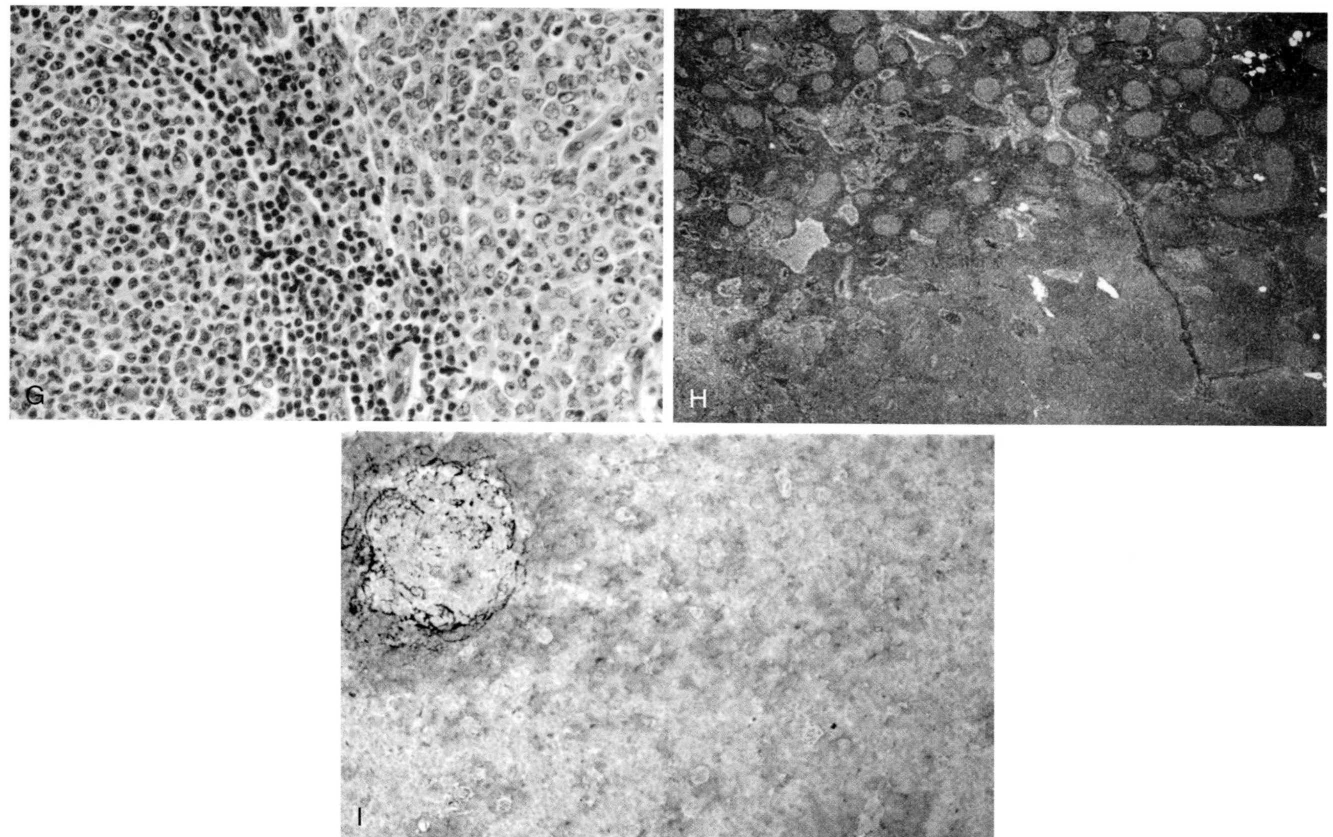

Figure 17-1, cont'd. **G,** In rare cases of predominantly low-grade FL, occasional follicles contain increased centroblasts, consistent with grade 3 FL. In such cases a diagnosis of FL grade 1-2 with focal areas of FL grade 3 (A or B) is appropriate. **H,** Areas of diffuse large B-cell lymphoma may be present in FL of any grade. **I,** In some cases, use of CD21 or CD23 immunostaining to highlight follicular dendritic cells may be useful to detect diffuse areas (immunoperoxidase stain for CD21).

In most cases of FL the centrocytes are relatively small, and the few centroblasts stand out sharply against the monotonous background of centrocytes. In some cases, however, the centrocytes are larger and may be almost as large as centroblasts. In these cases the centrocytes may appear more pleomorphic, with more deeply indented or multilobated-appearing nuclei; the centroblasts also appear atypical, with a variable nuclear size and shape, increased heterochromatin, and binucleate or multinucleated forms.

Mitotic activity is low in most cases of FL, and a "starry sky" pattern, with phagocytic histiocytes, is absent. However, in cases with increased numbers of centroblasts, mitoses are more numerous and, rarely, phagocytosis of nuclear debris may be seen. Polarization, as seen in reactive follicles, is rare in FL, although in some cases centroblasts may be more numerous in one area of the follicle than another, creating an impression of polarization.

FL rarely contains an appreciable number of plasma cells, which can be useful in its differentiation from reactive hyperplasia; however, rare reported cases of FL contain neoplastic plasma cells.[37] The neoplastic plasma cells are found in both the follicles and the interfollicular region and contain monotypic immunoglobulin. Many of these cases might now be considered examples of marginal zone lymphomas of mucosa-associated lymphoid tissue (MALT), nodal, or splenic types.[38,39]

In rare cases of FL the neoplastic centrocytes have large cytoplasmic vacuoles, either clear or eosinophilic, giving them the appearance of signet ring cells (see Fig. 17-1F).[40] In most of these cases cytoplasmic immunoglobulin can be demonstrated in the signet ring cells. Cases with clear cytoplasm typically express cytoplasmic immunoglobulin (Ig) G, with a predominance of lambda light chain, whereas those with periodic acid–Schiff–positive eosinophilic globules in the cytoplasm or nucleus more commonly express IgM.[40,41] On ultrastructural examination, the clear inclusions are large, membrane-bound vacuoles containing multiple tiny, coated vesicles, whereas the eosinophilic inclusions consist of dilated rough endoplasmic reticulum filled with electron-dense material, presumably immunoglobulin.[42] Clinically, FL with a signet ring cell morphology does not differ from typical FL. Most cases are classified as grade 1 or 2.

In addition to neoplastic cells, neoplastic follicles contain follicular dendritic cells (FDCs); their nuclei are similar in size to centroblast nuclei, but they have delicate nuclear membranes and central, small, eosinophilic nucleoli. FDCs are often binucleate, and the two nuclei are typically apposed to each other, with flattening of the adjacent nuclear membranes (see Fig. 17-1C). In contrast to centroblasts, their cytoplasm does not stain blue with the Giemsa stain. Small T cells are also present in neoplastic follicles; these are usually less numerous than in reactive germinal centers, but occasionally they may be very numerous.

Grading

FLs have variable numbers of centroblasts, and the clinical aggressiveness of the lymphoma increases with the number of centroblasts.[43] It has repeatedly been shown that an individual pathologist can effectively predict outcome in FL by grading according to the proportion of large cells, but this is difficult to reproduce among groups of pathologists.[44,45] Several studies have suggested that the "cell counting" method of Mann and Berard is more reproducible and better at predicting prognosis than other methods of grading FL.[44-46] In this method, the centroblasts (large nucleolated cells) per 40× microscopic high-power field (hpf) are counted (10 to 20 hpf in different randomly selected follicles). A case with up to 5 centroblasts/hpf is grade 1, 6 to 15 centroblasts is grade 2, and greater than 15 centroblasts is grade 3 (see Fig. 17-1B, D, and E).[43] Using a standard 0.159 mm^2 hpf, the international study of the REAL classification found that a cutoff of 15 centroblasts/hpf significantly predicted overall and disease-free survival in FL.[47] Approximately 80% of FLs are grade 1 (40% to 60%) or grade 2 (25% to 35%). Because there is no appreciable difference in clinical behavior between grades 1 and 2, the WHO classification now combines them into a "low-grade" category (Table 17-3).

Using these numerical cutoffs, the spectrum of grade 3 FL ranges from cases with 16 large cells/hpf to those in which the majority of cells in the follicle are centroblasts.[48] Some studies suggest that cases with solid sheets of centroblasts are biologically distinct from those with a mixture of centrocytes and centroblasts.[49] For this reason, the WHO classification recommends subdividing grade 3 FL: grade 3A, with more than 15 centroblasts/hpf, but centrocytes are still present; and grade 3B, with solid sheets of centroblasts (see Fig. 17-1D and E). Grade 3B cases are often associated with areas of DLBCL. Differences in genetic features and clinical behavior have led to the suggestion that grade 3A FL may be more indolent and genetically more closely related to low-grade FL, whereas grade 3B cases are more closely related to DLBCL. However, these studies have typically included cases of grade 3B FL with DLBCL.[49-53] One recent study found that although grade 3B FL had a distinctive gene expression profile, it was closer to that of grades 1 to 3A FL than to that of DLBCL.[54] Thus, all grades are currently still classified as FL.

The proliferation fraction using immunohistochemical staining for Ki-67 typically mirrors grade, with grade 1-2 cases having a proliferation fraction of less than 20%, and grade 3 greater than 30%. One study suggested that the Ki-67 fraction was less useful than the histologic grade in predicting outcome.[55] Two recent studies found that some histologically low-grade cases had a high proliferation fraction.[56,57] In one study, patients with a high proliferation fraction (>40%) had a survival more similar to that of grade 3 FL than to typical grade 1-2 FL.[57] Thus, the WHO suggests (but does not mandate) that Ki-67 staining be used as an adjunct to grading. The presence of a high Ki-67 fraction should not change the histologic grade; such cases are reported as "grade 1-2 with a high proliferation fraction," with a note that this may portend a more aggressive course than suggested by the grade (see Table 17-3).

Table 17-3 **World Health Organization Grading of Follicular Lymphoma**

Grade	Definition
Grade 1-2 (low grade)*	0-15 centroblasts/hpf†
Grade 1	0-5 centroblasts/hpf†
Grade 2	6-15 centroblasts/hpf†
Grade 3	>15 centroblasts/hpf†
Grade 3A	Centrocytes present
Grade 3B	Solid sheets of centroblasts
Reporting of Pattern	**Proportion Follicular (%)**
Follicular	>75
Follicular and diffuse	25-75‡
Focally follicular	<25‡
Diffuse	0§
Diffuse areas containing >15 centroblasts/hpf are reported as diffuse large B-cell lymphoma‡ with follicular lymphoma (grade 1-2, 3A, or 3B)	

*Cases of grade 1-2 follicular lymphoma with a proliferation fraction >40% may be reported as "follicular lymphoma grade 1-2 with a high proliferation fraction."
†hpf, high-power field of 0.159 mm^2 (40× objective). If using an 18-mm field-of-view ocular, count 10 hpf and divide by 10; if using a 20-mm field-of-view ocular, count 8 hpf; if using a 22-mm field-of-view ocular, count 7 hpf for an equivalent area and divide by 10 to get the number of centroblasts/0.159 mm^2 hpf.
‡Give approximate percentages in report.
§If the biopsy specimen is small, a note should be added that the absence of follicles may reflect sampling error.

The relative proportion of centrocytes and centroblasts may vary from one follicle to another in a given case. Multiple sections must be examined, and the proportion of large cells is estimated based on a representative sample of follicles. Rarely, individual follicles or parts of the node may show an abrupt transition from a predominance of centrocytes (grade 1-2) to a predominance of centroblasts (grade 3) (see Fig. 17-1G). In such cases it is appropriate to give the predominant grade (grade 1-2) with a separate diagnosis of grade 3 (A or B), giving the relative proportions of each.

Areas of DLBCL may also be found in lymph nodes showing FL (see Fig. 17-1H); this is more common in grade 3B cases but can occur in other grades. In such cases the primary diagnosis should be DLBCL (see Table 17-3) with a secondary diagnosis of FL and an estimate of the proportion of each. Occasional patients with FL have divergent histologic features in lymph nodes taken simultaneously from different sites, showing a variation in grade or progression to DLBCL.[58]

Pattern

Lymph nodes are typically enlarged, with complete effacement of the architecture by neoplastic follicles. The follicles are typically uniform in size; closely packed; lack a mantle zone, "starry sky" pattern, or polarization; and are evenly distributed throughout the lymph node, obliterating sinuses and extending outside the capsule (Fig. 17-2A). Neoplastic follicles may range in size from no larger than a primary follicle to much larger than the average reactive follicle; although usually round, they may be irregular and serpiginous (see Fig. 17-2B), mimicking floridly reactive hyperplastic follicles. Within a given tumor, the follicles are likely to be relatively

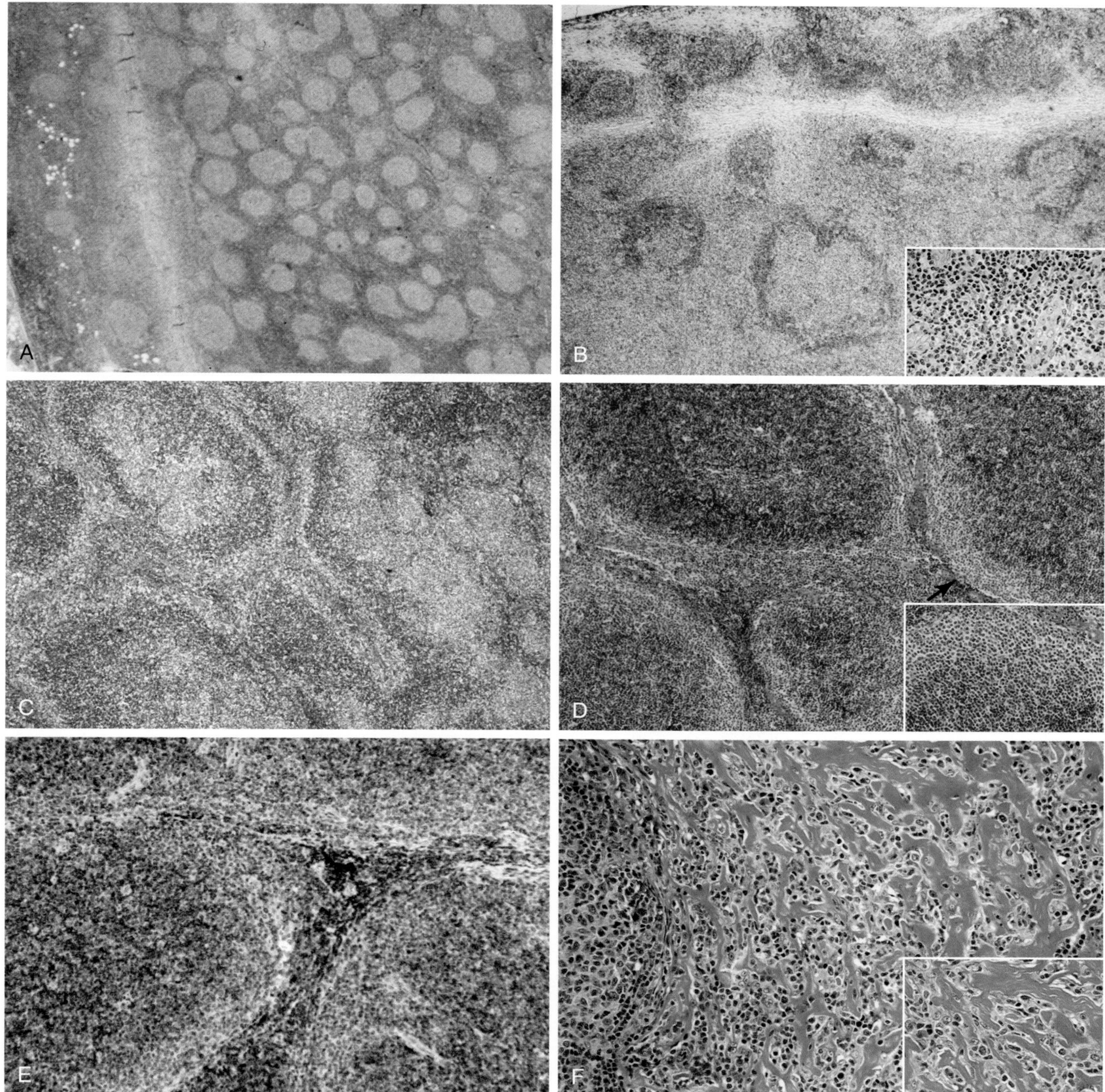

Figure 17-2. Morphologic patterns of follicular lymphoma (FL). A, In a typical case, the relatively uniform follicles are slightly larger than most reactive follicles. Note the extension of neoplastic follicles beyond the capsule (*left*), with concentric bands of fibrosis. **B**, Some cases of FL are composed of irregularly shaped follicles with focally prominent mantle zones. This example has prominent interfollicular involvement, and fibrosis extends beyond the capsule. Interfollicular regions (*inset*) contain predominantly small centrocytes, and high endothelial venules may be numerous. **C**, The floral variant of FL shows broken up follicles within a mantle zone of small lymphocytes, resembling progressively transformed germinal centers or nodular lymphocyte-predominant Hodgkin's lymphoma. **D**, In FL with marginal zone differentiation, a band of pale-staining cells is present outside the mantle zone, forming a marginal zone (*arrow*). The cells in the marginal zone have centrocyte-like nuclei but more abundant cytoplasm (*inset*). **E**, Cells in the marginal zone are often negative for CD10 and BCL6, whereas cells in the follicle and interfollicular regions are positive (immunoperoxidase stain for CD10). **F**, Diffuse area in low-grade FL contains prominent sclerosis; the follicle is at *left*. *Inset* shows a predominance of centrocytes with distorted, elongated nuclei.

Continued

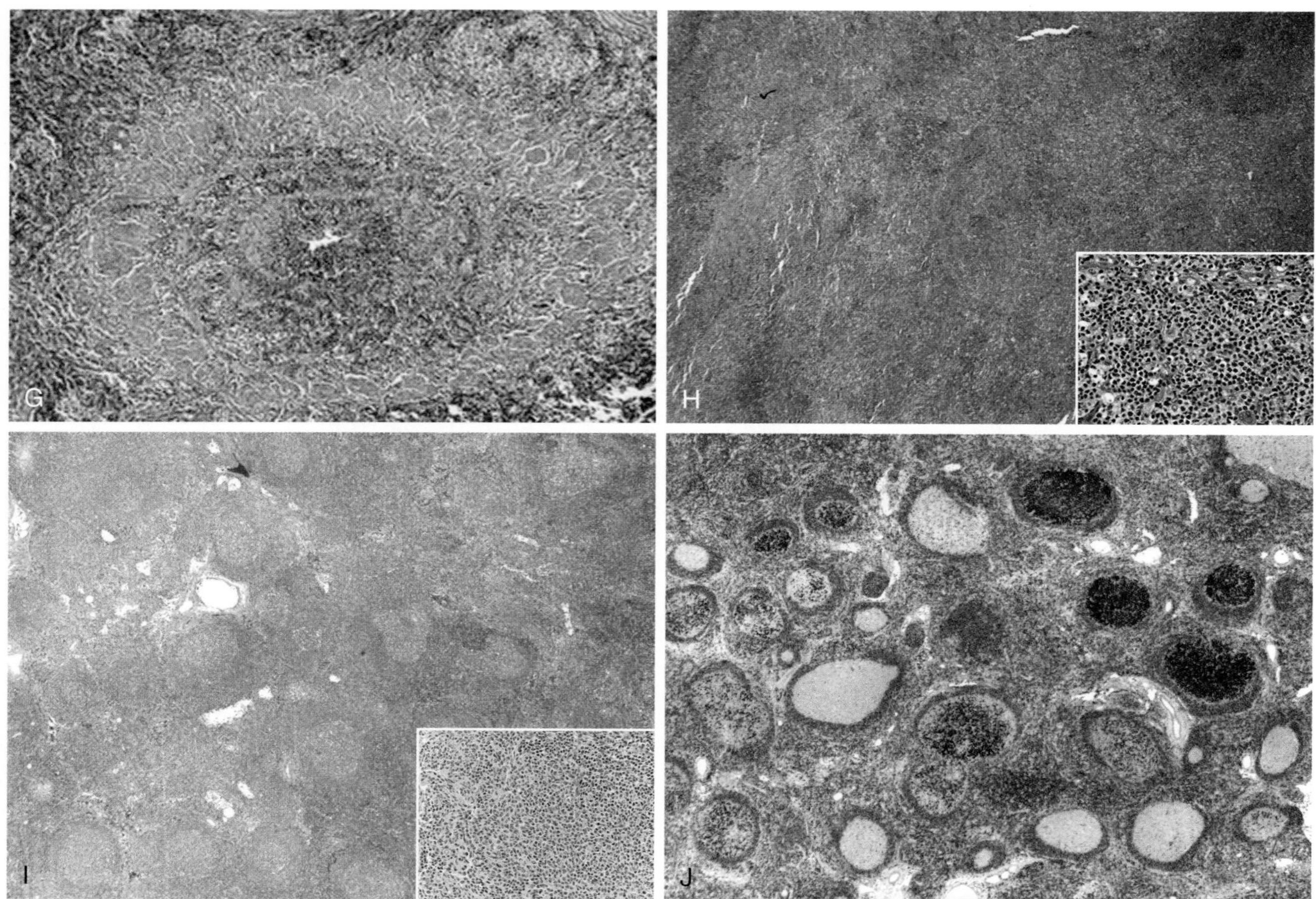

Figure 17-2, cont'd. G, Neoplastic lymphoid cells infiltrate the wall of a small vein, with compression of the lumen. **H,** Diffuse FL shows no areas with follicle formation. *Inset* shows a mixture of centrocytes and centroblasts. **I,** A lymph node partially involved by FL contains scattered monomorphous-appearing follicles, among other typical reactive follicles with preserved mantle zones. *Inset* shows a neoplastic follicle at higher magnification. **J,** BCL2 stain shows strongly positive cells in some follicles.

uniform and monotonous, but in some cases there is marked variation in size from one follicle to another. In other cases the follicles may appear irregularly mottled, resembling progressively transformed germinal centers; this usually occurs in cases with increased large cells and has been called the *floral variant* of FL (see Fig. 17-2C).[59,60]

Neoplastic follicles usually lack mantle zones, but in some cases partial or complete mantle zones may be present around all or some of the follicles (see Fig. 17-2B).[61] In some FLs the outer cells of the follicles may resemble marginal zone or monocytoid B cells, with nuclei similar to centrocytes but with more abundant, pale cytoplasm (see Fig. 17-2D and E). These cells may form partial or complete "marginal zones" around some or most of the follicles in a given case, and they may have an interfollicular and perisinusoidal distribution, resembling nodal involvement by extranodal MALT-type marginal zone lymphoma or nodal marginal zone lymphoma. This phenomenon should not be regarded as a "composite lymphoma" with follicular and monocytoid B-cell lymphoma, as has been suggested by some authors[62,63]; rather, it should be considered evidence of intratumoral differentiation.[64] Marginal zone B cells in cases of FL with marginal zone differentiation share the same genetic abnormalities as the neoplastic follicles.[65] In one study, the presence of significant marginal zone or monocytoid B-cell areas in FL was associated with a significantly worse prognosis compared with cases lacking this feature.[66]

Subcapsular and medullary sinuses are typically obliterated, but sinuses may be partially or completely preserved. Extracapsular extension is common but not universal; when it occurs, the capsule may be visible as a band of fibrous tissue within the tumor. Successive levels of extracapsular extension may appear as concentric parallel bands of fibrosis in the extranodal tissue (see Fig. 17-2A and B). In most cases the follicles are closely packed, with absence of the normal T zones. The interfollicular region may contain numerous small blood vessels of the high endothelial venule (HEV) type but is poor in transformed lymphocytes and plasma cells and usually contains neoplastic centrocytes.[61,67] In occasional cases, interfollicular involvement is prominent, leading to widely spaced follicles (see Fig. 17-2B). This interfollicular involvement is not considered to constitute a diffuse area: a diffuse area is defined as an area completely lacking follicles.

Sclerosis is common and may be present surrounding the follicles, in diffuse areas, or, less often, within the follicles.[68] It is more marked in areas in which the infiltrate is becoming diffuse, which can be a useful feature in distinguishing FL from follicular or diffuse lymphoid hyperplasia. In diffuse areas with sclerosis, the neoplastic centrocytes may be spindle shaped, resembling fibroblasts (see Fig. 17-2F). Centrocytes are often more numerous in sclerotic areas than in other areas; thus, in difficult cases, careful examination of the cells in areas of sclerosis is useful in establishing the diagnosis.

Occasional cases of FL may have amorphous, eosinophilic, extracellular, periodic acid–Schiff–positive material deposited in an irregular fashion within the follicle centers.[69,70] The nature of this material is not clear; Chittal and colleagues[70] found that ultrastructurally it contained membrane fragments, and on immunohistochemistry it contained many antigens found in and on the neoplastic cells (CD45, CD22, immunoglobulin). Others have speculated that it represents the deposition of antigen-antibody complexes on the processes of FDCs, analogous to the deposits often seen in reactive follicles.[69] However, in reactive follicles, extracellular immunoglobulin deposition is rarely massive enough to be conspicuous by light microscopy, whereas in the few lymphomas that exhibit this phenomenon, it may be impressive. Thus, although uncommon and by no means diagnostic, massive extracellular deposition of amorphous material within follicles should raise the question of lymphoma.

Vascular invasion is surprisingly common in FL, both within involved lymph nodes and in pericapsular veins.[9] Centrocytes infiltrate through the walls of small and even larger veins, accumulating within the intima (see Fig. 17-2G). Vascular invasion may be useful in distinguishing FL from hyperplasia. Perhaps as a consequence of this invasion, total infarction of the lymph node may occur.[9] The diagnosis can be confirmed in totally infarcted nodes by careful evaluation of the cells preserved in the extranodal tissue and by reticulin stains, which demonstrate the follicular pattern throughout the infarcted area; molecular genetic analysis can occasionally demonstrate immunoglobulin gene rearrangement in infarcted tissue, and immunohistochemistry may be used to document that the cells are $CD45^+$ and $CD20^+$, although nonspecific staining of necrotic tissue by these antibodies can be a problem.[71-73]

Diffuse Areas in Follicular Lymphoma

A diffuse area in FL is defined as an area that lacks evidence of neoplastic follicles and contains a mixture of cells similar to that seen within the neoplastic follicles (see Fig. 17-2H). Involvement of the interfollicular region by neoplastic cells is not considered evidence of a diffuse pattern. Although the prognostic importance of diffuse areas is debatable, the WHO Clinical Advisory Committee recommends that they be quantified. The WHO classification therefore recognizes three categories of grade 1-2 FL, covering the most clinically important subgroups: follicular (>75% follicular), follicular and diffuse (25% to 75% follicular), predominantly diffuse (<25% follicular), and diffuse (0% follicular) (see Table 17-3). Diffuse areas in low-grade (grade 1-2) FL are not thought to be of prognostic significance; however, diffuse areas composed predominantly of centroblasts (grade 3) are diagnosed as DLBCL (see Table 17-3).

Diffuse Follicular Lymphoma

Rare lymphomas composed of both centrocytes and centroblasts have a purely diffuse pattern, equivalent to diffuse centroblastic-centrocytic lymphoma in the Kiel classification (see Fig. 17-2H). In some of these cases it is likely that focal follicular areas are present and that the purely diffuse pattern is the result of a sampling problem. The frequency of these cases is difficult to determine because they are combined with a variety of other lymphomas in the diffuse "mixed" categories of the Rappaport classification and the working formulation. Lennert[9] reported that only 4% of centroblastic-centrocytic lymphomas in the Kiel registry were entirely diffuse and commented that these were often follicular in other lymph nodes. Studies using the Kiel classification suggest that purely diffuse cases of centroblastic-centrocytic lymphoma have a significantly worse prognosis than those with a follicular or follicular and diffuse pattern.[74]

In the WHO classification, diffuse FL is defined as a diffuse lymphoma composed of both centrocytes and centroblasts in which centrocytes predominate (grade 1-2, low grade). A diffuse lymphoma with a predominance of large follicle center cells (>15 centroblasts/hpf; grade 3) should be classified as DLBCL.

The diagnosis of diffuse FL should be made with caution, after other diffuse lymphomas have been excluded and when sufficient tissue is available to exclude FL. Immunophenotyping studies are essential to show that both small and large cells are B cells (to exclude T-cell–rich large B-cell lymphoma) and that the immunophenotype is consistent with FL ($CD10^+$, $BCL6^+$, $BCL2^+$, $CD5^-$, $CD43^-$, cyclin $D1^-$). If possible, molecular genetic analysis for evidence of *BCL2* rearrangement is useful to confirm this diagnosis. However, cases of predominantly diffuse FL lacking *BCL2* rearrangement, often with deletions at 1p36 and presentation at an early stage with large inguinal tumors, have been described.[75]

Partial Nodal Involvement

In some cases of FL the nodal architecture may be largely or partially preserved, with residual reactive germinal centers; this phenomenon is reportedly associated with a lower stage at diagnosis.[76] In other cases there may be widely spaced, monomorphous follicles surrounded by a relatively normal-appearing interfollicular region, without evidence of extrafollicular neoplastic cells (see Fig. 17-2I). This pattern appears to reflect the homing of neoplastic cells to preexisting reactive follicles, with follicular colonization by tumor cells.[77] This phenomenon may occur in lymph nodes with obvious FL elsewhere in the node, in adjacent nodes, or, rarely, in patients without evidence of overt lymphoma (see "Intrafollicular Neoplasia [In Situ Follicular Lymphoma]" later).[78,79]

Morphology in Sites Other Than Lymph Nodes

Spleen

Splenic involvement by FL typically produces uniform enlargement of white pulp, resembling reactive hyperplasia both on gross examination and at low magnification.[58] This phenomenon has been postulated to reflect the neoplastic cells' ability to "home" to normal B-cell regions (Fig. 17-3A). The white pulp follicles in FL are increased in number as well as size and show a monomorphous infiltrate of centrocytes and centroblasts, similar to that in lymph nodes. The marginal zone may be preserved, making it difficult to differentiate FL from splenic marginal zone lymphoma (see Fig. 17-3B). The red pulp typically contains numerous small follicles, but diffuse red pulp involvement is uncommon.

Bone Marrow

Bone marrow involvement by FL is seen as large, usually circumscribed nodules adjacent to bony trabeculae (see Fig. 17-3C).[58] This feature is useful in distinguishing nodules of lymphoma from benign lymphoid aggregates, which are usually central within marrow spaces rather than paratrabecular; however, occasional paratrabecular lymphoid aggregates can be seen in apparently healthy individuals.[58] Infiltrates that appear to hug or wrap around bony trabeculae are highly suspicious for FL, in contrast to those that simply touch the trabeculae. Marrow aggregates of FL are typically composed predominantly of small centrocytes (see Fig. 17-3D), with only rare centroblasts; the cellular composition may not reflect that of the lymph node, which may contain larger centrocytes and more centroblasts. Marrow involvement by identical cells can be seen in cases of diffuse large cell lymphoma—so-called discordant bone marrow histology.[80] Thus, lymphomas cannot be accurately subclassified based on their appearance in the bone marrow because this may not reflect the appearance of nodal tumor.

Peripheral Blood

Most patients with FL have small numbers of circulating neoplastic cells without an elevated lymphocyte count, which can be detected by flow cytometry or molecular genetic analysis to detect the t(14;18).[81-83] Approximately 10% of patients with FL have an elevated lymphocyte count with circulating centrocytes, which are usually slightly larger than small lymphocytes and have a nuclear cleft (see Fig. 17-3F).[25,84] The morphology of the circulating cells is similar in follicular and mantle cell lymphoma, and some cleaved cells may be seen in occasional patients with chronic lymphocytic leukemia. Immunophenotyping and often lymph node biopsy are typically necessary for correct subclassification.

Histologic Transformation

Patients with FL may develop a more aggressive B-cell lymphoma sometime during the course of their disease. The magnitude of this risk is difficult to assess because not all patients undergo repeat biopsy before repeat therapy. Gall and associates[6] found that six of eight autopsied cases showed some degree of progression from lower to higher grade, although only one case progressed to a diffuse high-grade lymphoma. Rappaport and associates[7] analyzed sequential biopsies or autopsies in 104 of their FL cases. Thirty-seven percent showed no change in cytology or pattern, 30% showed progression to a diffuse pattern without change in cytology, and 44% showed an increase in large cells with or without a diffuse pattern. The frequency of progression was highest in the "mixed" category, with 49% progressing to a large-cell type, most with a diffuse pattern. In addition, 86% of the cases of "nodular reticulum cell type" progressed to a diffuse pattern. More recent studies have shown an actuarial risk of transformation of approximately 20% at 8 years.[85-87] Transformation is usually to DLBCL (Fig. 17-4A), most commonly with cells resembling centroblasts but occasionally with anaplastic CD30⁺ cells.[88]

Cases of transformation to high-grade lymphoma resembling Burkitt's lymphoma (high-grade B-cell lymphoma, unclassifiable, intermediate between Burkitt's lymphoma and DLBCL) (see Fig. 17-4B) or precursor B-cell lymphoblastic leukemia or lymphoma have been reported,[89-94] typically with acquisition of a translocation involving the *MYC* gene on chromosome 8 ("double hit") (see Fig. 17-4C and D).[91-93] The high-grade tumors are typically clonally related to the preexisting FL.[94-97] Both *p53* mutations and *MYC* gene rearrangement have been associated with transformation in FL.[89,90,98,99]

FL may precede, follow, or occur simultaneously with Hodgkin's lymphoma.[100-104] The occurrence of both Hodgkin's lymphoma and FL in the same tissue is relatively rare but may occur (see Fig. 17-4E-G).[100] In two studies, single-cell analysis of neoplastic cells from the Hodgkin's lymphoma component and the FL component of composite or sequential lymphomas demonstrated identical immunoglobulin heavy-chain gene rearrangements in the two tumors; both showed somatic mutations, consistent with derivation from a common germinal center cell precursor.[105,106] Divergent patterns of somatic mutation indicated that the two tumors originated from a common precursor but diverged at the germinal center centroblast stage, with the FL continuing to acquire new somatic mutations.

Recently, several cases of histiocytic-dendritic cell tumors in patients with a history of FL were reported in which identical *IGH* and *BCL2* gene rearrangements were found in both tumors.[107] Loss of *PAX5* has been shown in animal models to result in dedifferentiation of B cells to precursors that can then differentiate into T cells or myeloid cells.[108-110] This finding in a mature B-cell neoplasm suggests that neoplastic B cells may exhibit lineage plasticity and give rise to secondary nonlymphoid tumors.

IMMUNOPHENOTYPE

FL B cells express pan-B antigens (CD19, CD20, CD22, CD79a, PAX5) and surface immunoglobulin with light-chain restriction (Table 17-4; Fig. 17-5A). In more than 50% of cases, the surface immunoglobulin is mu heavy chain, with a minority also expressing delta; a large minority express gamma heavy chains, and rare cases express alpha heavy chain.[111] The frequency of immunoglobulin heavy-chain class switching is higher in FL than in other low-grade lymphomas, consistent with the observation that immunoglobulin heavy-chain class switching normally occurs in the germinal center. Most cases express the germinal center–associated protein CD10 (see Fig. 17-5B); CD10 expression is often stronger in the follicles than in reactive germinal centers.[67,111,112] FL also invariably expresses nuclear BCL6 protein in at least a proportion of the tumor cells.[113] In normal germinal centers, virtually all cells are BCL6⁺, whereas only a variable proportion of cells are BCL6⁺ in FL (see Fig. 17-5C). Both CD10 and BCL6 may be downregulated in interfollicular neoplastic cells and in areas of marginal zone differentiation.[67,111,112] A novel marker of germinal center cells—GCET-1, also known as *centerin*—was discovered by gene expression analysis; it is consistently detected in FL and other lymphomas of germinal center B-cell derivation.[114]

FL is typically CD5⁻ and CD43⁻.[115-117] Rare cases of CD5⁺ FL have been reported.[118] Most CD43⁺ cases are grade 3 with diffuse areas.[117] MUM1/IRF4 is typically not expressed,

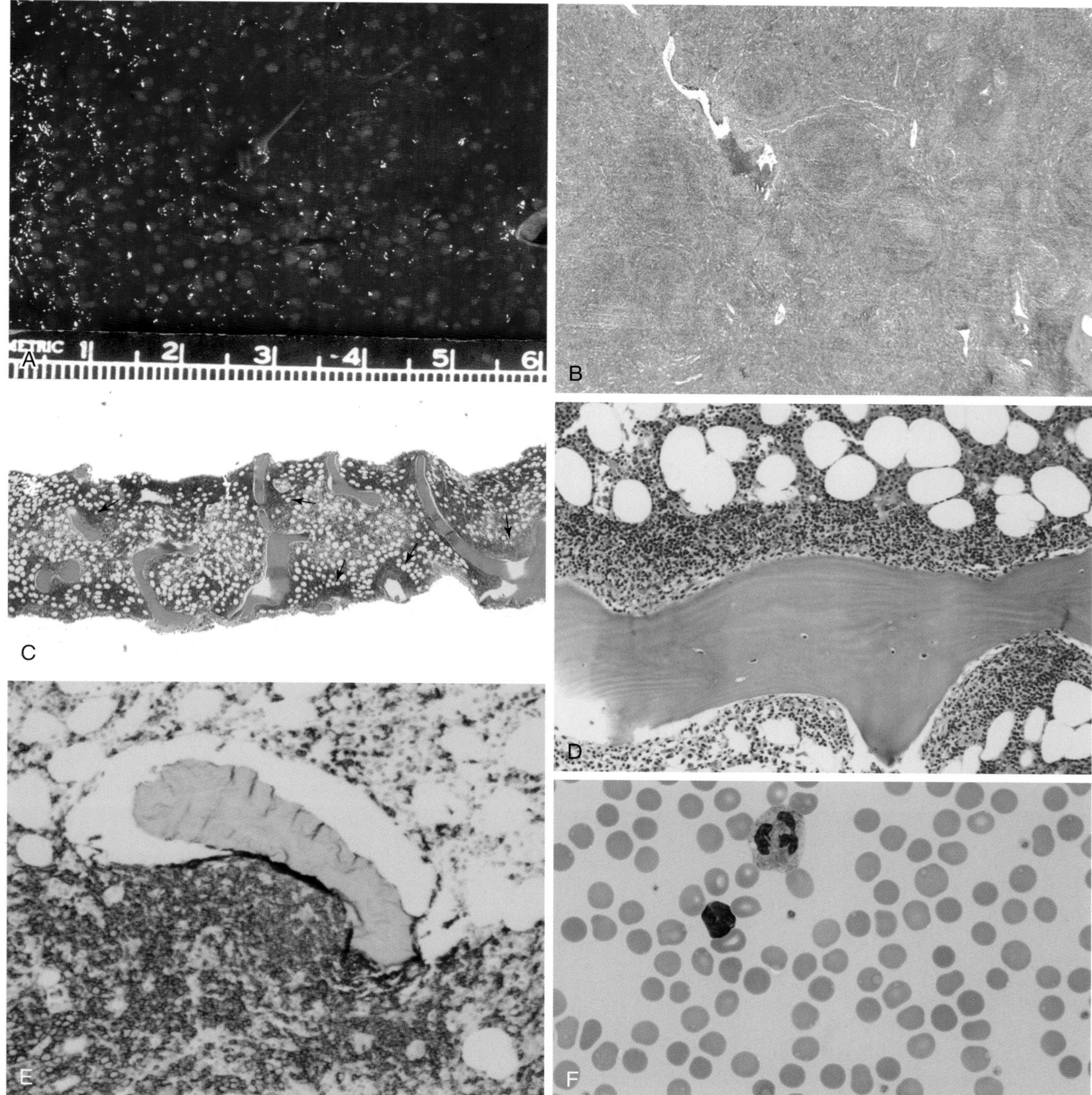

Figure 17-3. Appearance of follicular lymphoma (FL) in the spleen and bone marrow. A, In this gross photograph of a spleen involved by FL, the white pulp follicles are increased in size and number, and most are relatively round. **B**, In a low-power photomicograph of FL in the spleen, white pulp follicles are enlarged and increased in number; preserved marginal zones are present around some of the neoplastic follicles. **C**, In this bone marrow trephine biopsy, a broad cuff of neoplastic lymphoid cells surrounds many bony trabeculae (*arrows*). Residual normal hematopoietic marrow is present away from the bone and is recognizable as areas with a normal distribution of fat. **D**, At higher magnification, there is a predominance of centrocytes. **E**, Immunoperoxidase stain for CD20 confirms that they are B cells. **F**, Peripheral blood smear in a patient with FL shows circulating centrocytes with deep nuclear clefts (Wright-Giemsa stain). (**C** to **F**, Courtesy of Dr. Michael Kluk, Massachusetts General Hospital.)

Table 17-4 **Small B-Cell Neoplasms: Immunophenotypic and Genetic Features**

Neoplasm	sIg; cIg	CD5	CD10	CD23	CD43	Cyclin D_1	BCL6	IGV-Region Genes	Genetic Abnormality
Follicular lymphoma	+; –	–	+/–	–/+	–	–	+	Mutated, IH	t(14;18); *BCL2*R
Mantle cell lymphoma	+; –	+	–	–	+	+	–	70% unmutated, 30% mutated	t(11;14); *CCND1*R
Extranodal and nodal marginal zone lymphoma	+; +/–	–	–	–/+	–/+	–	–	Mutated, IH?	Trisomy 3; t(11;18) (extranodal)
CLL/SLL	+; –/+	+	–	+	+		–	50% unmutated, 50% mutated	Trisomy 12; 13q deletions
Lymphoplasmacytic lymphoma	+; +	–	–	–	–/+	–	–	Mutated	
Splenic marginal zone lymphoma	+; –/+	–	–	–	–	–	–	50% mutated, 50% unmutated	7q31-32 deletions

cIg, cytoplasmic immunoglobulin; CLL/SLL, chronic lymphocytic leukemia–small lymphocytic lymphoma; IGV, immunoglobulin variable region; IH, intraclonal heterogeneity; R, rearranged; sIg, surface immunoglobulin.

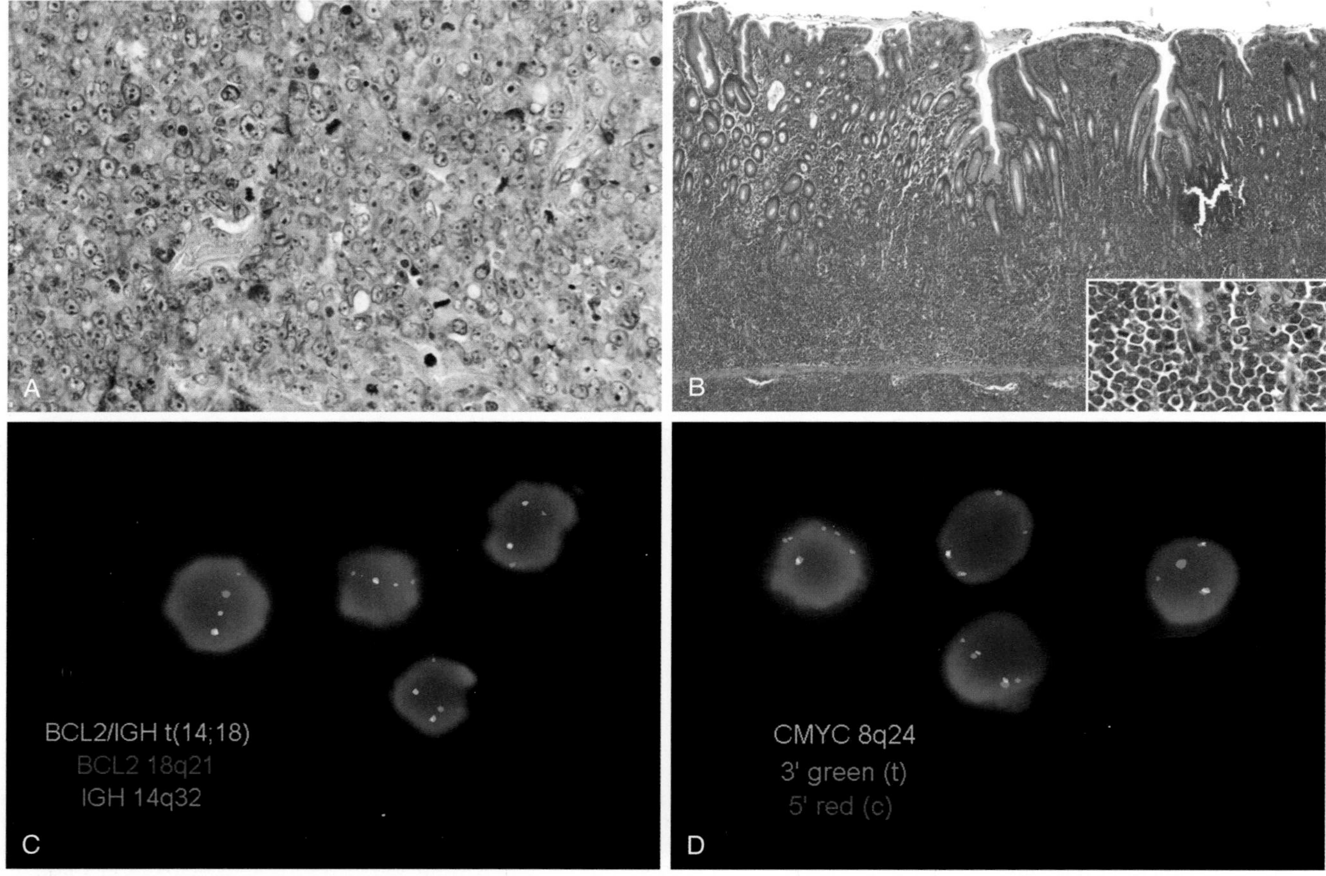

Figure 17-4. Transformed follicular lymphoma (FL). A, Most cases of transformed FL are diffuse large B-cell lymphoma (DLBCL); in this case the cells resemble centroblasts and immunoblasts (Giemsa stain). **B,** Occasional cases of FL transform to high-grade B-cell lymphoma intermediate between DLBCL and Burkitt's lymphoma. This patient with a history of FL grade 1-2 developed a gastric mass; resection showed a diffuse lymphoma extending from the lamina propria to the serosa. At higher magnification (*inset*), the cells are monotonous, of medium size, and resemble Burkitt's lymphoma. **C** and **D,** These cases are typically associated with translocation of *MYC* as well as *BCL2*.

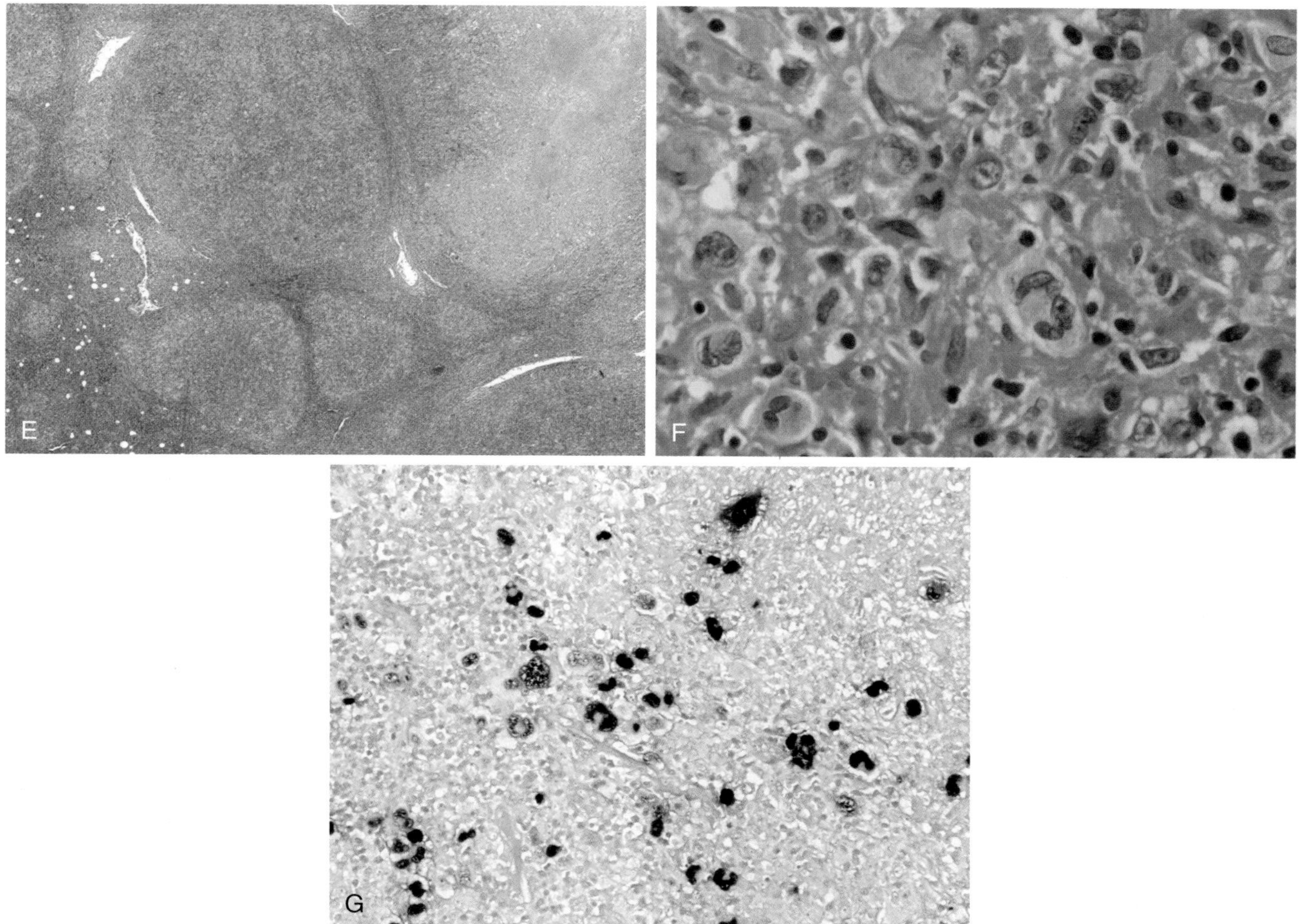

Figure 17-4, cont'd. E, Classic Hodgkin's lymphoma arising in FL shows FL on the *left* and a pale area of histiocytes and necrosis on the *upper right*. **F,** At higher magnification, Reed-Sternberg cells are seen. **G,** The Reed-Sternberg cells are positive for CD15 and CD30 (not shown) and for Epstein-Barr virus–encoded RNA (EBER). (**B,** Courtesy of Dr. Olga Kolman, Department of Pathology, Massachusetts General Hospital. **C** and **D,** Courtesy of Dr. Paola dal Cin, Cytogenetics Laboratory, Massachusetts General Hospital and Brigham and Women's Hospital.)

although occasional cases of grade 3 FL that lack CD10 and BCL2 and express MUM1/IRF4 have been reported.[119,120] FL typically expresses the CD95/Fas protein.[121] FL also expresses costimulatory molecules CD80 and CD86 and CD40.[67,122] Expression of these antigens is weak compared with that of normal germinal center B cells.[122]

About 75% of the cases express BCL2 protein (see Fig. 17-5D)[123]; the frequency is highest (85% to 97%) in grade 1-2 cases and as low as 50% to 75% in grade 3 cases.[124,125] Expression of BCL2 protein is highly predictive of the presence of a *BCL2* translocation; however, some cases of FL with *BCL2* rearrangement have mutations in the *BCL2* gene that affect detection of the protein by the commonly used antibody, resulting in a false-negative result.[126]

Neoplastic follicles contain many elements of the germinal center microenvironment.[127] Nodular aggregates of FDCs outline the neoplastic follicles, demonstrated by monoclonal antibodies to CD21 or CD23 (see Fig. 17-5E and F). Expression of CD21 and CD23 is variable, and some FLs may express one and not the other; thus, staining for both may be necessary. In diffuse areas of FL, FDCs are absent (see Fig. 17-11); this may be useful in distinguishing diffuse FL from mantle cell and marginal zone lymphomas, in which large, irregular aggregates of FDCs are present even in areas that appear diffuse on routine staining.[30,111] Neoplastic follicles also contain follicular-type T cells (positive for CD3, CD4, CD57, PD1, and CXCL13), which are usually less numerous in neoplastic than reactive follicles (see Fig. 17-5G) and are randomly distributed; this contrasts with the crescentic arrangement at the junction with the mantle zone that characterizes reactive follicles.[128,129] Varying numbers of FoxP3$^+$ T-regulatory cells and CD68$^+$ histiocytes are present, and the number of tumor-infiltrating T-regulatory cells, PD1$^+$ follicular T-helper cells, and CD68$^+$ macrophages has been reported to predict clinical prognosis in some[130-139] but not all[140] studies.

Most cases of low-grade FL have a proliferation fraction with Ki-67 of less than 15%; however, rare cases have a high (>40%) proliferation fraction (see Fig. 17-5H and I) and may behave more like grade 3 FL.[57]

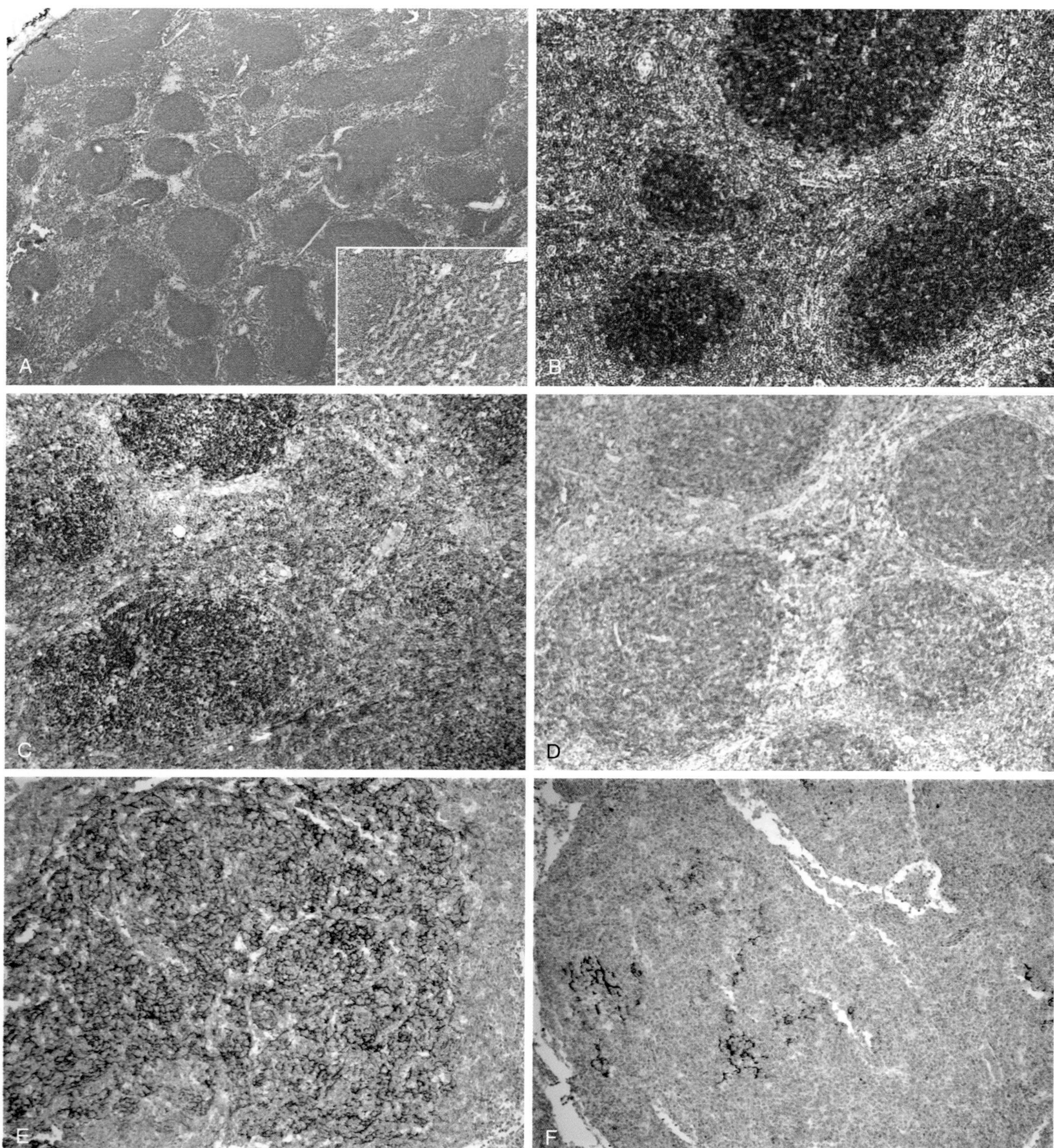

Figure 17-5. Immunohistochemistry of follicular lymphoma (FL) using immunoperoxidase stains in paraffin sections. A, FL stained for CD20 shows that $CD20^+$ B cells are present both within and between follicles (*inset*). **B**, FL immunostained for CD10 shows positive cells largely confined to follicles; interfollicular neoplastic cells may downregulate CD10. **C**, FL stained for BCL6 shows positive cells both within and between follicles. **D**, Immunoperoxidase stain for BCL2 in FL shows strong, uniform positivity within follicles. **E**, Follicular dendritic cells associated with neoplastic follicles are highlighted by CD21. **F**, In this case, CD23 highlights only rare follicular dendritic cells.

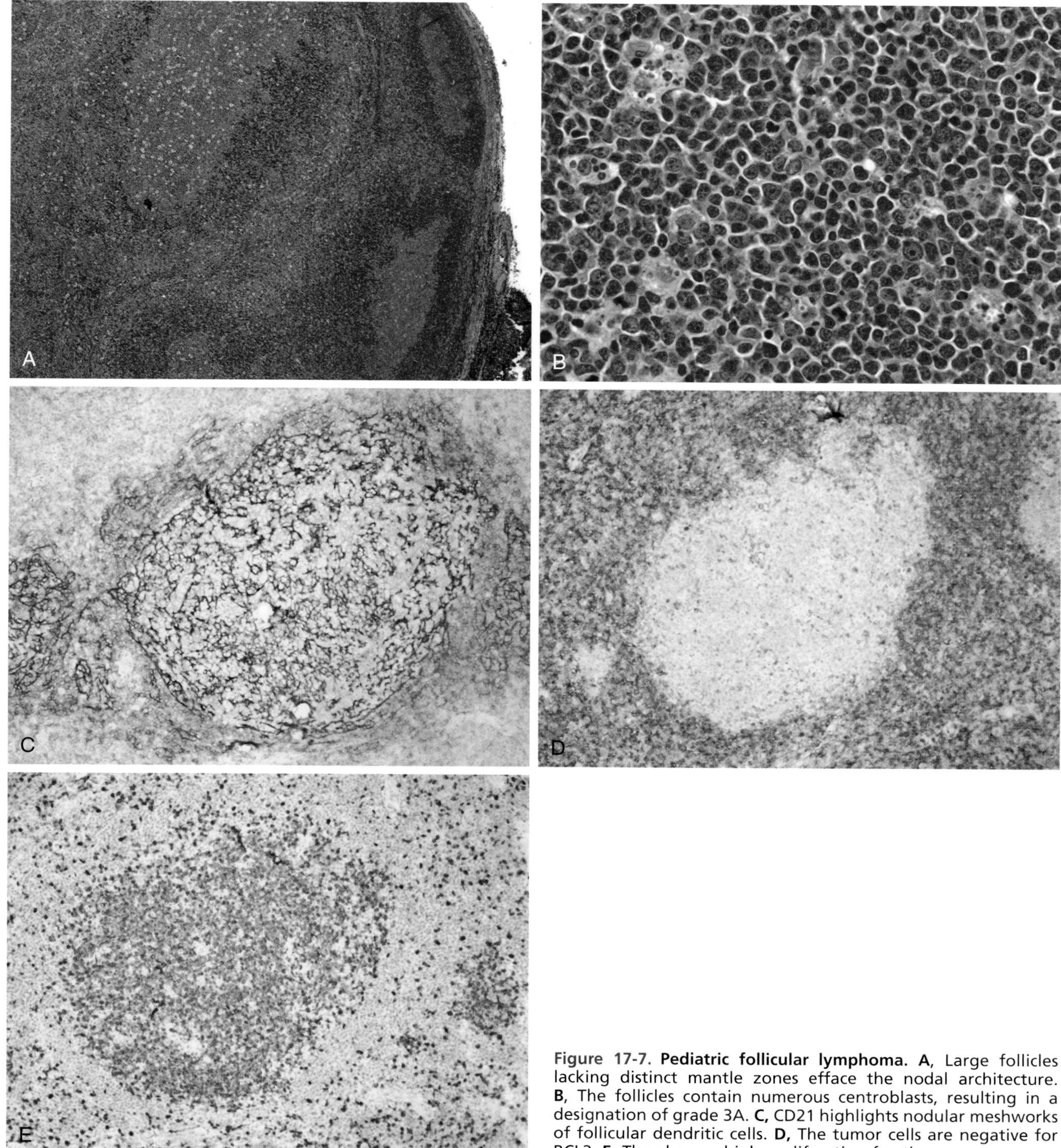

Figure 17-7. Pediatric follicular lymphoma. A, Large follicles lacking distinct mantle zones efface the nodal architecture. **B,** The follicles contain numerous centroblasts, resulting in a designation of grade 3A. **C,** CD21 highlights nodular meshworks of follicular dendritic cells. **D,** The tumor cells are negative for BCL2. **E,** They have a high proliferation fraction.

other genetic abnormalities to result in overt, progressive malignancy. Rarely it may represent the earliest evidence of a true FL that will progress to overt lymphoma. The term *in situ* may seem contradictory when applied to cells that have trafficking capabilities, but it refers to the fact that the cells occupy preexisting follicles rather than forming true neoplastic follicles. Because of the risk of diagnosing patients with lymphoma prematurely, the WHO classification suggests the term *intrafollicular neoplasia*, analogous to the recently adopted convention with regard to epithelial neoplasms (*intraepithelial neoplasia*).[1] In such cases a diagnosis of FL should not be made; the pathology report should indicate that the significance of the finding is unknown and that clinical evaluation for evidence of overt FL elsewhere is suggested.

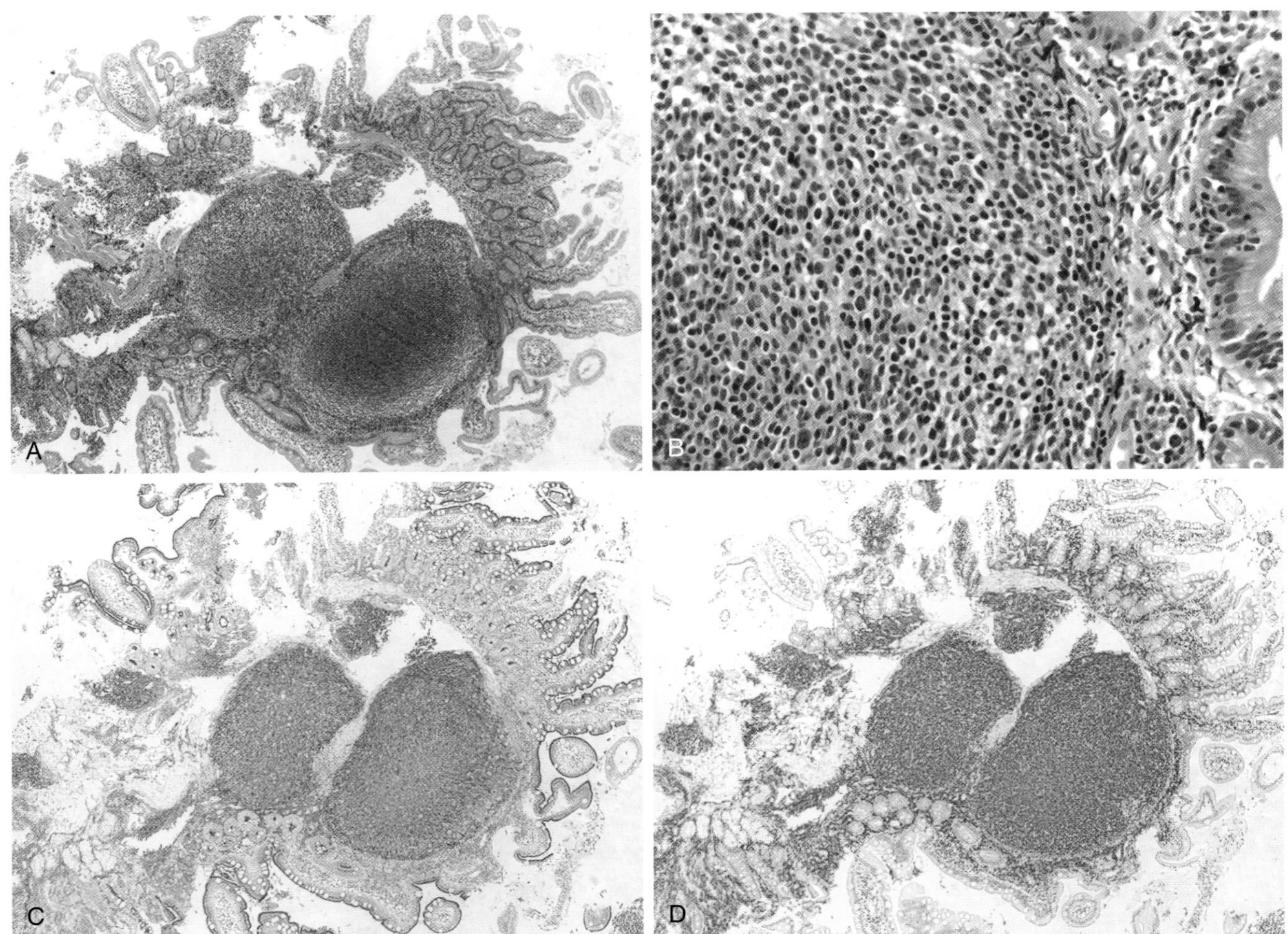

Figure 17-8. Follicular lymphoma of the duodenum. A, At low magnification, monomorphous follicles lacking mantle zones are present in the lamina propria. **B,** At higher magnification, there is a monotonous population of centrocytes. **C** and **D,** The cells are positive for CD10 (**C**) and BCL2 (**D**).

DIFFERENTIAL DIAGNOSIS

See Box 17-2.

Follicular Hyperplasia

Reactive follicular hyperplasia is the major differential diagnosis in cases of FL. In the vast majority of cases, typical architectural and cytologic features permit the diagnosis of FL based on morphologic criteria alone.[7,209] In difficult cases, immunophenotyping and, occasionally, molecular genetic studies can be helpful in establishing a diagnosis.

Box 17-2 *Differential Diagnosis of Follicular Lymphoma*

- Follicular hyperplasia
- Progressive transformation of germinal centers
- Other small B-cell lymphomas
  - Small lymphocytic lymphoma
  - Mantle cell lymphoma
  - Marginal zone lymphoma
- Hodgkin's lymphoma
  - Nodular lymphocyte-predominant Hodgkin's lymphoma
  - Nodular sclerosis classical Hodgkin's lymphoma

Morphologic Criteria

Pattern. Effacement of the normal architecture by closely packed, relatively uniform follicles that lack a mantle zone and extend outside the nodal capsule is diagnostic of FL (Table 17-6). Close packing of follicles, even focally—particularly if the follicles in this area are small and uniform—is highly suggestive of lymphoma. If the follicles are widely spaced, the interfollicular region should be examined at high magnification for the presence of centrocytes. Although transformed cells (immunoblasts and occasionally centroblasts) can be seen in the interfollicular regions of reactive nodes, centrocytes are virtually never found outside germinal centers in normal lymph nodes. Extension of follicles outside the capsule in association with concentric bands of sclerosis is a helpful feature (see Fig. 17-2A). Capsular fibrosis often occurs in lymphadenitis, with small lymphocytes and plasma cells

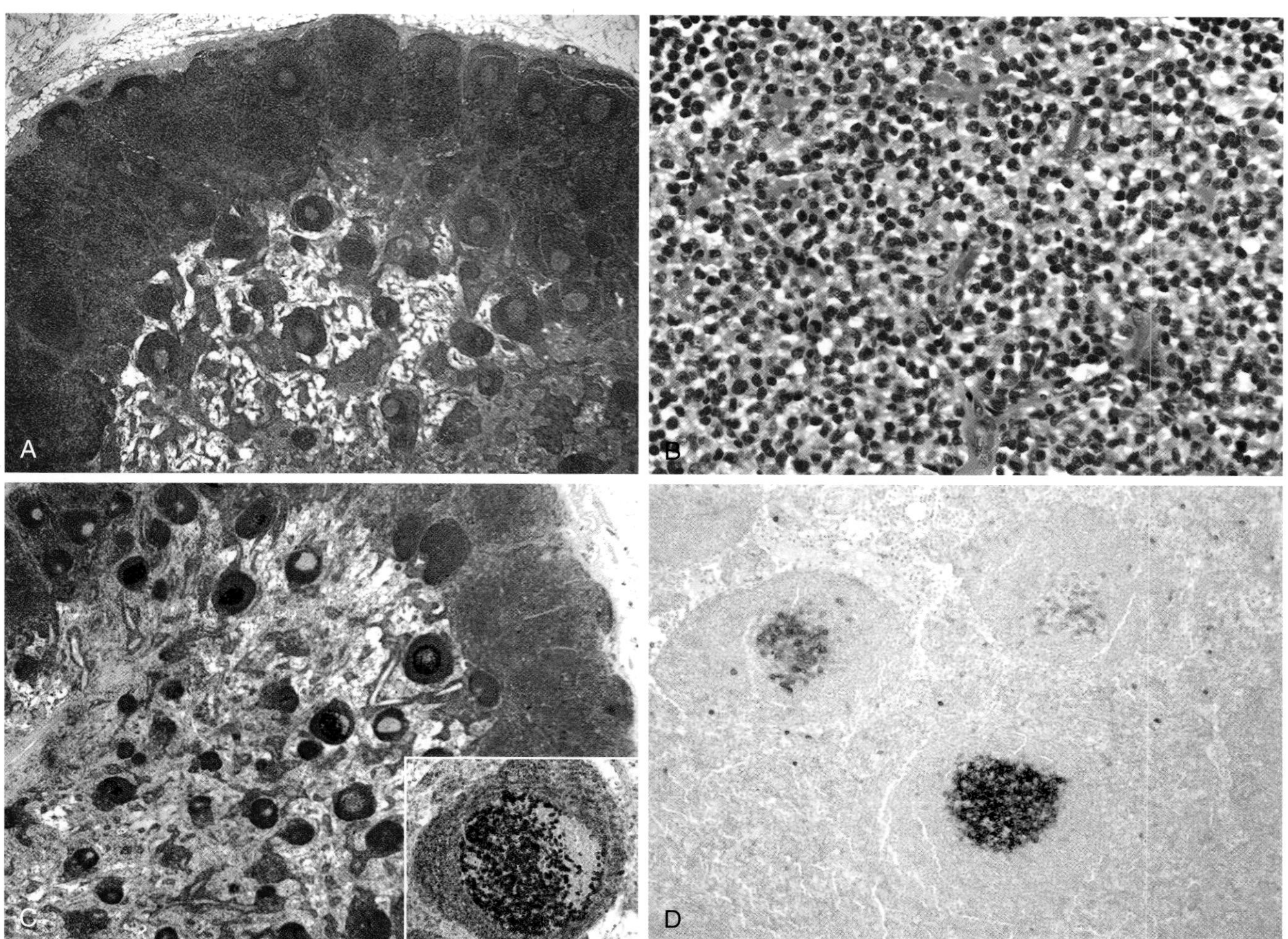

Figure 17-9. Intrafollicular neoplasia (follicular lymphoma in situ). The lymph node architecture is preserved (**A**), with reactive-appearing follicles (**B**). Immunohistochemistry for BCL2 (**C**) reveals occasional follicles containing strongly positive cells. The *inset* shows that some follicles are only partially involved. The BCL2^{+} follicles tend to express CD10 (**D**) more strongly than ordinary reactive follicles.

Table 17-6 **Histologic Features Useful in Distinguishing Follicular Lymphoma (FL) from Follicular Hyperplasia**

Characteristic	Specificity for FL	Frequency in FL
Centrocytes predominate in follicles	Diagnostic	High
Centrocytes present between follicles	Diagnostic	High
Vascular invasion by centrocytes	Diagnostic	Moderate
Close packing of follicles	Highly suggestive	High
Diffuse areas or sclerosis	Highly suggestive	Moderate
Follicles extend beyond nodal capsule	Highly suggestive	High
Mantle zone absent	Suggestive	High
"Starry sky" cells absent in follicles	Suggestive	High
Mantle zone present	Not helpful	Low
Some reactive follicles present	Not helpful	Low
Size, shape, uniformity of follicles	Not helpful	—
"Cracking" artifact or compression of reticulin	Not helpful	—

present in perinodal fat, but follicles with germinal centers are rarely seen outside the capsule. Sclerosis within the lymph node, particularly in diffuse areas, is also suggestive of lymphoma; areas of sclerosis should be scrutinized at high magnification for the presence of centrocytes. Finally, transmural invasion of the walls of small or medium-sized veins by centrocytes, either within the node or in perinodal tissue, is highly suggestive of lymphoma (see Fig. 17-2G).

Cytology. The cases that are difficult to diagnose are typically grade 3, in which the increased number of centroblasts more closely approximates the normal germinal center. In these cases the absence of phagocytic tingible body macrophages, low mitotic rate, lack of polarization, crowding of follicles, and lack of a mantle zone are helpful features. In some FLs the centroblasts or large centrocytes have a cytologically atypical appearance, with hyperchromatic or abnormally shaped nuclei. The cytology of the interfollicular, extranodal, and diffuse areas in these cases can be essential in establishing the diagnosis.

Immunophenotyping. In distinguishing benign from malignant lymphoid infiltrates, the most reliable criterion is immunoglobulin light-chain restriction, which is best evaluated by immunohistochemistry on frozen sections or in cell suspensions by flow cytometry. Evidence of light-chain restriction (kappa or lambda) within the follicles is usually diagnostic of lymphoma. However, clonal B cells have been reported within some follicles in cases of apparent reactive hyperplasia,[210] and clonal CD10⁺ B cells may be detected by flow cytometry in cases of florid follicular hyperplasia in children.[202] Thus, these results must be analyzed in the context of the morphologic appearance.

Immunohistochemical staining for BCL2 protein is the most useful technique for distinguishing FL from follicular hyperplasia on paraffin sections. Sections must be examined together with sections stained for CD20 and CD3 because numerous BCL2⁺ T cells may be present in both reactive and neoplastic follicles; staining of these cells should not be misinterpreted as BCL2 expression by neoplastic cells. In many cases the neoplastic follicle center cells express BCL2 more strongly than do the surrounding mantle zone or interfollicular cells; in some cases, however, staining of FL cells may be faint and restricted to a subset of cells—usually centrocytes. BCL2 staining should be interpreted together with BCL6, CD10, or FDC staining because expression of BCL2 by non–germinal center B cells is not indicative of lymphoma. Unfortunately, BCL2 positivity is less common in grade 3 FL—making it difficult to differentiate it from reactive hyperplasia—so the absence of BCL2 does not exclude lymphoma.[124]

Expression of CD10 or BCL6 by follicles is not a criterion for malignancy because it is also expressed by normal germinal center cells.[111] CD10 is typically expressed more strongly in neoplastic than reactive germinal centers, and BCL6 may be expressed by fewer cells in FL than in follicular hyperplasia. Detection of CD10⁺ or BCL6⁺ cells in the interfollicular region is suggestive of FL. However, rare normal interfollicular cells may be BCL6⁺, and interfollicular neoplastic cells may lack CD10 or express it more weakly than those within the follicles.[67,111] Assessment of the proliferation fraction using Ki-67 may be helpful because in reactive follicles the vast majority of the cells are in cycle, whereas even in grade 3 FL the proliferation fraction is rarely greater than 60%.

Molecular Genetic Analysis

Southern blot or PCR analysis for either immunoglobulin or *BCL2* rearrangements can be more sensitive for detecting small clonal populations than conventional immunophenotyping and may also prove clonality in immunoglobulin-negative or BCL2 protein–negative tumors. Southern blot analysis requires fresh tissue and detects immunoglobulin gene rearrangements in the vast majority of FLs.[153] PCR analysis is less sensitive, with only about 65% of FLs showing *IGH* clonal rearrangements; this lack of sensitivity has been attributed to the failure of consensus primers to bind because of extensive somatic mutations in the immunoglobulin genes in FL. In one study, 89% of FL cases had the t(14;18) translocation by cytogenetic analysis, 75% had *BCL2* rearrangement by Southern blot, and 65% had *BCL2* rearrangement detectable by PCR.[153] Thus, PCR analysis has a significant false-negative rate for the detection of both immunoglobulin and *BCL2* rearrangement. In addition, *BCL2* rearrangement can be detected in some normal tonsils and lymph nodes, so the detection of a small clonal population by this technique is not diagnostic of malignancy.[211]

Other Lymphomas

Other lymphomas with a nodular or follicular pattern may resemble FL. These include mantle cell lymphoma, marginal zone lymphoma, occasionally small lymphocytic lymphoma, and, rarely, Hodgkin's lymphoma.

Small B-Cell Lymphomas

Morphologic Features. The morphologic features of small B-cell lymphomas are summarized in Table 17-7. Chronic lymphocytic leukemia–small lymphocytic lymphoma (CLL/SLL) typically has a pseudofollicular pattern in lymph nodes; this can be mistaken for a true follicular pattern, resulting in confusion with FL. In general, pseudofollicles are uniform in size and shape and evenly spaced throughout the node, like bacterial colonies on a culture dish, exhibiting a "cloudy sky" pattern. They are poorly demarcated from the surrounding infiltrate, so they seem to "disappear" at progressively higher magnifications. They contain cells with predominantly round nuclei and show a subtle gradation from small lymphocytes to prolymphocytes to paraimmunoblasts, in contrast to the sharp dichotomy between centrocytes and centroblasts in FL. Sclerosis and extranodal extension are uncommon in CLL/SLL.

Cases of mantle cell lymphoma may have a vaguely nodular or, rarely, a true follicular pattern. In most cases the follicular

Table 17-7 Small B-Cell Neoplasms: Histologic Features Useful in the Differential Diagnosis

Neoplasm	Pattern	Small Cells	Transformed Cells
Follicular lymphoma	Follicular ± diffuse areas, rarely diffuse	Centrocytes (cleaved)	Centroblasts
Mantle cell lymphoma	Diffuse, vaguely nodular, mantle zone, rarely follicular	Similar to centrocytes (cleaved, rarely round or oval, may be large)	None
Marginal zone B-cell lymphoma	Diffuse, interfollicular, marginal zone, follicular colonization	Heterogeneous: round (small lymphocytes), cleaved (centrocyte-like, marginal zone, monocytoid B cells), plasma cells	Centroblasts Immunoblasts
CLL/SLL	Diffuse with pseudofollicles	Round (occasionally cleaved)	Prolymphocytes Paraimmunoblasts
Lymphoplasmacytic lymphoma	Diffuse; no pseudofollicles	Round (may be cleaved) Plasma cells	Centroblasts Immunoblasts

CLL/SLL, chronic lymphocytic leukemia–small lymphocytic lymphoma.

pattern is only focal, with large diffuse areas. In contrast to FL, which always contains a mixture of neoplastic centroblasts and centrocytes, mantle cell lymphoma contains a monotonous population of small cells that resemble centrocytes, with virtually no blast cells. Occasional centroblasts can be seen in areas of partially overrun follicles. In many cases foci of preserved germinal centers surrounded by a mantle zone of atypical cells can be found; this appearance would be unusual in FL. In many cases of mantle cell lymphoma there are single epithelioid histiocytes that are nonphagocytic. Mantle cell lymphoma often has a higher mitotic rate than FL. The character of the blood vessels may also provide a clue to the diagnosis. In mantle cell lymphoma the small vessels usually are not of the high endothelial venule type; they have flat endothelial cells and often have eosinophilic sclerosis of their walls. In contrast, in diffuse areas of FL the small vessels usually are of the high endothelial venule type and do not show prominent sclerosis. Compartmentalizing fibrosis, which is commonly seen at least focally in diffuse FL, is rare in mantle cell lymphoma. Finally, diffuse areas of FL frequently contain large numbers of small, reactive T lymphocytes, whereas mantle cell lymphoma contains many fewer reactive cells.

Marginal zone lymphomas may have a partially follicular pattern, owing to the presence of follicles that have been "colonized" by neoplastic marginal zone cells. Typically these follicles are widely spaced in a background of interfollicular marginal zone cells, but occasionally they may be numerous and mimic FL. In addition, FL may have marginal zone differentiation, mimicking marginal zone lymphoma. Marginal zone B cells have centrocyte-like nuclei but more abundant cytoplasm; however, occasional FLs may have cells with relatively abundant cytoplasm. Marginal zone lymphoma also enters the differential diagnosis of diffuse FL because both contain a mixture of small cells with irregular nuclei and large centroblasts or immunoblasts. Problems can also arise when biopsy specimens are small and a mixed population of centrocyte-like and centroblast-like cells is present without an obvious pattern. Features favoring marginal zone lymphoma include a predominant interfollicular infiltrate, irregular follicles, foci of reactive-appearing follicles, abundant cytoplasm, and plasmacytoid differentiation. Features favoring FL include monomorphism; round, uniform, and closely packed follicles; sclerosis; and vascular invasion.

Immunophenotype. The immunophenotypic and genetic features of small B-cell lymphomas are summarized in Table 17-4. Mantle cell lymphoma and CLL/SLL characteristically express IgM, IgD, CD5, and CD43; most cases are $CD10^-$. In contrast, FL is usually IgD^-, IgG^+ or IgM^+, and $CD5^-$; 50% to 80% of cases are $CD10^+$.[115] With antibodies to FDCs, follicular areas in FL are highlighted by concentric aggregates of FDCs, whereas diffuse areas show few if any FDCs; in contrast, both mantle cell lymphomas and many marginal zone lymphomas show large, irregular FDC aggregates throughout the tumors, even in areas that are diffuse on routine sections.[111,212] Staining for BCL2 may highlight residual negative reactive follicles in mantle cell lymphoma and marginal zone lymphoma, whereas follicle centers are typically positive in FL. Note that BCL2 staining of the extrafollicular neoplastic cells is not helpful in the differential diagnosis of small B-cell lymphomas because all are positive. Finally, staining for cyclin D1 shows nuclear staining in virtually all mantle cell lymphomas but is negative in FL.[213] This is particularly useful in the rare cases of $CD5^-$ mantle cell lymphoma.[214]

Immunophenotyping can be useful in the differential diagnosis between FL and marginal zone lymphoma with follicular colonization, but it requires careful interpretation because of the complex architecture of these neoplasms. The most useful antigens are CD10, BCL6, and BCL2; all must be assessed with respect to $CD21^+$ or $CD23^+$ FDC aggregates, which define the follicular areas. In FL most of the cells within the FDC aggregates should be $BCL2^+$, $CD10^+$, and $BCL6^+$, whereas in marginal zone lymphoma they are heterogeneous. Noncolonized follicles are $BCL2^-$, $CD10^+$, and $BCL6^+$; partially colonized follicles have an admixture of $BCL2^+$, $CD10^-$, and $BCL6^-$ neoplastic cells and $BCL2^-$, $CD10^+$, and $BCL6^+$ follicle center cells; and completely colonized follicles are typically $BCL2^+$, $CD10^-$, and $BCL6^-$. Expression of CD10 or BCL6 by extrafollicular B cells (away from FDC aggregates) supports follicle center lymphoma, whereas $CD10^-$, $BCL6^-$ extrafollicular cells favor marginal zone lymphoma.[113,212,215] MUM1/IRF4 is helpful if positive because most FLs are MUM1/IRF4 negative and some marginal zone lymphomas are positive. The presence of light-chain–restricted plasma cells also favors a diagnosis of marginal zone lymphoma.

Genetic Analysis. The *BCL2* gene rearrangement characteristic of FL is not found in mantle cell, small lymphocytic, or marginal zone lymphoma. The *CCND1* gene rearrangement is detectable by PCR in about 40% of mantle cell lymphomas and not in FL (see Table 17-4).

Hodgkin's Lymphoma

Rarely, cases of FL with interfollicular sclerosis may resemble nodular sclerosis classical Hodgkin's lymphoma. This confusion occurs in cases with very atypical large centrocytes and centroblasts that may resemble mononuclear or diagnostic Reed-Sternberg cells. In these cases the binucleate centroblasts do not have the abundant cytoplasm and multilobated nuclei of typical lacunar cells, and the background cells are centrocytes rather than the lymphocytes, eosinophils, and plasma cells of nodular sclerosis Hodgkin's lymphoma. Nonetheless, in some cases, immunohistologic studies may be required to distinguish the two: Hodgkin's lymphoma is $CD15^+$, $CD30^+$, $CD45^-$ or $^+$, and $CD20^-$ or $^+$; FL is $CD15^-$, $CD30^-$ or $^+$, $CD45^+$, $CD20^+$, $CD10^+$, $BCL6^+$, and Ig^+.

Occasionally, FL and nodular lymphocyte-predominant Hodgkin's lymphoma may resemble each other. This problem is most common in the so-called floral variant of FL. In this morphologic variant of grade 3 (large cell) FL, numerous small, polyclonal B cells are present both around and within the nodules of large, neoplastic follicle center B cells (see Fig. 17-2C). On morphologic examination, the size and shape of the follicles are useful: those of FL tend to be more uniform and smaller than the very large, variably shaped follicles of nodular lymphocyte-predominant Hodgkin's lymphoma. In addition, centrocytes are much more numerous in the nodules of FL than in those of Hodgkin's lymphoma. The nodules in both cases are true follicles with $CD21^+$ FDCs and a predominance of B cells. The small B cells in nodular lymphocyte-predominant Hodgkin's lymphoma are $BCL2^+$ but $CD10^-$ and $BCL6^-$ because they are mostly of the mantle zone type. BCL2 positivity of the large cells may be helpful because the neoplastic cells of this type of Hodgkin's lymphoma are typically BCL2$^-$. Demonstration of *IGH* rearrangement by Southern blot or PCR or demonstration of *BCL2* rearrangement strongly favors a diagnosis of FL in this setting.

CONCLUSION

FL is a distinctive tumor that reproduces most of the morphologic, immunophenotypic, and genetic features of the lymphoid germinal center. The biologic behavior of the tumor is ordained by a chromosomal translocation resulting in activation of a gene, *BCL2*, that confers a survival advantage on nonproliferating neoplastic cells, averting the rapid cell death that is the fate of most normal germinal center cells. Unlike normal germinal center cells, the neoplastic cells do not remain confined to the germinal center but migrate to other follicles, peripheral blood, and bone marrow; they home to follicular areas, resulting in a tumor that shows widespread involvement of lymphoid tissues. The diagnosis in most cases is relatively straightforward, relying on morphologic evidence of uncontrolled accumulation of centrocytes, accompanied by rare self-renewing centroblasts. Clinically, FL is an indolent malignancy with a long median survival that is unaffected by treatment in most cases; the pace of the disease is predictable to some extent based on the number of centroblasts in the neoplastic follicles. When a threshold of more than 15 centroblasts/hpf is reached, aggressive combination chemotherapy can result in improved survival. Transformation to an aggressive lymphoma may occur when additional chromosomal translocations or mutations cause the activation of oncogenes or the inactivation of suppressor genes, resulting in increased proliferation. New variants, including pediatric and duodenal FL, have recently been recognized, and they seem to be clinically localized and indolent. The diagnosis is usually straightforward, but morphologic clues, immunophenotyping, and genetic studies can help make the diagnosis in difficult cases.

Pearls and Pitfalls

- In distinguishing FL from reactive follicular hyperplasia, the presence of follicles outside the lymph node capsule, particularly with concentric bands of fibrosis, points to FL. Interfollucular centrocytes and vascular invasion by centrocytes, as well as diffuse areas with sclerosis, are also clues to FL. In difficult cases the morphology of the interfollicular areas can be more useful than that of the follicles.
- In distinguishing FL from mantle cell lymphoma, FL follicles always contain centroblasts. Mantle cell lymphoma may have a follicular pattern, but centroblasts are typically absent.
- In distinguishing FL (with or without marginal zone differentiation) from marginal zone lymphoma, immunophenotyping is essential. Attention must be directed at the immunophenotype of cells associated with FDC meshworks as well as interfollicular cells (especially CD10, BCL6, and BCL2). Remember that FL may involve extranodal sites.
- Occasional cases of FL may have an irregular distribution of centroblasts, resembling polarization, and may have preserved mantle zones, mimicking reactive follicles.
- The category of FL now includes purely diffuse cases, so a diagnosis of "follicular lymphoma grade 1-2, diffuse pattern" may be made.
- Any diffuse area in FL that has sufficient centroblasts to warrant designation as grade 3 (A or B) should receive a separate diagnosis of DLBCL—there is no such thing as "FL grade 3 (A or B), diffuse pattern."
- FL may transform into a high-grade lymphoma that resembles Burkitt's lymphoma; such cases typically have both *BCL2* and *MYC* rearrangement and should be classified as B-cell lymphoma intermediate between Burkitt's lymphoma and DLBCL (not as Burkitt's lymphoma).
- Some cases of FL may be negative for BCL2 by immunohistochemistry but still have *BCL2-IGH* rearrangement; PCR should be considered in cases of BCL2$^-$ FL.
- Pediatric-type FL (BCL2$^-$) typically behaves in an indolent fashion and should be diagnosed with caution—overdiagnosis may be more harmful than underdiagnosis. Some pediatric cases of follicular hyperplasia may have clonal CD10$^+$ B-cell populations detected by flow cytometry; it is not known whether these cases are early FL or simply reactive clones.
- BCL2 staining on reactive-appearing lymph nodes may disclose partial involvement of follicles by strongly BCL2$^+$ cells that are clonal (intrafollicular neoplasia or FL in situ); the clinical behavior of such cases is not predictable, and a diagnosis of lymphoma should generally not be made.
- Some cases of FL grade 1-2 may have a high proliferation index (>40%); these cases should be signed out as "FL grade 1-2 with a high proliferation index," not upgraded to FL grade 3 (grading is still based on morphology).

References can be found on Expert Consult @ www.expertconsult.com

Chapter 18

Extranodal Marginal Zone Lymphoma: MALT Lymphoma

Peter G. Isaacson

CHAPTER OUTLINE

In classifying non-Hodgkin's lymphomas, considerable attention has been paid to architectural, cytologic, and functional similarities between the various lymphomas and normal lymphoid tissue, exemplified by the peripheral lymph node. However, studies of extranodal lymphomas, particularly gastrointestinal lymphomas (accounting for the majority), suggest that their clinicopathologic features are related not to lymph nodes but to the structure and function of mucosa-associated lymphoid tissue (MALT).[1,2]

The anatomic distribution and structure of lymph nodes are adapted to deal with antigens carried to the node in afferent lymphatics, which drain sites at various distances from the node. Permeable mucosal sites, such as the gastrointestinal tract, are particularly vulnerable to pathogens and antigens because they are in direct contact with the external environment, and specialized lymphoid tissue—MALT—has evolved to protect them. MALT includes gut-associated lymphoid tissue, nasopharyngeal lymphoid tissue (tonsils), and other less well characterized aggregates of lymphoid tissue related to other mucosae. Gut-associated lymphoid tissue serves as the paradigm for MALT.

HISTOLOGY AND IMMUNOLOGY OF MUCOSA-ASSOCIATED LYMPHOID TISSUE

MALT in the gastrointestinal tract comprises four lymphoid compartments that include organized collections of lymphoid tissue. When concentrated in the terminal ileum, these collections form Peyer's patches; lamina propria lymphocytes, plasma cells, and accessory cells; intraepithelial lymphocytes; and mesenteric lymph nodes. MALT lymphomas essentially recapitulate the features of Peyer's patches.

PEYER'S PATCHES

Organized lymphoid nodules are distributed throughout the small intestine, the appendix, and the colorectum. These nodules are concentrated in the terminal ileum, where they collectively form *Peyer's patches*, the generic term applied to this compartment of MALT. Peyer's patches are unencapsulated aggregates of lymphoid cells that bear a certain resemblance to lymph nodes (Fig. 18-1A). Each Peyer's patch

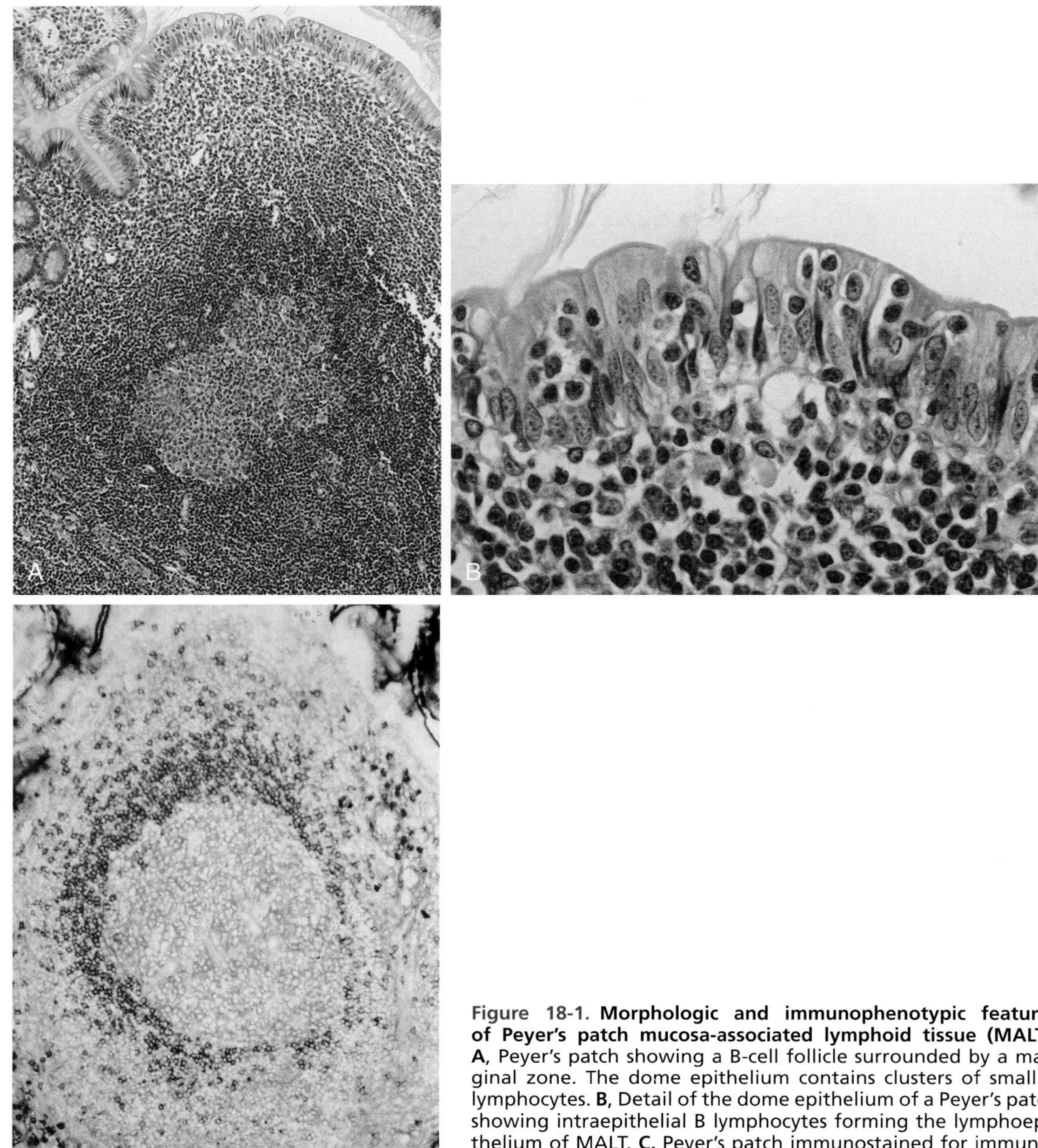

Figure 18-1. Morphologic and immunophenotypic features of Peyer's patch mucosa-associated lymphoid tissue (MALT). **A,** Peyer's patch showing a B-cell follicle surrounded by a marginal zone. The dome epithelium contains clusters of small B lymphocytes. **B,** Detail of the dome epithelium of a Peyer's patch showing intraepithelial B lymphocytes forming the lymphoepithelium of MALT. **C,** Peyer's patch immunostained for immunoglobulin (Ig) D (*brown*) and CD20 (*blue*). The IgD$^+$ mantle zone is surrounded by an IgD$^-$ (IgM$^+$), CD20$^+$ marginal zone.

nodule consists of B- and T-cell areas and associated accessory cells. The B-cell area comprises a germinal center surrounded by a mantle zone of small B lymphocytes, which is broadest at the mucosal aspect of the follicle. Surrounding the mantle zone is a broad marginal zone in which most of the cells are small to intermediate-sized B lymphocytes with moderately abundant, pale-staining cytoplasm and nuclei with a slightly irregular outline, leading to a resemblance to centrocytes. The marginal zone extends toward the mucosal surface, and some marginal zone B cells enter the overlying dome epithelium, where they form the lymphoepithelium, which is a defining feature of MALT (see Fig. 18-1B). Immunohistochemical studies of Peyer's patches have shown that the B-cell follicles are identical to those of lymph nodes.[3-5] In contrast to the immunoglobulin (Ig) M$^+$ and IgD$^+$ mantle zone, the peripheral marginal zone cells are IgM$^+$ but IgD$^-$ (see Fig. 18-1C). Lateral to the deep aspect of the B-cell follicle is a T-cell zone in which high endothelial venules are prominent, equivalent to the paracortical T-zone of the lymph node.

DEFINITION OF MALT LYMPHOMA

MALT lymphoma is an extranodal lymphoma comprising morphologically heterogeneous small B cells, including marginal zone (centrocyte-like) cells, cells resembling monocytoid cells, small lymphocytes, and scattered immunoblast and centroblast-like cells. There is plasma cell differentiation in a proportion of cases. The infiltrate is in the marginal zone of reactive B-cell follicles and extends into the interfollicular region. In epithelial tissues the neoplastic cells typically infiltrate the epithelium, forming lymphoepithelial lesions.[6]

MALT lymphomas arise in a wide variety of extranodal sites (Box 18-1), but curiously, most of these are not sites where MALT is normally present, such as the terminal ileum or the tonsils. One could question whether the term *MALT* is appropriate for lymphomas, such as those of the orbit, that do not arise in mucosal or epithelial tissues; however, their close association with mucosal tissue, together with their histology, immunophenotype, and genetic and clinical properties, tend to support their classification as MALT lymphomas.

EPIDEMIOLOGY

MALT lymphoma accounts for 7% to 8% of all B-cell lymphomas and at least 50% of primary gastric lymphomas.[7,8] Most cases occur in adults, with a median age of 61 years and a slight female predominance that is most marked in salivary gland and thyroid MALT lymphomas. There is a higher incidence of gastric MALT lymphoma in northeastern Italy, probably related to a high prevalence of *Helicobacter pylori*–associated gastritis in that region.[9] A special subtype of small intestinal MALT lymphoma known as *immunoproliferative small intestinal disease* (IPSID) occurs in the Middle East, parts of the Indian subcontinent, and the Cape region of South Africa.[10]

ETIOLOGY

MALT lymphomas only rarely arise from native MALT; they usually arise from MALT that has been acquired as a result of a chronic inflammatory disorder (see later) at sites normally devoid of MALT, such as the stomach, salivary gland, lung, thyroid, and ocular adnexa. MALT lymphomas of the salivary gland and thyroid, organs normally containing no lymphoid tissue, are always preceded by lymphoepithelial (myoepithelial) sialadenitis (LESA),[11-13] usually associated with Sjögren's syndrome and Hashimoto's thyroiditis, respectively. Histologic and immunohistochemical studies of the heavy lymphoid infiltrate that characterizes these two conditions have shown a remarkable resemblance to Peyer's patches. This is most graphically illustrated with reference to LESA. In this condition, lymphoid tissue accumulates around dilated salivary gland ducts and forms, in effect, small Peyer's patches, complete with a germinal center, mantle, small marginal zone, and, significantly, lymphoepithelium comprising collections of intraepithelial B cells (Fig. 18-2A). This lymphoid tissue, known as *acquired MALT*, is also a feature of Hashimoto's thyroiditis; and it has been identified in fetal and neonatal lung from infants with pulmonary infections of an undetermined nature.[14] It is also seen in a condition termed *follicular bronchiolitis*,[15] which is associated with various autoimmune disorders, including Sjögren's syndrome. It is worth emphasizing that native MALT, in the form of bronchus-associated lymphoid tissue, is not present in normal lung. Likewise, lymphoid tissue is not present in normal stomach, the most common site of MALT lymphoma; here too, MALT is commonly acquired, almost always subsequent to infection with *H. pylori,* which precedes the development of most cases of gastric MALT lymphoma.[16] Other infectious organisms have been implicated as etiologic agents of MALT lymphoma (see later).

Certain common factors relating to the acquisition of MALT may be relevant to the development of lymphoma at these sites. In most instances, autoimmunity seems to play an important role in the underlying disease. MALT accumulates in relation to columnar epithelium and appears to receive antigenic stimuli either from the epithelium itself or, like physiologic MALT, from antigens that enter the lymphoid tissue across the epithelium, rather than from antigens carried in afferent lymphatics. The functional characteristics of this acquired MALT and the degree to which it resembles normal MALT have not been investigated. Likewise, the factors that, in a small number of cases, result in the transformation of reactive MALT into lymphoma that recapitulates many of its normal morphologic and functional properties remain speculative.

Box 18-1 *Localization of MALT Lymphoma*

- Gastrointestinal tract
  - Stomach
  - Intestine (including immunoproliferative small intestinal disease)
- Salivary glands
- Respiratory tract
  - Lung, pharynx, trachea
- Ocular adnexa
  - Conjunctiva, lacrimal gland, orbit*
- Skin
- Thyroid
- Liver
- Genitourinary tract
  - Bladder, prostate, kidney
- Breast
- Thymus
- Rare sites

*Not mucosal.

Infectious Agents

Helicobacter pylori and Gastric MALT Lymphoma

Several lines of evidence suggest that gastric MALT lymphoma arises from MALT acquired as a consequence of *H. pylori* infection. *H. pylori* can be demonstrated in the gastric mucosa of the majority of cases of gastric MALT lymphoma.[17] The first study in which this association was examined showed that the organism was present in more than 90% of cases. Subsequent studies have shown a lower incidence,[18] but also that the density and detectability of *H. pylori* decrease as lymphoma evolves from chronic gastritis.[19] A subsequent case-control study showed an association between previous *H. pylori* infection and the development of primary gastric lymphoma.[20] More compelling evidence confirming the role of *H. pylori* in the pathogenesis of gastric lymphoma has been obtained from studies that detected the lymphoma B-cell clone in the chronic gastritis that preceded the lymphoma,[19] as well as from a series of in vitro studies showing that lymphoma growth could be stimulated in culture by *H. pylori* strain-specific T cells when crude lymphoma cultures were exposed to the organism.[21] Finally, following the initial study by Wotherspoon and coworkers,[22] several groups have confirmed that

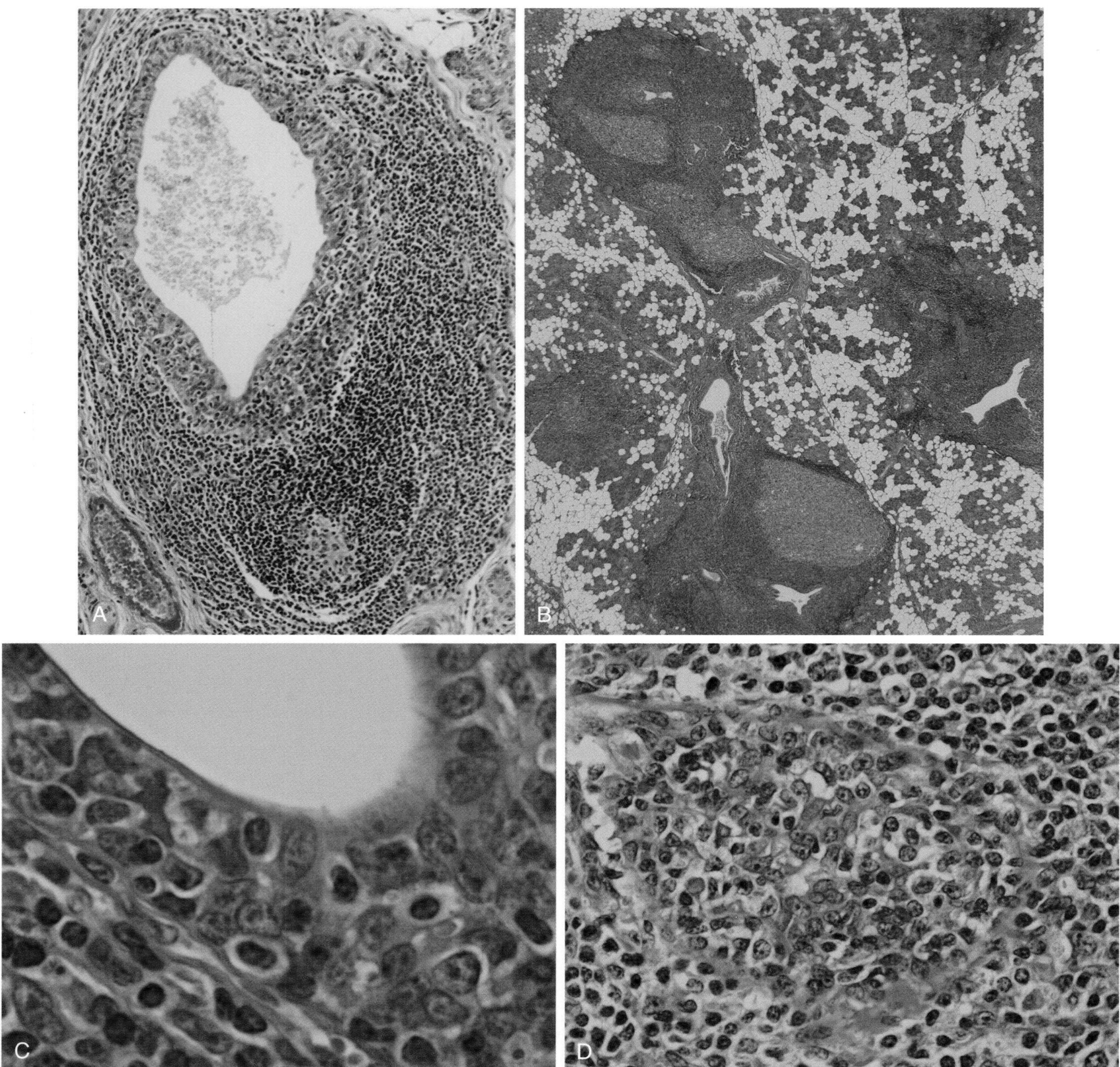

Figure 18-2. Lymphoepithelial sialadenitis (LESA)—acquired MALT. A, Peyer's patch–like lymphoid infiltrate in LESA. **B**, LESA of the parotid. Multiple Peyer's patch–like lymphoid infiltrates surround dilated ducts. **C**, High magnification of the lymphoepithelium in LESA. The lymphocytes have pale-staining cytoplasm and slightly irregularly shaped nuclei. **D**, Fully developed lymphoepithelial lesion in LESA.

eradication of *H. pylori* with antibiotics results in regression of gastric MALT lymphoma in 75% of cases (see later).[23]

Campylobacter jejuni and Immunoproliferative Small Intestinal Disease

Unlike gastric MALT lymphomas, relatively few cases of IPSID (which is rare, in any case) have definitively been shown to respond to broad-spectrum antibiotics.[24] Moreover, the presumptive organism linked to IPSID remains unknown. In 2004 Lecuit and associates,[25] based on a single case report, suggested that *Campylobacter jejuni* may play the same role in IPSID as *H. pylori* does in gastric MALT lymphoma. Isaacson and colleagues, in an unpublished polymerase chain reaction (PCR) study, confirmed an association between *C. jejuni* and IPSID but also detected the organism in other small intestinal lymphomas. To date, no laboratory study on the effects of *C. jejuni* on IPSID cells has been reported, and further studies on the effects of *C. jejuni* eradication are awaited.

Borrelia burgdorferi and Cutaneous MALT Lymphoma

In 1991 Garbe and colleagues[26] first described four cases of cutaneous lymphoma, later characterized as MALT lymphomas, associated with *Borrelia burgdorferi* infection. In 1997

Kutting and associates[27] reported clinical cures of two cases of cutaneous MALT lymphoma following eradication of *B. burgdorferi* using the antibiotic cefotaxime. Several additional reports have followed from Europe,[28] but similar success has not been reported from the United States.

Chlamydia psittaci and Ocular Adnexal MALT Lymphoma

A single case of an association between a chlamydial organism and a conjunctival MALT lymphoma was described by Yeung and coworkers[29] in 2004. Later that year Ferreri and colleagues,[30] in a PCR study, reported an association between *Chlamydia psittaci* and ocular adnexal MALT lymphoma in 80% of cases and went on to demonstrate the complete response of four cases following eradication of *C. psittaci* using doxycycline.[31] Similar studies by other groups have been largely negative, but Ferreri's group repeated its results in other cases (personal communication), interestingly, including cases in which they could not detect *C. psittaci*. They explain other groups' inability to repeat their results as being due to epidemiologic differences. This is supported by the large study of Chanudet and coworkers,[32] who investigated the presence of *C. psittaci* in 142 cases of ocular adnexal MALT lymphoma from six different countries. They found an overall prevalence of 22%, with the lowest prevalence in the United Kingdom (12%) and the highest in Germany (47%).

Establishing an Etiologic Link

To establish that a microorganism causes a particular disease, Koch's postulates should be fulfilled. Koch's postulates, slightly modified in relation to lymphoma in humans, can be summarized as follows:

1. The organism is demonstrable in every case (including histology and PCR).
2. The organism can be isolated and grown in pure culture.
3. The disease can be produced anew by infecting a healthy host.
4. The disease can be cured by eliminating the organism.

Clearly, only *H. pylori* satisfies these postulates to any significant extent with regard to gastric MALT lymphoma. Although *C. jejuni, B. burgdorferi* and *C. psittaci* are tempting targets, much more biologic and clinical research remains to be done before Koch's postulates are fulfilled.

HISTOPATHOLOGY OF ACQUIRED MALT

Tissues in which MALT lymphomas occur seem to mount a stereotypic response to certain known and unknown agents with the accumulation of lymphoid tissue that forms Peyer's patch–like structures. The two sites in which this is best illustrated are the salivary gland and the stomach.

Salivary Gland Acquired MALT (Lymphoepithelial Sialadenitis)

Apart from the intrasalivary gland lymph nodes, especially in the parotid, normal salivary glands contain no organized lymphoid tissue. Lymphoid tissue may accumulate in the salivary glands as a result of chronic inflammation of varying causes. Chronic inflammation following long-standing sialolithiasis is one example in which numerous lymphoid follicles may be present around dilated ducts that often contain a purulent exudate. This appearance is quite different from the chronic inflammation associated with established Sjögren's syndrome. In the earlier phase of this condition, isolated salivary ducts are dilated and surrounded by a lymphoid infiltrate that contains lymphoid follicles and recapitulates the structure of Peyer's patches (see Fig. 18-2B). Small, focal B-cell aggregates are characteristically seen in the duct epithelium, reminiscent of the dome epithelium of the Peyer's patch. These B cells are slightly larger than typical small lymphocytes of the mantle zone; they often have more abundant pale-staining cytoplasm and nuclei with an irregular outline (see Fig. 18-2C). The cytologic appearance and immunophenotype (see later) of these cells suggest that they are marginal zone B cells. Plasma cells are also present and tend to concentrate around the duct. As the disease progresses the ducts condense, with partial or complete loss of their lumens, and form lymphoepithelial lesions that consist of cohesive aggregates of duct epithelium containing variable numbers of marginal zone B lymphocytes (see Fig. 18-2D),[11,33] often associated with atrophy or, not infrequently, fatty replacement of acinar tissue. These Peyer's patch–like lesions may fuse to form larger islands of lymphoid tissue, and some of the lymphoepithelial islands may develop into cystic structures, resulting in a multicystic gland. Not all patients with this pattern of lymphoid infiltration in salivary glands are necessarily suffering from Sjögren's syndrome. Identical changes have been described in patients with a variety of other autoimmune diseases and sometimes in those with no evidence of an associated disorder.[34] Hence the generic terms *benign lymphoepithelial lesion* and *myoepithelial sialadenitis* are now more appropriately termed *lymphoepithelial sialadenitis.*[13] The histologic border between LESA and lymphoma is blurred, and it can be difficult to differentiate between them (see later). Whenever a diagnosis of LESA is made, the question of lymphoma remains open, to a certain extent.

Immunohistochemistry shows that the germinal centers are immunophenotypically identical to those in the Peyer's patches and lymph nodes. They are surrounded by $CD20^+$, IgM^+, IgD^+ mantle zone cells that express polytypic light chains (Fig. 18-3). The infiltrate of small lymphocytes present between the follicles is composed principally of $CD3^+$ T cells, which tend to concentrate around the B-cell follicles and are often accompanied by polytypic plasma cells. In some cases, large numbers of T cells are present and may even outnumber the B cells. Immunoglobulin gene rearrangement studies show a polyclonal B-cell population.

Helicobacter pylori Gastritis

Because of its ability to withstand a low pH, *H. pylori* is the one organism, apart from some other rare *Helicobacter* species, that can survive in the human gastric mucosa. The prevalence of *H. pylori* gastritis in any given population varies from 20% to 100%, depending on the locality and the age cohort. With some exceptions, the prevalence of gastric MALT lymphoma is related to that of *H. pylori* gastritis. Typically, infection results in active chronic inflammation with B-cell follicles and the formation of a lymphoepithelium by B-cell infiltration of glands immediately adjacent to the follicles (Fig. 18-4A)[35]—features of acquired MALT. Between the follicles the gastric

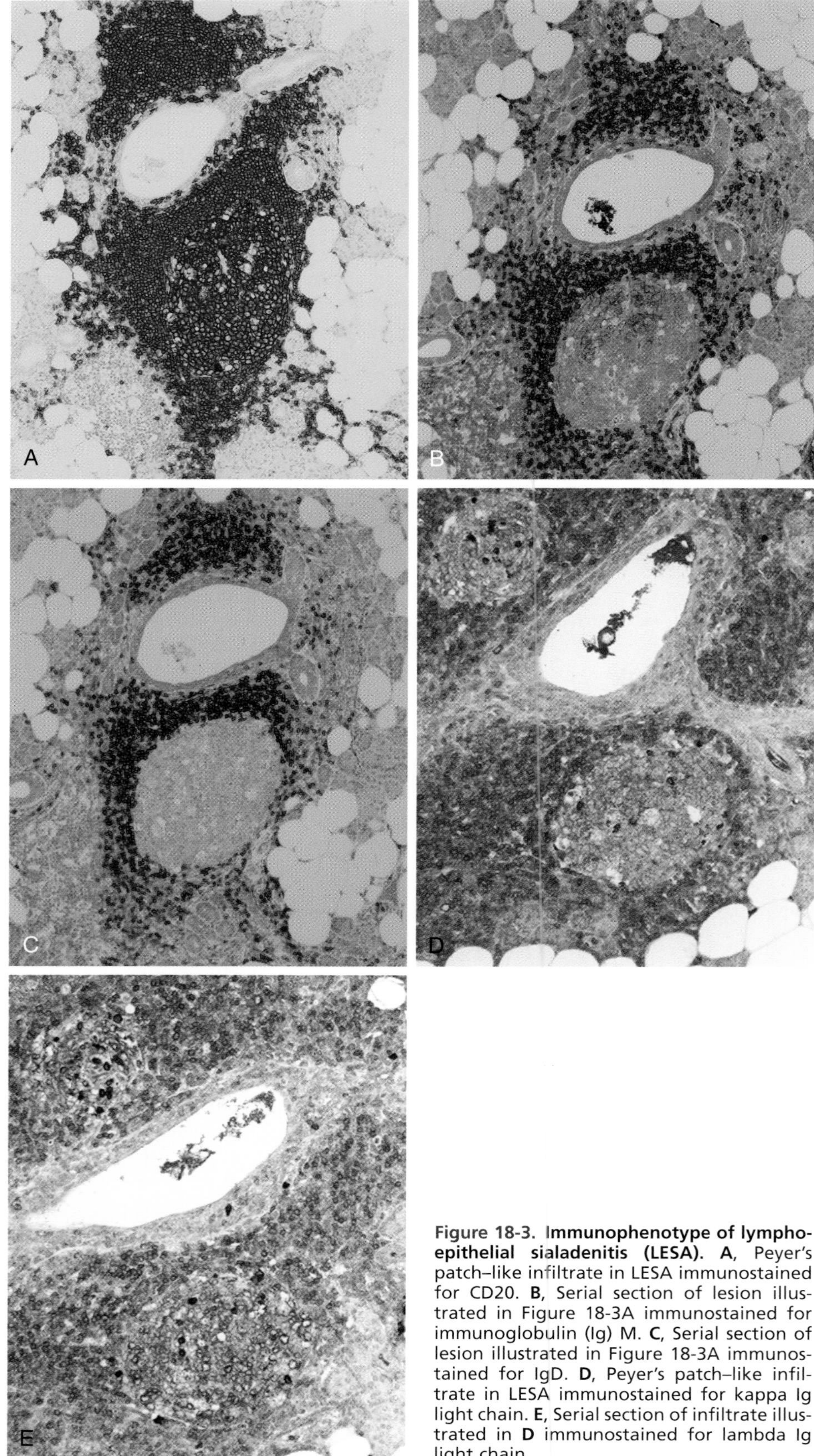

Figure 18-3. Immunophenotype of lymphoepithelial sialadenitis (LESA). A, Peyer's patch–like infiltrate in LESA immunostained for CD20. **B**, Serial section of lesion illustrated in Figure 18-3A immunostained for immunoglobulin (Ig) M. **C**, Serial section of lesion illustrated in Figure 18-3A immunostained for IgD. **D**, Peyer's patch–like infiltrate in LESA immunostained for kappa Ig light chain. **E**, Serial section of infiltrate illustrated in **D** immunostained for lambda Ig light chain.

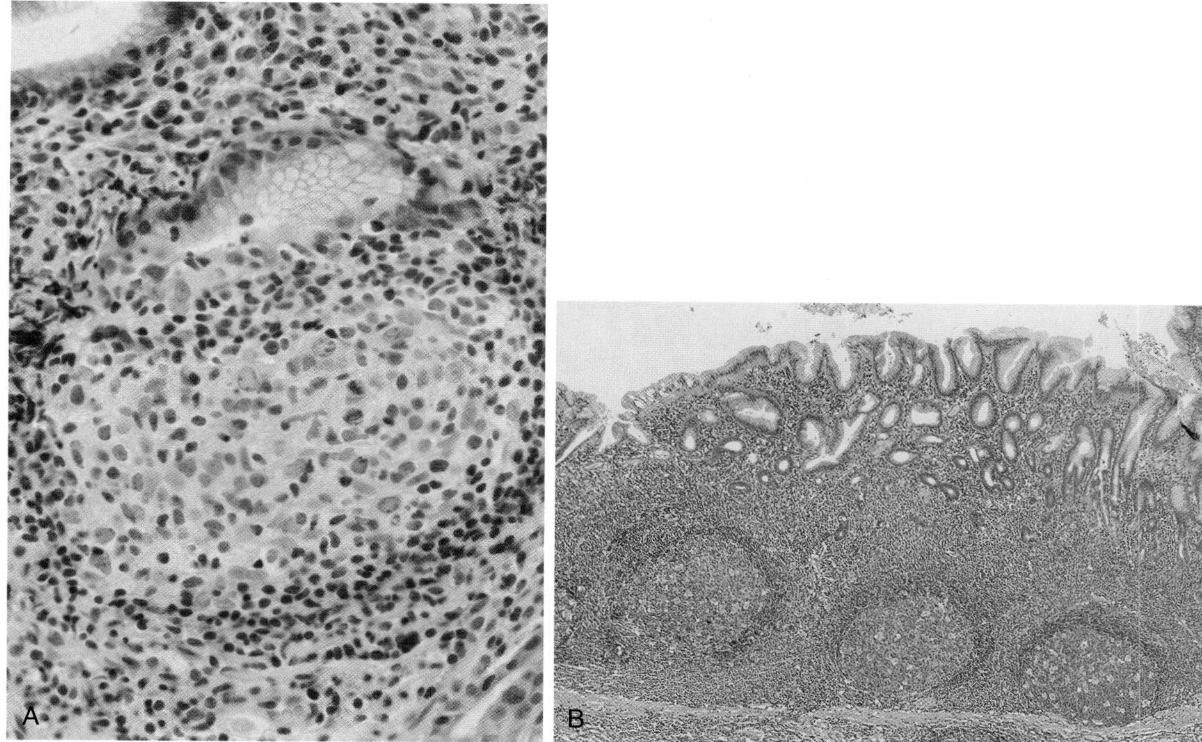

Figure 18-4. Architectural features in acquired and neoplastic MALT. A, Gastric acquired MALT in a case of *Helicobacter pylori* gastritis. Note the lymphoepithelium adjacent to the B-cell follicle. **B,** Gastric MALT lymphoma. The lymphoma infiltrates the lamina propria and the marginal zones around reactive follicles.

mucosa is infiltrated by T lymphocytes, plasma cells, macrophages, and occasional collections of neutrophils. The lymphoid infiltrate may be extremely florid and is sometimes difficult to distinguish from MALT lymphoma, especially when there are large, fused sheets of mantle zone cells in biopsy fragments.

Immunohistochemistry is useful in delineating the B-cell follicles and distinguishing the IgM^+, IgD^+ mantle zone cells from the IgM^+, IgD^- MALT lymphoma cells. Staining for immunoglobulin light chains can be useful in detecting monoclonal B cells and plasma cells in some cases of MALT lymphoma; however, the presence of polyclonal plasma cells does not exclude the diagnosis. PCR analysis normally reveals a polyclonal B-cell population in gastritis, but there are reports of spurious monoclonality detected in gastric biopsies from patients with *H. pylori* gastritis.[36] When the test is properly performed and interpreted, this is extremely uncommon,[37] but it is noteworthy that in patients with gastritis who later developed MALT lymphoma, the identical monoclonal B-cell population has been detected in both lesions.[19]

PATHOLOGY OF MALT LYMPHOMA

Macroscopic Appearance

Macroscopically, MALT lymphomas, although sometimes forming obviously tumorous masses, are frequently indistinguishable from the inflammatory lesions that underlie the acquisition of MALT from which the lymphoma arises. Gastric MALT lymphoma, for example, may form a single dominant mass but often results in only slightly raised congested mucosa, with superficial erosions indistinguishable at endoscopy from chronic gastritis. MALT lymphomas are typically multifocal, with small, even microscopic foci of lymphoma scattered throughout the organ involved. Each of these foci is clonally identical.[38]

Histopathology

Although there are some differences determined by the site of origin, the histology of MALT lymphoma is essentially stereotypic in that, like acquired MALT, the lymphoma recapitulates the histology of Peyer's patches, especially in the early stages of disease.[39] The neoplastic B lymphocytes infiltrate around reactive B-cell follicles, external to a preserved follicular mantle, in a marginal zone distribution; they spread out to form larger confluent areas that eventually overrun some or most of the follicles (see Fig. 18-4B). Like marginal zone B cells, the neoplastic cells have pale cytoplasm with small to medium-sized, slightly irregularly shaped nuclei containing moderately dispersed chromatin and inconspicuous nucleoli. These cells have been called *centrocyte-like* because of their resemblance to germinal center centrocytes. The accumulation of more abundant pale-staining cytoplasm may lead to a monocytoid appearance of the lymphoma cells; in some cases, the cells more closely resemble small lymphocytes (Fig. 18-5A to C). Scattered large cells resembling centroblasts or immunoblasts are usually present, but these are in the minority and do not form confluent clusters or sheets. Plasma cell differentiation is present in up to a third of cases (see Fig. 18-5D) and in gastric lymphomas tends to be maximal beneath the surface gastric epithelium.

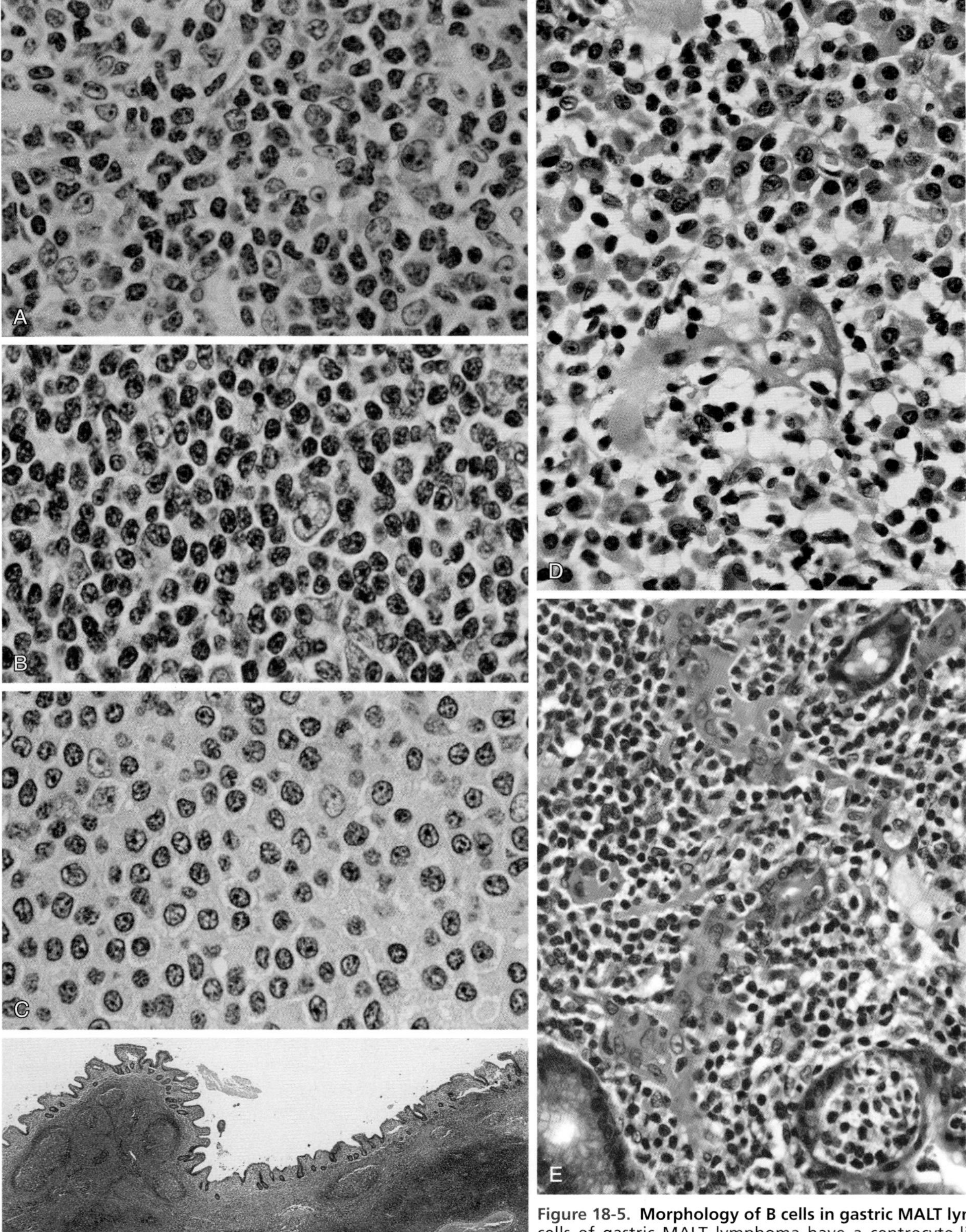

Figure 18-5. **Morphology of B cells in gastric MALT lymphoma. A**, The cells of gastric MALT lymphoma have a centrocyte-like appearance, with irregularly shaped nuclei. **B**, The tumor cells in this MALT lymphoma more closely resemble small lymphocytes. Note the presence of occasional transformed cells. **C**, The neoplastic cells in this MALT lymphoma have acquired more abundant pale-staining nuclei, leading to a monocytoid appearance. **D**, Plasma cell differentiation in a case of gastric MALT lymphoma. A lymphoepithelial lesion is present below. **E**, The tumor cells in this gastric MALT lymphoma form prominent lymphoepithelial lesions, with distortion and eosinophilic degeneration of gastric glandular epithelium. **F**, The neoplastic cells in this MALT lymphoma encircle reactive B-cell follicles (*upper left*) and have replaced follicles, leading to a nodular appearance below.

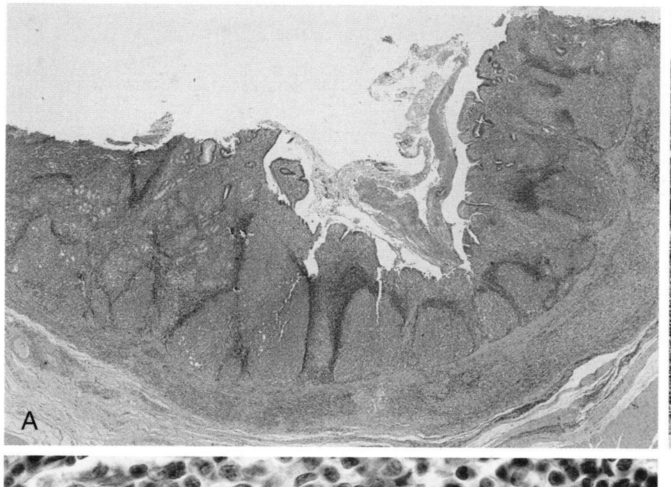

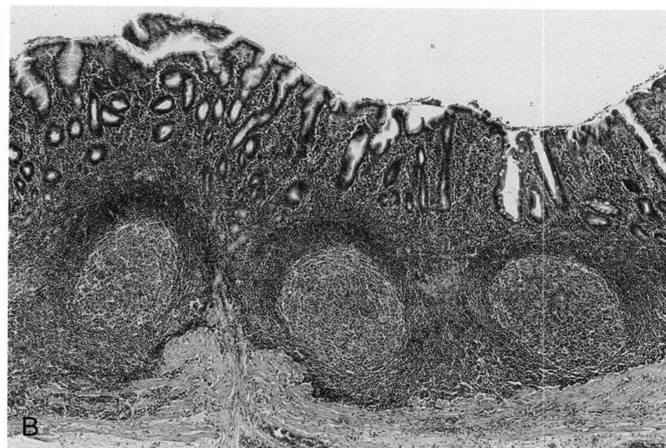

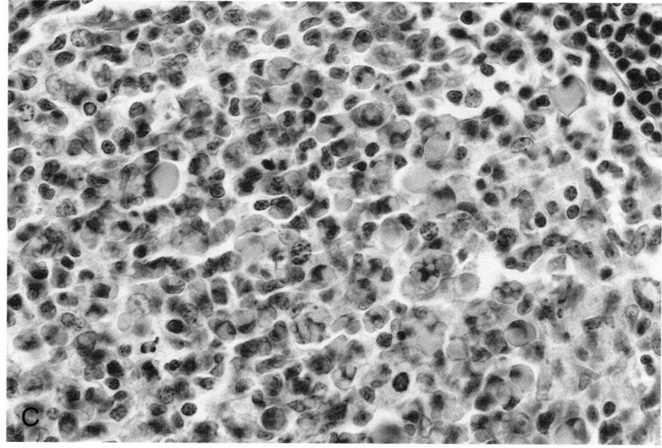

Figure 18-6. MALT lymphoma: relationship to B-cell follicles. A, The germinal centers of reactive B-cell follicles are colonized by transformed MALT lymphoma cells, resulting in an appearance simulating follicular lymphoma. **B,** The germinal centers of these reactive follicles are colonized by MALT lymphoma cells that have undergone plasmacytoid differentiation. **C,** Higher magnification of the germinal centers showing the cells stuffed with eosinophilic immunoglobulin.

Glandular epithelium is often invaded and destroyed by discrete aggregates of lymphoma cells, resulting in the so-called lymphoepithelial lesions (see Fig. 18-5D and E). These are defined as aggregates of three or more neoplastic marginal zone lymphocytes within glandular epithelium, preferably associated with distortion or necrosis of the epithelium. In gastric MALT lymphoma these lesions are often accompanied by eosinophilic degeneration of the epithelium. Lymphoepithelial lesions, although highly characteristic of MALT lymphoma, especially gastric lymphoma, are not pathognomonic. In some MALT lymphomas, such as those of the small and large intestine, they are difficult to find.

The lymphoma cells sometimes specifically colonize germinal centers of the reactive follicles (see Fig. 18-5F).[40] Usually this results in a vaguely nodular or follicular pattern. In some cases the lymphoma cells specifically target germinal centers, where they may undergo blast transformation (Fig. 18-6A) or plasma cell differentiation (see Fig. 18-6B and C). The presence of transformed blasts confined to preexisting germinal centers is not considered evidence of transformation to large B-cell lymphoma.

Like other low-grade B-cell lymphomas, MALT lymphoma may undergo transformation to diffuse large B-cell lymphoma.[41] Transformed centroblast- or immunoblast-like cells are present in variable numbers in MALT lymphoma (Fig. 18-7A), and there is some evidence that grading of MALT lymphoma according to the number of transformed cells has subtle clinical relevance.[42] However, only when solid or sheet-like proliferations of transformed cells are present should the lymphoma be considered to have transformed to diffuse large B-cell lymphoma (see Fig. 18-7B). This transformation may or may not result in complete overgrowth of the preceding MALT lymphoma. The current recommendation is that such cases are best designated diffuse large B-cell lymphoma; the presence or absence of concurrent MALT lymphoma and the relative proportions of both should be documented.[43]

Morphology of Gastric MALT Lymphoma Following Eradication of *Helicobacter pylori*

Approximately 75% of gastric MALT lymphomas respond to the eradication of *H. pylori*, with regression of the tumor over a period of up to 18 months.[22] Repeated endoscopy with biopsy is necessary to determine whether the lymphoma is responding (Fig. 18-8). The endoscopic appearance may revert within 6 months of the eradication of *H. pylori*, or it may take as long as 2 years. There is often a noticeable change in the histologic appearance of the biopsy within a few weeks, with gradual clearance of the lymphoma in the following months. Initially, the inflammatory infiltrate accompanying the lymphoma disappears, with an empty-appearing eosinophilic lamina propria that may contain lymphoid aggregates (Fig. 18-9). These aggregates are composed of small B

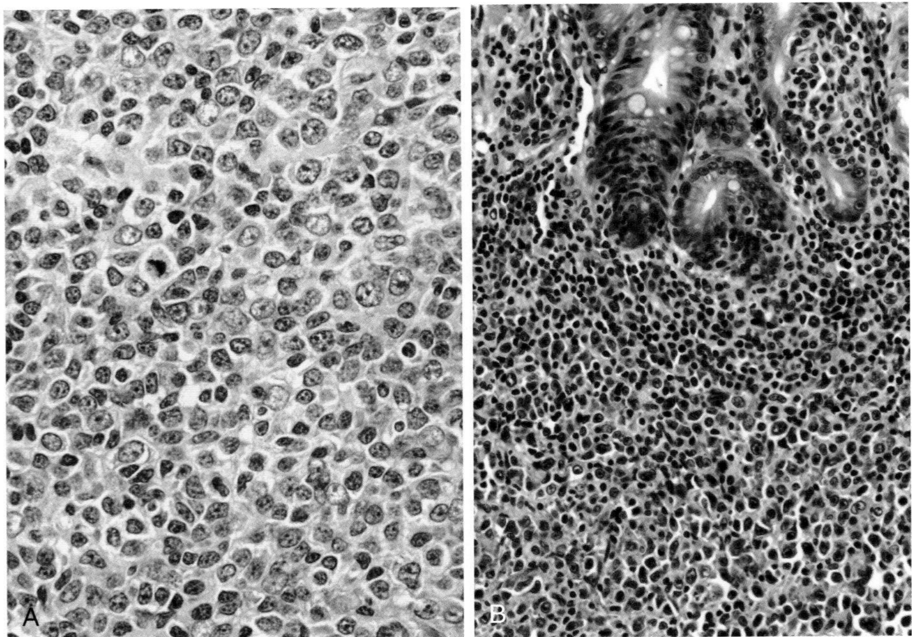

Figure 18-7. Transformation of MALT lymphoma. A, Although there are numerous transformed cells in this MALT lymphoma, they do not form confluent sheets; therefore, it is not considered to have transformed. **B,** Gastric MALT lymphoma (*above*) has transformed into diffuse large B-cell lymphoma (*below*).

lymphocytes without transformed blasts and gradually become smaller over time. Immunohistochemistry shows that they contain few accompanying T cells and have a markedly reduced proliferation fraction compared with the original lymphoma. Such aggregates may not disappear altogether and may persist for long periods at the base of the mucosa or in the submucosa. In up to 59% of cases, B-cell monoclonality can still be demonstrated using PCR,[44] suggesting that eradication of the bacteria has repressed but not eliminated the lymphoma clone, which is still represented in the lymphoid aggregates. The fate of these small aggregates is not completely known, but it is assumed that they eventually disappear. PCR analysis may reveal persistence of the neoplastic clone after the disappearance of morphologic evidence of lymphoma; however, the clinical significance of this finding is not clear. It is important not to make a diagnosis of persistent lymphoma based on molecular analysis alone in the absence of good histologic evidence.

Dissemination

The frequency and pattern of dissemination of MALT lymphoma vary with the site of disease. Thus, most gastric MALT lymphomas are at stage 1 when they present, between 4% and 17% have disseminated to regional lymph nodes, and approximately 10% have disseminated to the bone marrow at the time of diagnosis.[45] More than 90% of salivary gland MALT lymphomas present at stage 1, whereas 44% of pulmonary MALT lymphomas have disseminated to mediastinal lymph nodes at the time of diagnosis.[46] Approximately 20% of lymphomas of the ocular adnexa are beyond stage 1 at diagnosis.[47] In one study that grouped all MALT lymphomas together regardless of the site of origin, the disease had disseminated beyond the site of origin in 34% of cases.[48] MALT lymphomas tend to disseminate to other sites where MALT lymphomas occur. Gastric MALT lymphomas, for example, tend to disseminate to the small intestine, salivary gland, and lung.

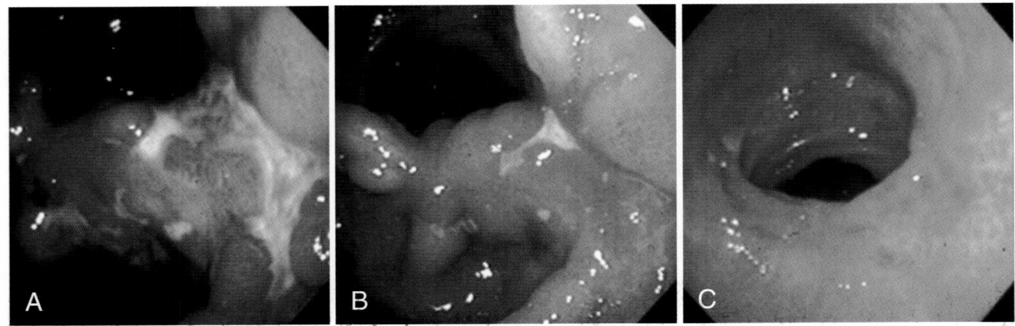

Figure 18-8. Serial endoscopic images of a gastric MALT lymphoma before (**A**), 2 weeks after (**B**), and 10 months after (**C**) eradication of *Helicobacter pylori* with antibiotics. The lymphoma has regressed completely after 10 months. (Courtesy of Dr. Naomi Uemara, Hiroshima, Japan.)

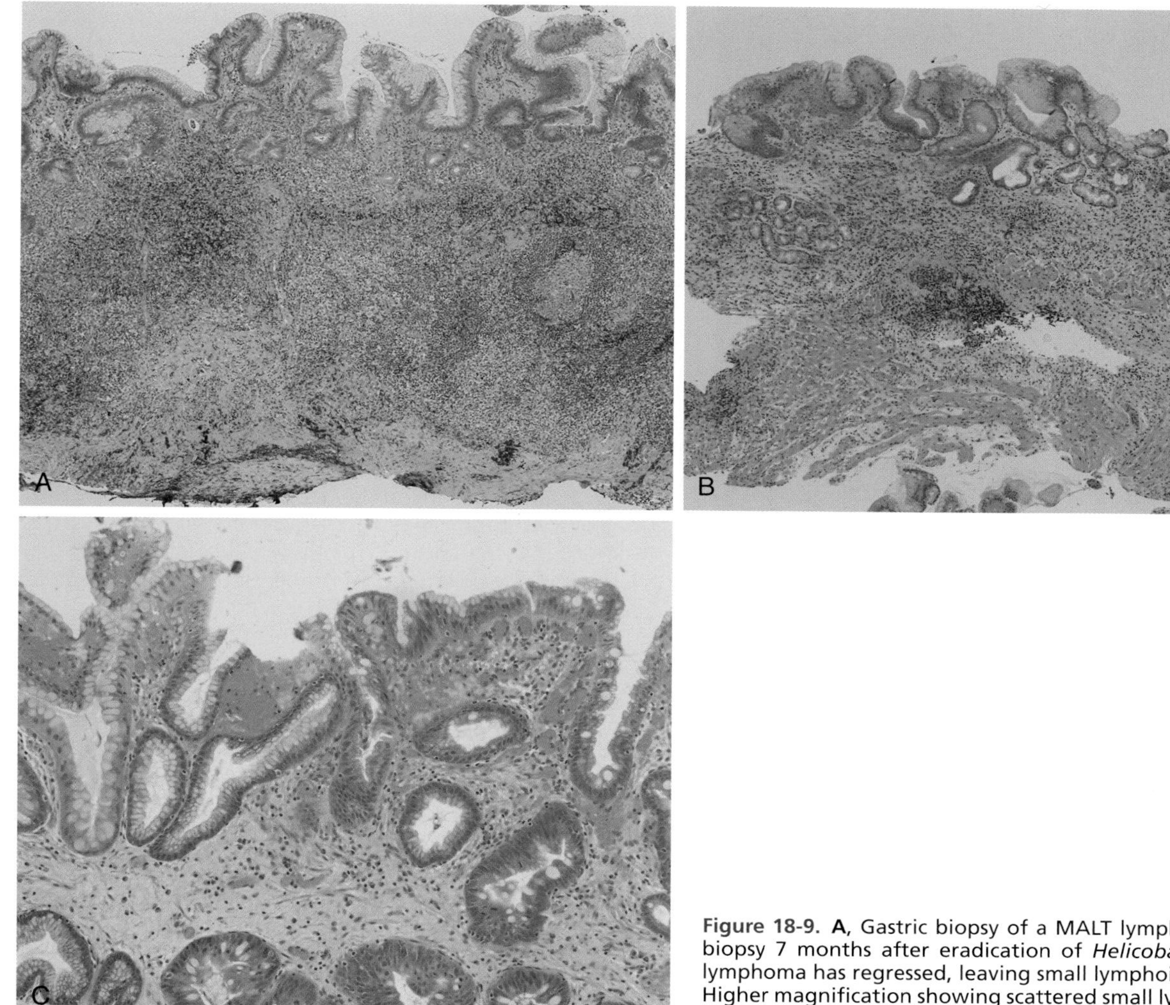

Figure 18-9. **A**, Gastric biopsy of a MALT lymphoma. **B**, Repeat biopsy 7 months after eradication of *Helicobacter pylori*. The lymphoma has regressed, leaving small lymphoid aggregates. **C**, Higher magnification showing scattered small lymphocytes in an empty-appearing lamina propria.

When MALT lymphomas disseminate to lymphoid tissue, including lymph nodes and spleen, they specifically invade the marginal zone (Fig. 18-10). This can lead to a deceptively benign or reactive appearance, especially in mesenteric lymph nodes, where a marginal zone is normally present. Immunohistochemistry for immunoglobulin light chains can be very helpful in discriminating normal marginal zone from disseminated MALT lymphoma. Subsequently, the lymphoma in the marginal zones expands to form more obvious sheets of interfollicular lymphoma. Occasionally, follicular colonization in involved lymph nodes can lead to an appearance that simulates follicular lymphoma (Fig. 18-11).

IMMUNOHISTOCHEMISTRY

The immunophenotype of MALT lymphoma essentially recapitulates that of marginal zone cells. The B cells are CD20, CD79a, CD21, and CD35 positive and CD5, CD23, and CD10 negative. CD43, indicative of a neoplastic phenotype, is expressed in approximately 50% of cases, and expression of CD11c is variable. The tumor cells typically express IgM, less often express IgA or IgG, are IgD^-, and show immunoglobulin light-chain restriction. A significant intratumoral population of $CD3^+$, predominantly $CD4^+$ T cells is characteristic. Expanded meshworks of follicular dendritic cells are typically detected with antibodies CD21 and CD23, corresponding to follicles that are colonized or overrun by the lymphoma cells. Variable numbers of $BCL6^+$, $CD10^+$ follicle center cells may be seen in these areas, whereas the neoplastic cells are negative for these antigens.

GENETIC FEATURES OF MALT LYMPHOMA

Antigen Receptor Genes

In the B cells of MALT lymphoma, immunoglobulin heavy- and light-chain genes are rearranged and show somatic mutation of their variable regions, consistent with a post–germinal center memory B-cell derivation.[49] Ongoing mutations are thought to occur in most cases.[50] Because of the difficulty in distinguishing between acquired MALT and MALT lymphoma, particularly in small biopsy specimens (see later), there has been a tendency to rely on molecular evidence of monoclonality detected by PCR for the diagnosis of lymphoma. This technique may fail to detect monoclonality in

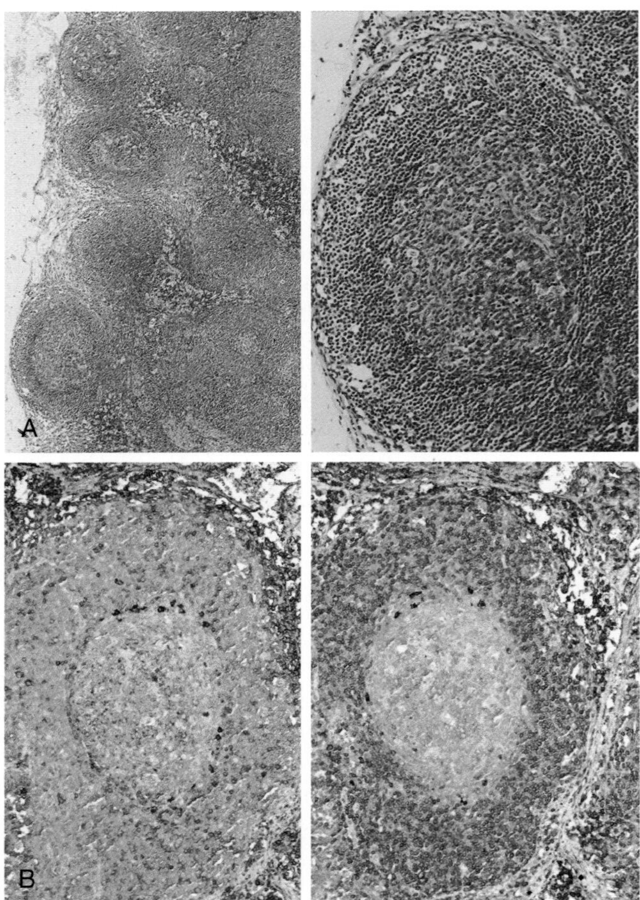

Figure 18-10. **A**, Gastric lymph node from a case of MALT lymphoma showing prominent marginal zones (*left*). Higher magnification of a single follicle (*right*). **B**, Immunostaining of a single follicle for kappa (*left*) and lambda (*right*) immunoglobulin light chain; the marginal zone lymphocytes show lambda light-chain restriction, indicative of involvement by lymphoma.

up to 15% of cases of overt lymphoma and thus produce false-negative results.[51] There are also reports of apparently spurious monoclonality in biopsies of acquired MALT, such as gastric biopsies showing only chronic gastritis, with no histologic evidence of malignancy.[36,52,53] The frequency of this spurious monoclonality varies among laboratories,[37] which suggests that technique may be a factor. These findings emphasize that MALT lymphoma should not be diagnosed in the absence of clear histologic evidence (Table 18-1). This point is underlined by the frequent finding of persistent monoclonality in small, residual, clinically insignificant lymphoid aggregates that persist following the eradication of *H. pylori* for the treatment of MALT lymphoma.

Genetic Abnormalities

A number of genetic abnormalities have been described in MALT lymphoma, including trisomies 3, 12, and 18 and the specific chromosomal translocations t(11;18)(q21;q21), t(1;14)(p22;q32), and t(14;18)(q32;q21) (Table 18-2).

The translocation t(11;18) involves the *API2* and *MALT1* genes and generates a functional API2-MALT1 fusion product.[54-56] The others, t(1;14) and t(14;18), juxtapose the *BCL10* and *MALT1* genes, respectively, to the immunoglobulin gene locus in 14q32, leading to deregulated expression of the oncogene.[57-60] The oncogenic activities of the three chromosome translocations are linked by the physiologic role of BCL10 and MALT1 in antigen receptor–mediated nuclear factor-κB (NF-κB) activation.[61] The incidences of the three chromosomal translocations are markedly variable in MALT lymphomas of different sites,[62,63] but they are always mutually exclusive.[61] Among the three translocations, t(11;18) is the most frequent, occurring most often in MALT lymphomas from the lung (40%) and stomach (30%), at a moderate rate in those from the ocular adnexa (15%), and rarely in those from the salivary gland, thyroid, and skin.[64-66]

There is growing evidence that t(11;18)-positive cases are distinct from other MALT lymphomas, including those with t(1;14) or t(14;18). Cases of t(11;18)-positive MALT lymphoma rarely undergo high-grade transformation,[67,68] even though the translocation is significantly associated with advanced-stage disease and lack of response to *H. pylori* eradication.[69,70] Cytogenetically, t(11;18)-positive tumors usually

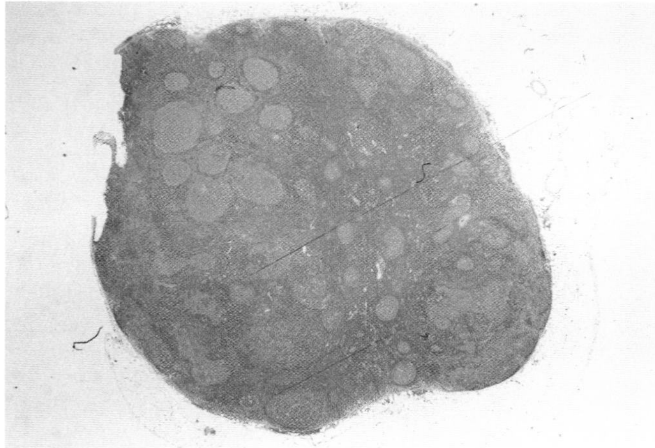

Figure 18-11. Lymph node involved by disseminated gastric MALT lymphoma with follicular colonization.

Table 18-1 Use of Histology Score to Differentiate Gastric MALT Lymphoma from Chronic Gastritis

Score	Interpretation	Histology
0	Normal	Occasional plasma cells
1	Chronic active gastritis	Lymphocyte clusters, no follicles
2	Follicular gastritis	Prominent follicles, no lymphoepithelial lesions
3	Suspicious, probably reactive	Follicles, occasional adjacent lymphoepithelial lesions, no diffuse infiltrate
4	Suspicious, probably lymphoma	Follicles, diffuse marginal zone cell infiltrate, no lymphoepithelial lesions
5	MALT lymphoma	Follicles, diffuse marginal zone cell infiltrate, lymphoepithelial lesions present

Table 18-2 Frequency (%) of Cytogenetic Alterations in MALT Lymphomas at Different Sites

Site	t(11;18)(q21;q21)	t(14;18)(p14;q32)	t(3;14)(p22;q32)	t(1;14)(p22;q32)	+3	+18
Stomach	6-26	0	0	0-5	11	6
Intestine	12-56	0	0	0-13	75	25
Ocular adnexa	0-10	0-25	0-20	0	38	13
Salivary glands	0-5	0-16	0	0-2	55	19
Lung	31-53	6-10	0	2-7	20	7
Skin	0-8	0-14	0-10	0	20	4
Thyroid	0-17	0	0-50	0	17	4

do not show other chromosomal aberrations, such as trisomies 3 and 18, which are frequently seen in t(11;18)-negative tumors, including those positive for t(1;14) and t(14;18).[71] Furthermore, t(11;18) MALT lymphomas do not exhibit microsatellite alterations and show markedly fewer chromosomal gains and losses than do translocation-negative tumors.[70]

A fourth translocation, t(3;14)(p14;q32) involving *IGH* and *FOXP1,* has recently been described in MALT lymphomas of the thyroid, ocular adnexa, and skin.[72] It is uncertain whether this translocation, like those described earlier, also affects the NF-κB pathway.

The t(11;18) can be detected in paraffin-embedded tissue by reverse transcription PCR; fluorescence in situ hybridization (FISH) is useful for demonstrating all four characteristic translocations. In cases positive for t(11;18), as well as 20% of translocation-negative cases, BCL10 protein is upregulated in the nucleus, where it stains weakly. In the much rarer t(1;14) cases, nuclear BCL10 is expressed intensely in both the nucleus and the cytoplasm. The significance of these findings is unknown.

POSTULATED CELL OF ORIGIN

The architectural features of MALT lymphoma, particularly early cases, show quite clearly that the neoplastic cells are infiltrating the marginal zone around B-cell follicles. In non-neoplastic lymphoid tissue a prominent marginal zone is present in the spleen, Peyer's patches, and mesenteric lymph nodes. This allows a comparison of the cytology and immunophenotype of normal marginal zone cells with those of MALT lymphoma (Fig. 18-12). Cytologically, MALT lymphoma cells bear a close resemblance to marginal zone cells. Both are slightly larger than small lymphocytes and have a slightly irregular nuclear outline and moderate amounts of pale-staining cytoplasm. Interestingly, in both Peyer's patches and LESA, collections of marginal zone cells are found within the dome and ductal epithelium, respectively. The immunophenotypes of cells of the marginal zone and MALT lymphoma are virtually identical, with both expressing CD20 and other pan–B-cell antigens, CD21, CD35, and IgM but not IgD.

CLINICAL COURSE

MALT lymphomas are among the most indolent of all lymphomas and have a good prognosis, regardless of stage. Five- and 10-year overall survival rates exceeding 80% are the rule, although progression-free survival may be somewhat lower.[48] Transformation to diffuse large B-cell lymphoma results in a significantly lower survival of approximately 50% at 5 years.[73]

Preferred treatment modalities differ according to the site of origin and vary from "watch and wait" for most salivary gland MALT lymphomas to radiotherapy or chemotherapy for those arising elsewhere.

The treatment of gastric MALT lymphoma has attracted considerable attention since the initial published report that the lymphoma may regress following eradication of *H. pylori* with antibiotics. The follow-up of MALT lymphoma patients following eradication of *H. pylori* is rather complex, requiring repeated gastroscopy with biopsy. In addition, it would be extremely useful to be able to identify the approximately 25% of cases of gastric MALT lymphoma that do not respond to

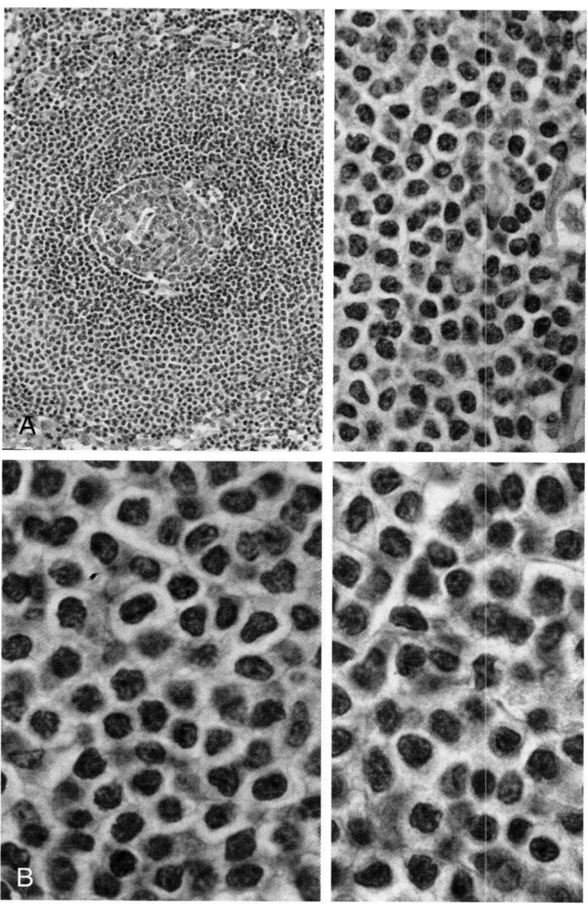

Figure 18-12. A, Reactive mesenteric lymph node with a prominent marginal zone (*left*) and illustrated at higher magnification (*right*). **B,** Marginal zone cells from the mesenteric lymph node (*left*) compared with the cells of a gastric MALT lymphoma (*right*).

eradication of *H. pylori*. Studies using endoscopic ultrasonography suggest that if the tumor has invaded beyond the submucosa, it is less likely to respond.[74,75] Likewise, cases that have transformed to large B-cell lymphoma are unlikely to respond, although there are reports of complete regression in such cases.[76,77]

More recently, following the cloning of t(1;14) and t(11;18) breakpoints, these translocations were shown to have a bearing on response to *H. pylori* eradication. Present in up to 40% of cases, t(11;18)(q21;q21) is strongly associated with failure to respond to eradication of *H. pylori*. Interestingly, both t(1;14) and t(11;18) are associated with nuclear expression of BCL10 protein, which is particularly intense in t(1;14)-positive cases. Moreover, the frequency of both t(11;18)(q21;q21) and nuclear BCL10 expression is significantly higher in tumors that have invaded or disseminated beyond the stomach (78% and 93%, respectively) than in those confined to the stomach (10% and 38%).[78] These findings partly explain the results based on endoscopic ultrasonography and suggest that both t(11;18)(q21;q21) and BCL10 nuclear expression are associated with failure to respond to *H. pylori* eradication and with more advanced stages of MALT lymphoma. Therefore, before embarking on *H. pylori* eradication as definitive therapy, the pertinent genotypic investigations should be carried out.

DIFFERENTIAL DIAGNOSIS

Reactive versus Neoplastic MALT

The distinction between acquired MALT, the precursor of MALT lymphoma, and MALT lymphoma in the early stages of evolution often gives rise to diagnostic difficulty. This is particularly true of gastric and salivary gland MALT lymphoma. Gastric MALT acquired as a consequence of *H. pylori* infection comprises reactive B-cell follicles without an identifiable marginal zone. The lamina propria around the follicles is infiltrated by a mixture of inflammatory cells, including plasma cells and T lymphocytes. A lymphoepithelium can be seen adjacent to the follicles (see Fig. 18-4A) and can mimic the lymphoepithelial lesion characteristic of MALT lymphoma (Fig. 18-13). In the presence of these intraepithelial B cells immediately adjacent to follicles, the absence of a diffuse infiltrate of IgM^+ B lymphocytes external to the IgD^+, IgM^+ mantle zone cells is very helpful in distinguishing such cases from MALT lymphom. In both Sjögren's syndrome and LESA, Peyer's patch–like lymphoid infiltrates are present in the salivary gland, usually the parotid. Here too, the ductal epithelium is infiltrated by B cells (see Fig. 18-2A to C). The earliest sign of lymphoma is an extension of the intraepithelial B cells around the duct, the lumen of which is often partly obliterated by epithelial cells, to form halo-like infiltrates around the duct (Fig. 18-14).[79] The cells constituting the halos are IgM^+ and show immunoglobulin light-chain restriction.

In the distinction between acquired MALT and MALT lymphoma, demonstration of clonality by virtue of light-chain restriction, either by immunohistochemistry (frozen or paraffin sections) or by flow cytometry, can be diagnostic. Coexpression of CD43 by B cells is a useful hint that the B-cell population is neoplastic. Use of PCR of immunoglobulin heavy-chain genes to discriminate reactive lymphoid infiltrates from MALT lymphoma is controversial, but there is no doubt that, properly performed, a positive PCR result is strong evidence of lymphoma.

MALT versus Other Small B-Cell Lymphomas

Because of differences in clinical behavior and management, it is important to differentiate MALT lymphoma from the other small B-cell lymphomas that may present in or involve extranodal sites (Table 18-3). These include mantle cell lymphoma, lymphocytic lymphoma (chronic lymphocytic leukemia), and follicular lymphoma. The need to distinguish between MALT lymphoma and lymphoplasmacytic lymphoma involving extranodal sites can also arise.

The cytologic features of mantle cell lymphoma can closely simulate those of MALT lymphoma, to the extent that occasional lymphoepithelial lesions may be present. However, the absence of transformed blasts together with expression of CD5, IgD, and, importantly, intranuclear expression of cyclin D1, a consequence of t(11;14), can distinguish mantle cell lymphoma. Small lymphocytic lymphoma (chronic lymphocytic leukemia) is characterized by small, round lymphocytes, usually with peripheral blood lymphocytosis and often with

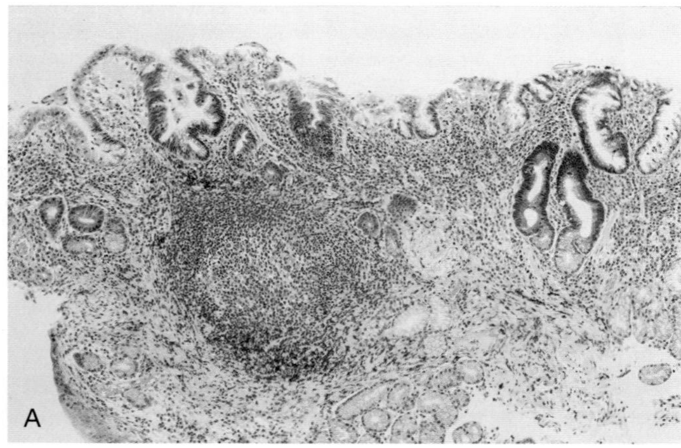

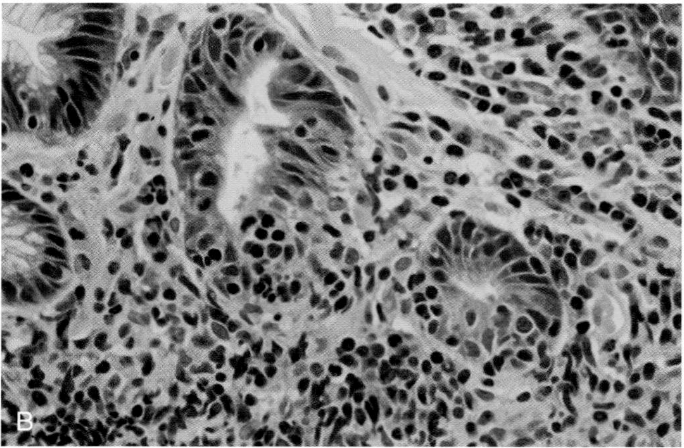

Figure 18-13. A, *Helicobacter pylori* gastritis with a prominent follicle adjacent to gastric glands. **B,** High magnification of gastric glands adjacent to the follicle shows infiltration of glandular epithelium by small lymphocytes, mimicking a lymphoepithelial lesion.

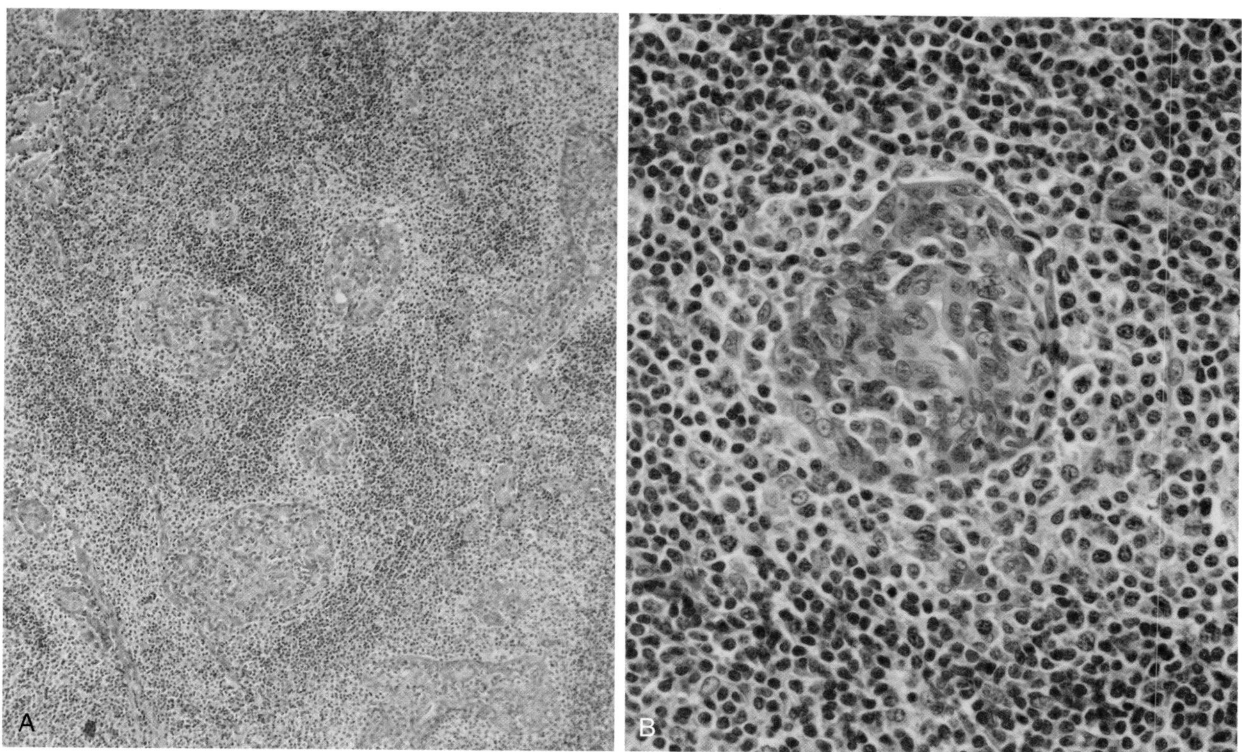

Figure 18-14. Early MALT lymphoma of the parotid gland evolving from lymphoepithelial sialadenitis. A, Lymphoma cells form "halos" around lymphoepithelial lesions. **B**, High magnification of the lymphoma cells constituting the halos.

Table 18-3 Differential Diagnosis of MALT Lymphoma and Other Lymphomas

	MALT	Mantle Cell	Follicular	CLL
Follicles	+	+	+	±
LELs	+	±	±	±
Cytology	CCL	CCL	CC	Occasional CCL
Ig	M^+, D^-	M^+, D^+	$M^\pm$, $D^\pm$	M^+, D^+
CD20	+	+	+	+
CD5	–	+	–	+
CD10	–	–	+	–
Cyclin D1	–	+	–	–

CC, centrocyte; CCL, centrocyte-like; CLL, chronic lymphocytic leukemia; Ig, immunoglobulin; LEL, lymphoepithelial lesion.

pseudofollicles, although these may be difficult to appreciate in extranodal sites. Expression of CD5, CD23, and IgD without nuclear cyclin D1 provides further distinction from MALT lymphoma. Finally, follicular lymphoma, which may arise extranodally, can be difficult to distinguish from MALT lymphoma with follicular colonization. The transformed MALT lymphoma cells within follicles may closely resemble centroblasts but are typically negative for CD10 and BCL6 (nuclear), in contrast to the cells of follicular lymphoma, which usually express both antigens both within and between follicles. Assessment of these antigens, together with stains for follicular dendritic cells such as CD21 or CD23, is useful. Cytogenetic and molecular genetic analysis to detect t(11;18) and t(14;18) or *BCL2* rearrangement is also helpful. Finally, MALT lymphoma with plasmacytic differentiation can be distinguished from lymphoplasmacytic lymphoma if the characteristic architecture is identified and marginal zone B cells are present; in cases lacking such features, the clinical picture—evidence of bone marrow involvement or a paraprotein—may be helpful.

Pearls and Pitfalls

- MALT lymphomas occur in acquired MALT and generally not in preexisting lymphoid tissue.
- Antigen drive plays a key role in most MALT lymphomas, although in some cases the initiating antigen has not been identified.
- PCR studies for *IGH@* rearrangement are generally useful for the distinction of reactive hyperplasia from MALT lymphoma; however, both false-positives and false-negatives may occur.
- Demonstration of light-chain restriction in a MALT lesion is useful in the distinction of acquired MALT and MALT lymphoma; CD43 coexpression is somewhat less sensitive.
- Gastric MALT lymphomas with (t[1;14] or t[11;18]) fail to respond to antibiotics as the sole therapeutic modality.
- MALT lymphomas may disseminate late to lymph nodes, and in many cases the distinction between primary and secondary marginal zone lymphomas in lymph nodes is difficult. A careful clinical history is key.

References can be found on Expert Consult @ www.expertconsult.com

Chapter 19

Primary Cutaneous B-Cell Lymphoma

Lyn McDivitt Duncan

CHAPTER OUTLINE

Cutaneous B-cell lymphomas account for approximately 25% of cutaneous lymphomas, with the remainder being of T-cell origin. Cutaneous B-cell lymphomas are generally less aggressive than their nodal counterparts, with 5-year disease-specific survivals of nearly 100% for primary cutaneous follicle center lymphoma (PCFCL) and cutaneous extranodal marginal zone B-cell lymphoma. The 5-year survival for diffuse large B-cell lymphoma (DLBCL) approaches 50%. These three primary cutaneous B-cell lymphomas account for more than 90% of the B-cell lymphomas involving the skin. This chapter focuses on the primary cutaneous B-cell lymphomas that arise in the skin without evidence of extracutaneous disease at presentation (Box 19-1). The prior requirement that the patient exhibit no evidence of extracutaneous disease for 6 months has been removed because, in practical terms, a diagnosis is best determined at the time of presentation.[1] Secondary involvement by a variety of B-cell lymphomas may occur, and the more common manifestations of secondary involvement are discussed briefly.

Although some primary cutaneous B-cell lymphomas show morphologic and even immunophenotypic overlap with B-cell lymphomas arising in lymph nodes, significant differences in clinical presentation and outcome initially justified their separation.[2] Subsequent studies have provided additional evidence supporting the recognition of some primary cutaneous B-cell lymphomas as distinct entities. The case is most strongly made for PCFCL, which lacks the characteristic *BCL2/IGH@* translocation of nodal follicular lymphoma. In contrast, although primary cutaneous marginal zone lymphoma (PCMZL) has some distinctive clinical features, it overlaps with other extranodal marginal zone lymphomas of mucosa-associated lymphoid tissue (MALT) in terms of its phenotype and genotype. Similarly, primary cutaneous large B-cell lymphoma (PCLBCL)–leg type shares many immunophenotypic and genomic features with the activated B-cell (ABC) type of DLBCL.

Not surprisingly, these distinctions have led to controversy over whether there should be independent classification systems for cutaneous lymphomas.[2] On the one hand, it is important that all specialists dealing with the diagnosis and treatment of lymphomas speak the same language; different terms should not be used for the same disease entity in different anatomic sites.[3] On the other hand, the unique clinical behavior of many cutaneous lymphomas needs to be recognized in order to provide appropriate clinical management.[2,4] Fortunately, there has been a meeting of the minds with the publication of the World Health Organization–European Organization for Research and Treatment of Cancer (WHO-EORTC) classification of cutaneous lymphomas.[1,5] This consensus provides a unified approach to the diagnosis, classification, and management of cutaneous lymphomas.

CLINICAL FEATURES AND CLINICAL PRESENTATION

Although primary cutaneous T-cell lymphomas have distinctive clinical presentations, most primary cutaneous B-cell lymphomas are relatively similar to one another (Table

Box 19-1 *B-Cell Lymphomas That Commonly Present in the Skin*

- Primary cutaneous extranodal marginal zone lymphoma of mucosa-associated lymphoid tissue (MALT lymphoma)
- Primary cutaneous follicle center lymphoma
- Primary cutaneous large B-cell lymphoma–leg type
- Primary cutaneous large B-cell lymphoma–other
  - T-cell–rich large B-cell lymphoma
  - Intravascular large B-cell lymphoma
- Plasmacytoma (see Chapter 25)
- Plasmablastic lymphoma (see Chapter 22)
- B-lymphoblastic leukemia/lymphoma (see Chapter 41)

19-1).[1,6] Cutaneous B-cell lymphomas rarely ulcerate and usually present as one or more erythematous papules or nodules that may coalesce to form plaques. The various subtypes of tumors show some regional predilection: PCFCL more commonly arises on the scalp or upper back, PCMZL usually occurs on the extremities, and the more aggressive PCLBCL–leg type usually arises on the lower leg.

EPIDEMIOLOGY

Primary cutaneous B-cell lymphomas are primarily tumors of adults, although PCMZL may also be seen in the pediatric age group (see later). In contrast to cutaneous T-cell lymphomas, which are relatively more common in blacks, cutaneous B-cell lymphomas show the highest incidence rate in non-Hispanic whites.[7] For most subtypes, the incidence rates in blacks are half those in non-Hispanic whites. Primary cutaneous B-cell lymphomas are relatively uncommon in Asian countries; in the United States, a decreased incidence was shown among Pacific Islanders and Hispanic whites.[7,8] Notably, the low incidence of cutaneous B-cell lymphomas overall in Pacific Islanders did not translate into a low incidence of aggressive B-cell lymphomas, including DLBCL.[7] These findings suggest differences in pathogenesis among the various subtypes of cutaneous B-cell lymphoma.

Table 19-1 General Principles in the Diagnosis and Management of Primary Cutaneous Lymphomas

	T-Cell Neoplasms	B-Cell Neoplasms
Clinical	Distinctive clinical manifestations often contribute to diagnosis	Similarity in clinical appearance among subtypes Site more helpful than appearance of lesion
Histologic	Epidermotropism often present Grenz zone usually absent Usually diffuse and/or perivascular	Epidermotropism absent Minimal epidermal changes Grenz zone present More commonly nodular
Immunophenotype	Immunophenotype important in disease definition	Immunophenotype contributes to disease definition
Gene rearrangements	*TCR* rearrangement detectable in most tumors False-positives may occur	Immunoglobulin gene rearrangement detected in only 50% of cutaneous B-cell lymphomas False-positives exceedingly rare
Treatment	Treatment dependent on tumor type and stage	Treatment dependent on subtype and number of lesions

HISTOPATHOLOGY

Malignancies of T lymphocytes frequently show epidermotropism, in contrast to B-cell lymphomas, in which the tumor cells spare the epidermis and are usually separated from it by a grenz zone.

IMMUNOPHENOTYPE

Some observers have proposed that cutaneous lymphomas develop in the setting of a persistent inflammatory reaction or immune dysregulation.[9-11] This hypothesis has been applied to T-cell proliferations in the setting of connective tissue disease, chronic actinic dermatitis (actinic reticuloid), and lymphomatoid drug eruptions; it has also been used to explain the development of cutaneous B-cell lymphomas in the setting of *Borrelia* infection and tattoos.[12,13] As with T-cell lymphomas, an aberrant B-cell immunophenotype supports the diagnosis of lymphoma, as may be seen in light-chain restriction or coexpression of CD43 and CD20. Because the responder cell in cutaneous inflammatory processes is usually a T cell, most nonneoplastic cutaneous infiltrates are composed almost exclusively of T cells. Thus, when B cells constitute greater than 75% of the dermal infiltrate, a diagnosis of cutaneous B-cell lymphoma is favored.[14] However, dense reactive T-cell infiltrates are frequently present in cutaneous lymphoma; in some cases of B-cell lymphoma, the neoplastic B cells may represent only a minor component of the dermal lymphocytic infiltrate.

GENE REARRANGEMENT

The Southern blot method of detecting immunoglobulin gene rearrangements may yield negative results if the tumor cells represent less than 5% of the sample.[15] Even techniques based on polymerase chain reaction (PCR) are reported to be positive in only 50% of cutaneous B-cell lymphomas. As with any diagnostic tool, genetic results should be interpreted in the context of the clinical, histologic, and immunophenotypic findings of the case.[13,16-18]

TREATMENT AND PROGNOSIS

Most cutaneous B-cell lymphomas have a similar treatment algorithm. Patients with solitary or localized tumors are usually treated with excision or radiation therapy, or both; solitary low-grade tumors may also be treated with injection of high-dose steroids, intralesional interferon-α, or rituximab. Patients with multifocal or disseminated cutaneous lymphoma may be treated with chemotherapy; single-agent chemotherapy is given to patients with more indolent tumors, and multiagent chemotherapy is occasionally administered to those with biologically aggressive lymphomas.[19,20] In general, cutaneous lymphomas are more indolent than their nodal counterparts. PCMZL and PCFCL usually remain localized to the skin and are often cured by local therapy.[21,22] PCLBCL–leg type is more often associated with eventual extracutaneous lymphoma and has a high relapse rate following local radiation therapy. Thus, current recommendations are that all such patients receive systemic multiagent chemotherapy, with or without rituximab.[22] However, even PCLBCL–leg type has a better disease-free survival rate than does nodal DLBCL.[23] This may be related to the usually low score employing the International Prognostic Index at presentation.[24]

CLASSIFICATION OF PRIMARY CUTANEOUS LYMPHOMA

It is now widely recognized that there are many distinct B-cell and T-cell lymphomas that occur as primary tumors of the skin. In 1994 the Revised European American Lymphoma (REAL) classification was published,[25] and shortly thereafter the EORTC Cutaneous Lymphoma Program Project Group published a classification scheme specifically for primary cutaneous lymphoma.[2] One of the aims of the EORTC report was to define primary cutaneous tumors and draw attention to those lymphomas with clinical behavior that would not have been predicted using classification schemes designed for nodal lymphomas (Table 19-2).[2,6] Since then, the International Agency for Research and Cancer published the WHO classification—*Pathology and Genetics of Tumours of Haematopoietic and Lymphoid Tissues*—which incorporated some of the EORTC recommendations, such as that PCFCL be distinguished from nodal follicular lymphoma.[26] Nevertheless, even in the 2001 WHO classification, PCFCL was not listed as a distinct disease entity, and there was no consensus as to the designation of those primary cutaneous B-cell lymphomas composed of large centrocytes and centroblasts. In conjunction with the development of WHO's *Pathology and Genetics of Skin Tumours*,[27] a group of pathologists and dermatologists representing the WHO and EORTC classification committees met in Zurich in 2004 to review the classification of follicular lymphoma and large B-cell lymphoma of the skin. The two groups reached agreement on the classification of these lymphomas, and a consensus document was published.[1] Most recently, *WHO Classification of Tumours of Haematopoietic and Lymphoid Tissues* was published, which formally incorporates the conclusions of these discussions.[28]

An understanding of how the terms *primary* and *secondary* have been applied to cutaneous lymphomas is critical to an understanding of the classification schemes. Most observers use the term *secondary cutaneous lymphoma* to describe lymphomas that develop in the skin as a secondary manifestation of a lymphoma arising primarily at a site other than skin. At present, the most broadly accepted definition of *primary cutaneous lymphoma* is a lymphoma arising in the skin without evidence of extracutaneous lymphoma at the time of initial presentation and staging.[29,30]

Table 19-2 Classifications of Mature B-Cell Lymphomas That Occur as Primary Skin Tumors: Changes in Terminology

REAL Classification (1994)	EORTC Classification (1997)	WHO Classification (2008)
Extranodal marginal zone B-cell lymphoma of MALT type	Marginal zone lymphoma (immunocytoma)	Primary cutaneous marginal zone lymphoma
Follicular lymphoma	Follicle center cell lymphoma (head and trunk)	Primary cutaneous follicle center lymphoma
Diffuse large B-cell lymphoma (subset)	Follicle center lymphoma	Primary cutaneous follicle center lymphoma
Diffuse large B-cell lymphoma (subset)	Large B-cell lymphoma of the leg	Primary cutaneous large B-cell lymphoma–leg type
Diffuse large B-cell lymphoma (subset)	Intravascular large B-cell lymphoma	Intravascular large B-cell lymphoma
Extranodal marginal zone B-cell lymphoma of MALT type	Plasmacytoma	Primary cutaneous marginal zone lymphoma

EORTC, European Organization for Research and Treatment of Cancer; MALT, mucosa-associated lymphoid tissue; REAL, Revised European American Lymphoma; WHO, World Health Organization.

B-CELL LYMPHOMAS OF THE SKIN

Of all cutaneous lymphomas, approximately 25% are thought to be of B-cell lineage.[31-33] The estimated annual incidence of primary cutaneous B-cell lymphomas in Europe is 0.2 per 100,000.[33] The vast majority of these patients have PCFCL and PCMZL, with a minor cohort of patients having large B-cell lymphomas. Other forms of cutaneous B-cell lymphoma represent rare but distinct clinical entities.

Primary Cutaneous Marginal Zone Lymphoma

Definition

All extranodal marginal zone lymphomas (EMZLs) share certain common features and are defined as neoplastic proliferations of small B cells, including marginal zone (centrocyte-like) cells, monocytoid B cells, lymphoplasmacytoid cells, and plasma cells. PCMZL shares these features with extranodal lymphomas of the MALT type. Other terms have been used as synonyms in the literature, including *monocytoid B-cell lymphoma* and *lymphoma of skin-associated lymphoid tissue*.[34-40] Primary cutaneous immunocytoma and cutaneous lymphoid hyperplasia with monotypic plasma cells are considered variants of PCMZL.[2,6,13,41-43]

Epidemiology

Cutaneous marginal zone lymphoma affects both men and women, with a median age of 50 years and a range of 24 to 77 years.[44] In a recent population-based study from the United States, the incidence rate in whites and non-Hispanic whites was substantially higher than that seen in blacks and Asians/Pacific Islanders.[7] Because of the predominance of T-cell lymphomas in the skin, PCMZL is rare among all cutaneous lymphomas. PCMZL is estimated to account for approximately 25% of primary cutaneous B-cell lymphomas, second only to follicular lymphoma.[29,34,39,45] Cases from earlier reports that were classified as immunocytoma[41,42,46,47] or grouped with low-grade B-cell lymphomas[6] likely represent PCMZL. Owing to differences in terminology, some authors estimate that PCMZL accounts for much more than 25% of primary cutaneous B-cell lymphomas,[48] whereas others, using more rigid diagnostic criteria, report it as a more rarely occurring tumor.[2] In some instances, cutaneous involvement occurs secondarily in patients with EMZL arising in other sites.[49] PCMZL has been reported in the pediatric age group.[50]

Etiology

The cause of most PCMZLs remains unclear. Several authors have proposed the existence of skin-associated lymphoid tissue that, with persistent antigenic stimulation, may give rise to neoplastic proliferations of marginal zone B cells.[51,52] Similar to the *Helicobacter pylori* story for gastric MALToma, *Borrelia burgdorferi* has been proposed as an etiologic agent in the development of PCMZL in Europe.[30,53-57] A few case reports even describe the resolution of lesions following antibiotic therapy. Interestingly, no association between *Borrelia* and PCMZL has been identified in reports from the United States and Asia.[58-60] Other settings in which PCMZL has been described include tattoos, vaccination sites, and insect bites (not related to tick-borne illness).

Clinical Features

EMZLs occur at many sites, including the skin, lung, orbit, salivary gland, thyroid, breast, trachea, prostate, kidney, gallbladder, and uterine cervix.[29,34,39] PCMZL shows a predilection for the trunk and upper extremities.[29,34,60-66] It usually presents as a deep red or violaceous, infiltrated papule, plaque, or nodule (Fig. 19-1). Tumors may be multiple or may present as a confluent plaque or erythematous papules. Patients with PCMZL do not have B symptoms and have normal serum levels of lactate dehydrogenase and β_2-microglobulins.[67] A rare association of EMZL, including cases with cutaneous involvement, is Waldenström's macroglobulinemia, with resulting hyperviscosity syndrome. Thus, it has been suggested that serum protein electrophoresis is a reasonable part of the laboratory evaluation of patients with EMZL.[68]

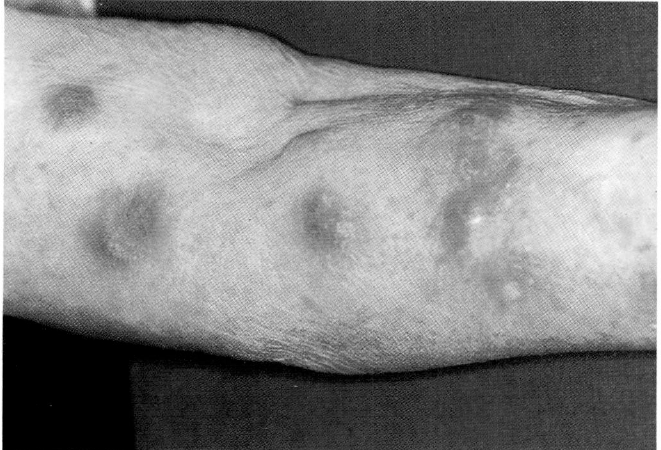

Figure 19-1. Clinical appearance of primary cutaneous marginal zone lymphoma. Firm red or violaceous nodules are present on the forearm. (Courtesy of Christian A. Sander, MD, Abteilung für Dermatologie, Hamburg, Germany.)

Histopathology

The histologic features of PCMZL, as in other sites, often include reactive germinal centers surrounded by a proliferation of marginal zone cells, plasma cells, and admixed reactive T lymphocytes.[14,34,35,37] The infiltrate is centered in the mid-dermis, often extending to the subcutaneous tissue. The neoplastic B cells are centrocyte-like cells with small, cleaved nuclei and pale cytoplasm. The foci with plasmacytic differentiation may contain plasma cells with intranuclear pseudoinclusions of immunoglobulin, termed *Dutcher bodies*. In patients undergoing serial biopsies, increasing degrees of plasmacytic differentiation may be seen over time.[69] Follicular colonization—the infiltration of reactive lymphoid follicles by neoplastic B cells—may be present.[60] Invariably there is a reactive T-cell infiltrate admixed with the neoplastic B cells. The T-cell infiltrate may be sparse or extremely dense; in some cases the T cells outnumber the neoplastic B cells.[42,70]

Gastric EMZLs characteristically display infiltrations of glandular epithelium termed *lymphoepithelial lesions*. This finding is less common in PCMZL and, when present, is observed in the epithelium of the hair follicles. The epidermis is usually free of lymphocytes and is separated from the underlying dermal tumor by a grenz zone of uninvolved papillary dermis (Fig. 19-2).

Immunophenotype

The neoplastic marginal zone cells usually have a $CD20^+$, $CD22^+$, $CD5^-$, $CD10^-$, $CD23^-$, $BCL6^-$ immunophenotype.[51,59,71,72] Monotypic plasma cells usually express CD138, CD79a, and MUM-1/IRF4 but not CD20. Nearly 70% of cases have plasmacytic differentiation, and cytoplasmic light-chain restriction is identified by immunohistochemistry or in situ hybridization.[14,34,44] The monotypic plasma cells are often most prominent immediately beneath the epidermis, and a similar subepithelial distribution is characteristic of EMZL in other sites, such as the stomach or conjunctiva. Scattered large $CD30^+$ cells also may be observed.[44] In contrast to most EMZLs, in which mu heavy-chain expression is found, PCMZLs often show evidence of heavy-chain class switching, with expression of immunoglobulin (Ig) G, IgA, or IgE.[73] In addition, the inflammatory environment differs from that of other EMZLs, in that *CXCR3* is not expressed, and T-helper 2 cells appear to predominate. These findings suggest possible differences in pathogenesis.

The staining pattern when B- and T-cell stains are compared is deceptively benign, with central zones of B cells and surrounding T cells. In cases with colonized follicles, $BCL6^-$, $BCL2^+$, $CD10^-$ neoplastic cells are observed admixed with $BCL6^+$, $BCL2^-$, $CD10^+$ follicle center cells, often with disrupted $CD21^+$, $CD23^+$ follicular dendritic cell meshworks.[71]

Genetics

Clonal rearrangement of immunoglobulin heavy-chain genes is detected using PCR-based techniques in 70% of PCMZLs. BCL2 protein expression is common in PCMZL but is not associated with the follicular lymphoma translocation involving *BCL2/IGH@*, t(14;18)(q32;q21).[74] Streubel and colleagues[51] suggested that postfollicular differentiation in the setting of antigenic stimulation may lead to genetic instability

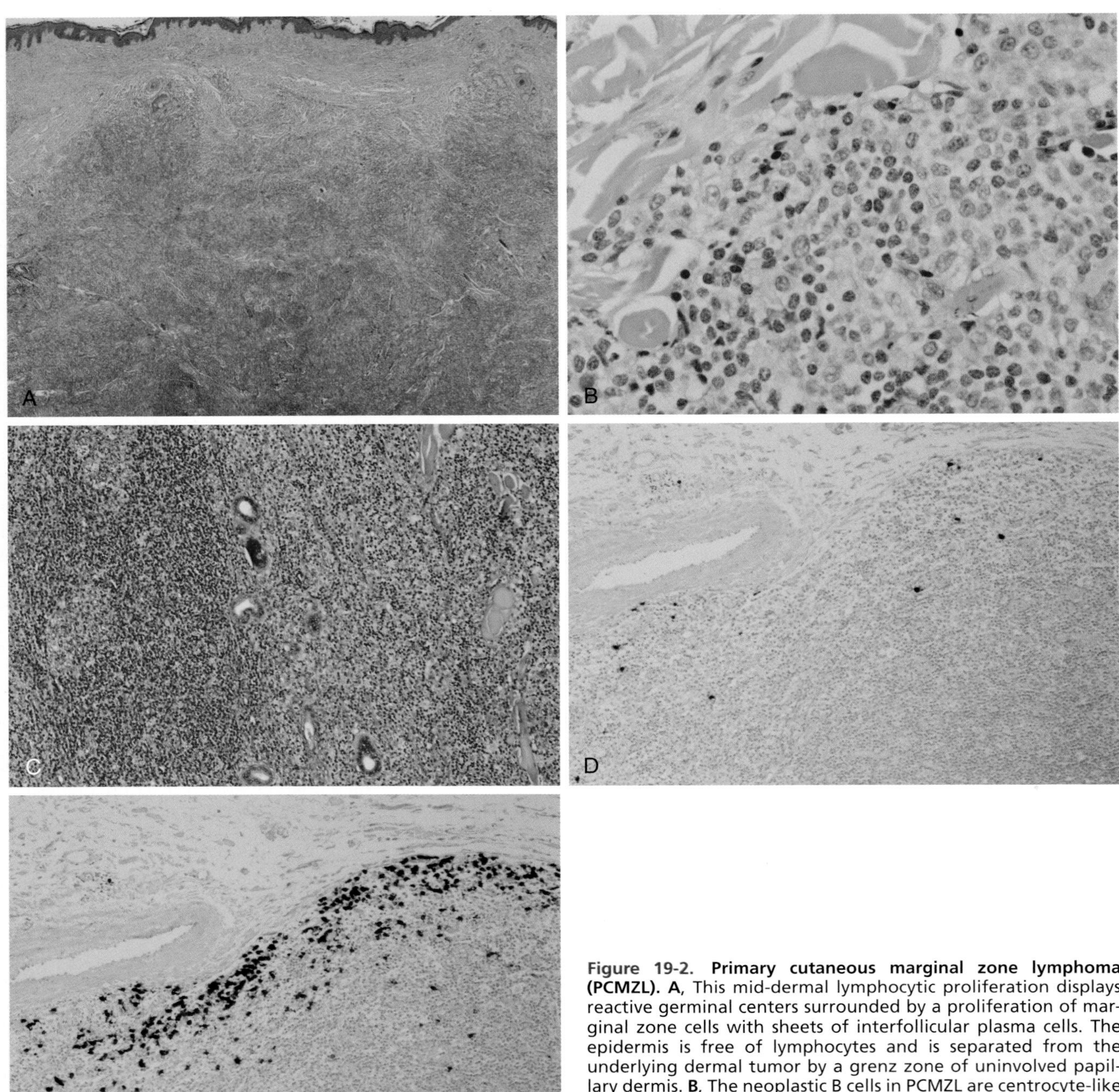

Figure 19-2. Primary cutaneous marginal zone lymphoma (PCMZL). A, This mid-dermal lymphocytic proliferation displays reactive germinal centers surrounded by a proliferation of marginal zone cells with sheets of interfollicular plasma cells. The epidermis is free of lymphocytes and is separated from the underlying dermal tumor by a grenz zone of uninvolved papillary dermis. **B,** The neoplastic B cells in PCMZL are centrocyte-like cells with small, cleaved nuclei and amphophilic cytoplasm. **C,** Periadnexal marginal zone cells with scattered plasma cells. **D** and **E,** Rare kappa light-chain–positive plasma cells (**D**) compared with lambda light chain (**E**).

and resultant abnormal genetic phenotypes, including trisomy 13, trisomy 18, p16 deletion, t(1;14)(p22;q32), and t(11;18)(q21;21). A t(14;18)(q32;q21) translocation in a subset of PCMZLs[44,51] results in juxtaposition of the *MALT1* gene located at chromosome 18q21 with the *IGH@* gene at chromosome 14q32. A study of 24 cases of EMZL in Asia revealed fusion of the apoptosis inhibitor-2 (*API2*) gene with the MALT lymphoma–associated translocation gene (*MALT1*), t(11;18)(q21;q21) in no cutaneous cases, and *BCL10* mutation in only one case.[59] Interestingly, 10 of 24 cases showed nuclear staining for BCL10 protein, in contrast to the cytoplasmic BCL10 staining that is characteristic of normal marginal zone B cells. BCL10 nuclear expression has been correlated with t(1;14)(p22;q32) at other tissue sites of marginal zone lymphoma.[75-79] Further work to determine the possible relationship between antigenic switches and particular genetic rearrangements in PCMZL is ongoing.[80] Inactivation of *p15* and *p16* genes, most commonly as a result of promoter hypermethylation, has been observed in PCMZL as well as in PCFCL and PCLBCL.[81]

Postulated Normal Counterpart

Marginal zone lymphoma is thought to recapitulate a post–germinal center memory B cell,[25] with somatic hypermutation and postfollicular differentiation.[51,82,83]

Clinical Course

PCMZLs are usually clinically indolent; however, up to 30% of patients diagnosed with PCMZL experience extracutaneous relapse,[34,44,45,63,84] most commonly at other extranodal sites such as the breast, salivary gland, and orbit. This clinical behavior is similar to that of EMZL at other sites and is still associated with an excellent prognosis.[29,34,35,37-39,84] Although rare, transformation to large cell lymphoma has been reported.[44,63]

Patients with PCMZL have been effectively treated with external beam irradiation, radiotherapy, intralesional interferon, and local injection of steroids.[44,51,60] A role for antibiotic therapy in the management of PCMZL has yet to be documented.[85] Patients with disseminated disease may receive more aggressive treatment, including rituximab and chemotherapy.[51] The 5-year disease-specific survival rate is close to 100%.

Differential Diagnosis

The differential diagnosis of PCMZL includes cutaneous lymphoid hyperplasia (CLH) and PCFCL. CLH is a benign reactive proliferation in the skin that probably arises secondary to continued antigenic stimulation (e.g., arthropod bite, autoimmune disease, drugs, tattoos, infectious agents). Synonyms for CLH include *pseudolymphoma, lymphocytoma cutis, lymphadenosis benigna cutis, pseudolymphoma of Spiegler-Fendt,* and *lymphadenoma granulosa.* Because of overlap in the clinical presentation and histologic features, it is likely that some cutaneous low-grade B-cell lymphomas were diagnosed as CLH in the past.[12,86] CLH with monotypic plasma cells is problematic.[61] Because of the morphologic and immunophenotypic features in common with PCFCL, these lesions have been regarded more recently as PCMZL. However, the clinical course is typically indolent, and there is often only a single lesion. Clonality by PCR may be absent. Therefore, a conservative approach to management may be appropriate, such as surgical excision and "watch and wait."

CLH and PCMZL affect females more often than males and present with single or multiple slow-growing cutaneous nodules on the face, arms, or trunk. Both entities are characterized by a dermal lymphocytic infiltrate, grenz zone, reactive follicles, and admixed inflammatory cells (Table 19-3). Marginal zone cells and confluent sheets or zones of monotypic plasma cells in the interfollicular regions and around the superficial vascular plexus support a diagnosis of PCMZL.[14] In contrast, epidermal atrophy or hyperplasia, exocytosis, spongiosis, and hyperkeratosis are seen in the majority of cases of CLH and only rarely in PCMZL. The more common occurrence of epidermal changes in CLH may be the result of an ongoing local inflammatory response to external antigen. Recognition of PCMZL and the finding that reactive lymphoid follicles are more commonly observed in PCMZL than in CLH have led to a revision of the historical dictum that the presence of lymphoid follicles favors a benign diagnosis.[87] In cases with inconspicuous follicles on hematoxylin-eosin stain, stains for BCL2 and CD21 are useful in identifying focal nonstaining areas and aggregates of follicular dendritic cells, respectively.[71] The presence of a bottom-heavy infiltrate, although traditionally thought to favor a diagnosis of lymphoma, is not diagnostic. A superficial dermal or top-heavy infiltrate may be observed in cutaneous B-cell lymphomas, whereas hypersensitivity reactions to injected antigens and lymphomatoid drug reactions may both show deep dermal, bottom-heavy lymphoid infiltrates. Although the presence of a grenz zone, eosinophils, or neutrophils is not a statistically significant distinguishing feature, aggregates of eosinophils or abundant neutrophils with nuclear dust should lead to the consideration of a diagnosis other than PCMZL.

PCR detects clonal rearrangement of immunoglobulin heavy-chain genes in only 30% to 50% of B-cell lymphomas.[88] More often, immunohistochemistry demonstrates monotypic cytoplasmic expression of light chains by plasma cells in PCMZL.[34] An infiltrate of at least 75% B cells and coexpression of CD43 and CD20 also support a diagnosis of B-cell lymphoma.[14,89]

In PCMZL the proliferation of marginal zone B cells may be minimal and inconspicuous. It is possible that cases reported as reactive lymphoid hyperplasia with monotypic plasma cells represent cutaneous marginal zone lymphomas with inconspicuous marginal zone B cells.[13,43]

Table 19-3 Histologic and Immunophenotypic Features of Cutaneous Lymphoid Hyperplasia and Primary Cutaneous B-Cell Lymphomas

	Cutaneous Lymphoid Hyperplasia	Primary Cutaneous Marginal Zone Lymphoma	Primary Cutaneous Follicle Center Lymphoma
Epidermal change	+/–	–	–
Eosinophils and neutrophils	+/–	–/+	–
Plasma cells (zones)	–	+/–	–
Marginal zone cells (sheets)	–	+	–
Dutcher bodies	–	+	–
Light-chain–restricted plasma cells	–	+	–
Light-chain–restricted follicles	–	–	+
Lymphoid follicles	–/+	+/–	+/–
Grenz zone	+	+	+
Immunophenotype	Mixed T and B Clonality not shown	$CD20^+$, $CD79a^+$, $CD10^-$, $BCL6^-$, $BCL2^{+/-}$	$CD20^+$, $CD79a^+$, $CD10^{+/-}$, $BCL6^+$, $BCL2^{-/+}$

There is also considerable overlap in the histologic appearance of PCFCL and PCMZL. A predominantly nodular or follicular pattern is observed in most PCFCLs. However, PCFCL may be entirely diffuse or display diffuse areas, and the majority of PCMZLs have some follicles that, when colonized, may mimic PCFCL. A predominance of small cells with irregular, somewhat cleaved nuclei characterizes both tumors. Moreover, anti-CD21 immunostaining highlights follicular dendritic cell meshworks, indicating true follicular structures in both PCFCL and PCMZL.

A combination of immunostaining for BCL6, CD10, and BCL2 yields distinct patterns of staining in the follicular and extrafollicular regions of PCFCL and PCMZL (Table 19-4). Distinguishing neoplastic follicles of PCFCL from reactive or colonized follicles of PCMZL may be difficult, because BCL6 and CD10 are expressed by both reactive and neoplastic follicles, and BCL2 is often negative in PCFCL.[71,90] In cases of PCMZL with colonized follicles, BCL6, CD10, BCL2, and CD21 may allow the distinction of colonized follicles (BCL6 and CD10 negative) from reactive follicles (BCL6 and CD10 positive). The colonized follicles, which typically correspond to nodular areas on hematoxylin-eosin sections, display tight, nodular aggregates of $CD21^+$ follicular dendritic cells, similar to neoplastic follicles or reactive germinal centers, but they contain distinct clusters of $BCL6^-$, $BCL2^+$ neoplastic B cells, in addition to clusters of $BCL6^+$, $BCL2^-$ germinal center cells. The other pattern observed in PCMZL is that of expanded, colonized meshworks of follicular dendritic cells corresponding to areas that appear diffuse or only vaguely nodular on routine sections, with only scattered $BCL6^+$ cells; most cells are $BCL6^-$. It remains unclear whether the $BCL6^+$ cells in the dispersed dendritic cell meshworks of PCMZL represent residual follicle center cells or blast transformation. Neoplastic follicles in PCFCL, in contrast, contain a uniform population of neoplastic $BCL6^+$ cells, and in those cases expressing BCL2, it is uniformly expressed by cells within the follicles. In contrast to PCFCL, $BCL6^+$ and $CD10^+$ cells are never seen in interfollicular and diffuse areas devoid of $CD21^+$ cells in PCMZL.

Primary Cutaneous Follicle Center Lymphoma

Definition

PCFCL is characterized by a mixture of centrocytes and centroblasts with a follicular, follicular and diffuse, or diffuse pattern. Tumors with a diffuse pattern composed entirely of centroblasts are excluded.

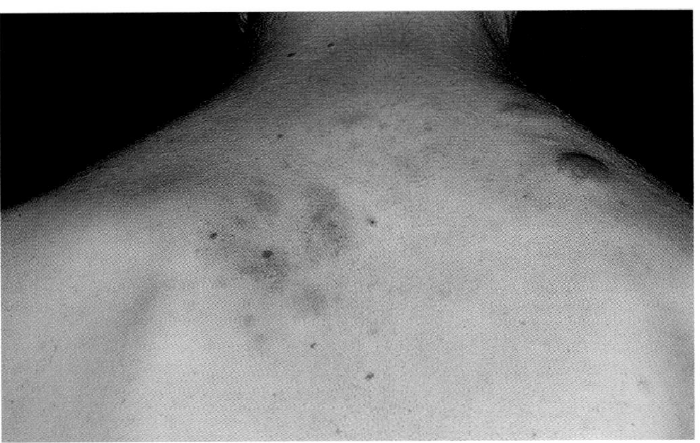

Figure 19-3. Clinical appearance of primary cutaneous follicle center lymphoma. A large, firm nodule is present on the upper back, with multiple smaller satellite nodules. (Courtesy of Christian A. Sander MD, Abteilung für Dermatologie, Hamburg, Germany.)

Epidemiology

PCFCL is the most common B-cell lymphoma that occurs as a primary lymphoma of the skin.[2,69] PCFCL is a tumor of adults, with a median age of 65 years, and it affects slightly more men than women.[66] In a population-based study from the United States, the highest incidence was in whites (Hispanic or non-Hispanic), with the lowest incidence in blacks and Asians/Pacific Islanders.[7]

Etiology

The cause of PCFCL is not known. There are significant geographic and racial differences in the incidence of nodal follicular lymphoma among different populations,[91] and as noted earlier, some of these racial and ethnic differences appear to hold true for PCFCL.[7]

Clinical Features

PCFCL most commonly presents in the head and neck region, often involving the scalp. The trunk, particularly the upper back, is often involved (Fig. 19-3). However, almost any cutaneous site can be affected.[61-63] PCFCL presents as multiple or solitary erythematous cutaneous papules, nodules, or plaques.[62,66,92-94] A common pattern is a larger central nodule surrounded by smaller satellite nodules in the same anatomic region.

Histopathology

PCFCL is characterized by a mid-dermal and subcuticular admixed proliferation of centrocytes and centroblasts in a

Table 19-4 Immunostaining in Primary Cutaneous Follicle Center and Marginal Zone Lymphomas

	PC Follicle Center Lymphoma		*PC Marginal Zone Lymphoma*		
Marker	Neoplastic Follicles	Interfollicular Areas	Reactive Follicles	Colonized Follicles	Interfollicular Areas
CD21	+F	–	+F	+F, disrupted	–
BCL6	+	+/–	+	–/+	–
CD10	+	–/+	+ (weak)	–	–
BCL2	–/+	–/+	–	+/–	+
IgD	Mantle zones absent or disrupted		Mantle zones may be present		

F, follicles; Ig, immunoglobulin; PC, primary cutaneous.

follicular, follicular and diffuse, or diffuse pattern. Usually the centrocytes are more plentiful than the centroblasts, and there is an admixed benign T-cell infiltrate of variable density. The centrocytes have small, medium-sized, or large cleaved or irregular nuclei with dispersed chromatin, inconspicuous nucleoli, and scant cytoplasm. Large centrocytes are generally more plentiful in diffuse PCFCL. Centroblasts have large, round nuclei with peripherally located basophilic nucleoli and a rim of basophilic cytoplasm. Although centroblasts are typically present, by definition, they do not form confluent sheets in PCFCL.

The infiltrate often appears as expanded, irregularly shaped lymphoid follicles in the dermis. Occasionally the neoplastic cells appear to spill out of the follicles and surround aggregates of benign small lymphocytes, termed *inside-out follicles* by some observers (Fig. 19-4). Sclerosis is often present, and the atypical cells may appear to dissect among the collagen bundles. Numerous admixed small lymphocytes are often present, but plasma cells are typically absent. Other inflammatory cells, including eosinophils and granulocytes, are sparse, but admixed histiocytes may be present.

Grading

Grading of PCFCL according to the number of centroblasts, as is done with nodal follicular lymphoma, has not been shown to have clinical relevance. The notation of the pattern—follicular, follicular and diffuse, or diffuse—is optional in the diagnosis.

Immunophenotype

Immunohistochemical stains or in situ hybridization for kappa and lambda light chains typically do not reveal light-chain restriction of the neoplastic centrocytes and centroblasts on paraffin sections because there is no plasmacytoid differentiation. The characteristic immunophenotype is $CD20^+$, $BCL6^+$, $BCL2^-$ or dimly positive; expression of CD10 is variable; and cells are $CD5^-$, $CD43^-$, MUM-1/$IRF4^-$.[71] Cases with a follicular pattern are more likely to be $CD10^+$, whereas diffuse PCFCLs are typically $CD10^-$. In contrast to nodal follicular lymphomas, almost all of which are $BCL2^+$, less than 30% of PCFCLs express the BCL2 protein.[95,96] Although faint or partial BCL2 staining may be seen in some cases, it is typically weaker than

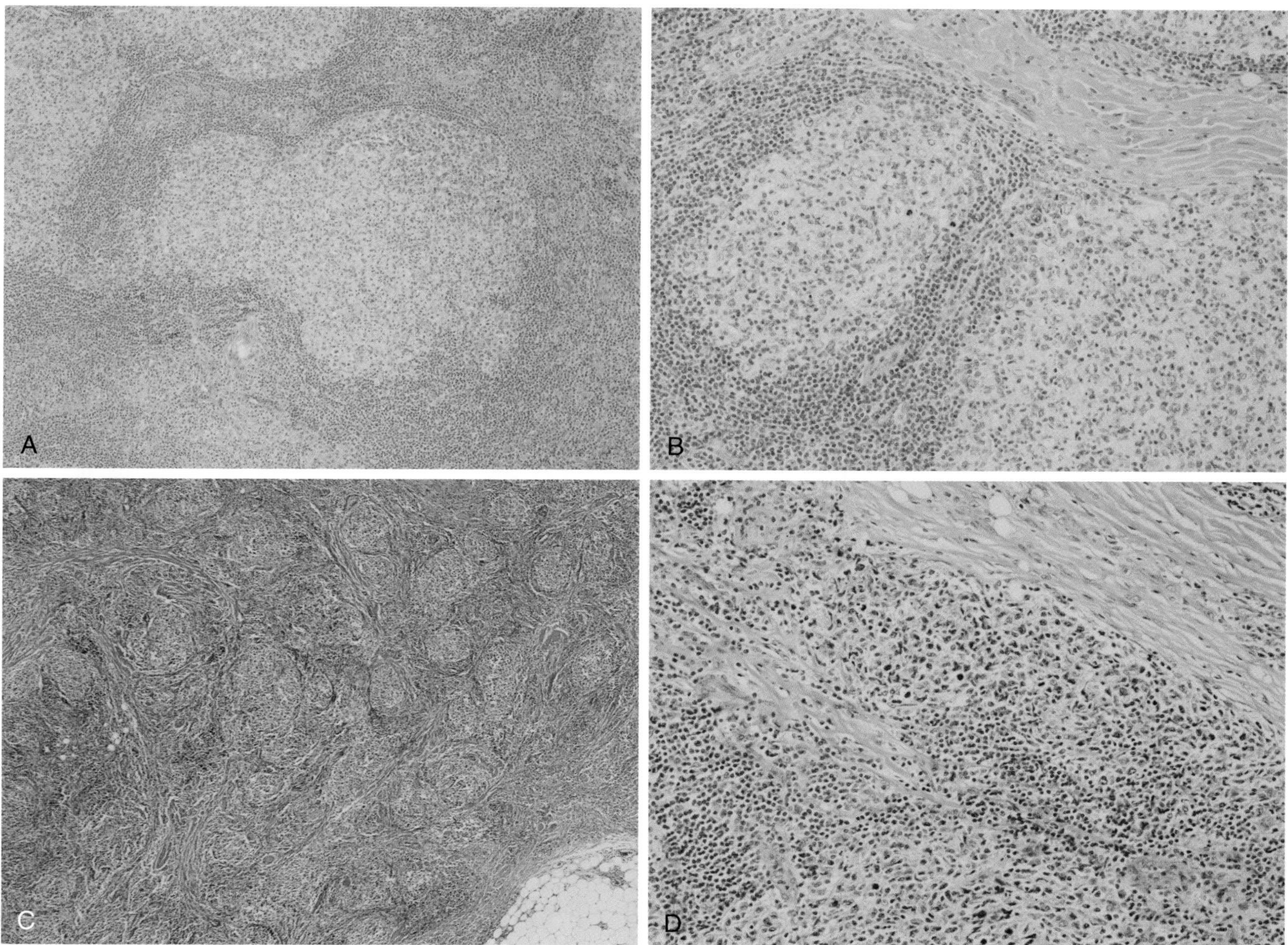

Figure 19-4. Primary cutaneous follicle center lymphoma. A, Expanded, irregularly shaped lymphoid follicles. **B,** The neoplastic cells appear to spill out of the follicles and surround aggregates of benign small lymphocytes, termed *inside-out follicles.* **C,** A pan-dermal and subcuticular admixed proliferation of centrocytes and centroblasts is present in a follicular and diffuse pattern. **D,** Centrocytes and centroblasts form aggregates in the reticular dermis without intervening zones of small lymphocytes.

that of normal T cells in the infiltrate; strong BCL2 staining should give rise to consideration of PCLBCL–leg type or secondary involvement by nodal follicular lymphoma. Because BCL2 protein is normally present on most T cells and B cells (except for the B cells in reactive follicle centers), and because the neoplastic cells in PCFCL are often $BCL2^-$, a negative BCL2 staining pattern of follicles with the remaining lymphocytes staining positively for BCL2 does not allow a distinction between a reactive and a neoplastic process in the skin. $CD21^+$, $CD23^+$, $CD35^+$ follicular dendritic cells may be detected forming nodular meshworks in follicular areas.[97]

Genetics

PCFCL typically lacks the t(14;18) observed in nodal follicular lymphoma[61,95,98,99]; however, some studies have found evidence of the translocation by fluorescence in situ hybridization.[61,65,95,96] Finding the translocation should lead to staging for evidence of extracutaneous follicular lymphoma, but it does not exclude PCFCL. PCR techniques detect clonal rearrangement of immunoglobulin genes in approximately 50% of cases. By comparative genomic hybridization, chromosomal imbalances were rare.[100]

Postulated Normal Counterpart

The postulated normal counterpart is a germinal center B cell, with a predominance of large and small centrocytes.

Clinical Course

PCFCLs rarely spread to lymph nodes, spleen, or bone marrow, unlike the majority of nodal follicular lymphomas.[6,61,93] The estimated 5-year survival rate for patients with PCFCL is greater than 97%.[2,69] Excision and radiation therapy are effective for localized lesions. If several lesions are present in the same region or more widely scattered, radiotherapy of multiple lesions may be employed. In patients with extensive cutaneous disease, systemic rituximab is recommended as the initial approach. Intralesional rituximab has also been used. Combination chemotherapy is not recommended unless unusual clinical circumstances suggest an aggressive clinical behavior.[85] An EORTC study suggested that PCFCLs presenting on the lower leg had a more aggressive clinical course than those presenting on the head, neck, or trunk.[19]

Differential Diagnosis

When PCFCL has a prominently follicular architecture, the differential diagnosis includes PCMZL, CLH, and secondary involvement by follicular lymphoma. When PCFCL has a diffuse pattern of growth, the differential diagnosis includes PCLBCL–leg type (see later).

Both PCMZL and PCFCL are predominantly localized to the head, trunk, or upper extremities.[6,29,34,62,64,84,93,101] Both tend to be localized to the skin at diagnosis and to have a low risk of dissemination to lymph nodes or bone marrow.[29,34,101] PCFCL and PCMZL also have overlapping morphologic features. PCFCL may have a partially follicular pattern,[62] and PCMZL typically contains reactive or colonized follicles; thus, B-cell follicles can be found in both lymphomas. Factors that make it difficult to distinguish the neoplastic follicles in PCFCL from the reactive follicles in PCMZL include the lack of BCL2 protein expression and *BCL2* gene rearrangement in the majority of PCFCLs[61,95] and the occasional presence of follicular colonization in PCMZL.[102]

Nodal follicular lymphoma may involve the skin as a secondary site, and occasionally this is the initial biopsy site. In nodal follicular lymphoma the follicular architecture is usually more pronounced, and the neoplastic follicles strongly express CD10 and BCL2. Fluorescence in situ hybridization for *BCL2/IGH@* is positive in the great majority of cases (>75%).[103] A mixture of centrocytes and centroblasts (grade 1 to 2) is seen in most secondary follicular lymphomas.

Diffuse Large B-Cell Lymphoma–Leg Type

Definition

PCLBCL–leg type is defined as a diffuse monomorphic proliferation of large transformed B cells, most commonly arising on the lower leg (Table 19-5). Immunophenotypic criteria are helpful in making an accurate diagnosis because the vast majority of cases express BCL2 and MUM-1/IRF4, exhibiting an ABC phenotype.

Epidemiology

PCLBCL–leg type occurs late in life, with more than 80% of tumors occurring in patients older than 70 years. It is more common in females than in males, in contrast to most other

Table 19-5 WHO-EORTC Criteria for PCFCL and PCLBCL–Leg Type

	PCFCL	PCLBCL–Leg Type
Histopathology	Predominance of centrocytes that are often large, especially in diffuse lesions Centroblasts may be present, but not in confluent sheets Pattern may be follicular, follicular and diffuse, or diffuse Continuum, without distinct categories or grades Sclerosis often present Numerous T cells	Predominance of large to medium-sized B cells with round, vesicular nuclei; prominent nucleoli; and basophilic cytoplasm Cells resemble centroblasts or immunoblasts Little stromal reaction; confluent destructive growth pattern Few T cells
Phenotype	$BCL2^{-/+}$; staining is weak when present $BCL6^{+/-}$ $CD10^{+/-}$ $MUM\text{-}1^-$	$BCL2^+$; staining is strong and present in most neoplastic cells $BCL6^{-/+}$ $CD10^-$ $MUM\text{-}1^+$
Clinical features	Middle-aged adults, male > female In most cases, lesions localized on head or upper trunk Tumor nodules, sometimes with satellite lesions Rarely multifocal lesions	Often elderly, female > male Lesions localized on leg, most often below knee May be multifocal or bilateral

EORTC, European Organization for Research and Treatment of Cancer; PCFCL, primary cutaneous follicle center lymphoma; PCLBCL, primary cutaneous large B-cell lymphoma; WHO, World Health Organization.

Chapter 20

Nodal Marginal Zone Lymphoma

Elaine S. Jaffe

CHAPTER OUTLINE

DEFINITION

Nodal marginal zone lymphoma (NMZL) is a primary nodal B-cell neoplasm derived from post–germinal center B cells. This lymphoma shares morphologic and immunophenotypic similarities with other marginal zone lymphomas, particularly extranodal marginal zone lymphoma (EMZL) of mucosa-associated lymphoid tissue (MALT) type and splenic marginal zone lymphoma (SMZL). Thus, secondary lymph node involvement by EMZL and SMZL should be excluded to establish the diagnosis with certainty. NMZL may show some evidence of plasmacytic differentiation, but generally less than that seen in lymphoplasmacytic lymphoma (LPL), which is often included in the differential diagnosis.

EPIDEMIOLOGY, ETIOLOGY, AND COFACTORS

NMZL is a relatively uncommon lymphoma, accounting for only 1.5% to 1.8% of all lymphoid neoplasms.[1,2] It is primarily a lymphoma of adults, but a pediatric variant of the disease exists, with some distinguishing morphologic and clinical features. The median patient age is between 50 and 60 years, with a female predominance in some but not all series.[3-6] An association with hepatitis C infection has been suggested in some studies[6,7] but is lacking in others.[3] These discrepant results may relate to overlap among a variety of B-cell neoplasms and different diagnostic criteria. The distinction among NMZL, EMZL, and SMZL can be difficult, and hepatitis C has been linked to EMZL and SMZL as well.[8-11] Alternatively, these differences could relate to different risk factors in different patient populations or geographic regions.

Underlying autoimmune disease has been implicated in a variety of EMZLs, including Sjögren's syndrome and Hashimoto's thyroiditis.[12] However, a history of autoimmune disease is lacking in most patients with NMZL. Nodal involvement may be prominent in many patients with salivary gland MALT lymphoma, with a predominance of monocytoid B cells.[13] Therefore, a careful clinical history is important in the evaluation of these cases. Both autoimmune hemolytic anemia and cryoglobulinemia have been reported in a subset of patients with NMZL.[3,14] However, the incidence is much less than that seen with LPL. As noted, the distinction between LPL and NMZL is not always straightforward, and some series of NMZL appear to contain a high proportion of cases with plasmacytic features that others might classify as LPL.[1,3]

CLINICAL FEATURES

The majority of patients present with generalized peripheral lymphadenopathy,[2,3,6] although two series found a higher proportion of localized stage I or II disease.[4,5,15] B symptoms are present in a minority. Clinical evaluation should be undertaken to rule out secondary nodal involvement by EMZL or SMZL, given the significant overlap in the morphologic features in lymph nodes.[15] Most investigators require the absence of extranodal sites of disease (other than bone marrow, liver, or spleen) in making the diagnosis.[4] Similarly, patients presenting with marked splenomegaly and bone marrow involvement with only minimal lymphadenopathy most likely fall into the category of SMZL. These imprecise diagnostic criteria make it difficult to compare clinical features and outcome.

Bone marrow involvement is relatively uncommon in most series, occurring in less than half the patients.[6] Peripheral blood involvement is generally rare, and the presence of circulating cells should at least raise the suspicion of other forms of B-cell neoplasia, including SMZL, splenic lymphoma with villous lymphocytes, and atypical chronic lymphocytic leukemia (CLL). According to the International Prognostic Index (IPI) or the modified Follicular Lymphoma IPI (FLIPI), most patients are in the low-risk or low-intermediate–risk groups.[6] Elevations in lactic dehydrogenase can be seen but are usually modest.

Although plasmacytoid differentiation can be observed histologically, it is uncommon to find monoclonal gammopathy in the serum.[14] One exception was the French series reported by Traverse-Glehen and colleagues,[3] in which 33% of patients had an M component or monoclonal spike. These distinctions may relate to differences in diagnostic criteria and the overlap between NMZL and LPL in tissue biopsies.

MORPHOLOGY

Cytologic Features

NMZLs are characterized by a parafollicular or interfollicular infiltrate of neoplastic B cells partially effacing the lymph node architecture. The neoplastic cells are heterogeneous in appearance and have been described as monocytoid, centrocyte-like, and plasmacytoid.[3,15] These smaller cells are usually admixed with a variable number of transformed cells or blasts. Monocytoid cells have round to irregular nuclei with condensed nuclear chromatin, inconspicuous nucleoli, and abundant pale cytoplasm with distinct cytoplasmic membranes. This cell type is commonly seen in MALT lymphomas associated with Sjögren's syndrome, and a dominant population of monocytoid cells should prompt a clinical evaluation for EMZL either concurrently or sometime in the distant past. Late relapses of EMZL have been described, sometimes many years after the primary diagnosis.[12,15] Centrocyte-like cells resemble their counterparts in EMZL. These small to medium-sized cells have coarsely clumped chromatin, irregular nuclei, and sparse cytoplasm. Plasmacytoid cells exhibit varying degrees of plasmacytoid differentiation. They are often slightly larger than the other cell types present, with an ample rim of basophilic cytoplasm. The nuclear chromatin is generally more dispersed than that of mature plasma cells, and small nucleoli may be present. Dutcher bodies may be seen but are generally less common than in LPL. Larger lymphoid cells or blasts, reminiscent of centroblasts, are present in variable proportions but should not constitute the majority of cells present. The overall impression is that of a heterogeneous population of cells that are medium in size, generally round but irregular, and lacking the monotony seen in some other B-cell lymphomas such as CLL or mantle cell lymphoma.

Other inflammatory cells, particularly epithelioid histiocytes, may be present. However, well-formed granulomas are usually absent. Eosinophils may be noted, particularly in cases with plasmacytoid differentiation.[16]

Architectural Features

In lymph nodes, the neoplastic cells have a marginal zone pattern of infiltration.[3,15] The residual follicles can be expanded, regressed, or, in some instances, colonized by neoplastic cells. These different patterns may correlate to some extent with the nature of the neoplastic cells in different variants. Campo and associates[15] described a "MALT type" of NMZL in which the follicles are generally well preserved, with reactive germinal centers and intact lymphoid cuffs (Fig. 20-1). In this histologic variant, monocytoid B cells are generally abundant. In almost 50% of these cases, further investigation discloses evidence of EMZL at some point in the patient's history (Fig. 20-2).

In the "splenic type" of NMZL described by Campo and colleagues,[15] residual lymphoid follicles are typically regressed, lacking well-formed germinal centers. The mantle cuff might be present but is usually attenuated (Fig. 20-3). The cellular infiltrate is very heterogeneous, comprising all the cell types described earlier. The term *splenic type* was applied to this subset because the tumor cells are typically weakly immunoglobulin (Ig) D positive, resembling the phenotype of SMZL. In addition, the lymph nodes show some resemblance to cases of SMZL with regional lymph node involvement.[17] However, in most of these cases, no connection to SMZL is shown.

Many cases do not correspond cleanly to either subtype. They have an overall polymorphic cellular composition—the polymorphic subtype of NMZL (Table 20-1). Follicles may be absent or partially preserved and may show prominent regressive features (Fig. 20-4). In these cases, follicular colonization is more common, and plasmacytoid differentiation is often present, either within or outside the follicles. Eosinophils may be abundant and tend to correlate with plasmacytoid differentiation.

Follicular colonization can be a prominent feature in NMZL, and extensive infiltration of residual follicles may impart a nodular or follicular growth pattern, mimicking follicular lymphoma.[18] Follicular colonization has also been described in EMZL.[19] In some cases the cytology of the cells within the colonized follicles may be different from that of the cells in the perifollicular zone. No definite pattern emerges,

Table 20-1 Comparison of Histologic Patterns in Nodal Marginal Zone Lymphoma

Feature	MALT Type	Splenic Type	Polymorphic Type
Hyperplastic germinal centers	++	+/–	+
Prominent mantle zones	++	–	–/+
Intrafollicular T cells	–	++	+
IgD expression	–	+	+/–
Plasmacytoid differentiation	–	+/–	++
Risk of extranodal disease	++	–	–

Ig, immunoglobulin; MALT, mucosa-associated lymphoid tissue.

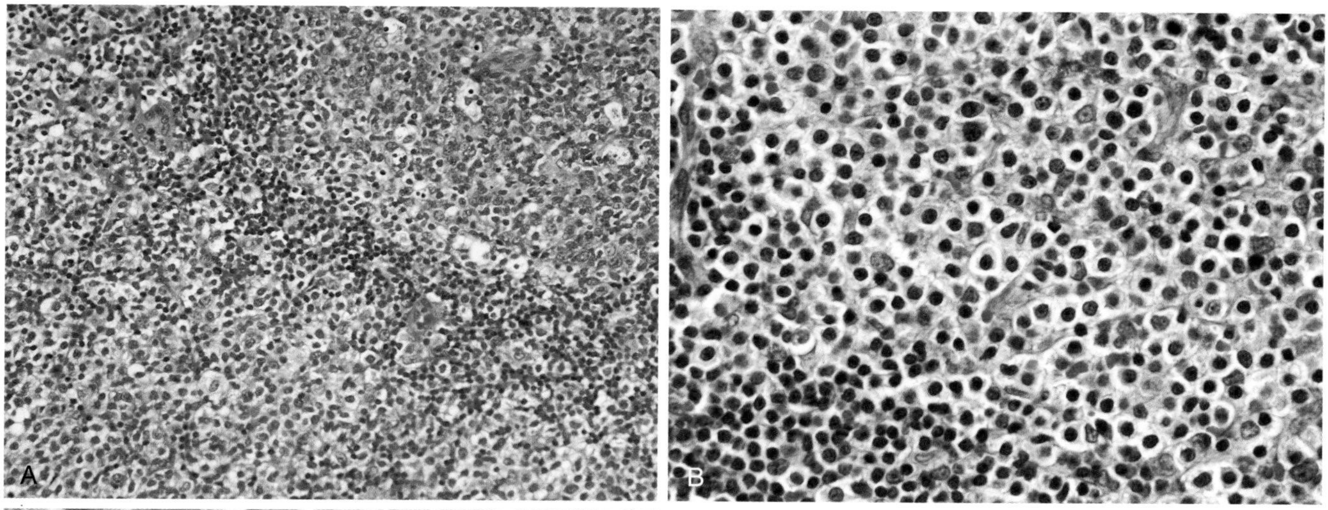

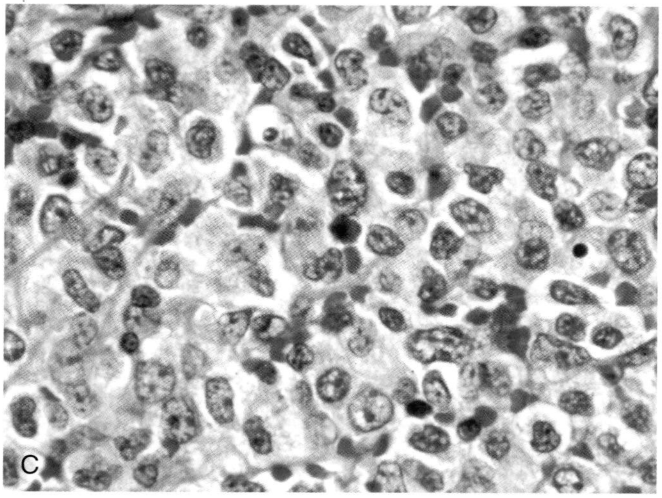

Figure 20-1. Nodal marginal zone lymphoma, mucosa-associated lymphoid tissue type. A, In this variant, reactive lymphoid follicles are well preserved, usually with an intact lymphoid cuff. **B**, The neoplastic cells have abundant clear cytoplasm with a monocytoid appearance. **C**, The cells may have irregular nuclei, and admixed blasts are few.

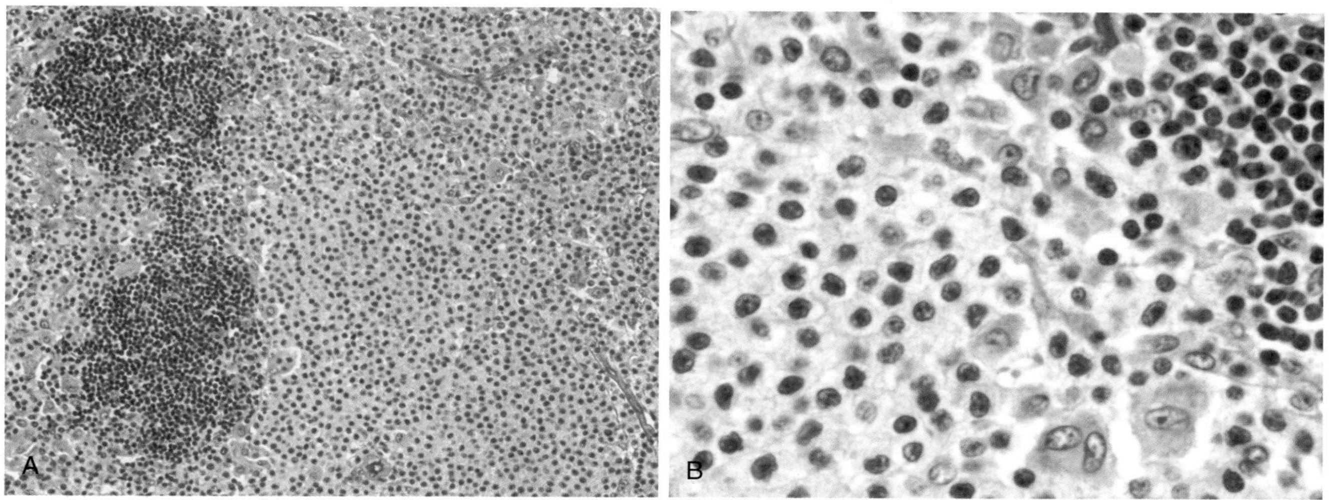

Figure 20-2. Secondary extranodal marginal zone lymphoma in the lymph node of a patient with Sjögren's syndrome. A, The histologic features closely resemble those of mucosa-associated lymphoid tissue–type nodal marginal zone lymphoma. **B**, The cells have abundant clear cytoplasm and distinct cytoplasmic membranes.

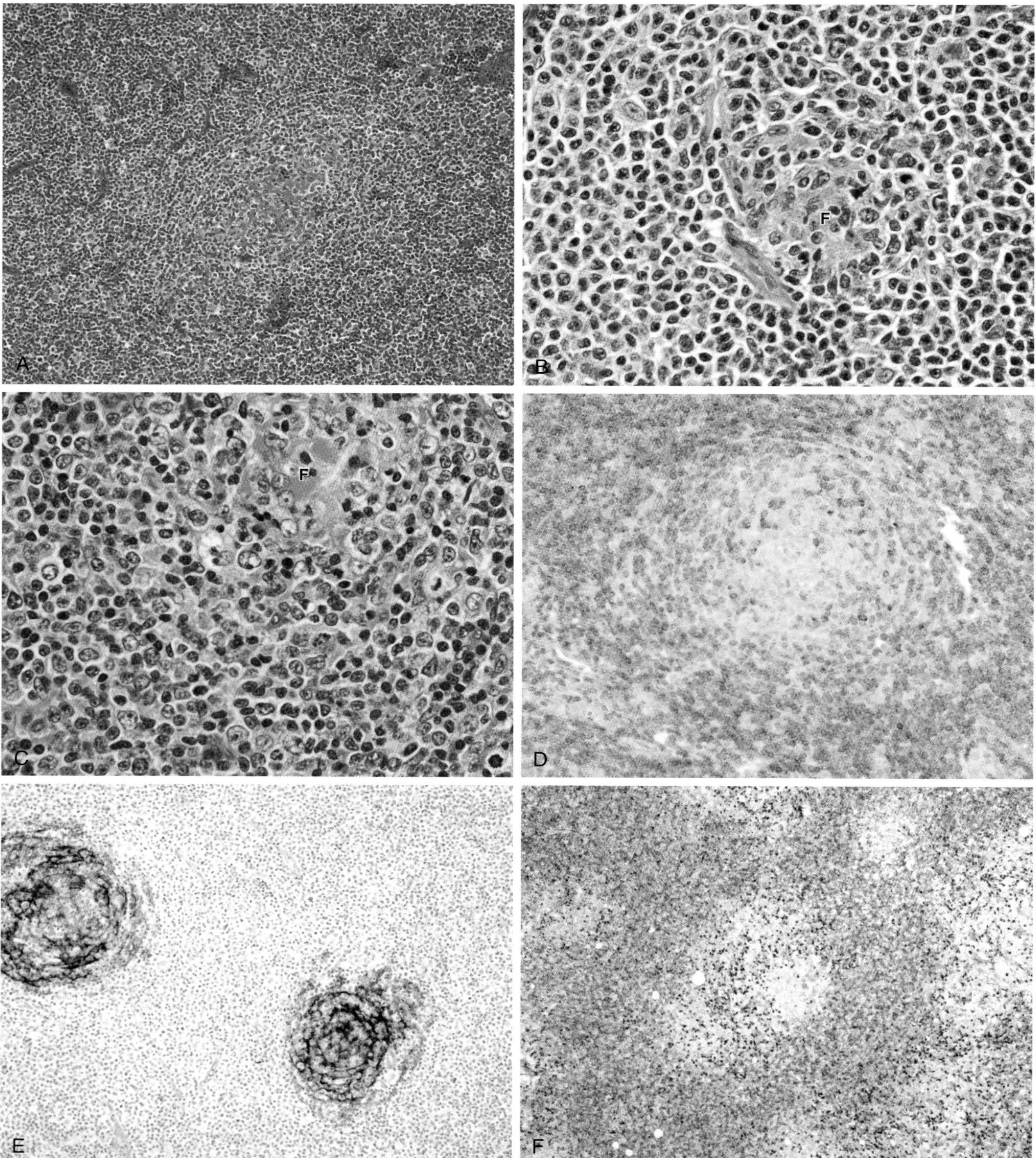

Figure 20-3. Nodal marginal zone lymphoma, splenic type. A, Atypical lymphoid cells surround and replace regressed germinal centers. **B**, A small regressed follicle is present in the center (F). The surrounding cells are slightly irregular, with a rim of pale cytoplasm. **C**, In this example, a higher proportion of blastic cells is present. A regressed follicle is shown (F). **D**, With BCL2 immunostain, the neoplastic marginal zone cells are weakly BCL2$^+$, whereas the regressed follicle is negative. **E**, CD21 immunostain highlights follicular dendritic cells in the regressed follicle center. **F**, With IgD immunostain, the neoplastic cells are weakly IgD$^+$, and the disrupted mantle cells are strongly IgD$^+$.

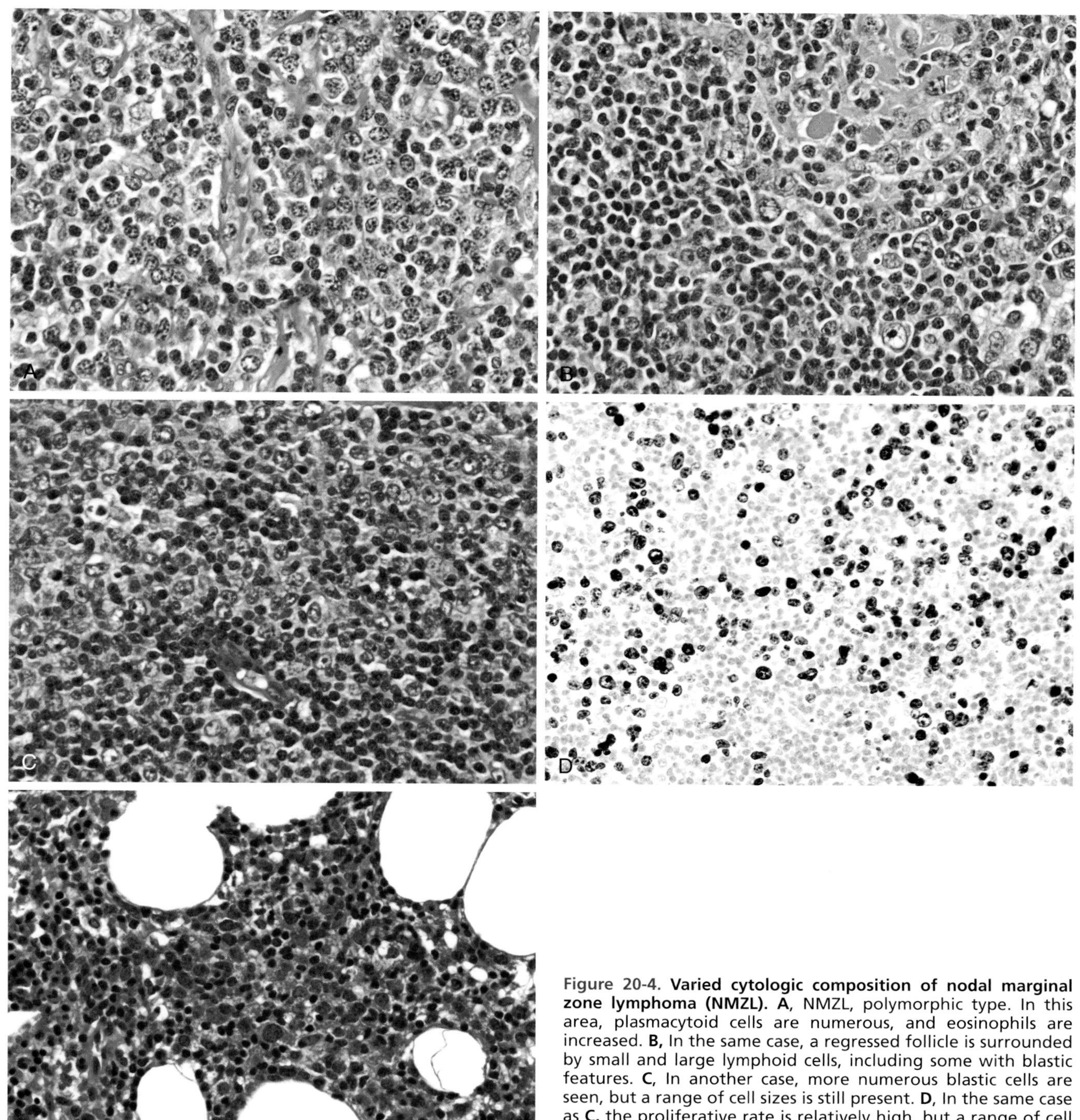

Figure 20-4. Varied cytologic composition of nodal marginal zone lymphoma (NMZL). A, NMZL, polymorphic type. In this area, plasmacytoid cells are numerous, and eosinophils are increased. **B,** In the same case, a regressed follicle is surrounded by small and large lymphoid cells, including some with blastic features. **C,** In another case, more numerous blastic cells are seen, but a range of cell sizes is still present. **D,** In the same case as **C,** the proliferative rate is relatively high, but a range of cell sizes is present (MIB-1). **E,** Bone marrow involvement in NMZL. A large cluster of lymphoid cells is present in a nonparatrabecular localization.

but plasmacytoid differentiation is often prominent in the colonizing cells. In some cases a higher proportion of blastic cells is noted within the colonized follicles.

In some cases, particularly in the pediatric variant of NMZL, hyperplastic germinal centers with expanded and irregular configurations may be seen. In pediatric cases these abnormal follicles resemble the disrupted follicles of progressive transformation of germinal centers.[20] Other authors have described these follicles as "floral" in nature, terming these cases the *floral variant* of NMZL.[21] The follicles, despite their unusual appearance, do not appear to be neoplastic because they regain expression of BCL6 and CD10 and are negative for BCL2 protein. This unusual morphologic variant of NMZL is most common in children and young adults but can also occur in older age groups.[20,21] Interestingly, most of these cases present with isolated nodal sites of stage I disease and do well with conservative therapy following simple excision of the nodal mass.

Other Anatomic Sites

The appearance of NMZL in other anatomic sites is not well described. Bone marrow involvement occurs in a minority of patients. Bone marrow infiltration generally consists of loose nonparatrabecular aggregates or, in some cases, interstitial infiltration.[22] One study also noted paratrabecular aggregates in some cases.[3] As noted earlier, peripheral blood involvement is rare. Involvement of other extranodal sites usually leads to a consideration of the diagnosis of EMZL.

Grading

There is no established grading system for NMZL, although considerable variation in the proportion of blastic cells or proliferating cells (as measured by Ki-67) may be seen. In general, the proportion of blastic cells is less than 20% of the total cell population.[14] Some authors have reported cases with foci of large cell transformation, but the clinical significance of these foci has not been shown.[1] In a subsequent study, the Lyon group noted that a number of cases contained more than 20% blastic cells and suggested that this feature might account for the more aggressive clinical course in that series.[3] However, the investigators were unable to relate outcome to the proportion of large cells or histologic progression. Specifically, there was no difference in survival between the groups with greater than 20% and less than 20% large cells. Nathwani and coworkers[2] reported a relatively high frequency (20%) of transformation to diffuse large B-cell lymphoma in NMZL, but the criteria for transformation were not delineated. Moreover, no difference in survival for those patients who had "transformed" was shown. One study from Japan found a poorer overall survival for cases of NMZL containing a component of diffuse large B-cell lymphoma, but overall, there was no difference in survival for the four histologic subtypes identified: splenic type, floral type, MALT type, and MALT type plus diffuse large B-cell lymphoma.[23] My practice is to perform Ki-67/MIB-1 staining in cases of NMZL and to note in the report if the proliferation rate is especially high (>50% of the nucleated cells), but it is not clear that different therapeutic approaches benefit this subset of cases.[14]

IMMUNOPHENOTYPE

NMZLs are mature B-cell lymphomas that express CD20, CD19, and CD79a but in most cases lack CD5, CD23, CD10, and BCL6. CD43 is positive in up to 50% of cases.[15] BCL2 protein is generally weakly positive. IgD is a helpful marker in highlighting the presence of a residual mantle cuff, which often illuminates the pattern of infiltration by the neoplastic cells. The neoplastic cells in the MALT type of NMZL are almost invariably negative for IgD, whereas variable to weak expression for IgD can be observed in 25% to 50% of NMZLs overall.[3,5,15] Although older studies had hypothesized a relationship between NMZL and normal monocytoid B cells,[24] the immunophenotype of NMZL differs from that of normal monocytoid B cells, arguing against a true association.[5,25]

Plasmacytoid differentiation is seen in NMZL in approximately 50% of cases. When present, the plasmacytoid cells may express MUM-1/IRF4, but usually only a subset of the cells with plasmacytoid features, either morphologically or immunophenotypically, are MUM-1/IRF4$^+$.[5,26] Overall, 25% to 50% of cases express this marker by immunohistochemistry, which first appears in late centrocytes and is thought to indicate commitment to the post–germinal center program.[27] Traverse-Glehen and colleagues[3] reported a much higher incidence of positivity for MUM-1/IRF4 by flow cytometry, which might reflect the greater sensitivity of this technique. CD38, another marker associated with plasmacytoid differentiation, was positive in 41% of cases in one study.[5]

Cytoplasmic immunoglobulin expression can be detected in cells exhibiting morphologic evidence of plasmacytoid differentiation and often in the blastic cells, which display a rim of basophilic cytoplasm. In most cases the cells are IgM$^+$, but IgG and IgA expression, indicative of heavy-chain class switching, has been reported in a small minority.[3] There is a strong bias toward the expression of kappa light chain over lambda light chain; in contrast, in EMZL, kappa and lambda are expressed in a ratio similar to that of normal B cells.[3,5] The distribution of plasmacytoid cells varies within lymph nodes. The plasmacytoid component is usually admixed with other cell types, but in some cases, plasmacytoid cells preferentially colonize germinal centers.

The neoplastic cells are generally negative for CD21 and CD23 by immunohistochemistry. However, these markers are useful in highlighting the distribution of residual follicular dendritic cell (FDC) meshworks. In contrast to follicular lymphomas, in which FDCs highlight the expanded follicular structures, in NMZL the FDCs are typically present in tight clusters, indicative of regressed follicles.[15] In exceptional cases with marked follicular colonization, the FDC meshworks may be expanded.[18] These latter cases can be distinguished from follicular lymphoma because the colonizing cells are negative for the germinal center–associated markers CD10 and BCL6 (Fig. 20-5).

There are limited data concerning other prognostic markers in NMZL. As noted earlier, staining for Ki-67/MIB-1 usually stains 20% or fewer of the neoplastic cells. However, clinical data correlating a higher proliferative rate with differences in clinical outcome do not exist.[3] Many low-grade B-cell lymphomas have alterations in the apoptosis pathway, leading to prolonged survival of the neoplastic cells. One study identified strong expression of survivin in approximately 40% of cases, with those patients having considerably decreased survival.[5] The same authors identified loss of active caspase E and increased expression of cyclin E as negative prognostic factors. Activation of the nuclear factor-κB (NF-κB) pathway has been implicated in most cases of EMZL.[28] However, NMZLs lack nuclear expression of BCL10 and do not show evidence of NF-κB activation, based on negative staining for NF-κB p65.[5]

GENETICS AND MOLECULAR FINDINGS

NMZLs show clonal rearrangement of the *IGH@* genes, as expected for any clonal B-cell neoplasm. During B-cell development, and as part of the maturation of the high-affinity antibody response, most B cells enter the germinal center and undergo somatic hypermutation (SHM) of the immunoglobulin variable region genes.[29] The detection of mutations in these genes is taken as evidence of transit through the germinal center, and germinal center neoplasms show evidence of ongoing mutations. NMZLs are heterogeneous with respect to SHM frequency. Most studies have shown evidence of SHM,[3,5,30-33] but rare cases are unmutated.[3,30] Conconi and

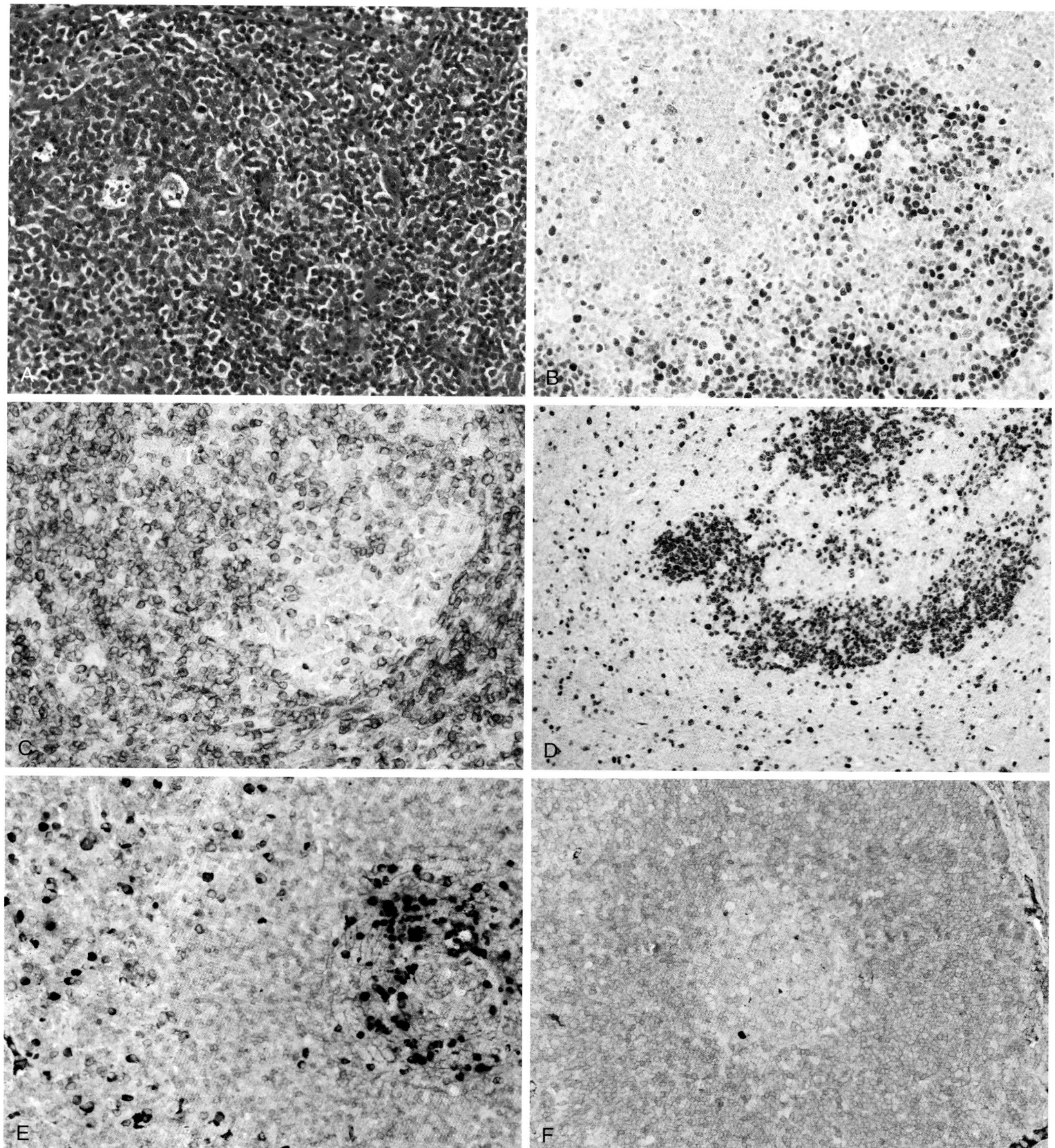

Figure 20-5. Follicular colonization in nodal marginal zone lymphoma (NMZL). A, Germinal center at *left* is partially infiltrated and replaced by neoplastic cells. "Starry sky" macrophages are noted within the disrupted germinal center. **B**, With BCL6 immunostain, the residual germinal center cells are BCL6$^+$, whereas infiltrating NMZL cells are BCL6$^-$. **C**, With BCL2 immunostain, the infiltrating NMZL cells are BCL2$^+$, whereas normal germinal center cells are BCL2$^-$. **D**, Residual germinal center is highlighted by a high proliferation rate with MIB-1. The surrounding neoplastic cells have a low proliferation rate. **E**, In another case, the cells colonizing the germinal center show plasmacytoid differentiation and are lambda light-chain restricted. Cells outside the germinal center also show light-chain restriction. **F**, Kappa is negative in corresponding areas.

associates[30] postulated that NMZL may arise from different subsets of marginal zone B cells, with representatives from virgin B cells that are unmutated, memory B cells with SHM, and even germinal center B cells with ongoing mutations. Most cases, however, do not show evidence of antigen selection.[14] The presence or absence of SHM might correlate with immunophenotype, as Conconi's group found that the only unmutated case was IgD+. The numbers are small, but two studies found selected usage of *VH4* and *VH3* gene segments, respectively.[3,5] Another study found differences in *VH* gene usage between those NMZLs associated with hepatitis C and those lacking this association, with the preferential usage of *VH1-69* in the former group.[31] Notably, *VH1-69* is preferentially used by both normal B cells and neoplastic B cells responding to the E2 viral antigen.[34] The B-cell receptors of selected B-cell lymphomas were shown to bind the hepatitis C viral envelope protein, implicating the virus in lymphoma pathogenesis.[35]

Consistent cytogenetic aberrations have not been identified in NMZL.[14] Numerical abnormalities are most common, with reports of +3, +7, +12, and +18 being most frequent.[14,36] Both duplication of chromosome 3 and gains in several regions, as identified by comparative genomic hybridization, have been reported.[37] A more recent study employing array comparative genomic hybridization identified gains in 3q11-q29 in two of nine cases of NMZL and confirmed the frequent presence of trisomy 3.[38] Other newly identified imbalances in NMZL included gains in 6p and deletions in 1p36 and 19q13.2. Notably, the genetic and genomic changes in NMZL differ from those reported in EMZL and LPL, providing additional evidence for a distinction among these disorders.[38,39] One exception to this statement is the recent report of both somatic mutations and genomic deletions of the NF-κB–negative regulator *TNFAIP3* (A20) in at least some cases of all marginal zone lymphoma types, including 18% of EMZLs, 8% of SMZLs, and 33% of NMZLs. Interestingly, this aberration provides evidence for constitutive NF-κB activation in all types of MZL.[40]

POSTULATED CELL OF ORIGIN

NMZLs are heterogeneous and are thought to be related to different subsets of marginal zone or memory B cells.[30] The morphologic, immunophenotypic, and genetic heterogeneity of these lymphomas is likely a reflection of the involvement of different B-cell subsets found within the marginal zone.[10] Marginal zone B cells can be both IgD positive and negative. They can show low levels of SHM, indicative of a pre–germinal center stage of maturation, or high levels of SHM.[41] In animal models a variety of cell types populate the marginal zone, including recirculating virgin B cells that can expand by a T-independent mechanism, and memory B cells generated in germinal centers. A direct relationship of NMZL to the parasinusoidal monocytoid B cells seen in *Toxoplasma* lymphadenitis has not been suggested in most studies.[25]

CLINICAL COURSE AND PROGNOSTIC FACTORS

NMZL is considered an indolent or "low grade" B-cell lymphoma. However, the 5-year overall survival is somewhat less than that seen for follicular lymphoma and CLL, two of the most common low-grade B-cell neoplasms. Most studies have reported 5-year overall survival in the range of 55% to 75%, with better outcomes in more recent series, possibly reflecting the increased use of rituximab.[3,5,14,23] The complete remission rate is approximately 50%, with progression-free or event-free survival at 5 years generally between 30% and 40%.[14] Because most patients are in the low or low-intermediate IPI risk groups, the IPI has not been especially useful as a prognostic marker; however, the FLIPI appears to be more predictive.[4,6]

As noted earlier, biologic markers have shown some promise in predicting outcome in NMZL. These include negative staining for survivin and active caspase 3 and increased expression of cyclin E, all of which are associated with a more aggressive clinical course.[5] However, these results are all from a single study and have yet to be confirmed. The role of Ki-67/MIB-1 is controversial as a predictive factor.

PEDIATRIC NODAL MARGINAL ZONE LYMPHOMA

Morphology and Immunophenotype

NMZL presenting in the pediatric age group has distinctive morphologic and clinical features, and in the 2008 World Health Organization classification it is delineated as a separate entity or variant (Table 20-2).[42] In affected lymph nodes the atypical cells have a predominantly interfollicular distribution, with marked expansion of the marginal zone (Fig. 20-6). The infiltrate is polymorphic, composed of monocytoid cells, centrocyte-like cells, and plasma cells.[20,43] Blasts are usually present but few in number—no more than two or three per high-power field. A characteristic feature, seen in most pediatric cases (70%), is follicular expansion, sharing some features with progressive transformation of germinal centers. The appearance of these atypical follicles is similar to that of the floral variant of NMZL.[21] In contrast to typical progressive transformation of germinal centers, the peripheral rims of the follicles are irregular, with blurring and disruption by the atypical proliferation in the marginal zone. The overall size of the follicles is expanded; the fragmented and irregular mantle zones are best visualized with stains for IgD. In some cases the atypical follicles show evidence of follicular colonization.

Plasmacytoid differentiation is best documented by stains for cytoplasmic immunoglobulin, and atypical cells showing light-chain restriction are seen in both the marginal zones and

Table 20-2 Comparison of Adult and Pediatric Nodal Marginal Zone Lymphoma (NMZL)

Feature	Adult NMZL	Pediatric NMZL
Male-to-female ratio	1:1	5:1 (higher in those <18 yr)
Median age (yr)	50-60	16
Stage	III-IV in up to 50%	Usually I
Sites of involvement	Peripheral LNs Bone marrow −/+	Cervical LNs
Prognosis	Moderately aggressive	Excellent Conservative management advised
Follicular hyperplasia with PTGC-like changes	−	+

LN, lymph node; PTGC, progressive transformation of germinal centers.

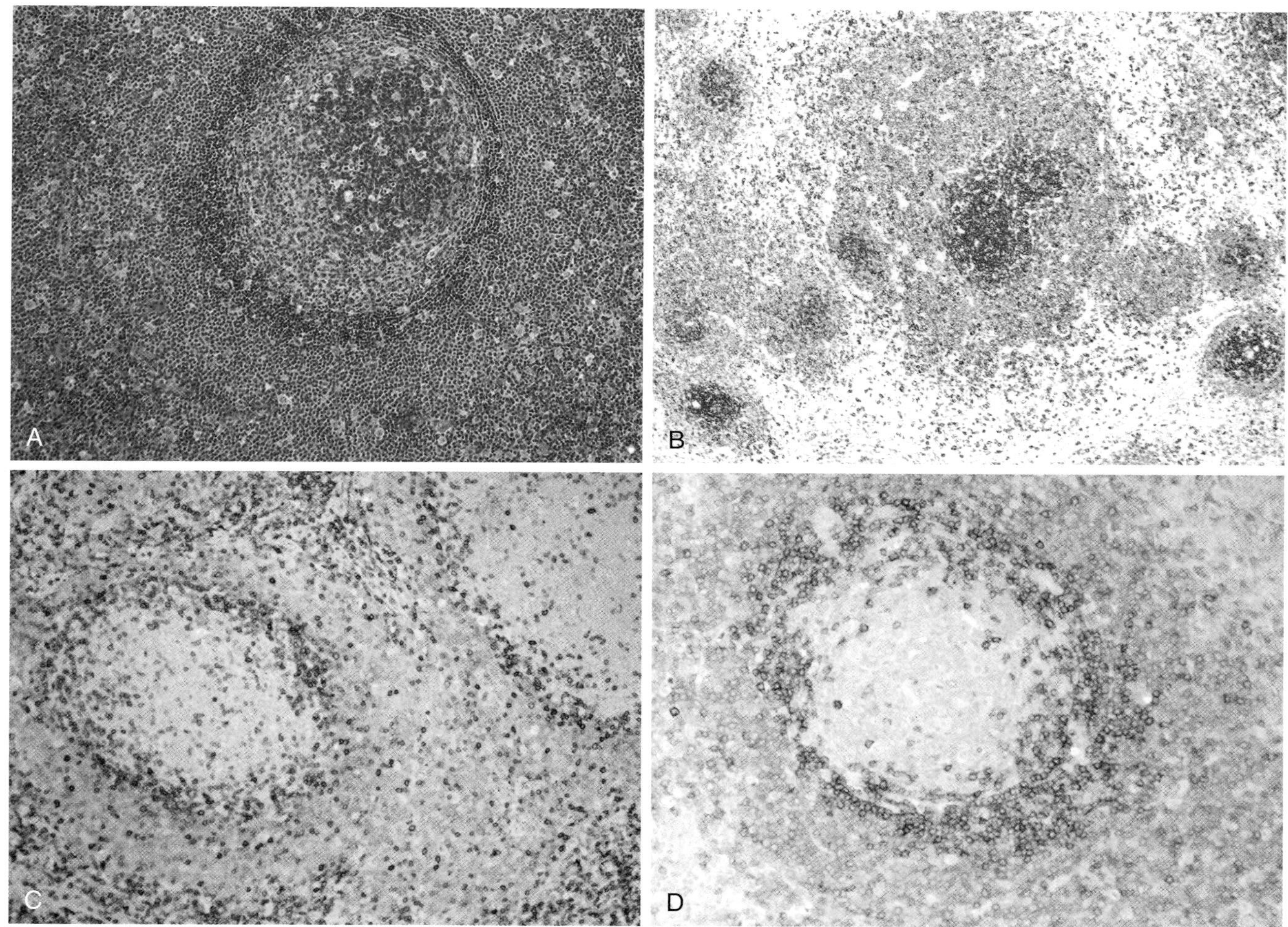

Figure 20-9. Chronic lymphocytic leukemia–small lymphocytic lymphoma (CLL/SLL) with a parafollicular marginal zone pattern. A, Reactive follicle is surrounded by a rim of CLL cells, resembling an expanded marginal zone. **B,** CLL cells show dim CD20 expression, contrasting with more intense staining of follicular B cells. **C,** CLL cells show dim CD5 expression. There is a thin rim of $CD5^+$ T cells at the periphery of the germinal center. **D,** The thin mantle cuff is strongly IgD^+, whereas the CLL cells are dimly IgD^+.

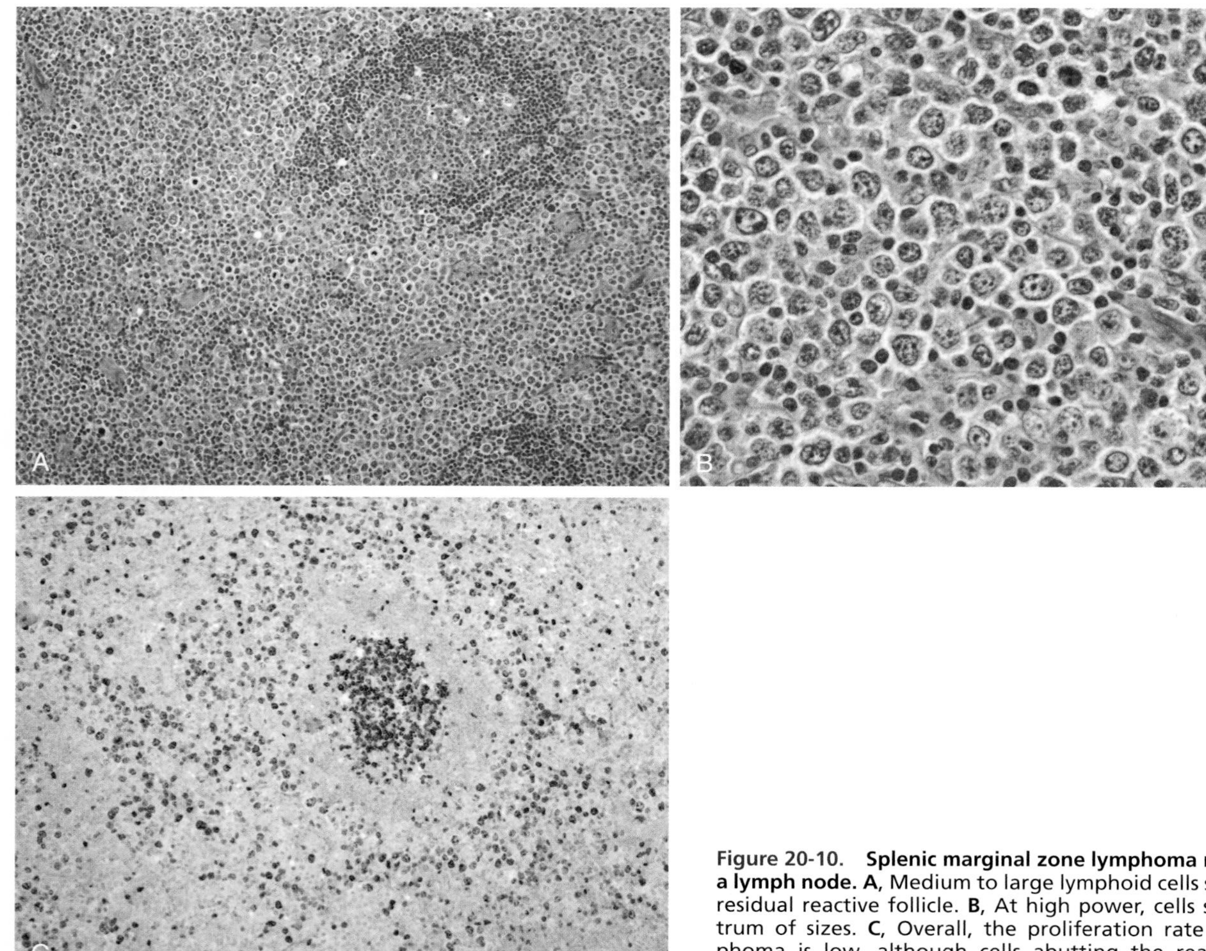

Figure 20-10. Splenic marginal zone lymphoma recurrence in a lymph node. **A**, Medium to large lymphoid cells surround the residual reactive follicle. **B**, At high power, cells show a spectrum of sizes. **C**, Overall, the proliferation rate of the lymphoma is low, although cells abutting the reactive follicle show a somewhat higher proliferation rate (MIB-1/Ki-67).

Pearls and Pitfalls

- NMZL is most often a diagnosis of exclusion, after other low grade B-cell lymphoma subtypes have been ruled out.
- In NMZL with prominent monocytoid B cells (MALT type), the diagnosis of secondary EMZL should be considered and ruled out clinically.
- Both NMZL and LPL may show plasmacytoid differentiation.
  - NMZL contains many different cell types—polymorphic cytology.
  - LPL contains few cell types—monomorphic cytology.
- NMZL with follicular colonization may closely mimic follicular lymphoma.
- The proportion of "blastic" or transformed cells varies widely, but no grading of NMZL is required or recommended.
- The pediatric variant of NMZL usually presents with localized, stage I disease and may be managed conservatively, following surgical excision of the nodal mass.

References can be found on Expert Consult @ www.expertconsult.com

Chapter 21

Mantle Cell Lymphoma

Elias Campo, Pedro Jares, and Elaine S. Jaffe

CHAPTER OUTLINE

DEFINITION

Mantle cell lymphoma (MCL) is defined in the World Health Organization (WHO) classification as a B-cell neoplasm composed of monomorphic small to medium-sized lymphoid cells with irregular nuclei that morphologically resemble centrocytes but often have slightly less irregular nuclear contours. Neoplastic transformed cells (centroblasts), paraimmunoblasts, and pseudofollicles are absent. The tumor cells are of a B-cell phenotype coexpressing CD5.[1] This neoplasm is genetically characterized by 11q13 translocations and rearrangement of the BCL1 region, leading to a constant overexpression of cyclin D1, which plays an important pathogenetic role in tumor development. These genetic and molecular aberrations have been crucial in recognizing MCL as a distinct disease entity and establishing precise diagnostic criteria, which in turn have allowed the identification of a broader spectrum of morphologic and clinical manifestations in MCL patients.[2]

MCL includes the previously recognized centrocytic lymphoma in the Kiel classification,[3] as well as different subtypes of B-cell lymphomas identified in the American literature under the terms *lymphocytic lymphoma of intermediate differentiation*,[4] *intermediate lymphocytic lymphoma*,[5] and *mantle zone lymphoma*.[6] The evolution in the knowledge and conceptual understanding of this lymphoma is an example of how a multidisciplinary approach to the study of these neoplasms, including morphology, phenotype, genetics, and molecular biology, can lead to a better definition of a disease.[2,7] The biologic behavior of most MCLs is very aggressive, and few patients are considered cured or achieve long survival with current therapeutic protocols. New strategies are needed to overcome the resistance of this aggressive lymphoma to conventional treatments.

EPIDEMIOLOGY AND CLINICAL MANIFESTATIONS

MCL represents 2.5% to 10% of all non-Hodgkin's lymphomas and occurs in elderly men (male-to-female ratio, 1.6 to 6.8:1) with a median age of approximately 60 years (range, 29 to 85 years) (Table 21-1). The reason for this male predominance is unknown. The mean annual incidence of this lymphoma has been estimated at 0.42 per 100,000 (range, 0.38 to 0.49), with a mean of 0.7 for men and 0.2 for women.[8] Similar to chronic lymphocytic leukemia (CLL), MCL may occur in families, associated with other lymphoid neoplasms.[9] More than 70% of patients present with stage IV disease with generalized lymphadenopathy and bone marrow involvement; bulky disease and B symptoms are less common (see Table 21-1).[10-20] Hepatosplenomegaly is relatively frequent, and massive splenomegaly is observed in 30% to 60% of cases. Pathologic splenic rupture may be the initial presentation of MCL.[21] Some patients have prominent splenomegaly with minimal or absent peripheral lymphadenopathy. This presentation is usually associated with peripheral blood involvement, and the differential diagnosis with other lymphoid leukemias may be difficult.[22,23]

Extranodal involvement is frequent in MCL. Tumor infiltration in more than two extranodal sites is observed in 30% to 50% of patients. However, an extranodal presentation without apparent nodal involvement occurs in only 4% to 15% of cases. Gastrointestinal involvement has been reported in 10% to 25% of patients, either at presentation or during the course of the disease. A peculiar manifestation of this involvement is lymphomatoid polyposis, in which multiple lymphoid polyps are identified in the small and large bowel. These patients may present with abdominal pain and melena.[24] Asymptomatic involvement of the gastrointestinal tract with no macroscopic lesions is very common, but detection of this microscopic infiltration rarely modifies the clinical management of patients.[25] Central nervous system involvement occurs in 10% to 20% of patients. In contrast to other extranodal sites, central nervous system involvement usually appears late in the clinical course and is associated with resistant disease or generalized relapse, with ominous significance.[26,27] Clinical manifestations include paraparesis, diplopia, and facial palsy. These patients frequently have advanced-stage disease, extensive infiltration in other extranodal localizations, and a leukemic phase. Other extranodal sites commonly involved are Waldeyer's ring, lung, and pleura (5% to 20%). Less common localizations are skin, breast, soft tissue, thyroid, salivary gland, peripheral nerve, conjunctiva, and orbit.[10,20]

Peripheral blood involvement at diagnosis varies among studies, depending in part on the disease definition. Conventional examination may detect leukemic involvement at diagnosis in 20% to 70% of patients. Atypical lymphoid cells may be observed in the peripheral blood in the absence of lymphocytosis,[16] and they may be detected by flow cytometry in virtually all patients.[28] Some patients present with leukemic involvement and no or minimal nodal disease.[23] Leukemic involvement may also appear during the evolution of the disease and may represent a manifestation of disease progression.[29,30] Some patients present with a very aggressive leukemic form mimicking acute leukemia. These cases have blastoid morphology; complex karyotypes, occasionally with 8q24 anomalies; and a very rapid evolution, with a median survival of only 3 months.[31-33]

Anemia and thrombocytopenia occur in 10% to 40% of patients, and high lactate dehydrogenase and β_2-microglobulin levels are detected in approximately 50% of cases. A monoclonal serum component, usually at low levels, has been reported in 10% to 30% of patients.[12,20,34] However, the immunoglobulin isotype is different in the serum and tumor cell surface in some cases. A second neoplasm detected before, concomitant with, or after the diagnosis of MCL has been reported in 12% to 21% of patients, with a certain predominance of urinary tract tumors; this suggests that patients with MCL may have an increased incidence of second malignancies.[10,35]

Table 21-1 Clinical Characteristics of Mantle Cell Lymphoma at Presentation

Characteristic	Percentage of Patients (Range)
Median age: 60 yr (range, 29-85 yr)	—
Male-to-female ratio: 3:1 (range, 1.6-6.8:1)	—
Sites of involvement	
Generalized lymphadenopathy	80 (75-87)
Bone marrow	71 (53-82)
Spleen (splenomegaly)	51 (27-59)
Liver (hepatomegaly)	20 (11-35)
Gastrointestinal tract	16 (9-24)
Waldeyer's ring	9 (2-18)
Lung/pleura	9 (2-17)
Peripheral blood	39 (24-53)
Bulky disease (≥10 cm)	18 (5-25)
Poor performance status	24 (6-51)
B symptoms	28 (14-50)
Elevated lactate dehydrogenase	37 (16-55)
Elevated β_2-microglobulin	52 (50-55)
Stage III-IV	81 (72-89)

POSTULATED CELL OF ORIGIN

MCL is derived in most cases from a subset of naïve pre–germinal center B cells expressing CD5. Human $CD5^+$ B cells are present in fetal lymphoid tissues and blood and decrease with age. In adults, $CD5^+$ B cells circulate in small numbers and localize in primary follicles and mantle zones of secondary follicles. Owing to the topologic distribution of tumor cells surrounding naked germinal centers and the positivity for alkaline phosphatase, early studies suggested a relationship between this tumor and cells of the primary lymphoid follicle or the mantle cells of secondary follicles.[36] However, CD5 expression in MCL is very high, resembling the intensity observed in fetal B cells, in contrast to the low levels detected in the subset of adult follicular mantle cells.[37] MCLs also maintain the expression of different genes normally expressed in naïve and follicular mantle zone cells, such as TCL-1,[38] tyrosine phosphatase SHP1,[39] and the polycomb group member BMI1.[40,41]

Most MCLs have few or no somatic mutations in immunoglobulin variable region heavy-chain (*IGHV*) genes, confirming an origin from pre–germinal center cells. However, somatic hypermutations are detected in 15% to 40% of MCLs, indicating that some tumors originate in cells that have undergone the influence of the mutational machinery of the follicular germinal center. The rate of mutations in MCL is lower than that in other lymphoid neoplasms such as CLL or follicular lymphoma, suggesting a weaker influence of the germinal center microenvironment.[42] A biased use of the *IGHV3-21*, *IGHV3-23*, and *IGHV4-34* genes has been detected in MCL, suggesting that these tumors may originate from specific subsets of B cells. However, in contrast to CLL, tumors with *IGHV3-21* genes occur mainly in unmutated MCLs, show a tendency for longer patient survival,[43,44] and seem to have fewer genomic imbalances.[45] Contrary to CLL, the mutational status of the *IGVH* genes in MCL does not correlate with survival or zeta-associated protein-70 (ZAP-70) expression.[44,46] Interestingly, MCLs with a leukemic, non-nodal clinical presentation, which are associated with longer survival, have frequent mutated *IGVH* genes.[23]

MORPHOLOGY

The architectural and cytologic features of MCL have a broader spectrum than was recognized in early descriptions of the tumor. Although these pathologic characteristics are distinctive of MCL, the similarities between some morphologic variants and other non-Hodgkin's lymphomas may require the use of ancillary studies to clarify the differential diagnosis (Table 21-2).

Table 21-2 Major Diagnostic Features in Mantle Cell Lymphoma

Morphology	Description
Architectural pattern	Mantle zone, nodular, or diffuse
Cytologic variants	
Classic	Monotonous proliferation of small to intermediate-sized lymphoid cells Nucleus with slightly cleaved contour and absence of nucleolus Small cell variant with rounded nuclei, mimicking chronic lymphocytic leukemia Absence of centroblasts, prolymphocytes, or paraimmunoblasts
Blastoid	Intermediate-sized cells Round nuclei with finely dispersed chromatin Inconspicuous nucleoli Very high mitotic index
Pleomorphic	Intermediate-sized to large cells Irregular nuclei with dispersed chromatin and possible small nucleoli High mitotic index
Small cell	Small, round lymphocytes with more clumped chromatin Absence of prolymphocytes, paraimmunoblasts, and proliferation growth centers
Marginal zone–like	Tumor cells with broad, pale cytoplasm Nucleus may have typical or blastoid morphology
Other features	Dispersed "pink" histiocytes without apoptotic bodies (occasional classic "starry sky" pattern in blastoid variants) Hyalinized small vessels
Immunophenotype	B-cell markers with coexpression of CD5 and CD43 Constant cyclin D1 positivity Usually negative for CD10, BCL6, CD23, MUM-1
Genetic	Constant t(11;14)(q13;q32) Complex karyotypes in blastoid variants Tetraploid clones in pleomorphic and blastic variants

Architectural Patterns

Nodal involvement by MCL usually results in effacement of the architecture, with three possible growth patterns: mantle zone, nodular, or diffuse (Fig. 21-1). The mantle zone pattern is characterized by expansion of the follicle mantle area by tumor cells surrounding a reactive "naked" germinal center.[6,14] This pattern may be associated with partial preservation of the nodal architecture, and it may be difficult to distinguish from follicular or mantle cell hyperplasias.[47] Transitional areas between nodular and diffuse patterns are common, but in rare cases, nodularity is prominent, leading to a misinterpretation of follicular lymphoma.[29] However, some nodules may be solid, without evidence of residual germinal centers, representing the malignant counterpart of primary follicles. Alternatively, the nodular pattern may be due to a massive infiltration and obliteration of the original germinal center by tumor cells. In some cases, cyclin D1 staining may help identify initial infiltration or colonization of reactive germinal centers, which may correspond to early stages of a nodular pattern (Fig. 21-2). Residual germinal centers can also be seen in tumors with a more diffuse pattern, although in these cases, they may be identified only focally.

Cytologic Variants

Classic (common or typical) MCLs are characterized by a monotonous proliferation of small to medium-sized lymphoid cells with scant cytoplasm, variably irregular nuclei, evenly distributed condensed chromatin, and inconspicuous nucleoli (Fig. 21-3). Large cells with abundant cytoplasm or prominent nucleoli are rare or absent; when present, they may correspond to reactive centroblasts of residual germinal centers overrun by lymphoma cells. Occasional cases may show a predominance of small lymphocytes with rounded nuclei (see Fig. 21-3). This variant may be difficult to distinguish from chronic lymphocytic leukemia–small lymphocytic lymphoma (CLL/SLL). However, proliferation centers (growth centers) or isolated prolymphocytes and paraimmunoblasts are absent in MCL. No differences in clinical behavior have been observed between this small cell variant and classic cases, but it is important to recognize this variant to avoid the misdiagnosis of CLL. Proliferative activity in classic and small cell MCL varies from case to case but is usually lower than 1 to 2 mitoses per high-power field. However, some tumors with a classic morphology may show a relatively high mitotic index, similar to the blastoid variants, and these patients may have an aggressive clinical course.[48,49] Scattered epithelioid histiocytes with eosinophilic cytoplasm are relatively common, but well-formed microgranulomas are not usually seen (Fig. 21-4). These histiocytes generally do not contain phagocytosed apoptotic bodies. Nuclei of follicular dendritic cells with the typical features of overlapping nuclei, delicate nuclear membranes, and an "empty" chromatin appearance are

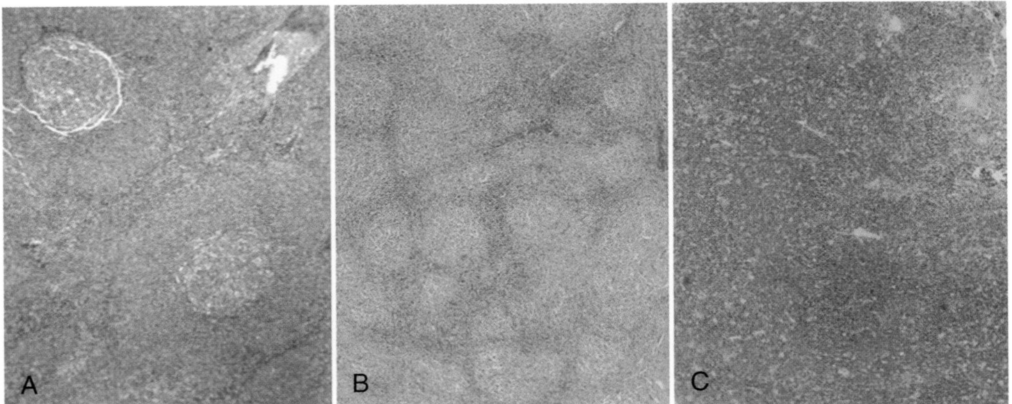

Figure 21-1. Architectural patterns in mantle cell lymphoma. A, Mantle zone pattern: the tumor cells expand the mantle cell cuff surrounding a reactive germinal center. **B,** Nodular pattern: the nodules are composed of tumor cells without evidence of residual germinal centers. **C,** Diffuse pattern: the lymph node is diffusely infiltrated by tumor cells.

frequently identified. In some cases, hyalinized small vessels may be seen scattered throughout the tumor.

More aggressive variants of MCL may have a morphology that ranges from a monotonous population of cells resembling lymphoblasts (blastoid variant) to a more pleomorphic appearance with larger irregular cells resembling diffuse large B-cell lymphoma (see Fig. 21-3). These variants may represent the ends of a morphologic spectrum; transitional areas between these subtypes may be observed, and some tumors have very discordant cytology, with areas of pleomorphic cells intermingled with others having a classic morphology.[42,50] These cytologic variants have the same phenotype and genetic alterations, including 11q13 translocations and cyclin D1 overexpression, as classic MCL, indicating that they correspond to the same entity.[51,52]

Blastoid MCL is characterized by a monotonous population of medium-sized lymphocytes with scant cytoplasm, rounded nuclei with finely dispersed chromatin, and inconspicuous nucleoli.[51] These cases may resemble lymphoblastic lymphoma or nodal involvement by acute myeloid leukemias. The mitotic index is very high, with more than 2 to 3 mitoses per high-power field. Histiocytes with tingible bodies and a "starry sky" pattern may be seen.

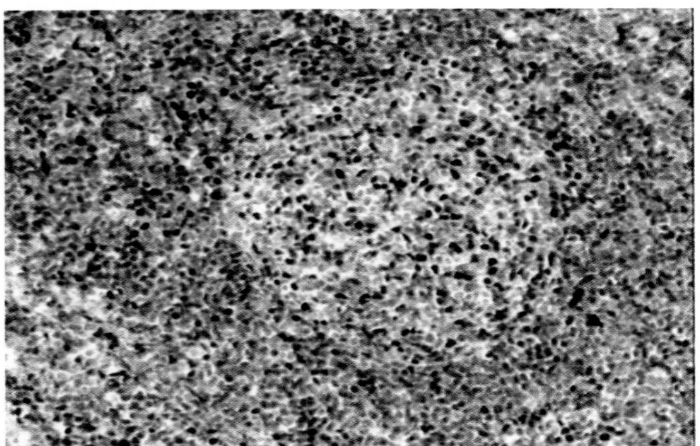

Figure 21-2. Colonization of a reactive germinal center by tumor cells highlighted by cyclin D1 staining.

MCLs with a more pleomorphic or large cell morphology were initially designated in the Kiel classification as *anaplastic centrocytic lymphomas* or *centroblastic lymphomas of the centrocytoid subtype*.[53,54] These tumors are composed of a more heterogeneous population of large cells with ovoid or irregular, cleaved nuclei; finely dispersed chromatin; and small, distinct nucleoli (see Fig. 21-3). The mitotic index is high but usually lower than in blastic cases. In some cases mitotic figures may show a striking hyperchromatic staining, with an apparently high number of chromosomes. This finding is usually associated with the presence of tetraploid clones.[55] This pleomorphic variant may be difficult to distinguish from large cell lymphomas. However, the nuclear characteristics of cleaved contours, finely dispersed chromatin, and discordance between the large nuclei and relatively small nucleoli may suggest a mantle cell origin. Ancillary studies are mandatory in these cases to confirm the diagnosis. Some leukemic MCLs, described as *prolymphocytic variants* of MCL, may in fact represent leukemic forms of the pleomorphic subtype of MCL.[56-59]

Some cases may have a variable number of cells with more abundant pale cytoplasm, mimicking monocytoid B cells (Fig. 21-5).[60] The nucleus of these cells may have a blastoid or classic morphology, but the peculiar cytoplasm may raise the possibility of marginal zone lymphomas or hairy cell leukemia. In some cases, these monocytoid-like cells may even expand to the marginal zone of lymphoid follicles, outside an apparently preserved mantle zone. CD5 and cyclin D1 positivity is crucial in the diagnosis of this variant. Some rare cases of MCL may have a clonally related plasma cell differentiation.[61]

Bone Marrow and Peripheral Blood

Bone marrow infiltration, independent of peripheral blood involvement, occurs in 50% to 91% of patients[16,62,63] and is detected more frequently in core biopsies than in aspirates.[64] Bilateral biopsies may account for the higher bone marrow involvement in some series.[64] The pattern of infiltration may be nodular, interstitial, or paratrabecular, with most biopsies exhibiting a combination of these. Isolated paratrabecular aggregates are rare. In some cases diffuse infiltration of the marrow may be seen. The degree of infiltration does not seem

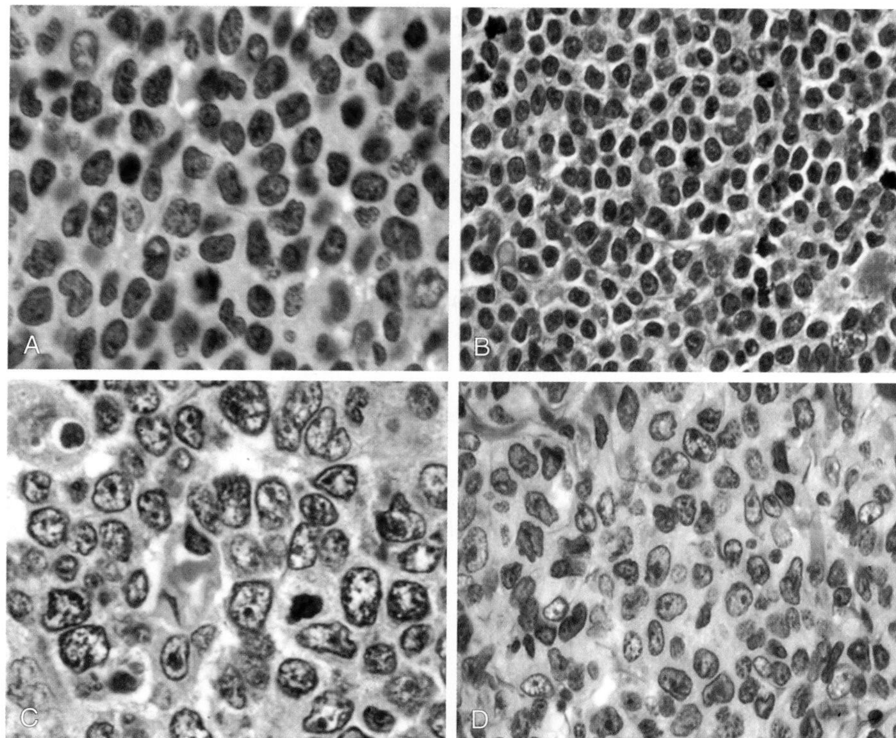

Figure 21-3. Cytologic variants of mantle cell lymphoma (MCL). A, Typical or classic MCL is characterized by small to medium-sized lymphocytes with irregular nuclei, condensed chromatin, and scant cytoplasm. **B,** The small cell variant is composed of small lymphocytes with rounded nuclei, simulating chronic lymphocytic leukemia. However, prolymphocytes and paraimmunoblasts are absent. **C,** In the blastoid variant, the tumor cells are medium-sized lymphocytes with rounded nuclei, finely distributed chromatin, inconspicuous or very small nucleoli, and a high mitotic index. **D,** The pleomorphic variant is composed of large cells with very irregular nuclei.

to correlate with the histologic variants of MCL identified in lymph node biopsies, architectural patterns, or patient survival.[64] Immunohistochemical stains, including cyclin D1 and p27, can be used in the differential diagnosis of bone marrow biopsies to distinguish MCL from other small cell lymphomas.[63,65]

The tumor cells' cytologic appearance in peripheral blood and bone marrow aspirates is similar to the spectrum seen in tissue samples (Fig. 21-6). Circulating cells in most MCLs usually show a mixture of small to medium-sized cells with scant cytoplasm, prominent nuclear irregularities, and reticular chromatin. Some cells may have rounded nuclei, but the chromatin does not have the clumped appearance seen in CLL. Leukemic blastoid MCL may mimic acute leukemia, with medium to large cells, a high nuclear-to-cytoplasmic ratio, fine dispersed chromatin, and relatively small or inconspicuous nucleoli. A number of studies have reported cases of leukemic MCL with very large atypical cells and prominent nucleoli that seem to correspond to a leukemic phase of the pleomorphic variant of MCL.[56-58] In fact, some of these cases have hyperdiploid karyotypes[56] and have been associated with a pleomorphic variant of MCL in the lymph nodes.[59] Cases previously diagnosed as B-prolymphocytic leukemia carrying the t(11;14) translocation and cyclin D1 overexpression are now considered leukemic MCL.[1]

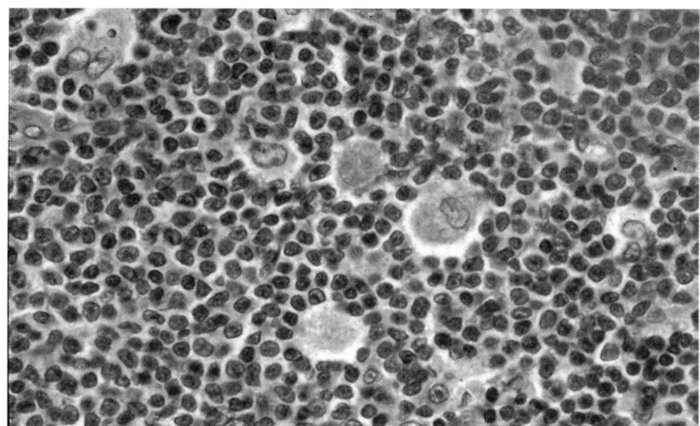

Figure 21-4. Classic variant of mantle cell lymphoma with scattered histiocytes with eosinophilic cytoplasm.

Spleen

Macroscopically, splenic involvement by MCL shows a generalized micronodular pattern that is occasionally associated with perivascular infiltration. Histologically, the differential diagnosis of MCL and other small cell lymphomas in the spleen may be difficult.[22,66,67] White pulp nodules are enlarged, with variable involvement of the red pulp. Residual "naked" germinal centers are found in 50% of cases. Tumor cells show a similar monotonous morphology as in other locations. Interestingly, some cases may exhibit a marginal zone–like area at the periphery of the nodules, comprising cells with more abundant pale cytoplasm.[67]

Gastrointestinal Tract

A common manifestation of gastrointestinal disease is lymphomatoid polyposis, in which multiple lymphoid polyps are identified in the small and large bowel (Fig. 21-7). These may be associated with large tumor masses, usually ileocecal, and regional lymphadenopathy.[24,68,69] Although this clinicopathologic presentation is relatively characteristic of MCL, it can also be caused by other non-Hodgkin's lymphomas, particularly follicular lymphoma and marginal zone lymphoma of the

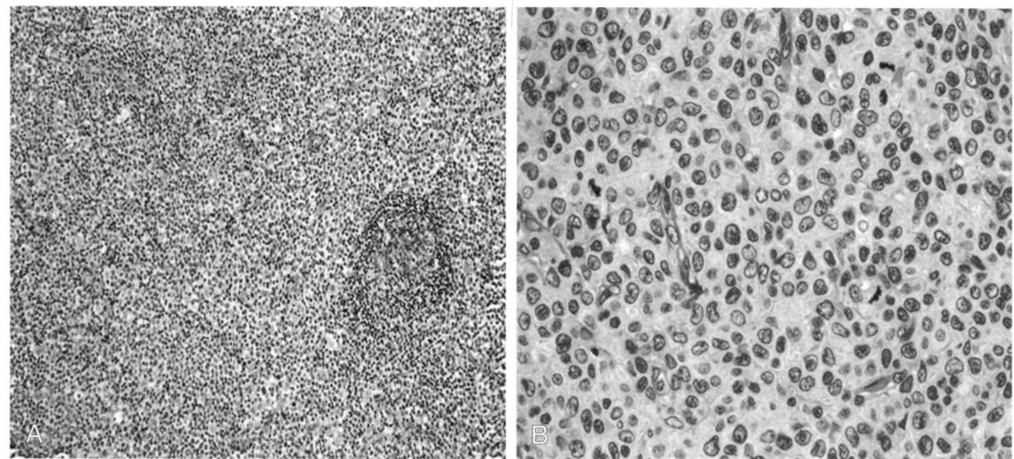

Figure 21-5. Mantle cell lymphoma with a marginal zone pattern. A, Tumor cells expand the marginal zone area outside an apparent preserved mantle cuff. In some of these cases, cyclin D1 staining may show that this mantle area is composed of tumor cells with less cytoplasm. **B,** Tumor cells in the marginal zone area have abundant pale cytoplasm, resembling monocytoid cells.

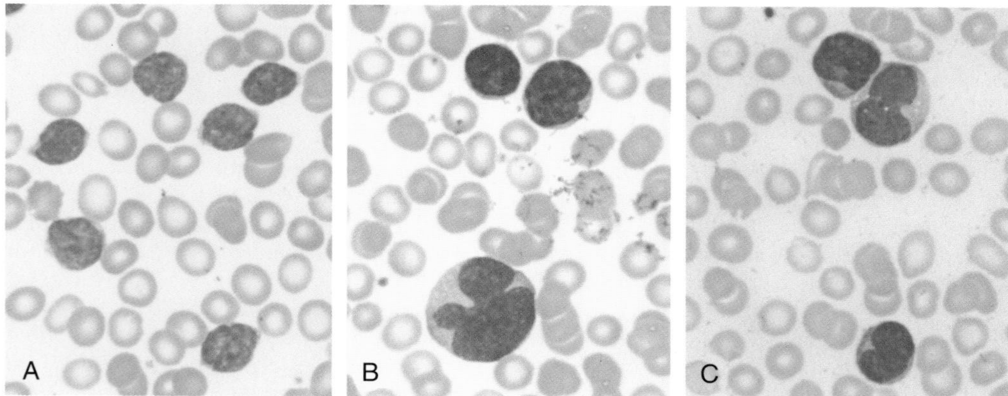

Figure 21-6. Cytologic spectrum of tumor cells in peripheral blood smears of leukemic mantle cell lymphoma. A, Tumor cells in classic variant are small lymphocytes with slightly indented or cleaved nuclei, condensed chromatin, and scant cytoplasm. **B,** Blastoid variant may show a mixture of small atypical cells and larger pleomorphic tumor cells with irregular nuclei. **C,** In other cases, all atypical cells have a more blastic morphology, with finely dispersed chromatin and inconspicuous nucleoli (Giemsa stain).

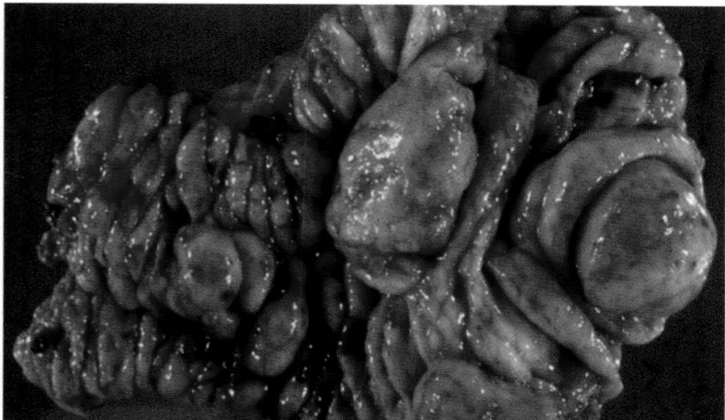

Figure 21-7. Mantle cell lymphoma involving the intestine with multiple lymphomatous polyposis. Small polyps are associated with larger tumor masses. (Courtesy of Dr. T. Alvaro, Hospital Verge de la Cinta, Tortosa, Spain.)

mucosa-associated lymphoid tissue (MALT) type.[69,70] Cyclin D1 expression and BCL1 rearrangement are useful for the differential diagnosis of these tumors.[68] Gastrointestinal involvement without the macroscopic appearance of polyposis may also occur.[71] In these cases, superficial ulcers, large tumor masses, and diffuse thickening of the mucosa are common macroscopic findings. Microscopic infiltration of gastrointestinal mucosa by MCL without gross lesions is very common.[25] In some cases glandular infiltration by tumor cells may mimic lymphoepithelial lesions, making the distinction between MCL and marginal zone lymphomas difficult. However, the scarcity of these lesions and the monotonous character of the lymphoid infiltrate should suggest a diagnosis of MCL.[71] Interestingly, MCLs, as well as other non-Hodgkin's lymphomas involving gastrointestinal mucosa, express $\alpha_4\beta_7$-integrin, a homing receptor that binds to mucosal addressin cell adhesion molecule-1 (MAdCAM-1), which is selectively expressed in endothelial cells of mucosa.[72]

Histologic Progression

Studies of sequential biopsies have shown that the histologic pattern of MCL remains relatively stable.[10,51,73] In some cases, obliteration of residual germinal centers and nodular progression to a more diffuse pattern may be observed in serial biopsies.[10,73] Interestingly, some cases may show an oscillating course, with changing patterns during the evolution of the disease.[15] Increased numbers of large blastic cells and mitotic figures may be seen in 20% to 25% of patients. However, most blastoid MCLs are detected at diagnosis, and cytologic progression from classic MCL to a pure blastoid variant is relatively uncommon in sequential biopsies,[10] although it may be detected more frequently at autopsy.[15] A clonal relationship has been demonstrated in occasional cases of progression from classic to blastoid MCL.[74] In some cases tumor progression is associated with the development of an overt leukemic phase.[29,30]

Composite Mantle Cell Lymphoma and Other Lymphoproliferative Disorders

A few cases of MCL associated with a second malignant lymphoma at the same site have been reported. The MCL component has been found with follicular lymphoma,[75] CLL/SLL,[75] plasmacytoma,[76] multiple myeloma,[77] and Hodgkin's lymphoma.[78,79] The two components are recognized by the different morphology and distinct phenotype of the two lymphomas. Molecular studies have identified unrelated clonal rearrangements in these tumors, suggesting distinct clonal origins. However, two cases showed a common clone-specific *IGH* rearrangement in the MCL and the second lymphoma, suggesting the unusual evolution of a single malignant clone resulting in two morphologically, phenotypically, and molecularly distinct lymphomas.[78]

IMMUNOPHENOTYPE

MCL is a mature B-cell neoplasm expressing the B-cell markers CD19, CD20, CD22, and CD79a (Fig. 21-8; Table 21-3). Surface immunoglobulins are usually of moderate to strong intensity, with frequent coexpression of immunoglobulin (Ig) M and IgD and, in contrast to other B-cell lymphomas, a particular tendency to express lambda light chain more frequently than kappa (see Table 21-3). The residual germinal centers seen in these tumors are always polyclonal. A peculiar characteristic of MCL, similar to CLL/SLL, is coexpression of the T-cell–associated antigen CD5 in virtually all cases (see Fig. 21-8). However, occasional bona fide CD5$^-$ MCLs may be seen. In addition, CD43 is frequently expressed in these two lymphoid malignancies, but other T-cell antigens are usually negative. CD8[80] and CD7[81] positivity by flow cytometry has been reported in isolated cases of MCL. CD23 is usually negative in MCL, whereas this antigen is expressed in virtually all cases of CLL/SLL.[82,83] Rare cases of blastoid MCL have been reported to be CD23$^+$,[83] and dim CD23 expression may be detected by flow cytometry in a number of MCLs.[84] CD10 and BCL6, two cell markers associated with follicular center cells and follicular lymphomas, and MUM-1/IRF4, an antigen related to late stages of B-cell and plasma cell differentiation, are usually negative in MCL. However, occasional cases may show BCL6 staining, and CD10 positivity has been documented in some cases.[85-87]

Overexpression of cyclin D1 is a constant and highly specific phenomenon in MCL associated with genetic

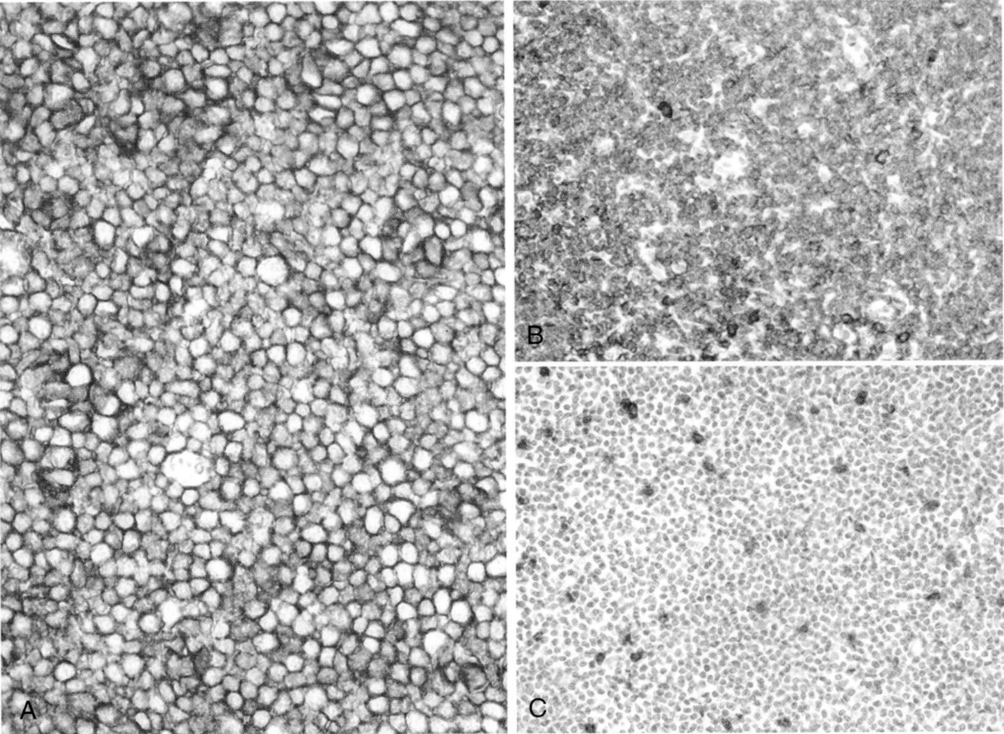

Figure 21-8. Mantle cell lymphoma immunophenotype. Tumor cells are strongly positive for CD20 (**A**), with coexpression of CD5 (**B**). CD3 is positive only in scattered reactive T cells (**C**) (immunoperoxidase stain).

Table 21-3 **Immunophenotype of Small Cell Malignant Lymphomas**

Diagnosis	Ig*	CD20	CD3	CD5	CD43	CD23	CD10	BCL6	Cyclin D1	IRF4/MUM-1	Annexin A_1
CLL	M/D	+	–	+	+	+	–	–	–	+/–†	–
MCL	M/D/λ	++	–	+	+	–	–	–	+	–	–
FL	M/G	++	–	–	–	–	+	+	–	–	–
LPL	M	++	–	–	+	–	–	–	–	+	–
MALT	M	++	–	–	–/+	–	–	–	–	+/–‡	–
SMZL	M/D	++	–	–	–	–	–	–	–	+/–‡	–
HCL	G/λ	++	–	–	–	–	–	–	–/+	–	+

*Kappa more commonly expressed than lambda, except as indicated.
†Positivity in occasional prolymphocytes and paraimmunoblasts.
‡Positivity in cells with plasmacytoid differentiation.
CLL, chronic lymphocytic leukemia; FL, follicular lymphoma; HCL, hairy cell leukemia; Ig, immunoglobulin; LPL, lymphoplasmacytic lymphoma; MALT, marginal zone B-cell lymphoma of mucosa-associated lymphoid tissue; MCL, mantle cell lymphoma; SMZL, splenic marginal zone lymphoma.

rearrangement of the *BCL1* locus (see later).[52,88,89] The development of different monoclonal antibodies has allowed the immunohistochemical detection of cyclin D1 in routine fixed and paraffin-embedded material, which is very useful for the diagnosis of this tumor (Fig. 21-9; see also Fig. 21-2).[63,90,91] However, this technique may be difficult to perform, and different protocols using heating methods and overnight incubation have been proposed.[92] A recently developed rabbit monoclonal antibody seems to provide more consistent cyclin D1 staining.[93] Bone marrow trephine biopsies may require particular attention.[94] In addition to immunohistochemistry, other strategies to detect cyclin D1 overexpression have been developed, including reverse transcription polymerase chain reaction (RT-PCR) on fresh-frozen material[95] or paraffin-embedded tissue and quantitative RT-PCR.[96] These alternative methods may be useful when routine immunohistochemistry is not successful or cannot be easily applied, such as in leukemic lymphoproliferative disorders or fine-needle aspirates. With sensitive methods, cyclin D1 overexpression is detected in virtually all MCLs.

Cyclin D1 is always detected in the cell nucleus, although the intensity may vary from cell to cell and case to case, probably reflecting parameters such as messenger RNA (mRNA) and protein stability as well as interaction with other proteins (see Fig. 21-9). Cyclin D1 is also detected in the nuclei of histiocytes, endothelial cells, and epithelial cells, providing an important internal positive control. In addition to MCL, cyclin D1 is expressed in 25% of multiple myelomas with the t(11;14) translocation, amplification of the gene, or without apparent structural alterations of the gene.[97] Low levels of cyclin D1 are also detected in hairy cell leukemia[98,99] and in cells of the proliferation centers in CLL, but this expression is not associated with *BCL1* rearrangement.[100] Cyclin D1 expression has been reported in occasional cases interpreted as splenic marginal zone lymphoma.[60,101] However, most of these tumors are negative by either Northern blot or immunohistochemical analysis.[102,103]

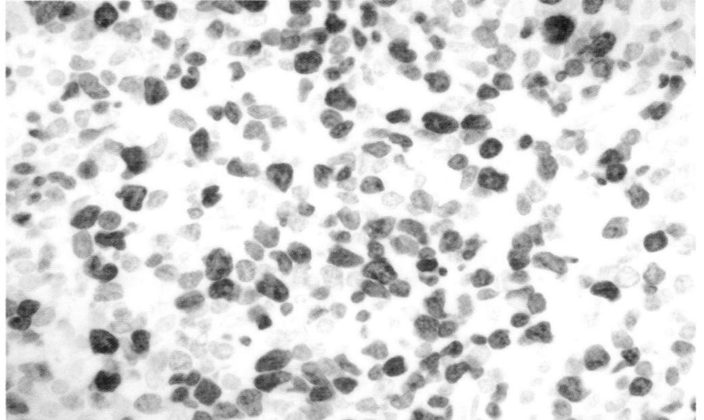

Figure 21-9. In mantle cell lymphoma, cyclin D1 is expressed in the nucleus of the cells with variable intensity (immunoperoxidase stain).

Immunohistochemical detection of the cyclin-dependent kinase (CDK) inhibitor $p27^{Kip1}$ is also useful in the differential diagnosis of MCL. Expression of $p27^{Kip1}$ in non-Hodgkin's lymphomas is usually inversely related to the proliferation activity of the cells. Thus, it is strongly expressed in CLL, follicular lymphomas, and marginal zone lymphomas, but it is negative or weakly expressed in large cell lymphomas. In MCL, p27 staining is independent of the proliferative rate and is usually negative in classic MCL and positive in blastoid variants.[104] Hairy cell leukemia is also negative or very weakly positive.[65] The mechanisms involved in this peculiar $p27^{Kip1}$ staining pattern in MCL and hairy cell leukemia are not fully understood (see later), but this staining pattern may be useful in the differential diagnosis of these tumors, particularly when cyclin D1 staining fails.[65]

Ki-67 staining with MIB-1 is helpful to assess the proliferative activity of these tumors, and a significant correlation among mitotic index, Ki-67 labeling, and S-phase has been found in MCLs.[105] In general, Ki-67 labeling is low in classic MCL and high in blastoid variants.[51,105] However, some cases with a classic morphology may have a relatively high Ki-67 index.[49]

MCL usually contains a prominent meshwork of follicular dendritic cells, which are more variable in frequency and distribution in diffuse cases than in nodular cases. In nodular cases, two different patterns of follicular dendritic cells have been recognized. A dense and concentric meshwork of cells may represent colonization of preexisting follicular centers by tumor cells, whereas a loose and irregular pattern may correspond to expansion of primary follicles.[106] Cyclin D1 staining may identify early infiltration of germinal centers by tumor cells.

CYTOGENETIC FINDINGS

The characteristic cytogenetic alteration in MCL is t(11;14)(q13;q32), although variant translocations involving the 11q13 breakpoint have been reported.[107] This translocation is detected by conventional cytogenetics in up to 65% of MCLs. However, using fluorescence in situ hybridization (FISH), it can be found in virtually all cases of MCL.[108-110] Initial studies reported t(11;14) in other lymphoproliferative disorders, but most of these tumors were likely misdiagnosed and probably represented MCL.[7] However, t(11;14) translocations have been identified in 5% of multiple myelomas.[7,111] B-prolymphocytic leukemia was defined before MCL was identified as a distinct entity, and a recent study revisiting these cases found that most B-prolymphocytic leukemias with t(11;14) probably correspond to MCL.[112] Molecular analysis of this translocation in MCL and multiple myeloma suggests that the mechanism in these tumors may be different, with an error in the V-D-J recombination in MCL and in the switch recombination process in myeloma.[113] In addition, cyclin D1 gene amplification without translocation has been documented in cases of multiple myeloma but not in MCL.[97]

Cytogenetic studies, including conventional analysis, FISH, comparative genomic hybridization, and array-based analysis, have revealed a high number of secondary chromosomal alterations in MCL.[114] A number of the genes targeted by these alterations have been identified or highly suggested (Table 21-4). The most common secondary alterations are losses of chromosomes 1p, 6q, 8p, 9p, 10p, 11q, 13, and 17p and gains in 3q, 7p, 8q, 12q, 18q, and Xq. Losses of chromosome 8p have been associated with a leukemic presentation in some studies[115] but not in others.[116-118] Blastoid variants have more complex karyotypes and more high-level DNA amplifications than classic variants.[31,55,119] In addition, certain chromosomal imbalances such as gains of 3q, 7p, and 12q and losses of 17p are significantly more frequent in blastoid than classic variants. Interestingly, tetraploidy is more frequent in pleomorphic (80%) and blastoid (36%) variants than in classic MCLs (8%).[55] Chromosome 8q24 alterations, including t(8;14)(q24;q32) and variants, have been identified in occasional blastoid MCLs with a very aggressive clinical course.[33,120] Recent studies using single nucleotide polymorphism arrays have identified frequent uniparental disomies in MCL that may be an alternative mechanism for the inactivation of mutated tumor suppressor genes such as *p53* at 17p21.[118]

MOLECULAR CHARACTERISTICS

Translocation (11;14)

The t(11;14) translocation juxtaposes the immunoglobulin heavy-chain joining region in chromosome 14 to a region on 11q13 designated BCL1 (B-cell lymphoma/leukemia 1). Other breakpoints far away from the original cloned region were also identified (Fig. 21-10). Most rearrangements (30% to 55%) occur in a region known as the *major translocation cluster* (MTC), whereas up to 10% to 20% of cases may have breakpoints in other distal regions. The MTC breakpoints occur within a relatively small region of around 80 base pairs on chromosome 11 and in the 5′ area of one of the immunoglobulin JH regions on chromosome 14, making it possible to detect this translocation by PCR techniques.[42]

Table 21-4 Commonly Altered Chromosomal Regions in Mantle Cell Lymphoma Detected by Comparative Genomic Hybridization[119,200] and Array-Based Genomic Analysis[118,156,164,167,201-204]

Chromosome Region*	Frequency (%)	Suggested Target Genes†	Functional Process
Gains			
3q25-qter	32-70	*ECT2, SERPINI2,* ?	?
4p12-13	57	?	?
7p21-22	16-34	*CARD11, GPR30, ETV1*	?
8q21-qter	16-36	***MYC***	Cell growth, proliferation, apoptosis
9q22	16-31	*SYK, GAS1, FANCC*	Cell signaling
10p11-12	12-24	*BMI1*	Cell cycle, DNA damage response, antisenescence
11q13.3	14	***CCND1***	Cell cycle
12q13	3-30	***CDK4***	Cell cycle
13q31.3	5-11	***[C13orf25]***	?
18q11-q23	18-55	***BCL2***	Antiapoptosis
Losses			
1p13-31	18-52	*GCLM, CDC14A, DPYD, CDKN2C, FAF1*	?
2q13	17	***BCL2L11***‡	Proapoptosis
6q23-q27	18-38	*TNFAIP3, IFNGR1*	
8p21-pter	17-34	*TNFRSF10A, FRSF10B, TNFRSF10C, TNFRSF10D, DLGAP2*	?
9p21-p22	18-41	***CDKN2A, ARF1,*** *MOBKL2B*‡	Cell cycle, DNA damage response
9q21-qter	18-45	*CDC14B, FANCC, GAS1*	?
10p14-p15	18-31	*PRKCQ, KIN*	?
11q22-q23	16-59	***ATM***	DNA damage response
13q13.3-q34	25-70	*RFP2, ING1, LIG4, TNFSF13B, DLEU1, DLEU2*	?
17p13-ter	25-70	***TP53***	Cell cycle, DNA damage response, antisenescence
22q11-q12	17-50	*UCRC, PRAME*	?

*Minimal altered regions vary slightly among different studies.
†Confirmed target genes are in bold.
‡Homozygous deletions of this gene have been identified in mantle cell lymphoma cell lines but not in primary tumors.[156]

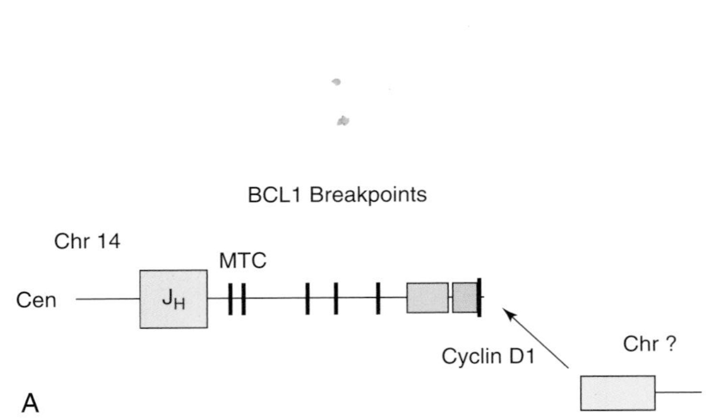

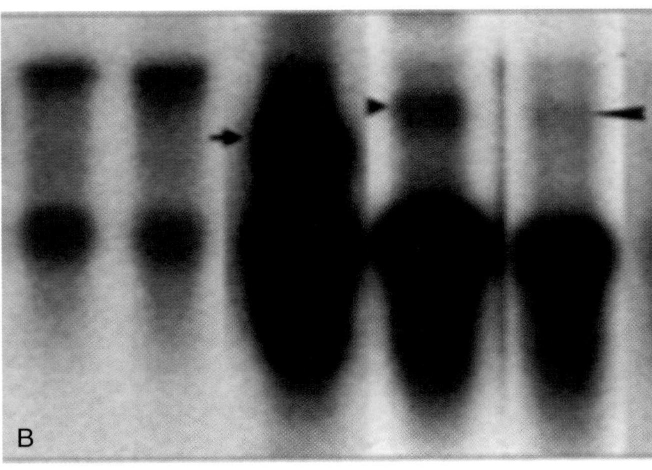

Figure 21-10. **A,** Schematic representation of the t(11;14) translocation. This translocation juxtaposes the immunoglobulin J_H region to the BCL1 region of chromosome 11q13. Cyclin D1 is the gene activated by this translocation. Most of the breakpoints occur in a region known as the *major translocation cluster* (MTC), but other breakpoints have been described between the MTC and the cyclin D1 gene. In some cases a second breakpoint occurs in the 3′ untranslated region of cyclin D1. **B,** Northern blot of cyclin D1 shows two transcripts of 4.5 and 1.5 kb. Tumors with a second rearrangement in the 3′ untranslated region of the gene express an aberrant shorter transcript instead of the 4.5-kb message (*arrows*).

Studies of a chromosome 11 inversion, inv(11)(p15;q13), in parathyroid adenomas led to the characterization of a new gene designated *PRAD-1,* which was considered the candidate oncogene activated by t(11;14).[121,122] It is located approximately 120 kb downstream of the original *BCL1* locus, and no other transcriptional units have been identified between the gene and the breakpoints. Analyses of the *PRAD-1* sequence showed a high homology with other cyclins, and it was recognized as a novel member of the cyclin D1 family involved in G_1 regulation. The gene was then renamed *CCDN1*, or cyclin D1.[122]

Cyclin D1 Messenger RNA Transcripts and Polymorphism

Cyclin D1 is not normally expressed in lymphocytes or myeloid cells, but it is constantly expressed in MCLs, indicating an important role in the pathogenesis of this lymphoma.[52,88,89] Messenger RNA studies have shown the expression of two major transcripts of 4.5 and 1.5 kb. Both transcripts contain the whole coding region of the gene and differ in the length of the 3′ untranslated region. Some MCLs express aberrant transcripts of altered sized instead of the 4.5-kb message (see Fig. 21-10). Interestingly, tumors with aberrant transcripts show very high levels of expression.[52,89] Molecular analyses of these cases have shown the loss of AUUUA destabilizing sequences at the 3′ region, which results in an increased half-life of cyclin D1 truncated transcripts. These anomalous truncated messages are due to rearrangements at the 3′ region of the gene, which usually coexist with a regular 5′ breakpoint on the same allele,[107,123,124] or to genomic microdeletions and point mutations at this 3′ UTR region.[125] Although it is not clear what role these shorter transcripts could have in MCL, their expression correlates with high levels of cyclin D1 mRNA, increased proliferation, and poor survival of patients,[125-127] suggesting that these secondary events in the 3′ region of the gene may be important in disease progression. Gains and amplifications of the translocated allele have been observed in some tumors that also have high levels of cyclin D1 expression.[118]

The cyclin D1 gene has a frequent polymorphism in the final codon of exon 4 that may modify the splice donor signal between exon and intron 4, thus generating a transcript variant, called *transcript b*, coding for a shorter protein missing the whole exon 5. The alternative transcript and protein are expressed in several normal and neoplastic tissues, including MCLs.[128] Although this single nucleotide polymorphism has been associated with increased cancer risk or poor outcome in other tumors, it does not seem to have an impact in MCL.[129] In addition, despite evidence of the tumorigenic role of this isoform,[130] its implication in MCL pathogenesis is not clear because human MCL cells express mostly the canonical cyclin D1a isoform and only low levels of cyclin D1b mRNA.[131]

Cyclin D1 Oncogenic Mechanisms

Cyclin D1 may function as an oncogene cooperating with other oncogenes, generally *MYC* and *RAS*.[132] However, the oncogenic mechanisms of cyclin D1 are not well understood. Cyclin D1 participates in the control of the G_1 phase by binding to CDK4 and CDK6. The complexes phosphorylate retinoblastoma protein, leading to the inactivation of its suppressor effect on cell cycle progression.[133] Hyperphosphorylation of retinoblastoma protein releases important transcription factors, such as E2F, that participate in the regulation of other genes involved in cell cycle progression. In MCL, retinoblastoma protein seems to be normally expressed in all cases, and no mutations in functional domains have been detected.[134] However, it is hyperphosphorylated, particularly in blastoid variants with high proliferative activity.[105] Concordantly, E2F overexpression is detected in a high number of MCLs.[135] These findings suggest than cyclin D1 may play a role in these tumors by overcoming the suppressive effect of retinoblastoma protein.

MCL may also have impaired control of late G_1 phase and G_1- to S-phase transition. This step is regulated by the cyclin

Chapter 22

Diffuse Large B-Cell Lymphoma

Alexander C. L. Chan and John K. C. Chan

Diffuse large B-cell lymphoma (DLBCL) is an aggressive lymphoma. In contrast to indolent (low-grade) lymphoma, the survival curve typically shows an initial downward slope followed by a plateau, indicating the potential curability of a significant proportion of patients who achieve remission (Fig. 22-1).

In previous classifications, such as the Kiel classification and the working formulation,[1,2] two major types of DLBCL were recognized: centroblastic (large noncleaved cell) and immunoblastic lymphomas. Practicing pathologists often agonized over the distinction between these two categories, a problem compounded by the fact that large noncleaved cell lymphoma was considered an intermediate-grade lymphoma, whereas immunoblastic lymphoma was a high-grade lymphoma in the working formulation.

In view of the low intraobserver and interobserver reproducibility in distinguishing between centroblastic (large noncleaved cell) and immunoblastic lymphomas, a single category of DLBCL was created to encompass both entities in the Revised European American Lymphoma (REAL) classification and the 2001 World Health Organization (WHO) classification.[3,4] It was recognized, however, that DLBCL is a heterogeneous category from which clinically relevant entities or variants might be delineated.[4,5] Currently, many clinicopathologic variants, distinct subtypes, and distinct disease entities are recognized (Box 22-1), although they account for only a minority of all DLBCLs. The remaining cases are referred to as DLBCL, not otherwise specified (DLBCL-NOS) in the 2008 WHO classification.[5]

DEFINITION

DLBCL is a diffuse proliferation of large or medium-sized neoplastic B cells with a nuclear size greater than or equal to that of a histiocyte nucleus, or more than twice the size of a small lymphocyte (Fig. 22-2).[5] Cases not conforming to the defined subtypes and entities are given the diagnostic label DLBCL-NOS.

EPIDEMIOLOGY

DLBCL is the most common type of non-Hodgkin's lymphoma, accounting for 31% of all cases according to an international multicenter study.[6] There is no significant difference in the incidence of this lymphoma among different ethnic and racial groups,[7] except for certain specific subtypes of DLBCL (see subsequent sections). In some populations, such as Asians, DLBCL accounts for a higher percentage of all non-

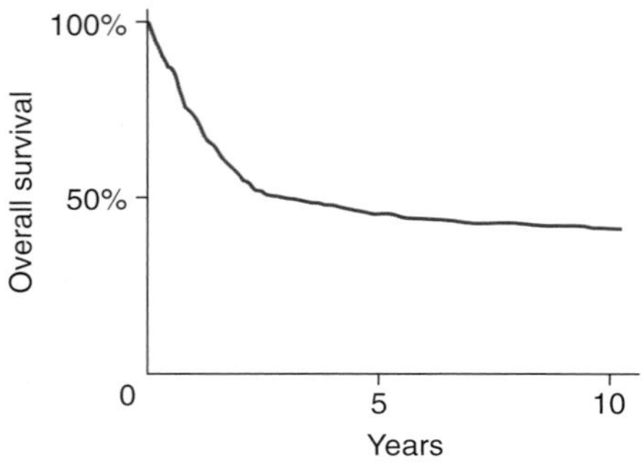

Figure 22-1. Idealized survival curve of diffuse large B-cell lymphoma. An initial downward slope is followed by a plateau, indicating curability in a proportion of patients.

Hodgkin's lymphomas than in the United States and western Europe (>40%), but this can be explained by a lower incidence of follicular lymphoma in these populations.[8,9]

The median age of patients is 64 years,[6] but patients of any age can be affected.[10,11] There is a slight male predominance (male-to-female ratio of 1.2:1).[6]

ETIOLOGY

Most patients with DLBCL have no known underlying risk factors. A minority of cases occurs in the setting of congenital immunodeficiency or acquired immunodeficiency, such as human immunodeficiency virus (HIV) infection, transplantation, methotrexate treatment in patients with rheumatoid arthritis, and fludarabine treatment in patients with low-grade B-cell lymphoma.[12,13] These cases are commonly associated with Epstein-Barr virus (EBV). EBV$^+$ DLBCL can also supervene in angioimmunoblastic T-cell lymphoma as a result of the immune dysfunction secondary to the neoplastic process.[14,15] EBV$^+$ DLBCL of the elderly, which occurs in patients without evidence of overt immunodeficiency, is believed to result from the subtle immunologic deterioration that occurs as part of the aging process.[16,17]

Rare extranodal cases of DLBCL are associated with chronic inflammation or irritation, such as postmastectomy lymphedema,[18] chronic suppurative inflammation in bone and skin,[19] previous surgery and metallic implants,[20,21] juxta-articular soft tissues in patients with long-standing rheumatoid arthritis,[22] and long-standing pyothorax.[23] Some of these cases are associated with EBV[19,21,23] and are considered a distinct entity (DLBCL associated with chronic inflammation) in the 2008 WHO classification.[24]

Most DLBCLs arise de novo, but some cases transform from an underlying low-grade lymphoma, such as follicular lymphoma, chronic lymphocytic leukemia–small lymphocytic lymphoma, lymphoplasmacytic lymphoma, marginal zone lymphoma, or nodular lymphocyte-predominant Hodgkin's lymphoma (NLPHL). Some cases of DLBCL occur synchronously or metachronously with classical Hodgkin's lymphoma.[25]

CLINICAL FEATURES

Patients present with rapidly enlarging lymph nodes or tumor masses in extranodal sites. About 30% of cases present in extranodal sites, and 71% have extranodal involvement during the course of the disease.[26] Common primary extranodal sites include the gastrointestinal tract (especially the stomach) and Waldeyer's ring, but practically any organ can be involved, including the skin, central nervous system, mediastinum, and bone.[27] Extranodal lymphomas of specific sites, especially of the skin and central nervous system, show distinctive clinical and biologic features (see Chapters 19, 61, and 62).

Approximately half the patients present with early-stage (stage I-II) disease, and one third have B symptoms.[26] Bone marrow involvement occurs in 16%,[26] and it may show concordant or discordant histology (see Prognostic Factors for the clinical significance).

MORPHOLOGY

Involved lymph nodes or tissues show complete or partial effacement of architecture by diffuse infiltrates of lymphoma

Box 22-1 ***Diffuse Large B-Cell Lymphoma: Variants, Subtypes, and Other Entities***

DLBCL, Not Otherwise Specified
- Common morphologic variants
  - Centroblastic
  - Immunoblastic
  - Anaplastic
- Rare morphologic variants
- Molecular subgroups
  - Germinal center B-cell–like
  - Activated B-cell–like
- Immunohistochemical subgroups
  - CD5$^+$ DLBCL
  - Germinal center B-cell–like
  - Non–germinal center B-cell–like

DLBCL Subtypes
- T-cell/histiocyte-rich large B-cell lymphoma
- Primary DLBCL of the central nervous system (see Chapter 62)
- Primary cutaneous DLBCL, leg type (see Chapter 19)
- EBV$^+$ DLBCL of the elderly

Other Lymphomas of Large B Cells
- Primary mediastinal (thymic) large B-cell lymphoma
- Intravascular large B-cell lymphoma
- DLBCL associated with chronic inflammation
- Lymphomatoid granulomatosis (see Chapter 23)
- ALK$^+$ large B-cell lymphoma
- Plasmablastic lymphoma
- Large B-cell lymphoma arising in HHV8-associated multicentric Castleman's disease (see Chapter 56)
- Primary effusion lymphoma (see Chapter 56)
- HHV8- and EBV-associated germinotropic lymphoproliferative disorder (not listed in the WHO classification)

Borderline Cases
- B-cell lymphoma, unclassifiable, with features intermediate between DLBCL and Burkitt's lymphoma (see Chapter 24)
- B-cell lymphoma, unclassifiable, with features intermediate between DLBCL and classical Hodgkin's lymphoma

ALK, anaplastic lymphoma kinase; DLBCL, diffuse large B-cell lymphoma; EBV, Epstein-Barr virus; HHV8, human herpesviruus 8; WHO, World Health Organization.
From Swerdlow SH, Campo E, Harris NL, et al, eds. *WHO Classification of Tumours of Haematopoietic and Lymphoid Tissues.* Lyon, France: IARC; 2008.

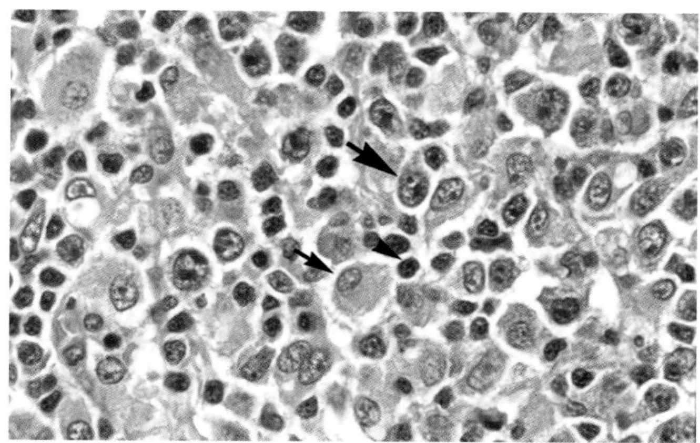

Figure 22-2. Diffuse large B-cell lymphoma: nuclear size assessment. In this example with numerous admixed histiocytes and lymphocytes, the interspersed histiocytes (with abundant eosinophilic cytoplasm) can conveniently be used as "rulers" for measuring the size of lymphoma cells. The lymphoma cells (*large arrow*) are considered large because their nuclei are slightly larger than those of the histiocytes (*small arrow*). The neoplastic cells are more than twice the size of the small lymphocytes (*arrowhead*).

cells, often with coagulative necrosis and permeation into the surrounding tissues (Figs. 22-3 and 22-4). Uncommonly, the lymphoma shows an interfollicular or sinusoidal pattern of nodal involvement (see Fig. 22-3B; Box 22-2). Exceptionally, the tumor cells form deceptively cohesive nodules, mimicking carcinoma (see Fig. 22-4B). There may be a "starry sky" appearance imparted by interspersed histiocytes with phagocytosed cell debris (Fig. 22-5). Sclerosis may be present, especially in mediastinal and retroperitoneal tumors (Fig. 22-6).[28] The lymph nodes may show coexisting low-grade lymphoma, such as follicular lymphoma, chronic lymphocytic leukemia (CLL), or NLPHL (Fig. 22-7).

At extranodal sites, in addition to forming tumor masses the lymphoma cells commonly infiltrate in an interstitial pattern, resulting in wide separation and loss of the normal specialized structures, such as gastric glands, salivary acini, seminiferous tubules, and thyroid follicles (Fig. 22-8). Infiltration into the epithelium can occur, and mucosal ulceration is common. An underlying extranodal marginal zone lymphoma of mucosa-associated lymphoid tissue (MALT) may be present.

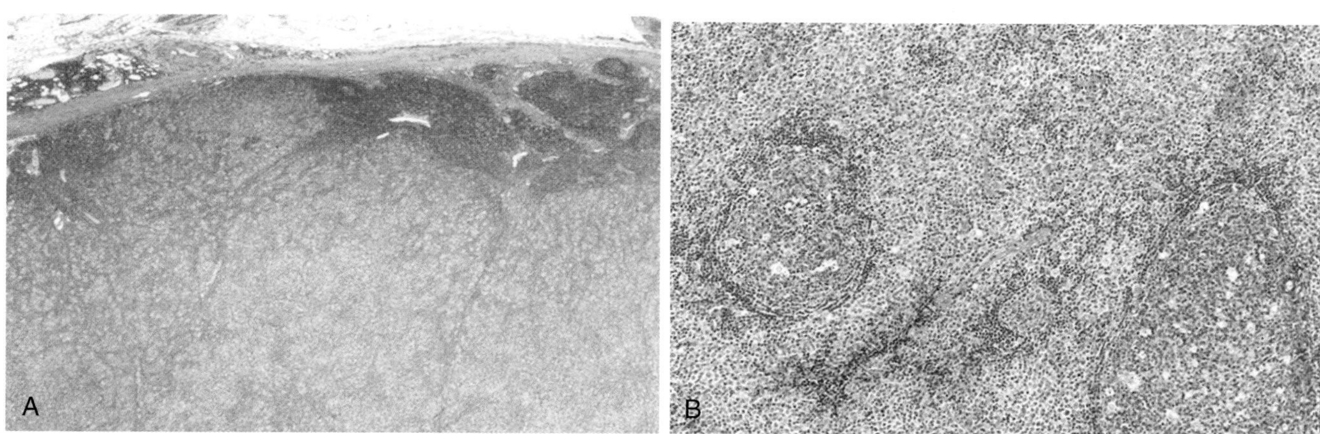

Figure 22-3. Nodal diffuse large B-cell lymphoma. A, The lymph node architecture is effaced by a diffuse lymphomatous infiltrate, with spillover into the perinodal tissue (*upper left field*). Some residual lymph node tissue is seen (*upper right field*). **B,** In this example, the lymphoma selectively involves the interfollicular zone, mimicking reactive lymphoid hyperplasia. Features supportive of a diagnosis of lymphoma include erosion of the mantles of the reactive follicles and a monotonous interfollicular cellular infiltrate.

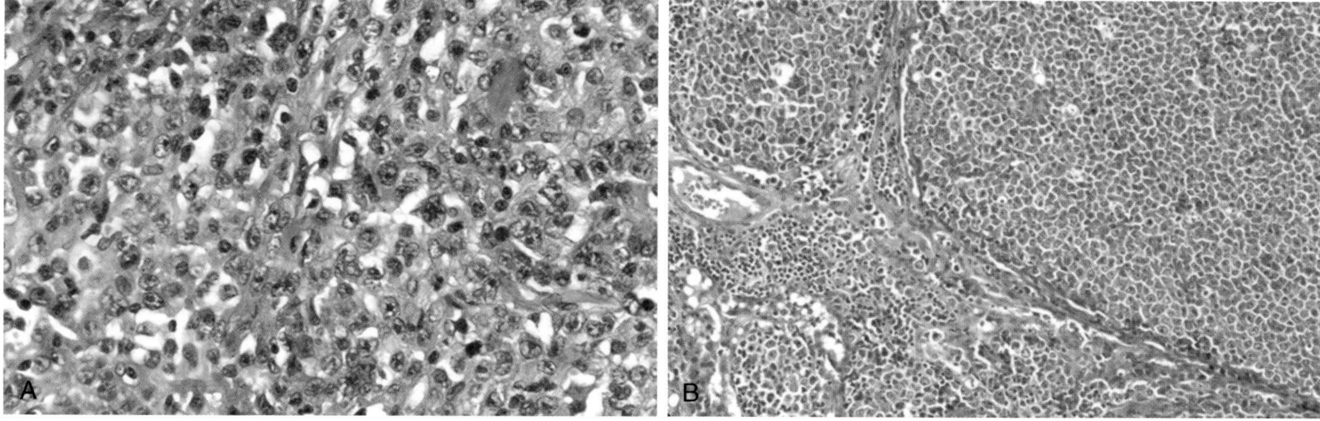

Figure 22-4. Nodal diffuse large B-cell lymphoma. A, In most cases the infiltrate comprises noncohesive neoplastic cells growing in a diffuse pattern. **B,** Sometimes the lymphoma cells form nodules or islands that exhibit a sharp interface with the stroma, mimicking carcinoma because of the pseudocohesive appearance.

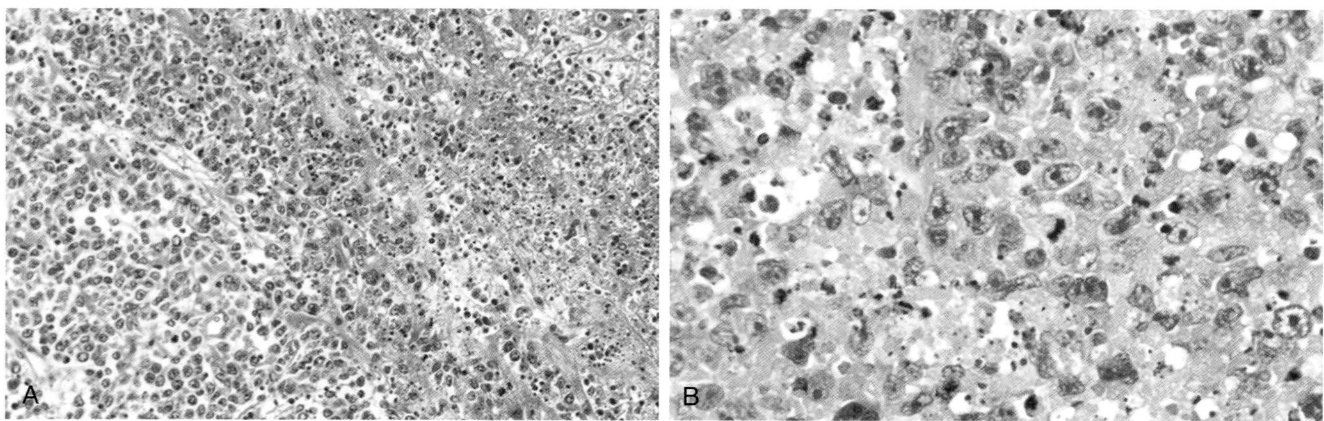

Figure 22-5. Diffuse large B-cell lymphoma. A, Coagulative necrosis (*right field*) is a fairly common finding. **B,** There may be abundant karyorrhectic debris among the lymphoma cells, mimicking Kikuchi's lymphadenitis.

Box 22-2 *Differential Diagnoses of Large Cell Neoplasms with a Prominent Sinusoidal Pattern of Nodal Involvement*

- Diffuse large B-cell lymphoma (DLBCL)
  - Sinusoidal DLBCL, $CD30^+$
  - Microvillous DLBCL
  - ALK^+ large B-cell lymphoma
  - DLBCL, not otherwise specified (uncommon)
- Anaplastic large cell lymphoma, ALK^+
- Anaplastic large cell lymphoma, ALK^-
- Histiocytic neoplasms or tumor-like conditions
  - Langerhans cell histiocytosis
  - Rosai-Dorfman disease
  - Histiocytic sarcoma (uncommon)
- Metastatic nonhematolymphoid malignancies (e.g., melanoma, carcinoma, germ cell tumor)

ALK, anaplastic lymphoma kinase.

Cytologically, DLBCL comprises large to medium-sized lymphoid cells with the morphologic features of centroblasts (large noncleaved cells), immunoblasts, or cells with intermediate features. Centroblasts have round to oval vesicular nuclei, multiple membrane-bound small nucleoli, and a thin rim of amphophilic cytoplasm (Fig. 22-9); they can show multilobated or angulated nuclei (see Fig. 22-9B and C).[29] Immunoblasts have round or oval vesicular nuclei; a single large, centrally located nucleolus; and a broad rim of basophilic cytoplasm (Fig. 22-10). The immunoblasts sometimes exhibit plasmacytoid features, with eccentrically located nuclei and paranuclear hof. Nonetheless, the lymphoma cells may not conform to these classic cell types, exhibiting hybrid features of centroblasts and immunoblasts, a huge cell size, a predominantly medium cell size, irregular nuclear foldings, elongated nuclei, voluminous cytoplasm in a cell with nuclear features of a centroblast, or clear cytoplasm (Figs. 22-11 and 22-12).

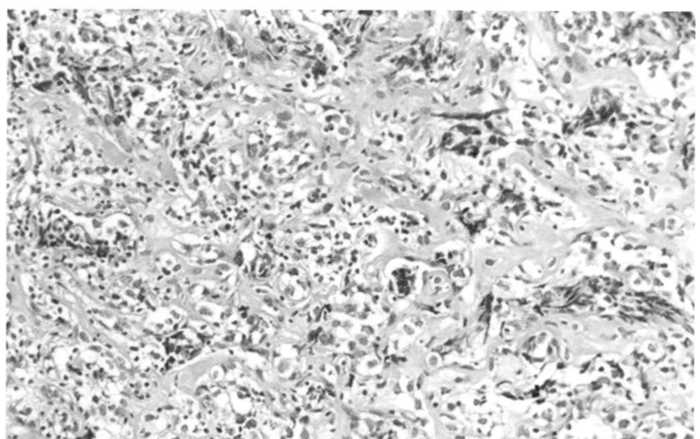

Figure 22-6. Diffuse large B-cell lymphoma with sclerosis. Thin sclerotic bands delineate the tumor into irregular packets. Lymphoma cells entrapped in the sclerotic areas often exhibit retracted cytoplasm or crush artifacts.

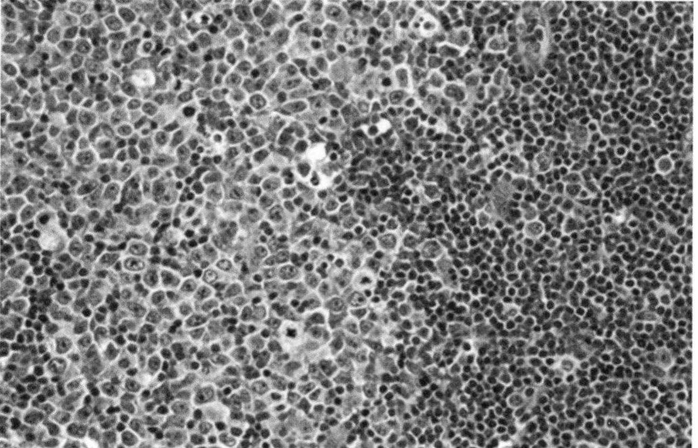

Figure 22-7. Diffuse large B-cell lymphoma arising in chronic lymphocytic leukemia (Richter's syndrome). The *left field* shows diffuse sheets of large lymphoma cells. The *right field* shows the preexisting chronic lymphocytic leukemia, comprising monotonous small lymphocytes; these cells are confirmed to be neoplastic by a $CD20^+$, $CD5^+$, $CD23^+$ immunophenotype (not shown).

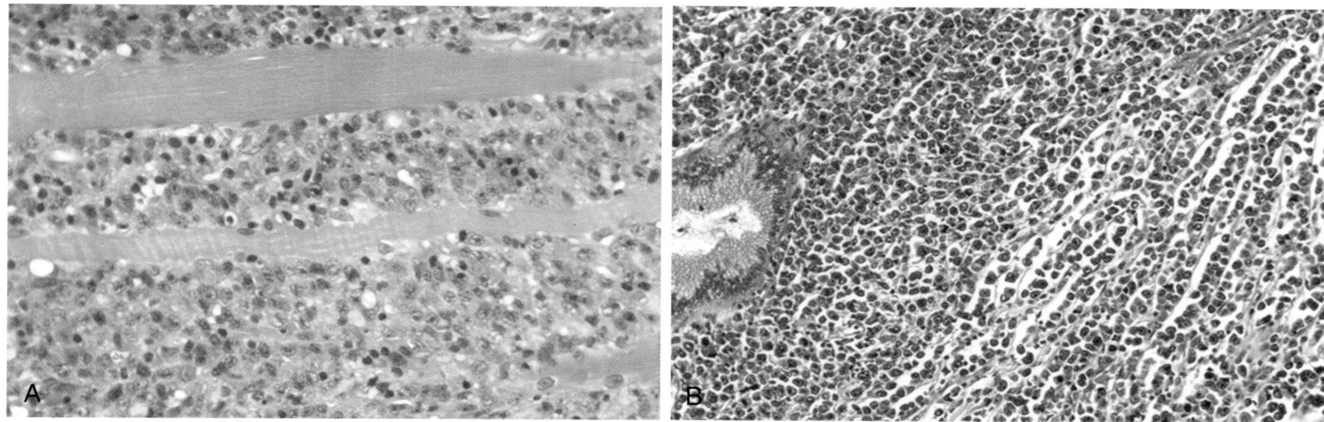

Figure 22-8. Extranodal diffuse large B-cell lymphoma. A, The interstitial infiltrate splits up and destroys the skeletal muscle fibers. **B,** In the fibrous stroma (uterine cervix in this example), a single-file pattern of infiltration can be seen.

Cytologic subclassification of DLBCL is optional. Lymphomas with greater than 90% immunoblasts are considered the *immunoblastic variant*, whereas those with less than 90% immunoblasts are considered the *centroblastic (large noncleaved cell) variant* (Fig. 22-13).[5] However, it can be difficult to decide whether a lymphoma cell is a centroblast or an immunoblast, and most DLBCLs contain a mixture of the two cell types or cells with intermediate features. The *anaplastic variant* comprises cells with bizarre pleomorphic nuclei, often with multinucleated forms, and abundant cytoplasm (Fig. 22-14).[30,31] It should not be confused with anaplastic large cell lymphoma, which is a T/null-cell neoplasm.[32] It may also mimic metastatic carcinoma because of the cellular pleomorphism, cohesive growth, or sinusoidal infiltration. This variant behaves no differently than conventional DLBCL.[32] Occasional cases of DLBCL show plasmacytic maturation, with lymphoma cells admixed with variable numbers of neoplastic mature-looking plasma cells (Fig. 22-15).

In DLBCL there can be variable numbers of reactive cells in the background, such as small lymphocytes (mostly T

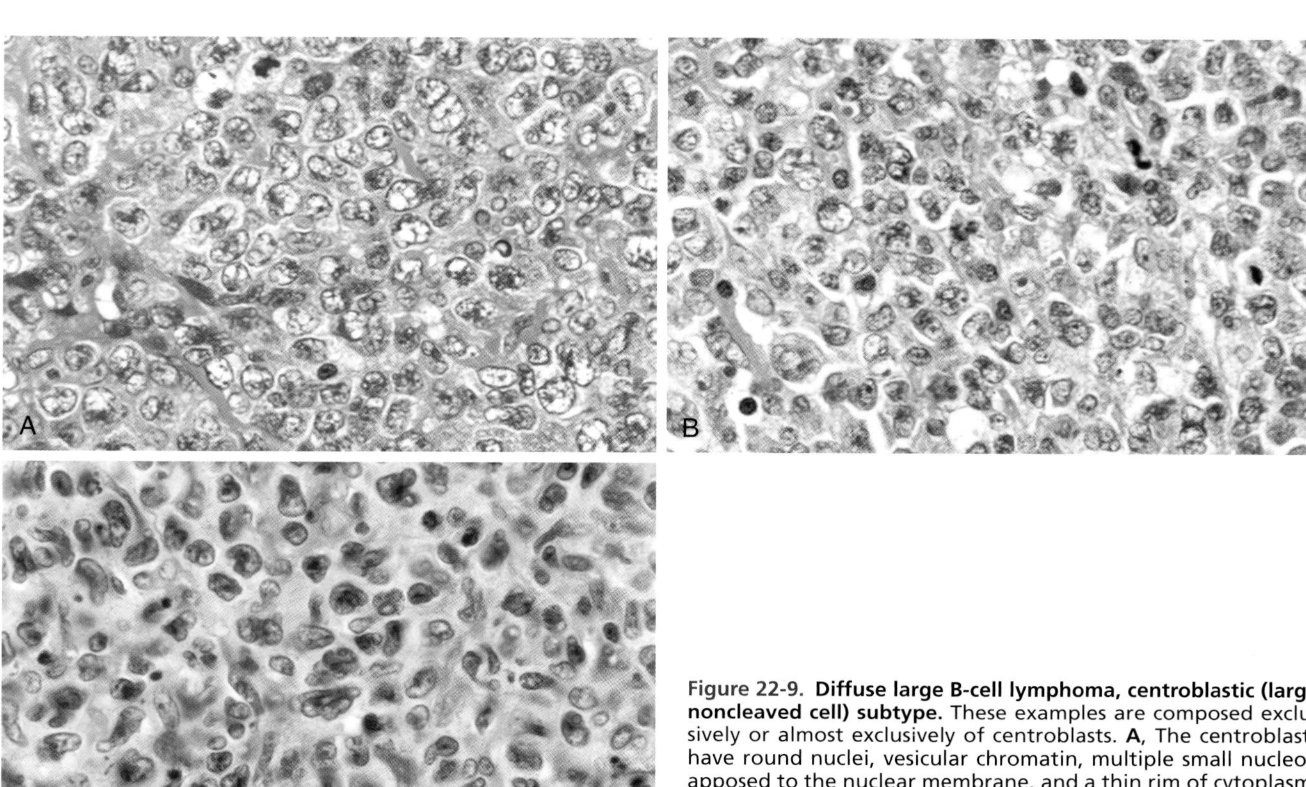

Figure 22-9. Diffuse large B-cell lymphoma, centroblastic (large noncleaved cell) subtype. These examples are composed exclusively or almost exclusively of centroblasts. **A,** The centroblasts have round nuclei, vesicular chromatin, multiple small nucleoli apposed to the nuclear membrane, and a thin rim of cytoplasm. **B,** Many cells have multilobated nuclei, resembling flowers with several petals. **C,** The large lymphoma cells show angulated or cleaved nuclei. The small nucleoli are obscured by the nuclear foldings.

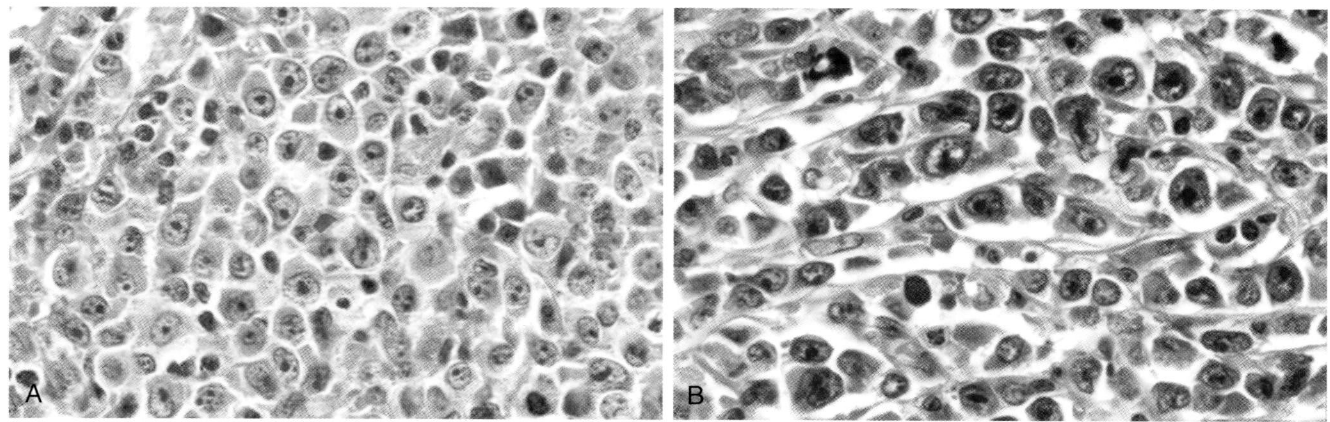

Figure 22-10. Diffuse large B-cell lymphoma, immunoblastic subtype. A and **B,** Practically all the large lymphoma cells show round or oval nuclei, prominent central nucleoli, and a broad rim of amphophilic cytoplasm.

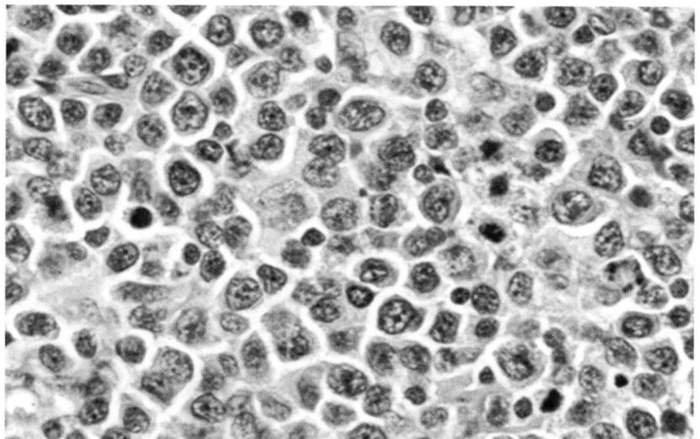

Figure 22-11. Diffuse large B-cell lymphoma comprising medium-sized cells. In the past, this case might have been classified as small noncleaved cell lymphoma, but it does not fulfill the current diagnostic criteria for Burkitt's or atypical Burkitt's lymphoma.

cells), plasma cells, histiocytes, and polymorphs. In rare cases, coalescing small clusters of epithelioid histiocytes are present, mimicking lymphoepithelioid T-cell lymphoma (Lennert's lymphoma) (Fig. 22-16).[33] Occasional cases may present initially with lymph node infarction (Fig. 22-17).[34,35]

Some uncommon or histologically deceptive morphologic variants are listed in Table 22-1 (Figs. 22-18 to 22-21).[36-49] A summary of the clinical, morphologic, immunophenotypic, and genetic features of DLBCL is presented in Box 22-3.

IMMUNOPHENOTYPE

DLBCLs express CD45 and various pan-B markers, including CD20, CD22, CD79a, and PAX5 (Fig. 22-22). However, CD20 expression is lost in 60% of recurrent tumors from patients treated with rituximab (anti-CD20 chimeric antibody).[50] Monotypic surface or cytoplasmic immunoglobulin (Ig) can frequently be demonstrated (IgM > IgG > IgA), and cytoplasmic immunoglobulin can sometimes be demonstrated

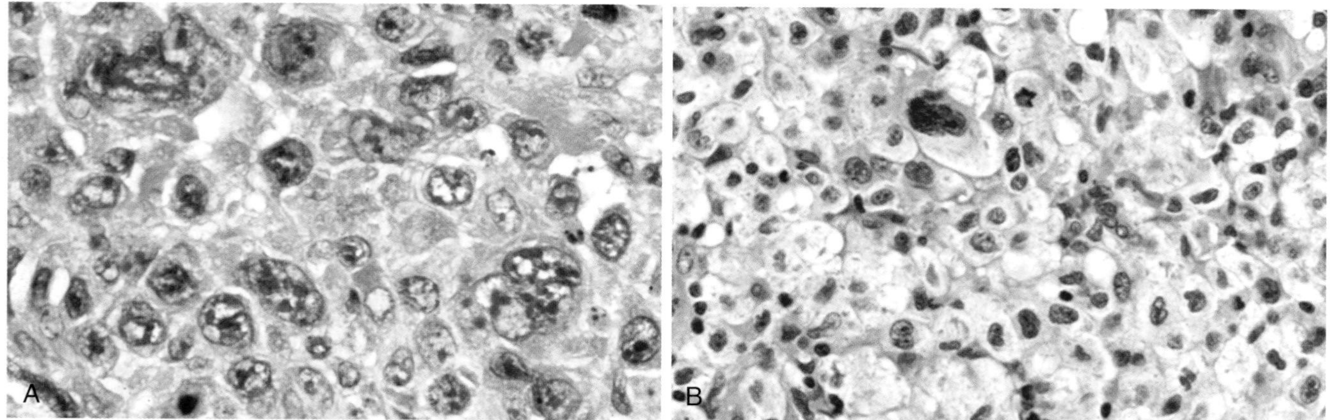

Figure 22-12. Diffuse large B-cell lymphoma with cells that are difficult to classify. A, All the cells are much larger than the usual immunoblasts or centroblasts, and some cells are huge and bizarre. **B,** In this example, the lymphoma cells have voluminous clear cytoplasm.

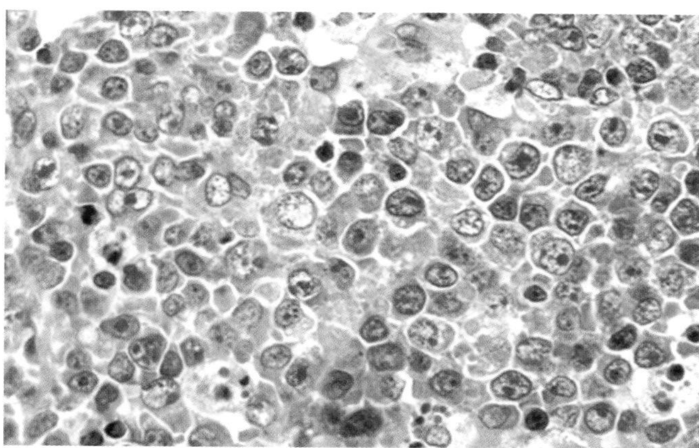

Figure 22-13. Diffuse large B-cell lymphoma, centroblastic subtype. Immunoblasts are present in addition to centroblasts; there are also many cells with an indeterminate appearance between the two cell types.

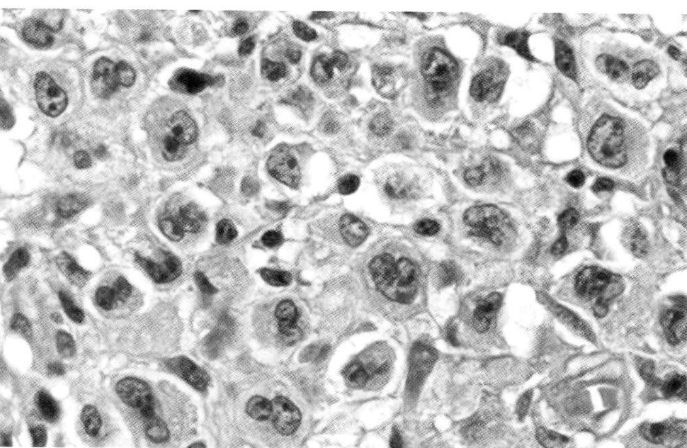

Figure 22-14. Diffuse large B-cell lymphoma, anaplastic subtype. The lymphoma cells are very large, with indented or irregularly folded nuclei and abundant cytoplasm, resembling those seen in T/null-cell anaplastic large cell lymphoma.

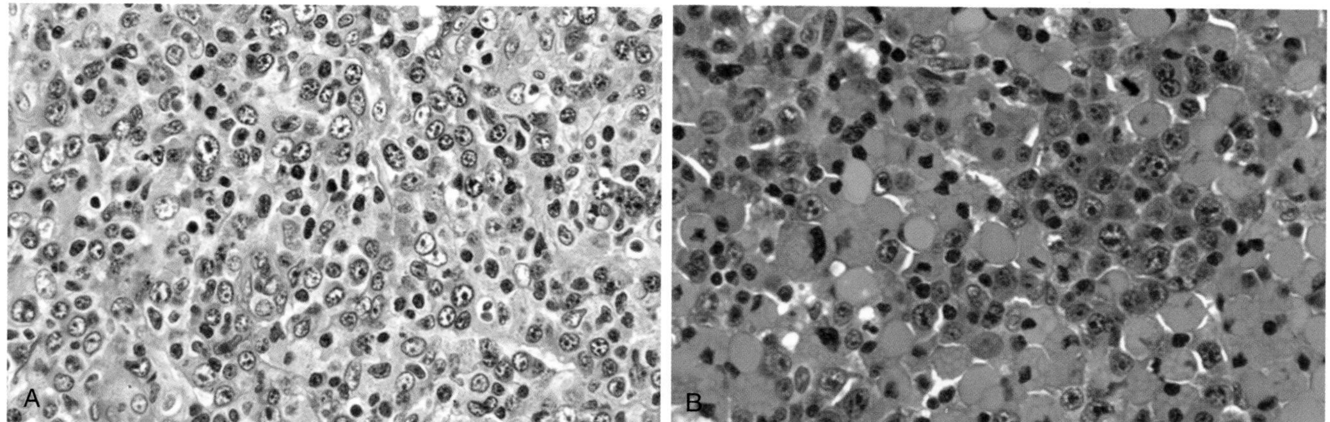

Figure 22-15. Diffuse large B-cell lymphoma with plasma cell differentiation. A, In this example, the large lymphoma cells show a gradual transition to plasmablasts and atypical plasma cells. This appearance is similar to that seen in the polymorphic type of posttransplant lymphoproliferative disorder. **B,** In this example, the large lymphoma cells show an abrupt transition to plasma cells, which are engorged with brightly eosinophilic globules of immunoglobulin.

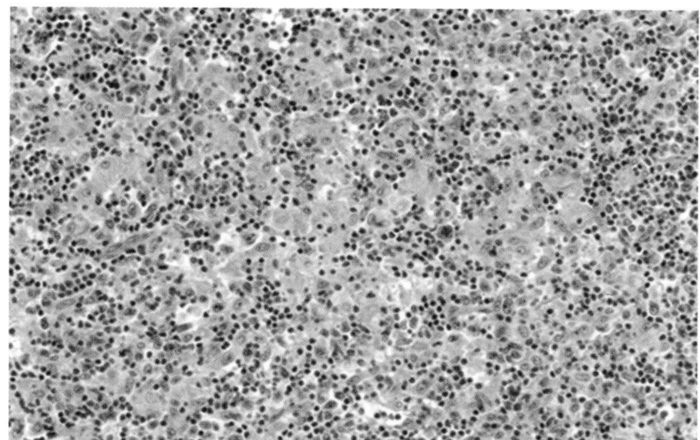

Figure 22-16. Diffuse large B-cell lymphoma with many interspersed small clusters of epithelioid histiocytes, reminiscent of Lennert's (lymphoepithelioid) T-cell lymphoma.

as well. Pan-T markers are negative, although CD3 is very rarely expressed.[51]

CD10 expression occurs in 20% to 40% of cases.[52-61] CD10 expression is useful in identifying the subset of DLBCL with a germinal center (GC) B-cell expression profile, and this marker is often expressed in cases carrying t(14;18).[62] The reported positivity rate for BCL6 protein is highly variable because the criteria for positive staining vary greatly from study to study.[52,54,59,63-67] Overall, approximately 60% of cases are BCL6$^+$ when only those with large aggregates of positive tumor cells are considered positive.[67] About 50% of cases express BCL2 protein,[59-61,68-74] and a higher frequency is observed in nodal than in extranodal tumors.[75]

A minority of DLBCLs express the activation marker CD30, usually in a heterogeneous pattern, affecting some to most of the neoplastic cells.[30] CD5 is expressed in approximately 10% of cases (Box 22-4; also see the subsequent section on de novo CD5$^+$ DLBCL).[76] Some cases express post-GC or plasma cell–

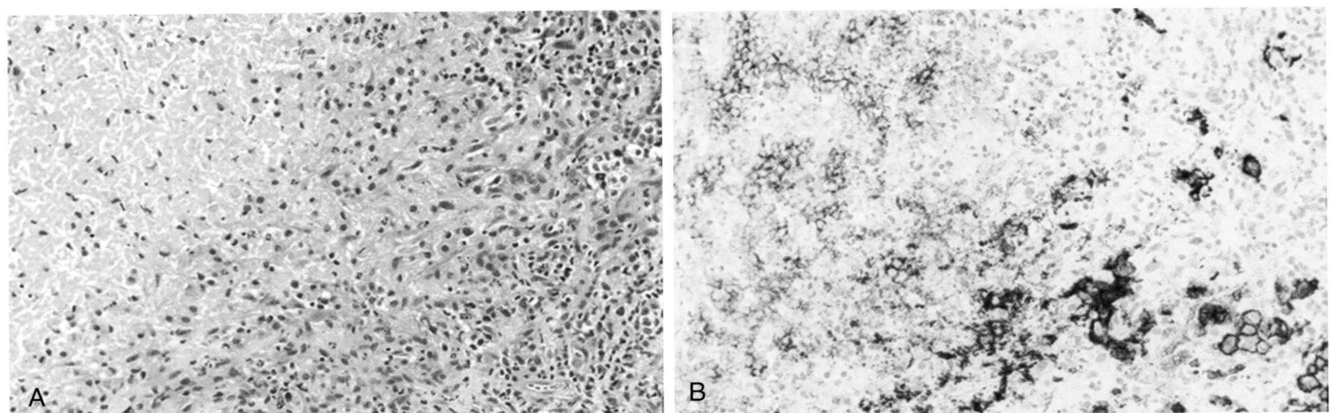

Figure 22-17. Diffuse large B-cell lymphoma presenting as lymph node infarction. A, The entire lymph node consists of necrotic material surrounded by a rim of fibrogranulation tissue. **B,** Immunostaining for CD20 shows that this antigen is still preserved in the necrotic cells (*left field*). Immunostaining for CD20 in necrotic tissue may be nonspecific, so viable cells must be shown to stain to ascertain that the staining is specific. A small number of viable lymphoma cells (more strongly stained) are also highlighted within the fibrogranulation tissue.

associated markers such as CD38, VS38, and IRF4/MUM-1, but CD138 expression is seen almost exclusively in cases showing morphologic evidence of plasmacytic differentiation, such as plasmablastic lymphomas.[59,77] Ki-67 staining usually shows a high proliferation index (>20%, but often <80%), although some cases may show an index approaching 100%.[78-82]

A simple immunophenotyping approach (the Hans algorithm) designed to distinguish GC B-cell–like (GCB) and non-GCB subgroups has gained wide popularity and is depicted in Table 22-2.[83] Nonetheless, correlation of immunophenotypic grouping and gene expression profiling results is not complete.[83]

GENETICS

DLBCLs have rearranged immunoglobulin heavy- and light-chain genes (*IGH@*, *IGK@*, and *IGL@*) and germline T-cell receptor (TCR) genes. The immunoglobulin heavy-chain variable region gene (*IGHV@*) is hypermutated, with some cases showing ongoing somatic mutations.[84,85]

Table 22-1 Morphologic Variants of Diffuse Large B-Cell Lymphoma (DLBCL)

Morphologic Variant	Main Pathologic Features	Tumors with Which It Might Be Confused
Myxoid stroma[37,38]	Sheets, cords, or single lymphoma cells suspended in abundant myxoid stroma	Various types of myxoid sarcomas, such as extraskeletal myxoid chondrosarcoma, myxofibrosarcoma
Spindle cell morphology[39,40]	Lymphoma cells have a spindly appearance due to spontaneous cellular spindling or molding by collagen; predilection for skin	Various types of spindle cell sarcomas, spindle cell carcinoma, desmoplastic melanoma
Signet ring cell morphology[41,42]	Lymphoma cells have cytoplasmic vacuoles, which may be due to immunoglobulin accumulation or aberrant membrane recycling	Signet ring cell carcinoma, liposarcoma
Fibrillary matrix or rosette formation[43,44]	Lymphoma cells associated with a prominent fibrillary matrix or rosette formation; because the fibrillary material is formed by interdigitating cytoplasmic processes (hence rich in cell membrane materials), it typically shows strong staining for leukocyte markers	Neural tumors, such as neuroblastoma, primitive neuroectodermal tumor
Abundant crystal-storing histiocytes[45]	Lymphoma cells intermixed with histiocytes having ingested crystallized immunoglobulin	Rhabdomyoma
Marked tissue eosinophilia[46]	Lymphoma cells intermixed with numerous eosinophils	Hodgkin's lymphoma, peripheral T-cell lymphoma
Microvillous DLBCL[47,48]	Presence of numerous microvillous projections on ultrastructural examination; may show prominent sinusoidal growth pattern (see Box 22-2); CD20^{+}, CD30^{-}, EMA^{-}, CD56$^{+/-}$	Anaplastic large cell lymphoma (CD20^{-}, CD3$^{+/-}$, CD30^{+}, EMA$^{+/-}$, ALK$^{+/-}$, CD56$^{-/+}$)
Sinusoidal CD30^{+} DLBCL[49]	Sinusoidal growth pattern (see Box 22-2); CD20^{+}, CD30^{+}, EMA$^{-/+}$, ALK^{-}	Anaplastic large cell lymphoma (CD20^{-}, CD3$^{+/-}$, EMA$^{+/-}$, ALK$^{+/-}$); microvillous DLBCL (CD30^{-}); ALK^{+} DLBCL (CD30^{-}, ALK^{+}); metastatic carcinoma (cytokeratin +); metastatic melanoma (S-100^{+})

ALK, anaplastic lymphoma kinase; EMA, epithelial membrane antigen.

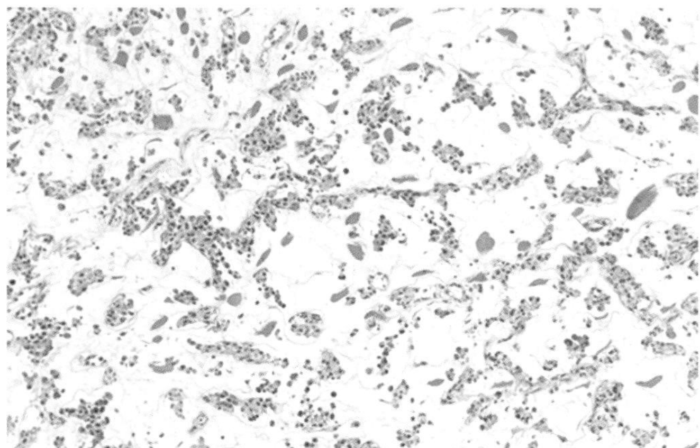

Figure 22-18. Diffuse large B-cell lymphoma with abundant myxoid stroma, mimicking extraskeletal myxoid chondrosarcoma.

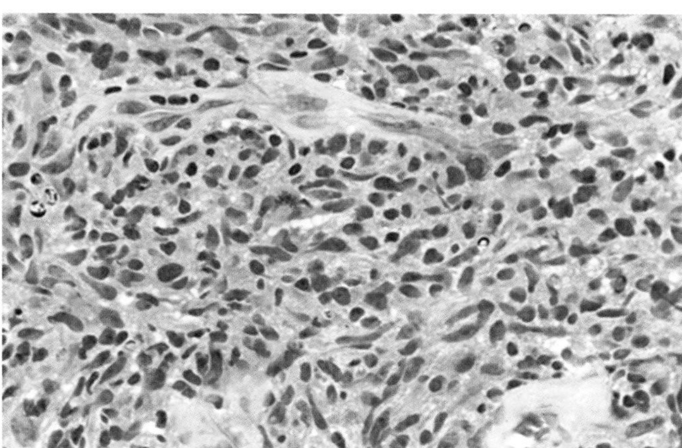

Figure 22-19. Diffuse large B-cell lymphoma with spindly lymphoma cells. Nucleoli are usually not obvious unless the cells are examined under high magnification.

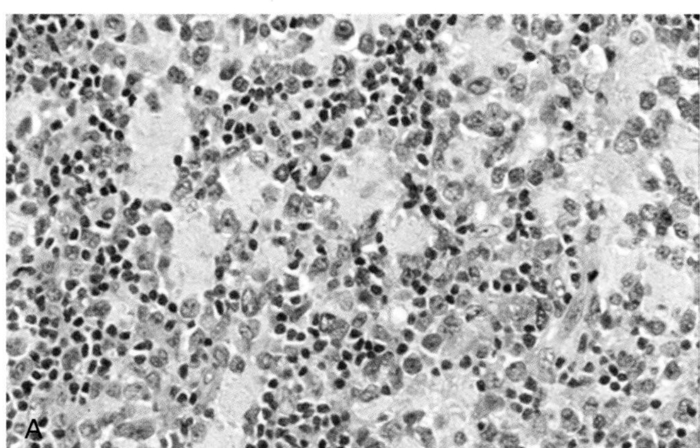

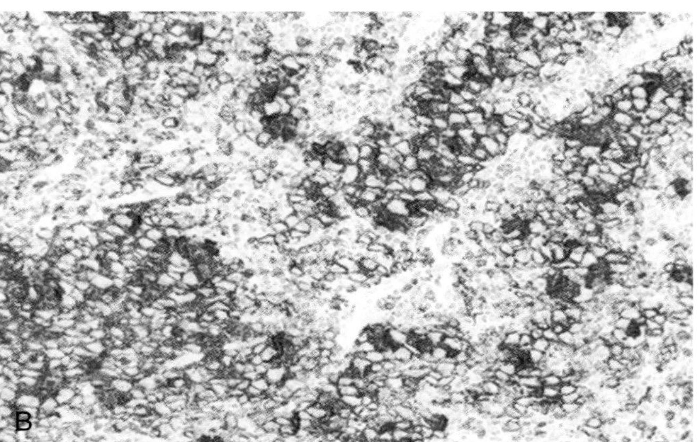

Figure 22-20. Diffuse large B-cell lymphoma with fibrillary matrix. A, The large lymphoma cells are associated with abundant eosinophilic fibrillary matrix. **B,** The matrix is actually formed by cell membrane materials from the lymphoma cells, as attested to by positive CD20 immunostaining.

Box 22-3 *Major Diagnostic Features of Diffuse Large B-Cell Lymphoma*

Clinical Features

- Median age: 64 years
- Slight male predominance
- Presents with rapidly growing nodal (70%) or extranodal (30%) tumor
- B symptoms in one third of cases
- Stage distribution: I, 25%; II, 29%; III, 13%; IV, 33%
- Potentially curable: when treated by standard chemotherapy, complete remission can be achieved in two thirds of patients, with two thirds of them remaining relapse-free on long-term follow-up; the overall survival rate is 46%, but in recent years survival has improved by about 20% with the addition of rituximab to the chemotherapy regimen

Morphology

- Diffuse proliferation of large to medium-sized lymphoid cells, which can be indistinguishable from normal centroblasts or immunoblasts or can exhibit overt atypical features such as irregular nuclear foldings, coarse chromatin, giant size, or bizarre nuclei
- May be associated with an underlying low-grade lymphoma
- Optional cytologic subclassification
  - Centroblastic (roundish vesicular nuclei with multiple peripheral small nucleoli; may be multilobated)
  - Immunoblastic (>90% immunoblasts with a single, centrally located, prominent nucleolus and abundant basophilic cytoplasm)
  - Anaplastic (markedly pleomorphic tumor cells, with frequent CD30 expression)
- Uncommonly, can show a variety of deceptive growth patterns (e.g., myxoid change, fibrillary matrix, spindly cells); see Table 22-1

Immunophenotype

- Positive for pan-B markers (e.g., CD20, CD22, CD79a, PAX5)
- Positive for surface or cytoplasmic immunoglobulin
- $BCL6^+$ in ≈60%
- $CD10^+$ in ≈40%
- $CD5^+$ in ≈10%
- $CD30^+$ in ≈10%
- $BCL2^+$ in ≈50%
- Ki-67 index: >20% (mean, 55%)

Molecular Features

- Clonally rearranged immunoglobulin genes
- *BCL2* rearranged in ≈20%
- *BCL6* rearranged in ≈30%
- *BCL6* mutated in ≈70%
- *MYC* rearranged in <10%
- Usually Epstein-Barr virus negative, except in the setting of immunodeficiency

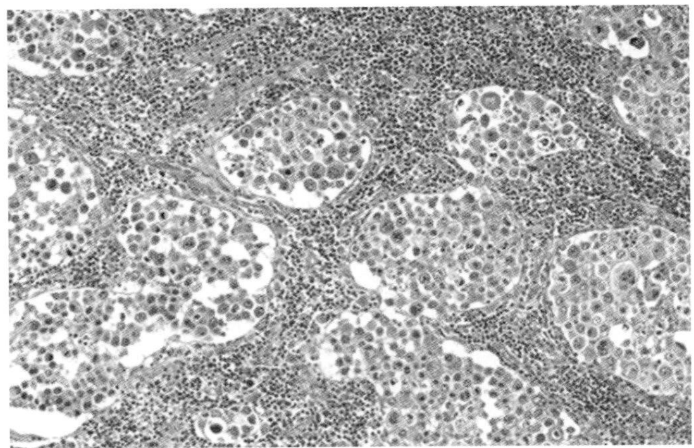

Figure 22-21. Sinusoidal CD30+ diffuse large B-cell lymphoma. The lymphoma cells are confined within the distended sinuses of the lymph node.

Box 22-4 *Major Differential Diagnoses of Diffuse Large B-Cell Lymphoma (DLBCL) with CD5 Expression*

- Mantle cell lymphoma, blastoid or pleomorphic variant
- Paraimmunoblastic variant of chronic lymphocytic leukemia
- DLBCL arising in chronic lymphocytic leukemia (Richter's syndrome)
- Intravascular large B-cell lymphoma
- Splenic DLBCL
- De novo CD5+ DLBCL

The pathogenesis of DLBCL is complex because it involves at least two different pathways: a transformation pathway and a de novo pathway. Approximately 20% of cases of DLBCL show *BCL2* rearrangement due to t(14;18)(q32;q21), a hallmark of follicular lymphoma.[86] Such cases may have transformed from a known or occult follicular lymphoma or may have evolved to DLBCL without a precursor phase of follicular lymphoma. Additional genetic alterations, such as *TP53* mutation, are required for transformation to DLBCL. *BCL6* and perhaps other unidentified genes play an important role in the de novo pathway. *BCL6* (3q27) rearrangement, which is found in some follicular lymphomas, occurs in about 30% of DLBCLs.[87-89] The translocation partner can be the immunoglobulin genes, most commonly in the form of t(3;14)(q27;q32), or other genes. *BCL6* somatic mutation is a common event in DLBCL (73% of cases) and is unrelated to the presence or absence of *BCL6* gene rearrangement.[90,91] It is a marker for cells that have been through the GC and is thus commonly observed in various types of B-cell lymphomas corresponding to the GC or post-GC stage of differentiation,

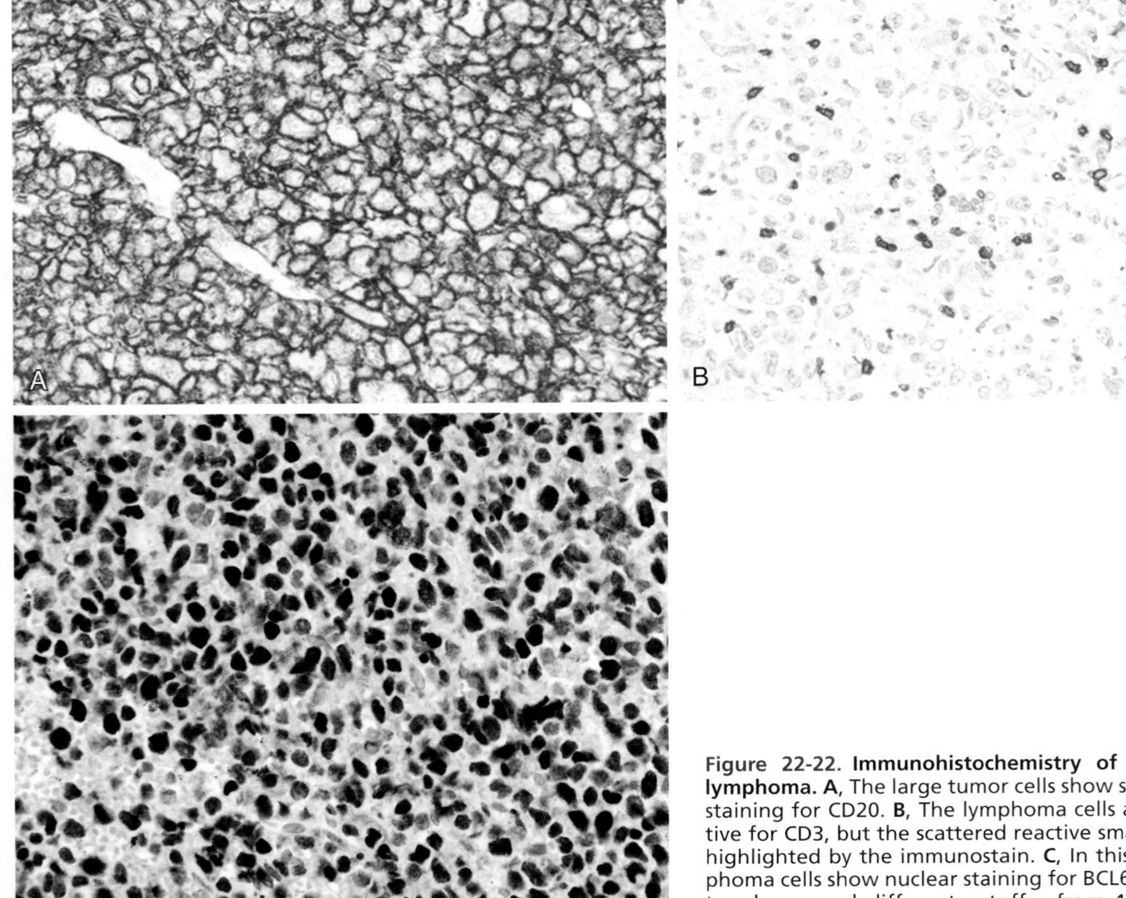

Figure 22-22. Immunohistochemistry of diffuse large B-cell lymphoma. A, The large tumor cells show strong cell membrane staining for CD20. **B,** The lymphoma cells are not immunoreactive for CD3, but the scattered reactive small T lymphocytes are highlighted by the immunostain. **C,** In this example, most lymphoma cells show nuclear staining for BCL6. Different investigators have used different cutoffs—from 10% to 60% positive cells—to consider a case positive.

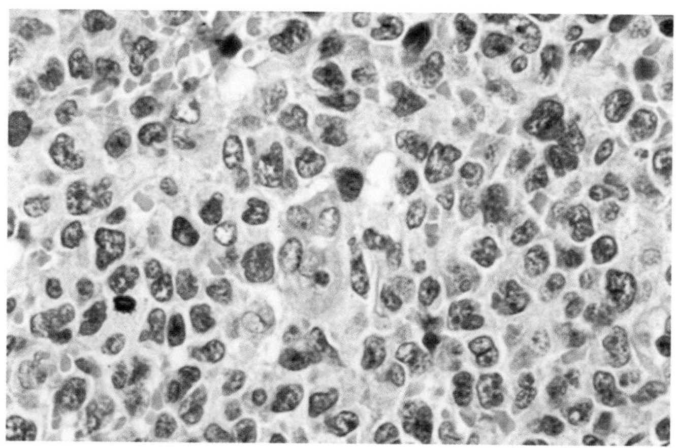

Figure 22-23. Pleomorphic or blastoid mantle cell lymphoma. The medium-sized to large lymphoma cells can lead to a misdiagnosis of diffuse large B-cell lymphoma. Staining for cyclin D1 is essential in such cases.

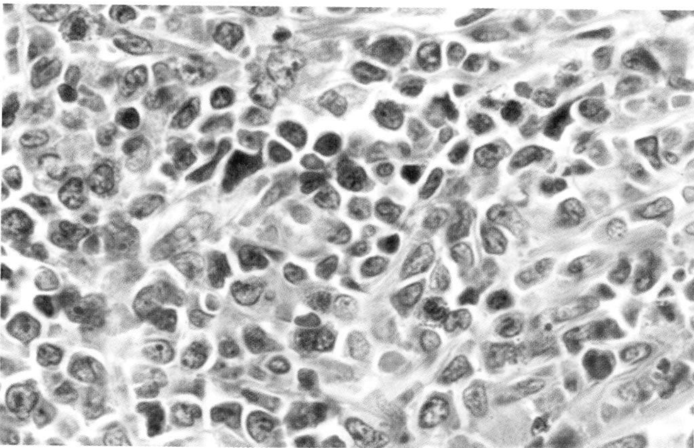

Figure 22-25. Myeloid sarcoma is an important differential diagnosis of diffuse large B-cell lymphoma. Clues to the correct diagnosis include the presence of interspersed eosinophilic myelocytes and the eosinophilic instead of amphophilic quality of the cytoplasm (which may have recognizable granules).

diagnosis can be confirmed by immunostaining for myeloperoxidase, lysozyme, CD34, and CD117.

The cells of histiocytic sarcoma are usually larger than those of DLBCL; most important, the cytoplasm is eosinophilic rather than amphophilic or basophilic. Diagnosis requires the expression of histiocytic markers (e.g., CD68, CD163) and the lack of pan-B, pan-T, and dendritic cell markers.

In the syncytial variant of nodular sclerosis or lymphocyte-depleted classical Hodgkin's lymphoma, distinction from DLBCL can be difficult. The presence of eosinophils favors classical Hodgkin's lymphoma, and syncytial nodular sclerosis Hodgkin's lymphoma almost always shows prominent coagulative necrosis. Uniform strong CD20 immunoreactivity and immunoglobulin expression favor a diagnosis of DLBCL, whereas negative or heterogeneous staining for CD20 and positive EBV-LMP1 expression favor a diagnosis of Hodgkin's

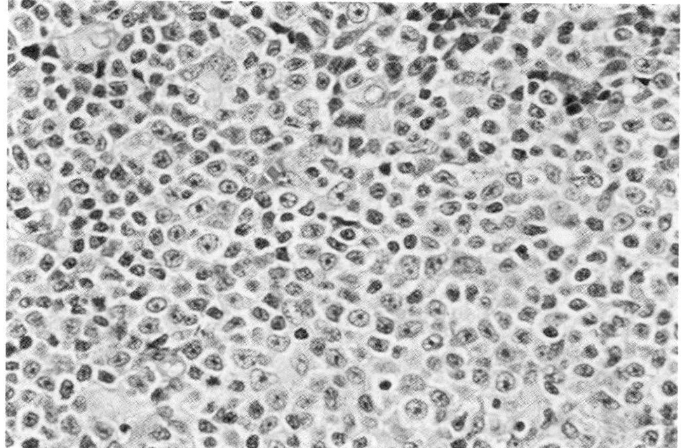

Figure 22-24. Paraimmunoblastic variant of chronic lymphocytic leukemia. The paraimmunoblasts differ from immunoblasts by being smaller and having paler cytoplasm. In addition, there are often admixed small lymphocytes and prolymphocytes, as characteristically seen in chronic lymphocytic leukemia.

lymphoma. Staining for the B-cell transcription factors Oct-2 and BOB.1 can be useful; one or the other is often lacking in classical Hodgkin's lymphoma, even when CD20 is expressed, whereas both are usually expressed in DLBCL.

In florid reactive immunoblastic proliferations such as infectious mononucleosis, other viral infections (including cytomegalovirus infection), drug reactions, and postvaccination reactions, the lymph node shows partial effacement of nodal architecture and infiltration by many large lymphoid cells, closely mimicking DLBCL (Fig. 22-26).[200-202] Necrosis is common, and Reed-Sternberg–like cells are occasionally found, especially around the necrotic foci. In contrast to DLBCL, the large activated cells apparently show transition and maturation into plasmablasts and plasma cells, and they usually do not show significant nuclear atypia such as irregular or twisted nuclear outlines. Immunohistochemically, the large cells in infectious mononucleosis consist of a mixture of B cells and T cells, and the B cells are polytypic.[200,203] Because there is a mixture of B cells at various stages of maturation toward plasma cells, CD20 staining is heterogeneous (with staining lost in late plasmablasts and plasma cells) (Fig. 22-27). Many cells are immunoreactive for EBV-LMP1. Correlation with clinical findings and serology helps one to arrive at the correct diagnosis.

In Kikuchi's lymphadenitis, the lymph nodes are usually small (<2 cm). The lymph nodes show patchy, nonexpansile karyorrhectic foci commonly associated with many large lymphoid cells. In contrast to DLBCL, the proliferated cells in Kikuchi's lymphadenitis consist of histiocytes ($CD68^+$, myeloperoxidase positive), plasmacytoid dendritic cells ($CD68^+$, $CD123^+$, myeloperoxidase negative), and cytotoxic $CD8^+$ T cells, with very few $CD20^+$ B cells.[204,205] Some of the histiocytes are typically packed with phagocytosed materials, compressing the nuclei into a thin crescent (crescentic histiocytes).[206]

Extramedullary hematopoietic tumor, with aggregates of megakaryocytes and immature erythroid and myeloid precursors, can be mistaken for DLBCL. Clues to the correct diagnosis include the identification of megakaryocytes and recognizable normoblasts (Fig. 22-28).

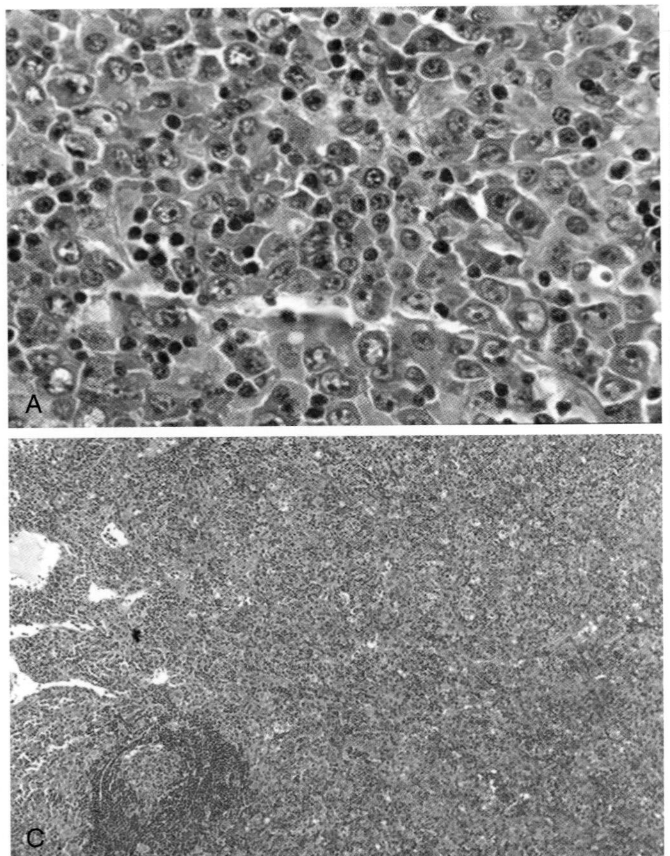

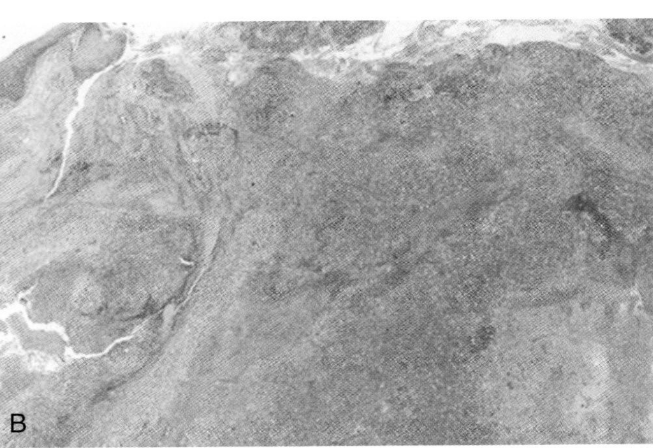

Figure 22-26. Infectious mononucleosis. A, Large lymphoid cells are present in an alarming number, raising the serious consideration of large cell lymphoma. Usually the large cells do not exhibit frank atypia and show a transition into recognizable plasmablasts and plasma cells. **B,** The tonsil is commonly involved and usually exhibits ulceration and necrosis. **C,** An important clue to the correct diagnosis of infectious mononucleosis is partial preservation of the normal lymph node architecture—sinuses and lymphoid follicles are seen in the *left field.*

SUBTYPES AND DISTINCT DISEASE ENTITIES

Four DLBCL subtypes and eight distinct disease entities are recognized in the latest 2008 WHO classification (see Box 22-1).[5] Some of these are discussed here, and the rest are covered in other chapters.

De Novo CD5$^+$ Diffuse Large B-Cell Lymphoma

Definition

De novo CD5$^+$ DLBCL is a subgroup with CD5 expression. It is still unclear whether it represents a distinct clinicopathologic entity or merely an immunophenotypic variant of DLBCL associated with adverse prognostic features.

Epidemiology

About 10% of all de novo DLBCLs express CD5.[52,76,144,207,208] The median age of patients is in the seventh decade. There is a slight female predominance (male-to-female ratio of 1:1.2), in contrast to the slight male predominance in CD5$^-$ DLBCL (male-to-female ratio of 1.4:1).[76]

Clinical Features

De novo CD5$^+$ DLBCL can involve nodal and extranodal sites, and it is associated with aggressive clinical features.[76] A high proportion of patients have high IPI scores, more than 60% of patients have stage III or IV disease, and 75% have extranodal involvement. The most frequently involved extranodal site is the bone marrow. A proportion of patients has intravascular large cell lymphoma or shows a splenic presentation.[207,209,210]

Morphology

Morphologically, de novo CD5$^+$ DLBCL is indistinguishable from DLBCL-NOS (Fig. 22-29). Most cases have a centroblastic appearance, and 19% have an intravascular or intrasinusoidal growth pattern (thus this group includes a subset of intravascular large B-cell lymphomas).[76] Selective involvement of the interfollicular zone is observed in a minority of cases. In the spleen, the infiltrate tends to be localized to the red pulp.[207] Four morphologic variants—common-monomorphic, giant cell–rich, polymorphic, and immunoblastic—have been described.[211]

Immunophenotype

The lymphoma cells express pan-B markers and CD5 (see Box 22-4).[76] They are usually CD10$^-$.[76] BCL2 and BCL6 are expressed in more than 80% of cases.[52] They are not related to CLL or mantle cell lymphoma because they are usually CD23$^-$ and cyclin D1 negative.[76,207,212,213]

Genetics

The immunoglobulin heavy- and light-chain genes are clonally rearranged,[212] accompanied by somatic hypermutation of the *IGHV@* gene.[213,214] There is a lower rate of ongoing somatic

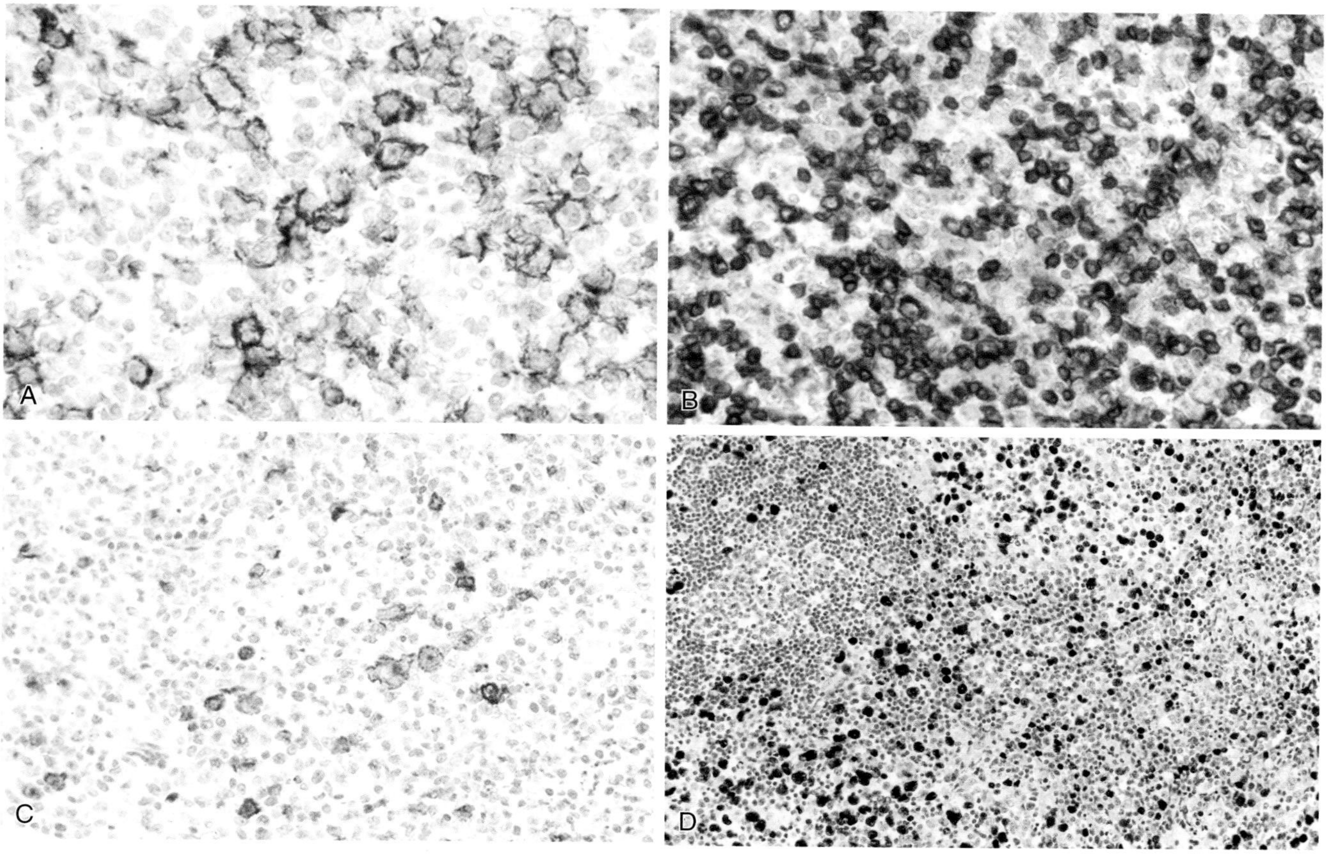

Figure 22-27. Immunohistochemistry of infectious mononucleosis. A, Although many CD20+ cells are often present, the intensity of staining in the large cells is often heterogeneous, indicating that some large cells are plasmablasts (weak or negative for CD20). The B cells are polytypic on staining for immunoglobulin (not shown). **B**, There are often many CD3+ cells, including some large ones. **C**, A proportion of cells stain for EBV-LMP1. **D**, A greater number show nuclear labeling for Epstein-Barr virus–encoded RNA (EBER) on in situ hybridization.

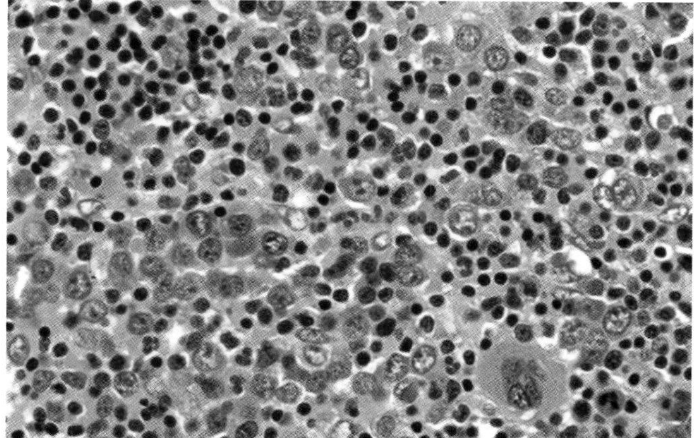

Figure 22-28. Extramedullary hematopoietic tumor. The histologic appearance can lead to a misdiagnosis of diffuse large B-cell lymphoma. Clues to the correct diagnosis include the finding of megakaryocytes (*lower right field*) and islands of erythroblasts, which can look superficially like lymphocytes (*upper left field*). The large cells are in fact immature cells of the myeloid and erythroid series.

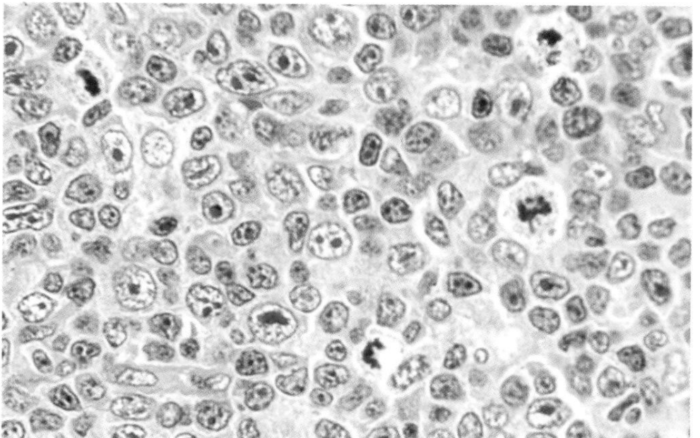

Figure 22-29. De novo CD5+ diffuse large B-cell lymphoma. Morphologically, it cannot be distinguished from conventional diffuse large B-cell lymphoma.

mutation of the *IGHV@* gene compared with CD5⁻ DLBCL.[208] *BCL2* is not rearranged, but *BCL6* is rearranged in about 40% of cases.[212] Cytogenetics and comparative genomic hybridization studies have shown preferential aberrations affecting 8p21 and 11q13; gains of 10p14-15, 19q13, 11q21-24, and 16p; and losses of 1q43-44 and 8p23, compared with CD5⁻ DLBCL.[215-217] Different gene expression profiles are observed between de novo CD5⁺ and CD5⁻ DLBCLs; the former overexpress β_1-integrin (CD29) or CD36 adhesion molecules, with CD29 overexpressed in the tumor cells and CD36 overexpressed in the vascular endothelium.[218] A CD5 signature has also been identified.[219]

Postulated Cell of Origin

The presence of somatic hypermutation of *IGHV@*, together with a low rate of ongoing somatic hypermutations and lack of CD10 expression, suggests post-GC B-cell differentiation.[76,208,213,214,220] Nonetheless, a minority of cases (20%) show a nonmutated immunoglobulin gene, suggesting pre-GC B-cell differentiation.[221] Overall, 82% of cases are classified immunophenotypically as non-GCB DLBCLs according to the Hans algorithm.[211]

Clinical Course

De novo CD5⁺ DLBCL is associated with a worse outcome compared with CD5⁻ DLBCL (5-year survival rate of 34% to 38% versus 50%),[52,76,211] and it is prone to central nervous system recurrence.[211] CD5 expression remains a significant poor prognostic factor for patients treated with rituximab plus CHOP.[222] Although CD5 expression is not an independent prognostic indicator, it is a marker for biologic aggressiveness that is associated with other unfavorable clinical parameters. One group recently reported that the common (monomorphic) variant represents a subgroup of CD5⁺ DLBCLs with a better prognosis.[211]

Differential Diagnosis

The most important differential diagnosis is the pleomorphic variant of mantle cell lymphoma, composed of medium-sized or large pleomorphic cells with irregularly folded nuclei. However, there are often areas with typical morphologic features of mantle cell lymphoma; the cytoplasm is generally scanty, even in the large cells; nucleoli are often inconspicuous; and cyclin D1 is positive.

For DLBCL complicating CLL (Richter's syndrome), there is a known history of CLL or evidence of CLL infiltrate in the biopsy in the form of monotonous small lymphocytes admixed with prolymphocytes and paraimmunoblasts, along with a pan-B⁺, CD5⁺, CD23⁺ immunophenotype.

The paraimmunoblastic variant of CLL can resemble de novo CD5⁺ DLBCL, but the tumor cells are medium-sized rather than large, and there are intermixed prolymphocytes and neoplastic small lymphocytes.

T-Cell/Histiocyte-Rich Large B-Cell Lymphoma

Definition

T-cell/histiocyte-rich large B-cell lymphoma (THRLBCL) is a variant of DLBCL associated with a prominent component of reactive T cells and usually histiocytes.[223-230] It is controversial whether THRLBCL represents a distinct clinicopathologic subtype or merely a morphologic variant of DLBCL.[231,232] Lymphomatoid granulomatosis shows some morphologic and immunophenotypic similarities with THRLBCL but is a separate entity.

Epidemiology

Similar to conventional DLBCL, the median age of patients with THRLBCL is in the sixth to seventh decades, but children may also be affected.[233] There is a slight male predominance (male-to-female ratio of 1.7:1).[227,234]

Etiology

No etiologic factors have been identified. The rich T-cell infiltrate may be related to interleukin-4 production by the lymphoma cells and histiocytes.[235] Tumor cell apoptosis, perhaps mediated by cytotoxic CD8⁺ T cells, may partly explain the relatively low number of neoplastic cells.[236] The small proportion of cases reported with EBV positivity[232,237-241] may correspond to other entities.[223]

It has been suggested that at least a proportion of cases are pathogenetically related to NLPHL.[242,243] Some patients have a prior history of NLPHL,[224] but such cases are often interpreted as the diffuse growth of NLPHL rather than THRLBCL, even though they are morphologically indistinguishable.

Clinical Features

THRLBCL is predominantly a nodal disease, but extranodal sites can also be involved.[234] Compared with conventional DLBCL, THRLBCL more frequently presents with high-stage disease (about two thirds in stage III-IV),[227,228,234] and bone marrow involvement is more common (32% to 62%, versus 16% in conventional DLBCL) (Box 22-6).[26,234,244] Splenomegaly is more frequent (25%).[234]

Morphology

The lymph node usually shows complete effacement of its architecture by a diffuse polymorphic cellular population. The large neoplastic cells, which should account for less than 10% of the cellular population, are dispersed singly, without the formation of discrete aggregates or sheets, in a background of small lymphocytes. The presence of a focal component of NLPHL on morphologic or immunohistochemical assessment excludes a diagnosis of THRLBCL.

The large cells can show the morphology of centroblasts, immunoblasts, large cells indeterminate between centroblasts and immunoblasts, pleomorphic large cells with irregularly folded nuclei, LP (or L&H) cells, or Reed-Sternberg cells (Fig. 22-30). The small lymphocytes in the background (reactive T cells) are either normal looking or mildly atypical, with a slightly larger size and mild nuclear foldings (see Fig. 22-30). In addition, variable numbers of histiocytes, epithelioid histiocytes, eosinophils, and plasma cells may be present. Fine trabecular fibrosis is common in the background.[232] In the histiocyte-rich subgroup, abundant nonepithelioid histiocytes are present, whereas plasma cells and eosinophils are usually scanty.[229,245]

Although different involved sites show similar histologic features in most cases, features of conventional DLBCL may be identified during the course of the disease in some cases.[246] Splenic involvement is characterized by a micronodular pattern, with the micronodules showing a cellular composi-

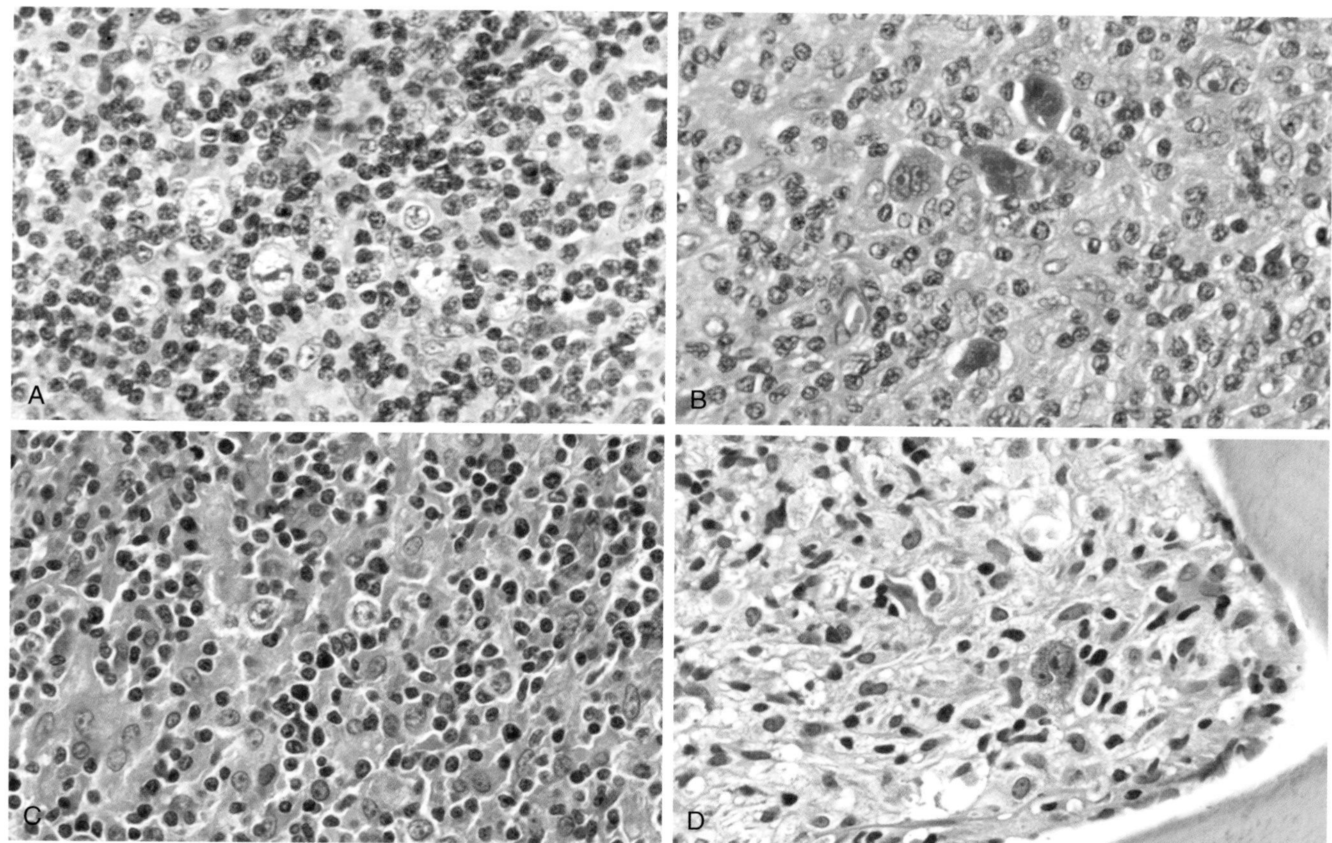

Figure 22-30. T-cell/histiocyte-rich large B-cell lymphoma. A, Large lymphoid cells are scattered singly among small lymphocytes. **B,** Large cells, some resembling Reed-Sternberg cells, occur in a background of slightly activated small lymphoid cells. **C,** This example is rich in small T lymphocytes and histiocytes in the background. **D,** T-cell/histiocyte-rich large B-cell lymphoma with bone marrow involvement. Note the scattered large atypical cells in a background of small lymphoid cells and histiocytes.

tion similar to that of other sites of involvement and lacking follicular dendritic cell meshworks.[247] A summary of THRLBCL is presented in Box 22-6.

Immunophenotype

The scattered large neoplastic cells express pan-B markers, and light-chain restriction is demonstrable in some cases (Fig. 22-31A).[225,227,248] They are frequently negative for CD15 and CD30.[224,225,227,240,246,248,249] The high CD30 positivity rate (up to 40%) reported in a recent series may be related to the use of more sensitive antigen-retrieval methods.[245] CD5 and CD10 are usually negative.[225,245] BCL2 is expressed in 40% of cases, and BCL6 in 40% to 60%.[242,245] EMA expression is variable, ranging from 3% to 100% of cases, with an overall rate of about 30%.[224,227,230,240,245,246,248]

The small cells in the background are overwhelmingly T cells (CD3$^+$), predominantly the CD8$^+$ cytotoxic type (see Fig. 22-31B).[236] In contrast to NLPHL, there are no rosettes of follicular T cells (CD57$^+$, PD-1$^+$) around the large neoplastic cells.[250] The cases reported to have many CD57$^+$ small lymphocytes may represent the diffuse variant of NLPHL.[242,245] Small reactive B cells should be rare.[245]

Genetics

THRLBCL has clonally rearranged immunoglobulin genes and germline TCR genes.[238,248,251-253] A hypermutated *IGHV@* gene and ongoing somatic mutations can be demonstrated in some cases.[254,255] *BCL2* rearrangement is present in about one fourth of cases.[224,227] Many cases fall into the "host response" subgroup of DLBCLs as defined by gene expression profiling.[256]

Postulated Cell of Origin

Demonstration of a hypermutated immunoglobulin gene with ongoing somatic mutations and *BCL2* rearrangement in some cases supports a GC stage of differentiation in a proportion of cases.[254,255] Comparative genomic hybridization has shown similar as well as distinct cytogenetic features in THRLBCL and NLPHL, suggesting a possible link between the two entities.[257]

Clinical Course

THRLBCL is an aggressive lymphoma, with a 3-year overall survival of 46%.[234] The poor outcome is probably related to the often advanced stage of disease at diagnosis. However, THRLBCL and conventional DLBCL, when matched for IPI, have similar outcomes after chemotherapy.[258] A primary cutaneous counterpart has been reported with a more favorable outcome.[259]

Differential Diagnosis

The main differential diagnoses and their distinguishing features are listed in Table 22-5. In some examples of

Box 22-6 *Major Diagnostic Features of T-Cell/Histiocyte-Rich Large B-Cell Lymphoma*

Definition
- Neoplastic large B cells should be dispersed singly and should not form discrete aggregates or sheets
- Background with abundant reactive T cells and usually histiocytes
- Absence of known or a recognizable component of NLPHL (which can be focal or subtle)

Clinical Features
- Age: older adults (sixth to seventh decades)
- Male-to-female ratio 1.7:1
- Nodal or extranodal involvement
- Usually advanced stage at presentation (two thirds, stage III and IV)
- Bone marrow involvement very common (60%)
- Prognosis: controversial; some studies report a poor prognosis, whereas others show no difference compared with comparable-stage conventional DLBCL

Morphology
- Diffuse infiltrate of scattered large neoplastic B cells that may resemble centroblasts, immunoblasts, LP (L&H) cells, or Reed-Sternberg cells
- Background cells include small T cells (which can show mild atypia), often with histiocytes, plasma cells, and eosinophils

Immunophenotype
- Large cells: pan-B^+, $CD30^-$, $CD15^-$, $EMA^{+/-}$, $BCL6^{+/-}$
- Background small cells: $CD3^+$, TIA-1^+
- There should be no large B cells residing within nodules of small B cells, which would indicate a diagnosis of NLPHL

Molecular Features
- Clonally rearranged immunoglobulin genes
- Germline TCR genes
- EBV usually negative

DLBCL, diffuse large B-cell lymphoma; EBV, Epstein-Barr virus; EMA, epithelial membrane antigen; NLPHL, nodular lymphocyte-predominant Hodgkin's lymphoma; TCR, T-cell receptor.

THRLBCL, many of the large cells resemble reactive immunoblasts, making it difficult to distinguish from reactive lymphoid hyperplasia. In THRLBCL, definite atypia (e.g., enlarged nuclei, irregular nuclear folding) can usually be recognized in at least a small proportion of the large cells after a careful search, and the pattern of uniform scattering of solitary large cells in a small lymphoid cell background is very unusual for a reactive process. Furthermore, in reactive lymphoid hyperplasia, the large lymphoid cells more often occur in patchy aggregates, show transition to plasmablasts and plasma cells, exhibit heterogeneous staining for CD20 owing to the presence of B cells in different stages of maturation, and show polytypic staining for immunoglobulin light chains.

The lymphocyte-rich and mixed cellularity types of classical Hodgkin's lymphoma can simulate THRLBCL.[230,260,261] Reed-Sternberg cells are either negative for pan-B markers or show heterogeneous staining if positive. They are frequently $CD30^+$ and $CD15^+$ and are more likely to harbor EBV.

In NLPHL with an extensive diffuse component, the presence of scattered large LP (L&H) cells with a B-cell phenotype in a background of small T lymphocytes is practically indistinguishable from THRLBCL.[240] Patients with NLPHL are younger (30 to 50 years), and most patients (80% to 95%) present with early-stage (I-II) disease.[262] Histologically, a nodular pattern is usually identified at least focally, with follicular T-cell rosettes around the tumor cells as demonstrated by CD57 or PD-1.[250] Although the small lymphocytes within the nodules are mostly B cells, those in the diffuse areas are mostly T cells. These T cells infrequently express the cytotoxic marker TIA-1.[240]

THRLBCL may also be confused with peripheral T-cell lymphoma because the activated T cells in the background of THRLBCL can show mild atypia. In peripheral T-cell lymphoma, the T cells show a more prominent degree of cytologic atypia, and the atypia involves lymphoid cells of various sizes. The larger cells within the infiltrate do not stand out distinctly as a separate population, as they do in THRLBCL, and there is a transition with the smaller atypical cells. Immunophenotypically, the large atypical cells express pan-T rather than pan-B markers. Nonetheless, confusion can arise because some peripheral T-cell lymphomas, especially angioimmunoblastic T-cell lymphoma, can be accompanied by a reactive large B-cell proliferation, which is often EBV driven.[263-266] Careful correlation between immunostaining and morphology reveals that although some large atypical cells are $CD20^+$, most atypical medium-sized and large cells are $CD20^-$ and $CD3^+$. Genotyping is confirmatory in difficult cases because THRLBCL has rearranged immunoglobulin genes,[238,248,251-253]

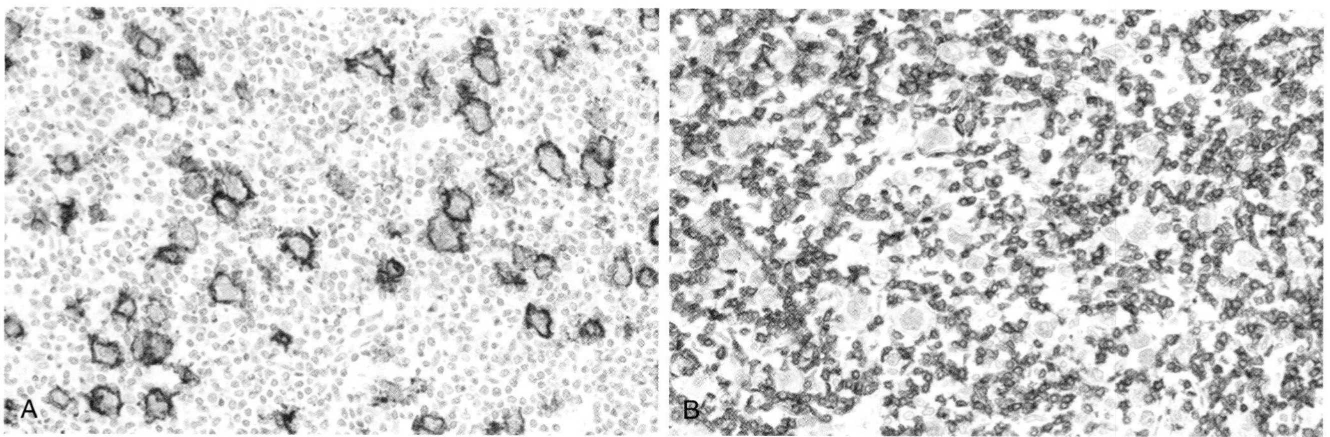

Figure 22-31. Immunohistochemistry of T-cell/histiocyte-rich large B-cell lymphoma. A, CD20 immunostain selectively highlights the dispersed large cells. **B,** Numerous small $CD3^+$ T lymphocytes are present in the background.

Table 22-5 Comparison of T-Cell/Histiocyte-Rich Large B-Cell Lymphoma, Peripheral T-Cell Lymphoma, Classical Hodgkin's Lymphoma, and Nodular Lymphocyte-Predominant Hodgkin's Lymphoma

Feature	T-Cell/Histiocyte-Rich Large B-Cell Lymphoma	Peripheral T-Cell Lymphoma	Classical Hodgkin's Lymphoma	Nodular Lymphocyte-Predominant Hodgkin's Lymphoma
Most commonly affected age group	6th-7th decades	7th decade	Bimodal age distribution: 2nd to 3rd decade and 6th decade onward	4th-5th decades
Site of disease	Nodal or extranodal	Nodal or extranodal; extranodal involvement common	Predominantly nodal	Predominantly nodal
Stage	Advanced stage (III-IV) in 67% of cases	Advanced stage (III-IV) in 80% of cases	Advanced stage (III-IV) in 50% of cases	Advanced stage (III-IV) in 10% of cases
Morphology of large cells	Variable appearance	Variable appearance; nuclei often show irregular foldings	Reed-Sternberg cells and variants	LP (L&H) cells with popcorn-like nuclei, often occurring within nodules of small lymphocytes
Morphology of small cells	Reactive T cells appear as small lymphocytes or mildly activated cells	Often atypical lymphocytes that commonly show a continuum through medium-sized to large cells	Mostly nonactivated small lymphocytes	Mostly nonactivated small lymphocytes
Immunophenotype	Large cells: CD20$^+$, CD30$^{-/+}$, CD15$^-$, Oct-2$^+$, BOB.1$^+$ Small cells: CD3$^+$ (many TIA-1$^+$)	Large and smaller cells: CD3$^+$, but some EBV$^+$ large B cells may be scattered	Large cells: CD30$^+$, CD15$^{+/-}$, CD20$^{-/+}$ (heterogeneous staining if +), Oct-2$^-$, BOB.1$^-$ Small cells: CD3$^+$	Large cells: CD20$^+$, CD30$^-$, CD15$^-$, Oct-2$^+$, BOB.1$^+$ Small cells: CD20$^+$ in nodular areas, with CD57$^+$ PD1$^+$ CD3$^+$ cells rosetting around LP (L&H) cells; many CD3$^+$ small cells in diffuse areas, sometimes within nodules, and usually TIA-1$^-$
Genotype	Rearranged immunoglobulin genes; germline TCR genes	Rearranged TCR genes; immunoglobulin genes usually germline	Immunoglobulin and TCR genes frequently germline (whole tissue DNA)	Immunoglobulin and TCR genes frequently germline (whole tissue DNA)
EBV association	Very rare	Uncommon, but EBV$^+$ B cells can be found in some cases, especially angioimmunoblastic T-cell lymphoma	Common (≈40%; higher in nonwhite populations)	Very rare

EBV, Epstein-Barr virus; TCR, T-cell receptor.

whereas peripheral T-cell lymphoma has rearranged TCR genes.

Lymphomatoid granulomatosis also features large atypical B cells in a background of reactive T cells, but it always presents in extranodal sites (most commonly lung and skin), and EBV is almost always positive (see Chapter 23).

EBV$^+$ Diffuse Large B-Cell Lymphoma of the Elderly

Definition

EBV$^+$ DLBCL of the elderly, originally known as *senile EBV-associated B-cell lymphoproliferative disorder*, is an EBV-associated clonal B-cell proliferation occurring in patients older than 50 years without any known immunodeficiency or prior lymphoma.[16,17] It is believed to result from immunologic deterioration related to the aging process.[267] Rare cases may occur in younger patients, but the possibility of an undiagnosed underlying immunodeficiency must be excluded. By definition, other well-defined EBV-associated disorders (e.g., infectious mononucleosis, lymphomatoid granulomatosis, primary effusion lymphoma, plasmablastic lymphoma, DLBCL associated with chronic inflammation) are not included in this category.

Epidemiology and Etiology

Although this entity has been reported almost exclusively in Asians,[16,115,268,269] it can definitely occur in other populations. Further studies are required to determine whether this lymphoma type is more prevalent in Asians. It has a frequency of 8% to 10% among all DLBCLs in those without a documented history of immunodeficiency.[267] The EBV positivity rate among DLBCLs increases with age, with a peak (20% to 30%) at older than 90 years.[267]

Clinical Features

The median age is 71 years, and the male-to-female ratio is 1.4:1. Extranodal presentation with or without nodal disease is common (70%), frequently involving skin, lung, tonsil, and stomach.[17] The clinical outcome is poor, with a median survival of 2 years and an overall 5-year survival of about 25%.[115,268] Unfavorable prognostic factors include B symptoms and age older than 70 years.[268]

Pathology

Histologically, the lymph node or extranodal site shows architectural effacement by an abnormal diffuse lymphoid infiltrate, often with prominent coagulative necrosis. The infiltrate includes many large cells that may have the morphology of centroblasts, immunoblasts, Reed-Sternberg–like cells, and highly pleomorphic cells. The two morphologic subtypes recognized, which have no clinical significance, are the large cell lymphoma subtype, characterized by monotonous sheets of large cells, and the polymorphic subtype, characterized by many admixed reactive cells such as small lymphocytes, plasma cells, histiocytes, and epithelioid histiocytes.[17,267]

Immunophenotypically, the tumor cells usually express pan-B markers, but rare cases may lack CD20 expression. CD10 and BCL6 are commonly negative, and IRF4/MUM-1 is frequently positive. There is variable CD30 expression, and CD15 is negative.[17] By definition, the tumor cells contain EBV, with Epstein-Barr virus–encoded RNA (EBER) positivity being demonstrated in the majority of tumor cells. LMP1 and EBNA2 are expressed in 94% and 28% of cases, respectively.[267] Clonal immunoglobulin gene rearrangement is demonstrable.

The presence of Reed-Sternberg–like cells and the reactive cellular component in the polymorphic subtype may suggest classical Hodgkin's lymphoma. In contrast to the latter, EBV^+ DLBCL of the elderly much more commonly involves extranodal sites (e.g., skin, gastrointestinal tract, lung), geographic necrosis is more frequent, CD20 is positive, and CD15 is consistently negative.[267,268,270]

Primary Mediastinal (Thymic) Large B-Cell Lymphoma

Definition

Primary mediastinal (thymic) large B-cell lymphoma (PMLBCL) is a distinct subtype of DLBCL of putative thymic B-cell origin. By definition, the major bulk of tumor is confined to the anterior mediastinum at presentation.[3,271]

Epidemiology

PMLBCL accounts for 2.4% of all non-Hodgkin's lymphomas.[6,7] Most patients are in the third decade of life (median age, 37 years),[6,272-274] but children can also be affected.[275] There is a female predominance, with a female-to-male ratio of 2:1.

Etiology

No etiologic factor has been identified. This lymphoma type does not appear to arise from thymic extranodal marginal zone lymphoma of MALT.

Clinical Features

Patients present with symptoms related to the large anterior mediastinal mass, such as superior vena cava obstruction, dyspnea, and chest discomfort.[28,276-278] Rare patients may be asymptomatic. The tumor can invade the chest wall, sternum, pericardium, pleura, and lung.[277,279-282]

Most patients present with early-stage disease (66% stages I and II).[6] Bone marrow involvement is uncommon (2%).[282] Unlike other DLBCLs, it is not associated with an elevated serum β_2-microglobulin level, despite the presence of bulky disease[283]; this may be related to the lack of expression of HLA class I molecules in PMLBCL.[284] The serum lactate dehydrogenase level is frequently elevated (76% of cases).[282]

Morphology

The tumor exhibits a diffuse infiltrate of large or medium-sized lymphoma cells with a highly variable appearance. The lymphoma cells can have a centroblastic, immunoblastic, anaplastic, unclassifiable, or Reed-Sternberg–like appearance. The nuclei are round or multilobated. Cytoplasm is often abundant and not uncommonly (40% of cases) shows clearing (Figs. 22-32 and 22-33A).[28,277,280,282,285-289] Sometimes the lymphoma cells assume a spindly morphology (see Fig. 22-33B). Rare cases exhibit a marked tropism for preexisting GCs.[290]

Sclerosis is common, ranging from delicate collagen fibers surrounding individual or groups of lymphoma cells ("compartmentalization") to broad septa of dense collagen (Fig. 22-34).[28,279,282] Occasionally there is identifiable remnant thymic epithelium, which can show atrophy, hyperplasia, or cystic change (Fig. 22-35).[280,291] A summary of PMLBCL is presented in Box 22-7.

Immunophenotype

PMLBCL expresses pan-B markers.[279,286,289,292,293] However, most cases do not express surface or cytoplasmic immunoglobulin, despite expression of CD79a (a component of a heterodimer associated with surface immunoglobulin) and the immunoglobulin transactivating factors Oct-2 and BOB.1.[286,288,293-296] Because messenger RNA transcripts of switched immunoglobulin heavy chain can be detected in PMLBCL,[297] the reason behind the immunoglobulin-negative immunophenotype remains unexplained.

PMLBCL is negative for CD21 and frequently expresses CD23 (70% of cases), similar to the asteroid B cells normally found in the medulla of the thymus (Fig. 22-36).[292-294,298-301] The tumor shows defective major histocompatibility complex (MHC) antigen expression.[302] Although previous studies reported infrequent staining for CD10 and CD30,[293,294] more recent studies show CD10, BCL6 and CD30 expression in 21% to 32%, 55% to 100%, and 69% to 86% of cases, respectively.[296,303-305] Two rare cases expressing human chorionic gonadotropin have been reported.[306]

MAL gene (on chromosome 2q) expression, which can be demonstrated by molecular methods or immunohistochemistry, occurs in 70% of cases but is extremely rare in other DLBCLs, supporting the distinctive nature of this lymphoma type.[307,308] Although the underlying molecular mechanism for *MAL* gene expression in PMLBCL is currently unknown, this feature can potentially serve as a specific marker for this entity.

Genetics

PMLBCL shows clonally rearranged immunoglobulin heavy- and light-chain genes and germline TCR genes.[309] There is no *BCL1* or *BCL2* rearrangement. *BCL6* rearrangement occurs in only 6% of cases, whereas *BCL6* mutation is reported in 10% to 70% of cases.[91,296,310,311] Rearrangements or point mutations in the *MYC* gene have been detected in occasional cases.[311,312] EBV is almost always negative.[282,311,312]

Comparative genomic hybridization shows a frequent gain of chromosomal material involving 9p, 12q, and Xq,[313,314] and array comparative genomic hybridization has revealed addi-

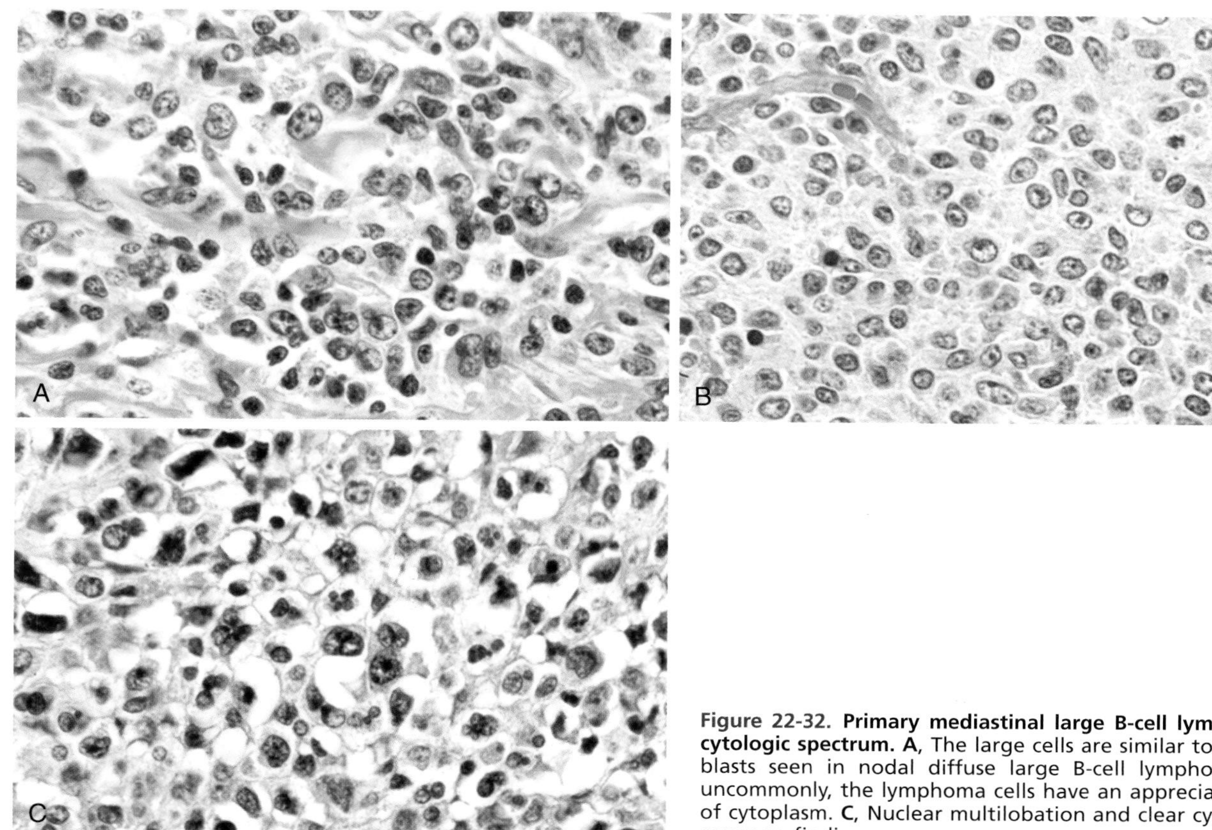

Figure 22-32. Primary mediastinal large B-cell lymphoma: the cytologic spectrum. A, The large cells are similar to the centroblasts seen in nodal diffuse large B-cell lymphoma. **B,** Not uncommonly, the lymphoma cells have an appreciable amount of cytoplasm. **C,** Nuclear multilobation and clear cytoplasm are common findings.

tional chromosomal gains and losses of other regions: gains involving 2p, 7q, and 9q, and losses involving 1p.[315,316] The most frequently observed gain in material on chromosome 9p may involve *JAK2*, *PDL1*, *PDL2*, and *SMARCA2* genes.[317] Activation of interleukin-4–induced gene 1 (*FIG1*) and *STAT6*, which may or may not be mediated through the overexpression of *JAK2*, has been observed in a majority of cases and may play a role.[318,319]

Some cases show high-level amplifications at 2p involving the *REL* proto-oncogene.[304,313,320,321] Nuclear accumulation of REL protein is common in PMLBCL, which may or may not be associated with gain or amplification of *REL*.[321] Combined nuclear REL expression and cytoplasmic TRAF1 expression, features indicating activation of the nuclear factor-κB signaling pathway, may be helpful for distinguishing PMLBCL from other DLBCLs.[322] Anomalies of the *TP53* and *CDKN2A* genes are detected in a minority of cases.[310,311]

Of interest, PMLBCL shows a gene expression profile that is much closer to that of classical Hodgkin's lymphoma than conventional DLBCL.[317,323]

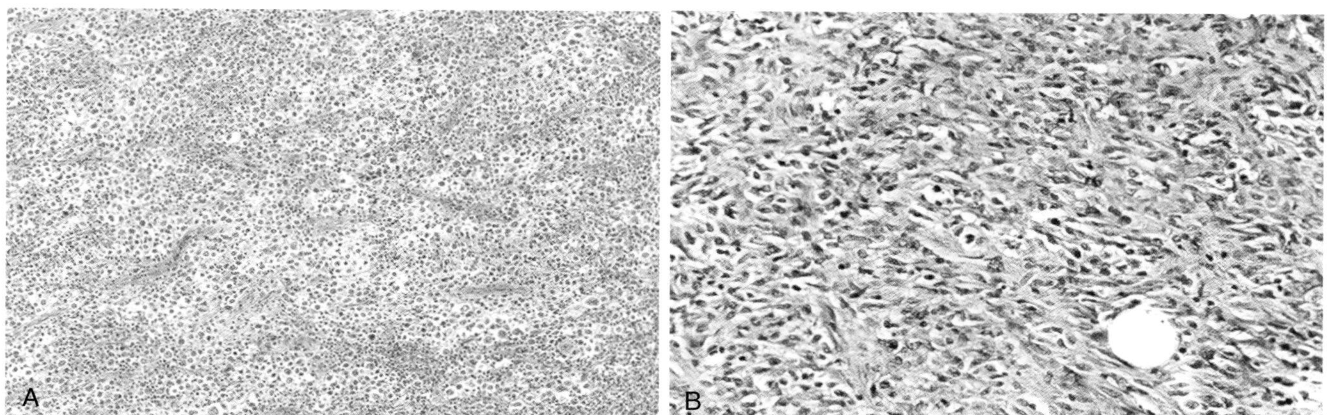

Figure 22-33. Primary mediastinal large B-cell lymphoma: unusual appearances. A, The presence of clear cells demarcated by fibrovascular septa produces an appearance reminiscent of germinoma. **B,** Spindly lymphoma cells are sometimes prominent.

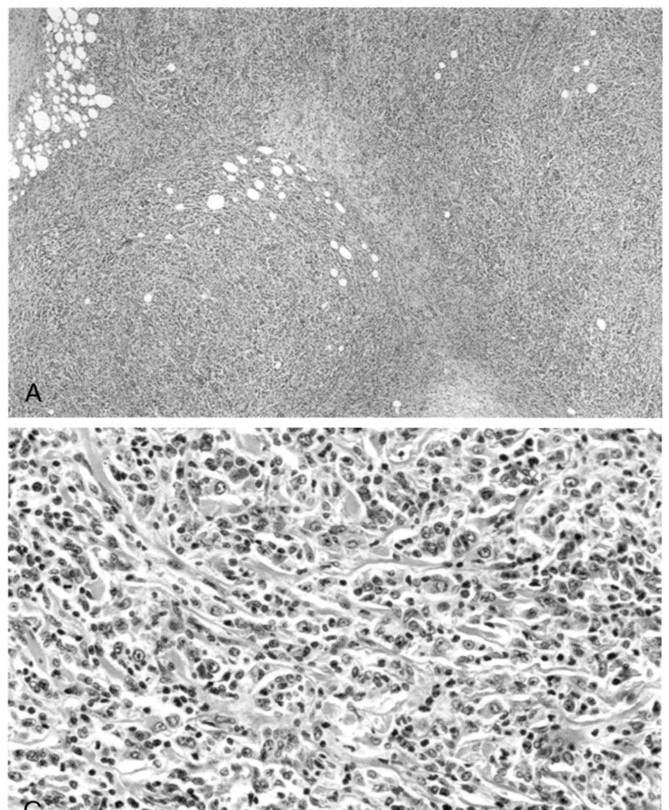

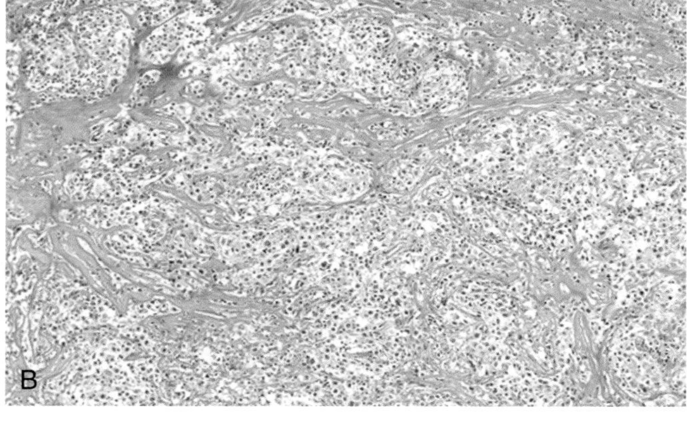

Figure 22-34. **Primary mediastinal large B-cell lymphoma: patterns of sclerosis. A,** Broad sclerotic bands traverse the tumor to produce large tumor nodules. **B,** Thinner sclerotic bands demarcate the tumor into packets. **C,** Delicate collagen fibrils are found within the tumor.

Postulated Cell of Origin

Addis and Isaacson[279] first suggested a thymic B-cell origin for PMLBCL based on the tumor location, frequent lack of nodal involvement, and presence of residual thymic tissue in some cases. Subsequently, a distinctive population of $CD21^-$ thymic B cells was identified in the normal thymus, and these cells (particularly the population with asteroid morphology) are considered the normal counterpart for PMLBCL.[298,299,301]

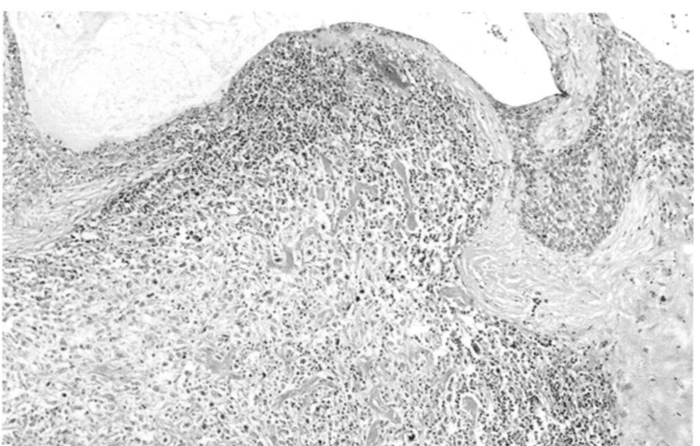

Figure 22-35. **Primary mediastinal large B-cell lymphoma.** In this example, there is proliferation of the residual thymic epithelium and formation of cysts lined by thymic epithelium.

Earlier studies reported a low frequency of *BCL2* and *BCL6* rearrangements (0% and 4% to 6%, respectively, compared with 20% to 30% and 35%, respectively, for conventional DLBCL), suggesting that PMLBCL is a distinct entity, unrelated to GC differentiation, as is a proportion of conventional DLBCLs.[310,311] Recent studies, however, show frequent BCL6 expression, *BCL6* mutation, and occasional CD10 expression in PMLBCL, raising the possibility of a GC or post-GC stage of differentiation.[296,303,304] The high load of somatic mutations in the immunoglobulin gene in PMLBCL also supports a late GC or post-GC stage of differentiation, but the absence of ongoing mutation favors the latter.[297]

What has been reported under the category of PMLBCL probably represents heterogeneous entities, including lymphoma of true thymic origin and lymphoma of mediastinal nodal origin.[324] The latter would be expected to be similar to DLBCL involving peripheral lymph nodes. This can explain why a specific immunophenotype and *MAL* gene expression are not identified in all cases. Similarly, gene expression profiling shows that a minority of clinical PMLBCL cases lack the characteristic molecular signature of PMLBCL.[317]

Clinical Course

The standard treatment is multiagent chemotherapy and rituximab, with or without radiotherapy, and the cure rate is 50% to 80%.[325-331] Although the older literature suggested a worse prognosis for PMLBCL compared with conventional DLBCLs, recent studies have shown similar or even better clinical outcomes.[6,282,331-333] The improved survival may be

Box 22-7 *Major Diagnostic Features of Primary Mediastinal Large B-Cell Lymphoma (PMLBCL)*

Distinctive Clinical Features (versus DLBCL-NOS)
- Young adult: median age 37 years (versus 64 years)
- Female predominance: male-to-female ratio 1:2 (versus 1.2:1)
- Symptoms related to anterior mediastinal mass (e.g., superior vena cava obstruction, dyspnea)
- Bulky disease (>10 cm) in 52% of cases (versus 30%)
- Early-stage (I and II) disease in 66% of cases (versus 54%)
- Marrow involvement very rare (3% versus 17%)
- Lactate dehydrogenase often elevated (75%), but β_2-microglobulin not elevated
- Survival not substantially different when treated with chemotherapy ± radiotherapy
- Relapse tends to occur in extranodal sites (e.g., gastrointestinal tract, kidney, adrenal, ovary, central nervous system)

Morphology
- Large or medium-sized lymphoma cells
- The following features are more common in PMLBCL than in DLBCL-NOS but are neither specific nor invariably present: clear cell change, prominent sclerosis

Immunophenotype
- Pan-B$^+$, CD3$^-$
- Immunoglobulin frequently negative
- BCL6$^+$ in ≈60%
- CD10$^+$ in ≈25%
- CD23$^+$ in ≈70%
- CD30$^+$ in ≈70%
- Deficient MHC molecule expression

Molecular Features
- Clonally rearranged immunoglobulin genes
- *BCL2* and *BCL6* genes usually not rearranged
- *BCL6* gene mutation in ≈70%
- *MAL* gene frequently expressed (70%)
- EBV$^-$

DLBCL-NOS, diffuse large B-cell lymphoma, not otherwise specified; EBV, Epstein-Barr virus; MHC, major histocompatibility complex.

due to the use of more aggressive chemotherapy, adjuvant radiotherapy, or rituximab.[274,278,328,330,333,334]

Poor prognostic indicators include pleural effusion, pericardial effusion, increased number of involved extranodal sites, positive posttreatment gallium scan, high serum lactate dehydrogenase level, low performance score, and high IPI score.[281,329,332,335] The histologic appearance is of no prognostic significance,[280] but loss of the MHC class II gene and protein expression is a poor prognostic indicator.[336] Cases with the molecular signature of PMLBCL are associated with better clinical outcomes than the GCB and ABC subgroups of DLBCLs.[317]

At the time of recurrence, PMLBCL has a tendency to spread to unusual extranodal sites, such as the kidney, central nervous system, adrenal gland, liver, pancreas, gastrointestinal tract, and ovary.[272,274,337,338]

Differential Diagnosis

By definition, the tumor bulk in PMLBCL is in the anterior mediastinum, thus excluding other nodal or extranodal DLBCLs that secondarily involve the mediastinum. The main differential diagnoses are listed in Table 22-6 (see also Pearls and Pitfalls at the end of this chapter).

The most important differential diagnosis for PMLBCL is nodular sclerosis Hodgkin's lymphoma. Similarities include occurrence in young patients, predominant anterior mediastinal location, large tumor cells, and sclerosis. The problem distinguishing the two is compounded by the fact that some PMLBCLs express CD30, and some cases of nodular sclerosis Hodgkin's lymphoma express pan-B markers. Nodular sclerosis Hodgkin's lymphoma is associated with an inflammatory background, most commonly eosinophils, and the tumor cells express CD30 and CD15 but not CD45. Although pan-B markers may be expressed in Reed-Sternberg cells, the expression is usually heterogeneous, in contrast to the uniformly strong staining in PMLBCL. Reed-Sternberg cells are usually negative for the immunoglobulin transactivating factors Oct-2 and BOB.1, contrasting with their consistent expression in PMLBCL.[296,339] EBV, when present, strongly favors a diagnosis of nodular sclerosis Hodgkin's lymphoma over PMLBCL.[261] Composite or metachronous cases of PMLBCL and nodular sclerosis Hodgkin's lymphoma have been described,[25,272,340,341] with demonstration of the same clone in the two different components in at least some cases.[341] The link between PMLBCL and classical Hodgkin's lymphoma is further supported by similarities in the gene expression profiles of the two entities[317,323] and the existence of occasional cases of MAL-expressing nodular sclerosis Hodgkin's lymphoma.[308,342]

Cases with intermediate features (e.g., mediastinal gray zone lymphoma)[341,343] are categorized as B-cell lymphoma, unclassifiable, with features intermediate between DLBCL and classical Hodgkin's lymphoma in the 2008 WHO classification.[344] These borderline cases include tumors with overlapping histologic features and transitional immunophenotypes; cases resembling PMLBCL morphologically but with CD15 expression or EBV association, in the absence of CD20 expression; and cases with the appearance of nodular sclerosis Hodgkin's lymphoma but uniformly strong expression of CD20 and other B-cell markers, in the absence of CD15 expression.[344] The most frequent histologic finding is a variable microscopic appearance in different areas, with sheets of tumor cells ranging from centroblast-like to lacuna-like or Hodgkin-like, in a diffusely fibrotic stroma. Inflammatory

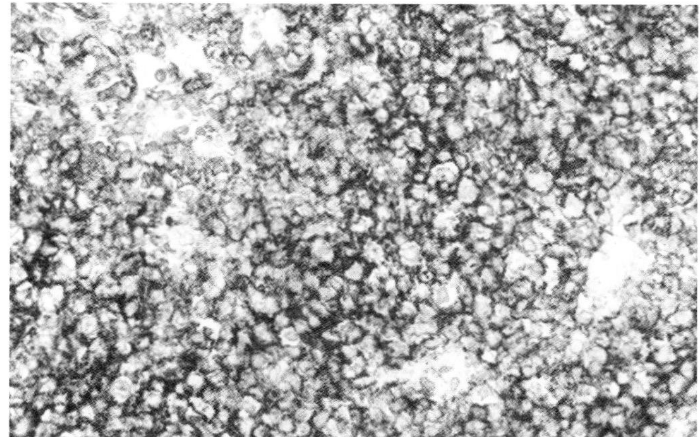

Figure 22-36. Primary mediastinal large B-cell lymphoma. The tumor cells show strong membrane staining for CD23, a marker recently shown to be frequently expressed in this lymphoma type.

Table 22-6 Differential Diagnosis of Primary Mediastinal Large B-Cell Lymphoma (PMLBCL)

Entity	Features Favoring Diagnosis of That Entity	Features Favoring Diagnosis of PMLBCL
DLBCL-NOS	Accompanied by disease in sites other than anterior mediastinum	Predominant mass in anterior mediastinum at presentation CD23 or MAL expression Immunoglobulin expression commonly absent
Nodular sclerosis Hodgkin's lymphoma, syncytial variant	Many eosinophils in background Necrosis common with dense sheets of large tumor cells $CD45^-$, $CD30^+$, $CD15^{+/-}$, pan-$B^{-/+}$ (heterogeneous if +), Oct-2^-, BOB.1^- EBV^+ in >35%	Clear cell change fairly common $CD45^+$, pan-B^+, $CD30^{+/-}$, $CD15^-$, Oct-2^+, BOB.1^+ EBV very rare
Anaplastic large cell lymphoma	Hallmark cells Pan-B^-, pan-$T^{+/-}$ $EMA^{+/-}$, $ALK^{+/-}$ Cytotoxic markers +/–	Sclerosis much more common Pan-B^+, pan-T^- EMA^-
Mediastinal seminoma	Almost exclusively male Nuclei often round Glycogen ++ $CD45^-$, Oct-$3/4^+$, placental alkaline phosphatase +, $CD117^+$	Although cells may have clear cytoplasm, nuclei are often lobated or folded Glycogen – $CD45^+$, pan-B^+, $CD117^-$
Thymic carcinoma	Cohesive growth; sharp interface with desmoplastic stroma May exhibit squamous or squamoid features Cytokeratin +	Although tumor may show packeting pattern, diffuse permeative growth in at least some areas Cytokeratin –, $CD20^+$
Thymic carcinoid	Nests of tumor cells separated by rich vasculature May form rosettes Cytokeratin +, neuroendocrine markers +	Although tumor may show packeting pattern, sclerotic septa are relatively avascular Cytokeratin –, $CD45^+$, neuroendocrine markers –

ALK, anaplastic lymphoma kinase; DLBCL-NOS, diffuse large B-cell lymphoma, not otherwise specified; EBV, Epstein-Barr virus; EMA, epithelial membrane antigen.

infiltrate is usually sparse, and coagulative necrosis is common. These borderline cases frequently express CD45, CD20, CD79a, Oct-2, and BOB.1, in addition to the Hodgkin's lymphoma markers CD30 and CD15. MAL expression is observed in a significant proportion of these cases.[341] These borderline cases show a more aggressive behavior than PMLBCL or classical Hodgkin's lymphoma.[344] The optimal treatment protocol remains controversial.

Anaplastic large cell lymphoma shares similarities with PMLBCL, including the presence of many large lymphoid cells and CD30 immunoreactivity. However, the former has a T-cell or null cell phenotype ($PAX5^-$), often with the expression of cytotoxic markers, and it may express ALK.[345]

PMLBCL can mimic mediastinal seminoma when there is tumor packeting and the presence of clear cells. However, seminoma occurs exclusively in males, shows round but not multilobated nuclei, and expresses placental alkaline phosphatase, CD117, and Oct-3/4 but not CD45 and pan-B markers.

Thymic carcinoma and neuroendocrine tumor may enter into the differential diagnosis if the biopsy sample is small and crushed. Both express cytokeratin and are negative for CD45 and pan-B markers.

Intravascular Large B-Cell Lymphoma

Definition

Intravascular large B-cell lymphoma (IVLBCL), also known as *intravascular lymphomatosis* or *angiotropic lymphoma*, is a rare subtype of DLBCL in which the lymphoma cells reside predominantly or exclusively within the lumens of blood vessels, with no or few circulating neoplastic cells in the peripheral blood.[346,347] In the past, an endothelial origin was speculated (hence the term *malignant angioendotheliomatosis*), but there is now no doubt that it is a lymphoid neoplasm.[348-351]

Epidemiology

IVLBCL is a rare lymphoma occurring predominantly in older patients in the sixth to seventh decades of life.[348,352] A variant associated with hemophagocytic syndrome has been reported mostly in Asian populations (see later).

Etiology

There is no known etiologic factor. The lymphoma cells' propensity to be localized in the lumens of blood vessels may be partly explained by the lack of expression of CD29 (β_1-integrin) and CD54 (ICAM-1), both of which are important for transvascular lymphocyte migration.[353]

Clinical Features

IVLBCL can involve any organ but is most common in the central nervous system, skin, kidney, lung, adrenal, and liver.[348,352,354] Patients commonly present with fever; nonspecific, nonlocalizing neurologic symptoms; or skin lesions. The neurologic symptoms are often bizarre, owing to the presence of multiple sites of infarct resulting from vascular occlusion. Patients may have one or more of the four neurologic syndromes: multifocal cerebrovascular events, spinal cord and roots lesions, subacute encephalopathy, and peripheral or cranial neuropathy.[355] The cutaneous manifestations are nonspecific, most commonly consisting of nodular, subcutaneous, firm masses or plaques, with or without hemorrhage.[356] Overlying telangiectasia may be prominent, and there may be ulceration. The trunk and extremities are frequently involved sites. Some patients may present with disease limited to the

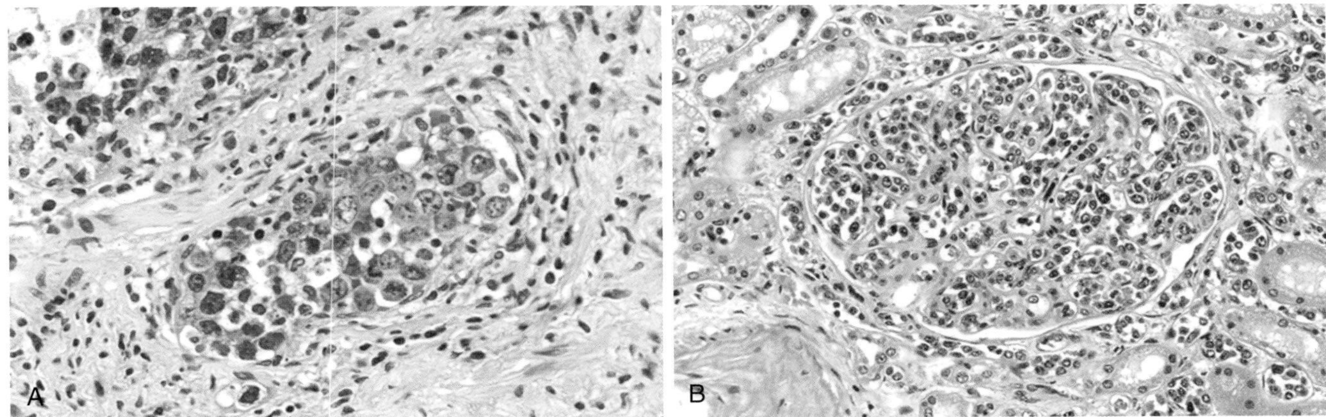

Figure 22-37. Intravascular large B-cell lymphoma. A, The noncohesive lymphoma cells are confined within medium-sized blood vessels. **B,** Lymphoma cells distend the capillaries of the glomeruli and the renal parenchyma.

skin (cutaneous variant), and they seem to have a better outcome.[354]

Uncommon presentations include interstitial lung disease,[357] pulmonary small vessel disease,[358] adrenal insufficiency,[359,360] minimal change disease of the kidney,[361] thrombotic microangiopathy,[362] and epididymal mass.[363] IVLBCL may be diagnosed by renal biopsy,[364,365] testicular biopsy,[366] marrow aspiration and biopsy,[210] or nerve and muscle biopsy,[367] and it may be an incidental finding in the prostate.[368,369] Association with autoimmune diseases has been observed in some patients,[352] and cases have been identified in patients with acquired immunodeficiency syndrome (AIDS).[370,371] IVLBCL may involve preexisting tumors, such as hemangioma,[372] lymphangioma,[373] renal cell carcinoma,[374] angiolipoma,[375] and Kaposi's sarcoma.[371]

Histologic marrow involvement is infrequent,[352] and peripheral blood involvement is very rare.[376] Nonetheless, the frequent demonstration of immunoglobulin gene rearrangement by polymerase chain reaction in histologically negative bone marrow samples suggests that subtle marrow involvement is in fact common.[377]

An Asian variant associated with hemophagocytic syndrome (also known as *malignant histiocytosis-like B-cell lymphoma*) has been described, mostly from Japan.[378-383] Interestingly, cases reported in Western series have been of Asian or Caribbean origin.[384] The patients are elderly and present with fever, hepatosplenomegaly, hemophagocytic syndrome with anemia and thrombocytopenia, marrow involvement, and disseminated intravascular coagulation. They usually lack lymphadenopathy, mass lesions, neurologic abnormalities, or skin lesions. There is no association with EBV or human T-lymphotropic virus-1.[378,382]

Morphology

Histologically, large or medium-sized abnormal lymphoid cells are found within the lumens of small or intermediate-sized blood vessels (Fig. 22-37).[350,352] They can have a centroblastic, immunoblastic, or unclassifiable appearance. They sometimes palisade along the luminal side of blood vessels, mimicking angiosarcoma (Fig. 22-38). They can appear deceptively cohesive, resembling islands of carcinoma (Fig. 22-39). The lymphoma cells may be entrapped within organized fibrin thrombi, and there may be superimposed florid endothelial hyperplasia. The vascular occlusion can result in tissue infarction and hemorrhage (Fig. 22-40). Some cases may have an extravascular component.[348,350,352]

The lymphomatous involvement is usually obvious morphologically, but it may be focal and subtle, requiring the help of immunohistochemistry to highlight the lymphoma cells.

Immunophenotype

The lymphoma cells express CD45 and pan-B markers (Fig. 22-41).[348,350] A small proportion of cases express CD5, CD10, and BCL6 (22% each),[209,210,348,373] and the CD5$^+$ cases are negative for CD23 and cyclin D1.[373] CD5 expression is not associated with any specific clinical feature. There may be apparent expression of factor VIII–related antigen owing to passive absorption into the tumor cells.[385] The reported finding of prostatic acid phosphatase expression requires confirmation.[386] A rare case with coexpression of myeloperoxidase has also been reported.[387] The immunophenotype of the Asian variant associated with hemophagocytic syndrome is similar to that of the usual IVLBCL.[380]

Rare cases of intravascular lymphoma are of T-cell,[363,388-390] NK-cell,[390-392] or true histiocytic lineage,[393,394] and there is a

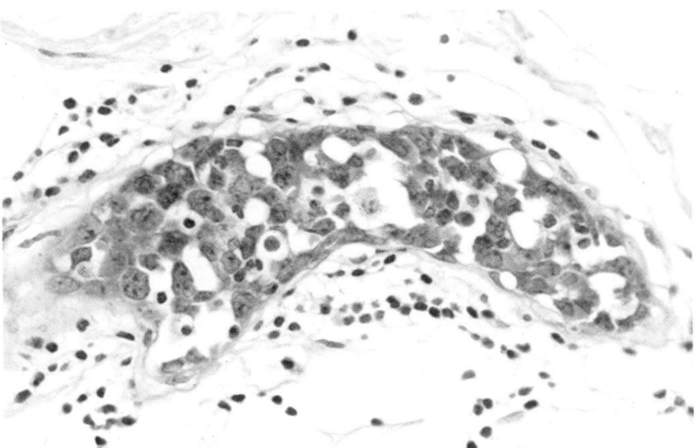

Figure 22-38. Intravascular large B-cell lymphoma involving subcutaneous tissue. Palisading of tumor cells along the luminal side of the blood vessel results in an angiosarcoma-like appearance.

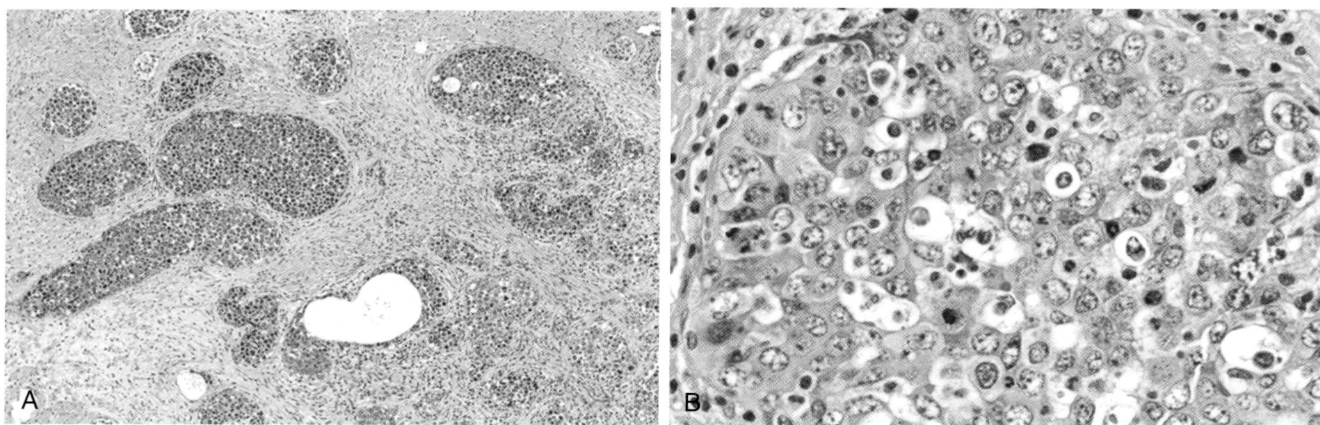

Figure 22-39. Intravascular large B-cell lymphoma mimicking carcinoma. A, In the prostate, plugging of the blood vessels by tumor cells results in a pattern reminiscent of islands of carcinoma. **B,** This island resembles high-grade carcinoma because of the apparently cohesive growth and the presence of gland-like spaces.

frequent association with EBV.[363,390-392,395] Such cases would not be classified IVLBCL.

Genetics

IVLBCL shows immunoglobulin gene rearrangement.[351,396] The *BCL2* gene is not translocated.[348] Cytogenetic abnormalities involving 8p21, 19q13, 14q32, and chromosome 18 have been reported in the Asian variant associated with hemophagocytic syndrome.[380,381] EBV association is uncommon,[348] but it has been reported in AIDS patients.[371]

Postulated Cell of Origin

IVLBCLs are derived from peripheral B cells, with the majority (83%) showing a non-GC immunophenotype according to the Hans algorithm.[397]

Clinical Course

The poor outcome of IVLBCL in the older literature is related in part to the failure to make a correct antemortem diagnosis.[352] Complete remission and long-term survival can be achieved in patients treated with aggressive combination chemotherapy.[354,398] Rare cutaneous cases with a prolonged clinical course have also been reported.[354,399] The clinical behavior of the Asian variant with hemophagocytic syndrome is aggressive, with a median survival of only 7 months.[380,397] The addition of rituximab has significantly improved the clinical outcome in both recent Western and Asian series.[400,401]

Differential Diagnosis

In acute leukemia, intravascular collections of blast cells can be seen. The blasts usually have fine chromatin, and cytoplasmic granules may be present in the myeloid type. Immunohistochemically, blasts in acute myeloid leukemia usually express myeloperoxidase but not pan-B or pan-T markers, whereas those in acute lymphoblastic leukemia express terminal deoxynucleotidyl transferase (TdT) with pan-B or pan-T markers. IVLBCL is always TdT^-.

The lumens of the lymphatic channels adjacent to inflamed tissue (e.g., acute appendicitis) are sometimes packed with reactive activated lymphoid cells. However, these lymphoid cells are smaller and do not have the atypical nuclear features of IVLBCL.

In patients with carcinomatosis, clusters of carcinoma cells may be lodged in the small lymphovascular channels. The

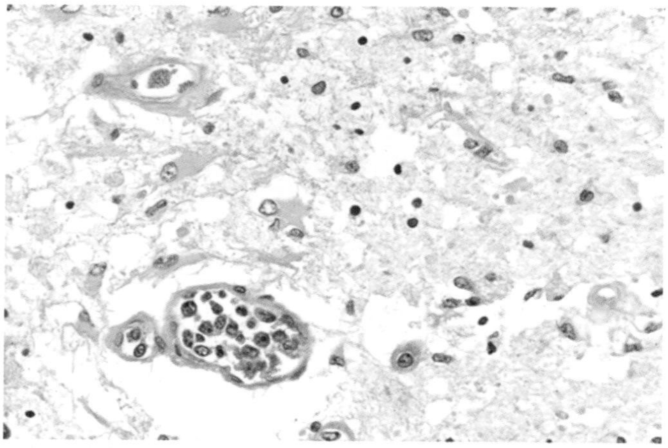

Figure 22-40. Intravascular large B-cell lymphoma involving the brain. The blood vessels are filled with large lymphoma cells. The surrounding brain parenchyma shows rarefaction due to ischemia from the vascular occlusion.

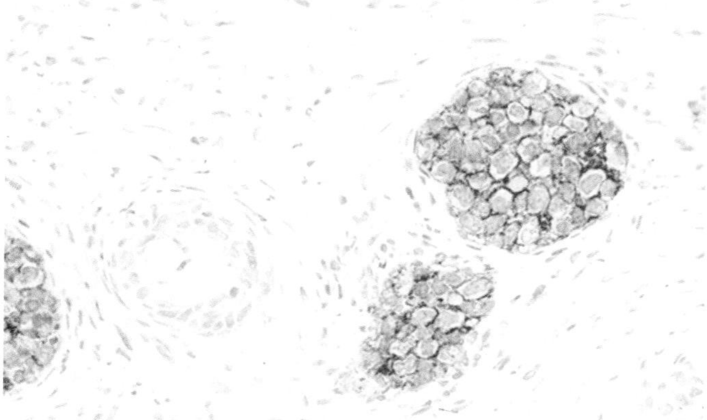

Figure 22-41. Immunohistochemistry of intravascular large B-cell lymphoma. The neoplastic cells within the blood vessels are selectively highlighted by CD20 immunostain.

tumor cells are generally cohesive, and they are cytokeratin positive and CD45⁻.

Diffuse Large B-Cell Lymphoma Associated with Chronic Inflammation

Definition

DLBCL associated with chronic inflammation occurs in the context of long-standing chronic inflammation and is associated with EBV. It usually involves body cavities or narrow spaces. Pyothorax-associated lymphoma represents the prototype of this form of DLBCL.[24]

Pyothorax-Associated Lymphoma

Epidemiology. Pyothorax-associated lymphoma is a pleura-based, mass-forming, EBV-associated DLBCL occurring in patients with long-standing pyothorax resulting from artificial pneumothorax for the treatment of pulmonary tuberculosis or tuberculous pleuritis.[23,402,403] It is a rare lymphoma more commonly found in Japan, but it has also been described in the West.[403-407] The higher incidence in Japan is explained by the more popular use of artificial pneumothorax for the treatment of pulmonary tuberculosis in the past.[23]

Patients are commonly in the seventh decade of life, with a striking male predominance (male-to-female ratio of 12.3:1).[403]

Etiology. Pyothorax-associated lymphoma is consistently associated with EBV.[23,402,403,406,408-411] The EBV shows a type III latency pattern, with expression of EBNA-2 and LMP1.[407,410,412-414] It has been postulated that chronic pyothorax may provide a local immunodeficient environment for EBV-infected B cells to proliferate and undergo malignant transformation.[409] There is no association with human herpesvirus 8 (HHV8).[407,408]

Clinical Features. Patients have a long history of chronic pyothorax and may present with chest pain, cough, dyspnea, or tumor in the chest wall. The median interval between the occurrence of pyothorax and the onset of lymphoma is 37 years (range, 20 to 64 years).[403] Imaging studies show pleura- or lung-based tumor masses, and the ribs may be involved. The outcome is poor, with overall 5-year survival of only 20% to 35%.[403,415] For patients who can achieve complete remission, a 5-year survival of 50% can be attained.[403]

Morphology. Pyothorax-associated lymphoma is characterized by a diffuse and destructive infiltrate of large lymphoma cells that are histologically indistinguishable from conventional DLBCLs (Fig. 22-42).[402] The cytoplasm can show plasmacytoid features.[407]

Immunophenotype. The lymphoma cells express CD45 and pan-B markers.[402] They usually exhibit a CD10⁻, BCL6⁻, IRF4/MUM-1⁺, CD138⁺ immunophenotype, suggesting a late GC or post-GC stage of differentiation.[407] Rare cases aberrantly express T-lineage markers such as CD2, CD3, or CD4 in addition to pan-B markers.[407,416,417] Pyothorax-associated lymphoma of a T-cell phenotype has also been reported rarely.[403]

Genetics. Pyothorax-associated lymphoma exhibits immunoglobulin gene rearrangement. The hypermutated *IGHV@* gene does not show ongoing somatic mutations.[409,418] Mutations of *TP53,* most commonly at dipyrimidine sites, are detected in 71% of cases,[23,402] and *MYC* amplification is found in 80%.[413] The gene expression profile is distinct from that of nodal DLBCL, with interferon-inducible 27 (*IFI27*) being one of the most differentially expressed genes.[419]

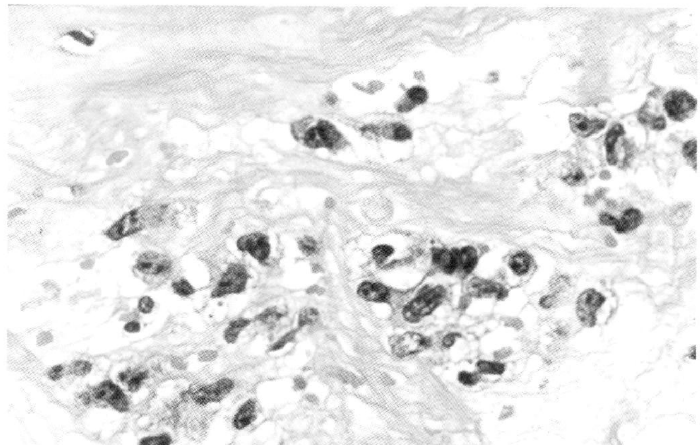

Figure 22-42. Pyothorax-associated lymphoma (diffuse large B-cell lymphoma associated with chronic inflammation). In this example, the large lymphoma cells are enmeshed in fibrin and sclerotic stroma.

Differential Diagnosis. Primary effusion lymphoma is a type of DLBCL that occurs in HIV-infected patients (see Chapter 56). It is consistently associated with HHV8 and commonly coinfected by EBV.[420,421] In contrast to pyothorax-associated lymphoma, the lymphoma cells are suspended in the effusion fluid instead of forming solid tumor masses. The neoplastic cells are often larger and exhibit a more pleomorphic or anaplastic appearance. Primary effusion lymphoma shows a plasmablastic immunophenotype and is frequently negative for conventional pan-B markers, but it expresses CD138 and CD30. It shows a restricted EBV latency pattern, with expression of EBNA1 in all cases, but low LMP1 and LMP2A levels.[422]

Plasmacytoma arising from ribs or vertebrae may secondarily involve the pleura or lung. The anaplastic form can mimic pyothorax-associated lymphoma, and features favoring a diagnosis of plasmacytoma include a history of multiple myeloma, background of smaller neoplastic plasma cells, and immunophenotype of CD20⁻, CD138⁺, and IRF4/MUM-1⁺.

Nonhematolymphoid malignancies (e.g., carcinoma, sarcoma, malignant mesothelioma) may show diffuse growth, mimicking pyothorax-associated lymphoma, but they are negative for CD45 and express their respective specific markers.

Other Inflammation-Associated Lymphomas

Other chronic inflammatory or suppurative conditions in which EBV-associated DLBCL may supervene include chronic osteomyelitis, chronic skin ulcer, metallic implant, and surgical mesh placement.[19,21,423] The interval between the onset of chronic inflammation or the implantation of exogenous materials and malignant lymphoma is usually more than 10 years, although this can be shorter. EBV⁻ cases of DLBCL occurring around chronically inflamed joints of patients with rheumatoid arthritis are pathogenetically unrelated to this group of lymphomas.[22]

The lymphoma arises at a site of chronic inflammation, often the skin, bones, joints, or soft tissues. The presenting symptom is usually pain or a mass lesion. The morphologic and immunophenotypic features are no different from those of pyothorax-associated lymphoma.

ALK⁺ Large B-Cell Lymphoma

Definition

This is an aggressive variant of DLBCL with ALK expression. It was first reported by Delsol and coworkers[157] in 1997 and has been nicknamed *Delsol's tumor*.[424]

Clinical Features

Patients' median age is 36 years (30% occur in the pediatric age group), with a male predominance (male-to-female ratio of 3:1).[425] They commonly present with high-stage nodal disease. There is no association with immunosuppression. Despite multiagent chemotherapy, most patients die of the tumor, and the overall median survival for high-stage (III-IV) patients is 11 months.[425]

Pathology

The tumor cells have an immunoblastic or plasmablastic appearance, and sinusoidal infiltration is common (Fig. 22-43; see Box 22-2). They can appear deceptively cohesive and thus may be misinterpreted as carcinoma cells. The frequency of expression of the various immunophenotypic markers is as follows: CD45, 71%; CD20, 3% (weak and focal); CD79a, 16%; EMA, 100%; CD30, 6% (weak and focal); kappa or lambda light chain, 90% (most often IgA); CD138, 100%; CD4, 64%; and CD57, 40%.[425] By definition, this lymphoma expresses ALK, with staining frequently confined to the cytoplasm, usually in a granular pattern. Cytokeratin expression has rarely been described, adding to the possible confusion with metastatic carcinoma, especially in combination with EMA positivity.[425]

Upregulation of the *ALK* gene is mainly due to the presence of t(2;17)(p23;q23), which leads to fusion of the *CLTC* (clathrin) gene with the *ALK* gene.[426,427] Rare cases with t(2;5)(p23;q35) (*NPM-ALK*) translocation and nuclear and cytoplasmic expression of ALK have also been reported.[428,429] All cases are EBV⁻. ALK⁺ large B-cell lymphoma should be distinguished from ALK⁺ anaplastic large cell lymphoma (of T/null-cell phenotype), plasmablastic lymphoma, and DLBCL with a sinusoidal growth pattern.

Plasmablastic Lymphoma

Definition

Plasmablastic lymphoma is a DLBCL with morphologic and immunophenotypic features of plasmablasts.[430] Specific subtypes of DLBCLs with a plasmablastic immunophenotype, such as primary effusion lymphoma, ALK⁺ large B-cell lymphomas, and HHV8⁺ germinotropic lymphoproliferative disorder, are not included in this category.

Clinical Features

This lymphoma occurs predominantly in the setting of immunodeficiency, most commonly HIV infection, but also iatrogenic immunosuppression among organ transplant recipients and those with autoimmune diseases.[431-434] Plasmablastic lymphoma has a predilection for the oral cavity, but other sites can also be involved, such as the nasal cavity, gastrointestinal tract (including the anus), skin, bone, soft tissue, and lung.[433,435-439] This lymphoma can also occur in patients without immunodeficiency, who present with disease in a lymph node or extranodal site.

There is a striking male predominance, with most patients in the fourth and fifth decades of life. In the original series, about 70% of patients presented with stage I disease, but spread to other sites (e.g., abdomen, retroperitoneum, bone) may occur during the clinical course.[431] Subsequent series showed a higher proportion of patients with more advanced disease.[433] The prognosis is generally poor: more than three quarters of patients die of the disease at a median interval of 6 to 7 months.[431,433,435]

Pathology

Histologically, there is a diffuse infiltrate of large lymphoma cells associated with a "starry sky" pattern. The cells appear cohesive and have a squared-off appearance, with eccentric

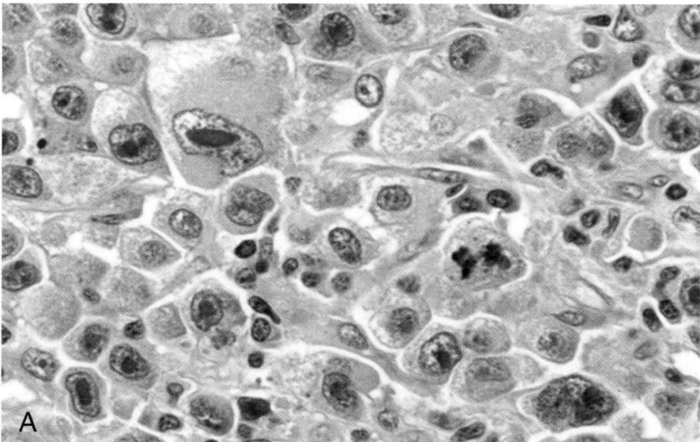

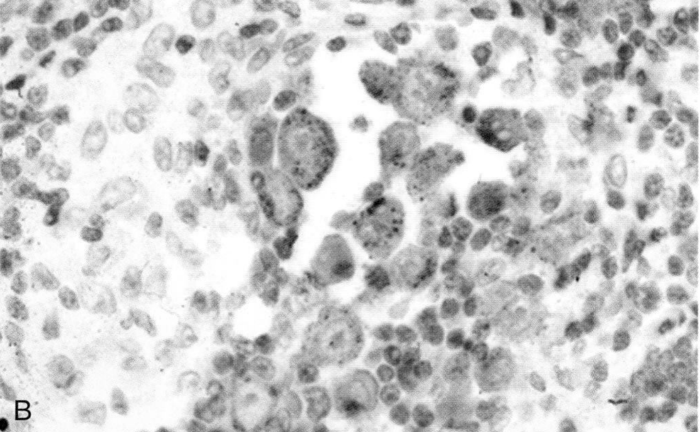

Figure 22-43. ALK⁺ large B-cell lymphoma. A, Typically, the cells are very large, with vesicular nuclei, inclusion-like nucleoli, and voluminous cytoplasm. **B,** They show granular cytoplasmic immunostaining for the ALK protein. Note the intrasinusoidal localization of the neoplastic cells. (Courtesy of Georges Delsol, University of Toulouse, Toulouse, France.)

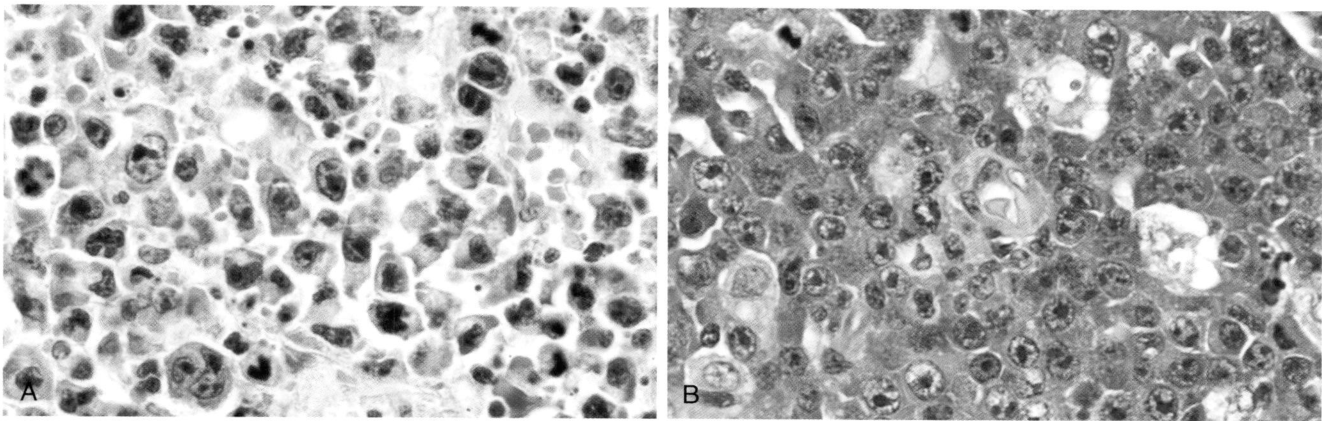

Figure 22-44. Plasmablastic lymphoma. A, Plasmablastic lymphoma in the colon of an HIV-positive subject. The lymphoma cells exhibit prominent nucleoli and abundant plasmacytoid cytoplasm. **B,** Plasmablastic lymphoma involving the lymph node of an immunocompetent subject. The neoplastic cells are apparently "frozen" at the stage of plasmablasts, without further maturation.

nuclei; single, centrally located, prominent nucleoli or multiple peripheral nucleoli; abundant basophilic cytoplasm; and paranuclear hof (Fig. 22-44). Maturing plasma cells are sometimes seen. Mitotic activity is brisk, and apoptotic bodies are numerous.

The immunophenotype is similar to that of plasma cells: $CD45^-$, $CD20^-$, $CD79a^{+/-}$, and $PAX5^-$ (Fig. 22-45). The tumors express plasma cell–associated markers, such as CD38, CD138, IRF4/MUM-1, and VS38c, and variably express immunoglobulin. They are associated with a high proliferation (Ki-67) index (>90%). BCL6 expression is mostly negative or only focally positive.[431,433,435,436] There is clonal immunoglobulin gene rearrangement. EBV is positive in 75% of cases, and HHV8 is negative.[431-433,435,436]

Differential Diagnosis

The most important differential diagnosis is anaplastic (plasmablastic) plasmacytoma because of the similar histology and immunophenotype. Although the absence of smaller neoplastic cells with plasmacytic differentiation was originally thought to be a feature that could distinguish plasmablastic lymphoma from plasmacytoma,[431] it is now recognized that these cells are present in some cases.[433,435] Whether CD56 expression can be used to favor a diagnosis of plasmacytoma is controversial.[433,436] The clinical picture (immunodeficiency, oral involvement, absence of multiple myeloma), high proliferation index, and frequent EBV association are features supporting a diagnosis of plasmablastic lymphoma over anaplastic plasmacytoma. In some cases a firm distinction cannot be made, and a descriptive diagnosis such as "plasmablastic neoplasm, indeterminate between plasmablastic lymphoma and anaplastic plasmacytoma" may be given. Further workup, such as serum paraprotein assay and marrow examination, may help resolve the diagnostic dilemma.

The "starry sky" pattern, the squared-off appearance of the tumor cells, and the high proliferation index may suggest a diagnosis of Burkitt's lymphoma. In contrast to plasmablastic lymphoma, the cells of Burkitt's lymphoma are medium-sized; do not usually show plasmacytic differentiation; are positive for CD45, CD20, and BCL6; and are negative for CD138 and VS38c.

In DLBCL-NOS, the tumor cells do not show such prominent basophilic cytoplasm and are usually $CD45^+$ and $CD20^+$. Although rare cases may show a proliferation index approaching the range in plasmablastic lymphoma, the index is generally lower.

Large B-cell lymphoma arising in HHV8-associated multicentric Castleman's disease, seen most often in HIV-positive

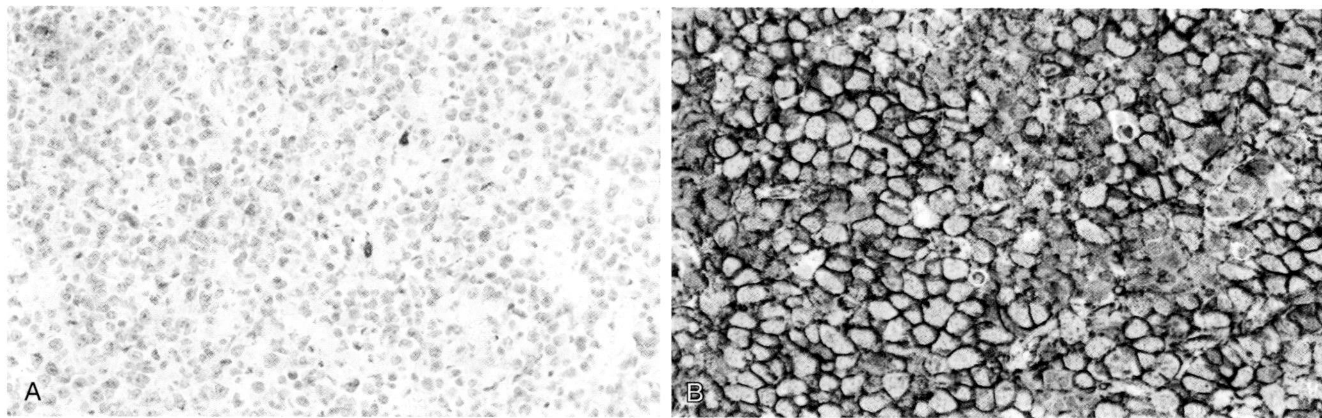

Figure 22-45. Immunohistochemistry of plasmablastic lymphoma. A, Typically the lymphoma cells lack immunoreactivity for CD20. There are scanty scattered small B lymphocytes in the background. **B,** The neoplastic cells show cell membrane immunostaining for CD138.

subjects, has also been termed *plasmablastic lymphoma* in the literature.[440-442] However, this is a distinct disease and should not be confused with the extranodal plasmablastic lymphomas. It shows predominantly nodal or splenic involvement, consistent association with HHV8 but not EBV, variable expression of CD20 and IgM with lambda light chain, and unmutated immunoglobulin variable region genes (see Chapter 56).

Primary effusion lymphoma, ALK⁺ large B-cell lymphoma, and HHV8- and EBV-associated germinotropic lymphoproliferative disorder are not classified as plasmablastic lymphoma, despite the presence of a plasmablastic immunophenotype.

HHV8- and EBV-Associated Germinotropic Lymphoproliferative Disorder

HHV8- and EBV-associated germinotropic lymphoproliferative disorder is a rare disorder occurring in immunocompetent adults who present with nodal enlargement.[443,444] Patients respond favorably to chemotherapy or radiotherapy. In one patient who had only lymph node excision for a single involved node, there was no relapse at 2 years.[444]

Histologically, the overall nodal architecture is preserved, but the GCs are expanded owing to partial or complete replacement by large clusters of plasmablasts, which can have bizarre nuclear features (Fig. 22-46). Histologic features of Castleman's disease are lacking. The plasmablasts are typically negative for CD20, CD79a, BCL2, CD10, and BCL6 but positive for IRF4/MUM-1 (see Fig. 22-46). Monotypic immunoglobulin light chain can be demonstrated. The neoplastic cells harbor both HHV8 and EBV (see Fig. 22-46D). Analysis of the immunoglobulin gene by polymerase chain reaction intriguingly shows an oligoclonal or polyclonal pattern—as a result, this lesion is termed *lymphoproliferative disorder* instead of *lymphoma*, despite the presence of significant cytologic atypia and monotypic immunoglobulin.[443,444]

A main differential diagnosis is large B-cell lymphoma arising in HHV8-associated multicentric Castleman's disease, which is also HHV8⁺; however, the patients are often HIV positive, plasmablasts are found preferentially in the mantle zone and express IgM and monotypic lambda chain, CD20 staining is variable, and EBV is usually negative (see Chapter 56). However, a recent EBV⁺ case was described in an HIV-positive patient, linking the two entities.[445]

Follicular lymphoma grade 3b is another mimicker of HHV8- and EBV-associated germinotropic lymphoproliferative disorder, owing to the presence of abnormal large cells localized in follicles. It is almost always immunoreactive for CD20 and BCL6 and lacks both HHV8 and EBV.

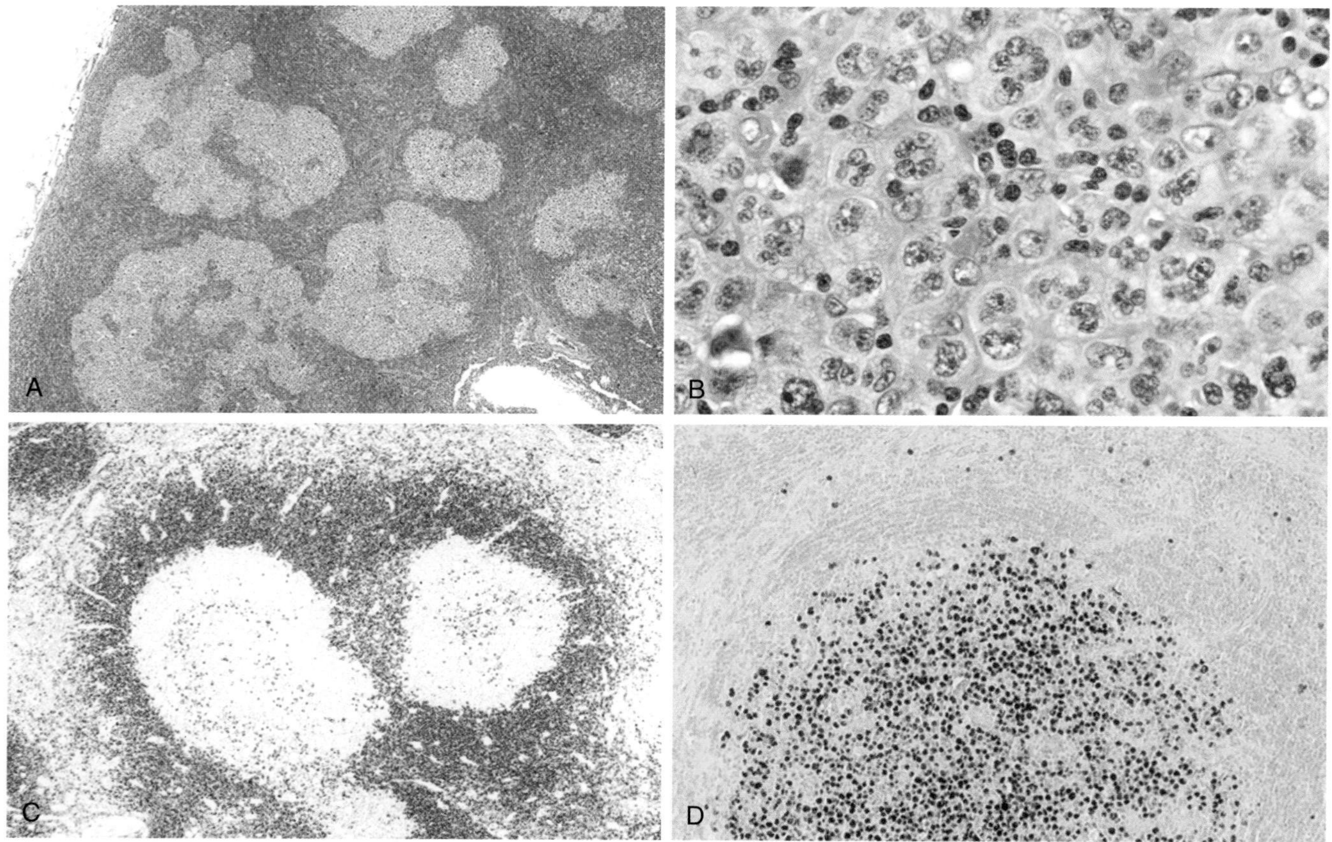

Figure 22-46. HHV8- and EBV-associated germinotropic lymphoproliferative disorder. A, The lymph node shows large, geographic-shaped germinal centers populated by large cells. **B,** The lymphoma cells possess round, multilobated or segmented nuclei and exhibit a considerable degree of nuclear pleomorphism. **C,** The mantle zone cells are immunoreactive for CD20, but the cells in the germinal centers are negative. **D,** In situ hybridization for EBER selectively labels the large lymphoid cells within the germinal centers.

Pearls and Pitfalls

Diffuse Large B-Cell Lymphoma (DLBCL)

- Although a diagnosis of DLBCL can be suspected by morphology, immunohistochemical confirmation is necessary because many types of lymphoma, leukemia, and nonhematolymphoid neoplasms can mimic DLBCL. In most circumstances, a simple immunohistochemical panel of CD20 and CD3 is sufficient to delineate the lineage.
- In young patients, reactive conditions (e.g., infectious mononucleosis, Kikuchi's lymphadenitis) must be seriously considered in the differential diagnosis. One should think twice and thrice before rendering a diagnosis of DLBCL in a patient younger than 20 years. Infectious mononucleosis in particular has to be suspected when the large cells show heterogeneous staining for CD20, there are many admixed large T cells, and Waldeyer's ring is involved.
- In young patients, Hodgkin's lymphoma, anaplastic large cell lymphoma, and Burkitt's lymphoma should also be seriously considered in the differential diagnosis.
- When bone marrow is involved, it is important to distinguish between involvement by large B-cell lymphoma and small cell or follicular lymphoma. The former is associated with a much worse prognosis.
- If DLBCL is EBV$^+$, consider underlying immunosuppression (e.g., posttransplant lymphoproliferative disorder, HIV-associated lymphoma, reversible methotrexate-associated lymphoproliferative disorder) and EBV$^+$ DLBCL of the elderly.
- If DLBCL is suspected but CD20 is negative, consider the possibility of prior rituximab therapy, ALK$^+$ large B-cell lymphoma, plasmablastic lymphoma, and anaplastic plasmacytoma. Apply additional B-lineage markers such as CD79a, PAX5, Oct-2, and BOB.1.

Primary Mediastinal Large B-Cell Lymphoma (PMLBCL)

- In the past, PMLBCL was often misdiagnosed as thymic carcinoma.
- A superior-anterior mediastinal mass in a young adult woman is most commonly caused by PMLBCL or nodular sclerosis Hodgkin's lymphoma. Mediastinal germ cell tumor and T-lymphoblastic lymphoma should also be considered in young male patients.
- CD30 expression is not helpful in distinguishing nodular sclerosis Hodgkin's lymphoma from PMLBCL. The histologic features and immunoprofile have to be taken into consideration to make the distinction. If the findings are indeterminate (e.g., CD30$^+$, CD15$^-$, CD20$^+$), lack of Oct-2 and BOB.1 staining and positive staining for EBV-LMP1 favor a diagnosis of nodular sclerosis Hodgkin's lymphoma.

References can be found on Expert Consult @ www.expertconsult.com

Chapter 23

Lymphomatoid Granulomatosis

Elaine S. Jaffe and Stefania Pittaluga

CHAPTER OUTLINE

DEFINITION AND BACKGROUND

Lymphomatoid granulomatosis (LYG), initially described by Liebow and colleagues,[1] is a rare extranodal Epstein-Barr virus (EBV)–associated B-cell lymphoproliferative disorder that shares similarities with posttransplant lymphoproliferative disorder (PTLD). Pathologically, LYG is characterized by an angiocentric and angiodestructive polymorphic lymphoid infiltrate that consists of lymphocytes, plasma cells, and atypical larger lymphoid cells that resemble immunoblasts or, less commonly, Hodgkin–Reed-Sternberg (HRS) cells. Well-formed granulomas are usually absent, making *lymphomatoid granulomatosis* something of a misnomer. The term was coined by Liebow and colleagues to distinguish it from Wegener's granulomatosis (WG), which it resembles clinically and radiologically in the lung. They considered LYG to be principally an angiodestructive disorder composed of lymphoreticular cells, and one that can progress to lymphoma.[1]

The infiltrate classically contains scattered EBV⁺ atypical B cells within a predominantly T-cell background.[2] Vascular changes are frequent, with lymphocytic infiltration of the vascular wall and variable necrosis. The disease is graded based on the number of atypical EBV⁺ B cells and the amount of necrosis (Box 23-1).[3,4]

Since its description more than 35 years ago, LYG has been an enigma. Because of the predominance of T cells within the lesions and the frequent cytologic atypia, it was first thought to be a form of T-cell lymphoma.[5] Other authors, in an attempt to unify the spectrum of clinical and histologic findings in LYG (and perhaps other related conditions), proposed that LYG was not a discrete clinicopathologic entity but a histologic response that could be encountered in the course of many diseases, including lymphoma.[6] It shares some clinical and histopathologic features with extranodal natural killer (NK)/T-cell lymphoma, nasal type, once termed *angiocentric lymphoma*,[7] and at one time was considered part of a common clinicopathologic entity called *angiocentric immunoproliferative lesion*.[8] The overlap with extranodal NK/T-cell lymphoma is explained by the common link to EBV, which appears to mediate the vascular damage common to many EBV⁺ lymphoproliferative disorders.[9]

Liebow and colleagues[1] first speculated on an association with EBV and noted features in common with some immunodeficiency disorders. The presence of EBV in LYG lesions was first noted by Katzenstein and Peiper[10] using polymerase chain reaction (PCR) technology.[10] Guinee and coworkers,[2,11] using in situ hybridization, showed that EBV was localized to B lymphocytes, although in some cases the number of EBV-infected cells is small. Moreover, EBV⁺ B cells may not be present in all sites, and some of the vascular lesions may be mediated by the effects of chemokines upregulated by EBV expression.[9] In lesions identified in the lung and other sites, most of the infiltrating lymphoid cells are secondary or reactive, presumably recruited in response to EBV. These cells are mainly T lymphocytes. The histologic grade of LYG is based on the respective proportions of the EBV-infected B cells, which may be monoclonal or oligoclonal, and the reactive component.[4] An associated immunodeficiency appears to be an intrinsic component of LYG, because clinical and laboratory evidence of defective T-cell function can be identified in most cases.[3,12] Moreover, the observed host response is ineffective in eradicating the EBV-infected clones.

The pathogenesis of the angiodestructive aspects of LYG is multifactorial. It involves both angioinvasion by infiltrating cells, mainly reactive T lymphocytes, and chemokine-mediated vascular damage. The responsible chemokines are induced by EBV. Therefore, EBV lies at the heart of LYG and

Box 23-1 *Major Diagnostic Features of Lymphomatoid Granulomatosis*

Proliferating Cells
- EBV⁺ B cells, positive for EBER
- LMP-1⁺ only in a subset of larger cells
- CD20⁺, CD79a⁺, PAX5⁺, CD30⁻/⁺, CD15⁻
- Cells vary in size
- *IGH@* genes clonal in high-grade cases

Background Reactive Cells
- CD3⁺ T cells, CD4 > CD8
- Plasma cells, histiocytes

Genotype
- B cells usually clonal by *IG* PCR in grades 2, 3
- Clonality indeterminate in grade 1
- EBV clonal by terminal repeat analysis
- T cells polyclonal

Sites of Involvement
- Lung, skin, kidney, liver, central nervous system
- Less common sites: adrenal, heart, peripheral nerve
- Not involved: lymph nodes, spleen, bone marrow

Risk Factors
- Underlying immunodeficiency; cause not apparent in most patients
- Wiskott-Aldrich, HIV infection, prior chemotherapy, iatrogenic immunosuppression

EBER, Epstein-Barr virus–encoded RNA; EBV, Epstein-Barr virus; HIV, human immunodeficiency virus; PCR, polymerase chain reaction.

is intrinsically linked to all aspects of its pathogenesis and pathophysiology.

EPIDEMIOLOGY

Although most cases of LYG occur in otherwise healthy patients, it occurs sporadically in patients with known underlying immunodeficiencies, both primary and secondary. LYG has been reported in association with Wiskott-Aldrich syndrome, human immunodeficiency virus (HIV) infection and acquired immunodeficiency syndrome (AIDS), and human T-cell leukemia virus infection, as well as secondary immunodeficiencies associated with chemotherapy and organ transplantation.[13-20] These observations suggested that all patients with LYG have some degree of immune compromise and led to the assessment of immune function in patients who did not have a history of immunodeficiency. One study of six patients reported the presence of profound immunologic abnormalities; four of five patients were anergic, and three of four patients tested had a significantly impaired in vitro response to common antigen stimulation and nonspecific mitogens.[12] Subsequent studies found evidence of impaired humoral and cell-mediated responses to EBV, suggesting that patients with LYG cannot effectively control EBV-induced B-cell proliferation because of either a generalized immunodeficiency or a more specific EBV-related immunodeficiency.[14,15] Studies of peripheral blood lymphocytes showed decreased total T cells with a more severe reduction of CD8⁺ cells.[3]

LYG usually presents in adulthood, although rare cases in children have been reported.[21] Most cases occur between the fourth and sixth decades of life. The male-to-female ratio is approximately 2:1.[4,22] No racial predisposition has been shown, but LYG appears to be primarily a disease of Western countries; there is no increase in Asians, in contrast to EBV⁺ T-cell and NK-cell lymphoproliferations.[23]

CLINICAL FEATURES

Most patients present with symptoms related to pulmonary involvement, which is the most frequently involved organ (Fig. 23-1). Most patients complain of cough, dyspnea, or chest pain on initial presentation.[22] Occasionally, an otherwise asymptomatic patient is found to have abnormalities on a routine chest radiograph. Systemic manifestations of fever, malaise, and weight loss are also common, occurring in 35% to 60% of patients.[24,25] The skin is the second most common organ affected by LYG (25% to 50%), presenting with cutaneous and dermal nodules, maculopapular rashes, macular erythema, and even ulcers.[26-28] Skin involvement is sometimes the initial manifestation of the disease, and it may also be an indication of relapse. In approximately 30% of patients, skin lesions develop later in the clinical course. Liver, kidneys, and central nervous system (CNS) are frequently involved (approximately 25% each). Renal and hepatic involvement is usually asymptomatic at presentation, and in the pre–computed tomography (CT) era, it often went undetected.[29] A higher incidence of renal and hepatic involvement is identified in autopsy series (up to 40%). Lymphadenopathy and splenomegaly are uncommon because lymphoid tissues are generally spared. The presence of lymph node involvement should raise questions regarding the diagnosis.

Radiographically, pulmonary disease is characterized by multiple nodules ranging in size from a few millimeters to several centimeters, with occasional cavities (Fig. 23-2). On occasion, pneumonic or mass-like lesions are seen. The lesions are most often bilateral in distribution and characteristically involve the mid and lower lung fields. In the case of small nodular lesions, increased lung markings or infiltrates may be the only findings on the chest radiograph, and a CT scan may be needed to adequately visualize the nodules. In a minority of cases, cavitation occurs within the nodules, and some patients may develop small pleural effusions. Advanced

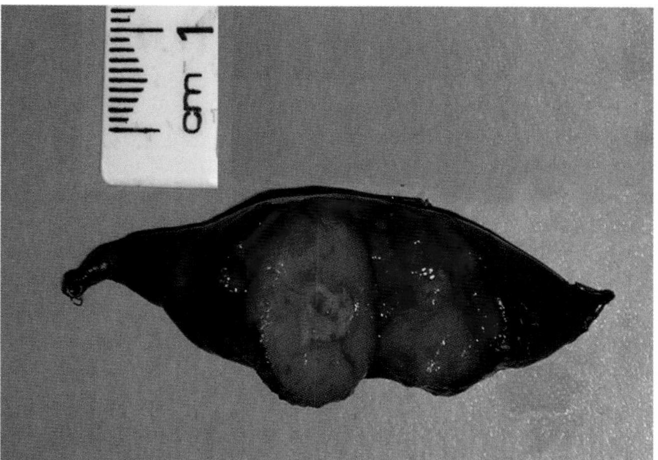

Figure 23-1. Pulmonary biopsy in a case of lymphomatoid granulomatosis. The lesion contains central necrosis surrounded by a firm, tan infiltrate, forming a discrete nodule.

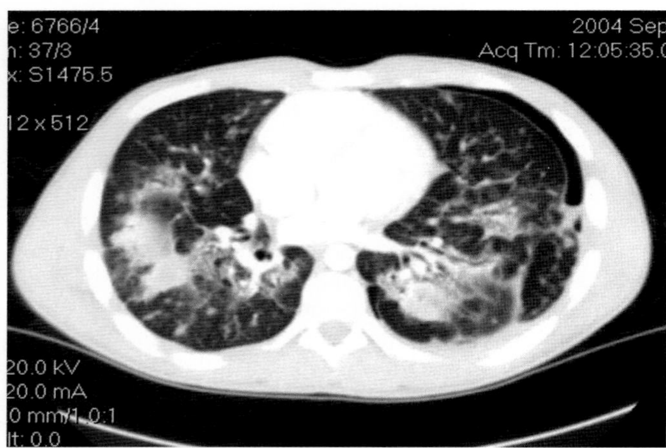

Figure 23-2. Magnetic resonance image of the lung in lymphomatoid granulomatosis. Pulmonary nodules, sometimes with central necrosis, are seen most often in the lower lung fields.

lung disease causes dyspnea, which may be debilitating. Massive hemoptysis occasionally occurs.

Patients with brain involvement may initially be asymptomatic, but symptoms such as confusion, dementia, ataxia, hemiparesis, and seizures, or cranial nerve signs such as diplopia, transient blindness, Bell's palsy, deafness, or vertigo, are likely to develop over time. In patients with clinical symptoms of CNS disease, the initial brain CT scan may show abnormalities such as a mass lesion or multiple cortical infarcts, or it may be normal.[30] The spinal fluid frequently has abnormal protein and glucose concentrations, and cytologically there are often increased small T lymphocytes, consistent with a reactive process. A cytologic diagnosis of LYG may be difficult to confirm. In only rare cases does the cerebrospinal fluid contain monoclonal B cells. Detection of EBV sequences by PCR is a more sensitive tool for the detection of CNS involvement.[31] It is important to emphasize that because some patients with CNS disease initially have no signs or symptoms, it is prudent to include a brain CT or magnetic resonance imaging scan and a lumbar puncture in the initial evaluation.

On initial presentation, the complete blood count is usually normal or only mildly abnormal: mild anemia occasionally occurs, and the white blood cell count is elevated in 30% of patients.[22] Approximately 20% have leukopenia or lymphopenia, or both; rarely, lymphocytosis is seen. Nonspecific abnormalities in serum immunoglobulin (Ig) are commonly seen. In one study of 32 patients, 47% had mild increases, usually in IgG or IgM, and in another study, 5 of 6 patients had abnormal immunoglobulin concentrations.[12,22] Although LYG lesions are characterized by vascular damage, it is not an inflammatory vasculitis in the classic sense, and tests for autoimmune disease, such as antinuclear antibody and rheumatoid factor, are generally negative. Laboratory tests of renal function, such as urinalysis, serum creatinine, and blood urea nitrogen, are typically normal at diagnosis in patients with renal involvement.[25] As expected, serologic evidence of prior EBV is found, but EBV viral loads in the serum or plasma are low.[32]

A striking clinical feature of LYG is its sparing of lymphoid tissues. However, up to 25% of patients develop an EBV$^+$ diffuse large B-cell lymphoma (DLBCL), and histologic progression may be associated with lymph node involvement. The bone marrow is usually uninvolved by LYG, although nonspecific changes may be observed, such as intertrabecular polymorphic lymphoid aggregates.

MORPHOLOGY

LYG produces nodular mass lesions in most affected organs, most commonly the lung, kidney, liver, and brain.[1,22] The nodules have a polymorphic cellular composition; in addition to the lymphocytes, which predominate, there are plasma cells, immunoblasts, and scattered histiocytes. Neutrophils, eosinophils, or well-formed granulomas are usually infrequent or absent. Reactive lymphoid follicles are generally absent. The EBV$^+$ B cells, which are the hallmark of LYG, vary in size and resemble lymphocytes, immunoblasts, and occasionally HRS cells (Fig. 23-3).[4] They may have deeply staining basophilic cytoplasm and a plasmacytoid appearance. Mummified cells with hyperchromatic nuclei may be seen.

Necrosis is relatively common in LYG, and the extent of necrosis roughly correlates with the grade (Fig. 23-4). The necrosis, which is infarct-like and coagulative, is often centered on altered vessels that show fibrinoid change, infiltration by lymphocytes and histiocytes, and sometimes fibrin thrombi. The necrotic lesions contain nuclear debris, but neutrophils are absent; this is a significant difference from the necrotizing lesions of WG.[33] The surrounding lymphoid infiltrates are nodular and usually efface the underlying architecture of the lung. The surrounding lung parenchyma may show more nonspecific inflammatory changes with perivascular collections of lymphoid cells. However, the diagnosis should not be based solely on a perivascular or interstitial pattern of lymphoid infiltration. Changes of organizing pneumonia are occasionally present but are not a usual feature.

The kidney, liver, and brain, if involved, show nodular infiltrates that are similar in composition to those of the lung. However, the cutaneous lesions, seen in approximately 50%

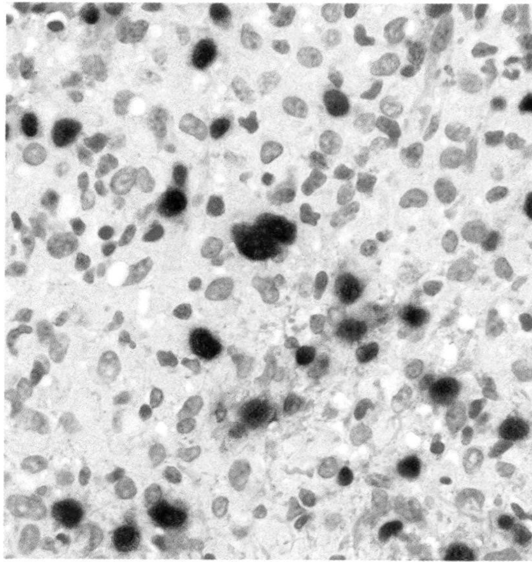

Figure 23-3. Epstein-Barr virus–encoded RNA (EBER) in situ hybridization, lung biopsy. EBER$^+$ cells vary in size, with some larger cells being polylobated, resembling Hodgkin cells.

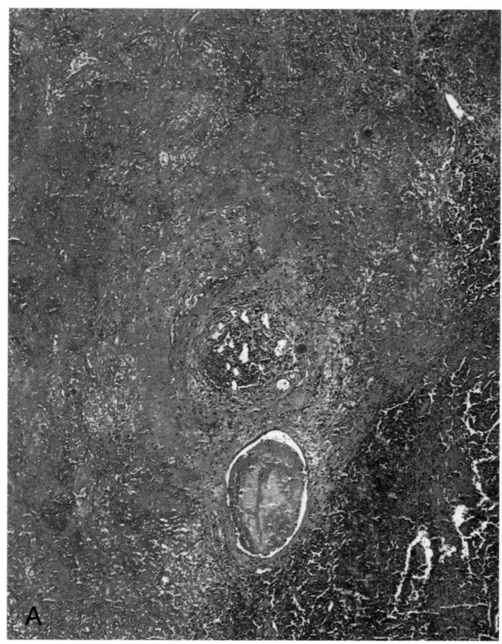

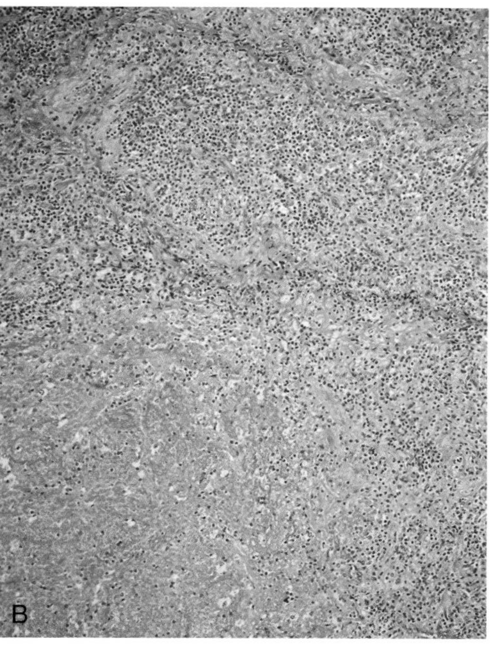

Figure 23-4. Vascular involvement in lymphomatoid granulomatosis. A, Necrotic nodules often contain occluded or damaged blood vessels surrounded by a dense lymphoid infiltrate. **B,** Vessels show medial and intimal infiltration by lymphocytes. Adjacent lung parenchyma is necrotic.

of patients, differ.[22,26] Patients most commonly exhibit subcutaneous or dermal nodules (Fig. 23-5). Fifteen percent of patients have more nonspecific plaque-like lesions with a sparse, superficial dermal periadnexal and perivascular lymphoid infiltrate reminiscent of lichen sclerosus et atrophicus. Characteristic lesions involve the subcutaneous tissue with a lymphohistiocytic infiltrate, with or without multinucleated giant cells (Fig. 23-6). Well-formed sarcoid-like granulomas or necrotizing granulomas are not seen. In some cases, particularly in larger lesions, a prominent vasculitic component, similar to that in the lung, may be seen. In such cases, necrosis may extend to the epidermis, with ulceration. In the dermis the infiltrate may have a periadnexal or perivascular-angiocentric distribution. Mild exocytosis of lymphocytes into the overlying epidermis may be present. EBV^+ cells are less often demonstrable in cutaneous lesions than in the lung, and they are usually identified in larger nodular lesions.[26,34]

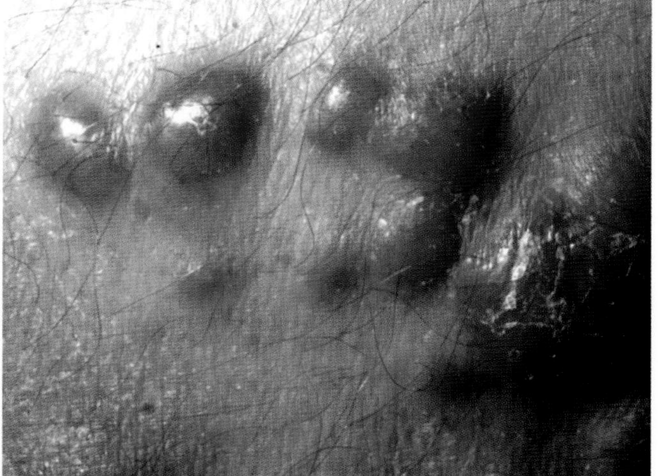

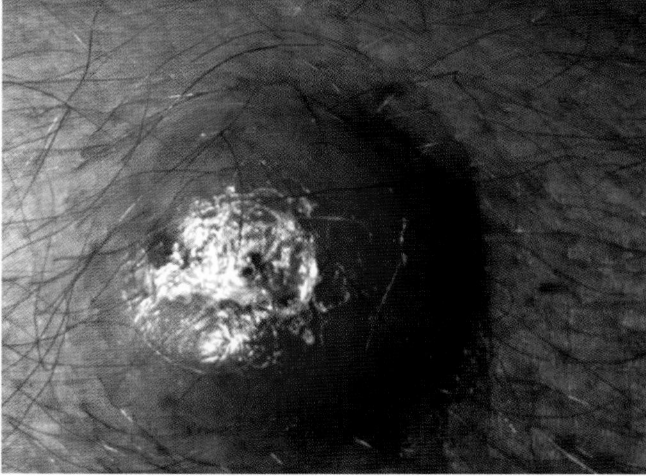

Figure 23-5. Cutaneous manifestations of lymphomatoid granulomatosis. Papulonodular lesions are common; larger nodules may show ulceration.

GRADING

The grading of LYG is based on the proportion of EBV^+ B cells relative to the reactive lymphocyte background.[4,11] Even early studies suggested that grading had prognostic relevance.[8,22] Grade 1 lesions contain a polymorphic lymphoid infiltrate without cytologic atypia. Large transformed lymphoid cells are absent or rare and are better appreciated by immunohistochemistry (Fig. 23-7). Necrosis is usually focal, when present. By in situ hybridization with an Epstein-Barr virus–encoded RNA (EBER) probe, EBV^+ cells number fewer than 5/high-power field. In some cases EBV^+ cells may be absent, but in this setting, the diagnosis should be made with caution, after studies to rule out other inflammatory or neoplastic conditions.

Grade 2 lesions contain occasional large lymphoid cells or immunoblasts in a polymorphic background. Small clusters may be seen, especially with CD20 staining. Necrosis is more common than in grade 1 lesions. In situ hybridization for EBV

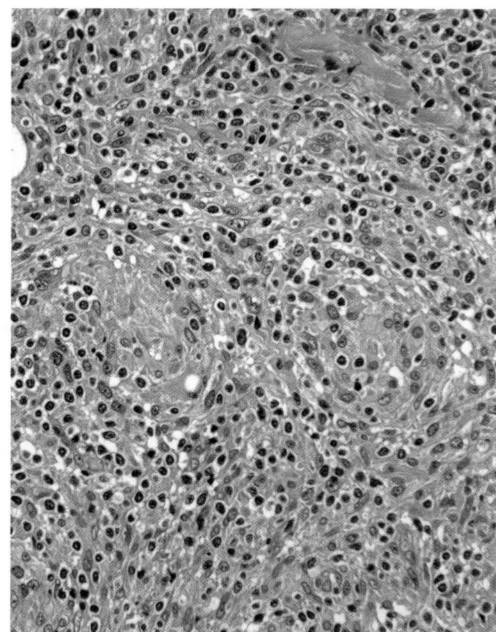

Figure 23-6. Cutaneous lesions are often characterized by subcutaneous lymphohistiocytic infiltrates with poorly formed granulomas.

readily identifies EBV+ cells, which usually number 5 to 20/high-power field. Variation in the number and distribution of EBV+ cells can be seen within a nodule or among nodules, and occasionally up to 50 EBV+ cells/high-power field are observed.

Grade 3 lesions still exhibit an inflammatory background but contain large, atypical B cells that are readily identified by CD20 and can form larger aggregates (Fig. 23-8). Markedly pleomorphic and Hodgkin-like cells are often present, and necrosis is usually extensive (Fig. 23-9). By in situ hybridization, EBV+ cells are extremely numerous (>50/high-power field), and focally they may form small confluent sheets. It is important to consider that in situ hybridization for EBV can be unreliable when large areas of necrosis are present, because of poor RNA preservation; additional molecular studies for EBV may be helpful. A uniform population of large, atypical EBV+ B cells without a polymorphic background should be classified as DLBCL and is beyond the spectrum of LYG as currently defined.

Grading should be based on a dominant mass lesion outside the skin. In addition, histologic grade may vary over time or from site to site. In general, histologic grade increases in patients with relapsed disease. Lesions in the CNS are often of high histologic grade.

IMMUNOPHENOTYPE

Although the hallmark of LYG is the presence of EBV+ B cells in an inflammatory background (Fig. 23-10),[2,35] the majority of the lymphocytes are T cells—a finding that originally led to speculation that LYG was a type of T-cell lymphoma.[5,8] CD4+ cells exceed CD8+ cells, but both are present. The smaller lymphocytes may show slight irregularity or atypia but lack convincing cytologic features of malignancy. T cells may be abundant within vascular lesions and may play a role in mediating vascular damage.[9] The larger EBV+ immunoblasts or pleomorphic large cells usually express B-cell markers such as CD20, PAX5, or CD79a, which can be detected in paraffin sections. LMP-1 is usually negative. Plasma cells can be abundant and may be polytypic or, less often, monotypic for light-chain expression.[36] Because of the polymorphic nature of the infiltrates and the frequent necrosis, flow cytometry is usually not informative for light-chain expression. Molecular studies are best used for the detection of clonality.[2,34,35] The large atypical cells may be CD30+; EBV has been shown to upregulate CD30 in B cells and B-cell lines.[37] However, CD15 is negative—a useful finding for the exclu-

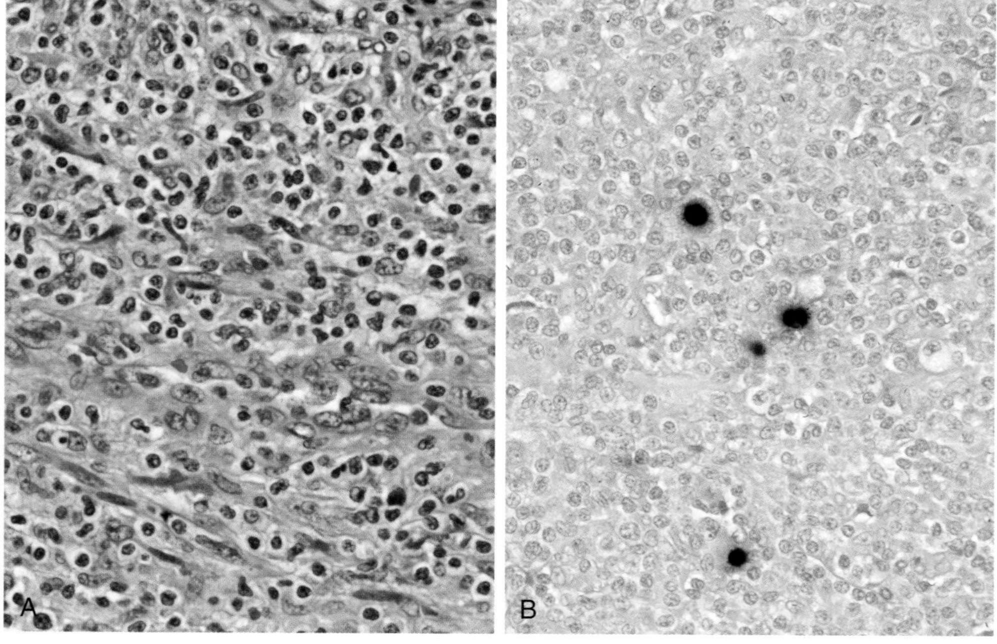

Figure 23-7. Grade 1 lymphomatoid granulomatosis. A, The infiltrate is composed mainly of small lymphocytes and histiocytes without significant atypia. The lumen of the infiltrated blood vessel is barely visible in the *center* of the field. **B,** EBER in situ hybridization of a grade 1 lesion shows only scattered positive cells.

Chapter 24

Burkitt's Lymphoma

Randy D. Gascoyne, Reiner Siebert, and Joseph M. Connors

CHAPTER OUTLINE

Denis Burkitt is credited with the pioneering work that led in 1958 to the first description of the clinical features of this unique tumor, the delineation of its geographic distribution, and the introduction of novel treatment protocols using chemotherapy.[1,2] The eponym *Burkitt's lymphoma* (BL) appropriately recognizes his enormous contribution. The initial descriptions of BL were of rapidly growing tumors in the jaws of children residing in the malarial belt of equatorial Africa.[3-6] This particular form of BL is typically associated with Epstein-Barr virus (EBV). Elsewhere in the world, the association with EBV is much more variable. In vitro studies using BL cell lines have been instrumental in advancing the field of hematopathology. The list of accomplishments includes the original descriptions of EBV itself, the first descriptions of the viral requirements for B-cell immortalization, and mapping of the *MYC* locus to chromosome 8.[7-9]

The nomenclature for this lymphoma entity has changed over the years. In the Rappaport classification, BL was called *undifferentiated lymphoma, Burkitt type.*[10] Lukes and Collins classified BL as small noncleaved follicular center cell lymphoma.[11] The working formulation for clinical usage, which separated lymphomas based on their survival characteristics, classified BL as a clinically high-grade lymphoma of the small noncleaved cell type.[12] Both the Rappaport classification and the working formulation separated undifferentiated or small noncleaved cell lymphomas into Burkitt and non-Burkitt types. The updated Kiel classification included BL as a distinct entity.[13] In the Revised European American Lymphoma (REAL) classification, BL was similarly considered a distinct lymphoma subtype, but the REAL proposal also included a provisional category of high-grade B-cell lymphoma, Burkitt-like, or Burkitt-like lymphoma.[14] The latter category recognized the existence of a small number of cases that challenged the distinction between BL and diffuse large B-cell lymphoma (DLBCL). These so-called gray zone or borderline cases (unclassifiable B-cell lymphoma, with features intermediate between DLBCL and BL) are now included in a new provisional category in the recent World Health Organization (WHO) classification and are discussed later.[15-17] The French-American-British classification of acute leukemia included a category of B-cell acute lymphoblastic leukemia (ALL), also known as *L3-ALL*.[18] In the majority of cases, L3-ALL is BL in leukemic phase.

In the WHO's new classification of hematopoietic and lymphoid tumors,[16] BL is considered a distinct lymphoid neoplasm with three clinical or epidemiologic types. Variations on the classic morphologic appearance are recognized, but distinct morphologic variants are not delineated.

DEFINITION

Burkitt's lymphoma is defined by the WHO as a highly aggressive lymphoid neoplasm, often presenting at extranodal sites or as an acute leukemia,[14,16,19,20] composed of monomorphic, medium-sized B cells with basophilic cytoplasm and a high mitotic rate. Translocations involving the *MYC* oncogene on chromosome 8 at band 8q24 are a constant feature. The frequency of EBV infection varies according to the epidemiologic subtype of BL (see later; Table 24-1).

EPIDEMIOLOGY

Three clinical variants of BL are recognized, with substantial differences in clinical presentation and anatomic localization of the primary tumor, subtle differences in morphology, and variable molecular genetics and biology.[16]

Endemic Burkitt's Lymphoma

BL is endemic in the malaria belt of equatorial Africa, which stretches from Senegal and Mauritania in the northwest to Tanzania and Mozambique in the southeast, and in Papua New Guinea. The areas of sub-Saharan Africa most implicated are those at altitudes with high annual rainfall and elevated temperatures, corresponding to regions endemic for malaria.[6] People living in urban areas are largely spared from BL. Endemic BL affects primarily young children, with a peak incidence in those aged 4 to 10 years and a 2:1 male-to-female predominance.[21] The tumors are most often extranodal, particularly involving the jaw, facial bones, and orbit. The majority of cases of endemic BL are EBV$^+$ and demonstrate distinct molecular *MYC* alterations at both the immunoglobulin heavy chain (*IGH*) and *MYC* loci (see Table 24-3).

Sporadic Burkitt's Lymphoma

This variant is seen throughout the world, commonly afflicting children and young adults.[22,23] It is uncommon in adults,

Table 24-1 Major Diagnostic Features of Burkitt's Lymphoma (BL) and Diffuse Large B-Cell Lymphoma (DLBCL)

Feature	Classic BL	Intermediate between BL and DLBCL	DLBCL
Architecture	Diffuse	Diffuse, rarely nodular	Diffuse
"Starry sky" pattern	Usually present	May be absent	Usually absent
Mitoses	Many	Many	Variable
Cytology	Monomorphic	Minimally pleomorphic	Variable
Nuclear shape	Round or oval	Some cells slightly irregular	Centroblasts predominate
Nuclear size	Intermediate	Intermediate, some admixed larger cells	Large cells
Nucleoli	Multiple (2-5), basophilic	May be single, central, and more prominent	Variable; centroblasts typically have 2-3 adjacent to nuclear membrane
Cytoplasm	Basophilic and often vacuolated; squared-off appearance present	Basophilic; vacuoles may be absent and may lack squared-off nuclear appearance	Basophilic to amphophilic and typically lacks vacuoles
Expression of CD19, CD20, CD22, CD79a	Positive	Positive	Most cases positive
CD10 expression	Positive	Positive	Variably positive; defines GCB subtype of DLBCL
BCL6 expression	Positive	Positive	Most cases positive
BCL2 expression	Negative	Variable; double-hit cases usually positive*	60%-70% positive, mostly within ABC subtype
Bright CD38	Positive	Variably positive	CD38 may be positive, but often dim
EBV-EBER	Positive (15%-30%)†	Negative	Usually negative
Cytogenetics	t(8;14) or variant t(2;8) or t(8;22), mostly simple karyotype	t(8;14) and other t(qq24), complex karyotype	
DNA content	Near diploid	Near diploid, may be complex	Complex karyotype often found
Molecular	*MYC* rearrangement to IG partner	*MYC* rearrangement to IG and non-IG partner, often accompanied by *BCL2* or *BCL6* rearrangement	*MYC* translocation in 5%-8% of de novo DLBCLs

*Some cases may lack staining with the Dako antibody (clone 124) but do stain with E17, an alternative antibody targeting a different epitope.
†Percentages apply to sporadic BL.
ABC, activated B-cell subtype; EBER, EBV-encoded RNA; EBV, Epstein-Barr virus; GCB, germinal center B-cell subtype.

accounting for only 1% to 2% of all lymphomas in Western Europe and North America.[24] It accounts for 30% to 50% of pediatric lymphomas. Sporadic BL is uncommon in those younger than 2 years. The median age of adult patients is approximately 30 years, and there is a male predominance of about 2:1 to 3:1. Some cases present in the elderly. Involvement of the gastrointestinal tract is common in sporadic BL, whereas involvement of the jaw or the orbit is unusual.[25] EBV is seen in less than 30% of reported cases, and in most Western countries it is found in 10% to 20%.[8] Sporadic BL can occur in people living in endemic regions and may account for some cases with atypical presentations or lack of EBV involvement. The breakpoint sites for both *IGH* and *MYC* are usually different from those encountered in endemic BL (see Genetics, Table 24-3, and Fig. 24-16).

The gray zone or borderline cases typically occur in an older age group compared with sporadic BL and present much more frequently as lymph node–based disease.[15,17,26-28] With the exception of immunodeficiency-related cases (particularly human immunodeficiency virus [HIV] infection), EBV is less commonly implicated.

Immunodeficiency-Associated Burkitt's Lymphoma

This variant of BL is seen primarily in association with HIV infection and accounts for approximately 30% to 40% of all acquired immunodeficiency syndrome (AIDS)–related cases of lymphoma.[29] Infection with EBV is seen in 25% to 40% of these cases.[30] Many cases demonstrate slightly atypical cytologic features and often exhibit plasmacytoid differentiation.[31,32] This variant of BL may also occur in other immunodeficiency states, including congenital disorders and iatrogenic causes such as the immunosuppression required following organ transplantation.[33] However, BL is uncommon in this setting.

ETIOLOGY AND PATHOGENESIS

The cause of BL is unknown. Chronic antigenic stimulation and the associated immune suppression that follow persistent malarial infection have been suggested as causative factors.[8,34] HIV infection has been similarly implicated.[35,36] Additionally, pesticide exposure in both adults and children has been noted.[37]

The most consistent factor implicated in the pathogenesis of BL is translocation of the *MYC* oncogene.[38] This gene is deregulated through either translocation or mutation in virtually all cases of BL.[39] Cumulative data from the literature suggest that *MYC* may fulfill at least two major roles: promoting cellular proliferation and downregulating the expression of human leukocyte antigen (HLA) class I molecules, thus allowing the tumor cells to evade host immune control.[36] Normal responses to *MYC* overexpression not only enhance cellular proliferation; *MYC* also promotes apoptosis. A number of genetic alterations may conspire to subvert the apoptotic signaling associated with *MYC*, including alterations in other genetic loci often found in BL cases (mutations or other aberrations in the *p53-MDM2-ARF* pathway), *MYC* mutations that abrogate apoptotic signaling, and possibly EBV infection.[40,41] Although a consistent finding in BL, *MYC* overexpression is insufficient on its own to induce lymphoma.[42,43] Overexpression of *MYC* in transgenic mice leads to a polyclonal expansion of precursor B cells, but monoclonal neoplasms do not develop for 6 to 9 months, almost certainly the result of additional genetic insults. These data in the aggregate suggest that although *MYC* is important for the development of BL, it may be only a cofactor or an initiating event that requires additional genetic alterations to express the full malignant phenotype.[42] Recent data suggest that within the category of DLBCL, *MYC* translocations or mutations may result from aberrant activity of the somatic hypermutation mechanism and thus may account for translocations that cannot be explained by mistakes in variable-diversity-joining (VDJ) or antibody class switch recombination.[44] Activation-induced cytidine deaminase (AID) is required for both class switch recombination and somatic hypermutation. It has recently been shown that AID is instrumental in promoting double-stranded DNA breaks in the promoter region of *MYC;* this, together with its creation of breaks in *IGH*, establishes the role of AID in promoting *IGH-MYC* translocation in neoplastic B cells.[45] The spatial proximity of these two loci within the nucleus may also play a role in promoting translocations.[46] A specific role for *MYC* in BL is difficult to reconcile, however, because *MYC* alterations can also be detected in DLBCL, rare lymphoblastic lymphomas, and follicular lymphoma.[47-53] Rare cases of BL appear to lack definable *MYC* translocations. Recent studies have suggested altered micro-RNA expression as a possible contributor to pathogenesis.[54]

EBV infection represents the second most frequent factor in the pathogenesis of BL. Importantly, neither of these factors has been shown to be specific or causative.[35,55-57] EBV is a nearly ubiquitous human herpesvirus that is capable of either transforming B cells or persisting within these cells in a latent state. Latent EBV infection is characterized by three different patterns of gene expression.[58,59] In latency pattern type I, which is characteristic of BL, the viral-associated genes expressed include *EBER-1, EBER-2,* and *EBNA-1*. In latency pattern II, which is characteristic of Hodgkin's lymphoma, peripheral T-cell lymphomas, and primary effusion lymphomas in the HIV setting, the viral genes expressed include *EBER-1, EBER-2, EBNA-1, LMP-1, LMP-2A,* and *LMP-2B*. In the type III latency pattern, seen in posttransplant lymphoproliferative disorders and lymphoblastoid cell lines, the full spectrum of latent viral genes are expressed, including *EBER-1, EBER-2, EBNA-1, 2, 3A, 3B,* and *3C,* and *LMP-1, 2A,* and *2B*.

Latent EBV infection with a type I pattern is associated with the vast majority of endemic BL, but importantly, it is not present in all cases.[58] These data suggest that EBV may not be critical to the pathogenesis or that another as yet unidentified virus is implicated. Moreover, EBV infection is seen in less than 30% of sporadic BL cases, although their morphologic and immunophenotypic features are identical to those of endemic BL.[8,60,61]

In support of EBV's role as an important causative agent in BL, most studies have shown evidence of a clonal infective event.[62,63] Using probes to the terminal repeat sequences of EBV, neoplastic cells harboring latent virus in the form of episomal DNA have a pattern on Southern blot analysis in keeping with infection of the malignant B cells before clonal expansion.[64] Contrasting with these data are recent in vitro studies of sequential clinical samples and corresponding cell lines in which EBV infection was shown to be a later event.[65]

The two main theories concerning the role of EBV in the pathogenesis of BL have much to do with the timing of infection in relation to translocation of the *MYC* oncogene.[66] In one hypothesis, EBV infection induces a polyclonal expansion of B cells with a "lymphoblastoid" pattern of latent EBV gene expression. Increased mitotic activity in this population increases the likelihood of an aberrant *MYC* rearrangement. Under these conditions, EBV may only potentiate tumor development by stimulating cellular proliferation, decreasing apoptotic signaling, or increasing genetic instability. The "hit and run" model, in which the virus does its damage and then is lost, fits with this concept and could explain why some cases of endemic BL are negative for latent EBV genomes.

The second hypothesis related to EBV suggests that infection by the virus occurs after the *MYC* translocation. This theory can be reconciled more easily with the pattern of latent EBV gene expression seen in BL, consisting of only *EBER-1*, *EBER-2*, and *EBNA-1* (latency type I).[59,63,65] This pattern of gene expression may offer a survival advantage, allowing an escape from immune surveillance because *EBNA-1* does not induce a potent cytotoxic T-cell response.[67] However, this theory is tenable only if the cell harboring the *MYC* translocation has no proliferative advantage or if only one cell led to the development of BL following EBV infection.

Perhaps more likely is an integrated model in which EBV infection demonstrating a lymphoblastoid pattern of gene expression (type III) produces a polyclonal B-cell expansion.[66] Given this background, perhaps *MYC* translocation occurs because of increased genetic instability secondary to EBV, resulting in a growth advantage for the cells, a concomitant downregulation of EBV latent genes, and a change in morphology from an immunoblastic appearance to one resembling BL. Although this seems to be a plausible theory, recent data suggest that forced expression of *MYC* in lymphoblastoid cell lines does not induce an EBV latency pattern switch from type III to type I.[68] In contrast, other data suggest that *MYC* and *EBNA-1* may cooperate in promoting lymphomagenesis.[67,69] Fundamental questions regarding the role of EBV and its contribution to the pathogenesis of BL remain largely unanswered. Overexpression of *E2F1* may also play a part in cell cycle deregulation in BL.[70] The precise role of holoendemic malaria and HIV infection as predisposing factors has yet to be firmly established.

CLINICAL FEATURES

The findings usually associated with the rapid growth of neoplastic cells typify virtually all cases of BL. Serious oncologic emergencies may develop, including bowel perforation, ureteric obstruction, or paraplegia secondary to paraspinal masses with cord compression. Involvement of the central nervous system (CNS) seems to be a risk associated with all three forms of BL.[71] Some unique clinical findings are associated with the different epidemiologic subtypes.

Endemic Burkitt's Lymphoma

Endemic BL involves extranodal sites, particularly the jaw and orbit, in approximately 50% of cases. The jaw and facial structures are involved in approximately 70% of cases in children younger than 5 years but in only 25% of those older than 14 years (Fig. 24-1).[21,72] The orbital involvement seen in endemic BL contrasts sharply with the North American experience with orbital lymphomas, where the majority of lymphomas involving the ocular adnexa are indolent B-cell lymphomas.[21,72] Other sites of involvement include the distal ileum, cecum, ovary, kidney, and breast.

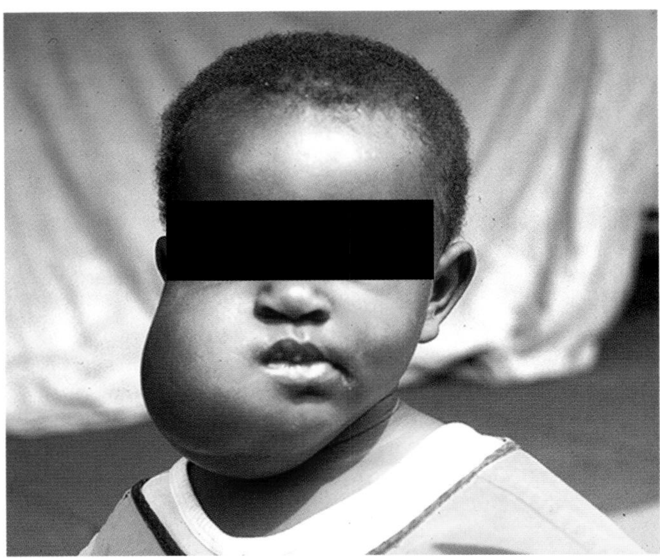

Figure 24-1. A young boy from South America with typical endemic Burkitt's lymphoma presenting in the mandible. (Courtesy Prof. Georges Delsol, Toulouse, France.)

Facial involvement by lymphoma may fill the sinuses or cause loosening of the teeth. Gross abnormalities of the orbit are common, as is involvement of cranial nerves.[71] Involvement of the bone marrow or presentation as acute leukemia is quite uncommon in endemic BL.[21,72] Patients may complain of abdominal pain, swelling, or a change in bowel habits.

Sporadic Burkitt's Lymphoma

In sporadic BL, involvement of the facial structures, in particular the jaw, is uncommon.[25] Eighty percent to 90% of cases present with involvement of intra-abdominal structures.[25] The ileocecal region is most commonly involved, but other sites include the appendix, ascending colon, and peritoneum.[25] Extra-abdominal sites include the ovary, kidney, and breast. Of note, bilateral breast involvement is a characteristic finding in BL, associated with the onset of puberty, pregnancy, or lactation. Patients may present with pleural effusions. Bone marrow involvement is more common than in endemic BL and is seen at some point in the course of the disease in almost every fatal case.[25,73] Although CNS involvement is uncommon at diagnosis, it develops eventually in most cases of sporadic BL unless effective CNS chemotherapy is given along with curative systemic chemotherapy.[74] Peripheral lymph node involvement is seen in only 10% to 15% of cases and is more common in adults than in children.[25] Involvement of Waldeyer's ring or the mediastinum is rare. Patients with advanced stage and/or bulky disease may have circulating neoplastic cells identified in the peripheral blood smear. A diagnosis of Burkitt's leukemia or L3-ALL is reserved for those cases with greater than 25% bone marrow involvement at diagnosis.

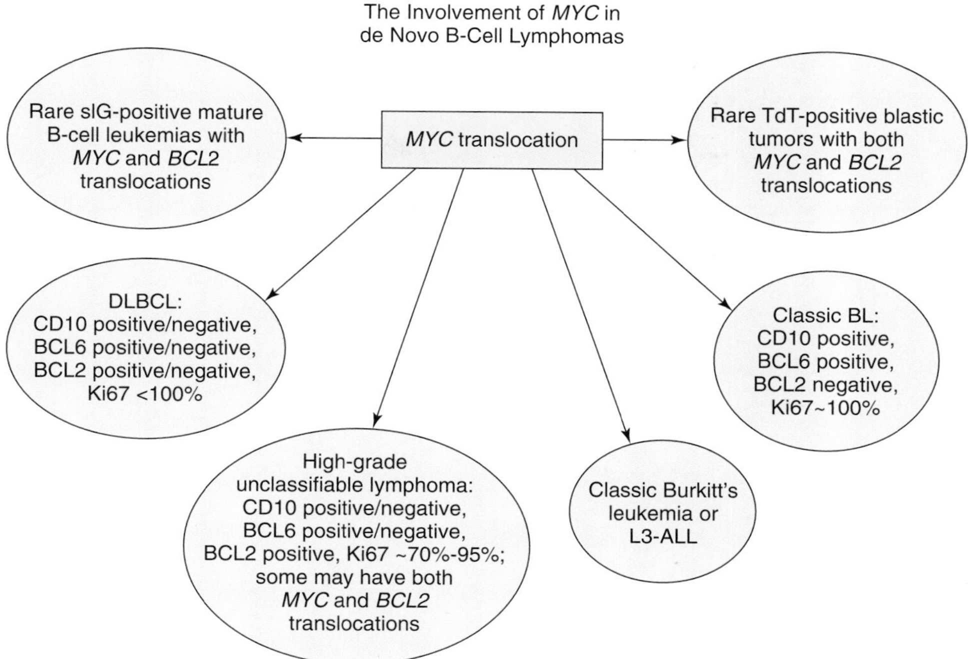

Figure 24-10. Schematic of the many morphologic and immunophenotypic manifestations of the *MYC* oncogene. Depicted are those disorders in which *MYC* has been implicated as a primary cytogenetic alteration or has been found coincident with other alterations in the karyotype of a de novo lymphoid neoplasm. *MYC* can result in a number of different histologic appearances, including classic Burkitt's lymphoma (BL), unclassifiable B-cell lymphoma with features intermediate between BL and diffuse large B-cell lymphoma (DLBCL), rare terminal deoxynucleotidyl transferase (TdT)–positive lymphoblastic lymphoma (LBL), B-cell acute lymphoblastic leukemia (L3-ALL), and so-called mature B-cell leukemia. *MYC* translocations can also occur as secondary events (not shown here), typically present at the time of histologic transformation; they result in high-grade histology, including unclassifiable B-cell lymphomas with features intermediate between DLBCL and BL and LBL. Secondary *MYC* alterations of this type have been described in follicular lymphoma, mantle cell lymphoma, myeloma, and splenic lymphoma with villous lymphocytes. The *longer arrows* indicate the common result of a *MYC* translocation in both children (BL) and adults (DLBCL). Classic BL may account for only one third of adults with *MYC* rearrangements detected in primary biopsy material. Dual-translocation cases with features suggesting LBL, including nuclear TdT expression, are best classified as LBL. Although not shown here, rare cases of DLBCL may mimic the immunophenotype of classic BL (see Fig. 24-14). Lacking knowledge of the status of the *MYC* gene, it is difficult to predict the clinical behavior of these tumors. sIg, surface immunoglobulin.

GENETICS

Burkitt Translocation Leading to *IGH-MYC* Juxtaposition and Its Light-Chain Variants

BL was the first lymphoma for which a recurrent chromosomal aberration was described. In 1972, marker chromosome 14 was identified in BL by Manolov and Manolova,[9] which was subsequently shown by Zech and collaborators[125] to be derived from a reciprocal translocation affecting the long (q-) arms of chromosomes 8 and 14. In typical BL the translocation t(8;14)(q24;q32) is present in approximately 75% to 80% of the cases, whereas its variants t(8;22)(q24;q11) and t(2;8)(p12;q24) are less frequent (Fig. 24-15).[38,63,121]

At the molecular level, t(8;14) and variants juxtapose the *MYC* gene located at chromosome region 8q24 next to one of the immunoglobulin gene (*IG*) loci, namely the *IGH@* locus at chromosome region 14q32, the *IGK* locus at 2p12, or the *IGL* locus at 22q11 (see Fig. 24-15). As a result of these translocations to the *IG* loci, control of normal *MYC* expression is lost, leading to constitutive expression of the protein throughout the cell cycle. *MYC* encodes a transcription factor that can function as both a transcriptional activator and a transcriptional repressor capable of inducing apoptosis as well as proliferation.[38,63,126] The *MYC* gene has been implicated in the genesis of DNA damage, the disruption of double-stranded DNA repair leading to increased chromosomal translocations, and the increased production of reactive oxygen species.[127-129] Novel technologies such as global promoter region microarrays have shed light on the vast number of downstream genes affected by *MYC* gene upregulation.[130] Constitutive *MYC* expression has also been shown to increase angiogenesis and lymphangiogenesis.[131]

The molecular breakpoints within the *MYC* locus at 8q24 depend on the translocation partners and show considerable interindividual variation.[132-134] In the case of classic t(8;14), the breakpoints in 8q24 typically lie within the centromeric (5′) part of the *MYC* locus. These have been classified according to the position of the chromosomal breakpoints relative to the *MYC* gene; translocations with breakpoints in the first (5′) exon or intron of *MYC* have been designated as class I, those with breakpoints immediately upstream of the gene as class II, and those with distant breakpoints as class III. In sporadic and immunodeficiency-associated BL, class I (and II) translocations are predominant, whereas in endemic African cases, class III translocations with breakpoints dispersed over several hundred kilobases upstream of the gene are most frequent (Fig. 24-16; Table 24-3).[38,63,135] The t(8;14) thus leads to activation of *MYC* on the der(14) chromosome

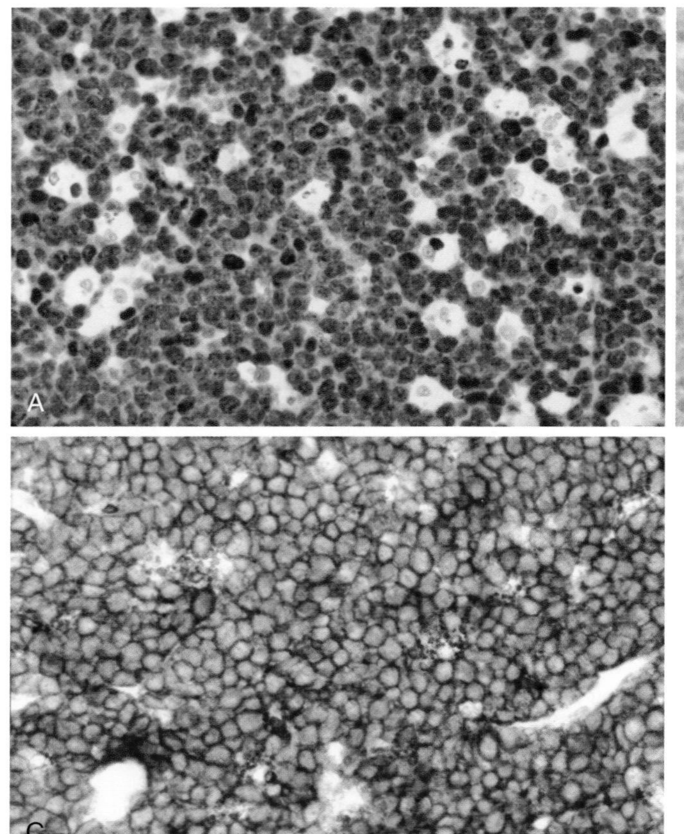

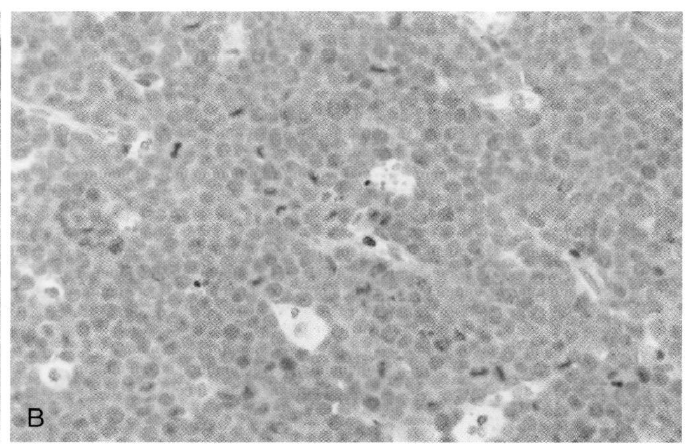

Figure 24-11. Immunostains of Ki-67 (**A**), BCL2 (**B**), and CD10 (**C**) in a case of classic Burkitt's lymphoma. Note that all cells are proliferating, as defined by positive Ki-67 staining, except the phagocytic histiocytes in the section. CD10 is strongly expressed by the malignant cells, and BCL2 is negative. Note several small, reactive lymphocytes in the section staining positively for BCL2.

containing the intact coding region of the gene. The breakpoints in the *IGH@* locus at 14q32 usually occur 5′ of the intron enhancer in a joining (J) or diversity (D) segment in endemic BL and 3′ of the intron enhancer in the switch mu region in sporadic and HIV-associated BL, suggesting that these translocations occur during an aberrant VDJ- or class switch–recombination process, respectively (see Table 24-3).[38,63,135] There is also evidence that Burkitt translocations might be the result of a misdirected somatic mutation.[136] Somatic and in part ongoing V_H mutations have been observed in some cases of BL. Similarly, mutations of the *MYC* gene are very frequent, particularly in endemic BL carrying t(8;14), presumably owing to somatic hypermutation driven by the immunoglobulin sequences juxtaposed to the *MYC* locus on the derivative chromosome 14.[44,136] Such mutations can alter *MYC* transcription or influence phosphorylation, stability, and activity of the protein.[38,63,126]

In contrast to the classic Burkitt translocation t(8;14), both variant translocations t(2;8) and t(8;22) lead to deregulation of *MYC* on the derivative chromosome 8, caused by

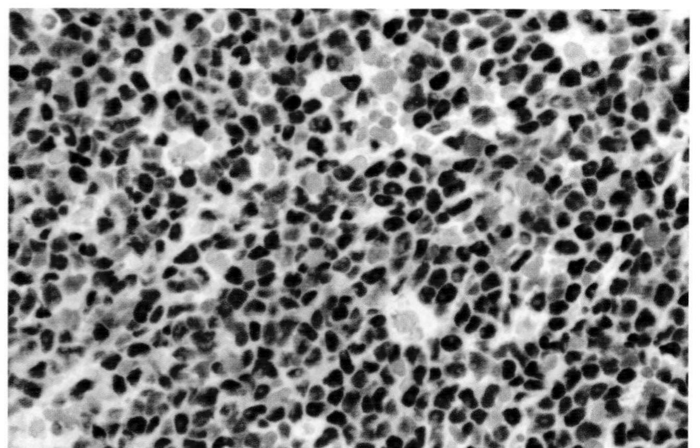

Figure 24-12. HIV-related case of Burkitt's lymphoma with latent Epstein-Barr virus infection. Section was subjected to in situ hybridization using probes for EBER (*brown*).

Table 24-2 Immunophenotypic and Molecular Features of AIDS-Related Lymphomas

Feature	AIDS BL	AIDS DLBCL	AIDS IBL
EBV infection (EBER positive)	30%	40%	90%
LMP-1 status	–	–	+
BCL6 expression	+	+	–
MUM-1/IRF4	–	–	+
CD138	–	–	+
MYC rearrangement	100%	Some	Some
BCL6 rearrangement	–	20%	–
p53 mutations	60%	Rare	Rare

AIDS, acquired immunodeficiency syndrome; BL, Burkitt's lymphoma; DLBCL, diffuse large B-cell lymphoma; EBER, EBV-encoded RNA; EBV, Epstein-Barr virus; IBL, immunoblastic lymphoma.

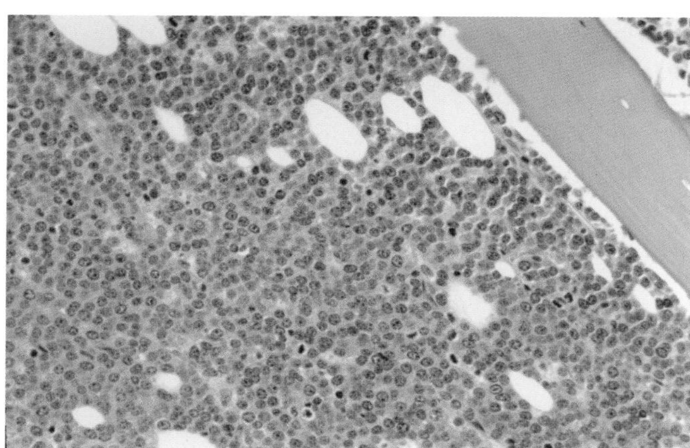

Figure 24-13. Bone marrow biopsy showing heavy infiltration with Burkitt's lymphoma. The packed bone marrow led to a diagnosis of B-cell acute lymphoblastic leukemia (L3-ALL).

juxtaposition next to the *IGK* and *IGL* genes, respectively (Fig. 24-17). The chromosome 8 breakpoints of these variants are located 3′ of *MYC* and can be dispersed over a region up to 2 Mb telomeric of the *MYC* gene (Fig. 24-18).[132] The breaks on chromosomes 2 and 22 occur usually 5′ of the *IGK* and *IGL* gene constant region segments, respectively.[38,63]

Importantly, *MYC* translocations are not restricted to BL. A range of 8q24 alterations targeting several partner chromosomes has been identified by novel molecular cytogenetic approaches in various B-cell neoplasms. For instance, in multiple myeloma, alterations affecting 8q24 have been described in 15% to 50% of cases.[137-139]

Non–*IG-MYC* Translocations

A steadily increasing number of *MYC* translocations to loci other than *IG* loci have been described as a result of FISH screening of lymphomas with features suggesting BL. These translocations have been termed *non–IG-MYC translocations,* and the most prominent seem to be t(8;9)(q24;p13) and t(3;8)(q27;q24).[28,105-107,140-142] The t(8;9) juxtaposes the *MYC* locus next to a region in 9p13 close to the *PAX5* gene, and the t(3;8) juxtaposes it to the *BCL6* locus at 3q27. The breaks in the *MYC* locus in these non–*IG-MYC* translocations occur mostly telomeric of *MYC,* similar to the light-chain variants of the Burkitt translocation. The exact mechanisms by which they deregulate *MYC* expression are still speculative, but a role for regulatory or promoter elements, as well as local changes in chromatin structure, is assumed. Remarkably, the non-*IG* translocations rarely if ever occur in typical BL but account for up to half the *MYC* translocations in intermediate or gray zone lymphomas.[94,121] Moreover,

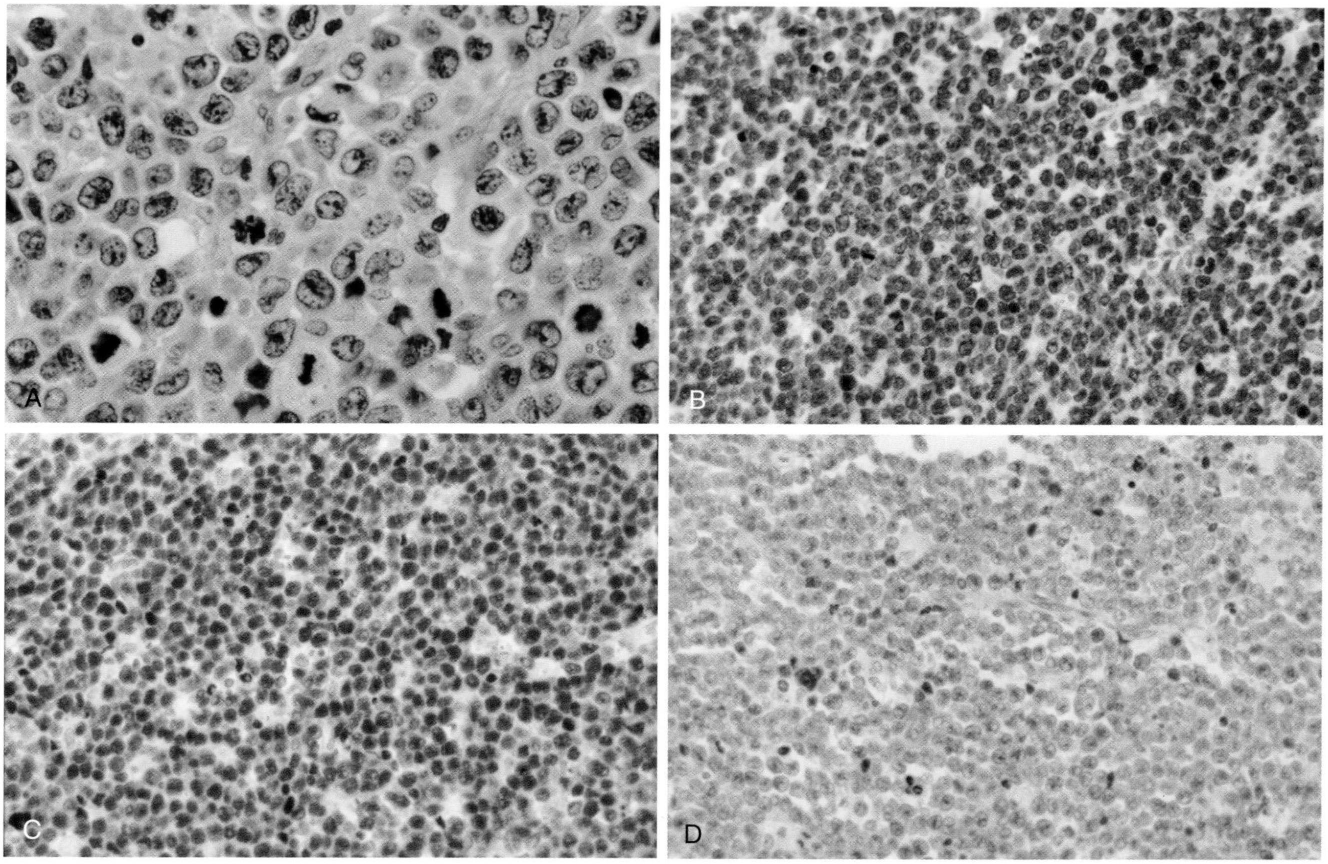

Figure 24-14. Hematoxylin-eosin stained section of diffuse large B-cell lymphoma with multilobated nuclei and a typical immunophenotype of classic Burkitt's lymphoma (**A**). The cells show 100% Ki-67 staining (**B**), strong nuclear expression of BCL6 (**C**), and absent BCL2 protein expression (**D**). Note the internal control staining of small lymphocytes. The cells in this case also express CD10 and CD43 (not shown). Information regarding the status of the *MYC* oncogene was not available.

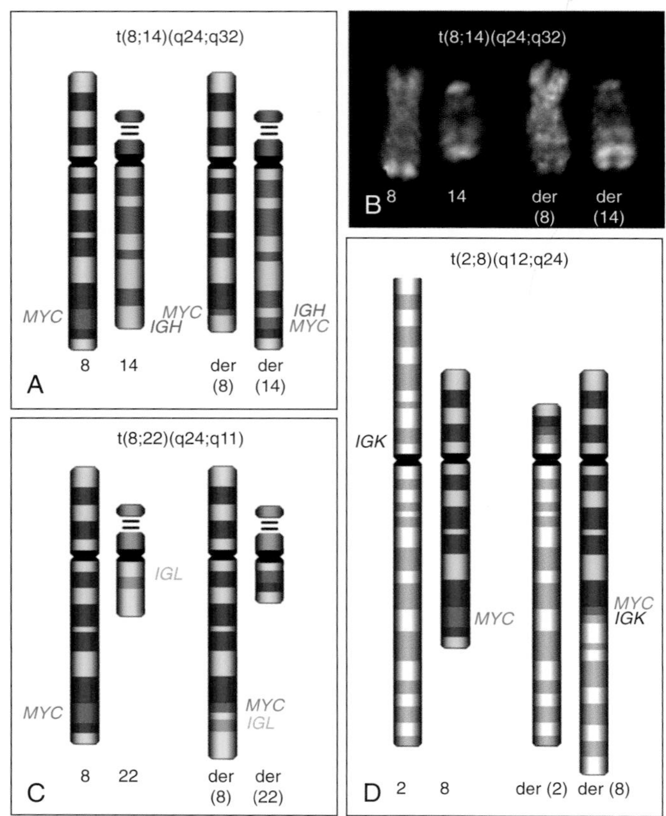

Figure 24-15. Schematic of the classic Burkitt translocation t(8;14) (**A** and **B**) and its variants t(8;22) (**C**) and t(2;8) (**D**). The involved chromosomes are highlighted by different colors. *Red* indicates the *MYC* locus at 8q24. The juxtaposition of *MYC* next to *IG* loci, leading to activation of the *MYC* gene, is indicated. Partial karyotype (fluorescence R-banding) shows normal and derivative chromosomes 8 and 14 from a lymphoma with classic Burkitt translocation.

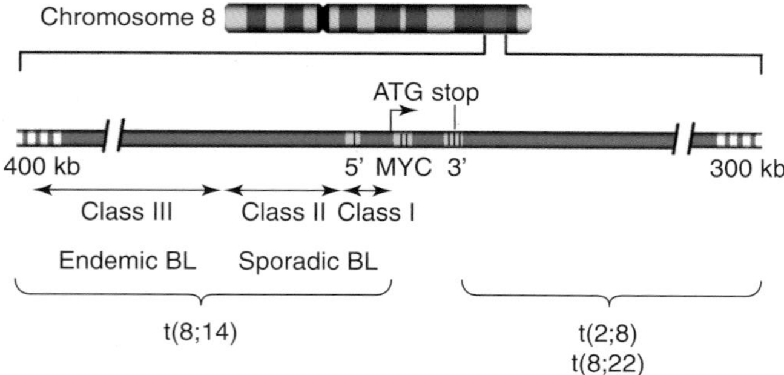

Figure 24-16. Illustration of the *MYC* locus at chromosome region 8q24 (not drawn to scale). The three exons of the *MYC* gene are indicated in *yellow*. The distribution of the various breakpoint regions is indicated below the map.

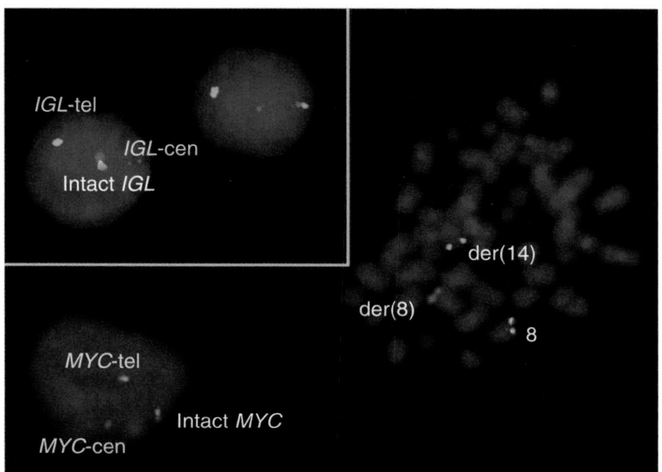

Figure 24-17. Detection of breakpoints in the *MYC* locus (*main figure*) and *IGL* locus (*inset*) using differently labeled probes flanking these loci. The *MYC* break-apart probe consists of a 5′ probe that begins less than 140 kb upstream of the 5′ end of *MYC* and extends 260 kb toward the centromere (*red*). The 3′ probe starts about 1 Mb 3′ of *MYC* and extends toward the telomere for approximately 400 kb (LSI MYC Dual Color, Break-Apart Rearrangement Probe; Vysis Inc., Downers Grove, IL). The *IGL* break-apart probe consists of differently labeled BAC clones flanking the *IGL* locus at 22q11.[163] The colocalization of one red and one green signal indicates intact *MYC* and *IGL* loci, respectively. The breakpoint in the *MYC* locus and the *IGL* locus in Burkitt's lymphomas caused by t(8;14) (*main figure*) and t(8;22) (*inset*), respectively, is indicated by separation of the red and green signals.

t(8;9)(q24;p13) is closely associated with the presence of t(14;18)(q32;q21) and *IGH-BCL2* juxtaposition. For the coexistence of a *MYC* breakpoint and a breakpoint affecting another typical lymphoma oncogene, such as *BCL2, BCL6,* or *CCND1*, the term *double hit* has been coined.[89,143] Nevertheless, this term is ambiguous, because a double hit could also mean the coexistence of *BCL2* and *BCL6* translocations, for example. Similarly, such double-hit lymphomas have been subsumed under the umbrella of *MYC*-complex lymphomas, which also contain *IG-MYC*–positive lymphomas with numerous secondary genetic aberrations.[121] Thus, it is probably more precise to call such coexistence *BCL2-/MYC*-break–positive lymphomas, for example. There is good evidence from cytogenetic and molecular cytogenetic investigations that the *MYC* gene can be quite promiscuous in B-cell lymphomas and that additional non–*IG-MYC* translocations will be characterized in the future.

Table 24-3 Characteristic Genetic Features of Burkitt's Lymphoma (BL)

Feature	Endemic BL	Sporadic BL	AIDS-Associated BL
Predominant *MYC* breakpoint in t(8;14)(q24;q32)	Far 5′ (centromeric) of *MYC* (class III)	Exon and intron 1 (class I) and 5′ (centromeric) of *MYC* (class II)	Exon and intron 1 (class I)
Predominant *IGH@* breakpoint in t(8;14)(q24;q32)	VDJ region	Switch region	Switch region
Somatic *IGH@* mutations	Yes	Yes	Yes
EBV positivity	>90%	5%-30%	25%-40%

AIDS, acquired immunodeficiency syndrome; EBV, Epstein-Barr virus.

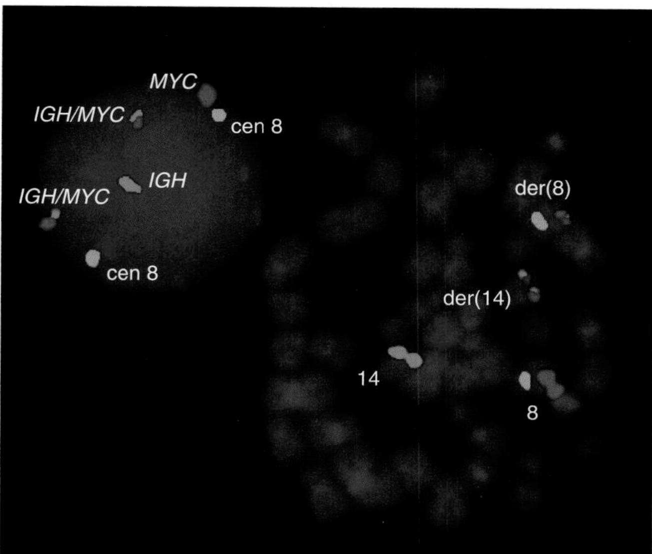

Figure 24-18. Detection of t(8;14) in a case of Burkitt's lymphoma using an *IGH-MYC* dual fusion probe. This probe is a mixture of a 1.5-Mb *IGH* probe (*green*) containing sequences homologous to essentially the entire *IGH* locus, as well as sequences extending about 300 kb beyond the 3′ end of the *IGH* locus, and a 750-kb large *MYC* probe (*red*) extending approximately 400 kb upstream of *MYC* and about 350 kb 3′ beyond *MYC*. The t(8;14) leads to fusion signals on both der(8) and der(14) chromosomes, in addition to isolated green and red signals on intact chromosomes 8 and 14, respectively. The multiple copies of chromosome 8 can be detected using an alpha satellite probe (*pink false color*) directed to the centromeric region of this chromosome (LSI IGH/MYC, CEP 8 Tri-color, Dual Fusion Translocation Probe; Vysis Inc., Downers Grove, IL).

Genetic Changes in Typical Burkitt's Lymphoma

With the exception of few cases discussed later, typical BL, both endemic and sporadic, always carries one of the three translocations leading to *IG-MYC* fusion: t(8;14)(q24;q32), t(2;8)(p12;q24), or t(8;22)(q24;q11), with t(8;14) being the most common. The Burkitt translocations are considered primary events in BL. They usually form part of a pretty simple karyotype; that is, no or very few additional chromosomal aberrations are detectable. Two recent comprehensive reviews showed that in more than half of typical BLs, no secondary aberrations can be identified at the cytogenetic level.[143,144] The most common secondary aberrations in this core subset (occurring in 44% of cases) are copy number gains involving 1q, 7, and 12 and losses involving 6q, 13q32-34, and 17p. Remarkably, it seems that gain of 1q is associated with a lack of other recurrent abnormalities, with a mostly random scattering of abnormalities in the other cases. There is some evidence that increasing chromosomal complexity is associated with poorer outcome in typical BL.[143,144] The pattern of chromosomal imbalances identified by conventional cytogenetic studies are in line with studies of BL using comparative genomic hybridization (CGH) and array CGH, which have been performed on much smaller series so far.[145,146] Nevertheless, it is remarkable that these studies have failed to identify novel cytogenetic, cryptic chromosomal imbalances in BL and have shown that the pattern of chromosomal imbalances in pediatric and adult typical BL is identical, despite the well-known differences in incidence.[147,148]

Do *MYC*-Negative Typical Burkitt's Lymphomas Exist?

There is ongoing discussion whether typical BL lacking either *MYC* translocation or *IG-MYC* fusion actually exists. Indeed, Hummel and coworkers[121] reported very rare cases of mature, aggressive B-cell lymphomas carrying the gene expression signature of BL but lacking a detectable *MYC* aberration. Similarly, Leucci and colleagues[54] reported a series of *MYC*-negative classic BLs showing an alternative pathogenetic mechanism involving micro-RNA deregulation. From a diagnostic point of view, it needs to be emphasized that none of the techniques currently used to diagnose genetic changes—that is, cytogenetics, FISH, polymerase chain reaction (PCR), or Southern blot—can unambiguously rule out all *MYC* translocations. In particular, cryptic insertions of *IG* into the *MYC* locus and vice versa, as well as far 5′ and 3′ breaks, might escape detection. However, it is notable that, independent of being defined by gene expression or morphology, BL lacking *MYC* or 8q24 aberrations shows a completely different, significantly more complex pattern of chromosomal imbalances than *IG-MYC*–positive typical BL.[121,143] Moreover, the age distribution seems to be different. Therefore, the diagnosis of *IG-MYC* negative Burkitt's lymphoma deserves special attention, although it should be made only if all other features except the lack of *IG-MYC* support this diagnosis.

Is *MYC* Translocation Specific to Burkitt's Lymphoma?

Translocation of the *MYC* oncogene, although characteristic of BL, is by no means specific. As detailed in Figure 24-10, *MYC* rearrangements are found in a number of de novo lymphomas. Moreover, *MYC* translocation as a secondary cytogenetic event is well described in many hematopoietic neoplasms. *MYC* translocation occurs in approximately 5% to 8% of newly diagnosed cases of de novo DLBCL and, in the era of CHOP treatment, was associated with inferior survival.[47-49,51-53,90,143,149,150] Surrogate markers such as a proliferation rate in excess of 95% may not accurately define these cases. Moreover, there is an imperfect relationship between a classic BL immunophenotype (CD10$^+$, BCL6$^+$, BCL2$^-$) and the presence of a *MYC* translocation in DLBCL.

Genetic Changes in B-Cell Lymphoma, Unclassifiable, with Features Intermediate between Diffuse Large B-Cell Lymphoma and Burkitt's Lymphoma

The 2008 WHO classification introduced B-cell lymphoma, unclassifiable, with features intermediate between DLBCL and BL, based on recent gene expression (see later) and genetic data.[94] The morphologic features are discussed earlier. From a genetic point of view, these cases are a "wastebasket" of diagnostically difficult mature, aggressive B-cell lymphomas that may have arisen by the acquisition of a *MYC* translocation as a secondary event. Because this category is intended to be used for primary diagnosis, not for the diagnosis of relapsed lymphoma, this clonal progression occurred, by definition, in the preclinical phase. However, genetically similar tumors can also be identified at relapse of another B-cell lymphoma.

In childhood and young adulthood, these intermediate cases are infrequent in comparison to older age groups; one can speculate that they might represent lymphomas originating as BL but exhibiting overlapping features with DLBCL secondary to the acquisition of chromosomal complexity.[121,148] Alternatively, in older age groups, cases with these features most often arise in the setting of a prior DLBCL or follicular lymphoma by the acquisition of *MYC* translocations and other secondary genetic events.[28] Correspondingly, the pattern of genetic aberrations in the latter group reflects that of follicular lymphoma and DLBCL, with a considerable number of cases harboring *BCL6* or *BCL2* breaks.[121] The intermediate lymphomas are enriched for *MYC* translocations, which are present in approximately half the cases; non–*IG-MYC* fusions account for roughly half these breaks. Lymphomas with double hits accumulate in this group. Karyotypes have frequently been described as *MYC* complex, based on the presence of double hits, non–*IG* translocations, and *IG-MYC* fusions and multiple secondary changes. In this regard, it should be noted that the definition of *complexity* depends on the resolution of the technique applied, and a cutoff should not be fixed.[121]

Diagnostic and Clinical Implications of Genetic Changes in Burkitt's Lymphoma and Intermediate Lymphomas

Although the presence of *MYC* translocations or their molecular counterparts are the "gold standard" for the diagnosis of BL, these alterations are not sufficient for diagnosis.[17,120,121,151] These and other changes affecting the *MYC* gene at 8q24 can be observed in other neoplasms, including follicular lymphoma, mantle cell lymphoma, multiple myeloma, DLBCL, and others.[137,152,153] In these malignancies, t(8;14) and variants frequently constitute secondary changes, which may be associated with aggressive morphologic and clinical features.

For a confident diagnosis of BL, a Burkitt translocation should be sought. Conventional cytogenetic analysis using chromosomal banding techniques is considered the gold standard for the analysis of BL. Besides the detection of diagnostic translocations, cytogenetic analyses can identify variant *MYC* translocations involving non-*IG* loci, as well as other characteristic primary chromosomal aberrations that may indicate the aggressive transformation of a variety of underlying low-grade non-Hodgkin's lymphomas. Moreover, chromosomal banding analysis is the only technique that provides a complete genomic overview of balanced and unbalanced secondary changes (Table 24-4).[39]

Nevertheless, in the routine setting, viable cells are often not available for cytogenetic analyses, in part owing to a low mitotic index or poor-quality metaphase spreads. Molecular methods such as Southern blot or PCR-based approaches can detect Burkitt-associated *MYC* alterations, but these methods require fresh or cryopreserved material. In addition, because there may be scattered breakpoints over several hundred kilobases for both *MYC* and *IG* loci, multiple probes or sequence-specific primers must be applied, making Southern blot and PCR analysis time-consuming and expensive. Nevertheless, long-distance PCR techniques using various sets of primers can reliably detect *IG-MYC* junctions in classic and variant

Table 24-4 Secondary Cytogenetic Alterations in Lymphomas with t(8;14)*

Aberration	Frequency (%)
dup (1q)	17
+7	13
+12	7
del(6)(q)	7
+3	6

*The most frequent recurrent secondary chromosomal changes according to Boerma EG, Siebert R, Kluin PM, Baudis M. *Leukemia*. 2009 Feb;23(2):225-34. Epub 2008 Oct 16 and Cytogenic evolution patterns in non-Hodgkin's lymphoma. Johansson B, Mertens F, Mitelman F. *Blood*. 1995 Nov 15;86(10):3905-14.

Burkitt translocations, making them potentially applicable to the development of quantitative PCR assays using clone-specific primers for monitoring minimal residual disease.[83,154-156]

The most robust technique currently available for the routine detection of the Burkitt translocation is interphase FISH, which can be applied to virtually every type of tissue.[157,158] In principle, two different types of FISH assays have been developed for use in BL: break-apart assays and fusion assays. Break-apart assays use differently labeled probes on both sides of the typical breakpoint regions in the *MYC*, *IGH@*, *IGK*, or *IGL* loci.[159-165] In cases with an intact locus, both signals are colocalized. A breakpoint within the locus leads to dissociation of the double-colored signal pair (see Fig. 24-17). For diagnostic use, the proper location of the probes applied to the typical breakpoints has to be assured. To detect all breakpoints in the loci affected, the differently labeled probes have to be physically separated by up to 1 Mb or more.[121] This can cause considerable spatial separation of the signals derived from both probes, even in cells without a breakpoint. The signal distance depends on the condensation of the nucleus and the size of the probes. If control experiments take these features of the assay into account, break-apart FISH performed on cell suspensions from live cells can reliably detect as few as 5% clonal cells containing the chromosomal breakpoint.[158]

Confirmation of a Burkitt translocation and exclusion of other aberrations affecting *MYC* or *IG* loci have to be performed by fusion assays using differently labeled probes spanning the respective loci.[166] The most reliable assays use probes spanning the breakpoints of both affected loci (see Fig. 24-18). With these probes, which produce a double fusion on the der(8) and der(14), respectively, the false positive rate is less than 1%, at least in bone marrow and peripheral blood samples.

From a diagnostic standpoint, it is best to perform conventional cytogenetic studies whenever possible if a diagnosis of BL or an intermediate lymphoma is being considered. Interphase FISH can supplement conventional cytogenetics to resolve chromosomal aberrations. FISH should be restricted to cases in which no material for cytogenetics can be obtained, despite appropriate efforts to do so. Considering the problems of insertions of *MYC* into *IG* (and vice versa) and the wide spreading of breakpoints, an *IG-MYC* fusion can be excluded only if well-designed *IGH@-MYC, IGL-MYC,* and *IGK-MYC* fusion probes have been applied. If these translocations have been ruled out, non–*IG-MYC* breaks can be detected using one or several (depending on the spread between the breaks) *MYC* break-apart probes. Moreover, *IGH@-BCL2* fusions and

Pearls and Pitfalls

- Beware that slight nuclear irregularity and variation in cell size and shape may be due to fixation or processing artifacts and do not preclude a diagnosis of BL. B5 fixation tends to make cells appear smaller and more frequently results in the appearance of a single, central nucleolus.
- Focal, weak BCL2 protein expression may rarely be encountered in classic BL.
- Most dual-translocation cases have a lower proliferation rate (Ki-67) than classic BL cases.
- Have a low threshold for performing *MYC* FISH studies.
- Remember that variant *MYC* translocations may not be detected with Southern blot or PCR; standard cytogenetic analysis or locus-specific FISH studies are required.
- The most commonly encountered de novo lymphoma (outside of endemic BL areas) with *MYC* translocation is DLBCL.
- If a diagnosis of BL is being considered and the results of cytogenetic studies are available, they should show either a classic *MYC* translocation as defined by t(8;14) or a variant translocation. Beware of three-way translocations and cryptic translocations. If other criteria of classic BL are met but *MYC* FISH is negative, the case may still be classified as BL.
- The reverse is not true: *MYC* translocation is not specific for BL and may be seen in a variety of different lymphoma subtypes. Beware of cases with both *MYC* and *BCL2* translocations, which much more frequently harbor variant translocations, including non-*IG* partners, and strongly express BCL2 protein in most cases.
- Most dual-translocation lymphomas will default to the category of unclassifiable B-cell lymphoma with features intermediate between DLBCL and BL.
- *MYC* translocations are found in 5% to 8% of de novo DLBCLs and may not be adequately treated with R-CHOP.

References can be found on Expert Consult @ www.expertconsult.com

Chapter 25

Plasma Cell Neoplasms

Robert W. McKenna and Steven H. Kroft

CHAPTER OUTLINE

DEFINITION

The plasma cell neoplasms and related disorders, sometimes referred to as immunosecretory disorders, are clonal proliferations of immunoglobulin-producing plasma cells or lymphocytes that make and secrete a single class of immunoglobulin or a polypeptide subunit of a single immunoglobulin that is usually detectable as a monoclonal protein (M protein) on serum or urine protein electrophoresis. Immunosecretory disorders may consist exclusively of plasma cells (plasma cell neoplasms) or a mixture of plasma cells and lymphocytes. Those with a mixture of plasma cells and lymphocytes are generally categorized as lymphomas. Most plasma cell neoplasms originate as bone marrow tumors, but they occasionally present in extramedullary sites.

CLASSIFICATION

Box 25-1 lists the categories of plasma cell neoplasms included in the World Health Organization (WHO) classification of tumors of hematopoietic and lymphoid tissues.[1]

PLASMA CELL MYELOMA (MULTIPLE MYELOMA)

Definition

Plasma cell myeloma is a bone marrow–based, multifocal plasma cell neoplasm associated with an M protein in serum or urine.[1] The bone marrow is the site of origin of nearly all myelomas, and in most cases there is disseminated marrow

Box 25-1 *World Health Organization Classification of Plasma Cell Neoplasms*

- Monoclonal gammopathy of undetermined significance (MGUS)
- Plasma cell myeloma
  - Asymptomatic (smoldering) myeloma
  - Nonsecretory myeloma
  - Plasma cell leukemia
- Plasmacytoma
  - Solitary plasmacytoma of bone
  - Extraosseous (extramedullary) plasmacytoma
- Immunoglobulin deposition diseases
  - Primary amyloidosis
  - Systemic light- and heavy-chain deposition diseases
- Osteosclerotic myeloma (POEMS syndrome)

From McKenna RW, Kyle RA, Kuehl WM, et al. Plasma cell neoplasms. In: Swerdlow SH, Campo E, Harris NL, et al, eds. *WHO Classification of Tumours of Haematopoietic and Lymphoid Tissues*. Lyon, France: IARC; 2008:200-213.

involvement. Other organs may be secondarily involved. The diagnosis of myeloma is made by a combination of clinical, morphologic, immunologic, and radiographic information. The disease spans a clinical spectrum from asymptomatic to highly aggressive disease. In some myelomas, manifestations of the deposition of abnormal immunoglobulin chains in tissues are the major clinical findings.[1]

Diagnostic Criteria

The usual findings in plasma cell myeloma are increased and abnormal bone marrow plasma cells or a plasmacytoma, together with an M protein in serum or urine. Frequently, lytic bone lesions are present. The minimal percentage of plasma cells and quantity of M protein necessary for diagnosis vary somewhat in different diagnostic systems.[1-4] The diagnostic criteria for symptomatic plasma cell myeloma adopted in the WHO classification are listed in Box 25-2.[1,5]

Epidemiology

Plasma cell myeloma (and its variants) is the predominant type of malignant immunosecretory disorder. Its incidence is approximately 4 cases per 100,000 persons per year in the United States.[6] Myeloma accounts for about 1% of malignant tumors and 10% to 15% of hematopoietic neoplasms.[7,8] It is more common in men than in women (1.4:1) and occurs twice as frequently in African Americans as in whites.[6] The risk of plasma cell myeloma is 3.7-fold higher for individuals with a first-degree relative with the disease.[9] Myeloma is not found in children and is rare in adults younger than 35 years; the incidence increases progressively after age 35, with approximately 90% of cases occurring in individuals older than 50 years. The median age at diagnosis is about 68 years.[10] In the past half century there has been a significant increase in the incidence of myeloma.[10] The reasons for this are uncertain, but the increased proportion of older individuals in the population and improved recognition and case reporting probably contribute to the higher incidence.

Box 25-2 *Diagnostic Criteria for Symptomatic Plasma Cell Myeloma*

- M protein in serum or urine*
- Bone marrow clonal plasma cells or plasmacytoma†
- Related organ or tissue impairment‡

*No minimal level of M protein is included in the criteria, but in most cases it is >30 g/L of IgG, >25 g/L of IgA, or >1 g/24 hours of urine light chain. However, some patients with symptomatic myeloma have lower levels.
†Monoclonal plasma cells usually exceed 10% of nucleated cells in the marrow; however, no minimal level is designated because about 5% of patients with symptomatic myeloma have <10% marrow plasma cells.
‡The most important evidence of related end-organ damage is a manifestation of one or more of the following: hypercalcemia, renal insufficiency, anemia, bone lesions (CRAB).
From International Myeloma Working Group. Criteria for the classification of monoclonal gammopathies, multiple myeloma and related disorders: a report of the International Myeloma Working Group. *Br J Haematol*. 2003;121:749-757.

Clinical Features

The most frequent symptom at presentation is bone pain in the back or extremities due to lytic lesions or osteoporosis. In advanced cases, vertebral collapse may cause loss of height. Weakness and tiredness, often related to anemia, are common complaints. Some patients present with infections, bleeding, or symptoms related to renal failure or hypercalcemia. Rarely, neurologic manifestations due to spinal cord compression or peripheral neuropathy lead a patient to seek medical attention. In asymptomatic individuals, the diagnosis of plasma cell myeloma occasionally follows the discovery of a serum M protein on protein electrophoresis. Physical findings are often nonspecific or lacking. Pallor is most common, followed by organomegaly. Palpable plasmacytomas are rare, but tenderness and swelling over the site of a pathologic fracture or plasmacytoma may be encountered. Tissue masses and organomegaly due to plasma cell infiltration or amyloidosis are found in a few patients. Skin lesions due to plasma cell infiltrates or purpura are observed in rare cases.

Laboratory Findings

Box 25-3 lists the diagnostic studies recommended by the International Myeloma Working Group for the assessment of patients suspected of having plasma cell myeloma.[5] The data obtained from these studies are the basis for clinicopathologic diagnostic criteria and provide important prognostic information.[1-5]

Assessment of the serum and urine for M protein is an essential component of the evaluation for suspected plasma cell myeloma. Agarose gel electrophoresis is the preferred method to screen for M proteins.[5] An M protein is found on serum protein electrophoresis in most patients with myeloma (Fig. 25-1). The total immunoglobulin is usually increased due to the M protein, but normal polyclonal immunoglobulins are commonly decreased. With serum protein electrophoresis, M protein may be undetectable in cases with low levels of monoclonal immunoglobulin (Ig), as commonly seen in IgD, IgE, and light-chain myeloma; hypogammaglobulinemia due to decreased normal polyclonal immunoglobulins may be the only abnormal finding. Urine protein electrophoresis on a concentrated urine specimen and immunoglobulin quantitation on a 24-hour urine collection should be performed in all cases of suspected myeloma (Fig. 25-2). Monoclonal light chains (Bence Jones protein) are found in some patients

Box 25-3 *Diagnostic Studies for Plasma Cell Myeloma*

- History and physical examination
- Complete blood count and leukocyte differential
- Peripheral blood smear examination
- Chemistry screen, including calcium and creatinine
- Serum protein electrophoresis and immunofixation
- Nephelometric quantification of immunoglobulins
- Urinalysis
- 24-hour urine collection for electrophoresis and immunofixation
- Bone marrow aspirate and trephine biopsy
  - Cytogenetics
  - Immunophenotyping
  - Plasma cell labeling index
- Radiographic skeletal bone survey (spine, pelvis, skull, humeri, femora)
- β_2-microglobulin, C-reactive protein, lactate dehydrogenase
- Measurement of free light chains

From International Myeloma Working Group. Criteria for the classification of monoclonal gammopathies, multiple myeloma and related disorders: a report of the International Myeloma Working Group. *Br J Haematol.* 2003;121:749-757.

without a serum M protein. Serum and urine immunofixation electrophoresis is the "gold standard" for characterizing heavy and light chains and for detecting small quantities of M protein, as may be seen in patients with light-chain amyloidosis, plasmacytoma, heavy-chain disease, and light-chain deposition disease and following treatment of myeloma (see Figs. 25-1 and 25-2). Immunofixation is capable of detecting an M protein level of 0.02 g/dL in serum and 0.004 g/dL in urine.[5] With immunofixation electrophoresis, an M protein is identified in the serum or urine in about 97% of myelomas.[5,8] Monoclonal light chains are found in the urine in approximately 75% of cases; in nearly two thirds of them, the light chains are kappa. A patient may have a negative urine electrophoresis when immunofixation of a concentrated urine specimen identifies a monoclonal light chain.[5] Light chains are reabsorbed by proximal renal tubules. Therefore, renal function plays a role in determining whether light chain is detectable in urine. Serum free-light-chain analysis provides a more sensitive method of detecting and monitoring light-chain disease and nonsecretory myeloma, as well as many cases of amyloidosis and solitary plasmacytoma.[5,11,12]

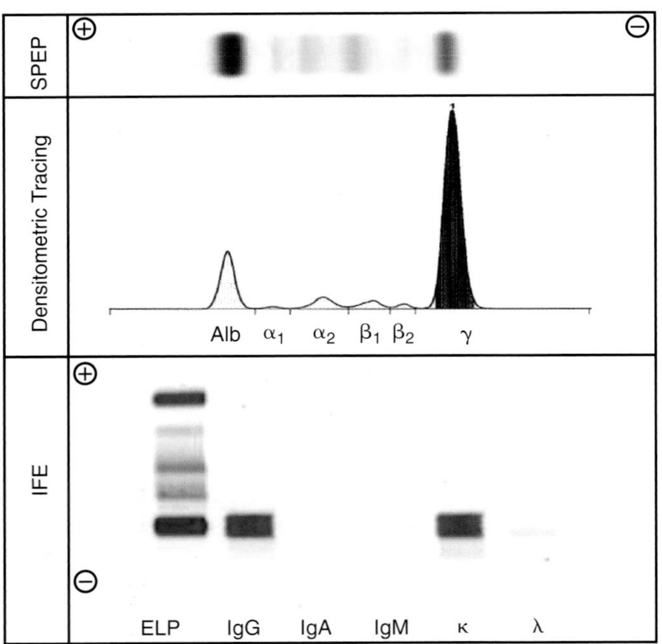

Figure 25-1. Serum electrophoresis from a 65-year-old man with plasma cell myeloma. There is a single large (8.1 g/dL) M protein peak on the densitometric tracing (*shaded area, middle panel*) on the serum protein electrophoresis pattern (SPEP). The M protein was identified by immunofixation electrophoresis (IFE) as IgGκ, located in the γ region of the electrophoresis (ELP) pattern. There were only 5% plasma cells in the marrow aspirate, but lytic bone lesions were present. The patient had a hyperviscosity syndrome, and his myeloma was refractory to therapy. (Courtesy of Drs. Frank H. Wians Jr. and Dennis C. Wooten, Department of Pathology, University of Texas Southwestern Medical Center, Dallas.)

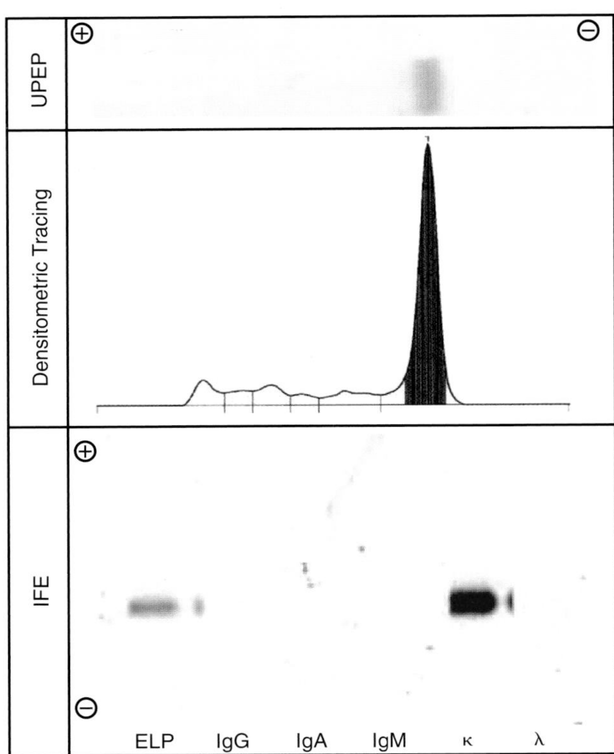

Figure 25-2. Urine electrophoresis from a 54-year-old man with light-chain-only plasma cell myeloma. The patient presented with right hip pain and a previously diagnosed lung plasmacytoma. Radiographic imaging revealed a right pubic ramus fracture and a lytic lesion. There was no M protein identified on serum protein electrophoresis. The patient's urine protein electrophoresis pattern (UPEP), using a sample (concentrated 100×) from his 24-hour urine specimen (total protein, 217 mg/24 hours), demonstrates a single M protein peak (140 mg/24 hours) on the densitometric tracing (*shaded area, middle panel*) in the γ region of the gel. The M protein was identified by immunofixation electrophoresis (IFE) as free kappa light chains. (Courtesy of Drs. Frank H. Wians Jr. and Dennis C. Wooten, Department of Pathology, University of Texas Southwestern Medical Center, Dallas.)

An IgG M protein is found in slightly more than half of patients with myeloma; about 20% have IgA, and only monoclonal light chains are found in almost 20%.[5] IgD, IgE, IgM, and biclonal myeloma, all of which are rare, constitute the remainder of M proteins; less than 3% of patients have non-

Table 25-1 **Monoclonal Immunoglobulins in Plasma Cell Myeloma**

Monoclonal Immunoglobulin	Approximate % of Cases
IgG	55
IgA	22
Light chain only	18
IgD	2
Biclonal	2
Nonsecretory	2
IgE	1
IgM	1

secretory myelomas. The average frequencies of the various M proteins in several large series of myeloma patients are shown in Table 25-1.[13-15] Kappa light chain is more common than lambda for all immunoglobulin types of myeloma except IgD. The quantity of serum M protein varies from undetectable to more than 10 g/dL. The median is approximately 5 g/dL for IgG myeloma and 3.5 g/dL for IgA. Approximately 40% of patients with symptomatic myeloma have an M protein level less than 3 g/dL.[5] In cases of light-chain myeloma, the serum M protein is very low or undetectable; the 24-hour urine protein may be mildly to markedly increased.

Anemia is present in about two thirds of patients at diagnosis.[5,13] Red cell indices are usually normocytic and normochromic. Leukopenia and thrombocytopenia are found in less than 20% of patients but frequently evolve as the disease progresses.[13] Patients occasionally present with leukocytosis or thrombocytosis. The erythrocyte sedimentation rate is variably increased and roughly related to the level of M protein.

Hypercalcemia is present in nearly one fifth of patients, and creatinine is elevated in one fifth to one third.[5,16] Hyperuricemia is found in more than half of patients.[13] Hypoalbuminemia is observed in patients with advanced disease.[2]

Radiographic Studies

Radiographic skeletal surveys reveal lytic lesions, osteoporosis, or fractures in 70% to 85% of myeloma patients at diagnosis.[5,13,16,17] In some cases all these changes are observed. The vertebra, pelvis, skull, rib, femur, and proximal humerus are most often affected. Computed tomography scans and, particularly, magnetic resonance imaging (MRI) are more sensitive than plain radiographs for detecting small bone lesions and extramedullary plasma cell infiltrates.[16,18] MRI findings may have prognostic significance in patients with myeloma; those with normal or only focal abnormalities on thoracolumbar MRI have a better treatment response and survival.[19]

Blood Smear and Bone Marrow Findings

Rouleaux formation is usually the most striking feature on blood smears and is related to the quantity and type of M protein (Fig. 25-3). The blood smear may show a faint purple background when the level of M protein is markedly elevated. Circulating nucleated red cells or a frank leukoerythroblastic reaction may be observed in some cases. Plasma cells are found on blood smears in approximately 15% of cases, usually in small numbers. They are more commonly observed in advanced stages of disease. Marked plasmacytosis is present in plasma cell leukemia, which is discussed later with the plasma cell myeloma variants.

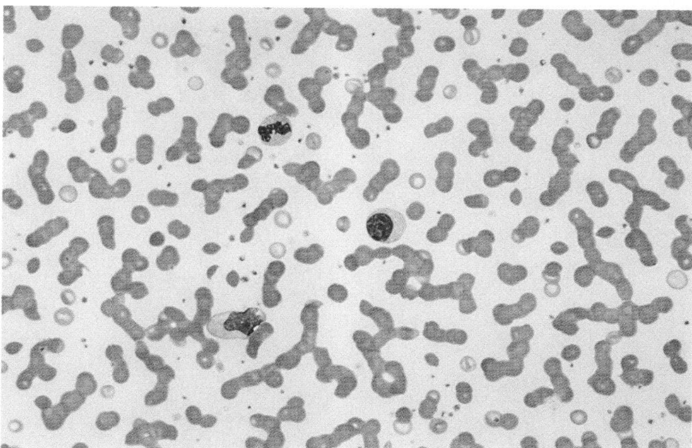

Figure 25-3. Increased rouleaux formation is seen in this blood smear from a patient with a large M protein. Marked rouleaux formation is often a clue to the diagnosis of a plasma cell neoplasm, but may also be observed in other conditions (Wright-Giemsa stain).

The bone marrow examination is the most important element of the diagnosis of plasma cell myeloma. A bone marrow examination is nearly always required to confirm the diagnosis of myeloma, even when there is substantial clinical, laboratory, and radiographic evidence. The bone marrow study also provides prognostic information and is useful to follow patients' response to therapy and to identify recurrent disease. The marrow is the major source of tissue for special studies such as immunophenotyping, cytogenetics, and thymidine labeling indices. In many cases the diagnosis can be made from the marrow examination alone.[20] Criteria for the morphologic diagnosis of myeloma are shown in Box 25-4.

Both aspirate smears and trephine biopsy sections are required for optimal evaluation. They are independently diagnostic in most cases, but in some patients a combination of findings in the two preparations leads to the diagnosis. The average number of plasma cells in the aspirate smears is 20% to 36% (Fig. 25-4).[13,15] In about 5% of cases of symptomatic myeloma, the plasma cells number less than 10%.[5,15] This may be owing to a suboptimal marrow aspirate or to the frequently focal nature of lesions and the uneven distribution of myeloma in the marrow. The neoplastic plasma cells vary from normal appearing with mature features to blast-like cells barely recognizable as plasma cells. The atypical features that characterize many cases of myeloma encompass changes in both the

Box 25-4 *Criteria for the Morphologic Diagnosis of Myeloma*

Findings on Random Bone Marrow Biopsy

- Atypical plasma cells with morphologic appearance outside the range of a reactive process
- Infiltrative sheets of plasma cells on sections
- Nearly 100% plasma cells on a hypercellular aspirate or section
- Less useful criteria include multinucleation of plasma cells and lack of predilection for vascular structures

From Dick FR. Plasma cell myeloma and related disorders with monoclonal gammopathy. In: Koepke JA, ed. *Laboratory Hematology.* New York: Churchill-Livingstone; 1984:445-481.

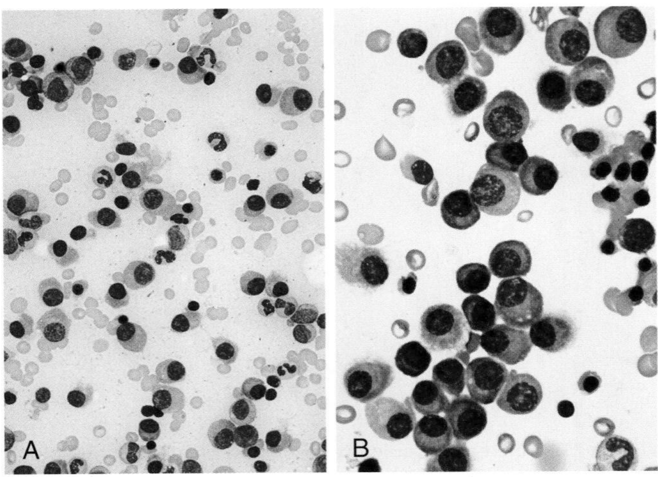

Figure 25-4. Bone marrow aspirate smears from two patients with plasma cell myeloma are heavily infiltrated with moderately atypical plasma cells. One marrow smear **(A)** contains 30% plasma cells, and the other **(B)** more than 50%. In both cases the diagnosis of myeloma can be made on the basis of extensive marrow plasmacytosis. Both patients had an IgGκ serum M protein greater than 3.5 g/dL (Wright-Giemsa stain).

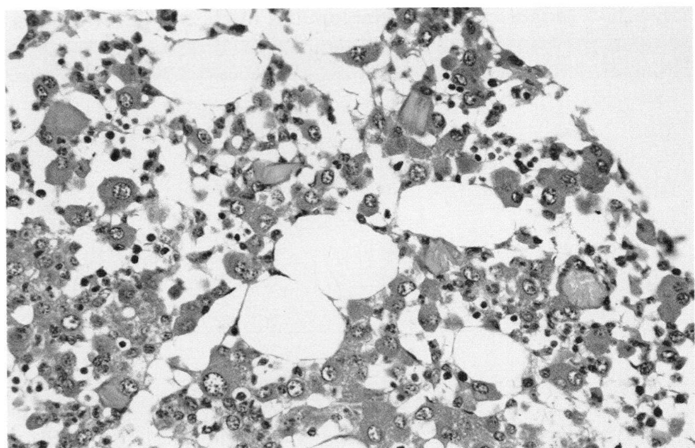

Figure 25-6. Bone marrow biopsy section from a patient with plasma cell myeloma. Many of the plasma cells contain cytoplasmic crystalline inclusions.

nucleus and the cytoplasm. The myeloma cells are often larger than normal plasma cells but may be normal sized or small. Moderate to abundant basophilic cytoplasm is usual. An array of cytoplasmic changes is observed, including fraying and shedding of the cytoplasmic edges, vacuoles, granules, and cytoplasmic inclusions. The nucleus is larger than normal in most cases, and the chromatin is less condensed; nucleoli are variably prominent.

Various types of cytoplasmic and nuclear inclusions are observed in myeloma cells and may distort the cytoplasm. Cytoplasmic crystals are found occasionally in myeloma and are a common finding in adult Fanconi syndrome (Figs. 25-5 and 25-6).[21] Except in adult Fanconi syndrome, in which the light-chain type is invariably kappa, crystals have no obvious relationship to the immunologic type of myeloma.

Multiple dark-staining cytoplasmic inclusions are observed in rare cases of myeloma (Fig. 25-7). These are often associated with large pleomorphic plasma cells. Multiple small, Russell body–type, hyaline intracytoplasmic and intranuclear inclusions are relatively common (Fig. 25-8). In contrast to hyaline intranuclear inclusions, Dutcher-type nuclear inclusions are pale staining, single, and generally large (Fig. 25-9). In some cases cytoplasmic inclusions resemble the Buhot plasma cell structures found in patients with mucopolysaccharidosis. Phagocytic plasma cells are observed in a minority of cases of myeloma; rarely, erythrophagocytosis is striking.[22]

Approximately 2% of myelomas are distinguished by marked nuclear lobation and convolution.[15,23] In some cases these cells are mixed with other easily recognizable plasma cells, but in others they constitute a relatively uniform population and may be difficult to recognize as myeloma cells (Fig. 25-10). Small plasma cells predominate in some myelomas, and in approximately 5% of cases the plasma cells have a distinctly lymphoid appearance (Fig. 25-11). In one study 20% of the cases with lymphoid morphology were IgD myelomas.[15] Overall, attempts to relate morphologic characteristics to monoclonal immunoglobulin type have failed, except for a small number of cases of IgA myeloma with markedly pleomorphic, large, multinucleate plasma cells; flaming plasma

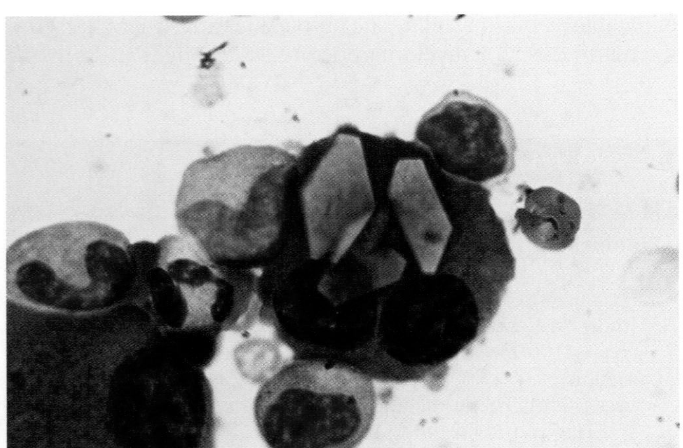

Figure 25-5. Bone marrow aspirate smear from a 68-year-old man with IgG myeloma shows a large binucleate plasma cell containing large cytoplasmic crystals (Wright-Giemsa stain).

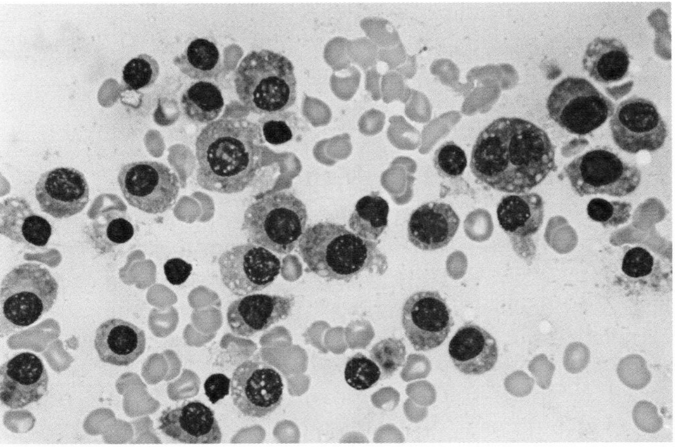

Figure 25-7. Cytoplasm of neoplastic plasma cells contains numerous irregular, variably eosinophilic inclusions (Wright-Giemsa stain).

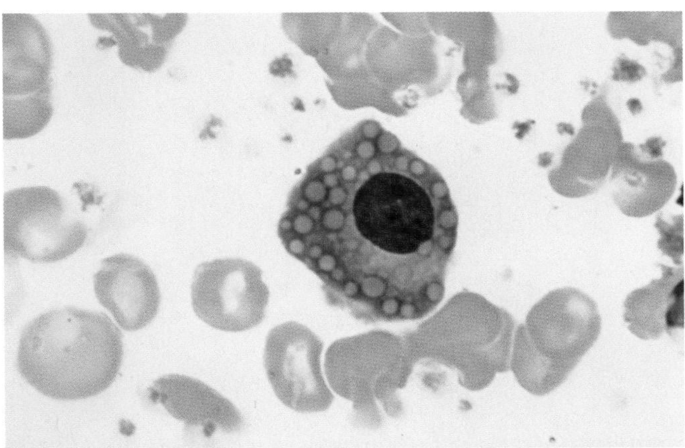

Figure 25-8. Plasma cell with multiple cytoplasmic hyaline inclusions (Russell bodies) in a bone marrow aspirate from a patient with plasma cell myeloma (Wright-Giemsa stain).

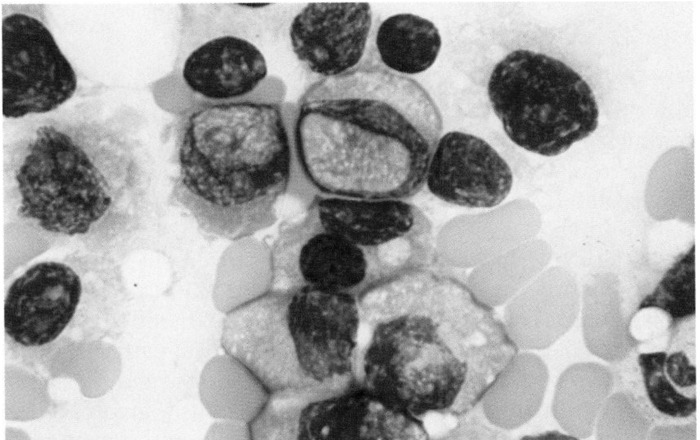

Figure 25-9. Bone marrow smear from a patient with IgA myeloma. Large nuclear inclusions (Dutcher bodies) are present in two of the plasma cells (Wright-Giemsa stain).

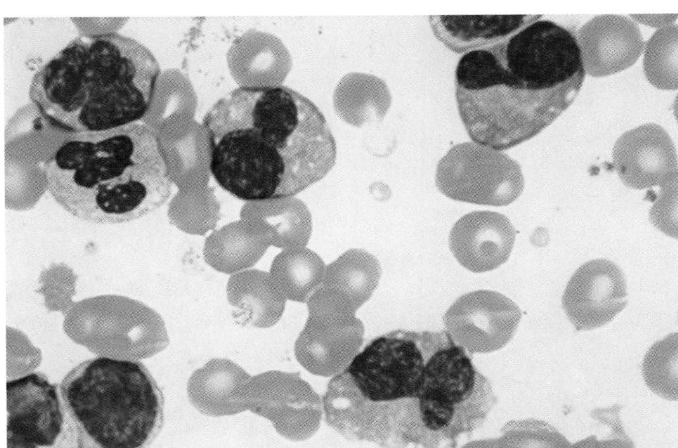

Figure 25-10. Bone marrow smear from a patient with light-chain-only myeloma. The nuclei of the plasma cells show striking irregularity and convolution. Most of the plasma cells in this case manifested these lobulated or monocytoid-type nuclei. The neoplastic cells in myelomas of this type may be difficult to recognize as plasma cells (Wright-Giemsa stain).

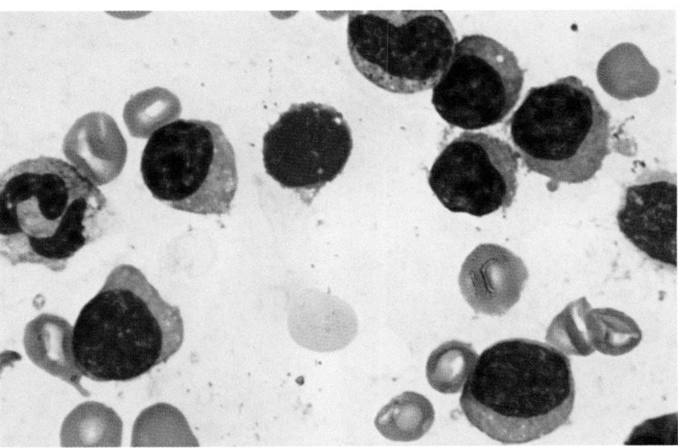

Figure 25-11. Lymphoid-appearing myeloma. Marrow aspirate smear from a 72-year-old man with lytic bone lesions and a seurm IgGλ M protein of 3.2 g/dL. The myeloma plasma cells have cytologic features in common with plasmacytoid lymphocytes (Wright-Giemsa stain). Often, myelomas with this type of morphology express CD20 and *cyclin D1*, and have a t(11;14)(q13;q32).

cells; and cells with pale, frayed, and fragmented cytoplasm (Fig. 25-12). Intranuclear inclusions are found in about 20% of cases of IgA myeloma, much more frequently than in the other immunologic types (see Fig. 25-9).[15]

Based on their cytologic features, myelomas have been classified as mature, intermediate, immature, and plasmablastic (Figs. 25-13 to 25-16).[24] Patients with plasmablastic myeloma have a median survival of 10 months, compared with 35 months for the other types. There appears to be no significant difference in survival among the other three types. Other classifications have been proposed that include three to six cytologic types.[25,26]

Histopathology

The diagnostic yield of trephine biopsies is often directly related to the size and number of specimens. Focal lesions

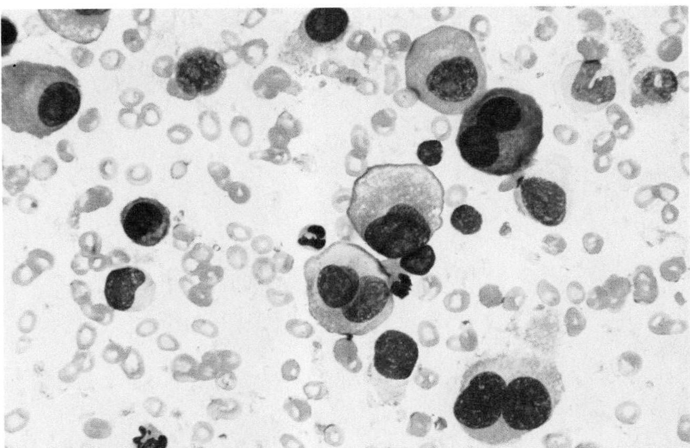

Figure 25-12. IgA myeloma. Bone marrow aspirate smear heavily replaced by large pleomorphic plasma cells. Most have a relatively low nuclear-to-cytoplasmic ratio and abundant light blue cytoplasm. Several large double-nucleated plasma cells are present. One plasma cell has a red cytoplasmic margin, and another has light pink cytoplasm. The patient had a large IgA serum M protein (Wright-Giemsa).

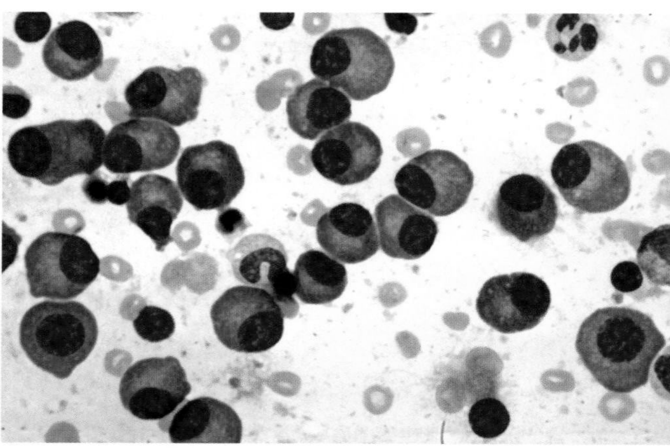

Figure 25-13. Mature-type myeloma. Bone marrow aspirate smear from a 58-year-old woman with extensive marrow replacement with plasma cell myeloma. The plasma cells have cytologic features approximating those of mature plasma cells (Wright-Giemsa stain). (Courtesy of Dr. Patrick C. J. Ward, Department of Pathology, University of Minnesota, Duluth.)

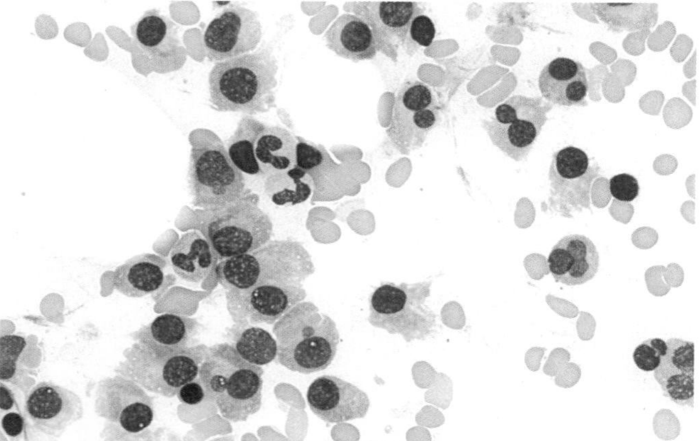

Figure 25-14. Intermediate-type myeloma. Marrow smear from a patient with extensive involvement with myeloma. The plasma cells exhibit features intermediate between mature and immature types of myeloma. They have moderately dispersed chromatin and occasional small nucleoli; several have lobated nuclei, and two are binucleate (Wright-Giemsa stain).

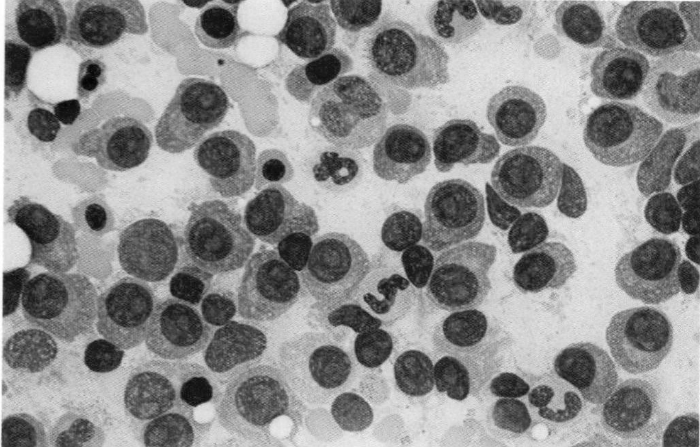

Figure 25-15. Immature-type myeloma. The plasma cells in this marrow smear are immature. They have prominent nucleoli and less dense chromatin than those in Figure 25-13. The marrow is extensively replaced with myeloma. A marrow biopsy section from this patient is illustrated in Figure 25-20 (Wright-Giemsa stain).

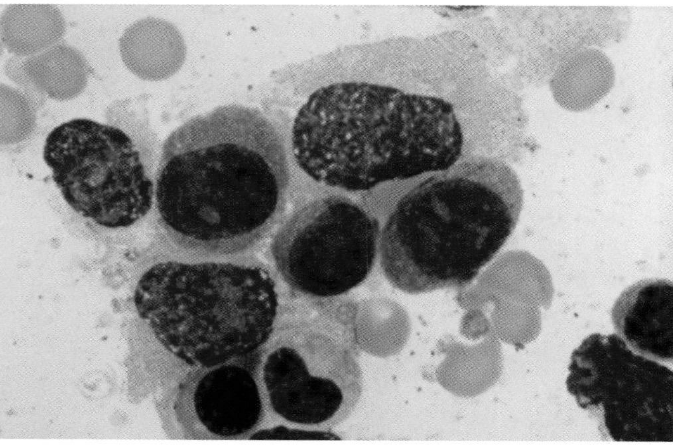

Figure 25-16. Plasmablastic myeloma. Marrow aspirate smear from a patient with plasma cell myeloma shows atypical plasma cells with a high nuclear-to-cytoplasmic ratio. The nuclei have dispersed chromatin and contain small nucleoli. The plasma cells show features of an immature- to plasmablastic-type myeloma. A marrow biopsy section from this patient is illustrated in Figure 25-21 (Wright-Giemsa stain).

may be irregularly distributed and widely spaced. Occasionally only one or two small myeloma lesions are found in a trephine biopsy, with no evidence of a plasma cell infiltrate in the remainder of the section or in specimens from the contralateral posterior iliac spine. The pattern of the plasma cell infiltrate may be interstitial, focal, or diffuse (Figs. 25-17 to 25-19).[15,25] The extent of marrow involvement varies from an apparently small increase in plasma cells to complete replacement. The pattern of involvement is directly related to the extent of disease. With interstitial and focal patterns, there is generally considerable sparing of the marrow and preservation of normal hematopoiesis. With diffuse involvement, expansive areas of the marrow are replaced, and hematopoiesis may be markedly suppressed. There is typically a progression from interstitial and focal disease in early myeloma to diffuse involvement in advanced stages of the disease.[25]

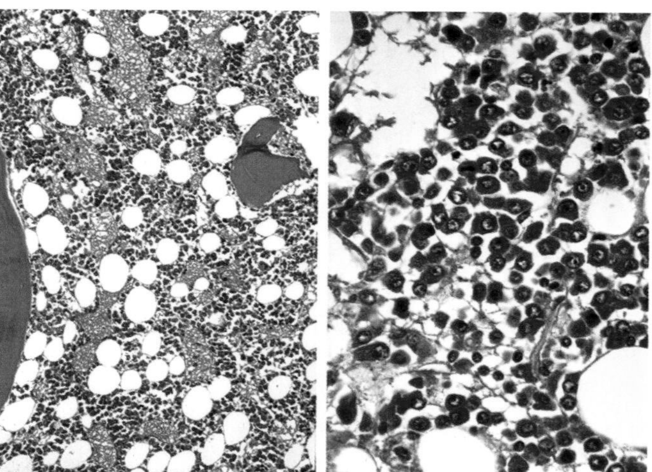

Figure 25-17. Bone marrow trephine biopsy section from an elderly man with myeloma shows an interstitial pattern of bone marrow involvement (*left*). The overall marrow architecture is preserved, but normal hematopoiesis is decreased. The higher magnification (*right*) shows plasma cells in clusters.

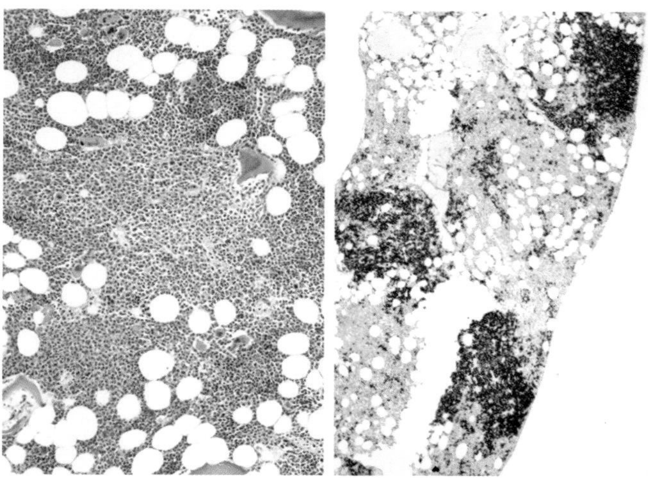

Figure 25-18. Focal plasma cell myeloma lesions are scattered throughout the marrow, with mostly normal hematopoietic tissue between lesions (*left*; hematoxylin-eosin). An immunostain for lambda light chain more clearly illustrates the predominantly focal pattern (*right*).

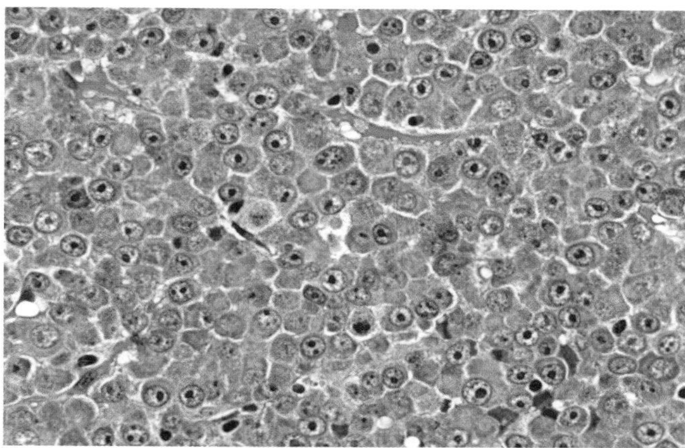

Figure 25-20. Immature-type plasma cell myeloma. High magnification of a section of bone marrow from a patient with myeloma shows large vesicular nuclei, large eosinophilic nucleoli, and a moderate amount of eosinophilic cytoplasm. (A marrow aspirate smear from this patient is illustrated in Figure 25-15.)

A staging system has been proposed based on the percentage of marrow space replaced by myeloma in marrow trephine biopsies.[25,27] In stage I, less than 20% of the marrow is replaced; in stage II, 20% to 50%; and in stage III, more than 50%. The extent of involvement in biopsy sections usually reflects the overall tumor burden. There appears to be good correlation among histologic stage, clinical stage, and prognosis.[25]

Myelomas with atypical plasma cell morphology may be difficult to recognize in trephine biopsies (Figs. 25-20 to 25-22). Plasmablastic myeloma and cases with lymphoid-appearing plasma cells, plasma cells with lobulated nuclei, or markedly pleomorphic plasma cells are particularly problematic. Cytologic examination of the cells in aspirate smears is often essential for diagnosis in these cases. Occasionally, cytoplasmic inclusions in the myeloma cells are the most striking feature of the bone marrow section. The inclusions are often found in large plasma cells that are distorted by crystalline or globular material. The globular inclusions may be strongly positive with periodic acid–Schiff stain.

In approximately 9% of myelomas, the bone marrow lesions show reticulin or collagen fibrosis.[15,28] In many of these cases, the fibrosis is extensive. A disproportionate number of fibrotic myelomas produce monoclonal light chains only.[28] Coarse fibrosis has been correlated with diffuse marrow involvement and aggressive disease.[25]

Clinical Variants

The three variants of plasma cell myeloma recognized in the WHO classification have clinical or biologic characteristics

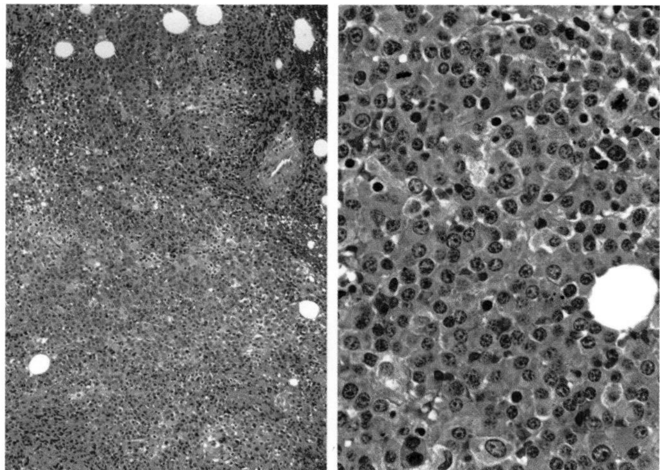

Figure 25-19. Bone marrow biopsy from a patient with advanced plasma cell myeloma. There is diffuse and extensive marrow involvement and no identifiable normal hematopoiesis in this section. The myeloma cells have mature- to intermediate-type cytologic features. (Courtesy of Dr. Patrick C. J. Ward, Department of Pathology, University of Minnesota, Duluth.)

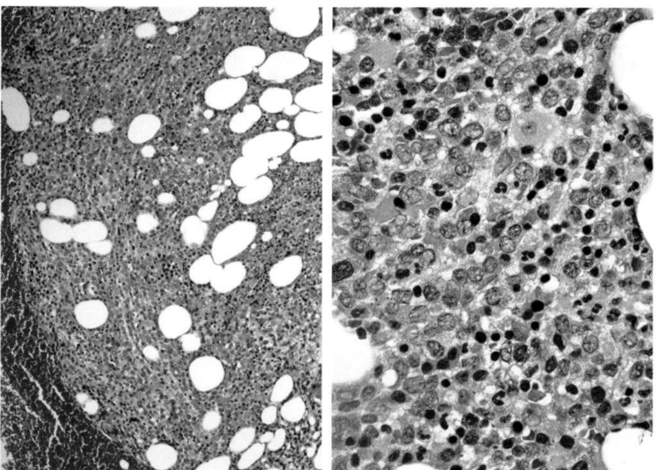

Figure 25-21. Plasmablastic-type plasma cell myeloma. There is heavy interstitial involvement with myeloma. The neoplastic plasma cells are poorly differentiated, with a high nuclear-to-cytoplasmic ratio and dispersed chromatin; some contain a small nucleolus. Their cytologic features resemble blasts or possibly a small blue cell tumor. (A marrow aspirate smear from this patient is illustrated in Figure 25-16.) (Courtesy of Dr. Patrick C. J. Ward, Department of Pathology, University of Minnesota, Duluth.)

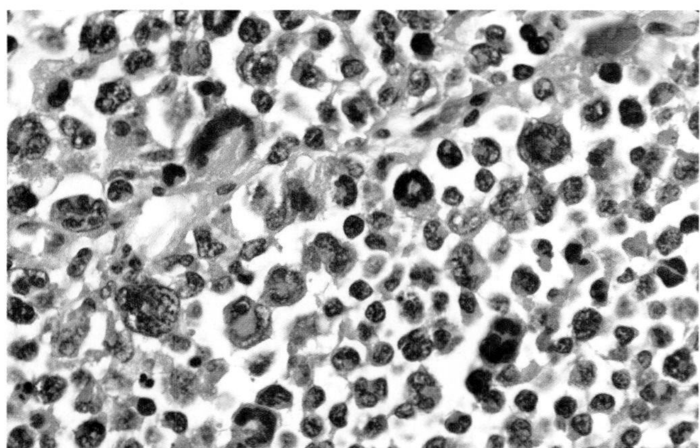

Figure 25-22. Trephine biopsy section from a patient with a poorly differentiated polymorphic (anaplastic) plasma cell myeloma. There is little cytologic evidence of myeloma in this field. The cells stained positively for CD138 and exhibited kappa light-chain restriction by immunohistochemical staining. There was a 6.5 g/dL IgG serum M protein. This type of myeloma must be differentiated from a polymorphic lymphoma and from metastatic tumors such as anaplastic carcinoma and malignant melanoma. (Courtesy of Dr. Patrick C. J. Ward, Department of Pathology, University of Minnesota, Duluth.)

that differ from those of typical plasma cell myeloma. They are nonsecretory myeloma, asymptomatic (smoldering) myeloma, and plasma cell leukemia.

Nonsecretory Plasma Cell Myeloma

Nonsecretory myeloma accounts for about 3% of plasma cell myelomas.[1,5] In these rare cases the neoplastic plasma cells appear to lack the capacity to secrete immunoglobulin, and there is no M protein in either the serum or the urine by immunofixation analysis.[29-31] In about two thirds of these patients, however, elevated serum free light chains or an abnormal free-light-chain ratio is detectable.[11] Monoclonal light chains are demonstrated in the cytoplasm of the myeloma cells in about 85% of cases by immunohistochemical staining. In 15% no staining is detected, suggesting that immunoglobulin is not produced (nonproducer myeloma).[5] The cytologic and histologic features, immunophenotype, and genetics of nonsecretory myeloma appear to be similar to those of other myelomas. The clinical features of nonsecretory myeloma are also generally similar to those of other plasma cell myelomas, except for a lower incidence of renal insufficiency and hypercalcemia and less depression of normal polyclonal immunoglobulin. Treatment, response to therapy, and survival appear to be similar as well.[5]

Asymptomatic Plasma Cell Myeloma (Smoldering Myeloma)

Patients with asymptomatic plasma cell myeloma manifest the diagnostic criteria for myeloma, except there is no related end-organ damage or tissue impairment (Box 25-5).[1,5] There is often no disease progression for prolonged periods without therapeutic intervention.[1,32-35] Patients with Durie-Salmon stage I disease are included in this category; in some series, so are those with asymptomatic solitary plasmacytoma of bone in which only MRI reveals additional abnormalities.[1,2,5,35] About 8% of patients with plasma cell myeloma are initially asymptomatic, and the incidence of asymptomatic myeloma seems to have increased in recent years.[32,35] Patients with asymptomatic plasma cell myeloma must be followed closely, because most eventually become symptomatic.

The median level of serum M protein in patients with asymptomatic plasma cell myeloma is about 30 g/L; the majority have between 10% and 20% bone marrow plasma cells. Approximately 50% of patients have monoclonal light chains in urine, and polyclonal immunoglobulins are decreased in more than 80%.[32] Plasma cells are cytologically atypical in marrow aspirate smears, and focal aggregates of plasma cells or interstitial infiltration, or both, are found in trephine biopsy sections.[33] The immunophenotype and genetics appear to be similar to those of other myelomas.

Asymptomatic myeloma behaves clinically like monoclonal gammopathy of undetermined significance (MGUS), but it is much more likely to progress to symptomatic myeloma.[7,32,35] The cumulative probability of progression to symptomatic myeloma or amyloidosis is 73% at 15 years, with a median time to progression of 4.8 years.[32] Patients with greater than 10% plasma cells and greater than 30 g/L of M protein have the highest rate of progression to symptomatic myeloma.[1,32] Median survival after the development of symptomatic myeloma is about 3.5 years. There is no apparent advantage in terms of response rate or survival for asymptomatic patients treated before progression to symptomatic myeloma.[35]

Plasma Cell Leukemia

Plasma cell leukemia (PCL) is a myeloma in which the number of neoplastic plasma cells in the blood is greater than 20% of the total leukocytes, or the absolute plasma cell count exceeds 2.0×10^9/L.[1,36-39] PCL may be primary, present at the time of initial diagnosis, or secondary, evolving during the course of disease in a patient with previously diagnosed myeloma; approximately 60% of cases are primary.[37-40] Primary PCL is found in approximately 2% to 5% of cases of myeloma.[1,36-39,41]

Most of the usual clinical and laboratory abnormalities associated with other myelomas are found in patients with PCL, but there are several features that distinguish it. The median age at diagnosis is younger in patients with PCL; lymphadenopathy, organomegaly, and renal failure are significantly more common; and lytic bone lesions and bone pain are less common.[37] Anemia is present in 80% of cases of PCL, and thrombocytopenia in 50%.[38,39] Nucleated red cells are frequently observed in blood smears. The total leukocyte count may be in the normal range but is usually elevated and may be as high as 100×10^9/L.

Box 25-5 *Diagnostic Criteria for Asymptomatic (Smoldering) Myeloma*

- M protein in serum at myeloma levels (≥30 g/L)

and/or

- 10% or more clonal plasma cells in bone marrow
- No related organ or tissue impairment (end-organ damage or bone lesions) or myeloma-related symptoms

From International Myeloma Working Group. Criteria for the classification of monoclonal gammopathies, multiple myeloma and related disorders: a report of the International Myeloma Working Group. *Br J Haematol.* 2003;121:749-757.

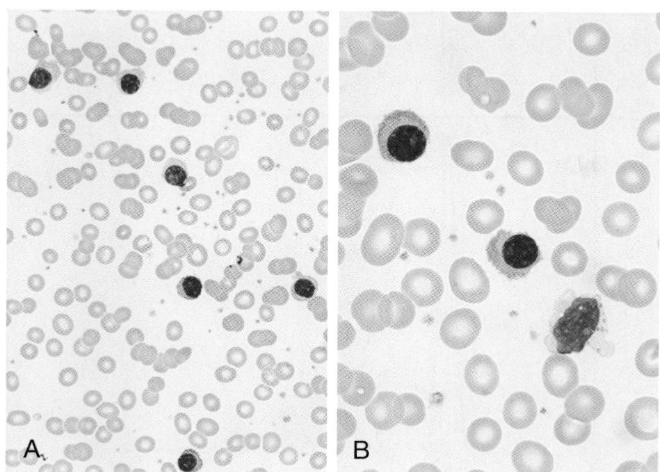

Figure 25-23. A, Blood smear from a 68-year-old man with plasma cell leukemia. The total blood leukocyte count is mildly elevated. There are 50% plasma cells, most of which are small and difficult to distinguish from plasmacytoid lymphocytes. The marrow is diffusely replaced. The M protein in this case is kappa light chain only. **B,** Higher magnification of the same blood smear shows two small plasma cells and a large granular lymphocyte (Wright-Giemsa stain).

The cytologic characteristics of the leukemic plasma cells span most of the morphologic spectrum found in other myelomas, but large and pleomorphic plasma cells are unusual. The leukemic cells vary from normal appearing to some that are barely recognizable as plasma cells. Often, many of the plasma cells are smaller than usual, with relatively little cytoplasm, and they may resemble plasmacytoid lymphocytes (Fig. 25-23).[15] Cases with these features may be difficult to distinguish from lymphoplasmacytic lymphoma on blood smear examination. The immunophenotype of the neoplastic cells in most cases of PCL differs from that of other plasma cell myelomas by the lack of CD56 expression (Fig. 25-24; see the section on immunophenotype). Monoclonal immunoglobulins of all types have been reported in PCL. However, higher proportions of light-chain-only, IgE, and IgD myelomas present as PCL compared with IgG or IgA myelomas; PCL is found in approximately 20% of cases of the rare IgE myeloma.[36,38,42] An abnormal karyotype is more frequently found in PCL than in other myelomas, and there is a higher incidence of unfavorable cytogenetics.[41]

Treatment is similar to that for other advanced myelomas. Patients with PCL have more aggressive disease, a poor response to therapy, and a significantly shorter survival than patients with more typical myelomas.[37-39,41]

Etiology and Pathogenesis

Exposure to toxic substances and radiation has been associated with an increased incidence of plasma cell myeloma.[43,44] Chronic antigenic stimulation from chronic infection or other disease may also be a predisposing factor.[44] Most patients with myeloma, however, have no identifiable exposure history or known chronic antigenic stimulation.

There is convincing evidence that plasma cell myeloma results from a disorder of an early hematopoietic cell that is manifested at a mature stage of B-cell development.[27,45] Part of the evidence supporting this view is the presence, in nearly all cases of myeloma, of monoclonal blood lymphocytes immunophenotypically and genetically related to the neoplastic bone marrow plasma cells.[45]

Recent information on the molecular genetics of plasma cell myeloma has greatly enhanced the understanding of its pathogenesis (see later discussion on genetics). The bone marrow microenvironment is also important in the pathogenesis and progression of myeloma.[14,46] Cytokines and growth factors and the functional consequences of direct interaction

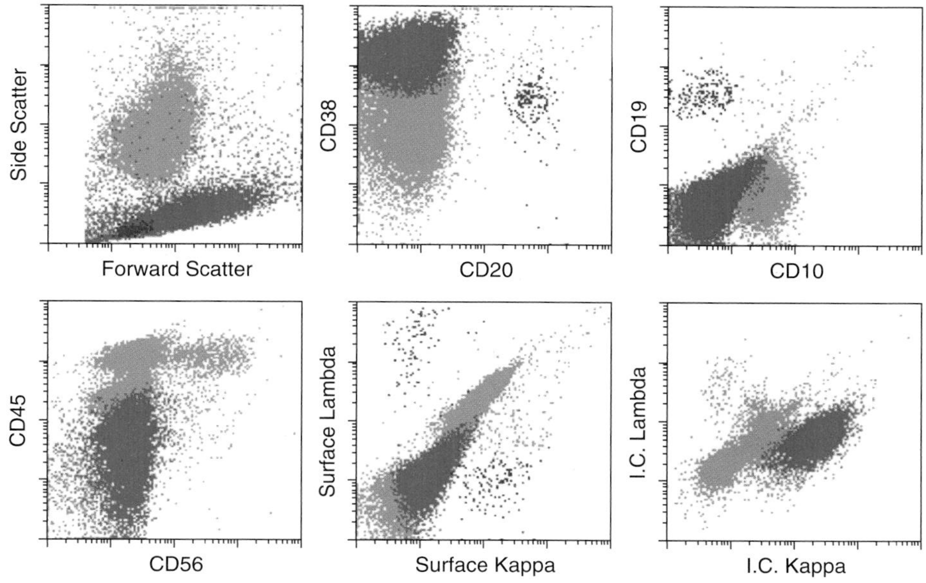

Figure 25-24. Flow cytometry histograms of plasma cell leukemia. The leukemic plasma cells (*red*) exhibit strong expression of CD38; are CD20, CD19, and CD10 negative; and express dim partial CD45. The plasma cells lack surface light chains but have intracytoplasmic (I.C.) kappa light-chain restriction. Unlike most myelomas, but typical of plasma cell leukemia, the neoplastic plasma cells are CD56 negative. Normal B lymphocytes are *blue*.

of bone marrow stromal cells with neoplastic plasma cells are major constituents that influence the pathophysiology of myeloma.[46] Several pieces of evidence point to the involvement of interleukin-6 (IL-6) as a factor in the pathogenesis of plasma cell myeloma. IL-6 appears to support the survival and expansion of myeloma cells by stimulating cell division and preventing programmed cell death. IL-6, along with IL-1b and tumor necrosis factor-α (TNF-α) and other cytokines, have osteoclastic activating properties that lead to lytic lesions through a complex mechanism involving the RANKL pathway.[47] These cytokines may also affect hematopoiesis.

Monoclonal Gammopathy of Undetermined Significance: A Precursor Lesion of Plasma Cell Myeloma

Definition

Monoclonal gammopathy of undetermined significance (MGUS) refers to the presence of a monoclonal immunoglobulin in the serum or urine of a patient in whom there is no evidence of plasma cell myeloma, amyloidosis, Waldenström's macroglobulinemia, or other lymphoproliferative disorder or any other disease known to produce monoclonal immunoglobulins. In most cases patients do not develop malignant plasma cell neoplasms during their lifetimes, but in a significant minority of cases there is eventual progression to a malignant immunosecretory disease. IgM MGUS is usually associated with a lymphoplasmacytic proliferation and can progress to lymphoma. Non-IgM MGUS has plasma cell features and may progress to a malignant plasma cell neoplasm. The diagnostic criteria for MGUS are listed in Box 25-6.[1,5]

Epidemiology

MGUS is the most common monoclonal gammopathy and is found in about 3% of persons older than 50 years and in more than 5% of those older than 70.[1,14,48-55] The incidence of MGUS is twice as high in African Americans as in whites, roughly paralleling the incidence of plasma cell myeloma.[55,56] At least 60% of individuals with MGUS are male.[14,54-56]

Etiology

No cause or association with any specific disease has been identified for MGUS.[55] However, because of the advanced age of many patients at the time of its recognition, underlying health problems are relatively common. Cardiovascular disease, cancer, connective tissue disorders, dermatologic diseases, endocrinopathies, liver disease, and neurologic diseases have all been described in patients with MGUS.[54] M protein is often identified during the evaluation for one of these disorders.[49] Transient oligoclonal and monoclonal gammopathies have been described in young patients following renal and allogeneic bone marrow transplants; there is a correlation with graft-versus-host disease in bone marrow transplant recipients.[15,57]

Box 25-6 *Diagnostic Criteria for Monoclonal Gammopathy of Undetermined Significance*

- M component less than myeloma levels
- Marrow plasmacytosis <10%
- No lytic bone lesions
- No myeloma-related symptoms

From McKenna RW, Kyle RA, Kuehl WM, et al. Plasma cell neoplasms. In: Swerdlow SH, Campo E, Harris NL, et al, eds. *WHO Classification of Tumours of Haematopoietic and Lymphoid Tissues*. Lyon, France: IARC; 2008:200-213.

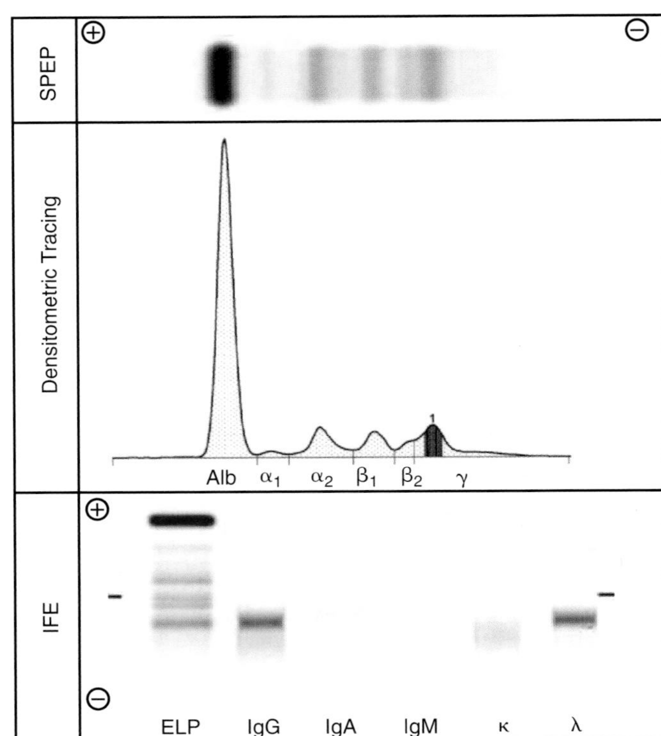

Figure 25-25. Serum electrophoresis from a 73-year-old man with monoclonal gammopathy of undetermined significance. The patient has no clinical, hematologic, or imaging evidence of a plasma cell dyscrasia, except for a persistent, modest (0.4 g/dL), single M protein peak on the densitometric tracing (*shaded area, middle panel*) of the serum protein electrophoresis pattern (SPEP). The M protein was identified by immunofixation electrophoresis (IFE) as IgGλ, located in the β_2 region of the electrophoresis (ELP) pattern. (Courtesy of Drs. Frank H. Wians Jr. and Dennis C. Wooten, Department of Pathology, University of Texas Southwestern Medical Center, Dallas.)

Clinical and Laboratory Features

Patients are asymptomatic as pertains to the monoclonal gammopathy. Other than the M protein and a mild increase in bone marrow plasma cells, there are no consistent or specific clinical findings. Abnormal laboratory studies in individuals with MGUS usually reflect a coexisting disease. The typical laboratory and radiographic abnormalities associated with a malignant plasma cell neoplasm are not observed in MGUS. The M protein is found on serum protein electrophoresis in most cases (Fig. 25-25). The quantity of the M protein is less than 3 g/dL; the median is about 1.7 g/dL.[15,49] In patients with a very low quantity of M protein, immunofixation electrophoresis is required for detection (see Fig. 25-25). Normal serum polyclonal immunoglobulins are decreased in about 40% of cases.[15,49,50] Light chains (Bence Jones protein) are present in the urine in small quantities in up to 28% of cases; in most, the quantity of urinary protein is less than 1 g/24 hours.[15,49,50]

The distribution of monoclonal heavy- and light-chain types generally reflects the normal quantitative distribution of immunoglobulin-producing cells, except for a disproportionate increase in the frequency of IgM. In 67% to 75% of cases the monoclonal heavy chain is IgG. IgM is found in about 15% of cases, IgA in 10% to 14%, and 2% to 3% are biclonal gammopathies; the light chain is kappa in 54% to 63%.[5,15,49,54] Only rare cases of IgD and light-chain-only MGUS have been reported.[58] However, some studies suggest that up to 20% of cases of MGUS may be light chain only, detectable only with the serum free-light-chain assay.[14,52]

Blood and Bone Marrow Findings

There are no specific blood findings associated with MGUS. Rouleaux formation may be increased in patients with M protein levels on the high side of the range. When blood count abnormalities or other changes on blood smears are found, they are usually related to a coexisting disease.

Approximately half the patients with MGUS have a mild increase in plasma cells in marrow aspirate smears, but clonal plasma cells are less than 10% (median, 3%).[5,15] Plasma cell morphology is typically normal, but mild changes, including cytoplasmic inclusions and nucleoli, may be observed. In trephine biopsy sections, the marrow is generally normocellular. The level of plasma cell infiltration in the biopsy sections is low. Plasma cells may be evenly scattered throughout the marrow or found in small clusters. Clustering of plasma cells is most common in cases with an increased percentage of plasma cells. An immunohistochemical stain for CD138 facilitates the assessment of plasma cell number and distribution on bone marrow trephine biopsies. Detection of light-chain restriction by kappa and lambda stains on biopsy sections is often difficult because the clone may be small and in a background of normal plasma cells. In a minority of cases there is a distinctively monoclonal pattern with an excess of either kappa- or lambda-staining plasma cells; the ratio of light-chain excess is less than in plasma cell myeloma.[59,60]

In MGUS two populations of plasma cells are frequently identified by flow cytometry: a polyclonal population with a normal immunophenotype (brightly positive for CD38, positive for CD19 and negative for CD56) and an aberrant monoclonal population most often CD19 negative and either CD56 positive or negative.[53,61] The monoclonal population may also manifest other aberrant antigen expression.[53,61,62]

The genetics of MGUS is discussed in the section on the genetics of plasma cell myeloma.

Clinical Course

In most individuals the clinical course of MGUS is stable, with no increase in M protein or other evidence of progression to a malignant plasma cell dyscrasia. In a substantial minority, however, there is eventual evolution to an overt plasma cell myeloma, amyloidosis, macroglobulinemia, or other malignant lymphoproliferative disorder. In one large study with a follow-up of 22 to 39 years, 57% of patients died of unrelated causes without progression of their monoclonal gammopathy; another 6% were living with no substantial increase in M protein; in 10% of cases the serum M protein increased to 3g/dL or more, but the patients did not require treatment and had no other changes in clinical status; and 27% developed a malignant plasma cell dyscrasia or lymphoproliferative disease.[63] The interval from diagnosis of MGUS to diagnosis of a malignant immunosecretory disease was 1 to 32 years (median, 10.4 years).[63] By actuarial analysis, the conversion of MGUS to a malignant plasma cell dyscrasia was 17% at 10 years and reached 33% at 20 years. In another large study, the actuarial probability for malignant transformation of MGUS was 6% at 5 years, 15% at 10 years, and 31% at 20 years.[64] The median survival for patients with MGUS is only slightly shorter than that of a comparable population in the United States, but the risk of progression is indefinite and persists even after more than 30 years.[63,65]

In patients who exhibit disease progression, the malignant diagnosis is plasma cell myeloma in 66% to 79% of cases, Waldenström's macroglobulinemia in 8% to 12%, and amyloidosis in 4% to 14%; 6% to 8% develop chronic lymphocytic leukemia (CLL) or other lymphoma.[50,63,64] The type and size of M protein and serum free-light-chain ratio are significant clinical risk factors.[5,50,64] Patients with IgM or IgA MGUS appear to be at greater risk of progression to a malignant disorder than those with IgG—37%, 32%, and 21%, respectively.[49,65] Risk of progression also appears to be higher for patients with M protein levels at the upper end of the spectrum, and an increasing serum M protein seems to be a reliable parameter for predicting disease progression.[49,64,66] In addition, the detection of DNA aneuploidy, a high fraction of bone marrow plasma cells with an abnormal immunophenotype, and decreased levels of polyclonal immunoglobulin are significant clinical risk factors.[53] MGUS should be considered a preneoplastic condition, and patients should be followed for evidence of progression indefinitely.[49,64,66]

Immunophenotype

Flow Cytometry

Immunophenotyping by flow cytometry is useful for diagnosing myeloma, identifying cases that may respond to therapeutic agents with specific membrane targets, and detecting minimal residual disease; in some cases the immunophenotype provides prognostic information.[67] Normal plasma cell populations and reactive plasma cell expansions express a polyclonal pattern of cytoplasmic immunoglobulin, CD19, strong CD38, and CD138 (syndecan-1). Neoplastic plasma cells also usually express strong CD38 and CD138, but in contrast to normal cells, they have monoclonal cytoplasmic immunoglobulin and are nearly always CD19$^-$; in addition, CD56 is aberrantly expressed in 67% to 79% of myelomas.[68-70] This abnormal antigen expression profile is virtually diagnostic of a plasma cell dyscrasia (Fig. 25-26).

Aberrant expression of antigens is found in nearly all cases of myeloma.[68,71-74] Neoplastic plasma cells may express CD56, CD117, CD20, CD52, or CD10, in decreasing order of frequency; occasionally, myeloid and monocytic antigens are found.[27,68,71,73-77] Aberrant antigen expression provides a basis for following patients for minimal residual disease by flow cytometry on bone marrow specimens (Fig. 25-27).[67,68,78] In the minority of patients whose myeloma cells express CD20 or CD52, there may be the potential for specifically targeted therapy using rituximab (CD20) and alemtuzumab (CD52).[68,71]

The CD56$^-$ subset (21% to 33%) of myelomas has more extensive marrow infiltration, lower osteolytic potential, higher β_2-microglobulin levels, more renal insufficiency,

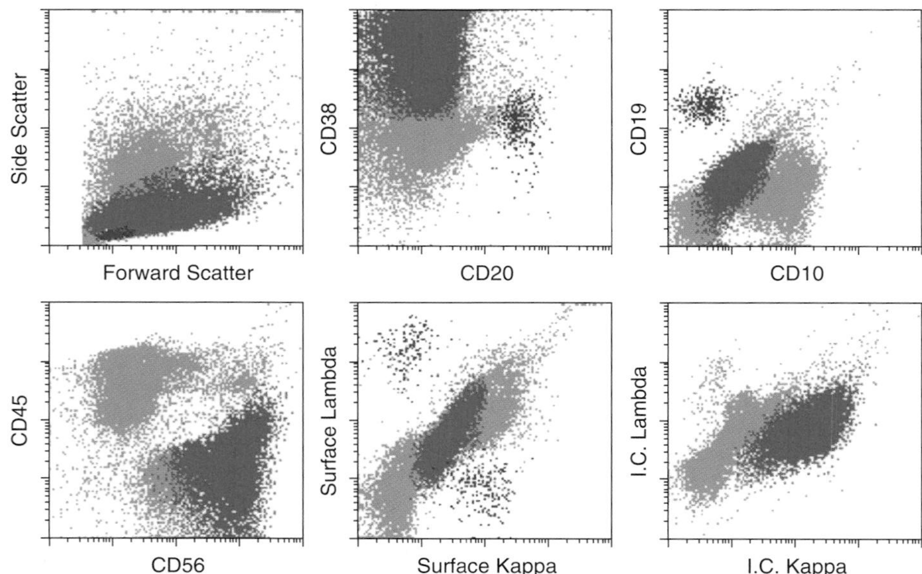

Figure 25-26. Flow cytometry histograms of plasma cell myeloma. The neoplastic plasma cells (*red*) have a typical myeloma immunophenotype. They exhibit strong expression of CD38; are negative for CD20, CD19, and CD10; and express CD56 and dim, partial CD45. The plasma cells lack surface light chains but have intracytoplasmic (I.C.) kappa restriction. Normal polyclonal B lymphocytes are *blue*.

more frequent plasmablastic morphology, and a tendency for malignant plasma cells to circulate in the blood.[69,70,79] About 80% of cases of PCL are CD56⁻ (see Fig. 25-24). Furthermore, CD56⁻ myelomas that do not present as PCL are more likely to develop a secondary PCL than are CD56⁺ cases.[69] Patients with CD56⁻ myeloma have a significantly shorter survival.[79]

Immunohistochemistry

Immunohistochemistry can supplement flow cytometry or provide the primary immunophenotypic assessment for plasma cell dyscrasias when a specimen is not obtained for flow cytometry or contains inadequate numbers of plasma cells for analysis. The following are indications for immunohistochemical stains on marrow biopsies or other tissues in the assessment of plasma cell dyscrasias:

- Assessing the quantity of plasma cells in marrow biopsies
- Identifying a monoclonal plasma cell proliferation
- Distinguishing myeloma from other neoplasms

Plasma cells may be difficult to recognize and quantify in suboptimally prepared sections and when they are distributed

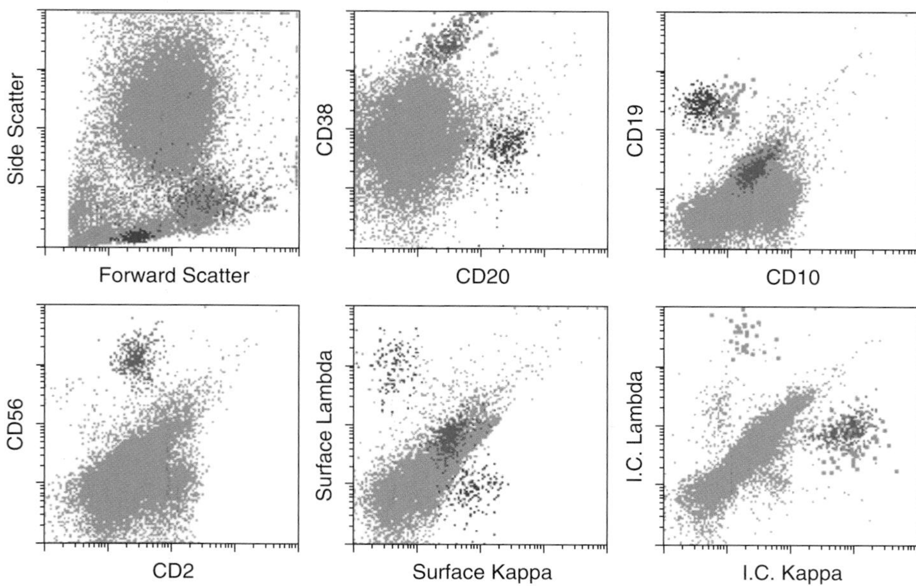

Figure 25-27. Flow cytometry histograms of bone marrow show minimal residual myeloma following autologous stem cell transplantation. A minute population of myeloma cells (*red*) is strongly expressing CD38 and is negative for CD20, CD19, CD10, and CD2. The neoplastic plasma cells are CD56⁺ and negative for surface light chains but exhibit intracytoplasmic (I.C.) kappa restriction. In contrast, the normal polyclonal plasma cells (*green*) are CD19⁺ and CD56⁻ and show a polyclonal pattern of intracytoplasmic light-chain expression. Normal polyclonal B lymphocytes are *blue*.

interstitially in the marrow. Stains for plasma cell–associated antigens, (e.g., CD138, CD38, CD79a, kappa, lambda) usually stain plasma cells brilliantly on biopsy sections, allowing easy quantification. Immunohistochemical stains for kappa and lambda light chains are useful in characterizing malignant plasma cell proliferations and differentiating them from reactive causes of increased plasma cells, such as connective tissue disorders, chronic liver disease, chronic infections, and metastatic tumors.[5] Normal or reactive plasma cells and myeloma plasma cells are both rich in cytoplasmic immunoglobulin and generally react strongly with antibodies to kappa or lambda light chains. In cases of myeloma, the plasma cells express a monoclonal pattern of reactivity.[59,80] In normal marrow and in reactive plasma cell proliferations, there is a polyclonal pattern of kappa- and lambda-staining plasma cells, usually with a slight to moderate kappa predominance (Fig. 25-28). In some cases of MGUS the kappa-to-lambda ratio is normal; in others it is skewed, but generally less so than in myeloma. In one large study a kappa-to-lambda staining ratio of 16:1 or higher on marrow biopsies distinguished myeloma from MGUS in nearly all instances; other investigators found a ratio of 8:1 to be as effective.[59,60] Neither the number of marrow plasma cells nor the quantity of M protein correlates well with the light-chain ratio.[60] Kappa and lambda stains are particularly useful in cases with a relatively low percentage of marrow plasma cells.

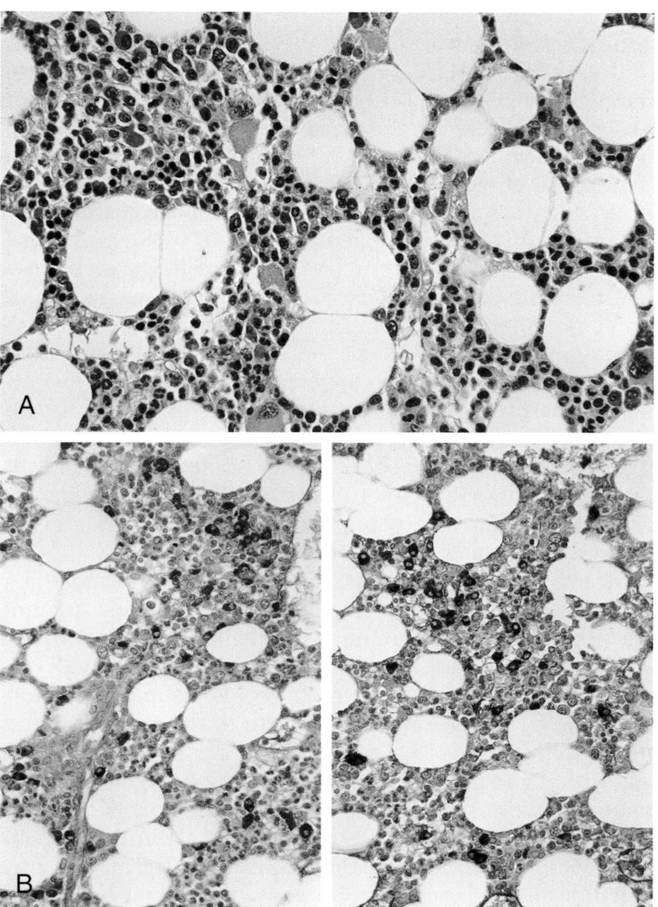

Figure 25-28. Reactive bone marrow plasmacytosis. A, Bone marrow biopsy section from a 59-year-old man with a lymphoma in the gastrointestinal tract. There were 10% plasma cells in the marrow aspirate. In this section, plasma cells appear to be increased but are mostly scattered in an interstitial pattern, with a few small clusters. **B,** Immunohistochemical stains for kappa and lambda light chains show a polyclonal staining pattern, consistent with a reactive plasmacytosis.

Immunohistochemistry is often helpful in differentiating an anaplastic or plasmablastic myeloma from other hematopoietic neoplasms and metastatic tumors. In addition to kappa and lambda, staining for CD138 (syndecan-1) and plasma cell–reacting pan–B-cell antigens such as CD79a is especially valuable in the differential diagnosis. CD138 reacts with normal plasma cells and is expressed in 60% to 100% of myelomas.[68,81,82] Generally, 70% to 100% of the neoplastic cells are positive in myeloma. CD138 appears to be plasma cell specific among normal hematopoietic cells in the marrow; however, other neoplastic B-cell disorders may react with some anti-CD138 antibodies.[83] CD79a is positive in the plasma cells in most cases of myeloma, but it is a pan–B-lymphocyte antigen and is found in most B-cell neoplasms. It may be helpful in distinguishing myeloma from non–B-cell hematopoietic neoplasms and metastatic tumors. Cyclin D1 is expressed in approximately 25% of cases of myeloma.[84,85] Strong nuclear expression generally correlates with the lymphoid-appearing type of myeloma and with the t(11;14)(q13;q32) cytogenetic abnormality (see later), whereas weak expression may be seen in association with other genetic abnormalities.[84]

Genetics

Abnormalities are found by conventional cytogenetics in about one third of cases of plasma cell myeloma.[86,87] Molecular cytogenetic analysis using fluorescence in situ hybridization (FISH) increases the frequency of cases with detectable genetic abnormalities to over 90%.[86,88-90] Both numerical and structural aberrations are found. Abnormalities of nearly every chromosome have been reported. Trisomies, whole or partial chromosome deletions, and translocations are most frequent; complex cytogenetic abnormalities are common.[87] Fifty-five percent to 70% of plasma cell myelomas have translocations involving the heavy-chain locus (*IGH@*) at chromosome 14q32.[89,91] In about 40%, one of five recurrent oncogenes is involved in these translocations. These are *cyclin D1* (11q13) in 15% to 18%, *C-MAF* (16q23) in 5%, *FGFR3/MMSET* (4p16.3) in 15%, *cyclin D3* (6p21) in 3%, and *MAFB* (20q11) in 2%.[88,92-94] The remaining myelomas are mostly hyperdiploid, with trisomies in the odd-numbered chromosomes; only infrequently do they have one of the five recurrent translocations involving *IGH@*.[89,90,95,96] Both the recurrent *IGH@* translocations and hyperdiploidy appear to be early events in the pathogenesis of myeloma. They are unified by the associated dysregulation and overexpression of one of the *cyclin D* genes (*D1, D2, D3*).[93,96,97]

The expression levels of *cyclin D1, D2,* and *D3* and the overexpression of oncogenes dysregulated by the five recurrent *IGH@* translocations can be determined by gene expression profiling. Plasma cell myeloma can be classified into eight groups using patterns of translocations and cyclin D expression (TC groups) (Table 25-2). These eight groups are based mostly on initiating or early pathogenic events.[94] Some of them may represent distinct biologic types of myeloma that require different approaches to therapy.[94]

Table 25-2 Translocation and Cyclin D Groups

Group	Primary Translocation	Gene	Cyclin D	Ploidy	Frequency (%)	Prognosis
6p21	6p21	*CCND3*	D3	NH	3	Good
11q13	11q13	*CCND1*	D1	D, NH	16	Good
D1	None	None	D1	H	34	Good
D1 + D2	None	None	D1 + D2	H	6	? Poor
D2	None	None	D2	H, NH	17	?
None	None	None	None	NH	2	? Good
4p16	4p16	*FGFR3/MMSET*	D2	NH>H	15	Poor
maf	16q23	*c-maf*	D2	NH	5	Poor
	20q11	*mafB*			2	

D, diploid; H, hyperdiploid; NH, nonhyperdiploid.
Data from Bergsagel PL, Kuehl WM. Molecular pathogenesis and a consequent classification of multiple myeloma. J Clin Oncol 2005:23:6333-6338.

Another molecular classification identifies seven groups of myeloma, based on unsupervised clustering of tumors by gene expression profiles.[98] The groups are similar but differ somewhat from the TC groups. One of these seven molecular groups is defined by progression events that lead to increased proliferation.

Monosomy or partial deletion of chromosome 13 (13q14) also appears to be an early event in pathogenesis and is the single most common structural abnormality by conventional cytogenetics.[88,89] By FISH analysis, del(13) is found in more than 40% of myelomas and 70% of PCLs. Activating mutations of *K-* or *N-RAS* are present in about 30% to 40% of myelomas and probably represent an early event in progression. In some patients they may mediate the MGUS-to-myeloma transition.[89,99] There are several other recurrent genetic changes associated with disease progression. These include gains of chromosome 1q and loss of 1p, deletion or mutation of p53 (17p13), translocations involving c-*MYC* or *N-MYC*, secondary *IGH@* or *IGL* translocations, inactivation of *p18INK4c* or *RB1*, mutations of genes that result in activation of the nuclear factor-κB pathway, and mutations of *FGFR3* in tumors with t(4;14).[1,88,92,94,96,100-103]

Karyotypic abnormalities are rarely reported in MGUS. However, molecular cytogenetic studies using FISH have demonstrated both numerical and structural abnormalities in most patients.[89-91,104-107] The abnormalities in non-IgM MGUS are similar to those in plasma cell myeloma, but with a different prevalence. Aneuploidy has been demonstrated by image analysis of Feulgen-stained specimens in more than 60% of cases of MGUS, and most of these have numerical abnormalities by FISH, hyperdiploidy being most common.[105] Abnormalities of 14q32 and del(13), the most frequent structural abnormalities in myeloma, have also been identified in MGUS in a substantial percentage of cases.[91,104,108] In two studies of large numbers of patients, 47% and 46% of cases of MGUS and smoldering myeloma, respectively, had 14q32 rearrangements; del(13) was found in 23% and 50% of cases, respectively. The t(11;14)(q23;q32) is present in 15% to 25% of MGUS, t(4;14)(p16.3;q32) in 2% to 9%, and t(14;16)(q34q23) in 1% to 5%.[91,107] About 40% of MGUS cases have hyperdiploidy, with chromosomal trisomies similar to those in myeloma.[90] Compared with myeloma, activating *K-* and *N-RAS* mutations are much less frequent in MGUS—about 30% to 40% in myeloma versus 5% in MGUS.[99] No obvious clinical or biologic correlations with cytogenetic abnormalities have been identified in MGUS.[104,107]

Genetic findings have proved to be an important indicator of prognosis in myeloma (see the later section on prognostic features).

Differential Diagnosis

The most common differential diagnosis among the plasma cell neoplasms is early myeloma versus MGUS or a reactive bone marrow plasmacytosis. In most cases this is not difficult to distinguish because the composite clinical and pathologic findings required for a diagnosis of myeloma are lacking in MGUS and in reactive plasma cell proliferations.

Patients with MGUS have a serum M protein level of less than 3 g/dL of IgG or 2 g/dL of IgA, little or no protein in the urine, less than 10% plasma cells in the bone marrow, and no anemia, hypercalcemia, renal failure, or osteolytic lesions. Only when the M protein level or percentage of marrow plasma cells is at the high extreme for MGUS is the distinction from asymptomatic myeloma problematic. In many cases immunohistochemical stains for kappa and lambda light chains on marrow biopsies are helpful. There is a plasma cell light-chain excess in the vast majority of myelomas, usually exceeding 16:1; in MGUS the ratio is less than 16:1 in more than 90% of cases.[59] In some patients, differentiation of early myeloma and MGUS is not possible at the initial evaluation. Close observation and monitoring for evidence of progression to overt malignancy must be continued indefinitely.

Reactive bone marrow plasmacytosis of 10% or more may occur in several conditions, including viral infections, immune reactions to drugs, autoimmune disorders such as rheumatoid arthritis and lupus, and acquired immunodeficiency syndrome (AIDS). Reactive plasmacytosis is distinguished from myeloma by the lack of an M protein in the serum or urine in most instances. The plasma cells are generally mature appearing, and stains for kappa and lambda light chains on marrow sections show a polyclonal plasma cell staining pattern (see Fig. 25-28). Systemic polyclonal immunoblastic proliferations are the most difficult reactive plasma cell proliferations to distinguish from myeloma morphologically. The disorder is uncommon and usually presents as an acute systemic illness with fever, lymphadenopathy, and hepatosplenomegaly; anemia and thrombocytopenia are present in most patients. Autoimmune manifestations are often present. The leukocyte count is usually elevated, with large numbers of plasma cells, immunoblasts, and reactive lymphocytes, and there is eosinophilia and neutrophilia in some cases

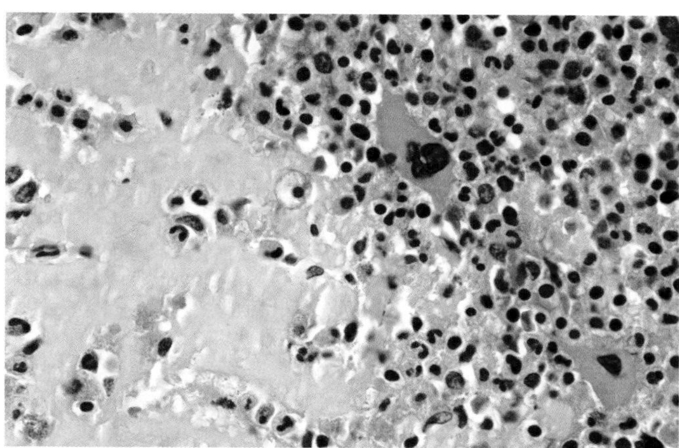

Figure 25-37. Trephine biopsy section from a patient with amyloidosis. There are large deposits of amyloid adjacent to and incorporating normal hematopoietic cells. The amyloid in this case replaced extensive portions of bone marrow. (Courtesy of Dr. Patrick Ward, Department of Pathology, University of Minnesota, Duluth.)

Other Tissues. Amyloid is found in many other tissues and organs, including subcutaneous fat, kidney, heart, liver, gastrointestinal tract, and peripheral nerves. Blood vessel walls and basement membrane are most commonly affected. Organ parenchyma may become massively replaced by amyloid deposits as the disease progresses. Subcutaneous fat aspiration and rectal biopsy are each diagnostic in approximately 80% of cases when adequate tissue is obtained.[157,164,165] Skin biopsies are diagnostic in approximately half the cases; gingival biopsy is less commonly positive.[157,165,166] Renal biopsy is diagnostic in well over 90% of cases but carries a greater risk than the other procedures and is usually unnecessary. Similarly, liver biopsy is diagnostic in most cases but should be avoided if possible because of associated bleeding complications. Cardiac involvement can be documented by endomyocardial biopsy in a high percentage of cases.[166]

An additional method for diagnosing and following patients with amyloidosis is scintigraphy with iodine-labeled serum amyloid P component (SAP).[167] SAP has specific binding affinity for amyloid fibrils. Iodine-labeled SAP is rapidly localized to amyloid deposits in vivo and is useful in identifying and quantitating amyloid deposition.[167]

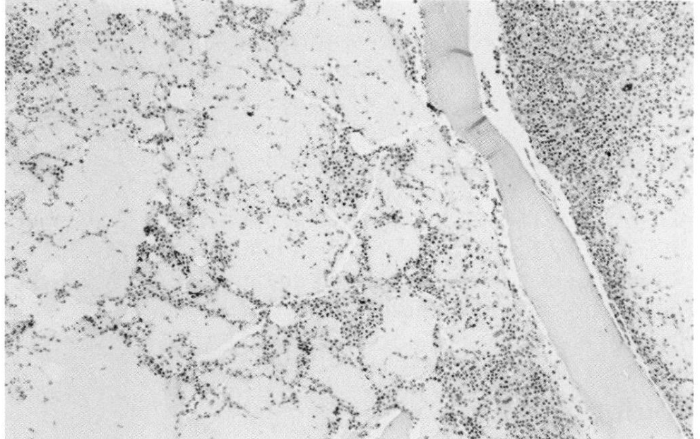

Figure 25-38. Bone marrow biopsy section from a patient with advanced primary amyloidosis shows extensive replacement of the marrow with deposits of amyloid.

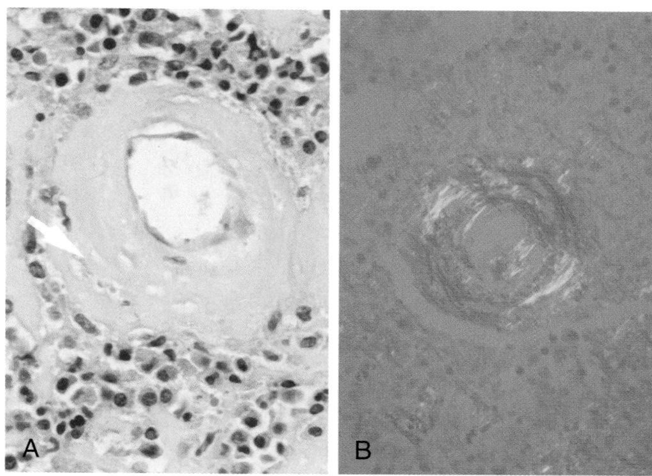

Figure 25-39. **A,** Trephine biopsy section from a patient with primary amyloidosis. The wall of the blood vessel in the center of the field is thickened by deposits of amyloid. There are also amyloid deposits and numerous plasma cells in the marrow adjacent to the vessel (hematoxylin-eosin). **B,** Congo red stain on the bone marrow section shows typical birefringence of amyloid in the vessel wall under polarized light.

Histochemistry, Immunohistochemistry, and Immunophenotype

Amyloid is moderately periodic acid–Schiff positive, stains metachromatically with crystal violet and methyl violet, and is fluorescent when reacted with thioflavin T.[159,168] The most useful cytochemical procedure in the diagnosis of amyloidosis is Congo red stain, which, under polarized light, produces a characteristic apple-green birefringence (Fig. 25-39). AL and AA amyloid may be distinguished by preincubation of biopsy sections with potassium permanganate followed by Congo red staining; AL amyloid retains its apple-green birefringence, but Congo red staining of AA is lost.[168] The technique requires careful interpretation, however, because in some cases of AL amyloidosis Congo red staining is reduced after permanganate treatment.[159]

The bone marrow plasma cells may show a monoclonal or, if the clone is small and masked by normal plasma cells, a polyclonal staining pattern with anti-kappa and anti-lambda light-chain antibodies.[168-170] The majority show a monoclonal pattern regardless of whether there is evidence of myeloma.[168-170] Monoclonal lambda staining is most common. The other immunophenotypic findings are similar to those of plasma cell myeloma.

Immunohistochemistry using antibodies to amyloid fibril or to AL kappa and lambda is definitive for distinguishing primary and secondary amyliodosis (AA) in less than half of cases. This is because of the presence of background normal immunoglobulins or loss of light-chain segments recognized by the antisera.[159,168,171] AA amyloid is recognized by immunohistochemistry in nearly all cases.[162]

Cytogenetics

The cytogenetic rearrangements reported in primary amyloidosis are similar to those in plasma cell myeloma, except for a much greater frequency of t(11;14) in amyloidosis (40%) than in myeloma (15% to 20%).[89,172,173]

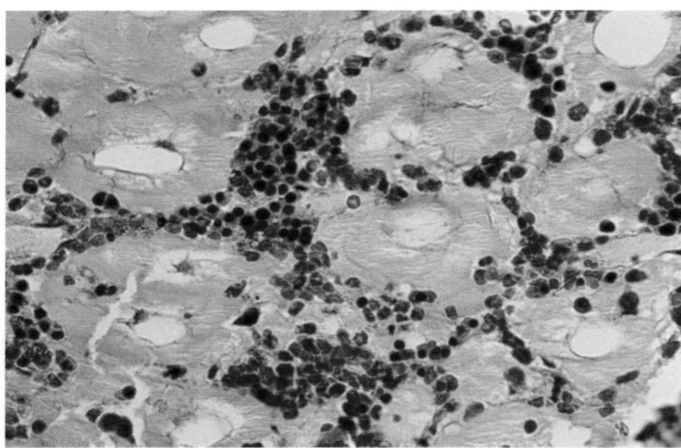

Figure 25-40. Biopsy specimen from an elderly man with advanced cancer and severe cachexia. There is extensive serous atrophy of fat, which bears a superficial resemblance to and could potentially be confused with amyloid.

Differential Diagnosis

The differential diagnosis of amyloidosis is quite limited. In some cases systemic non-AL amyloidosis, including hereditary types and AA amyloidosis, and light- or heavy-chain deposition disease must be distinguished from primary AL amyloidosis. Clinical findings and history are key to distinguishing AL amyloidosis from the other forms. Immunohistochemical studies using antibodies against the various amyloid fibril proteins can be performed and are particularly effective in identifying AA-type amyloid.[162] A Congo red stain or electron microscopic studies can differentiate AL amyloid and light- or heavy-chain deposition disease.

In the bone marrow, extensive extra-vessel deposits of amyloid may bear histologic resemblance to serous atrophy of fat (Fig. 25-40). The Congo red stain, clinical history, and laboratory findings should readily distinguish these two processes.

Treatment, Clinical Course, and Prognosis

Treatment of AL amyloidosis is aimed at controlling amyloid production and deposition in tissues by suppressing the clonal plasma cells. Chemotherapy agents and regimens similar to those for myeloma are used to treat amyloidosis. Improvement in clinical status is achieved in some patients, and survival has improved in recent years.[161] There is no treatment available that directly targets amyloid deposits. Colchicine is used to inhibit amyloid deposition. It has been effective in cases of amyloidosis in patients with familial Mediterranean fever and marginally effective in AL amyloidosis.[174,175] Supportive and symptomatic treatment for congestive heart failure, renal failure, and other manifestations related to amyloid deposition are important aspects of therapy.[159,160]

The median survival for patients with AL amyloidosis is nearly 2 years from diagnosis. Shorter survival is usual for patients who present with congestive heart failure (≈6 months). For patients whose only presenting clinical manifestation is peripheral neuropathy, the median survival is approximately 5 years.[160] Patients with myeloma and amyloidosis have a shorter survival than those without myeloma.[159,161] The most frequent cause of death is amyloid cardiac disease (≈40%).[160] Other less common causes of death include renal failure, infection, hemorrhage, intestinal obstruction, liver failure, and respiratory failure.

Findings associated with a poor prognosis are elevated urine creatinine, hepatomegaly, major weight loss, excretion of lambda light chains in the urine (versus kappa light chains or no M protein), β_2-microglobulin levels above 2.7 μg/mL, and large whole-body amyloid load on SAP scintigraphy.[160,162,176]

Systemic Light- and Heavy-Chain Deposition Diseases

There are three major types of these disorders: light-chain deposition disease, light- and heavy-chain deposition disease, and heavy-chain deposition disease.[177-180] These disorders are rare and differ from primary amyloidosis in the following ways: the amorphous material is nonfibrillary and lacks a β-pleated sheet configuration, does not stain with Congo red, and lacks a P-component.[175] In addition, light-chain deposits are most commonly kappa (80%), with overrepresentation of VκIV. Many organs may be involved with deposits, but the kidneys are most frequently affected. Liver, heart, nerves, and blood vessels are also commonly involved. Renal insufficiency, cardiac disease, and liver disease are all more common than in primary amyloidosis.[175] The monoclonal deposits appear as refractile eosinophilic material in glomerular and tubular basement membranes in renal biopsies. There is an M-component in about 85% of cases and increased plasma cells in the marrow in 50% to 60%. Most cases (≈55%) are associated with myeloma. Treatment is similar to that for amyloidosis, with limited success. Median overall survival for light-chain deposition disease is about 4 years. Prognosis is related to age, presence of myeloma, and light-chain deposition in extrarenal sites.[1,181]

OSTEOSCLEROTIC MYELOMA (POEMS SYNDROME)

Definition

Osteosclerotic myeloma is usually accompanied by a syndrome that includes *polyneuropathy, organomegaly, endocrinopathy, monoclonal* gammopathy, and *skin* lesions (POEMS).[1,182-186] Several other features are often present that are not included in the POEMS acronym: Castleman's disease, papilledema, edema, and serous effusions and thrombocytosis.[184,186,187] Most patients do not present with all the manifestations, and the number of features necessary for diagnosis is not clearly defined. Altered regulation leading to an imbalance of proinflammatory cytokines has been implicated in the pathogenesis of POEMS syndrome; vascular endothelial growth factor may be an important pathogenic factor in the disease.[188-192] Some patients with POEMS syndrome and multicentric Castleman's disease have been infected with human herpesvirus 8.[183,193] The pathophysiologic connection among POEMS syndrome, Castleman's disease, and osteosclerotic myeloma is not clearly defined, however.

Epidemiology

Osteosclerotic myeloma is rare, constituting 1% to 2% of plasma cell dyscrasias.[183] One half of patients with myeloma and peripheral neuropathy have osteosclerotic lesions.[194] The median age at diagnosis is about 51 years, but one third of patients are 45 years or younger; slightly more than 60% of patients are men.[184]

Clinical Features

Peripheral neuropathy is a prominent feature in most patients with osteosclerotic myeloma and a defining feature of POEMS syndrome. It is typically the initial symptom, but occasionally patients present with a plasma cell dyscrasia and later develop a neuropathy.[184] Organomegaly is present in at least half of patients. Hepatomegaly, splenomegaly, and lymphadenopathy are about equally common. Endocrinopathy, another defining feature of POEMS syndrome, is present in two thirds of cases. Hypogonadism is most common, followed by adrenal and thyroid function abnormalities. Skin changes are also found in about two thirds of patients; hyperpigmentation is the most frequent abnormality.[184]

Seventy-five percent to 85% of patients with osteosclerotic myeloma, with or without the other characteristic findings in POEMS syndrome, have an M protein by serum immunofixation electrophoresis. The quantity of the M protein is characteristically low (median, 1.1 g/dL).[184] In all cases the light chain is lambda; the heavy chain is about equally distributed between IgA and IgG. A urine M protein is found by immunofixation electrophoresis in less than half of patients.

Other recurrent and relatively common clinical findings in POEMS syndrome include Castleman's disease, edema and serous cavity effusions, papilledema, thrombocytosis, weight loss, fatigue, clubbing, bone pain, and arthralgias. Occasionally patients present with or develop pulmonary hypertension, congestive heart failure, thrombosis, and renal failure.

Radiographic bone abnormalities are found in nearly all cases. These vary from single sclerotic lesions in about half of cases to more than three lesions in one third of cases.[184] Many patients have mixed sclerotic and lytic lesions; purely lytic changes are rare.

Blood and Bone Marrow Findings

A variety of abnormal blood counts are found in patients with POEMS syndrome. These include thrombocytosis in 54% to 88% of patients and polycythemia in 12% to 19%.[184,186,187] In some patients blood counts are normal. There are no specific or recurrent morphologic changes in blood smears.

Directed bone marrow biopsies show features of plasmacytoma, but with marked osteosclerotic changes in bone trabeculae. There is typically paratrabecular fibrosis with entrapped plasma cells (Figs. 25-41 to 25-45).[1] The plasma cells may appear elongated due to distortion by small bands of connective tissue. The bone marrow away from the osteosclerotic plasmacytomas is usually normal appearing and contains less than 5% plasma cells.[183] In a minority of patients with more generalized osteosclerotic myeloma, greater than 10% plasma cells may be found in random marrow aspiration and trephine biopsies.[186]

Other Tissues

Two thirds of patients with lymphadenopathy have changes consistent with the plasma cell variant of Castleman's disease.[184]

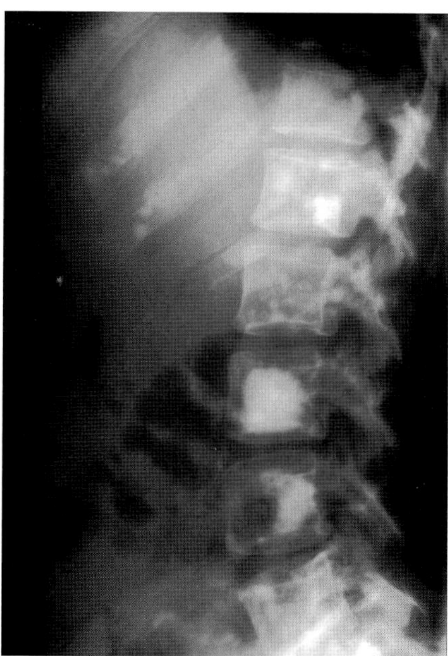

Figure 25-41. Radiograph of the spine in a patient with POEMS syndrome. There are numerous osteoblastic lesions of vertebral bodies and ribs. Lytic changes are also present. (Courtesy of Dr. Patrick C. J. Ward, Department of Pathology, University of Minnesota, Duluth.)

Immunophenotype and Genetics

Immunohistochemical stains reveal either IgA or IgG cytoplasmic immunoglobulin. Virtually all cases are lambda light-chain restricted.[184,186] There is little information available on the genetics of POEMS syndrome.

Treatment, Clinical Course, and Prognosis

Radiotherapy alone or combined with surgery is the most common therapy for localized osteosclerotic lesions. For more

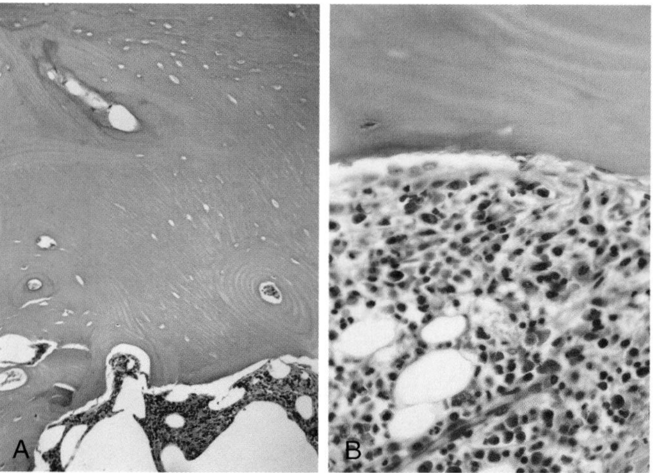

Figure 25-42. Osteosclerotic lesion in a patient with POEMS syndrome. The biopsy is of an osteosclerotic vertebral lesion in a patient with polyneuropathy and a serum IgAλ M protein. **A,** Low magnification shows markedly thickened bone. **B,** A plasma cell proliferation adjacent to the bone is appreciated at higher magnification, and osteoblasts line the bony surface.

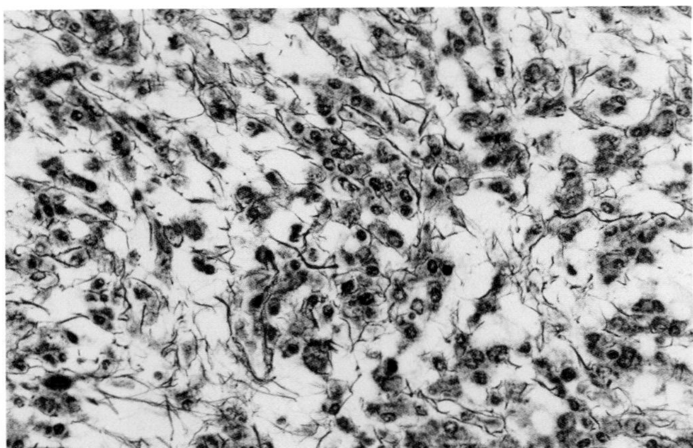

Figure 25-43. Reticulin stain of a plasma cell lesion in POEMS syndrome. There is a moderate increase in reticulin, with fibers weaving around clusters of plasma cells (Wilder's reticulin stain).

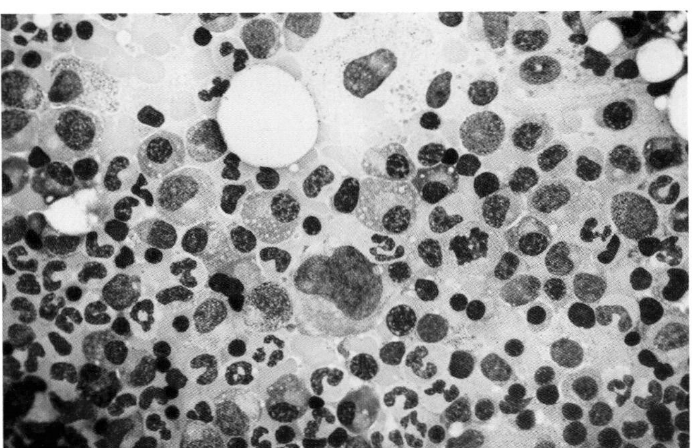

Figure 25-45. Bone marrow aspirate from a patient with POEMS syndrome and multiple osteosclerotic bone lesions. There are increased plasma cells. They appear relatively mature, and many contain cytoplasmic vacuoles (Wright-Giemsa stain).

generalized osteosclerotic myeloma, chemotherapy regimens similar to those for other myelomas are used. Most patients experience at least some response to therapy. When the plasma cell neoplasm responds to treatment, the other elements of POEMS syndrome improve or even disappear over a period of several weeks.[184,186]

Osteosclerotic myeloma is a more indolent disease than typical plasma cell myeloma. Overall, median survival is up to 165 months, with 60% of patients surviving 5 years.[183,184] Patients often develop additional features of POEMS syndrome over time. The prognosis is better for patients with solitary lesions. Patients who experience a good response to therapy have a better median survival; those with edema, effusions, and fingernail clubbing have a poorer survival. The number of presenting major features of POEMS syndrome does not appear to affect survival.[184] The most common causes of death are cardiorespiratory failure and infection.

HEAVY-CHAIN DISEASE

The heavy-chain diseases are clonal immunosecretory disorders that manifest as lymphomas or chronic lymphoproliferative disorders. The corresponding neoplasms are discussed in detail in other chapters. The major features of the heavy-chain diseases are briefly described here.

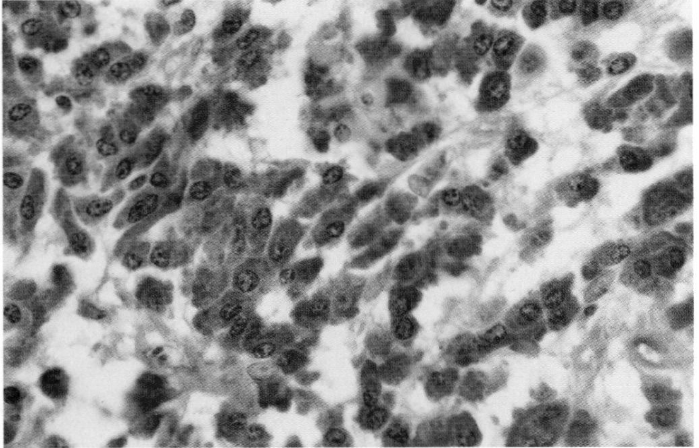

Figure 25-44. Lambda light-chain staining of a plasma cell lesion from a patient with POEMS syndrome. There is a marked predominance of plasma cells staining for lambda light chain.

Definition

Heavy-chain diseases are a group of syndromes characterized by the production of an M protein composed of incomplete heavy chains of IgG, IgA, or IgM type and no light chains. The protein abnormality is usually associated with a lymphoma or CLL.[195-197]

Epidemiology

There are no reliable data on incidence, but all the heavy-chain diseases are rare. Alpha-chain disease is the most common and is encountered at least 3 or 4 times more frequently than gamma chain disease and 10 times more often than mu chain disease. It is probable that heavy-chain diseases are underdiagnosed.

Gamma Chain Disease

The median age at diagnosis of gamma chain disease is 60 years; it is equally distributed between men and women.[197-199] Weakness, fatigue, and fever are the most frequent presenting symptoms; autoimmune phenomena are common (26% of cases).[200,201] Hepatomegaly, splenomegaly, and lymphadenopathy are each found in about 60% of patients.[198,201] Routine serum protein electrophoresis may show hypogammaglobulinemia but may fail to identify an M protein. Immunofixation is necessary for diagnosis and reveals an incomplete gamma chain without a light chain.[198] Urine protein is usually less than 1 g/24 hours.[198] Anemia is present in more than half of patients; leukopenia and thrombocytopenia are also relatively common. Atypical lymphocytes and plasma cells may be found on blood smears. The bone marrow is involved by a lymphoproliferative disorder in two thirds of patients.[198,201]

Involved tissues show no consistent histopathologic pattern. A majority of patients with gamma chain disease have a malignancy similar to Waldenström's macroglobulinemia

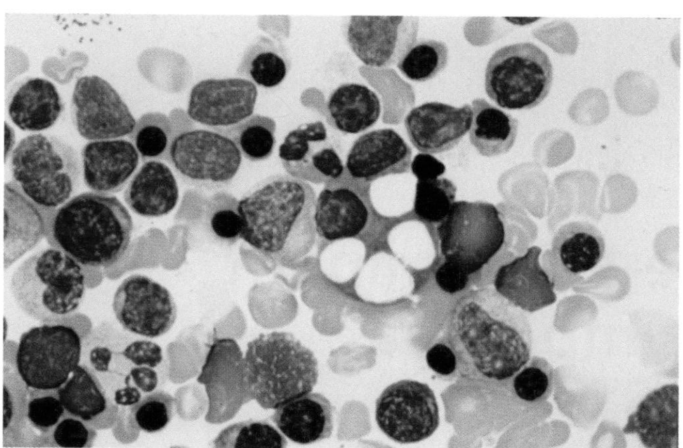

Figure 25-46. Plasma cells in mu heavy-chain disease. A plasma cell with several large, clear cytoplasmic vacuoles is illustrated. This type of plasma cell is characteristic but not pathognomonic of mu heavy-chain disease (Wright-Giemsa stain).

(lymphoplasmacytic lymphoma). In about 15% of cases there is a predominance of plasma cells in the lesions. Occasionally gamma chain disease is associated with CLL or a large cell lymphoma. In some cases there is no obvious evidence of a lymphoproliferative disorder.[198,201] The clinical course varies from asymptomatic and stable to an aggressive malignant process. Median survival is about 1 year.[196,201]

Mu Chain Disease

Mu chain disease is a very rare clonal B-cell neoplasm in which the mu heavy chain produced by the neoplastic cells lacks a variable region.[196,197] In more than half the patients with mu chain disease the proliferative cells produce monoclonal light chains that do not assemble with the heavy chain.[202] The light chains are excreted in the urine as Bence Jones protein.

The median age at diagnosis of mu chain disease is 48 years.[203,204] The majority of patients have a long history of CLL (or CLL-like lymphoproliferative disorder). The disorder differs from most cases of CLL by the high frequency of hepatosplenomegaly and the rarity of lymphadenopathy. Occasionally patients present with lymphoma, immunoblastic transformation of CLL, myeloma, or amyloidosis. Two thirds of patients with mu chain disease have characteristic vacuolated plasma cells in the bone marrow (Fig. 25-46). The plasma cells are typically mixed with small lymphocytes exhibiting features characteristic of CLL. The clinical course of mu chain disease is indolent and slowly progressive.

Alpha Chain Disease

Alpha chain disease is a variant of extranodal marginal zone lymphoma of MALT.[197,205] The disease is characterized by the secretion of defective alpha chains. It affects primarily young individuals, with a peak incidence in the second and third decades of life. There is a remarkably uniform clinical picture of severe malabsorption, chronic diarrhea, and abdominal pain and distention.[195,205-207] Enlarged mesenteric lymph nodes can often be palpated. Hepatosplenomegaly and lymphadenopathy are rare. The lymphoproliferative disorder associated with alpha chain disease involves the gastrointestinal tract, mainly the small intestine and mesenteric lymph nodes, and shows the characteristic features of MALT lymphoma. The lamina propria is heavily infiltrated with lymphoid cells, many at the plasma cell stage. The bone marrow is usually normal, but alpha chain–secreting plasma cells may be identified. The disease is responsive to antibiotic therapy in its early stages, but if untreated, it progresses to an aggressive lymphoma in most instances.

Waldenström's Macroglobulinemia

Waldenström's macroglobulinemia, an immunosecretory disorder usually associated with a lymphoplasmacytic lymphoma and production of IgM M protein, is discussed in Chapter 14 on chronic lymphoproliferative diseases.

Pearls and Pitfalls

Pearls

- Diagnosis of plasma cell neoplasms requires integration of clinical, morphologic, radiographic, and laboratory findings (especially serum and urine protein studies).
- Serum and urine immunofixation electrophoresis is the "gold standard" for characterizing the heavy and light chains of a monoclonal immunoglobulin and for detecting small quantities of M protein.
- Immunohistochemical stains are valuable for assessing the quantity of plasma cells in marrow biopsies, identifying a monoclonal plasma cell proliferation, and distinguishing myeloma from other neoplasms.
- Patients with MGUS must be followed indefinitely for evolution to a malignant plasma cell dyscrasia. Increasing size of the serum M protein is the most reliable parameter for predicting disease progression.
- Cytogenetic abnormalities have important prognostic significance in plasma cell myeloma and should be evaluated in all cases.
- A careful search, including MRI, should be carried out before making a diagnosis of solitary plasmacytoma of bone.

Pitfalls

- M protein may be undetectable with serum protein electrophoresis in cases with low levels of monoclonal immunoglobulin, as is common in IgD, IgE, and light-chain-only myeloma.
- Focal marrow myeloma lesions may be missed in random biopsies. The diagnostic yield can be directly related to the size and number of specimens.
- Extraosseous plasmacytoma must often be distinguished from lymphoplasmacytic lymphoma and marginal zone lymphoma with extreme plasma cell differentiation.
- Diagnosis of amyloidosis on marrow examination may be problematic. Amyloid deposition is often minimal or absent, the percentage of plasma cells is low, and their cytologic features are normal.

References can be found on Expert Consult @ www.expertconsult.com

Chapter 26

Nodular Lymphocyte-Predominant Type of Hodgkin's Lymphoma

Çiğdem Atayar and Sibrand Poppema

CHAPTER OUTLINE

DEFINITION

The nodular lymphocyte-predominant subtype of Hodgkin's lymphoma (NLPHL) is recognized as a separate entity in the World Health Organization (WHO) classification. This reflects the fact that there are clear and consistent histologic, epidemiologic, immunologic, and genetic differences between NLPHL and the other, so-called classical Hodgkin's lymphomas (CHLs). NLPHL is an indolent germinal center (GC) B-cell malignancy, representing a nodular proliferation comprising a minority of large neoplastic centroblasts with multilobated nuclei, the so-called popcorn or lymphocyte-predominant (LP) cells (formerly called *L & H cells, for lymphocytic and/or histiocytic Reed-Sternberg cell variants),* and a majority of reactive lymphocytes and histiocytes.

HISTORICAL BACKGROUND

Several schemes have been used to classify Hodgkin's lymphoma (HL) since 1947.[1] Jackson and Parker[1] identified three subtypes termed *Hodgkin's paragranuloma, Hodgkin's granuloma,* and *Hodgkin's sarcoma.* Hodgkin's paragranuloma was characterized by obliteration of the normal lymph node architecture by abundant small lymphocytes, among which Hodgkin Reed-Sternberg (HRS) cells were present as single cells or in small groups. In a study of follicular lymphomas, Hicks and associates[2] described a nodular variant of paragranuloma.

In the classification of HL proposed by Lukes and Butler in 1966, six subgroups were identified.[3] At the Rye conference on the staging of Hodgkin's disease,[4] the six subclasses of Lukes and Butler were reduced to four, combining their lymphohistiocytic nodular and lymphohistiocytic diffuse types into one class designated *lymphocyte predominant.* This so-called Rye classification was in widespread use until the 1990s.

In 1979 Poppema and coworkers[5-7] published a series of three papers on the histology, immunophenotype, and epidemiology of the nodular and diffuse lymphocyte-predominant subtype of Hodgkin's disease, indicating that NLPHL was a separate entity. In these papers, the association between progressively transformed germinal centers (PTGCs) and NLPHL was established, as well as the first documented cases of transition to diffuse large B-cell lymphoma (DLBCL). Further, it was established that NLPHL and its diffuse variant (nodular paragranuloma and diffuse paragranuloma) did not transform to other subtypes. In the 1980s, clinical studies delineated important differences in immunophenotype and clinical course between NLPHL and CHL.

A more formal distinction between NLPHL and CHL was proposed by the International Lymphoma Study Group in the Revised European American Lymphoma (REAL) classification.[8] This proposal was adopted by the WHO classification,[9] which emphasizes that NLPHL is biologically distinct from CHL. A category of lymphocyte-rich CHL (LRCHL) was proposed in the REAL classification as resembling the lymphocyte-predominant HL of the Rye classification, based on the abundance of normal lymphocytes, but being biologically and clinically more closely related to CHL. A nodular form of LRCHL was described by Ashton-Key and colleagues,[10] which they termed *follicular Hodgkin's lymphoma*. Both nodular and diffuse forms of LRCHL are included in the WHO classification and are discussed more fully in Chapter 27.

EPIDEMIOLOGY

NLPHL accounts for 3% to 8% of HLs in Western countries.[11,12] In some series, up to half the cases may in fact have been LRCHL. NLPHL occurs in all age groups, with a peak incidence in the fourth decade, in contrast to a peak incidence in the third decade for the nodular sclerosis subtype (Fig. 26-1).[7,13] There is a male preponderance of 2.4:1, different from the slight preponderance of female patients with the nodular sclerosis type. There are no significant differences between cases that are exclusively nodular and those with prominent diffuse areas.

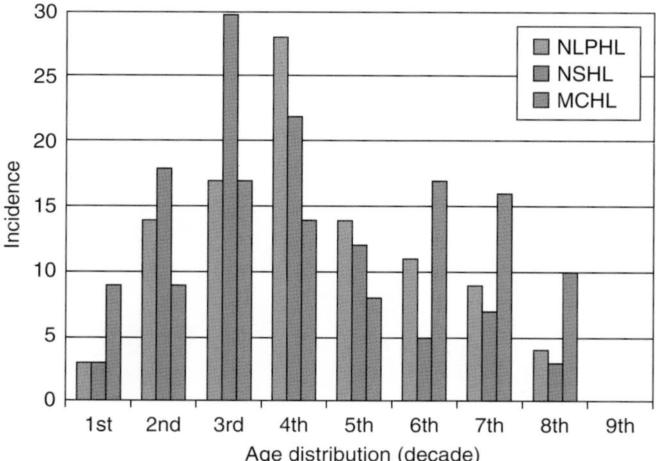

Figure 26-1. Age distribution of nodular lymphocyte-predominant Hodgkin's lymphoma (NLPHL; *n* = 206), nodular sclerosis Hodgkin's lymphoma (NSHL; *n* = 398), and mixed cellularity Hodgkin's lymphoma (MCHL; *n* = 293) in a series of cases from the Lymph Node Registry in Kiel, Germany, 1978. Note the peak incidence of NLPHL in the fourth decade, versus the peak incidence of NSHL in the third decade.

There are several indications that HL may have an infectious cause,[14,15] and there is extensive evidence that Epstein-Barr virus (EBV) plays a role in a major subset of CHL.[16,17] The published data regarding the association between NLPHL and EBV appear to be confusing. Although some investigators, especially in developing countries, reported positive cases,[18-21] most others found only negative cases.[22,23] A consensus review of NLPHL cases revealed that all were negative for EBV genomes, and the plausible explanation for the discordant data is the inclusion of LRCHL cases in the series that found EBV$^+$ cases.[24] Early EBV infection, as seen in developing countries, may be an alternative explanation for the occurrence of rare EBV$^+$ NLPHL in some series.[20] A possible role for other viruses, including human herpesvirus 6, has been studied,[25] but no other viruses have been demonstrated to date.

Immune responses to HL may be influenced by interindividual genetic variations. There have been numerous suggestions that HL is influenced by the human leukocyte antigen (HLA) class II region, and specifically by alleles at the HLA-DPB1 locus (DPB1*0301 associated with susceptibility, and DPB1*0201 with resistance),[26,27] although the relative risks associated with these alleles were small. Taylor and colleagues[28] also found that susceptibility to NLPHL is associated with the DPB1*2001 allele. Only rare familial cases of NLPHL have been reported to date.[29] The risk of HL in young adults decreases with an increasing number of C alleles at position −174 in the interleukin-6 promoter.[30] A significant excess of G alleles at this position was observed in young adults with NLPHL.[31] Although CHL is seen with increased frequency in human immunodeficiency virus (HIV)–infected patients, a risk for NLPHL has not been observed.[32]

CLINICAL FEATURES

Patients usually present with isolated lymphadenopathy of long duration. There is frequent involvement of cervical and axillary nodes, with less frequent inguinal or femoral nodal involvement. Mediastinal NLPHL is an unusual finding (7%).[13,33] The most frequently involved primary extranodal sites include the tonsil, parotid gland, and soft tissue. The liver and spleen are common extranodal sites of high-stage node-based disease. B symptoms are uncommon and are found in only 10% of patients.[33] Bone marrow involvement by NLPHL is extremely rare (2.5%) and is associated with aggressive clinical behavior and a poor prognosis.

NLPHL typically presents as early-stage disease, with slow progression and an excellent outcome with standard therapy. Approximately 20% of patients have advanced disease at the time of presentation.[13] Recurrences develop in a relatively high percentage (≈21%), regardless of original clinical stage, and multiple recurrences (27%) are not uncommon.[13] In 65% of cases the recurrence is local or regional, in 23% the recurrence is in a different region, and in 12% the disease is generalized.

NLPHL does not transform to other subtypes of HL.[5] Transformation to DLBCL has been reported to occur in 3% to 10% of cases.[5,34] Less commonly, NLPHL and DLBCL are seen in the same site as composite lymphoma.[35,36] The issues of transformation to DLBCL and the potential relation to T-cell/histiocyte-rich B-cell lymphoma (T/HRBCL) are discussed later.

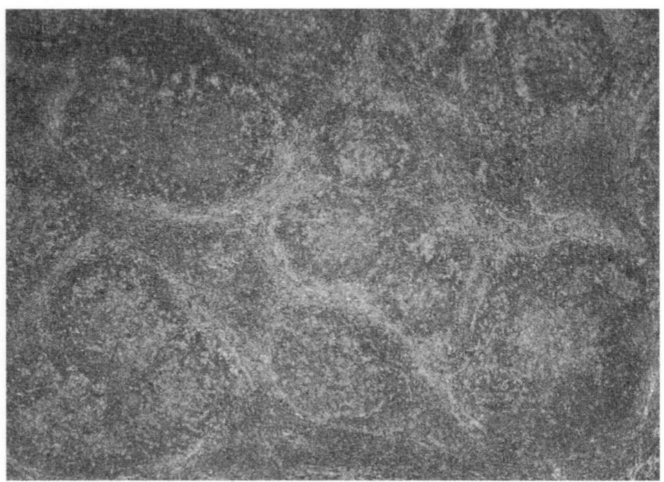

Figure 26-2. The normal lymph node architecture is replaced by nodules containing predominantly small lymphocytes.

MORPHOLOGY

At low magnification, complete obliteration of the lymph node architecture is usually evident. In some cases a compressed rim of normal lymphoid tissue with reactive follicles is present in the periphery of the node, usually sharply demarcated from the tumor tissue. Fan and associates[37] described six immunoarchitectural patterns of NLPHL: classic B-cell-rich nodular; serpiginous nodular; nodular with prominent extranodular LP cells; T-cell-rich nodular; diffuse T/HRBCL-like; and diffuse with a B-cell–rich pattern. A mixture of patterns in a single biopsy is more commonly observed than a single, pure pattern. Neoplastic cells are found both within and outside the macronodules (Fig. 26-2).[5,6] The nodularity created by loose aggregates of follicular dendritic cells (FDCs) is generally easily appreciated in routine hematoxylin-eosin slides, but it may be visualized by immunohistochemistry. The nodules vary in size, but they are mostly large. A diffuse growth pattern can be seen focally; rarely, it may predominate.

The predominant cell population in the nodules is small lymphocytes. The presence of histiocytes and LP cells leads to a "moth-eaten" appearance (Fig. 26-3). The number of epithelioid histiocytes varies, and in some cases they are the most conspicuous cells. This feature led to the original term *lymphohistiocytic type of Hodgkin's disease*. In some cases, groups of epithelioid cells may form a ring in a circular pattern around the nodules (Fig. 26-4).

Scattered FDC nuclei can be identified; in some cases multinucleated, Warthin-Finkeldey–type giant cells are seen. These are most likely FDC multinucleated variants (Fig. 26-5). The cellular composition of the nodules may vary within the same lymph node: nodules with a predominance of lymphocytes can be seen together with nodules showing a large proportion of epithelioid histiocytes.

Occasionally, only a small number of LP cells are present; more often, they can be found with little difficulty. In rare cases, they form large clusters and are the most conspicuous cell type within some nodules. The clinical significance of this variation is not known. Classic HRS cells are not required to make a diagnosis of NLPHL, but neoplastic cells resembling classic HRS cells are not as infrequent as previously reported in the literature.[5,24] The identification of classic HRS cells should always prompt careful immunohistochemical evaluation to exclude the possibility of LRCHL with a nodular pattern. However, it is also recognized that in some cases of NLPHL the LP cells may mimic classic HRS cells while retaining the immunophenotype of LP cells.

The compressed internodular areas contain small lymphocytes and high endothelial venules. Plasma cells and eosinophils are characteristically scarce or absent. In some cases of NLPHL there is a nodular sclerotic stromal reaction, particularly in large nodal masses. Because a documented history of long-term nodal enlargement is available in some of these cases, it is possible that this represents a chronic-phase tissue reaction to the NLPHL.

Lymphocyte-Predominant Cells

LP cells are large cells, with nuclei larger than those of normal centroblasts (see Fig. 26-5). Owing to their complex lobation, the term *popcorn cells* has been widely used. The nucleoli are medium-sized, generally basophilic, and smaller than those of classic HRS cells. The cytoplasm of LP cells is relatively sparse. In Giemsa-stained tissue sections and in Wright-

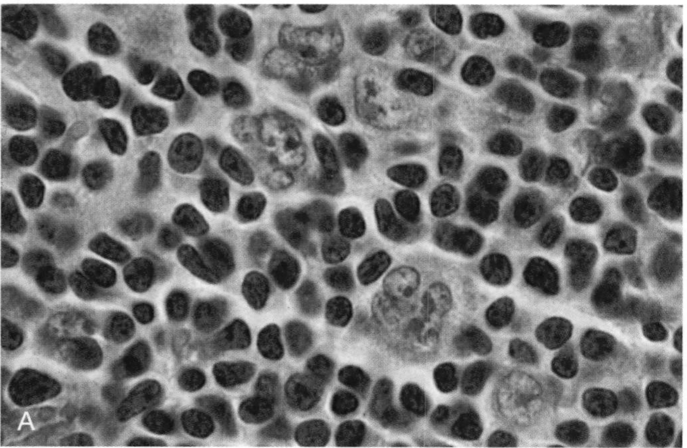

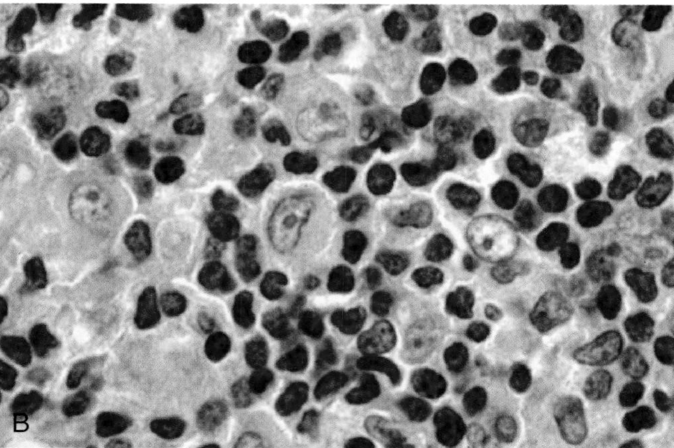

Figure 26-3. A, Several LP-type HRS cells with multilobated nuclei and a small rim of cytoplasm can be seen. **B,** Several histiocytes with prominent cytoplasm are present. Both cell types are surrounded by small lymphocytes.

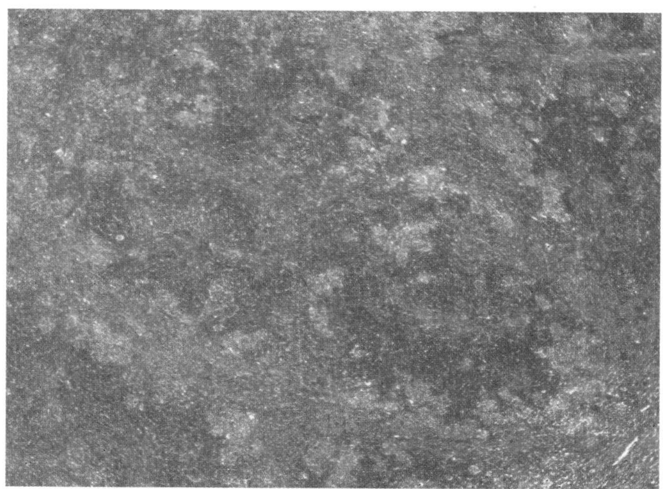

Figure 26-4. Sometimes the nodules of nodular lymphocyte-predominant Hodgkin's lymphoma are surrounded by clusters of epithelioid histiocytes.

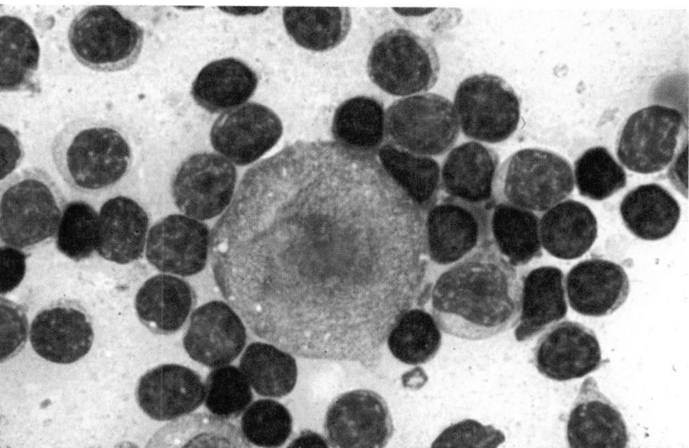

Figure 26-5. Imprint of lymph node with nodular lymphocyte-predominant Hodgkin's lymphoma showing an LP cell surrounded by rosetting activated lymphocytes.

stained imprints or smears, the cytoplasm may be moderately basophilic.

Diffuse Variant

The absence of criteria by which a diffuse variant of NLPHL (D-LPHL) can be distinguished from T/HRBCL with available methodologies has led to some controversy over whether the former actually exists.[38] An argument in favor of the existence of D-LPHL is that many cases of NLPHL have diffuse areas and other cases transform to a diffuse morphology. Therefore it appears likely that there are also primary diffuse variants.[39] The presence of numerous LP cells outside the nodules may predict for progression to a diffuse T/HRBCL-like pattern.[37] Metachronous occurrence of D-LPHL after NLPHL has been described.[40]

A precise definition of D-LPHL does not exist in the literature, but it is defined arbitrarily as a lymphoma with cytologic characteristics of NLPHL but lacking evidence of a nodular growth pattern either morphologically or with adjunctive immunophenotypic studies. In a review of a large series of patients with LPHL by the European Task Force on Lymphoma, only 2% of the cases were without nodular areas.[41] In the largest series of NLPHL cases reviewed, only 7 cases out of 219 (3%) closely resembled T/HRBCL by the presence of loosely distributed neoplastic cells in a background infiltrate of lymphocytes without evidence of nodularity.[24]

A majority of the diffuse cases in older studies would likely be included in the nodular type today, owing to the ability to demonstrate the presence of an FDC meshwork by immunohistochemistry. Other cases, especially those without supportive evidence from immunohistochemical studies, could be examples of LRCHL.

The major diagnostic features of NLPHL are summarized in Table 26-1.

IMMUNOPHENOTYPE

Lymphocyte-Predominant Cells

Lymphocyte Signaling Molecules

LP cells stain with anti–leukocyte common antigen (LCA/CD45) antibodies as well as CD45RA (KiB3), CD45RB, and CD45RC, but not CD45RO (UCHL1) reagents, in contrast to most classic HRS cells (Table 26-2).[42,92] There is consistent staining for pan–B-cell markers such as CD20 (L26) (Fig. 26-6A), CD22, MB2, CDw75 (LN1), and CD79a in frozen and paraffin tissue sections of NLPHL cases.[44-48,93] This profile differs from that of HRS cells in CHL, which typically show CD20 expression in only a subset of neoplastic cells and cases.[94,95] L26 recognizes a cytoplasmic portion of the CD20 molecule and is present in greater abundance than surface CD20. CD79a is usually positive but varies in intensity.[24] LP

Table 26-1 Major Diagnostic Features of Nodular Lymphocyte-Predominant Hodgkin's Lymphoma

Feature	LP Cells	Background Cells
Morphology	Nuclei larger than centroblasts, hyperlobated nuclei, medium-sized nucleoli, sparse basophilic cytoplasm	Follicles with predominantly small lymphocytes, together with histiocytes and LP cells; "moth-eaten" appearance
Immunophenotypic features	$CD45^+$, $CD20^+$, $CD15^-$, $CD30^-$, $BCL6^+$, AID^+, $BSAP^+$, Oct-2^+, BOB.1^+, PU.$1^{+/-}$, MUM-$1^{+/-}$, T-$bet^{+/-}$, $HGAL^+$, $BCL2^-$, $p53^-$, $CD10^-$, $CD138^-$, EBV^-	Predominantly $CD4^+$ T cells; $CD4^+$, c-Maf^+, $CD57^+$, PD-1^+ T-cell rosettes around LP cells are present; low ratio of TIA-1^+ to $CD57^+$ T cells
Genetic and molecular findings	Clonal immunoglobulin gene rearrangements; ongoing mutations; *BCL6* rearrangements in half of cases; *BCL2* translocation usually not detected	Polyclonal B and T cells

AID, activation-induced cytidine deaminase; EBV, Epstein-Barr virus; HGAL, human germinal center–associated lymphoma protein; LP, lymphocyte predominant.

Table 26-2 **Antigen Expression of Lymphocyte-Predominant Cells**

Antigen	Significance	Findings
Lymphocyte Signaling Molecules		
CD45 (LCA)	All leukocytes Tyrosine phosphatase activity	Positive[43]
CD45RA (KIB3)	B cells, T-cell subsets, monocytes	Positive[43]
CD45RB	Thymocytes, T cells	Positive
CD45RC	B cells, $CD8^+$ T cells	Positive
CD45RO (UCHL1)	Thymocytes, monocytes, macrophages, granulocytes	Negative
CD20 (L26)	B cells (not plasma cells)	≈100% positive[44-48]
MB2	B cells (not plasma cells)	Positive[44-48]
CDw75 (LN1)	GC cells	Positive[44-48]
CD79A (MB1)	Pan–B cell	Positive, but lower than CD20[24]
CD19	B cells (not plasma cells)	Negative[49]
CD40	B cells, dendritic cells, macrophages	Positive[50]
CD70	Activated B and T cells, receptor for CD27	Positive[50]
CD80	GC blasts and APC, receptor for CD28 and CTLA-4	Positive[50]
CD86	GC blasts and APC, receptor for CD28 and CTLA-4	Positive[50]
MHC II (TAL1B5)	Control of immune responses through presentation of peptide antigens to T cells	Positive
CD74 (LN2)	B cell, invariant chain of MHC II	Positive
CD30 (Ki1/Ber H2)	Activated T and B cells	Generally negative[24]
CD15 (Leu M1)	Myeloid cells	Negative[24]
J chain	B cell	≈60% positive[51,52]
IgG, IgM, IgA, IgD	B cell	Variably positive
Igκ, Igλ	B cell	Variably positive
FREB	Leukocyte Fc receptor family, GC B cell	Positive[53]
AID	Essential for SHM and CSR in GC B cells	Positive[54]
GCET1	GC B cells	Positive[55]
HGAL (GCET2)	GC B cells	Positive[56]
SWAP70	B cells, specificity for the switch regions upstream of the constant region Ig genes	Positive[57]
CD10	GC B cells	Negative[58,59]
Signaling Intermediates		
NTAL	Adapter protein, linker for activation of B cells	Positive[60]
CD138 (SDC1)	Post-GC terminal B cells, epithelial cells	Negative[61]
LYN kinase	B-cell intracellular signaling molecule	Usually negative[62]
JAK2	B-cell intracellular nonreceptor tyrosine kinase	Positive[63]
Transcription Factors and Regulators		
Oct-1	Ig gene TF	Positive[64]
Oct-2	Ig geneTF	Positive[64]
BOB.1	Essential for response of B cells to antigens and formation of GC	Positive[64]
BSAP/PAX5	B-cell development and differentiation	Positive[64]
ID2	Negative regulation of E2A and PAX5	Positive[65]
PU.1	Ig gene TF	Variably positive[66,67]
MUM-1	Subset of GC B cells, plasma cells	Inconsistently positive[68]
BCL6	TF expressed in GC cells	Positive[69]
BLIMP1	GC B cells showing plasma cell differentiation, plasma cells	Negative[70]
FOXP1	Mantle zone, some GC B cells	Negative[71]
T-bet	Th1 cell development, role in Ig class switching	Half of cases positive[72]
GATA3	Th2 cell development	Negative[72]
GATA2	Development of hematopoiesis	Negative[73]
c-Maf	Th2 cells, responsible for tissue-specific expression of IL-4	Negative[72]
NFATc1	Normal homeostasis and differentiation	Usually cytoplasmic positive[74]
REL (c-Rel)	NF-κB family member, antiapoptotic activity, function in lymphopoiesis	Negative >> positive[75]
RELA	NF-κB family member, antiapoptotic activity, function in lymphopoiesis	Positive[76]
BAFF-R (TNFRSF13C)	Mantle zone B cells, subset of GC B cells	Weakly positive or negative[77]
JUNB	Component of AP1 transcription complex involved in cell proliferation and apoptosis	Negative[78]
Cell Cycle Proteins		
Ki-67 (MKI67)	Marker of proliferation	Positive
PCNA	Proliferating cells	Positive[79]
TOP2A	Cell proliferation marker	Positive[80]

Table 26-2 Antigen Expression of Lymphocyte-Predominant Cells (Continued)

Antigen	Significance	Findings
Tumor Suppressors and Apoptosis-Related Proteins		
CASP3	CD95-mediated apoptosis	Negative[81,82]
c-FLIP	Competitive negative regulator of Fas-induced death	Negative >> positive[83]
p53	Apoptosis-related protein	Negative[84]
TP73L (p63)	Subset of GC B cells	Positive[85]
BCL2	Represses cell death by apoptosis	Negative[22]
BAX	Promotes cell death by apoptosis	Positive[86]
A20	Inhibits cell death by apoptosis induced by TNF	Variably positive[87]
TRAF1	Downstream component in CD30 signaling pathway	Negative[75]
Structural Proteins and Adhesion Molecules		
Vimentin	Intermediate filament	Negative[88]
Fascin	Actin bundling protein, dendritic cell marker	Negative[89]
CD44H	Mediates adhesion of leukocytes	Negative[90]
EMA	Epithelial cells, plasma cells	Variably positive[91,92]

AID, activation-induced cytidine deaminase; APC, antigen presenting cell; AP1, activator protein-1; BAFF-R, B-cell activating factor receptor; CSR, class switch recombination; EMA, epithelial membrane antigen; FREB, Fc receptor homologue expressed in B cells; GC, germinal center; GCET, germinal center B-cell expressed transcript; HGAL, human germinal center–associated lymphoma protein; Ig, immunoglobulin; IL, interleukin; MHC, major histocompatibility complex; NFAT, nuclear factor of activated T cells; NF-κB, nuclear factor-κB; NTAL, non–T-cell activation linker; PCNA, proliferating cell nuclear antigen; SHM, somatic hypermutation; SWAP70; switch-associated protein-70; TF, transcription factor; TNF, tumor necrosis factor; TOP2A, topoisomerase II alpha enzyme.

cells commonly lack CD19.[49] LP-type cells also stain for CD40, CD70, CD80, CD86, HLA class II, and CD74 (the invariant chain of HLA class II).[50,96] All these are also expressed on normal GC blasts, with the exception of CD70, which is the receptor for CD27. In normal GCs, CD70 expression appears to be confined to GC blasts expressing only immunoglobulin (Ig) D, which can be seen sporadically in clusters in GCs of tonsil.

CD30 (Ki-1, Ber-H2) staining is usually negative.[58,97,98] In a few cases, weak, usually cytoplasmic staining of LP cells can be discernible. The NLPHL-derived cell line DEV also expresses CD30, albeit less intensely than the CHL-derived cell lines.[99] Thus, expression of CD30 should not totally exclude a diagnosis of NLPHL.[100] In contrast, strongly CD30$^+$ parafollicular immunoblasts located outside the B-cell nodules are more commonly identified and represent a potential diagnostic pitfall.[58] LP cells are typically negative for CD15 (Leu M1), but CD15 may be expressed in a subset of neoplastic cells in otherwise typical cases.[24]

LP cells, in contrast to other types of HRS cells, produce J chain, a 15-kD polypeptide essential for linking to the tailpieces of multimeric immunoglobulin molecules (see Fig. 26-6B).[51,52] Because J chain is not present in serum, the demonstration of J chain in LP cells cannot be the result of phagocytosis or endocytosis but indicates immunoglobulin production, providing the first definitive proof of the B-cell origin of LP cells. In paraffin sections LP cells infrequently express demonstrable cytoplasmic IgG, IgM, and IgA. However, strong expression for only IgD is identified in a subset of cases, most often young males with cervical lymph node involvement.[101] Fc receptor homologue expressed in B cells (FREB) is a member of the family of Fc receptors for IgG. It is expressed predominantly in normal GC B cells, mantle zone cells, and a majority of NLPHL cases.[53] Activation-induced cytidine deaminase (AID) is indispensable for class switch recombination and somatic hypermutation of immunoglobulin genes. In keeping with the notion that LP cells represent transformed GC B cells showing evidence of somatic hypermutation, AID is consistently expressed in LP cells.[54] New markers of GC derivation, such as GC B-cell expressed transcript 1 (GCET1),[55] human GC-associated lymphoma protein (HGAL-GCET2),[56] and switch-associated protein-70

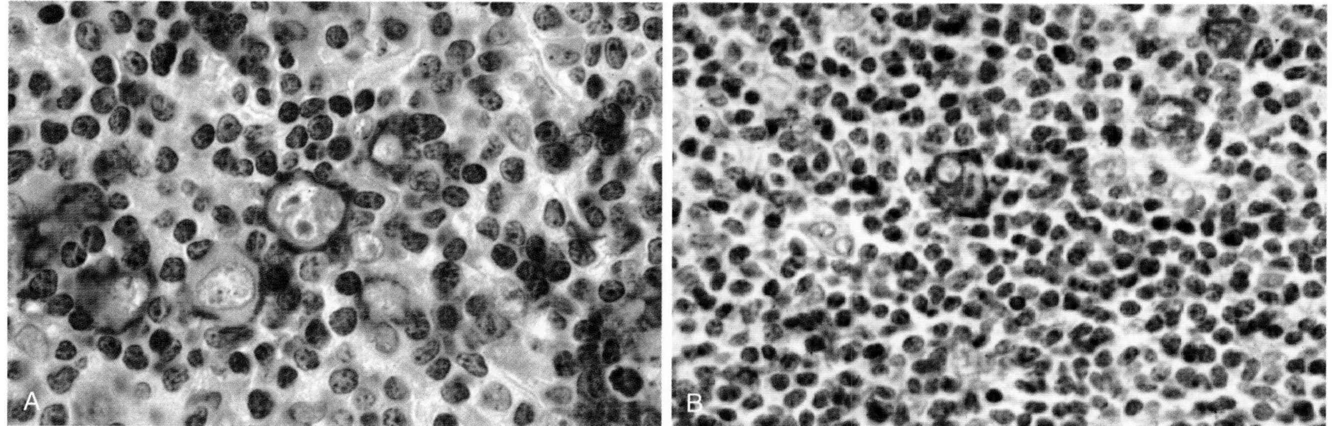

Figure 26-6. Immunohistologic stain for CD20 (L26) shows positive membrane staining of several LP-type HRS cells (**A**), and stain for J chain shows positive cytoplasm in an LP-type HRS cell (**B**).

(SWAP70),[57] are also expressed in the majority of NLPHL cases. However, another GC B-cell marker, CD10, is negative.[59]

Signaling Intermediates

Recently, the expression of a new group of molecules called *transmembrane adapter proteins* that are involved in receptor signaling in immune cells has been investigated.[60] Among the seven transmembrane adapter proteins known to date, LP cells express only the non–T-cell activation linker that is also expressed in most B cells and B-cell neoplasms.[60] This linker functions as a negative regulator of early stages of B-cell receptor signaling. Syndecans (SDC) are transmembrane proteoglycans that play an important role in cell-matrix and cell-cell interactions, as well as modulating receptor activation.[102] In hematopoietic cells, SDC1 is expressed only in B cells at pre-B and plasma cell differentiation stages.[103] LP cells are SDC1$^-$, in accordance with their derivation from GC B cells.[59,61]

In most CHL cases, several receptor tyrosine kinases are expressed, whereas none are detected in 50% of NLPHL cases. Receptor tyrosine kinase A, which is essential for the survival of memory B cells, was in fact expressed in only 30% of NLPHLs in one study.[104] JAK2, an intracellular non–receptor tyrosine kinase that transduces cytokine-mediated signals via the JAK2/STAT pathway, is expressed in most NLPHL cases.[63]

Transcription Factors and Regulators

Transcription factors regulating the expression of immunoglobulin genes and other genes important for B-cell development (e.g., BSAP/PAX5, Oct-1, Oct-2, BOB.1) are consistently expressed in LP cells.[64] ID2, which is uniformly expressed in the HRS cells of CHL and likely represses B-cell–specific gene expression by inactivating E2A (and perhaps also PAX5), is also aberrantly expressed in LP cells and might contribute to the reduced expression of some B-cell genes.[65] PU.1 is reported to be variably expressed in NLPHL but absent in both CHL and T/HRBCL.[66,67] PU.1 staining is stronger in reactive macrophages and myeloid elements than in LP cells, and PU.1$^+$ histiocytes may be confused morphologically with LP cells. MUM-1-IRF4 cooperates with PU.1 as a transcriptional regulator in lymphoid cells.[105] Similar to the variable expression of PU.1 in LP cells, MUM-1 is inconsistently expressed in LP cells.[68] MUM-1$^+$ cells in reactive lymph nodes consist of plasma cells and a small fraction of B cells located in the light zone of the GC.[106] BCL6 positivity in B cells indicates derivation from GC B cells. In normal GC B cells, MUM-1 function can be blocked by BCL6.[107] Therefore, expression of MUM-1 and BCL6 are accepted as mutually exclusive in normal GC B cells. Unlike the situation in normal GC B cells, BCL6 is consistently present in LP cells, together with inconsistent expression of MUM-1.[59,61] BLIMP1 (PRDM1) is a transcriptional repressor that affects multiple key target genes for the terminal differentiation of B cells along the plasma cell lineage.[108] However, it is negative in both CHL and NLPHL.[70]

Expression of FOXP1 has been demonstrated in normal activated B cells using genomic scale expression profiling.[109,110] The physiologic role of FOXP1 in lymphocytes is unclear. It is expressed in DLBCL of the activated B-cell type[111] but is negative in both CHL and NLPHL.[71] T-bet (TBX21) is expressed in CD4$^+$ T lymphocytes committed to T-helper-1 (Th1) T-cell development[112] and in a subset of T-cell non-Hodgkin's lymphomas. The role of T-bet in B-lymphocyte development is not well understood, but it may participate in immunoglobulin class switching.[113] In reactive lymphoid tissues, the vast majority of B cells do not express T-bet,[114] whereas the neoplastic cells of NLPHL and CHL are positive.[72] However, other T-cell transcription factors such as GATA3, MAF (c-Maf), and GATA2 are not expressed in LP cells.[72] The absence of GATA transcription factors in LP cells is not surprising, because PU.1 expression inhibits the expression of the genes that encode GATA factors.[115] In T cells, nuclear factor of activated T cells (NFAT) is required for effector differentiation, whereas in B cells, NFAT regulates both normal homeostasis and differentiation.[116] NFATc1 normally resides in the cytoplasm but relocates to the nucleus when activation of the pathway leads to its dephosphorylation. LP cells show cytoplasmic NFATc1 staining in most cases and nuclear NFATc1 staining in some cases, whereas in classic HRS cells, NFATc1 is expressed in only a minority of cases.[74]

Nuclear factor-κB (NF-κB) plays a key role in the regulation of immune and inflammatory responses, functions as a potent inhibitor of apoptosis, and is involved in the malignant transformation of different cell types.[117] Depending on the stimulus, the duration of stimulation, and the cellular context, the NF-κB family members p50, p52, p65 (RELA), RELB, and REL (c-Rel) form different homo- or heterodimers. The constitutive activation of the NF-κB pathway is involved in the proliferation and survival of HRS cells in CHL.[118] REL (c-Rel) generally is not expressed in LP cells,[75] but NF-κB p65 subunit RELA is observed in all cases of NLPHL.[76] The physiologic and clinical significance of nuclear RELA expression in LP cells is currently undefined. B-cell activating factor receptor (BAFF-R) is required for the NF-κB alternative activation pathway.[119] Although most cases of B-cell lymphoproliferative disorders (78%) are BAFF-R$^+$, NLPHL exhibits weak to negative staining for BAFF-R,[77] which may imply that the NF-κB alternative activation pathway is not involved in LP cells. The activator protein-1 (AP1) family of transcription factors has been implicated in the control of proliferation, apoptosis, and malignant transformation. JUNB is a transcription factor belonging to the AP1 family that binds to the CD30 promoter. In classic HRS cells, CD30 overexpression has been attributed to the constitutive expression of JUNB.[120] LP cells are negative for JUNB, which is consistent with a CD30$^-$ phenotype.[78]

Cell Cycle Proteins

Immunostains for proliferation-associated nuclear proteins such as Ki-67 or proliferating cell nuclear antigen are positive in the LP cells, indicating that they are in cycle.[121] The topoisomerase II alpha enzyme (TOP2A), which controls and alters the topologic states of DNA during transcription and is the target for several chemotherapeutic agents, shows a high level of immunohistochemical expression in LP cells.[80] High TOP2A expression in LP cells might correlate with a favorable outcome in patients with NLPHL treated with TOP2A inhibitors such as doxorubicin or epirubicin.

Tumor Suppressors and Apoptosis-Related Proteins

Caspase 3 (CASP3), which is important for CD95-/Fas-mediated apoptosis, is not expressed at detectable levels in NLPHL, similar to low-grade non-Hodgkin's lymphomas.[81,82] The competitive negative regulator of Fas-induced apoptosis,

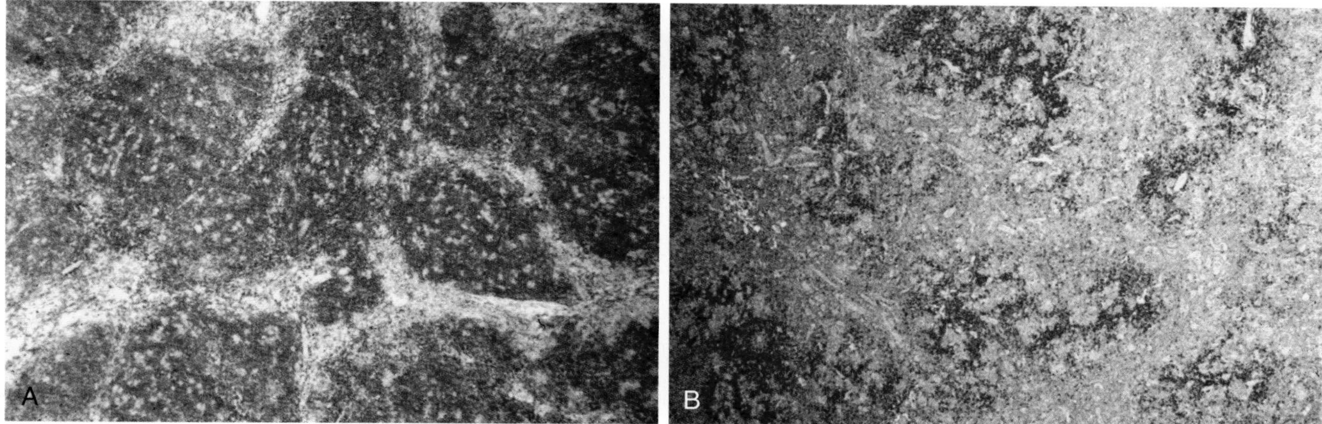

Figure 26-7. Immunohistologic stains for CD20 (L26) show a large majority of positive-staining small B lymphocytes in the nodules (**A**) and a minority that stain positively in another case (**B**).

c-FLIP, was found to be expressed in a lower proportion (32%) of NLPHL cases compared with CHL (81%) or DLBCL (93%) cases.[83] In contrast to CHL, p53 is not expressed in NLPHL.[84] Tumor protein p73-like (TP73L), or p63, is a member of a newly discovered family of proteins related to the tumor suppressor p53.[122] In p63 knockouts, severe developmental abnormalities are exhibited, but there is no increased cancer susceptibility, in contrast to p53 knockouts.[123] This p63 is expressed in a subset of GC B cells and in NLPHL, but not in CHL.[85]

The balance between BCL2 and BAX is important for the induction of programmed cell death; when BCL2 predominates, apoptosis is inhibited, whereas when levels of BAX are increased, the cell initiates the apoptotic machinery.[124] BCL2 overexpression is not present in LP cells,[22] but BAX is expressed in LP cells in all cases of NLPHL.[86]

A20 and TRAF1 are two antiapoptotic components of the intracellular signaling pathway of the tumor necrosis factor receptor (TNFR) family. CD30 stimulation induces A20 and TRAF1 expression.[87] A20 but not TRAF1 is expressed in NLPHL, although in variable numbers of LP cells.[75,87] Because most NLPHL cases are CD30$^-$, it is plausible that stimulation of another member of the TNFR family, such as CD40, may also control A20 expression in LP cells.[125]

Structural Proteins and Adhesion Molecules

Vimentin[88] and fascin,[89] usually positive in classic HRS cells, are not expressed by LP cells. Staining for CD44H shows variable membranous and Golgi area reactivity in the neoplastic cells of all CHLs but is negative in NLPHL.[90] Expression of epithelial membrane antigen by LP cells has been reported in several studies.[91,92] However, it is often identified in only a small proportion of neoplastic cells, and in many cases it is negative. Thus, it is generally not a diagnostically useful marker.

Background Cells

The LP cells usually reside in the background of small B cells, most of which derive from the follicular mantle and are IgM and IgD positive.[126,127] These lymphocytes are also positive for CD20, CD21, CD22, and CD45RA (Ki-B3) and negative for CD45RB (MT3) (Fig. 26-7; Table 26-3).[5,44,46,48,69,114,127-131] The expression of CD23 is relatively strong, which has also been noted in PTGCs. Over time, the proportion of small background B cells tends to decrease, and in multiple-relapse cases B cells may be few in number.

Immunohistochemical studies indicate that the number of T cells in the nodules of NLPHL is highly variable, ranging from a minority to a vast majority of cells.[44] In one study, flow cytometric analysis identified a mean of 61% T cells in five NLPHL cases.[132] Even if few, the T cells usually form rosettes around the LP cells. There are indications that the proportion of T cells in the nodules increases over time, and especially in recurrences, a high proportion of T cells can be found. A significant proportion of such T cells has a distinctive immunophenotype: c-Maf$^+$, CD2$^+$, CD3$^+$, CD4$^+$, PD1$^+$, CD57$^+$.[44,114,127,129,133,134] The characteristic T cells usually directly surround the LP cells in rosettes or collarettes (Fig. 26-8).[48] The staining intensity for CD57 varies, and it may represent an activation antigen on GC T cells. It is important to note that all anti-CD57 monoclonal reagents are of the mouse IgM subclass, and that this may result in suboptimal staining when secondary reagents are used that are geared toward detecting mouse IgG.

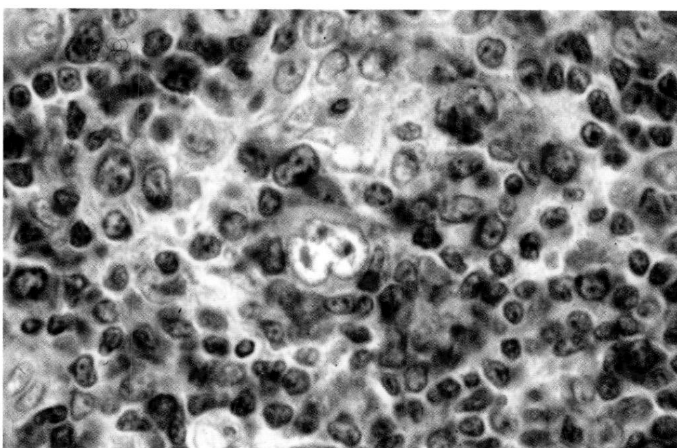

Figure 26-8. LP cells surrounded by an almost complete rosette of CD57$^+$ lymphocytes, with several other CD57$^+$ lymphocytes in the area. Note the dot-like cytoplasmic staining in the CD57$^+$ lymphocytes.

Table 26-3 Antigen Expression of Background Cells in Nodular Lymphocyte-Predominant Hodgkin's Lymphoma

Antigen	Significance	Findings
Background T Lymphocytes		
CD2	T cells, thymocytes, NK cells	Positive[44,127]
CD3	T cells, thymocytes	Positive[44,127]
CD4	Th and Tr cells	Positive[48]
CD45RA	B cells, naïve T cells, monocytes	Negative[48]
CD45RO	B-cell subsets, T-cell subsets	Positive[48]
CD57	NK cells, GC Th cells	Positive[48]
PD1	GC T cells	Positive[129]
CD69	Early activation marker	Positive[44,48]
CD134	Early activation marker	Positive
CD38	Persistent activation marker	Negative
MHC II	Control of immune responses through presentation of peptide antigens to T cells	Negative[48]
CD25	Activated T and B cells and monocytes IL-2R	Negative[48]
CD71	Activated leukocytes, function as transferrin receptor	Negative[48]
CD40L	Activated T-cell subset ligand for CD40	Negative[69]
TIA-1	Cytotoxic T cells and NK cells	Negative or few cells positive[130]
BCL6	GC Th cells	Positive[131]
c-Maf	Th2 cells, responsible for tissue-specific expression of IL-4	Positive[114]
T-bet	Th2 cell development, role in Ig class switching	Predominantly negative[114]
GATA3	Th2 cell development	Predominantly negative[114]
MUM-1	Subset of GC B cells, plasma cells	Positive
Background B Lymphocytes		
CD20 (L26)	B cells (not plasma cells)	Positive[44]
CD21	Mature B cells, FDCs	Positive
CD22	B cells (not plasma cells)	Positive
CD23	Mantle zone B cells, T cells, macrophages, platelets, eosinophils	Positive
CD45RA (KIB3)	B cells, T-cell subsets, monocytes	Positive[128]
CD45RB(MT3)	Thymocytes, T cells	Negative[128]
IgM	Bright on B cells in mantle and marginal zone	Positive[5,44,46]
Follicular Dendritic Cell Meshwork		
IgD	Bright on mantle zone B cells	Positive[5,44,46]
CD21	Mature B cells, FDCs	Positive[5,44]
CD35	FDC marker, C3b rec	Positive[5,44]
FDC	FDC marker	Positive[5,44]
CD23	Mantle zone B cells, T cells, macrophages, platelets, eosinophils	Negative[5,44]
CD21L (R4/23)	FDC marker	Positive[5,44]

FDC, follicular dendritic cell; GC, germinal center; Ig, immunoglobulin; IL, interleukin; MHC, major histocompatibility complex; NK, natural killer.

CD4$^+$ CD57$^+$ T cells are normally present exclusively in GCs and are mostly confined to the light zones, where centrocytes and cells with plasmacellular differentiation predominate (Fig. 26-9).[135] They are not present in the early phases of GC reactions, when proliferating small centroblasts predominate. Nor are they the population of CD4$^+$ T cells that can be identified in a sharp rim at the border of the GC and mantle zone. These "rim cells" are CD40L$^+$ and are absent in the nodules of NLPHL and PTGCs. CD4$^+$ CD57$^+$ T cells in reactive GCs express the chemokine receptor CXCR5, similar to the small B lymphocytes, and are attracted by the chemokine CXCL13 produced by FDCs. Interestingly, it has been shown that the CD4$^+$ CD57$^+$ T cells themselves also produce high amounts of CXCL13 upon activation, in contrast to extrafollicular T cells.[136] Their messenger RNA profile is consistent with a T-regulatory-1 (Tr1) type of cell.[132] The majority of cases of NLPHL can be shown to contain a mature nonneoplastic T-cell population with dual expression of CD4 and CD8 (CD4$^+$ CD8$^+$) constituting 10% to 38% of T cells; these may reflect an activated or reactive T-cell subset and should not lead to a misdiagnosis of T-cell lymphoma.[137] NLPHLs bearing this population do not differ from other NLPHLs in terms of clinical, histologic, or immunohistochemical features.

The FDCs predominant within the macronodules are CD21$^+$ and CD35$^+$ but CD23$^-$, thus resembling the FDCs of the mantle zone and not those of the GC (Fig. 26-10). They do not carry immunoglobulin complexes. The major interaction between FDCs and B cells appears to be mediated by the CD11a/CD18 (LFA1) and CD54 (ICAM-1) pathway.[138]

Diffuse Variant

Like the nodular variant, the diffuse variant contains numerous LP cells that react with pan–B-cell reagents. However, in contrast to the nodular variant, small B lymphocytes are sparse. The predominant cells are small T lymphocytes that are CD4$^+$, with a considerable proportion of CD57$^+$ T cells participating in the T-cell rosettes around the LP cells. When there is an absence of CD57$^+$ cells, a diagnosis of T/HRBCL

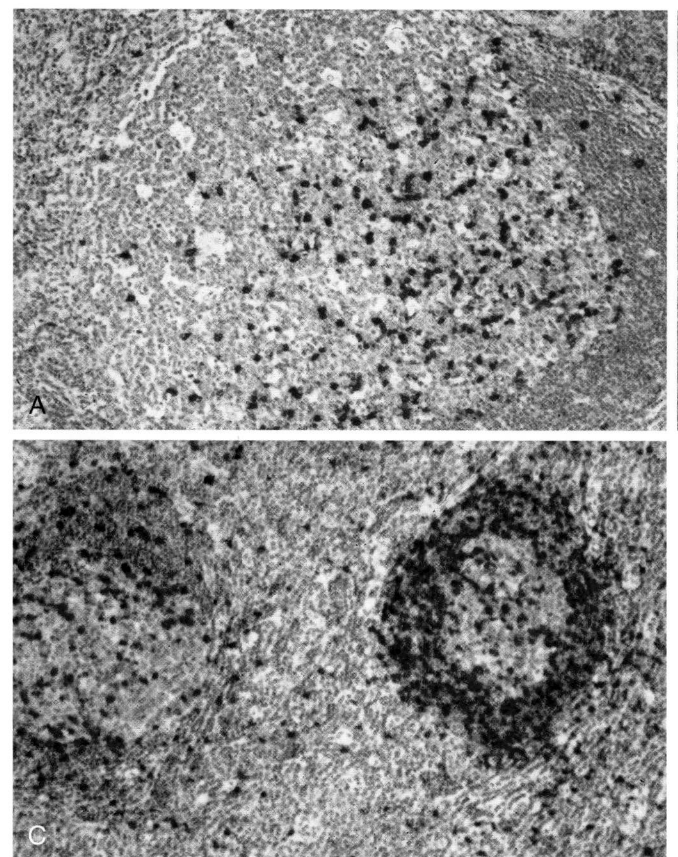

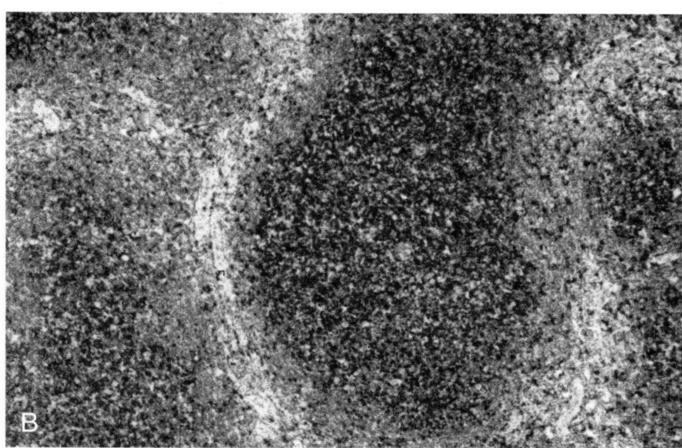

Figure 26-9. Immunohistologic stains for CD57 show positive lymphocytes in the light zone of a normal secondary follicle (**A**) and an increased number of positive lymphocytes in progressively transformed germinal centers (**B**) and in the mantle zone of a morphologically normal secondary follicle in a case of follicular hyperplasia with progressively transformed germinal centers (**C**).

should be considered. In accord with the absence of a nodular pattern, FDCs cannot be demonstrated with CD21 antibodies.

GENETICS AND MOLECULAR FINDINGS

Cytogenetic Findings

Few cytogenetic data on NLPHL are available. All cases studied have a complex karyotype with more than three numerical or structural abnormalities, but most are in the diploid range (46 to 49 chromosomes); tetraploidy, often seen in CHL, is rare.[139,140] With conventional cytogenetics, significant imbalances involve chromosomes 1, 4, 7, 9, and 13.[140] In contrast, comparative genomic hybridization has shown a high number of genomic imbalances (average, 10.8 per case) involving all chromosomes except for 19, 22, and Y, indicating a high level of complexity.[141] Gains of 1, 2q, 3, 4q, 5q, 6, 8q, 11q, 12q, and X and loss of chromosome 17 were identified in 36.8% to 68.4% of the analyzed cases. Particularly interesting was the frequent overrepresentation of chromosome arm 6q, a region frequently deleted in DLBCL. The cytogenetic analysis of the NLPHL-derived cell line DEV revealed a 48, XY, +X, t(3;7)(q13;p21), der(3)t(3;14)(p14;q32)t(3;22)(q27;q11.2), +12, der(14)t(3;14)(p14;q32), der(22)t(3;22)(q27;q11.2) karyotype.[95] Using array comparative genomic hybridization, a 3-Mb homozygous deletion was identified in the 17q24 region.[99] However, by combined immunofluorescence for CD20 and fluorescence in situ hybridization (FICTION), the 17q24 deletions could not be confirmed in 11 primary cases of NLPHL. Although Franke and colleagues[141] also showed deletion of chromosome 17 in their studies of NLPHL, it is unclear whether 17q24 deletion is important for the pathogenesis of NLPHL

Immunoglobulin Gene Rearrangement Studies

As in other forms of HL, the relative paucity of LP cells in NLPHL has made biologic studies difficult. Studies using in

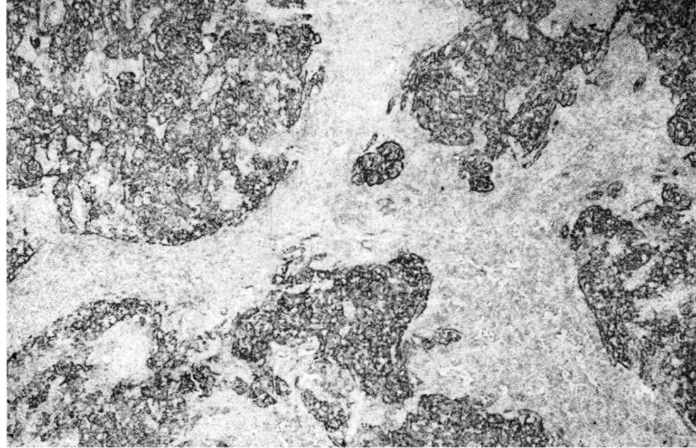

Figure 26-10. Immunohistologic stain for CD21 demonstrates loose nodular aggregates of follicular dendritic cells in nodular lymphocyte-predominant Hodgkin's lymphoma.

situ hybridization to detect Igκ or Igλ messenger RNA yielded variable results.[142-144] Although light-chain restriction was documented in a high percentage of cases in some reports,[143,144] other studies failed to demonstrate the presence of light-chain messenger RNA.[142,145] Southern blot studies were of limited use in showing immunoglobulin gene rearrangement, given their relatively low sensitivity and the rarity of LP cells in involved tissues.[146,147] Polymerase chain reaction (PCR) studies on total tissues also yielded conflicting results.[148-150] These discrepancies result from PCR's limited sensitivity owing to the large numbers of reactive B cells present in NLPHL. All recent PCR-based studies of multiple microdissected LP cells from individual patients have demonstrated the presence of monoclonal immunoglobulin gene rearrangements.[151-153] Monoclonality has been shown in multiple nodules, multiple paraffin blocks, and multiple lymph nodes from the same patient. NLPHL exhibited ongoing mutations within clonal rearranged gene segments, with intraclonal diversity in the majority of cases. Ongoing mutations are normally confined to GC B cells. This agrees with the finding that the immunoglobulin gene sequences are translated into functional membrane immunoglobulin expression and are therefore subject to antigen selection.

Oncogene Rearrangement Studies

Recurrent rearrangements of the *BCL6* gene are detected in approximately half the cases of NLPHL analyzed by interphase fluorescence in situ hybridization[154] and by FICTION.[155] *BCL6* aberrations in NLPHL target immunoglobulin as well as nonimmunoglobulin loci, similar to those found in DLBCL.[155,156] The NLPHL-derived cell line DEV shows a *BCL6* rearrangement with a break in the *BCL6* alternative breakpoint region.[99] FICTION analysis revealed no breaks in the *BCL6* alternative breakpoint region in 12 NLPHL cases, suggesting that such breaks may not be common in primary cases of NLPHL.[99] *BCL2* gene rearrangements have been investigated and detected in a small number of cases.[147,157] It is not clear whether the rearrangement was present in LP cells or, more likely, in bystander B cells. Because LP cells generally do not express BCL2 protein, *BCL2* translocation probably does not play a role in the pathogenesis of NLPHL. The proto-oncogene *BIC* (B-cell integration cluster), or pre–miR-155, and mature miR-155, which is now considered an onco–micro-RNA,[158] are highly expressed in NLPHL as well as CHL.[159,160] Similar to DLBCL and CHL tumor cells, LP cells are also targeted by aberrant somatic hypermutation in at least one of the four proto-oncogenes encoding signal transducers and transcription factors involved in B-cell development and differentiation—*PIM1*, *PAX5*, *RhoH/TTF*, and *c-Myc*—which may be relevant for B-cell lymphomagenesis.[161] The suppressors of cytokine signaling (*SOCS*) are involved in the regulation of cellular proliferation, survival, and apoptosis via cytokine-induced JAK/STAT signaling, and aberrant activities of JAK/STAT signaling pathways have been observed in several hematologic malignancies. Mutations in *SOCS* of either somatic or germline origin were observed in micromanipulated tumor cells in 50% of NLPHLs; however, activating mutations in exon 12 of *JAK2*, which are frequent in myeloproliferative diseases, were not observed.[63] *SOCS1* mutations may contribute to high JAK2 expression and activation of the JAK2/STAT6 pathway.

T-Cell Receptor Gene Rearrangement Studies

The T-cell receptor (TCR) V-beta chain gene repertoire of rosetting T cells was studied in two cases of NLPHL.[162] There was no evidence of clonal restriction or selection of V-beta receptor gene expression. Trumper and associates[163] examined rosetting complexes of a single NLPHL case by single-cell analysis for the *TCR-γ* gene. They found clonal *TCR-γ* sequences in two independent experiments analyzing 7 and 10 different rosetting complexes. These findings have not yet been confirmed by other studies, although as noted earlier, rare cases of T-cell lymphoma have been seen in patients with NLPHL.[36]

RELATION TO PROGRESSIVELY TRANSFORMED GERMINAL CENTERS

Follicular hyperplasia with PTGCs is a benign disorder of unknown pathogenesis. It is diagnosed most often in the second decade of life, with a male predominance. Patients present with an asymptomatic, solitary enlarged lymph node in the cervical region.[164] Histologically, the PTGC follicles are much larger than normal follicles and have expanded mantles, which intrude on the GC. The PTGC follicles are scattered in a background of follicular hyperplasia (Fig. 26-11A). They share with NLPHL the nodular motif of disrupted GCs with increased numbers of small B lymphocytes and dispersed centroblasts; thus they may mimic NLPHL both cytologically and by the presence of large numbers of T cells, including CD4⁺ CD57⁺ cells. However, in PTGCs the T cells are dispersed, whereas in NLPHL the T cells are in clusters surrounding the LP cells.[92] Prominent FDCs and multinucleated Warthin-Finkeldey–type giant cells can also be seen in PTGCs. Immunophenotypic studies of PTGCs show polyclonal IgM^+ IgD^+ lymphocytes; FDCs; and increased numbers of $CD4^+$ $CD57^+$, c-Maf^{+}[114] and $CD4^+$ $CD8^{+}$[137] T cells. In fact, the only difference between PTGCs and the nodules of NLPHL is the absence of LP cells (see Fig. 26-11B).

Early studies suggested an association between PTGCs and NLPHL.[5] All possible combinations were encountered, with PTGCs preceding or following NLPHL or occurring in separate lymph nodes at the same time. Since then, many other studies have confirmed this association.[165,166] The frequent association and the structural similarity between PTGCs and the nodules of NLPHL suggest that PTGCs are a precursor of NLPHL or, alternatively, that PTGCs and NLPHL are manifestations of an abnormal follicular center reaction based on B- or T-cell defects. Patients having concurrent PTGCs and different types of immunodeficiencies have been reported.[167] Importantly, no study has convincingly shown that the presence of a few PTGCs in a case of reactive follicular hyperplasia actually carries an increased risk for the development of NLPHL. Moreover, the progressive transformation of GCs is not a clonal process.[168] However, it is important to note that in cases in which the absence of LP cells precludes a diagnosis of NLPHL, a high incidence of NLPHL is found in subsequent biopsies. Confluent areas of PTGCs should raise the index of suspicion and mandate careful sectioning of the entire lymph node biopsy to rule out focal NLPHL.

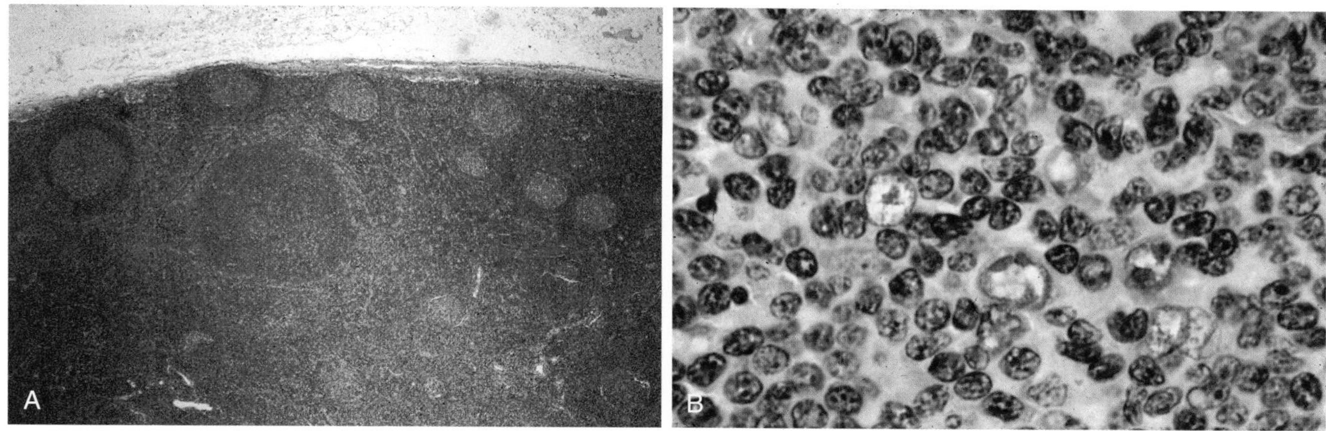

Figure 26-11. **A,** Lymph node with follicular hyperplasia and progressively transformed germinal center. **B,** At higher magnification, a predominance of small lymphocytes and a few centroblasts can be identified.

Differential Diagnosis

PTGCs differ histologically from NLPHL in that LP variants are absent. Epithelioid histiocytes are absent in the expanded follicles, but may form a necklace-like reaction around them, as sometimes seen in NLPHL. In contrast to NLPHL, in which complete obliteration of the lymph node with only a rim of displaced normal tissue is generally present, the lymph node is not totally involved in PTGCs. There is virtually always associated florid follicular hyperplasia. A combination of pan-B and pan-T antigens can be a useful adjunct to morphology in distinguishing NLPHL from PTGCs.[92] Immunostains for CD20, BOB.1 and especially Oct-2 may be useful in highlighting the LP cells. Stains for CD3 and CD57 may highlight rosettes around LP cells, which are not seen in PTGCs.

Association with Autoimmune Lymphoproliferative Syndrome

Autoimmune lymphoproliferative syndrome (ALPS) is generally caused by a mutation in genes associated with apoptosis, such as *FAS*, *FASL*, *CASP8*, and *CASP10*. As a result, the normal homeostasis of T and B lymphocytes is disturbed, and a proliferation of polyclonal T lymphocytes occurs. The proliferating T cells are positive for TCR$\alpha\beta$ or TCR$\gamma\delta$, or both, but they lack both CD4 and CD8; hence they are termed *double-negative* T cells. Individuals with germline mutations in the *FAS* gene have a high risk of developing non-Hodgkin's (14×) as well as Hodgkin's (51×) lymphomas, particularly NLPHL.[169] The occurrence of NLPHL has now been reported in two families with ALPS. Moreover, the reactive lymph nodes of patients with ALPS may show PTGCs.[167] The common link may be the CD57$^+$ T cells that are typically increased in the nodules of NLPHL and PTGCs and are also the proliferative cell population in ALPS.

TRANSFORMATION TO DIFFUSE LARGE B-CELL LYMPHOMA

In some relatively large series of NLPHL, between 3% and 10% of the patients developed DLBCL, suggesting that there is indeed an underlying abnormal clone of B cells, most likely the LP cells, that can further transform to DLBCL (Fig. 26-12).[5,35] Nodules with an almost pure population of LP-type cells can be seen in otherwise classic cases of NLPHL, suggesting that this is an intermediate stage in histologic progression. Hansmann and colleagues[170] found 14 cases of DLBCL among a series of 537 cases of NLPHL (about 3%). By RNA in situ hybridization, it was shown that both LP cells and DLBCL cells express the same type of immunoglobulin light-chain messenger RNA.[171] A clonal relationship between DLBCL arising from NLPHL and the initial tumor could be established by PCR analysis.[171,172] Ohno and associates[173] provided direct evidence by single-cell analysis and through sequence analysis of the IgH CDRIII that the LP cells were clonally related to the DLBCL cells in two cases of NLPHL with associated DLBCL. No EBV genome or EBV-related antigens have been demonstrated in the vast majority of NLPHL or in NLPHL-related DLBLCL.

There is controversy regarding the prognosis of DLBCL arising in NLPHL. The studies reported in the literature suffer from too few cases and limited follow-up, precluding a firm conclusion. In the study of Ohno and associates,[173] two cases of NLPHL with associated DLBCL showed aggressive behavior, in contrast to the previously published findings that patients with DLBCL arising from NLPHL had a good prognosis, with overall and event-free survival similar to that of de novo NLPHL.[35,174] Recent publications suggest that patients with DLBCL arising in NLPHL have a prognosis similar to those with de novo DLBCL and should be treated aggressively.[173,175] Although progression from NLPHL to DLBCL has been well established, fewer cases with an initial presentation of DLBCL before NLPHL have been reported.[37,176] It is uncertain whether the DLBCL and NLPHL in these cases are clonally related. These DLBCLs had an indolent course, and subsequent NLPHL developed at the same site, which may favor the conclusion that DLBCL and NLPHL are related processes. Some rare cases of concurrent NLPHL and therapy-unrelated T-cell lymphomas have been reported.[36] In all likelihood, these two diseases cannot be clonally related, but development of T-cell lymphoma may be related to the prominent and possibly important initiating role of T cells in the disturbed GC reaction of NLPHL.

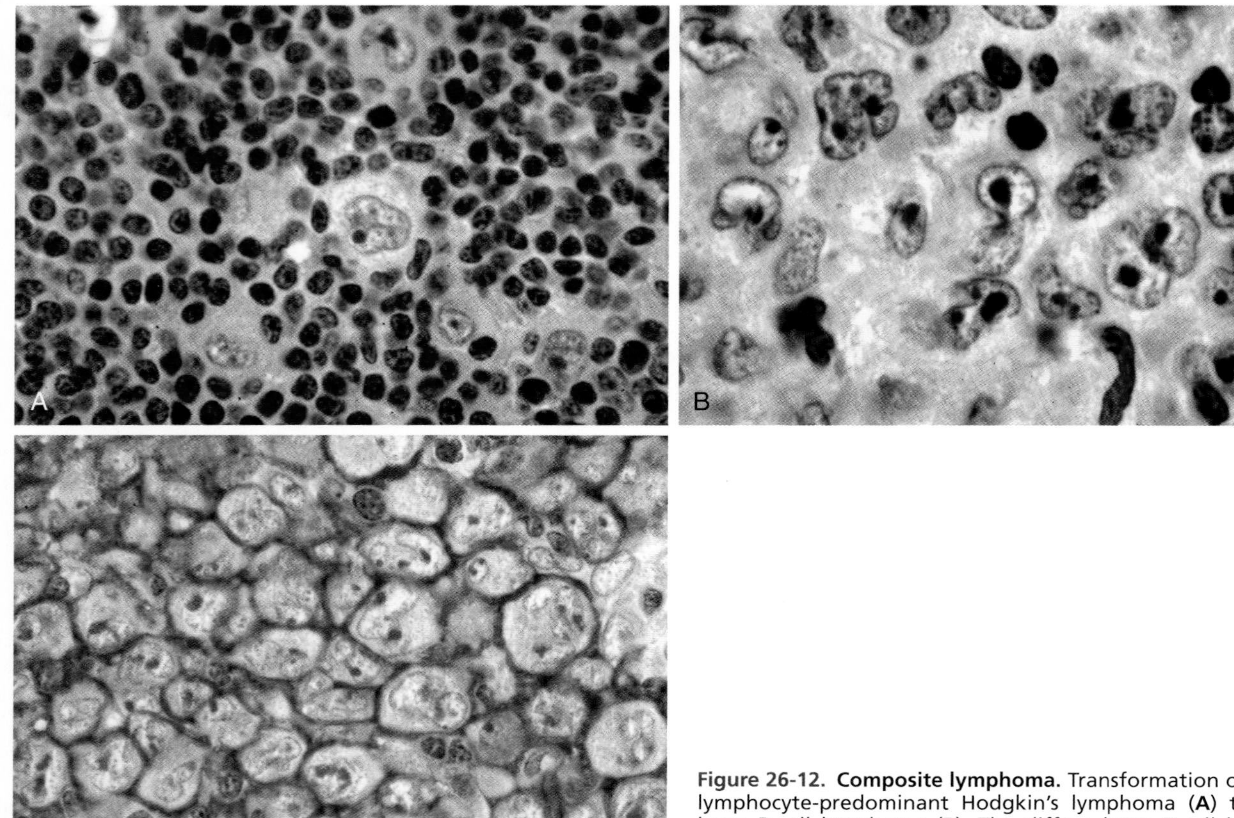

Figure 26-12. Composite lymphoma. Transformation of nodular lymphocyte-predominant Hodgkin's lymphoma **(A)** to diffuse large B-cell lymphoma **(B)**. The diffuse large B-cell lymphoma cells stain for CD20 **(C)**.

RELATION TO T-CELL/HISTIOCYTE-RICH B-CELL LYMPHOMA

Malignant lymphoma with features of T/HRBCL is the most common subtype of non-Hodgkin's lymphoma that develops after NLPHL.[176] T/HRBCL is characterized by a neoplastic population of large B cells scattered in a reactive background of T lymphocytes and histiocytes.[177] In the WHO classification, T/HRBCL is a subtype of DLBCL and may represent more than one disease entity (see Chapter 22). However, the prototype category of T/HRBCL is largely similar to the diffuse variant of NLPHL. In such cases, NLPHL and T/HRBCL may be the two extremes of a single spectrum of disease, or alternatively, T/HRBCL could be a transformation of NLPHL. It is still unresolved whether primary and secondary T/HRBCL can be distinguished.

Early studies suggested that T/HRBCL with LP-type tumor cells might be related to NLPHL (the so-called paragranuloma-like T/HRBCL) (Fig. 26-13).[176,178,179] Moreover, several authors reported that NLPHL and T/HRBCL could be seen as composite lymphomas, as metachronous lymphomas, or in multiple members of the same family.[176] Nevertheless, some T/HRBCL cases diagnosed following NLPHL may lack LP-type cells. Although several morphologic features of T/HRBCL are identical to those of NLPHL, clinically, most patients with T/HRBCL have advanced disease.[177,179]

Single-cell studies revealed ongoing mutations in T/HRBCL similar to NLPHL.[180] The BCL6 protein, which is normally present in GC cells, is frequently expressed in LP cells and also in the tumor cells of T/HRBCL. It has been proposed that the distinction between NLPHL and T/HRBCL can be made in difficult cases by demonstrating *IGH2* or *IG light* chain clonality.[181] However, because NLPHL can progress to diffuse NLPHL or transform to DLBCL, the distinction between these entities is predictably vague. Both CD79a and BCL2 are more frequently expressed in T/HRBCL than in NLPHL.[22,182] The neoplastic cells of T/HRBCL are leukocyte-specific phosphoprotein (LSP1) positive and generally PU.1$^-$,[66,67,178] with some exceptions[183]; in contrast, LP cells are mostly LSP1$^-$ with variable PU.1 expression.[67] Expression of FREB in the majority of NLPHLs but not in T/HRBCL might also aid in the differential diagnosis.[53] The T-cell rosettes typical of NLPHL are not seen in T/HRBCL (Fig. 26-14).[114,129] Some suggest that the expanded meshworks of FDCs in NLPHL are a useful feature for the differential diagnosis, but diffuse areas of NLPHL may lack FDC meshworks. Relative proportions of TIA-1$^+$ or granzyme B–positive T cells and CD57$^+$ PD1$^+$ T cells are thought to be useful in the differential diagnosis; a high TIA-1$^+$– or granzyme B–positive–to–CD57$^+$ ratio supports a diagnosis of T/HRBCL, and a low ratio supports a diagnosis of NLPHL.[130,178] However, the practical use of this ratio is limited because an absolute number has not been defined.

The question remains whether NLPHL can transform into T/HRBCL. Loss of the nodular growth pattern and of CD57$^+$ T cells would be epiphenomena, but a change in malignant potential of the neoplastic B-cell clone would be the significant change. Theoretically, there are two possibilities. First, the LP cells might undergo a further transformation. Second,

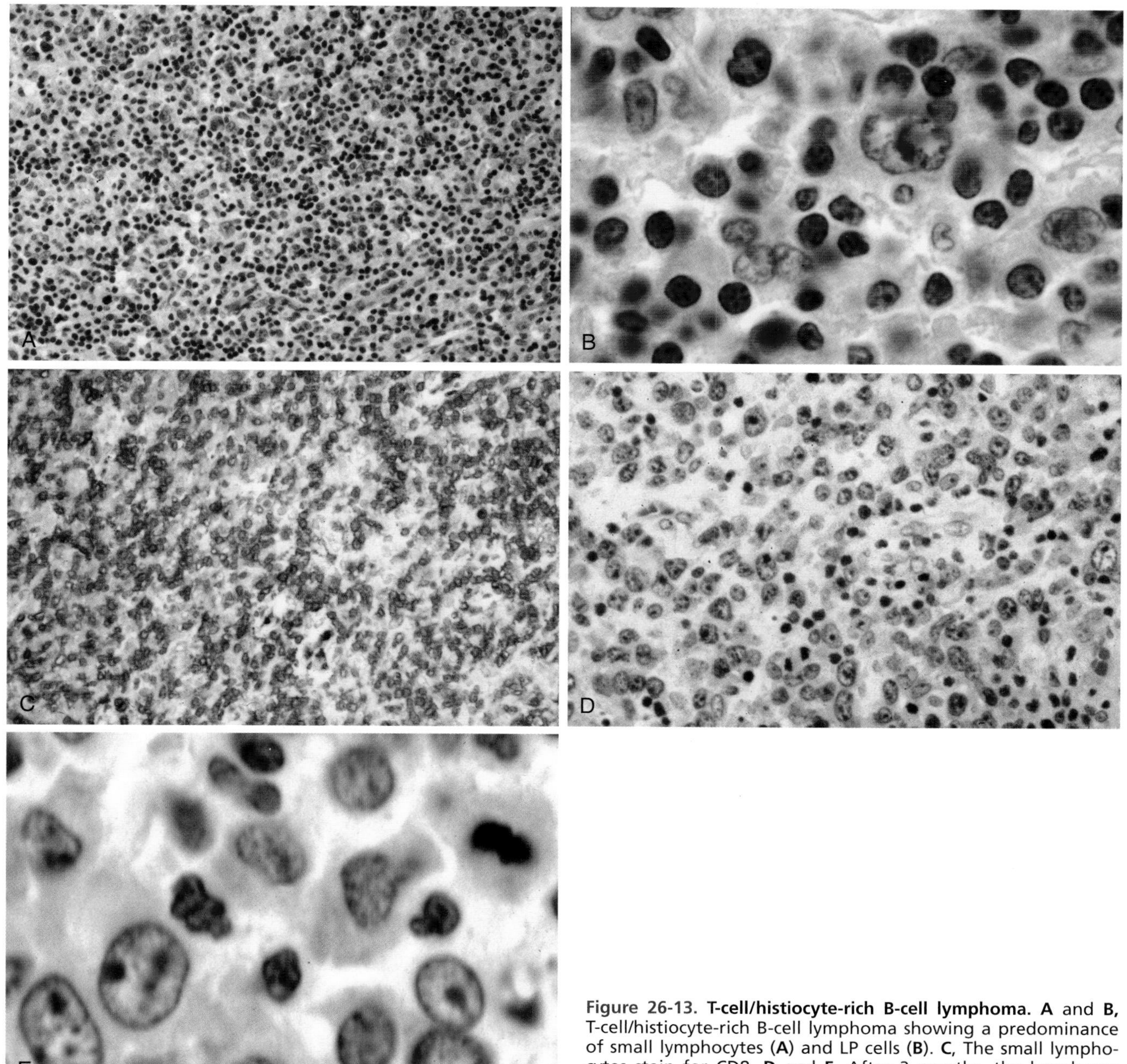

Figure 26-13. T-cell/histiocyte-rich B-cell lymphoma. A and B, T-cell/histiocyte-rich B-cell lymphoma showing a predominance of small lymphocytes (**A**) and LP cells (**B**). **C,** The small lymphocytes stain for CD8. **D** and **E,** After 3 months, the lymphoma recurred as diffuse large B-cell lymphoma.

the LP cells and the neoplastic cells of T/HRBCL might have a common precursor, and T/HRBCL would then be the result of a second transforming event. By applying comparative genomic hybridization after single-cell microdissection,[141] significantly fewer genomic imbalances were detected in T/HRBCL (5.6 per tumor) than in NLPHL (11.6 per tumor).[184] Gains of 4q and losses of 19/19p were observed in almost half the cases of both disorders. However, many other genomic changes that are frequently overrepresented in NLPHL were seen only sporadically in T/HRBCL. Considering the presence of common chromosomal imbalances, some as yet unspecified genes located on 4q or chromosome 19 may be affected in GC ancestors of both entities. Based on the cytogenetic changes in the two disorders, a straightforward progression from NLPHL to T/HRBCL is unlikely. It is therefore of great interest to identify differences in gene expression between LP cells and the tumor cells of T/HRBCL to establish what determines the dramatically different behavior of these morphologically similar tumor types.

OTHER DIFFERENTIAL DIAGNOSES

Follicular Lymphoma

Both architectural and cytologic features contribute to the difficulty of distinguishing NLPHL from the floral type of follicular lymphoma, which also has very large nodules. In low-grade follicular lymphoma, centrocytes are admixed with

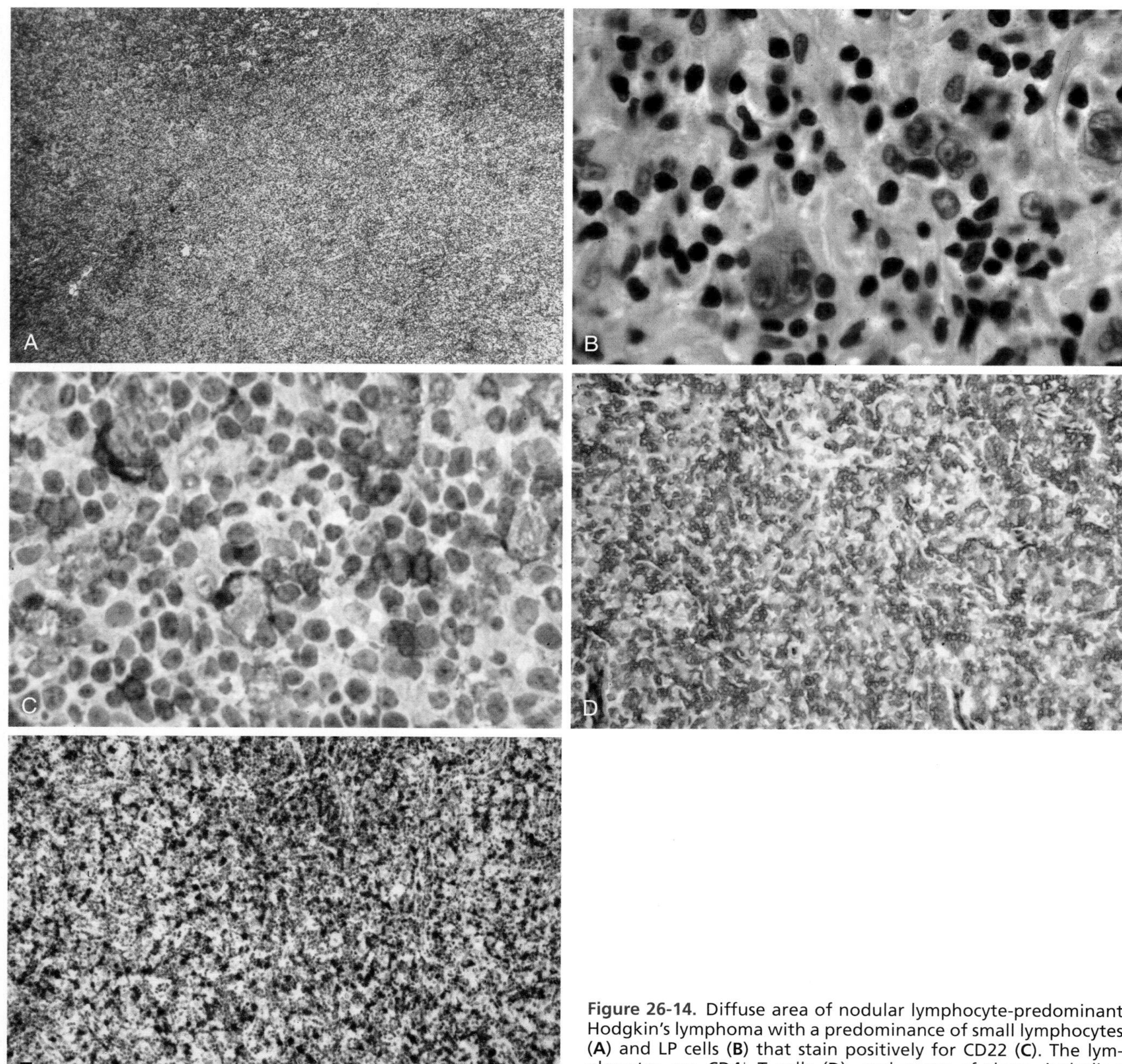

Figure 26-14. Diffuse area of nodular lymphocyte-predominant Hodgkin's lymphoma with a predominance of small lymphocytes (**A**) and LP cells (**B**) that stain positively for CD22 (**C**). The lymphocytes are CD4+ T cells (**D**), and many of them, including rosetting cells, also stain for CD57 (**E**).

varying numbers of centroblasts that are CD45+ and CD20+ and resemble LP cells in some cases. However, the presence of characteristic LP cells with polylobated nuclei, delicate nuclear membranes, and inconspicuous nucleoli helps identify and distinguish NLPHL from follicular lymphoma. In grade 1 follicular lymphoma, all cells have irregular cleaved nuclear outlines and condensed nuclear chromatin, whereas the nuclei of the background cells in NLPHL are mostly round, but also may include some irregular nuclei. Ancillary studies can be performed if a morphologic diagnosis is not evident. The small cells of follicular lymphoma have a distinctive phenotype, being CD10+ monoclonal B cells, readily distinguished from the B cells in NLPHL.

Lymphocyte-Rich Classical Hodgkin's Lymphoma

In the absence of immunohistochemical information, LRCHL is the major morphologic mimic of NLPHL.[38] In a study of 426 cases that were morphologically interpreted as NLPHL, 115 (27%) were reclassified as LRCHL.[13,185,186] On hematoxylin-eosin stains, the presence of regressed GCs is a characteristic feature of LRCHL, distinct from the expanded macrofollicles of NLPHL. NLPHL and LRCHL patients have similar clinical characteristics,[186] except that LRCHL patients tend to be older.[187] Immunohistochemical stains are now considered essential for the distinction of LRCHL from NLPHL

Table 26-4 Differential Diagnosis of Nodular Lymphocyte-Predominant Hodgkin's Lymphoma

	Morphologic Features		*Immunophenotypic and Molecular Features*	
Disease	**Tumor Cells**	**Background**	**Tumor Cells**	**Background**
PTGCs	No LP-type HRS cells, but centroblasts are present	Nodules with broken-down interface between mantle zone and GCs Lymph node is usually not totally replaced in PTGCs; association with florid follicular hyperplasia	No reactivity with EMA	$CD20^+$ or $CD30^+$ immunoblasts, irregular broken-up $CD20^+$ nodules; $CD57^+$, $PD1^+$, c-Maf^+ T cells, but no prominent T-cell rosettes
LRCHL	Classic HRS cells	Diffuse or nodular variant	$CD15^+$, $CD30^+$, $CD45^-$, $CD20^{+/-}$, EMA^-, EBV^+ (≈50%)	$CD57^-$, $PD1^+$, loose $CD21^+$ FDC meshwork
FL	Small cleaved cells together with large centroblasts	Generally smaller nodules Lymphocytes in nodules are atypical	$CD20^+$, $CD10^+$ (60%), $BCL2^+$	*BCL2* gene rearrangement is usually present
T/HRBCL	Centroblasts or immunoblasts or popcorn cells	Diffuse pattern	$CD20^+$, EMA^+, $CD15^-$, $CD30^-$, LSP^+, $FREB^-$	Few background B cells; no $CD57^+$, $PD1^+$, c-Maf^+ T-cell rosettes; high TIA-1^+-to-$CD57^+$ ratio

EBV, Epstein-Barr virus; EMA, epithelial membrane antigen; FDC, follicular dendritic cell; FL, follicular lymphoma; GC, germinal center; HRS, Hodgkin Reed-Sternberg; LP, lymphocyte predominant; LRCHL, lymphocyte-rich classical Hodgkin's lymphoma; LSP, leukocyte-specific phosphoprotein; PTGC, progressively transformed germinal center; T/HRBCL, T-cell/histiocyte-rich B-cell lymphoma.

(Table 26-4). The most important difference is the nature of the HRS cells (Fig. 26-15). In LRCHL these are of the classic type, expressing CD30 consistently, CD15 frequently, and EBV-encoded RNA (EBER) in around 40% of cases; they express CD20 in only some cases,[186] and then always in only a subset of HRS cells.

TREATMENT

Patients with NLPHL respond well to standard treatment for HL, but the treatments considered standard for other HL subtypes may represent overtreatment for most patients with NLPHL, particularly for those with early-stage disease. Therefore, the optimal treatment of NLPHL remains controversial. Different treatment modalities have been evaluated in stage IA NLPHL patients. Thirty percent of the patients remained in complete remission after lymphadenectomy alone. Overall event-free survival was 90% with combined-modality treatment and 42% with "watch and wait."[188] Thus "watch and wait" cannot be recommended in stage IA NLPHL patients. Involved field radiotheraphy is effective and is regarded as standard in stage IA NLPHL. Rituximab (anti-CD20 antibody) has excellent activity in previously untreated and relapsed NLPHL.[189] An undesirable consequence of treatment with rituximab might be the selection of $CD20^-$ tumor cell subclones, which can result in a $CD20^-$ recurrent lymphoma.[190] Using anti-CD79a as a B-cell marker and PCR clonality studies to analyze different IgH regions can help overcome the diagnostic problems with such recurrent tumors. For advanced-stage NLPHL, regimens currently used for the treatment of B-cell non-Hodgkin's lymphoma, including R-CVP (rituximab, cyclophosphamide, vincristine, prednisone), R-CHOP (rituximab, cyclophosphamide, hydroxydaunomycin [doxorubicin], Oncovin [vincristine], prednisone), or even rituximab alone, are all reasonable options. ABVD (Adriamycin [doxorubicin], bleomycin, vinblastine, dacarbazine), highly effective in CHL, is less effective in advanced-stage NLPHL. Therefore, for treatment purposes, NLPHL can be considered closer to B-cell lymphomas.

PROGNOSIS

With pathologic staging and standard treatment, mortality from NLPHL is low; nearly all deaths are cardiac related or due to a secondary tumor.[13] The prognosis of NLPHL is related primarily to stage and patient age at diagnosis, and survival ranges from 40% to 99%.[176] Life expectancy of patients with stage I NLPHL is about the same as that of the general population. Patients with splenic involvement (stage IIIS) or with stage IV have a poor prognosis with current therapies.

Regula and coworkers[40] compared the clinical course of NLPHL and D-LPHL in a series of 73 patients. The diffuse cases had a course similar to other types of HL, with relapse and only two deaths due to HL. Those with the nodular type showed significantly more relapses, which occurred independent of stage or treatment and were evenly distributed temporally up to 10 years after initial therapy. These cases were diagnosed before the recognition of LRCHL, so the clinical results may have been influenced by the inclusion of some cases of CHL. Bodis and associates[191] reported that patients with a diffuse pattern had a significantly greater rate of freedom from relapse than those with a nodular pattern. Among the immunoarchitectures described by Fan and associates,[37] the presence of a T/HRBCL-like diffuse pattern was an independent predictor of recurrent disease; however, this result was limited by a short follow-up period for patients without recurrent disease. In other studies,[13,192-194] no difference in relapse rate between nodular and diffuse cases was found, although unusually long intervals to relapse were observed in two patients with a nodular histology.[193] Histologically, the majority of relapse patients have persistence of NLPHL. Importantly, despite relatively frequent late relapses, NLPHL still maintains an indolent course. The main risk factor related to poor outcome is advanced stage.

CONCLUSION

NLPHL is a rare B-cell lymphoma of GC derivation. NLPHL differs from CHL in histologic and clinical presentation.

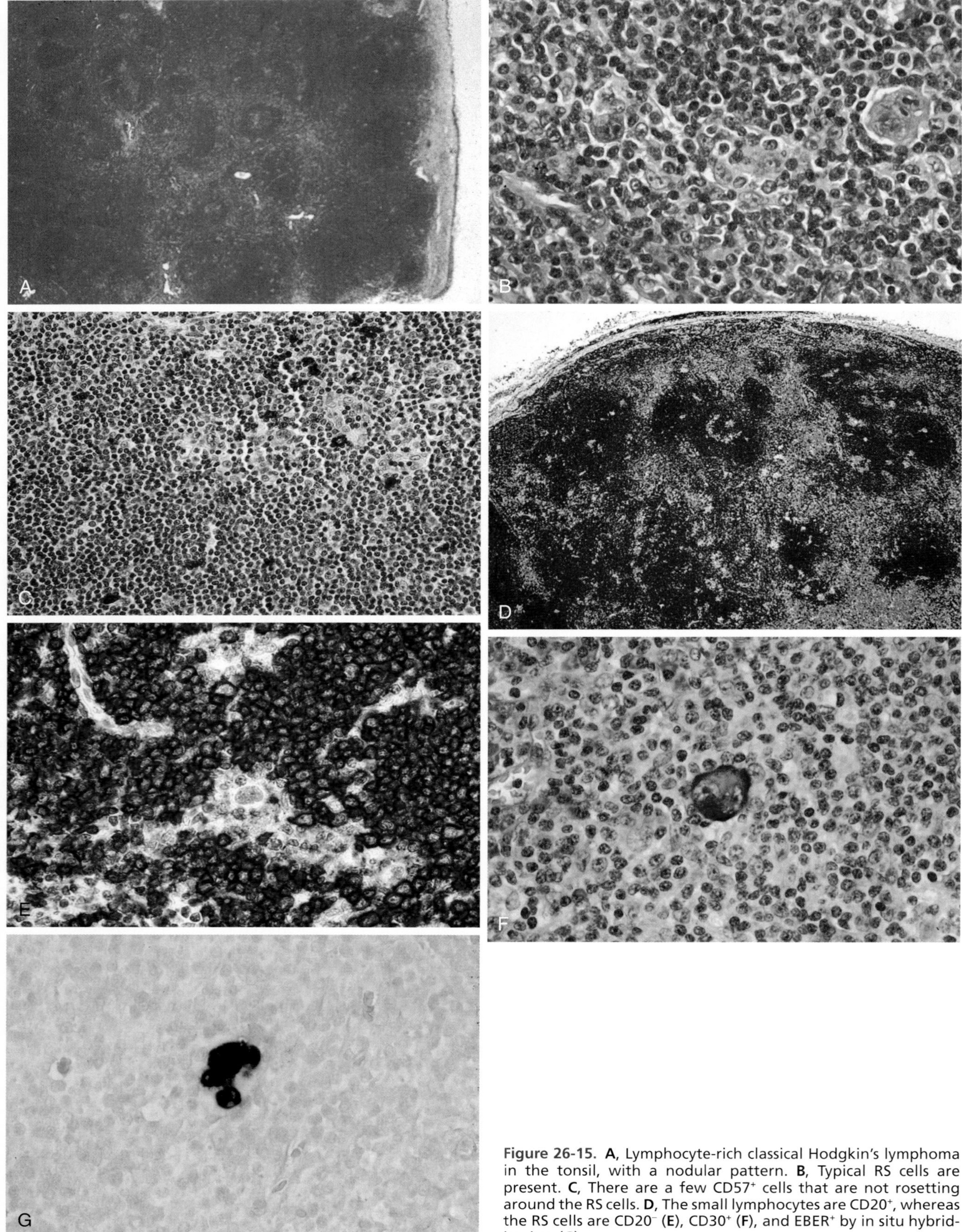

Figure 26-15. **A**, Lymphocyte-rich classical Hodgkin's lymphoma in the tonsil, with a nodular pattern. **B**, Typical RS cells are present. **C**, There are a few CD57^{+} cells that are not rosetting around the RS cells. **D**, The small lymphocytes are CD20^{+}, whereas the RS cells are CD20^{-} (**E**), CD30^{+} (**F**), and EBER^{+} by in situ hybridization (**G**).

Nevertheless, both subtypes have a key characteristic in common with other subtypes of HL: the interaction of a majority of reactive lymphocytes with a minority of transformed lymphoid cells. Although isolated PTGCs may not be a true risk factor for subsequent NLPHL, they are associated with the disease in many cases. NLPHL transforms relatively frequently to DLBCL; nodules with increased numbers of LP-type HRS cells may represent a transitional phase. In some cases of NLPHL with coexistent DLBCL, a clonal relation has been demonstrated by immunoglobulin gene analysis. Clinically, NLPHL has a good prognosis, despite the fact that there are frequent relapses, including relapses in distant sites. However, some cases progress to involve the spleen and bone marrow, findings usually associated with a poor outcome.

Several questions remain unanswered. What is the functional significance of the $CD4^+$ $CD57^+$ T cells in the pathogenesis of NLPHL and PTGCs? What are the mechanisms of transformation to DLBCL? Is T/HRBCL a biologically distinct disease, or does it represent progression of NLPHL? What type of molecular genetic abnormalities underlies the spectrum from NLPHL to T/HRBCL? Long-term studies will be required to answer these questions.

Pearls and Pitfalls

- Neoplastic cells with classic RS cell morphology are not required for diagnosis, but they are also not as infrequent as previously reported.
- Despite a morphologic resemblance to HRS cells, the phenotype is that of LP cells.
- Eosinophils, plasma cells, and neutrophils are rarely observed in an NLPHL background.
- NLPHL cases are generally negative for EBV.
- $CD20^+$ centroblasts must be distinguished from LP cells in the differential diagnosis of PTGCs and NLPHL. These centroblasts are not surrounded by $CD57^+$ rosettes.
- $PU.1^+$ histiocytes may be confused morphologically with LP cells.
- The most useful markers for diagnosis in paraffin sections are CD20, Oct-2, IgD, CD3, and CD57.
- The presence of $CD4^+$ $CD8^+$ T cells should not lead to a misdiagnosis of T-cell lymphoma.

References can be found on Expert Consult @ www.expertconsult.com

Chapter 27

Classical Hodgkin's Lymphoma

Falko Fend

CHAPTER OUTLINE

DEFINITION

Classical Hodgkin's lymphoma (CHL) is a clonal, malignant lymphoproliferation originating from germinal center B cells.[1,2] In contrast to most other lymphomas, the malignant cells usually represent only a small minority, between 0.1% and 2%, of the total cellular population of involved tissues. A histopathologic diagnosis of CHL is based on the identification of diagnostic Reed-Sternberg (RS) cells in an appropriate inflammatory background. Although many cases of CHL can, in principle, be diagnosed on the basis of morphology alone, current diagnostic criteria include the characteristic immunophenotype of the neoplastic population. RS cells and variants express the CD30 and CD15 antigens in the majority of cases, lack the common leukocyte antigen CD45, and show an inconsistent and heterogeneous expression of lineage-specific lymphoid markers.[3,4]

CLASSIFICATION

In contrast to non-Hodgkin's lymphomas (NHLs), the classification of Hodgkin's lymphoma (HL) has remained remarkably constant (Box 27-1). Notwithstanding the significant progress in delineating the antigenic profile and the origin of the neoplastic cells of HL, the majority of cases are classified much as they were 30 years ago, after the development of the Rye classification.[5-7] This underlines the paramount importance of morphology for the correct diagnosis of this neoplasm.

The change in terminology from *Hodgkin's disease* to *Hodgkin's lymphoma* was first proposed in the Revised European American Lymphoma (REAL) classification[8] and reflects our better understanding of the nature and histogenesis of this lymphoproliferation. After decades of controversy as to whether HL represents an infectious, immunologic, or neoplastic disorder, the success of radiotherapy and multimodal

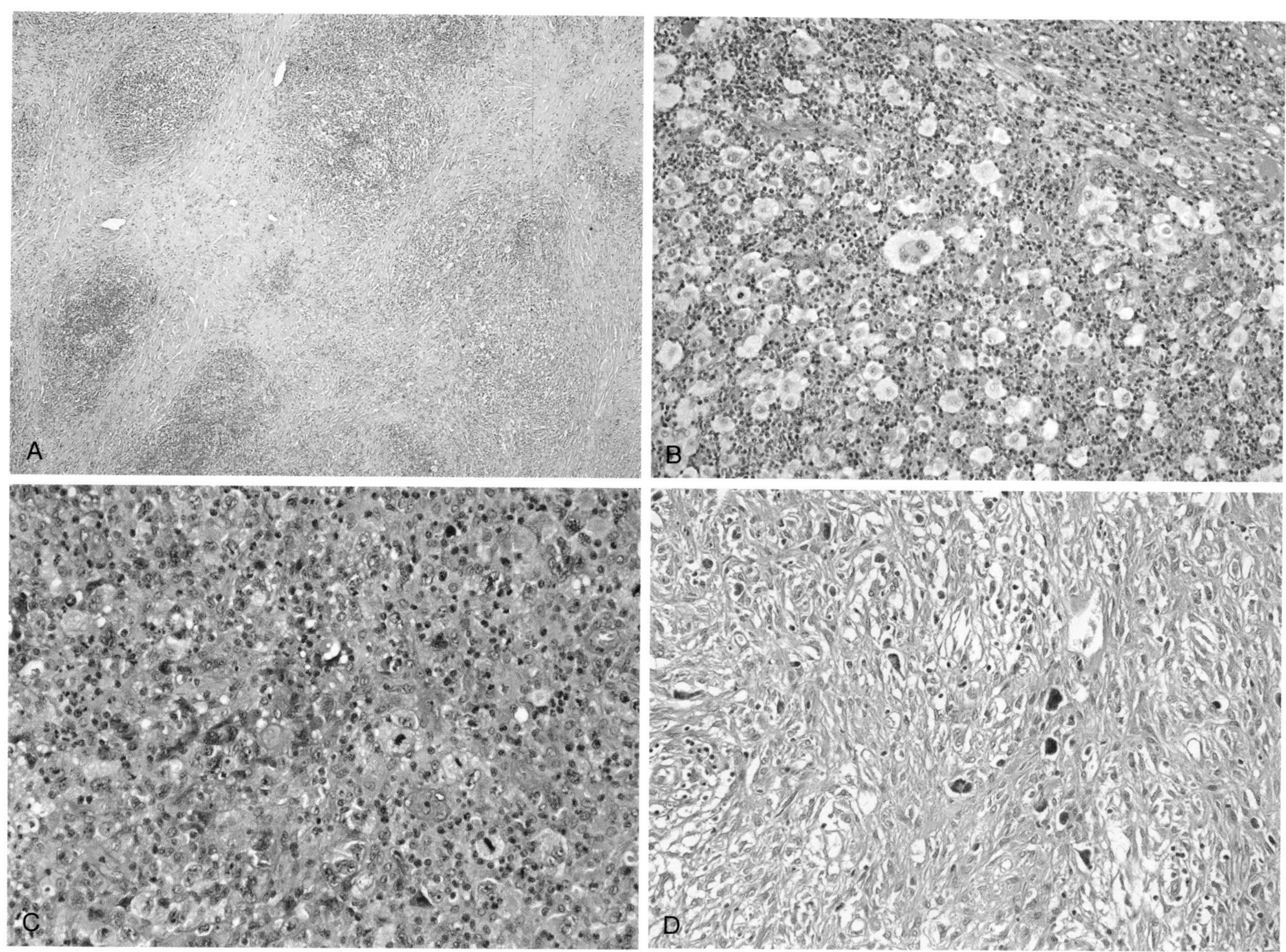

Figure 27-2. Morphology of classical Hodgkin's lymphoma (CHL). A, Nodular sclerosis CHL. Cellular nodules are separated by concentric bands of mature collagen. **B,** Close-up of cellular nodule shows numerous lacunar cells with clear cytoplasm intermingled with lymphocytes, neutrophils, and eosinophils. Note collagen bands rimming the nodule. **C,** Nodular sclerosis CHL grade II. Confluent sheets of neoplastic cells with partly anaplastic features, intermingled with a minority of inflammatory cells. This morphology is consistent with the so-called syncytial variant of CHL. **D,** Lymphocyte-depleted CHL, diffuse fibrosis subtype. Neoplastic Reed-Sternberg and Hodgkin cells in a hypocellular background with histiocytes and fibroblasts. This case lacks nodularity and ordered collagen bands.

try is highlighted by the fact that approximately 30% of the cases submitted as NLPHL to two multicenter studies were reclassified as LRCHL, mostly based on immunophenotypic findings.[61,98] The reactive background consists of small immunoglobulin (Ig) M$^+$ and IgD$^+$ B cells, typical for the mantle zone of follicles (see Fig. 27-4B). Appropriate stains reveal a fine, expanded meshwork of follicular dendritic cells and highlight the nodular architecture of the infiltrate. The neoplastic cells are frequently rimmed by CD3$^+$ T cells that lack CD57 and PD1, markers of follicular T cells.[3,61,98,103-105]

The second variant of LRCHL, which was initially described as a provisional entity in the REAL classification,[8] shows an interfollicular or diffuse growth pattern with classic RS cells in a background of small lymphocytes that, in contrast to those in the nodular pattern, are predominantly of a T-cell phenotype. B-cell follicles are either pushed aside or, rarely, absent. In the past, such cases were described as *interfollicular Hodgkin's disease*.[106]

For now, it is still unclear whether LRCHL really represents a biologically distinct subtype of CHL or, in some cases, is an early phase of either mixed cellularity or nodular sclerosis CHL. Although the clinical features of LRCHL seem to be sufficiently distinct from other types of CHL to warrant its separation,[70] more information on its morphologic spectrum will enhance the differentiation from other subtypes.

Lymphocyte-Depleted Classical Hodgkin's Lymphoma

This is the least frequently diagnosed subtype of CHL, constituting about 1% of patients in recent series. Many cases from earlier series probably represented aggressive NHL or would today be classified as nodular sclerosis CHL grade II.[107] In the original classification of Lukes and Butler, two types of lymphocyte depletion were recognized; these were subsequently combined in the Rye classification.[6,7] The diffuse fibrosis type shows a hypocellular infiltrate with disordered, diffuse reticulin fibrosis and atypical cells, including RS cells and a sparse, heterogeneous background population (see Fig. 27-2D). The presence of organized collagen bands mandates a diagnosis of nodular sclerosis CHL. The reticular variant is

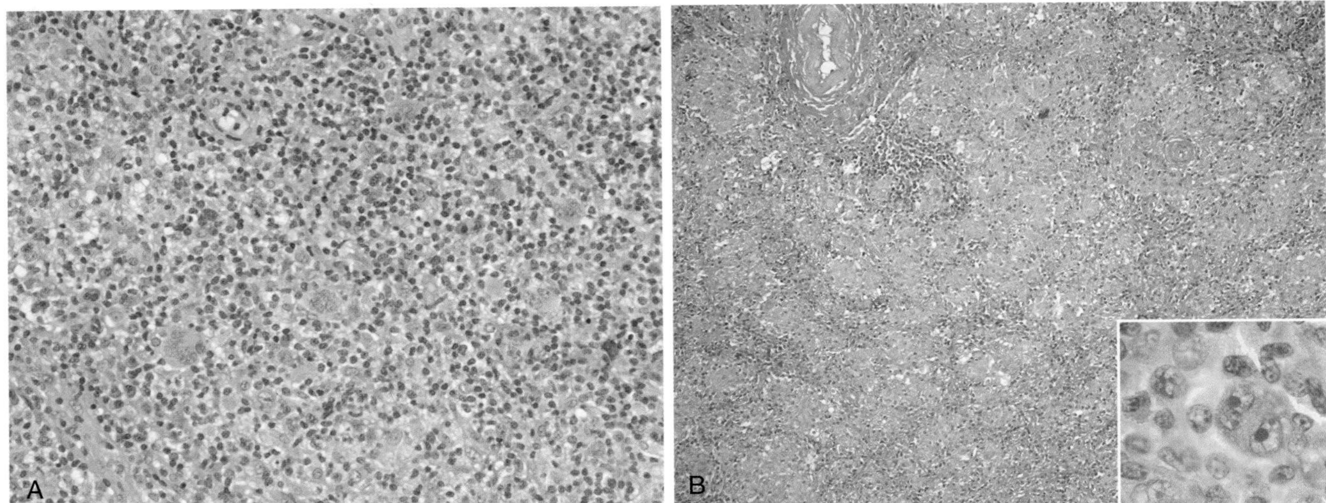

Figure 27-3. Mixed cellularity classical Hodgkin's lymphoma (CHL). A, The lymph node contains a mixed population of lymphocytes, plasma cells, eosinophils, histiocytes, and easily recognizable Reed-Sternberg (RS) cells and variants. **B,** Histiocyte-rich mixed cellularity CHL containing confluent sheets of epithelioid cell granulomas with rare interspersed RS cells (*inset*). If areas of more typical mixed cellularity CHL are missing, non-Hodgkin's lymphoma with epithelioid cell granulomas (e.g., so-called Lennert's lymphoma) or even reactive conditions may be considered.

characterized by sheets of atypical cells, including many bizarre, anaplastic RS cells. Immunohistochemical demonstration of a characteristic CHL phenotype is required for the sometimes difficult exclusion of large cell lymphomas, especially ALCL.[4,8]

Classical Hodgkin's Lymphoma, Unclassified, and Unusual Morphologic Patterns

All cases that cannot be confidently placed in any of the four categories described should be designated CHL, unclassified. Small biopsy specimens or biopsies from extranodal sites, partial lymph node involvement, unusual histologic features, or poor technical quality may preclude subtyping. Partial involvement by CHL is frequently found, especially if a smaller node from the periphery of a lymph node conglomerate is removed. The infiltrate usually resides in the interfollicular area in a background of T cells, with preserved or regressed germinal centers. This interfollicular pattern frequently falls into the LRCHL category.[8,61,106] RS cells of CHL may occur in monocytoid B-cell clusters, and an accompanying monocytoid B-cell reaction can be observed in a small minority of cases.[108,109] Rarely, sinusoidal involvement by RS cells and variants can mimic ALCL.

Relapsed CHL usually retains the initial histologic subtype but may show morphologic progression, especially at previously treated sites, with an increase in the number and pleomorphism of tumor cells.[110] These cases are sometimes designated the lymphocyte-depleted subtype, but assignment of the histologic subtype should be based on initial pretherapy biopsies. In patients with suspected relapses of CHL, the possibility of a secondary neoplasm should always be considered if the morphologic and phenotypic criteria for a diagnosis of CHL are not met. Similarly, persistent mass lesions after treatment for CHL may occasionally prompt a biopsy. Frequently, only hyalinized scar tissue can be identified. A diagnosis of residual CHL should be made only if Hodgkin cells can be identified unequivocally by morphology and immunophenotype.

Diagnostic Criteria for Extranodal Sites

The criteria for a diagnosis of CHL in an extranodal organ depend in part on whether the patient has an established diagnosis of CHL at a nodal site. In liver and bone marrow biopsies obtained for staging purposes in patients with CHL, identification of a mixed cellular infiltrate with occasional atypical mononuclear cells is regarded as sufficient for a diagnosis of involvement by CHL, because diagnostic RS cells are lacking in most small tumor foci.[111] Demonstration of CD30 or CD15 expression by the large cells further supports the diagnosis. In the liver, the infiltrate usually involves the portal triads. In the bone marrow, focal fibrosis detected by reticulin stains is an ominous sign and should prompt further examinations such as step sectioning and immunohistochemistry.

As mentioned earlier, the thymus is frequently involved in mediastinal disease, which is almost always of the nodular sclerosis subtype. Thymic CHL can be associated with a prominent reactive proliferation of thymic epithelium intermingled with neoplastic cells and the development of epithelial cysts, sometimes leading to a misdiagnosis of thymoma or multilocular inflammatory thymic cyst.[77,78] This error can be avoided by generous sampling of the lesion and appropriate immunohistochemical studies.

In contrast to patients with known CHL, great caution is required before establishing a primary diagnosis of CHL in an extranodal site, and subtyping is often not possible. Stage IE is extremely rare in CHL, and many cases from older studies probably represented extranodal NHL simulating HL. Therefore, immunohistochemical confirmation of the diagnosis is mandatory in primary extranodal CHL to rule out morphologic mimics.

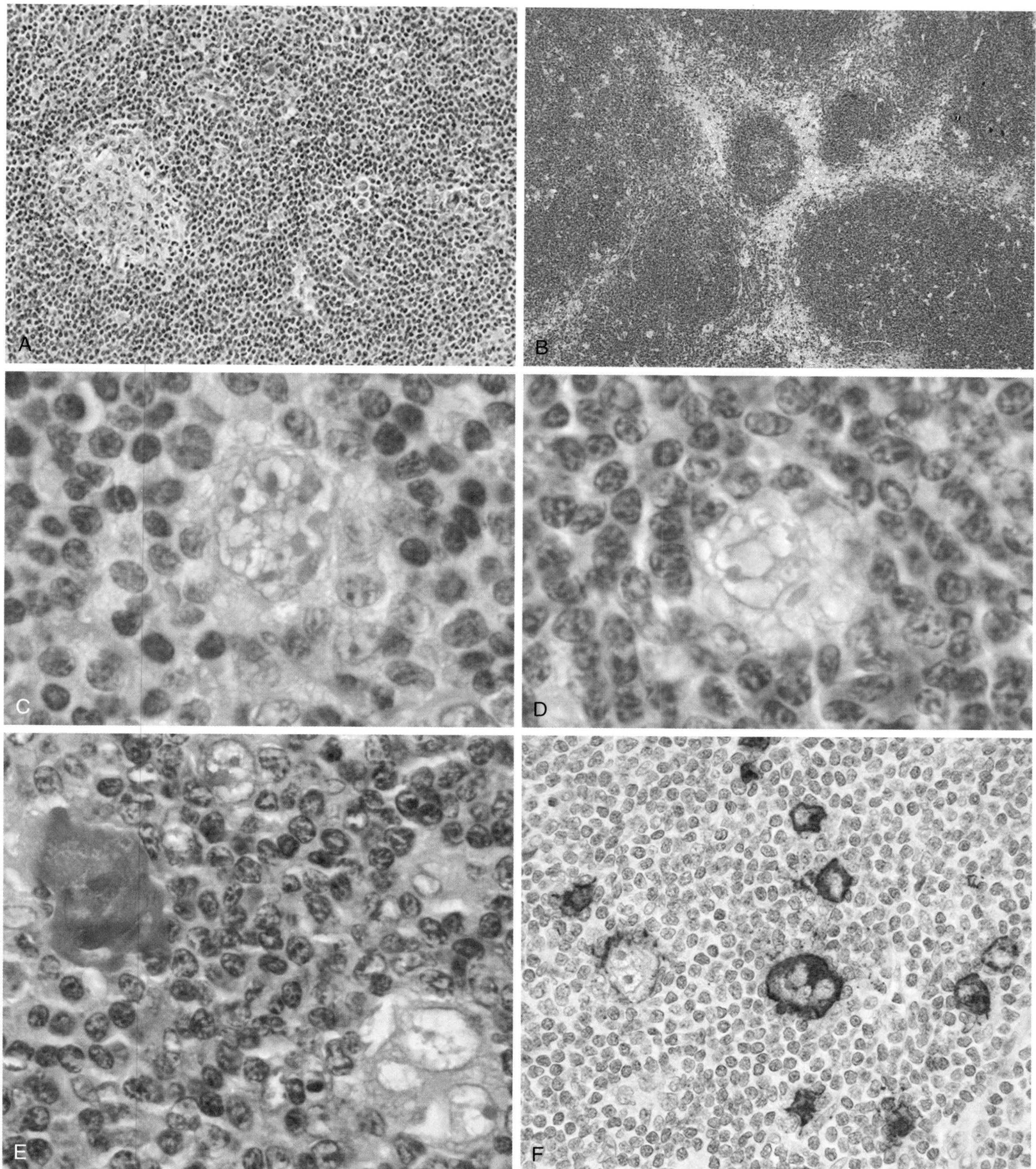

Figure 27-4. Lymphocyte-rich classical Hodgkin's lymphoma (CHL), nodular variant. A, The lymph node is dominated by small lymphocytes arranged in a nodular pattern, frequently with atrophic germinal centers. The tumor cells are found in the expanded mantle zones of these B-cell nodules. **B,** Immunohistochemistry for CD20 highlights the nodular pattern with a predominance of B cells. **C** to **E,** The morphologic spectrum of neoplastic cells in lymphocyte-rich CHL varies from classic Reed-Sternberg (RS) cells (**E**) to cells resembling the LP (L & H) cells of nodular lymphocyte-predominant Hodgkin's lymphoma (**C** and **D**). **F,** Immunohistochemistry for CD15 reveals strong positivity of the neoplastic cells, including a classic binucleate RS cell.

Table 27-2 Major Diagnostic Features: Phenotype and Molecular Features

	Positive	Negative
Immunophenotype	CD30 (>90%)	CD45
	CD15 (75%-85%)	CD43
	BSAP (PAX5)	EMA
	IRF4/MUM-1	Cytokeratin
	Fascin	ALK1
	Vimentin	CD79a (rarely +)
	CD25	J chain
	HLA-DR (Ia)	T-cell markers (rarely +)
	CD40	BOB.1
	CD20 –/+	Oct-2 –/+
	LMP-1 (20%-50%)	TIA-1, granzyme B –/+
Genotype	Clonally rearranged immunoglobulin genes detectable by single-cell PCR in >95% of cases, but inconsistently in bulk tissue analysis	
	Clonal EBV infection in 20%-50+% of cases (MC > NS)	
	Absence of t(14;18), t(2;5) and variants as well as other NHL-specific translocations	
	Complex, hyperdiploid karyotype	
	Recurrent amplification of 2p by CGH	

ALK, anaplastic lymphoma kinase; CGH, comparative genomic hybridization; EBV, Epstein-Barr virus; EMA, epithelial membrane antigen; MC, mixed cellularity; NHL, non-Hodgkin's lymphoma; NS, nodular sclerosis; PCR, polymerase chain reaction.

IMMUNOPHENOTYPE

Owing to the unique features of CHL, both the phenotype of the neoplastic cells and the antigenic profile of the reactive background population are of diagnostic importance. Despite the significant morphologic variability among the four subtypes of CHL, the immunophenotype of the neoplastic cells is quite constant. The most important antigens of diagnostic relevance are summarized in Table 27-2. RS cells and variants express various activation-associated antigens, including CD30,[112,113] CD25 (interleukin [IL]-2 receptor alpha chain)[114] CD40,[115] CD71 (transferrin receptor), and HLA-DR, as well as antigens normally found on such diverse cell types as lymphocytes, granulocytes, and follicular dendritic cells.[3,4,51] They characteristically lack the common leukocyte antigen CD45 and show inconstant and heterogeneous expression of some B-cell or, rarely, T-cell markers. The immunophenotype of CHL may be difficult to assess owing to the immersion of the neoplastic RS cells in an abundant reactive infiltrate, especially for markers expressed by most or all nonneoplastic cells in the immediate vicinity, such as CD45 or T-cell markers. Another potential source of confusion is the cytoplasmic uptake of serum proteins, such as immunoglobulins, by RS cells.[116]

The most reliable and most frequently used markers for CHL are the CD30 and CD15 antigens. CD30 is a member of TNF–nerve growth factor (NGF) receptor superfamily of cytokine receptors.[117] CD30 is expressed on RS cells and variants in the vast majority of cases of CHL (85% to 96%).[113,118-121] Staining is membranous and cytoplasmic, with frequent dot-like accentuation in the perinuclear area, corresponding to the Golgi field (Fig. 27-5A). In contrast, the LP cells of NLPHL usually lack CD30 staining.[61,98] CD30 is expressed in a variety of NHLs, most notably ALCL,[113,122,123] but also in a subset of peripheral T-cell NHL, unspecified, and in some large B-cell lymphomas.[3,124] Some nonhematopoietic neoplasms, such as embryonal carcinoma, frequently express the CD30 antigen.[125,126] Perifollicular blasts in reactive lymph nodes are often positive for CD30 and should not be interpreted as interfollicular HL.[113] In general, the greater sensitivity of immunohistochemistry achieved by heat-induced antigen retrieval has significantly increased the range of lesions that can express antigens with "restricted" reactivity, such as CD30; thus, a careful evaluation of positivity is required in the context of morphology.

CD15, detected in paraffin sections by the Leu M1 or other antibodies, is an antigen of late granulopoiesis and is found in 75% to 85% of cases of CHL, although staining may be weaker than CD30 and restricted to a subset of the neoplastic cells (see Figs. 27-4F and 27-5B).[120,127-131] The staining pattern is otherwise similar to that of CD30. The reactivity in RS cells is occasionally obscured by large numbers of granulocytes in cases of nodular sclerosis (see Fig. 27-5B). The expression of CD15 is useful for differentiating RS cells from $CD30^+$ reactive blasts or RS-like cells in conditions such as infectious mononucleosis, which usually are $CD15^-$.[132,133] A notable exception are cytomegalovirus-infected cells, which show CD15 expression and may simulate Hodgkin cells by virtue of their eosinophilic nuclear inclusions.[134] In neoplastic disorders other than CHL, coexpression of CD15 and CD30 is infrequent.[122,135-137]

Not surprising in light of the B-cell derivation of CHL, expression of pan–B-cell markers—mainly CD20—can be found in a percentage of cases of CHL.[3,61,120,129,138] CD20 positivity of RS cells has been reported in less than 20% to 80% of cases[138] (the difference probably related to technical factors), with the majority of reports being in the 20% to 40% range. Improvements in antigen retrieval techniques are most likely the cause for an apparent increase in CD20 expression in recent years. In contrast to most B-cell lymphomas, notably T-cell/histiocyte-rich large B-cell lymphoma (THRLBCL) and NLPHL, CHL usually shows weaker staining restricted to a subpopulation of neoplastic cells (see Fig. 27-5C). CD79a is detected infrequently in CHL,[61,139,140] and J chain is always absent, whereas IRF4/MUM-1, a late B-cell marker, is often found.[61,141-143] Another B-cell–restricted antigen found in the cells of 90% of CHLs is the PAX5 gene product B-cell–specific activator protein (BSAP), whereas other B-cell transcription factors such as Oct-2, BOB.1, and PU.1 are either lacking or only partly expressed.[144-149] The expression profile of B-cell transcription factors and B-cell antigens is helpful in the differential diagnosis.[146] PAX5 is usually weaker than in reactive B cells, and strong expression of both BOB.1 and Oct-2 is very unusual for CHL and should prompt the consideration of a B-cell lymphoma unclassifiable, with features between DLBCL and CHL.

Several antigens related to follicular dendritic cells are expressed by RS cells in varying percentages of cases, among them CD21 and the intermediate filaments restin and fascin.[150-153] The latter is a useful diagnostic marker for HL owing to its consistent and intense staining of neoplastic cells.[153]

Positivity of RS cells for diverse T-cell antigens such as CD3, CD4, CD45RO, CD43, and T-cell receptor β in a minority of cases has been described by several groups using various approaches to circumvent the difficulties of interpreting T-cell antigen expression due to the surrounding T cells.[114,154-157] In addition, cytoplasmic staining for the cytotoxic granule-associated proteins TIA-1, granzyme B, or perforin, antigens

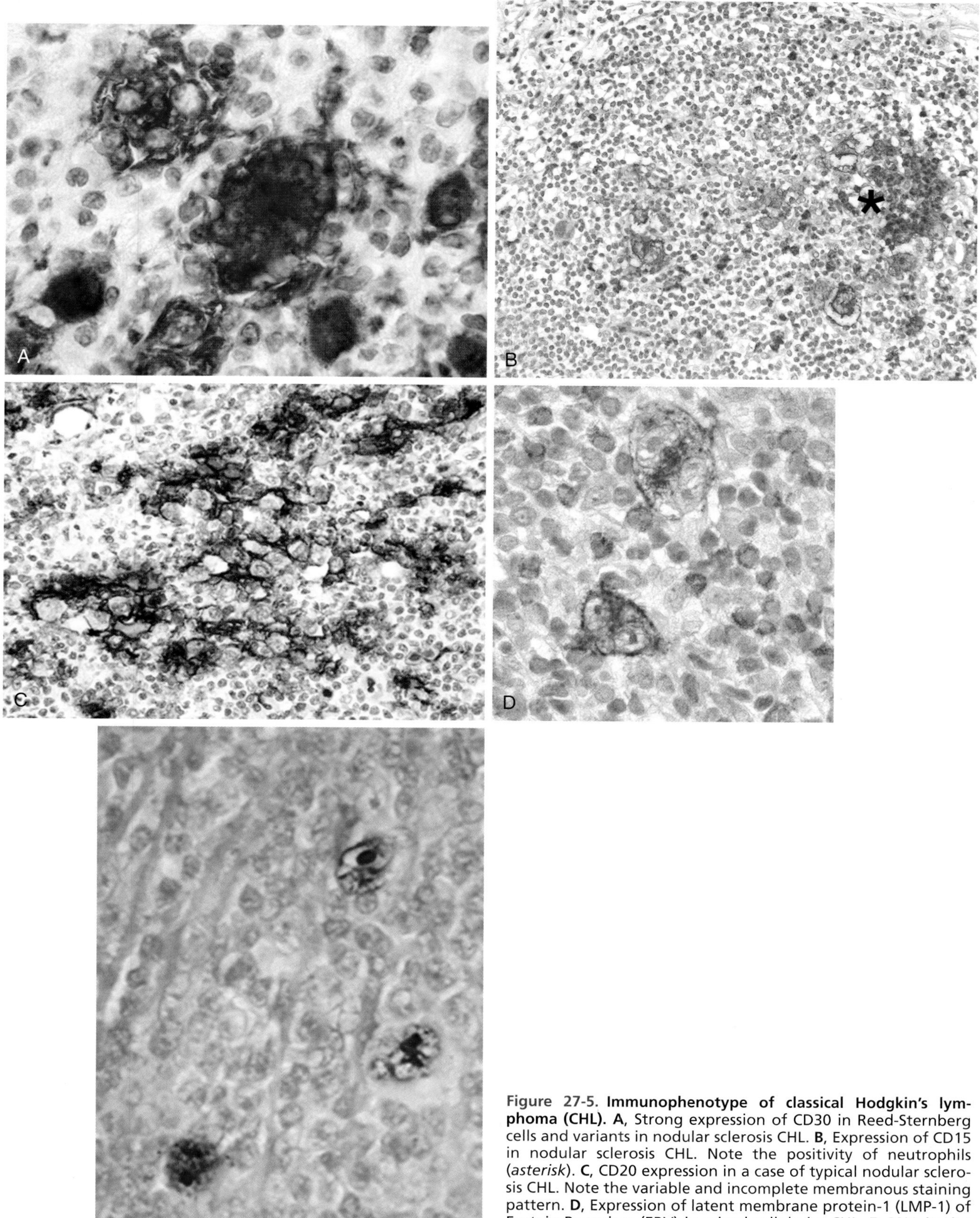

Figure 27-5. Immunophenotype of classical Hodgkin's lymphoma (CHL). A, Strong expression of CD30 in Reed-Sternberg cells and variants in nodular sclerosis CHL. **B**, Expression of CD15 in nodular sclerosis CHL. Note the positivity of neutrophils (*asterisk*). **C**, CD20 expression in a case of typical nodular sclerosis CHL. Note the variable and incomplete membranous staining pattern. **D**, Expression of latent membrane protein-1 (LMP-1) of Epstein-Barr virus (EBV) in mixed cellularity CHL. **E**, RNA in situ hybridization for EBV-encoded RNAs (EBERs) in a case of EBV^+ CHL, with strong nuclear staining restricted to the neoplastic large cells.

expressed by activated cytotoxic T cells and natural killer cells and neoplasms derived thereof, has been found in approximately 10% to 20% of cases of CHL.[11,122,158,159] Staining is usually weak and heterogeneous. Epithelial membrane antigen (EMA) and the anaplastic lymphoma kinase (ALK)-1 protein are constantly absent from RS cells of true CHL.[69,122,160-162] The absence of the common leukocyte antigen CD45 is a useful diagnostic hallmark of CHL and helps separate it from various NHL mimics as well as from NLPHL.[128,131] Similar to other types of tumors, RS cells frequently lack expression of HLA class I antigens, a potential mechanism of immune evasion.[163]

As mentioned earlier, the LMP-1 protein of EBV is expressed in approximately 25% to 50% of CHLs, depending on histologic subtype and patient characteristics.[21,39-41] The staining is membranous and cytoplasmic, and usually all or most neoplastic cells are positive (see Fig. 27-5D). In situ hybridization for EBERs shows concordance with LMP-1 immunohistochemistry if the nuclear reactivity of only RS cells (and not of rare small lymphocytes) is considered positive (see Fig. 27-5E).[36]

The phenotype of RS cells is usually constant during the course of the disease. Major variations in antigen expression in multiple biopsy sites or recurrences from the same patient are infrequent, especially with the use of heat-induced antigen retrieval.[164]

The reactive background lymphocytes of CHL, with the exception of the nodular pattern of LRCHL, are predominantly T cells. The majority express CD4, belong to the memory compartment, and show signs of activation.[165] However, their phenotype and cytokine profile are more consistent with immunosuppressive regulatory T cells, emphasizing the fact that the inflammatory response in CHL is an inadequate response to the tumor.[74,75a] The T cells surrounding the neoplastic cells express costimulatory molecules and CD30 and CD40 ligands, possibly contributing to the survival of the RS cells.[51,166] Numbers of CD8$^+$ cytotoxic T cells are low in CHL, except in patients with HIV infection. A helpful diagnostic criterion is the rarity of CD57$^+$ T cells in CHL (including the nodular variant of LRCHL), in contrast to NLPHL.[61,167,168] The nodular pattern of LRCHL is characterized by a predominance of B-cell follicles with expanded mantle zones, containing a fine meshwork of dendritic cells. Residual B-cell follicles and follicular dendritic cells can also be identified in a significant percentage of other subtypes, mainly nodular sclerosis CHL.[169]

GENETICS AND MOLECULAR FINDINGS

Immunoglobulin and T-Cell Receptor Genes

With optimized techniques of single-cell procurement and analysis, clonal immunoglobulin heavy-chain gene rearrangements can be demonstrated in the vast majority of cases of CHL, independent of the expression of B-cell markers such as CD20.[10,11,170-172] Only rare cases of CHL, even among cases preselected for T-antigen expression, have been shown to contain clonally rearranged T-cell receptor genes, suggesting their derivation from T cells.[155,173] Because some peripheral T-cell lymphomas may mimic CHL both morphologically and immunophenotypically, attributing cases with rearrangements of the T-cell receptor genes to CHL is controversial.[137] Somehow surprising in light of the molecular findings in primary cases, almost half the established CHL-derived cell lines have a T-cell phenotype and genotype.[9]

Despite the presence of rearranged immunoglobulin genes, and in contrast to NLPHL, CHL lacks immunoglobulin expression on the messenger RNA and protein level.[172,174] Several reasons for this lack of immunoglobulin transcription have been proposed. In some cases of CHL analyzed by single-cell PCR, so-called crippling mutations of the rearranged immunoglobulin heavy-chain genes leading to a premature stop codon, or mutations of the immunoglobulin promoter region, have been found, aborting immunoglobulin transcription.[1,175] Interestingly, most cases with crippling mutations are EBV$^+$, indicating EBV's role in the survival of these cells.[2] In contrast, CHL lacks expression of the B-cell transcription factors Oct-2 and PU.1 and the coactivator BOB.1/OBF.1, which are indispensable for immunoglobulin gene transcription.[147-149] Irrespective of its cause, the lack of immunoglobulin transcription indicates a breakdown of the normal regulatory mechanisms of apoptosis in CHL, given that immunoglobulin expression is a prerogative for the survival of B cells under normal circumstances.

Despite the progress concerning the histogenesis and clonality of CHL, molecular techniques still play a minor role in its practical diagnosis. In bulk tissue extracts of CHL, detection of B-cell clonality by Southern blot analysis or PCR using consensus primers is successful in only a minority of cases and usually yields weak clonal bands, reflecting the paucity of neoplastic cells.[11,176] Newer techniques such as the BIOMED-2 primer set seem to increase clonality detection rates in CHL, requiring caution in the interpretation of results.[177] Nevertheless, the presence of a major clonal B-cell or T-cell population, as evidenced by a strong clonal band in PCR or Southern blot assays, clearly favors a diagnosis of NHL over CHL and can be useful for NHL cases that simulate CHL morphologically, such as some peripheral T-cell NHLs, including ALCL or low-grade B-cell NHL with RS-like cells.[122,178,179]

Cytogenetics

Because of the small percentage of neoplastic cells in involved tissues and the difficulties in growing them in culture, cytogenetic examination of CHL has proved difficult. Several studies demonstrated recurrent chromosomal aberrations and aneuploidy of RS cells, but classic cytogenetics is prone to underestimate the amount of alterations.[180-182] Although the IgH locus at 14q32 is involved in CHL, recurrent translocations typical for NHL are absent.[11,176] Combining immunophenotypic identification of RS cells and molecular cytogenetics, chromosomal aberrations and hyperdiploidy have been detected in 100% of cases of CHL.[183] Comparative genomic hybridization of isolated RS cells after random genomic amplification has been used to quantify gains and losses of chromosomal material, leading to the identification of a commonly amplified region on 2p13 containing the *REL* oncogene. *REL* encodes a part of the Rel-A/NF-κB complex, which is constitutively activated in CHL.[184-186]

Alterations of Proto-oncogenes and Tumor Suppressor Genes

The limitations of molecular studies mentioned earlier extend to analyses of oncogenes and tumor suppressor genes.

Although initial PCR studies demonstrated BCL2 rearrangements in tissues involved by CHL,[187] subsequent investigations failed to find evidence of this translocation in neoplastic cells.[188] It is likely that positive PCR results stem from rare nonneoplastic "bystander" B cells carrying this translocation, which can also be found in healthy subjects. Likewise, detection of the t(2;5) translocation in CHL by reverse transcriptase PCR reported in an initial study could not be confirmed in subsequent analyses.[189,190] Currently, the presence of t(2;5) or one of its variants is regarded as specific for ALK$^+$ ALCL.[122] Although p53 protein is frequently expressed by RS cells, mutations of the *p53* gene are rare.[191,192] With the exception of mutations of the NF-κB inhibitor IκB in a subset of cases, there is only limited information on specific recurrent alterations in other tumor-related genes.[193]

Gene Expression Profile

Recently, large-scale screening strategies such as complementary DNA library sequencing and complementary DNA array hybridization have been used to study the expression profile of CHL-derived cell lines or primary RS cells.[194-196]

Despite the presence of clonal IgH gene rearrangements in CHL, the downregulation of most B-cell antigens and the virtual lack of a B-cell–specific gene expression profile justify the separation of CHL from B-cell NHL.[12,195] In part, this phenotype may be due to epigenetic silencing of B-cell–specific transcription factors through promoter region methylation.[197] The survival of the neoplastic cells of CHL despite the lack of a functional B-cell receptor and B-cell program indicates a profound deregulation of apoptotic pathways, which is also evidenced by the constitutive expression of antiapoptotic proteins such as BCL2, BCLxL, and c-FLIP.[2,198] Therefore, not surprisingly, expression profiling of CHL shows significant differences with most B-cell neoplasms, with the exception of mediastinal B-cell lymphoma, an entity exhibiting both morphologic and phenotypic overlap with CHL.

Other Molecular Alterations

A central feature of CHL is the constitutive activation of the NF-κB and AP-1 transcription factor families.[186,199] Signaling through members of the TNF-NGF receptor superfamily expressed by RS cells, such as CD30 and CD40 and also LMP-1, activates a complex intracellular signaling cascade involving TRAF1 and 2 (among other molecules), ultimately leading to NF-κB activation. The constitutively activated Rel-A/NF-κB complex induces transcription of various genes thought to play an important role in the evasion of apoptosis, survival, and proliferation of RS cells.[186,200] Deletions and mutations in the *IκBα* gene, an inhibitor of NF-κB, and amplifications of the locus of the *REL* oncogene may also contribute to the deregulation of this transcription factor.[184,185,201]

Furthermore, CHL shows aberrant activation of a variety of receptor tyrosine kinases, contributing to constitutive activation of several signaling cascades, including the Notch 1, PI3K/AKT, MAPK, STAT3, and STAT6 pathways.[2,202] The intense inflammatory response typical of CHL points to the involvement of disturbed immunologic pathways in disease pathogenesis.[200] As lymphoid cells in a constant state of activation, the neoplastic cells of CHL influence their surroundings with a wide range of secreted cytokines and chemokines.[51,203] Among the substances produced by RS cells, or in part by the accompanying reactive infiltrate, are TNF-α, transforming growth factor-β (TGF-β), IL-5, IL-6, IL-8, IL-10, IL-12, and IL-13, as well as the chemokines eotaxin, thymus- and activation-regulated chemokine (TARC), macrophage inflammatory protein (MIP1α), and others.[203] The majority of factors attract and activate Th2 cells and may contribute to a local suppression of cytotoxic T cells.[74,75,204] IL-5 and eotaxin are likely responsible for tissue eosinophilia.[205] TGF-β, found predominantly in nodular sclerosis CHL, is immunosuppressive and induces fibroblast proliferation and collagen formation, characteristic of this subtype.[206] The expression of some cytokines, such as IL-10, correlates with the EBV status of the disease.[207] In addition to attracting the inflammatory infiltrate and providing growth and survival stimuli to the neoplastic cells, the secreted cytokines are probably one of the reasons for the frequent presence of systemic symptoms.[51]

POSTULATED CELL OF ORIGIN

For most cases of CHL studied by single-cell analysis, the presence of clonally rearranged, somatically mutated immunoglobulin genes indicates a derivation from germinal center B cells incapable of immunoglobulin transcription.[10,11] However, the virtual lack of a B-cell expression profile underlines that the sum of genetic alterations of a neoplastic cell rather than its origin shapes its phenotype and clinical behavior.[195,196,200]

CLINICAL COURSE

The clinical course and prognosis of CHL have changed dramatically since the introduction of multimodal chemotherapy and radiotherapy. The natural history of the disease is characterized by slow but relentless tumor progression with extensive organ involvement, and in the past, many patients succumbed to infectious complications. Today, the overall cure rate for all patients is 80% to 85%. CHL is exquisitely sensitive to radiation, and complete remissions can be obtained by moderate doses in a majority of patients with early-stage (I and IIA) disease.[208] When used as the only therapeutic modality, radiotherapy is usually applied to the involved area and adjacent nodes (extended field). In advanced-stage disease, radiotherapy is combined with chemotherapy, especially if bulky disease is present.[208] Disease recurrence after isolated radiotherapy is more frequent than after chemotherapy or combined treatment. However, relapses occurring after primary radiotherapy achieve similar rates of remission as primary disease if treated systemically.[91]

Currently, multimodal therapeutic approaches combining less toxic, abbreviated chemotherapy regimens with limited radiotherapy are partly replacing conventional extended-field radiation for early-stage disease. The rationale of this approach is to reduce the frequency of late complications of radiotherapy without compromising the excellent cure rates.[91] Multiagent chemotherapies such as ABVD (Adriamycin [doxorubicin], bleomycin, vinblastine, dacarbazine) or newer regimens are the mainstay of treatment of advanced-stage HL. High-dose chemotherapy with autologous stem cell transplantation can be administered successfully to patients with primary progressive disease or early relapse, who have an extremely poor prognosis with conventional chemotherapy.[209] Experimental approaches using immunotoxins or radiolabeled antibodies directed against CD30 or other antigens are currently being tested for refractory disease.[209]

Given the high cure rate, complications of therapy, especially second malignancies, have gained importance. Patients cured of CHL have a significantly increased risk of secondary cancers, which are the main cause of death in long-term survivors.[210,211] Although common solid tumors such as carcinoma of the colon, breast, and lung are the most frequently encountered malignancies, the greatest increase in incidence is observed for acute nonlymphocytic leukemias, mainly as a result of alkylating agents. The cumulative incidence of secondary NHL after CHL is approximately 1% according to recent results—a lower rate than in earlier studies.[212,213] The majority of cases are DLBCLs, frequently at extranodal sites.[213,214] In general, the prognosis of secondary malignancies is poor.

Stage is the most important single prognostic factor in CHL. Nevertheless, in more than half the patients with disseminated disease (stage IV), complete remission can be achieved and is durable in a significant fraction of them.[209] Other clinical parameters of adverse prognostic significance include age, male sex, bulky mediastinal disease, and liver involvement, as well as anemia, leukocytosis, lymphopenia, hypoalbuminemia, and elevated lactate dehydrogenase.[209,215,216] Bone marrow involvement per se does not confer a worse prognosis compared with other patients with advanced disease.[68] Newer surrogates of disease activity, such as increased levels of soluble CD30 or cytokine levels, have prognostic relevance.[51,198,203] An important new prognostic factor is the use of positron emission tomography to evaluate the response to chemotherapy.[217] In contrast, the impact of histologic subtype and histologic grade in nodular sclerosis CHL has diminished. Although initial BNLI studies of large numbers of patients found grade II nodular sclerosis to be an indicator of poor response to therapy, increased relapse rates, and poor overall survival,[95,96] later studies showed mixed results.[218-220] Recent comparative data suggest that newer, more effective therapies tend to abolish the prognostic differences.[97]

In addition to morphology, a number of other features have been analyzed for their potential prognostic relevance. Tissue eosinophilia, lack of expression of CD15 and CD30, BCL2 expression, and presence of increased numbers of activated cytotoxic T cells are all associated with a worse prognosis,[120,198,219,221] whereas the presence of follicular dendritic cells is associated with a better prognosis.[222] The prognostic impact of EBV positivity and CD20 expression is controversial and may depend on the affected age group.[198,223-226]

DIFFERENTIAL DIAGNOSIS

Although most cases of CHL can now be safely classified on the basis of morphology and immunohistochemical features, distinction from various subtypes of NHL, reactive disorders, or even nonhematopoietic neoplasms can prove difficult. Some lymphoid neoplasms show a significant morphologic and phenotypic overlap with CHL, occasionally making a clear distinction impossible. Although some of these lesions probably represent true borderline cases between CHL and NHL, so-called gray zone lymphomas,[227] others are mere morphologic and phenotypic mimics. A broader group of NHLs may contain RS-like cells and may exhibit a pattern reminiscent of the reactive inflammatory background of CHL. However, immunohistochemical stains usually make the neoplastic character of the background population in these cases readily apparent. Furthermore, RS-like cells can occur in reactive disorders or even neoplasms of nonlymphoid origin and may lead to diagnostic difficulties, especially in small biopsy specimens.

Nodular Lymphocyte-Predominant Hodgkin's Lymphoma (Nodular Paragranuloma)

Studies of the German Hodgkin's Lymphoma Study Group and the European Task Force on Lymphoma have helped refine the criteria for differentiating CHL and NLPHL.[13,61,98] Using morphology alone, many cases of nodular LRCHL will be misclassified as NLPHL. NLPHL is characterized by nodular structures reminiscent of progressively transformed germinal centers, whereas the nodules in LRCHL consist of expanded follicle mantles with atrophic or residual germinal center remnants.[61,103] The morphology of the neoplastic cells is of limited value because LP cells can occur in both entities, so immunophenotyping is of paramount importance for the differential diagnosis. Strong and homogeneous expression of CD20, CD79a, J chain, and B-cell transcription factors, as well as expression of EMA and CD45, supports a diagnosis of NLPHL, whereas the neoplastic cells of LRCHL are usually positive for CD30 and CD15 and may be infected with EBV.[146] The small numbers of CD30$^+$ blasts frequently observable in NLPHL mostly represent nonneoplastic perifollicular immunoblasts rather than LP cells.[61] Both entities usually show a predominance of B cells in the background population and contain follicular dendritic cell networks. However, increased numbers of CD57$^+$ T cells are characteristic for NLPHL and rare in CHL (Table 27-3).[61,98,167,168]

Diffuse Large B-Cell Lymphoma and Variants

The differentiation of CHL from DLBCL is usually straightforward by morphology and is easily confirmed by immunohistochemistry, even in cases with occasional RS-like giant cells in a background of more conventional immunoblasts or centroblasts. However, some subtypes of DLBCL exhibit morphologic, phenotypic, and probably biologic overlap with CHL. These include primary mediastinal large B-cell lymphoma, THRLBCL, and EBV$^+$ DLBCL of the elderly. For cases with transitional morphologic features and an ambiguous immunophenotype, the new category of B-cell lymphoma unclassifiable, with features intermediate between DLBCL and CHL, has been included in the new WHO classification. Of note, this category should not be used as a "wastebasket" for otherwise typical cases of either DLBCL or CHL with an occasional aberrant expression of phenotypic markers; it is appropriate only for cases that truly take an intermediate position between the two entities.[14,179,227,228a]

Primary mediastinal (thymic) large B-cell lymphoma (PMLBCL) is a clinically and phenotypically distinct form of NHL. It presents with bulky mediastinal disease and is characterized by a diffuse proliferation of medium-sized to large blasts often with clear cytoplasm, sometimes resembling

Table 27-3 Differential Diagnosis: Classical Hodgkin's Lymphoma (CHL), Nodular Lymphocyte-Predominant Hodgkin's Lymphoma (NLPHL), and T-Cell/Histiocyte-Rich Large B-Cell Lymphoma (THRLBCL)

	CHL	NLPHL	THRLBCL
Architecture	Nodular (NS and LR) Diffuse (MC)	Nodular	Diffuse
Neoplastic cells	Classic RS cells Lacunar cells (NS)	LP (L & H) cells	Atypical large blasts, RS-like cells may occur
Phenotype	$CD15^+$, $CD30^+$, $CD20^{-/+}$, $CD45^-$, EMA^-, $PAX5^+$ (weak), $CD79a^-$, J $chain^-$, Oct-$2^{-/+}$, $EBV^{+/-}$	$CD20^+$, $CD79a^+$, Oct-2^+, J $chain^+$, $CD45^+$, $EMA^{+/-}$, $CD30^-$, $CD15^-$, BOB.1^+, EBV^-	$CD20^+$, $CD79a^+$, EMA^+, $CD45^+$, light chain restriction, $CD30^-$, $CD15^-$, EBV^-
Background	T cells (NS and MC) Small B cells (LR nodular) $FDC^{+/-}$ (LR, some NS)	B cells, CD57/PD-1^+ cells, FDC^+	T cells, no small B cells, no FDCs, rare CD57/PD-1^+ cells
Genotype (whole tissue)	Usually polyclonal (B and T cells), minority B-cell clone	Polyclonal	Often monoclonal (B cell)

EBV, Epstein-Barr virus; EMA, epithelial membrane antigen; FDC, follicular dendritic cell; LP lymphocyte predominant; LR, lymphocyte rich; MC, mixed cellularity; NS, nodular sclerosis; RS, Reed-Sternberg.

lacunar cells. Many cases show a dense meshwork of collagen fibers rather than concentric fibrosis.[229] Although distinction from CHL is usually possible by virtue of the architecture and morphology of the infiltrate, as well as its strong and homogeneous staining for CD20 and other B-cell markers, many cases also express the CD30 antigen and may be confused with CHL.[124] In addition, some tumors show overlapping features between PMLBCL and CHL, with nodularity of the infiltrate; dominance of cells resembling lacunar cells; appearance of RS-like cells, with sparse inflammatory cells; common expression of CD20 and CD79a, as well as CD30 and sometimes CD15; and lack of CD45. The transcription factors BOB.1, Oct-2, and PAX5 are usually positive, with variable BCL6 reactivity.[228] These cases, which are more common in young males, probably represent true gray zone lymphomas, indicating that a biologic continuum between these two entities may exist.[228] Mediastinal gray zone lymphomas account for the majority of cases in the category of unclassifiable B-cell lymphoma, intermediate between DLBCL and CHL. The frequent amplification of the *REL* oncogene in both CHL and PMLBCL, expression of the MAL protein characteristic for PMLBCL in a subgroup of CHLs, and significant similarities in gene expression compared to conventional nodal DLBCL also favor this hypothesis.[184,196,230,231] Some patients may have tumors with features of a composite lymphoma, with areas of both morphologically and immunologically typical nodular sclerosis CHL and PMLBCL in the same biopsy. In some patients these two components may be diagnosed sequentially at different times.[227,232] These composite or sequential tumors must be diagnosed as such, indicating both histologic components; they should not be included in the category of B-cell lymphomas unclassifiable, with features intermediate between DLBCL and CHL. Treatment of borderline cases is an unresolved issue. A higher relapse rate in patients with CHL initially treated for high-grade NHL was observed in a retrospective study.[232] However, regimens for aggressive B-cell lymphomas have been used successfully in mediastinal gray zone lymphoma.

THRLBCL is a DLBCL characterized by a minority of large blasts of B-cell origin in a background of reactive T cells and histiocytes. THRLBCL usually exhibits a diffuse growth pattern. Some of the tumor cells may resemble classic RS cells, but a resemblance to LP cells is more common (Fig. 27-6A). The neoplastic cells of THRLBCL usually stain strongly for CD20 and other B-cell markers, as well as BCL6 (see Fig. 27-6B); they frequently express EMA but usually lack CD30 and CD15 (see Table 27-3).[105] Rare cases with classic RS cells and an ambiguous phenotype may fall into the unclassifiable B-cell lymphoma group mentioned earlier.[14] Whether cases with a $CD20^+$, $CD15^-$, $CD30^-$ phenotype classified as CHL in the German Hodgkin's Lymphoma Study Group are related to these cases needs to be investigated.[120]

Anaplastic Large Cell Lymphoma

ALCL, initially identified by virtue of its strong reactivity with antibodies against the CD30 antigen,[113] shows some morphologic and phenotypic similarities to CHL.[233] Tumor cells of ALCL may resemble RS cells or mononuclear variants, but they are usually smaller than the neoplastic cells of CHL and often show bean-shaped or horseshoe-shaped nuclei ("hallmark" cells) rather than the round nuclei of Hodgkin cells. Furthermore, ALCL usually grows in cohesive sheets and frequently involves lymph node sinuses—rare features in CHL. Immunophenotypically, expression of T-cell antigens, cytotoxic molecules, EMA, ALK-1 protein, and CD45 supports a diagnosis of ALCL, whereas expression of CD15, CD20, and BSAP/PAX5 suggests CHL (Table 27-4).[122,123,145-147,160,161] The presence of a clonal T-cell rearrangement or t(2;5) is generally

Table 27-4 Differential Diagnosis: Classical Hodgkin's Lymphoma (CHL) and Anaplastic Large Cell Lymphoma (ALCL)

	CHL	ALCL
Architecture	Nodular or diffuse	Diffuse or sinus involvement
Neoplastic cells	Lacunar cells, classic RS cells	Mononuclear cells predominate, "hallmark" cells, some RS-like cells
Phenotype	$CD30^+$, $CD15^+$, $CD20^{-/+}$, LMP-$1^{+/-}$, $PAX5^+$, T-cell markers negative, $ALK1^-$, EMA^-	$CD30^+$, $CD15^{-/+}$, $CD20^-$, $CD4^+$, $CD45^{+/-}$, LMP-1^-, $PAX5^-$, T-cell markers often positive, $ALK1^{+/-}$, EMA^+
Genotype	Usually polyclonal (B and T cells)	Clonal T-cell rearrangement (80%-90%)

ALK, anaplastic lymphoma kinase; EMA, epithelial membrane antigen; LMP, latent membrane protein; RS, Reed-Sternberg.

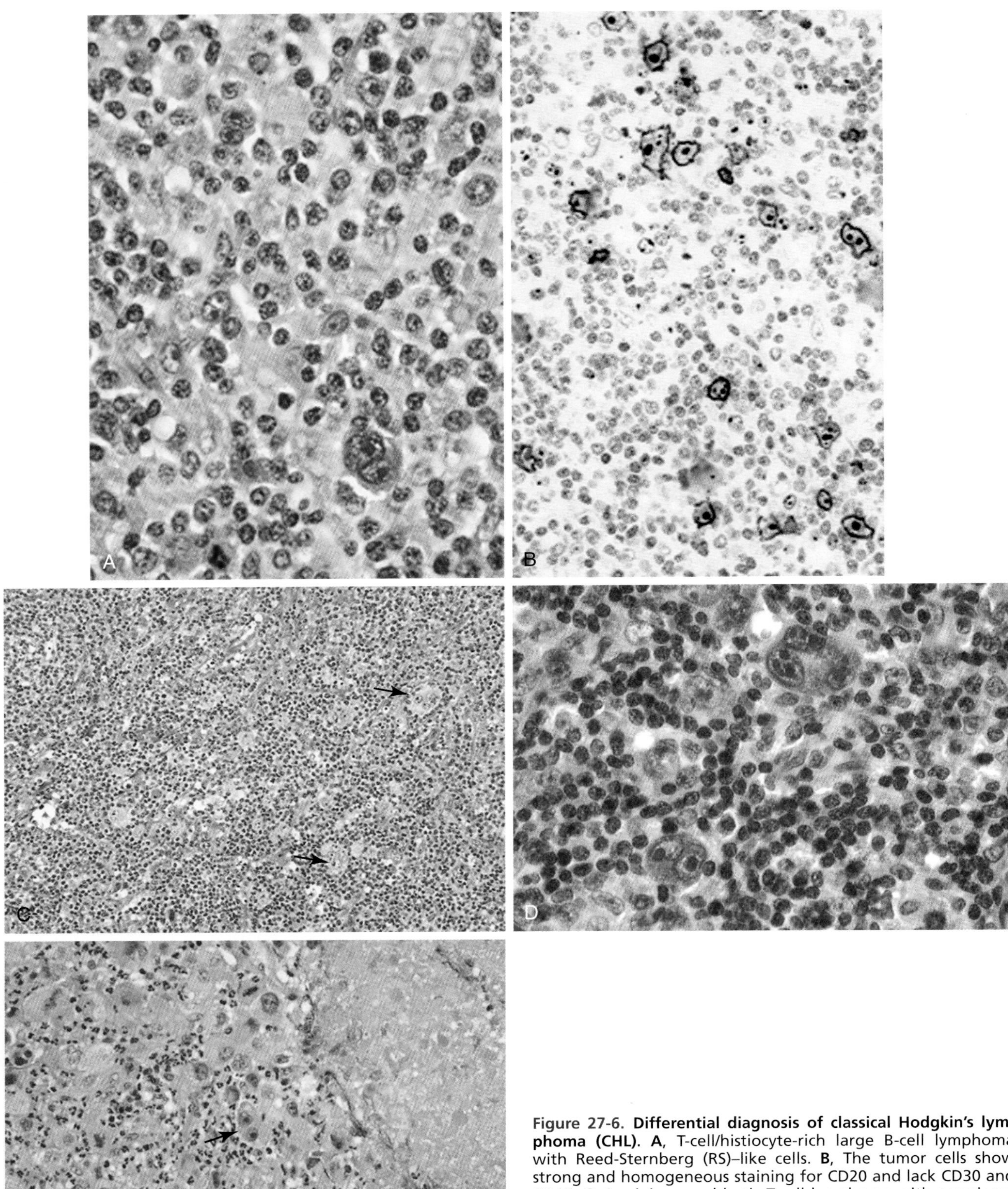

Figure 27-6. Differential diagnosis of classical Hodgkin's lymphoma (CHL). **A**, T-cell/histiocyte-rich large B-cell lymphoma with Reed-Sternberg (RS)–like cells. **B**, The tumor cells show strong and homogeneous staining for CD20 and lack CD30 and CD15. **C**, Angioimmunoblastic T-cell lymphoma with occasional Epstein-Barr virus–positive RS-like cells (*arrows*) of B-cell phenotype (CD20$^+$, CD30$^+$). **D**, Hodgkin-like posttransplant lymphoproliferative disorder with occasional RS cells in a polymorphous B-cell proliferation. **E**, Mediastinal lymph node biopsy of anaplastic large cell carcinoma with occasional RS-like cells (*arrow*).

thought to exclude CHL.[122,189,190] Cases previously described as ALCL, Hodgkin-like and included as a provisional entity in the REAL classification exhibit confluent sheets of neoplastic cells and sometimes sinus involvement, but they have architectural features of nodular sclerosis CHL, such as nodular growth and concentric collagen bands.[8,234] Most of these cases are now thought to represent either grade II nodular sclerosis CHL or lymphocyte-depleted CHL. Only rare cases of ALCL with a nodular growth pattern resemble nodular sclerosis CHL, and they are readily diagnosed with immunohistochemical studies, including ALK staining.[235] Based on recent data, the category of ALCL, Hodgkin-like was dropped from the WHO classification because these two entities can be readily distinguished with appropriate studies.[236]

Other Subtypes of Non-Hodgkin's Lymphoma and Composite Lymphomas

RS-like cells can occur in a wide range of NHLs of both B- and T-cell types. Among B-cell lymphoid neoplasms, this phenomenon is most frequently encountered in chronic lymphocytic leukemia (CLL). In most cases, RS-like cells are present singly or in small clusters in the background of morphologically and phenotypically classic CLL ($CD5^+$, $CD20^+$, $CD23^+$). They frequently express CD30 and sometimes CD15, may coexpress CD20, and are usually infected by EBV ($EBER^+$, LMP-1^+).[179,237,238] These cases may represent precursor lesions for CHL, which has an increased incidence in patients with CLL and occasionally presents as a composite lymphoma.[179,237] Indeed, a clonal relationship between the two populations has been shown for some but not all cases studied by single-cell PCR.[239,240] These cases, which have also been designated *Hodgkin-like Richter's transformation*, arise more commonly from CLL with mutated immunoglobulin genes and seem to carry a better prognosis than conventional Richter's syndrome.[241] Transformed B cells with RS-like morphology, as well as true composite lymphomas with separate areas of both CHL and B-cell NHL, have also been observed in other B-cell NHL subtypes, most frequently follicular lymphoma.[179,242-244] In some cases, a common clonal origin has been demonstrated by molecular studies.[2,245]

Peripheral T-cell lymphomas frequently show a polymorphic inflammatory background with eosinophils, neutrophils, plasma cells, and histiocytes and may contain RS-like giant cells.[178,246-248] In some neoplasms, such as nodal peripheral T-cell lymphoma, not otherwise specified, and transformed mycosis fungoides, RS-like cells show coexpression of CD30, CD15, and T-cell markers and probably represent transformed cells of the malignant clone. Usually they form part of a continuum of small to medium-sized and large blasts.[136,137,179] In contrast, RS-like cells in angioimmunoblastic T-cell lymphoma and adult T-cell lymphoma/leukemia are EBV-transformed, nonclonal B cells and are probably the result of an underlying local immune dysregulation (see Fig. 27-6C).[178,248] Because the background population of neoplastic T cells in cases of T-cell NHL with RS-like giant cells can sometimes show only minimal cytologic atypia, detailed immunophenotyping and molecular studies may be necessary for the distinction from CHL.[178]

The occurrence of true CHL in patients with T-cell NHL has been observed most frequently in mycosis fungoides.[179] Although an initial case report demonstrated a common clonal T-cell origin for both lymphomas, probably representing large cell transformation of the initial T-cell clone, most subsequent studies produced evidence of two clonally distinct neoplasms.[179,249,250]

Epstein-Barr Virus–Associated Lymphoproliferations in the Immunosuppressed Host

Solid organ or bone marrow transplant recipients, as well as patients receiving immunosuppressive therapies for various connective tissue diseases, are at risk for the development of EBV-driven lymphoproliferative disorders.[251,252] Both CHL and CHL-like lymphoproliferative disorder are included in the new WHO classification. The latter cases consist of a polymorphous proliferation of small to large lymphoid cells with frequent RS-like cells. True CHL in the posttransplant setting simulates sporadic CHL morphologically and phenotypically; it occurs late after transplantation and usually does not respond to a reduction in immunosuppression.[30] Morphologically, RS-like cells in HL-like posttransplant lymphoproliferative disorder are part of a continuum of lymphoid cells in various stages of transformation rather than embedded in a reactive background of small lymphocytes (see Fig. 27-6D).[253] They usually coexpress CD30 and CD20 but are $CD15^-$ and show EBV positivity with latency type III expressing EBNA2, in contrast to CHL.[21,49,251,252]

The category of EBV^+ DLBCL of the elderly, a new addition to the updated WHO classification, is a polymorphous proliferation of transformed large B cells with the common occurrence of RS-like large cells and areas of geographic necrosis.[254] EBV^+ DLBCL shows expression of B-cell markers, with common CD30 positivity but lack of CD15, and often exhibits the full range of EBV latency products, including LMP-1 and EBNA2, thus resembling posttransplant lymphoproliferative disorders. This disorder, which has so far been systematically described only in Asian countries, is believed to be the result of a deteriorated immune system caused by the aging process. In contrast to CHL, the majority of cases arise in extranodal sites and have a poor prognosis.[255,256]

Reactive Disorders

Reactive lymphadenopathies with a wide range of both infectious and noninfectious causes can exhibit RS-like cells. Infectious mononucleosis typically shows florid interfollicular hyperplasia, with at least partial preservation of the lymph node architecture. The paracortical proliferation may be dominated by variously sized immunoblasts or show a mixed cytology, with small lymphocytes and interspersed, frequently binucleate blasts closely resembling RS cells.[31,132] Necrosis may be present. The clinical picture and serologic findings are crucial in avoiding a misdiagnosis of CHL in such cases. Morphologically, the range of cell sizes and the marked cytoplasmic basophilia of many blasts are indicators of a reactive disorder. RS-like cells in infectious mononucleosis can express CD30 and LMP-1[257] but lack CD15 and frequently show CD20 expression.[132,133]

Other lymphadenitides of viral or unknown cause may occasionally mimic CHL, especially the interfollicular growth pattern.[258] Necrotizing lymphadenitides such as cat-scratch disease or Kikuchi's lymphadenitis may resemble the necrotic foci found in nodular sclerosis CHL. However, careful morphologic review and immunohistochemical stains demonstrate the absence of RS cells among the histiocytes rimming the necrotic areas.

Neoplasms of Nonlymphoid Origin

A large number of nonlymphoid neoplasms may resemble CHL morphologically, especially if only small biopsy specimens are available. In most instances, immunohistochemical studies resolve these cases. However, one should be aware of the potential pitfalls of a limited antibody panel. Both CD15 and CD30 can be expressed by a range of nonhematopoietic neoplasms, and reliance on a single positive marker may be perilous.[126,135] Lymph node metastasis of large cell undifferentiated carcinoma or melanoma may resemble the syncytial variant of nodular sclerosis CHL (see Fig. 27-6E), but it is usually easily differentiated by appropriate immunostainings for cytokeratins or S-100 protein and melanoma antigens, respectively. Undifferentiated nasopharyngeal carcinoma can resemble CHL both morphologically and clinically because the tumor frequently presents with cervical lymph node metastasis, whereas the primary tumor is often clinically unapparent.[259] Extragonadal germ cell tumors can simulate nodular sclerosis CHL with a mass lesion in the anterior mediastinum. The neoplastic cells of seminoma may resemble lacunar cells and sometimes exhibit a nodular growth pattern with concentric fibrosis, but demonstration of PLAP (placenta-like alkaline phosphatase) positivity resolves these cases. Inflammatory variants of sarcomas may contain RS-like cells, but these usually do not pose major diagnostic problems.

Pearls and Pitfalls

- The diagnosis of CHL requires the presence of RS cells in the appropriate cellular milieu and background.
- Expression of CD30 and CD15, although highly characteristic of CHL, can rarely be seen in other neoplasms, including both aggressive B-cell and T-cell lymphomas.
- Nodular sclerosis CHL is distinct from other forms of CHL in terms of its demographics and epidemiology, whereas the mixed cellularity and lymphocyte-depleted subtypes are closely related.
- LRCHL most often has a nodular growth pattern and is most likely to be confused with NLPHL morphologically.
- The existence of composite, synchronous, and metachronous occurrences of CHL and other B-cell lymphomas first suggested a B-cell origin for the neoplastic cells of CHL.
- CHL is a B-cell neoplasm in which the B-cell program is highly suppressed. In cases with CHL morphology but strong, homogeneous expression of B-cell markers, a diagnosis of unclassifiable B-cell lymphoma should be considered.

References can be found on Expert Consult @ www.expertconsult.com

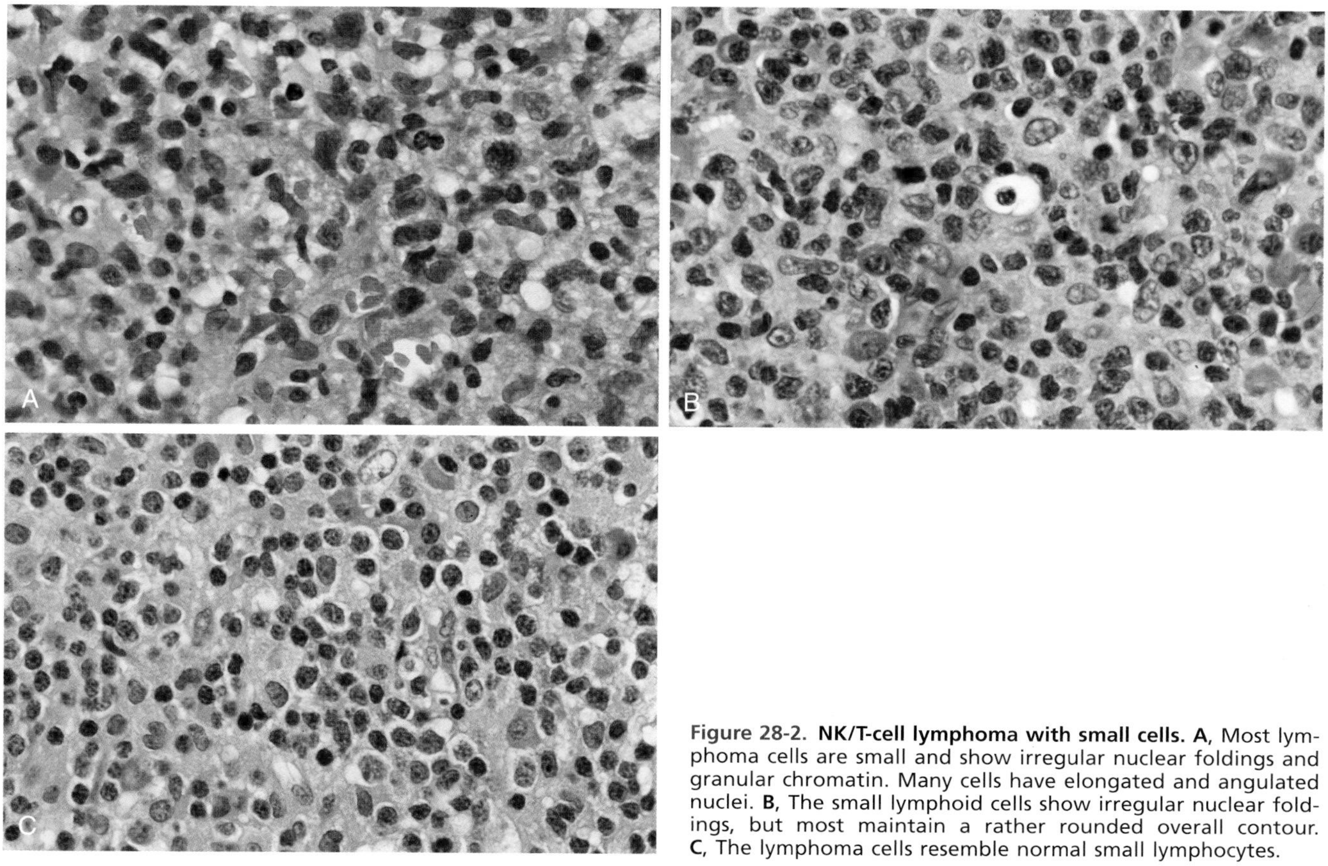

Figure 28-2. NK/T-cell lymphoma with small cells. A, Most lymphoma cells are small and show irregular nuclear foldings and granular chromatin. Many cells have elongated and angulated nuclei. **B,** The small lymphoid cells show irregular nuclear foldings, but most maintain a rather rounded overall contour. **C,** The lymphoma cells resemble normal small lymphocytes.

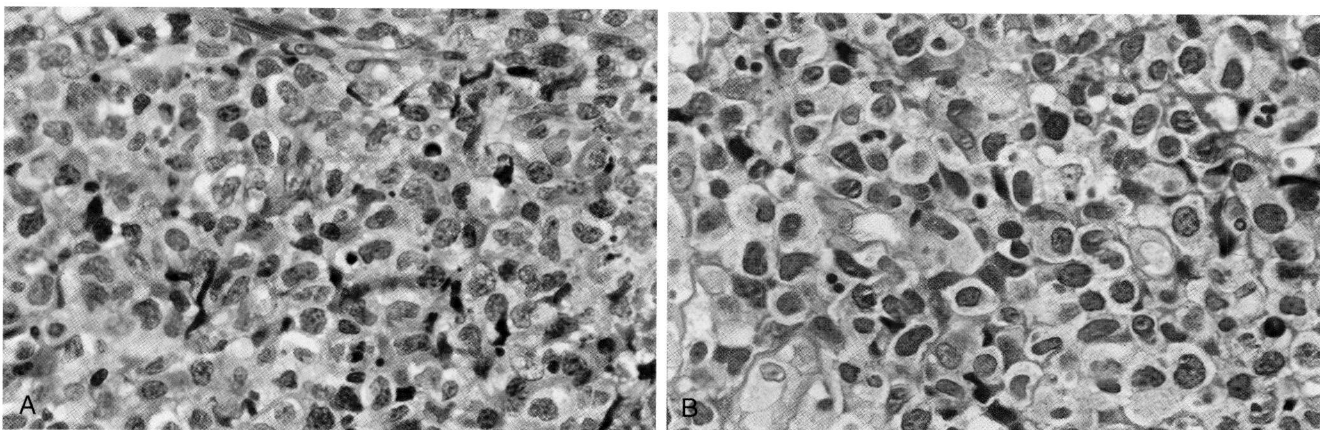

Figure 28-3. NK/T-cell lymphoma with medium-sized cells. A, The medium-sized cells show irregular nuclear foldings and scanty cytoplasm. Note the admixed apoptotic bodies. **B,** In this example, the medium-sized lymphoma cells possess a moderate amount of clear cytoplasm.

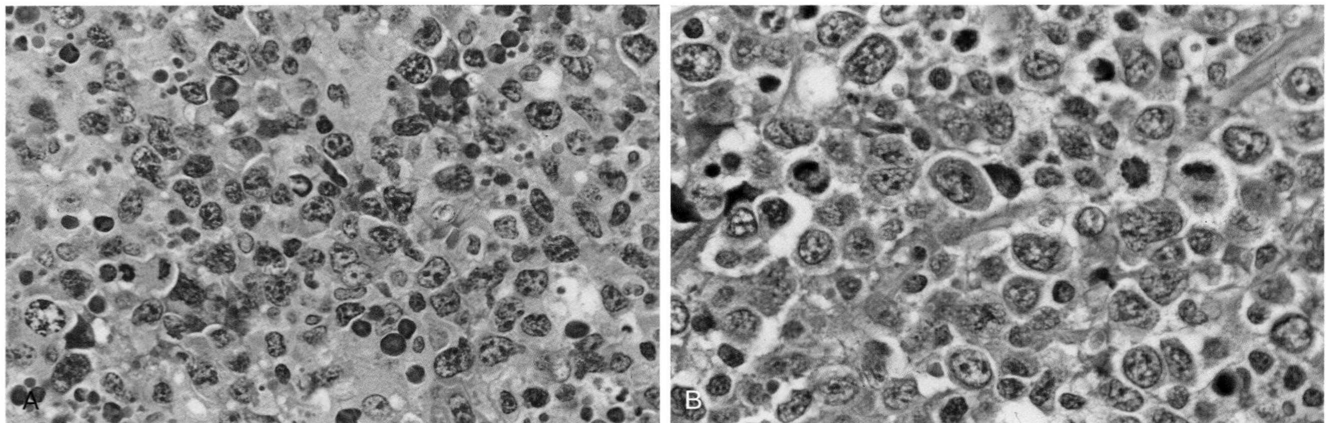

Figure 28-4. NK/T-cell lymphoma with large cells. A, The large cells show distinct nucleoli, and there are many intermingled apoptotic bodies. **B,** The cells are even larger in this example. The distinction from diffuse large B-cell lymphoma cannot be made on morphologic grounds alone.

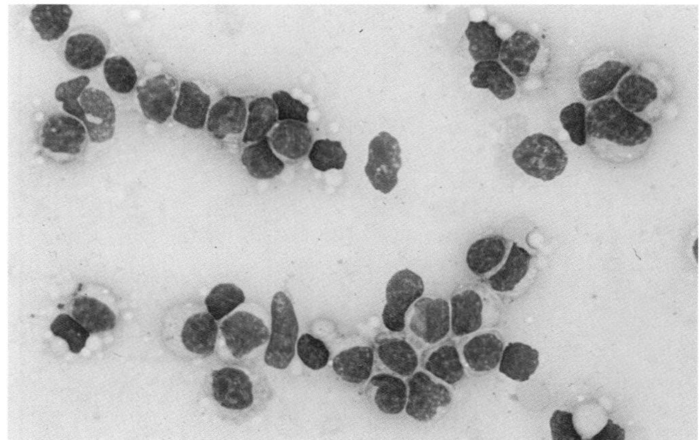

Figure 28-5. Nasal NK/T-cell lymphoma. Giemsa-stained touch preparation reveals medium-sized cells with pale cytoplasm. Some cells contain small numbers of fine azurophilic granules (where cytotoxic molecules are stored).

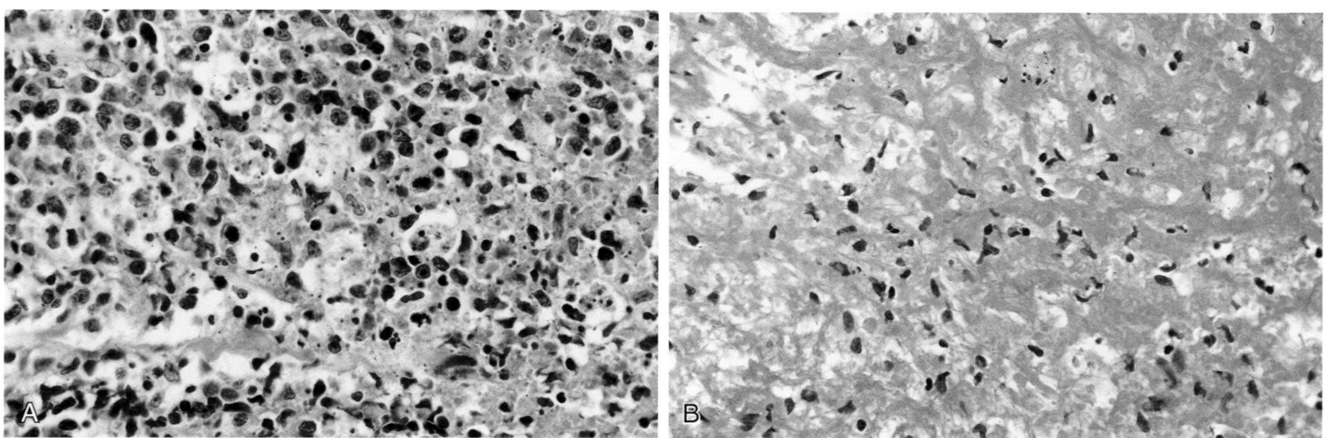

Figure 28-6. NK/T-cell lymphoma. A, Numerous apoptotic bodies (karyorrhectic debris) are found among the lymphoma cells. **B,** Extensive necrosis with fibrin deposition is a common finding.

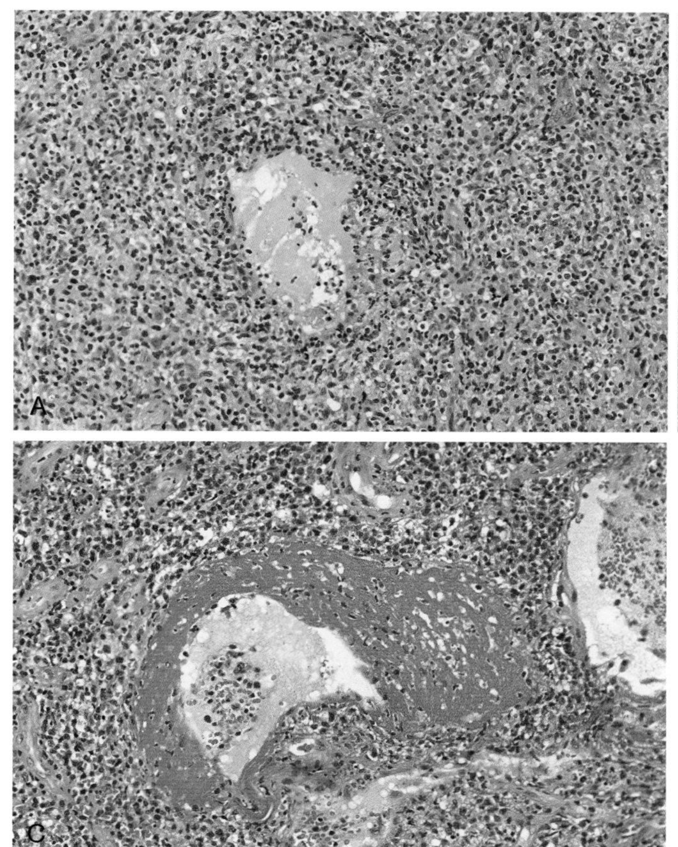

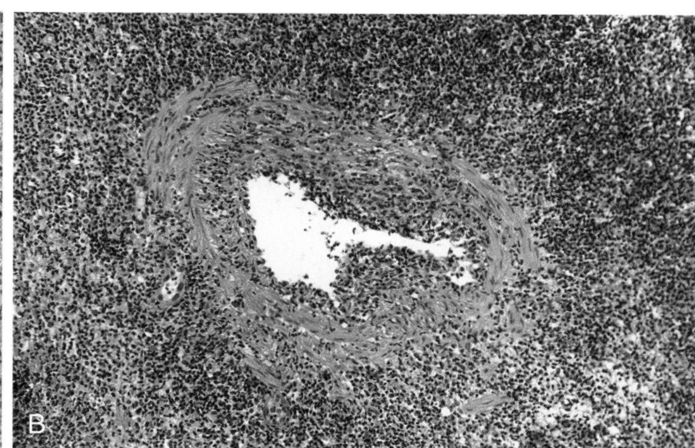

Figure 28-7. Vascular changes in nasal NK/T-cell lymphoma. A, The blood vessel wall is swarmed with lymphoma cells. This qualifies as angiocentric growth because the tumor cell density is much higher in the vessel wall compared with the surrounding involved tissue. **B,** In addition to the concentration of lymphoma cells around and in the wall of this blood vessel, there is infiltration of the intima. This qualifies as angiocentric growth. **C,** There is deposition of fibrinoid material in the blood vessel wall.

lymphoma disseminating to skin than in primary cutaneous NK/T-cell lymphoma.[108,109] In the subcutaneous tissue the lymphoma cells percolate among the adipocytes, producing a panniculitis-like picture (Fig. 28-12). The lymphoma cells can palisade around fat vacuoles, and fat necrosis is common.[13,110] Taken out of context, the histologic features may be indistinguishable from subcutaneous panniculitis-like T-cell lymphoma.

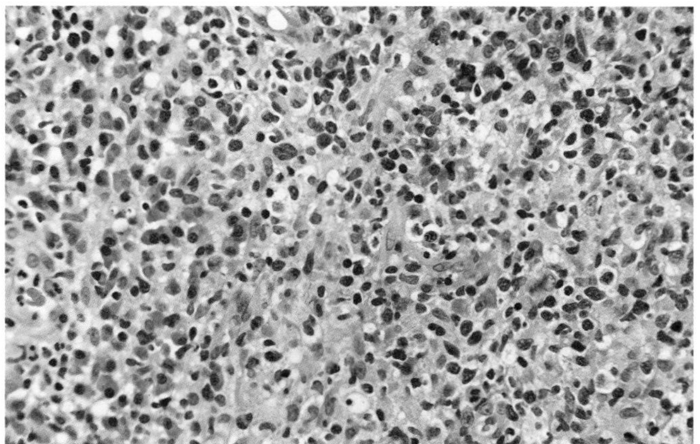

Figure 28-8. Nasal NK/T-cell lymphoma. Not uncommonly, the cellular infiltrate is polymorphic, with many intermingled acute and chronic inflammatory cells.

In the gastrointestinal tract there is usually transmural infiltration by lymphoma cells. Extensive coagulative necrosis, deep ulcers, and perforation are common (Fig. 28-13).[13,99,111]

In the testis there is infiltration of the interstitium by dense sheets of lymphoma cells, often accompanied by angiodestruction and necrosis.[89] The seminiferous tubules are lost, atrophic, or infiltrated by lymphoma cells (Fig. 28-14).

In the soft tissues there is a permeative growth, prominent destruction of skeletal muscle fibers, and invasion of the nerves (Fig. 28-15). Sometimes the muscle fibers show flocculent necrosis, invasion of the cytoplasm by lymphoma cells, or dropout of individual cells, leaving empty spaces.[97]

Grading

Cytologic grading of extranodal NK/T-cell lymphoma is optional because its value is controversial.[64,112,113] The International Peripheral T-Cell Lymphoma Project recently reported that the presence of greater than 40% transformed cells predicted a worse overall survival in nasal cases but not in extranasal cases.[27]

Immunophenotype

The prototypic immunophenotype of NK/T-cell lymphoma is $CD2^+$, surface $CD3^-$, cytoplasmic $CD3\varepsilon^+$, and $CD56^+$, although occasional cases may show minor deviations, such as lack of cytoplasmic CD3ε or CD56 expression (Fig. 28-16).[12,27,59,114-116] CD43 and CD45RO are commonly positive, and CD7 is

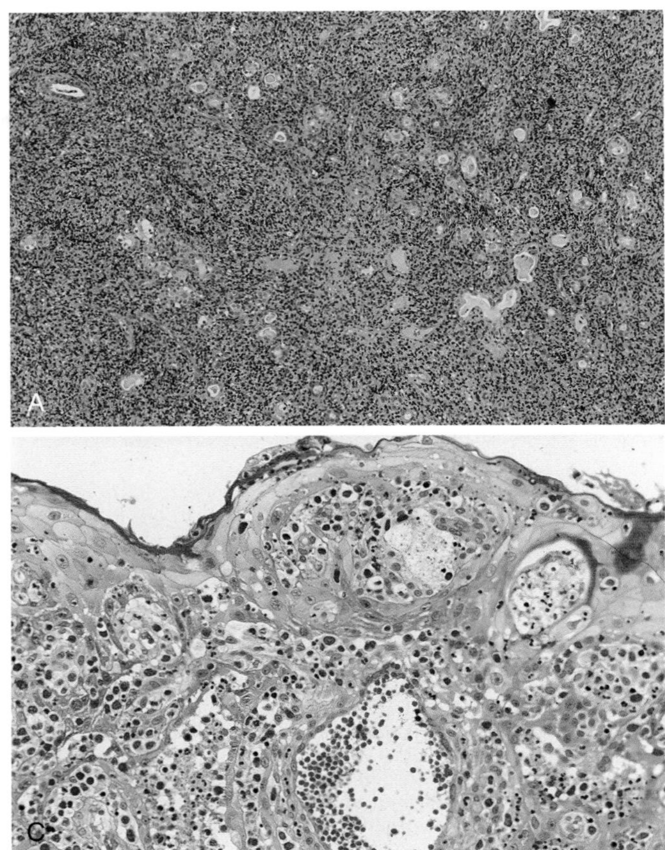

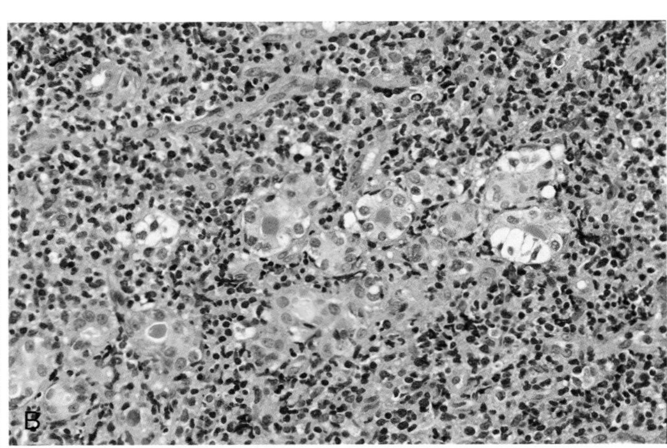

Figure 28-9. **Nasal NK/T-cell lymphoma. A**, Typically, the nasal mucosa is expanded by a dense lymphoid infiltrate. The mucosal glands, which normally occur as discrete lobules, are pushed apart by the lymphomatous infiltrate. **B**, The interstitial lymphomatous infiltrate causes separation of the mucosal glands, which not uncommonly exhibit clear cell change (possibly a manifestation of cellular injury). **C**, In this example, the surface epithelium shows squamous metaplasia and infiltration by lymphoma cells.

occasionally expressed. Other T-cell–associated antigens such as CD4, CD5, CD8, TCRαβ, and TCRγδ are usually negative (see Table 28-1).[1,12-16,27,117] Rare cases can exhibit aberrant expression of CD20.[118,119] Very few B cells are present in the background.

The only NK marker consistently expressed is CD56; CD16 and CD57 are almost always negative (see Table 28-1, Fig. 28-16C). In most cases, the expression of CD56 is consistent in the various sites of involvement and in relapses.

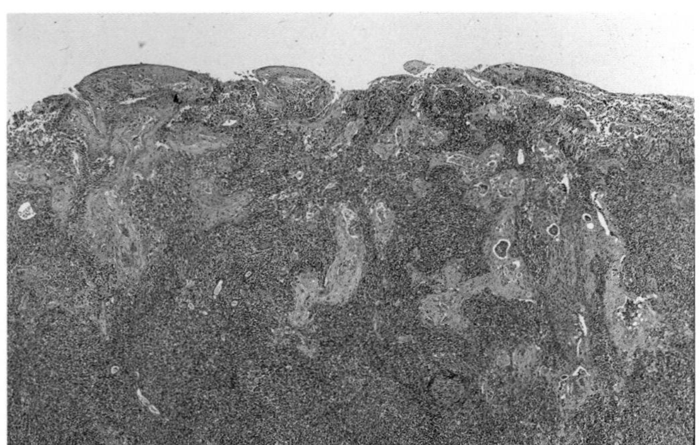

Figure 28-10. Nasal NK/T-cell lymphoma with florid pseudoepitheliomatous hyperplasia, mimicking squamous cell carcinoma.

However, in some cases a $CD56^+$ tumor may relapse as a $CD56^-$ tumor, or vice versa. The specificity of CD56 for NK/T-cell lymphoma is addressed in Pearls and Pitfalls (see later). Cytotoxic molecules such as TIA-1, granzyme B, and perforin are usually positive,[1,70,76,120] and they may mediate the tissue injury and cell death commonly observed in this lymphoma type.[121,122]

Similar to normal NK cells, both Fas (CD95) and Fas ligand (CD178) are frequently expressed,[123,124] and the Fas–Fas ligand system has been postulated to play a role in tumor apoptosis and vascular injury. A proportion of cases expresses human leukocyte antigen (HLA)-DR (≈40%) and CD25 (≈15%).[1,12] CD30 is positive in about half the cases, especially in those rich in large cells.[27,77] In contrast to anaplastic large cell lymphoma, CD30 expression is usually focal and not as intense. Frequent expression of cyclin-dependent kinase 6 and loss of CD44 have also been reported.[125]

The proliferative fraction as demonstrated by Ki-67 immunostaining is usually high (>50%), even for small cell–predominant lesions.[1] One study suggested that a high Ki-67 index (≥65%) is associated with a worse prognosis, and another reported that a Ki-67 index greater than 50% predicts worse overall survival for nasal but not extranasal NK/T-cell lymphoma.[27,126] Pearls and Pitfalls (see later) addresses the practical issues in the diagnosis of extranodal NK/T-cell lymphoma when only paraffin-embedded materials are available.

Most NK/T-cell lymphomas express the NK-cell receptor CD94/NKG2, but only some express KIRs.[14-16] NK-cell receptors are not specific for NK/T-cell lymphomas; they are also

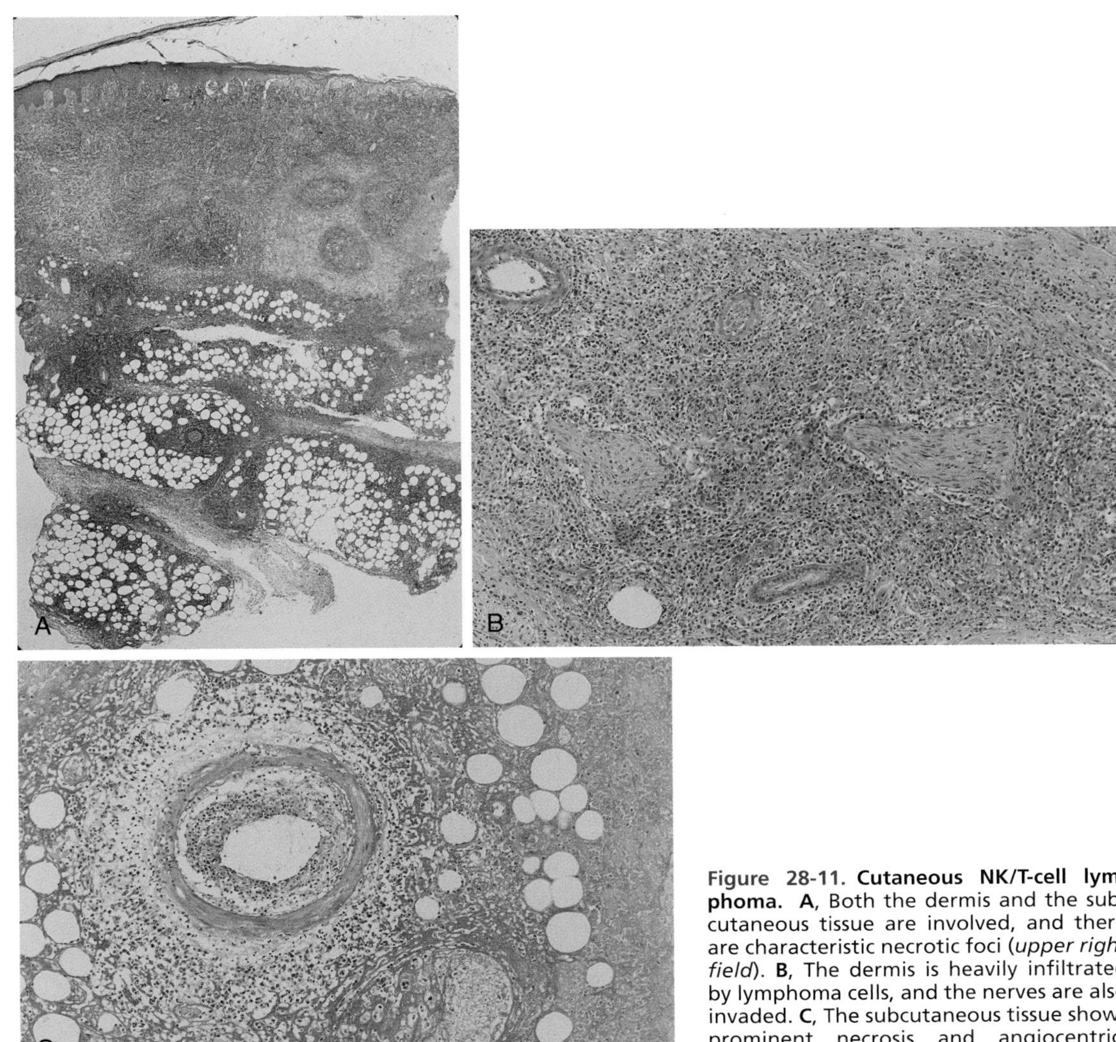

Figure 28-11. Cutaneous NK/T-cell lymphoma. A, Both the dermis and the subcutaneous tissue are involved, and there are characteristic necrotic foci (*upper right field*). **B**, The dermis is heavily infiltrated by lymphoma cells, and the nerves are also invaded. **C**, The subcutaneous tissue shows prominent necrosis and angiocentric-angiodestructive growth.

Figure 28-12. Cutaneous NK/T-cell lymphoma with involvement of subcutaneous tissue. A, The subcutaneous tissue shows infiltration by a mixture of atypical small, medium-sized, and large lymphoid cells. **B**, The lace-like infiltrate and rimming of fat vacuoles by lymphoma cells simulate the histologic features of subcutaneous panniculitis-like T-cell lymphoma.

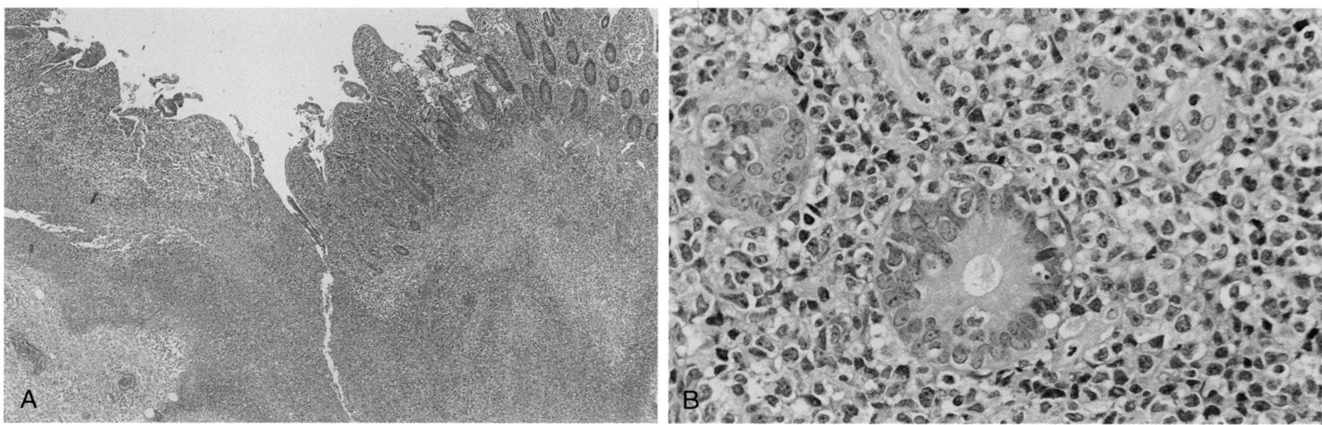

Figure 28-13. Primary NK/T-cell lymphoma of the gastrointestinal tract. A, The ileum shows infiltration by lymphoma, necrosis, deep ulceration, and perforation. **B,** The rectal mucosa shows dense interstitial infiltration by lymphoma cells with clear cytoplasm. There is also invasion of the crypt epithelium.

expressed by some cytotoxic T-cell lymphomas and hepatosplenic T-cell lymphomas. However, demonstration of a skewed NK-cell repertoire by flow cytometry using antibodies against KIRs, CD94, and NKG2A may imply a monoclonal NK-cell proliferation.[127]

Nasal lymphomas that are CD56⁻ but demonstrate a CD3ε⁺, cytotoxic molecule–positive, EBV⁺ phenotype are also included in the category of nasal NK/T-cell lymphoma.[43,128] Some of these cases are probably NK-cell lymphomas that have lost CD56 expression, whereas others are cytotoxic T-cell lymphomas, as evidenced by surface CD3 expression. Some of the latter express TCRαβ and some express TCRγδ.[124,129,130] One report suggested a high frequency of TCRγδ expression among nasal NK/T-cell lymphomas,[131] but a reinvestigation of that series of cases failed to confirm this observation.[132] The clinical features and morphology of the CD56⁻ group are indistinguishable from those of the CD56⁺ group.[27] Nasal lymphomas that show a CD3ε⁺, CD56⁻, cytotoxic molecule–positive, EBV⁻ phenotype are not included in this category and should be diagnosed as peripheral T-cell lymphoma, not otherwise specified.

Genetics and Molecular Findings

The TCR and immunoglobulin genes are in germline configuration in the majority of cases. A small proportion of cases shows rearrangement of the TCR genes—up to 38% in one series; the positive cases probably represent neoplasms of cytotoxic T cells rather than NK cells.[1,27,66,71,76,116,117,133,134]

There is a nearly consistent association with EBV (Fig. 28-17). Although some EBV⁻ cases have been reported, this phenomenon may be related to differences in criteria for case inclusion.[1,135] For example, in the recent International Peripheral T-Cell Lymphoma Project study, EBV positivity was an obligatory inclusion criterion.[27] It is prudent to require EBV positivity for confirmation of diagnosis in extranasal cases, because many types of peripheral T-cell lymphomas show morphologic and immunophenotypic overlap with NK/T-cell lymphoma. The EBV exists in a clonal episomal form in the tumor cells and shows a type II latency pattern.[70,136,137] It is usually of subtype A, with a high frequency of 30-bp deletion of the *LMP-1* gene.[70,136,137] Circulating plasma or serum EBV DNA levels are often elevated, and a high titer is correlated

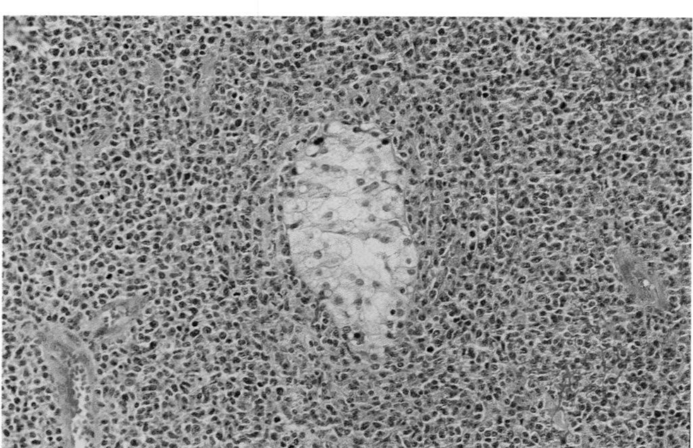

Figure 28-14. Primary testicular NK/T-cell lymphoma. The dense lymphomatous infiltration is accompanied by a striking loss of seminiferous tubules. The tubule in the *center* field shows multilayering of the basement membrane due to infiltration by lymphoma cells.

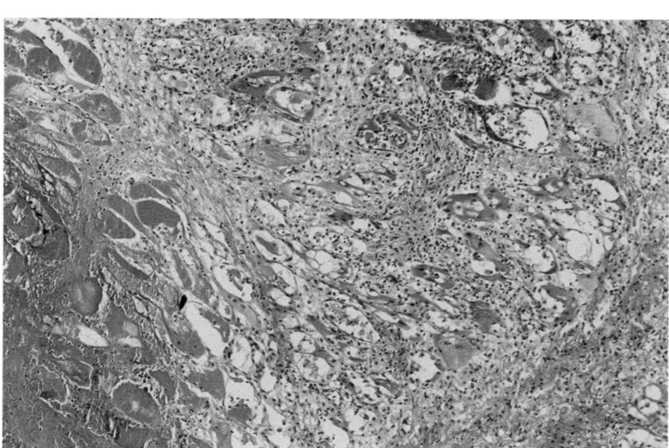

Figure 28-15. Primary soft tissue NK/T-cell lymphoma. There is interstitial infiltration by lymphoma, accompanied by prominent necrosis and destruction of skeletal muscle fibers.

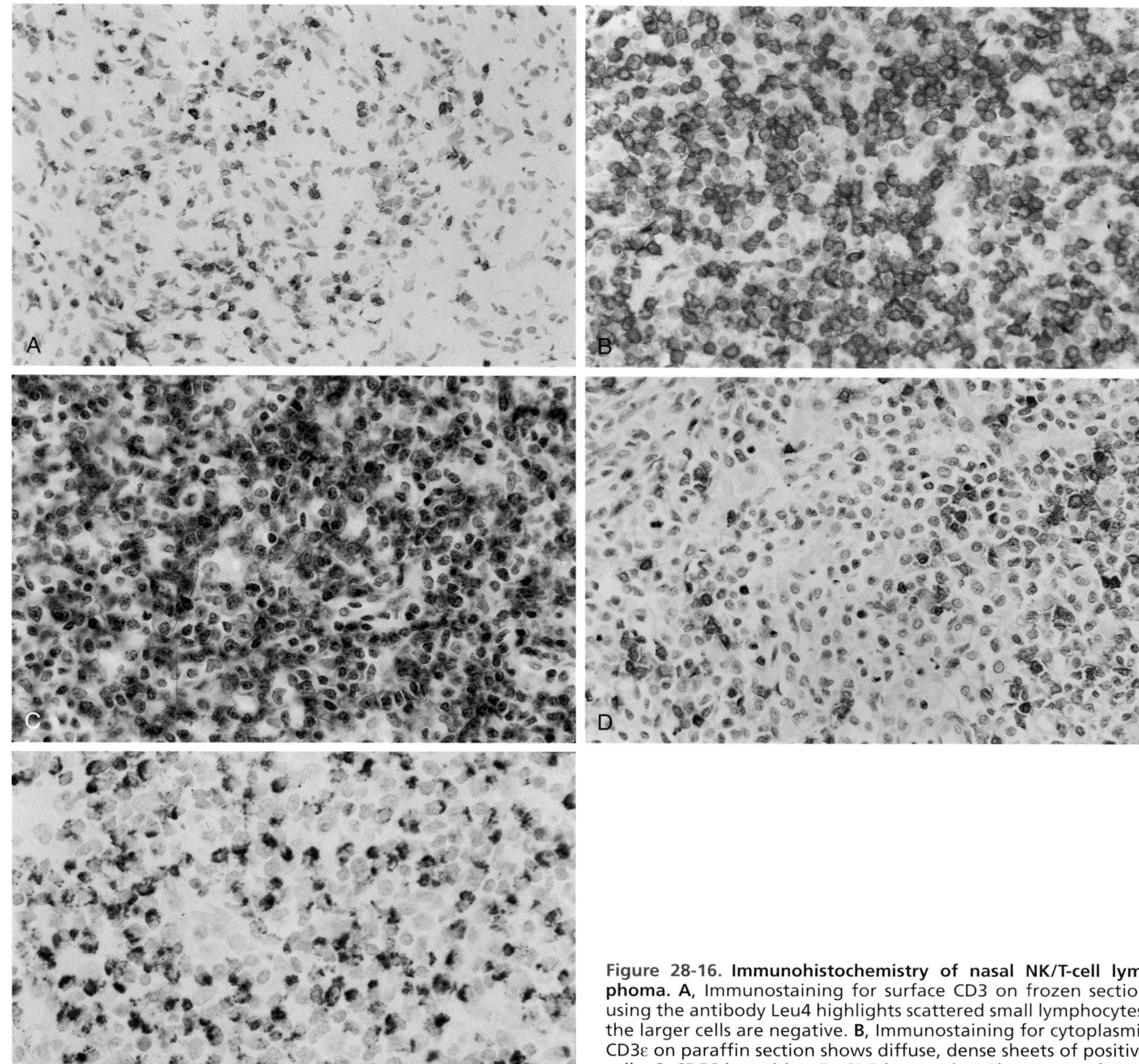

Figure 28-16. Immunohistochemistry of nasal NK/T-cell lymphoma. A, Immunostaining for surface CD3 on frozen section using the antibody Leu4 highlights scattered small lymphocytes; the larger cells are negative. **B,** Immunostaining for cytoplasmic CD3ε on paraffin section shows diffuse, dense sheets of positive cells. **C,** CD56 is positive. **D,** CD5 is negative. The scattered positive cells are admixed reactive T cells. **E,** Numerous cells show granular staining for the cytotoxic marker TIA-1.

with extensive disease, unfavorable response to treatment, and poor survival.[138,139]

Overexpression of p53 protein occurs in 45% to 86% of NK/T-cell lymphomas, whereas *p53* gene mutation is found in 24% to 62% of cases, with some variation in frequencies reported from different populations.[140-142] The *p53* mutation has been found to correlate with large cell morphology and advanced stage at presentation.[143] Mutations of the *β-catenin*, *K-Ras*, and *c-Kit* genes are detected in 22%, 14%, and 6%, respectively, but the significance is not clear.[142]

Promoter methylation leading to gene silencing commonly affects the *p73*, *retinoic acid receptor β*, and *death-associated protein kinase* genes. Demonstration of aberrant methylation of these genes by methylation-specific polymerase chain reaction (PCR) may be useful for monitoring minimal residual tumor after treatment, occult bone marrow metastasis, and early relapse.[144,145]

Demonstration of KIR repertoire restriction by reverse transcriptase PCR can support the monoclonal nature of NK/T-cell lymphoma. Taken together with germline TCR genes, this finding further confirms the true NK lineage of the lymphoma in most cases.[146] However, KIR repertoire restriction alone is not specific for NK-cell lymphomas and can also be observed in some T-cell lymphomas with a cytotoxic phenotype.

Complex chromosomal abnormalities have been found in extranodal NK/T-cell lymphomas.[104,147-150] The most common changes are 6q−, 2q+, 8p−, 11q−, 12q−, 13q−, 15q+, 17q+,

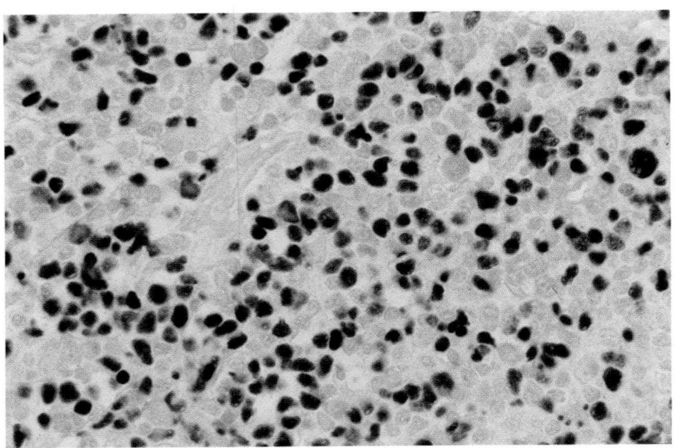

Figure 28-17. Nasal NK/T-cell lymphoma. In situ hybridization for Epstein-Barr virus–encoded RNA (EBER) labels the nuclei of most lymphoma cells.

and 22q+. Specific chromosomal translocations have not been identified, but translocations involving the 8p23 breakpoint have been reported in a number of cases.[151-153]

Postulated Cell of Origin

Lien and coworkers[125] proposed the normal counterpart to be an early NK/T bipotent progenitor cell based on the consistent expression of cyclin-dependent kinase 6, a marker of immature T cells and NK/T bipotent progenitors.[133] However, expression of CD94 suggests an origin from mature NK cells.[14] Cytotoxic T lymphocyte is likely the normal counterpart of some cases (which can be $CD56^+$ or $CD56^-$).

Clinical Course

Although patients with nasal NK/T-cell lymphoma usually present with localized disease, dissemination to various sites frequently occurs either early or late in the course of the disease.[64,154] Hemophagocytic syndrome may complicate the disease in some patients.[155,156] Radiotherapy, either alone or in combination with chemotherapy, is the single most important key to a successful outcome.[157-161] The overall response rate ranges from 60% to 83%, and the reported 5-year survival rate is 40% to 78%. Despite the high initial response rate, relapses are frequent, varying from 17% to 77%,[162,163] with 50% being reported most commonly.[154,164] Chemotherapy is the treatment of choice for stage III or IV disease.[165] Anthracyclin-based regimens such as CHOP (cyclophosphamide, hydroxydaunomycin, Oncovin [vincristine], prednisone) have traditionally been used, but the results are disappointing and the overall 5-year survival rate for advanced disease is only approximately 10%,[27,64,166] which may be due to frequent expression of a multidrug resistance gene (P-glycoprotein) by the tumor cells.[167] Recently, favorable clinical outcomes have been reported with DeVIC (dexamethasone, etoposide, ifosfamide, carboplatin) and L-asparaginase.[168-170] High-dose chemotherapy with autologous or allogeneic stem cell support is an alternative method of treatment, but the reported survival benefit requires further confirmation.[171-175] The prognostic significance of the nasal $CD56^-$ subgroup is currently unclear; one study suggested that $CD56^-$ lymphomas have a more favorable outcome than $CD56^+$ lymphomas, but the former group in that study was heterogeneous, including both $CD56^-$ NK/T-cell lymphomas and peripheral T-cell lymphomas, not otherwise specified.[64]

Extranasal NK/T-cell lymphoma usually presents as advanced disease or shows early dissemination in the small proportion of patients who present with early-stage disease. Chemotherapy is the mainstay of treatment, but the response is generally poor. The long-term survival rate for patients with this highly aggressive lymphoma is less than 10%, and the median survival is only 4.3 months.[13,27,64,100] Nonetheless, rare cases of primary cutaneous NK/T-cell lymphoma may pursue a protracted or waxing and waning clinical course; however, it is not possible to identify which cases will exhibit this less aggressive behavior.[1,109]

Differential Diagnosis

The main differential diagnoses are listed in Table 28-3. For lesions composed mostly of large lymphoid cells, it is easy to recognize their neoplastic nature; the problem is distinguishing them from diffuse large B-cell lymphoma and nonhematolymphoid malignancies. This problem can usually be readily solved by immunohistochemistry.

For lesions composed predominantly of small or mixed cells, distinction from reactive or inflammatory conditions can be very difficult (see Table 28-3). In extranodal sites, the normal small lymphocytes often appear mildly atypical, with slightly enlarged and irregularly folded nuclei; they thus overlap morphologically with the small neoplastic cells seen in NK/T-cell lymphoma (Figs. 28-18 and 28-19). The presence of some or all of the following morphologic features favors a diagnosis of lymphoma: (1) dense infiltrate causing separation or destruction of the mucosal glands, (2) prominent tissue necrosis and ulceration, (3) angioinvasion, (4) presence of mitotic figures in a small cell–predominant lymphoid infiltrate, (5) clear cells, and (6) significant population of atypical medium-sized cells with irregular nuclei (Fig. 28-20). The diagnosis can be confirmed by immunohistochemical demonstration of large groups or sheets of $CD3\varepsilon^+$, $CD56^+$ cells. If the infiltrate is $CD3\varepsilon^+$ and $CD56^-$, positive immunostaining for TIA-1 and in situ hybridization for EBV-encoded RNA (EBER) support the diagnosis. See Pearls and Pitfalls for the assessment of posttreatment biopsies (Fig. 28-21).

Wegener's granulomatosis is an important differential diagnosis for nasal NK/T-cell lymphoma. It is a much more common destructive lesion of the upper respiratory tract in Western populations. It shares many morphologic features with the nasal NK/T-cell lymphoma in the form of a mixed inflammatory infiltrate, ulceration, necrosis, and vasculitis or vasculitis-like lesions. The same features helpful for the distinction between NK/T-cell lymphoma and reactive or inflammatory conditions also apply here.

The unifying concept of *angiocentric immunoproliferative lesions* was proposed by Jaffe[176] in the 1980s for a family of extranodal lymphoid proliferations characterized by prominent angiocentric-angiodestructive growth, necrosis, and a polymorphic cellular infiltrate. It included benign lymphocytic vasculitis, polymorphic reticulosis, lymphomatoid granulomatosis, and angiocentric lymphoma. On immunostaining of frozen sections, many cells in the lesions expressed a T-lineage marker, so at the time, these entities were considered

Table 28-3 **Differential Diagnosis of Extranodal NK/T-Cell Lymphoma**

Entity	Features Favoring Diagnosis of Entity	Features Favoring Diagnosis of Extranodal NK/T-Cell Lymphoma
Reactive lymphoid hyperplasia	Nonexpansile and nondestructive infiltrate of mixed lymphoid cells No definite cytologic atypia On immunostaining, nodular aggregates of $CD20^+$ B cells are separated by many $CD3^+$ T cells that are $CD56^-$ $EBER^-$	Dense, expansile infiltrate causing distortion or destruction of mucosal glands Ulceration and tissue necrosis Presence of atypical cells—medium-sized cells, clear cells, or cells with significant nuclear irregularities More than occasional mitotic figures in a small lymphoid cell–predominant lesion Angiocentric and angioinvasive growth $CD3\varepsilon^+$, $CD56^+$; or $CD3\varepsilon^+$, $CD56^-$, TIA-1^+, $EBER^+$
Wegener's granulomatosis	White patients Antineutrophil cytoplasmic antibody positive Involvement of kidney and lung No definite cytologic atypia Granuloma formation with multinucleated giant cells Microabscesses or eosinophils in areas away from necrosis EBV^-	Asian or Latin American patients Presence of atypical cells Usually no granuloma Acute inflammatory cells usually confined to vicinity of ulcers EBV^+
Large B-cell lymphoma	Angiocentric growth uncommon $CD20^+$, $CD3\varepsilon^-$	Angiocentric and angioinvasive growth common $CD20^-$, $CD3\varepsilon^+$
Lymphomatoid granulomatosis	Predominantly affects lung; sometimes brain, skin, and kidney Large atypical tumor cells are $CD20^+$, $CD3^-$ B cells; background rich in reactive T cells	Asian or Latin American patients (lymphomatoid granulomatosis is extremely rare in these populations) Most commonly affects sinonasal areas; lung involvement extremely rare $CD3\varepsilon^+$, $CD20^-$
Subcutaneous panniculitis-like T-cell lymphoma	Subcutaneous nodules alone or almost exclusively subcutaneous involvement, with at most minimal dermal involvement Angiocentric growth less common Surface CD3/$Leu4^+$, $CD8^+$ (usually), $CD56^-$ (usually) EBV^- TCR genes rearranged	Skin nodules, often in multiple sites and commonly accompanied by other sites of disease Dermal involvement almost always present in addition to subcutaneous involvement Frequent angiocentric and angioinvasive growth Surface CD3/$Leu4^-$, $CD8^-$, $CD56^+$ (usually) EBV^+ TCR genes germline
Blastic plasmacytoid dendritic cell neoplasm (formerly blastic NK-cell lymphoma)	Monotonous infiltrate of medium-sized blastic cells with thin nuclear membrane and fine chromatin, morphologically reminiscent of leukemic infiltrate; nuclei commonly round or oval Angioinvasion and necrosis uncommon $CD56^+$, $CD4^+$, $CD123^+$, $TdT^{+/-}$, $CD3\varepsilon^-$ (usually) EBV^-	Monotonous or mixed infiltrate of lymphoma cells of variable sizes; nuclei often irregularly folded and more chromatin rich Angioinvasion and necrosis often prominent $CD56^+$ (usually), $CD4^-$, $CD123^-$, TdT^-, $CD3\varepsilon^+$ (usually) EBV^+
Squamous cell carcinoma	Often shows deep invasion Dysplastic or carcinoma in situ changes in surface epithelium	Squamous proliferation (pseudoepitheliomatous hyperplasia) limited to superficial zone of mucosa Lack of desmoplastic reaction Presence of atypical lymphoid cells between tongues of atypical squamous epithelium

EBER, EBV-encoded RNA; EBV, Epstein-Barr virus; TCR, T-cell receptor; TdT, terminal deoxynucleotidyl transferase.

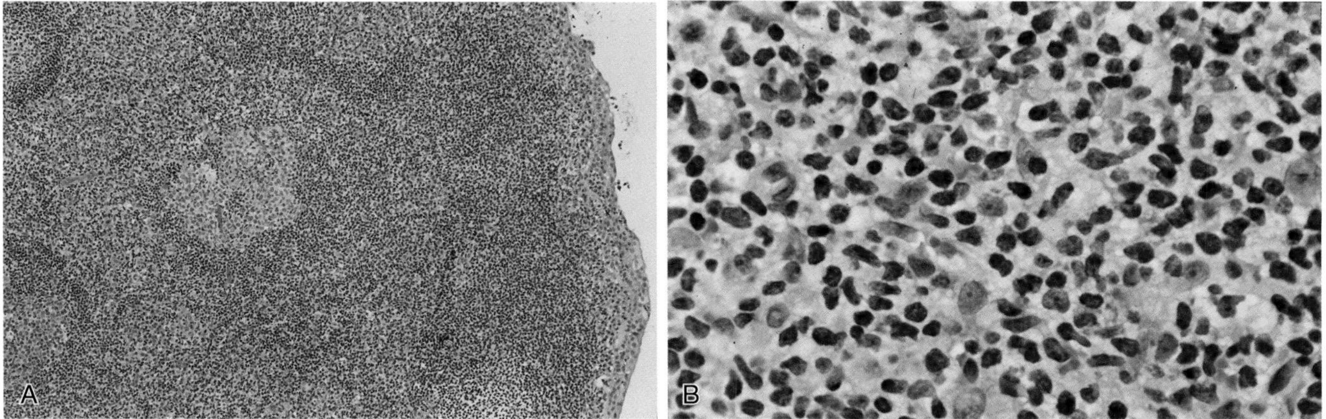

Figure 28-18. Nasopharyngeal mucosa with reactive lymphoid hyperplasia. A, The mucosa is rich in lymphoid cells, and reactive lymphoid follicles are present. **B**, Closer examination of the interfollicular zone shows that the small lymphoid cells are often slightly larger than small lymphocytes and can exhibit nuclear foldings. Thus there is cytologic overlap between mucosal reactive lymphoid cells and NK/T-cell lymphoma cells (compare with Fig. 28-2).

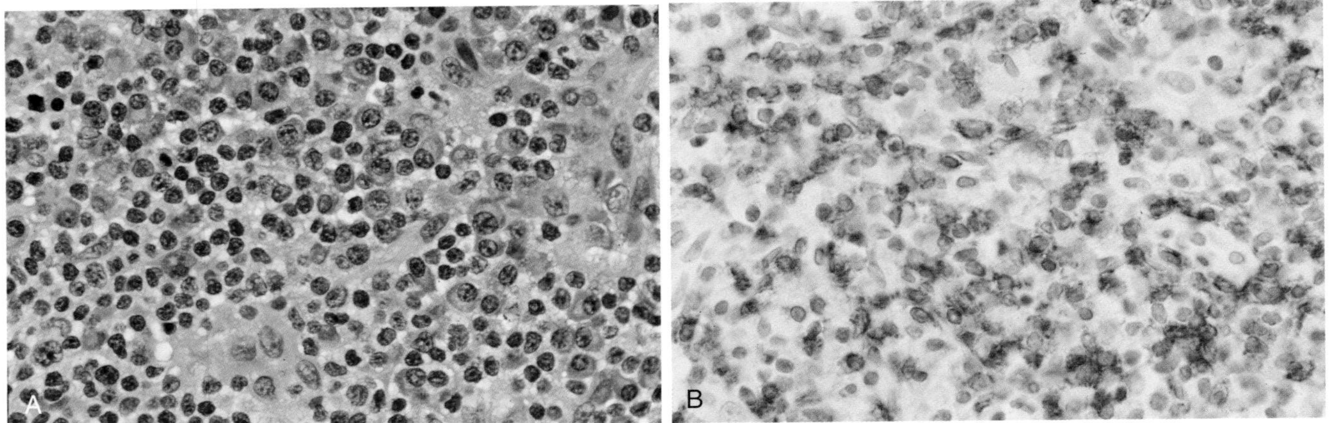

Figure 28-19. Nasal NK/T-cell lymphoma that is difficult to diagnose. A, The predominance of small lymphoid cells with round nuclei and admixed plasma cells suggests a benign lymphoid infiltrate. However, other features are suggestive of lymphoma, such as ulceration and loss of mucosal glands (not shown). **B,** Immunostaining shows many CD56$^+$ cells (which are also CD3ε$^+$), supporting a diagnosis of nasal NK/T-cell lymphoma. In the normal or reactive mucosa, CD56$^+$ cells are not present in such large numbers.

T-cell lymphoproliferative disorders. Studies in the past decade based on paraffin section immunohistochemistry (which permits much better cytomorphologic correlation) and molecular studies have shown that most examples of polymorphic reticulosis represent NK/T-cell lymphoma, whereas lymphomatoid granulomatosis represents a peculiar form of T-cell–rich large B-cell lymphoproliferative disorder with a strong association with EBV and a good response to interferon-α2b therapy.[177-179]

Herpes simplex infection of the nasopharynx can simulate nasal NK/T-cell lymphoma owing to the presence of a mass lesion, a dense lymphoid infiltrate with necrosis, and CD56 expression by the lymphoid cells.[180] The presence of scattered herpesvirus inclusions, lack of angioinvasion, expression of CD4 by the T-cell infiltrate, absence of EBV, and lack of TCR gene rearrangement support this diagnosis over NK/T-cell lymphoma.

Atypical proliferation of NK cells producing superficial erosions of the gastrointestinal tract has been reported in a patient with antigliadin antibodies but the absence of full-blown celiac disease.[181] These lesions are relatively circumscribed and superficial, and the CD56$^+$ NK cells are negative for EBER. The benign nature of the disease is further confirmed by the nonprogressive course and improvement with a gluten-free diet.

AGGRESSIVE NK-CELL LEUKEMIA

Definition

Aggressive NK-cell leukemia, also known as aggressive NK-cell leukemia/lymphoma, is a neoplasm of NK cells with primary involvement of the peripheral blood and bone marrow and a fulminant clinical course (Box 28-2).[24,182,183] It is often termed a *leukemia/lymphoma* because in contrast to the usual leukemias, neoplastic cells can be sparse in the peripheral blood and bone marrow.

This tumor shows many similarities with extranodal NK/T-cell lymphoma, such as the presence of azurophilic granules, immunophenotype (CD2$^+$, surface CD3$^-$, CD56$^+$), genotype (germline configuration of TCR gene), EBV association, and higher prevalence in Asian populations. However, the clinical

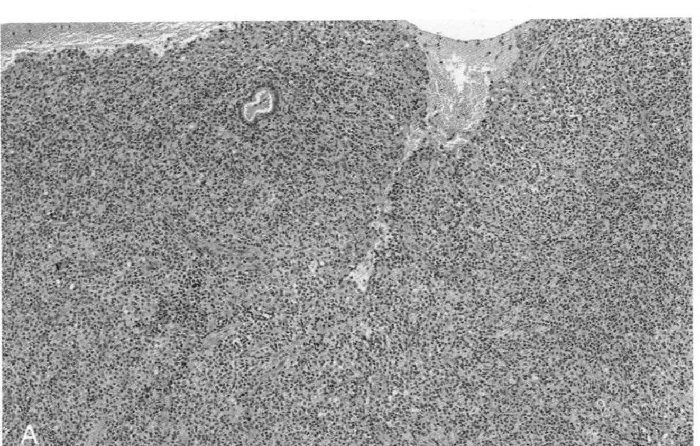

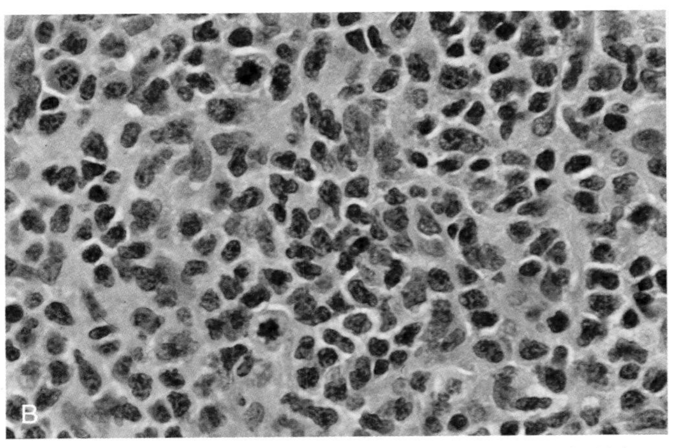

Figure 28-20. Nasal NK/T-cell lymphoma with histologic features supporting a diagnosis of lymphoma over reactive lymphoid hyperplasia. A, Extensive and dense lymphoid infiltrate with loss of mucosal glands. **B,** Definite cytologic atypia in the lymphoid cells supports a diagnosis of lymphoma. Compared with Figure 28-18, the cells are slightly larger and show more irregular nuclear foldings. Readily found mitotic figures in a small lymphoid infiltrate are another feature suggestive of lymphoma.

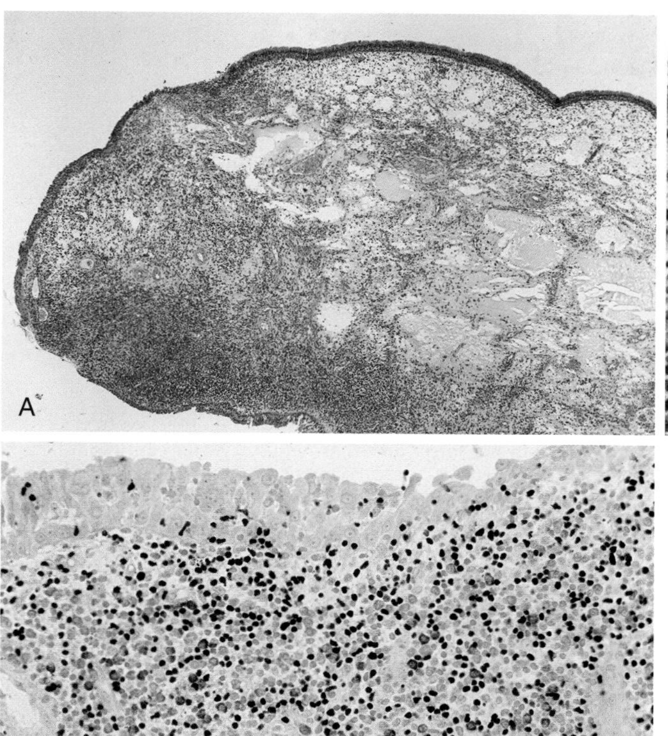

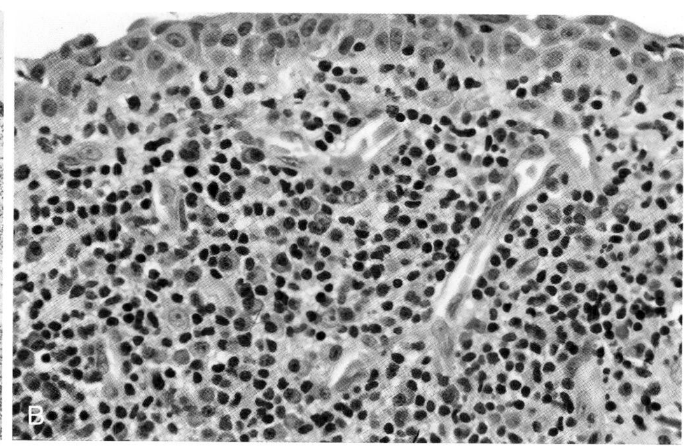

Figure 28-21. Nasal NK/T-cell lymphoma—posttreatment biopsy. A, The nasal mucosa appears hypocellular in most areas. **B,** In the more cellular areas, plasma cells are admixed with small lymphoid cells, suggesting a benign lymphoid infiltrate. **C,** Surprisingly, numerous $EBER^+$ cells are present, indicating residual disease.

Box 28-2 *Major Diagnostic Features of Aggressive NK-Cell Leukemia*

Clinical Features and Behavior

- More prevalent in Asians
- Age: teenage to middle age (mean, 39 years)
- Sex: male = female
- Presentation: ill patient with fever, constitutional symptoms, hepatosplenomegaly, generalized lymphadenopathy, and sometimes bleeding tendency
- Fulminant clinical course with cytopenia, coagulopathy, and multiorgan failure, often resulting in death within a few weeks

Morphology

- Peripheral blood or marrow smear: few to numerous large granular lymphocytes, many of which are atypical (e.g., irregular nuclear foldings, very large size) or immature (e.g., open chromatin, distinct nucleoli)
- Involved tissues: usually dense, permeative, and monotonous infiltrate of medium-sized lymphoid cells with prominent apoptosis; angiocentric growth and necrosis common

Immunophenotype and Genotype

- $CD3\varepsilon^+$, surface $CD3^-$, $CD56^+$, $CD16^{+/-}$, $CD57^-$, positive for cytotoxic molecules
- EBV^+
- TCR genes germline

features are very different. Aggressive NK-cell leukemia affects mainly young patients, and the prognosis is dismal.

Epidemiology and Etiology

The disease occurs with a much higher frequency in Asians compared with whites,[17] suggesting that ethnic factors play a role in disease susceptibility, similar to extranodal NK/T-cell lymphoma. It is strongly associated with EBV.[11,13,19,21,25,184-186] Rare cases may evolve from EBV-associated lymphoproliferative diseases[187,188] or nasal NK/T-cell lymphoma.[189] The rare cases of aggressive leukemia that arise from chronic lymphoproliferative disorder of NK cells are not associated with EBV,[190] and their relationship with aggressive NK-cell leukemia has yet to be clarified.

Patients are typically adolescents or young adults, but older patients can also be affected. The mean age is 39 years.[13,14,17-26,191] There is no sex predilection.

Clinical Features

The typical presentation is fever, hepatosplenomegaly, lymphadenopathy, and a leukemic blood picture.[13,14,17-26,191] Skin nodules are uncommon, but some patients may have a nonspecific rash. Patients are often very ill, and in some cases the disease may be complicated by hemophagocytic syndrome.[191,192] The serum lactate dehydrogenase level is often

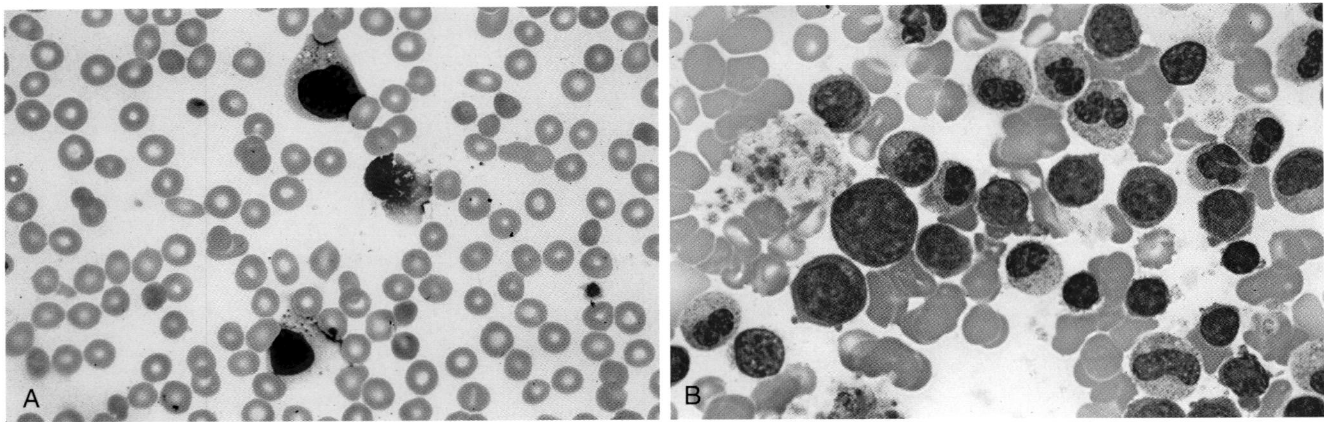

Figure 28-22. Aggressive NK-cell leukemia. A, In the peripheral blood smear, there are large granular lymphocytes with atypia. The cell in the *lower field* has small nucleoli, and the cell in the *upper field* has a large nucleolus. **B,** Buffy coat smear shows many lymphoid cells with immature nuclear chromatin, distinct nucleoli, and cytoplasmic granules. There are admixed immature cells of the granulocytic series.

markedly elevated, as is circulating Fas ligand.[193,194] It has been postulated that systemic shedding of large quantities of Fas ligand from the tumor cells may contribute to the multiorgan failure commonly seen in aggressive NK-cell leukemia. Binding of Fas ligand to Fas, which is normally expressed in many different types of normal cells, results in apoptosis of the Fas-bearing cells.

Morphology

Circulating leukemic cells range from scanty to abundant, accounting for less than 5% to greater than 80% of lymphocytes. The cells often exhibit a range of appearances in an individual case, from normal-looking large granular lymphocytes to immature and atypical-looking large granular lymphocytes (Fig. 28-22). They have round nuclei with condensed chromatin, or larger nuclei with mildly irregular foldings. In some cases nucleoli are prominent. The cytoplasm is moderate to abundant in amount and is lightly basophilic, with variable numbers of fine and occasionally coarse azurophilic granules. In the bone marrow, large granular lymphocytes constitute 6% to 92% of all nucleated cells.[26] Thus, the pattern of involvement ranges from diffuse interstitial to subtle and patchy (Fig. 28-23).[26]

In histologic sections there is a diffuse, destructive, and permeative infiltrate consisting of monomorphic cells with round or irregular nuclei, fairly condensed chromatin, and a thin to moderate rim of pale or amphophilic cytoplasm. Interspersed apoptotic bodies and zonal cell death are common (Fig. 28-24). Angioinvasive-angiodestructive growth is also frequently noted.[13,25]

Immunophenotype and Molecular Findings

The immunophenotype is identical to that of extranodal NK/T-cell lymphoma—CD2$^+$, surface CD3/Leu4$^-$, cytoplasmic CD3ε$^+$, CD56$^+$, and positive for cytotoxic markers—except that CD16 expression is seen in approximately half the cases (Fig. 28-25). CD57 is often negative (see Table 28-1).[13,14,17-25,27] The TCR genes are typically germline.

EBV is reported in approximately 90% of cases overall.[11,13,19,21,26,184,185,191,195] However, a diagnosis of aggressive NK-cell leukemia should be viewed with some skepticism if EBV is negative.

Although previous comparative genomic hybridization studies suggested similar genetic changes in aggressive NK-cell leukemia and extranodal NK/T-cell lymphoma, such as 3p+, 6q−, 11q−, and 12q+,[104,147] a more recent array-based comparative genomic hybridization study revealed significant differences between the two diseases.[150] For instance, 7p−, 17p−, and 1q+ are frequent in aggressive NK-cell leukemia but not in extranodal NK/T-cell lymphoma. The 6q− commonly found in the latter was not observed in aggressive NK-cell leukemia included in that series.

Clinical Course

The disease is almost invariably fatal, with a median survival of only 58 days.[26] Most patients die within days to weeks after presentation. The disease is frequently complicated by coagulopathy, bleeding, and multiorgan failure. Response to chemotherapy is usually poor.[195] There have been rare reports of successful bone marrow transplantation, but the disease almost always relapses.[13,17,18,24-26,175,191,196]

Differential Diagnosis

Aggressive NK-cell leukemia must be distinguished from the more common T-cell large granular lymphocytic leukemia, which is EBV$^-$ and frequently pursues an indolent clinical course.[23,197] Patients with T-cell large granular lymphocytic leukemia are generally older (mean age, 55 to 65 years) and commonly present with infection, hepatosplenomegaly, and pure red cell aplasia or neutropenia; there may be associated rheumatoid arthritis. Although both T-cell large granular lymphocytic leukemia and aggressive NK-cell leukemia are characterized by circulating lymphoid cells with azurophilic granules, the lymphoid cells in the former do not exhibit atypia or an immature appearance, as is commonly observed in the latter. T-cell large granular lymphocytic leukemia cells show a surface CD3$^+$,

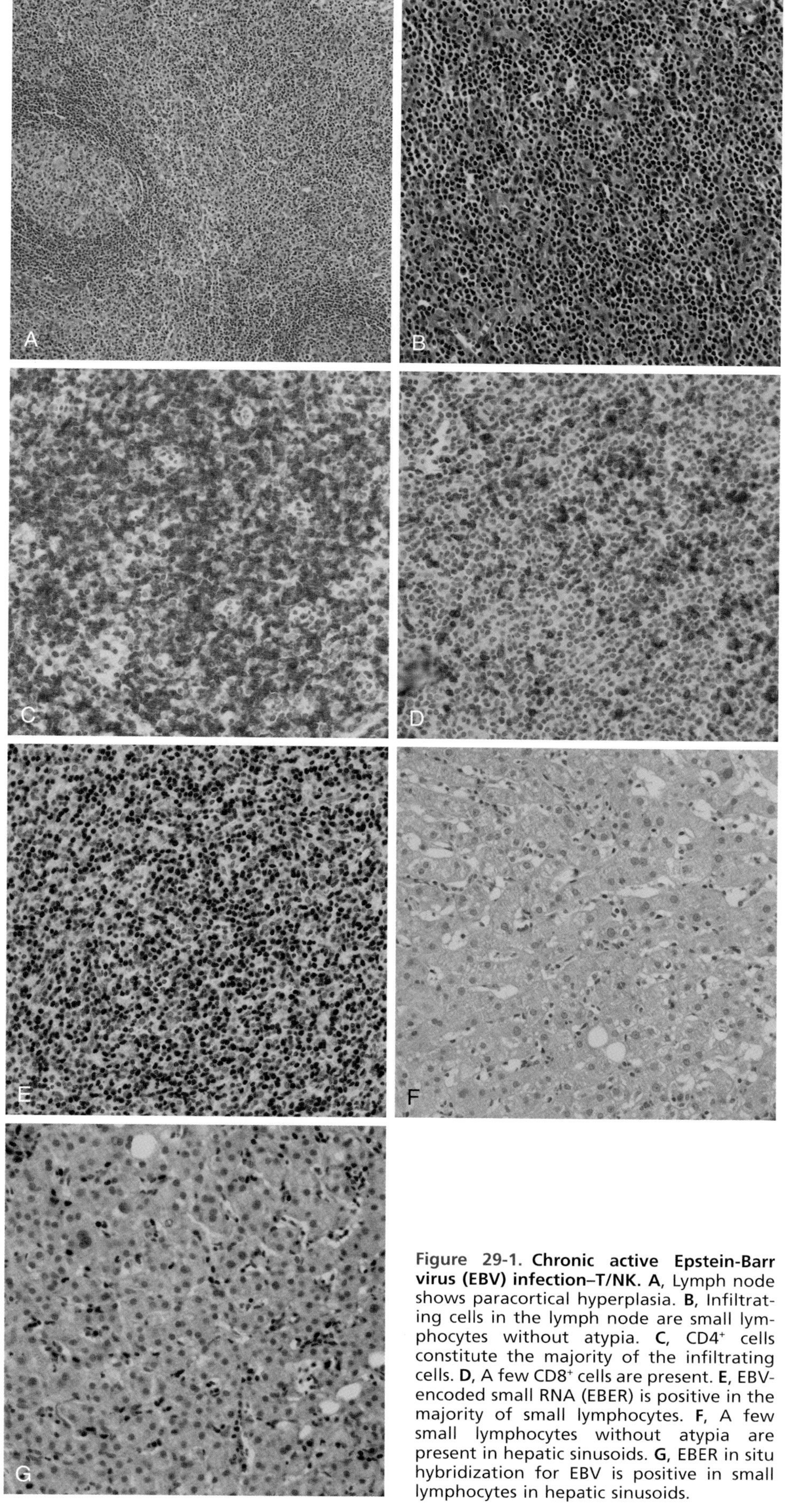

Figure 29-1. Chronic active Epstein-Barr virus (EBV) infection–T/NK. A, Lymph node shows paracortical hyperplasia. **B**, Infiltrating cells in the lymph node are small lymphocytes without atypia. **C**, $CD4^+$ cells constitute the majority of the infiltrating cells. **D**, A few $CD8^+$ cells are present. **E**, EBV-encoded small RNA (EBER) is positive in the majority of small lymphocytes. **F**, A few small lymphocytes without atypia are present in hepatic sinusoids. **G**, EBER in situ hybridization for EBV is positive in small lymphocytes in hepatic sinusoids.

Box 29-2 *Recommended Tests to Diagnose Chronic Active Epstein-Barr Virus Infection–T/NK and Related Diseases*

- In situ hybridization for EBER
- Immunostains for CD3, CD20, and CD56 combined with EBER in situ hybridization
- Immunostains for cytotoxic markers: TIA-1, granzyme B, perforin
- Viral load in peripheral blood
- EBV antibody titers
- EBV terminal repeat analysis
- T-cell receptor gene rearrangement

EBER, EBV-encoded small RNA; EBV, Epstein-Barr virus; NK, natural killer.

Postulated Cell of Origin

The postulated cells of origin are cytotoxic T or NK cells.

Prognosis and Predictive Factors

The prognosis of CAEBV-T/NK is variable. Some patients experience an indolent clinical course, but many patients die of the disease. The process may evolve from a polyclonal to a monoclonal proliferation of T or NK cells and eventually progress to overt lymphoid malignancy.[1,31] The main causes of death are hemophagocytic syndrome, multiple organ failure, and T- or NK-cell malignancy. The median survival is 78 months. Patients with a late onset of CAEBV-T/NK (older than 8 years), thrombocytopenia, and T-cell infection have significantly poorer outcomes.[5] Patients with T-cell CAEBV often present with high fever, lymphadenopathy, hepatosplenomegaly, and high titers of EBV-specific antibodies and experience rapid disease progression. Patients with NK-cell disease, in contrast, often have hypersensitivity to mosquito bites, rash, and high levels of IgE but do not necessarily have elevated EBV-specific antibody titers.[27] The 5-year survival rate of patients with T-cell CAEBV is 59%, whereas that for NK-cell disease is 87%.[5] B-cell neoplasms and Hodgkin's lymphoma can occur rarely.[32]

Differential Diagnosis

Because the infiltrating cells in CAEBV-T/NK are not atypical, it is easy to overlook the diagnosis. In situ hybridization for EBER is a valuable tool for recognizing the disease in the appropriate clinical setting.

Systemic EBV⁺ T-cell LPD or other clearly clonal proliferations must be distinguished from CAEBV-T/NK. In cases with a monoclonal population, the infiltrating cells tend to have increased cytologic atypia and include a higher proportion of EBV⁺ cells. Because distinction by morphology is difficult, demonstration of the clonality of EBV and EBV-infected T cells is necessary.

MOSQUITO BITE HYPERSENSITIVITY

Definition

Mosquito bite hypersensitivity is a cutaneous manifestation of chronic EBV infection characterized by intense local skin symptoms, including erythema, bullae, ulcers, and scar formation, and by systemic symptoms such as fever, lymphadenopathy, and liver dysfunction after mosquito bites.[33,34] It has a close association with CAEBV-T/NK and aggressive NK-cell leukemia occurring in children (Box 29-3).

Epidemiology

Mosquito bite hypersensitivity is very uncommon. Most cases have been reported from Japan,[33,35-38] with a few cases from Taiwan,[39,40] Korea,[41,42] and Mexico.[43]

Pathophysiology

Hypersensitivity to mosquito bites is not a simple allergic disease but a cutaneous manifestation of CAEBV of NK-cell lineage.[44] CD4⁺ T cells are mosquito antigen specific and proliferate in response to mosquito salivary gland extract.[45] When mosquito antigen–specific CD4⁺ cells are cocultured with EBV-carrying NK cells, EBV is activated, and NK cells express EBV lytic cycle antigens. The activation of NK cells latently infected by EBV and the subsequent CTL response seem to play a key role in the pathogenesis of the skin lesions and systemic symptoms of patients with mosquito bite hypersensitivity.[46,47] EBV-carrying NK cells may be preneoplastic cells, with a risk of the subsequent development of NK-cell lymphoma/leukemia through the oncogenic influence of latent EBV genes. In fact, EBV-infected NK cells are often oligoclonal or monoclonal by terminal repeat analysis.[33]

Box 29-3 *Major Diagnostic Features of Mosquito Bite Hypersensitivity*

Definition
- Cutaneous manifestation of chronic EBV infection activated by mosquito bite

Diagnostic Criteria
- Intense local skin symptoms, including erythema, bulla, ulcer, and scar formation, associated with systemic symptoms such as fever, lymphadenopathy, and liver dysfunction after mosquito bites

Clinical Features
- Most patients are in the first 2 decades of life, with a median age of 6.7 years
- Often high EBV load and NK-cell lymphocytosis
- Variable clinical course; some patients may develop hydroa vacciniforme, systemic symptoms of CAEBV, or NK-cell lymphoma/leukemia

Morphology
- Necrosis and ulceration of epidermis, with infiltration of neutrophils and small lymphocytes and fibrinoid necrosis of small blood vessels

Immunophenotype
- Cutaneous infiltration by CD4⁺ T cells, CD8⁺ T cells, and NK cells expressing cytotoxic molecules
- NK cells containing EBV in peripheral blood

CAEBV, chronic active EBV infection; EBV, Epstein-Barr virus; NK, natural killer.

Clinical Features

Most patients are in the first 2 decades of life, with a median age of 6.7 years.[48] Skin lesions at the site of the mosquito bite typically demonstrate erythema and bullae that subsequently become necrotic with ulceration and eventually heal with scarring (Fig. 29-2). Systemic symptoms, including fever and malaise, are common. Hematuria, proteinuria, and bloody stool may be seen, with laboratory evidence of anemia or hypoproteinemia. After recovery from the general symptoms, patients are symptom free until the next mosquito bite. Vaccination may cause a similar skin reaction at the injection site in some patients.[48] Patients show a high level of serum IgE, a high EBV load in the peripheral blood, and peripheral NK lymphocytosis (80% of patients).[33]

Complications in patients with hypersensitivity to mosquito bites commonly include CAEBV-T/NK, NK/T-cell lymphoma/leukemia, and hemophagocytic syndrome.[38,48,49] Sometimes hypersensitivity to mosquito bites is the first manifestation of clonal EBV⁺ NK-cell malignancy.[33]

Morphology

The skin at the mosquito bite site exhibits epidermal necrosis and ulceration. The dermis shows edema and infiltration of polymorphonuclear leukocytes, nuclear debris, and extravasated red blood cells, with fibrinoid necrosis of small blood vessels in the center of the lesion. The infiltrate of small lymphoid cells extends from the dermis to subcutaneous tissue in an angiocentric pattern.

Immunophenotype and Genetics

The infiltrating lymphoid cells are $CD4^+$ T cells, $CD8^+$ T cells, and NK cells that express cytotoxic molecules. EBV^+ cells constitute a minor population, accounting for 3% to 10% of infiltrating lymphocytes. EBV^+ cells may not be detected in the skin in the absence of NK lymphocytosis, despite a high viral load in the peripheral blood.[50]

Postulated Cell of Origin

NK cells are the postulated cell of origin.

Prognosis

The clinical course is variable. Some patients have a prolonged and indolent disease course that may be complicated with CAEBV-T/NK or HV-like eruptions. Half the patients die of hemophagocytic syndrome or aggressive NK-cell leukemia/lymphoma.[48] Rarely, patients with CAEBV develop monoclonal B-cell proliferations or Hodgkin's lymphoma, suggesting that EBV is targeting the cells of multiple lineages.

HYDROA VACCINIFORME

Definition

HV is a rare cutaneous manifestation of an EBV-associated polyclonal T/NK-cell LPD characterized by blistering photodermatosis in childhood that heals with vacciniform scarring (Table 29-2). It has been divided into two types based on the

Table 29-2 Major Diagnostic Features of Hydroa Vacciniforme (HV) and HV-Like T-Cell Lymphoma

Feature	*Hydroa Vacciniforme* Classic	*Hydroa Vacciniforme* Severe	HV-Like T-Cell Lymphoma
Epidemiology	Worldwide	Asia and Latin America	Asia and Latin America
Skin lesions	Sun exposed	Sun exposed and rarely unexposed	Sun exposed and rarely unexposed
	Vesiculopapular	Vesiculopapular and ulcerative; facial edema	Vesiculopapular and ulcerative; facial edema
Photoprovocation	Usually positive	Usually positive	Variable
Histopathology	Epidermal vesicles Superficial dermal infiltrates	Epidermal vesicles and ulcers Deeper dermal infiltrates No cytologic atypia	Epidermal vesicles and ulcers Deeper dermal infiltrates with angiocentricity and panniculitis Possible cytologic atypia
Phenotype	Cytotoxic $CD4^+$ or $CD8^+$ T cells	Cytotoxic $CD4^+$ or $CD8^+$ T cells	Usually $CD8^+$ cytotoxic T cells
$EBER^+$ cells	5%-50% of lymphocytes	5%-50% of lymphocytes	Majority of lymphoid cells
T-cell receptor	Polyclonal	Polyclonal	Monoclonal
Systemic symptoms*	Usually absent	Usually present	Present
Anti-EBV antibody profile	Usually normal	Often abnormal	Often abnormal
EBV DNA load in peripheral blood	Slightly high	High	High
Associated conditions	Usually absent	CAEBV-T/NK Mosquito bite hypersensitivity HPS (rare)	
Prognosis	Remission with photoprotection	Remissions and recurrences Progression to HV-like T-cell lymphoma in some patients	2-year survival rate <50%

*Fever, increased liver enzymes, lymphadenopathy.
CAEBV, chronic active EBV infection; EBER, EBV-encoded small RNA; EBV, Epstein-Barr virus; HPS, hemophagocytic syndrome; NK, natural killer.

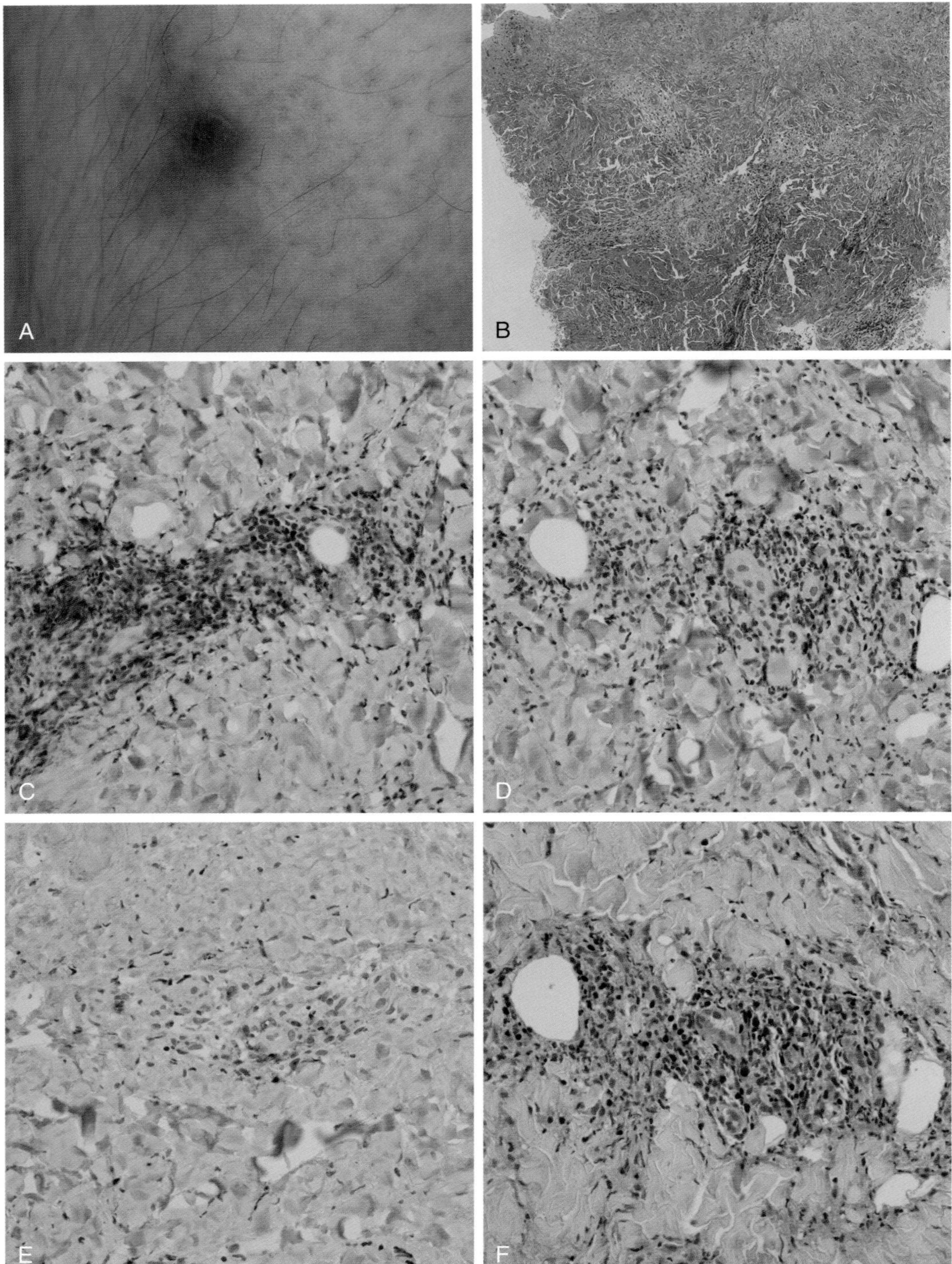

Figure 29-2. Mosquito bite hypersensitivity. A, Skin at the mosquito bite site shows epidermal necrosis and ulceration. **B**, Skin shows necrosis of the epidermis. Blood vessels in the deep dermis exhibit vasculitic changes, with fibrinoid necrosis and fibrin thrombi. **C**, Perivascular cellular infiltrates in the dermis are mainly CD3^{+} T cells. **D**, Some cells are CD8^{+}. **E**, CD56 stains scattered perivascular cells. **F**, Many perivascular cells are EBER^{+}. (**A,** Courtesy of Professor H. S. Kim, Chonnam National University.)

clinical features. The classic type is a self-limited disease characterized by the formation of vesicles on sun-exposed areas; it has a benign course, resolving in adolescence or young adulthood.[51,52] The severe type tends to exhibit more extensive skin lesions; systemic manifestations, including fever, hepatomegaly, and serologic abnormalities; and peripheral NK lymphocytosis. Severe HV often progresses to EBV-associated NK- or T-cell malignancy.[52]

Epidemiology

Classic HV occurs worldwide, independent of race.[51,53] Usually the disease is sporadic, but familial cases have been reported in identical twins and siblings.[54] Severe HV occurs predominantly in Asian children[2,53,55,56] and rarely in Western countries.[57]

Pathophysiology

The cause of classic HV is unknown, although ultraviolet radiation–induced delayed-type hypersensitivity to an endogenous cutaneous autoantigen has been suggested.[58] Identification of latent EBV infection in the cutaneous infiltrates of children with HV provided insight into the pathogenesis of HV and the relationship between the classic and severe forms. EBV was observed in both severe and classic HV in Asian[53,59] and Indian children.[60] A Japanese study reported that even classic HV patients showed slightly elevated levels of EBV DNA in peripheral blood mononuclear cells compared with normal healthy persons, whereas severe HV patients had markedly increased levels of EBV DNA associated with NK lymphocytosis and other complications.[52] These clinical observations suggest that classic HV and severe HV represent cutaneous manifestations of CAEBV-T/NK, with differences in clinical severity depending on host immunity.

In Western countries, the EBV status in HV has not been well studied, but one study documented a French patient with classic HV who had EBV-infected cells in the skin.[52] Other rare EBV$^+$ cases have been encountered in Caucasian children by the authors (personal communication). The high incidence of severe HV in persons of Asian descent may be ascribed to the influence of the patients' genetic background and may be linked to human leukocyte antigen (HLA) type, environmental factors, and immunologic tolerance because of early exposure to EBV infection.[61]

Clinical Features

Classic Hydroa Vacciniforme

HV usually presents in children younger than 10 years, but a minority of cases present in young adulthood.[51] The eruption is seasonal, usually occurring in spring or summer.[51,62] The skin lesions are characterized by recurrent vesicles and crust formation on the face and arms after sun exposure, and they typically heal with vacciniform scarring (Fig. 29-3). Lesions are inducible by sunlight exposure and, less commonly, by repeated exposure to broad-spectrum ultraviolet A or, less reliably, ultraviolet B irradiation.[63]

Severe Hydroa Vacciniforme

Unlike classic HV, the cutaneous lesions of severe HV can occur in exposed as well as unexposed sites and are frequently refractory to the wearing of sun protection. Severe HV shows necrotic papulovesicles, nodules, or facial swelling[64] and can recur for years.

Morphology

The characteristic histologic features of HV are epidermal reticular degeneration leading to spongiotic vesiculation. The dermis contains perivascular and periappendigeal lymphocytic infiltration. The histologic changes of severe HV are similar to those of classic HV, but the dermal infiltrates tend to be more extensive and deeper, reaching to the subcutaneous tissue.

Immunophenotype and Genetics

The majority of the infiltrating cells are CD4$^+$ or CD8$^+$ T cells[65]; NK cells are rare.[66] Most cells express cytotoxic molecules such as TIA-1 and granzyme B. The number of EBV$^+$ lymphocytes varies from 5% to 50% of infiltrating cells[53,64] and increases in the spring and summer; during periods of remission in autumn and winter, very few EBV$^+$ cells are present. EBV-containing cells do not express LMP-1. T-cell receptor gene rearrangements are polyclonal.[64]

Postulated Cell of Origin

The postulated cells of origin are cytotoxic T cells homing to the skin.

Prognosis

Most patients with classic HV show spontaneous remission; some are cured after protection from sunlight, but a few patients experience recurrent eruptions despite sun protection.[51] Classic HV can rarely progress to the severe form with age and finally develop into a cutaneous EBV$^+$ NK- or T-cell lymphoma.[52,67] Severe HV is often complicated by CAEBV-T/NK,[68] peripheral NK lymphocytosis, mosquito bite hypersensitivity, and virus-associated hemophagocytic syndrome.[3,52] About half the patients with severe HV develop EBV-associated NK/T-cell lymphoma in the skin or other organs 2 to 14 years after onset, and using the new WHO terminology, these cases would be classified as HV-like T-cell lymphoma.[2,4,9,69,70] Adverse prognostic factors include no spontaneous improvement with age, severe facial and lip swelling, systemic complications such as a high-grade fever and liver damage, dense lymphocytic infiltration containing atypical cells, increased EBV$^+$ cells, mosquito bite hypersensitivity, and abnormal EBV antibody titers suggestive of CAEBV.[52]

HYDROA VACCINIFORME–LIKE T-CELL LYMPHOMA

Definition

Hydroa vacciniforme–like T-cell lymphoma (HV-TCL) is an EBV-associated clonal, cutaneous T-cell LPD characterized by recurrent vesiculopapular eruptions mainly on the face and arms. It may be a progression of HV,[52,67] or it may occur as de novo disease.[69,71,72] This entity includes some cases of severe HV reported in the literature.[43]

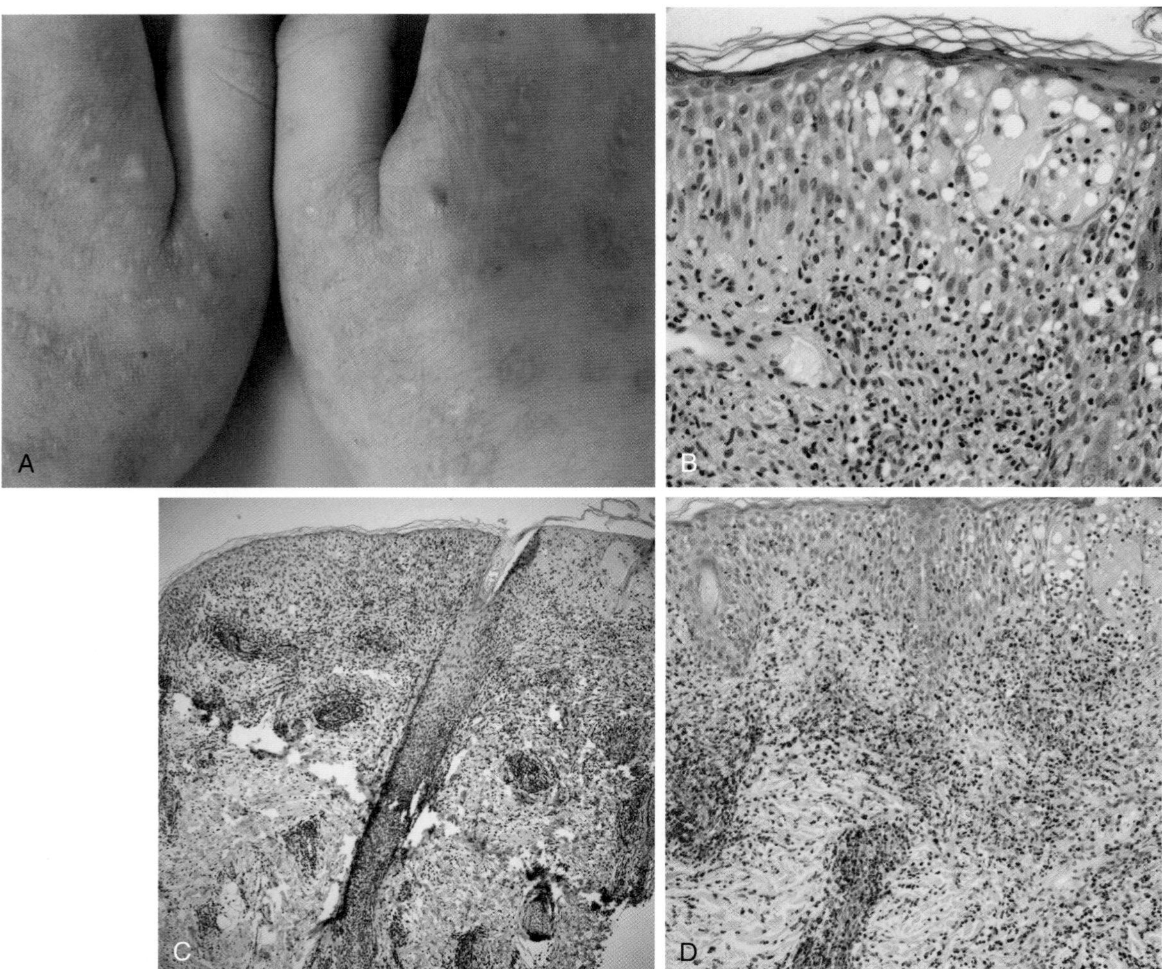

Figure 29-3. Hydroa vacciniforme, classic type. A, This 9-year-old girl has a papulovesicular skin eruption with vacciniform scarring of the hands and face (not shown). **B**, Skin shows epidermal reticular degeneration, leading to spongiotic vesiculation. The dermis contains a perivascular and periappendigeal lymphocytic infiltrate. **C**, Perivascular infiltrates are $CD3^+$ T cells. **D**, Approximately 50% of lymphocytes are $EBER^+$.

Epidemiology

HV-TCL has been reported under various names, including *severe HV*,[43] *edematous, scarring vasculitic panniculitis*,[43] *EBV-associated lymphoproliferative lesions presenting as recurrent necrotic papulovesicles of the face*,[69] and *angiocentric cutaneous T-cell lymphoma of childhood*.[72] The disease has been described mainly in Asia and Latin America, including Japan,[67] Korea,[70] Taiwan,[73-75] Mexico,[43,72] Peru,[71] and Guatemala.[76]

Clinical Features

Most patients are children,[71,73,75] with some cases occurring in young adults.[70] Patients present with fever, malaise, and a refractory, relapsing cutaneous rash involving the face and upper and lower arms, often accompanied by lymphadenopathy, hepatosplenomegaly, increased liver enzymes and lactate dehydrogenase,[71] and large granular lymphocytosis in the peripheral blood.[70] Cutaneous lesions are severe and disfiguring (Fig. 29-4) and go through stages of edema, vesicles, erythema, ulceration, and scars in sun-exposed and unexposed areas.[43,69,71] A seasonal variation in eruptions is characteristic, being worse in spring and summer and remitting in autumn and winter. Some patients have hypersensitivity to insect or mosquito bites.[43]

Morphology

The cutaneous lesion consists of degenerated and ulcerated epidermis and moderate to dense cellular infiltrates throughout the dermis and subcutaneous tissue. The infiltrates are composed of atypical lymphocytes with enlarged and hyperchromatic nuclei, frequently with an angiocentric and periadnexal arrangement and septal or lobular panniculitis. Reactive histiocytes may be admixed.

Immunophenotype and Genetics

Tumor cells are predominantly $CD8^+$ CTLs,[71,73] with a minority of $CD4^+$ cases.[75] Rare cases express CD56.[76] A variable number of $CD30^+$ cells can be seen.[72] In situ hybridization for EBER has been positive in all but one of the cases reported so far.[73] T-cell receptor gene rearrangement is monoclonal.

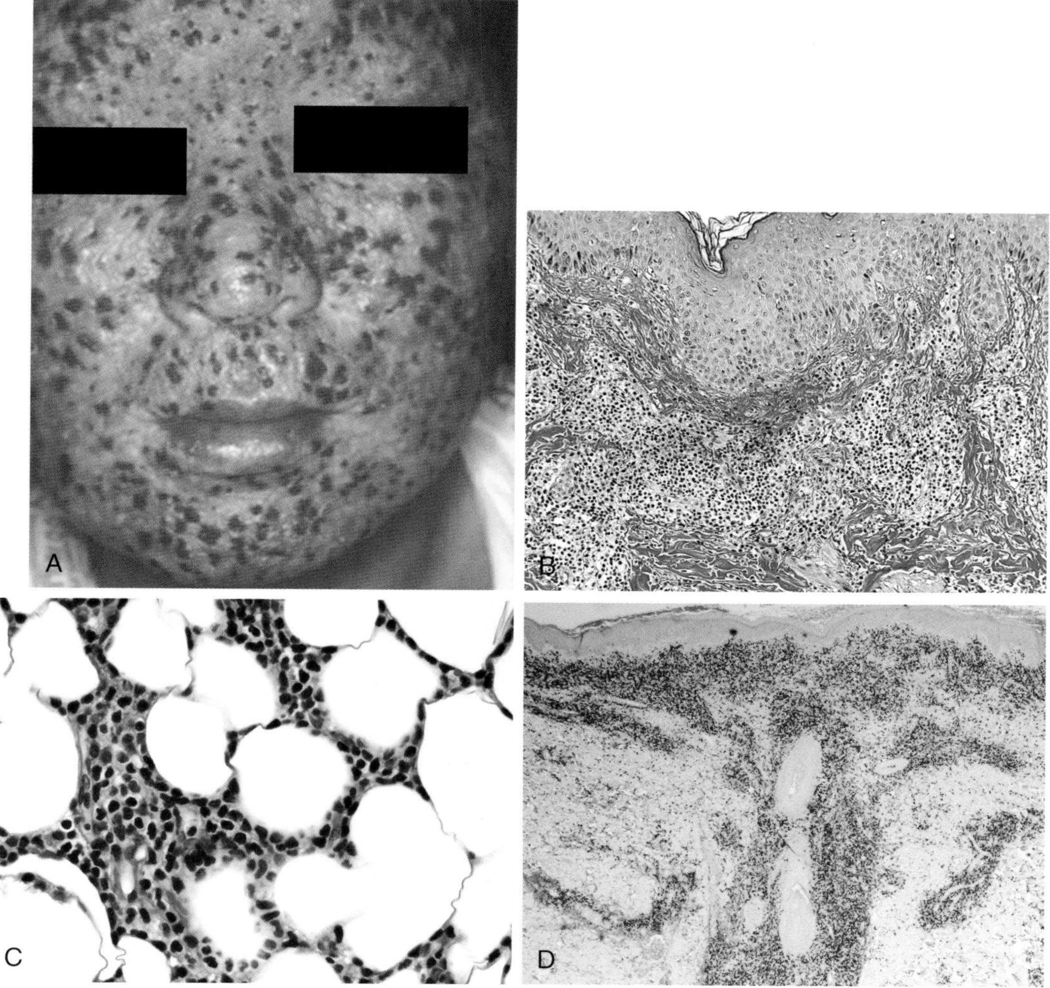

Figure 29-4. Hydroa vacciniforme–like T-cell lymphoma. A, This 24-year-old man with recurrent necrotic papulovesicles on the face for 6 years eventually developed a systemic EBV+ T-cell lymphoproliferative disease. **B,** Small to medium-sized lymphoid cells infiltrate the dermis. **C,** Infiltrate extends into subcutaneous tissue. **D,** Nearly all lymphoid cells are EBER+ (EBER in situ hybridization). (**A,** Courtesy of Professor K. H. Cho, Seoul National University.)

Postulated Cell of Origin

Cytotoxic T cells or rarely NK cells homing to the skin are the postulated cells of origin.

Prognosis

The prognosis is usually poor; the 2-year survival rate is 36%. Patients receiving chemotherapy or chemotherapy and radiation therapy have a partial response rate of 30%. Sepsis and liver failure are the main causes of death.[71] The clinical course may be indolent in patients with the NK-cell phenotype.[76]

Differential Diagnosis

The main differential diagnoses for HV-TCL are cutaneous NK/T-cell lymphoma and subcutaneous panniculitis-like T-cell lymphoma. Distinguishing extranodal NK/T-cell lymphoma is problematic because some cases may be of T-cell derivation. Characteristic, recurrent papulovesicular skin lesions, T-cell receptor gene rearrangement, and negativity for CD56 favor a diagnosis of HV-TCL over extranodal NK/T-cell lymphoma, nasal type.

Subcutaneous panniculitis-like T-cell lymphoma presents with deep subcutaneous nodules rather than vesiculopapular skin eruptions and is invariably negative for EBV.[77,78] Primary cutaneous gamma-delta T-cell lymphoma may appear clinically similar, and there may be dermal, epidermal, and subcutaneous involvement; the epidermis may be ulcerated. Primary cutaneous gamma-delta T-cell lymphoma is also negative for EBV.[79,80]

SYSTEMIC EPSTEIN-BARR VIRUS–POSITIVE T-CELL LYMPHOPROLIFERATIVE DISEASE

Definition

Systemic EBV+ T-cell LPD of childhood is a fulminant illness characterized by a clonal proliferation of EBV-infected T cells with an activated cytotoxic phenotype. It can occur shortly after primary acute EBV infection or develop in the clinical

Box 29-4 *Major Diagnostic Features of Systemic T-Cell Lymphoproliferative Disease of Childhood*

Definition
- Systemic clonal proliferation of EBV-infected T cells of an activated cytotoxic phenotype that occurs shortly after primary acute EBV infection or develops in the clinical setting of chronic active EBV infection; it usually has a rapid progression with multiple organ failure, sepsis, and death

Clinical Features and Behavior
- Prevalent in Asia and Latin America
- Children younger than 10 years and young adults
- Fulminant course lasting 1 or 2 months in cases of young children with primary acute EBV infection
- Fever, anemia, liver dysfunction, coagulopathy, rash, central nervous system symptoms, hepatosplenomegaly
- More prolonged survival in patients with chronic active EBV infection, but most patients die of disease within 1 year
- Causes of death are usually disseminated intravascular coagulation, multiorgan failure, and sepsis

Morphology
- Histiocytic erythrophagocytosis in bone marrow and secondary lymphoid organs
- Variable atypia in infiltrated lymphocytes

Immunophenotype and Genotype
- Predominantly cytotoxic $CD8^+$ T cells in cases of primary EBV infection
- Predominantly $CD4^+$ T cells or mixed $CD4^+/CD8^+$ or $CD8^+$ T cells in cases with chronic active EBV infection
- Monoclonal for EBV terminal repeat and T-cell receptor gene rearrangement

EBV, Epstein-Barr virus.

setting of CAEBV-T/NK. It is usually characterized by a rapid clinical progression, with multiple organ failure, sepsis, and death. A hemophagocytic syndrome is nearly always present (Box 29-4).

Epidemiology

Systemic EBV^+ T-cell LPD of childhood, which is most prevalent in Asia, is nearly always accompanied by a fulminant hemophagocytic syndrome. It has been described under a variety of names, including *fatal EBV-associated hemophagocytic syndrome*,[81] *fulminant EBV^+ T-cell LPD*,[82] *fulminant childhood hemophagocytic syndrome mimicking histiocytic medullary reticulosis*,[83] and *fatal hemophagocytic lymphohistiocytosis*.[84] Cases have been reported primarily from Taiwan[83,85,86] and Japan,[81,87] with a few cases from Korea[88] and Mexico.[82] The disease occurs most often in young children[89] and young adults.[90]

Systemic EBV^+ T-cell LPDs developing during the clinical course of CAEBV-T/NK have been described mainly in Japan,[1,31] with a few reports from Korea[91] and Western countries.[18] They occur mainly in teenagers,[1,91] young children, and adults.[1] There is no sex imbalance.

Pathophysiology

Hemophagocytic syndrome with a fulminant clinical course is the characteristic clinical picture of systemic EBV^+ T-cell LPD of childhood. The infection of T cells by EBV activates T cells to secrete Th1 cytokines such as tumor necrosis factor-α (TNF-α) and interferon-γ, which subsequently activate macrophages.[92] EBV LMP-1 activates the transcription factors nuclear factor-κB and JNK (c-Jun N-terminal kinase); this not only provides the molecular mechanism for LMP-1–induced cell proliferation and transformation but also confers resistance to TNF-α–mediated apoptosis via downregulation of TNF-α receptor 1 in the cytokine milieu of hemophagocytic syndrome.[93,94]

Clinical Features

Patients with systemic EBV^+ T-cell LPD developing after primary EBV infection present with a fulminant course lasting for 1 to 3 weeks and manifesting as fever, anemia, liver dysfunction, coagulopathy, rash, central nervous system symptoms, and hepatosplenomegaly with histiocytic erythrophagocytosis in the bone marrow and secondary lymphoid organs.[85] Generalized lymphadenopathy is not common. Viral serology is negative for EBNA antibody and positive for VCA IgG antibody, suggesting primary EBV infection.[95] VCA IgM is positive in only one third of systemic EBV^+ T-cell lymphomas after primary EBV infection.[96]

Systemic EBV^+ T-cell LPD arising in patients with a history of CAEBV-T/NK develops at a median of 35 months (range, 3 to 264 months) after the onset of CAEBV-T/NK. Before the development of T-cell LPD, patients experience intermittent or persistent fever of unknown origin, lymphadenopathy, or liver dysfunction over months or years, or HV-like skin eruptions occurring over months or several years.[1,88] The clinical course in these patients is somewhat more variable than that in patients with primary disease, but most patients eventually die of the disease.

Morphology

Hyperplasia of histiocytes and marked hemophagocytosis with increased numbers of small T lymphocytes are the most striking histologic changes in the bone marrow, spleen, and liver of young children with EBV^+ T-cell LPD occurring after primary EBV infection. The liver exhibits prominent portal as well as sinusoidal infiltrates of small lymphocytes with intracellular and intracanalicular cholestasis, steatosis, and focal necrosis. The histologic changes in the lymph nodes are variable; some cases show preserved architecture with open sinuses, whereas others may have diffuse effacement of the normal nodal architecture by infiltration with relatively homogeneous small, medium, or large lymphocytes with hyperchromatic nuclei and irregular nuclear contours. Epithelioid histiocytes, small granulomas, or necrosis may be present. The degree of cytologic atypia in the EBV^+ lymphocytes is variable, and in many cases the cytology is surprisingly bland (Fig. 29-5). The severe clinical manifestations usually alert one to the serious nature of the lymphoid proliferation.

Systemic T-cell LPDs that develop after a diagnosis of CAEBV-T/NK exhibit variable cytologic atypia, depending on the differentiation stage of the EBV-infected T cells.[11] The lymph node may show partial or total effacement of architecture, with polymorphic cellular infiltrates that include small to medium lymphocytes, plasma cells, and histiocytes with granulomas. Cytologic atypia of lymphocytes may not be

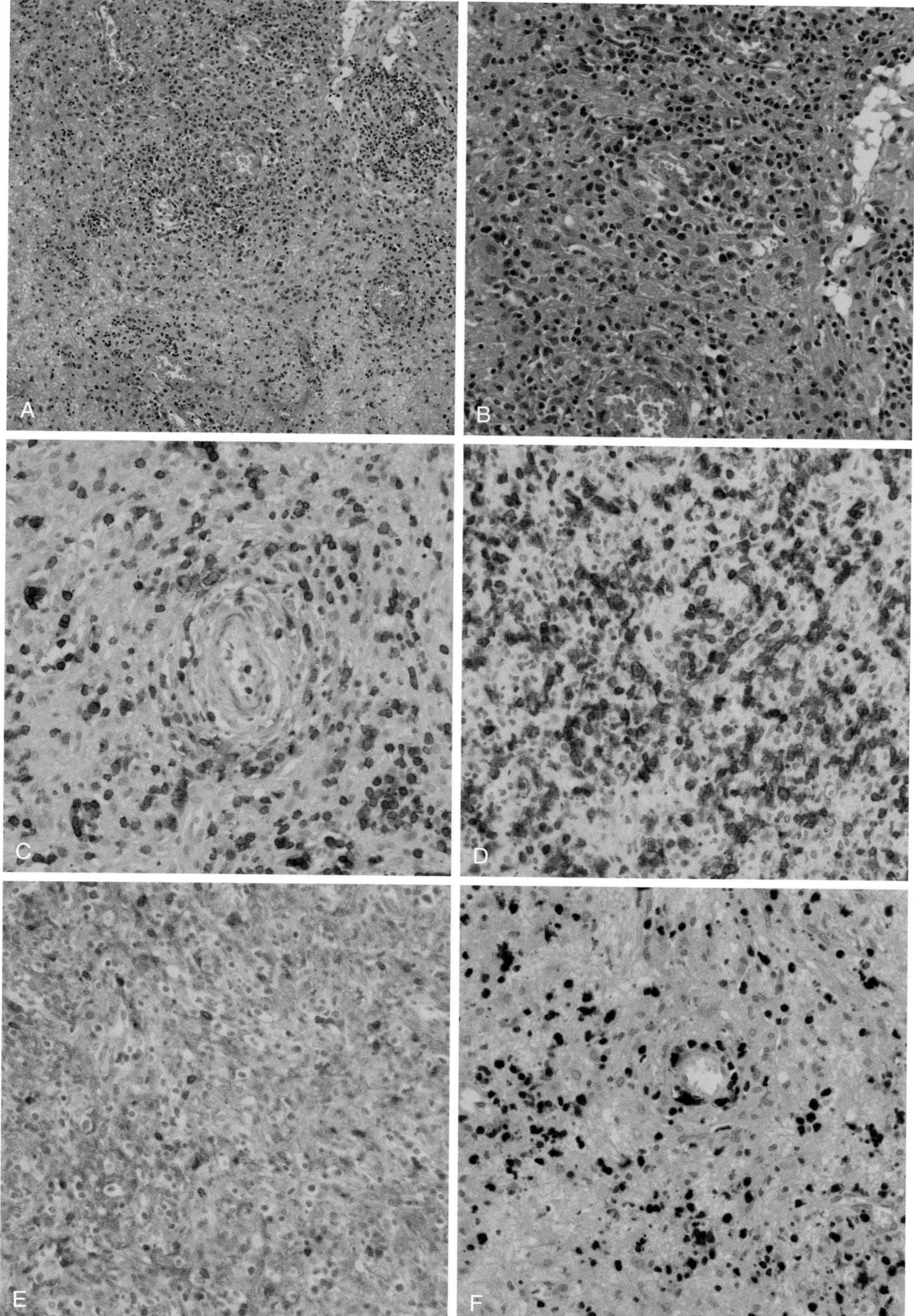

Figure 29-5. Systemic EBV⁺ T-cell lymphoproliferative disease of childhood. A 6-year-old girl presented with fever, hepatosplenomegaly, lymphadenopathy, and pancytopenia. **A,** Lymph node shows diffuse necrosis with a perivascular cellular infiltrate. **B,** Atypical lymphoid cells are present, and there is abundant apoptotic debris. **C-F,** Atypical lymphocytes in the lymph node are $CD3^+$, $CD8^+$, $CD4^-$, and $EBER^+$.

Continued

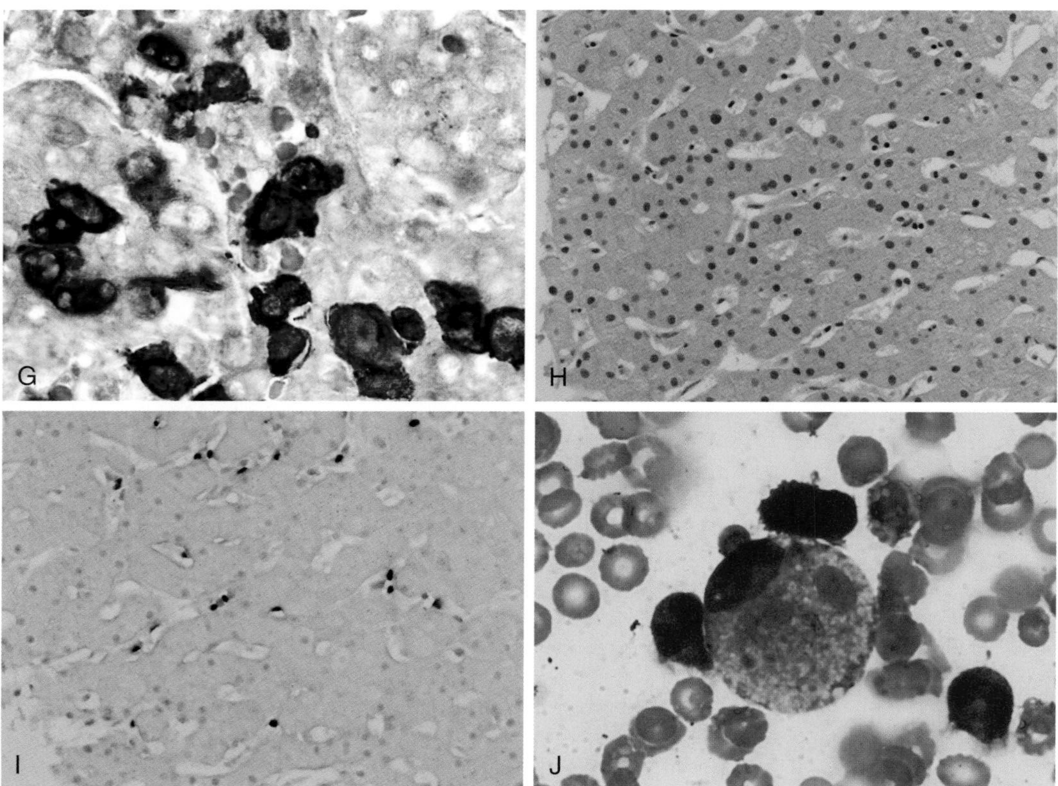

Figure 29-5, cont'd G, Atypical lymphoid cells in the spleen show membrane staining for CD3 and nuclear positivity with the EBER probe (double immunohistochemical and in situ hybridization reaction). **H** and **I,** A few small lymphocytes lacking significant atypia in the hepatic sinusoids are EBER⁺ (I). **J,** Hemophagocytic histiocytes are present in the bone marrow aspirate.

obvious. The atypical lymphoid cells are generally homogeneous in appearance, with round, hyperchromatic nuclei and inconspicuous nucleoli. In the skin biopsy the infiltrates are perivascular and periappendigeal in the upper dermis.

Immunophenotype and Genetics

The infiltrating cells in primary systemic EBV$^+$ T-cell LPD are predominantly CD8$^+$ cytotoxic alpha-beta T cells.[82,88] They are CD2$^+$, CD3$^+$, TIA-1$^+$, granzyme B$^+$, and CD56$^-$. Cases following CAEBV-T/NK infection show a more heterogeneous phenotype, mostly CD4$^+$,[18,31,82] or mixed CD4$^+$ and CD8$^+$ or CD8$^+$.[1]

EBV is clonal by terminal repeat analysis.[90] In situ hybridization for EBER shows striking positivity in the majority of small lymphoid cells that show minimal cytologic atypia, as well as in the obviously atypical cells. In situ hybridization for EBER and immunohistochemistry confirm EBV infection in T lymphocytes.

Postulated Cell of Origin

The postulated cells of origin are cytotoxic CD8 or CD4 T lymphocytes.

Clinical Course and Prognostic Factors

Young children with systemic EBV$^+$ T-cell LPD after primary EBV infection have a fulminant clinical course, with all patients dying within a few days to months of diagnosis. The rapidly progressive clinical course is similar to that of aggressive NK-cell leukemia.

Patients with systemic EBV$^+$ T-cell LPD that develops after CAEBV-T/NK may have a more prolonged clinical course, but most patients die of the disease within 1 year. Cause of death is usually disseminated intravascular coagulation, multiorgan failure, and sepsis.[1]

Differential Diagnosis

Aggressive NK-cell leukemia is very similar to systemic EBV$^+$ T-cell LPD arising in young children in terms of the fulminant clinical manifestations, presence of EBV in proliferating cells, and systemic hemophagocytosis. However, aggressive NK-cell leukemia is more common in adults (typically young adults), and the tumor cells express NK-cell markers, including CD56, and do not show clonal T-cell receptor gene rearrangement.[97]

Systemic EBV$^+$ T-cell LPD, arising either de novo or in the setting of CAEBV-T/NK, may show absent or minimal cytologic atypia. Such cases cause diagnostic problems, and the distinction from CAEBV may be difficult on morphologic grounds alone. In situ hybridization for EBER followed by clonality analysis is essential to avoid misdiagnosis.

Systemic EBV$^+$ T-cell lymphoma of the elderly is a rare, recently described disease that shares similar clinical and pathologic findings with the disease in children and young adults, but there are some differences.[88] Generalized lymphadenopathy is more common, patients have no history of CAEBV-T/NK, and hemophagocytosis or involvement of bone marrow at initial presentation is rare. Patients frequently have a history of hepatitis B or C virus infection, which suggests an underlying derangement of T-cell immunity against viral infection.

Pearls and Pitfalls

- Correct diagnosis of EBV⁺ lymphoproliferative diseases requires the integration of clinical, immunophenotypic, genotypic, and morphologic features.
- Chronic active EBV infection of T cells and NK cells includes a constellation of clinical syndromes that vary in their aggressiveness.
- Hydroa vacciniforme and mosquito bite hypersensitivity are cutaneous EBV-associated proliferations of T cells and NK cells in which cytokines and chemokines contribute to the homing of EBV-infected cells to sites of inflammation, leading to the characteristic symptoms.
- Definitive criteria for the distinction of hydroa vacciniforme and hydroa vacciniforme–like T-cell lymphoma are lacking, but clonality of the proliferating T cells favors the latter diagnosis.
- Systemic EBV⁺ T-cell lymphoproliferative disorder of childhood may appear deceptively benign cytologically, but it pursues an aggressive clinical course.

References can be found on Expert Consult @ www.expertconsult.com

Chapter 30

T-Cell Large Granular Lymphocytic Leukemia

Fan Zhou and Wing C. (John) Chan

CHAPTER OUTLINE

HISTORY AND CLASSIFICATION

Large granular lymphocytes (LGLs) exhibit distinct cytoplasmic azurophilic granules and can be divided into two basic types: T-cell large granular lymphocytes (T-LGLs) and natural killer (NK) cell large granular lymphocytes (NK-LGLs). T-LGLs are a subset of T lymphocytes expressing CD3, CD8, and CD57.[1,2] Leukemias derived from T-LGLs are classified as peripheral T-cell lymphoproliferative disorders (mature T-cell neoplasms). Large granular lymphocytic leukemias of the NK type often express the CD3$^-$, CD16$^+$, CD56$^+$ phenotype[3,4] and are classified as NK-cell lymphoproliferative disorders (mature NK-cell neoplasms).

The first probable cases of what is now termed *LGL proliferation/leukemia* can be found in a 1973 report by Lille and coworkers[5] in a series of 11 patients with "chronic lymphocytic leukemia (CLL) of T-cell origin." These cases were characterized by reactivity of the leukemic cells with antisera to T cells. In six of the cases, the lymphocytes had abundant cytoplasm and numerous cytoplasmic azurophilic granules, and these cells exhibited β-glucuronidase and acid phosphatase activities by cytochemistry.

Four years later McKenna and coworkers[6] reported a detailed clinicopathologic study on four patients with a lymphoproliferative disorder consisting of lymphocytes with abundant cytoplasm and many azurophilic cytoplasmic granules. These cells were considered to be T cells because they formed rosettes with sheep erythrocytes. These cells also expressed the Fc receptor. Electron microscopy showed that the granules had a characteristic structure consisting of bundles of microtubules surrounded by a limiting membrane. These structures have been termed *parallel tubular arrays*. A small fraction of normal peripheral blood lymphocytes (10% to 20%) has a similar morphology to the lymphocytes found in this lymphoproliferative disorder, and they can be separated from other lymphocytes using Percoll gradient centrifugation. It was found that almost all the NK and antibody-dependent cell-mediated cytotoxic activity resided in this cell population, and these lymphocytes were given the name *large granular lymphocytes*.[8,9]

Bom-van Noorloos and colleagues[10] reported two cases of LGL proliferation and examined the cytotoxic functions of the LGLs. The cells showed no NK activity but did have antibody-dependent cell-mediated cytotoxic activity. Because these cells express Fc receptor for immunoglobulin (Ig) G, the term *T-gamma lymphoproliferative disorder* has also been applied to this condition.[11] When monoclonal antibodies became available to study the LGL proliferation in the early 1980s, it came as a surprise that the vast majority of cases had the T-cell rather than the NK-cell phenotype.[12,13] The typical immunophenotype was CD2$^+$, CD3$^+$, CD8$^+$, CD4$^-$, T-cell receptor (TCR) αβ$^+$, CD16$^+$, CD57$^+$, and CD56$^-$. This observation explains why the LGL proliferations generally do not exhibit NK-cell activity, in contrast to normal peripheral blood LGLs.

However, NK activity can be induced in T-LGL proliferations by in vitro treatment with anti-CD3 monoclonal antibody.[14] A second major type of LGL proliferation, constituting about 10% to 20% of all such proliferations in Western countries, was later characterized.[12] The cells in this lymphoproliferation are NK cells and have NK functions.[15] Subsequently, many additional cases of LGL proliferation have been identified and reported.[15,16] Immunophenotypic, functional, and molecular studies have revealed significant heterogeneity among these cases, as described later.

DEFINITION

By definition, T-cell large granular lymphocytic leukemia (T-LGLL) must have a clonal proliferation of LGLs of the T-cell lineage. Large granular lymphocytic leukemia has been operationally defined as an increased LGL count of 2000/μL or greater in the peripheral blood. The LGL lymphocytosis should persist for more than 6 months without any identifiable cause that could induce reactive LGL proliferation. However, patients with LGL counts exceeding 2000/μL represent only a slight majority of cases of clonal T-LGL proliferation.[17] Some patients with lower LGL counts exhibit the typical manifestations of the disease. An LGL count of greater than 600/μL is well above the normal limit[18] and has been suggested as the minimal count for diagnosing T-LGLL. However, setting a lower limit is difficult because LGLs normally account for about 10% to 15% of the peripheral blood lymphocytes, and they are predominantly $CD3^-$ NK-LGLs.[18]

Morphologic criteria alone are obviously not sufficient for diagnosing T-LGLL, and all LGL proliferations should be immunophenotyped. Immunophenotyping is useful to differentiate T-LGL from NK-LGL proliferations. The immunophenotype of this leukemia is often indistinguishable from that of a reactive T-LGL lymphocytosis. To confirm the diagnosis of T-LGLL, T-cell clonality should be demonstrated. Clonal TCR gene rearrangement has been observed in patients with LGL counts less than 600/μL. These patients could be diagnosed with leukemia in an appropriate clinicopathologic and immunologic context.

A 6-month follow-up has been recommended to exclude a possible reactive LGL lymphocytosis. This practice is based on the assumption that LGL lymphocytosis may represent a proliferation in response to a certain stimulus that may resolve spontaneously when the stimulus is removed. However, in the proper clinical setting, the 6-month follow-up may not be essential when a monoclonal proliferation is clearly established by either polymerase chain reaction (PCR) or Southern blot analysis. Two questions may be raised: (1) Is a clonal expansion of T-LGLs sufficient to establish a malignant (leukemia) diagnosis? (2) What should we call a polyclonal or oligoclonal expansion of T-LGLs, and what is its relationship to a monoclonal proliferation? It has been clearly established that clonality does not automatically equate with malignancy or leukemia. Clonal expansions of $CD8^+$ T cells (especially the $CD57^+$ subset) can be detected in normal individuals,[19] especially in the setting of advanced age,[20] autoimmune diseases,[21] B-cell lymphoproliferative disorders,[22-24] post bone marrow transplantation,[25,26] and human immunodeficiency virus (HIV) infection.[27] In these cases, the "benign" clonal T lymphocytes are often $CD3^+$, $CD8^+$, and $CD57^+$, although cytoplasmic granules are not documented in all cases. Conversely, there are cases of T-LGL proliferation with polyclonal or oligoclonal TCR gene rearrangement. These patients may be otherwise indistinguishable from those with a monoclonal proliferation, and, by definition, the condition may be termed *T-LGL proliferation* or *lymphocytosis* but not *leukemia*. It is possible that these proliferations represent a phase of T-LGL expansion in response to a certain stimulus before the emergence of a dominant clone. During the course of proliferation of the T-LGLs, one or more secondary genetic alterations may occur, favoring the survival and proliferation of one or more selected clones and eventually resulting in a monoclonal process that we currently call *T-cell large granular lymphocytic leukemia*.

ETIOLOGY AND EPIDEMIOLOGY

T-LGLL is uncommon and represents less than 5% of chronic lymphocytic leukemia cases. Patients are often in their 50s or 60s, and the disease has been reported in diverse ethnic groups. Less than 10% of patients are younger than 40 years. Men and women are approximately equally involved.

The cause of T-LGLL is unclear. Epstein-Barr virus is often associated with aggressive NK-cell large granular lymphocytic leukemia but is rarely demonstrable in the T-cell type.[15,28] Antibodies to human T-lymphotropic virus 1 (HTLV-1) proteins p24 and p21 have been detected in the sera of a substantial proportion of patients; however, the genome of HTLV-1 or -2 and the related primate and bovine leukemia viruses are not identified by PCR.[29,30] It has been suggested that the antibodies are against some cross-reacting viral or cellular antigens and that the immune stimuli presumably provide a background for initiating and maintaining an antigen-driven proliferation of T-LGLs. An increased incidence of T-LGLL in organ transplant recipients and in patients with acquired immunodeficiency syndrome (AIDS), rheumatoid arthritis, and other autoimmune disorders suggests that a dysregulated immune system plays a role in the development of large granular lymphocytic leukemias.

CLINICAL FEATURES

Most patients with T-LGLL are middle-aged or elderly, with a median age of 55 years. The lymphoproliferation is typically indolent and nonprogressive, even on prolonged follow-up; a rare instance of spontaneous remission has been described. About two thirds of T-LGLL patients are symptomatic at the time of diagnosis. Clinical features are summarized in Table 30-1 and can be grouped into two major categories: hematologic disorders and autoimmune disorders.

Hematologic Manifestations

In the common type of T-LGLL, the vast majority of patients have cytopenia, especially neutropenia. Anemia is moderately common, and rare cases of pure red cell aplasia have also been observed. Thrombocytopenia is least common and occurs in up to 20% of cases[31]; it is usually mild and seldom leads to bleeding. Peripheral blood lymphocytosis is generally mild to moderate. Many patients do not have an absolute lymphocytosis, but the absolute number of LGLs is generally elevated to greater than 600/μL. Bone marrow involvement by T-LGLs is usually quite modest, with most patients having less than

Table 30-1 Clinical Manifestations and Laboratory Findings in T-Cell Large Granular Lymphocytic Leukemia

Frequency	Clinical	Laboratory
Common	Modest splenomegaly Infections Symptoms associated with anemia	Neutropenia Anemia Hypergammaglobulinemia Autoantibodies: ANA, RF β_2-microglobulinemia Clonal TCR gene rearrangement Bone marrow infiltrate LGL lymphocytosis
Moderately common	RA Mild hepatomegaly B symptoms	Absolute lymphocytosis Thrombocytopenia
Uncommon	Rash Associated conditions such as malignancy, AIDS, autoimmune diseases other than RA	Aplastic anemia PRCA Abnormal karyotypes Mixed proliferation of T- and NK-cell LGLs

AIDS, acquired immunodeficiency syndrome; ANA, antinuclear antibody; LGL, large granular lymphocyte; NK, natural killer; PRCA, pure red cell aplasia; RA, rheumatoid arthritis; RF, rheumatoid factor; TCR, T-cell receptor.

50% of lymphocytes in the marrow. Often, the degree of marrow infiltrate does not correlate with the severity of cytopenias.

The major causes of morbidity and mortality are the associated cytopenias. Marked neutropenia predisposes patients to bacterial infections. Skin infections are common, and occasional episodes of severe systemic infections such as sepsis and pneumonia occur during the course of the disease, leading to death in some patients. Patients may present with a perirectal abscess or a severe oropharyngeal infection. Anemia is common, and severe anemia, such as that seen in patients with associated pure red cell aplasia, can lead to serious morbidity. In rare cases, aplastic anemia is a presenting manifestation in T-LGLL patients.[32] The majority of T-LGLL patients do not have hypocellular bone marrow; more than 30% of the patients actually have hypercellular bone marrow. Occasionally T-LGLL is diagnosed in patients with myelodysplastic syndrome (MDS). Patients with T-LGLL and MDS may respond to immunosuppressive agents such as cyclosporine or antithymocyte globulin, but with a significantly lower response rate than those without MDS.[33] From a practical standpoint, one must be careful not to misdiagnose MDS in patients with T-LGLL. The morphologic criteria for MDS must be met.

Approximately half of T-LGLL patients have splenomegaly, and a few have hepatomegaly and lymphadenopathy. Patients with CD56$^+$ T-LGLL reportedly experience an aggressive clinical course, with B symptoms, rapidly increasing spleen size, extensive lymphadenopathy, and high LGL counts.[34] These clinically aggressive cases must be distinguished from hepatosplenic T-cell lymphoma.[35] Others have observed CD56$^+$ T-LGLL pursuing an indolent clinical course.[36]

Autoimmune Manifestations

Up to 30% of T-LGLL patients have clinical evidence of rheumatoid arthritis (RA). About one third of RA patients with neutropenia and up to 40% of patients with Felty's syndrome have a clonal proliferation of T-LGLs. Patients with RA and Felty's syndrome and patients with T-LGL proliferations plus RA have a high frequency (≈90%) of human leukocyte antigen (HLA)-DR4. The HLA-DR4 frequency in T-LGLL patients without RA is about 30%, which is around the normal frequency in the general population.[37] T-LGLL has also been reported in patients with other autoimmune diseases such as systemic lupus erythematosus, idiopathic thrombocytopenic purpura, pure red cell aplasia, Sjögren's syndrome, and autoimmune polyendocrinopathy syndrome types I and II.[31,38] Patients with T-LGLL frequently have autoantibodies, immune complexes, and hypergammaglobulinemia.[39,40]

Nonspecific Symptoms and Other Associated Conditions

A few patients may have a nonspecific erythematous or papular rash. Rarely, LGLs may infiltrate the deep dermis. A small percentage of patients (≈20%) may have overt systemic symptoms, including low-grade fever, fatigue, night sweats, and weight loss. Because T-LGLL can be associated with a variety of other diseases, patients may also present with clinical features of paroxysmal nocturnal hemoglobinuria, chronic lymphocytic leukemia, hairy cell leukemia, monoclonal gammopathy of unknown significance, or Hodgkin's lymphoma.[41,42] The natural history of T-LGL proliferations associated with B-cell leuekmias is generally benign, with no independent impact on the clinical course. Rarely, T-LGLL is seen in patients with solid tumors, including hepatocellular carcinoma.[43] It is not uncommon to find HIV patients with polyclonal or even monoclonal CD8$^+$ T-LGL proliferations.[27] Patients who have undergone renal, liver, and bone marrow transplants may also have T-LGLL or T-LGL proliferations.[44,45]

MORPHOLOGY AND LABORATORY STUDIES

There are generally no morphologic features that can differentiate clonal leukemic LGLs from polyclonal reactive LGL proliferations. A typical LGL has abundant light blue cytoplasm with fine or occasionally coarse azurophilic granules (Fig. 30-1). The nucleus has a round or slightly indented outline, with moderately condensed nuclear chromatin. Under the electron microscope, some of the azurophilic granules are composed of bundles of microtubules that may be perpendicular to each other—a characteristic ultrastructural appearance termed *parallel tubular arrays* (Fig. 30-2A).[12] However, these parallel tubular arrays are not unique to leu-

Chapter 31

T-Cell Prolymphocytic Leukemia

Anna Porwit and Miroslav Djokic

CHAPTER OUTLINE

DEFINITION

T-cell prolymphocytic leukemia (T-PLL) is an aggressive disease characterized by a proliferation of small to medium-sized lymphocytes with a postthymic phenotype usually involving blood, bone marrow, lymph nodes, spleen, and skin.[1,2] This leukemia was first described by Catovsky and coworkers[3] in reference to a patient who presented with cytologic features similar to B-cell prolymphocytic leukemia (B-PLL), but the cells were shown to bind sheep erythrocytes (E-rosette positive). A more detailed report was published in 1986 by Matutes and colleagues[4] comparing morphologic and clinical characteristics of 29 T-PLL and 33 B-PLL cases and defining the immunophenotype as consistent with mature T cells. In 1987 the same group reported an association of T-PLL with inv(14)(q11;q32) and trisomy for 8q.[5]

EPIDEMIOLOGY

T-PLL represents approximately 3% of all T-cell disorders.[6] This leukemia occurs mainly in the elderly (median age, 65 years; range, 33 to 91 years) and slightly more often in men (male-to-female ratio about 1.4:1).[7-9] An increased frequency has been found in patients with ataxia-telangiectasia, who also develop T-PLL at a younger age (26 to 43 years).[10]

CLINICAL FEATURES

Most T-PLL patients present with general symptoms: sweating, malaise, weight loss, or fever.[7-9,11,12] The median duration of symptoms is 2 months before diagnosis. In most patients, a high white blood cell count (>100 × 10^9/L in 72%), splenomegaly (79%), lymphadenopathy (46%), and enlarged liver (39%) are found.[7-9] One fourth of patients have skin lesions at diagnosis, mainly maculopapular rash, nodules, or (more seldom) erythroderma.[7,8,11-14] In 15% to 30% of patients, mainly those with high white blood cell counts, serous effusions are found at diagnosis. Serous effusions may also develop later in the course of the disease.[7,8,11,12] Central nervous system involvement is rare.[7,8] Thirty percent to 50% of patients present with anemia (hemoglobin <10 g/dL) or thrombocytopenia (<100 × 10^9/L), or both.[7,8,11,12] Usually there is no neutropenia or monocytopenia. Hyperuricemia and increased levels of lactate dehydrogenase are common. Other liver function tests may be mildly elevated, whereas serum immunoglobulin and renal biochemistry are normal.[7,8] Although serum from most Western T-PLL patients has tested negative for human T-lymphotropic virus (HTLV) types 1 and 2, in some Japanese patients DNA samples contained an HTLV-1 *TAX* sequence.[7,8,15] A single case of Epstein-Barr virus–related T-PLL has been described.[16]

MORPHOLOGY

Typical T-PLL cells in the peripheral blood are medium-sized lymphocytes with a high nuclear-to-cytoplasmic ratio and deeply basophilic cytoplasm without granules, often showing protrusions (Box 31-1; Fig. 31-1A). Ultrastructural studies show numerous ribosomes, polyribosomes, and profiles of rough endoplasmic reticulum, accounting for the cytoplasmic basophilia.[4,7,8,13] Nuclei are often irregular, with numerous short indentations, and they have moderately condensed chromatin and prominent nucleoli. Cytochemical staining for α-naphthyl-acetate esterase shows a characteristic dot-like pattern.[17]

In approximately 20% of cases the leukemic cells are smaller, the nuclei are round, and the nucleoli cannot be readily seen by light microscopy (see Fig. 31-1B), although they are easily detected by electron microscopy.[4,18] In some publications these cases are called a "small cell variant" of T-PLL. Because the clinical and cytogenetic features are similar, both variants of T-PLL probably belong in the same category.[11,18] Most cases included in publications on T-cell

Box 31-1 ***Major Features of T-Cell Prolymphocytic Leukemia***

Morphology
- Peripheral blood cytomorphology
  - Common variant: intermediate-sized lymphocyte with round or irregular nuclear contour, moderately condensed chromatin, prominent central nucleoli, abundant basophilic cytoplasm with protrusions, no granules
  - Small cell variant: small lymphocyte with round to mildly irregular nucleus, clumped chromatin with inconspicuous nucleolus, scant basophilic cytoplasm
- Bone marrow histomorphology: diffuse, solid sheets of lymphocytes effacing normal bone marrow architecture; less frequently, diffuse interstitial or nodular infiltrates with partially preserved architecture

Immunophenotype
- $CD2^+$, $CD3^+$, $CD5^+$; usually strongly $CD7^+$; TCRαβ
- $CD4^+/CD8^-$ (most common); $CD4^+/CD8^+$ or $CD4^-/CD8^+$ (less frequent)
- $TCL1^+$, $CD26^+$ (usually)
- NK-associated marker (CD16, CD56, CD57) negative
- Cytotoxic granule molecule (TIA-1, granzyme B) negative

Genetics
- *TCRβ, TCRγ* genes rearranged
- Rearrangement of *TCL1*, *TCL1β* in inv(14)(q11;q32.1) or t(14;14)(q11;q32.1)
- Rearrangement of *MTCP1* in t(X;14)(28;q11)
- Trisomy 8 or iso8q
- Mutations in *ATM* at 11q23

chronic lymphocytic leukemia show a typical morphology and immunophenotype and chromosomal changes that correspond to the small cell variant of T-PLL.[19-21] In rare cases, polylobated nuclei similar to those in adult T-cell leukemia/lymphoma are noted. In other cases, cerebriform nuclei, as seen in Sézary's syndrome, are described. These cases were previously designated *Sézary cell leukemia*.[13,22]

In bone marrow trephine biopsies there is usually increased cellularity, which varies from slightly hypercellular to a "packed" bone marrow. Patterns of infiltration may be nodular or interstitial, with leukemic cells constituting only part of the bone marrow cellularity, or diffuse infiltration with a dominance of leukemic cells (see Fig. 31-1C).[23] In some cases there is discordance between the blood and bone marrow involvement, and patients with marked leukocytosis may have surprisingly sparse marrow involvement.[24] There is often slight fibrosis, shown by an increase in the density of reticulin fibers. On trephine sections, T-PLL cells are small to medium-sized and relatively round, making them difficult to differentiate from the cells of other chronic lymphoproliferative disorders. Characteristic cytologic features are more noticeable on bone marrow imprints or smears that show an infiltration of cells similar to those in peripheral blood.[24]

Lymph nodes show a diffuse infiltration of leukemic cells. These cells are seen mostly in interfollicular areas, but they may also completely replace the normal architecture (Fig. 31-2A). Residual germinal centers may be present.[25] In paraffin sections, leukemic cells are medium-sized and rather monomorphic. Mitotic figures are easily identified, and Ki-67 (MIB-1) staining shows a high fraction of proliferating cells (usually 30% to 60%) (see Fig. 31-2B). Typical features, including prominent nucleoli and abundant cytoplasm, are more easily appreciated in imprints or fine-needle aspirates from the lymph nodes (see Fig. 31-2C).

Morphologic features of splenic involvement by T-PLL have been described by Osuji and associates.[26] The spleen is often grossly enlarged. T-PLL cells infiltrate the red pulp—both sinusoids and cords—and the white pulp shows signs of disruption due to infiltration of leukemic cells into the follicles (see Fig. 31-2D). The sinus pulp cord architecture is not distorted. Angioinvasion and infiltration of fibrous trabeculae are prominent. Leukemic cells infiltrate through the splenic capsule and into perisplenic fat tissue.[26]

In the liver T-PLL infiltrates are usually confined to portal tracts, with variable portal tract expansion and sinusoidal involvement.[14] T-PLL cells can be seen within the blood vessels of portal tracts.

Skin infiltrates are usually confined to the dermis (see Fig. 31-2E). The infiltrates sometimes extend into the subcutaneous adipose tissue. In rare cases, epidermotropism or a subcutaneous mass may develop.[14,25] Infiltrates are usually present around capillaries and skin appendages.[14] There is a variable degree of stromal edema surrounding the blood vessels, with minimal endothelial damage and few extravasated erythrocytes. In most skin infiltrates, round nuclei are seen. Only rare cases with Sézary-like cells have been found.[14] Progression to high-grade cutaneous $CD30^+$ large cell lymphoma, with chromosomal changes identical to those seen in blood T-PLL cells, has been described.[27] Rare cases of ocular involvement have been described presenting with panuveitis, retinal detachment, or perivascular conjunctival involvement.[28,29]

Reports on the morphology of other extramedullary sites involved by T-PLL are rare in the literature.[25] In a transbronchial biopsy from a T-PLL patient, small aggregates of leukemic cells were found in the bronchial mucosa. In another T-PLL patient, colon endoscopy showed superficial ulcers, and microscopic examination revealed infiltrates in the lamina propria, but without lymphoepithelial lesions.

IMMUNOPHENOTYPE

Almost all T-PLL cases are positive for CD7, usually with high intensity.[7,8,11,30,31] Leukemic cells are positive for cytoplasmic CD3, but membrane CD3 is negative in 20% of cases. The cells are usually positive for CD2, CD5, CD43, and CD26.[7,8,11,12,26] Most cases (≈60%) display a $CD4^+$, $CD8^-$ phenotype, but other cases display a $CD4^+$, $CD8^+$ phenotype (15% to 25%) or a $CD4^-$, $CD8^+$ phenotype (10% to 15%) (Fig. 31-3). There is no expression of natural killer (NK)–cell markers (CD56, CD57, CD16) or of the cytotoxic marker TIA-1, even in $CD8^+$ cases. However, perforin expression is noted in some cases.[26] T-cell activation markers such as CD25, CD38, and human leukocyte antigen (HLA)-DR are variably expressed.[7,8,12] TCL1 protein is present in most cases (Fig. 31-4).[12] Two cases of $CD103^+$ T-PLL have been described, but data on CD103 expression in larger series are not available.[31] Similarly, there are no published studies on ZAP-70 expression, but some cases may be positive.[32] Terminal deoxynucleotidyl transferase (TdT), CD1a, CD30, TRAP, anaplastic lymphoma kinase-1 (ALK-1), BCL6, and BCL3 are negative.[7,8,12,26,33] Data on BCL2 expression are not available in the

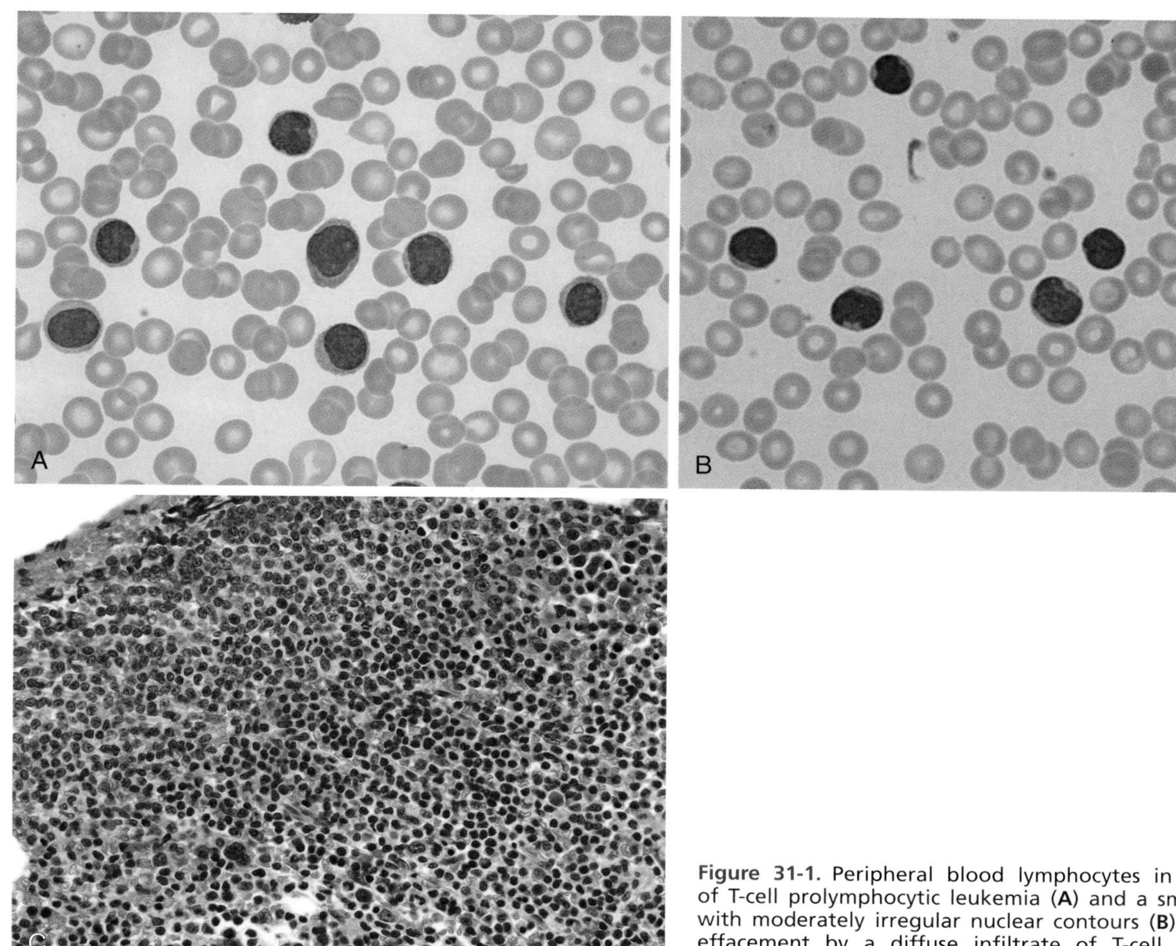

Figure 31-1. Peripheral blood lymphocytes in a typical case of T-cell prolymphocytic leukemia (**A**) and a small cell variant with moderately irregular nuclear contours (**B**). Bone marrow effacement by a diffuse infiltrate of T-cell prolymphocytic leukemia (**C**).

literature, but our own experience suggests that BCL2 is strongly positive (see Fig. 31-2F).

In a series of cases published by Garand and coworkers,[11] T-PLL cases with an initially indolent course were more often negative for CD45RO and CD38 compared with aggressive T-PLL. CD52 is found on T-PLL cells at a higher density than on normal B and T lymphocytes or in B-cell chronic lymphocytic leukemia, which may be the reason for the favorable response to treatment with anti-CD52.[34]

GENETICS AND MOLECULAR FINDINGS

Cytogenetic studies in T-PLL have found recurrent chromosomal abnormalities. In 90% of all cases, the Xq28 (*MTCP1*) or 14q32.1 (*TCL1* and *TCL1b*) regions are involved in translocations or inversions with *TCRA/D* at 14q11.[5,35] However, the frequency of these aberrancies may be lower in Japanese T-PLL patients.[36] *TCL1* and *MTCP1* have partial amino acid or nucleotide sequence similarity (41% identical and 61% similar).[37] A third member of this family, *TCL1b*, also shows similarities of structure and expression with *TCL1*. *TCL1b* has been located at 14q32.1.[38] In T-PLL, all three genes are activated and overexpressed by juxtaposition to the alpha-delta locus at 14q11. *TCL1* encodes for a predominantly cytoplasmic protein of 14 kD that is also found in small quantities in the nuclei of lymphoid cells.[39] The TCL1 protein binds to the D_3 phosphoinositide-regulated kinase AKT1, enhancing its activity and promoting its transport to the nucleus.[38] In T-PLL, T-cell receptor (TCR) stimulation leads to the rapid recruitment of TCL1, AKT, and tyrosine kinases to membrane-associated activation complexes.[40] It has also been shown that TCL1 protein expression confers resistance to activation-induced cell death and growth arrest in T-PLL cells and the TCL1-driven T-cell leukemia cell line SUP-T11 by inhibiting the ERK pathway, concomitant with and probably due to an impairment of PCKθ activation.[41]

TCL1 protein expression as shown by immunohistochemistry is normally observed in early T-cell progenitors and in the lymphoid cells of B lineage (both progenitors and mature lymphocytes, especially mantle zone cells), but not in mature T lymphocytes.[39,42] In T-PLL, a distinct positivity is found (see Fig. 31-4), but other postthymic T-cell lymphomas, including cutaneous T-cell lymphoproliferations, are negative.[12] In many B-cell tumors, both nuclear and cytoplasmic expression has been detected. However, lymphomas showing plasma cell differentiation, such as marginal cell lymphomas, mucosa-associated lymphoid tissue (MALT) lymphomas, and plasmacytomas, are mostly negative.[39,43] In B-cell tumors, no *TCL1* rearrangement is found, but an alternative mechanism of activation by loss of methylation of an *NotI* site adjacent to the

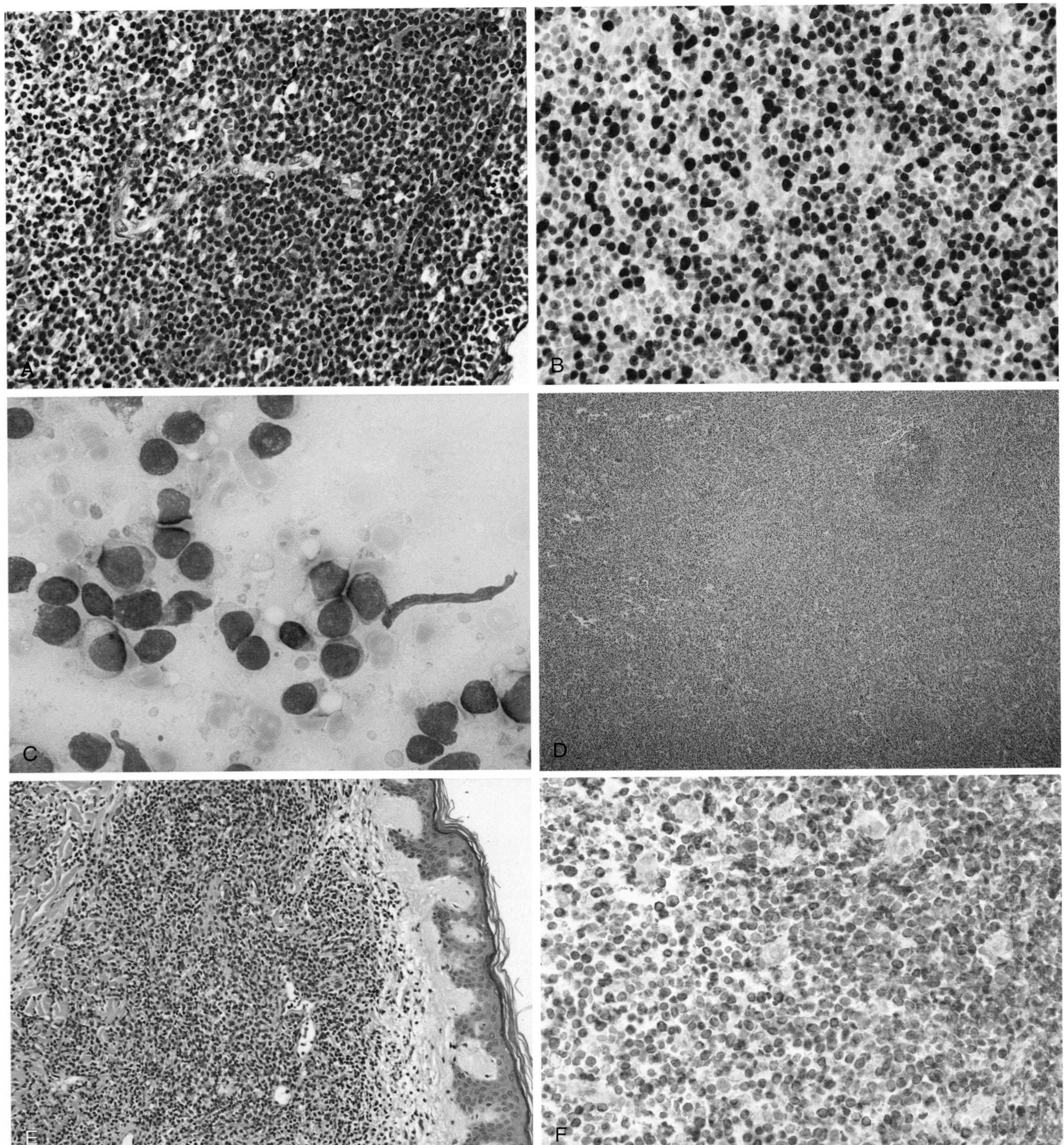

Figure 31-2. **A,** Core needle biopsy of a lymph node shows a diffuse infiltrate of T-cell prolymphocytic leukemia (T-PLL). **B,** Ki-67 immunostain shows high proliferative activity of T-PLL (estimated at 60%). **C,** Fine-needle aspirate smear from a lymph node shows prominent nucleoli and abundant cytoplasm of neoplastic cells. **D,** Effacement of splenic red pulp by diffuse T-PLL infiltrate. **E,** Heavy infiltrate in the skin involves primarily the dermis and subcutaneous soft tissues, with characteristic sparing of the epidermal layer. **F,** BCL2 shows uniformly strong expression in neoplastic cells of T-PLL.

TATA box in the *TCL1* promoter has been detected.[44] Transgenic mice, which overexpress either activated *TCL1* or *MTCP1* gene in T cells, develop mature T-cell leukemias.[45] Preleukemic T-cell populations have been observed in young mice, and T-cell leukemias, mostly CD4$^-$, CD8$^+$, developed by the age of 15 months.[46]

In most T-PLL cases, changes involving chromosome 14 are accompanied by other complex abnormalities. Unbalanced rearrangements of chromosome 8 have been reported frequently, mainly trisomy 8q; monosomy 8p, such as i(8)(q10); t(8;8)(p12;q11); or translocations involving 8p and other chromosomal partners.[47] Although rearrangement of

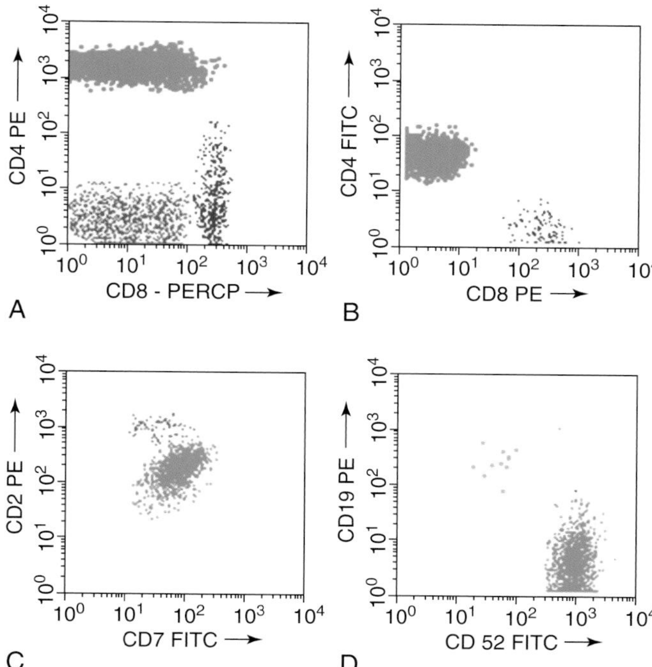

Figure 31-3. Flow cytometry results in T-cell prolymphocytic leukemia (T-PLL). A, Direct immunofluorescence with CD3FITC/CD4PE/CD8-PERCP. The CD3 gate shows a population of leukemic cells that are $CD4^{bright+}$, $CD8^{dim+/-}$ (*green dots*). **B,** The same antibody combination in another T-PLL case. Leukemic cells are $CD4^{+}$, $CD8^{-}$ (*green dots*). **C,** In the same case shown in figure **B,** the leukemic cells have weaker expression of CD2 (*green dots*) than do normal T cells (*red dots*). **D,** Strong expression of CD52 in a T-PLL case (*green dots*). Normal B cells (*blue dots*) are shown for comparison.

c-MYC has not been described, overexpression of c-MYC protein has been shown by flow cytometry.[48] Thus, additional copies of *c-MYC* may represent a secondary abnormality providing proliferative advantage.

Abnormalities of chromosome 11, including recurrent losses of the 11q21-q23 regions, have also been detected using fluorescence in situ hybridization (FISH) or loss of heterozygosity analysis. Biallelic inactivation (missense mutations) of the *ATM* gene located at 11q21-q23 was demonstrated in virtually all sporadic cases of T-PLL, suggesting that *ATM* has a tumor suppressor gene function.[49,50] Truncating mutations in the *ATM* gene are the main cause of ataxia-telangiectasia, a rare familial recessive disorder involving progressive neurologic disease, immunodeficiency syndrome, and chromosomal instability.[10] In patients with ataxia-telangiectasia, small clones harboring cytogenetic alterations involving 14q11 (AT clonal proliferations) may be seen several years before the onset of the T-PLL.[10] Knockout mice with a complete ataxia-telangiectasia–like phenotype consistently produce immature ($CD3^{-}$, $CD4^{+}$, $CD8^{+}$) T-cell thymic lymphomas that arise coincidentally with V(D)J recombination.[51] Development of these malignancies in knockout mice can be prevented by bone marrow transplantation, which replaces the ATM-deficient hematopoiesis.[52]

Other reported abnormalities detected by loss of heterozygosity analysis, FISH, or conventional cytogenetics include deletions of 12p13; deletions or translocations involving 6q, 13q14.3, or 17p; and monosomy 22.[8,18,53,54] Recent studies using an animal model suggested the *CDKN1B* gene encoding the p27KIP1 protein as a candidate target gene in the chromosome 12p13 deletion that causes CDKN1B haploinsufficiency.[55] Mapping of the 13q14.3 deletion revealed that the D13S25 region telomeric of the retinoblastoma (*RB-1*) gene is the most frequently deleted marker at 13q14.3.[56] Of the 13 T-PLL patients studied, 5 had the *p53* allele deletion, but none had *p53* mutation by direct sequencing. However, in 7 of 13 samples, p53 protein overexpression was noted. This suggests that nonmutational mechanisms are responsible for the accumulation of p53 protein.[57]

Most of these abnormalities were confirmed by comparative genomic hybridization analysis that showed an abnormal profile in virtually all cases, with several recurrent abnormalities present in each T-PLL case.[58,59] The number of chromosomal alterations was not related to morphologic characteristics or the clinical behavior of the disease. Combined single nucleotide polymorphism–based genomic mapping and global gene expression profiling showed that

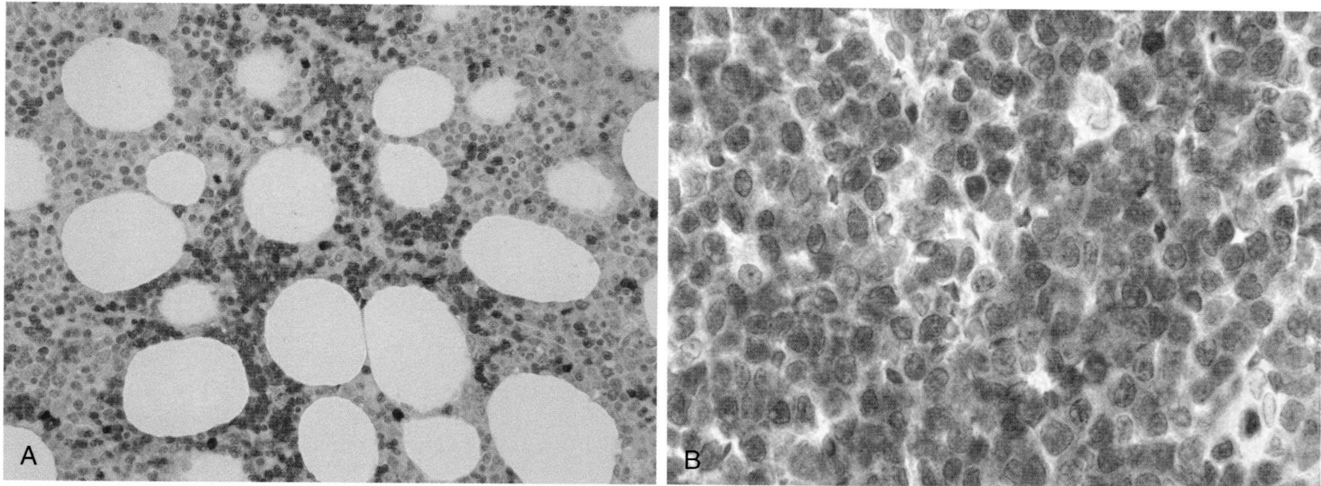

Figure 31-4. Strong nuclear and cytoplasmic staining is seen with anti-TCL1 antibody in bone marrow **(A)** and lymph node **(B)** infiltrated by T-cell prolymphocytic leukemia. (Courtesy of Dr. Elisabeth Hyjek, Department of Pathology, University of Chicago.)

several of the genes upregulated in T-PLL are involved in the regulation of transcription, nucleosome assembly, translation, and cell cycle control (e.g., Nijmegen breakage syndrome 1 [*NBS1*], *TCF7L, CCNB2, CCNB1, CCNG2, PFAS, PAICS, HIST1H2AE, HIST1H2B, HIST1H4G, ELF4EBP1, ELL3*). In contrast, various proapoptotic genes, such as *FAS, CASP1, CASP4, CASP8, STK17A,* and *TRAIL,* were downmodulated.[60]

Both $TCR\alpha$ and $TCR\beta$ genes are rearranged in most cases.[11,61] However, some cases with only $TCR\gamma\delta$ rearrangement have been described.[25,62,63] Pathologic restriction of the variable (V) region of beta chain use was detected by a broad array of antibodies and flow cytometry.[64]

POSTULATED CELL OF ORIGIN

The cell of origin of T-PLL is unclear, but immunophenotypic and *TCR* gene rearrangement studies suggest a T cell with a postthymic phenotype. Studies performed on transgenic mice, in which expression of p13MTCP1 was controlled by CD2 regulatory sequences and p13MTCP1 was overexpressed in the thymus and spleen, showed a high incidence of T-PLL–like leukemia. In CD2-p13MTCP1 mice, clonal T-cell populations in both the spleen and the liver emerged long before the onset of lymphocytosis, which suggests that the oncogenic activity of *MTCP1* is specific for a precise but as yet not clearly defined stage of T-cell differentiation.[46,65]

CLINICAL COURSE

The clinical course of T-PLL is usually aggressive, with progressive disease and median survival of 7 to 8 months from diagnosis. There is a poor response to treatment or early relapse after a short remission.[7,8,11] About one third of patients in a large French study and several separately described patients had an initially indolent clinical course, lower and stable leukocytosis, no anemia or thrombocytopenia, and no splenomegaly or skin changes.[11,66,67] The morphologic and cytogenetic characteristics of this group were similar to those of patients with aggressive disease. The stable phase had a median duration of 33 months (range, 6 to 103 months), but in seven patients it was longer than 5 years, and one patient survived for 15 years.[11,67] At progression, an aggressive clinical course was observed.

TREATMENT

Only rare T-PLL patients respond to single-agent therapy with alkylating drugs. Approximately 30% of patients achieve short-term remissions with combination chemotherapy, such as CHOP (cyclophosphamide, hydroxydaunomycin, Oncovin [vincristine], prednisone).[7-9] Pentostatin treatment produced better results, with a 40% overall response and 12% complete remission for a median duration of 6 months.[68] So far, the best treatment response has been achieved in patients treated with humanized anti-CD52 monoclonal antibody (alemtuzumab [Campath-1H]).[69-71] Most previously untreated patients achieved complete remission,[70] and in a previously treated group, a 37.5% complete remission rate was noted.[72] A combination of chemotherapy and alemtuzumab did not improve the overall results in a phase II study.[70] In responding patients, a rapid clearance of leukemia cells from peripheral blood was noted, and lymphadenopathy, splenomegaly, and skin infiltrates resolved in a majority of these patients. The disease was more resistant in patients with hepatomegaly, serous effusions, or bulky disease. However, no cures were achieved, even with alemtuzumab treatment. Most patients suffered relapse a median of 2 years after remission. In some of these patients a second complete remission may be achieved with alemtuzumab or stem cell transplantation (SCT) (Fig. 31-5).[70,72] The emergence of a CD52⁻ phenotype has been described as a mechanism for resistance to Campath-1H therapy.[73] Therefore, all eligible patients who respond to therapy should be considered for consolidation with SCT. Results from one study show that autologous SCT can increase disease-free survival, but one third of patients relapse.[74] Allogeneic SCT may be difficult to perform owing to patients' usually advanced age at diagnosis.[74]

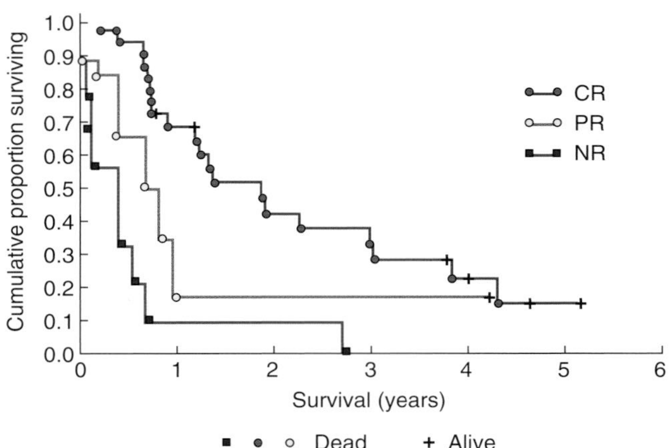

Figure 31-5. Results of treatment with alemtuzumab in T-cell prolymphocytic leukemia. CR, complete remission; NR, no remission; PR, partial remission. (Modified from Dearden C. Alemtuzumab in peripheral T-cell malignancies. *Cancer Biother Radiopharm.* 2004;19:391-398.)

DIFFERENTIAL DIAGNOSIS

With modern immunophenotyping by flow cytometry or immunostaining of paraffin tissue sections, the differentiation between B-PLL and T-PLL is rather straightforward owing to the presence of the monoclonal B cell (CD19 and CD20 positivity and light-chain restriction by flow cytometry, or PAX5, CD20 [L26], and CD79a expression by immunohistochemistry) or T-cell phenotype, respectively. Similarly, T-cell acute lymphocytic leukemia (T-ALL) can be easily distinguished from T-PLL by the expression of TdT or CD1a in T-ALL. The differential diagnosis between T-PLL and other mature T-cell leukemia/lymphomas (e.g., adult T-cell leukemia/lymphoma, mycosis fungoides–Sézary syndrome, large granular lymphocytic leukemia, and hepatosplenic T-cell lymphoma) may be more of a challenge because of highly overlapping morphology and partly overlapping immunophenotypes (especially if a limited panel of markers is applied). The main differentiating features helpful in obtaining the correct diagnosis are summarized in Table 31-1 and Pearls and Pitfalls. The most specific markers for T-PLL by immunophenotyping are CD26 and TCL1 protein expression, which are not detected in the other mature T-cell leukemia/lymphomas.[12] However, the most reliable diagnostic criteria for T-PLL are the specific genetic abnormalities described earlier.

Table 31-1 Differential Diagnosis of T-Cell Prolymphocytic Leukemia

	T-PLL	ATLL	MF-SS	LGLL	HSTCL
Lymphocytosis	Marked (usually >100 × 10^9/L)	Marked	Mild to moderate	Mild (usually <15 × 10^9/L)	No*
Peripheral blood morphology	Prolymphocytic (most common), small lymphocytic, cerebriform	Pleomorphic nuclei, multilobated ("flower cell")	Cerebriform nuclei	Large azurophilic granules (cytoplasmic)	Intermediate-large size
Pattern in bone marrow	Diffuse (common), interstitial, nodular	Patchy, sparse (rarely diffuse)	Uncommon in bone marrow; small focal or interstitial, eosinophilia	Interstitial (small clusters), intrasinusoidal	Intrasinusoidal, interstitial
Extramedullary involvement					
Hepatosplenomegaly	Common	Variable	Rare*	Common	Common
Lymphadenopathy	Variable	Common	Common	Rare	Rare
Skin	Variable (dermal infiltrates)	Common	Common	—	—
Effusions	>30%, usually pleural	Rare	Rare	Rare	Rare
Immunophenotype	$CD4^+/CD8^-$ (common); $CD4^+/CD8^+$, $CD4^-/CD8^+$	$CD4^+/CD8^-$	$CD4^+/CD8^-$	$CD4^-/CD8^+$ (common); $CD4^+/CD8^-$, $CD4^+/CD8^+$	$CD4^-/CD8^-$
	TCRαβ	TCRαβ	TCRαβ	TCRαβ	TCRγδ (common); TCRαβ (rare)
	$CD5^+$, $CD7^+$	$CD5^+$, usually $CD7^-$	$CD5^+$, usually $CD7^-$	CD7 variable	$CD5^-$, CD7 variable
	$CD26^+$	$CD26^-$, $CD25^{++}$	$CD26^-$	$CD26^-$	$CD26^-$
	NK marker negative, cytotoxic markers negative, $TCL1^+$	Cytotoxic markers negative	Cytotoxic markers negative	$CD57^+$, cytotoxic markers positive, $CD56^{+/-}$	$CD16^+$, $CD56^+$, TIA^+, perforin negative
Clinical course	Aggressive	Usually aggressive	Chronic	Indolent	Aggressive
Viral etiology	—	HTLV-1	—	—	—
Genetics	Rearrangements at 14q32.1 (*TCL1, TCL1β*), Xq28 (*MTCP1*), trisomy 8 or iso8q, 11q23 (*ATM*)	Clonal integration of HTLV-1	Complex karyotypes, no unique abnormalities	No unique abnormalities	iso7q, trisomy 8

*May occur late in disease course.

ATLL, adult T-cell leukemia/lymphoma; HSTCL, hepatosplenic T-cell lymphoma; HTLV-1, human T-lymphotropic virus type 1; LGLL, large granular lymphocytic leukemia; MF-SS, mycosis fungoides–Sézary syndrome; T-PLL, T-cell prolymphocytic leukemia.

Pearls and Pitfalls

- Peripheral blood lymphocytosis greater than $100 \times 10^9/L$ is common.
- Different cytomorphologic characteristics of neoplastic cells are described, but in a given case, the cells usually show a fairly high degree of cytologic monomorphism.
- Specific genetic abnormalities and immunologic phenotypes do not correlate with morphologic variants.
- Overexpression of TCL1 protein (or its functional homologues) and certain clinical features (e.g., markedly elevated lymphocyte count) provide a higher degree of diagnostic specificity than cytologic characteristics of neoplastic cells, histomorphologic patterns of bone marrow involvement, or immunophenotype.
- Even in cases with $CD8^+$ expression, the neoplastic cells do not express cytotoxic granule molecules.
- The characteristic pattern of splenic infiltration involves both red and white pulp, with effacement of normal splenic architecture.

References can be found on Expert Consult @ www.expertconsult.com

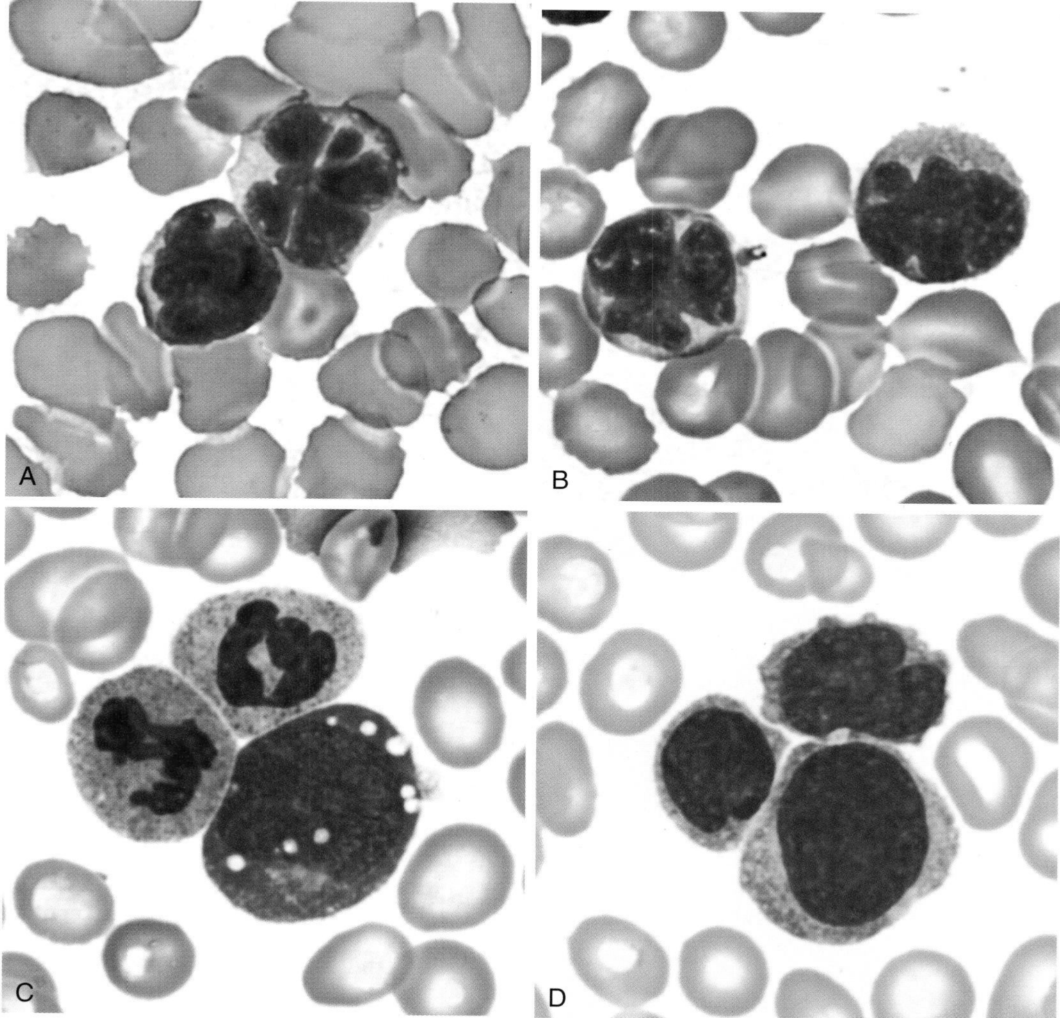

Figure 32-6. Peripheral blood findings in adult T-cell leukemia/lymphoma. Flower cells with markedly polylobated nuclei (**A** and **B**) are most common, but one can also see blast-like cells (**C**) and cells with rounder nuclear contours (**D**).

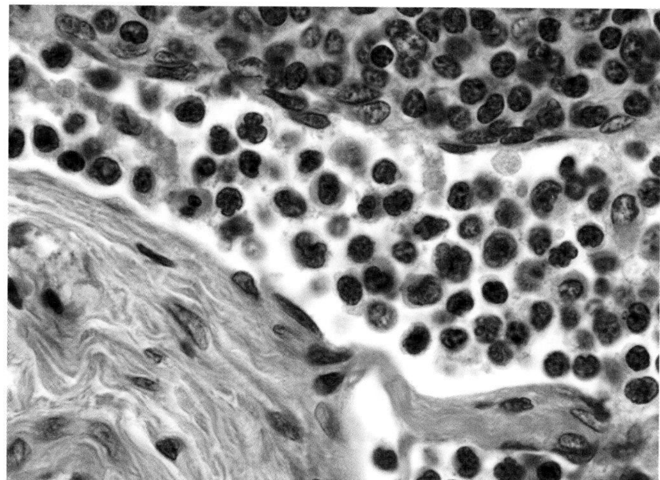

Figure 32-7. Lymph node in a patient with adult T-cell leukemia/ lymphoma. In the leukemic phase, dilated sinuses may contain atypical cells.

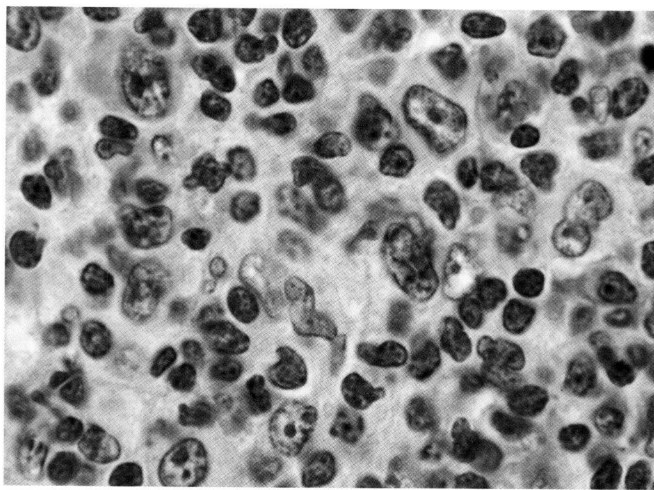

Figure 32-8. Lymph node in a patient with adult T-cell leukemia/ lymphoma. Small pleomorphic lymphoid cells may be admixed with larger blast-like cells with vesicular nuclei and prominent nucleoli.

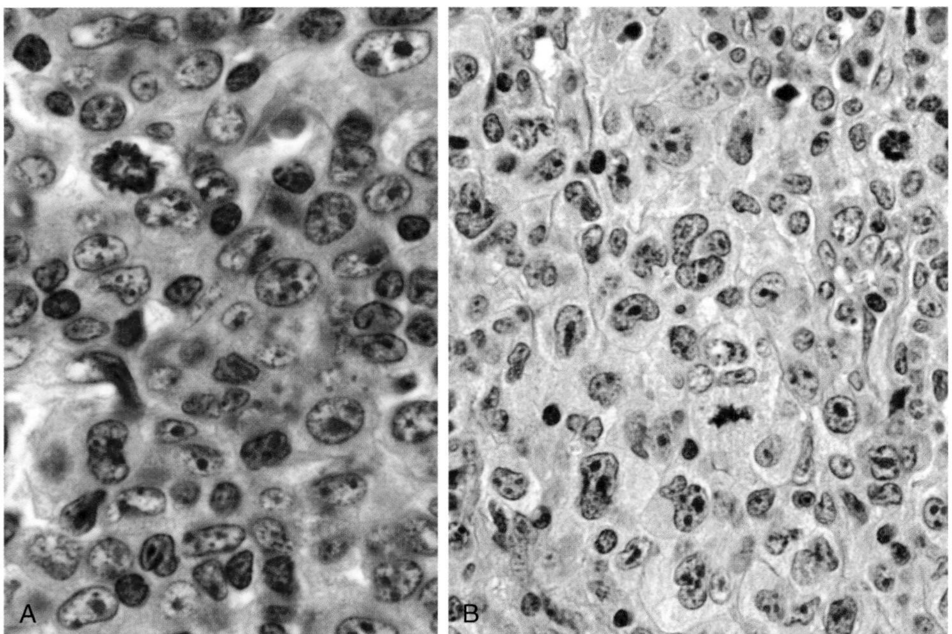

Figure 32-9. Lymph nodes in patients with adult T-cell leukemia/lymphoma. A, In this case, cells with blastic features predominate. The process may mimic a diffuse large B-cell lymphoma if immunohistochemical studies are not performed. **B,** Giant cells with pleomorphic nuclei may be present as well.

confluent, without numerous histiocytes or eosinophils. The smaller neoplastic cells usually predominate in the skin. In the smoldering and chronic types, cytologic atypia may be minimal. Hyperparakeratosis is variably present in the overlying epidermis. The skin lesions are clinically and histologically diverse and may mimic inflammatory disorders.[38]

Bone marrow involvement is typically not prominent. The marrow may contain patchy atypical lymphoid infiltrates. However, the degree of bone marrow infiltration is less than expected, given the marked lymphocytosis that may be present. Correlating with the clinical finding of hypercalcemia, there is often evidence of bone resorption and osteoclastic activity (Fig. 32-12).[39] Bone trabeculae may show evidence of remodeling, and in some patients, lytic bone lesions are present even in the absence of tumoral bone infiltration (Fig. 32-13).[19]

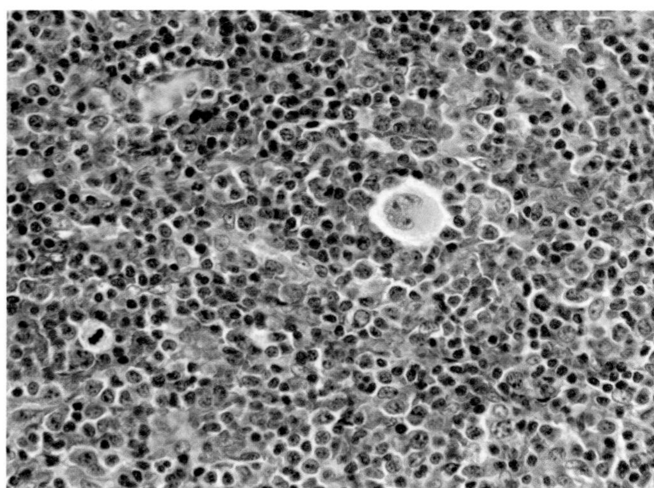

Figure 32-10. Lymph node in a patient with incipient adult T-cell leukemia/lymphoma. Cells resembling Hodgkin–Reed-Sternberg cells may be present, mimicking classical Hodgkin's lymphoma. The Hodgkin-like cells are Epstein-Barr virus–positive transformed B cells, and the background contains HTLV-1 T cells.

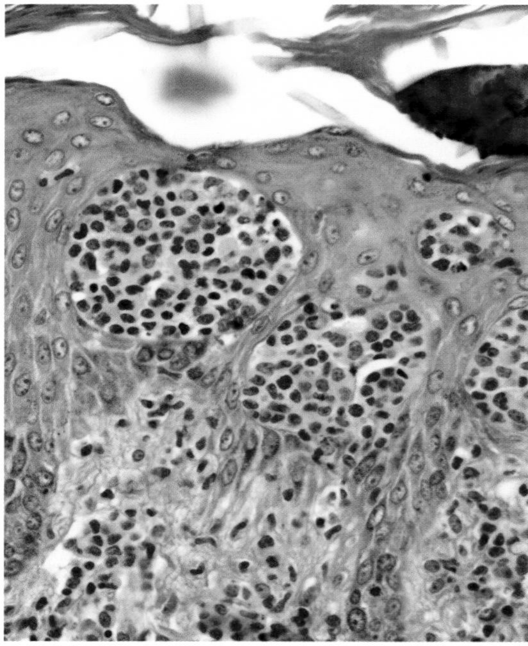

Figure 32-11. Skin biopsy specimen in adult T-cell leukemia/lymphoma. There is marked epidermotropism, with infiltration of the overlying epidermis.

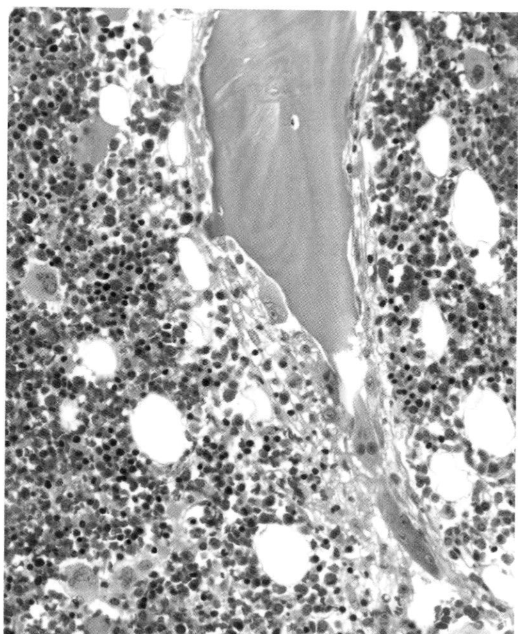

Figure 32-12. Bone marrow core biopsy in adult T-cell leukemia/lymphoma. The bone marrow space shows myeloid hyperplasia without identifiable tumor cells. However, the bone trabeculae show evidence of remodeling and increased osteoclasts.

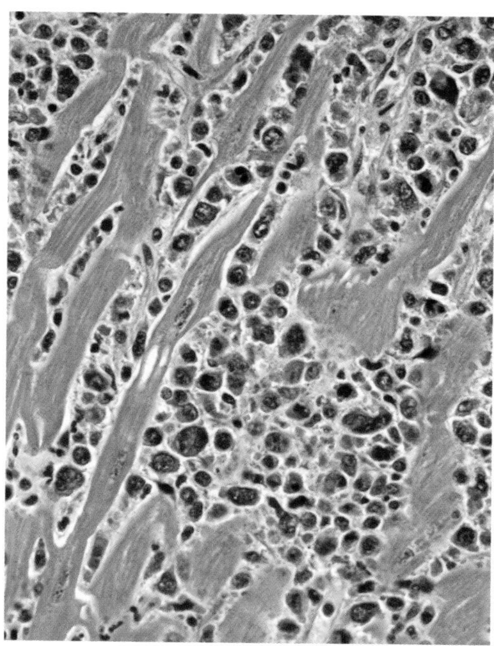

Figure 32-14. Cardiac involvement by adult T-cell leukemia/lymphoma.

Other frequent sites of involvement include the lung and cerebrospinal fluid. Correlating with a leukemic phase, the pulmonary infiltrates are generally patchy and interstitial, with no formation of tumor nodules. Cardiac involvement has been reported rarely and is always associated with concomitant pulmonary involvement (Fig. 32-14).[29]

Involvement of the central nervous system usually manifests as meningeal infiltration without nodular parenchymal lesions. Neoplastic cells may be detected in cytologic preparations of cerebrospinal fluid. However, rare cases with parenchymal tumor masses have been reported.[40] Central nervous system involvement is nearly always associated with widespread systemic disease, but rare cases with isolated central nervous system involvement have been reported.[23]

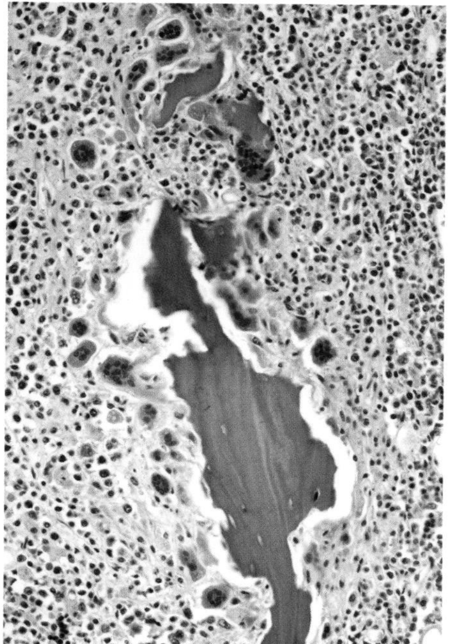

Figure 32-13. Lytic bone lesion in adult T-cell leukemia/lymphoma. Numerous osteoclasts surround bone trabeculae.

Although there is no formal cytologic grading system for ATLL, the neoplastic cells in the chronic and smoldering variants of the disease usually show minimal cytologic atypia, perhaps in keeping with the more indolent clinical course.

IMMUNOPHENOTYPE

The neoplastic cells, regardless of cytologic subtype, are $CD4^+$ alpha-beta T cells that strongly express the alpha chain of the interleukin-2 receptor (IL-2R) or CD25 (Fig. 32-15).[41] High levels of soluble IL-2R can also be found in the serum and correlate with disease activity.[42] CD7 is nearly always absent, but CD3 and other mature T-cell antigens (CD2, CD5) are usually expressed. CD52 is usually positive, a finding of clinical relevance for the use of anti-CD52 humanized antibody (alemtuzumab [Campath]) for treatment purposes. CD30 can be expressed in the larger blastic cells. Because many peripheral T-cell lymphomas have a $CD3^+$, $CD4^+$, $CD7^-$ immunophenotype, the most specific feature of ATLL is strong CD25 positivity. With enhanced antigen retrieval techniques, CD25 expression can be detected in formalin-fixed, paraffin-embedded tissue sections.[43] Because of its strong expression, CD25 has become a target of immunotherapy for ATLL.[41] Recent studies suggest that the cells of ATLL may be the equivalent of regulatory T (Treg) cells.[44,45] In one study, 68% of the cases tested were positive for FOXP3 in at least some of the neoplastic cells, although usually only a small minority. No other T-cell lymphoma subtype expresses this transcription

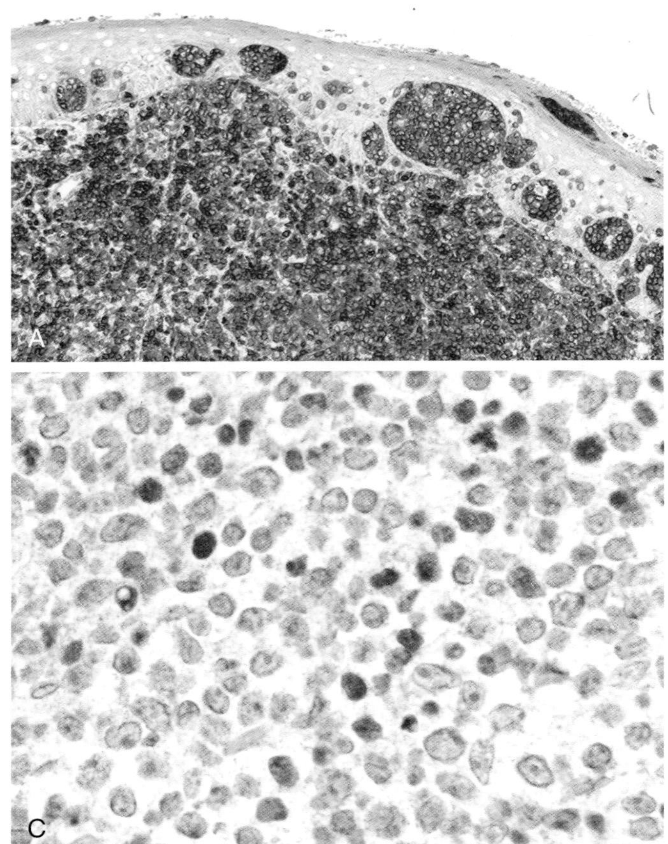

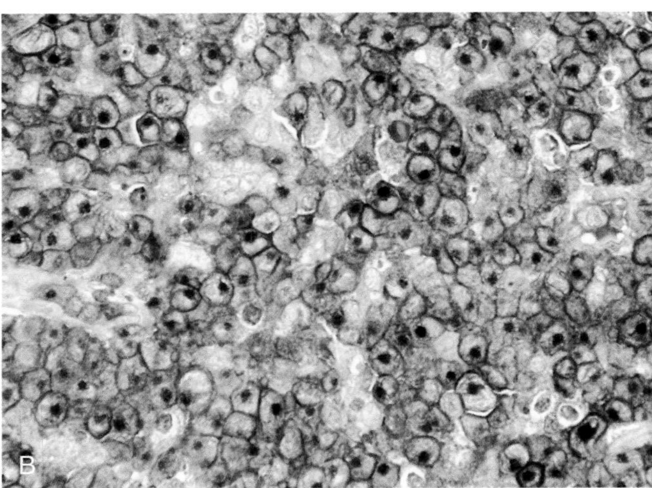

Figure 32-15. Immunohistochemistry of adult T-cell leukemia/ lymphoma. A, Skin biopsy shows positive staining for CD3 in epidermal and dermal lymphoid cells. **B,** Tumor cells show strong membrane and Golgi staining for CD25. **C,** A subpopulation of tumor cells is positive for FOXP3, with the larger atypical cells being negative. (**A - C,** immunoperoxidase with hematoxylin counterstain.)

factor, which is a hallmark of Treg cells, in conjunction with CD25 and CD4. This finding helps explain the immunodeficiency associated with ATLL. FOXP3-positive cases appear to be a lower grade, manifesting fewer cytogenetic abnormalities.[46]

GENETICS, MOLECULAR FINDINGS, AND ROLE OF HTLV-1

ATLL is a mature T-cell malignancy with clonal rearrangement of the T-cell receptor genes. In patients with acute or lymphomatous ATLL, there is evidence of a single dominant clone in all sites involved by the disease. HTLV-1 carriers do not show a dominant T-cell clone but may have oligoclonal T-cell expansion. The high-density expression of IL-2R renders these cells responsive to growth in response to cytokines both in vitro and in vivo.[47] Similarly, in the early phases of smoldering or chronic ATLL, more than one T-cell clone may be present, with emergence of a dominant clone at the time of progression.[48]

The HTLV-1 proviral DNA is clonally integrated into neoplastic T cells.[33] Patients with incipient ATLL or those with early-stage disease may contain T-cell clones with defective or partial viral integration.[49] Southern blotting techniques are useful to follow the clone, as the unique site of integration produces a distinctive band.[50] PCR techniques for HTLV-1 sequences can be used to quantify the viral load in the peripheral blood.[51,52] Patients with HAM/TSP do not have circulating T cells with clonal integration of the HTLV-1 virus. However, in keeping with the aberrant immune response to HTLV-1 involved in HAM/TSP, clonal and oligoclonal T-cell populations directed against the virus may be identified.[53]

HTLV-1 is the first human retrovirus shown to cause malignant transformation.[1] It contains the structural genes *gag*, *pol*, and *env* and a pX region at the 3′ end that encodes, among others, the regulatory proteins TAX and REX. The viral gene *TAX* plays a pivotal role in HTLV-1–initiated leukemogenesis. The TAX protein is a transcriptional activator of the viral long terminal repeat. TAX can act by transactivation to deregulate a variety of cellular genes, leading to activation of signal transduction,[54] deregulation of the cell cycle,[3] and induction of genetic instability resulting in multiple cytogenetic abnormalities.[55,56] TAX itself is oncogenic and can transform human T cells and rodent fibroblasts.[54]

TAX acts via several signal transduction pathways, including nuclear factor-κB (NF-κB), the CREB/ATF family (leucine zipper protein), serum response factor, and AP-1 families.[57] TAX can bind directly to several members of the NF-κB family of proteins.[58] TAX also binds to proteins that inhibit NF-κB, providing an alternative mechanism for NF-κB activation.

In addition, TAX can inactivate p53. Thus, although most cases of ATLL do not show p53 mutation or deletion, p53 is inactivated directly by TAX.[59] This promotes destabilization of the genome and the development of other genetic abnormalities. *TAX* also inhibits the cell cycle regulators p16 and INK4A, promoting continuous cellular proliferation of HTLV-1–infected cells.[58]

TAX plays a role in the effects mediated by IL-2 and IL-15. The alpha chain of IL-2R was the first gene shown to be upregulated by TAX.[60] TAX upregulates the expression of both IL-2 and IL-15, a relative of IL-2, providing a mechanism for an autocrine loop in HTLV-1–infected cells.[61] IL-15 uses the beta and gamma chains of IL-2R for signaling. TAX also upregulates IL-15Rα in ATLL cells.[61] Other cellular genes may be activated by TAX, such as *IL-6*; this activity may be responsible for the hypercalcemia characteristic of ATLL by promoting the secretion of parathormone-like substances, leading to osteoclastic activation.[62,63] The hypercalcemia of ATLL can be replicated in TAX transgenic mice.[64] Activation of NF-κB also appears to play a role in the production of osteoclast-activating factors.[63] Finally, ATLL cells express RANK ligand, which promotes the differentiation of hematopoietic precursors into osteoclasts.[13,65]

ATLL cells show numerous complex structural cytogenetic abnormalities affecting every chromosome pair. There are no recurrent cytogenetic changes, however, that are useful in making the diagnosis.[66,67] Structural abnormalities occur most frequently in chromosome 6. In six patients with chromosome 6 deletions, there were breakpoints at bands q11, q13, q16q23, q21q23, q22q24, and q23q24, and the presence of abnormalities in 6q appeared to correlate with a more aggressive clinical course.[66] Translocations are identified in about 10% of cases involving the T-cell receptor-$\alpha\Delta$ gene locus on 14q11.[68] Studies employing comparative genomic hybridization have confirmed the diversity and frequency of genetic changes.[69] Different genetic changes were observed in the acute and lymphomatous subtypes, suggesting that these two variants might proceed along different molecular pathways. The complexity of the cytogenetic abnormalities are likely mediated in large measure by TAX.[54,70,71] TAX impairs DNA repair mechanisms and represses the expression of DNA polymerase-β, an enzyme involved in base excision repair. TAX also represses nucleotide excision repair, which plays a critical role in repairing ultraviolet irradiation–induced damage.

Recent studies employing gene expression profiling identified overexpression of *BIRC5* (survivin), a gene that blocks apoptosis.[72] The antiapoptotic function of *BIRC5* may also play a role in the resistance of ATLL cells to chemotherapy.

Thus, although HTLV-1 infection does not lead directly to malignant transformation of T cells, it promotes the development of neoplastic transformation by a variety of mechanisms, including stimulation of T-cell growth, inhibition of T-cell death via apoptosis, deregulation of DNA repair mechanisms and promotion of chromosomal instability, and activation of signal transduction pathways. The *TAX* gene plays a role in most of these actions.

POSTULATED NORMAL COUNTERPART

ATLL cells are alpha-beta T cells that most closely resemble Treg cells. Treg cells play a major role in regulating the immune response, mainly by suppressing it. They require the transcription factor FOXP3 for functional development in the thymus gland[73] and have a $CD3^+$, $CD4^+$, $CD25^+$ phenotype. Although FOXP3 is not universally expressed in all cases of ATLL, it is expressed in some instances.[44,45]

CLINICAL COURSE

Acute and lymphomatous forms of ATLL have an aggressive clinical course, with a median survival of less than 1 year and a projected 4-year survival of only 5%.[74] Without treatment, most patients die within weeks to months; even with treatment, most remissions are short-lived.[6,19,75] As noted earlier, the expression of survivin may play a role in the resistance to chemotherapy.[72] Major prognostic indicators for acute ATLL include performance status, high lactate dehydrogenase, age (older than 40 years), more than three sites of disease, and hypercalcemia.[76] Other factors that appear to impact prognosis include thrombocytopenia, eosinophilia, and bone marrow involvement. Some molecular alterations are associated with a more aggressive clinical course, including *p16* gene deletion[77] and *p53* mutation.[78]

The clinical course is more protracted in patients with chronic or smoldering disease, but median survival is still less than 5 years for these patients. Prognostic factors of predictive value for chronic ATLL include high lactate dehydrogenase, low albumin, and high blood urea nitrogen levels.[76] Deletion of the *p16* gene in the chronic phase is also a negative prognostic factor, and gene deletion by comparative genomic hybridization correlates with an adverse prognosis.[77,79] Molecular alterations are also shown to occur during progression from chronic to acute-phase disease.[80]

Conventional chemotherapy regimens (doxorubicin based) have been largely ineffective, prompting the investigation of other agents such as deoxycoformycin (pentostatin), with limited success.[81] More intensive high-dose chemotherapy and bone marrow transplantation have been used in limited numbers of patients. Treatment-related mortality is very high, limiting the utility of this approach.[82] Because ATLL is caused by a retrovirus, there was speculation that drugs active against other retroviruses, such as human immunodeficiency virus (HIV), might have activity. Initial trials employing zidovudine (AZT) and α-interferon suggested some efficacy,[83,84] but the initial good outcomes were not reproduced in subsequent studies.[85] However, this regimen may have a role in patients with smoldering or chronic disease.[76] In another study, a combination of arsenic and α-interferon was used, with the suggestion that it might lead to the downregulation of *TAX*.[86] The efficacy of this approach has not been demonstrated in clinical trials. Promising results have been obtained in monoclonal antibody–based therapies directed against IL-2R, which is highly expressed in ATLL; the efficacy of humanized anti-tac, either unconjugated or labeled with yttrium 90,[41,87] was highest in patients with chronic or smoldering disease. Because ATLL has such a poor prognosis, clinical efforts to control ATLL have been largely directed at preventing infection in susceptible populations.

DIFFERENTIAL DIAGNOSIS

The differential diagnosis of acute and lymphomatous ATLL differs somewhat from that of chronic or smoldering ATLL (Table 32-2). The clinical picture of acute ATLL with hypercalcemia and systemic disease usually prompts consideration of the diagnosis. The diagnosis of ATLL may be less obvious in patients presenting with lymphoma and without hypercalcemia. ATLL cells have an immunophenotype that is relatively specific, so the combination of a T-cell malignancy expressing

Table 32-2 **Differential Diagnosis of Adult T-Cell Leukemia/Lymphoma (ATLL)**

Diagnosis	Clonal TCR	HTLV-1 Integration	CD25	Flower Cells
ATLL	+	+	++	+
Mycosis fungoides	+	–	–	–
T-PLL	+	–	–	–
ALCL	+	–	++	–
PTCL, NOS	+	–	–/+	–

ALCL, anaplastic large cell lymphoma; HTLV-1, human T-lymphotropic virus 1; PTCL, NOS, peripheral T-cell lymphoma, not otherwise specified; TCR, T-cell receptor; T-PLL, T-cell prolymphocytic leukemia.

CD3, CD4, and CD25 is highly suggestive. CD25 is expressed in other B-cell and T-cell malignancies, including hairy cell leukemia,[88] classical Hodgkin's lymphoma,[89] and anaplastic lymphoma kinase–positive anaplastic large cell lymphoma[43]; however, demonstration of a B-cell phenotype can readily exclude the diagnosis. Although anaplastic large cell lymphoma is usually positive for CD25, CD3 is often negative in the neoplastic cells. CD30 is strongly expressed in anaplastic large cell lymphoma, whereas usually only a minority of ATLL cells are CD30 positive. Serologic studies for antibodies to HTLV-1 or PCR studies for HTLV-1 viral sequences can be confirmatory.

To assist in epidemiologic studies of ATLL, a scoring system was proposed.[30] Clinical features counting as 1 point each are hypercalcemia, skin lesions, and a leukemic phase. Laboratory criteria, counting as 2 points each, include a T-cell phenotype, seropositivity for HTLV-1 or -2, expression of CD25 by tumor cells, and evidence of HTLV-1 or -2 sequences at the molecular level. A score of 5 or greater is a strong indication for a diagnosis of ATLL. It should be borne in mind that patients from endemic areas may be seropositive for HTLV-1 but develop other lymphomas, independent of viral positivity. Thus, demonstration of viral integration in the tumor cells is the strongest indication for a diagnosis of ATLL.

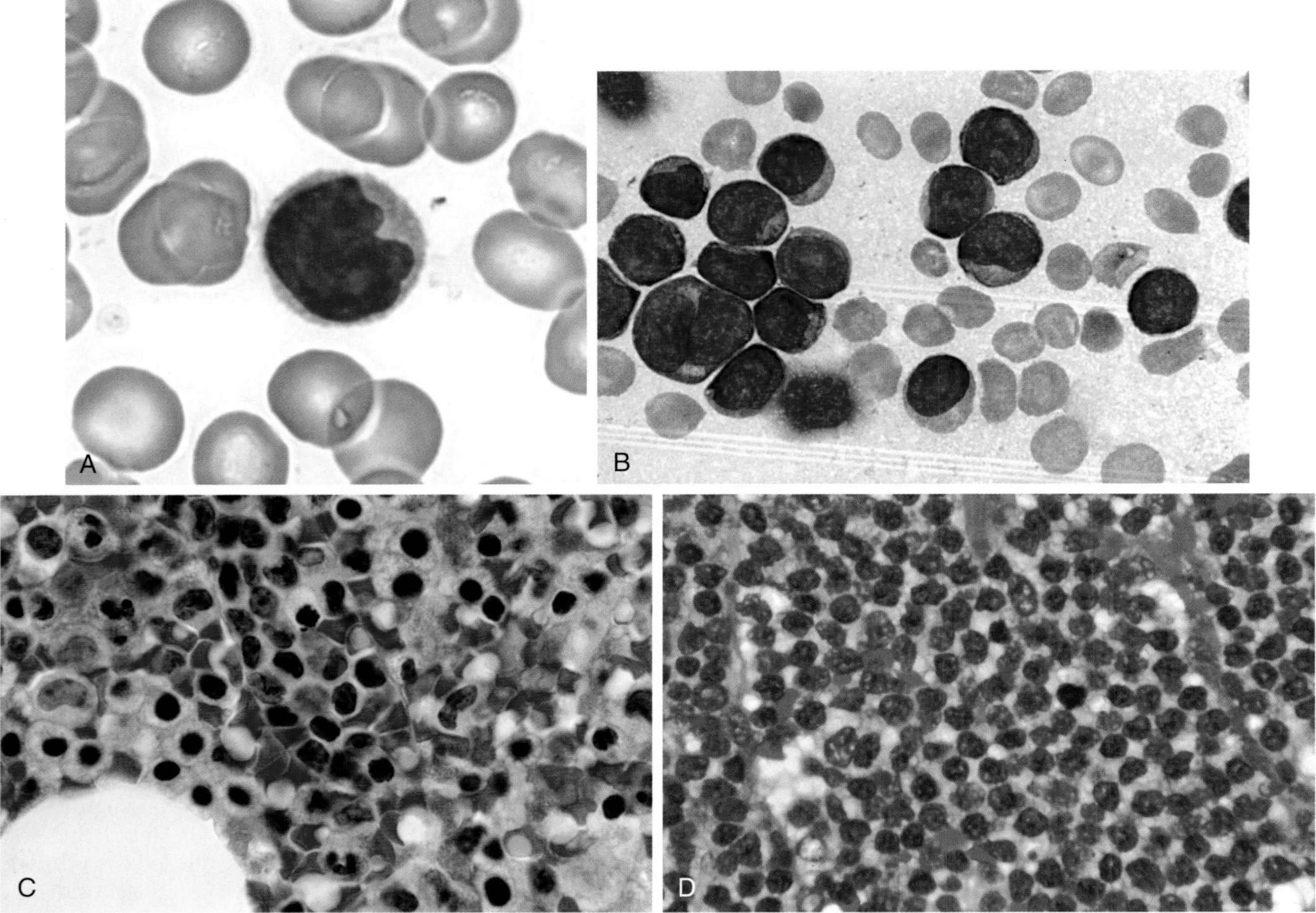

Figure 32-16. Differential diagnosis of adult T-cell leukemia/lymphoma (ATLL). A, Sézary cells show less nuclear hyperchromasia and more subtle nuclear changes. **B,** In T-cell prolymphocytic leukemia, lymphoid cells have round to oval nuclear contours and prominent nucleoli. **C,** The bone marrow is diffusely infiltrated, in contrast to ATLL, which typically shows minimal infiltration. **D,** T-cell prolymphocytic leukemia cells in the lymph node are round to slightly irregular, with central small nucleoli.

The differential diagnosis of chronic or smoldering ATLL is more diverse and includes mycosis fungoides and other cutaneous T-cell lymphomas, chronic dermatitis, and T-cell prolymphocytic leukemia. ATLL may show marked epidermotropism with Pautrier's microabscesses, mimicking mycosis fungoides. In distinction from mycosis fungoides, ATLL usually lacks an inflammatory background in the cutaneous lesions, with a higher density of neoplastic cells. Indeed, the first patient from which HTLV-1 was isolated was thought to have an aggressive form of mycosis fungoides.[1] In the peripheral blood, Sézary cells have less nuclear hyperchromasia and a cerebriform rather than a polylobated nuclear contour (Fig. 32-16). Further complicating the differential diagnosis was the suggestion in some studies that HTLV-1 sequences might be detected in the blood cells of some cases of otherwise typical cutaneous T-cell lymphomas.[90] Subsequent studies have largely ruled out a role for HTLV-1 in the pathogenesis of mycosis fungoides or Sézary syndrome.[91]

T-cell prolymphocytic leukemia can be $CD4^+$ or $CD8^+$, but CD25 is usually negative. CD7 is usually positive, in contrast to ATLL cells. The cells are typically round or slightly irregular and lack the pronounced nuclear irregularities of ATLL cells. In T-cell prolymphocytic leukemia, the bone marrow biopsy usually shows extensive infiltration, whereas ATLL usually shows less bone marrow involvement than expected, based on the degree of lymphocytosis. The bone marrow does not appear to be a site of proliferation for ATLL cells.

HTLV-2 is a retrovirus related to HTLV-1. It has not been clearly linked to any form of leukemia or lymphoma.[92] The molecular tests for HTLV-1 sequences also detect HTLV-2, so it may be necessary to rule out HTLV-2 infection in some cases. HTLV-2 has been found most often in intravenous drug users. Its clinical effects have been linked to a HAM/TSP clinical picture.

References can be found on Expert Consult @ www.expertconsult.com

Pearls and Pitfalls

- HTLV-1 seropositivity does not prove a diagnosis of ATLL. Patients from HTLV-1–endemic areas may have antibodies to HTLV-1.
- ATLL is associated with a broad cytologic spectrum. Most cytologic variants do not have clinical significance.
- The Hodgkin's-like form of ATLL may mimic classical Hodgkin's lymphoma. It represents an incipient form of ATLL in which HTLV-I–infected cells are sparse. Hodgkin's-like cells are Epstein-Barr virus–positive B cells.
- Smoldering and chronic forms of ATLL may resemble chronic dermatitis.

Chapter 33

Hepatosplenic T-Cell Lymphoma

Philippe Gaulard

CHAPTER OUTLINE

DEFINITION

Hepatosplenic T-cell lymphoma (HSTL) is an aggressive subtype of extranodal lymphoma characterized by a hepatosplenic presentation without lymphadenopathy and a poor outcome. The neoplasm results from a proliferation of nonactivated cytotoxic T cells, usually monomorphic and medium-sized, that exhibit a unique sinusoidal pattern of infiltration in the spleen, liver, and bone marrow. It is associated with a recurrent cytogenetic abnormality, the isochromosome 7q. Most cases are derived from the gamma-delta T-cell subset, and the gamma-delta T-cell phenotype has been part of the definition of the entity, which was initially named *hepatosplenic gamma-delta T-cell lymphoma* in the Revised European American Lymphoma (REAL) classification.[1] Recently, a few similar cases with an alpha-beta phenotype have been described, and the term *hepatosplenic T-cell lymphoma* is preferred in the current World Health Organization (WHO) classification.[2]

EPIDEMIOLOGY

HSTL is rare, with cases reported in both Western and Asian countries.[3-6] The disease represents less than 5% of all peripheral T-cell lymphomas. Its incidence might be underestimated, however, because the disease may mimic other conditions, and the diagnosis is sometimes difficult to establish. There is also difficulty in assessing the gamma-delta T-cell origin on routine specimens. HSTL is characterized by a male predominance and occurs in young adults, with a median age around 35 years.[3-7] Cases of HSTL in adolescents or children have been reported,[8-15] but it is relatively rare in older individuals.

ETIOLOGY

A number of cases have been reported in patients with immunologic manifestations or with a previous history of immune deficit, especially in patients receiving long-term immunosuppressive therapy for solid organ transplantation.[4,16,20,21a] In this context, HSTL is regarded as a late-onset posttransplantation lymphoproliferative disorder of host origin.[20] Occasional cases have been observed following acute myeloid leukemia or Epstein-Barr virus (EBV)–positive lymphoproliferative disorders, in patients with falciparum malaria,[4,21,22] or during pregnancy.[23] A few cases have been recently reported in patients with Crohn's disease treated with azathioprine.[24] The use of the anti–tumor necrosis factor agent infliximab along with azathioprine may increase the risk of HSTL in patients with inflammatory bowel disease, especially children.[25,26] From these observations and in view of the functional properties of normal gamma-delta T cells, it has been postulated that chronic antigen stimulation in the setting of an underlying immune defect might play a role in the pathogenesis of the disease. As an example, expansion of gamma-delta T cells is observed in the peripheral blood of renal allograft recipients,[27] and in vitro studies have shown that human gamma-delta T cells display an alloreactive response to various leukocyte antigen molecules.[28]

To date, no association with human T-lymphotropic virus 1 or 2, human immunodeficiency virus, human herpesvirus

8, or hepatitis C virus has been reported. One case has been reported in a patient positive for human herpesvirus 6.[29] The vast majority of cases do not show EBV association, with the exception of rare cases with cytologic features of transformation.[4,30,31]

CLINICAL FEATURES

The disease occurs mainly in young adults presenting with marked splenomegaly and most often hepatomegaly, but without lymphadenopathy. Most patients have B symptoms, including fatigue, fever, and weight loss, associated with abdominal pain, probably secondary to marked splenomegaly.[3-5,32,33]

Thrombocytopenia is almost always present and is associated with anemia or leukopenia in about half of patients. A few cases have been reported in which features of idiopathic thrombocytopenic purpura[3,34] or Coombs-negative hemolytic anemia[9] were the first symptoms of HSTL. An overt leukemic picture is rare at presentation, and lymphocytosis is uncommon. However, with careful examination of blood smears, a minor population of atypical lymphoid cells can be identified in some patients.[4,35] An association with hemophagocytic syndrome has occasionally been reported.[4,14,31] Abnormal liver function tests are an inconstant finding at presentation.

Computed tomography shows an absence of mediastinal and retroperitoneal lymphadenopathy. In my experience, owing to bone marrow involvement (see later), all patients have Ann Arbor stage IV disease. They also frequently have elevated serum lactate dehydrogenase levels and a performance status greater than 1. As a consequence, the majority of patients present with two to three adverse risk factors of the age-adjusted International Prognostic Index and fall into its high-risk group.[4]

MORPHOLOGY

Macroscopy

The spleen is enlarged (commonly weighing 1000 to 3500 g), with a homogeneous pattern and no gross lesions identifiable. The cut surface is homogeneous red-purple. Hilar lymph nodes are not enlarged.

Histology

The diagnosis of HSTL is based on histopathologic and immunohistochemical findings. In the past, the diagnosis was often made by examination of the spleen or liver biopsy, obtained at the time of splenectomy; less often the diagnosis was made by bone marrow biopsy. Because the histologic features in the bone marrow are now recognized as highly characteristic, bone marrow biopsy is the recommended diagnostic strategy, thus avoiding splenectomy for diagnosis. In addition, to establish expression of the gamma-delta T-cell receptor (TCRγδ), flow cytometry on bone marrow cell suspensions is advised. Alternatively, snap frozen material can be studied by immunohistochemistry. The neoplastic cells are monomorphic and medium-sized and located preferentially in the sinusoids of the liver, cords and sinuses of the splenic red pulp, and sinuses of the bone marrow.

Spleen

In the spleen the pattern of involvement is characterized by diffuse red pulp infiltration and preservation of the sinus and pulp cord architecture, whereas there is marked reduction or complete loss of the white pulp (Fig. 33-1A). The red pulp contains a more or less dense infiltration consisting of usually monomorphic, medium-sized lymphoid cells with round to oval or slightly irregular nuclei, slightly dispersed chromatin,

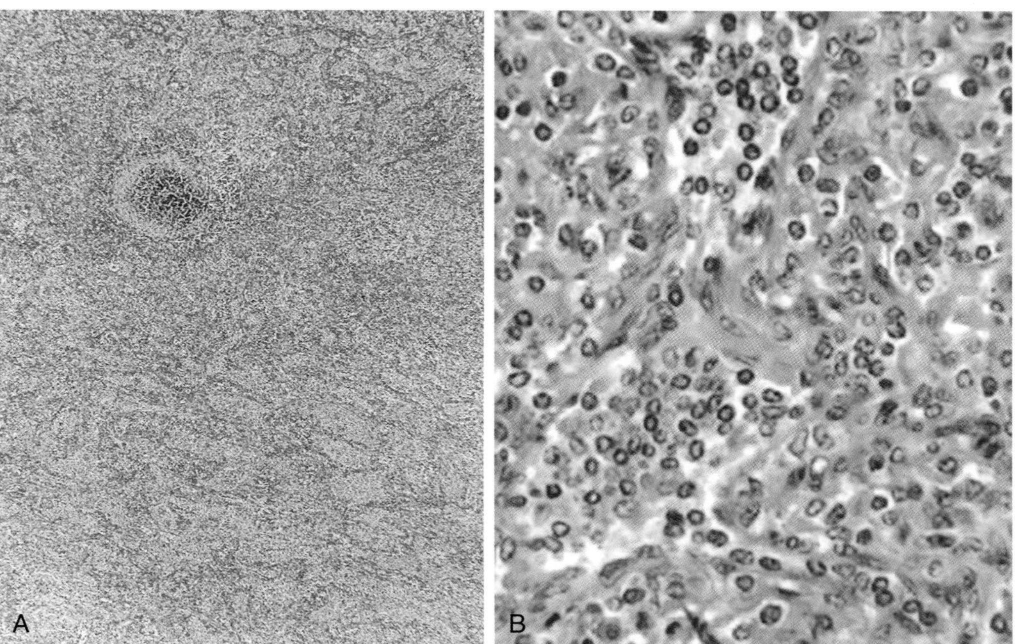

Figure 33-1. Histopathology of the spleen. A, At low magnification, the red pulp is expanded, whereas only a few atrophic nodules of white pulp are observed. **B,** At high magnification, note infiltration of the cords and sinuses by neoplastic medium-sized lymphoid cells.

and inconspicuous nucleoli. The cytoplasm is pale and seldom exhibits azurophilic granules on smears or imprints. Mitotic figures are rare. Pleomorphism is very limited within a single case. The atypical cells are present within the cords and, to a variable extent from case to case, within the sinuses of the red pulp (see Fig. 33-1B). Dilated sinuses filled with sheets of neoplastic cells can be observed. A few small lymphocytes may be admixed, but plasma cells are rare. Histiocytes may be numerous. Rare cases show features of hemophagocytosis at presentation or during the course of the disease.

Hilar Lymph Nodes

Although usually not significantly enlarged, hilar lymph nodes commonly show some involvement confined to the sinuses or perisinusoidal areas, without destruction of the normal lymph node architecture.[4,32,36]

Liver

Histologic involvement of the liver is quite constant. It results in hepatomegaly without nodules in more than half of patients at presentation. Liver infiltration shows a sinusoidal pattern in all cases (Fig. 33-2), which can lead to pseudopeliotic lesions.[37] A mild portal and periportal lymphomatous infiltrate may be observed, but it is not conspicuous.

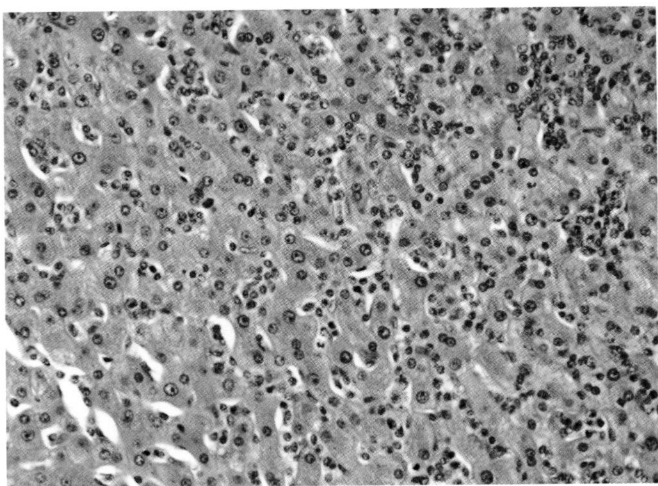

Figure 33-2. Histopathology of the liver. The neoplastic infiltrate is observed predominantly in the sinusoids.

Bone Marrow

According to the literature, bone marrow involvement is reported in about two thirds of patients. In fact, bone marrow involvement is nearly always present when trephine biopsies are carefully investigated by combined histologic and immunohistochemical studies.[4,35,38,39] Neoplastic cells selectively infiltrate and expand the bone marrow sinuses, a feature that is highly characteristic and thus a useful diagnostic criterion. The initial diagnostic bone marrow biopsy specimens are usually hypercellular, with trilineage hyperplasia, and may be misdiagnosed as myelodysplastic or myeloproliferative syndrome. The marrow lymphoma infiltration is discrete, often subtle, and may be difficult to recognize in routine hematoxylin-eosin–stained sections; immunohistochemistry is often required for its demonstration. There is an exclusively or predominantly sinusoidal infiltrate composed of atypical small to medium-sized lymphoid cells forming indian files or aggregates within more or less dilated sinuses, a pattern that is strongly highlighted by CD3 immunostaining (Fig. 33-3).[4,32,35,38,39] Together with the typical sinusoidal distribution in the bone marrow, the demonstration of a $CD3^+$, $CD5^-$, TIA1+ phenotype is characteristic of, if not specific for, HSTL.

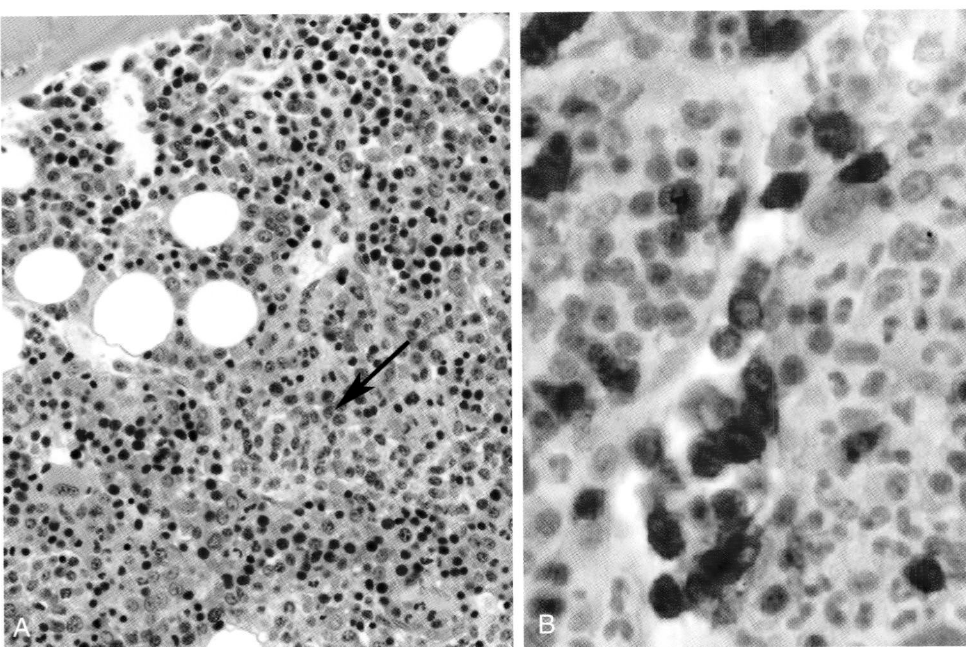

Figure 33-3. Histopathology of the bone marrow. A, The marrow is hypercellular. The *arrow* indicates the sinusoidal infiltrate composed of medium-sized lymphocytes. **B,** CD3 staining strongly highlights the sinusoidal infiltration.

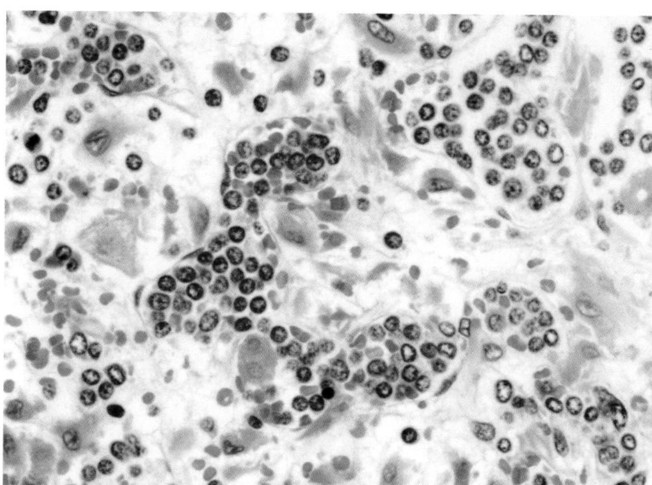

Figure 33-4. With disease progression, bone marrow involvement is more intense, and the neoplastic cells are larger, with blast-like features. Note the presence of a few histiocytes with erythrophagocytosis.

Additionally, careful examination of aspirate smears may identify a minor population of atypical lymphoid cells, which are sometimes described as blast-like cells and in some instances may contain fine cytoplasmic granules. Examination of bone marrow aspirates by flow cytometry enables the characterization of the gamma-delta origin of the neoplastic cells in most cases.

Cytologic Variants

Overall, the cytologic appearance at presentation shows little variation from patient to patient. Neoplastic cells are usually monomorphic small to medium-sized lymphocytes. Cytologic variation (e.g., more blastic or pleomorphic medium to large cells) has occasionally been observed at diagnosis but more often occurs with disease progression.[4,17,40,41] Histologic variants manifest a similar tissue distribution. However, during late stages of the disease, the pattern of bone marrow involvement has a tendency to become more extensive, diffuse, and interstitial, with expansion beyond the sinuses; in addition, the neoplastic cells become larger (Fig. 33-4).

IMMUNOPHENOTYPE

On paraffin sections, all cases disclose a $CD3^+$ T-cell phenotype, negative for B-cell–associated markers. The general pattern of expression of T-cell antigens is $CD3^+$, $CD2^+$, $CD5^-$, $CD7^{+/-}$, and $CD4^-/CD8^-$ or, more rarely, $CD4^-/CD8^+$ (Fig. 33-5). Most cases exhibit the CD56 natural killer (NK) cell–associated marker but are $CD57^-$. They may express CD16. All cases have a cytotoxic phenotype (see Fig. 33-5), as shown by the presence of granular cytoplasmic TIA-1 staining; this is usually of the nonactivated type, because the great majority of cases do not express the other cytotoxic molecules granzyme B and perforin.[32,42] Cytotoxic activity has been demonstrated in a few cases.[21] HSTL is negative for CD25 and CD30 activation antigens. Expression of killer immunoglobulin-like receptors (KIRs) and, to a lesser degree, CD94/NKG2A seems to be a common feature (see later).[43,44] On frozen sections, the majority of cases express TCRγδ, as shown by a $\beta F1^-/TCR\delta\text{-}1^+$ phenotype. Most, but not all, HSTLs of the gamma-delta type seem to derive from the subset of gamma-delta T cells having rearranged the *Vδ1* gene, as revealed by molecular studies and positive staining with the δTCS-1 antibody.[4,45-48] Gamma-delta HSTL expresses the serine protease granzyme M, a finding consistent with a derivation from lymphocytes involved in innate immunity.[49]

Recently, cases of HSTL with a TCRαβ phenotype ($\beta F1^+/TCR\delta\text{-}1^-$) have been reported.[9,39,50,51] On the basis of similar clinicopathologic and cytogenetic features, they are considered a variant of the more common gamma-delta form of the disease.[2] However, in view of the recent observation that the gamma-delta phenotype is an adverse prognostic factor in cutaneous T-cell lymphomas,[52,53] further studies are needed to determine whether alpha-beta and gamma-delta HSTLs should be regarded as separate subtypes in the future.

It is noteworthy that determination of the alpha-beta or gamma-delta T-cell origin may be difficult to establish in a number of cases because the expression of TCRγδ cannot be reliably investigated using monoclonal antibodies in routinely fixed, paraffin-embedded tissues. In routine practice, when frozen samples are not available, flow cytometric analysis of marrow aspirate smears is highly recommended.

GENETICS AND MOLECULAR FINDINGS

Molecular Studies

Irrespective of their gamma-delta or alpha-beta phenotype, HSTLs show a clonal rearrangement of the TCRγ gene, as demonstrated by polymerase chain reaction studies used in routine practice. Southern blot or polymerase chain reaction studies have demonstrated a rearrangement, usually biallelic, of the TCRδ chain,[4,46,48] in accordance with a genotype of gamma-delta T cells. Unproductive rearrangements of the beta chain have been reported in some HSTLs of gamma-delta T-cell origin, following the same observation in normal gamma-delta T cells.[46,47] In addition to the clonal rearrangement of the gamma chain, alpha-beta cases disclose a clonal rearrangement of the TCRβ chain genes.[9,51]

Recently, the gene expression profile of four cases of HSTL, including three with a gamma-delta phenotype, was reported. The HSTL signature was distinct from that of other T-cell lymphomas and was characterized by an overexpression of genes encoding KIR molecules.[54]

Cytogenetics

In conventional cytogenetic and fluorescence in situ hybridization studies published in more than 40 cases,[55] most gamma-delta HSTLs have been characterized by the presence of an isochromosome 7q (i[7][q10]) (Fig. 33-6).[10,11,14,17,33,44,55-59] This has occasionally been the sole karyotypic abnormality, suggesting that it plays a primary role in disease pathogenesis. In addition to trisomy 8 and loss of chromosome Y, an increased number of 7q signals has been found in progressive cases, indicating that the i(7)(q10) chromosome tends to multiply during evolution of the disease.[55] Recently, a ring chromosome 7 with amplification of a 7q31 sequence was reported.[11] Interestingly, i(7)(q10) has also been found in

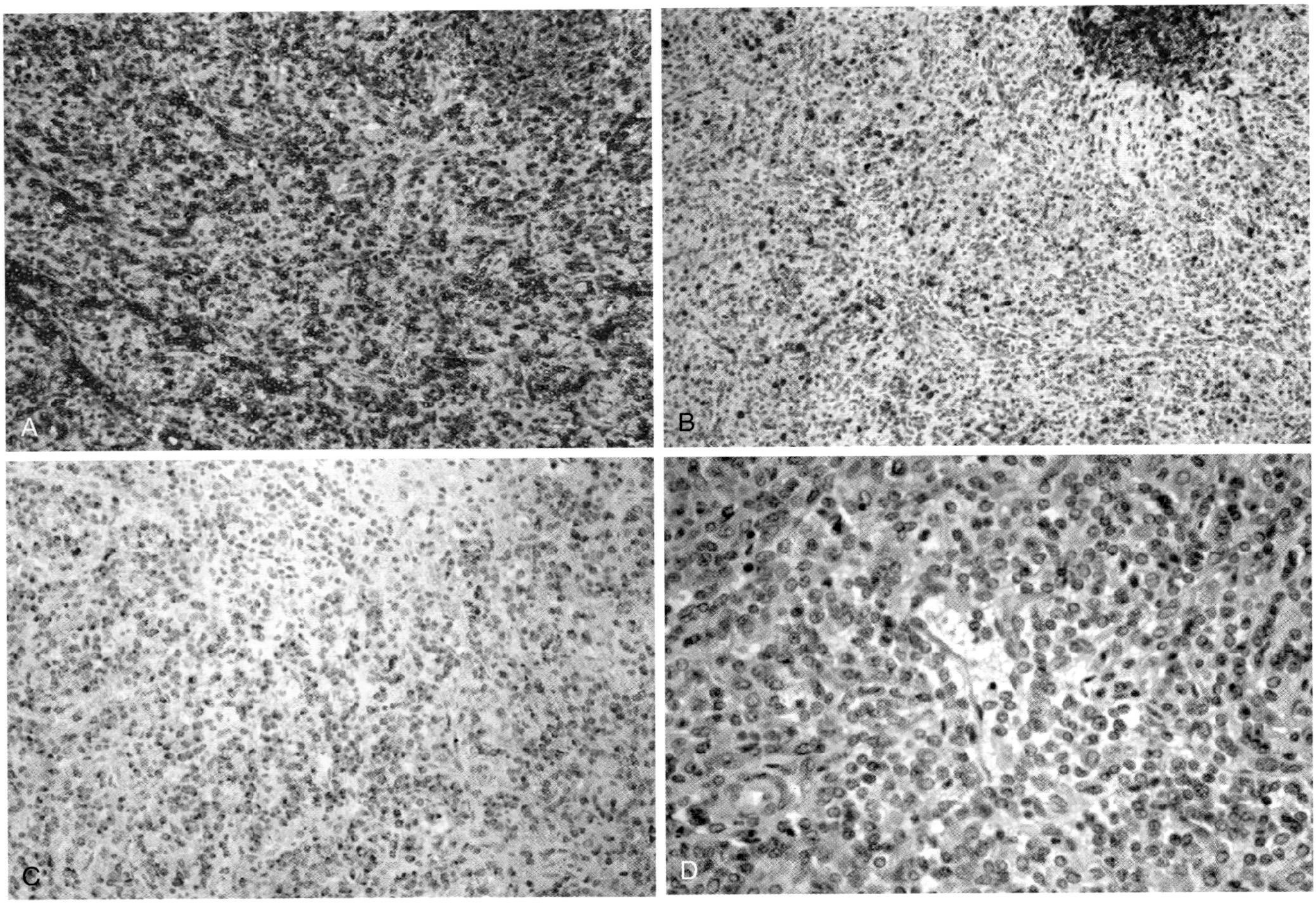

Figure 33-5. The characteristic immunophenotypic profile of hepatosplenic T-cell lymphoma is CD3+ (**A**), CD5− (**B**), with only scattered reactive CD5+ lymphocytes. Neoplastic cells have a nonactivated cytotoxic profile, with expression of TIA-1 (**C**) without granzyme B (**D**).

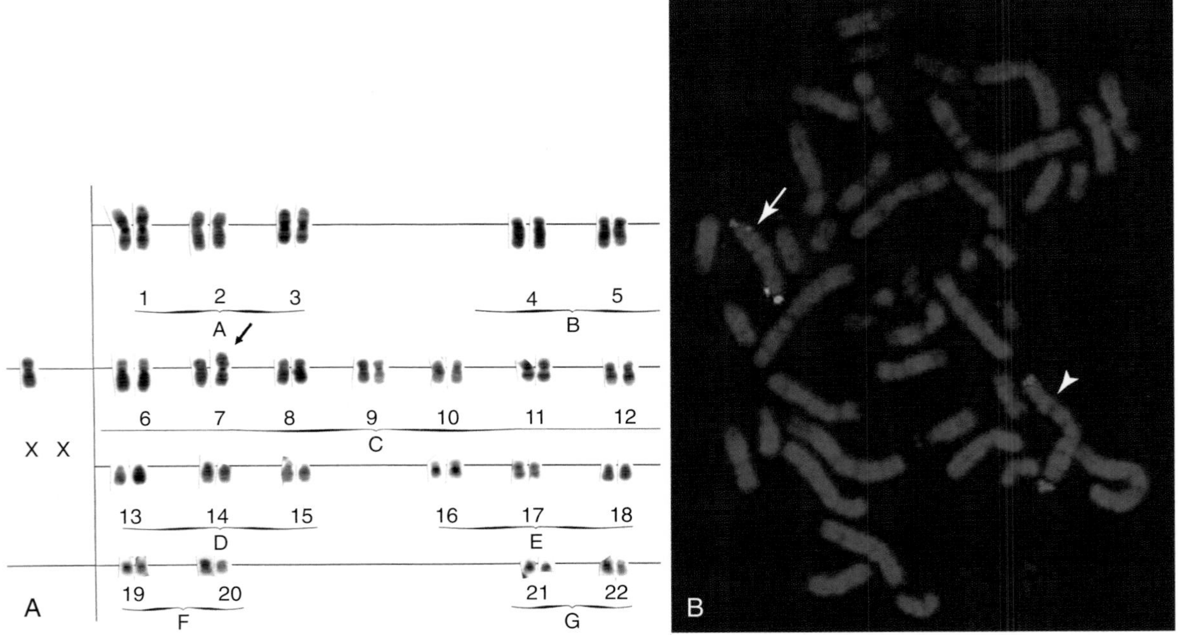

Figure 33-6. **Cytogenetics of gamma-delta hepatosplenic T-cell lymphoma. A,** Representative karyotype with isochromosome 7q (i[7][q10]) indicated by the *arrow*. **B,** Example of abnormal metaphase with i(7)(q10) after fluorescence in situ hybridization subtelomeric probes for 7p (*green*) and 7q (*red*). The *arrow* and *arrowhead* show normal chromosome 7 and i(7)(q10), respectively. Note i(7)(q10)-associated loss of the 7p signal and gain of the 7q signal. (Courtesy of Dr. Iwona Wlodarska, University of Leuven, Belgium.)

Chapter 34

Peripheral T-Cell Lymphoma, Not Otherwise Specified

Laurence de Leval, Elisabeth Ralfkiaer, and Elaine S. Jaffe

CHAPTER OUTLINE

DEFINITION

The category of peripheral T-cell lymphoma, unspecified, introduced in the Revised European American Lymphoma (REAL) classification in 1994,[1] was maintained in the 2001 World Health Organization (WHO) classification.[2] In the 2008 WHO monograph, this category is designated *peripheral T-cell lymphoma, not otherwise specified* (PTCL, NOS), an appellation reflecting the expectation of better specification or subdivision in the future.[3] It encompasses all mature T-cell neoplasms lacking specific features that would allow their categorization in any of the better-defined subtypes of post-thymic T-cell lymphoma/leukemia described in the WHO classification.[3] Hence, other categories of T-cell lymphoma must be excluded before a diagnosis of PTCL, NOS is established. It is recognized that this group is unlikely to constitute only one entity. However, reliable criteria for the distinction of specific clinicopathologic diseases within this broad group of neoplasms are not yet available.

EPIDEMIOLOGY AND ETIOLOGY

These tumors are rare overall but represent the most common PTCL category in North America and Europe, where they account for one third to one half of PTCLs. Conversely, they are relatively less common in Asia, where other PTCL subtypes (human T-lymphotropic virus 1–associated and Epstein-Barr virus [EBV]–associated natural killer [NK]/T-cell neoplasms) are more prevalent.[4-6]

The disease tends to affect older adults (median age, 60 years), but children can also be affected. There is a slight male predominance in most published series.[5,6]

The cause of the disease (or, more likely, diseases) is unknown. In a minority of cases, associations with other clinical conditions have been reported. For example, patients with the lymphoproliferative variant of the hypereosinophilic syndrome, a condition associated with a clonal proliferation of interleukin-5–producing T cells, carry an increased risk of developing T-cell lymphomas.[7,8] A subset of individuals with B-cell chronic lymphocytic leukemia harbor clonal populations of circulating T cells with a large lymphocytic granular morphology, which might be precursors to the development of cytotoxic T-cell lymphomas in rare patients.[9]

CLINICAL FEATURES

Most patients present with nodal involvement, but any site may be affected. A combination of nodal and extranodal involvement in one or several sites is frequently encountered. A majority of patients have advanced disease, with infiltrates

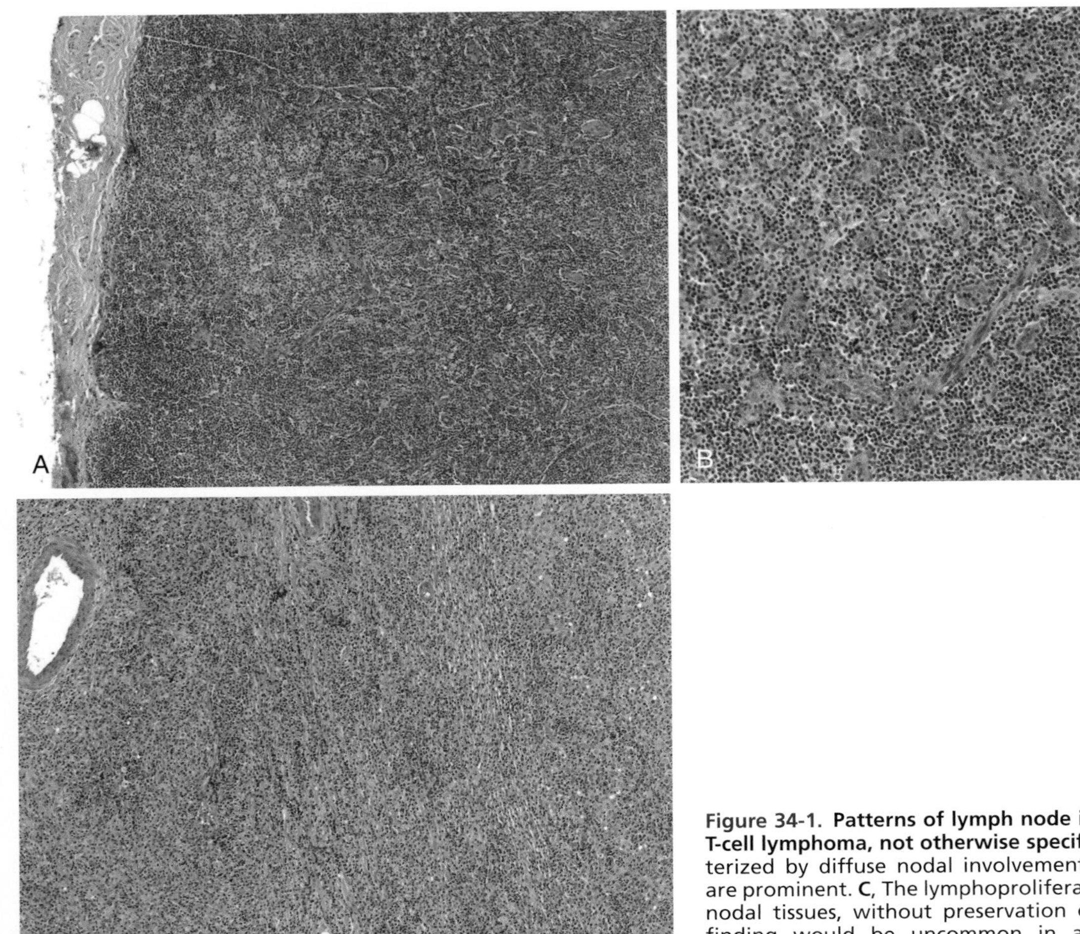

Figure 34-1. Patterns of lymph node involvement in peripheral T-cell lymphoma, not otherwise specified. A, This case is characterized by diffuse nodal involvement. **B,** Postcapillary venules are prominent. **C,** The lymphoproliferation extends into the perinodal tissues, without preservation of the cortical sinus. This finding would be uncommon in angioimmunoblastic T-cell lymphoma.

in the bone marrow, liver, spleen, and extranodal tissues, frequently including the skin.

Constitutional symptoms, poor performance status, and elevated lactate dehydrogenase levels are reported in 40% to 60% of cases, and about half of patients have an intermediate to high-risk International Prognostic Index (IPI). Blood eosinophilia, anemia, and thrombopenia are present at the time of diagnosis in a minority of patients. The occurrence of a hemophagocytic syndrome, often associated with a rapidly fatal course, has been reported in a few cases.[4,5,10-12]

MORPHOLOGY

Lymph Nodes

The morphologic spectrum of PTCL, NOS is extremely broad. Most commonly, the pattern of lymph node involvement is diffuse, but some cases present with an interfollicular or paracortical infiltrate (Fig. 34-1). The cytology is typically pleomorphic (variable tumor cell morphology), with most cases containing a mixed population of small and large cells (Fig. 34-2). Many cases consist predominantly of medium-sized or large cells with irregular nuclei, prominent nucleoli, and many mitotic figures.[1,13,14] Other cases—small pleomorphic T-cell lymphomas—have a predominance of atypical small cells with irregular nuclei. Irregular nuclear contours may provide a helpful hint to the neoplastic nature of infiltrates composed of predominantly small cells. In some cases there may be cells with clear cytoplasm, and Hodgkin–Reed-Sternberg (HRS)–like cells may be present. High endothelial venules are usually increased, and arborizing vessels are often abundant. Many cases have a polymorphic cellular composition, with an admixture of reactive cells, including small lymphocytes, eosinophils, histiocytes, B cells, and plasma cells. With relapse, tumors tend to retain similar morphologic features and patterns of nodal involvement, but some cases are characterized by histologic progression, with increased numbers of large cells.[15]

Bone Marrow and Extranodal Involvement

Bone marrow involvement by PTCL, NOS can be diffuse, usually with hypercellularity and extensive replacement of the normal hematopoietic tissue; alternatively, bone marrow involvement may be focal, usually in a nonparatrabecular localization. As in the lymph nodes, there is a broad cytomorphologic spectrum; the infiltrates are often pleomorphic and associated with prominent vascularity, increased reticulin fibrosis, and an admixed reactive inflammatory infiltrate.[16]

Splenic infiltrates may take the form of single or multiple discrete lesions, a micronodular pattern, or diffuse parenchymal involvement of the red and white pulps. Localization to

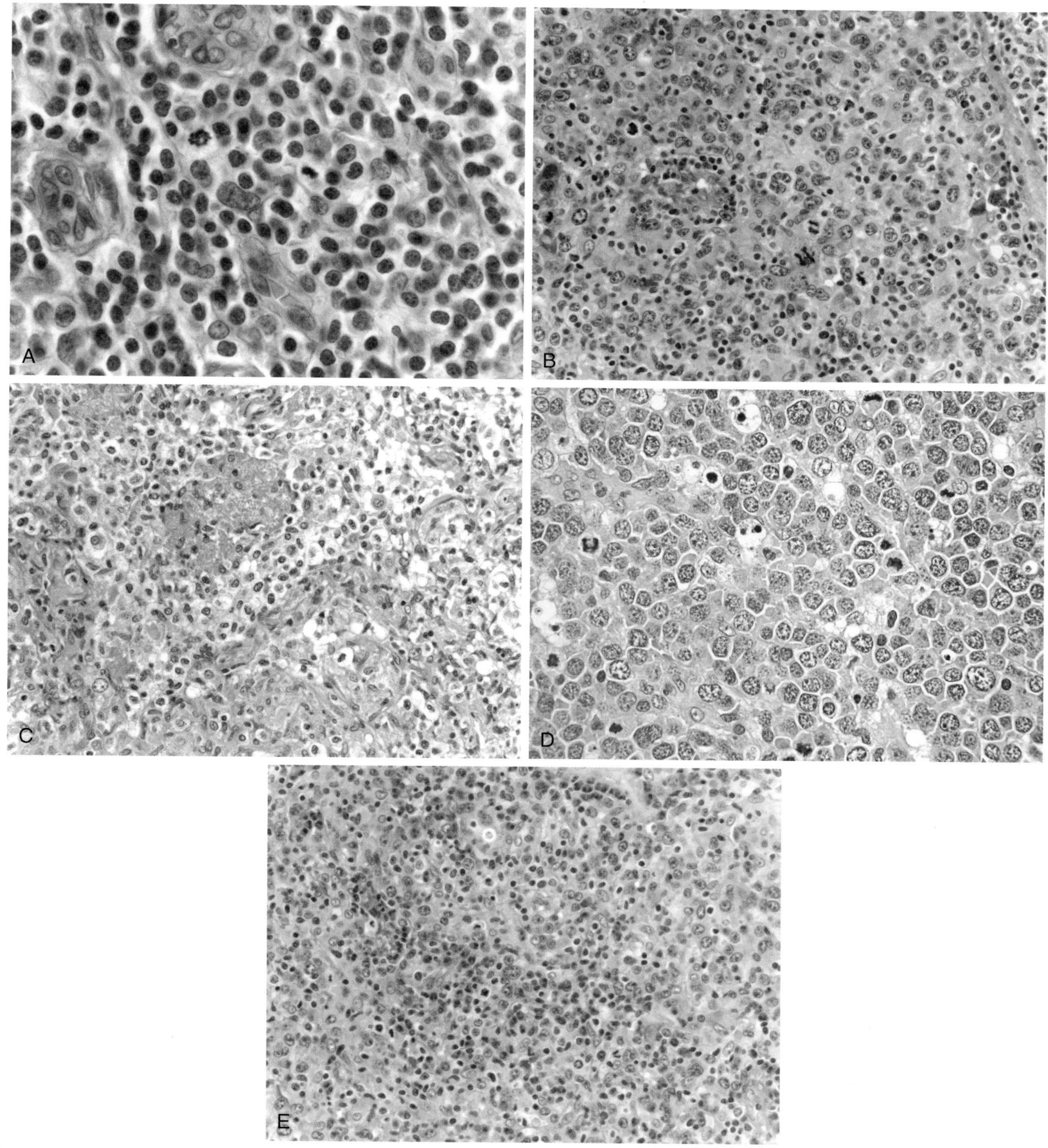

Figure 34-2. Cytologic spectrum of peripheral T-cell lymphoma, not otherwise specified (PTCL, NOS). A, PTCL, NOS composed predominantly of small cells, with scattered large transformed cells; note the presence of mitotic figures and nuclear irregularities. **B**, PTCL, NOS composed of pleomorphic medium to large cells and occasional Reed-Sternberg–like cells. **C**, PTCL, NOS involving the lung and composed of a dominant population of cells with clear cytoplasm. **D**, PTCL, NOS, monomorphic large cell type. **E**, Tissue eosinophilia is a common feature that may be prominent, as in this case.

Continued

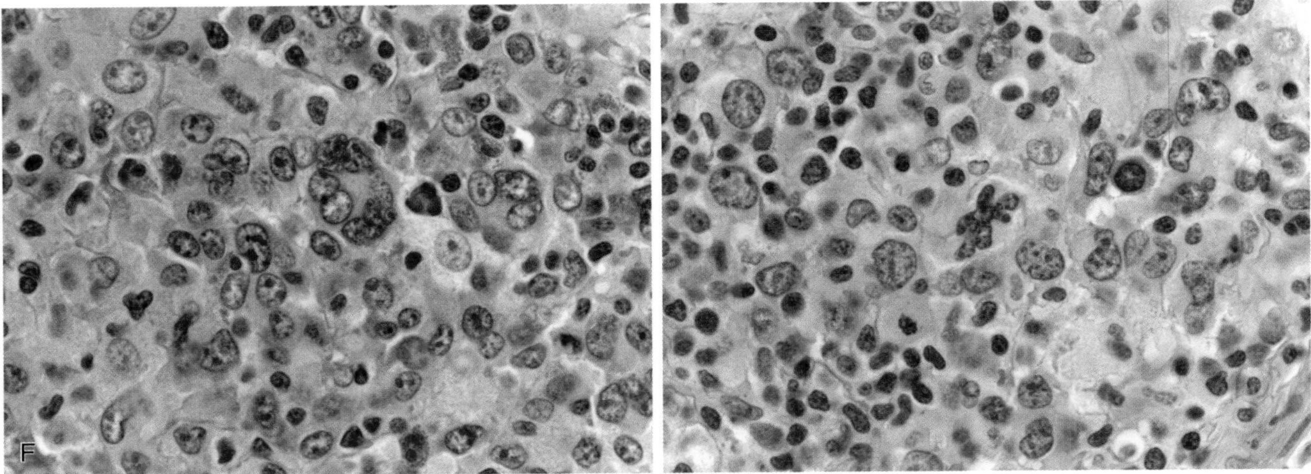

Figure 34-2, cont'd F, PTCL, NOS with giant Reed-Sternberg–like cells (*left*) and cells with markedly irregular nuclei (*right*).

T-cell–dependent regions, such as the periarteriolar lymphoid sheath or marginal zone, may be seen.

PTCL, NOS may manifest primarily in the skin, and cutaneous involvement is frequent in cases of systemic PTCL, NOS. Several provisional categories of primary cutaneous T-cell lymphoma are discussed in Chapter 40. The pattern of cutaneous infiltration is variable and may be diffuse, nodular, or band-like, and angiocentricity can be seen (Fig. 34-3).[17] Although epidermotropism is a more specific feature of mycosis fungoides and Sézary syndrome, it can be encountered in other forms as well.

GRADING

Some have proposed stratifying PTCL, NOS into prognostic categories according to morphology and size of the predominant neoplastic cellular population. In that scheme, small cell tumors were categorized as low grade, and mixed medium and large cell tumors and large cell tumors were deemed high grade.[14] However, most PTCLs, NOS follow an aggressive course, irrespective of histologic and cytologic features; therefore, grading of these tumors is not generally recommended or required.[3,12]

DIAGNOSTIC PITFALLS: VARIANTS

Three morphologic variants are recognized in the 2008 WHO classification. Two of them—the lymphoepithelioid and T-zone variants—were described as separate diseases at the time of the Kiel classification,[14] whereas the follicular variant has been recognized only recently.[18] These variants are rare and account for less than 5% of PTCLs in unselected series.[5,19] Identification of their specific features and their delineation from other cases of PTCL, NOS may be subtle, and distinction among them may be difficult.[20] Moreover, the feasibility of morphologic subclassification is hampered by inter- and intraobserver variability, and its prognostic significance and clinical relevance are not clear.[14,19-24] Nevertheless, it is useful for the pathologist to be familiar with these variants because they may be confused with other subtypes of lymphoma and with reactive processes.

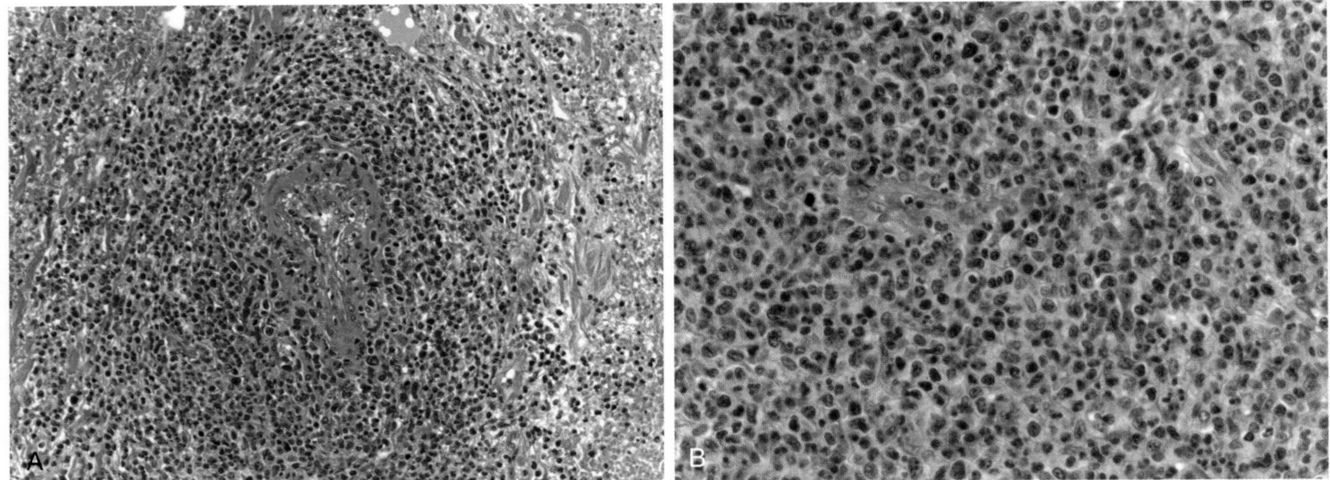

Figure 34-3. Peripheral T-cell lymphoma, not otherwise specified, involving the skin. A, The lymphoma cells show marked angiocentricity. **B**, This lymphoma, composed of medium to large cells, contains a prominent reactive infiltrate of eosinophils and scattered plasma cells.

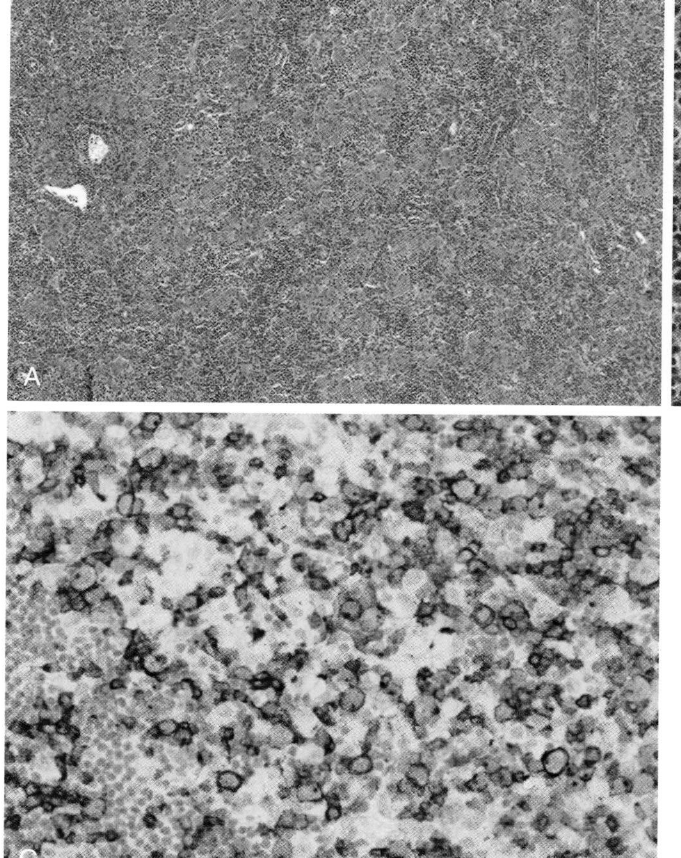

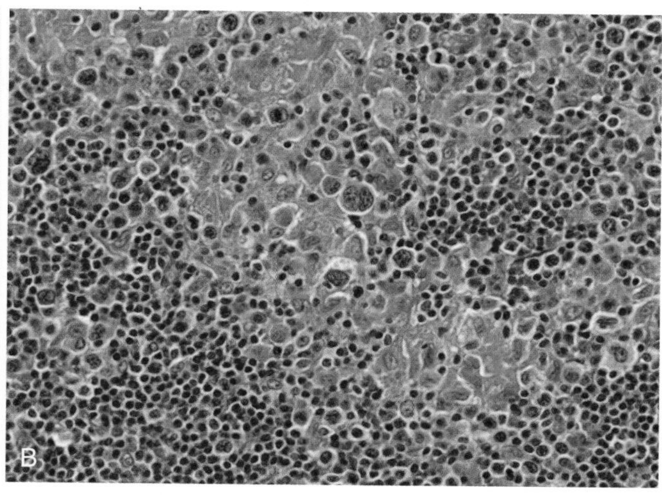

Figure 34-4. **Lymphoepithelioid variant of peripheral T-cell lymphoma, not otherwise specified (Lennert's lymphoma). A,** Diffuse nodal involvement by an infiltrate composed predominantly of pink epithelioid histiocytes, with a vaguely nodular or granulomatous appearance. **B,** The majority of lymphoma cells are small. A few are larger, sometimes with a Reed-Sternberg–like morphology. **C,** CD2 immunostaining highlights the small and large cells.

Lymphoepithelioid Variant (Lennert's Lymphoma)

The lymphoepithelioid variant, originally described by Lennert in 1952 as a variant of Hodgkin's disease (hence the eponym Lennert's lymphoma), is characterized by a prominent reactive infiltrate of epithelioid histiocytes distributed singly or, more typically, in small clusters (Fig. 34-4).[25] Most histiocytes are mononucleate, but multinucleate forms are occasionally seen. These cells may be so abundant that they obscure the neoplastic cells, which are small, atypical T cells with only slight nuclear irregularities.[14] The infiltrate is diffuse but may be interfollicular. In addition to the small atypical cells, some medium-sized or large cells are present, and some clear cells may be seen. HRS-like cells, eosinophils, and plasma cells are commonly seen as well.[26] Compared with other PTCLs, NOS, the lymphoepithelioid variant tends to remain confined to lymph nodes, with infrequent extranodal involvement,[27] and it may be associated with an overall better prognosis.

T-Zone Variant

T-zone lymphoma is characterized by a preserved architecture with residual, sometimes hyperplastic B-cell follicles and interfollicular lymphomatous involvement (Fig. 34-5).[14] The neoplastic infiltrate is composed of small to medium-sized T cells with only slight atypia, admixed with various reactive cells (eosinophils, plasma cells, histiocytes). Clear cells and occasional blastic cells may be seen. Distinction of this disease from a reactive lesion can be very difficult and usually requires investigation of the T-cell receptor (TCR) genes. Identification of an aberrant phenotype with antigen loss can be a helpful clue to the diagnosis.

Follicular Variant

This peculiar form of PTCL, NOS refers to a pattern of growth intimately related to follicular structures. The original description was of cases with a truly follicular pattern, mimicking follicular lymphoma.[18] The cytology is variable; some cases contain medium-sized cells with abundant clear cytoplasm, whereas others consist of cells resembling centrocytes and centroblasts (Fig. 34-6). The follicular variant also includes cases of T-cell lymphoma with a nodular paracortical or perifollicular growth pattern, similar to marginal zone lymphomas,[28-30] and T-cell neoplasms manifesting as cellular aggregates within expanded mantle zones.[31]

IMMUNOPHENOTYPE

Pan–T-cell–associated antigens (CD3, CD2, CD5, CD7) are positive, but aberrant T-cell phenotypes that lack one or several of these markers (most commonly CD5 or CD7) are

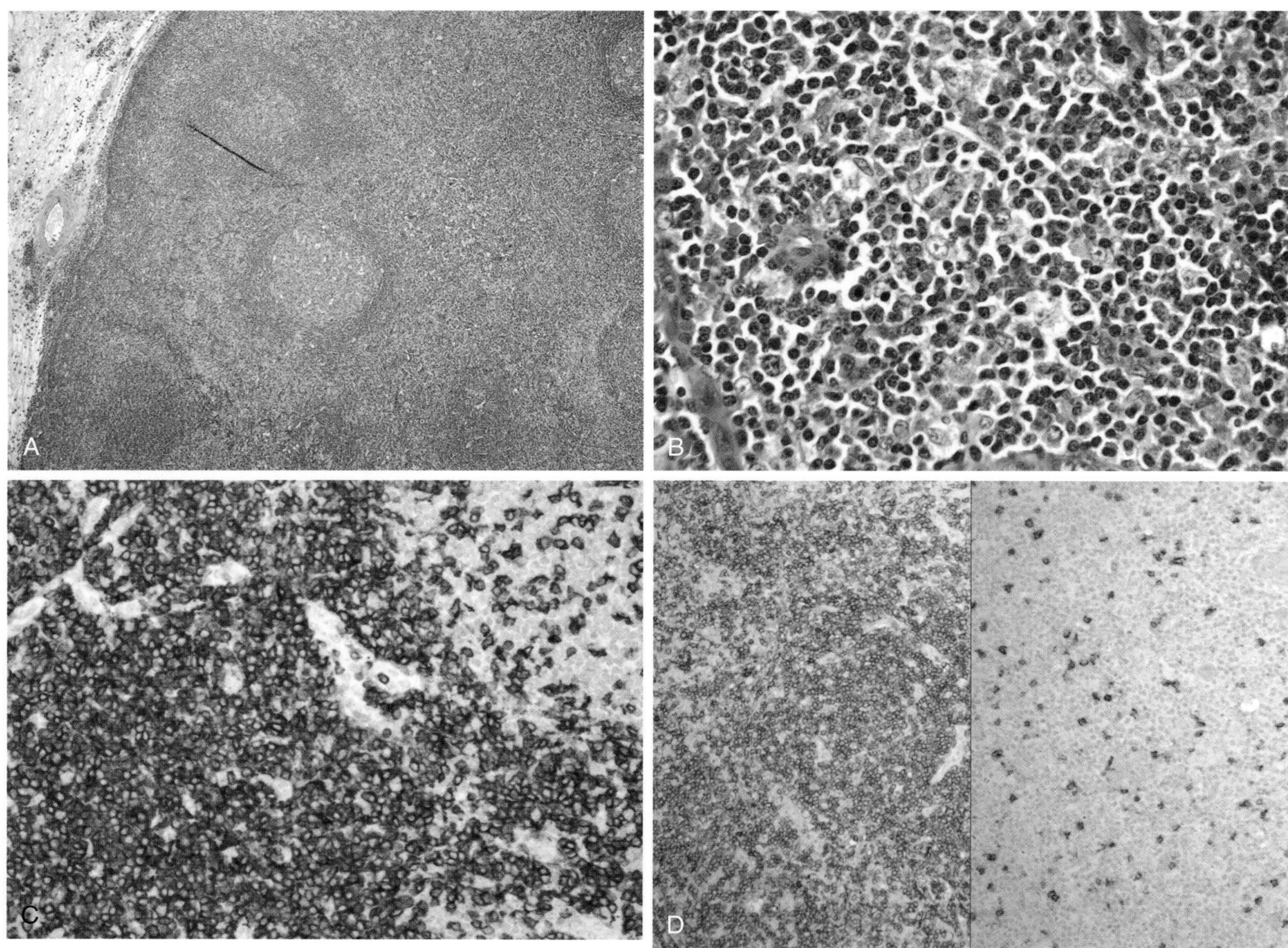

Figure 34-5. T-zone variant of peripheral T-cell lymphoma, not otherwise specified. A, Atypical lymphoid cells infiltrate the paracortex, with sparing of follicles. **B,** The majority of the lymphoid cells are small, with slight nuclear atypia. **C,** CD3 highlights nuclear irregularity in the lymphoid cells. **D,** The lymphoid cells are $CD4^+$ (*left*), with only infrequent admixed $CD8^+$ lymphocytes (*right*).

typically encountered (Fig. 34-7).[32,33] In more than 85% of cases, the neoplastic cells express TCRαβ ($TCR\beta F1^+$ by immunohistochemistry on paraffin sections), and a minority of cases are either of gamma-delta derivation ($TCR\delta F1^+$ by frozen section immunohistochemistry) or negative for both (TCR silent).[33-35] Most cases are single-positive $CD4^+$ or, less often, $CD8^+$ T cells, but a significant proportion of tumors are double negative or, more rarely, positive for both antigens.[32,33,36] Whether the expression of CD4 or CD8 is associated with any prognostic impact is unclear, but it has been suggested that $CD4^+$ cases tend to be associated with a better outcome, and a double-negative immunophenotype might be associated with an unfavorable prognosis.[33,36]

A subset of PTCLs, NOS has a cytotoxic immunophenotype. T-cell intracellular antigen-1 (TIA-1), a marker of cytotoxic T cells irrespective of their activation status, is detected in 30% to 40% of PTCLs, NOS; however, the expression of additional molecules (perforin and granzyme B), indicative of an activated cytotoxic phenotype, is usually less frequent or tends to be restricted to a smaller proportion of the tumor cells.[33,36-39] Expression of cytotoxic molecules tends to correlate with a $CD8^+$ phenotype.[36,39] In particular, most cases of lymphoepithelioid lymphoma appear to be derived from $CD8^+$ cytotoxic T cells.[26,36,38] Cytotoxic PTCLs, NOS are generally associated with several clinical features indicative of a poor prognosis.[39] A subset of nodal $CD8^+$ cytotoxic T-cell lymphomas composed of larger cells, with or without EBV infection, displays massive necrosis or apoptosis, is accompanied by disseminated intravascular coagulation or hemophagocytic syndrome, and pursues a very aggressive or fulminant course.[38,40,41] Such cases overlap with the systemic EBV^+ T-cell lymphomas seen mainly in children in Asian countries (see Chapter 29). Most cytotoxic PTCLs, NOS are tumors of alpha-beta derivation, and a smaller proportion are gamma-delta neoplasms. CD56 is expressed in rare cases, a phenomenon more commonly observed in extranodal cases.[36,39,42]

$CD4^+$ PTCLs, NOS are heterogeneous with respect to the expression of differentiation antigens and of chemokine receptor and activation markers, the expression of which varies in normal T cells according to their functional properties. A subset of $CD4^+$ PTCL, NOS corresponds to a central memory cell phenotype ($CD45RA^-$, $CD45RO^+$, $CD27^-$), suggesting derivation from a noneffector T-cell population.[43,44] It has been suggested that subclasses of PTCL, NOS might be delineated according to the expression markers associated

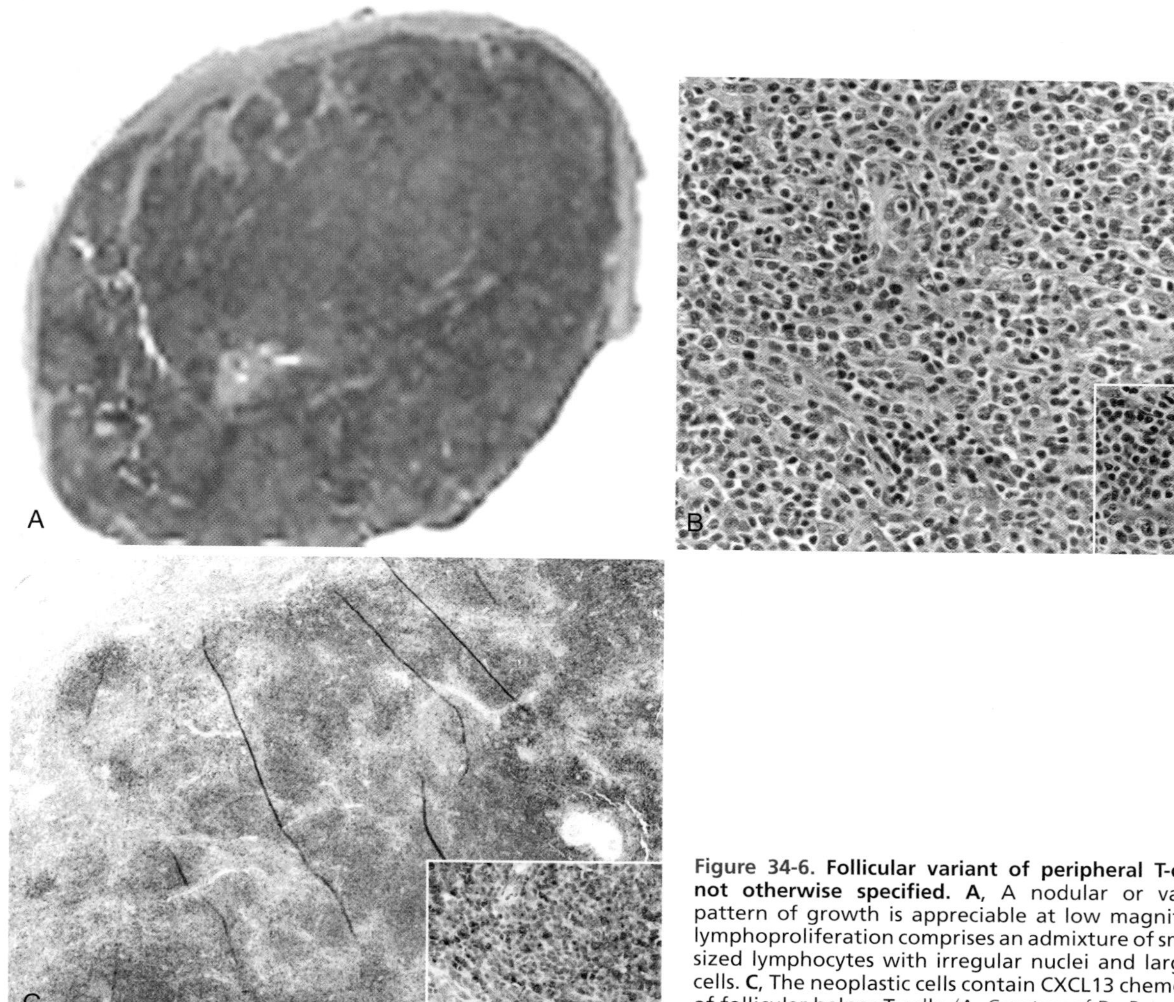

Figure 34-6. Follicular variant of peripheral T-cell lymphoma, not otherwise specified. A, A nodular or vaguely nodular pattern of growth is appreciable at low magnification. **B,** The lymphoproliferation comprises an admixture of small to medium-sized lymphocytes with irregular nuclei and large transformed cells. **C,** The neoplastic cells contain CXCL13 chemokine, a marker of follicular helper T cells. (**A,** Courtesy of Dr. Peter Banks, Celligent Diagnostics, Charlotte, North Carolina.)

with Th1 (CXCR3, CCR5, CD134/OX40, CD69, T-bet) or Th2 (CCR4, CXCR4, ST2[L]) differentiation.[45-48] One study from Japan suggested that cases with expression of CXCR3, CCR5, or ST2(L) may have a more favorable prognosis than those without expression of these molecules.[48,49] In another report by the same investigators, expression of CCR4, CCR3, and CXCR3 defined three nonoverlapping subgroups of PTCL, NOS that differed significantly in terms of outcome.[49] These findings need to be confirmed in other studies; however, this corroboration is hampered by the technical difficulty of assessing these markers, which are not used in routine practice.

PTCLs, NOS are generally negative for the transcription factor FOXP3, which is a marker of regulatory T cells.[50] Expression of CD10 and of follicular helper T-cell markers (BCL6, CXCL13, PD-1, SAP), which is typical of angioimmunoblastic T-cell lymphoma, is usually absent in PTCL, NOS. One exception is the follicular variant, which exhibits a follicular helper T-cell phenotype, suggesting a possible relationship to angioimmunoblastic T-cell lymphoma.[18,51,52]

The activation marker CD30, variably expressed, is often detected in occasional tumor cells; however, it can be more extensively expressed, especially in large cell variants.[36,39,53] Strong CD30 expression by a majority of tumor cells is seen occasionally, but anaplastic lymphoma kinase (ALK) expression is, by definition, absent. The differential diagnosis between ALK$^-$ anaplastic large cell lymphoma (ALCL) and PTCL, NOS expressing CD30 is controversial, and well-defined criteria have not been delineated. We advocate that the diagnosis of ALK$^-$ ALCL be reserved for cases with the morphology of ALCL and a cytotoxic phenotype, similar to that of ALK$^+$ ALCL. Coexpression of CD30 and CD15, a phenotype typically associated with classical Hodgkin's lymphoma, has been reported in some PTCLs, NOS, including a subset of cases that, by morphology, contained Reed-Sternberg–like cells, mimicking Hodgkin's lymphoma (Fig. 34-8).[54] The expression of CD15 appears to be indicative of a poor prognosis.[33,54]

B-cell markers usually highlight a small number of reactive B cells, but in some cases the B-cell component is extensive, ranging from isolated or small clusters of activated B cells to focally confluent transformed B cells that may partly obscure the neoplastic population.[55,56] In addition, a small proportion of PTCLs, NOS (≤5%) expresses CD20 (Fig. 34-9), as

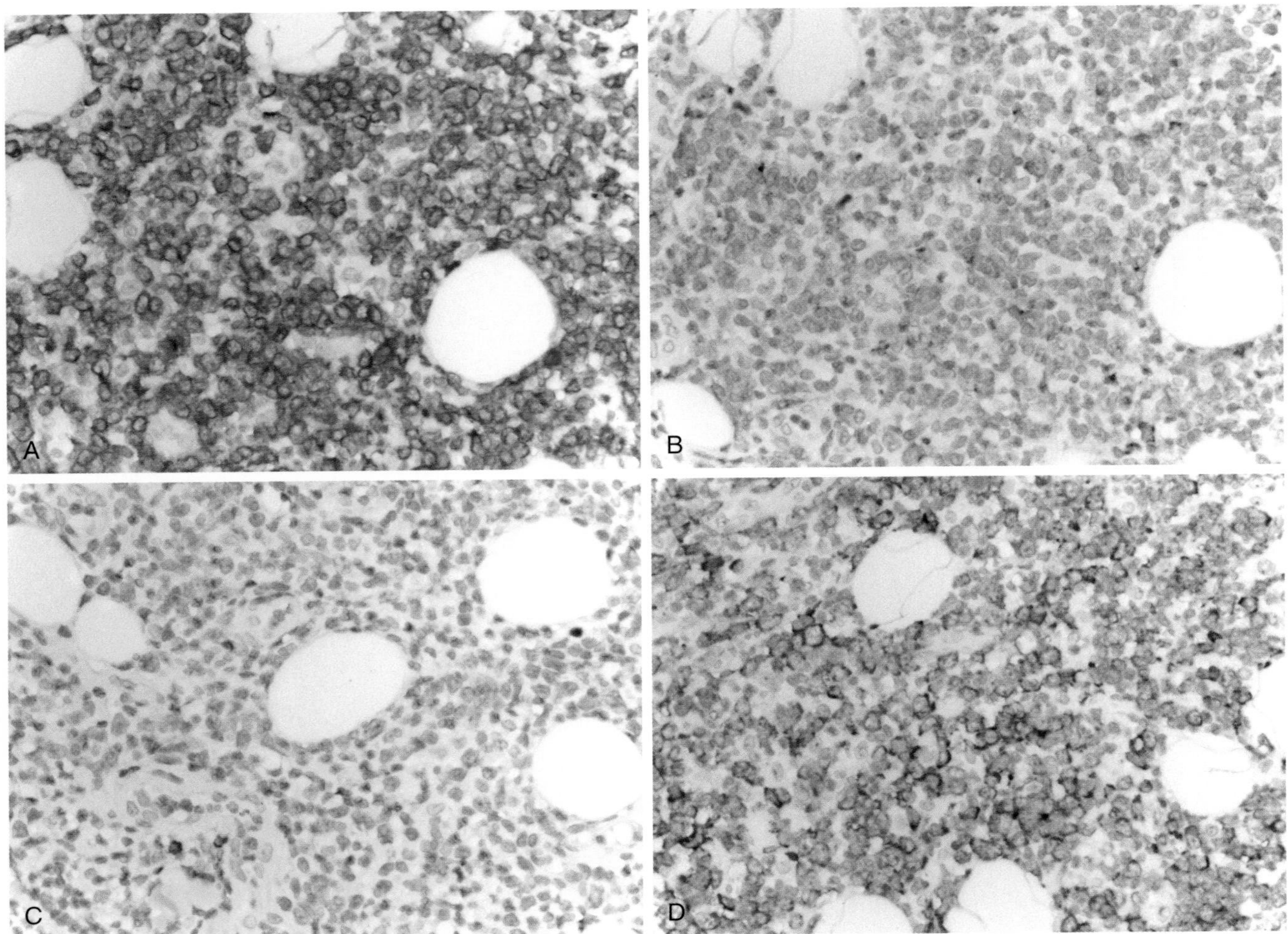

Figure 34-7. Aberrant T-cell antigen expression in peripheral T-cell lymphoma, not otherwise specified. A, The tumor cells are positive for CD3. **B,** They show marked downregulation of CD2 expression. **C,** They are negative for CD5. **D,** They show heterogeneous expression of CD7.

evidenced by immunohistochemistry or flow cytometry. The intensity of CD20 expression may be dimmer than that of normal B cells, and its distribution may be restricted to a subset of the neoplastic population, which is otherwise positive for pan–T-cell antigens. It is unclear whether CD20 expression in PTCL, NOS reflects derivation from a subset of $CD20^{dim}$ T cells that has undergone transformation or is a marker of the activation and proliferation of neoplastic T cells. There is no correlation with morphologic features, and the anatomic sites of disease involvement are variable. $CD20^+$ PTCL, NOS occurs predominantly in elderly males and pursues an aggressive course in many cases. Expression of other B-cell markers (CD19, CD79a, PAX5) has been documented in rare cases of PTCL, NOS, but the detection of more than one B-cell marker in an individual case is exceptional.[57-60]

EBV is detected in up to 50% of cases, and this finding correlates with a lower survival rate. In most instances, only a small number of cells are positive by in situ hybridization, and these represent mainly bystander B cells; less commonly, a variable fraction of tumor cells contains the virus. The EBV^+ B cells may assume Reed-Sternberg–like features, mimicking Hodgkin's lymphoma.[61-64] The development of EBV^+ large B-cell lymphomas, a relatively common event in angioimmunoblastic T-cell lymphomas, has also been described occasionally in PTCL, NOS.[55,56] Moreover, the occurrence of EBV^- clonal or monotypic B-cell proliferations with plasma cell differentiation, ranging from plasmacytomas to B-cell neoplasms with plasmacytic or plasmablastic differentiation, has been reported in association with PTCL, NOS.[65]

GENETICS

Antigen Receptor Genes

Clonally rearranged TCR genes can be demonstrated in most cases. Using the Biomed-2 multiplex protocols, the clonality detection rate is greater than 90% for both *TCRβ* and *TCRγ* targets and reaches 100% when both loci are interrogated.[66] Simultaneous detection of a clonal or oligoclonal immunoglobulin heavy-chain gene rearrangement has been reported in a variable proportion of cases (up to one third), usually but not always in association with the presence of EBV^+ B-cells or morphologic evidence of B-cell expansion, suggesting that this feature might not be helpful in the differential diagnosis with angioimmunoblastic T-cell lymphoma.[67]

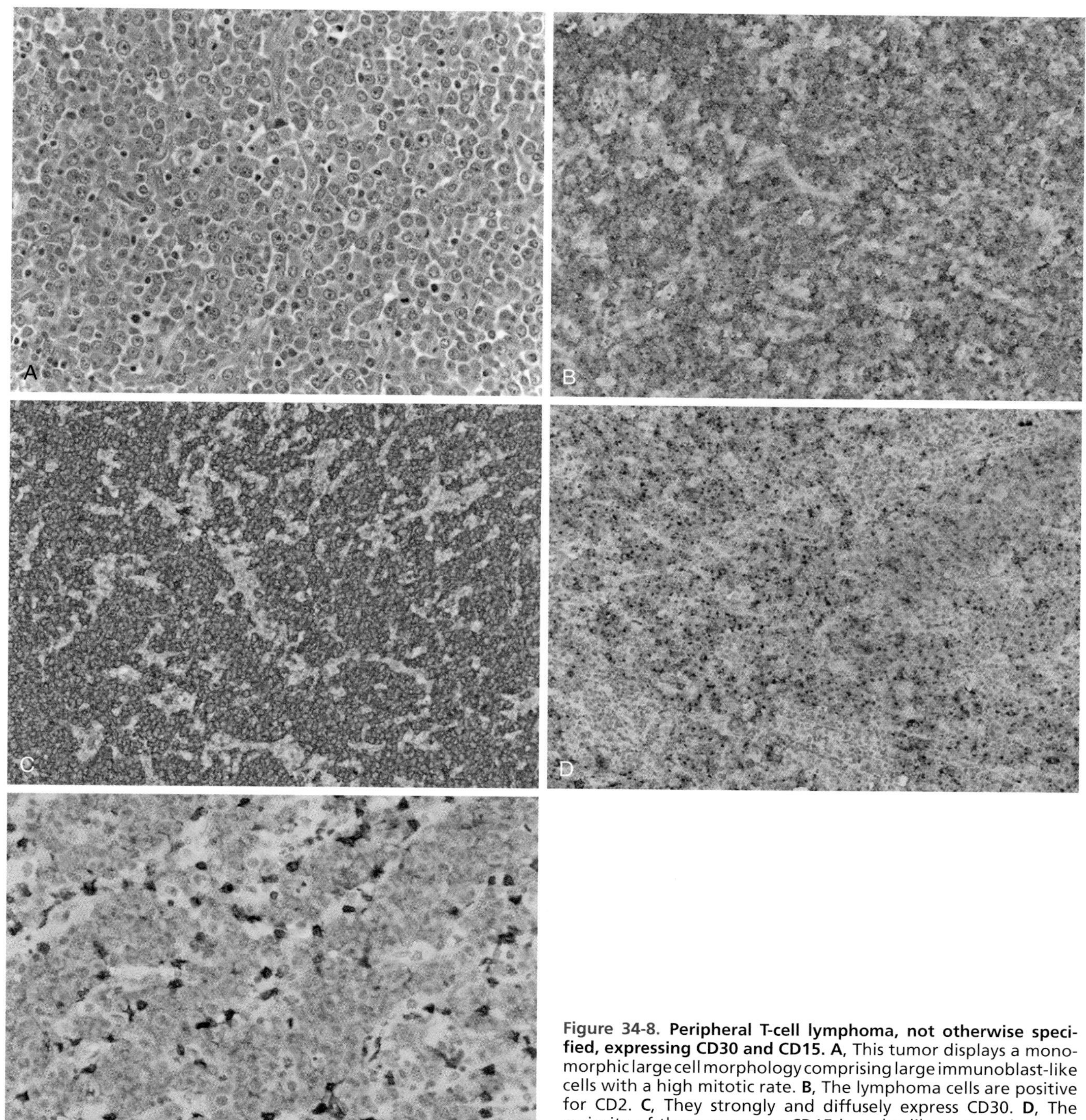

Figure 34-8. Peripheral T-cell lymphoma, not otherwise specified, expressing CD30 and CD15. A, This tumor displays a monomorphic large cell morphology comprising large immunoblast-like cells with a high mitotic rate. **B,** The lymphoma cells are positive for CD2. **C,** They strongly and diffusely express CD30. **D,** The majority of them coexpress CD15 in a dot-like paranuclear and membranous pattern. **E,** They show dim CD8 expression. Granzyme B, epithelial membrane antigen, and anaplastic lymphoma kinase were negative (not shown).

Genetic Abnormalities

By conventional cytogenetics, clonal aberrations comprising a vast number of different numerical and structural alterations have been described.[68-70] Trisomy 3 seems to be frequent in the lymphoepithelioid variant.[69] Complex karyotypes reportedly correlate with larger cell morphology[69] and an inferior outcome.[71]

Virtually all cases harbor genetic imbalances, with gains outnumbering losses. By comparative genomic hybridization,[71-73] recurrent gains have been observed in chromosomes 7q,[74] 8q,[73] 17q, and 22q, and recurrent losses in chromosomes 4q, 5q, 6q, 9p, 10q, 12q, and 13q. Zettl and colleagues[72] identified a group of nodal cytotoxic CD5^{+} PTCLs, NOS associated with deletions in chromosomes 5q, 10q, and 12q and a better prognosis. For a few altered loci, correlation

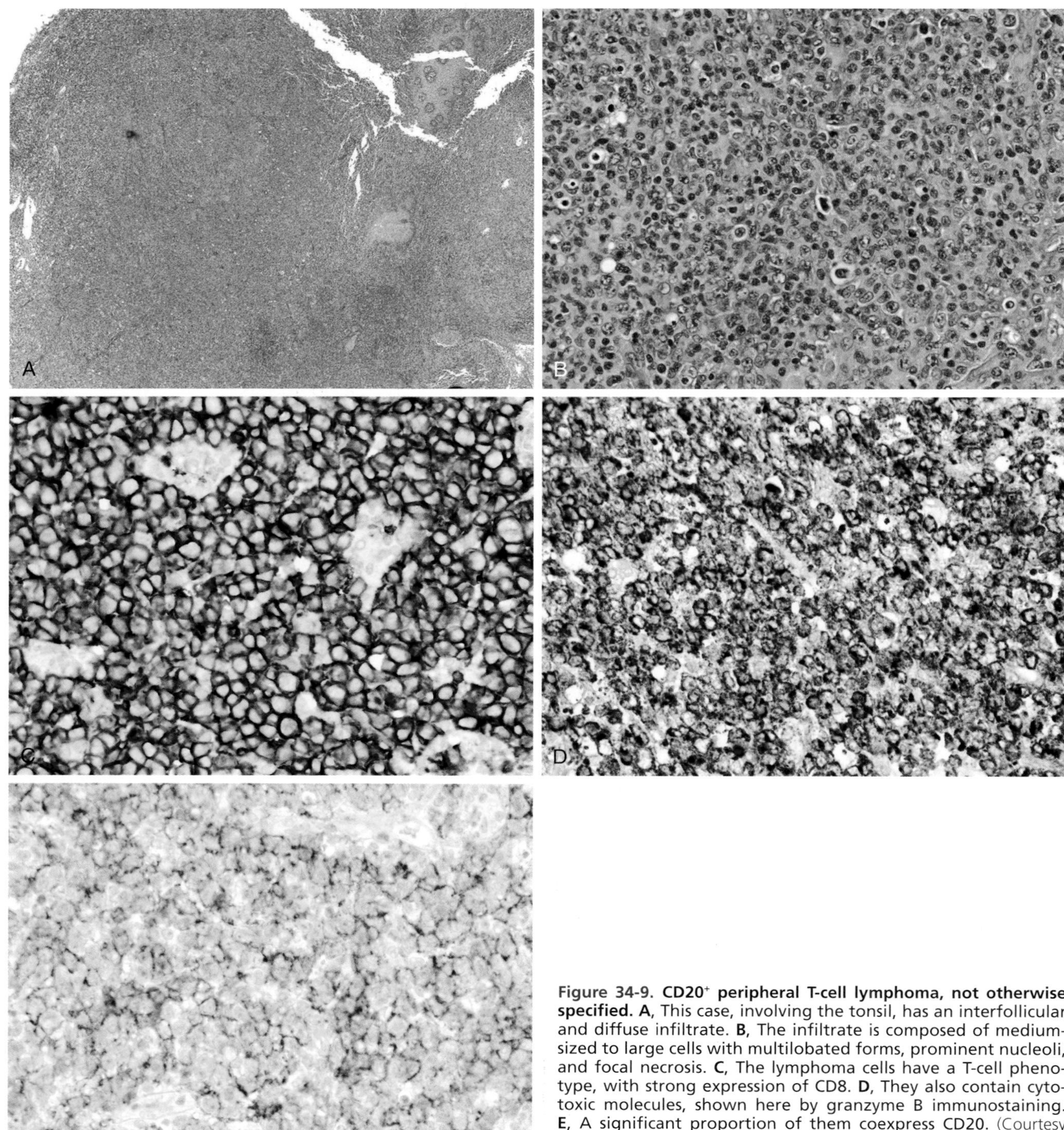

Figure 34-9. CD20[+] peripheral T-cell lymphoma, not otherwise specified. A, This case, involving the tonsil, has an interfollicular and diffuse infiltrate. **B**, The infiltrate is composed of medium-sized to large cells with multilobated forms, prominent nucleoli, and focal necrosis. **C**, The lymphoma cells have a T-cell phenotype, with strong expression of CD8. **D**, They also contain cytotoxic molecules, shown here by granzyme B immunostaining. **E**, A significant proportion of them coexpress CD20. (Courtesy of Aliyah Sohani and Judith Ferry, Massachusetts General Hospital, Boston.)

with deregulated gene expression has been demonstrated, and a few genes of interest have been highlighted. For example, gains at 7q have been found to target cyclin-dependent kinase 6,[74] those at 8q involve the *MYC* locus,[73] losses at 9p21 are associated with reduced expression of two inhibitors of cyclin-dependent kinases, and gains at 7p22 correlate with increased levels of CARMA1, a factor involved in the activation of nuclear factor-κB.[75]

Few recurrent chromosomal translocations have been described in PTCL, NOS. The t(5;9)(q33;q22) translocation that fuses the N-terminal region of *ITK* to the tyrosine kinase domain of *SYK* is found predominantly in association with the rare follicular variant of PTCL, NOS,[76] suggesting that the *SYK-ITK* fusion might define a distinct PTCL subtype. Chromosomal breaks involving the TCR gene loci (mostly the TCR alpha/delta loci at 14q11.2) have been reported in rare

the obvious pathogenetic role of EBV in a variety of other lymphomas, it is currently believed that the presence of EBV in AITL is not causative; it most likely reflects the underlying immunodeficiency that is characteristic of the neoplastic process, although a more direct role for EBV in driving the T-cell proliferation has been postulated.[20]

CLINICAL FEATURES

The clinical presentation of AITL is unique among malignant lymphomas, and the diagnosis is frequently suspected on clinical grounds. Most patients present with generalized peripheral lymphadenopathy, hepatosplenomegaly, and prominent systemic symptoms including fever, weight loss, and rash, often with pruritus.[13,14] One third of patients present with edema, especially in the upper extremities and face; pleural effusion; arthritis; and ascites. Polyclonal hypergammaglobulinemia and Coombs-positive hemolytic anemia are frequently present. Bone marrow is commonly involved. Approximately 30% of patients present with eosinophilia, and 10% present with plasmacytosis. Laboratory studies reveal the presence of cold agglutinins, circulating immune complexes, anti–smooth muscle and antinuclear antibodies, positive rheumatoid factor, and cryoglobulins. The evolution of the disease is often complicated by intercurrent infections with conventional and opportunistic microorganisms. There is no consensus regarding the best therapeutic approach to patients with AITL.[21] Patients may respond initially to steroids or mild cytotoxic chemotherapy, but progression usually occurs.

MORPHOLOGY

In contrast to other peripheral T-cell lymphomas, AITL displays some unique morphologic features in involved lymph nodes (Box 35-1).[22,23] At low magnification, the lymph node architecture is usually effaced. There is a polymorphic infiltrate of small to medium-sized lymphocytes intermingled with granulocytes, eosinophils, plasma cells, fibroblast-like dendritic cells, histiocytes, and epithelioid cells (Fig. 35-1) predominantly occupying the paracortical or interfollicular area. Occasionally a neoplastic T-cell population can be readily identified on morphologic grounds. In these cases there is an infiltration of atypical T cells characterized by round to irregular nuclear contours and broad, clear cytoplasm with distinct cell membranes (clear cells) (Fig. 35-2A). Cytologic atypia of the lymphoid cells, although frequently observed, is not a prerequisite for the diagnosis (see Fig. 35-2B). The proportion of atypical T cells may vary greatly from small foci to large confluent sheets, sometimes posing problems in the differential diagnosis with peripheral T-cell lymphoma, not otherwise specified (PTCL, NOS). Noteworthy is that medium-sized to large basophilic blasts of B-cell phenotype may be present, some of them reminiscent of Hodgkin cells (Fig. 35-3).[4,16,24]

The vast majority of AITL cases display a pronounced proliferation of cells with the phenotype of follicular dendritic cells (FDCs) localized outside the residual follicles, typically abutting the high endothelial venules (HEVs). Occasionally, remnants of follicles with concentrically arranged, onion-shaped FDC meshworks are present, giving them a "burned out" appearance (Fig. 35-4). In less obvious cases, FDC proliferation may be recognized only after immunohistochemical staining with antibodies directed against CD21, CD23, or CD35 antigens. Another diagnostic feature of the disease is extension of the infiltrate beyond the lymph node capsule into the perinodal fat, frequently sparing preserved cortical sinuses that appear to be "jumped over" by the tumor cells (Fig. 35-5). A key feature is the presence of numerous, frequently arborizing, postcapillary HEVs, which are also seen

Box 35-1 *Diagnostic Criteria of Angioimmunoblastic T-Cell Lymphoma*

Morphology
- Usually effaced lymph node architecture
- Perinodal extension of infiltrate, with sparing of sinuses
- Polymorphic infiltrate of lymphocytes, granulocytes, plasma cells, and immunoblasts
- T cells with abundant clear cytoplasm (clear cells)
- Proliferation of FDCs
- Proliferation of arborizing high endothelial venules

Immunophenotype
- Demonstration of FDC networks $CD21^+$, $CD23^+$
- $CXCL13^+$, $PD1^+$, $CD10^+$, $BCL6^+$, $CD4^+$ neoplastic T cells
- $CD3^+$, $CD5^+$, CD4 >> CD8 with no T-cell antigen loss
- EBV^+ B blasts

Molecular Genetics
- TCR gene clonally rearranged in 75% of cases (range, 70%-90%)
- IGH gene clonally rearranged in 12% of cases (range, 10%-20%)
- T_{FH} molecular signature

Cytogenetics
- Clonal chromosome aberrations in 89%
- Unrelated chromosome clones frequent (47%)
- +3, +5, additional X chromosome

EBV Positivity
- 50%-97% of cases by in situ hybridization
- $EBER^+$ B cells and rarely T cells

EBER, EBV-encoded small RNA; EBV, Epstein-Barr virus; FDC, follicular dendritic cell; IGH; immunoglobulin heavy chain; TCR, T-cell receptor; T_{FH}, follicular helper T cell.

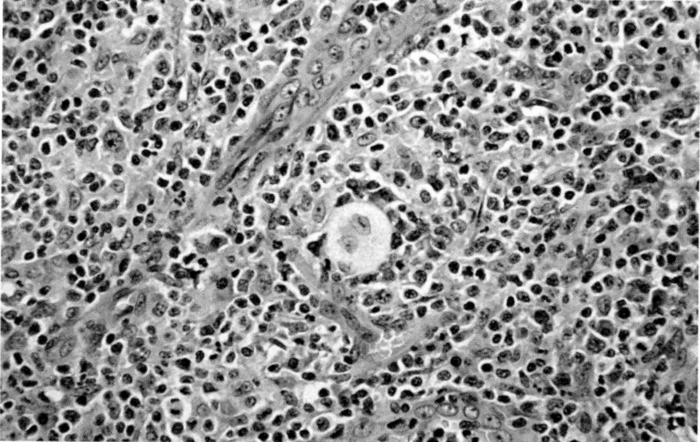

Figure 35-1. Typical morphology of angioimmunoblastic T-cell lymphoma. There is a polymorphic infiltrate of small to medium-sized lymphocytes with clear cytoplasm intermingled with eosinophils, plasma cells, fibroblast-like dendritic cells, histiocytes, and epithelioid cells.

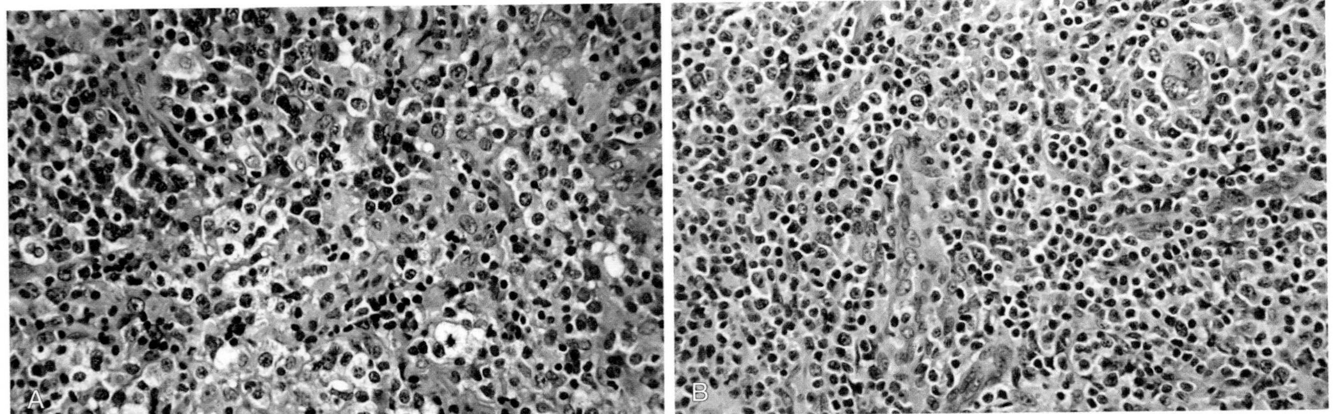

Figure 35-2. **Cytologic spectrum of neoplastic T cells in angioimmunoblastic T-cell lymphoma. A,** The infiltrate is composed of atypical T cells characterized by irregular nuclear contours and broad, clear cytoplasm with distinct cell membranes (clear cells). **B,** The neoplastic T cells are small to intermediate in size, with no atypia and clear cytoplasm.

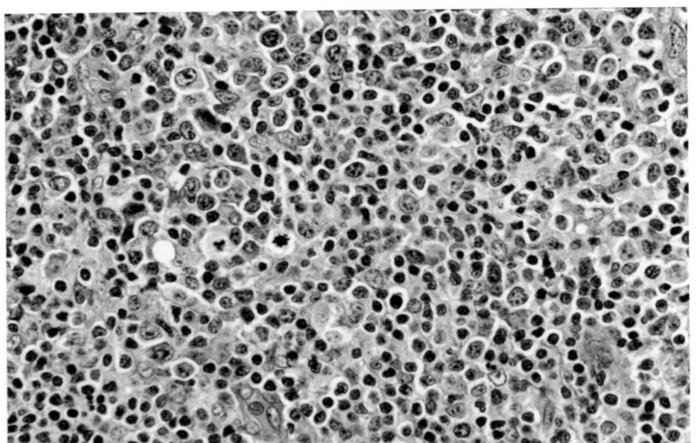

Figure 35-3. **Large B-cell blasts.** Intermingled with the neoplastic T cells are medium-sized to large basophilic blasts of B-cell phenotype, some of them reminiscent of Hodgkin cells.

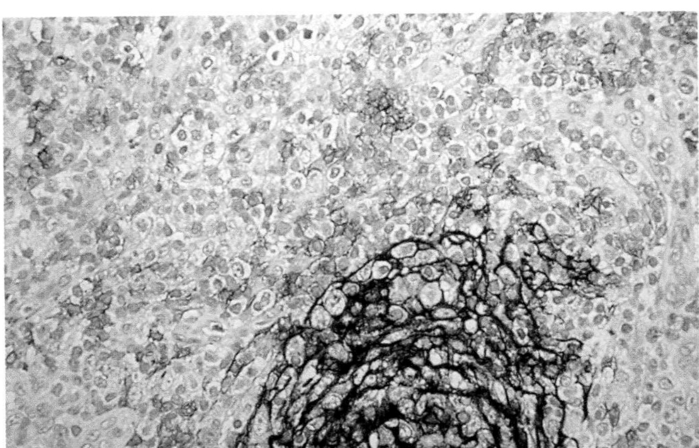

Figure 35-4. **Follicular dendritic cells highlighted with CD21 immunostaining.** A "burned out" germinal center with onion-shaped follicular dendritic cell meshworks is depicted. Note the proliferation of $CD21^+$ dendritic cells beyond the follicles.

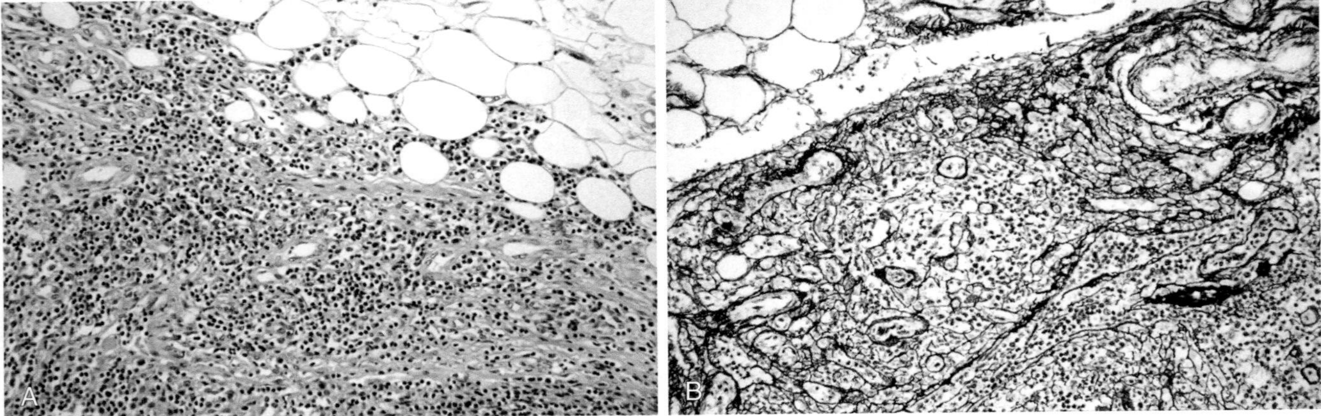

Figure 35-5. **Extension of the infiltrate beyond the capsule. A,** Infiltration into the fat, with preservation of the cortical sinuses that appear to be "jumped over" by the tumor cells. **B,** Gomori stain highlights the presence of open cortical sinuses, a diagnostic feature of angioimmunoblastic T-cell lymphoma.

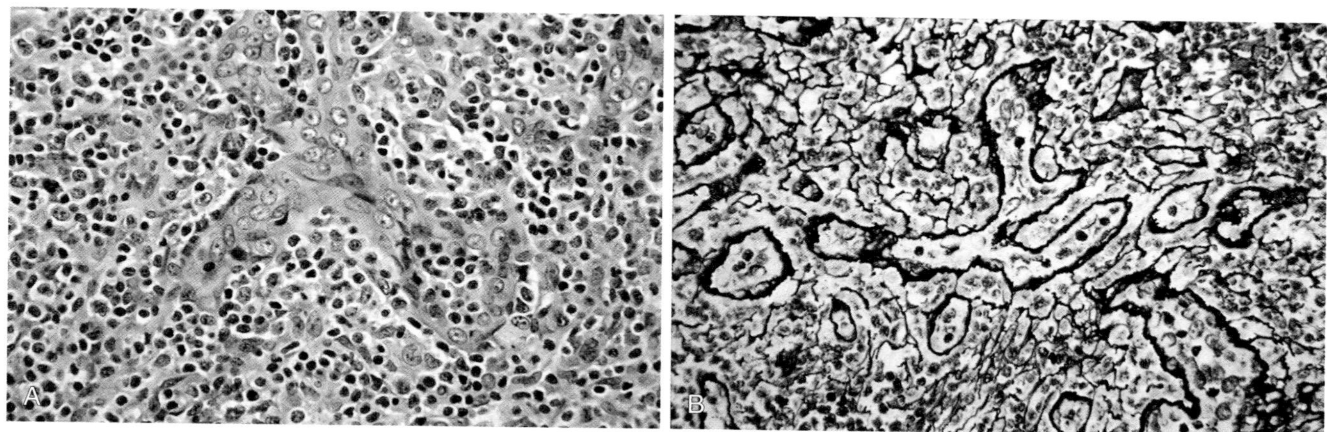

Figure 35-6. **A,** Arborizing high endothelial venules. **B,** Gomori stain highlights the presence of arborizing high endothelial venules, a characteristic finding in angioimmunoblastic T-cell lymphoma.

outside the lymph nodes in the perinodal infiltrate. The HEVs are best recognized in silver stains, such as Gomori silver impregnation, or in periodic acid–Schiff stains, highlighting both the conspicuous angioarchitecture and the thickened, hyalinized basement membranes of vessel walls (Fig. 35-6).[9] In the original description of AITL, the absence of reactive, hyperplastic B-cell follicles was thought to be a characteristic feature of the disease. However, it is now accepted that the architectural changes in AITL fall into three major patterns.[25-27] In pattern 1 (20% of cases) the lymph node architecture is preserved, with hyperplastic germinal centers (Fig. 35-7A). Pattern 2 (30% of cases) is characterized by the loss of normal

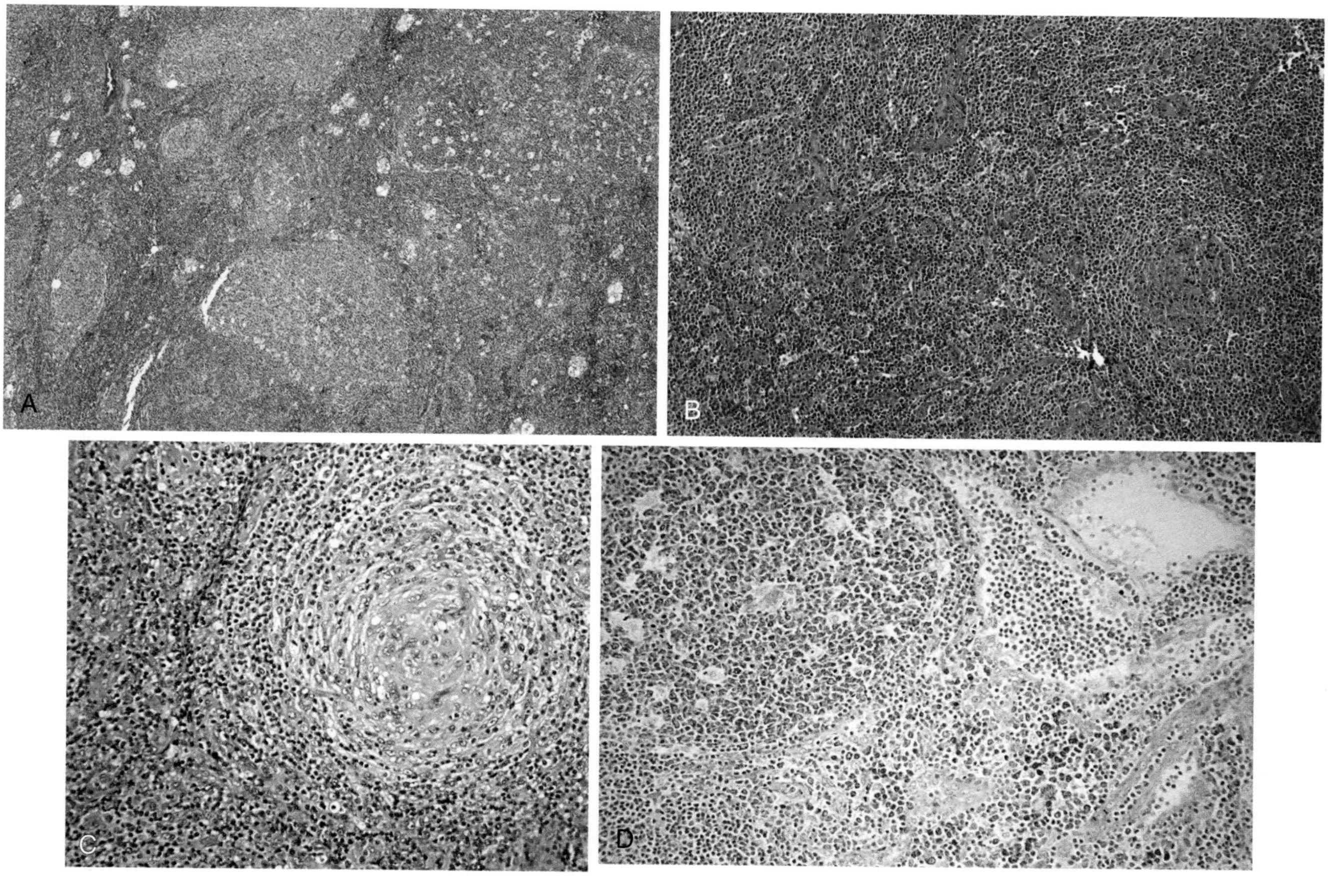

Figure 35-7. Histologic patterns of angioimmunoblastic T-cell lymphoma. A, Early case with hyperplastic follicles without a mantle zone and an expanded paracortical area (pattern 1). **B,** Case with "burned out" germinal centers, reminiscent of Castleman's disease, with paracortical expansion and proliferation of arborizing high endothelial venules (pattern 2). **C,** Higher magnification of a depleted, atrophic follicle with clear proliferation of follicular dendritic cells (pattern 2). **D,** Giemsa stain of a hyperplastic follicle with absence of a mantle zone and an expanded paracortical area (pattern 1).

architecture and the presence of occasional depleted follicles or "burned out" germinal centers (see Fig. 35-7B and C). In pattern 3 (50% of cases) the normal architecture of the lymph node is completely effaced, and no B-cell follicles are present. These patterns seem to represent different morphologic stages of the disease, with consecutive biopsies from the same patient showing a transition from pattern 1 to pattern 3 as the disease progresses.[25,26,28]

DIAGNOSTIC PITFALLS

Hyperplastic Germinal Centers

In a rare, possibly early, and difficult to diagnose morphologic stage of the disease, well-structured (hyperplastic) germinal centers with poorly developed mantle zones and sometimes ill-defined borders are still present (see Fig. 35-7D).[25] The specific morphologic alterations are confined to the interfollicular and pericapsular areas of the lymph node. These cases are remarkable because of their increased vascularity and occasional appearance of atypical T cells. An expanded CD21$^+$ FDC meshwork is very helpful in making the diagnosis (Fig. 35-8A), but this feature can be subtle or absent.[26] The presence of CD4$^+$ T cells (see Fig. 35-8B), with aberrant expression of CD10, BCL6, or programmed death 1 (PD1) in the outer rim of the germinal centers and paracortex, has been described as an important diagnostic feature (see Fig. 35-8C and D).[26] If this early stage of the disease is suspected, evidence of a clonal expansion of T cells should be obtained, and clinical features should be compatible with the diagnosis. In subsequent biopsies, some of these cases may show progression to typical AITL with effaced nodal architecture.[25,29]

Abundant Epithelioid Cell Reaction

Some cases of AITL may show a prominent admixture of epithelioid cells, obscuring the diagnostic morphologic features of the disease (Fig. 35-9A). According to Patsouris and coworkers,[30] the diagnosis of AITL relies on the presence of arborizing vessels and proliferating FDCs, in contrast to epithelioid cell–rich classical Hodgkin's lymphoma (containing classic Hodgkin and Reed-Sternberg [HRS] cells) and the lymphoepithelioid variant of PTCL, NOS (Lennert's lymphoma), in which these features are lacking.

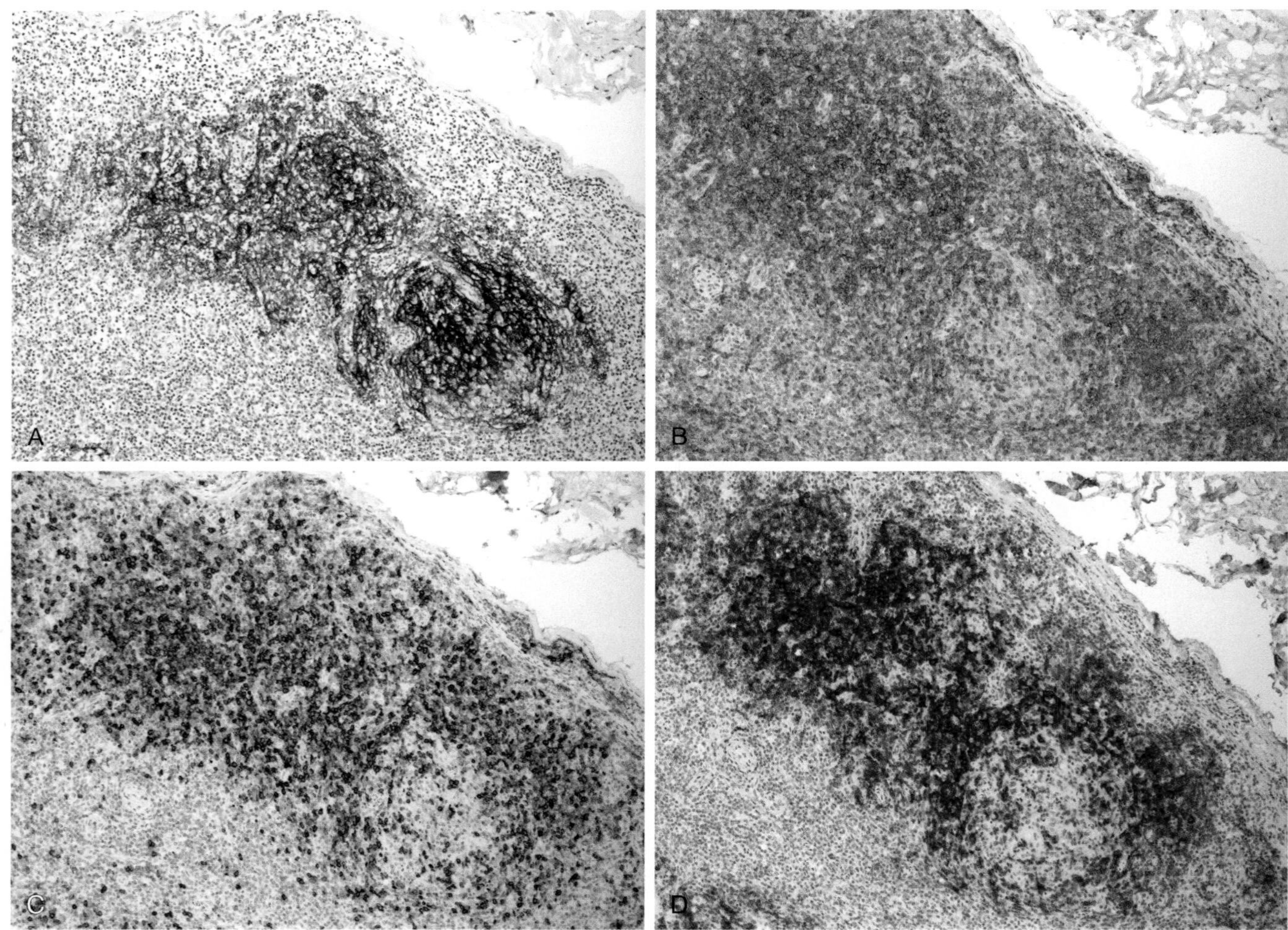

Figure 35-8. Angioimmunoblastic T-cell lymphoma with hyperplastic germinal centers and depleted follicles (pattern 1-2). A, Expanded CD21$^+$ follicular dendritic cell (FDC) meshwork extends from the depleted, atrophic follicle. **B,** CD4$^+$ T cells surrounding the depleted follicle and embedded in the meshwork of CD21$^+$ FDCs. **C,** The CD4$^+$ T cells are strongly positive for CD10. Note the absence of CD10 expression in the depleted follicle. **D,** The same cells are PD1$^+$.

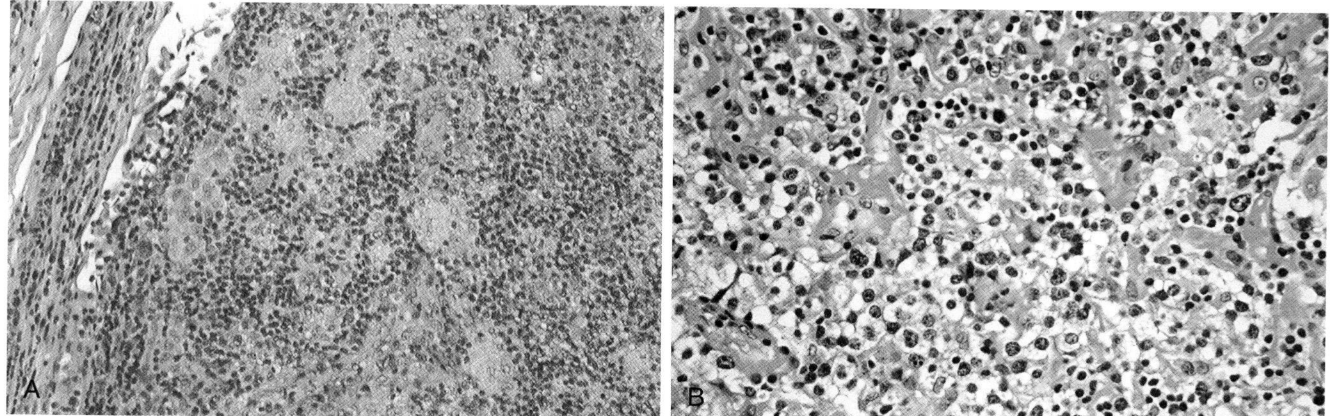

Figure 35-9. Pitfalls in the diagnosis of angioimmunoblastic T-cell lymphoma (AITL). A, AITL with abundant epithelioid reaction. Note the open cortical sinus, a characteristic diagnostic feature. **B,** AITL with sheets of large neoplastic T cells.

Sheets of Large Neoplastic T Cells

In some cases the neoplastic T-cell population becomes unusually predominant, forming sheets of medium-sized to large cells and obscuring the "inflammatory" background infiltrate commonly present in AITL (see Fig. 35-9B). Although clear-cut criteria have not been defined, we tend to classify these cases as high-grade variants of AITL, as long as the diagnostic features are still recognizable (e.g., hypervascularity, perinodal extension, FDC proliferation). Nevertheless, there seems to be an overlap with PTCL, NOS, which sometimes exhibits similarities to AITL. Owing to the lack of studies in the literature, it is not clear whether AITL can progress to PTCL, NOS composed of a uniform population of large, transformed T cells.

B-Cell Lymphoproliferation or B-Cell Lymphoma

There is clear evidence that large B-cell lymphomas may arise in AITL. These large B-cell lymphomas may be present at the initial diagnosis or develop over time.[31-33] It seems that in many if not all cases, the B-cell lymphoproliferation is triggered by EBV infection, which in turn is facilitated by the profound immunodeficiency associated with the disease and possibly by the additional immunosuppression induced by chemotherapy. Recent publications indicate that EBV-associated B-cell lymphoproliferations in AITL constitute a spectrum of alterations.[34-36] The histologic picture in these cases is characterized by the presence of large EBV$^+$ B blasts in an otherwise typical AITL (Fig. 35-10A). These blasts may have the appearance of immunoblasts or bear a resemblance to Hodgkin cells; they may be focally accentuated, diffusely scattered, or form confluent sheets indistinguishable from diffuse large B-cell lymphoma.[35] These B blasts are usually EBV-encoded small RNA (EBER) positive, CD20$^+$, CD30$^+$, CD15$^-$, and latent membrane protein-1 (LMP-1) positive or negative (see Fig. 35-10B to D).

Rare cases of AITL have been described with a monoclonal plasma cell population,[9] although it has been debated whether these cases represent true AITL or multicentric Castleman's disease.[37]

Reed-Sternberg–Like Cells

Rare cases show the presence of typical HRS cells with a classic immunophenotype (CD20$^{+/-}$, CD30$^+$, CD15$^+$, EBV$^+$) in an otherwise typical setting of AITL (Fig. 35-11).[29] In contrast to classical Hodgkin's lymphoma, molecular studies have revealed clonal rearrangements of the TCRγ chain gene and an oligoclonal pattern of immunoglobulin heavy-chain gene in the microdissected HRS-like cells. Preliminary data suggest that these patients are not at high risk of progression to classical Hodgkin's lymphoma.

IMMUNOPHENOTYPE

The infiltrating lymphocytes are predominantly T cells (CD3$^+$ and CD5$^+$), usually with an admixture of CD4 and CD8 cells. CD4$^+$ cells are thought to predominate in the majority of cases,[8,38] although CD8$^+$ T cells may constitute the majority of the lymphoid infiltrate in some cases.[39] Nevertheless, recent studies have shown that the neoplastic population in AITL corresponds to T cells with a CD4$^+$ phenotype (Fig. 35-12A).[26,40] In contrast to other types of T-cell lymphoma, loss of pan–T-cell antigen expression is an uncommon finding in AITL. B cells (CD20$^+$, CD79a$^+$) are found in varying numbers and are occasionally present in follicular aggregates. They are usually small cells but may become larger and activated, especially when infected with EBV. Immunoblasts may be null, T, or, more frequently, B cells and usually express CD30. The expression of EBV LMP can be demonstrated in 30% to 50% of cases, although in situ hybridization is more sensitive for detecting the viral genome.[18]

The proliferation of FDCs, a diagnostic hallmark of AITL, can be readily appreciated with immunohistochemical stains. CD21 highlights the disorganized and largely expanded meshworks of FDCs, usually surrounding HEVs in the vast majority of cases (see Fig. 35-12B). The exact nature of the CD21$^+$ cells with dendritic morphology has not been fully resolved. The abnormal proliferation is centered around the HEV and is rarely associated with B-cell follicles. It has been postulated that the CD21$^+$ cells are not true FDCs but activated fibroblastic reticulum cells that have upregulated the CD21 antigen.[41] Fibroblastic reticulum cells and FDCs are

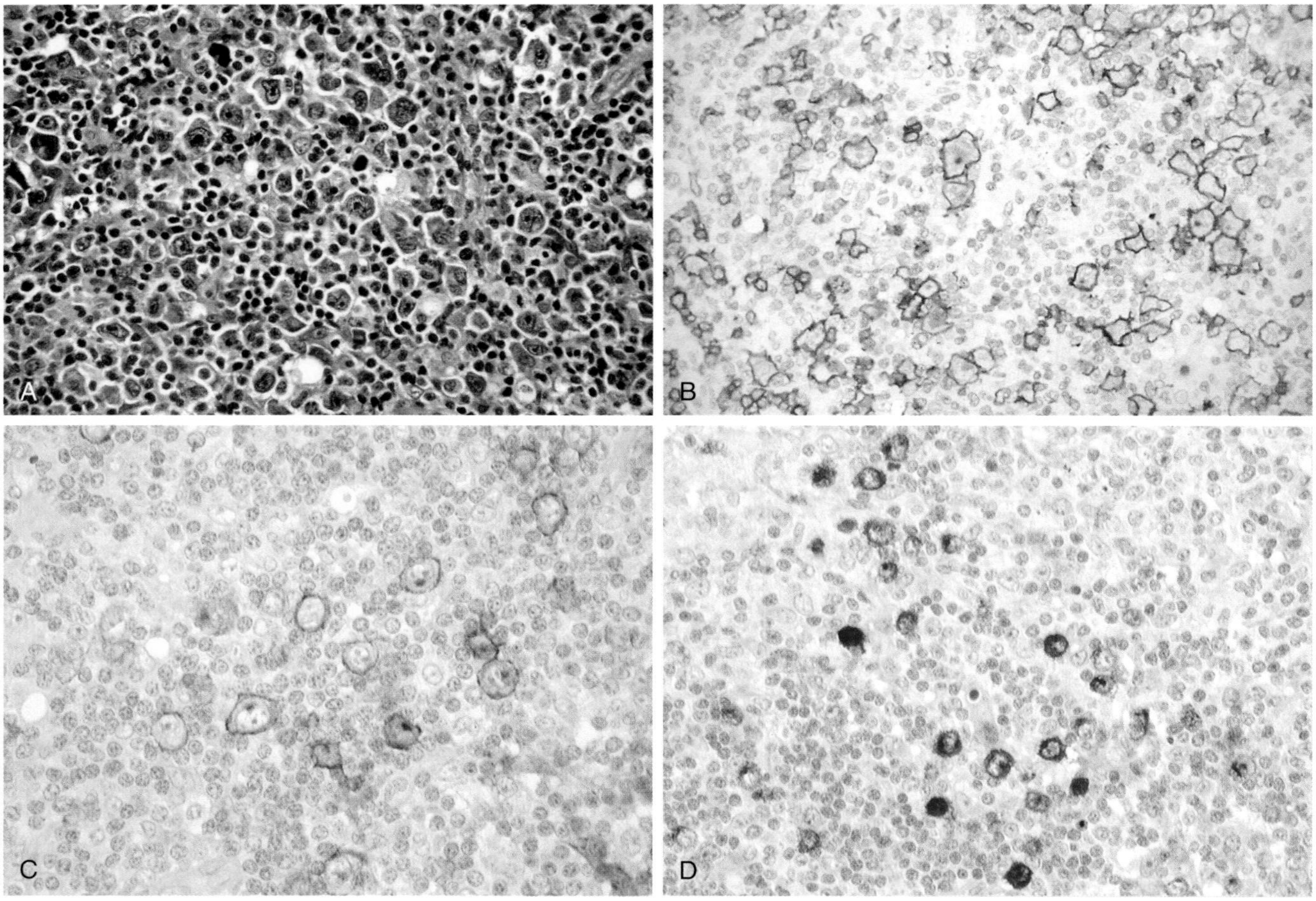

Figure 35-10. Angioimmunoblastic T-cell lymphoma (AITL) with B-cell lymphoproliferation. A, Proliferation of B-cell blasts in an otherwise typical AITL case. The B cells might resemble centroblasts, immunoblasts, or Hodgkin cells. **B,** CD20 staining highlights the spectrum of B-cell morphology in AITL. **C,** The B cells are positive for CD30. **D,** The B-cell blasts are EBV LMP-1^{+}.

both derived from mesenchyma rather than of hematopoietic origin.[42,43] Therefore, the histogenesis of the characteristic and diagnostically useful $CD21^{+}$ cells is not firmly established.

More recently, it has been shown that the neoplastic cells in a high proportion of AITL cases (80% to 90%) express CD10 and BCL6 in addition to CD4, similar to a particular subset of $CD4^{+}$ T cells normally found in reactive germinal centers—the T_{FH} cells.[26,44] The aberrant expression of CD10 seems to characterize the neoplastic T-cell population in AITL, which in the majority of cases corresponds to the clear cells seen with hematoxylin-eosin stains (see Fig. 35-12C). Furthermore, $CD10^{+}$ cells have been identified in only 10%

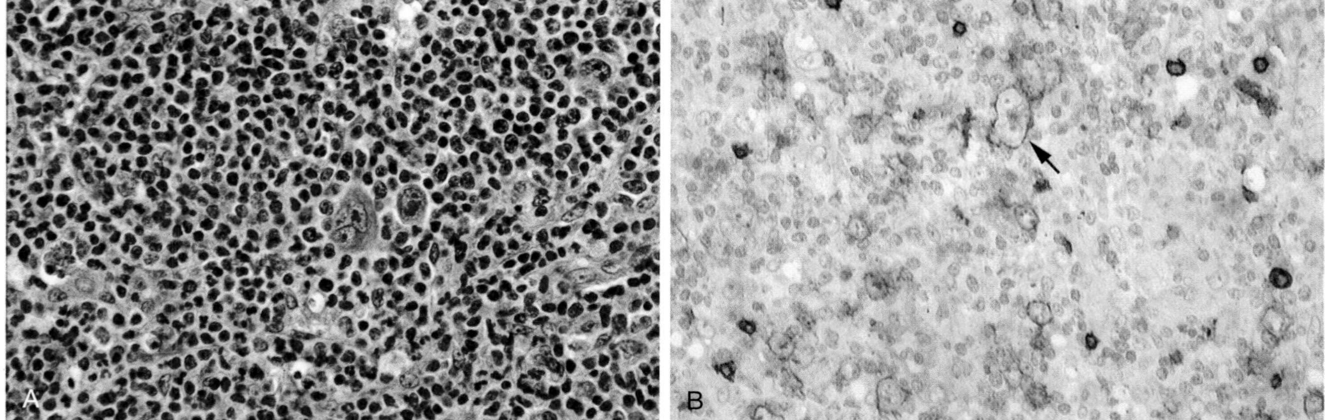

Figure 35-11. Angioimmunoblastic T-cell lymphoma with Reed-Sternberg–like cells. A, Reed-Sternberg–like cells are depicted. Note the minimal atypia of the surrounding neoplastic T cells. **B,** The Reed-Sternberg–like cells are $CD20^{+}$ (*arrow*).

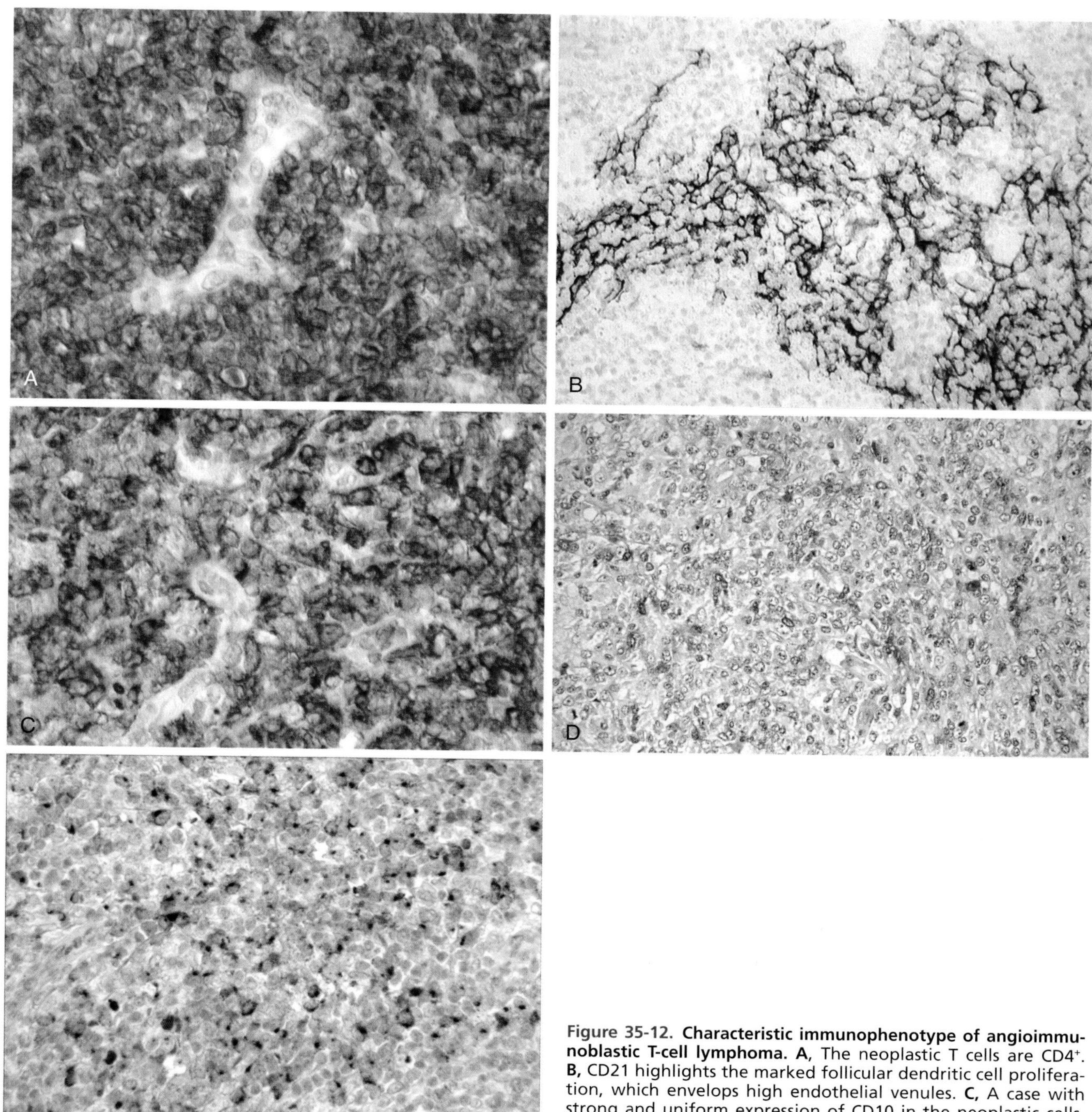

Figure 35-12. Characteristic immunophenotype of angioimmunoblastic T-cell lymphoma. A, The neoplastic T cells are CD4$^+$. **B,** CD21 highlights the marked follicular dendritic cell proliferation, which envelops high endothelial venules. **C,** A case with strong and uniform expression of CD10 in the neoplastic cells. **D,** CD10 expression in only a minority of the tumor cell population. **E,** The neoplastic T cells are strongly CXCL13$^+$.

to 20% of peripheral T-cell lymphomas, unspecified, and are absent in anaplastic large cell lymphoma, in other PTCLs, NOS, and in lymphoid hyperplasias.[45,46] Nonetheless, despite variation from case to case, the expression of CD10 in AITL is often weak, heterogeneous, and confined to a small population of tumor cells (see Fig. 35-12D), mostly the clear cells and the neoplastic cells around the residual follicles. More recently, Grogg and associates[47] reported strong expression of CXCL13 (a chemokine upregulated in the T_{FH} subset) in the vast majority of tumor cells (>80%) and in most cases of AITL (86%) (see Fig. 35-12E). The expression of CD10, BCL6, and CXCL13 represents an important adjunct in the diagnosis of AITL and provides further evidence that AITL derives from T_{FH}.[45,47] Additional markers of normal T_{FH} cells, including CXCR5, CD154, PD1, and SLAM-associated protein (SAP), have been demonstrated by immunohistochemistry to be expressed in the majority of AITL cases.[48,49] Although the expression of T_{FH} markers is characteristic of AITL, a recent study showed that 28% of PTCLs, NOS express at least two T_{FH} markers and display some AITL-like features, suggesting that the morphologic spectrum of AITL may be broader than previously thought and that the criteria distinguishing AITL and PTCL, NOS might be too strict.[50]

GENETICS

The availability of molecular techniques has led to significant progress in the understanding of the biology of AITL since its early description in the 1970s. The clonal expansion of T cells with rearranged TCR genes detectable in 75% of cases using Southern blot analysis or polymerase chain reaction strategies provides evidence that AITL is a form of peripheral T-cell lymphoma in the majority of cases.[6-8,22] Of note, in approximately 25% to 30% of cases, rearrangements of the immunoglobulin heavy-chain (*IGH@*) or light-chain genes coexist with rearrangements of the *TCRβ* or *TCRγ* genes, either at presentation or during the course of the disease.[28] In addition, a small group of cases (7%) with the morphology of AITL reveals clonal rearrangements of the *IGH@* genes alone. The presence of *IGH@* rearrangements is thought to be a manifestation of clonal expansion of EBV-infected B cells that are frequently identified in lymph nodes involved by AITL.[17] EBV is found mainly in two types of B cells in AITL: cells resembling memory B cells, which show relatively little tendency for clonal expansion, and cells resembling germinal center B cells, which are driven into massive proliferation and acquire somatic mutations during clonal expansion without selection for a functional B-cell receptor (immunoglobulin-deficient or "forbidden" clones).[51] Furthermore, diffuse large B-cell lymphomas have been reported to arise from these EBV-immortalized B-cell clones owing to either the inherent immunodeficiency of the disease or the transient suppression of the immune system after treatment.[31,35]

Cytogenetic studies have demonstrated a distinct pattern of chromosomal abnormalities in AITL lesions.[52] The most frequent cytogenetic abnormalities are trisomy 3, trisomy 5, and an additional X chromosome. By combining classic metaphase cytogenetics and interphase cytogenetics, 89% of AITL cases have been found to harbor aberrant chromosomal clones.[53] AITL shows a high load of cytogenetically unrelated clones and single cells with completely different karyotypes. This is a peculiar phenomenon, because unrelated chromosomal clones or oligoclones are an otherwise exceptional finding among lymphomas in general (47% in AITL versus 0.6% in general). Cytogenetic studies have demonstrated that clones can appear and disappear and new clones can emerge over time.[9,52] The significance of these findings is unclear. However, based on these results, previous[54] and more recent[15] studies have argued that AITL most likely starts as a deregulated immune response to antigenic stimulation, which involves T and B lymphocytes and may lead to multiple proliferating clones (oligoclones). Some of these clones may regress spontaneously, and some may progress and transform into malignant clones. Although the current belief is that AITL generally starts de novo as a peripheral T-cell lymphoma, it is possible that in some cases AITL represents a continuum whereby atypical and oligoclonal cell proliferations correspond to a precursor or preneoplastic lesion before the development of an overt malignant lymphoma.

Still unresolved is the nature of the 11% to 25% of cases of AITL reported to lack either clonal TCR or cytogenetic abnormalities. It is currently believed that these cases may represent early stages of a lymphoma with a minor oligoclonal T-cell population. One study using single target amplification of lymphocyte receptor gene rearrangements from single T cells confirmed the CD4$^+$ T-cell phenotype of the neoplastic cells.[40] However, in those cases with no clonal TCR rearrangement identified in whole-tissue DNA analysis, the authors were unable to demonstrate any minor clonal T-cell population even at a single cell resolution. Thus, despite the molecular analysis of single cells, it is still unclear whether these cases represent a prelymphomatous state or malignant lymphoma at its inception. Gene expression profiling studies have confirmed that the neoplastic cells in AITL show features of CD4$^+$ T_{FH}.[55] Furthermore, traces of the T_{FH} signature were also identified among CD30$^-$ PTCLs, NOS, suggesting again that the morphologic spectrum of AITL may be wider than previously thought.

CLINICAL COURSE AND PROGNOSIS

The clinical course of AITL is characterized by rapid progression in most patients; however, spontaneous remissions may occur.[13,14] The median survival is less than 3 years. The majority of deaths are due to infectious complications rather than progressive lymphoma, which makes AITL particularly difficult to treat with chemotherapy. Owing to the underlying immunodeficiency and abnormalities of T-cell function, in addition to the infectious complications, patients may develop expanded EBV$^+$ clones that lead to EBV$^+$ large B-cell lymphomas in rare cases.[17,31] The clinical course appears to correlate with the extent of systemic symptoms at presentation (rash, pruritus, edema, ascites). Because 90% of patients with AITL have stage III or IV disease at presentation, staging is not very useful in predicting clinical outcome for most patients.

Outside of lymph nodes, the most common sites of involvement are bone marrow and skin. Rash is a common presenting feature in many patients. In some cases the cutaneous infiltrates may show the characteristic phenotype of AITL, with aberrant expression of CD10.[56] Clonal T-cell gene rearrangement identical to the pattern in lymph nodes also may be found.[57] However, it is unlikely that a primary diagnosis of AITL can be made based on a skin biopsy alone.

Bone marrow involvement is characterized by nonparatrabecular lymphoid aggregates with a polymorphic cellular composition similar to that seen in lymph nodes. Aberrant expression of CD10 is again useful in the diagnosis.[58] Circulating CD10$^+$ T cells may be identified in the peripheral blood by flow cytometry.[44,59-60]

AITL may be associated with marked splenomegaly, but splenectomy is not indicated; therefore, the diagnosis is uncommonly made in the spleen. Because AITL is usually a systemic disease, the characteristic infiltrates may be seen in other sites of involvement, including the liver and lung.

DIFFERENTIAL DIAGNOSIS

Although the histopathologic features of AITL are well described, there is considerable morphologic overlap with atypical T-zone hyperplasia (paracortical hyperplasia) and PTCL, NOS (Table 35-1).[9,23] Atypical T-zone hyperplasia is usually associated with viral infections or with a hyperimmune reaction secondary to an autoimmune disease. An

Table 35-1 Differential Diagnosis of Angioimmunoblastic T-Cell Lymphoma

Feature	AITL	Atypical T-Zone Hyperplasia	PTCL, NOS	Classical Hodgkin's Lymphoma
Nodal architecture	Usually effaced	Preserved	Usually effaced	Usually effaced
Clear cells	Present	Absent	Frequent	Absent
FDC proliferation	Present	Absent	Absent	Absent
HEVs	Present	Absent	Occasional	Absent
HRS cells	Rare, B-cell phenotype	Absent	Rare, T-cell phenotype	Present, B-cell phenotype
Immunophenotype	CD4$^+$, CD10$^+$, PD1$^+$, CXCL13$^+$, BCL6$^+$ CD21$^+$ FDCs, EBV$^+$ B blasts	Mixed CD4/CD8 Scattered CD20$^+$ Variable CD30$^+$	CD4 > CD8, antigen loss (CD7, CD5)	CD15$^+$, CD30$^+$, CD20$^{-/+}$, LMP-1$^{+/-}$
Genotype	TCR and IGH genes rearranged Oligoclonal pattern	No rearrangements	TCR genes rearranged	Polyclonal IGH gene rearranged in HRS cells

+, nearly always positive; –/+ may be positive, but usually negative; +/–, may be negative, but usually positive.
AITL, angioimmunoblastic T-cell lymphoma; EBV, Epstein-Barr virus; FDC, follicular dendritic cell; HEV, high endothelial venule; HRS, Hodgkin–Reed-Sternberg; IGH, immunoglobulin heavy chain; LMP-1, latent membrane protein-1; PTCL, NOS, peripheral T-cell lymphoma, not otherwise specified; TCR, T-cell receptor.

important hint to the diagnosis of atypical T-zone hyperplasia is preservation of the lymph node architecture, with the presence of follicles and germinal centers and the lack of aberrant FDC proliferation. The paracortical area is expanded with a mixed infiltrate of medium-sized and small lymphoid cells without atypia. Not infrequently, the numerous plasma cells, immunoblasts, and activated lymphocytes may mimic the cellular composition of AITL. Immunophenotypic analysis reveals a mixed CD4-CD8 population with scattered CD20$^+$ cells and variable numbers of CD25$^+$ and CD30$^+$ cells. No TCR rearrangements are identified. Moreover, CD10$^+$ cells, if present, are confined to the follicles.

The differential diagnosis between AITL and PTCL, NOS, especially the T-zone variant, can be complicated. The cellular infiltrate in these entities may be similar, including the presence of small to medium-sized cells with little or no atypia and an inflammatory polymorphic background with eosinophils, plasma cells, and epithelioid histiocytes. Prominent HEVs, clusters of clear cells, and scattered HRS-like cells may be present in both entities. Morphologic features that favor the diagnosis of AITL are open, usually distended peripheral cortical sinuses; proliferation of FDCs highlighted by CD21; and prominent arborizing endothelial venules. The presence of CD10$^+$, BCL6$^+$, CXCL13$^+$, PD1$^+$ T cells, recently reported as a specific finding in AITL, also may be observed in PTCL, NOS.[26,45,47,49,50] Occasionally the presence of numerous EBV$^+$ B cells, some of which acquire HRS-like features, may mimic Hodgkin's lymphoma.[29] These cells have the immunophenotype of HRS cells (CD15$^+$, CD30$^+$, CD20$^+$) and harbor EBV (EBER and LMP-1). Because many cases of AITL show minimal cytologic atypia of T cells, the distinction from classical Hodgkin's lymphoma may be difficult. In contrast to classical Hodgkin's lymphoma, molecular studies reveal clonal rearrangements of the *TCRγ* chain gene in AITL. Finally, owing to the frequent occurrence of randomly scattered B blasts in AITL, T-cell/histiocyte-rich large B-cell lymphoma should be included in the differential diagnosis. In T-cell/histiocyte-rich large B-cell lymphoma, the background infiltrate is not as polymorphic as in AITL, expanded meshworks of FDCs do not occur, and the B blasts are generally CD30$^-$ and EBV$^-$. Molecular biology analysis shows monoclonal immunoglobulin heavy-chain rearrangements, and no TCR gene rearrangements are identified.

Pearls and Pitfalls

- The clinical presentation of AITL is an essential diagnostic feature—localized lymphadenopathy is rare.
- Although considered a T-cell lymphoma, B-cell or plasma cell proliferation is virtually always present in affected lymph nodes.
- In early phases, reactive follicular hyperplasia may be present, mimicking a reactive process.
- Highly characteristic histologic features include the following:
  - Prominent arborizing postcapillary high endothelial venules.
  - Extension of the infiltrate beyond the lymph node capsule into the perinodal fat, frequently sparing the preserved cortical sinuses, which are dilated.
- The most helpful routine immunophenotypic tools for diagnosis are inappropriate expression of CD21 and CD10 in extrafollicular dendritic cells and T cells, respectively.
- EBV$^+$ B cells are nearly always present and may evolve to EBV$^+$ large B-cell lymphoma or a mimic of classical Hodgkin's lymphoma.

References can be found on Expert Consult @ www.expertconsult.com

Chapter 36

Anaplastic Large Cell Lymphoma, ALK Positive and ALK Negative

Georges Delsol, Laurence Lamant-Rochaix, and Pierre Brousset

CHAPTER OUTLINE

DEFINITION AND BACKGROUND

Among the heterogeneous group of hematopoietic neoplasms with a predominant population of large cells, Stein and coworkers[1] recognized a subgroup of tumors with large cells exhibiting bizarre morphologic features and prominent sinusoidal invasion and expressing the Ki-1 antigen (now referred to as *CD30*). Based on the strong expression of this molecule, these tumors were designated *Ki-1 lymphoma*.[1] Because of the lack of strict morphologic criteria, some tumors were diagnosed as Ki-1 lymphoma simply because they consisted of large cells positive for the CD30 antigen, whatever their B-, T-, or null cell phenotype. Later, the term *Ki-1 lymphoma* was replaced by *anaplastic large cell lymphoma*. Although there was no clear consensus among pathologists with regard to the definition of *anaplastic*, and despite the fact that some of these tumors consist of small to medium-sized cells, the term *anaplastic large cell lymphoma* (ALCL) was incorporated into most classifications. Later it was discovered that a significant proportion of ALCLs are associated with the t(2;5)(p23;q35) translocation.[2] A major advance was made with the cloning of this translocation[3] and the production of antibodies detecting its gene product—anaplastic lymphoma kinase (ALK).[4] As a consequence, ALCLs were divided in two main categories—those positive for ALK protein and those lacking this marker. In the third edition of the World Health Organization (WHO) classification of hematopoietic neoplasms, ALK$^+$ and ALK$^-$ ALCLs were considered a single disease entity and were defined as lymphomas consisting of lymphoid cells that are usually large and have abundant cytoplasm and pleomorphic, often horseshoe-shaped nuclei.[5] The cells are CD30$^+$, and most cases express cytotoxic granule-associated proteins[6,7] and epithelial membrane antigen (EMA).[8] It became clear that although ALCLs expressing ALK are relatively homogeneous, cases with similar morphology and phenotype but lacking ALK expression are much more heterogeneous. ALCLs lacking ALK also differ from peripheral T-cell lymphomas, not otherwise specified (PTCL, NOS). In the fourth edition of the WHO classification, ALCL, ALK$^+$ is a distinct entity, and ALCL without ALK expression is a provisional entity. Primary systemic ALCL, both ALK$^+$ and ALK$^-$, must be distinguished from the primary cutaneous type of ALCL and from other

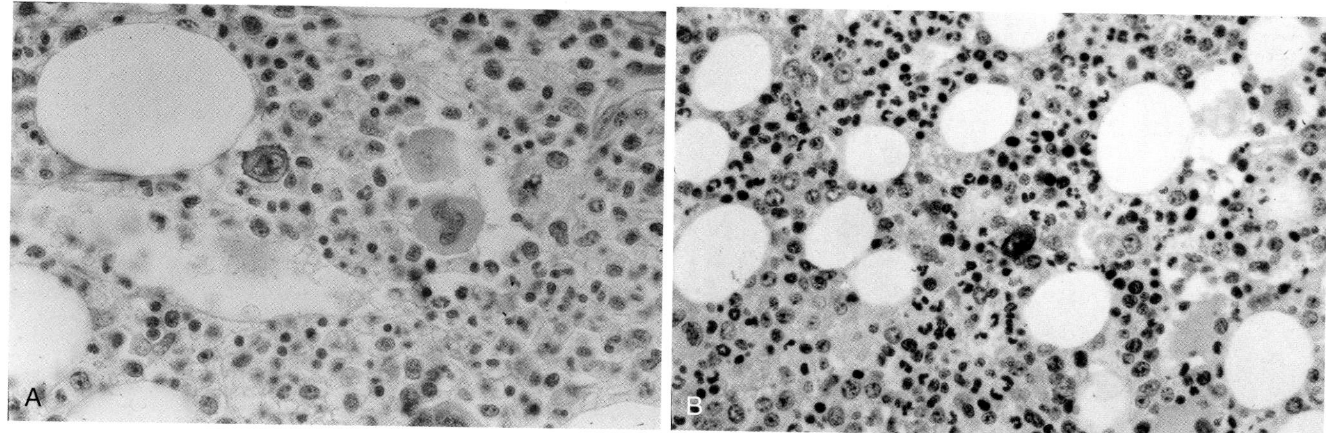

Figure 36-1. Although the bone marrow biopsy was considered to be uninvolved on standard histopathologic examination, immunohistochemistry shows scattered malignant cells strongly positive for CD30/Ber-H2 (**A**) and ALK1 antibody (**B**).

subtypes of T- or B-cell lymphoma with anaplastic features or CD30 expression.[9]

ANAPLASTIC LARGE CELL LYMPHOMA, ALK POSITIVE

Epidemiology

ALCL accounts for 5% of all non-Hodgkin's lymphomas and 10% to 30% of childhood lymphomas.[10] ALK$^+$ ALCL is most frequent in the first 3 decades of life and shows a slight male predominance.[11,12]

Etiology

No pathogenic factor has been demonstrated. However, in rare cases, an association with recent insect bites has been suggested.[13,13a] Occasional cases occur in human immunodeficiency virus (HIV)–positive patients or after solid organ transplantation.[14]

Clinical Features

The majority of patients (70%) with systemic ALCL present with advanced stage III to IV disease with peripheral or abdominal lymphadenopathy, often associated with extranodal infiltrates and involvement of the bone marrow.[10,12] Patients often show B symptoms (75%), especially high fever.[10,12,15] Several cases with a leukemic presentation have been reported.[16-18]

Primary systemic ALCL positive for the ALK protein frequently involves both lymph nodes and extranodal sites. Extranodal sites commonly include skin (26%), bone (14%), soft tissues (15%), lung (11%), and liver (8%).[10,12,15] Retinal infiltration responsible for blindness and placental involvement have also been reported.[19] Involvement of the gut and central nervous system is rare. However, occasional cases of primary ALCL in the stomach, bladder, or central nervous system have been observed[20] (authors' unpublished observations). Mediastinal disease is less frequent than in Hodgkin's lymphoma. The incidence of bone marrow involvement is approximately 10% when analyzed with hematoxylin-eosin but increases significantly (30%) when immunohistochemical stains for CD30, EMA, or ALK are used (Fig. 36-1).[21] This is due to the fact that bone marrow involvement is often subtle, with only scattered malignant cells that are difficult to detect by routine examination. Most patients have circulating antibodies against nucleophosmin (NPM)-ALK protein, and these antibodies may persist in patients who are apparently in complete remission.[22]

Morphology

The morphologic features of ALCL are wider than was initially described,[1] ranging from small cell neoplasms, which many pathologists might categorize as pleomorphic T-cell lymphomas, to tumors in which very large cells predominate.[11]

ALCLs positive for the ALK protein exhibit a broad morphologic spectrum.[11,23-27] However, all cases contain a variable proportion of large cells with eccentric horseshoe- or kidney-shaped nuclei, often with an eosinophilic region near the nucleus. These cells have been referred to as *hallmark cells* (Fig. 36-2A) because they are present in all morphologic patterns.[11] Although the hallmark cells are typically large, smaller cells with similar cytologic features may be seen and can greatly aid in making the diagnosis.[11] Depending on the plane of the section, some cells may appear to contain cytoplasmic inclusions. These are not true inclusions, however, but invaginations of the nuclear membrane. Cells with these features have been referred to as *donut cells* (see Fig. 36-2A).[28,29] In some cases the nuclei are round to oval, and the proliferation appears quite monomorphic (see Fig. 36-7A).

The tumor cells have more abundant cytoplasm than most other lymphomas. The cytoplasm may appear clear, basophilic, or eosinophilic. On lymph node imprints these cells show vacuolated cytoplasm (see Fig. 36-2B). Multiple nuclei may occur in a wreath-like pattern, giving rise to cells resembling Reed-Sternberg cells. The nuclear chromatin is usually finely clumped or dispersed, with multiple small basophilic nucleoli. Prominent inclusion-like nucleoli are relatively uncommon, aiding in the differential diagnosis with Hodgkin's lymphoma.[30]

ALCLs exhibit a very broad range of cytological appearances.[11,30,31] Five morphologic patterns are recognized in the fourth edition of the WHO classification.[32]

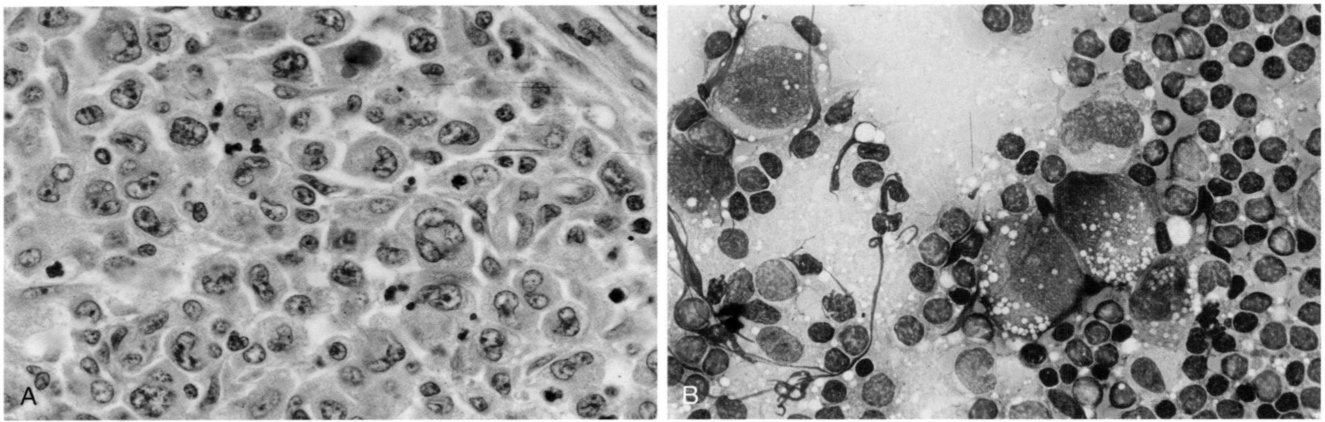

Figure 36-2. Anaplastic large cell lymphoma, common pattern. A, Predominant population of large cells with irregular nuclei. Note the large "hallmark" cells with eccentric kidney-shaped nuclei. One "donut" cell can be seen in this field. **B,** Lymph node imprint preparation shows lymphoma cells with vacuolated cytoplasm.

Anaplastic Large Cell Lymphoma, Common Pattern

ALCL, common pattern (70%) is composed predominantly of pleomorphic large cells with the hallmark features described earlier. Tumor cells with more monomorphic, rounded nuclei also occur, either as the predominant population or mixed with the more pleomorphic cells. Rarely, erythrophagocytosis by malignant cells may be seen. When the lymph node architecture is only partially effaced, the tumor characteristically grows within the sinuses and thus may resemble a metastatic tumor (Fig. 36-3). Tumor cells may also colonize the paracortex and often grow in a cohesive manner (Fig. 36-4).

Anaplastic Large Cell Lymphoma, Lymphohistiocytic Pattern

ALCL, lymphohistiocytic pattern (10%) is characterized by tumor cells admixed with a large number of histiocytes (Fig. 36-5A to C).[11,25,33,34] The histiocytes may mask the malignant cells, which are often smaller than in the common pattern (see Fig. 36-5D). The neoplastic cells often cluster around blood vessels and can be highlighted by immunostaining using antibodies to CD30 (see Fig. 36-5E and F), ALK, or cytotoxic molecules. Occasionally the histiocytes show signs of erythrophagocytosis. The histiocytes typically have finely granular eosinophilic cytoplasm and small, round uniform nuclei. Well-formed granulomas are absent, and clusters of epithelioid cells (as may be seen in the lymphoepitheloid cell variant of PTCL, NOS) are not seen.

Anaplastic Large Cell Lymphoma, Small Cell Pattern

ALCL, small cell pattern (10%) shows a predominant population of small to medium-sized neoplastic cells with irregular nuclei (Fig. 36-6A to C).[11,24,28] However, morphologic features vary from case to case, and cells with round nuclei and clear cytoplasm ("fried egg" cells) may predominate. Hallmark cells are always present and are often concentrated around blood vessels (see Fig. 36-6D).[11] Usually there is massive infiltration of the perinodal connective tissue. This morphologic variant of ALCL is often misdiagnosed as PTCL, NOS by conventional examination. When the blood is involved, atypical cells reminiscent of flower-like cells may be observed in smear prepa-

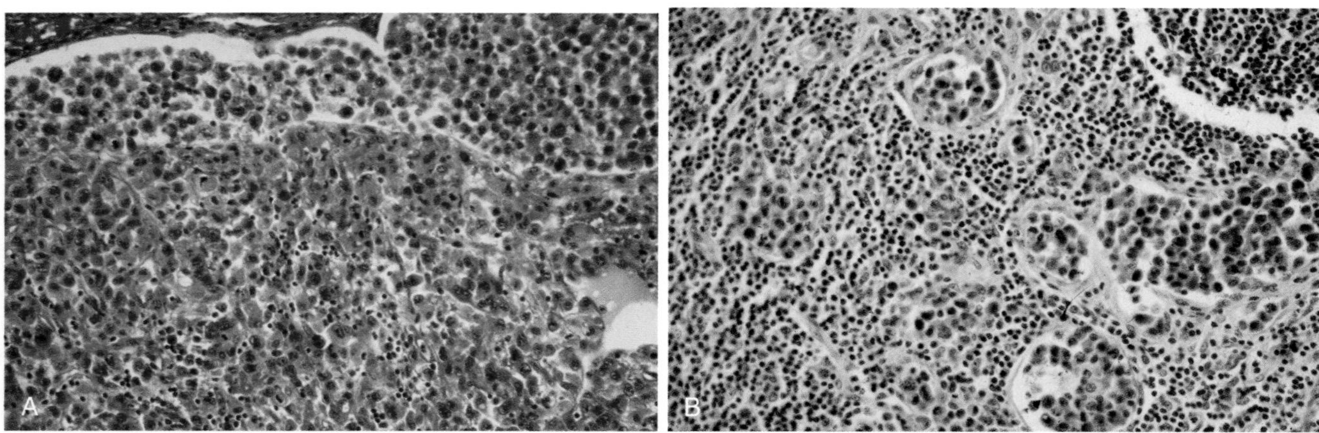

Figure 36-3. General features of anaplastic large cell lymphoma, common pattern. A, The lymph node architecture is obliterated by malignant cells, and intrasinusoidal cells are observed. **B,** In some cases the predominant sinusoidal growth pattern mimics a metastatic malignancy.

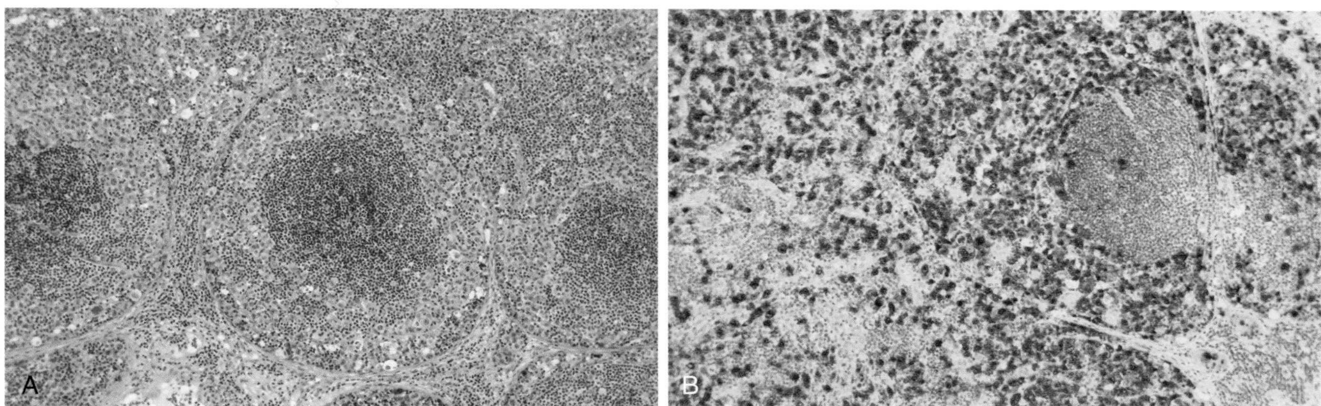

Figure 36-4. Anaplastic large cell lymphoma, common pattern. A, Classic case with a predominant perifollicular and paracortical pattern on hematoxylin-eosin stain. **B,** ALK1 staining.

rations.[16,17] It is likely that the small cell and lymphohistiocytic patterns are closely related.[9,29]

Anaplastic Large Cell Lymphoma, Hodgkin-Like Pattern

ALCL, Hodgkin-like pattern (1% to 3%) is characterized by morphologic features mimicking nodular sclerosis classical Hodgkin's lymphoma.[35] These cases show a vaguely nodular fibrosis associated with capsular thickening and a significant number of tumor cells resembling classic Reed-Sternberg cells associated with hallmark cells (see Fig. 36-7E). In the past, many tumors with similar features were referred to as *Hodgkin-like ALCL*. However, most cases designated as such were negative for ALK and were more likely variants of classical Hodgkin's lymphoma rich in Hodgkin cells or lymphomas with features intermediate between Hodgkin's lymphoma and diffuse large B-cell lymphoma—so-called gray zone lymphomas.[29,36] It must be stressed that CD30$^+$ lymphomas, with or without a sinusoidal growth pattern, should not be diagnosed as ALCL, Hodgkin-like unless they are positive for ALK. In cases negative for ALK protein, additional immunophenotypic and molecular studies usually permit their classification as aggressive B-cell or T-cell lymphomas, including the new WHO category of B-cell lymphoma, unclassifiable, with features intermediate between diffuse large B-cell lymphoma and classical Hodgkin's lymphoma.[37]

Anaplastic Large Cell Lymphoma, Composite Pattern

ALCL with a composite pattern accounts for 10% to 20% of cases. These cases have features of more than one pattern in a single lymph node biopsy. In addition, in some cases, a repeat biopsy taken at the time of relapse may reveal morphologic features that differ from those seen initially, suggesting that the morphologic patterns of ALCL are simply variations of the same entity.[11,24]

Other Histologic Patterns

Other histologic patterns may be seen, although they are not recognized as distinctive patterns in the WHO classification. They are often responsible for diagnostic difficulties. These include a giant cell–rich pattern (Fig. 36-7B), a sarcomatoid pattern (see Fig. 36-7C), and a "signet ring"–like pattern (see Fig. 36-7D). Some ALCLs may mimic a metastatic malignancy, with cohesive neoplastic cells encased within a dense fibrosis (see Fig. 36-7F). Some ALCLs may show a striking edematous or myxoid background, either focally or throughout the whole tissue section (see Fig. 36-7G). Tumors with such a morphology have been reported as hypocellular ALCL.[38] A "starry sky" appearance may also be observed, suggesting Burkitt's lymphoma on low-power magnification.

Immunophenotype

By definition, all ALCLs are positive for CD30. In most cases, virtually all neoplastic cells show strong CD30 staining on the cell membrane and in the Golgi region (Fig. 36-8A). In the small cell variant, the strongest immunostaining is seen in the large cells; smaller tumor cells may be only weakly positive or even negative for CD30.[11] In the lymphohistiocytic and small cell patterns, the strongest CD30 expression is also present in the larger tumor cells, which often cluster around blood vessels (see Figs. 36-5F and 36-6D).[11] The majority of ALCLs are positive for EMA.[8,11] The staining pattern for EMA is usually similar to that seen with CD30, although in some cases only a proportion of malignant cells is positive (see Fig. 36-8B).

The great majority of ALCLs express one or more T-cell or natural killer (NK)-cell antigens.[10,11,39] However, owing to the loss of several pan–T-cell antigens, some cases may have an apparent null-cell phenotype. Because no other distinctions can be found in cases with a T-cell versus null-cell phenotype, T/null ALCL is considered a single entity.[11,40] CD3, the most widely used pan–T-cell marker, is negative in more than 75% of cases.[11] This tendency for loss of CD3 is also seen in ALK$^-$ ALCL. CD5 and CD7 are often negative as well. CD2 and CD4 are more useful and are positive in a significant proportion of cases. CD43 is expressed in more than two thirds of cases, but this antigen lacks lineage specificity' (see Fig. 36-8C). Furthermore, most cases exhibit positivity for the cytotoxic-associated antigens TIA-1, granzyme B, and perforin (see Fig. 36-8D and E).[6,7] CD8 is usually negative, but rare CD8$^+$ cases exist. Occasional cases are positive for CD68/KP1 but not CD68/PGM1.

Tumor cells are variably positive for CD45 and CD45RO but strongly positive for CD25.[8] Blood group antigens H and

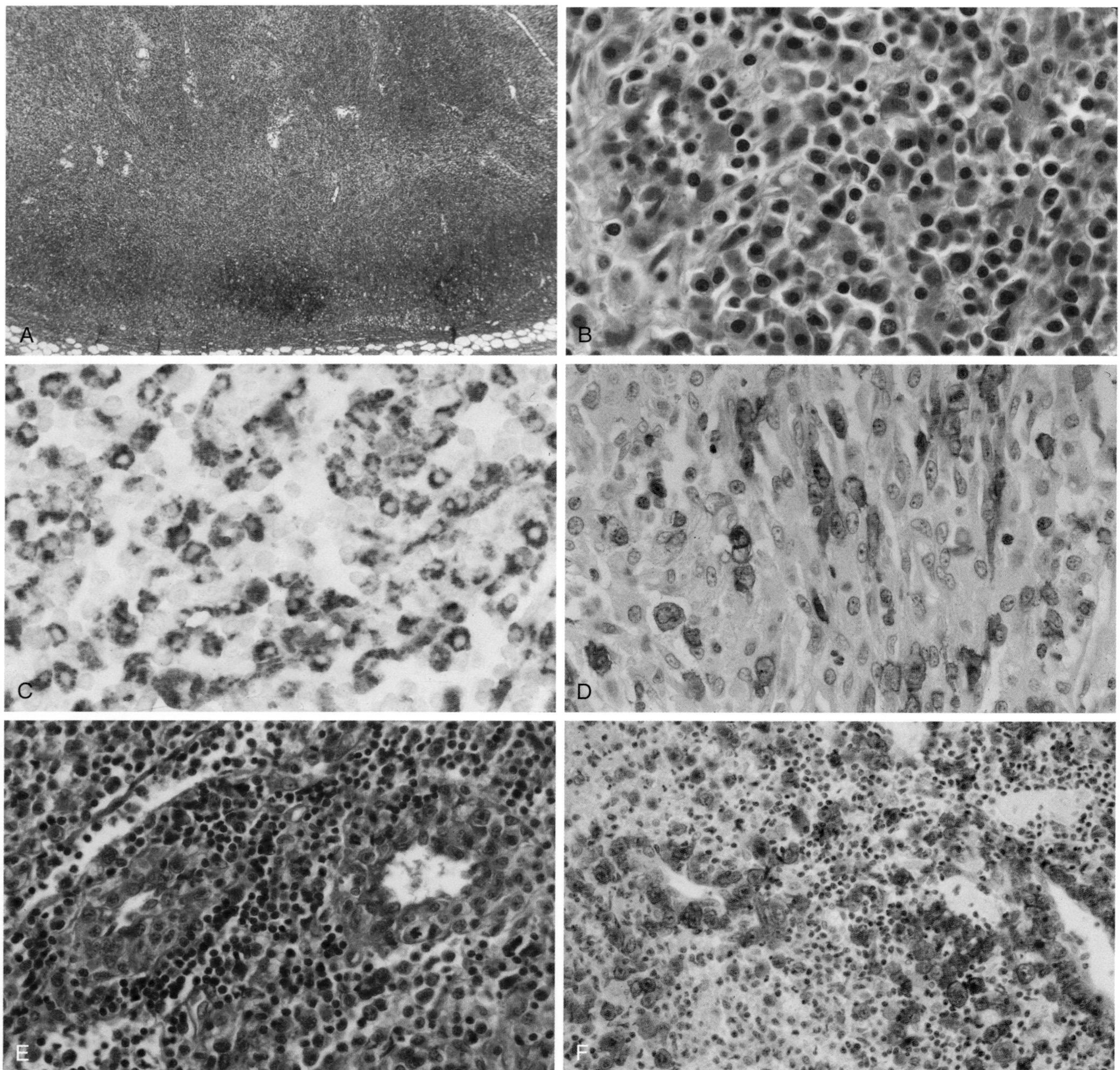

Figure 36-5. Anaplastic large cell lymphoma (ALCL), lymphohistiocytic pattern. A, At low power the infiltrate is mainly paracortical in distribution. **B**, On a high-power view, malignant cells are admixed with a predominant population of nonneoplastic histiocytes. The malignant cells may be extremely rare and difficult to detect on hematoxylin-eosin stain. **C**, Double immunostaining with CD68/KP1 (*brown*) and ALK1 (*blue*) confirms the paucity of malignant cells (blue nuclear staining). **D**, CD30 staining shows that the malignant cells vary in size, with some exhibiting a fibroblast-like morphology. **E** and **F**, Characteristically, the neoplastic cells often cluster around blood vessels and can be highlighted by immunostaining using antibodies to CD30. Such a perivascular pattern is also observed in ALCL, small cell variant.

Y (detected with antibody BNH.9) have been reported in more than 50% of cases (see Fig. 36-8F).[41] CD15 expression is rarely observed, and when present, only a small proportion of neoplastic cells is stained.[11] ALCLs are consistently negative for Epstein-Barr virus (EBV) (i.e., EBV-encoded small RNA [EBER] and latent membrane protein-1 [LMP-1]).[42] A study employing array technology to detect new genes expressed in ALCL found that clusterin is aberrantly expressed in all cases of systemic ALCL but not in primary cutaneous ALCL.[43] Most ALK$^+$ ALCLs are negative for BCL2 (see Fig. 36-8G).[44] A number of other antigens are expressed in ALCL, but they are not of diagnostic value. They include CD56[45-47]; SHP1 phosphatase[48]; BCL6, C/EBPβ, and serpinA1[49,50]; myeloid-associated antigens CD13 and CD33[51]; and p63.[52]

The ALK staining may be cytoplasmic, nuclear, and nucleolar, or it may be restricted to either the cytoplasm or, more rarely, the cell membrane (Fig. 36-9). ALK expression is virtually specific for ALCL because it is absent from all normal

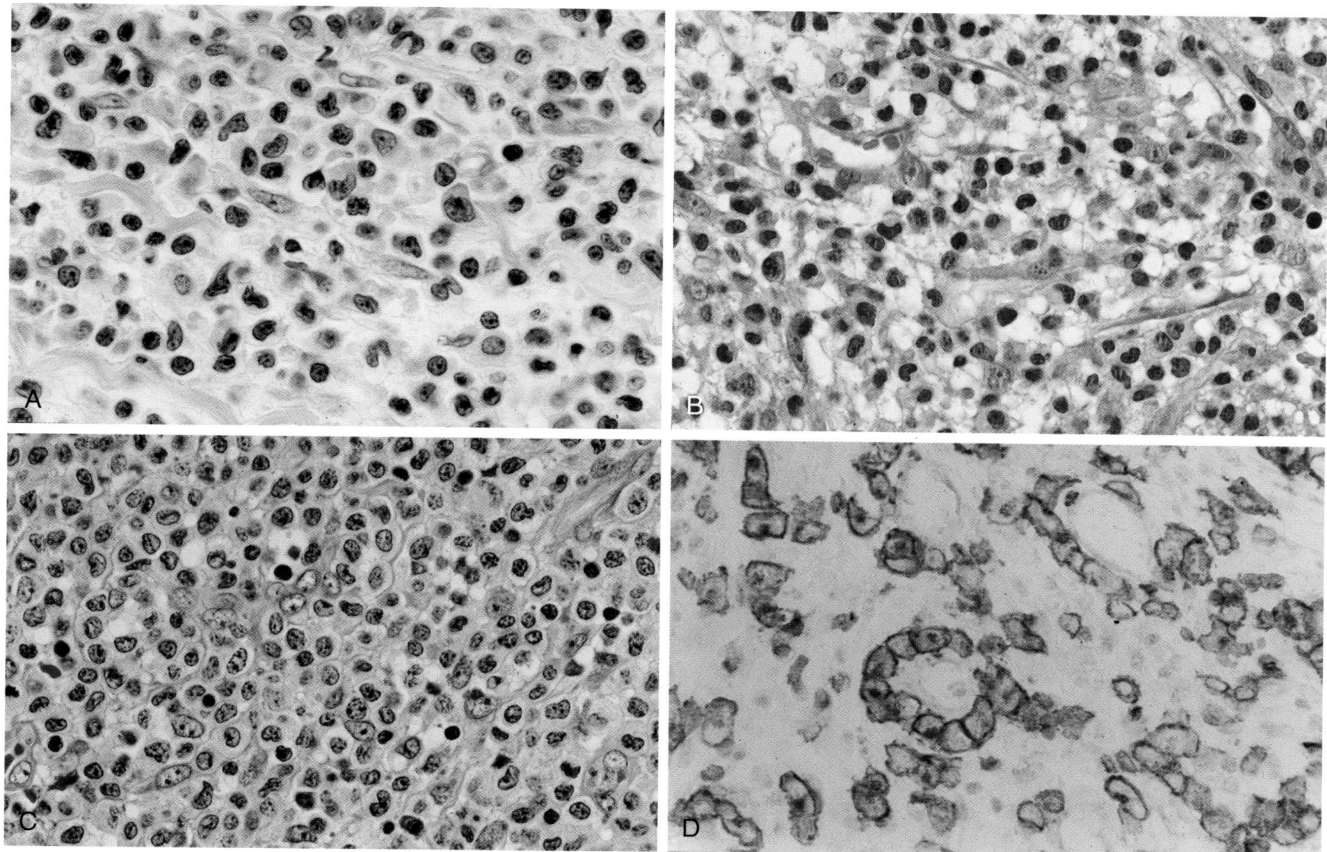

Figure 36-6. Anaplastic large cell lymphoma, small cell variant. A and B, Predominant population of small cells with irregular nuclei associated with scattered "hallmark" cells with kidney-shaped nuclei. **C,** This case exhibits a monomorphic population of small cells with clear cytoplasm ("fried egg" cells). **D,** In most cases the neoplastic cells are perivascular, a pattern that is highlighted by CD30 staining. Note that the large cells are strongly positive for CD30, whereas the small and medium-sized malignant cells are only weakly stained.

postnatal human tissues except for rare cells in the brain.[53] It is also absent from human lymphoid neoplasms other than ALCL, with the exception of ALK$^+$ large B-cell lymphomas (see Fig. 36-11)[54] and a novel form of ALK$^+$ histiocytosis seen in infancy.[55] It is important to note that in the small cell pattern and, to a lesser extent, in the lymphohistiocytic pattern, ALK staining may be restricted to scattered large cells. However, ALK staining performed without a nuclear counterstain reveals a large population of small cells showing restricted nuclear staining.

Genetics and Molecular Findings

Approximately 90% of ALCLs show clonal rearrangement of the T-cell receptor genes, irrespective of whether they express T-cell antigens.[6] The majority of ALCLs are associated with a reciprocal translocation, t(2;5)(p23;q35), which juxtaposes the gene at 5q35 encoding NPM, a nucleolar-associated phosphoprotein, with the gene at 2p23 coding for ALK, a receptor tyrosine kinase.[3,56] Polyclonal and monoclonal antibodies recognizing the intracellular portion of ALK react with both NPM-ALK protein and the full-length ALK protein, but no normal lymphoid cells express full-length ALK; as a consequence, immunostaining with anti-ALK has been used to detect ALCL cases carrying the t(2;5) translocation.[3,53,57] However, variant translocations involving *ALK* and other partner genes on chromosomes 1, 2, 3, 17, 19, and 22 also occur (Table 36-1).[37,58-65] All result in the upregulation of *ALK*, but the distribution of the staining varies, depending on the translocation. Classic t(2;5) leads to positive staining for ALK in the nucleolus, nucleus, and cytoplasm (see Fig. 36-9A and B).[66] In the variant translocations, often only cytoplasmic staining is observed (see Fig. 36-9C to E). In t(2;5)(p23;q35), the particular cytoplasmic, nuclear, and nucleolar staining can be explained by the formation of dimers between wild-type NPM and the fusion NPM-ALK protein. Wild-type NPM provides nuclear localization signals whereby the NPM-ALK protein can enter the nucleus.[66,67] The formation of NPM-ALK homodimers using dimerization sites at the N-terminus of NPM mimics ligand binding and is responsible for activation of the *ALK* catalytic domain (i.e., autophosphorylation of the tyrosine kinase domain of *ALK*), which is responsible for its oncogenic properties.

Besides t(2;5), at least 11 variant translocations involving the *ALK* gene at p23 have been recognized. In all these translocations the *ALK* gene is placed under the control of the promoter of genes that are constitutively expressed in lymphoid cells—hence the *ALK* gene expression. The most frequent variant translocation is t(1;2)(q25;p23),[59,60] in which the *TPM3* gene on chromosome 1 (which encodes a nonmuscular tropomyosin protein)[59] is fused to the *ALK* catalytic

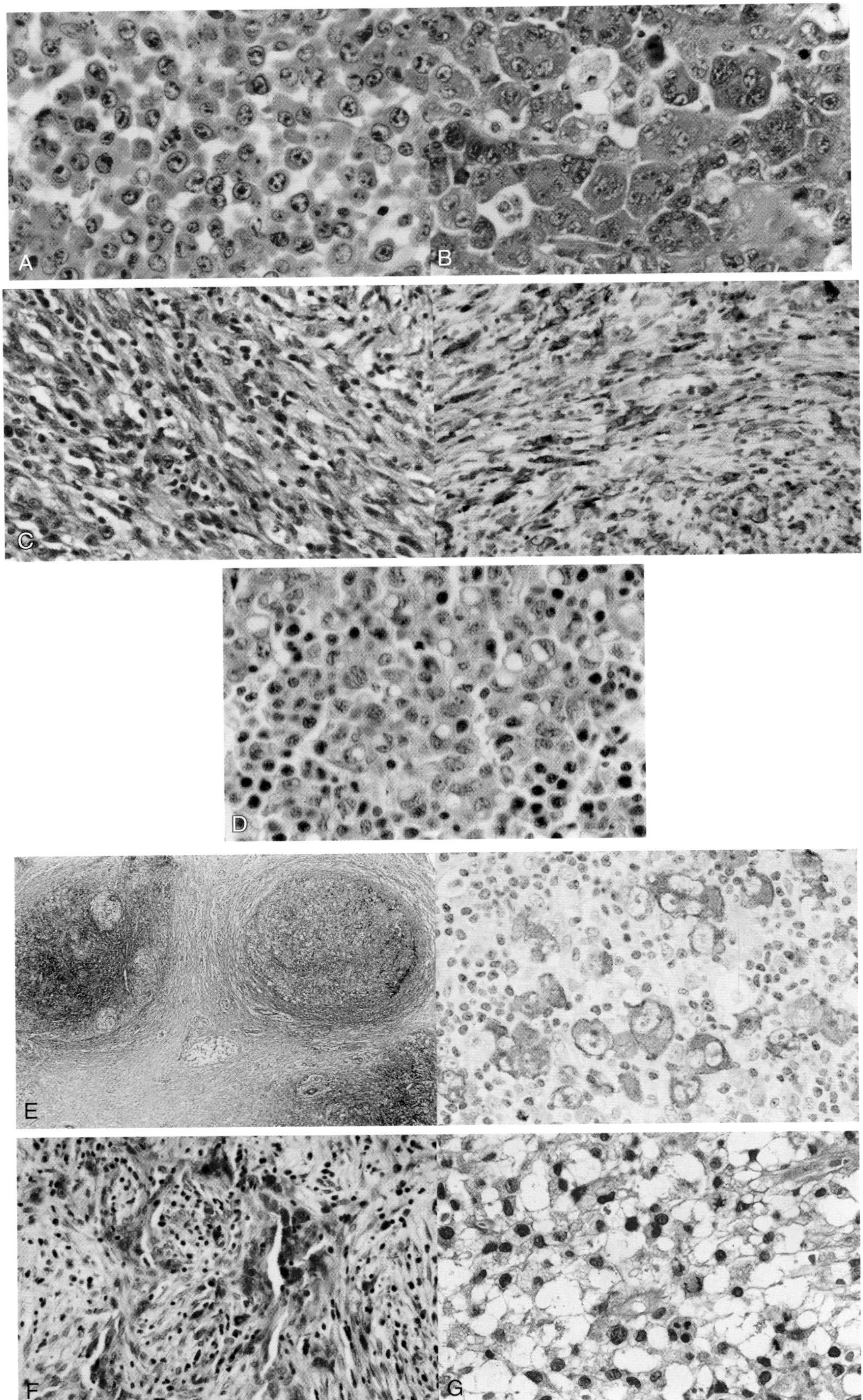

Figure 36-7. Other histologic patterns of anaplastic large cell lymphoma (ALCL). All these cases were positive for anaplastic lymphoma kinase (ALK) protein. **A**, ALCL exhibits monomorphic large cells with round nuclei. **B**, ALCL consisting of pleomorphic giant cells. **C**, ALCL with sarcomatous features (left: hematoxylin-eosin; right: CD30 staining). **D**, ALCL rich in "signet ring" cells. **E**, ALCL mimicking nodular sclerosis classical Hodgkin's lymphoma (left: hematoxylin-eosin; right: ALK staining). Cases of ALCL with this morphology are extremely rare. **F**, ALCL mimicking a metastatic malignancy. **G**, ALCL with edematous stroma. Tumors showing this morphology have been reported as hypocellular ALCL. (**G**, Courtesy of Dr. J. K. C. Chan, Hong Kong.)

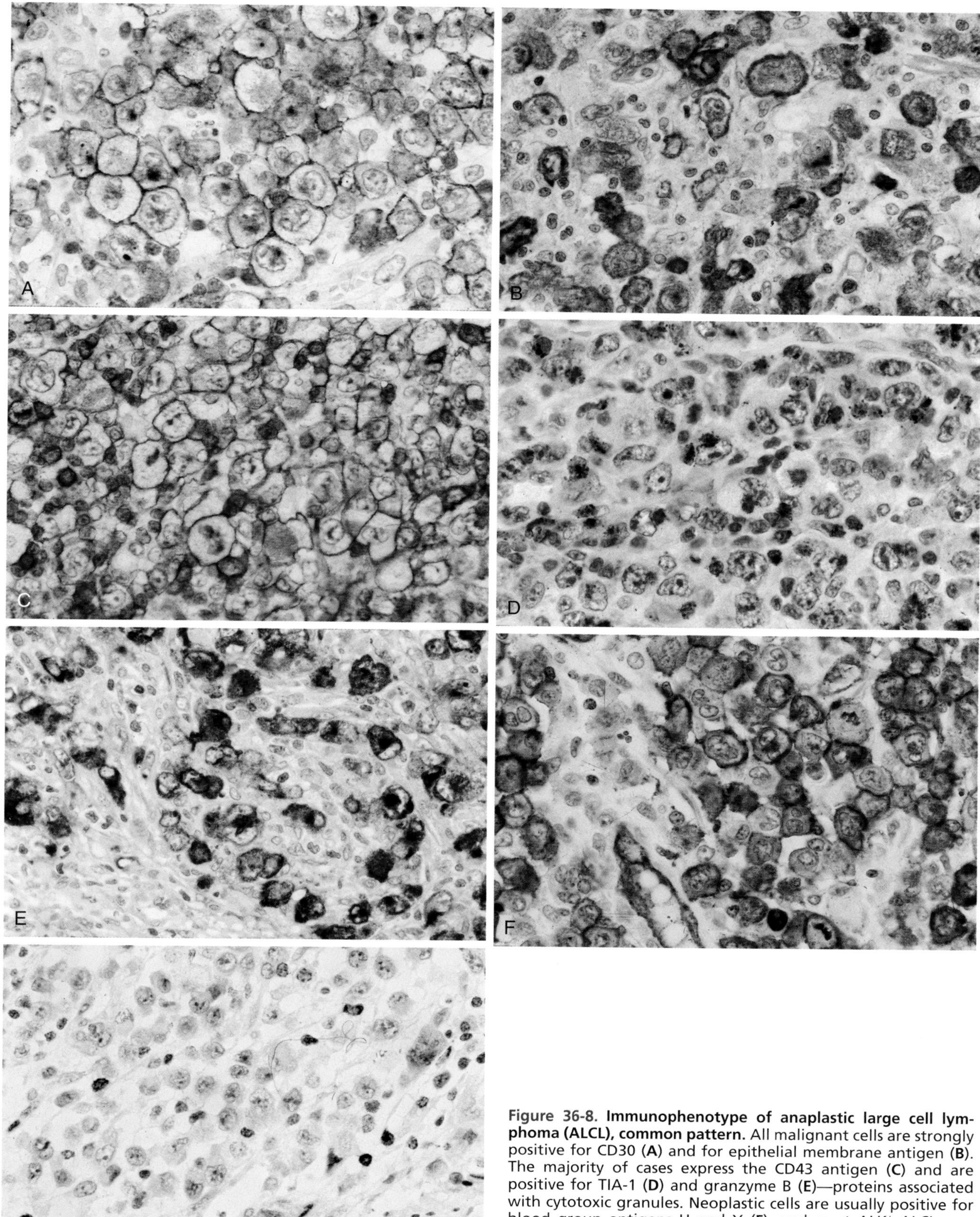

Figure 36-8. Immunophenotype of anaplastic large cell lymphoma (ALCL), common pattern. All malignant cells are strongly positive for CD30 (**A**) and for epithelial membrane antigen (**B**). The majority of cases express the CD43 antigen (**C**) and are positive for TIA-1 (**D**) and granzyme B (**E**)—proteins associated with cytotoxic granules. Neoplastic cells are usually positive for blood group antigens H and Y (**F**), and most ALK$^+$ ALCLs are negative for BCL2 (**G**). Note the positive small lymphocytes used as internal controls.

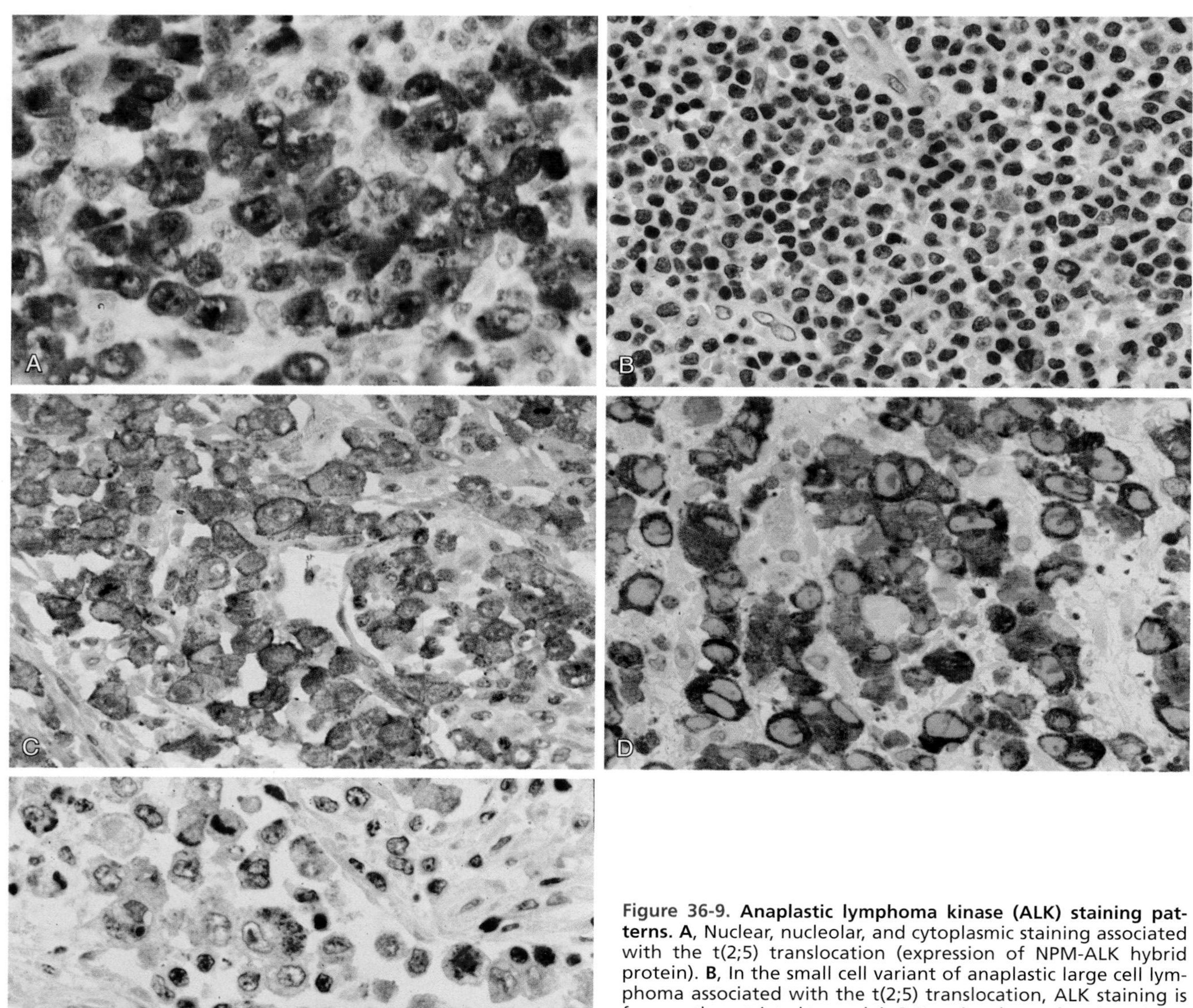

Figure 36-9. Anaplastic lymphoma kinase (ALK) staining patterns. A, Nuclear, nucleolar, and cytoplasmic staining associated with the t(2;5) translocation (expression of NPM-ALK hybrid protein). **B,** In the small cell variant of anaplastic large cell lymphoma associated with the t(2;5) translocation, ALK staining is frequently restricted to nuclei. **C,** Restricted cytoplasmic staining with enhanced membrane staining in a case associated with the t(1;2) translocation (expression of TPM3-ALK hybrid protein). **D,** Diffuse cytoplasmic staining in a case associated with the inv(2)(p23q35) (expression of ATIC-ALK). **E,** Finely granular cytoplasmic staining associated with the t(2;17) translocation (expression of CLTC-ALK hybrid protein).

domain. However, in cases associated with the t(1;2) translocation, which express the TPM3-ALK protein (104 kDa), ALK staining is restricted to the cytoplasm of malignant cells, and in virtually all cases there is stronger staining on the cell membrane (see Fig. 36-9C).[53,59] This staining pattern is found in 15% to 20% of ALK$^+$ ALCLs. Tropomyosins are known to form dimeric alpha-coiled coil structures that can induce dimerization of the chimeric TPM3-ALK protein and activation of the *ALK* catalytic domain (i.e., autophosphorylation of ALK protein).[59] The genes fused with *ALK* in t(2;3)(p23;q11)[58,60] and inv(2)(p23q35)[62,63] have recently been identified (see Fig. 36-9D). Two different fusion proteins of 85 and 97 kDa (TFG-ALK$_{short}$ and TFG-ALK$_{long}$) are associated with t(2;3)(p23;q11), which involves *TFG* (TRK-fused gene).[58] The inv(2)(p23q35) involves the *ATIC* gene (formerly known as *pur-H*), which encodes 5-aminomidazole-4-carboxamide-ribonucleotide transformylase-IMP cyclohydrolase (ATIC), which plays a key role in the de novo purine biosynthesis pathways.[62] In TFG-ALK$^+$ and ATIC-ALK$^+$ ALCLs, ALK staining is restricted to the cytoplasm in a diffuse pattern.[58,62]

Rare cases of ALCL show a unique granular ALK cytoplasmic staining pattern (see Fig. 36-9E).[61] In these cases, the *ALK* gene is fused to the *CLTC* gene, which encodes the clathrin heavy polypeptide (CLTC) that is the main structural protein of coated vesicles. The sequence of the fusion gene suggests that these tumors might have reciprocal translocations involving breakpoints at 17q11-qter and 2p23. In *CLTC-ALK*$^+$ ALCL, the implication of the clathrin heavy polypeptide in the hybrid protein accounts for the granular cytoplasmic staining pattern because the CLTC-ALK protein is involved in

Table 36-1 Genetic Abnormalities in ALK-Positive Lymphoma That Create Fusion Genes

Chromosomal Anomaly	*ALK* Partner	Molecular Weight of ALK Hybrid Protein	ALK Staining Pattern	Percentage*
t(2;5)(p23;q35)	*NPM*	80	Nuclear, diffuse cytoplasmic	84
t(1;2)(q25;p23)	*TPM3*	104	Diffuse cytoplasmic with peripheral intensification	13
inv(2)(p23q35)	*ATIC*	96	Diffuse cytoplasmic	1
t(2;3)(p23;q11)	TFG_{Xlong}	113	Diffuse cytoplasmic	<1
	TFG_{long}	97	Diffuse cytoplasmic	
	TFG_{short}	85	Diffuse cytoplasmic	
t(2;17)(p23;q23)	*CLTC*	250	Granular cytoplasmic	<1
t(2; X)(p23;q11-12)	*MSN*	125	Membrane staining	<1
t(2;19)(p23;p13.1)	*TPM4*	95	Diffuse cytoplasmic	<1
t(2;22)(p23;q11.2)	*MYH9*	220	Diffuse cytoplasmic	<1
t(2;17)(p23;q25)	*ALO17*	ND	Diffuse cytoplasmic	<1
Others†	?	?	Nuclear or cytoplasmic	<1

* Percentage of these variants in an unpublished series of 270 cases of ALK⁺ ALCL.
†Unpublished series of 270 cases of ALK⁺ ALCL.
ALCL, anaplastic large cell lymphoma; ALK, anaplastic lymphoma kinase; ND, not determined.

the formation of the clathrin coat on the surface of vesicles. Moreover, the process of clathrin coat formation mimics ligand binding; this allows the autophosphorylation of the carboxy-terminal domain of ALK protein, which is probably responsible for its oncogenic property.[61] In a single report, the moesin (*MSN*) gene at chromosome Xq11-12 was identified as a new *ALK* fused gene (MSN-ALK fusion protein) in a case of ALCL with a distinct ALK membrane-restricted pattern.[68] The particular membrane staining pattern of ALK is probably due to the binding properties of the N-terminal domain of moesin to cell membrane–associated proteins. In this case, the *ALK* breakpoint was different from that described in all other translocations and occurred within the exonic sequence coding for the juxtamembrane portion of ALK. In the recently reported translocation of dicentric (2;4)(p23;q33), the *ALK* partner was not identified.[69]

In a recent study, the supervised analysis by class comparison between ALK⁺ and ALK⁻ ALCL tumors provided distinct molecular signatures.[49] Among the 117 genes overexpressed in ALK⁺ ALCL, *BCL6, PTPN12* (tyrosine phosphatase), *serpinA1*, and *C/EBPβ* are the four overexpressed genes with the most significant *P* values.

Clinical Course and Prognostic Factors

The International Prognostic Index appears to be of some value in predicting outcome, although less so than in other types of lymphoma.[27,70] Overall, in multivariate analysis, three prognostic factors remain significant: mediastinal involvement, visceral involvement (defined as lung, liver, or spleen involvement), and skin lesions.[15] The most important prognostic indicator is ALK positivity, which has been associated with a favorable prognosis in series from North America, Europe, and Japan.[4,70,71] No differences have been found between NPM-ALK⁺ tumors and tumors showing variant translocations involving *ALK* and fusion partners other than *NPM*.[71] The overall 5-year survival of ALK⁺ ALCL varies from 70% to 80%, in contrast to less than 50% in ALK⁻ cases.[72] Relapses are not uncommon (30% of cases), but they often remain sensitive to chemotherapy.[73] Quantitative polymerase chain reaction for NPM-ALK in bone marrow and peripheral blood at diagnosis could identify patients at risk of relapse.[74]

ANAPLASTIC LARGE CELL LYMPHOMA, ALK NEGATIVE

ALK⁻ ALCL is less well characterized than the ALK⁺ type, and it is controversial whether tumors with morphologic and phenotypic features consistent with ALCL but negative for ALK should be considered a phenotypic variant of systemic ALCL or a different entity. We have no clear phenotypic or molecular markers to definitively answer this question. The clinical course of ALK⁺ compared with ALK⁻ ALCL suggests that the latter represents a different, possibly heterogeneous entity. However, there are also clinical data suggesting that ALK⁻ ALCL has a better prognosis than PTCL, NOS.[72] Some experienced pathologists think that ALK⁻ ALCL should simply be considered an anaplastic variant of PTCL, NOS, in light of its poor prognosis and partially overlapping phenotype.[29,75-77]

Definition

In the fourth edition of the WHO classification, ALK⁻ ALCL is a provisional entity defined as "a neoplasm that is not reproducibly distinguishable on morphological grounds from ALK-positive ALCL."[78] Lymphoma cells are uniformly positive for CD30 and express a T or null phenotype; a significant proportion of cases is positive for cytotoxic granule-associated proteins.

Epidemiology

Unlike ALK⁺ ALCL, the peak incidence of ALK⁻ ALCL is in adults (40 to 65 years),[10,77] with no clear male or female preponderance. Occasional cases have been reported in women with silicone breast prostheses placed for cosmetic reasons.[79] These tumors are localized to the seroma cavity, and appear to have an excellent prognosis with a low risk of spread. They probably constitute a distinct entity.[79a]

Clinical Features

Patients present with peripheral or abdominal lymphadenopathy or extranodal tumor; however, extranodal involvement is less common than in ALK^{+} ALCL.[10] Skin involvement must be distinguished from primary cutaneous ALCL; in a case with only cutaneous involvement, the presumptive diagnosis is primary cutaneous ALCL.

Morphology

Like ALK^{+} ALCL, ALK^{-} ALCL exhibits a broad spectrum of morphologic features. On morphologic grounds alone, some cases are strictly similar to ALCL, common pattern, including "hallmark" cells that typically grow within sinuses (Fig. 36-10A). Other cases consist of more pleomorphic cells with a high nuclear-to-cytoplasmic ratio (see Fig. 36-10B and C).[4,27,30,80] Morphologic features suggestive of aggressive classical Hodgkin's lymphoma (grade 2 nodular sclerosis or lymphocyte depleted) but not supported by immunophenotype may be observed. Of note, cases corresponding to ALCL, small cell pattern, are not recognized in the WHO classification because there are no phenotypic or molecular markers that allow the differentiation of ALK^{-} ALCL from PTCL, NOS expressing CD30.

Immunophenotype

In addition to homogeneous CD30 staining, more than half of all cases express one or more T-cell markers. Positive staining for CD3 is more common than in ALK^{+} ALCL. CD2 and CD4 are positive in a significant proportion of cases,

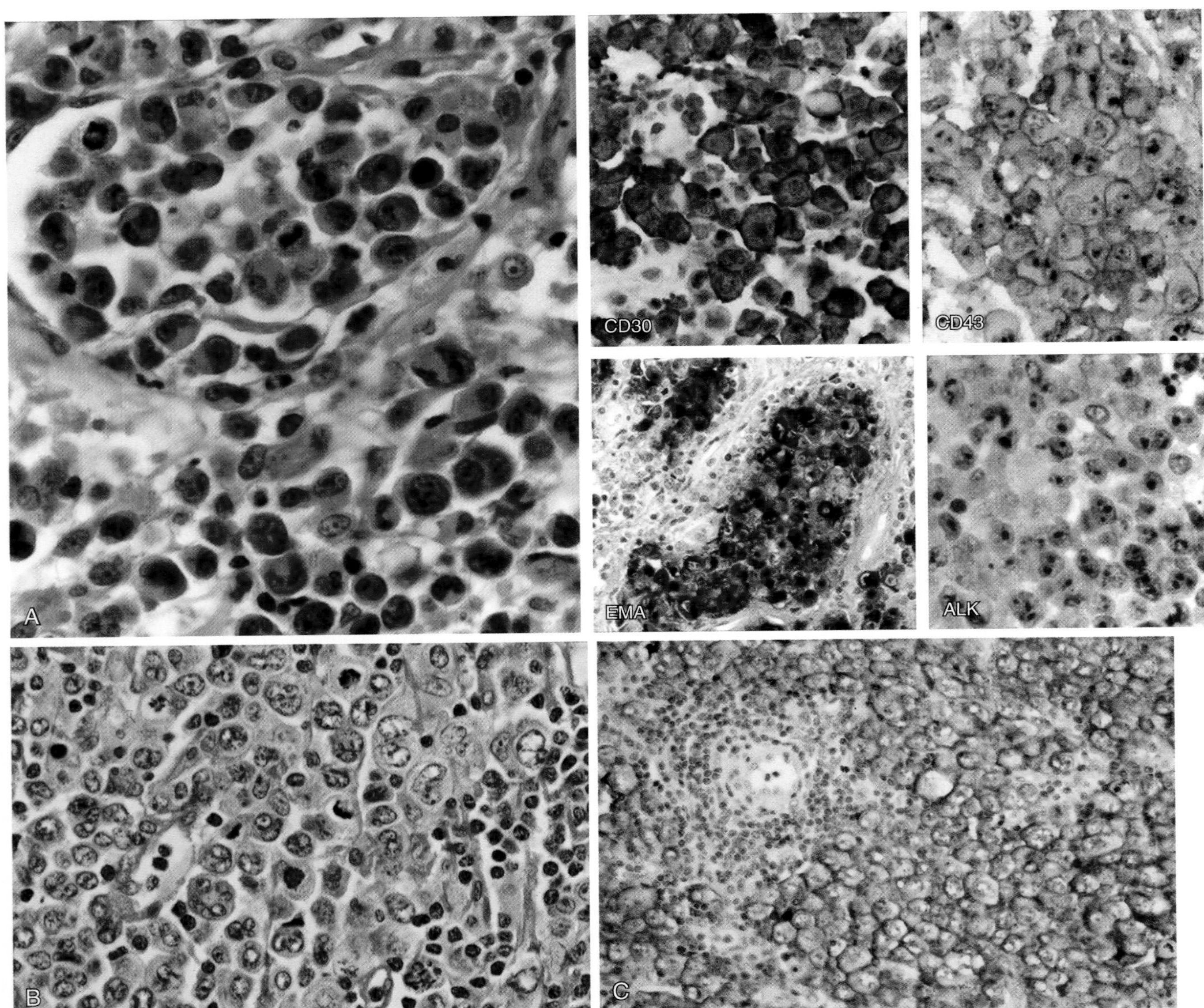

Figure 36-10. **A**, Anaplastic lymphoma kinase (ALK)-negative anaplastic large cell lymphoma (ALCL) showing morphologic and phenotypic features closely comparable to those observed in ALK^{+} ALCL. ALK staining was repeated twice and proved to be negative. Numerous "hallmark" cells grow within sinuses. The immunophenotype is similar to that of ALK^{+} ALCL in most respects: CD30^{+}, epithelial membrane antigen (EMA) positive, perforin positive, CD43^{+}, CD2^{+}. **B** and **C**, ALK^{-} ALCL consisting of more pleomorphic cells with a high nuclear-to-cytoplasmic ratio, strongly positive for CD30. The case shown in **B** was of T phenotype (CD3^{+} and CD4^{+}) but negative for EMA.

whereas CD8$^+$ cases are rare. As in ALK$^+$ ALCL, the loss of one or more T-cell markers is frequently noted. In cases with a null-cell phenotype, a diagnosis of Hodgkin's lymphoma rich in neoplastic cells must be excluded. PAX5 is a very useful marker in this setting because nearly all cases of Hodgkin's lymphoma and gray zone lymphoma express PAX5. In contrast to ALK$^+$ ALCL, expression of EMA is variable. Some pathologists tend to diagnose ALK$^-$ ALCL only in cases with typical morphologic features and coexpression of CD30 and EMA. The cytotoxic-associated markers TIA-1, granzyme B, and perforin are found in a significant proportion of cases. ALK$^-$ ALCL is consistently negative for EBV (i.e., EBER and LMP-1).[42]

Genetics and Molecular Findings

T-cell receptor genes are clonally rearranged in a majority of cases, regardless of whether they express T-cell antigens. No recurrent primary cytogenetic abnormalities have been described. However, some studies indicate that ALK$^-$ ALCL tends to differ from both PTCL, NOS and ALK$^+$ ALCL in terms of chromosome losses or gains.[81,82] In a recent study, patients with ALK$^-$ ALCL and complex chromosomal abnormalities were found to have significantly shorter overall survival.[83] The molecular signature of ALK$^-$ ALCL includes overexpression of *CCR7*, *CNTFR*, *IL22*, and *IL21* genes but does not identify the underlying oncogenic mechanism associated with these tumors.[49] In addition, these results do not provide definitive evidence of whether ALK$^-$ ALCL is more closely related to ALK$^+$ ALCL or to PTCL, NOS.[49,84,85]

Clinical Course and Prognostic Factors

The clinical outcome of conventionally treated ALK$^-$ ALCL is clearly poorer than that of ALK$^+$ ALCL.[86] In the recent study by Savage and coworkers,[72] the overall 5-year survival of patients with ALK$^-$ ALCL was only 49%, compared with 70% for those with ALK$^+$ ALCL. Furthermore, PTCL, NOS with high CD30 expression, which can be difficult to differentiate histologically from ALK$^-$ ALCL, has a poorer prognosis and a 5-year overall survival of 19%.

DIFFERENTIAL DIAGNOSIS OF ANAPLASTIC LARGE CELL LYMPHOMA

Even if the morphologic features of most ALCLs suggest the diagnosis, a definitive diagnosis cannot be made without immunohistochemistry. A major advance was made with the production of ALK1 and ALKc antibodies.[26,53] They are of critical diagnostic value in some ALK$^+$ ALCLs with unusual morphologic features. The diagnosis of ALK$^-$ ALCL is more difficult because of the lack of specific markers. As a consequence, all tumors consisting of large cells expressing the CD30 antigen need to be considered in the differential diagnosis (Table 36-2).

Anaplastic Large Cell Lymphoma, Common Pattern

ALCL, common pattern is easy to recognize in children. In adults the main differential diagnoses are metastatic malignancies because the majority of these ALCL cases exhibit a sinusoidal growth pattern. However, undifferentiated carcinomas usually express cytokeratin and EMA and are negative for the CD30 antigen. We have observed rare cases of carcinomas that are weakly positive for CD30. Metastasis from a melanoma may simulate ALCL, but most of these tumors are S-100$^+$, HMB45$^+$, PNL2$^+$, EMA$^{-/+}$, and CD30$^-$; however, rare cases positive for CD30 have also been reported.[87] Embryonal carcinoma expresses CD30, but morphologically it never mimics ALCL.[88] The most difficult problem in the differential diagnosis is represented by ALK$^-$ PTCL, NOS consisting of a predominant population of large cells, sometimes infiltrating lymphatic sinuses. Some of these tumors strongly express CD30 and may be positive for EMA.[89] In contrast to most ALCLs, these tumors are usually strongly positive for CD3 and may express BCL2 protein. However, the distinction between PTCL, NOS and ALK$^-$ ALCL is not clear-cut, and there is a tendency among hematopathologists to diagnose ALK$^-$ ALCL only if both the morphology and the phenotype are close to those of ALK$^+$ ALCL.[78] It should be noted that in extranodal nasal-type NK/T-cell lymphoma and enteropathy-associated T-cell lymphoma, a varying proportion of tumor cells expresses CD30.[9] Diffuse large B-cell lymphomas with anaplastic morphology may show the morphologic features, including a sinusoidal growth pattern, and the phenotypic features (CD30 positivity) of ALCL. In contrast to ALCL, these tumors express several B-cell antigens, and t(2;5) is not found in such cases.[90] However, some rare large B-cell lymphomas exhibit a predominant sinusoidal growth pattern and thus may simulate ALCL.

Mainly, two types of tumors deserve attention. The first is ALK$^+$ large B-cell lymphoma, which is now considered a distinct entity.[54] Morphologically, these tumors are composed of monomorphic large plasmablast- or immunoblast-like cells with large central nucleoli, and they have a tendency to invade lymphatic sinuses (Fig. 36-11A and B). At low magnification these tumors resemble ALCL, but they lack CD30. These lymphomas strongly express EMA (see Fig. 36-11C), as does ALCL, but they also contain intracytoplasmic immunoglobulin (usually IgA) of a single light-chain type. They often lack lineage-associated leukocyte antigens (CD3, CD20, CD79a), with the exception of CD4 and CD57 in some cases. These tumors weakly express or may even be negative for the leukocyte common antigen CD45. Occasional cases are positive for cytokeratin, which, in addition to EMA positivity and weak or negative staining for CD45, may lead to the misdiagnosis of carcinoma. Characteristically, lymphoma cells are strongly positive for ALK. In most cases the staining is restricted to the cytoplasm and is granular, indicating an association with CLTC-ALK protein.[32,91] ALK$^+$ diffuse large B-cell lymphoma typically follows an aggressive course. The other lymphomas exhibiting a sinusoidal growth pattern are either negative, such as so-called microvillous lymphomas, or positive for CD30.[92,93] However, these tumors are relatively easy to recognize by immunohistochemistry because they express B-cell antigens (CD20 and CD79a) and are negative for ALK.

The second type of tumor deserving attention is true histiocytic tumor, which is extremely rare. In a report based on the study of more than 900 lymphomas, there were only four true histiocytic tumors.[94] Histiocytic sarcomas usually consist

Table 36-2 Differential Diagnosis of Anaplastic Large Cell Lymphoma

Entity	Phenotype of Neoplastic Cells	Comments
ALCL, common type	CD30$^+$, EMA$^+$, ALK$^+$ (85%), CD45$^{-/+}$, CD3$^{-/+}$, CD43$^+$, CD2$^{-/+}$, CD4$^{-/+}$, CD5$^{-/+}$, CD7$^{-/+}$, CD8$^{-/+}$, cytotoxic proteins* +/–, BCL2$^-$ (most cases)	Sinusoidal growth pattern "Hallmark" cells
Metastatic malignancy		
Carcinoma	Cytokeratin +, EMA$^+$, CD30$^-$, CD45$^-$	Rare cases CD30$^+$
Melanoma	S-100$^+$, EMA$^{-/+}$, HMB45$^+$, PNL2$^+$, CD45$^-$	Weak CD30 staining has been reported
PTCL, NOS with predominantly large cells	CD30$^{-/+}$, EMA$^{-/+}$, ALK$^-$, CD3$^+$, CD2$^{-/+}$, CD4$^{-/+}$, CD5$^{-/+}$, CD7$^{-/+}$, CD8$^{-/+}$, cytotoxic proteins* +/–, BCL2$^+$	Rare cases with sinusoidal growth pattern and pleomorphic cells
Diffuse large B-cell lymphoma (DLBCL)		
ALK$^+$ DLBCL	CD30$^-$, EMA$^+$, ALK$^+$, CD20/CD79a$^-$, cytoplasmic IgA	Sinusoidal growth pattern Immunoblast or plasmablastic cells Full-length ALK
DLBCL, anaplastic variant†	CD30$^{-/+}$, EMA$^{-/+}$, ALK$^-$, CD20/CD79a$^+$	Some show a sinusoidal growth pattern but are ALK$^-$
Histiocytic sarcoma	CD30$^-$, EMA$^-$, ALK$^-$, CD68$^+$, CD163$^+$, lysozyme +	
ALCL, lymphohistiocytic	CD30$^+$, EMA$^+$, ALK$^+$, CD68$^-$, CD45$^{-/+}$, CD3$^{-/+}$, CD43$^+$, CD2$^{-/+}$, CD4$^{-/+}$, CD5$^{-/+}$, CD7$^{-/+}$, CD 8$^{-/+}$, cytotoxic proteins* +/–	Sinusoidal growth pattern may be absent, but perivascular pattern is observed in all cases Only reactive histiocytes are CD68$^+$
Lymphadenitis rich in histiocytes	CD30$^-$, EMA$^-$, ALK$^-$	Rare CD30$^+$ immunoblasts No perivascular pattern
ALCL, small cell variant	CD30$^+$, EMA$^+$, ALK$^+$, CD45$^{-/+}$, CD3$^+$ (most cases), CD43$^+$, CD2$^{+/-}$, CD4$^{+/-}$, CD5$^{+/-}$, CD7$^{+/-}$, CD8$^{+/-}$, cytotoxic proteins* +	Sinusoidal growth pattern may be absent, but perivascular pattern is observed in all cases Restricted nuclear ALK staining
PTCL, NOS with small to medium-sized cells	CD30$^{-/+}$, EMA$^{-/+}$, ALK$^-$, CD45$^{+/-}$, CD3$^+$ (most cases), CD43$^+$, CD2$^{-/+}$, CD4$^{-/+}$, CD5$^{-/+}$, CD7$^{-/+}$, CD8$^{-/+}$, cytotoxic proteins* +/–	Scattered CD30$^+$ cells may be observed, but without perivascular pattern
ALCL, other‡	CD30$^+$, EMA$^+$, ALK$^+$, CD45$^{-/+}$, CD3$^{-/+}$, CD43$^+$, CD2$^{-/+}$, CD4$^{-/+}$, CD5$^{-/+}$, CD7$^{-/+}$, CD8$^{-/+}$, cytotoxic proteins* +/–, BCL2$^-$ (most cases)	Sinusoidal growth pattern "Hallmark" cells Rare cases of ALK$^+$ ALCL may show CD15$^+$ paranuclear staining
Hodgkin's lymphoma	CD30$^+$, EMA$^-$, CD15$^{+/-}$, ALK$^-$, CD45$^-$, CD3$^-$, PAX5$^-$, CD43$^-$, CD20$^{-/+}$ (heterogeneous staining), EBV/LMP-1$^{+/-}$ (60%), BCL2 variable	Rare sinusoidal growth pattern No perivascular pattern
Inflammatory myofibroblastic tumors	CD30$^-$, EMA$^-$, ALK$^+$ (cyt)	ALCL with sarcomatous morphology is always CD30$^+$, EMA$^+$, and ALK$^+$
Rhabdomyosarcoma	CD30$^-$, EMA$^-$, ALK$^{-/+}$ (cyt), desmin +	Rare cases of rhabdomyosarcoma may show rare cells positive for CD30 and EMA

*Perforin, TIA-1, granzyme B.
†Rare cases of DLBCL show a predominant sinusoidal growth pattern but are negative for ALK.
‡Includes giant cell, sarcomatous, hypocellular; rare cases may resemble Hodgkin's lymphoma at low-power magnification.
ALCL, anaplastic large cell lymhoma; ALK, anaplastic lymphoma kinase; (cyt), cytoplasmic; EBV, Epstein-Barr virus; EMA, epithelial membrane antigen; PTCL, NOS, peripheral T-cell lymphoma, not otherwise specified.

of large cells with moderate or abundant cytoplasm and pleomorphic nuclei with prominent nucleoli. Morphologically malignant-appearing cells are positive for CD68 (KP1 and PGM1) and CD163, macrophage-associated antigens, and for lysozyme. Like normal histiocytes or macrophages, true histiocytic sarcomas react with CD4 but are negative for all other T-cell and B-cell markers. These cells are negative for CD1a and S-100. Recognition of these tumors is important because of their poor prognosis in the majority of cases. Similar morphologic and phenotypic features are seen in monoblastic leukemias, which can be reliably distinguished from histiocytic sarcomas only by the clinical presentation (i.e., bone marrow involvement). Rare cases of aggressive mastocytosis may consist of large cells reminiscent of "hallmark" cells and express the CD30 antigen. They are positive for CD117, CD4, and CD68 antigens. Acid toluidine blue shows the characteristic metachromatic granules, but in malignant cases, granularity may be sparse. Immunohistochemistry for mast cell tryptase is the preferred diagnostic tool.[95]

Anaplastic Large Cell Lymphoma, Lymphohistiocytic Pattern

ALCL, lymphohistiocytic pattern may be extremely difficult to recognize and is commonly misdiagnosed as histiocyte-rich lymphadenitis. One must keep in mind that the lymph node architecture is obliterated in these lesions, a feature that is rare in reactive processes. As described earlier, malignant cells are difficult to identify because they are obscured by large numbers of reactive histiocytes associated with varying numbers of plasma cells. The key to the diagnosis is immunohistochemistry using CD30 and ALK-reactive antibodies; this highlights the malignant cells scattered among the histiocytes and typically concentrated around blood vessels.[11,96]

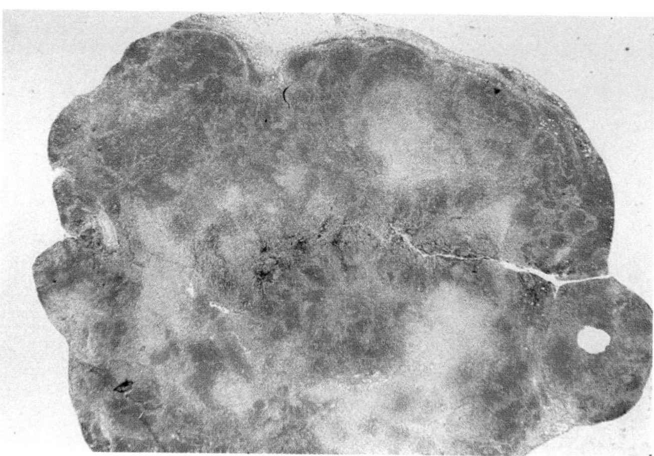

Figure 37-10. Areas of necrosis without evidence of lymphoma in a mesenteric lymph node from a case of enteropathy-associated T-cell lymphoma.

Table 37-1 Properties of Classic and Type II Enteropathy-Associated T-Cell Lymphoma (EATL)

	Classic EATL	Type II EATL
Frequency	80%-90%	10%-20%
Morphology	Variable	Monomorphic small cell
Immunophenotype		
CD8	Negative (20% positive)	Positive
CD56	Negative	Positive
HLA-DQ2/-DQ8	90% positive	30%-40% positive*
Genetics		
+9q31.3 or −16q12.1	86%	83%
+1q32.2-q41	73%	27%
+5q34-q35.2	80%	20%
+8q24 (*MYC*)	27%	73%

*Corresponds to the frequency in the normal white population.

thelial lymphocytes are, however, phenotypically heterogeneous.[20-22] Most are cytotoxic T cells that express CD3 and CD8 and have rearranged TCR beta chain genes. There is a minority population of $CD4^-$, $CD8^-$ intraepithelial lymphocytes with rearranged gamma-delta but not beta chain genes. These gamma-delta T cells constitute 10% to 15% of intraepithelial lymphocytes in normal mucosa; their concentration may increase to 30% in patients with celiac disease. Finally, a third population of $CD56^+$ cells accounts for a very small fraction of intraepithelial lymphocytes that is virtually undetectable in immunostained paraffin sections (unpublished observations).

CLINICAL COURSE

The clinical course of EATL is very unfavorable, except in a minority of cases in which resection of a localized tumor has been followed by long remission. In most cases the lymphoma involves multiple segments of intestine, rendering resection impossible, or it has already disseminated beyond the mesenteric lymph nodes or out of the abdomen. Chemotherapy, sometimes with bone marrow transplantation, may result in temporary remission of the disease.

REFRACTORY CELIAC DISEASE

Some cases of celiac disease become unresponsive to a gluten-free diet or may be unresponsive de novo. The term *refractory celiac disease* or, more commonly, *refractory sprue* has been used for these cases.[23] Although EATL may occur more or less immediately after the onset of refractory celiac disease, other cases persist as refractory celiac disease for many years without the emergence of overt lymphoma. Nonspecific inflammatory ulcers of the small intestinal mucosa, identical to those that occur in EATL, are often present in refractory celiac disease and are termed *ulcerative jejunitis* (Fig. 37-11).[24] Studies of TCR genes in both EATL and refractory celiac disease have now elucidated the relationship between the two conditions.[25]

Using PCR followed by sequence analysis of TCRγ genes, Murray and associates[17] showed that a T-cell population in the "uninvolved" enteropathic small intestinal mucosa adjacent to EATL shared the same monoclonal TCRγ

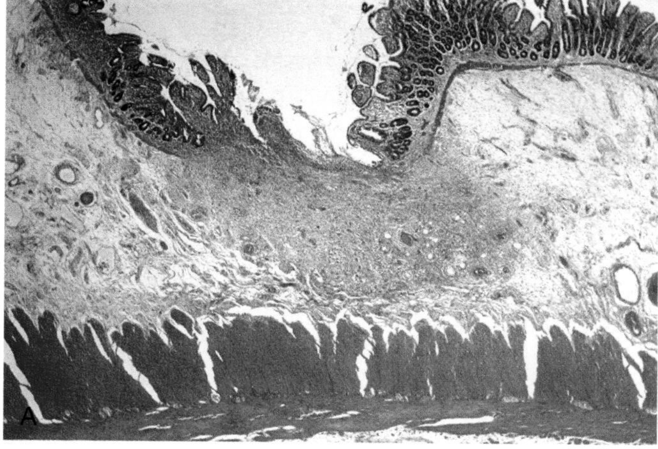

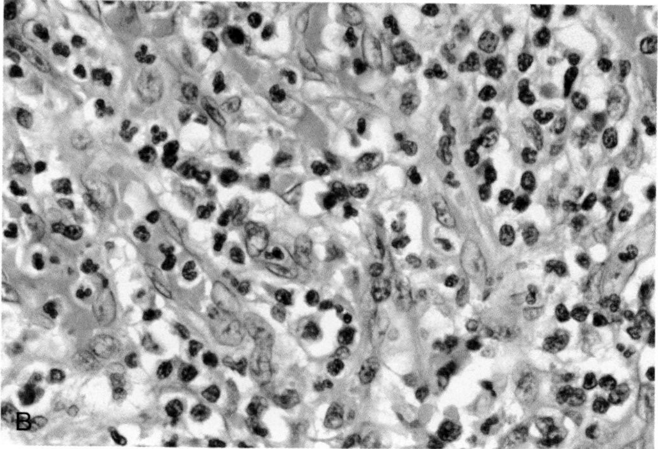

Figure 37-11. A, Shallow mucosal ulcer in a case of enteropathy-associated T-cell lymphoma. **B,** High magnification of the ulcer base shows no evidence of lymphoma.

rearrangement as the lymphoma. Ashton-Key and colleagues[25] confirmed this finding and, further, showed TCRγ monoclonality in the nonspecific "inflammatory" ulcers accompanying EATL, as well as in the ulcers and intervening mucosa of refractory sprue. In cases in which lymphoma subsequently developed, the same clone could be detected in the malignant cells by PCR and sequence analysis. Cellier and coworkers[26] investigated cases of refractory sprue and showed that monoclonal populations of T cells were present in the small intestinal mucosa; this monoclonal population was composed of phenotypically abnormal CD3⁻ (CD3ε⁺), CD4⁻, CD8⁻ intraepithelial lymphocytes. Cellier and coauthors later compiled the clinical and laboratory features of refractory sprue.[27] Importantly, they definitively clarified the relationship between celiac disease and refractory sprue by showing the presence of celiac disease–specific antiendomysial or antigliadin antibodies in most cases, as well as other characteristics of celiac disease, including a previous response to gluten withdrawal or the *HLADQA1*0501* and *DQB1*0201* phenotype.[6] Additionally, they showed that in all truly refractory cases, the intraepithelial lymphocytes were monoclonal or expressed an abnormal immunophenotype, or both.

These studies raise several questions regarding the significance of the presence of a monoclonal T-cell population in the small intestine. First, where exactly do these cells reside, and what is their phenotype? Second, what is the link, if any, between the different complications of celiac disease characterized by monoclonal populations of T cells in enteropathic mucosa? Third, is clonality synonymous with neoplasia or even malignancy? And finally, what are the implications of such a population for patient management?

Bagdi and coworkers[28] showed that in double-stained (CD8 and CD3) preparations of sections of small intestine from patients with refractory celiac disease and monoclonal T-cell populations in the small intestinal mucosa, there was a marked decrease in the proportion of CD8⁺ intraepithelial lymphocytes (Fig. 37-12). Moreover, in cases of EATL, the cytologically bland intraepithelial lymphocytes in the intervening mucosa shared the immunophenotype and genotype of the lymphoma. Specifically, in CD56⁺ cases (type II EATL), these lymphocytes also expressed CD56 (Fig. 37-13). Interestingly, these clonal and immunophenotypically aberrant intraepithelial lymphocytes were often present in the crypt epithelium, in contrast to uncomplicated celiac disease, where they are confined to the surface epithelium. Moreover, these cells were widely distributed throughout the gastrointestinal tract from stomach to anus.

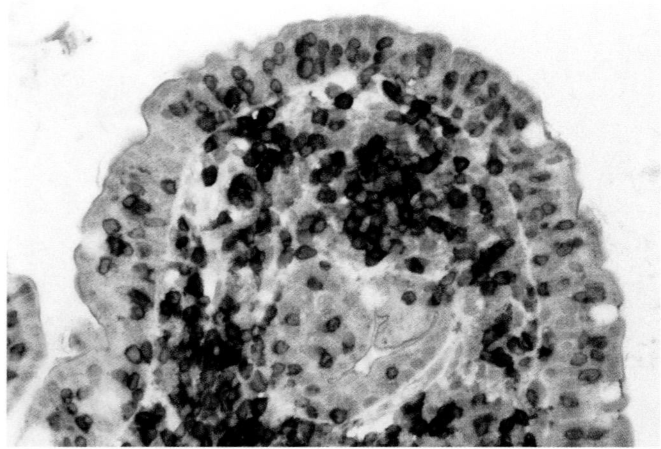

Figure 37-12. Small intestinal mucosa from a case of refractory celiac disease double-immunostained for CD8 (*brown*) and CD3 (*blue*). There is an excess of CD3⁺, CD8⁻ intraepithelial lymphocytes.

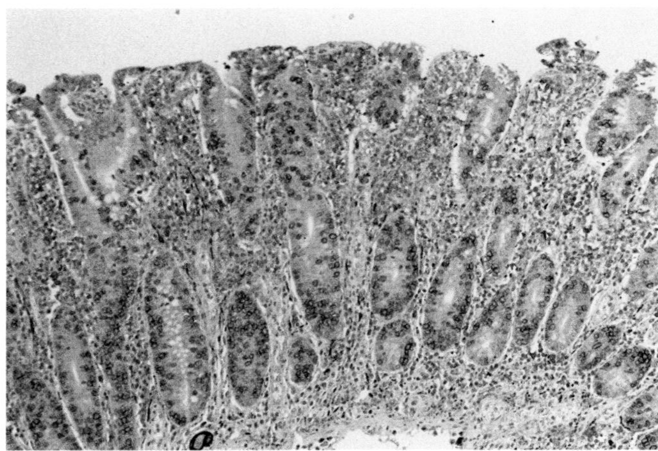

Figure 37-13. CD56⁺ intraepithelial lymphocytes in the nonlymphomatous mucosa from a case of CD56⁺ enteropathy-associated T-cell lymphoma. The CD56⁺ cells extend into the crypt epithelium.

It therefore seems safe to conclude that the monoclonal intraepithelial lymphocytes in patients with refractory sprue are neoplastic, even though they are not cytologically abnormal and do not form tumor masses. The accumulation of phenotypically aberrant monoclonal intraepithelial lymphocytes appears to be the first step in the genesis of EATL. Patients with refractory celiac disease or ulcerative jejunitis are therefore suffering from a neoplastic T-cell disorder, possibly involving most of the gastrointestinal tract. Treatment of these patients, most of whom have severe, unremitting malabsorption, is difficult. It is uncertain whether chemotherapeutic regimens appropriate for lymphoma have anything to offer in these cases, or whether new strategies must be devised. Further cellular and molecular investigations are indicated, particularly to establish the precise relationship between the neoplastic intraepithelial lymphocytes and the cells of fully developed EATL.

CLASSIC AND TYPE II ENTEROPATHY-ASSOCIATED T-CELL LYMPHOMA: VARIANTS OF THE SAME DISEASE?

Before the era of immunophenotyping, it was assumed that the rare tumors composed of uniform small round cells reflected the variation in cytomorphology that characterized EATL. These cases were also associated with villous atrophy, crypt hyperplasia, and intraepithelial lymphocytosis of the uninvolved mucosa. It later became clear that the immunophenotype of the tumor cells in this variant (CD3⁺, CD8⁺, CD56⁺) was different from that of most cases of EATL, and although they shared many clinical features and some genetic properties, there were also distinct differences (see Table 37-1). Subsequently, doubt has been raised about the association between type II EATL and celiac disease because it occurs in populations in which celiac disease is unknown.[29,30]

Table 37-2 Differential Diagnosis of Enteropathy-Associated T-Cell Lymphoma and Other Intestinal T-Cell Lymphomas

	Classic EATL	EATL Type II	Extranodal NK/T-cell	CD4⁺	ALCL
Morphology	Pleomorphic large cells	Monomorphic small cells	Monomorphic small cells	Monomorphic small cells	Pleomorphic large cells
Phenotype	$CD3^+$, $CD4^-/CD8^-$	$CD3^+$, $CD4^-$, $CD8^+$, $CD56^+$	$CD3^{+/-}$, $CD4^-$, $CD8^-$, $CD56^+$	$CD3^+$, $CD4^+$, $CD8^-$	$CD3^{-/+}$, $CD8^-$, $CD4^+$, $CD30^+$
Genetics	TCR rearrangement	TCR rearrangement	TCR germline	TCR rearrangement	TCR rearrangement
Mucosa	Villous atrophy	Villous atrophy	Villous atrophy in involved areas	Normal	Normal
IELs	Increased $CD4/8^-$	Increased $CD8^+$	Increased in involved areas $CD4/CD8^-$	Normal	Normal
EBV	–	–	+	–	–

ALCL, anaplastic large cell lymphoma; EATL, enteropathy-associated T-cell lymphoma; EBV, Epstein-Barr virus; IEL, intraepithelial T lymphocyte; NK, natural killer; TCR, T-cell receptor.

In light of these differences, it has been suggested that type II EATL is in fact a different disease.[7]

OTHER T-CELL LYMPHOMAS UNASSOCIATED WITH ENTEROPATHY

$CD56^+$ extranodal natural killer (NK)/T-cell lymphoma of the nasal type typically arises in the upper respiratory tract, but it frequently spreads to the gastrointestinal tract and may also arise there as a primary tumor (Table 37-2).[20] The lymphoma involves multiple sites, forming tumor masses. Typically, it also infiltrates long segments of intestinal mucosa, where it is associated with villous atrophy. However, unlike type II EATL, with which NK/T-cell lymphoma is often confused, villous atrophy is seen only in mucosa infiltrated by lymphoma; the villous architecture of uninvolved mucosa is normal. Moreover, the cells in this tumor almost invariably contain Epstein-Barr virus–encoded RNA (EBER). A closely related entity is primary cutaneous gamma-delta T-cell lymphoma, which typically presents with cutaneous disease but also has a high incidence of mucosal involvement; some cases may present primarily in the intestine.[31-33]

Carbonnel and coworkers[34] and Svrcek and aassociates[35] described a distinctive intestinal T-cell lymphoma composed of small $CD4^+$ lymphocytes widely distributed throughout the lamina propria of the intestinal mucosa. In common with EATL, this suggests a specific derivation from native gut lymphoid tissue—in this case, the lamina propria rather than the intraepithelial T cells. These cases are characterized by a slow, relentless course and prolonged survival—an unusual feature for T-cell lymphomas.

There are numerous isolated case reports of a wide variety of T-cell lymphomas arising in the gastrointestinal tract, but they are not recognized clinicopathologic entities. Among these, $CD30^+$ anaplastic large cell lymphoma (both anaplastic lymphoma kinase [ALK] positive and negative) may closely simulate EATL, which itself can present as a $CD30^+$ tumor. However, unlike anaplastic large cell lymphoma, EATL is usually not positive for epithelial membrane antigen; nor is it ever ALK^+. Anaplastic large cell lymphoma is usually $CD4^+$ rather than $CD8^+$, and it is not associated with celiac disease or villous atrophy.

Pearls and Pitfalls

- EATL is the most common (but not the only) intestinal T-cell lymphoma.
- EATL is a disease largely restricted to individuals of northern European origin.
- EATL may be the first clinical manifestation of celiac disease.
- EATL is characterized by a very broad morphologic spectrum.
- The diagnosis of EATL is facilitated by examination of adjacent uninvolved mucosa.

References can be found on Expert Consult @ www.expertconsult.com

Chapter 38

Mycosis Fungoides and Sézary Syndrome

Philip E. LeBoit

CHAPTER OUTLINE

Mycosis fungoides and Sézary syndrome are two closely related conditions in which neoplastic T cells infiltrate the skin and circulate in the peripheral blood. Both conditions are neoplasms that typically have a mature helper T-cell phenotype and a propensity to colonize the epidermis. Because individual patients can have discrete cutaneous lesions at one point in time and erythroderma with circulating neoplastic cells at another time, some advocate the term *cutaneous T-cell lymphoma* to describe what they consider to be a single disease.[1] However, the delineation of a variety of other distinct clinicopathologic entities that are also cutaneous T-cell lymphomas[2] has, in my opinion, rendered this term imprecise and obsolete. For example, the skin may be the only site involved by anaplastic large T-cell lymphoma.

This chapter covers mycosis fungoides and its many variants and Sézary syndrome. Other primary cutaneous T-cell lymphoproliferative disorders are considered elsewhere in this text.

MYCOSIS FUNGOIDES

Definition

Mycosis fungoides is a T-cell lymphoma in which lymphocytes infiltrate the epidermis in its early stages, resulting in flat, often slightly scaly lesions (patches); eventually, lymphocytes acquire the ability to proliferate in the dermis (forming plaques and nodules) and in internal organs. Most cases of mycosis fungoides have a T-helper phenotype, but clinically and histopathologically identical infiltrates can be seen in which T suppressor cells or even B cells are present. My view, which is not shared by all workers, is that the clinical evolution of patches to plaques and tumors is what determines whether a patient has the disease mycosis fungoides, not a specific immunophenotype. If a patient has indolent patches in which there are epidermotropic $CD8^+$ T cells, there is no harm in labeling that patient as having mycosis fungoides. Indeed, in many centers, immunophenotypic studies are not routinely performed, and patients are treated with excellent results. The term *mycosis fungoides* does not apply, however, to a disease caused by infection with the retrovirus human T-lymphotropic virus 1 (HTLV-1), despite the clinical and pathologic resemblance of some cases; that condition is referred to as *adult T-cell leukemia/lymphoma*. The major diagnostic features of mycosis fungoides are listed in Box 38-1.

Epidemiology

Mycosis fungoides is largely a disease of middle-aged and older people. However, as clinicians and pathologists have become more adept at recognizing its early stages, more cases in young adults and even in children have come to light. The

Box 38-1 *Key Diagnostic Features of Mycosis Fungoides*

- Clinical presentation: progression from patches to plaques and tumors
- Histopathologic features: from sparse perivascular to band-like (lichenoid) to diffuse dermal lymphocytic infiltrates, coupled with variable infiltration of the epidermis and variable cytologic atypia
- Immunohistochemical features: $\beta F1^{+}$, $CD3^{+}$, $CD4^{+}$, $CD8^{-}$ immunophenotype is most common, but variations in otherwise typical disease occur and have little meaning
- Genotypic findings: clonality common but not obligatory by PCR-based gamma chain gene rearrangements

incidence of mycosis fungoides in a population is certainly affected by the number of dermatologists in the community, their interest in and awareness of the disease, and their threshold for diagnosis. An interesting observation is that the incidence of mycosis fungoides rose rapidly in the early 1980s,[3] coincident with the delineation of criteria for the diagnosis of patch-stage disease by Sanchez and Ackerman.[4] Following the publication of their paper, many pathologists began to diagnose mycosis fungoides based on infiltrates they might have previously regarded as parapsoriasis en plaques or inflammatory conditions such as spongiotic dermatitis. The increased incidence of mycosis fungoides in the United States seems to reflect a rise in the detection and diagnosis of early patch-stage disease.

Etiology

A number of investigators have tried to link mycosis fungoides to environmental exposures, without success. Studies to determine whether common inflammatory skin diseases such as atopic dermatitis, chronic allergic contact dermatitis, or psoriasis give rise to mycosis fungoides are undermined by several factors. Early patches of mycosis fungoides can resemble these diseases clinically, so a patient with a 20-year history of "atopic dermatitis" preceding mycosis fungoides might have had patches of mycosis fungoides that were simply not recognized as such. Early patch-stage lesions of mycosis fungoides can resemble various inflammatory conditions under the microscope, so that even "biopsy-proven" psoriasis may not be that disease at all.

Several studies have sought the presence of a virus in the cells of mycosis fungoides. In the 1970s, interest centered on the identification of viral particles in skin biopsy samples of mycosis fungoides by electron microscopy.[5] More recently, interest has focused on a possible role for HTLV-1, the retrovirus that causes adult T-cell leukemia/lymphoma, in mycosis fungoides.[6] An initial study seemed to identify partial viral transcripts in the cells of mycosis fungoides, but further investigation has not borne this out in most cases. Another theory related to infection is that mycosis fungoides is an abnormal response to bacterial superantigens.[7]

Clinical Features

Mycosis fungoides is largely defined by the clinical features of its early stages. Requisite to this definition is an initial presentation as flat, scaly lesions or patches. These first appear in areas of the skin that are best protected from sunlight—the buttocks and groins of both sexes and the breasts of women. Subtle wrinkling, slight erythema, telangiectases, and either hypo- or hyperpigmentation are variable findings. Often, the patches are so subtle that patients do not notice them for some time, and both patients and their physicians may attribute the condition to dry skin or atopic dermatitis.

Patches are generally round or oval, although they are sometimes finger-shaped or digitate (Fig. 38-1). Their size can range from about 1 cm to more than 10 cm. Some clinicians use the terms *small plaque parapsoriasis* to refer to small patches (smaller than an adult palm) and *large plaque parapsoriasis* to refer to larger lesions of patch-stage mycosis fungoides. Those who believe that mycosis fungoides begins as an inflammatory condition that may regress often employ the term *parapsoriasis*. This usage is based on the work of the French dermatologist Brocq in the late 19th and early 20th centuries. He envisaged a complex relationship among psoriasis, eczema, seborrheic dermatitis, the conditions now known as pityriasis lichenoides acuta and chronica, and mycosis fungoides.[8] In my opinion, the term *parapsoriasis* is invalid scientifically, although it may have some functional utility, in that it is shorthand for "I don't know whether this is an early patch of mycosis fungoides or not." This dilemma is better expressed in clear language, however. Confounding this already confusing situation is the habit of some dermatologists to use *parapsoriasis* to refer to pityriasis lichenoides, an inflammatory disease.

Digitate or finger-shaped patches may occur by themselves or with the conventional lesions of mycosis fungoides. This has led some observers to conclude that the condition formerly called *digitate dermatosis* is in fact a form of mycosis fungoides.[9] Because the prognosis of patients with only digitate lesions is excellent, and the histopathologic findings are often paltry, others question the usefulness of labeling patients with digitate dermatosis as having mycosis fungoides.[10] The first documented report of a patient with digitate dermatosis evolving into conventional mycosis fungoides did not appear until recently, pointing out the importance of at least recognizing that patients with this condition have a different prognosis.[11]

In some patients with preexisting patches of mycosis fungoides, and in others who claim that they never had such patches, areas of the skin can become thin and wrinkled and marked by macules of hypo- and hyperpigmentation, along with telangiectases. This appearance is known as *poikiloderma* or *poikiloderma vasculare atrophicans*. It appears to be a manifestation of regression of patch-stage mycosis fungoides.

The large majority of patients with mycosis fungoides who have patches over a small area of skin at presentation prove to have an indolent condition that, even if untreated, seldom becomes more than a cosmetic problem. In a minority of such patients, disseminated patches arise. Over time, plaques (raised, flat, and indurated lesions) may supervene, followed by tumors (Fig. 38-2). Most of the literature written before 1980 applies to these unfortunate patients with plaques and tumors, because the patch stage was not widely recognized before that time. Many of these early studies reported a grim prognosis for patients with mycosis fungoides, and the more recent decline in mortality[12] seems to be due to recognition of the disease at an earlier stage rather than better treatments.

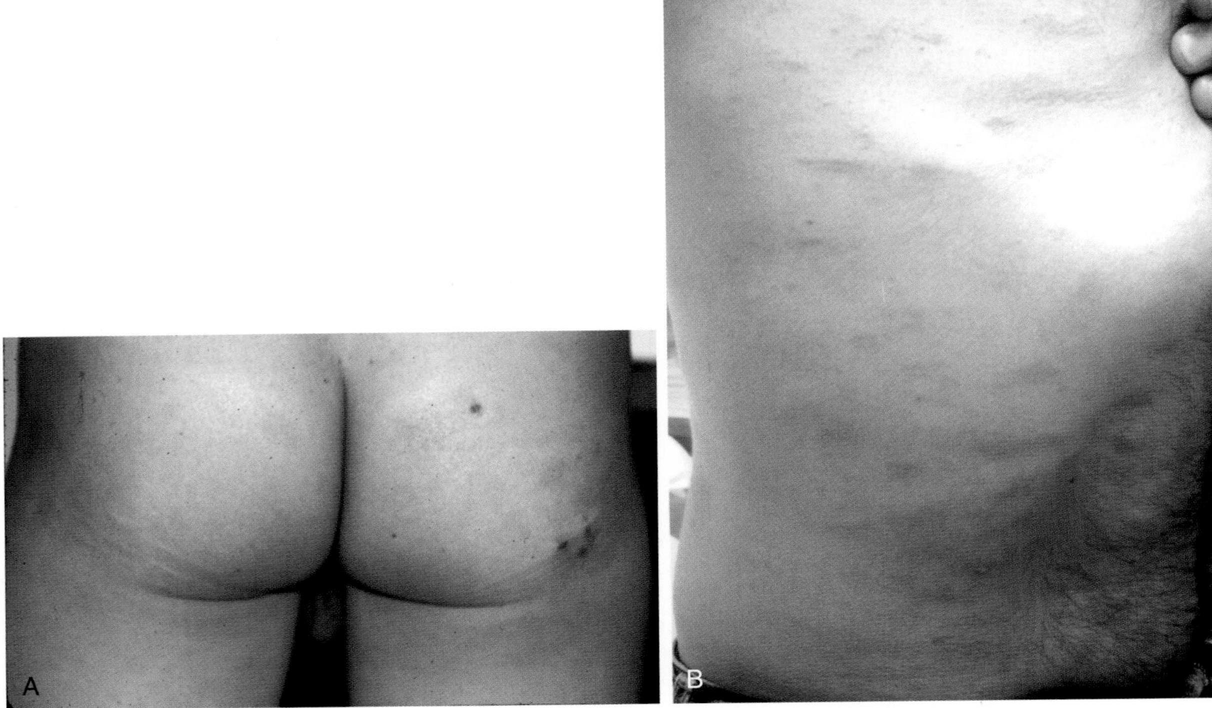

Figure 38-1. Patches of mycosis fungoides often arise on double-clothed areas, and the lesions may recede with light exposure. **A**, Classic patches are often the size of a palm or larger. **B**, Digitate lesions of mycosis fungoides are so called because they are finger-shaped patches, often aligned along Langer's lines.

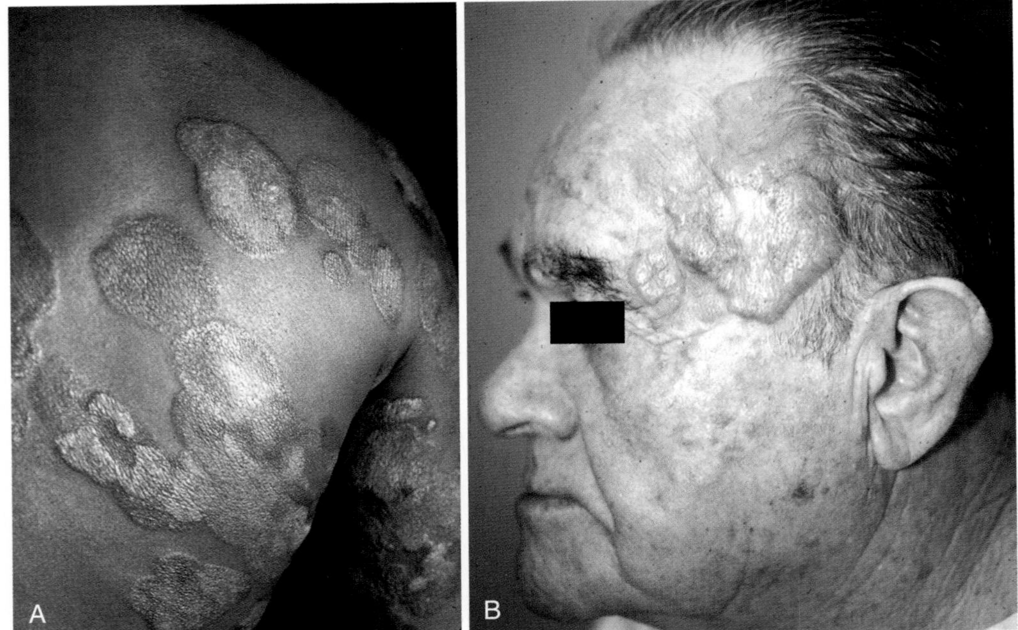

Figure 38-2. **A**, Plaques of mycosis fungoides often have a polycyclic appearance. **B**, Tumors are more elevated above the skin surface. By the time tumors supervene, sun-exposed skin, such as the face, is often involved.

Plaques of mycosis fungoides are usually raised, varying shades of red to red-brown, and scaly. They are often polycyclic, with clearing in the center (see Fig. 38-2A). They sometimes ulcerate, but not as much as nodules or tumors do. Nodules or tumors of mycosis fungoides are often plum colored and are clinically indistinguishable from nodules and tumors of other cutaneous lymphomas. Only a careful examination that detects patches can distinguish the tumors of mycosis fungoides from those of other T-cell lymphomas. Tumors of mycosis fungoides are raised, are often smooth, and frequently ulcerate (see Fig. 38-2B). These fungating lesions resulted in the name *mycosis fungoides*, attributed to the disease by Alibert.[13]

Follicular mucinosis can occur within lesions of mycosis fungoides, usually in plaques or tumors. In this process, mucin is aberrantly produced by follicular epithelial cells and collects in the interstices between them. The follicles lose their hair. The clinical result is a swollen or puffy-appearing pink lesion that, if situated in hair-bearing skin, is alopecic. The term *alopecia mucinosa* was initially coined to refer to an inflammatory condition in which plaques of alopecia are present on the hair-bearing skin of young persons, with mucin accumulating in the affected follicles. Some recent studies suggest that this distinction may not be valid and that alopecia mucinosa may be an indolent form of mycosis fungoides.[14,15] Studies of T-cell receptor gene rearrangements have found clonal populations in about the same number of cases of both idiopathic alopecia mucinosa and mycosis fungoides with follicular mucinosis. Patients in whom alopecia mucinosa is the dominant finding often have lesions that prominently involve the skin of the face, unlike those of conventional mycosis fungoides. The face is typically the last area involved in conventional disease, which is often sensitive to ultraviolet light, resulting in a propensity to initially involve so-called double-clothed areas.

Another alternative morphologic expression, based on follicular involvement, is folliculotropic mycosis fungoides. Patients with this condition may have disseminated papules centered around hair follicles, a finding that can be appreciated with the use of a hand lens. This variant may have a less favorable prognosis.[16,17]

Morphology

There is vast variability in the histopathologic appearance of mycosis fungoides, especially in patch-stage disease. This reflects the fact that early lesions may be composed largely of nonneoplastic cells, exerting their influence via cytotoxicity and cytokine production and in ways not yet appreciated.

The early patches of mycosis fungoides feature lymphocytes that are not morphologically abnormal, in contrast to those found in inflammatory skin diseases. Therefore, identification of a section as representing mycosis fungoides, either definitely or possibly, requires attention to the histopathologic pattern of the infiltrate.

The earliest patches of mycosis fungoides feature small lymphocytes around venules of the superficial plexus; some are scattered interstitially in the papillary dermis, with only a few within the epidermis (Fig. 38-3). When the cells of mycosis fungoides enter the epidermis, they usually elicit spongiosis or edema between keratinocytes. The degree of spongiosis is usually less than that seen when the same number of lymphocytes enter the epidermis in an inflammatory skin disease. The tendency of the cells of mycosis fungoides to colonize the epidermis is referred to as *epidermotropism*. This term is also used to connote that there are areas of the epidermis that have only slight spongiosis and many lymphocytes. *Exocytosis* describes the migration of inflammatory cells into the epidermis and is a more neutral term. Because the term *epidermotropism* presupposes the ultimate diagnosis, it is best avoided.

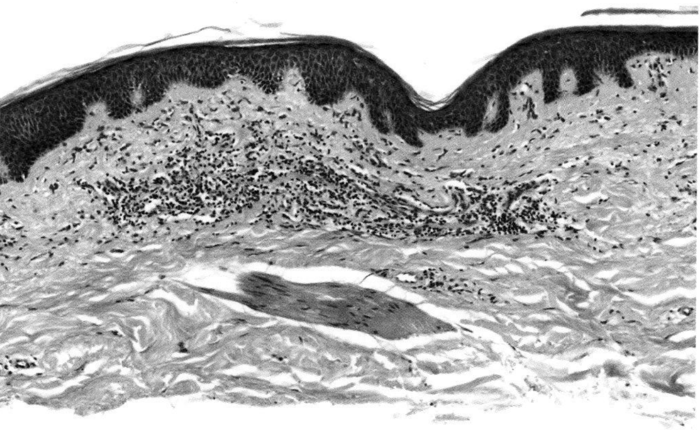

Figure 38-3. Early patch of mycosis fungoides featuring a psoriasiform lichenoid pattern, with small lymphocytes in a band in the papillary dermis and only a few in the epidermis. An unequivocal diagnosis is not possible at this stage.

In early patch-stage disease, mycosis fungoides is often not recognizable with certainty. As the patches develop, the papillary dermis becomes fibrotic. The collagen bundles of the papillary dermis are usually fine and haphazardly oriented. This meshwork changes to one in which there are coarse fibers sometimes likened to "pink fettuccini." At the same time, rete ridges begin to elongate, usually only slightly and very evenly. Their bases remain rounded, unlike in many interface dermatitides. Lymphocytes may lodge in the basal layer of the epidermis, with only slight vacuolar changes and few necrotic keratinocytes.[18]

The papillary dermal lymphocytic infiltrate often becomes band-like, at least in foci. The combination of elongated rete ridges with rounded bases and band-like lymphocytic infiltrates is known as a *psoriasiform lichenoid pattern*; if spongiosis is also present, it is referred to as a *spongiotic psoriasiform lichenoid pattern*. If the lymphocytes engaged as a host response to the neoplasm kill keratinocytes that constitute rete ridges, the epidermis may become thin and flat based—an *atrophic lichenoid pattern*. These three patterns should raise the pathologist's suspicion that he or she may be dealing with a lesion of mycosis fungoides, because only a few inflammatory skin diseases share these patterns (Box 38-2).

As the infiltrates of mycosis fungoides become dense and band-like in the papillary dermis, they also begin to exhibit cells with atypical nuclei (Fig. 38-4). Cells of patch-stage mycosis fungoides have slightly larger nuclei than those of lymphocytes in inflammatory conditions, with an irregular nuclear contour—the so-called cerebriform lymphocyte (Fig. 38-5). An important caveat is that if nuclear atypia is used as a criterion for the differential diagnosis between a patch of mycosis fungoides and an inflammatory condition, the atypia must be unmistakable. Many pathologists can convince

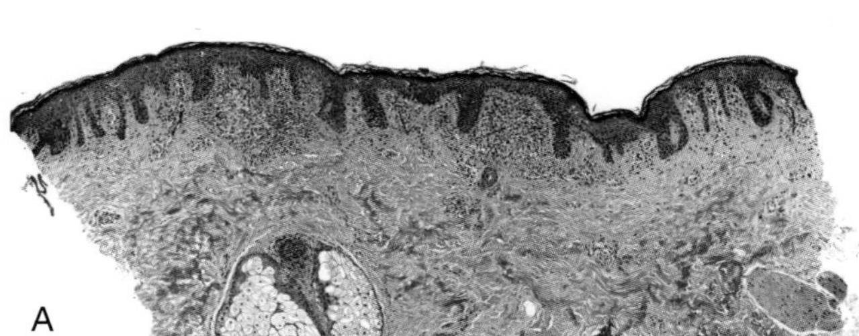

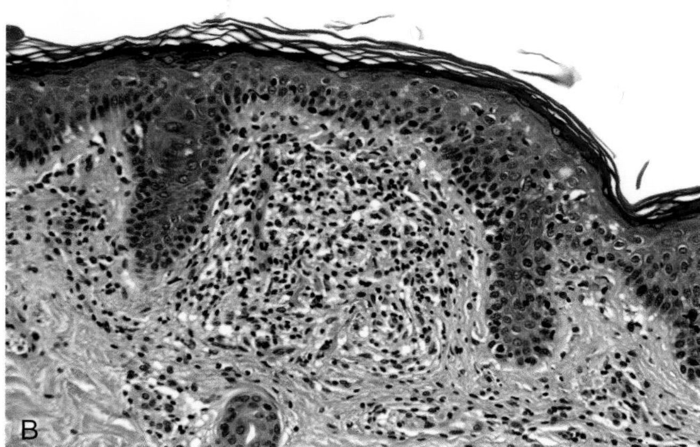

Figure 38-4. **A,** Later patch of mycosis fungoides, again with a psoriasiform lichenoid pattern. **B,** In this lesion (unlike that in Fig. 38-3), many lymphocytes infiltrate the epidermis, with only scant spongiosis. Those in the epidermis have slightly larger and darker nuclei than those in the dermis.

themselves that the nuclei of lymphocytes are atypical by staring at them for too long under an oil immersion lens.

Some patches of mycosis fungoides feature epidermal atrophy, in concert with a patchy lichenoid lymphocytic infiltrate. The papillary dermis is often markedly fibrotic and contains telangiectases and melanophages, corresponding to the clinical picture of poikiloderma vasculare atrophicans. In such atrophic patch-stage lesions, it may be difficult to demonstrate a sufficient number of lymphocytes in the epidermis to rule out an inflammatory disease with an atrophic lichenoid pattern (see Box 38-2).

Plaques of mycosis fungoides are raised and palpable on clinical examination. This correlates with the presence of lymphocytes in the reticular dermis, not only around vessels but also interspersed between reticular dermal collagen bundles (Fig. 38-6). This finding occurs beneath an epidermis and papillary dermis displaying the changes described earlier for fully developed patches of mycosis fungoides. Although lymphocytes with atypical nuclei are few in early patches and more numerous in late ones, they almost always constitute a significant percentage of the infiltrate in plaques. Similarly, aggregations of lymphocytes, termed Pautrier's microabscesses or collections, are rare in patches but common in plaques. (Interestingly, this distinctive clue to the diagnosis of mycosis fungoides was discovered not by Pautrier but by Darier.[19]) Plaques may also feature "transformed" cells (Fig. 38-7). The atypical lymphocytes of patches have scant cyto-

Box 38-2 *Common Patterns of Patch-Stage Mycosis Fungoides and the Inflammatory Skin Diseases That Share Them*

Psoriasiform Lichenoid Pattern
- Mycosis fungoides, patch stage
- Secondary syphilis (usually superficial and deep, with many plasma cells and histiocytes)
- Lichenoid purpura (extravasated erythrocytes and siderophages)
- Lichen striatus (linear eruption of papules in a child or teenager)
- Early lesions of lichen sclerosus et atrophicus
- Surface of some lesions of morphea
- Drug reaction (one pattern among many)

Spongiotic Psoriasiform Lichenoid Pattern
- Mycosis fungoides, patch stage
- Urticarial stage of bullous pemphigoid
- Drug reactions (one pattern among many)
- Allergic contact dermatitis (rarely; so-called lichenoid contact dermatitis)
- Chronic photoallergic dermatitis (actinic reticuloid)

Atrophic Lichenoid Pattern
- Mycosis fungoides, atrophic patch stage
- Atrophic lichen planus
- Lichenoid purpura
- Regression of melanoma, Bowen's disease, superficial basal cell carcinoma
- Centers of lesions of porokeratosis (sometimes)
- Poikilodermatous lesions of dermatomyositis

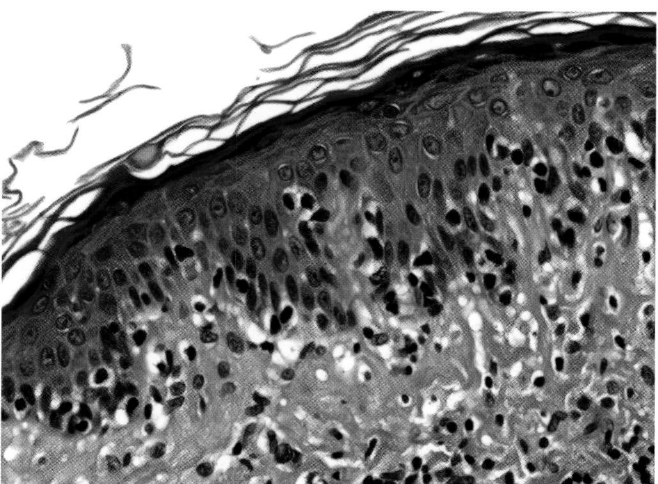

Figure 38-5. Lymphocytes in the epidermis of a patch of mycosis fungoides with scant cytoplasm and large hyperchromatic nuclei. Small halos are present around some of them.

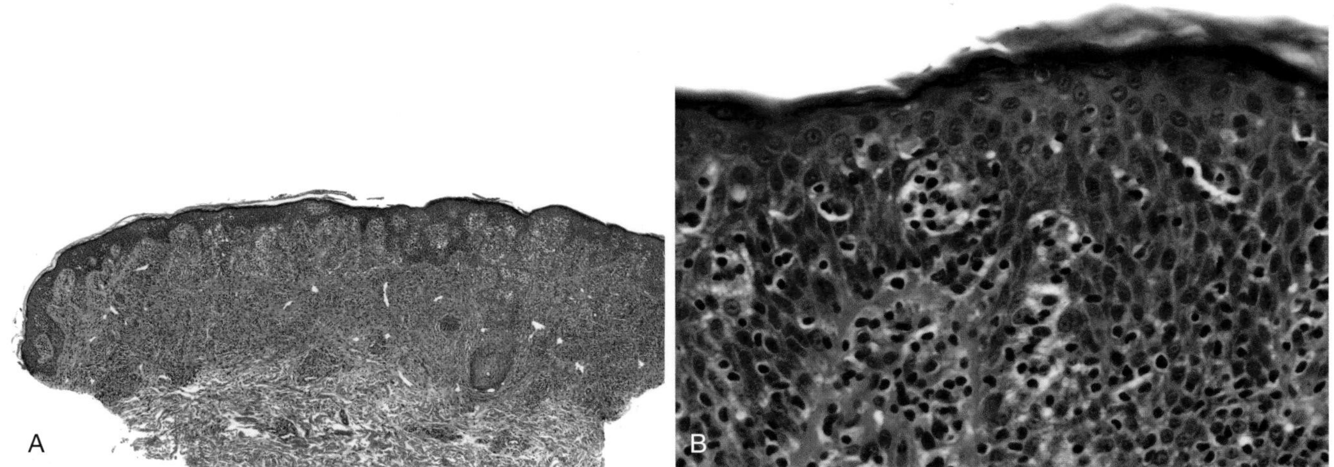

Figure 38-6. **A,** Plaque-stage mycosis fungoides features infiltration of the superficial reticular dermis. **B,** In this case, there are prominent collections of lymphocytes (Pautrier's microabscesses) in the epidermis as well.

plasm and irregular, sometimes cerebriform lymphocytes. In plaques (and tumors), transformed lymphocytes have large vesicular nuclei, large nucleoli, and some discernible cytoplasm. In contrast to patches, which lack eosinophils and plasma cells, plaques and tumors of mycosis fungoides often have many of these cells. This might correlate with a shift from Th1 to Th2-like cytokine production as lesions change from patches to plaques.

Follicular mucinosis is found more frequently in plaques than in patches and tumors of mycosis fungoides (Fig. 38-8). Follicular mucinosis is the aberrant production of mucopolysaccharides by follicular keratinocytes. The result is the distention of intercellular spaces in the outer root sheath. In well-balanced hematoxylyin-eosin–stained sections, the mucin can be detected as tiny basophilic granules. Keratinocytes adjacent to the widened spaces are often elongated, and the spines connecting them appear stretched. Follicles involved in this manner usually have infiltrates of lymphocytes around and within them. In some cases the lymphocytes do not infiltrate the epidermis and are not sufficiently atypical to establish a diagnosis of mycosis fungoides on cytologic grounds alone, even though patients may have clinically obvious mycosis fungoides.

Nodules or tumors of mycosis fungoides acquire their clinical features by virtue of lymphocytic infiltrates that are present as nodules or diffusely replace the reticular dermis (Fig. 38-9). Transformed cells can be present in nodules of mycosis fungoides.[20,21] Their appearance ranges from cells with large round or slightly oval vesicular nuclei and scant cytoplasm to cells with large oval vesicular nuclei, large nucleoli, and abundant cytoplasm, similar to the cells of anaplastic large cell lymphoma. Some pathologists classify mycosis fungoides as having undergone large cell transformation only if cells four times the size of normal lymphocytes constitute 25% of the infiltrate or form nodules.[20] This usually occurs in advanced disease and may have an adverse prognostic impact.

Anaplastic large cells may predominate to such an extent that only the clinical identification of patches or plaques at

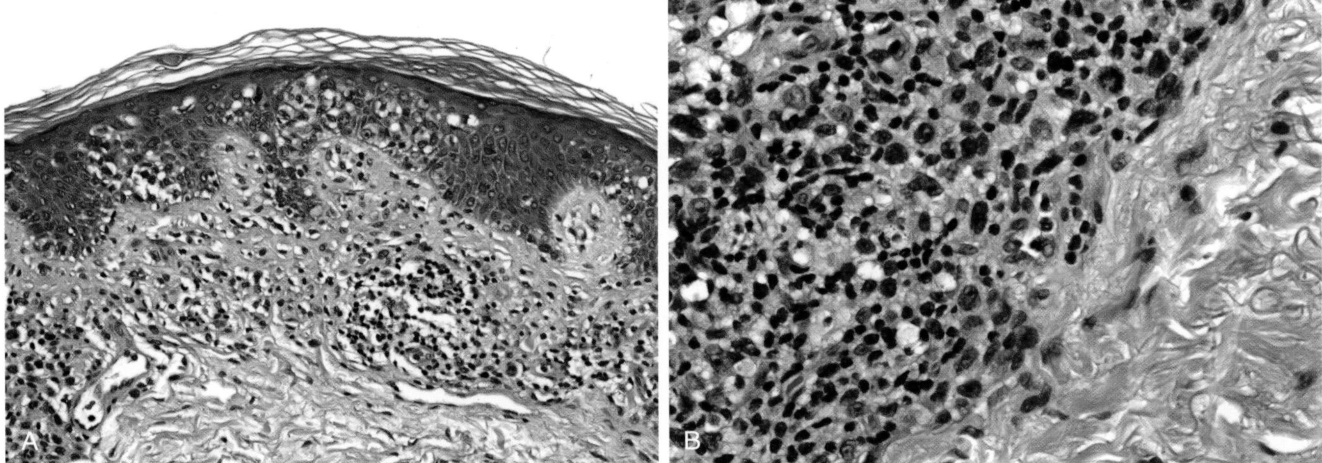

Figure 38-7. **A,** Thin plaque of mycosis fungoides with large cell transformation. **B,** Although the infiltrate is sparser than that of the plaque in Figure 38-6, many lymphocytes have large, vesicular nuclei with prominent nucleoli. Large cell transformation may confer an adverse prognosis in some clinical contexts.

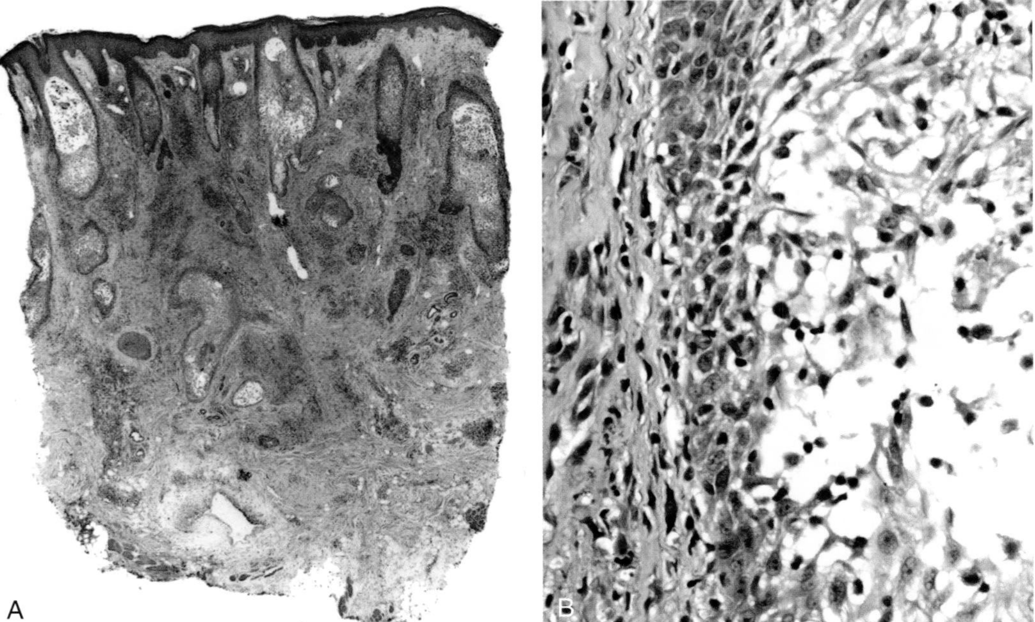

Figure 38-8. Follicular mucinosis in mycosis fungoides. A, Note that the infiltrates surround pilosebaceous units and spare the epidermis and papillary dermis. **B,** Spaces between keratinocytes are markedly widened due to the accumulation of mucin.

other sites allows the distinction from anaplastic large cell lymphoma. Although lymphocytes home to the epidermis in patch- and plaque-stage lesions, some tumors of mycosis fungoides completely lack intraepidermal lymphocytes. The loss of dependence on an epidermal environment for cellular proliferation in the skin occurs apace with the cells' capacity to lodge in internal organs in mycosis fungoides.

Grading

Although biopsy interpretation is critical in establishing a diagnosis of mycosis fungoides, little prognostic information can be gleaned from histopathologic sections. Whether a patient has patches, plaques, or tumors can be determined clinically (there are a few pitfalls, however, such as mistaking lesions elevated by comedones for nodules). The finding of transformed lymphocytes in plaques and tumors of mycosis fungoides has an adverse effect on survival in some studies and little effect in others. One study showed that follicular mycosis fungoides—cases in which the epidermis was largely spared and hair follicles bore the brunt of infiltration by lymphocytes, with or without follicular mucinosis—has a less favorable prognosis than more routine presentations.[16] Folliculotropic lesions are small papules and can be suspected clinically, but their occurrence should be confirmed by pathologic examination.

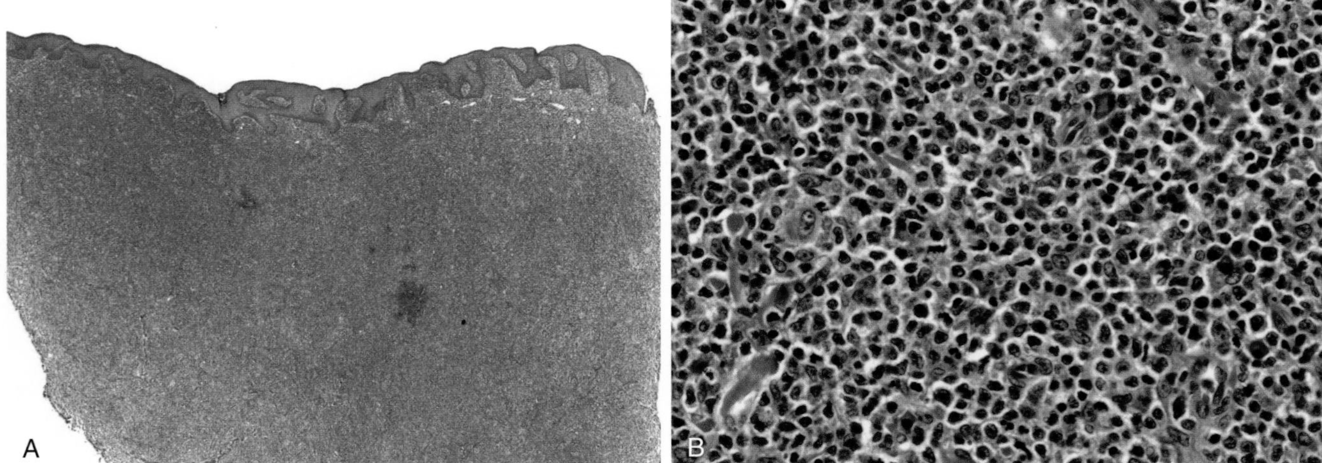

Figure 38-9. A, Mycosis fungoides tumor with diffuse infiltration of the dermis. There may be a variety of cytomorphologic findings in the lymphocytes of tumor-stage lesions, but large cerebriform cells or cells with large vesicular nuclei usually predominate. **B,** Unlike in patches, eosinophils and plasma cells are commonly present in tumors, and the epidermis is often spared.

Immunophenotype

The cells of mycosis fungoides are mature helper T cells in the large majority of cases, with a βF1⁺, CD3⁺, CD4⁺, CD8⁻ phenotype. Patches of mycosis fungoides usually have neoplastic cells that express the normal panoply of T-cell antigens, such as CD2 and CD5, but may not express CD7.[22] Some papers refer to a "loss" of CD7, whereas others view mycosis fungoides as a neoplastic expansion of the normally occurring (but minority population) of CD7⁻ helper T cells. Whether the finding of large numbers of CD3⁺, CD4⁺, CD7⁻ cells in a cutaneous infiltrate is diagnostic of mycosis fungoides is controversial. There are practical impediments to the implementation of this finding as a diagnostic criterion, even if it were a scientifically valid concept. Staining for CD7 is most reliable in frozen sections, where it is difficult to discern morphologic features. There are commercially available antibodies to CD7 that react with paraffin-embedded sections,[23] and some groups have published results suggesting that staining may be helpful in the diagnosis. One limitation is that fixation in formalin for longer than 24 hours seems to abolish staining. This makes the technique difficult to use in laboratories that receive outpatient specimens. Also, the neoplastic population may be in the minority in many patches of mycosis fungoides, making it difficult to assess cell phenotype.

As noted earlier, a variety of immunophenotypes can occur in patients who, on clinical grounds and by conventional histopathologic examination, seem to have mycosis fungoides. These include CD8⁺ and even CD56⁺ immunophenotypes. How common this situation is depends on how many cases are tested with these antibodies. CD8⁺ cases usually have a cytotoxic immunophenotype. CD56⁺ cases are rarer and can have several different immunophenotypes.[24]

Plaques and tumors of mycosis fungoides often have other aberrations—diminished expression of CD5, CD2, or even CD3—but by the time these findings are present, the diagnosis can be easily established by routine methods. A cytotoxic phenotype with TIA-1 and granzyme B expression can occur in later stage lesions.[25]

CD30 is an antigen expressed on the cells of Hodgkin's lymphoma and by those of anaplastic large cell lymphoma. Its presence is not specific, and it is also expressed by lymphocytes that have been stimulated by antigen in infectious and inflammatory conditions. CD30⁺ cells occur in some plaques of mycosis fungoides, but mostly in tumors that have anaplastic large cells. There seems to be no prognostic significance to CD30 expression in mycosis fungoides when it is detected in patches.[26]

Genotype

Mycosis fungoides cells have undergone rearrangement of their T-cell receptor genes. Clonal rearrangement of the alpha-beta T-cell receptor genes is present in the vast majority of cases and can be detected by Southern blot using fresh or frozen specimens. Rearrangement of the gamma chain gene is also present in the great majority of cases and can be detected using polymerase chain reaction (PCR). Various modifications of PCR have been used to enhance its specificity. Because PCR can detect the presence of even 1% clonal cells, there is significant risk that the blind application of this technique may lead to the misdiagnosis of inflammatory skin diseases of various kinds as mycosis fungoides. It is therefore important that PCR be applied judiciously to cases in which mycosis fungoides is compatible clinically and suspected microscopically.

A recent modification of PCR testing has enabled analysis of the T-cell receptor beta chain gene. This may prove to be more specific, but only a few studies of inflammatory skin diseases and simulators of cutaneous lymphoma have been performed with this technique.[27]

Postulated Cell of Origin

Because patches of mycosis fungoides have a CD3⁺, CD4⁺, CD8⁻ phenotype in the large majority of cases, the cell of origin is most likely the lymphocytic population with similar findings in peripheral blood. These are activated, mature helper T cells. Recently, attention has been given to the role of T regulatory cells in several inflammatory skin diseases and in mycosis fungoides. It appears that these cells, which are positive for CD25 and FOXP3, may play a role in mycosis fungoides, but whether the disease derives from them is still an open question.[28]

Clinical Course

As noted earlier, patients with patches of mycosis fungoides often have indolent disease for many years; if the condition is limited to less than 10% of the body surface, life span is often unaffected.[29] Those with more extensive patches are more likely to develop plaques and tumors as well as internal disease. Patients with disseminated plaques, tumors, or both may develop internal disease. This can take the form of adenopathy, hepatosplenomegaly, or infiltrates in other organs that can be detected only by biopsy or necropsy. The most serious effects are on the immune system, however. Although the peripheral helper T-cell counts of patients with mycosis fungoides may be nearly normal or high, those with advanced disease often have diminished numbers of functional T-helper cells. Those in the blood may be neoplastic cells, which cannot respond effectively to infection. In its terminal stages, mycosis fungoides results in death from immunodeficiency.[30]

Differential Diagnosis

A number of conditions simulate mycosis fungoides clinically, pathologically, or both. Knowledge of the differential diagnosis of mycosis fungoides is critical for recognition of its patch stage; it is less important in more advanced stages.

The skin diseases that simulate the patch stage of mycosis fungoides result in macules or patches of slightly inflamed, scaling skin. These include forms of spongiotic dermatitis, such as allergic contact or nummular dermatitis; pityriasis rosea; and interface dermatitides, such as lichenoid drug eruptions. Spongiotic dermatitis usually has perivascular rather than band-like infiltrates in the superficial dermis, as well as areas with abundant spongiosis without many lymphocytes. A helpful feature in some cases is the presence of eosinophils. Early patches of mycosis fungoides seldom have more than a few eosinophils. Although spongiotic dermatitides may lack eosinophils entirely, many cases have eosinophils in both the dermis and (if one looks carefully) the

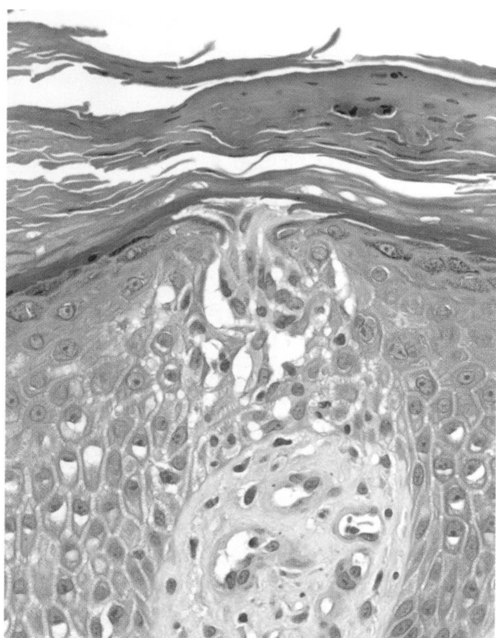

Figure 38-10. Vase-shaped collection of Langerhans cells in spongiotic dermatitis.

epidermis. Early patches of mycosis fungoides practically never have eosinophils in the epidermis.

One pitfall posed by the spongiotic dermatitides is the presence of collections of pale staining mononuclear cells in the epidermis (Fig. 38-10). These collections, composed of Langerhans cells and their monocytic precursors, have a heterogeneous composition.[31] Their cells have pale cytoplasm and reniform vesicular nulcei. True Pautrier's microabscesses or collections in mycosis fungoides are compactly arranged aggregations in which lymphocytes predominate. The cells have scant cytoplasm, and the nuclei are darker than in so-called Langerhans cell pustules. Another clue is the shape of the aggregations. True Pautrier's microabscesses are round, whereas their spongiotic counterparts often have a vase-like shape, with everted lips on the epidermal surface.[31] In the rare case when immunohistochemistry is used to distinguish between Pautrier's microabscesses and Langerhans cell pustules, the former are composed mostly of cells that stain for CD3, and the latter are composed of cells that stain for either CD1a or CD68. A CD1a⁺ Langerhans cell is usually found at the center of each Pautrier's microabscess.

Interface dermatitides are a clinically diverse group of diseases in which lymphocytes obscure the dermoepidermal junction. The consequences of this infiltration include vacuolar change, an alteration in the shape of rete ridges (they become serrated or recede entirely), and cytotoxic damage to keratinocytes, visible as dyskeratotic cells in the epidermis and as colloid bodies when these descend into the papillary dermis. Small foci with these findings commonly occur in mycosis fungoides. They are seldom the dominant feature in all lesions of a single patient, although there is a rare variant in which such changes occur (Fig. 38-11).[32] It cannot be overemphasized, however, that a single biopsy from a patient with mycosis fungoides can show an interface pattern and that several biopsies must be done if mycosis fungoides is suspected clinically.[33] Pathologists unfamiliar with lichen planus, lichenoid drug eruptions, lichenoid keratoses, and even densely infiltrated lesions of lupus erythematosus may mistake these lesions for mycosis fungoides owing to numerous lymphocytes in the lower part of the epidermis in such cases. Lichenoid keratoses may present a particular diagnostic challenge because they can feature many lymphocytes in the epidermis.[34]

There are several inflammatory diseases that cause a psoriasiform lichenoid pattern or a psoriasiform lichenoid spongiotic pattern—the most common patterns in patches of mycosis fungoides. In some cases lymphocytes even lie in the basal layer of the epidermis in a linear fashion ("beads on a string"), without the same degree of vacuolar change or number of necrotic keratinocytes seen in most interface dermatitides. Luckily, many of these conditions do not simulate mycosis fungoides clinically. Lichen striatus, for example, causes linearly arranged papules along Blaschko's lines in children and adolescents more often than in adults.[35] Lichen sclerosus et atrophicus has an inflammatory phase that can mimic mycosis fungoides, but solitary lesions of mycosis fungoides on the skin of the genitalia essentially do not occur. Extragenital lichen sclerosus may present problems in this regard, especially if sampled by a thin shave biopsy.[36]

Among the most treacherous entities with a psoriasiform lichenoid pattern are members of a group of conditions

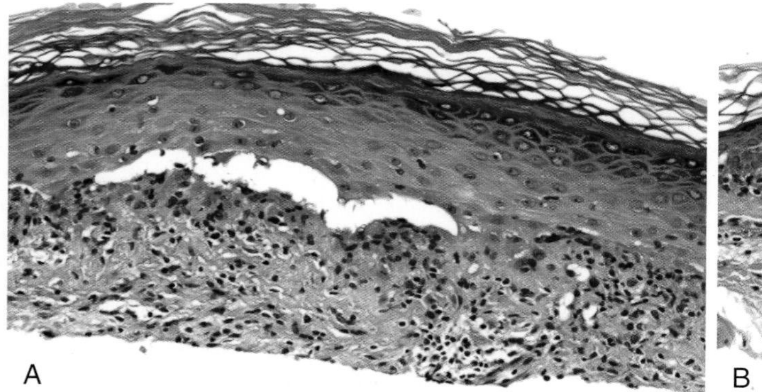

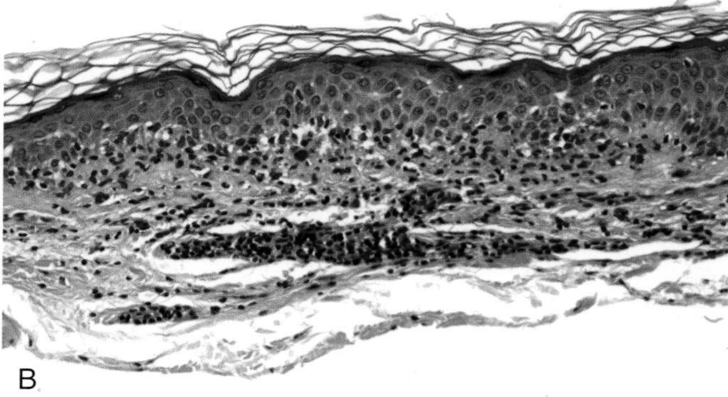

Figure 38-11. A, The lichenoid variant of mycosis fungoides is easily mistaken for an interface dermatitis. Clefts may be present at the dermoepidermal junction, and there may be wedge-shaped foci of hypergranulosis, as in lichen planus. **B,** Another area features a more characteristic pattern.

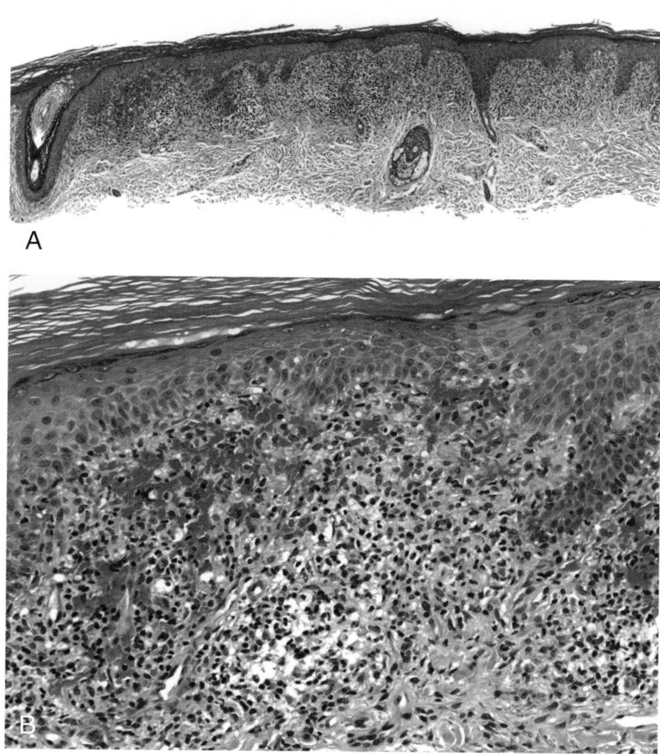

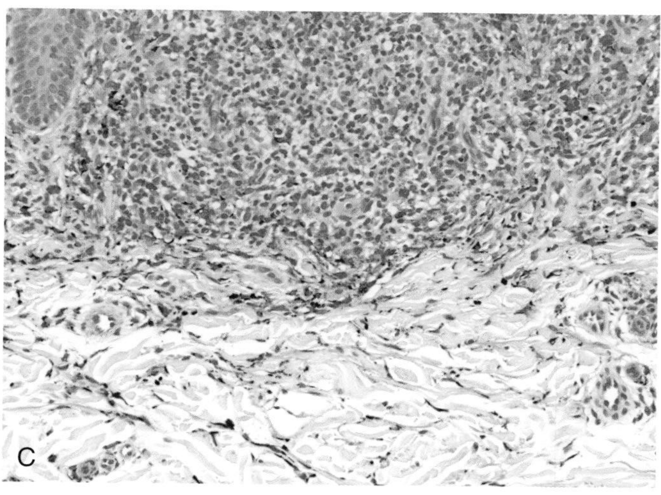

Figure 38-12. Lichenoid purpura can simulate mycosis fungoides because of its psoriasiform lichenoid pattern (**A**). Many extravasated erythrocytes are often present (**B**), resulting in the deposition of siderophages, which can be highlighted by Perls stain (**C**).

termed *persistent pigmented purpuric dermatitis*.[37,38] These diseases usually affect the skin of the legs, resulting in red to rust or golden brown macules, papules, and sometimes plaques. They are caused by infiltrates of lymphocytes that somehow induce venules to leak red blood cells into the dermis. Over time, siderophages accumulate. Two forms—lichenoid purpura of Gougerot and Blum and lichen aureus—have dense, band-like infiltrates of lymphocytes, sometimes in a fibrotic and thickened papillary dermis (Fig. 38-12). Because lesions of mycosis fungoides can become purpuric, it is possible for the lichenoid variants of persistent pigmented purpuric dermatitis to have all the features of purpuric mycosis fungoides except for the striking cytologic atypia. To the extent that there may be edema of the papillary dermis in persistent pigmented purpuric dermatitis, the conditions can be distinguished histopathologically.

Whether the close histomorphologic similarities between mycosis fungoides and persistent pigmented purpuric dermatitis indicate a biologic relationship is an unanswered question. One of the first cases of lichen aureus reported in North America turned out to be mycosis fungoides.[39] Clonality can be present in many cases of persistent pigmented purpuric dermatitis using PCR-based methods, making that technique less useful for telling the conditions apart. The clinical picture—whether lesions are mostly on the legs or disseminated—can be more helpful than histopathologic or immunophenotypic findings. Patients with clinically typical lichen aureus show no significant tendency to progress to mycosis fungoides, despite the finding of clonality in about half the cases.[40]

Although children only rarely develop mycosis fungoides, there are several pitfalls in diagnosing such cases. Mycosis fungoides in children seems to result in hypopigmentation in a disproportionate number of cases[41]; so-called hypopigmented mycosis fungoides can be mistaken for vitiligo, pityriasis alba, and pityriasis lichenoides chronica, and vice versa. Vitiligo usually has symmetrically distributed lesions (unlike those of mycosis fungoides), with a tendency to affect flexural skin. One problem is that biopsy specimens from the edge of the lesion, especially in so-called trichrome vitiligo, can feature many lymphocytes among keratinocytes of the basal layer. Rebiopsy of the center of the lesion should show a picture devoid of lymphocytes and with a lack of melanocytes. Pityriasis alba is a spongiotic dermatitis that results in pale, slightly scaly lesions. There are superficial lymphocytic infiltrates with a touch of spongiosis. The lymphocytes do not align themselves along the junction and are no larger than their dermal counterparts. The dermal papillae should be edematous, not fibrotic. Pityriasis lichenoides chronica is an interface dermatitis, and vacuolar change coupled with single necrotic keratinocytes at the junction should be present.

A recently described condition, annular lichenoid dermatitis of youth,[42] may simulate mycosis fungoides by virtue of large, annular lesions and a tendency for lymphocytes to be clustered at the bases of rete ridges. Although the clusters of lymphocytes can resemble those of mycosis fungoides in terms of size, the shapes of the rete ridges are distinctive. They are square based in annular lichenoid dermatitis of youth, and the cells in the basal layer are squamous rather than cuboid. In the only large series to date on this condition, clonal T-cell

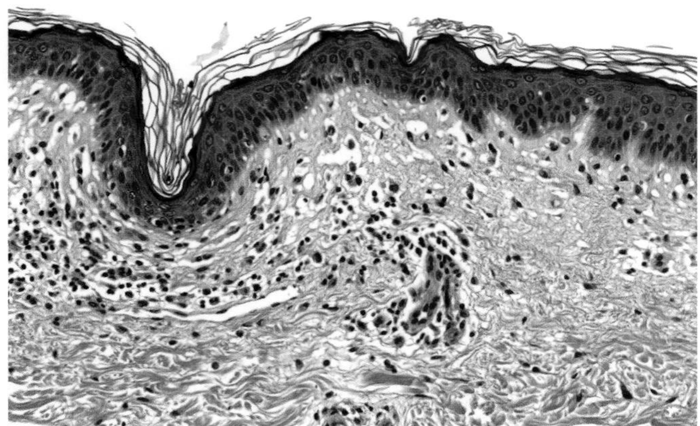

Figure 38-13. In the atrophic patch stage of mycosis fungoides, there are often very few lymphocytes within the epidermis, making a specific diagnosis problematic, especially with small biopsy specimens.

populations were not present. The immunophenotype is usually CD8+ and cytotoxic.[43]

The atrophic or poikilodermatous patch stage of mycosis fungoides is imitated by several conditions in which the epidermis is thinned by an interface dermatitis (Fig. 38-13). These include the atrophic variant of lichen planus (and, rarely, atrophy from a lichenoid drug eruption), poikilodermatomyositis, atrophic centers of lesions of porokeratosis (a condition in which a clone of abnormal keratinocytes migrates centrifugally, sometimes leaving atrophy in its wake), and, occasionally, atrophic lesions of persistent pigmented purpuric dermatitis. There are other rare forms of poikiloderma, such as the congenital Rothmund-Thomson syndrome.[44] Similar histopathologic changes also result from regression of melanoma if little pigment is present and from regression of Bowen's disease, superficial basal cell carcinoma, and solar lentigo (so-called lichen planus–like keratosis). In all these conditions, and in atrophic patches of mycosis fungoides, lymphocytes of the host response to a neoplasm destroy the keratinocytes of rete ridges, resulting in epidermal atrophy. It may not be possible to distinguish between atrophic mycosis fungoides and these conditions unless many lymphocytes reside in the basal layer of the epidermis. This may require extensive sampling.

Another important mimic of mycosis fungoides is lymphomatoid allergic contact dermatitis.[45] In this unusual type of allergic contact dermatitis, many more lymphocytes are attracted to the epidermis than normally; sometimes the lymphocytes are cytologically atypical. Although a distinction between conventional spongiotic dermatitis and mycosis fungoides is usually possible without recourse to clinical information, in some cases of lymphomatoid contact dermatitis, the clinical history is key.

Drug eruptions can also simulate the patch stage of mycosis fungoides. Diphenylhydantoin can cause a systemic illness in which adenopathy is accompanied by an eruption resembling mycosis fungoides. This may also occur without any systemic symptoms. The clinical history is one key to making this diagnosis. Other drugs can cause hypersensitivity reactions that mimic the patches of mycosis fungoides, even digitate ones.[46]

For the most part, the plaque and tumor stages of mycosis fungoides are simulated by other lymphomas, not by inflammatory conditions. One exception is the recently described interstitial type of mycosis fungoides.[47] Interstitial mycosis fungoides usually has scant lymphocytes in the epidermis and papillary dermis in comparison with conventional plaque-stage disease. Its hallmark is the finding of strands of lymphocytes positioned between collagen bundles in the reticular dermis. Clinically, it may resemble some dusky lesions of morphea or granuloma annulare, and it can be very difficult to distinguish from the former.

Tumors of mycosis fungoides may be impossible to distinguish from those of other T-cell lymphomas without recourse to clinical examination. The infiltrates of peripheral T-cell lymphomas can present in the skin or with systemic disease.[48] The infiltrates are predominantly dermal. Because some lymphocytes can infiltrate the epidermis in peripheral T-cell lymphomas, a pathologist with no knowledge of the clinical picture cannot differentiate a plaque or tumor of mycosis fungoides from a nodule of peripheral T-cell lymphoma. Only the presence of patches elsewhere on the patient's body allows these conditions to be distinguished. A tumor of mycosis fungoides in which anaplastic large lymphocytes predominate and diffusely express CD30 can be an exact replica of anaplastic large cell lymphoma, but the patient has a much worse prognosis. Again, the clinical examination is key.

One variant of primary cutaneous lymphoma, CD4+ small/medium T-cell lymphoma (formerly called CD4+ small/medium pleomorphic T-cell lymphoma), is particularly problematic to distinguish pathologically from mycosis fungoides. Usually, very few lymphocytes are present in the epidermis. The differential diagnosis is a tumor of mycosis fungoides with little epidermal involvement and a predominance of smaller cells. The number of B cells in this condition is substantial and has been attributed to a proliferation of follicular center T cells.[49-51] Primary cutaneous CD4+ small/medium T-cell lymphoma usually presents as a single plaque or nodule, although more than one may be present. It is imperative to perform a full-body skin examination before making the diagnosis. The prognosis is excellent, compared with that of tumor-stage mycosis fungoides.

Variants

The various effects of the cells of mycosis fungoides on the different constituents of the skin, the effects of host inflammatory cells responding to the neoplastic ones, and the disturbed microenvironment of cytokines, chemokines, and the like account for the prodigious differences in the clinical and microscopic appearance of mycosis fungoides lesions. The cells of mycosis fungoides, which usually home to the epidermis, can also localize in other sites.

Follicular Mycosis Fungoides

The hair follicles can become a magnet for the cells of mycosis fungoides (Fig. 38-14). This reaction is usually accompanied by the accumulation of mucopolysaccharides between keratinocytes in the outer root sheath. The resulting histopathologic pattern, follicular mucinosis, is not specific for mycosis fungoides and can occur as an incidental finding. The term *alopecia mucinosa* refers to follicular mucinosis in multiple follicles, resulting in hair loss. As noted earlier, it is contro-

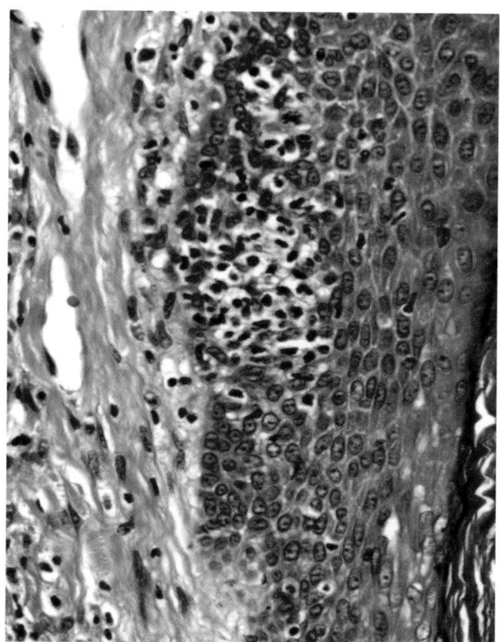

Figure 38-14. In follicular mycosis fungoides, lymphocytes may home to the follicular epithelium rather than to the epidermis.

versial whether alopecia mucinosa is an inflammatory condition or an indolent form of mycosis fungoides.[52]

Lesions of mycosis fungoides presenting with alopecia mucinosa feature variably dense perifollicular infiltrates of lymphocytes and, notably, eosinophils; lymphocytes within the follicular epithelium; mucin in the widened spaces between keratinocytes; and plugging of follicular ostia by compact hyperkeratosis. The interfollicular epidermis is usually spared, and most of the lymphocytes are relatively small, making an outright diagnosis of lymphoma difficult.

In a minority of patients with follicular lesions, little or no excess mucin accumulates. The follicular papules that result can clinically simulate keratosis pilaris or other follicular diseases. Regardless of whether mucin is present, these patients seem to have a less favorable prognosis than those with conventional mycosis fungoides.[16,17,53]

Mycosis Fungoides with Cysts and Comedones

Some patients with follicular mycosis fungoides, with or without follicular mucinosis, have lesions in which large comedones or even follicular cysts develop.[54,55] This probably results from occlusion of the follicular infundibulum by the infiltrates of mycosis fungoides. This complication is disfiguring but may respond to treatment of the disease. The prognosis is the same as that for follicular mycosis fungoides.

Bullous Mycosis Fungoides

In this rare variant, the cells of mycosis fungoides replace basal keratinocytes to the extent that cohesion between the epidermis and dermis is compromised, and trivial shearing forces result in clinical vesiculation. Usually the diagnosis can be made by examining areas that have not vesiculated.[56]

Syringotropic Mycosis Fungoides

Lymphoma cells' tropism for secretory glands is exemplified by the epimyoepithelial islands formed in some low-grade B-cell lymphomas, such as marginal zone lymphoma (although not in the skin). Some patients with mycosis fungoides have dense infiltrates of lymphocytes around eccrine secretory coils in addition to infiltrates elsewhere in the dermis and epidermis (Fig. 38-15).[57] A more purely syringotropic variant of mycosis fungoides in a patient who also had folliculotropic infiltrates was initially described as *syringolymphoid*

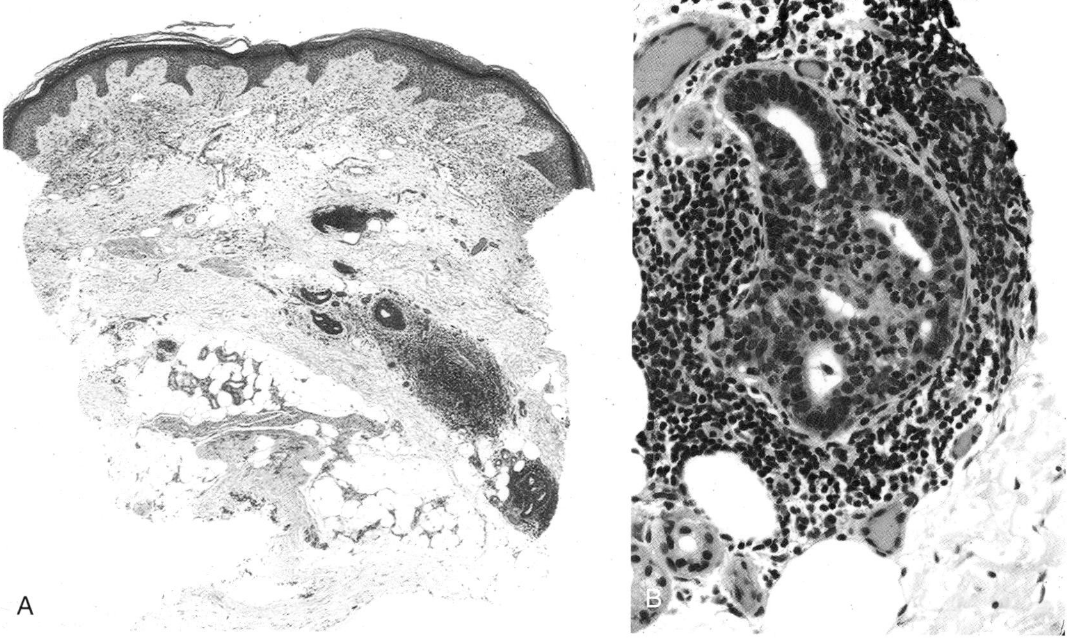

Figure 38-15. **A**, Syringotropic mycosis fungoides features dense infiltrates of lymphocytes around the eccrine secretory coils. **B**, There may be hyperplasia of the epithelial and myoepithelial cells, similar to that in epimyoepithelial islands.

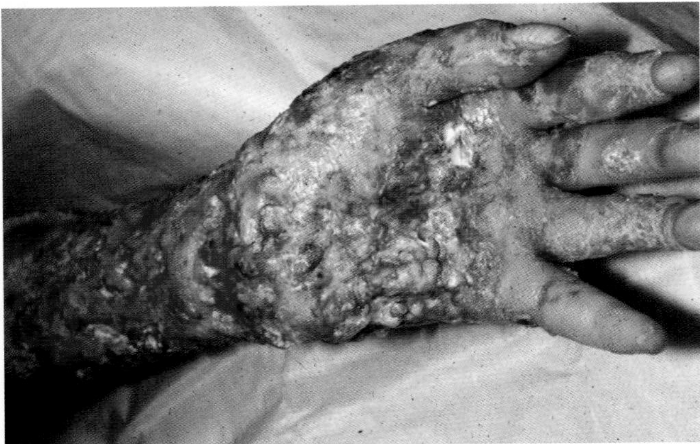

Figure 38-16. Woringer-Kolopp disease, or pagetoid reticulosis, presents as verrucous plaques on acral skin. (Courtesy of Dr. Sabine Kohler, Stanford University.)

hyperplasia with alopecia.[58] The cutaneous lesions are often small papules and may be accompanied by anhidrosis. Most authors accept that this condition is a variant of mycosis fungoides rather than an inflammatory disease.[59] This variant is too rare to know with certainty whether its prognosis is different from that of more common forms, but in a review of 15 cases published before 2004, its behavior seemed unremarkable.[60]

Pagetoid Reticulosis

Although the bullous and syringotropic variants have lymphocytes that ignore the epidermis in favor of adnexal epithelium, in pagetoid reticulosis the lymphocytes' attraction to the epidermis is exaggerated. The affected skin is usually on the extremities, so the clinical lesions are warty, hyperkeratotic plaques on the hands and feet (Fig. 38-16). Pagetoid reticulosis was initially described by Woringer and Kolopp in two children; subsequent reports have highlighted that it occurs in younger patients than is usual for mycosis fungoides. It also differs from conventional mycosis fungoides by its failure to disseminate in the vast majority of cases.

Its histopathologic hallmark is verrucous epidermal hyperplasia, coupled with infiltrates of lymphocytes that have cytologic atypia and are disproportionately situated in the epidermis (Fig. 38-17).[61] The immunophenotype includes $CD4^+$ or $CD8^+$ T cells and a propensity for the cells to be $CD30^+$ and, in some cases, to lack CD45 (leukocyte common antigen).[62] Its prognosis is far better than that of conventional mycosis fungoides. Many patients achieve durable remissions by local therapeutic means, such as excision of lesions or radiation therapy.

Another entity that shares the moniker pagetoid reticulosis is the Ketron-Goodman variant of mycosis fungoides, with striking epidermotropism and disseminated lesions. Some examples of this condition have a $CD4^-$, $CD8^-$ (primitive T-cell) phenotype.[63] Some of these cases may be $CD8^+$ aggressive epidermotropic lymphoma, sometimes termed *Berti's lymphoma.*[64]

Granulomatous Mycosis Fungoides

There are many lymphomas, both cutaneous and nodal, that have foci in which histiocytes predominate. Plaques and tumors of mycosis fungoides can contain such foci in the

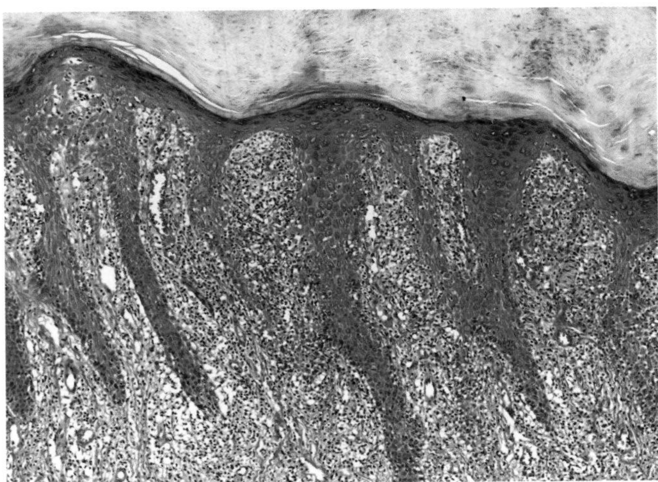

Figure 38-17. Histopathologic findings in pagetoid reticulosis include verrucous epidermal hyperplasia with infiltration of the epidermis, similar to or even more pronounced than that seen in conventional mycosis fungoides.

reticular dermis. The findings can range from loose clusters of histiocytes to scattered giant cells to well-formed granulomatous tubercles (Fig. 38-18). The plaques and tumors of granulomatous mycosis fungoides usually do not have a distinct appearance.

In the initial description of granulomatous mycosis fungoides, the authors noted that their patient had survived longer than expected. Fourteen years later, their patient was still alive and had had granulomatous mycosis fungoides for nearly 3 decades.[65] Their conclusion, that the prognosis of granulomatous mycosis fungoides is more favorable than that of conventional mycosis fungoides, has not been confirmed by other studies.[66,67] There may be a variety of causes of granulomatous infiltrates in mycosis fungoides: lymphocytes may attract histiocytes, giant cells may appear as antigens on elastotic fibers (similar to the foci that resemble actinic gran-

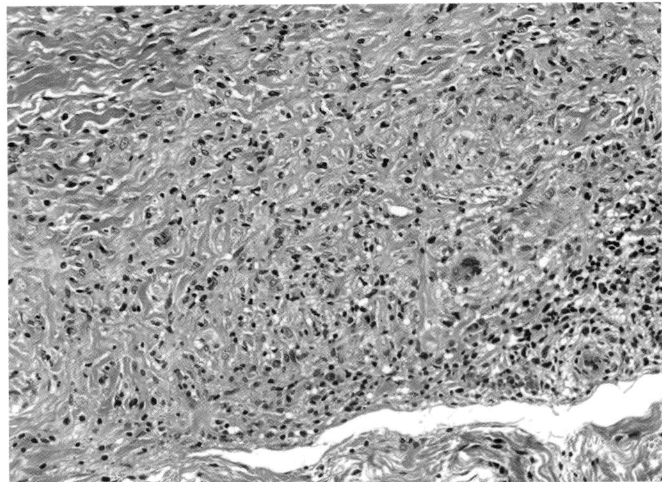

Figure 38-18. Granulomatous mycosis fungoides is not distinctive clinically, but its histopathologic findings include many histiocytes, sometimes multinucleated, interspersed with lymphocytic infiltrates in the dermis.

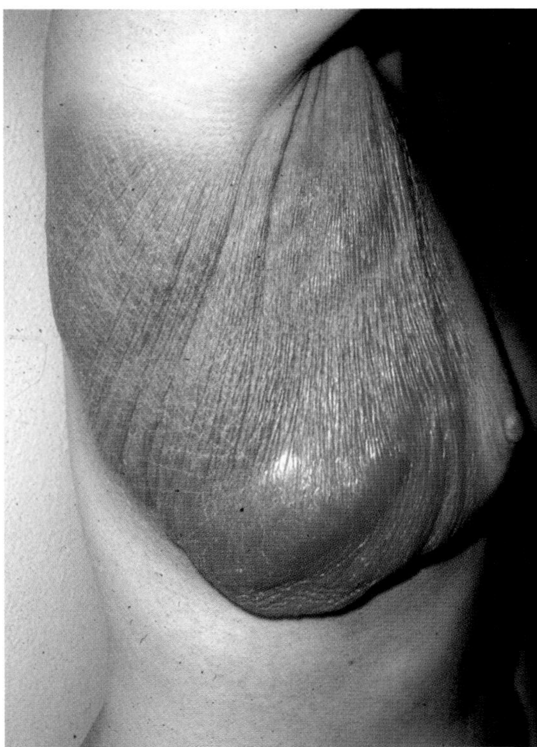

Figure 38-19. Granulomatous slack skin typically presents with pendulous masses in the axilla and groin.

uloma in many inflammatory diseases in sun-damaged skin), or keratin or mucin from leaky follicles, may incite a granulomatous reaction. A reanalysis of the data seems to be prudent before reaching firm conclusions about the prognosis of this variant.

Granulomatous Slack Skin

Granulomatous slack skin is a peculiar condition in which the cells of an epidermotropic T-cell lymphoma attract histiocytes, which in turn digest elastic tissue and lead to the formation of large sac-like skin folds. The disease affects younger patients than is usual for mycosis fungoides, with most cases beginning in young adulthood. The usual sites of involvement are the axilla and groin (Fig. 38-19). Hodgkin's lymphoma has reportedly developed in several patients with granulomatous slack skin.[68,69] However, it is uncertain whether the lymphoma that develops in the internal organs of patients with granulomatous slack skin is truly Hodgkin's lymphoma or is a large T-cell lymphoma, given that the reported cases were not comprehensively worked up by current standards.

The most striking histopathologic feature of granulomatous slack skin is involvement of the dermis and subcutaneous lobules by tuberculoid granulomas—clusters of histiocytes and giant cells surrounded and infiltrated by small lymphocytes.[70-72] The tubercles tend to be discrete and spaced at regular intervals throughout the infiltrate (Fig. 38-20). The giant cells sometimes contain elastic fibers in specially stained sections, indicating that they are responsible for the profound elastolysis that occurs in this condition and leads to the distinctive pendulous skin folds.

Only when one examines the epidermis and papillary dermis is it evident that granulomatous slack skin is related to mycosis fungoides. Indeed, the changes in the superficial part of the biopsy can be identical to those of mycosis fungoides. Immunophenotypic studies have been performed in only a few cases, but they indicate a $CD4^+$, $CD7^-$ T-cell population, like that of mycosis fungoides. Gene rearrangement studies have shown clonality in almost all cases tested to date.

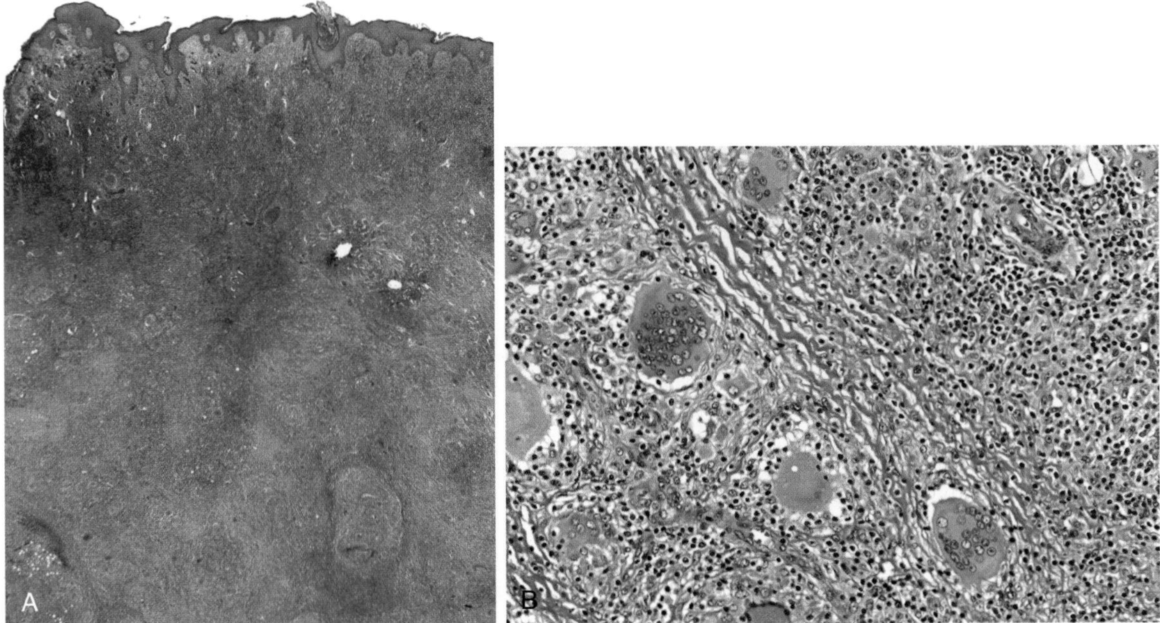

Figure 38-20. Granulomatous slack skin usually shows a dense, diffuse infiltrate of small lymphocytes throughout the dermis (**A**), with infiltration of the epidermis similar to that seen in mycosis fungoides and large histiocytic giant cells that enact elastophagocytosis (**B**).

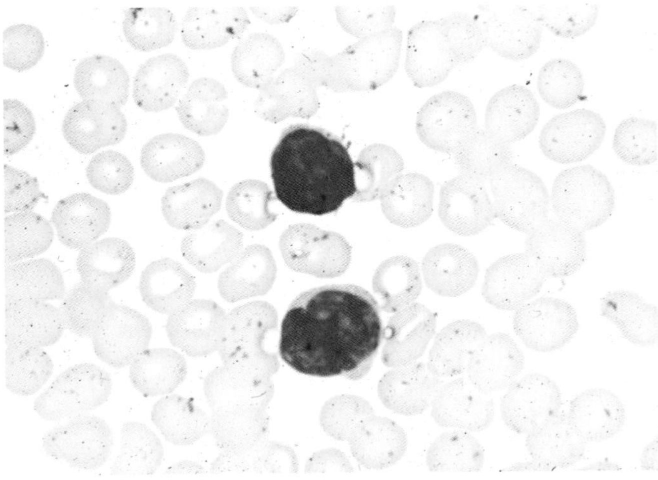

Figure 38-21. Sézary cells in a peripheral blood smear. Recognition of these cells is no longer critical for the diagnosis since the advent of clonality studies and flow cytometry.

SÉZARY SYNDROME

Definition

Sézary syndrome is the leukemic counterpart of mycosis fungoides. The classic features include circulating Sézary cells (lymphocytes with abnormally convoluted nuclei; Fig. 38-21), erythroderma (diffuse reddening of the skin; Fig. 38-22), hyperkeratosis of the palms and soles, and lymphadenopathy. Because many of these features can supervene in patients with mycosis fungoides, some advocate the term *erythrodermic cutaneous T-cell lymphoma*. Criteria for the diagnosis of Sézary syndrome include the presence of a peripheral blood lymphocytosis, a T-cell clone in the peripheral blood, an elevated CD4/CD8 ratio (>10), and immunophenotypic abnormalities. When strictly defined, Sézary syndrome is quite rare.

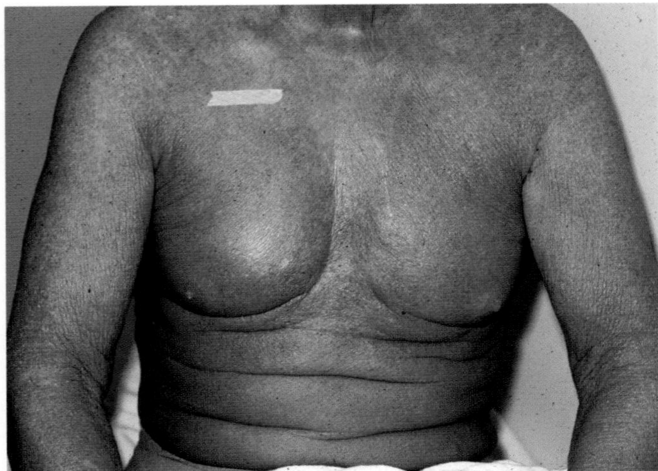

Figure 38-22. Sézary syndrome presents with erythroderma—diffuse red skin. The term *erythroderma* is often overused by clinicians; it should refer to confluent erythema, not just widespread erythematous lesions.

Epidemiology

Like mycosis fungoides, Sézary syndrome is a disease of the middle-aged and elderly. When strictly defined—requiring true erythroderma rather than just disseminated lesions—it is much less common than mycosis fungoides.

Etiology

There are no known risk factors for Sézary syndrome (other than mycosis fungoides). As is the case with mycosis fungoides, a link to HTLV-1 has been proposed but is far from proved.

Immunophenotypic Features

The majority of cases of Sézary syndrome are $CD3^+$, $CD4^+$, $CD8^-$, $CD7^-$ neoplasms consisting of mature helper T cells, similar in these respects to mycosis fungoides. The finding of a predominant phenotype in the peripheral blood by flow cytometry favors the diagnosis of Sézary syndrome, especially when buttressed by clonality. One must remember that in skin biopsies, an elevated CD4/CD8 ratio is not as specific.[73] The phenotype in a given patient is sufficiently stable that flow cytometry can be used to monitor response to therapy.[74]

Genotypic Features

Sézary syndrome has long been known to be a clonal T-cell proliferation.[75] Unlike mycosis fungoides, in which biopsy specimens are full of nonneoplastic cells, Sézary syndrome has a sufficient number of circulating neoplastic cells to prove the diagnosis in most cases. Chromosomal abnormalities can be identified in Sézary syndrome, but no one abnormality is found in a preponderance of cases.[76] Analysis using comparative genomic hybridization has shown differences between Sézary syndrome and mycosis fungoides.[77]

Clinical Features

The salient clinical features of Sézary syndrome—erythroderma, palmar and plantar hyperkeratosis, and lymphadenopathy—were first noted by Sézary and Bouvrain in their original report. Erythroderma is a clinical sign in which the entire skin becomes red and sometimes scaly. It has also been called the "red man" effect. In erythroderma due to lymphoma, the skin can become doughy as well. There are many other causes of erythroderma besides Sézary syndrome, but its presence in a middle-aged or older patient should evoke a differential diagnosis that includes lymphoma. Hyperkeratosis of the palms and soles leads to red, scaly, and sometimes fissured skin. The nails may be lost or become dystrophic. Generalized lymphadenopathy is often present in patients with Sézary syndrome.

Histopathologic Features

Biopsy of the skin is often the first step in the diagnosis of Sézary syndrome, but it can be a frustrating exercise (Fig. 38-23). Many patients with Sézary syndrome have skin changes that resemble those of mycosis fungoides; however, even if repeated biopsies are done, only about half have find-

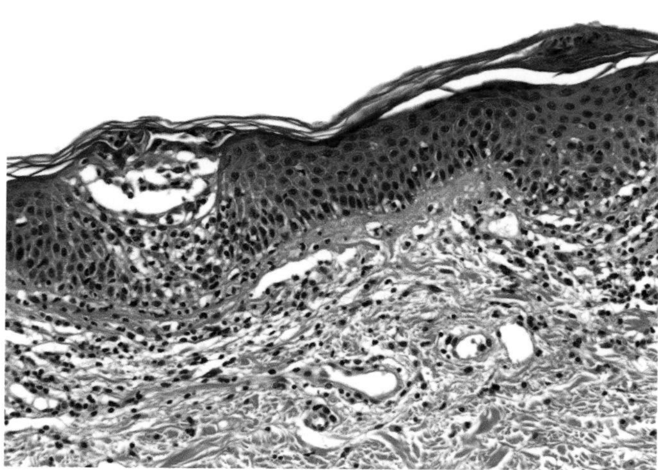

Figure 38-23. The histopathologic findings in Sézary syndrome often fall short of being diagnostic. In this example, there is too much spongiosis for an outright diagnosis without knowing the clinical and peripheral blood findings.

ings that would not be diagnostic of mycosis fungoides. There is often more spongiosis than in diagnostic samples of mycosis fungoides, and the lymphocytes are often small.

Differential Diagnosis

Because of the many inflammatory conditions that cause erythroderma, and because of the lack of diagnostic changes in the biopsies of many patients with Sézary syndrome, one must approach the differential diagnosis of erythroderma with great caution. The most common causes of erythroderma, aside from Sézary syndrome, include psoriasis, pityriasis rubra pilaris, generalized allergic contact dermatitis, and drug eruptions. In some patients the erythroderma resolves spontaneously, and its cause is never determined. In general, the histopathologic features of erythrodermic presentations of inflammatory skin diseases are those of the underlying condition.

The findings in erythrodermic psoriasis resemble those of early patches of psoriasis rather than well-developed plaques. The rete ridges are slightly elongated; keratinocytes have pale cytoplasm; and dilated, tortuous vessels are prominent in edematous dermal papillae and may even appear to touch the undersurface of the epidermis. Small mounds of parakeratosis, both with and without neutrophils, may be present.

Pityriasis rubra pilaris shares many features with psoriasis, but it presents with diffuse orange-red skin. The palms and soles of affected patients are often thickened by cornified material that has been likened to carnauba wax. Biopsies of pityriasis rubra pilaris often show slight psoriasiform epidermal hyperplasia, an epidermis with a gently undulating surface, and lamellar hyperkeratosis containing scattered parakeratotic nuclei.

Erythrodermic allergic contact dermatitis represents a generalized response to a contactant. Its features are essentially those of a conventional spongiotic dermatitis. There may be more of a tendency for the inflammatory cells in the papillary dermis to have a band-like pattern than in conventional allergic contact dermatitis.

Erythrodermic drug eruptions have a variety of histopathologic presentations. These include the findings of spongiotic dermatitis, interface dermatitis, or, rarely, psoriasiform dermatitis.

Pearls and Pitfalls: Diagnosing Early Mycosis Fungoides

- Diagnosis during the patch stage is optimal but may not influence survival.
- Overdiagnosis of mycosis fungoides can be emotionally traumatic to patients.
- Immunophenotypic studies are usually not essential for diagnosis and do not provide prognostic information.
- Genotypic studies are useful for confirming the diagnosis only if mycosis fungoides is clinically and pathologically plausible.
- There are myriad inflammatory skin diseases, and many can simulate mycosis fungoides clinically and pathologically. The diagnosis of mycosis fungoides is best established with the collaboration of a knowledgeable clinician, unless the histopathologic findings are unequivocal.

References can be found on Expert Consult @ www.expertconsult.com

Chapter 39

Primary Cutaneous CD30-Positive T-Cell Lymphoproliferative Disorders

Marshall E. Kadin

CHAPTER OUTLINE

DEFINITION

Three types of primary cutaneous CD30⁺ lymphoproliferative disorders (LPDs) are recognized in the World Health Organization classification: primary cutaneous anaplastic large cell lymphoma (C-ALCL), lymphomatoid papulosis (LyP), and borderline lesions. These entities represent a continuous spectrum of lesions that are not clearly demarcated by clinical appearance or histology in some instances.[1,2] LyP occurs as multiple recurrent, often centrally necrotic, papulonodular lesions up to 2 cm in diameter; the lesions regress spontaneously, usually in 4 to 6 weeks, leaving a hyper- or hypopigmented scar.[3,4] C-ALCL commonly presents as one to several tumors greater than 2 cm in diameter, often localized, but occasionally multicentric.[2,4,5] The tumors of primary C-ALCL frequently ulcerate. Partial or complete regression occurs at diagnosis or relapse in up to 42% of these tumors.[6] Borderline lesions are intermediate in size, clinical appearance, and histology and usually persist for several months if not treated (Fig. 39-1; Table 39-1).[7]

Primary cutaneous CD30⁺ T-cell LPDs present in the skin without extranodal manifestations for at least 6 months.[6] Primary cutaneous CD30⁺ LPDs must be distinguished from systemic ALCLs with secondary cutaneous manifestations as well as progression from other cutaneous lymphomas such as mycosis fungoides or Sézary syndrome. Secondary CD30⁺ cutaneous lesions generally have a poorer prognosis than primary cutaneous CD30⁺ LPDs.[6,8]

EPIDEMIOLOGY

The peak incidence of LyP is in the fifth decade, although children younger than 10 years and patients up to 80 years old can be affected.[9,10] The male-to-female ratio for LyP patients from ten published series is 3:2.[6,8,11-19] For primary C-ALCL the male-to-female ratio is 2.5:1. Primary C-ALCL can occur in children; therefore, not all cases of C-ALCL in children should be considered secondary manifestations of systemic ALCL.[23] Lack of anaplastic lymphoma kinase (ALK) expression favors primary C-ALCL (see later).

Our LyP registry data revealed an interesting bimodal distribution of patients at age of diagnosis. Most patients younger than 19 years were male, and most of those aged 19 or older at diagnosis were female. Ten of 85 LyP patients who completed a questionnaire had immune thyroiditis.[10] All patients with thyroiditis were women older than 20 years, and none had developed a malignant lymphoma. The prevalence of thyroiditis in this cohort was significantly higher (11%) than in the U.S. general population (791.7 per 100,000; $P < .0001$). Two thirds of 35 patients who developed LyP in childhood (younger than 18 years) had atopy, which is significantly more than the expected prevalence (relative risk, 3.1; 95% confidence interval [CI], 2.2-4.3).[9] Fletcher and colleagues[23] reported four cases of primary cutaneous CD30⁺ LPDs (one LyP, three C-ALCLs) in young adult patients with active atopic eczema since early childhood. These results from separate medical centers show an association between primary

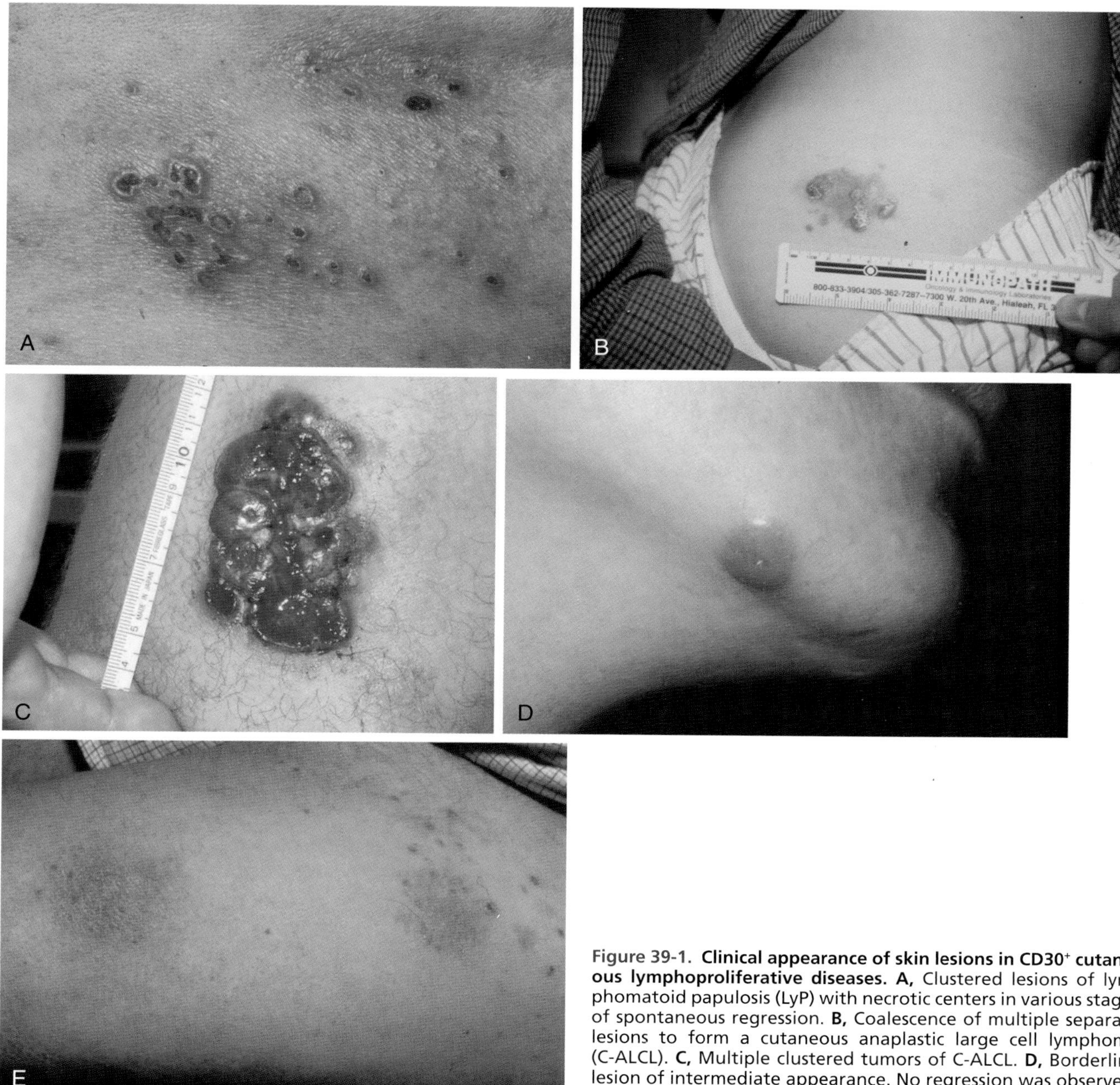

Figure 39-1. Clinical appearance of skin lesions in $CD30^+$ cutaneous lymphoproliferative diseases. A, Clustered lesions of lymphomatoid papulosis (LyP) with necrotic centers in various stages of spontaneous regression. **B,** Coalescence of multiple separate lesions to form a cutaneous anaplastic large cell lymphoma (C-ALCL). **C,** Multiple clustered tumors of C-ALCL. **D,** Borderline lesion of intermediate appearance. No regression was observed. **E,** Coexistent lesions of LyP and patch-stage mycosis fungoides.

cutaneous $CD30^+$ LPDs and atopy. Further studies are needed to determine whether there is a causal link between these two conditions.

A remarkable association between LyP and other lymphomas occurs in 10% to 20% of patients. The most common lymphomas are mycosis fungoides, Hodgkin's lymphoma, and ALCL.[6,12,15,21,24-27] A case-control study revealed that of 57 LyP patients, 3 had Hodgkin's lymphoma, 3 had non-Hodgkin's lymphoma, 10 had mycosis fungoides, and 4 had nonlymphoid malignancies (1 brain tumor, 2 lung cancers, 1 breast cancer).[16] In addition, 4 patients had received radiation therapy 8 to 40 years before the onset of LyP. None of 67 age- and gender-matched controls had any history of radiation or lymphoid or nonlymphoid malignancy. A Dutch study of 118 LyP patients found that 23 (19%) had lymphomas (11 mycosis fungoides, 10 C-ALCL, 2 Hodgkin's lymphoma).[6] In addition to lymphomas, prospective follow-up of our 57 LyP case-control patients revealed a high frequency of nonlymphoid malignancies (10 of 57; 18%). The relative risk of developing lymphoid and nonlymphoid malignancies in this cohort of patients over 8.5 years of follow-up was 13 (95% CI, 2.2-44) and 3.1 (95% CI, 1.206-6.47), respectively.[17] The factors that predispose these patients to develop malignancies are unknown. Possible risk factors based on small case series include age at onset or years at risk for LyP,[9,28] male gender,[29] and histologic subtype. For example, Dutch investigators found that patients with type C LyP have an increased risk of developing malignant lymphoma, whereas none of seven

Table 39-1 Major Distinguishing Features of CD30⁺ Primary Cutaneous Lymphoproliferative Disorders

	LyP	ALCL	Borderline Lesions
Clinical	Crops of papules with central necrosis; spontaneous regression	One to several ulcerating nodules or tumors; occasional partial regression	Intermediate-size nodules (1-2 cm); tendency for slow regression
Histology	Early lesions have superficial dermal perivascular infiltrates Neutrophils in blood vessels Atypical large cells scattered and concentrated around blood vessels, surrounded by inflammatory cells Fully developed lesions show wedge-shaped infiltrate	Dense dermal infiltrate, generally sparing epidermis; some exocytosis of atypical lymphocytes possible; infiltrate extends into and often involves subcutis Confluent sheets of large atypical cells Inflammatory cells confined to periphery, except for numerous PMNs in neutrophil-rich variant	Clusters or sheets of large atypical cells usually confined to dermis, but sometimes extending focally into subcutis Admixture of inflammatory cells Often a spectrum of cerebriform and large RS-like cells
Immunophenotype	$CD30^+$, $CD4^+$, LCA^+, TIA-1^+	$CD30^+$, $CD4^+$, LCA^+, TIA-1^+	$CD30^+$, $CD4^+$, LCA^+, TIA-1^+
Genetics	Absence of t(2;5) Diploid or aneuploid Polyclonal, oligoclonal, or monoclonal by TCR gene analysis	Absence of t(2;5) except in rare cases, primarily in children Complex aneuploid karyotype Clonal by TCR analysis	Absence of t(2;5) No data on cytogenetics Clonal by TCR gene analysis

ALCL, anaplastic large cell lymphoma; LCA, leukocyte common antigen; LyP, lymphomatoid papulosis; PMN, polymorphonuclear leukocyte; RS, Reed-Sternberg; TCR, T-cell receptor.

patients with pure type B lesions had or developed a malignant lymphoma.[29] Clinical manifestations of mycosis fungoides or Hodgkin's lymphoma can occur before, after, or simultaneous with LyP. In nearly all cases, LyP lesions precede the development of C-ALCL.[29]

ETIOLOGY

The etiology of LyP and C-ALCL is unknown. A viral origin was initially suspected but has not been confirmed.[30-33] Human T-lymphotropic virus 1 (HTLV-1); herpesviruses 6, 7, and 8; and Epstein-Barr virus (EBV) could not be detected in primary skin lesions or in cell lines derived from CD30⁺ cutaneous lymphomas.[30-36]

A possible mechanism for LyP in some women of childbearing age is an alloimmune reaction to fetal cells. Cells in the fetal-maternal circulation can persist in the tissues of postpartum women, a phenomenon known as *fetal microchimerism*. Hashimoto's thyroiditis, common in adult female LyP patients, is associated with microchimerism.[37,38] Fetal microchimerism has also been proposed as a mechanism for the pathogenesis of scleroderma.[39]

CD30 expression is a hallmark of LyP and C-ALCL.[40-42] CD30 is a "late" activation antigen maximally expressed 72 hours after lymphocyte activation in vitro.[43] Engagement of CD30 by its natural ligand CD30L (CD156) can lead to sustained proliferation, cell cycle arrest, or apoptosis, depending on the target cell, its state of differentiation, and environmental costimulatory signals.[44-47] CD30 cross-linking of ALCL cell lines clonally derived from LyP causes upregulation of nuclear factor-κB (NF-κB) and ERK/MAP kinases, promoting cell survival and proliferation.[48] CD30 activation also enhances the expression of FLICE-like inhibitory protein, which protects lymphocytes from apoptosis induced by Fas/CD95.[49] Our studies suggest that the level of CD30 transcription is genetically determined, rendering some individuals more or less susceptible to CD30⁺ LPDs, including primary cutaneous LPDs.[50] This might explain LyP patients' increased risk of developing Hodgkin's lymphoma and ALCL. LyP patients also have a significantly increased risk of both lymphoid and nonlymphoid malignancies, suggesting an as yet undefined genetic defect that is not limited to lymphoid cells.[17]

CLINICAL FEATURES

LyP lesions appear as small self-healing papules, often with a necrotic center (see Fig. 39-1A). Patients may experience itching and, less often, fever or other systemic symptoms. LyP lesions often appear in clusters and recur in the same region of the body. In a few patients, continual eruptions of papulonodules histologically typical of LyP occur in a well-circumscribed area, equivalent to limited plaque mycosis fungoides.[51] The extremities, trunk, and particularly the buttocks are affected. Lesions occur infrequently on the face, palms, soles, and anogenital areas and only rarely on mucous membranes.[52-54] These clinical observations raise the possibility that cytokines or chemokines released from epidermal keratinocytes or Langerhans cells may contribute to the development of LyP.

LyP lesions occur in crops, often with long lesion-free intervals. Many patients experience the development of new lesions while others are regressing, and lesions may be continuous. LyP lesions often reoccur in the original site. In some women, LyP lesions appear to be modulated by the menstrual cycle or develop during pregnancy.[55] LyP lesions can coalesce to form one or more large lesions indistinguishable from C-ALCL (see Fig. 39-1B). In other patients, one or a few lesions grow progressively to form a primary C-ALCL without prior LyP lesions (see Fig. 39-1C). Large lesions often ulcerate centrally and show some degree of spontaneous regression, even after 2 to 3 months. In borderline lesions, the distinction between C-ALCL and LyP cannot be established (see Fig. 39-1D); however, in most patients, follow-up clarifies the lesion type.

Regional lymphadenopathy can develop and likely represents the local spread of tumor cells (Fig. 39-2). The prognosis does not appear to be affected by regional lymphadenopathy.[6] Regional lymph node enlargement can also represent dermatopathic lymphadenopathy. No staging system has been developed for primary cutaneous CD30⁺ LPDs; the staging system used for mycosis fungoides is not appropriate.

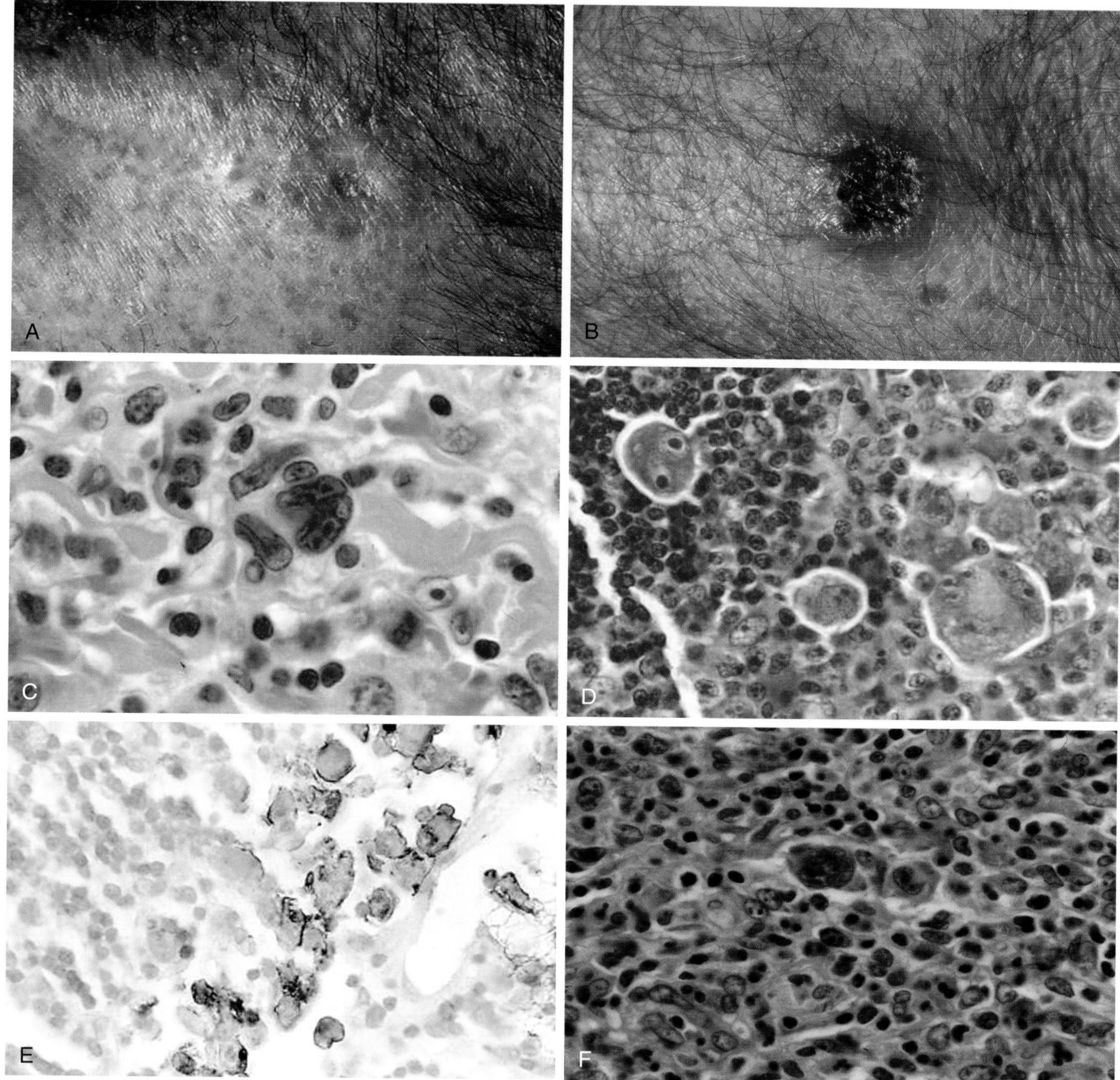

Figure 39-2. CD30⁺ T-cell lymphoproliferative disease and malignant lymphoma in a lymph node. A, Cluster of lymphomatoid papulosis (LyP) lesions. **B,** Ulcerated cutaneous anaplastic large cell lymphoma. **C,** Anaplastic large cell in skin. **D,** Coexistent lymph node with Reed-Sternberg or Reed-Sternberg–like cells. **E,** Staining of tumor cells for CD15. **F,** In a different patient with LyP, bizarre multinucleated cells are surrounded by eosinophils in a lymph node. Such cases raise the differential diagnosis of Hodgkin's lymphoma versus anaplastic large cell lymphoma.

The development of systemic symptoms of fatigue, fever, weight loss, night sweats, or bone pain should raise the possibility of systemic lymphoma complicating LyP. In these individuals, more extensive staging with imaging of the chest and abdomen should be done. Abdominal or intrathoracic lymphadenopathy should be regarded as highly suspicious for malignant lymphoma. I have noted bone lesions in several LyP patients who developed systemic CD30⁺ ALCL (Fig. 39-3).

Extensive staging procedures are generally not warranted for asymptomatic patients with LyP or clinically localized primary C-ALCL. Bone marrow examination is not recommended owing to the low frequency of involvement. A Sézary preparation or flow cytometry of the peripheral blood is not indicated in patients with uncomplicated primary cutaneous CD30⁺ LPDs. A chest radiograph is recommended to exclude asymptomatic mediastinal lymphadenopathy, which can be a presenting feature of Hodgkin's lymphoma. A summary of recommendations for the management of patients with primary cutaneous CD30⁺ LPDs has been compiled by the Dutch Cutaneous Lymphoma Group.[6] More recent

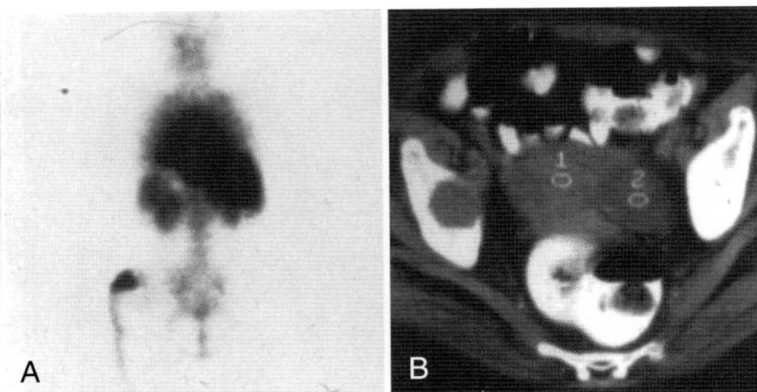

Figure 39-3. Bone lesions in two patients with cutaneous anaplastic large cell lymphoma secondary to lymphomatoid papulosis. A, Bone scan shows an area of increased activity in the right ileum. B, Computed tomography scan shows a large, round lytic lesion in the ileum of a second patient.

discussions of management decisions based on experience has been compiled at Stanford and Beth Israel Deaconess Medical Center in Boston and Roger Williams Medical Center in Providence, RI.[56,56b]

The development of persistent patch, plaque, or scaly erythematous lesions; hair loss; or onychodystrophy can indicate the presence of mycosis fungoides complicating LyP (see Fig. 39-1E). This would necessitate the use of a systemic approach to therapy (e.g., psoralen with ultraviolet A [PUVA] or ultraviolet B, topical nitrogen mustard or carmustine, bexarotene, total skin electron beam therapy, extracorporeal photoimmunotherapy), depending on the stage of disease.[56,56b]

MORPHOLOGY

LyP lesions vary in appearance, depending on their stage of development at the time of biopsy (Fig. 39-4). Early lesions reveal mainly perivascular and superficial dermal accumulations of atypical lymphoid cells surrounded by variable numbers of inflammatory cells. Neutrophils within the lumens of blood vessels are a nearly constant feature of LyP. Surrounding the large atypical cells are variable numbers of neutrophils, eosinophils, and small lymphocytes (see Fig. 39-4A). Few to many neutrophils often percolate through the epidermis, accounting for the pustular appearance of LyP lesions. Macrophages and plasma cells generally are not prominent. Fully developed or late lesions are often wedge shaped, sometimes extending into the deep dermis with little or no involvement of the subcutis. Hair follicles and sweat glands may be infiltrated by atypical cells. Other unusual histopathologic patterns associated with LyP include follicular mucinosis; myxoid stroma[57]; epidermal vesicle formation[11]; granulomatous eccrinotropic,[58] angiocentric,[59] syringosquamous metaplasia; and a band-like rather than wedge-shaped distribution of lymphoid cells.[11] The atypical cells often concentrate around and can be found within the lumens of blood vessels.

LyP comprises three main histologic types, with some overlapping features (Table 39-2; see also Fig. 39-4).[4,6,60,61] Type A may resemble Hodgkin's lymphoma because of the presence of large Reed-Sternberg–like cells with prominent, often eosinophilic nucleoli (see Fig. 39-4H). These cells are surrounded by variable numbers of inflammatory cells. In some lesions the atypical cells resemble immunoblasts with amphophilic to basophilic cytoplasm, slightly eccentric nuclei, and conspicuous but usually not huge nucleoli. When such cells are confluent or occur in sheets confined to the dermis, with relatively few inflammatory cells, the lesion is classified as LyP type C (see Fig. 39-4J). Type B lesions resemble mycosis fungoides (see Fig. 39-4I). The predominant cell is a mononuclear cell with nuclear irregularities, sometimes cerebriform, without prominent nucleoli. Mitoses are infrequent. Epidermotropism is often present. Neutrophils and other inflammatory cells are not abundant. There is some controversy over whether LyP type B lesions represent a papular variant of mycosis fungoides.[62] It is not uncommon to find LyP lesions that contain a spectrum of cerebriform cells to larger immunoblasts or Reed-Sternberg–like cells with abundant inflammatory cells. These lesions can be referred to as type A/B to indicate a hybrid or mixed histology.[4,22,63,64]

C-ALCL occurs as an extensive dermal infiltrate, usually sparing the epidermis, and is composed almost entirely of large anaplastic cells (Fig. 39-5). The deep part of the lesion usually extends into the subcutis. Inflammatory cells are less frequent than in LyP; they are often nearly absent or confined to the lesion's periphery. An exception is the neutrophil-rich variant of C-ALCL, in which a confluence of neutrophils may obscure the appearance of the large atypical cells.[65,66]

Mitoses are common among the large atypical cells in LyP and especially in C-ALCL (see Figs. 39-4 and 39-5). Several studies indicate a high ratio of apoptotic cells to dividing cells in LyP. A significantly higher apoptotic index is found in LyP (12.5%) than in $CD30^+$ large T-cell lymphoma (3.1%).[67] The high rate of apoptosis in LyP can be attributed in part to the low expression of BCL2[68,69] and the high expression of the proapoptotic protein BAX.[70] The proportion of $CD30^+$ cells expressing death receptor apoptosis pathway mediators FADD and cleaved caspase 3 is significantly higher in primary cutaneous $CD30^+$ LPDs than in systemic ALCL.[71]

Borderline lesions contain an extensive infiltrate or sheets of atypical cells with focal extension into the subcutis, making them difficult to distinguish from LyP type C or C-ALCL.

IMMUNOPHENOTYPE

The usual immunophenotype of the large atypical cells in LyP is that of activated helper T lymphocytes expressing CD4 and lymphocyte activation antigens such as CD30, CD25, CD71, and HLA-DR.[40-42] Other T-cell antigens (e.g., CD3, CD2, CD5, CD7) are often not expressed, resulting in an aberrant T-cell phenotype (Fig. 39-6) characteristic of postthymic T-cell malignancies. A natural killer cell phenotype for the large atypical cells was noted in 10% to nearly 50% of cases in one study,[11] but in none of 18 cases in another study.[72] In one series one third of cases had a $CD8^+$ phenotype.[11] $CD8^+$ LyP can be confused with aggressive epidermotropic $CD8^+$ cytotoxic T-cell lymphoma.[73]

In most cases the atypical cells express cytotoxic proteins, including TIA-1, granzyme B, and perforin (see Fig. 39-6).[74] ALK is negative, leukocyte common antigen (LCA; CD45) is characteristically expressed, and CD15 is usually absent in LyP. This profile helps distinguish LyP and ALCL from Hodgkin's lymphoma.[75] C-ALCL also displays an activated T-cell phenotype, with frequent expression of cytotoxic molecules. CD30 must be expressed by at least 75% of large cells.[29] Epithelial membrane antigen (EMA) and ALK staining is usually absent in C-ALCL, in contrast to systemic ALCL.[76,77] Rare cases of C-ALCL are associated with a cytoplasmic variant of ALK (Fig. 39-7).[78] Homeobox gene *HOXC5* is often expressed.[79]

GENETICS AND MOLECULAR FINDINGS

DNA cytophotometry has shown that LyP cells may be diploid, hypertetraploid, or aneuploid. Willemze and associates found that aneuploidy is associated with a type A histology.[12,80,81] Cytogenetic studies of regressing lesions in LyP have demonstrated either a normal karyotype or numerical and structural abnormalities of chromosomes 7, 10, and 12. The t(2;5) (p23;q35) translocation has not been found.[82] All cases of C-ALCL have demonstrated multiple complex karyotypic abnormalities.[83] The t(2;5) translocation has been described only rarely in C-ALCL.[84] Nested polymerase chain reaction (PCR) and in situ hybridization demonstrated cases with nucleophosmin (NPM)-ALK RNA transcripts in one series,[85] but these findings were not supported by ALK protein expression and therefore are of uncertain pathogenetic significance.

Allelic deletion at 9p21-22, causing inactivation of the *p16* tumor suppressor gene, has been reported in some C-ALCLs.[86] Comparative genomic hybridization confirmed the presence

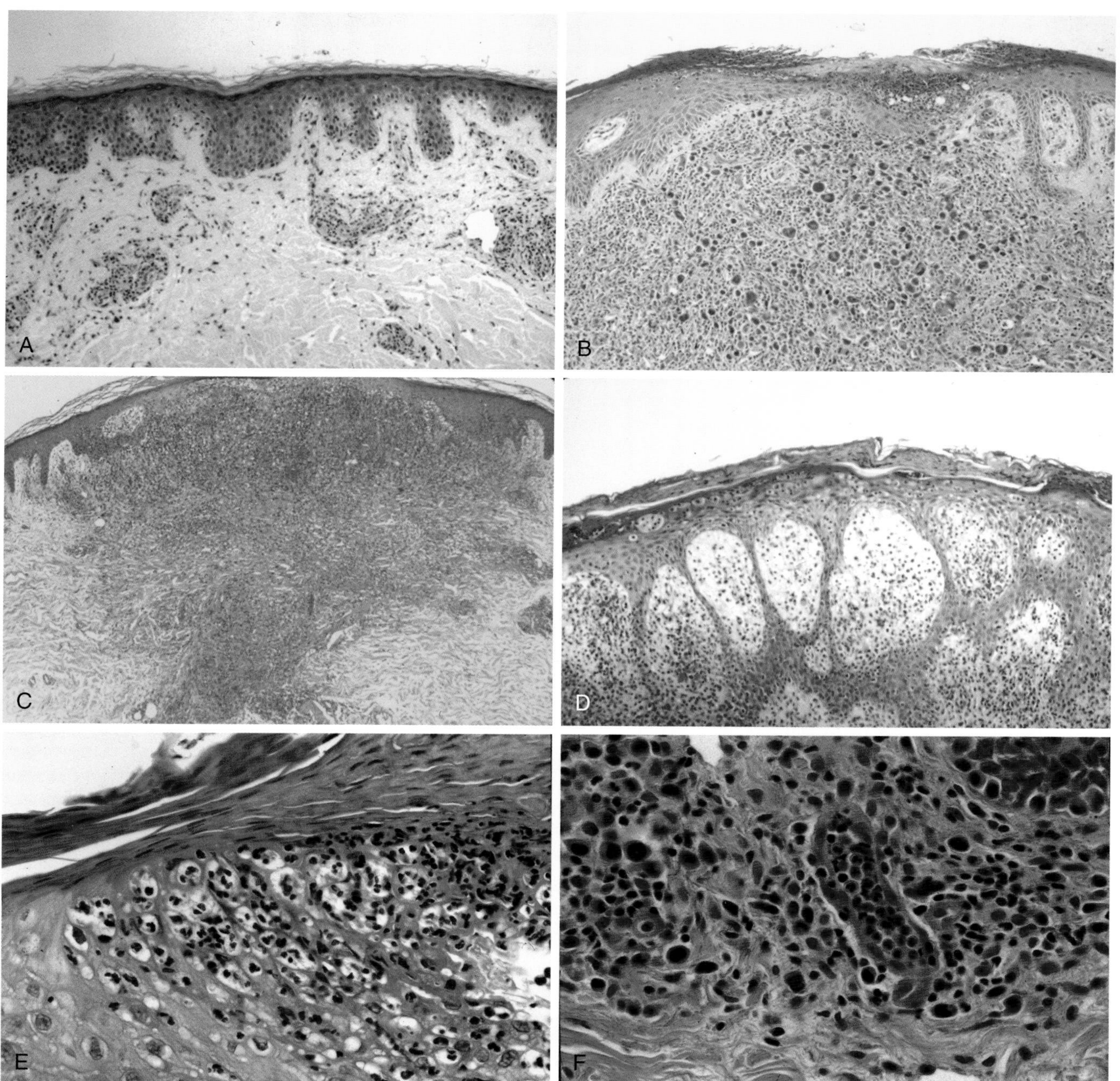

Figure 39-4. Histology of lymphomatoid papulosis (LyP). A, Early lesion with a perivascular accumulation of atypical lymphocytes. **B,** Erosion of the epidermis and scattered anaplastic cells in LyP. **C,** Fully developed wedge-shaped lesion. **D,** Parakeratosis, acanthosis, and edema of the papillary dermis. **E,** Neutrophil exudate in the epidermis. **F,** Collection of neutrophils in a dermal venule surrounded by anaplastic cells, characteristic of LyP.

Continued

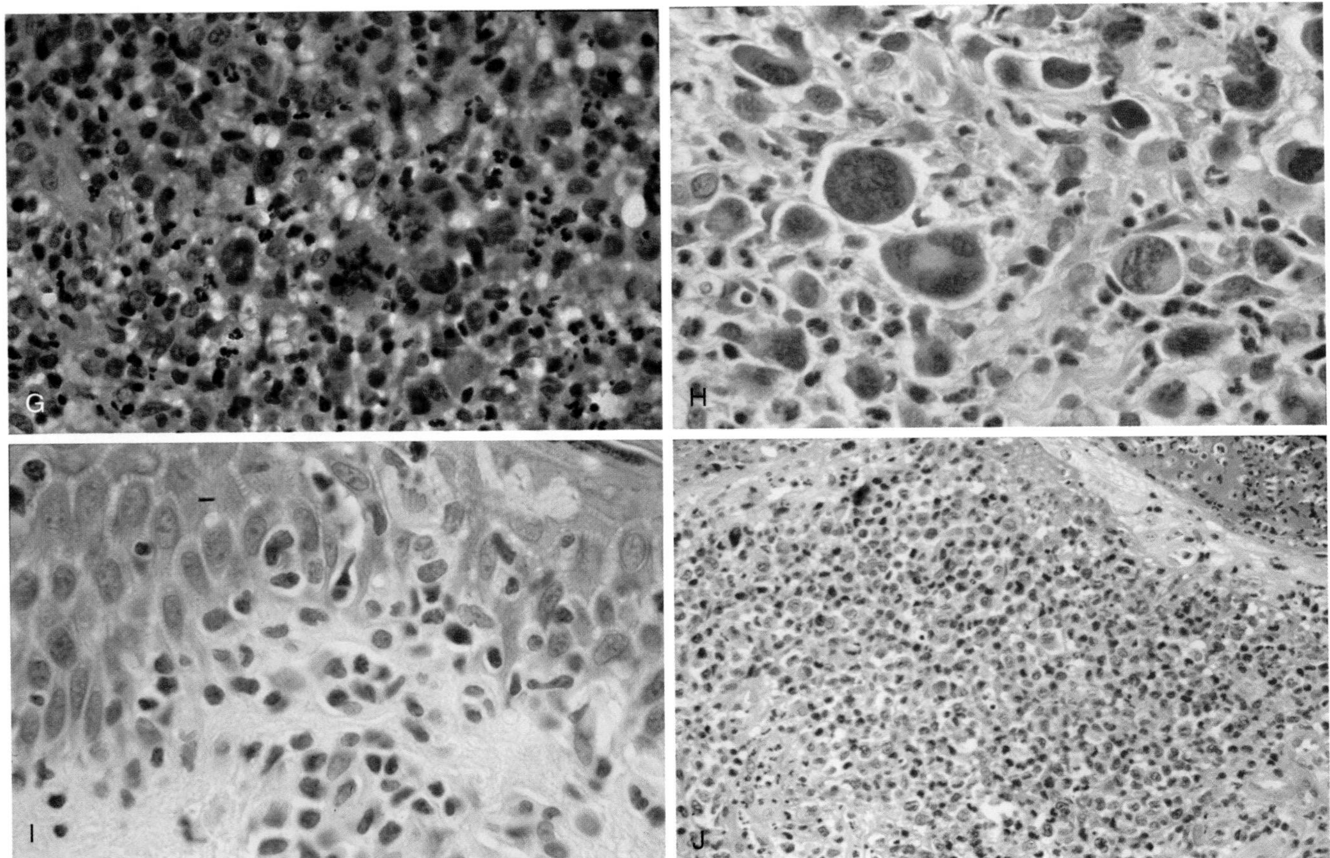

Figure 39-4, cont'd. G, Minority of large, atypical cells and abnormal mitosis surrounded by numerous neutrophils and eosinophils in LyP. **H,** LyP type A with Reed-Sternberg–like cells surrounded by inflammatory cells. Apoptotic bodies are present. **I,** LyP type B with epidermotropic cerebriform cells. **J,** LyP type C with sheets of large cells in the dermis.

of multiple chromosomal imbalances in C-ALCL.[87] The most common regions of oncogene amplification involved CTSB (8p22), RAF1 (3p25), REL (2p12p12), and JUNB (19p13.2). Immunohistochemical amplification of JUNB was confirmed in C-ALCL and LyP.[87,88]

Clonal rearrangements of the T-cell receptor (TCR) beta or gamma chain genes have been detected in nearly all C-ALCLs and in most individual lesions of LyP.[20-23,89,90] The frequency of clonal rearrangements in LyP varies from 40% to 100%, depending on the method used. Weiss and associates[89] reported clonal or oligoclonal T-cell populations detected by Southern blot in LyP. In one patient studied at multiple sites, different clonal populations were detected. Using Southern blot, Whittaker and coworkers[63] reported clones in most type B and mixed type A/B lesions but in no pure type A lesions of LyP. Using a more sensitive PCR approach with variable region–specific primers, Chott and colleagues[20] found dominant T-cell clones in 9 of 11 LyP patients. In several patients the same clone was detected in LyP lesions of different histologic types. A single-cell analysis of $CD30^+$ cells in LyP demonstrated that they were monoclonal in each of the 11 patients evaluated.[91] One patient who had progressed from LyP to C-ALCL had the same dominant clone detected in all lesions. However, another study found that clonal cells reside in the $CD30^-$, $CD3^+$ smaller cell compartment.[92] Humme and coworkers[93] performed molecular genetic analysis of skin lesions and blood of LyP patients by combining TCRγ PCR and beta-variable complementarity-determining region 3 (CDR3) spectratyping. They were able to detect a clonal T-cell population in 36 of 43 skin samples (84%) and in 35 of 83 blood samples (42%). Comparison of skin and blood demonstrated different T-cell clones, suggesting the

Table 39-2 Comparison of Histologic Subtypes of Lymphomatoid Papulosis

	Type A	Type B	Type C
Cytology	Immunoblasts, sometimes Reed-Sternberg–like cells	Cerebriform cells	Immunoblasts, sometimes a spectrum of cerebriform cells and immunoblasts
Inflammatory cells	Numerous	Infrequent	Few to moderate
Mitoses	Frequent	Infrequent	Frequent
Clinical regression	4-6 wk	8 wk	Slow and incomplete

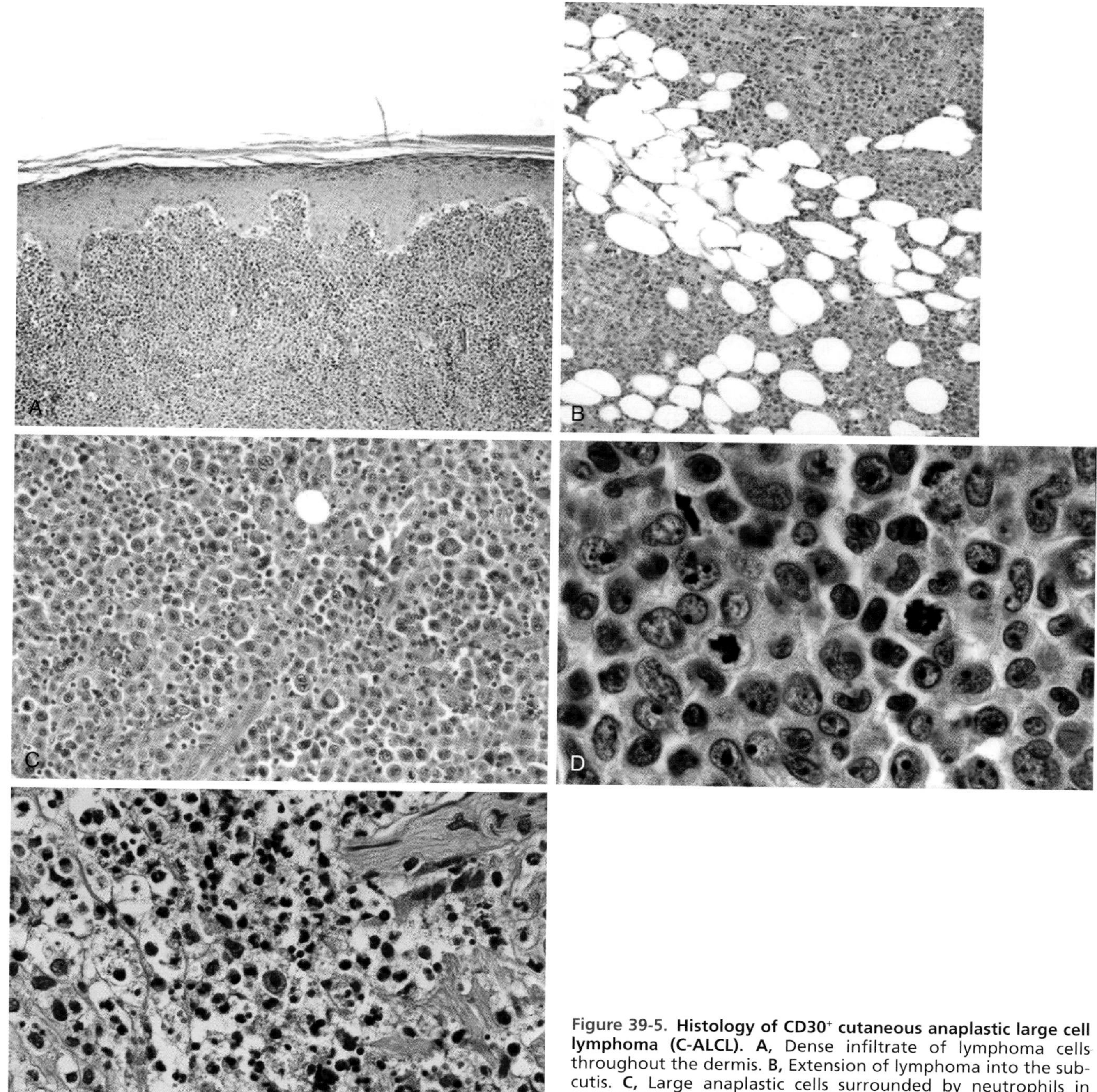

Figure 39-5. Histology of CD30⁺ cutaneous anaplastic large cell lymphoma (C-ALCL). A, Dense infiltrate of lymphoma cells throughout the dermis. **B,** Extension of lymphoma into the subcutis. **C,** Large anaplastic cells surrounded by neutrophils in C-ALCL. **D,** Large cells with pleomorphic, anaplastic morphology. **E,** Neutrophil-rich C-ALCL. Note the isolated lymphoma cell with a nucleolus at the *center*.

unrelated nature of the clonal T cells in the skin and blood. Moreover, CDR3 spectratyping revealed a restricted T-cell repertoire in the blood, suggesting T-cell stimulation by an unknown antigen. Thus, the exact nature of the clonal cells in LyP is still unsettled.

The dominant T-cell clone is often detected in the associated T-cell lymphoma that develops in LyP patients.[20,21,22,94-97] Finally, it appears that C-ALCL may evolve from a polyclonal to oligoclonal and eventually monoclonal T-cell proliferation over time.[98]

POSTULATED CELL OF ORIGIN

The cell of origin for LyP and C-ALCL is an activated helper T lymphocyte ($CD4^+$) expressing cytotoxic proteins.[42,64,74] In vitro studies of the cytokine profile of these cells point to a predominant Th2 type according to the classification of Mosmann and associates.[99] The tumor cells secrete interleukin (IL)-4, IL-6, and IL-10 but not interferon (IFN)-γ or IL-2. This is consistent with the usual functional profile of $CD30^+$ T lymphocytes.[100] The Th2 profile of LyP cells has justified the

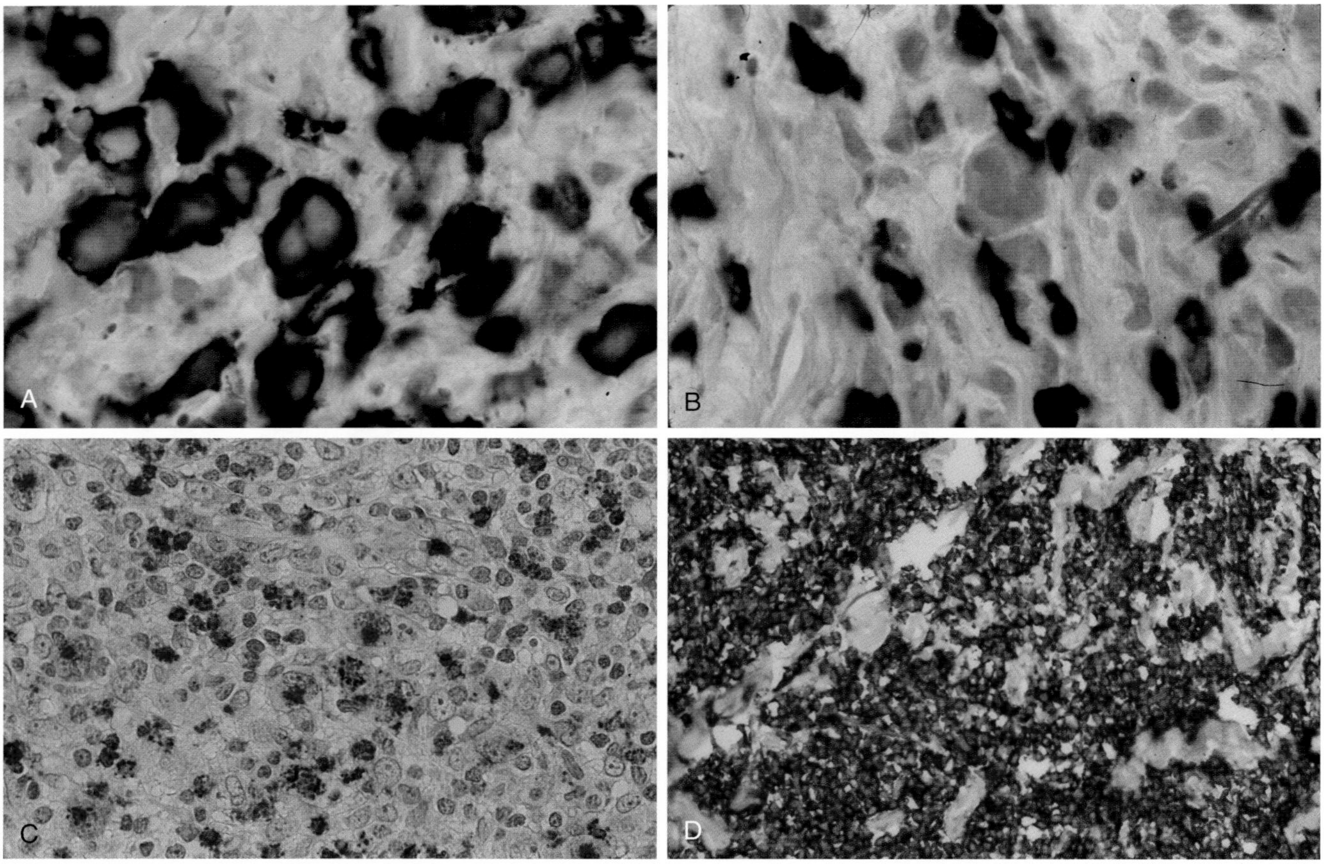

Figure 39-6. Immunohistochemistry of CD30⁺ cutaneous lymphoproliferative disorders. A, CD30 expression on atypical cells in lymphomatoid papulosis (LyP). **B,** CD3 expression on small T lymphocytes but not on atypical cells in LyP. Aberrant expression of T-cell antigens is common on large atypical cells in LyP. **C,** Staining for TIA-1 in large atypical cells of LyP. **D,** CD30 stains nearly all cells in cutaneous anaplastic large cell lymphoma.

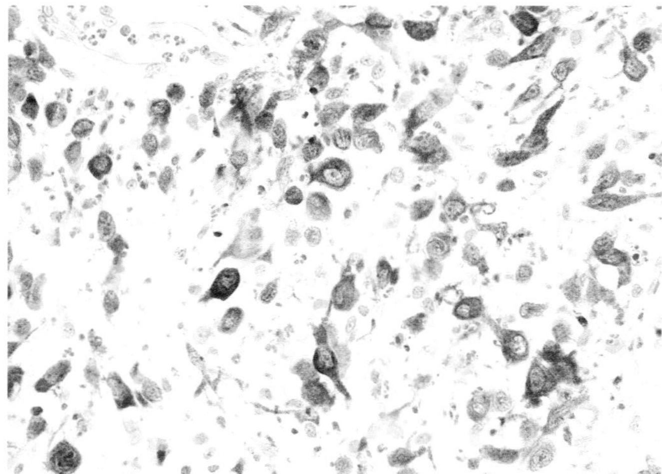

Figure 39-7. Cytoplasmic variant of anaplastic lymphoma kinase (ALK) in cutaneous anaplastic large cell lymphoma. Note the absence of staining over the nuclei of tumor cells. ALK was confirmed to be activated (phosphorylated) in this case.

use of IFN-γ in the treatment of primary cutaneous $CD30^+$ LPDs.[101] Alternatively, the $CD30^+$ cells in LyP and C-ALCL can have a phenotype ($CD4^+$, $CD25^{high}$, $CD45RO^+$, surface transforming growth factor-β [TGF-β] positive) consistent with induced regulatory T cells that can suppress proliferation and cytokine production of $CD25^-$ T cells, at least in part by the action of the inhibitory cytokine TGF-β.[102] The suppressor activity of natural regulatory T cells[103] requires cell contact and is mediated by granzyme B, a property of $CD30^+$ cells in LyP.[74] In contrast to natural regulatory T cells, the $CD30^+$ cells in LyP lack the *FOXP3* gene.

CLINICAL COURSE

There is often a long delay before the correct diagnosis of LyP is made. LyP usually follows a chronic course, with intermittent lesion-free periods. For most patients, LyP is a lifelong disease. In some patients, particularly children, the disease may spontaneously remit.[104] Most patients with LyP do not require treatment, at least not initially. If lesions are numerous, cause unsightly scarring, or occur on the face, hands, or other cosmetically undesirable areas, treatment with PUVA or low-dose oral methotrexate (starting at 10 to 25 mg/week) is most effective; 90% of patients treated with methotrexate achieve a significant reduction in lesions.[105] PUVA accelerates photoaging of the skin and increases the risk of skin cancer.[106] Bexarotene is an RXR (retinoid X receptor)-selective retinoid that decreases the number or duration of LyP lesions when given orally or applied as a gel.[107] High-potency steroids applied topically have minimal benefit. These treatments suppress LyP, but the lesions are likely to recur when treatment is stopped. Importantly, treatment is unlikely to prevent the development of lymphoma, particularly mycosis fungoides or Hodgkin's lymphoma, but it may inhibit the progression to C-ALCL.[6] No definite risk factors for tumor progression have been identified.[6] However, mutations of receptors for the lymphocyte growth inhibitory cytokine TGF-β,[108-110] high expression of *BCL2* genes,[68] and expression of the cytoskeletal protein fascin[111] have been associated with progression of LyP to C-ALCL.

Progression of LyP to C-ALCL appears to be associated with an altered response to CD30 signaling. Although CD30L expression is quantitatively increased in regressing CD30$^+$ skin lesions,[112] CD30 ligation in C-ALCL cell lines that have progressed from LyP causes increased cell proliferation, associated with activation of NF-κB.[48] CD30 ligation of NPM-ALK cell lines (e.g., Karpas 299) causes growth arrest by upregulation of cell cycle inhibitor p21 and accumulation of Rb (retinoblastoma) protein in the unphosphorylated state.[46,47] Thus, CD30 signaling plays an important role in the biology of LyP and ALCL.

X-irradiation is an effective treatment for nonregressing skin lesions complicating LyP or C-ALCL.[6] An observation period of 2 to 3 months is usually recommended before resorting to irradiation, because some lesions regress spontaneously. Multiagent chemotherapy has no role in LyP or localized C-ALCL. However, a regimen of cyclophosphamide, hydroxydaunorubicin, Oncovin (vincristine), and prednisone or prednisolone (CHOP) is effective chemotherapy for multifocal C-ALCL and is essential in cases with extracutaneous spread.[6,8]

Sites of relapse in C-ALCL are unpredictable and may be either local or distant in the skin. Extracutaneous spread is often to the bony skeleton (see Fig. 39-3).[110] Regional lymph nodes in proximity to large skin lesions are most often involved. Patients with C-ALCL or Hodgkin's lymphoma may relapse with LyP after primary systemic therapy.[56,56b]

There is a tendency to treat LyP and C-ALCL too aggressively. This is due to the high-grade histopathology, with many large atypical cells and high mitotic rate; frequent clinical recurrences; and most clinicians' lack of familiarity with the natural history of the disease. Because of the diagnosis of recurrent high-grade lymphoma, many clinicians resort to systemic and even high-dose ablative chemotherapy with peripheral stem cell rescue or bone marrow transplantation. Unfortunately, such aggressive approaches are not curative and should therefore be avoided because they produce unwarranted toxicity and limit future treatment options, particularly if the patient develops an extracutaneous lymphoma. The worst prognostic feature for patients with primary cutaneous CD30$^+$ LPDs is extracutaneous spread.[6,8] Spontaneous regression is associated with a good prognosis.[8]

DIFFERENTIAL DIAGNOSIS

Several neoplastic and nonneoplastic lesions may mimic primary cutaneous CD30$^+$ LPDs either clinically or histologically (Table 39-3).

Systemic Anaplastic Large Cell Lymphoma

Systemic ALCL is associated with extranodal disease in 40% of cases, and the skin is the most common extranodal site.[113-115] Secondary skin lesions of systemic ALCL and C-ALCL can be histologically similar. Clinical features that favor primary C-ALCL are spontaneous regression, localized skin lesions, absence of lymphadenopathy, and age older than

Table 39-3 Differential Diagnostic Features of CD30$^+$ Primary Cutaneous Lymphoproliferative Disorders

	Systemic ALCL	Hodgkin's Lymphoma	Mycosis Fungoides	Pityriasis Lichenoides	Arthropod Bite	Scabies
Clinical	Generalized lymphadenopathy Lack of spontaneous regression	Advanced disease generally has multifocal lymphadenopathy, splenomegaly Deep-seated tumors in primary cutaneous Hodgkin's lymphoma	Scaling, erythematous patches or plaques; lack of central necrosis Spontaneous regression can occur, causing arcuate lesions	Younger age Central hemorrhage Not associated with lymphoma	History of exposure	Itchy lesions Responds to treatment with Kwell
Histopathology and immunophenotype	Lack of epidermotropism and cerebriform cells	Classic RS cells, CD15$^+$, LCA$^-$	Epidermotropism of cerebriform cells Lack of inflammatory cells and RS-like cells	Necrosis of keratinocytes Extravasation of erythrocytes Lack of RS-like cells	Punctum, insect parts may be identified Polymorphic inflammation CD30$^+$ cells may be present	Presence of mite in histologic sections CD30$^+$ cells and B cells present
Genetics	t(2;5) frequently present Clonal TCR	Triploidy and tetraploidy Absence of t(2;5) Absence of TCR gene clonality except in rare cases	Lack of t(2;5) Complex karyotype TCR clonal or oligoclonal in all cases	Diploid; no chromosomal abnormalities TCR genes clonal in up to 50% of cases	No abnormalities	No abnormalities

ALCL, anaplastic large cell lymphoma; LCA, leukocyte common antigen; RS, Reed-Sternberg; TCR, T-cell receptor.

30 years. Pathologic and immunophenotypic features that favor primary C-ALCL are cerebriform cells in the epidermis and superficial dermis, absence of t(2;5) and ALK staining,[116] absence of EMA staining,[76] and expression of cutaneous lymphocyte antigen.[76] The combined clinical, histologic, and immunophenotypic features usually permit the distinction between systemic ALCL and primary C-ALCL.

Systemic Hodgkin's Lymphoma

Hodgkin's lymphoma can involve the skin as a secondary site. This is usually a consequence of direct obstruction from regional lymph nodes and occurs only in advanced disease, when the diagnosis of Hodgkin's lymphoma is obvious.[117] Cutaneous lesions of secondary Hodgkin's lymphoma most commonly occur on the trunk. Hodgkin's lymphoma occurs with increased frequency in LyP patients and can appear before or after the clinical manifestations of LyP.[21,29,118] LyP can persist or recur following successful chemotherapy of Hodgkin's lymphoma and has no known adverse prognostic significance; therefore, the distinction of LyP from cutaneous Hodgkin's lymphoma is clinically important.[118] Clinically, LyP lesions regress, whereas those of secondary Hodgkin's lymphoma do not. LyP can be distinguished from Hodgkin's lymphoma by the expression of LCA and T-cell antigens and the absence of CD15 and EBV-associated antigens.[32,75,119]

Primary Cutaneous Hodgkin's Lymphoma

Primary cutaneous Hodgkin's lymphoma is rare and usually presents as deep dermal lesions producing tumors on the

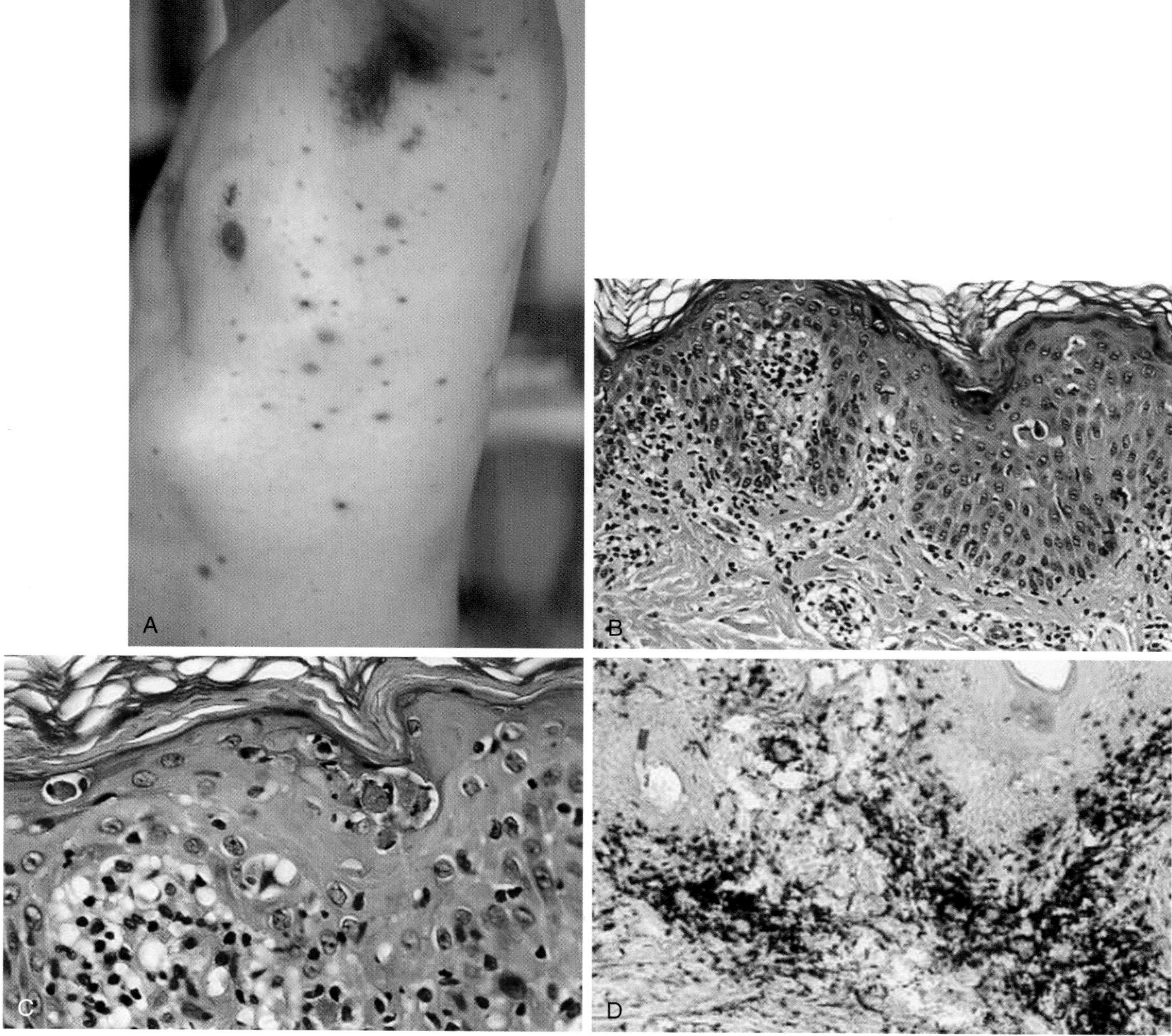

Figure 39-8. Pityriasis lichenoides et varioliformis acuta. A, Clinical photograph of centrally necrotic lesions on the thorax. **B,** Histology showing a lichenoid lymphoid infiltrate. **C,** Necrotic keratinocytes. **D,** Prevalence of CD8⁺ cells.

extremities or trunk.[75,119] The skin lesions contain classic Reed-Sternberg cells that have a CD15+, LCA− phenotype and may be positive for EBV-associated antigens (e.g., LMP-1).[119] Lesions of primary cutaneous Hodgkin's lymphoma do not regress. Patients with primary cutaneous Hodgkin's lymphoma appear to have a significant risk of developing nodal Hodgkin's lymphoma.[75,119]

Mycosis Fungoides

Mycosis fungoides can occur before, after, or simultaneous with LyP.[22,29,51,97] Mycosis fungoides lesions are usually scaling, erythematous patches or plaques that can be readily distinguished from LyP. However, mycosis fungoides can also present with small papular lesions that closely resemble LyP.[62,120] I favor an interpretation of mycosis fungoides rather than LyP type B for papulosquamous lesions that display histologic features of mycosis fungoides, whether they are persistent or spontaneously regressing.[62] Mycosis fungoides lesions can be readily distinguished morphologically from LyP type A by the absence of Reed-Sternberg–like cells and neutrophils and from type C by the absence of clusters or sheets of large CD30+ cells.

Pityriasis Lichenoides

Pityriasis lichenoides et varioliformis acuta (PLEVA) can be indistinguishable from LyP clinically and histologically (Fig. 39-8).[121] PLEVA tends to occur in patients younger than 30 years, is often not recurrent, and is not associated with an increased risk of developing malignant lymphoma.[122] Similar to LyP, clonality of T cells can be found in many PLEVA cases.[123] However, PLEVA usually lacks the large, atypical Reed-Sternberg–like cells of LyP type A and has few neutrophils or eosinophils. PLEVA shows damage of individual keratinocytes with focal keratinocyte necrosis and extravasation of erythrocytes. Neutrophils in blood vessels characteristic of LyP are lacking in PLEVA. The lichenoid lymphoid infiltrate in PLEVA lacks the frequent CD30+ cells found in LyP and contains a predominance of CD8+ cells, whereas CD4+ cells predominate in LyP.[124] Pityriasis lichenoides chronica can be more difficult to distinguish from LyP clinically. However, the lack of large, atypical CD30+ cells, neutrophils, and eosinophils favors pityriasis lichenoides chronica.

Arthropod Bite

LyP can be confused with arthropod bites clinically and histologically. One report found that CD30+ cells were absent in arthropod bites,[125] but this finding has not been confirmed.[126] A clinical history and follow-up may be necessary to exclude arthropod bite from the differential diagnosis of primary cutaneous CD30+ LPDs. Nodular scabies in the genital region can closely resemble LyP clinically. Scabies lesions often contain CD30+ immunoblasts surrounded by inflammatory cells, usually eosinophils.[127] The key distinction is demonstration of the offending mite in scabies (Fig. 39-9).

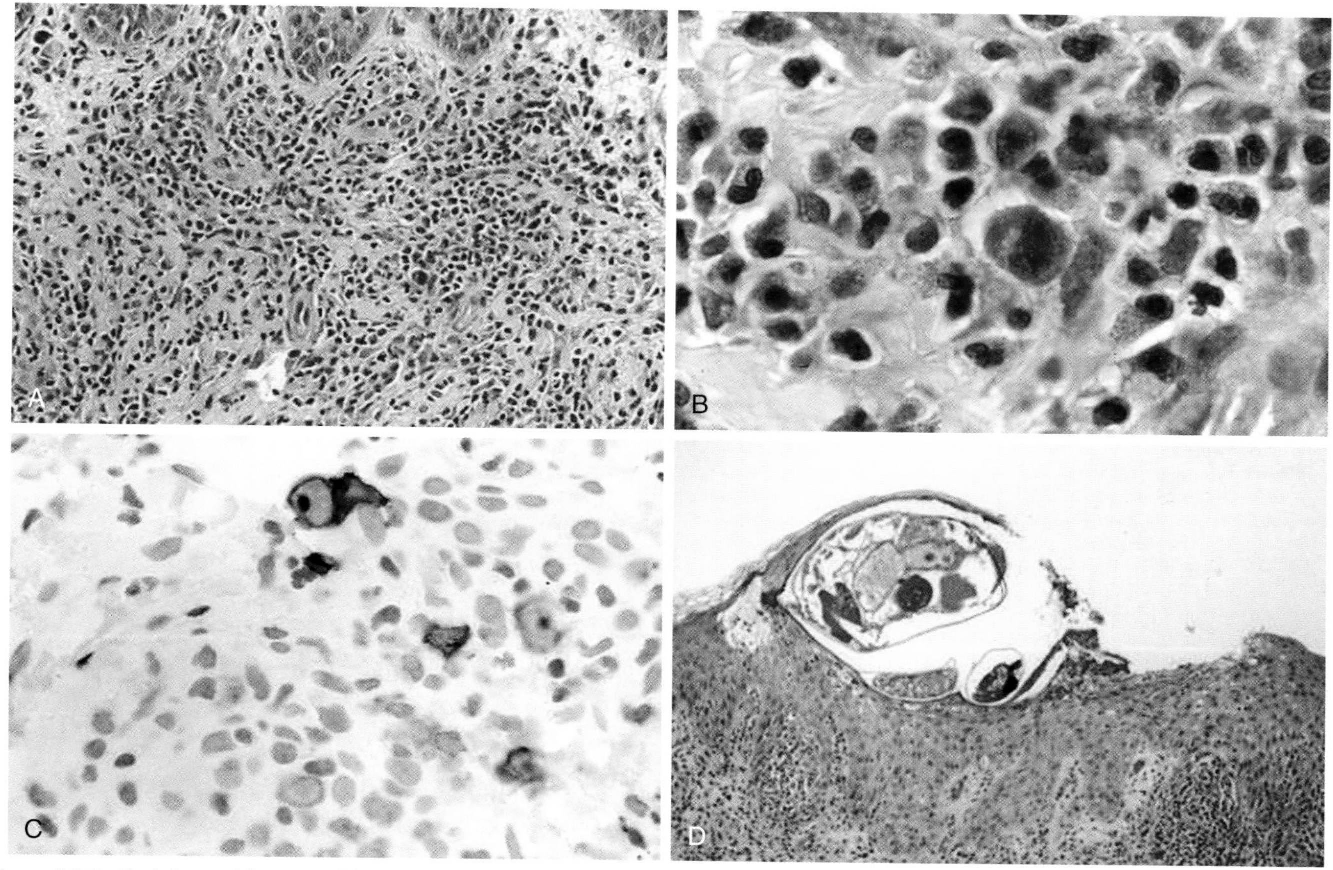

Figure 39-9. Nodular scabies resembling lymphomatoid papulosis. A, Dense dermal and perivascular infiltrate. **B,** Large atypical cell surrounded by eosinophils. **C,** CD30 stain of large atypical cells. **D,** Mite (*Sarcoptes scabiei* var. *hominis*) embedded in the epidermis.

OTHER SKIN CONDITIONS WITH CD30-POSITIVE LARGE CELLS

Several other cutaneous disorders that contain significant numbers of CD30$^+$ cells can enter into the differential diagnosis of primary cutaneous CD30$^+$ LPDs. These include atopic dermatitis, molluscum contagiosum, herpes simplex infection, herpes varicella-zoster, tuberculosis, milker's nodule, leishmaniasis, syphilis, lymphomatoid drug eruption, and hydroa-like lymphoma.[128-133] In most cases the correct diagnosis can be established by clinical history, physical examination, and laboratory tests.

Pearls and Pitfalls

- LyP and C-ALCL can coexist and probably represent a continuum of lesions.
- Histologic distinction of LyP from lymphoma can be extremely difficult, making clinical correlation imperative. The diagnosis is often obvious when one sees the patient.
- The correct diagnosis of LyP is essential to avoid overtreatment.
- ALK expression has not been reported in LyP that has not progressed to lymphoma.
- LyP and C-ALCL can occur in children. In addition, some cases of ALK$^+$ ALCL may present with isolated cutaneous disease (without evidence of systemic disease for longer than 6 months).
- Consider the diagnosis of scabies in genital lesions resembling LyP in children.
- Edema of the papillary dermis can be prominent in LyP and distinguishes it from PLEVA.
- Allow up to 3 months for spontaneous regression of CD30$^+$ skin lesions in the absence of extracutaneous disease.
- Low-dose methotrexate therapy is well tolerated and effective in more than 90% of LyP patients in the absence of preexisting liver disease. Local application of corticosteroids may cause regression of individual lesions.
- Suppression of LyP is usually temporary and does not prevent the development of mycosis fungoides or Hodgkin's lymphoma.
- The histologic distinction of C-ALCL and systemic ALCL can be difficult. The absence of EMA and ALK expression and the expression of cutaneous lymphocyte antigen favor C-ALCL.
- Regional lymph node involvement is usually not associated with aggressive disease in patients with CD30$^+$ primary cutaneous LPDs.

References can be found on Expert Consult @ www.expertconsult.com

Chapter 40

Primary Cutaneous T-Cell Lymphomas: Rare Subtypes

Lyn McDivitt Duncan and Shimareet Kumar

CHAPTER OUTLINE

CUTANEOUS T-CELL LYLMPHOMAS

Cutaneous T-cell lymphomas (CTCLs) account for approximately 70% of all cutaneous lymphomas (Table 40-1), with the vast majority being mycosis fungoides and its variants (see Chapter 38). This chapter focuses on four relatively uncommon types of CTCL that have been identified as distinct clinical entities with characteristic clinical and pathologic features. Subcutaneous panniculitis-like T-cell lymphoma (SPTCL) and primary cutaneous gamma-delta T-cell lymphoma are two distinct entities involving mainly the subcutaneous tissue. Although initially included in the same category, these tumors are now considered two different diseases with different clinical impacts.[1] Primary cutaneous $CD8^+$ aggressive epidermotropic cytotoxic T-cell lymphoma and primary cutaneous $CD4^+$ small/medium T-cell lymphoma remain provisional entities in the recent World Health Organization classification; more information is needed before they can be considered distinct diseases.[1] The diagnosis of these rare forms of CTCL requires the exclusion of mycosis fungoides and other T-cell lymphomas presenting in the skin. The differential diagnosis may be established based on the clinical and pathologic features of these tumors (Table 40-2).

Clinical Features

CTCLs have distinctive clinical presentations.[2] Mycosis fungoides has an indolent clinical course, usually with progression over many years from erythematous patches to infiltrated plaques and ultimately, in some patients, to tumor

Table 40-1 T-Cell Lymphomas and Leukemias That Occur in the Skin

Disease	Percentage of All Cutaneous Lymphomas
Primary Cutaneous T-Cell and NK-Cell Lymphomas	
Mycosis fungoides	44
Mycosis fungoides variants and subtypes	6
Sézary syndrome	3
Primary Cutaneous CD30⁺ Lymphoproliferative Disorders	
Primary cutaneous anaplastic large cell lymphoma	8
Lymphomatoid papulosis	12
Extranodal NK/T-cell lymphoma, nasal type	<1
Hydroa vacciniforme–like lymphoma	<1
Subcutaneous panniculitis-like T-cell lymphoma	1
Primary cutaneous gamma-delta T-cell lymphoma	<1
Primary cutaneous CD8⁺ aggressive epidermotropic T-cell lymphoma*	<1
Primary cutaneous CD4⁺ small/medium pleomorphic T-cell lymphoma*	2
Primary cutaneous peripheral T-cell lymphoma, unspecified	2
Secondary T-Cell Neoplasms	
Adult T-cell leukemia/lymphoma	–
T-cell prolymphocytic leukemia	–

*Provisional entity.[1]

formation.[3-5] This is a tumor of older adults and most commonly involves the skin of sun-protected sites. In contrast to mycosis fungoides, most other forms of T-cell lymphoma, including SPTCL and CD4⁺ small/medium T-cell lymphoma, usually present as tumor nodules without a preceding patch or plaque stage. Indeed, if only nodules are present, the diagnosis is most likely not mycosis fungoides but another form of CTCL. SPTCL has a predilection for the lower extremities, whereas CD4⁺ small/medium T-cell lymphoma most commonly arises on the skin of the face, neck, or upper trunk, and CD8⁺ aggressive epidermotropic cytotoxic T-cell lymphoma presents with generalized skin lesions.

Histomorphology

Malignancies of T lymphocytes frequently show epidermotropism, in contrast to B-cell lymphomas, in which the tumor cells spare the epidermis and are usually separated from it by a grenz zone. Of the T-cell lymphomas, primary cutaneous CD4⁺ small/medium T-cell lymphoma and SPTCL are characterized by the absence of epidermotropism. The cytologic features of the CTCLs are wide ranging. Mycosis fungoides, CD8⁺ aggressive epidermotropic cytotoxic T-cell lymphoma, and CD4⁺ small/medium T-cell lymphoma are all composed predominantly of small to medium-sized lymphocytes with convoluted nuclear contours, dense nuclear chromatin, and scant cytoplasm. The neoplastic T cells observed in SPTCL, extranodal natural killer (NK)/T-cell lymphoma, and cutaneous gamma-delta T-cell lymphoma are usually medium-sized to large cells with densely clumped nuclear chromatin. Immunophenotyping is helpful in distinguishing many of these tumors, particularly those with overlapping histologic features.

Immunophenotype

Some observers have proposed that cutaneous lymphomas develop in the setting of a persistent inflammatory reaction or immune dysregulation.[6-8] This hypothesis has been applied not only to T-cell proliferations in the context of connective tissue disease, chronic actinic dermatitis (actinic reticuloid), and lymphomatoid drug eruptions but also to the development of cutaneous B-cell lymphomas associated with *Borrelia* infection and tattoos.[9,10]

In T-cell lymphomas, an aberrant immunophenotype supports the diagnosis of lymphoma. This is most commonly observed in mycosis fungoides, in which one or more pan–T-cell antigens (CD2, CD5, CD7) may be absent. In general, the loss of CD7 is so common in reactive T-cell infiltrates that the loss of this marker alone is not helpful in making a diagnosis of T-cell lymphoma. The presence of a nonepidermotropic dense dermal or subcutaneous T-cell infiltrate should prompt an immunophenotyping panel that includes the T-cell markers CD3, CD4, CD8, and CD30, as well as CD56 and the pan–B-cell marker CD20 to determine the density of B cells. Tumors with a cytotoxic phenotype (CD8⁺, TIA-1⁺, perforin positive, granzyme B positive) and the CD56⁺ NK/T-cell tumors have a more aggressive clinical course than do CD4⁺, CD8⁻, CD56⁻ tumors.[11,12]

Gene Rearrangements

Clonal rearrangement of the T-cell receptor (TCR) genes is characteristic of CTCLs. With the advent of very sensitive polymerase chain reaction (PCR) technologies, the detection of clonally rearranged TCR has also been described in drug eruptions and other reactive processes. As with any diagnostic tool, the genetic results should be interpreted in the context of the clinical, histologic, and immunophenotypic findings.[10,13-15]

Treatment and Prognosis

Therapies for these rare forms of CTCL include surgical excision and radiotherapy for localized tumors and multiagent chemotherapy for tumors with a more aggressive clinical course. SPTCL and primary cutaneous CD4⁺ small/medium T-cell lymphoma are both associated with a relatively good prognosis (80% 5-year survival); cutaneous gamma-delta T-cell lymphoma and primary cutaneous CD8⁺ aggressive epidermotropic cytotoxic T-cell lymphoma are aggressive tumors with median survivals of 15 months and 32 months, respectively.

SUBCUTANEOUS PANNICULITIS-LIKE T-CELL LYMPHOMA

Definition

SPTCL is a lymphoma of mature cytotoxic T-cell derivation that involves the subcutaneous fat in a manner reminiscent of panniculitis.[16-18] It is composed of atypical lymphoid cells of different sizes, frequently associated with fat necrosis. Although cases of both alpha-beta and gamma-delta phenotypes were included in this category in earlier studies,[16-18] it is now evident that the two phenotypes are quite distinct

Table 40-2 Differential Diagnosis of Lymphomas Involving Skin and Subcutaneous Tissue

Lymphoma	Clinical Presentation	Histologic Features	Immunophenotype			Molecular Findings
			T-Cell Markers	Cytotoxic Proteins	EBV	
SPTCL	Subcutaneous nodules, HPS, dissemination rare, indolent clinical course	Neoplastic lymphocytes rim individual fat cells, prominent karyorrhexis, histiocytes, vascular infiltration	$CD3^+$, $CD8^+$, $CD4^-$, $\beta F1^+$	+	–	TCR R
Primary cutaneous gamma-delta T-cell lymphoma	Cutaneous nodules, often ulcerated; HPS; frequent dissemination with aggressive clinical course	Dermal and epidermal involvement in addition to subcutaneous involvement; in the latter, rimming with karyorrhexis identical to SPTCL is common	$CD3^+$, $CD4^-$, $CD8^-$, $CD56^+$, $TCR\delta\text{-}1^+$	+	–	TCR R
$CD8^+$ aggressive epidermotropic cytotoxic T-cell lymphoma	Localized or multiple papules, nodules, and tumors; central necrosis or ulceration; aggressive clinical course	Pagetoid epidermotropism, destruction of adnexal structures	$CD3^+$, $CD8^+$, $\beta F1^+$, $CD5^-$, $CD56^-$	+	–	TCR R
$CD4^+$ small/medium T-cell lymphoma	Solitary or localized lesions on head, neck, and trunk; indolent clinical course	Monotonous small cell infiltrate in dermis with no epidermotropism	$CD3^+$, $CD4^+$, $CD8^-$, $\beta F1^+$, $PD1^+$	–	–	TCR R
Extranodal NK/T-cell lymphoma, nasal type	Skin involvement with tumors, disseminated disease common, HPS	Tumor cells sheet out, angiocentric pattern, necrosis	$sCD3^-$, $cCD3^+$, $CD4^-$, $CD8^-$, $CD56^+$	+	+	TCR G
Mycosis fungoides	Cutaneous patches, plaques, tumors	Dermal and epidermal involvement, marked epidermotropism with Pautrier's microabscesses, cerebriform cells	$CD3^+$, $CD4^+$, $CD8^-$, $\beta F1^+$	–	–	TCR R
ALCL, systemic type	Nodal and extranodal involvement, skin and soft tissues commonly involved	Diffuse infiltrate, hallmark cells identified	$CD3^+$, $CD4^+$, $CD8^-$, $CD30^+$, EMA^+, $ALK\text{-}1^+$	+	–	TCR R t(2;5)
C-ALCL	Cutaneous tumor, often solitary; surface ulceration	Diffuse infiltrate, pleomorphic cells, multinucleate giant cells, RS-like cells	$CD3^+$, $CD4^+$, $CD8^-$, $CD30^+$, EMA^-	+	–	TCR R

ALCL, anaplastic large cell lymphoma; ALK, anaplastic lymphoma kinase; c, cytoplasmic staining; C-ALCL, primary cutaneous anaplastic large cell lymphoma; EBV, Epstein-Barr virus; EMA, epithelial membrane antigen; G, germline; HPS, hemophagocytic syndrome; R, rearranged; RS, Reed-Sternberg; s, surface or membrane staining; SPTCL, subcutaneous panniculitis-like T-cell lymphoma; TCR, T-cell receptor.

in terms of their histologic features and clinical behavior; therefore, the term *SPTCL* is now restricted to cases with the alpha-beta phenotype.[1] Lymphomas of gamma-delta derivation involving the subcutaneous tissue are believed to represent a different clinical entity; they often involve the dermis and epidermis in addition to the subcutis and pursue a more aggressive clinical course (see later).[1,12,17,19-21]

This entity encompasses the majority of cases previously described in the literature as *cytophagic histiocytic panniculitis*[22,23] and *fatal panniculitis*,[24] as well as some reported as *malignant histiocytosis*.[25]

Epidemiology

SPTCL affects men and women, adults and children, with a median age of onset of 35 years. Although there is a slight predominance of tumors in women and the suggestion of an association with lupus erythematosus, the relationship of this tumor to autoimmune disease remains unclear.[18,20,21,26]

Etiology

The disease is sporadic in the majority of cases, and no specific etiologic factors have been identified. The tumors may exhibit histologic features that overlap with subcutaneous lupus (lupus profundus, lupus panniculitis), and SPTCL may present with a clinical syndrome of fever, polyarthritis, and pericarditis that mimics an autoimmune disease.[26,27] The lesions have also been associated with rheumatoid arthritis,[28] inflammatory bowel disease,[20,29] tuberculosis,[20] sites of ethnic scarification,[30,31] and after transplantation.[32,33] These associations have led some to propose causes related to chronic antigen exposure and immune dysregulation.[34-36] Despite the suggestion that immunosuppression may play a role in SPTCL, there is no association with Epstein-Barr virus (EBV) or *Borrelia* infection.[17,18,26] Cases previously described as EBV⁺ likely represent other tumor types, such as NK/T-cell lymphoma, nasal type.[37,38]

Clinical Features

Patients present with solitary or multiple nodules or plaques, usually on the lower extremity. The upper extremities and trunk may also be involved. The tumors may be small or measure several centimeters in diameter, but they rarely ulcerate. The indurated appearance may lead to the clinical diagnosis of an abscess, and tumors may undergo incision and drainage without resolution. This tumor may be associated with systemic symptoms, including fever, fatigue, and weight loss. Hemophagocytic syndrome is a rare complication associated with an aggressive clinical course; it is less common than in the gamma-delta T-cell tumors.[19,26]

Morphology

This tumor is characterized by a dense, predominantly subcutaneous infiltrate of small to medium-sized T cells, with occasional large lymphocytes and many histiocytes (Fig. 40-1). The lymphoid atypia is variable from case to case and may be subtle or readily evident. There is usually minimal involvement of the overlying epidermis and dermis. The individual adipocyte spaces show rimming by neoplastic lymphocytes with enlarged nuclei, clumped chromatin, and scant cytoplasm. Macrophages containing cellular debris are characteristically present, with associated fat necrosis and karyorrhexis. In rare cases the histiocytes may aggregate to form granulomas; however, this is not a dominant finding.[16,17,39,40] Erythrophagocytosis by histiocytes is rarely observed in the subcutaneous infiltrates but may be present. Vascular invasion is common and may be associated with regions of necrosis.[12,17,18]

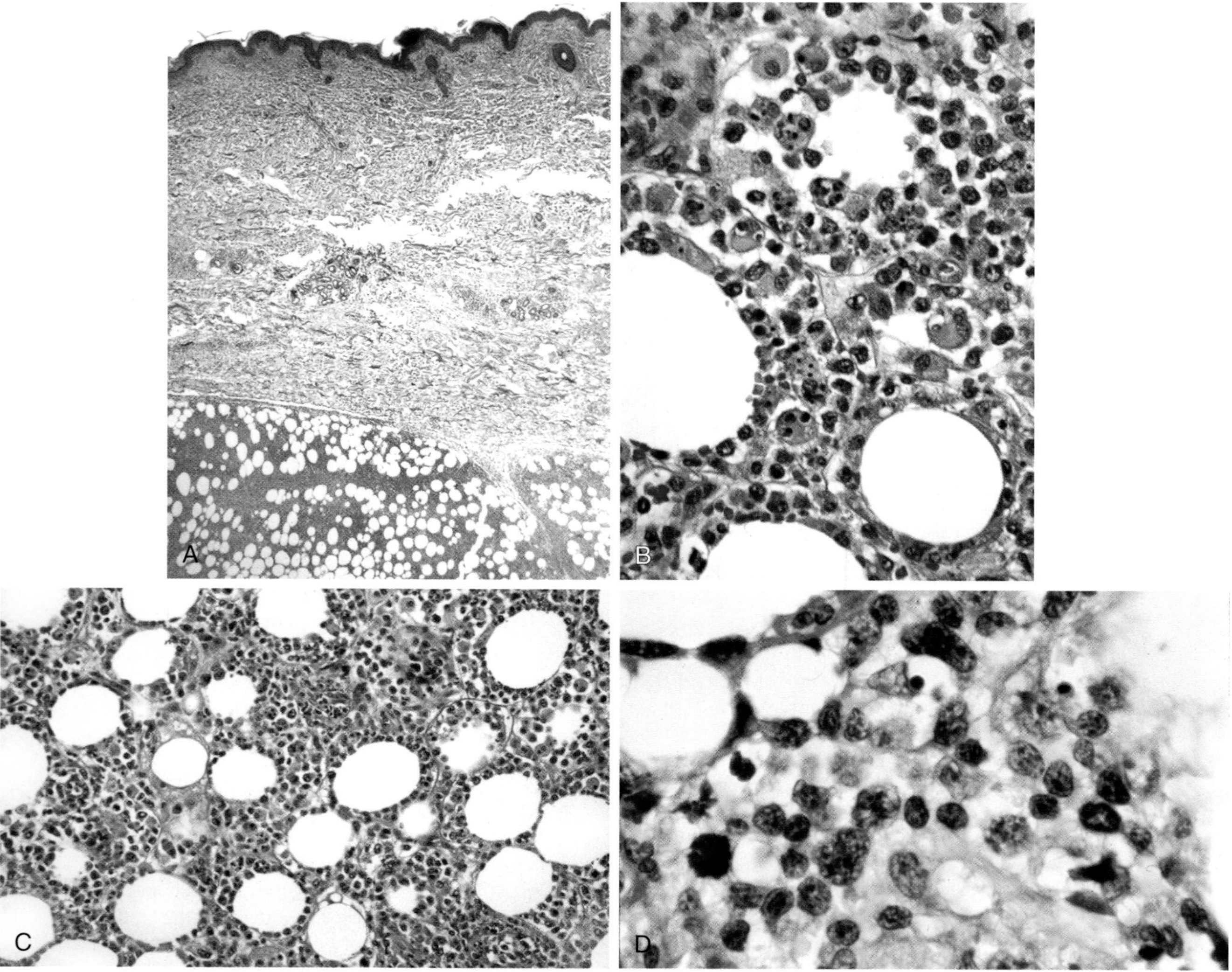

Figure 40-1. Subcutaneous panniculitis-like T-cell lymphoma. A, The malignant lymphoid infiltrate is localized to the subcutaneous tissue, without involvement of the overlying dermis and epidermis. **B,** The infiltrate is composed of neoplastic lymphocytes and admixed benign histiocytes. **C,** Neoplastic lymphocytes rim individual fat spaces in a lace-like pattern, reminiscent of panniculitis. **D,** The neoplastic lymphoid cells are medium sized, with hyperchromatic nuclei and occasional cells with prominent nucleoli. Scattered mitoses are present. (Courtesy Dr. E. Jaffe, Bethesda, MD)

Immunophenotype

The tumor cells of SPTCL have a mature alpha-beta cytotoxic T-cell phenotype, characteristically $CD3^+$, $CD8^+$, $CD4^-$, and $\beta F1^+$ (Fig. 40-2). The cytotoxic proteins granzyme B, TIA-1, and perforin are usually present. These tumors only rarely express CD56 or CD30. Cases may rarely coexpress CD4 and CD8,[18] but the absence of both CD4 and CD8 suggests a gamma-delta T-cell lymphoma.[12] Granzyme M may be helpful in distinguishing alpha-beta from gamma-delta tumors; it is positive more often in gamma-delta lymphomas and negative in alpha-beta SPTCL (see Table 40-2).[39]

Genetics

Clonal rearrangement of TCR genes is detected in most cases. These tumors are negative for EBV.

Clinical Course

The 5-year disease-specific survival is estimated at 80%, with dissemination to lymph nodes and other organs a rare event.[16,17,41] Local recurrences may occur over a period of several years, but the disease remains confined to the subcutis in most patients. There have been reports of PCR detection of T cells clonally identical to the SPTCL in peripheral blood and bone marrow, supporting the idea that circulating cells may be present in some patients without detectable tumors at noncutaneous sites.[29,42]

Hemophagocytic syndrome may occur, and if it does, the prognosis is poor; it is the cause of death in the majority of cases.[16,26,43,44] Rarely, hemophagocytic syndrome may respond to aggressive chemotherapy.[16] Although hemophagocytosis is rarely observed in the subcutaneous tumors, histiocytes containing phagocytosed erythrocytes may be evident in bone marrow aspirate smears and in the sinuses of lymph nodes (Fig. 40-3).

Prior reports of a rapidly fatal course of SPTCL in the absence of hemophagocytic syndrome were related to the inclusion of gamma-delta T-cell tumors, which demonstrated a worse prognosis.[21,45] Multiagent chemotherapy has been the treatment of choice for these tumors, but recent studies indicate that cyclosporine, steroids, and chlorambucil may be effective.[29,41,46]

Differential Diagnosis

The differential diagnosis of SPTCL includes other forms of lymphoma involving the subcutaneous fat (see Table 40-2), lupus profundus (Table 40-3), and reactive panniculitis in the setting of a drug reaction or injected antigen. Immunophenotyping may be helpful in distinguishing this tumor from other forms of lymphoma (see Table 40-2). The absence of CD4, CD8, and βF1 supports the diagnosis of a gamma-delta T-cell

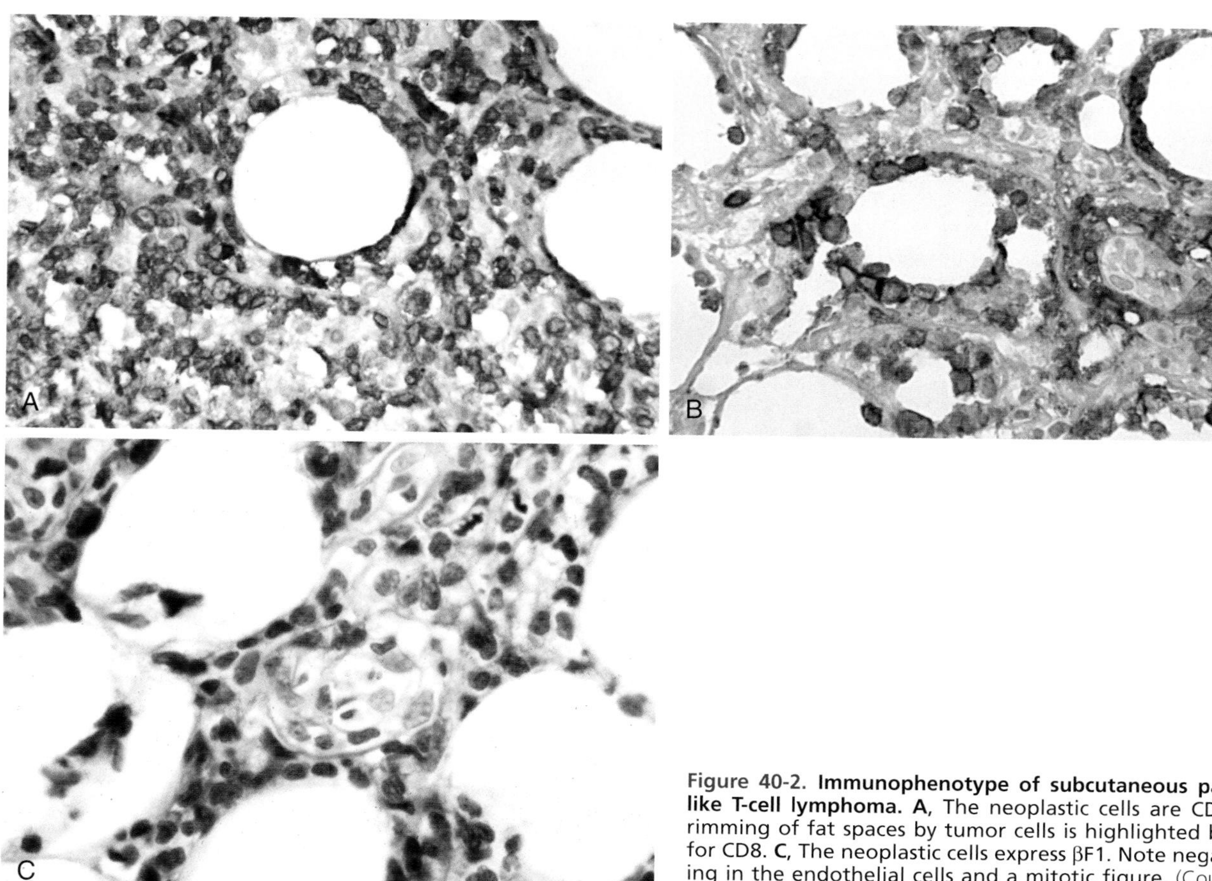

Figure 40-2. Immunophenotype of subcutaneous panniculitis-like T-cell lymphoma. A, The neoplastic cells are $CD3^+$. **B,** The rimming of fat spaces by tumor cells is highlighted by staining for CD8. **C,** The neoplastic cells express βF1. Note negative staining in the endothelial cells and a mitotic figure. (Courtesy Dr. E. Jaffe, Bethesda, MD)

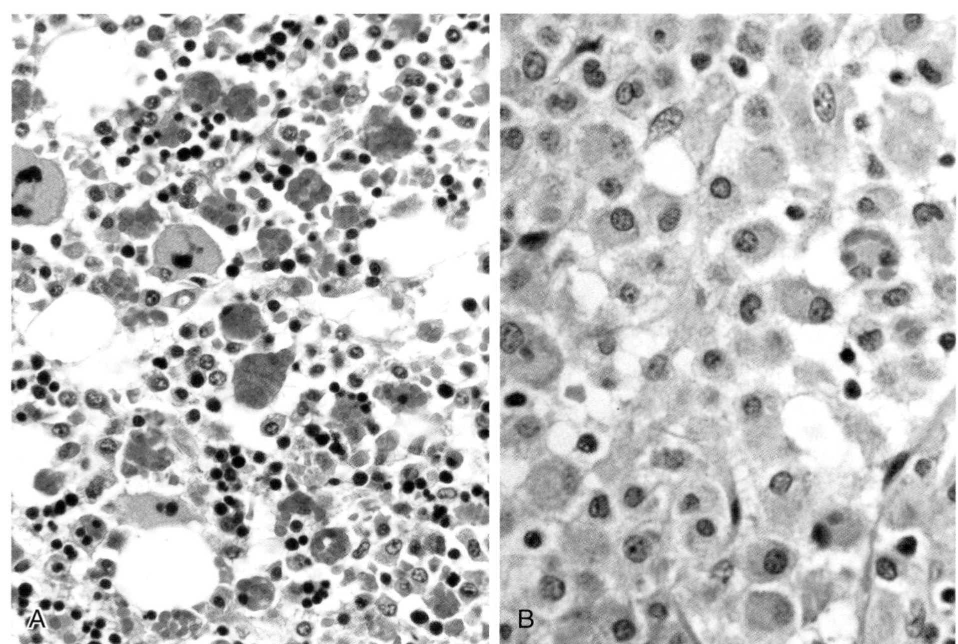

Figure 40-3. Hemophagocytic syndrome in subcutaneous panniculitis-like T-cell lymphoma. Hemophagocytosis in a bone marrow core biopsy (**A**) and a lymph node (**B**).

lymphoma. Tumors with a gamma-delta phenotype have a worse prognosis and are diagnosed as cutaneous gamma-delta T-cell lymphoma rather than SPTCL. Gamma-delta T-cell lymphomas more often display periadnexal and epidermal involvement than do alpha-beta tumors. In addition to gamma-delta T-cell lymphoma, a subcutaneous lymphoma expressing CD56 may represent extranodal NK/T-cell lymphoma, nasal type. These tumors do not express surface CD3 but stain positively for cytoplasmic CD3, and in situ hybridization for EBV (EBV-encoded RNA [EBER]) is positive. Also, angioinvasion and filling of the fat lobules rather than rimming of the adipocyte spaces are more common with NK/T-cell lymphoma involving the subcutis. $CD30^+$, $CD4^+$, $CD8^-$ tumors also tend to overrun the adipocyte spaces and should be included in the group of $CD30^+$ anaplastic large cell lymphomas. Unlike SPTCL, $CD30^+$ anaplastic large cell lymphomas usually are ulcerated and diffusely involve the dermis.

Table 40-3 Differentiation between Subcutaneous Panniculitis-Like T-Cell Lymphoma and Lupus Profundus

Feature	Lupus Profundus	Subcutaneous Lymphoma
Diffuse infiltration of fat lobules by atypical medium-sized lymphocytes	+	+
Fat necrosis	+	+
Histocytes containing cellular debris	+	+
Lymphoid follicles	+	–
Eosinophilic hyaline change of fat ("honeycomb")	+	–
Hyaluronic acid deposition ("mucin")	+	–
Epidermal changes (atrophy, vacuolar interface change, follicular plugs)	+	–
Erythrophagocytosis	–	+
Rimming of adipocytes by atypical T cells	–	+
CD8	+	+
CD56	–	–
CD30	–	–

The most challenging diagnostic problem is often differentiating lupus profundus and SPTCL (see Table 40-3).[20,47,48] Both processes are characterized by a dense proliferation of enlarged lymphocytes in subcutaneous lobules, with sparing of the interlobular septa and debris-laden macrophages (Fig. 40-4). Lupus characteristically exhibits infiltrates of plasma cells, reactive lymphoid follicles, lymphocytic vasculitis, and eosinophilic hyalinization of the fat, with a distinctive honeycomb-like appearance (see Fig. 40-4). The presence of characteristic epidermal changes of lupus, including epidermal atrophy and vacuolar alteration of basal layer keratinocytes, and increased dermal and subcutaneous connective tissue mucin deposits also support the diagnosis of lupus.[49] Occasionally, however, these distinguishing findings may be absent (see Table 40-2). Erythrophagocytosis and rimming of adipocyte spaces by markedly atypical medium-sized lymphocytes with chromatin clumping favor a diagnosis of lymphoma. Nevertheless, the degree of cytologic atypia observed in SPTCL is variable, and multiple biopsies may be necessary before a definitive diagnosis can be made.[16,26,47]

Very rarely the differential diagnosis may include reaction to a drug. In this case the tumor cells are mostly small, with rare medium-sized cells, and a lymphocytic vasculitis may be present; the features of lupus and the characteristic rimming of fat spaces by atypical lymphocytes are absent. The differential diagnosis may also include reaction to an arthropod bite; however, the bite is usually remembered when it leads

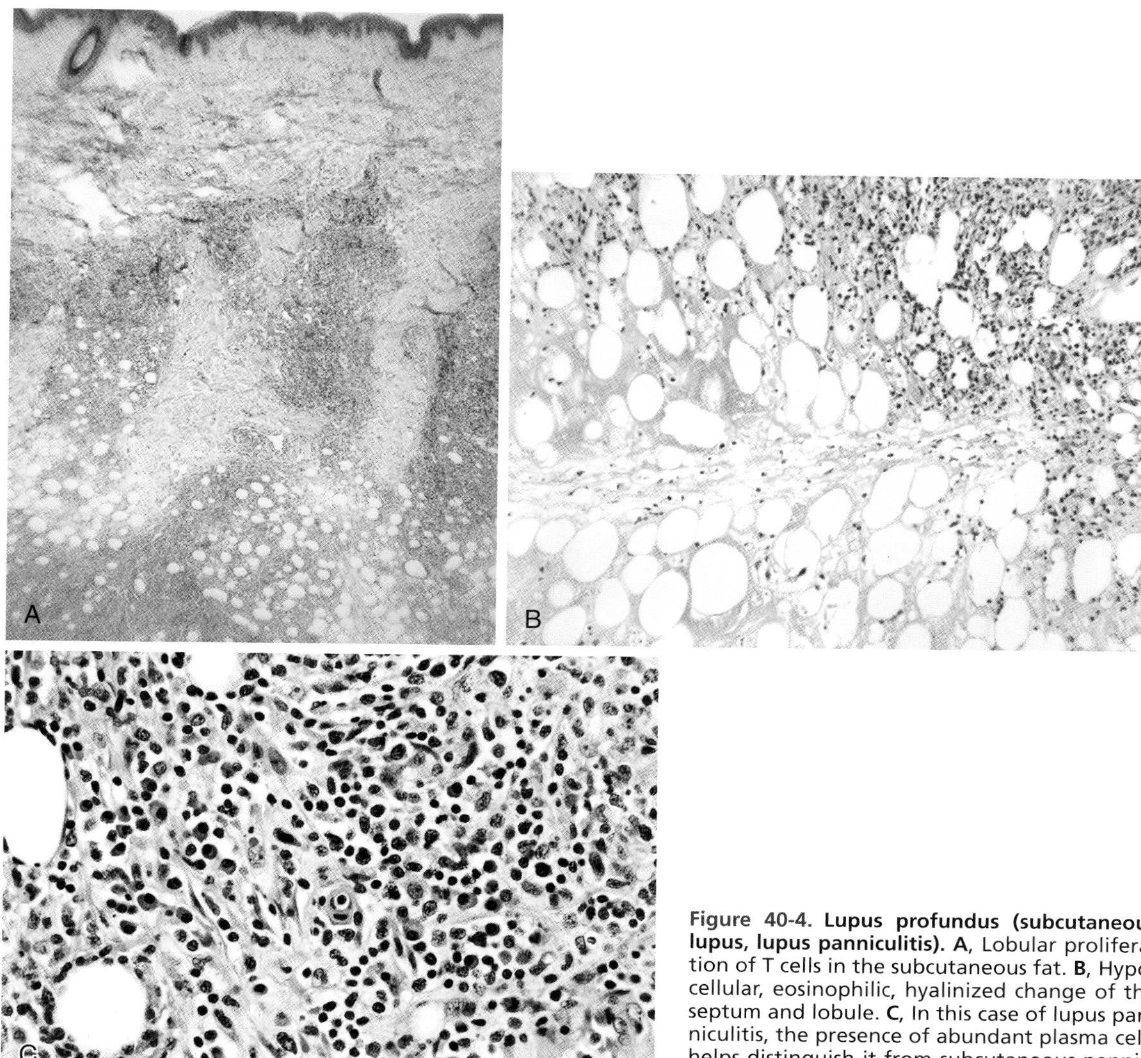

Figure 40-4. Lupus profundus (subcutaneous lupus, lupus panniculitis). A, Lobular proliferation of T cells in the subcutaneous fat. **B,** Hypocellular, eosinophilic, hyalinized change of the septum and lobule. **C,** In this case of lupus panniculitis, the presence of abundant plasma cells helps distinguish it from subcutaneous panniculitis-like T-cell lymphoma.

to a large tumoral lesion. Such reactions usually have a mixed inflammatory infiltrate with a lymphocytic panniculitis, scattered neutrophils, and numerous eosinophils.

PRIMARY CUTANEOUS GAMMA-DELTA T-CELL LYMPHOMA

Definition

This rare form of CTCL is characterized by a proliferation of mature activated gamma-delta T cells with a cytotoxic phenotype. These tumors include cases previously considered SPTCL with a gamma-delta phenotype. Gamma-delta mucosal T-cell lymphomas may be related to this entity, but more studies are needed to determine their potential relationship.[45,50,51]

The cell of origin is the mature and activated cytotoxic gamma-delta T cell of the innate immune system. The distribution of gamma-delta tumors involving mainly skin and mucosal sites seems to follow the normal distribution of gamma-delta T cells.

Epidemiology and Clinical Features

This tumor occurs most commonly in young adults, with a median age of 40 years. Women are affected more commonly than men. Overall this tumor accounts for less than 1% of CTCLs.

Gamma-delta T-cell lymphomas most commonly present with multiple lesions on the extremities, particularly the thighs and buttocks, and as infiltrated plaques or ulcerated subcutaneous nodules. Involvement of the mucosa and extension to other extranodal sites are common, but the lymph nodes, spleen, and bone marrow are usually spared.[34] Patients with subcutaneous tumors may develop hemophagocytic syndrome, which is associated with a poor prognosis. B symptoms are present in most patients. Nearly 50% of patients develop elevated liver enzymes and leukopenia, and these findings are also associated with a poor prognosis.[52]

This tumor is clinically aggressive, with a median survival of slightly more than 1 year. Gamma-delta T-cell lymphoma is resistant to radiotherapy and to multiagent chemotherapy. Patients with involvement of the subcutaneous fat have a worse prognosis than those with tumors limited to the epidermis and dermis.[21,45]

Morphology

Cutaneous gamma-delta T-cell lymphoma may be histologically heterogeneous, with an epidermotropic, dermal, or predominantly subcutaneous infiltrate (Fig. 40-5). One or more patterns may be observed in a single biopsy. Alternatively, biopsies from the same patient may show different infiltrative growth patterns. Epidermotropism may be prominent and display a pagetoid distribution, or it may be minimal. In subcutaneous tumors the neoplastic gamma-delta T cells rim the fat spaces, a finding similar to that in alpha-beta SPTCL.[41] However, the gamma-delta tumors also show dermal and epidermal infiltrates. The tumor cells are medium to large lymphocytes with coarsely clumped chromatin; large cells with blastic vesicular nuclei and prominent nucleoli are infrequent (see Fig. 40-5). Angioinvasion and apoptosis and necrosis with cellular debris are also commonly observed (see Fig. 40-5).

Immunophenotype

The tumor cells express the T-cell markers CD3 and CD2 but are negative for βF1 and usually double negative for CD4 and CD8, although CD8 may be present in some cases. CD7 may be expressed, but CD5 is negative. CD56 and the cytotoxic proteins (granzyme B, granzyme M, TIA-1, perforin) are strongly positive.[41] The tumor cells express the TCR

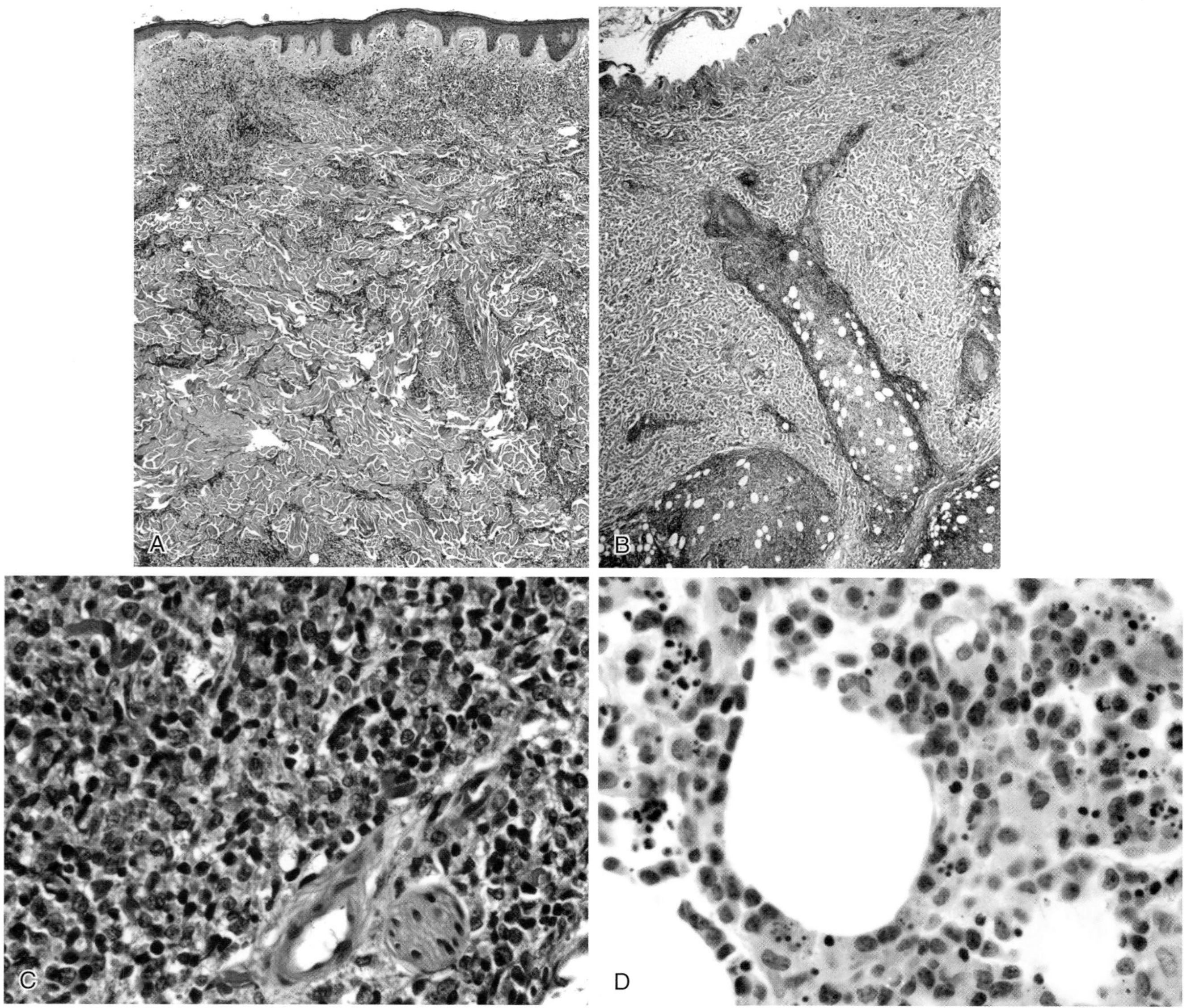

Figure 40-5. Cutaneous gamma-delta T-cell lymphoma exhibits three prominent patterns: epidermotropic, dermal, and subcutaneous. **A**, This case displays a predominantly dermal infiltration by medium to large lymphocytes. **B**, This case shows subcutaneous and dermal involvement with a periadnexal and perivascular distribution. **C**, Medium and large lymphocytes, some with prominent nucleoli, are observed. Many cases display a prominence of cells with coarse, clumped chromatin. **D**, Subcutaneous tumors may show rimming of fat spaces and histiocytes containing cellular debris.

delta chain, but its detection usually requires either frozen tissue or flow cytometry studies. If this staining is not available, the absence of βF1 may serve as a surrogate for the gamma-delta phenotype, provided other diagnostic criteria are fulfilled.[53]

Genetics

Clonal rearrangement of the TCRγ and TCRδ genes is observed. Although TCRβ may be rearranged or deleted, it is not expressed. These tumors are negative for EBV.

Differential Diagnosis

This tumor must be distinguished from other forms of CTCL that may have a $CD56^+$, $CD8^-$ immunophenotype, including the $CD4^+$, $CD56^+$ blastic plasmacytoid dendritic cell neoplasm. These tumors involve the dermis and may extend to the subcutaneous tissue but usually spare the epidermis. Angioinvasion and necrosis are not present. The tumor cells have irregular nuclei with finely dispersed chromatin and usually stain positively for CD123 and TCL1. Although mycosis fungoides and SPTCL may resemble gamma-delta T-cell lymphoma on hematoxylin-eosin–stained tissue sections, immunophenotyping aids in arriving at the correct diagnosis; the presence of CD56, absence of βF1, and presence of TCRδ support the diagnosis of cutaneous gamma-delta T-cell lymphoma.

The differential diagnosis also includes lupus panniculitis; both processes may exhibit a dense lymphoid and histiocytic infiltrate overrunning the subcutaneous fat lobules, with lymphoid atypia and fat necrosis (see Table 40-3). Hyalinization of the fat lobule, germinal center formation, plasma cells, and dermal and subcutaneous deposits of connective tissue mucin (hyaluronic acid) are common findings in lupus panniculitis but are usually not observed in subcutaneous lymphoma (see Fig. 40-4). Nevertheless, there is significant overlap, and cases originally diagnosed as lupus panniculitis may be recategorized as gamma-delta T-cell lymphoma as the clinical course progresses.[54]

PRIMARY CUTANEOUS CD8-POSITIVE AGGRESSIVE EPIDERMOTROPIC CYTOTOXIC T-CELL LYMPHOMA

Definition

This uncommon form of CTCL is characterized by an epidermotropic $CD8^+$ proliferation of cytotoxic T cells and an aggressive clinical course.[55,56]

Epidemiology and Clinical Features

This tumor occurs in adults and accounts for less than 1% of CTCLs. $CD8^+$ aggressive epidermotropic cytotoxic T-cell lymphoma manifests as eruptive papules or nodules that are frequently ulcerated or as hyperkeratotic patches and plaques.[56-61] The cutaneous lesions may be localized or generalized. Patients may develop extracutaneous spread to the lung, testis, oral mucosa, and central nervous system, but the lymph nodes are typically not involved.[56,59] The degree of cytologic atypia and size of the tumor cells do not appear to have prognostic significance. This tumor is clinically aggressive, with a median survival of less than 3 years.[56]

Morphology

$CD8^+$ aggressive epidermotropic cytotoxic T-cell lymphoma is characterized by a dense, intraepidermal epidermotropic infiltrate of cytologically atypical $CD8^+$ cells; the pattern has been termed *pagetoid* because of its resemblance to Paget's disease of the breast (Fig. 40-6). There may be epidermal ulceration, dyskeratotic keratinocytes, mild spongiosis, and subepidermal edema, occasionally with blister formation. The epidermotropic tumor cells may extend down adnexal structures. Acanthosis and hyperkeratosis are commonly observed.[56,60,61] The tumor cells have small to medium-sized pleomorphic or large blastic nuclei. In addition to the infiltration of adnexal structures, the tumor cells may be distributed in an angiocentric pattern, sometimes with angioinvasion.

Immunophenotype

The tumor cells are $CD8^+$, $CD3^+$, granzyme B positive, TIA-1^+, perforin positive, $βF1^+$, $CD45RA^{+/-}$, $CD45RO^-$, $CD7^{-/+}$, $CD2^{-/+}$, $CD4^-$, and $CD5^-$ (see Fig. 40-6). Rarely these tumors may express CD15 or CD30.[62,63]

Genetics

Clonal rearrangement of TCR genes is found. These tumors are negative for EBV.

Differential Diagnosis

The diagnosis of $CD8^+$ aggressive epidermotropic cytotoxic T-cell lymphoma requires a combination of clinical, histologic, and immunophenotypic findings (see Table 40-2). Other forms of CTCL may be derived from $CD8^+$ cytotoxic T cells and must be distinguished from this tumor.[12] CTCLs that may have a $CD8^+$ immunophenotype include mycosis fungoides and rare variants of $CD30^+$ lymphoproliferative disorders; these tumors are identified by the clinical presentation, clinical behavior, and extent of epidermotropism. A prolonged clinical course with plaques and patches is characteristic of mycosis fungoides but is not observed in $CD8^+$ aggressive epidermotropic cytotoxic T-cell lymphoma. $CD30^+$ tumors usually present as solitary nodules, frequently with ulceration; this clinical presentation and the expression of CD30 help distinguish the rare $CD8^+$, $CD30^+$ CTCL from $CD8^+$ aggressive epidermotropic cytotoxic T-cell lymphoma. Cases classified in the past as the Ketron-Goodman variant of pagetoid reticulosis likely represent either $CD8^+$ aggressive epidermotropic cytotoxic T-cell lymphoma or gamma-delta T-cell lymphoma. Clinical features of $CD8^+$ aggressive epidermotropic cytotoxic T-cell lymphoma may resemble gamma-delta T-cell lymphoma; phenotyping allows the distinction of these two tumors. In contrast to $CD8^+$ aggressive epidermotropic cytotoxic T-cell lymphoma, gamma-delta T-cell lymphoma is usually $CD56^+$ and lacks CD4, CD8, and βF1. Gamma-delta T-cell lymphoma often presents with disseminated plaques and ulcerated nodules on the extremities. Although the infiltrates of gamma-delta T-cell lymphoma may display epidermotropism, they may also involve the dermis and

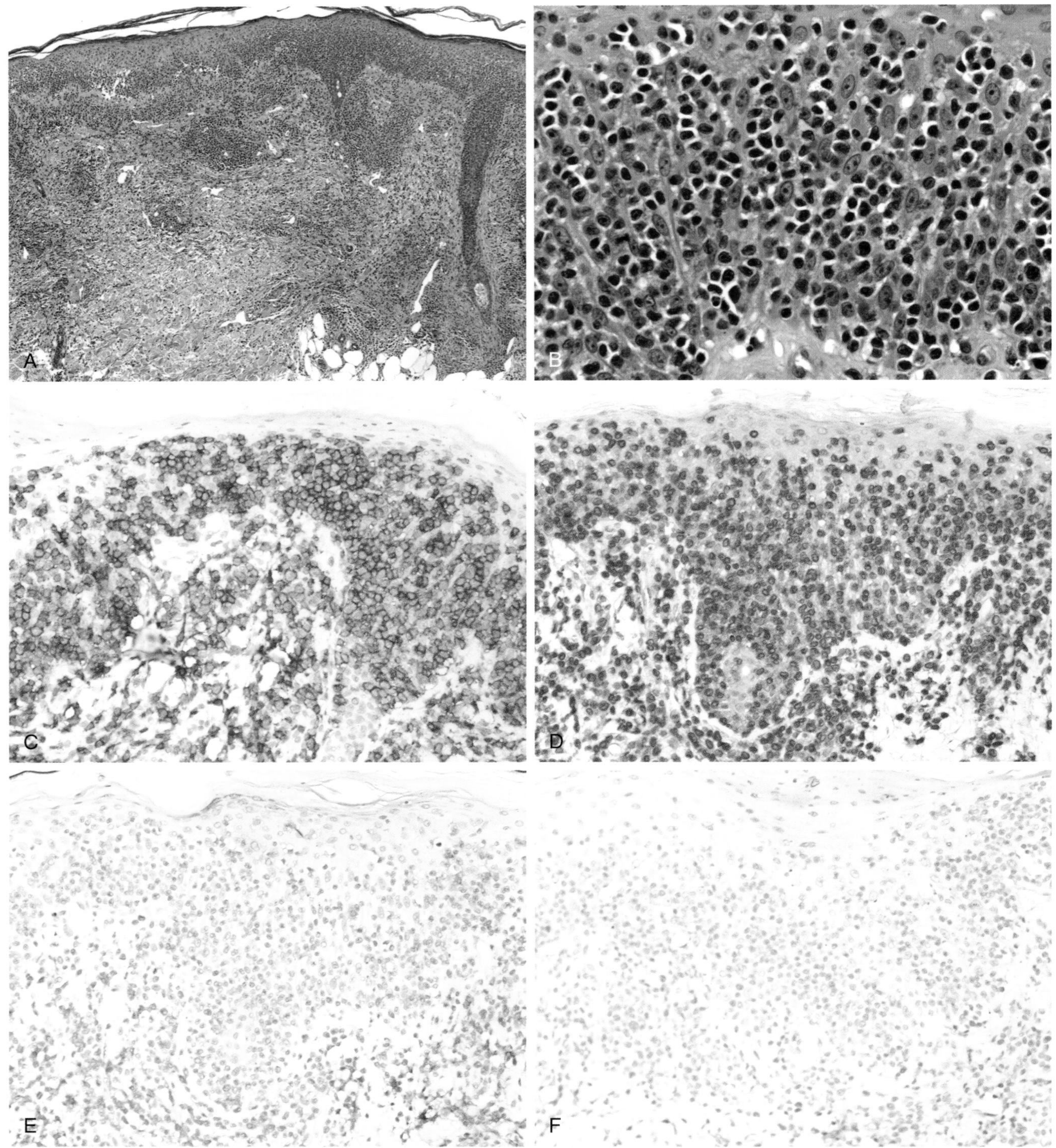

Figure 40-6. Primary cutaneous CD8[+] aggressive epidermotropic cytotoxic T-cell lymphoma. A, There is extensive epidermotropism with an associated dermal infiltrate. **B,** The epidermotropic lymphocytes have densely chromatic nuclei and irregular nuclear contours; the pattern of individual cell infiltration resembles Paget's disease. **C–F,** The tumor cells are positive for CD8 (**C**) and CD3 (**D**) but negative for CD4 (**E**) and CD56 (**F**).

subcutaneous fat. CD8+ aggressive epidermotropic cytotoxic T-cell lymphoma may occasionally involve the subcutaneous fat in a pattern similar to that of SPTCL. These CD8+ tumors share a βF1+ phenotype, with the expression of cytotoxic proteins. The prominent epidermotropism is helpful in identifying CD8+ aggressive epidermotropic cytotoxic T-cell lymphoma; epidermal involvement is rare in SPTCL.

PRIMARY CUTANEOUS CD4-POSITIVE SMALL/MEDIUM T-CELL LYMPHOMA

Definition

This tumor is characterized by a dense dermal, minimally epidermotropic infiltrate of CD4+ small to medium-sized pleomorphic lymphocytes, with no clinical history of patches or plaques. This provisional entity does not include tumors that express CD8.[1,11]

Epidemiology and Clinical Features

Primary cutaneous CD4+ small/medium T-cell lymphoma occurs in adults and is rare, accounting for approximately 2% of CTCLs. It usually appears as a solitary plaque or nodule on the face, neck, or upper trunk. The tumor may also present as localized or multiple lesions. Involvement of the lower extremities is uncommon, and by definition, there should be no history of the patches characteristic of mycosis fungoides.[11,63-66]

These tumors have a favorable prognosis, with a 5-year survival rate of more than 80%.[11,63-67] Patients with solitary or localized tumors have a better prognosis than those with multiple generalized tumors.[68,69] Rapidly growing tumors with large lesions and the presence of ulceration have been associated with extracutaneous dissemination and a worse prognosis.[68] Surgical excision or local radiotherapy is the most common treatment.

Morphology

The tumors show a dense dermal infiltrate of small to medium-sized pleomorphic lymphocytes, occasionally with extension into the subcutaneous fat (Fig. 40-7).[11,64-70] Epidermotropism is not a characteristic finding but may be present focally. Scattered large neoplastic lymphocytes constituting less than 30% of the tumor may be observed in rare cases. Scattered B cells

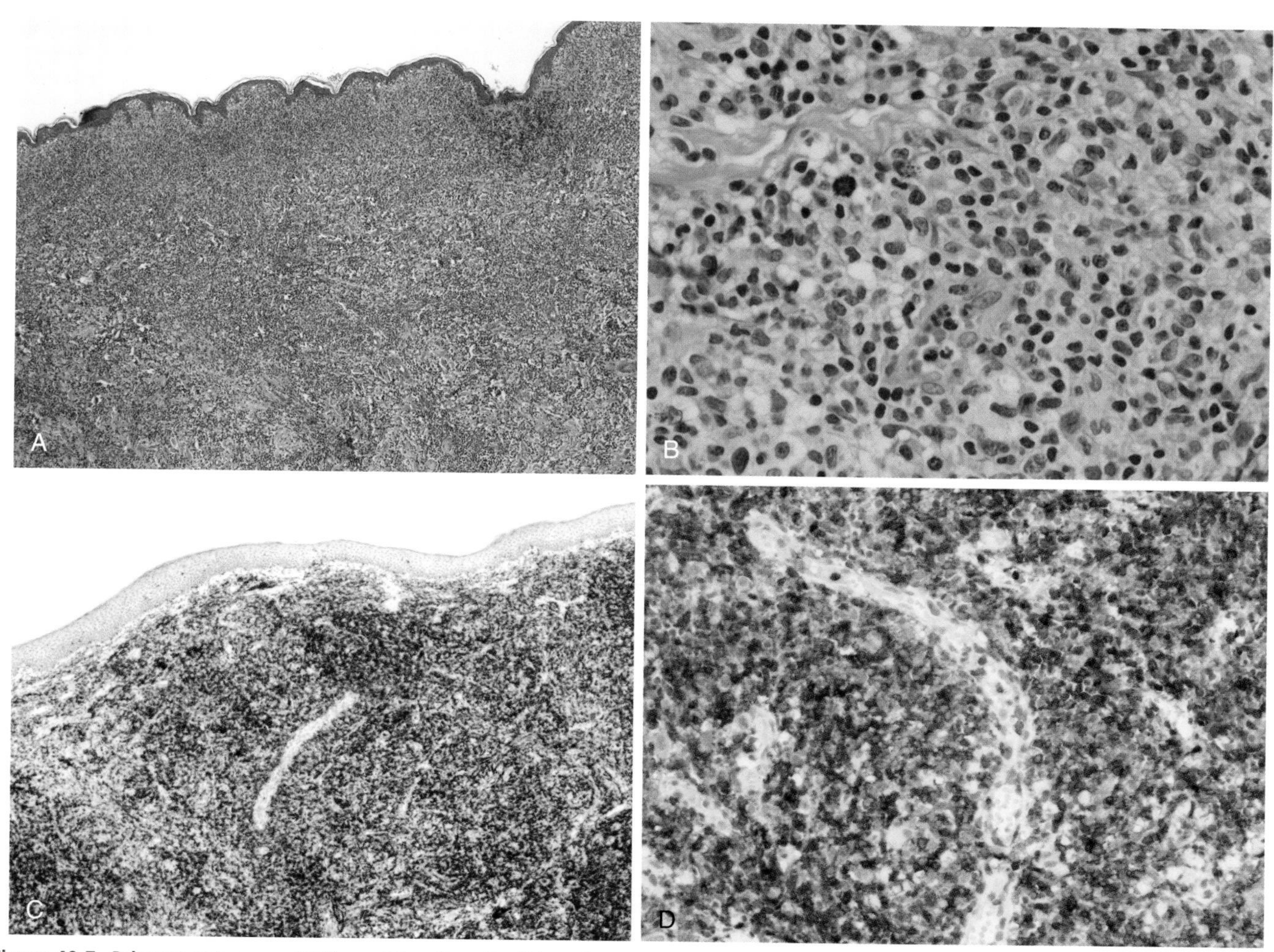

Figure 40-7. Primary cutaneous CD4+ small/medium T-cell lymphoma. A and B, Diffuse dermal involvement by irregular small to medium-sized cells with atypical mitotic figures. **C and D,** The cells express CD3 **(C)** and CD4 **(D)**. (Courtesy of Dr. E. Campo and Dr. A. Garcia, Hospital Clinic, University of Barcelona.)

(sometimes numerous), plasma cells, and histiocytes are often present.[68-70] Some cases, particularly those presenting with multiple lesions, reportedly contain numerous eosinophils.[68] The extent of infiltration by CD8⁺ T cells and the proliferation rate vary in these tumors and may be related to disease progression.[68] Tumors with a significantly higher proliferation rate, as evaluated by Ki-67 staining, and with a lower number of infiltrating CD8⁺ T cells are associated with more rapidly evolving tumors and extracutaneous dissemination.[68]

Immunophenotype

The tumor cells have a βF1⁺, CD3⁺, CD4⁺, CD8⁻, CD30⁻ phenotype (see Fig. 40-7). There is occasional loss of pan–T-cell markers. As a rule, cytotoxic proteins are not expressed. The larger cells seem to express the follicular T-helper cell–associated antigen PD1.[70]

Genetics

Clonal rearrangement of TCR genes is present. These tumors are negative for EBV.

Differential Diagnosis

The differential diagnosis often includes a reactive lymphoid hyperplasia, particularly in those cases with mixed infiltrates that include histiocytes and eosinophils. This distinction can be particularly difficult when the degree of atypia in the neoplastic cells is similar to that observed in activated T cells in drug reactions or other reactive processes. Additionally, loss of pan–T-cell antigens is rare in CD4⁺ small/medium T-cell lymphoma. Although some authors require clonal TCR rearrangement for the diagnosis of lymphoma, sensitive PCR-based technologies can reveal clonal rearrangement in reactive T-cell infiltrates as well. In the absence of drug exposure, the presence of a cytologically atypical proliferation of slightly enlarged small to medium-sized CD4⁺ T cells, loss of T-cell markers, and clonal TCR rearrangement support the diagnosis of lymphoma.

Because of the clinically significant difference in prognosis, CD4⁺ small/medium T-cell lymphoma must be distinguished from other forms of CTCL that generally have a more aggressive course (see Table 40-2). CD4⁺ small/medium T-cell lymphoma is distinguished from mycosis fungoides by the presence of papules and nodules in the absence of the characteristic patch stage of mycosis fungoides. The tumor cells of CD4⁺ small/medium T-cell lymphoma infiltrate the dermis and subcutis with little epidermotropism, in contrast to mycosis fungoides, which is characterized by a band-like epidermotropic infiltrate.[69]

The differential diagnosis also includes peripheral T-cell lymphoma, unspecified. Cases with greater than 30% large pleomorphic tumor cells should be classified as peripheral T-cell lymphoma, unspecified, and patients should be evaluated for the possibility of secondary lymphoma. These cases with more than 30% large cells tend to follow an aggressive clinical course.[67]

Pearls and Pitfalls

Pearls

- The differential diagnosis of a primary cutaneous lymphoma with infiltration of the subcutaneous tissue includes NK/T-cell lymphoma, subcutaneous panniculitis-like lymphoma, and primary cutaneous gamma-delta T-cell lymphoma.
- A subcutaneous lymphoma expressing CD56⁺ may represent extranodal NK/T-cell lymphoma or primary cutaneous gamma-delta T-cell lymphoma. In situ hybridization for EBV helps in the differential diagnosis, being positive in the NK/T-cell lymphomas and negative in the gamma-delta tumors.
- Angioinvasion and filling of the fat lobules rather than rimming of the adipocyte spaces are more common in NK/T-cell lymphoma than in subcutaneous panniculitis-like lymphoma.
- Patients with CD8⁺ aggressive epidermotropic cytotoxic T-cell lymphoma and gamma-delta T-cell lymphoma may develop extracutaneous spread, but the lymph nodes are generally not involved.
- In contrast to CD8⁺ aggressive epidermotropic cytotoxic T-cell lymphoma, gamma-delta T-cell lymphoma is usually CD56⁺ and lacks CD4, CD8, and βF1.
- CD4⁺ small/medium T-cell lymphoma is distinguished from mycosis fungoides by the presence of papules and nodules in the absence of the characteristic patch stage of mycosis fungoides.
- The tumor cells of CD4⁺ small/medium T-cell lymphoma infiltrate the dermis and subcutis with little epidermotropism, in contrast to mycosis fungoides, which is characterized by a band-like epidermotropic infiltrate.
- Cases that resemble CD4⁺ small/medium T-cell lymphoma but have greater than 30% large pleomorphic tumor cells should be classified as peripheral T-cell lymphoma, unspecified; these tumors tend to follow an aggressive clinical course, in contrast to the good prognosis associated with CD4⁺ small/medium T-cell lymphoma.

Pitfalls

- The presence or absence of epidermotropism is not useful in making the diagnosis of gamma-delta T-cell lymphoma. Epidermotropism may be prominent and display a pagetoid pattern, as in CD8⁺ aggressive epidermotropic cytotoxic T-cell lymphoma, or it may be minimal.
- In subcutaneous tumors the neoplastic T cells may rim the fat spaces, but this finding is not specific for either gamma-delta tumors or subcutaneous panniculitis-like lymphoma.
- In some cases it may be impossible to distinguish lupus panniculitis from subcutaneous panniculitis-like lymphoma.

References can be found on Expert Consult @ www.expertconsult.com

Chapter 41

Precursor B- and T-Cell Neoplasms

Frederick Karl Racke and Michael J. Borowitz

CHAPTER OUTLINE

CLASSIFICATION OF PRECURSOR LYMPHOID NEOPLASMS

Precursor lymphoid neoplasms encompass acute lymphoblastic leukemias (ALLs) and lymphoblastic lymphomas (LBLs), generally of either B- or T-cell origin. The majority of ALLs are derived from precursor B cells, and the majority of LBLs possess a precursor T-cell phenotype. In general, ALLs and LBLs comprising precursor B cells are considered biologically equivalent, as is the case with precursor T-cell ALL and T-cell LBL. The distinction between lymphoma and leukemia is somewhat arbitrary. If there is significant blood or bone marrow involvement, the term *ALL* is used. If the tumor involves primarily an extramedullary site with little or no blood or bone marrow involvement, the term *LBL* is preferred. Conventionally, blood or bone marrow involvement by 25% or more blasts has been used as the cutoff between LBL and ALL, although it is generally conceded that this distinction bears little clinical or biologic significance. However, precursor B-cell tumors are biologically and clinically distinct from precursor T-cell neoplasms, and they are discussed separately. Moreover, because the diagnosis of ALL automatically implies that a tumor is derived from a lymphoid precursor, the term *precursor* is now considered redundant as part of the diagnosis, and these diseases may be referred to as *B-cell ALL* and *T-cell ALL*.

B-CELL LYMPHOBLASTIC LEUKEMIA/ LYMPHOBLASTIC LYMPHOMA

Definition

B-cell ALL/LBL is a clonal hematopoietic stem cell disorder with evidence of early B-cell differentiation. The disease is characterized by the presence of a rapidly proliferating population of immature blasts, with minimal morphologic evidence of differentiation. Defining these tumors generally requires immunophenotypic demonstration of B-cell lineage antigen expression. For example, more than 95% of cases express CD19 and HLA-DR.[1] Further, nearly all show clonal rearrangement of the immunoglobulin heavy-chain gene.[2,3]

Epidemiology

ALL is the most common malignancy in children. It accounts for 80% of childhood leukemias but only about 20% of adult acute leukemias. Most cases occur in children younger than 6 years, with the majority being B-cell ALL.[4] The peak incidence is approximately 4 to 5 cases per 100,000 between 2 and 5 years of age; the incidence decreases thereafter until age 50 years, when it begins to climb slightly again. ALL more commonly affects whites than blacks. B-cell LBL is less common, accounting for only about 10%

of LBLs.[5] B-cell LBL is also a disease of young individuals, with the majority of cases occurring in those younger than 20 years.[6,7]

Etiology

The etiology of B-cell (and T-cell) ALL is unknown. A number of recent studies have suggested a prenatal origin of the genetic events predisposing to the development of leukemia; others have demonstrated the presence of clone-specific antigen receptor gene rearrangements, consistent with an in utero origin of at least a portion of childhood ALLs.[8,9] Further, identical leukemia-specific translocations and antigen receptor gene rearrangements have been documented in monozygotic twins with B-cell ALL.[10] Although the specific genetic and environmental factors that predispose to ALL are not well defined, certain factors, such as exposure to ionizing radiation, and certain genetic diseases, such as trisomy 21 and ataxia-telangiectasia, have been associated with the development of ALL.[11,12] Also, rare cases of ALL following chemotherapy have been documented; these often possess rearrangements involving the *MLL* gene on chromosome 11q23.[13]

Clinical Features

The typical clinical presentation of B-cell ALL (Box 41-1) relates to the development of cytopenias secondary to the replacement of normal bone marrow by leukemic blasts. Clinical manifestations include weakness and pallor due to anemia, petechiae and bruising secondary to thrombocytopenia, and fever despite granulocytopenia. It is important to note that ALL patients may present with low, normal, or elevated peripheral white blood cell counts. Thus, patients with unexplained pancytopenia may warrant a bone marrow examination to exclude leukemia. In addition, hepatosplenomegaly or lymphadenopathy may be present at diagnosis, and there may be organ dysfunction due to leukemic infiltration. Bone or joint pain is also common, particularly in children, and is due to intramedullary growth of the leukemic cells. B-cell LBL typically presents with skin or lymph node involvement with or without peripheral blood or bone marrow involvement.[6] In contrast to T-cell LBL, it rarely involves the mediastinum.

Box 41-1 ***Major Clinical and Diagnostic Features of Acute Lymphoblastic Leukemia***

- Twenty percent or greater lymphoblasts in bone marrow or peripheral blood*
- Immunophenotypic evidence of either early B (80%) or early T (20%) differentiation
- Absence of significant myeloid differentiation
- Anemia, thrombocytopenia, and granulocytopenia (common)
- Clinical features that include fatigue, bleeding, bone pain, fever, lymphadenopathy, organomegaly, and central nervous system involvement

*The conventional cutoff to consider a case acute lymphoblastic leukemia rather than lymphoblastic lymphoma is the finding of 25% or more blasts in the blood or bone marrow. This is important for some treatment protocols.

Morphology

The morphologic examination of peripheral blood or bone marrow remains an essential part of the diagnosis of ALL. Blasts in B-cell ALL can be heterogeneous. Previous classification schemes attempted to subdivide ALL on the basis of cytologic features, including nuclear-to-cytoplasmic ratio, nucleoli, nuclear membrane contours, and cell size. However, aside from distinguishing the more mature Burkitt's leukemia/lymphoma (previously considered ALL, L3) from precursor B-cell ALL, subdividing ALL on the basis of morphology alone has little prognostic value and has been supplanted by immunophenotypic, cytogenetic, and molecular subclassification. Nevertheless, recognition of lymphoblasts is important to initiate the appropriate diagnostic evaluation. On a peripheral blood or bone marrow smear, lymphoblasts range from small, round blasts with high nuclear-to-cytoplasmic ratios, relatively condensed chromatin, and inconspicuous nucleoli to larger cells with an increased amount of blue-gray to blue cytoplasm, irregular nuclei with dispersed chromatin, and variably distinct nucleoli. Cytoplasmic vacuoles may be present; this finding does not automatically indicate Burkitt's leukemia/lymphoma.

Several morphologic variants of B-cell ALL have been described. The first, the so-called hand-mirror cell leukemia, displays a distinctive morphology characterized by the presence of an asymmetric cytoplasmic projection called a *uropod*, which typically sits atop an umbilicated nucleus.[14,15] Although the cause of this unusual morphology is uncertain, it has been suggested that immune complexes contribute to the formation of uropods.[14,15] The presence of hand-mirror cells does not appear to be associated with any particular subtype of ALL, nor does it independently affect prognosis. The second, less common morphologic variant is granular ALL. In this disorder, the blasts contain azurophilic cytoplasmic granules that do not contain myeloperoxidase but can contain acid phosphatase or acid esterase activity, suggesting a lysosomal origin.[16] Rarely, cases of B-cell ALL may be associated with peripheral blood eosinophilia that is so marked it obscures the lymphoblasts; the lymphoblasts themselves are not morphologically distinctive. Although the eosinophils are not part of the neoplastic clone, patients with ALL and eosinophilia often have symptoms related to the toxic effects of eosinophil degranulation, particularly cardiac disease. This unusual manifestation is often associated with the chromosomal abnormality t(5;14)(q31-33;q32), which juxtaposes the interleukin-3 (*IL3*) gene with the immunoglobulin heavy-chain (*IGH@*) gene on chromosome 14.[17-19]

The histopathologies of B-cell ALL and LBL are indistinguishable; the distinction is based on the distribution of tissue involvement. In ALL the bone marrow is almost always hypercellular, with replacement of normal marrow elements by a diffuse infiltrate of immature cells (Fig. 41-1). High-power examination reveals morphologic heterogeneity similar to that observed on smear preparations, ranging from small blasts with fine chromatin and inconspicuous nucleoli to more heterogeneous cells with irregular nuclei and more abundant cytoplasm. Occasionally, tingible body macrophages accompany the infiltrate, imparting a "starry sky" appearance. However, the tingible body macrophages are usually not as abundant as in Burkitt's lymphoma and may occur only focally. With B-lineage ALL, there can be significant organ

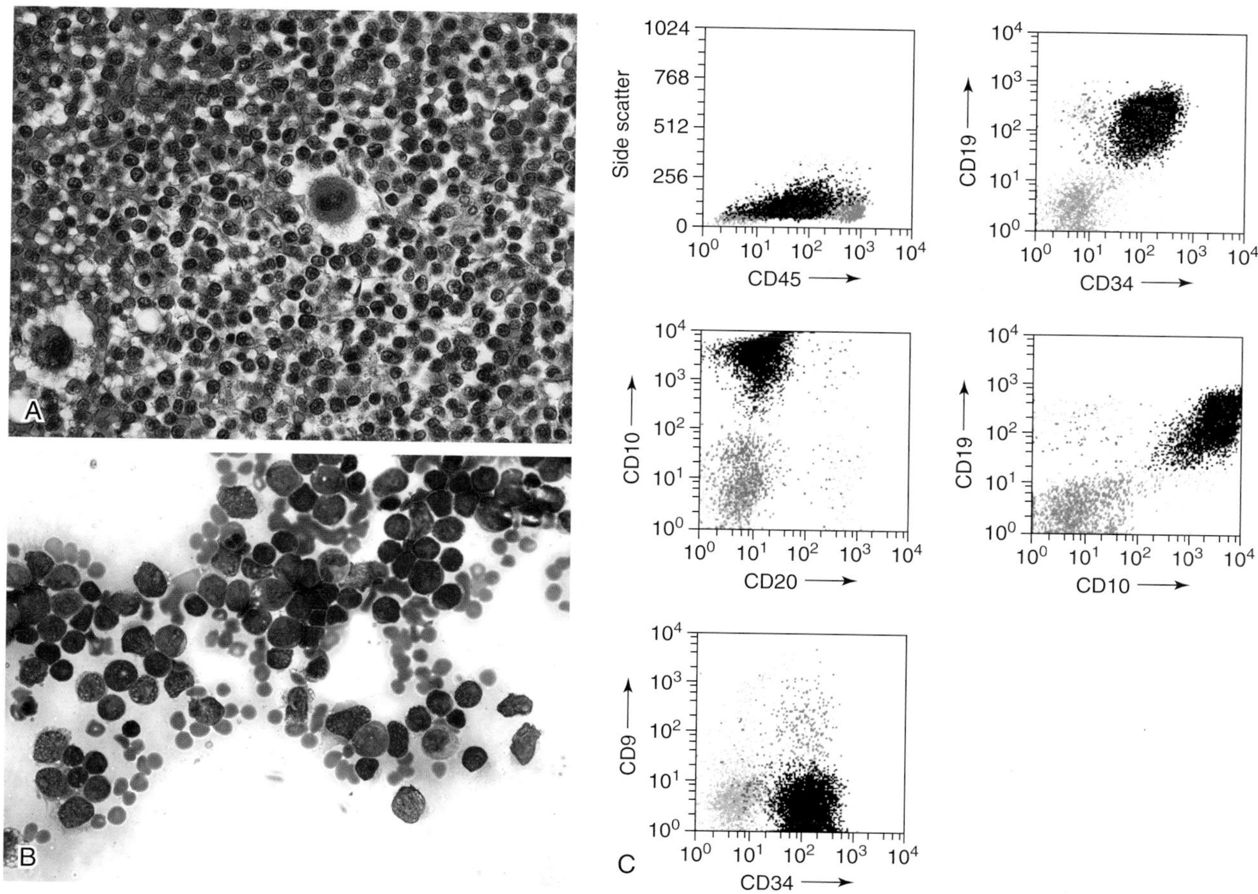

Figure 41-1. B-cell acute lymphoblastic leukemia (ALL). A, Bone marrow infiltrated by an interstitial immature lymphoblast population. **B,** Accompanying bone marrow aspirate shows an increase in immature blasts. **C,** Multiparametric flow cytometry demonstrates the blasts to be CD19⁺, CD34⁺, CD10⁺, CD9⁻, and CD20⁻, a phenotype highly correlated with the t(12;21) translocation in childhood ALL.

involvement, with the liver, spleen, kidneys, gonads, and central nervous system (CNS) being common sites. B-cell LBL is diagnosed when there is an extramedullary tumor of lymphoblasts but less than 25% lymphoblasts in the blood or bone marrow. It is found most often in extranodal sites, most commonly skin or bone. Lymph nodes are less commonly involved and may demonstrate a paracortical distribution, with preservation of follicles. Hepatic involvement is typically sinusoidal, whereas splenic disease involves the red pulp.

Immunophenotype

B-cell ALL is defined by evidence of B-cell differentiation. Normal precursor B cells exist in variable numbers, normally in the bone marrow. These undergo a reproducible pattern of antigen expression during normal B-cell differentiation. In contrast, B-cell ALL almost always demonstrates an aberrant antigen profile that is incompatible with normal B-cell differentiation; this usually permits a distinction between malignant and reactive precursor B cells.[20] Nearly all cases of B-cell ALL express CD19, cytoplasmic CD79a, terminal deoxynucleotidyl transferase (TdT), and HLA-DR. CD10 is present in most, but not all, cases. Surface expression of CD22 is weak but consistent, and CD20 is usually variable, with about a fourth of cases completely negative. Cytoplasmic CD22 is a very sensitive marker for B-cell ALL, but it may also be detected in acute myeloid leukemia (AML),[21] with possible weak expression of CD19 and TdT. CD79a has been suggested as both a sensitive and a specific marker of B-lineage ALL, although it is seen in a significant fraction of cases of T-cell ALL/LBL.[22] PAX5 is more specific than CD79a, although it may be seen in some cases of AML.[23] Although immunoglobulin heavy-chain gene rearrangements occur relatively early in B-cell development, and B-cell ALLs show clonal rearrangements by molecular analysis, almost all fail to express surface immunoglobulin. Additional antigenic markers have been useful in characterizing B-lineage ALL. These include CD24, CD34, and CD9, all of which are expressed in the majority of cases.[1,24] It should be noted that among B-cell neoplasms, CD34 and TdT are uniquely expressed in lymphoblastic lesions and have particular significance in classifying these lesions. CD45, or the leukocyte common antigen, fails to be expressed in roughly 10% to 20% of cases and typically shows considerable variability in expression in the remaining cases.[25,26] It is important to appreciate that Ewing's sarcoma may resemble LBL. The antigen CD99, which is expressed by Ewing's sarcoma, is also expressed by most hematopoietic tumors that express TdT.[27-29] Thus, expression of CD99 coupled with lack of CD45 expression does not exclude LBL; additional lymphoid markers as well as TdT may

Table 41-1 **Major Molecular and Immunophenotypic Features of Acute Lymphoblastic Leukemia (ALL)**

Subtype	Molecular Lesion	Immunophenotype*
Precursor B-cell ALL with 11q23 translocations	*MLL* fusion with protein, with gain-of-function transcriptional activity	CD19+, CD22+, CD79a+,TdT+, CD9+, **CD10−, CD24−, CD15/65+**
Precursor B-cell ALL with t(12;21)	*ETV6-RUNX1* (*TEL-AML1*) fusion protein that represses normal *RUNX1* transcription	CD19+, CD22+, CD79a+, CD10+, TdT+, CD34+, CD20+/−, **CD9−**
Precursor B-cell ALL with t(9;22)	*BCR-ABL1* fusion protein that leads to aberrant tyrosine kinase activity	CD19+, CD22+, CD79a+, CD10+, TdT+, CD34+, CD20+/−, CD9+
Pre-B-cell ALL with t(1;19)	Oncogenic fusion protein of transcription factors *TCF3* (*E2A*) and *PBX1*	CD19+, CD22+, CD79a+, CD10+, TdT+, **CD34−**, CD20+/−, CD9+
Early pro-T-cell ALL†	Aberrant overexpression of *LYL1* oncogenic transcription factor	**CD4−, CD8−**, cCD3+, CD34+, TdT+
Early cortical T-cell ALL	Aberrant overexpression of *TLX1* (*HOX11*) oncogenic transcription factor	CD4+, CD8+, cCD3+, CD1a+, CD10+, TdT+
Late cortical T-cell ALL	Aberrant overexpression of *TAL1* oncogenic transcription factor	CD4+, CD8+, cCD3 high, TCRα/β+
Medullary T-cell ALL	Unknown	**CD4+ or CD8+**, sCD3+, TCRα/β+, CD1a−

*Boldface denotes immunophenotypic feature characteristic of that particular molecular lesion.
†Molecular and phenotypic correlates adapted from Ferrando AA, Neuberg DS, Staunton J, et al. Gene expression signatures define novel oncogenic pathways in T cell acute lymphoblastic leukemia. *Cancer Cell.* 2002;1:79.
c, cytoplasmic; s, surface; TCR, T-cell receptor; TdT, terminal deoxynucleotidyl transferase.

be necessary to exclude LBL. Finally, expression of myeloid antigens, including CD13, CD33, and CD15, but not myeloperoxidase, is found in about 10% to 15% of childhood B-cell ALLs[30] and in roughly 25% of adult cases.[31,32] However, the myeloid-blast–associated antigen CD117 is rarely present.[33]

Distinct clinical subgroups of B-cell ALL are accompanied by unique patterns of antigen expression. Some of these are associated with distinct molecular or cytogenetic defects and have distinct clinical characteristics (Table 41-1). For example, *pre-B-cell ALL* is distinguished from other cases of B-cell ALL by the expression of cytoplasmic immunoglobulin mu heavy-chain without surface immunoglobulin.[34] About 25% of cases of pre-B-cell ALL harbor a specific t(1;19) translocation, discussed in more detail later. *Transitional pre-B-cell ALL* is another distinct immunologic subset of B-cell ALL with differentiation characteristics that are intermediate between pre-B-cell ALL and Burkitt's leukemia/lymphoma. In transitional pre-B-cell ALL, surface immunoglobulin mu heavy chain is expressed, but immunoglobulin light chain is not.[35] This neoplasm lacks the typical L3 morphology of Burkitt's leukemia/lymphoma and does not possess translocations involving the *MYC* oncogene. It also possesses the immature markers CD34 and TdT, which are usually absent in more mature B-cell leukemias. These tumors must be distinguished from Burkitt's leukemia/lymphoma because they respond well to ALL-type therapy. In addition, rare cases of ALL with non-L3 morphology express both immunoglobulin heavy and light chain and lack the *MYC* translocation characteristic of Burkitt's leukemia/lymphoma. Although there have been no systematic studies of this rare subgroup, in practice, such patients are treated similarly to other B-cell ALL patients.

Genetics and Molecular Findings

Nearly all cases of B-cell ALL have rearrangement of the immunoglobulin heavy-chain gene.[3] However, immunoglobulin heavy-chain gene rearrangement can also occur in T-cell ALL as well as in AML, limiting the utility of this test as a marker of lineage commitment. Immunoglobulin light-chain rearrangement can also occur and is thought to be a more specific marker of B-cell differentiation.[36,37] Unlike the more mature B-cell lymphoproliferative disorders, translocations activating oncogenes in B-cell ALL rarely involve immunoglobulin loci.

B-lineage ALL is increasingly being defined by specific genetic abnormalities associated with specific phenotypes and clinical behaviors; most of these are incorporated into the most recent World Health Organization classification of B-cell ALL (Box 41-2). Risk stratification may be used to identify patients for whom low-intensity therapy will likely be curative, thus avoiding complications of more aggressive treatment, as well as to identify patients needing more intensive therapy. Moreover, as epitomized by ALL with *BCR-ABL1*, some of the genetic abnormalities may provide clues leading to specific targeted therapy. Thus, it is useful to consider these common recurrent molecular and cytogenetic abnormalities individually.

Quantitative Chromosomal Abnormalities

It has long been known that hyperdiploidy with greater than 50 chromosomes is a strong predictor of durable response to therapy in childhood ALL. These patients account for about

Box 41-2 *Classification of Acute Lymphoblastic Leukemias*

- B-lymphoblastic leukemia/lymphoma with recurrent genetic abnormalities
  - t(9;22)(q34;q11.2); *BCR-ABL1*
  - t(v;11q23); *MLL* rearranged
  - t(12;21)(p13;q22); *ETV6-RUNX1* (*TEL-AML1*)
  - t(5;14)(q31;q32); *IL3-IGH@*
  - t(1;19)(q23;p13.3); *TCF3-PBX1* (*E2A-PBX1*)
  - Hyperploidy (>50 chromosomes)
  - Hypoploidy (<46 chromosomes)
- B-lymphoblastic leukemia/lymphoma, not otherwise specified
- T-lymphoblastic leukemia/lymphoma, not otherwise specified

From Swerdlow SH, Campo E, Harris NL, et al, eds. *WHO Classification of Tumours of Haematopoietic and Lymphoid Tissues.* Lyon, France: IARC Press; 2008.

25% of cases of childhood ALL and often possess other favorable features, including lower peripheral white blood cell count and age between 2 and 10 years.[38,39] Hyperdiploidy confers a good prognosis independent of these other indicators and predicts a favorable response regardless of peripheral white blood cell count.[40] The good prognosis associated with hyperdiploidy appears to be due to the addition of specific chromosomes. Trisomies involving chromosomes 4, 10, and 17 confer the best prognosis[41,42]; patients with hyperdiploid ALL lacking particularly favorable trisomies do not fare well. Children with ALL having hyperdiploidy with 47 to 50 chromosomes account for 10% to 15% of cases and do not have a favorable prognosis.[38] Hypodiploidy also occurs, usually due to the loss of one chromosome, an unbalanced translocation, or the formation of dicentric chromosomes. Patients with hypoploidy with fewer than 44 chromosomes have a particularly unfavorable outcome.[43]

Qualitative Abnormalities of Chromosome Structure

There are a number of well-characterized chromosomal translocations associated with B-cell ALL. In children the most common molecular abnormality is t(12;21)(p13;q22), which is observed in roughly 25% of childhood B-cell ALLs but only 3% of adult cases.[44] This translocation produces an abnormal fusion protein between the Ets family transcription factor *ETV6* (*TEL*) and the DNA-binding subunit of the core binding factor complex *RUNX1* (*AML1*). Both these transcription factors appear to be necessary for hematopoiesis,[45,46] and transduction of the *ETV6-RUNX1* fusion protein into mouse hematopoietic stem cells has recently been shown to induce ALL.[47] It is important to note that detection of this translocation event frequently requires the use of specialized techniques such as fluorescence in situ hybridization or reverse transcriptase polymerase chain reaction because there is generally a balanced cryptic translocation that is unapparent when using classic karyotyping.[48] Interestingly, B-cell ALLs harboring this translocation often possess a characteristic immunophenotype: expression of CD34, partial expression of CD20, and, in particular, little or no expression of CD9.[49] Several studies have suggested that the presence of the t(12;21) translocation confers an improved event-free survival, but the good prognosis of this disease has been questioned by some groups that suggest these patients are at increased risk for late relapse.[50] Although this point remains controversial, the unusual demonstration of clonally identical t(12;21) leukemias arising years apart in monozygotic twins has led to the hypothesis that t(12;21) is an early event in leukemogenesis,[8] raising the interesting question of whether late relapses might be new second leukemias derived from a dormant leukemic precursor.

In adults the most frequently observed chromosomal abnormality is t(9;22)(q34;q11), or the Philadelphia (Ph) chromosome. This translocation, present in about 25% of adult and 3% to 5% of childhood B-cell ALLs,[44] involves the *ABL1* oncogene on chromosome 9 and the guanosine triphosphate–binding protein BCR on chromosome 22. The resultant fusion protein has abnormal tyrosine kinase activity, leading to disturbances in proliferation, survival, and adhesion.[51] Although the *BCR-ABL1* fusion protein is also found in chronic myelogenous leukemia, in about 70% of cases of *BCR-ABL1*$^+$ ALL, the expressed protein is only 190 kDa, rather than the 210 kDa typically seen in chronic myelogenous leukemia, reflecting less contribution of the *BCR* gene to the fusion protein.[52] Philadelphia chromosome positivity is associated with a poor prognosis in both children[53,54] and adults.[55]

Recurrent chromosomal abnormalities involving the chromosome 11q23 locus have been observed in B-cell ALL and have prognostic significance.[56] The most common of these is t(4;11)(q21;q23). These leukemias frequently involve chromosome 4q21 but may also partner chromosome 11q23 with chromosome 1p32 or 19p13. The molecular lesion involves aberrant regulation of the homeotic regulator mixed lineage leukemia (*MLL*) gene. ALLs with t(4;11) tend to occur in infants and often present with high white blood cell counts, organomegaly, and CNS involvement and have a poor prognosis. These lymphoblastic leukemias have a unique phenotype that distinguishes them from other B-cell ALLs. They characteristically express CD19 but lack CD10 and CD24.[57] They have a propensity to coexpress the myeloid antigens CD15 and CD65,[58] prompting the *mixed lineage leukemia* moniker. In fact, recent gene expression profiling studies suggest that *MLL* leukemias are different from other B-cell ALLs and AMLs and may warrant classification as a distinct leukemic process.[59] Although t(4;11) leukemia confers a poor prognosis, there is some controversy as to whether leukemias that use alternative fusion partners with *MLL* have an equally poor outcome.

As mentioned earlier, t(1;19)(q23;p13) is associated with pre-B-cell ALL and is much less commonly seen in B-cell ALL without cytoplasmic mu expression. The chromosomal lesion generates a fusion protein between the bHLH transcription factor *E2A* (also known as *TCF3*) and *PBX1*, generating a potent oncogenic fusion protein. The pre-B-cell ALLs associated with the *TCF3-PBX1* translocation display a characteristic immunophenotype expressing CD19, CD10, homogeneous CD9, and partial CD20 and completely lacking CD34.[60] Although the presence of t(1;19) was once thought to confer a poor prognosis, with current intensive therapies, the outcome in these children is comparable to that in those with similar risk factors.[61,62]

Recent advances in microarray-based technology have allowed the interrogation of copy number alterations and loss of heterozygosity at high resolution. These approaches have led to the recognition of frequent abnormalities in genes involved in B-cell differentiation in more than 60% of B-cell ALLs.[63] Frequently involved genes are lymphoid transcription factors such as *PAX5*, *IKZF1*, and *EBF1*. There are significant differences in the frequency of copy number alterations among the genetic subtypes of B-cell ALL. For example, *MLL*-rearranged B-cell ALLs possess relatively few copy number alterations, whereas *ETV6-RUNX1*$^+$ and *BCR-ABL1*$^+$ ALLs have, on average, six or more. Interestingly, nearly all cases of Ph$^+$ B-cell ALL possess deletions of *IKZF1*[63]; moreover, *IKZF1* deletions may be seen in the absence of *BCR-ABL1* and appear to confer a very poor prognosis.[64]

Normal Counterpart

The normal counterpart for B-cell ALL is the normal precursor B cell that resides within the bone marrow. These cells, also known as *hematogones,* are seen with increased frequency in children and tend to decrease with age. However, hematogone content can vary widely, especially during hematopoietic regeneration. Hematogones possess a very reproducible pattern of antigen acquisition that helps distinguish them from ALL. The earliest hematogones express dim CD45 with low right-angle light scatter, CD19, CD10, CD34, CD38, and TdT. These cells lack CD20 and surface immunoglobulin expression and express dim CD22. As the cells mature, CD20 is acquired, and early antigens such as CD34 and CD10 are lost. Because of the reproducible nature of antigen expression on normal precursor B cells, muliparametric flow cytometry can reliably distinguish normal from leukemic precursor B cells in most cases.[65]

Clinical Course

In general, B-cell ALL of childhood has become a disease with a high cure rate, whereas adults with B-cell ALL fare more poorly. Prognosis, however, hinges on the presence or absence of increasingly well-characterized genetic and molecular abnormalities. Children with leukemias harboring the *ETV6-RUNX1* translocation or possessing more than 50 chromosomes have a long-term event-free survival rate of 85% or greater. However, those with the t(4;11) translocation or the *BCR-ABL1* fusion fare considerably worse, with long-term event-free survival of less than 30%. The reason for the different clinical outcomes in these subtypes remains unknown. However, new insights into the molecular and cellular biology of these subtypes may help tailor subgroup-oriented therapies. The development of small molecule inhibitors directed against specific kinases—such as imatinib mesylate for *BCR-ABL1*[66] and, more recently, inhibitors of FLT3,[67] a receptor kinase overexpressed in certain cases of ALL, including those with 11q23 translocations[59]—raises hope that targeted therapies may be developed that improve treatment outcomes or reduce treatment sequelae. Also, the repressive effects of *ETV6-RUNX1* on normal *RUNX1 (AML1)* transcription can potentially be reversed by small molecule inhibitors of histone deacetylase enzymes.[68,69] Finally, it is likely that a better understanding of pharmacogenomics will help explain the sensitivities of certain individuals to particular therapeutic regimens. Genes encoding enzymes involved in drug metabolism and molecular transporters may not only guide therapeutic strategies but also predict the risk for developing ALL. This has already been borne out for folate-metabolizing enzymes: polymorphisms in methylenetetrahydrofolate reductase are associated with a reduced risk for the development of ALL.[70] Increased sensitivity of *MLL-AFF1* (also known as *MLL-AF4*) leukemias to high-dose cytarabine has been linked to increased expression of hENT1, which transports cytarabine into the cell.[71] Further understanding of the genetic polymorphisms of drug-metabolizing enzymes will almost certainly aid in the understanding of factors involved in both the development and the treatment of ALL.

Early response to therapy is also an important prognostic factor. How rapidly a patient clears morphologically evident disease during induction predicts long-term outcome.[72] More recently, it has become apparent that the presence of minimal residual disease (MRD) at levels below that of morphologic detection is also a strong prognostic factor,[73,74] and these measurements are playing an increasing role in risk stratification. More sensitive methods to precisely quantitate response to chemotherapy have advantages over morphologic evaluation to assess early response, which is much more subjective. MRD may be measured by flow cytometry[73] or by polymerase chain reaction.[74] The latter can be used to look for unique fusion transcripts, where as few as 1 leukemic cell per 1 million cells can sometimes be detected. However, such techniques are applicable to only a subset of ALL cases. Polymerase chain reaction directed against antigen receptor genes is more cumbersome and expensive because it requires the production of patient-specific probes or primers, but this method can detect MRD at a level approaching 1 cell in 100,000 in more than 90% of cases. Flow cytometry can readily achieve sensitivities of 1 in 10,000 in 95% of cases. There is evidence, particularly in childhood ALL, that thresholds of MRD as low as 0.01% discriminate between those with a high probability of cure and those with a considerably higher rate of relapse.[73] In fact, day 29 marrow MRD was the most important prognostic variable in a multivariate analysis of outcome in children with ALL. When a combination of favorable risk factors is combined with MRD negativity, it is possible to identify a group of patients that account for 12% of all patients who are almost certain to be cured with limited therapy.[75] Such distinctions should allow improved risk stratification to dictate future therapy.

Differential Diagnosis

The differential diagnosis generally includes a number of hematopoietic tumors that may possess blast-like morphology, as well as a small number of undifferentiated or primitive nonhematopoietic tumors (Table 41-2). Immunophenotypic

Table 41-2 Differential Diagnosis of Acute Lymphoblastic Leukemia

Tumor	Distinguishing Features
Acute myeloid leukemia with minimal differentiation	Myeloid phenotype
Acute leukemias of ambiguous lineage	Coexpression of myeloid and lymphoid antigens or evidence of both myeloid and lymphoid differentiation
Lymphoid blast crisis of chronic myelogenous leukemia (CML)	History of antecedent CML, Ph^+
Chronic lymphocytic leukemia	Condensed nuclear chromatin, mature B-cell phenotype
Prolymphocytic leukemia	Lower nuclear-to-cytoplasmic ratio, prominent nucleolus, mature B-cell phenotype
Blastic variant of mantle cell lymphoma	Mature B-cell phenotype, t(11;14), cyclin D1 expression
Large B-cell lymphoma	Larger cells; mature B-cell phenotype
Burkitt's lymphoma/leukemia	More prominent nucleoli; prominent basophilic cytoplasm; mature B cell phenotype, t(8;14)
Small, round blue cell tumors (including Ewing's sarcoma, neuroblastoma, embryonal rhabdomyosarcoma, medulloblastoma)	Cohesive growth, absence of lymphoid markers
Reactive proliferations of normal precursor B cells (hematogones)	Indistinct or absent nucleoli, normal continuum of B-cell antigen acquisition during differentiation

analysis is often required to distinguish among these neoplasms.

T-CELL LYMPHOBLASTIC LYMPHOMA/ LYMPHOBLASTIC LEUKEMIA

Definition

Like precursor B-cell tumors, T-cell lymphoblastic lesions are clonal hematopoietic stem cell disorders, but they are characterized by an immature T-cell, rather than B-cell, phenotype. Operationally, identification of T-cell antigen expression is required for the diagnosis of T-cell lymphoblastic tumors. Morphologically, T-cell ALL and T-cell LBL are indistinguishable, being composed of variably sized blasts with finely dispersed chromatin and indistinct nucleoli. Compared with B-cell lesions, the blasts in T-lymphoblastic tumors tend to be more heterogeneous in terms of size and nuclear morphology, although there is considerable overlap. As with precursor B-cell tumors, the distinction between T-cell ALL and T-cell LBL is based more on convention than on any biologic differences.

Epidemiology

Perhaps because the thymus is the major site of normal T-cell development, the majority of T-cell LBLs are found in the mediastinum. T-lymphoblastic tumors account for only about 15% of childhood ALLs but nearly 90% of LBLs. LBLs are more common in late childhood and account for about a third of all pediatric cases of non-Hodgkin's lymphoma; they constitute only a small percentage of adult cases. Both T-cell ALL and T-cell LBL show a male predominance.

Etiology

Although specific genetic disturbances are involved in T-lymphoblastic lesions, the underlying etiologic factors are unknown.

Clinical Features

Patients with T-cell ALL typically present with high tumor burdens, including high peripheral white cell counts (>50,000/μL), organomegaly, and peripheral lymphadenopathy. Children with T-cell ALL are typically older than those with B-cell ALL. The presence of a mediastinal mass is highly associated with a T-cell phenotype in ALL. Like patients with B-cell ALL, those with T-cell ALL may present with anemia, thrombocytopenia, organomegaly, and bone pain, although they are less frequently leukopenic.

Patients with T-cell LBL also have high tumor burdens, evidenced by advanced stage or bulky disease. In patients with mediastinal involvement, the mass is often quite large, leading to compromise of regional anatomic structures. This may manifest with clinical symptoms such as dyspnea due to airway obstruction, dysphagia due to esophageal compromise, or superior vena cava syndrome. Pulmonary and cardiac function may also be compromised by the presence of pleural or pericardial effusions.

Morphology

Like precursor B-cell lesions, the morphologic characteristics of T-cell ALL and T-cell LBL are identical. Moreover, distinguishing T-cell lesions from B-cell lesions by morphology alone is impossible. Cytologically, lymphoblasts range from small, round blasts with high nuclear-to-cytoplasmic ratios, relatively condensed chromatin, and inconspicuous nucleoli to larger cells with increased amounts of blue-gray to blue cytoplasm, irregular nuclei with dispersed chromatin, and variable numbers of distinct nucleoli (Fig. 41-2). Cytoplasmic vacuoles are seen occasionally. Typically, T-cell lymphoblasts tend to have more cytologic heterogeneity and more nuclear convolutions; in some cases the nuclear convolutions are quite prominent, leading to the subclassification of a convoluted variant. However, because no phenotypic, molecular, or clinical differences have been correlated with this morphology, such subclassification has no obvious benefit.

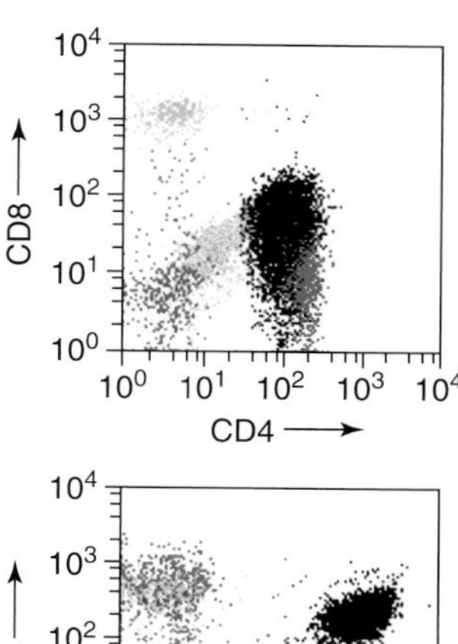

Figure 41-2. T-cell acute lymphoblastic leukemia. A, Bone marrow aspirate shows a predominant population of heterogeneous blasts with a range of sizes. **B,** Multiparametric flow cytometry shows a population of abnormal T cells (*black*) expressing CD4, CD8, CD1a, and CD5. Residual normal CD4+ T cells (*green*) and CD8+ T cells (*yellow*) are also present.

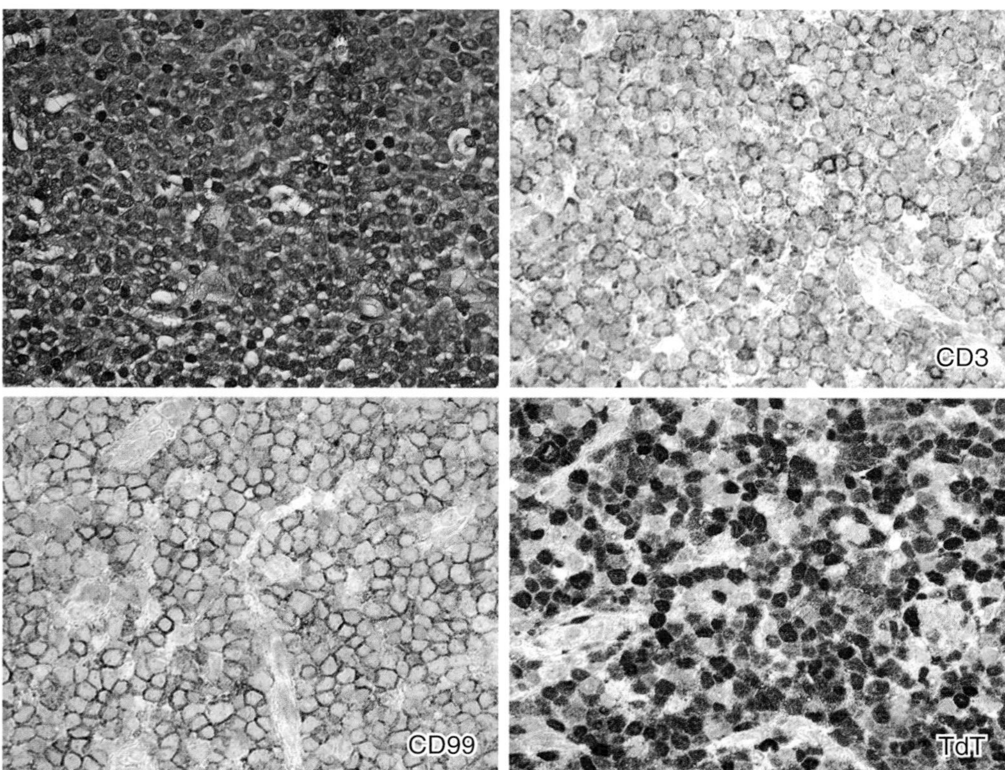

Figure 41-3. T-cell lymphoblastic lymphoma. Mediastinal mass shows malignant lymphoblasts with dispersed chromatin. The tumor expresses CD3, CD99, and terminal deoxynucleotidyl transferase (TdT) as indicated.

Histologically, T-cell LBL is a diffuse infiltrative process that occasionally involves lymph nodes in an interfollicular pattern but more commonly diffusely replaces the nodal architecture (Fig. 41-3). Frequently the tumor extends through the capsule, infiltrating the perinodal fat. T-cell LBL tends to be a proliferative process with numerous mitotic figures. Rapid cell turnover can give rise to a "starry sky" appearance due to the presence of tingible body macrophages, but rarely does this pattern predominate to the extent seen in Burkitt's lymphoma.

Immunophenotype

Precursor T-cell malignancies can express markers associated with T-cell differentiation and maturation in almost any combination, although an understanding of phenotypic changes associated with normal T-cell maturation is helpful in understanding malignant phenotypes. The common lymphoid progenitors express TdT, CD34, and HLA-DR. Other early markers include CD7, which can be expressed on some myeloid precursors,[76] and CD2, which is on dendritic cell precursors[77]; however, expression of cytoplasmic CD3 is generally considered the first definitive marker of T-cell lineage commitment. Early T-cell precursors first enter the thymus at the corticomedullary junction and proceed to the outer cortex, acquiring CD5 and CD1 and losing HLA-DR. These are the so-called double-negative thymocytes, which lack expression of CD4 and CD8. At this stage, the T-cell receptor (TCR) chains remain in a germline configuration. TCR gene rearrangement then occurs, with the sequential rearrangement of the delta, gamma, beta, and finally alpha chains. This allows the development of a functional TCR to permit thymic education through both positive and negative selection. The common thymocyte represents the major thymic population. The CD4, CD8 double-positive thymocytes that successfully engage major histocompatibility complex (MHC)-I are destined to be CD8^{+} T cells, and those that engage MHC-II will become CD4^{+} T cells. TdT continues to be expressed throughout cortical thymic development and is lost as the thymocytes enter the medullary phase of maturation. Because precursor T-cell tumors resemble their normal thymic counterparts, knowledge of the normal patterns of antigen expression that highlight the uniqueness of thymocytes can be helpful in the recognition of T-cell ALL. For example, expression of TdT and CD1 on T cells outside the thymus does not normally occur; when seen, this indicates an abnormal population.

In some cases T-cell ALL has a more primitive immunophenotype than T-cell LBL, perhaps reflecting either an earlier thymocyte or even a bone marrow precursor. Many of these cases express antigens commonly seen in AML. This includes CD7, which appears to be the most sensitive antigen for T-cell ALL; however, as noted earlier, it is frequently expressed in AML, including some cases of myeloperoxidase-negative AML.[78] TdT, although present in up to 20% of AML cases, can distinguish between AML and T-cell ALL when intensity is considered. Expression of CD117, or c-Kit, is thought to be a relatively specific marker for myeloid differentiation; however, CD117 is occasionally seen in T-cell ALL as well.[79] CD117 expression is observed in very early normal T-cell precursors before TCR rearrangement. At this stage it is coexpressed with CD135,[80] also known as the *FLT3* receptor. Interestingly, activating mutations in the *FLT3* receptor, the most common genetic abnormality seen in AML,[81] were found only in T-cell ALL cases expressing c-Kit.[82] A recent clinical study of so-called early T-cell precursor ALL demonstrated that such patients have a particularly poor prognosis. In that study, these cases were identified by their distinctive immunophenotype (CD1a⁻, CD8⁻, CD5^{dim}, with stem cell or myeloid antigen expression).[83]

Because myeloid antigen expression is so common, a definitive distinction between AML and T-cell ALL may be difficult. HLA-DR may be helpful because it is expressed in virtually all CD7$^+$ AMLs but in only a small portion of T-cell ALLs. CD2 expression can vary in T-cell ALL, and decreased CD2 expression was found to correlate with a reduced event-free survival,[84] but it is not T-cell specific. T-cell antigens such as CD1, CD3, and CD8 show high specificity but are expressed in less than half of cases. Of all the markers, cytoplasmic CD3 appears to be the most reliable marker for establishing T-cell lineage and is expressed by virtually all precursor T-cell neoplasms; however, intensity is important because it may be weakly expressed in some cases of AML, whereas it is bright in T-cell ALL.

Most T-cell LBLs have a phenotype resembling a late cortical thymic phenotype, with expression of cytoplasmic CD3, TdT, and both CD4 and CD8. An important point is that virtually all precursor T-cell tumors have aberrant patterns of antigen expression that distinguish them from normal thymocytes. These changes include loss of pan–T-cell markers and aberrant coexpression of B-cell antigens (CD24, CD9, CD21) or myeloid antigens (CD13, CD33). Recognition that precursor T-cell tumors have an abnormal immunophenotype has proved to be useful on the rare occasion when an ectopic thymus is sent for flow cytometric analysis.[85]

Genetics and Molecular Findings

As mentioned previously, during normal T-cell development there is an ordered rearrangement of TCR chain loci, starting with the delta chain, followed by gamma and beta, and finally, if gamma and delta fail to generate a competent rearrangement, TCRα. Precursor T-cell tumors often show patterns of TCR gene rearrangement that reflect this. As such, the most primitive T-cell ALL may have no rearranged TCR genes or only TCRγ. TCRα often remains in a germline configuration, except for tumors with the most mature phenotypes. Although TCR rearrangements are a vital step in T-cell development, there is significant lineage infidelity at the molecular level. TCR rearrangements are frequently observed in B-cell ALLs. Less frequent is the rearrangement of *IGH@* loci in precursor T-cell tumors; *IGL@* locus rearrangement is almost never observed in precursor T-cell neoplasms.

In addition to the demonstration of TCR gene rearrangements, a number of nonrandom chromosomal translocations have been consistently observed in precursor T-cell tumors. Unlike precursor B-cell lesions, which rarely involve the immunoglobulin loci, these translocations frequently involve the TCR loci on chromosomes 7 and 14.[86] Most of the rearrangements involve transcription factors, suggesting that disruption or inappropriate regulation of these factors contribute to leukemogenesis; many of these same transcription factors can be dysregulated by mechanisms other than translocation. One factor in particular, *SCL* or *TAL1*, is a commonly targeted factor in precursor T-cell neoplasms. *TAL1* is overexpressed in roughly 60% of T-cell ALLs. These include cytogenetically apparent translocations between chromosomes 1 and 14, which occur in roughly 3% of cases,[87] and interstitial deletions of the 5′ UTR (untranslated region) of *TAL1*, which is estimated to occur in as many as 25% of cases.[88] Curiously, *TAL1*, which is important for erythroid and megakaryocytic lineage development, is not normally expressed in lymphoid differentiation.[89] Other transcription factors identified in T-cell ALL–related translocations include the homeobox protein *TLX1* (*HOX11*), potential transcriptional regulatory proteins rhombotin 1 and 2, c-*MYC*, and others. In addition to the involvement of transcription factors, translocations involving chromosomes 1p34 and 7q34 place the SRC family protein tyrosine kinase *LCK* adjacent to the TCRβ enhancer region.[90] *LCK* appears to be important for thymopoiesis; overexpression of *LCK* in transgenic mice induces lymphoid malignancies, including thymic tumors.[91] Finally, *NUP214-ABL1* fusions leading to a constitutively activated tyrosine kinase are reported to occur in roughly 4% to 6% of adult T-cell ALLs.[92] These tend to reside in episomes and are usually undetectable by classic cytogenetic analysis.

Microarray analyses have also shed light on the molecular pathogenesis of T-cell ALL. Using oligonucleotide arrays, Ferrando and colleagues[93] showed that five T-cell oncogenic transcription factors are frequently and aberrantly expressed in T-cell ALL. Further, overexpression of particular oncogenes correlated with defined stages of normal thymopoiesis may predict clinical outcome. *TLX1*, for example, correlates with an early cortical thymocyte and has an improved clinical outcome compared with other T-cell ALLs.[93,94] This may relate to the lack of antiapoptotic genes, such as *BCL2*, at this stage of T-cell development. However, the related homeobox protein *TLX3* (*HOX11L2*) does not appear to be associated with a favorable prognosis and may actually be less favorable, although there is some controversy about this.[95,96] Similarly, less favorable outcomes are associated with overexpression of *TAL1* and *LYL1*, which resemble late cortical and early pro-T-cell stages, respectively. The relationship of some of these molecular lesions to immunophenotype and stage of T-cell maturation is shown in Table 41-1.

Recently, mutations in the *NOTCH1* gene have been implicated in the pathogenesis of a significant subset of T-cell ALLs.[97,98] Although rare cases with a t(7;9) translocation involving *NOTCH1* had previously been described, point mutations, insertions, and deletions in the *NOTCH1* gene, all leading to an increase in signaling, have been found in more than half of cases of T-cell ALL, including those in all the molecular subgroups noted earlier,[98] suggesting that these mutations play a central role in pathogenesis. Of interest, the increased *NOTCH1* signaling associated with these mutations is dependent on the downstream activity of gamma secretase,[97] suggesting that gamma secretase inhibitors might play a role in the treatment of T-cell ALL.

A rare but unique syndrome of T-cell LBL associated with tissue or peripheral blood eosinophilia and a concomitant or subsequent myeloid malignancy has been recognized.[99] It is usually associated with translocations involving the fibroblast growth factor receptor-1 (*FGFR1*) gene on chromosome 8p11, most often as t(8;13)(p11;q12) involving *ZMYM2* (*ZNF198*), a gene on chromosome 13 that encodes a protein with a zinc finger–related motif.[100] This fusion likely leads to activation of the *FGFR1*-associated tyrosine kinase.

Normal Counterpart

The normal counterpart of T-cell ALL/LBL is thought to be the precursor T cells that arise from bone marrow–derived hematopoietic stem cells that migrate to the thymus, where they develop. As noted earlier, these precursor cells possess unique antigen expression patterns that clearly distinguish them from more mature extrathymic T cells.

Clinical Course

Children with T-cell ALL generally have a more aggressive clinical course than those with B-cell ALL.[101,102] This is largely due to the presence of higher-risk clinical features. T-cell ALL tends to occur in older children, and patients have higher white blood cell counts. These patients also have a higher incidence of CNS involvement and were recently shown to have a higher incidence of MRD. Many centers consider T-cell ALL to be more aggressive independent of traditional risk factors. Adults with T-cell ALL may actually fare better than those with B-cell ALL, which likely reflects the relatively high incidence of Ph^+ disease in the adult population.

The majority of patients with LBL have advanced disease, evidence of B symptoms, and high lactate dehydrogenase levels. In contrast to T-cell ALL, there is typically preservation of peripheral blood counts, presumably owing to the lack of bone marrow replacement. Bone marrow or testicular involvement by LBL is strongly correlated with CNS disease. Historically, LBL has been an aggressive disease associated with poor survival in response to standard lymphoma therapy. More recently, however, because of the limited success of standard therapy and the increasing recognition of the biologic similarities between T-cell ALL and LBL, trials in pediatric centers have used more intensive treatments modeled after ALL therapy. Using these regimens, dramatic improvements in outcome were seen,[103] particularly for low-stage LBL. Studies in adult patients with T-cell LBL indicate that they too can benefit from ALL-type regimens.[104] Another important therapeutic strategy is CNS prophylaxis, given the high rate of CNS relapse in patients who do not receive it. Because local recurrence is also a major indication of treatment failure, inclusion of mediastinal radiotherapy may play a role in preventing relapse, particularly in adult patients.

Although intensified ALL-type therapy seems to have improved the outcome in T-cell LBL, there are no clear prognostic factors that predict remission or survival. Identification of such clinical or biologic parameters is critical for risk stratification, in particular when deciding whether hematopoietic stem cell transplantation is warranted. The role of newer diagnostic modalities such as positron emission tomography scanning may play a role in risk stratification.

Table 41-3 Differential Diagnosis of Lymphoblastic Lymphoma

Tumor	Distinguishing Features
Myeloid sarcoma	More distinct cytoplasm, eosinophilic myelocytes, myeloid phenotype
Lymphocytic thymoma	Presence of abnormal cytokeratin+, thymic epithelial cells
Small lymphocytic lymphoma	Condensed nuclear chromatin, mature B-cell phenotype
Blastic variant of mantle cell lymphoma	Mature B-cell phenotype, t(11;14), cyclin D1 expression
Large B-cell lymphoma	Large cells, more prominent nucleoli, mature B-cell phenotype
Burkitt's lymphoma	More prominent nucleoli, distinct cytoplasmic rim, mature B-cell phenotype, t(8;14)
Small, round blue cell tumors (including Ewing's sarcoma, neuroblastoma, embryonal rhabdomyosarcoma, medulloblastoma)	Cohesive growth, absence of lymphoid markers
Ectopic thymus	Indistinct or absent nucleoli, normal continuum of T-cell antigen acquisition during differentiation, normal epithelium

Differential Diagnosis

The differential diagnosis of T-cell and B-cell ALL is similar (see Table 41-2), and that for LBL (Table 41-3) generally includes similar lesions that are likely to present as tumor masses. Immunophenotypic analysis is the key to distinguishing among these neoplasms.

CONCLUSION

Precursor lymphoid neoplasms are aggressive tumors that require immediate diagnosis and treatment. However, with appropriate intensive therapy, these malignancies are curable, particularly in the pediatric population. Greater understanding of the biology of lymphoblastic tumors will undoubtedly lead to more tailored therapy, in terms of both risk stratification and the development of targeted therapeutic agents.

Pearls and Pitfalls: Diagnosis of Acute Lymphoblastic Leukemia (ALL)

Pearls

- Precursor B-cell neoplasms generally present as leukemias, and precursor T-cell neoplasms generally present as lymphomas; if leukemic, the latter are associated with significant tissue involvement. Mediastinal masses in patients with ALL are seen almost exclusively with precursor T-cell neoplasms.
- Precursor lymphoid tumors recapitulate certain aspects of normal precursor lymphoid maturation. However, because of the reproducible nature of antigen acquisition in normal precursors, virtually all neoplastic populations can be reliably distinguished from normal precursors by multiparametric flow cytometry.
- For B-cell ALL, the presence of hyperdiploidy or *ETV6-RUNX1* fusion confers a favorable prognosis in childhood, whereas *BCR-ABL1* fusion or *MLL* rearrangement confers an unfavorable prognosis.
- Bone marrow and testicular involvement by lymphoblastic lymphoma is associated with central nervous system involvement.

Pitfalls

- Precursor lymphoid tumors may lack common leukocyte antigen (CD45) and express O13 (CD99) so that this profile does not distinguish them from Ewing's sarcoma. Inclusion of other lymphoid markers and TdT may be helpful in discriminating between these alternatives.
- Expression of CD79a, commonly used as a B-cell marker, may occasionally be expressed on T-cell tumors, including precursor T-cell neoplasms.
- Expression of myeloid antigens such as CD13, CD33, and CD15 occurs commonly in B-cell ALL and does not imply that the tumor is biphenotypic (see Chapter 42).
- The presence of $CD19^+$, $CD10^+$ cells in the marrow, even in significant numbers, does not necessarily establish a diagnosis of B-cell ALL because these cells must be distinguished from normal B-cell precursors (hematogones).
- The *ETV6-RUNX1* translocation is almost always cytogenetically inapparent and requires fluorescence in situ hybridization of reverse transcriptase polymerase chain reaction to identify cryptic translocations.

References can be found on Expert Consult @ www.expertconsult.com

Chapter 42

Acute Leukemias of Ambiguous Lineage

Edward G. Weir and Michael J. Borowitz

CHAPTER OUTLINE

Standard classification criteria for acute leukemia derive from the morphologic, cytochemical, and immunophenotypic characterization of bone marrow specimens and are designed to identify optimal therapy and predict prognosis.[1-4] Based on these criteria, most cases of acute leukemia can be unequivocally assigned to the myeloid or B-lymphoid lineage, and fewer to the T-lymphoid lineage. However, a small but heterogeneous subset of leukemias cannot be clearly identified with recognized patterns of myeloid or lymphoid ontogeny. Despite sophisticated methods of immunophenotypic analysis, the lack of widely accepted criteria for recognizing and defining these leukemias has hindered our understanding of their biology and the establishment of standard therapeutic protocols.

Leukemias that fall into this category have been given many different names, including *undifferentiated leukemia*, *biphenotypic leukemia*, *mixed lineage leukemia*, and *hybrid leukemia*, among others. By convention, they are now most commonly referred to as *acute leukemia of ambiguous lineage* (ALAL), as proposed by the World Health Organization (WHO) classification of hematolymphoid malignancies.[5] In this chapter we describe the identifying characteristics and clinical features of different types of ALAL, with a focus on immunophenotypic profiles.

DEFINITION

Many cases of ALAL are composed of blasts that have a rudimentary or hematopoietic "stem cell" phenotype, which is characterized by the failure to express lineage-defining features of differentiation. These acute leukemias with primitive phenotypes are commonly referred to as *acute undifferentiated leukemias* (AULs). Other cases of ALAL demonstrate a multiplicity of antigens that are associated with two or, rarely, three different lineages and may be referred to as *mixed phenotype acute leukemias* (MPALs).

Terminology referring to MPAL has been confusing, and terms such as *mixed lineage* or *dual lineage leukemia*, *hybrid leukemia*, *biphenotypic leukemia*, and *bilineal leukemia* have all been used. MPAL is most clearly recognized in two variations. Some cases have a single dominant population of blasts that express antigens in combinations that preclude definitive lineage assignment; these have been referred to as *biphenotypic leukemias*. Other cases of MPAL are recognized as having more than one population of blasts, each of which exhibits an unequivocal, lineage-specific pattern of differentiation. This latter group has traditionally been referred to as *bilineal leukemia* to convey the presence of two disparate populations of blasts. However, many cases of MPAL present with overlapping features of both biphenotypic and bilineal leukemia; that is, they are characterized by the presence of two disparate populations of blasts, one or (rarely) both of which demonstrate a complex pattern of antigen expression that lacks lineage specificity. Furthermore, cases classified as either biphenotypic or bilineal at diagnosis may relapse as the other. Owing to this immunophenotypic ambiguity, and because these variations lack significant clinical distinction, it is reasonable to combine them into a single category of MPAL. The classification of ALAL as recently proposed by the WHO is shown in Box 42-1.

EPIDEMIOLOGY AND ETIOLOGY

Collectively, this heterogeneous subset of leukemias of ambiguous lineage accounts for less than 3% of all acute leukemias.[6,7] They occur in patients of all ages, although those with t(9;22) are more common in adults than in children, and

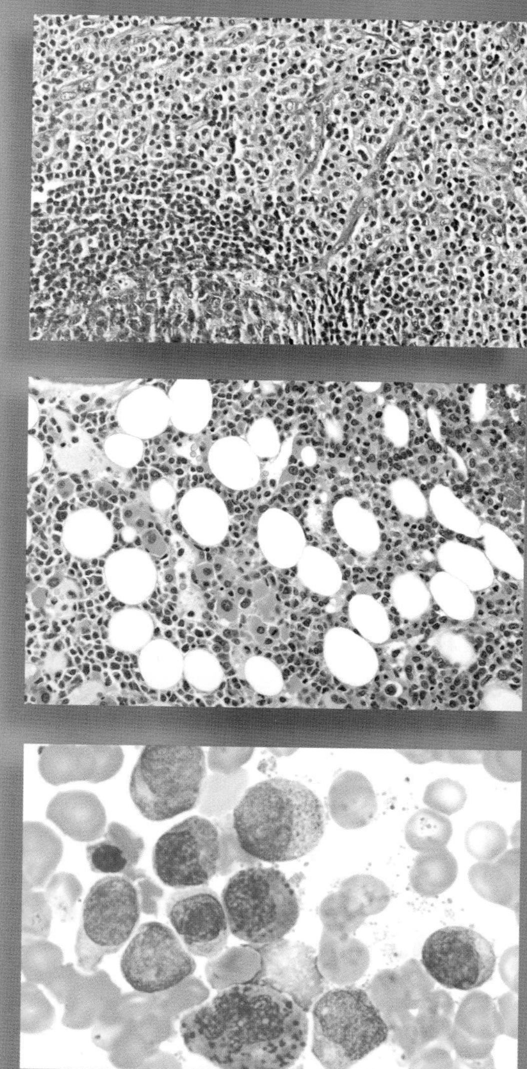

PART IV

Myeloid Neoplasms

Chapter 43

Principles of Classification of Myeloid Neoplasms

Daniel A. Arber and James W. Vardiman

CHAPTER OUTLINE

The fourth edition of the World Health Organization's classification of myeloid neoplasms, *WHO Classification of Tumours of Haematopoietic and Lymphoid Tissues*,[1] is used in this book. The principles of the WHO classification have been described elsewhere,[2,3] and the process for developing this consensus classification is summarized in Chapter 13. Briefly, the classification relies on a combination of clinical, morphologic, immunophenotypic, genetic, and other biologic features to define specific disease entities—a logical approach similar to that followed by a clinician and a pathologist working together to reach a diagnosis in a patient suspected of having a myeloid neoplasm. The relative contribution of each feature varies, depending on the case. Only through familiarity with the classification system and with the criteria for each entity can the appropriate studies be chosen to arrive at an accurate diagnosis in an expedient manner. Although perhaps overused as an example of the prototype for the classification of myeloid neoplasms, chronic myeloid leukemia (CML) symbolizes the utility of the WHO approach. This leukemia is recognized mainly by its clinical and morphologic features and is consistently associated with a specific genetic defect, the *BCR-ABL1* fusion gene. This abnormality leads to the production of a constitutively activated protein tyrosine kinase that interacts with a number of different cellular pathways to influence the proliferation, survival, and differentiation of neoplastic cells. The protein is sufficient to cause the leukemia, but it also provides a target for therapy that has prolonged the lives of thousands of patients with this disease.[4] The diagnosis of CML, however, is not based on any single parameter. There are other myeloid leukemias that mimic its clinical presentation and morphology, and the *BCR-ABL1* fusion is seen not only in CML but also in some cases of acute lymphoblastic leukemia and mixed phenotype acute leukemia. Thus, CML is a perfect model for the integration of all pieces of relevant information to define an entity in a classification scheme. Furthermore, there are still mysteries regarding CML, so there is still more to learn (see Chapter 46).

As the focus in all neoplasms turns increasingly to the genetic infrastructure of malignant cells and to molecular abnormalities that may be targets for therapeutic agents, it is only natural that more genetic and molecular data are incorporated into the diagnostic algorithms or nomenclature of classification schemes. The previous (third) edition of the WHO classification included, for the first time in any widely used system, genetic information as criteria for the diagnosis of not only CML but also some subtypes of acute myeloid leukemia (AML).[5] In the nearly 8 years that elapsed between the third and fourth editions of the WHO classification, a number of significant genetic abnormalities were discovered that are associated with subgroups of myeloid neoplasms or with specific disease entities within the subgroups. In some instances, such as malignant eosinophilia associated with rearrangements involving *PDGFRA* or *PDGFRB*, the genetic defect (coupled with the morphology and clinical findings) is the major criterion for naming the disease and for selecting specific targeted therapy (see Chapter 49). In other instances, such as the *BCR-ABL1*-negative myeloproliferative neoplasms (MPNs) that are often but not invariably associated with the *JAK2* V617F mutation, the presence of the genetic defect is an objective criterion that identifies the myeloid proliferation as neoplastic. Additional criteria are necessary to define the specific disease associated with the mutated *JAK2* and to distinguish it from other MPNs that share the same mutation (see Chapter 46). Therefore, although the latest WHO classification scheme incorporates genetic abnormalities, a multidisciplinary approach is still required for the classification of myeloid neoplasms. This multidisciplinary approach succeeds in defining many distinct disease entities that cannot be adequately identified by relying on morphology or clinical features alone. Such a limited approach to the myeloid neoplasms is no longer adequate, and in many cases a diagnosis is not complete until the results of all studies have been correlated, often requiring amended pathology reports.

New entities and new diagnostic criteria for old entities in the WHO classification scheme are based mainly on published clinical and scientific studies that have been widely quoted and their significance widely acknowledged. However, to accommodate recent data that have not yet "matured," the classification includes a number of "provisional entities." These are newly described or characterized disorders that are clinically or scientifically important and should be considered in the classification, but additional studies are needed to clarify their significance. Many of these will likely be incorporated as full entities in future editions, and their presence emphasizes that the classification is ever-changing.

EVALUATION OF MYELOID NEOPLASMS

Myeloid neoplasms are serious, often life-threatening disorders, and their diagnosis requires a concerted and serious effort by the clinician and the pathologist to thoroughly and carefully evaluate the clinical, morphologic, immunophenotypic, and genetic data. Too often, a diagnosis is based on insufficient knowledge of the clinical and laboratory information and, particularly, on inadequate diagnostic specimens. Although the proper collection and processing of blood and bone marrow specimens is addressed in Chapter 3, Box 43-1 emphasizes additional guidelines when assessing specimens from patients suspected of having myeloid neoplasms. One rule of thumb is that morphology is a key criterion in the diagnosis of all myeloid neoplasms, even those in which there is a closely associated genetic defect or characteristic immunophenotypic profile. If the specimen is not adequate to evaluate morphologically, a new specimen should be obtained.

The WHO criteria apply to initial peripheral blood and bone marrow specimens obtained before any definitive therapy (including growth factor therapy) for the suspected hematologic neoplasm. Morphologic, cytochemical, and immunophenotypic features are used to establish the lineage of the neoplastic cells and to assess their maturation. The blast percentage remains a practical tool for subcategorizing myeloid neoplasms and judging their progression. A myeloid neoplasm with 20% or more blasts in the blood or bone marrow is considered to be AML when it occurs de novo, evolution to AML if it occurs in the setting of a previously diagnosed myelodysplastic syndrome (MDS) or MDS/MPN, or blast transformation in a previously diagnosed MPN. Furthermore, a gradually increasing blast count at any level is usually associated with disease progression. Blast percentages should be derived, when possible, from 200-cell leukocyte differential counts of the peripheral blood smear and 500-cell differential counts of all nucleated bone marrow cells on cellular bone marrow aspirate smears stained with Wright-Giemsa or a similar stain. Blasts are defined using the criteria recently proposed by the International Working Group on Morphology of Myelodysplastic Syndrome[6] and as outlined in Box 43-1. Determination of the blast percentage by flow cytometry assessment of CD34$^+$ cells is not recommended as a substitute for visual inspection; not all leukemic blasts express CD34, and hemodilution and other processing artifacts can produce misleading results. The detection of more

Box 43-1 *Evaluation of Myeloid Neoplasms*

Specimen Requirements

- Peripheral blood and bone marrow specimens obtained before any definitive therapy for the suspected myeloid neoplasm
- Peripheral blood and cellular marrow aspirate smears or touch preparations stained with Wright-Giemsa or similar stains
- Bone marrow biopsy at least 1.5 cm long and at right angles to the cortical bone for all cases, if feasible
- Bone marrow specimens for complete cytogenetic analysis and, when indicated, for flow cytometry, with an additional specimen cryopreserved for molecular genetic studies; the latter studies should be performed based on initial karyotypic, clinical, morphologic, and immunophenotypic findings

Assessment of Blasts in Peripheral Blood and Bone Marrow Specimens

- Determine the blast percentage in peripheral blood and cellular bone marrow aspirate smears by visual inspection
- Count myeloblasts, monoblasts, promonocytes, megakaryoblasts (but not dysplastic megakaryocytes) as blasts when determining blast percentage for diagnosis of AML or blast transformation; count abnormal promyelocytes as "blast equivalents" in acute promyelocytic leukemia
- Proerythroblasts are not counted as blasts except in rare instances of "pure" acute erythroleukemia
- Flow cytometric assessment of CD34$^+$ cells is not recommended as a substitute for visual inspection; not all blasts express CD34, and artifacts introduced by specimen processing may result in erroneous estimates
- If the aspirate is poor or marrow fibrosis is present, immunohistochemistry on biopsy sections for CD34 may be informative if blasts are CD34$^+$

Assessment of Blast Lineage

- Multiparameter flow cytometry (at least three colors) is recommended; the panel should be sufficient to determine lineage as well as aberrant antigen profile of the neoplastic population
- Cytochemistry, such as myeloperoxidase or nonspecific esterase, may be helpful, particularly in AML, NOS, but it is not essential in all cases
- Immunohistochemistry on bone marrow biopsy may be helpful; many antibodies are now available for the recognition of myeloid and lymphoid antigens

Assessment of Genetic Features

- Complete cytogenetic analysis of bone marrow at initial diagnosis
- Additional studies, such as fluorescence in situ hybridization or reverse transcriptase polymerase chain reaction, should be guided by clinical, laboratory, and morphologic information
- Mutational studies for mutated *NPM1*, *CEBPA*, and *FLT3* are recommended in all cytogenetically normal AMLs; mutated *JAK2* should be sought in *BCR-ABL1* negative MPNs, and mutational analysis for *KIT*, *NRAS*, *PTNP11*, and so forth should be performed as clinically indicated

Correlation and Reporting of Data

- All data should be assimilated into one report that states the WHO diagnosis

AML, acute myeloid leukemia; MPN, myeloproliferative neoplasm; NOS, not otherwise specified.

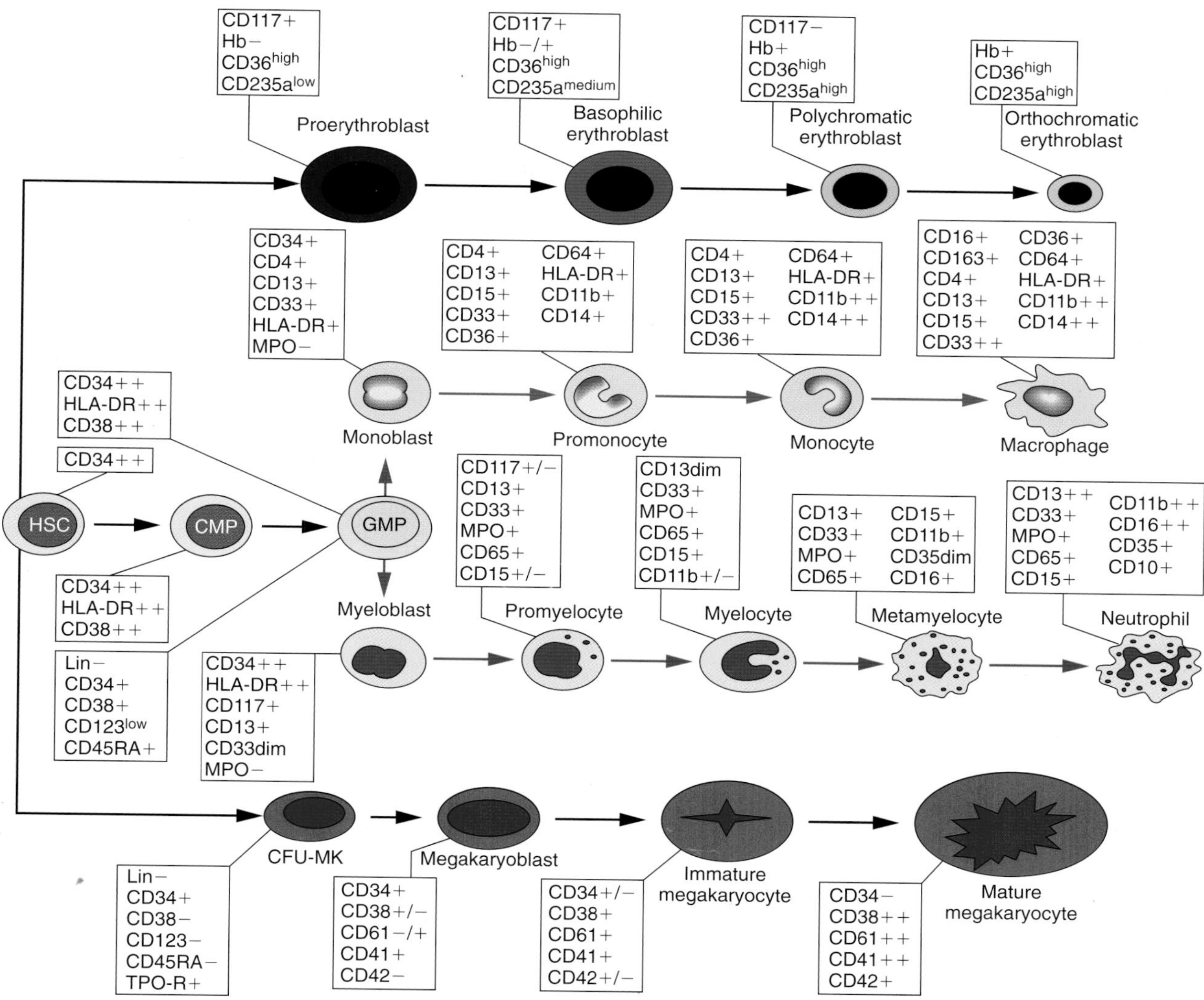

Figure 43-1. Antigen expression at various stages of normal myeloid differentiation. (Courtesy of Dr. Anna Porwit, Karolinksa University Hospital, Stockholm.)

CD34+ cells by flow cytometry than expected from the morphologic evaluation, however, requires a reassessment of both specimens to resolve the discrepancy. Such reassessment may identify unusually small blasts that were initially confused with lymphocytes, or it may show erythroid hyperplasia that, after red blood cell lysis of the flow cytometry specimen, resulted in a falsely elevated CD34 count. For acute leukemia, multiparameter flow cytometry (three or more colors) with CD45 versus side scatter gating is the method of choice for determining the blast lineage as well as for detecting aberrant antigenic profiles that may prove useful for disease monitoring. Figure 43-1 demonstrates antigens expressed at various levels of normal myeloid differentiation. These can be detected by flow cytometry or by immunohistochemistry on bone marrow biopsy specimens. However, asynchronous expression of maturation-associated antigens by neoplastic myeloid cells is not uncommon and is best determined by flow cytometric analysis.[7]

Although a bone marrow biopsy is not required for diagnosis in every patient with a myeloid neoplasm (particularly if the patient is frail and there are few treatment options available), an adequate biopsy provides the most accurate assessment of marrow cellularity, topography, stromal changes, and maturation patterns of the various lineages, and it can be invaluable in detecting residual disease following therapy. In addition, the biopsy provides material for the immunohistochemical detection of antigens that can be diagnostically and prognostically useful, particularly if marrow aspirate smears are poorly cellular.[8]

A complete cytogenetic analysis of bone marrow cells is essential during the initial evaluation for establishing a baseline karyotype; thereafter, repeat analyses are recommended as needed to judge the response to therapy or detect genetic evolution. Additional genetic studies should be guided by the results of the initial karyotype and by the suspected diagnosis based on the clinical, morphologic, and immunophenotypic studies. In some cases, reverse transcriptase polymerase chain reaction or fluorescence in situ hybridization may detect variants of well-recognized cytogenetic abnormalities or submicroscopic abnormalities not detected by routine karyotyping, such as the *FIP1L1-PDGFRA* rearrangement found in some myeloid neoplasms associated with eosinophilia,[9] or detection of the *BCR-ABL1* fusion in about 5% to 10% of cases of CML when the Philadelphia chromosome is not found by routine cytogenetic studies. Molecular studies may also prove useful in emergency situations while awaiting routine cytogenetic results, such as detection of *PML-RARA* fusion in cases of acute promyelocytic leukemia. In addition, gene mutations are increasingly being recognized as important diagnostic and prognostic markers in myeloid neoplasms (as will become apparent in the chapters that follow). These include mutations of *JAK2, MPL,* and *KIT* in MPN[10-15]; *NRAS, KRAS, NF1, RUNX1,* and *PTPN11* in MDS/MPN[16-21]; *NPM1, CEBPA, FLT3, RUNX1, KIT, WT1,* and *MLL* in AML[22-26]; and *GATA1*[27] in myeloid proliferations associated with Down syndrome. In some cases, if there is reason to suspect a specific neoplasm, the mutational analysis should be done "up front" in the evaluation of diagnostic specimens; for example, in suspected cases of *BCR-ABL1*-negative MPNs, detecting the *JAK2* V617F mutation can substantiate the diagnosis of a clonal myeloproliferation. In other cases, cryopreservation of a portion of the blood or marrow specimen allows future testing guided by the morphologic, clinical, and cytogenetic findings. Although over- and underexpression of genes can affect the prognosis in some myeloid neoplasms,[23] at the present time, analysis of gene dosage by quantitative reverse transcriptase polymerase chain reaction (other than the quantitative assessment of *BCR-ABL1* fusion transcripts in the monitoring of patients with CML) is not practical on a daily basis, nor have gene expression arrays been introduced into routine use.

WHO CLASSIFICATION

The WHO classification of myeloid neoplasms is shown in Box 43-2. The term *myeloid* includes all cells belonging to the granulocytic (neutrophil, eosinophil, basophil), monocyte/macrophage, erythroid, megakaryocytic, and mast cell lineages.

In general, the diseases are stratified into neoplasms comprising precursor cells (blasts) with minimal if any maturation (i.e., AML) and those in which there is maturation, either effective or ineffective, in the myeloid lineages. Each subgroup includes entities that are clinically or nosologically relevant and are defined using the WHO principles. Table 43-1 lists the major subgroups of myeloid neoplasms and their characteristics at diagnosis. Each subgroup is described in detail in the following chapters, but some brief comments regarding the rationale for the classification and the major changes from previous schemes are provided here.

Box 43-2 *WHO Classification of Myeloid Neoplasms*

Myeloproliferative Neoplasms (MPNs)

- Chronic myelogenous leukemia, *BCR-ABL1* positive
- Chronic neutrophilic leukemia
- Polycythemia vera
- Primary myelofibrosis
- Essential thrombocythemia
- Chronic eosinophilic leukemia, not otherwise specified
- Mastocytosis
- MPN, unclassifiable

Myeloid and Lymphoid Neoplasms Associated with Eosinophilia and Abnormalities of *PDGFRA*, *PDGFRB*, or *FGFR1*

- Myeloid and lymphoid neoplasms associated with *PDGFRA* rearrangement
- Myeloid neoplasms associated with *PDGFRB* rearrangement
- Myeloid and lymphoid neoplasms associated with *FGFR1* abnormalities

Myelodysplastic/Myeloproliferative Neoplasms (MDS/MPNs)

- Chronic myelomonocytic leukemia
- Atypical chronic myeloid leukemia, *BCR-ABL1* negative
- Juvenile myelomonocytic leukemia
- Myelodysplastic/myeloproliferative neoplasm, unclassifiable
- Provisional entity: Refractory anemia with ring sideroblasts and thrombocytosis

Myelodysplastic Syndrome (MDS)

- Refractory cytopenia with unilineage dysplasia
  - Refractory anemia
  - Refractory neutropenia
  - Refractory thrombocytopenia
- Refractory anemia with ring sideroblasts
- Refractory cytopenia with multilineage dysplasia
- Refractory anemia with excess blasts
- MDS with isolated del(5q)
- MDS, unclassifiable
- Childhood MDS
  - Provisional entity: refractory cytopenia of childhood

Acute Myeloid Leukemia and Related Neoplasms

- Acute myeloid leukemia (AML) with recurrent genetic abnormalities
  - AML with t(8;21)(q22;q22); *RUNX1-RUNX1T1*
  - AML with inv(16)(p13.1q22) or t(16;16)(p13.1;q22); *CBFB-MYH11*
  - Acute promyelocytic leukemia with t(15;17)(q22;q12); *PML-RARA*
  - AML with t(9;11)(p22;q23); *MLLT3-MLL*
  - AML with t(6;9)(p23;q34); *DEK-NUP214*
  - AML with inv(3)(q21q26.2) or t(3;3)(q21;q26.2); *RPN1-EVI1*
  - AML (megakaryoblastic) with t(1;22)(p13;q13); *RBM15-MKL1*
  - Provisional entity: AML with mutated *NPM1*
  - Provisional entity: AML with mutated *CEBPA*
- AML with myelodysplasia-related changes
- Therapy-related myeloid neoplasms
- AML, not otherwise specified
  - AML with minimal differentiation
  - AML without maturation
  - AML with maturation
  - Acute myelomonocytic leukemia
  - Acute monoblastic/monocytic leukemia
  - Acute erythroid leukemia
    - ■ Pure erythroid leukemia
    - ■ Erythroleukemia, erythroid/myeloid
  - Acute megakaryoblastic leukemia
  - Acute basophilic leukemia
  - Acute panmyelosis with myelofibrosis
- Myeloid sarcoma
- Myeloid proliferations related to Down syndrome
  - Transient abnormal myelopoiesis
  - Myeloid leukemia associated with Down syndrome
- Blastic plasmacytoid dendritic cell neoplasm

From Swerdlow SH, Campo E, Harris NL, et al, eds. *WHO Classification of Tumours of Haematopoietic and Lymphoid Tissues*. Lyon, France: IARC; 2008.

INCIDENCE

The incidence of MDS increases dramatically with age, forming an exponential curve that begins to rise noticeably by the early 40s (Fig. 44-1).[1,11-19] MDS (especially low-grade subtypes) may be subtle and difficult to diagnose, even in experienced hands. MDS has been confused in the historical literature with other discrete diseases, such as de novo AML with a low blast count (so-called MDS with favorable cytogenetics).[20] There has been disagreement whether to include some cases of cytopenias with dysplasia under the umbrella of MDS (e.g., Pearson's syndrome and hematopoietic dysplasia in acquired immunodeficiency syndrome [AIDS]). The potential for misdiagnosis is high. The list of differential diagnoses for MDS (discussed later) is long, and definitive diagnosis may be difficult. Many elderly patients receive only supportive treatment for possible MDS, without an explicit diagnosis. The underlying biology of MDS remains largely unknown, with disagreement over whether MDS is truly neoplastic. At least in part for these reasons, many national cancer epidemiology programs have failed to record cases of MDS. Despite these limitations, it is evident that the incidence of MDS overall exceeds that of AML.[15-19,21] MDS appears to precede or be pathogenetically related to about half of AML cases (including the large majority of AML in the elderly), and demographic studies of MDS patients indicate that 10% to 40% of MDS cases (estimated average, about 20%) actually progress to AML.[1] In several restricted regional and national studies, the incidence of MDS in children appears to be in the range of 0.05 to 0.2 cases per 100,000 per year.[22-24] The exact incidence in young adults is uncertain but low, appearing to approximate that in children. The incidence of MDS exceeds 25 cases per 100,000 per year by age 70 and may be considerably higher.[15-19,22-24] With the noted data limitations, the median age at onset of MDS is estimated to be at least 65 to 70 years. As the elderly population increases, it is predictable that both absolute case numbers and the median age of MDS patients will rise. MDS is more common in males, with a male-to-female ratio approaching 2:1, although at least one subset of MDS (5q– syndrome) is largely restricted to elderly women.

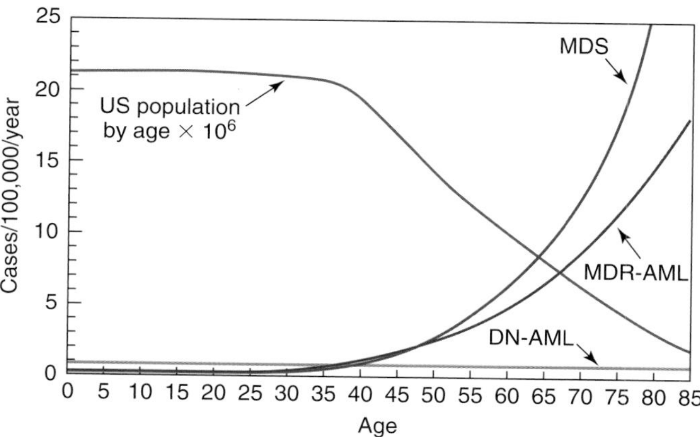

Figure 44-1. Age incidence of myelodysplastic syndrome (MDS) for the population at risk. These curves are approximations (estimated from references 1, 11-18, and 22-24). Population-based incidence data are insufficient to describe the exact relationship between MDS and MDS-related acute myeloid leukemia (MDR-AML) curves. The exact slope of the de novo acute myeloid leukemia (DN-AML) curve is uncertain; some data suggest a slight upslope with progressive age.[17]

CLINICAL FEATURES

MDS typically presents with symptoms and signs related to single or multiple peripheral blood cytopenias: anemia (weakness, pallor), thrombocytopenia (petechiae, bleeding), and neutropenia (recurrent infections).[25-28] Occasional patients are recognized when asymptomatic cytopenias are noted during a routine complete blood count or when increased blasts, dysplastic morphology, or clonal cytogenetic abnormalities are identified in studies of peripheral blood or bone marrow obtained for other purposes.

LABORATORY FEATURES

Peripheral Blood Parameters

Patients typically present with anemia—usually normocytic to slightly macrocytic, but occasionally microcytic—and may display dual populations of red blood cells (RBCs), with one being normocytic or microcytic and hypochromic, and the second being macrocytic.[25,27,28] These findings should be interpreted with the transfusion history in mind. The anemia may be isolated, or it may coexist with neutropenia or thrombocytopenia. Less commonly, patients present with isolated neutropenia or thrombocytopenia. The cytopenias vary in severity. Although reticulocyte production is typically low in MDS, the reticulocyte count may be spuriously elevated in some patients owing to retained debris in circulating RBCs rather than increased RBC production.[29,30] This may cause diagnostic confusion with hemolytic anemia.

Microscopic Features in Peripheral Blood and Bone Marrow

Despite peripheral cytopenias, marrow is typically hypercellular to packed in MDS.[31-34] Less commonly, it is normocellular, and in a small percentage of cases it is hypocellular. The origin of the name MDS is an unusual set of dysplastic morphologic features found in hematopoietic cells in the marrow and peripheral blood (Table 44-1; Figs. 44-2 to 44-4). Some features are best seen in mature cells in peripheral blood, such as large or abnormally granulated platelets or basophilic stippling and poikilocytosis in RBCs. Others occur in immature precursors and are best seen in marrow; however, immature hematopoietic precursors (nucleated RBCs, immature granulocytes, megakaryocyte nuclei, mononuclear megakaryocytes) are frequent in peripheral blood and may show the same anomalies. The morphologic abnormalities are distinctive, but most are neither unique to nor pathognomonic for MDS. Nor are they a sine qua non for diagnosis, because incontrovertible cases of MDS may lack dysplastic morphologic features. Nevertheless, morphologic dysplasia is usually helpful in establishing the diagnosis of MDS. Erythroid hyperplasia is typical. Marrow blasts are increased in high-grade MDS, frequently with circulating blasts. The blasts are typically myeloblasts but may be other types, including monoblasts and megakaryoblasts. Similarly, AML evolving from MDS may be characterized by a variety of myeloid blast types. Some cases of MDS

Table 44-1 **Dysplastic Morphologic Features of Myelodysplastic Syndrome**

	Peripheral Blood	Bone Marrow
RBCs and precursors	Aniso- and poikilocytosis* Dual RBC populations Basophilic stippling Siderocytes	Cloverleaf nuclei and variations Megaloblastoid change Multinuclearity Vacuolated erythroblasts Internuclear bridging Pyknotic nuclei Irregular hemoglobinization of precursors Howell-Jolly bodies Periodic acid–Schiff–positive precursors Ring sideroblasts, or abnormal sideroblasts with large or multiple siderosomes
Granulocytes and precursors	Acquired (pseudo) Pelger-Huët anomaly Hypogranularity Hypersegmentation Ring nuclei	Megaloblastoid change Hypogranularity Myeloperoxidase deficiency Abnormal localization of immature precursors† Nuclear-cytoplasmic asynchrony Pseudo–Chédiak-Higashi granules
Platelets and megakaryocytes	Large, vacuolated, or hypogranular platelets	Small mononuclear megakaryocytes Larger megakaryocytes with multiple small nuclei Hypolobated megakaryocytes Large megakaryocytes with large hyperchromic nuclei

*Numerous abnormal forms may be seen, including ovalocyte, elliptocyte, teardrop, target, and fragmented forms.
†In normal marrow, immature myeloid precursors are located adjacent to bony trabeculae and blood vessels. In myelodysplastic syndrome, they may be abnormally located in the center of marrow spaces, hence the descriptive name *abnormal localization of immature precursors*. This finding is not completely specific; for example, it can also be seen in regenerating marrow after an aplastic event.
RBC, red blood cell.
See references 29-34.

and MDR-AML have a mix of blast types. Minor levels of dysplastic features may be encountered in patients who do not have MDS. There have been attempts to quantify dysplastic features in MDS; however, although experienced observers can generally agree on the presence of significant dysplasia in a marrow sample, quantitation of dysplastic features is inherently variable among observers for several reasons: the subtlety of some dysplastic features, the observer's experience and other human variables, differing significance and subjective weighting of specific dysplastic features (e.g., basophilic stippling of erythroid precursors versus internuclear bridging), and gaussian variation in sampling. The WHO classification recommends that 10% of cells in a lineage demonstrate dysplastic features to be considered significant.[2,9] This guideline should be applied with an understanding of the previous comments.

Auer rods have been described in MDS patients.[2,9,35,36] Given the historical confusion of MDS and AML with a low blast count (the latter often having t[8;21], which typically has frequent Auer rods) and the additional difficulty of definitively separating high-grade MDS and MDR-AML, the literature must be read with caution.[20] Auer rods are uncommon in MDS. They were used in the French-American-British (FAB) classification of MDS to upgrade cases to refractory anemia with excess blasts in transformation (RAEB-T); RAEB-T has been deleted in the WHO classification of MDS, but Auer rods are used to upgrade cases to RAEB-2 (see later).[2,9,37] The validity of this usage of Auer rods has been challenged.[38]

Extramedullary Manifestations

Granulocytic sarcomas (chloromas) have been reported uncommonly in patients with MDS. Given the difficulties of distinguishing MDS and AML, some reported cases are questionable. Organomegaly and skin infiltrates (including Sweet's syndrome) are described uncommonly in MDS.[39,40] Given that MDS in the older literature included diseases now classified as myelodysplastic/myeloproliferative neoplasms and AML with a low blast count, and given that tissue infiltrates and organomegaly are frequent in these settings, such reports must be treated with caution.[20] Nevertheless, tissue myeloid infiltrates do occur in a minority of definite cases of MDS. If a tissue infiltrate in this setting consists predominantly of blasts, progression to MDR-AML should be diagnosed.

Cytogenetic Abnormalities

MDS is characterized by a recurring set of clonal cytogenetic abnormalities, as well as nonrecurring clonal abnormalities and multiple complex abnormalities (Box 44-1).[9,41-43] The large majority of identified genetic abnormalities in MDS consist of loss or gain of large segments of chromosomes, the most frequent being –7, 5q– or –5, and +8. These deletions may represent in part occult unbalanced translocations.[44] It is presumed that they correspond to the loss or gain of function of critical genes, but most of the genes in question remain unidentified. An uncommon set of translocations also occurs with low frequency in MDS. It is important to emphasize that all these cytogenetic abnormalities appear to be secondary events; 60% of patients have normal cytogenetics at presentation, and the abnormalities may appear or disappear over time with genetic progression of the disease.[4,5] MDS cytogenetic abnormalities are shared with MDR-AML. It is essential that cases with cytogenetic abnormalities characteristic of de novo AML (see first footnote, Box 44-2) not be considered MDS; if clinically symptomatic, such cases should be considered de novo AML, regardless of marrow or blood blast percentages.[20]

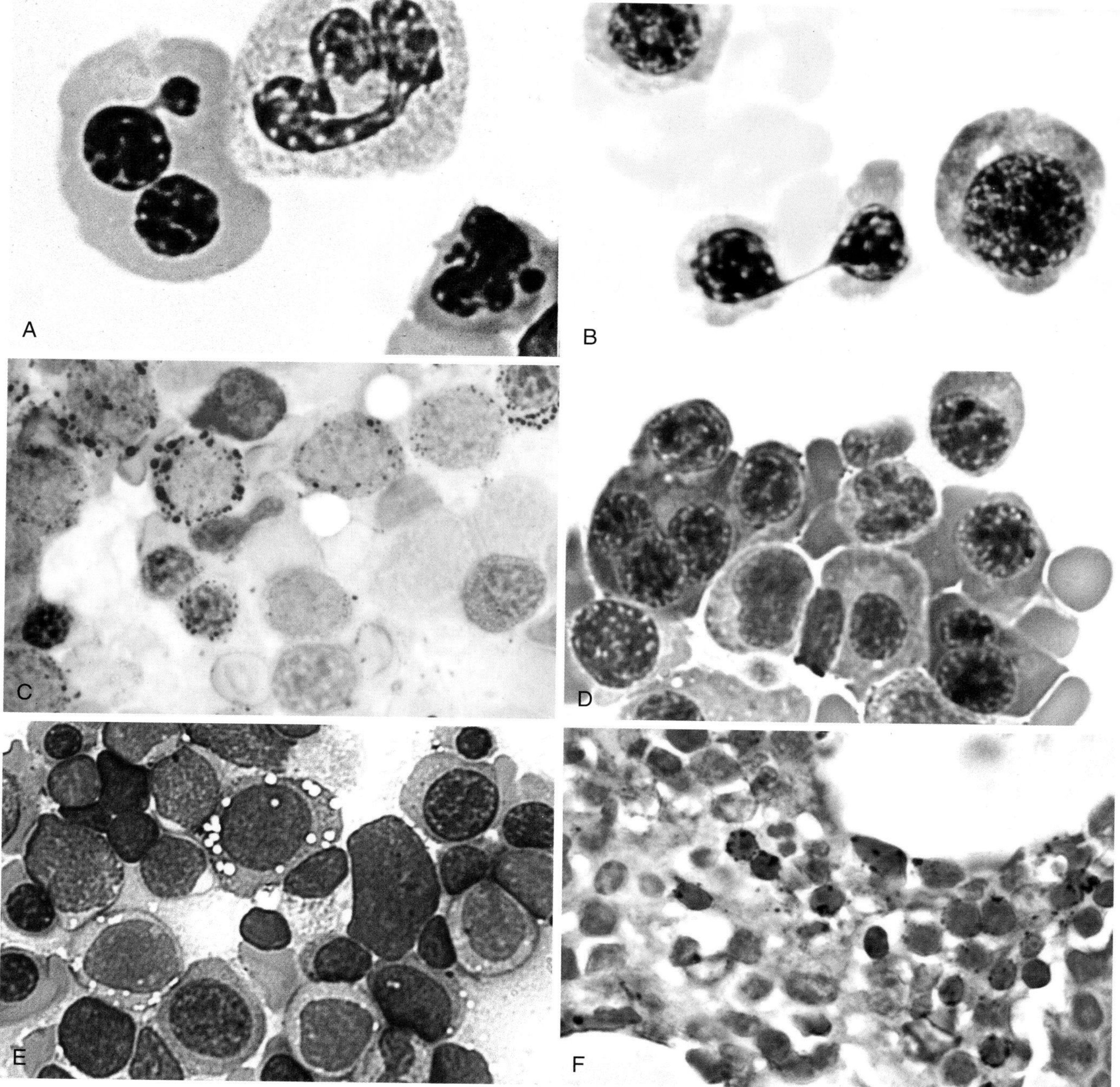

Figure 44-2. Dysplastic features of erythroid precursors in bone marrow aspirate smears in myelodysplastic syndrome. A, Erythroid precursors with abnormal nuclear lobulation. **B,** Internuclear bridge in erythroid precursors (note the pointed nuclei at the base of the bridge). **C,** Periodic acid–Schiff–positive erythroblasts (note the coarse granular positivity in immature precursors and the finer granular positivity in more mature precursors). **D,** Multinucleation and megaloblastoid change in erythroid precursors. **E,** Erythroblasts containing cytoplasmic vacuoles. **F,** Ring sideroblasts (Prussian blue stain).

Other Biologic Abnormalities and Assessments

Clonality

Clonal hematopoiesis is a hallmark of MDS.[41-43,45,46] At least in the subsets of MDS that progress to AML, clonal hematopoiesis involves all three lineages of myeloid precursors (erythroid, granulocytic, megakaryocytic). Studies demonstrating this have included Lyon hypothesis–based tests (glucose-6-phosphate dehydrogenase and human androgen receptor gene assay in females) and cytogenetic fluorescence in situ hybridization (FISH) assays using informative numerical cytogenetic abnormalities.

Loss of Function in Hematopoietic Cells

A variety of losses of function (or abnormal function) have been described in hematopoietic cells in random MDS patients. Some, such as loss of myeloperoxidase function in neutrophil precursors or accumulation of iron in

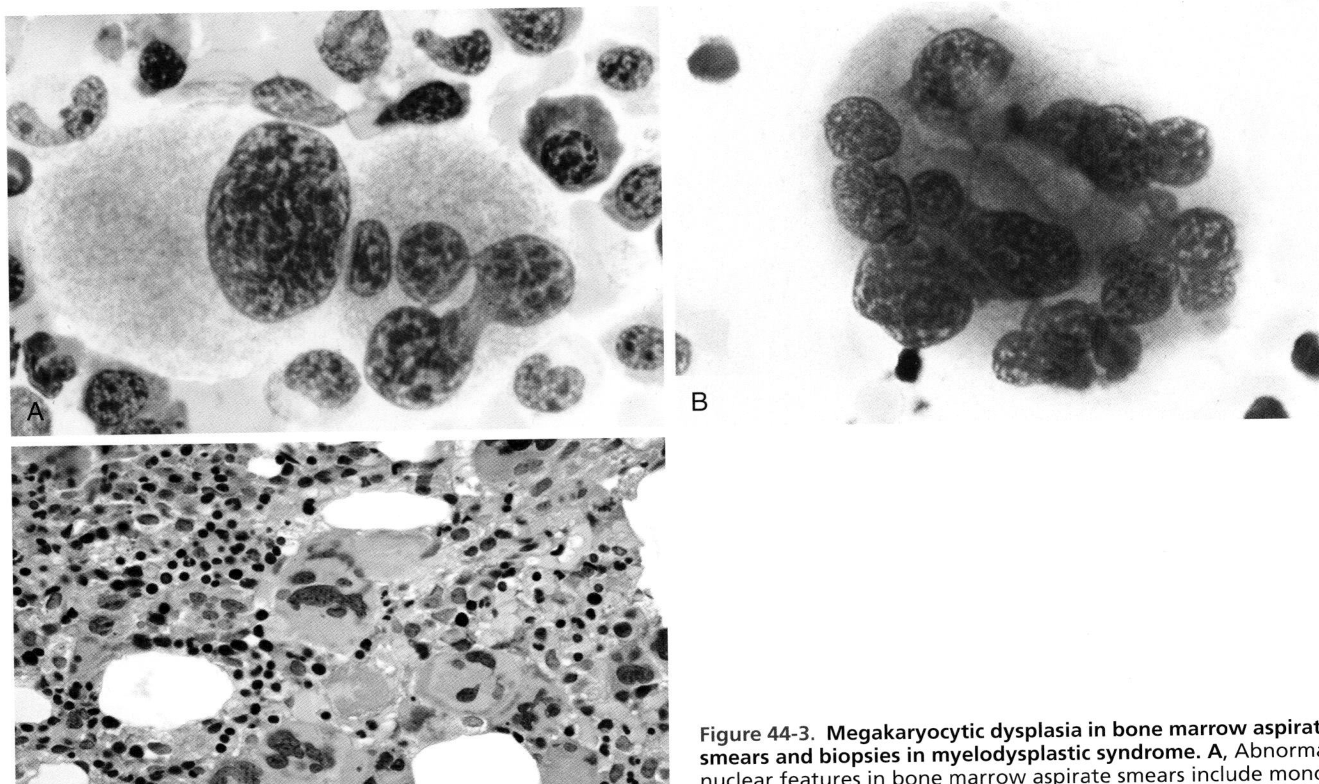

Figure 44-3. Megakaryocytic dysplasia in bone marrow aspirate smears and biopsies in myelodysplastic syndrome. A, Abnormal nuclear features in bone marrow aspirate smears include monolobate and multiple separate small nuclei. **B,** Hyperlobation of megakaryocytic nuclei. **C,** Clustered dysplastic megakaryocytes in a bone marrow biopsy.

Box 44-1 *Cytogenetic Abnormalities in Myelodysplastic Syndrome*

- Gain or loss of chromosomal material
  - −7, 7q−
  - 5q−, −5
  - +8
  - +21, −21
  - 17p−, −17
  - −20, 20q−
  - 11q−, +11
  - −Y
  - 9q−
  - +6
  - 12p−
  - 13q−
- Uncommon translocations and inversions
  - t(3;3)(q21;q26), inv3(q21q26), t(3;21)(q26;q22) and other 3q21 and 3q26 translocations
  - t(1;7)(p11;p11)
  - t(2;11)(p21;q23)
  - t(11;16)(q23;p13)
  - i(17)q, unbalanced and dicentric translocations at 17p
- Any acquired clonal cytogenetic abnormality in hematopoietic cells, except characteristic de novo acute myeloid leukemia (AML) translocations*
- Complex abnormalities (multiple cytogenetic abnormalities, excluding those characteristic of de novo AML)

*Common de novo AML translocations: t(15;17), t(8;21), inv(16) or t(16;16), t(9;11), t(11;19), t(11;17), t(8;16), t(1:22).
See references 41-43.

mitochondria in erythroid precursors (ring sideroblasts), may be of diagnostic value.[32] Others, such as loss of bactericidal ability in neutrophils,[47-49] acquired pyruvate kinase deficiency in red cells,[50,51] acquired hemoglobin H disease,[52] or loss of hemostatic function in platelets,[53] may have clinical significance. Still others, such as the appearance of paroxysmal nocturnal hemoglobinuria anomalies such as a positive Ham test,[54] spurious reticulocytosis,[29,30] increased hemoglobin F,[55] or changes in blood group antigen expression,[56] are perplexing and may cause diagnostic confusion (see the later discussion of differential diagnosis). Some of these abnormalities may correlate with significant clinical abnormalities such as hemolysis. The cause of these recurring loss of function abnormalities is uncertain; they may be the result of a random mutator phenotype or epigenetic silencing of transcription of an unknown cause. For most of the anomalies it is difficult to conjecture a contribution to disease progression in MDS.

Flow Cytometric Analysis

The potential use of flow cytometry for the diagnosis of MDS is the focus of ongoing investigations (see Chapter 5).[57-63] When analyzed with panels of antibodies to track differentiation of hematopoietic cells, marrow samples from MDS patients frequently demonstrate abnormal maturation patterns in myeloid, monocytic, and erythroid precursors. This approach requires the use of a large panel of antibodies to ensure a high level of sensitivity, but it provides good correlation of aberrant differentiation with morphologic dysplasia in MDS. Hematopoietic precursors in MDS may also demon-

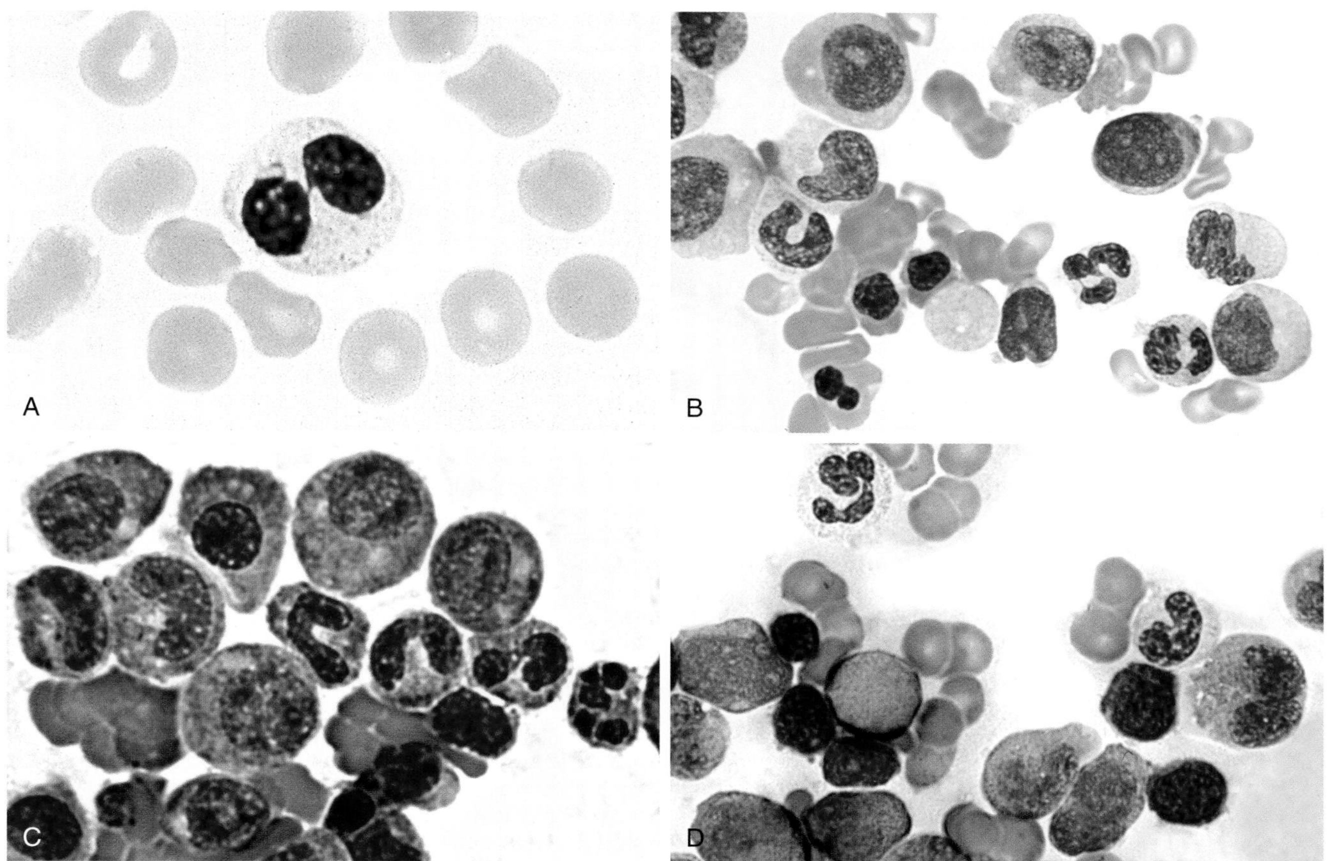

Figure 44-4. Granulocytic dysplasia in peripheral blood and bone marrow aspirate smears in myelodysplastic syndrome. A, Hypogranular and pseudo–Pelger-Huët cell with bilobed nucleus in peripheral blood smear. **B** and **C,** Asynchronous maturation of granulocytes (**B**) and megaloblastoid change, including hyposegmented nuclei (**C**), in bone marrow aspirate smears. **D,** Myeloperoxidase-negative granulocytes (yellow is positive) in bone marrow aspirate smear (myeloperoxidase stain, Giemsa counterstain).

strate lineage aberrant antigen expression. It should be noted that there are only limited data on the possible differential diagnostic problems related to this application of flow cytometry in MDS. Similar abnormalities may be seen in marrow recovering from chemotherapy or with growth factor stimulation, common clinical situations in patients with a potential diagnosis of MDS. This use of flow cytometry works best with larger panels of antibodies and more sophisticated multicolor instrumentation than are currently in general use. For these reasons, such flow cytometric data are not yet generally available and are better viewed as corroborative rather than diagnostic in MDS. As more experience is acquired and more sophisticated instrumentation becomes widely available, this situation may change.

Finally, flow cytometry is effective for quantifying and characterizing hematopoietic blasts in MDS, with several caveats. One is that hypogranular neutrophils may merge into a typical blast display gate because of decreased side scatter (hypogranularity), leading to a significant overestimate of blast numbers. A second is that preparation of samples for flow cytometry in a clinical setting typically includes lysis of RBCs (to remove enucleated mature red cells); however, this step also removes most nucleated red cells, thus decreasing the denominator for calculation of the blast percentage and artificially raising the final blast percentage. Third, the sample sent for flow analysis may be hemodiluted, leading to an underestimate of marrow blast numbers. For these reasons, correlation with morphology remains essential for the quantitation of blasts.

Apoptosis and Cell Cycle Analysis

Numerous reports using a variety of assays have described increased ex vivo apoptosis in patients with MDS, including a coordinated burst of DNA digestion occurring several hours earlier in MDS marrow than in control marrow.[64-66] The significance of these observations is uncertain. The apoptosis may affect a large percentage (>50%) of marrow cells, yet uric acid (an obligate by-product of in vivo cell death and degradation) levels are generally not increased in MDS. The appearance of a strong DNA ladder ex vivo suggests instead that actual cell death may be triggered and coordinated by the removal of marrow cells from their normal milieu. Paradoxically, the antiapoptotic protein BCL2 is also overexpressed in some patients with MDS.[67] Cell cycle analyses, predominantly in vitro studies based on DNA content, have reported increased cells in the S and G_2 phases of the cell cycle in some patients with MDS.[64,66,68,69] Possible pathogenetic implications of these data are discussed later. These findings are not uniform among reports, and these studies are not currently used for the diagnosis of MDS.

Molecular Biologic Abnormalities

The genetic events that initiate MDS are not known. However, some mutations acquired after the initiation of MDS that may contribute to its progression to MDR-AML have been identified. These include *NRAS*, *CSF1R* (*c-FMS*), and *FLT3* activating mutations and overexpression of *KIT* (all of which drive the proliferation of hematopoietic progenitors), as well as dysregulation of *EVI1* (which competitively blocks GATA1 DNA binding, thus interfering with the differentiation of hematopoietic progenitors).[70-76] Changes that occur earlier in MDS have also been identified, but their contribution to progression is unclear. *TP53* mutations may be present, especially in therapy-related disease, and loss of one *TP53* allele in MDS with 17p– may contribute to disease progression.[77,78] *CSF3* (granulocyte colony-stimulating factor [G-CSF]) receptor mutations are associated with progression of Kostmann's syndrome (severe congenital neutropenia) to MDS or AML.[79] BCL2 is overexpressed in some cases of MDS but is not mutated.[67] The membrane pump MDR1 is overexpressed and functional in a high percentage of MDS patients, especially those with therapy-related MDS and MDR-AML, and it may contribute to resistance to chemotherapy in these patients.[80] Silencing of expression of the *CDKN2B* (*p15*) gene by methylation has been described and may contribute to disease progression.[81] Shortening of telomeres is found in some MDS patients and may be associated with progression to AML.[82-84]

DIAGNOSIS

Diagnosis of MDS is complicated by the lack of understanding of its pathogenesis and by the absence of tests to confirm the diagnosis with absolute specificity. We are left with a set of diagnostic features that all appear to be secondary to the underlying disease process and neither completely sensitive nor completely specific. Because of these limitations and the numerous clinical situations that can mimic MDS, clinicopathologic correlation is essential for an accurate diagnosis. Given these ambiguities, diagnosis may be influenced by therapeutic considerations. Because the only curative treatment of MDS is allogeneic hematopoietic stem cell transplantation, therapeutic goals (and diagnostic implications) differ by age. In the elderly, who cannot tolerate allogeneic transplantation, therapeutic goals tend to be supportive or limited to noncurative intervention (e.g., hypomethylating agents, cytotoxic chemotherapy); in patients who would receive only supportive care anyway, a specific diagnosis may not be required. In patients younger than 60 years, however, in whom allogeneic transplantation is an option, the need for an accurate diagnosis and subclassification is critical and obvious. Minimal diagnostic criteria for MDS have been proposed and are listed in Box 44-2.[85]

Application of these diagnostic criteria must take into account the clinical context of a case, because many of these abnormalities may be present in other settings. Abnormalities should be stable over several weeks at least. Recovery from marrow aplasia of any cause may include transient elevation of myeloblasts above 5% in the marrow. Clonal cytogenetic abnormalities in the marrow may be transient in some clinical settings, such as aplastic anemia, some congenital marrow failure syndromes, and nutritional deficiencies (folate, vitamin B_{12}).[86-89] AML with a low blast count may mimic MDS, with increased blasts between 5% and 20% but with cytogenetic abnormalities characteristic of de novo AML (see first footnote, Box 44-2).[20] Recent exposure to chemotherapy may cause megaloblastoid or dysplastic morphology, discounting their significance in this clinical setting.

Box 44-2 *Minimal Criteria for a Diagnosis of Myelodysplastic Syndrome*

- Absence of de novo acute myeloid leukemia cytogenetic abnormalities*
- At least two of the following:
  - Sustained unexplained anemia, neutropenia, or thrombocytopenia
  - Dysplastic morphology in erythroid, granulocyte, or megakaryocyte or platelet lines (at least bilineage, except in RCUD, RARS, and 5q– syndrome)†
  - Acquired, sustained clonal cytogenetic abnormality in hematopoietic cells
  - Increased blasts (≥5% of marrow cells)

*t(15;17), t(8;21), inv(16) or t(16;16), t(9;11), t(11;19), t(11;17), t(8;16), t(1:22).
†By definition, refractory cytopenia with unilineage dysplasia (RCUD) and refractory anemia with ring sideroblasts (RARS) have unilineage dysplasia, and 5q– syndrome may have unilineage dysplasia.
See reference 85.

To evaluate a potential case of MDS, the minimal requisite studies are a complete blood count with differential and peripheral smear examination, Wright-Giemsa–stained bone marrow aspirate smear, hematoxylin-eosin–stained biopsy section, iron stain on either a smear or a particle section, flow cytometric evaluation (to characterize blasts, if increased on morphologic examination), and cytogenetic analysis that includes both karyotyping and FISH analysis for common abnormalities in MDS. The iron stain should not be performed on the biopsy specimen because decalcification leaches iron from the sample; staining an aspirate smear works best for the detection of ring sideroblasts. Additional studies may be helpful. Periodic acid–Schiff stain of an aspirate smear may show abnormal positivity in erythroid precursors. Myeloperoxidase stain may show myeloperoxidase-negative maturing granulocytes. Reticulin stain may demonstrate reticulin fibrosis in marrow that cannot be aspirated. A variety of other tests may be useful in specific clinical situations, such as vitamin B_{12}, folate, pyridoxine, and copper levels.

Other tests cited earlier might be useful in the diagnosis of MDS but are either not readily available or not validated for clinical use in this context, or the abnormalities they identify may be so uncommonly encountered in MDS as to have limited utility. For example, demonstration of marrow clonality by means other than cytogenetics could be helpful in evaluating potential MDS patients, but it is not available in clinical laboratories. Paroxysmal nocturnal hemoglobinuria–like abnormalities, impaired microbial killing by neutrophils, platelet function abnormalities, and other acquired functional abnormalities in hematopoietic cells may be seen in MDS, but most are relatively infrequent, and testing to support a diagnosis of MDS is often not available or not pursued unless prompted by specific clinical findings.

CLASSIFICATION

Myelodysplastic Syndrome–Related Disease versus De Novo Acute Myeloid Leukemia

In clinical practice, the most critical distinction among the acute myeloproliferative diseases is, perhaps surprisingly, not the separation of MDS from AML but the separation of MDS-related disease (MDS and MDR-AML) from de novo AML (AML with recurrent genetic abnormalities in the WHO classification).[1,2,9] Current treatments for high-grade MDS and MDR-AML are frequently similar, including hypomethylating agents and chemotherapy, with allogeneic stem cell transplantation being the only curative option. In both MDS and MDR-AML, aggressive chemotherapy may lead to prolonged, life-threatening cytopenias and subsequent complications, generally with a limited effect on overall survival. In contrast, aggressive cytotoxic chemotherapy may induce long-term, complete remissions in cases of de novo AML, and patients tend to tolerate chemotherapy better than those with MDS-related disease. The distinction of de novo AML from MDS and MDR-AML is currently based on history and clinical presentation, cytogenetics and molecular genetics, morphology (background dysplasia), and, if all else fails, the patient's age (see Fig. 44-1). It is hoped that advances in our understanding of these diseases will lead to more objective methods of making this distinction in all cases.

Stages of Myelodysplastic Syndrome

Low-grade MDS can be a relatively stable disease, both clinically and genetically, with a low or absent rate of progression to high-grade MDS or AML.[90] In contrast, other cases of MDS appear to have a mutator phenotype, are characterized by progressive and complex genetic abnormalities, and tend to progress to higher grades of MDS and MDR-AML.[4,5] Thus, three stages of MDS-related disease can be defined: low-grade MDS (nonprogressive subtypes), high-grade MDS, and MDR-AML. These stages exhibit different biologic features and have different outcomes.

Low-Grade versus High-Grade Myelodysplastic Syndrome

Low-grade and high-grade MDS differ in terms of median survival (6 to 8 years or longer versus 6 to 30 months), rate of progression to MDR-AML (0% to 10% versus 25% to 60%), lineages with dysplastic morphology (restricted lineage dysplasia in low-grade MDS), and percentage of myeloid blasts in the peripheral blood (<1% in low-grade MDS) and bone marrow (<5% in low-grade MDS).[2,7-10,26,37,91-94] It is clear that these differences reflect variations in the biologic processes of the disease, but the differences are not understood. Therefore, separation of low-grade and high-grade MDS is based on the percentage of blasts in bone marrow and peripheral blood and lineage involvement with dysplasia. As our understanding of the biology of MDS improves, criteria to subclassify MDS will evolve.

High-Grade Myelodysplastic Syndrome versus MDS-Related Acute Myeloid Leukemia

As noted earlier, the distinction between high-grade MDS and MDR-AML is often less critical than the accurate differentiation of MDS-related disease and de novo AML. Once this latter distinction is made, the general direction of treatment can be established. There are, however, biologic differences between high-grade MDS and MDR-AML and some differences in treatment protocols. Historically, the distinction between high-grade MDS and MDR-AML was based on the marrow blast percentage; if the threshold of 30% was exceeded, the diagnosis was AML. This threshold was incorporated in the FAB classification, and MDS with 20% to 30% marrow blasts was designated RAEB-T.[37] In the 2001 WHO classification of MDS, the threshold for separating MDS and MDR-AML was decreased to 20%, and the diagnostic category of RAEB-T was eliminated[2]; this revision was retained in the 2008 WHO classification.[9,10] This change generated discussion and disagreement in the literature,[3,95,96] centered on the ambiguity of distinguishing MDS from MDR-AML based on a single observation of the blast percentage.[97]

An alternative approach is based on the disease characteristics of MDS versus AML. MDS is a marrow failure syndrome, with ineffective hematopoiesis, whereas AML is characterized by the dysregulated hyperproliferation of blasts. Blastic nuclear morphology per se does not prove proliferation; rather, it only indicates dissociation of DNA from histones (dispersed chromatin), which can occur in circumstances other than replication of DNA. Knockout of histone deacetylase in a transgenic mouse model results in blastic nuclear morphology without proliferation.[98,99] Dispersed ("blastic") chromatin is commonly seen in MDS in cells with mature cytoplasmic features (nuclear-cytoplasmic asynchrony), a finding inconsistent with cell proliferation. In this context, some cases with a blast percentage of 20% to 30% continue to behave like MDS, with predominant marrow failure and cytopenias, whereas other cases behave like AML, with rapid proliferation of blasts. This distinction has definite clinical ramifications because the principal therapeutic approach to AML remains cytotoxic chemotherapy using drugs that block cell proliferation. A disease characterized by marrow failure, such as MDS, is unlikely to respond well to cytotoxic chemotherapy, but AML might. It may not be possible to reliably distinguish proliferation versus marrow failure with a single marrow examination, but serial examination may allow this distinction (Fig. 44-5). If the marrow blast percentage remains stable or rises slowly over time to exceed a threshold (whether 20% or 30%), the underlying disease process has not changed, and the case represents persistent MDS, even if the blast percentage eventually exceeds 30%. If the blast percentage rises abruptly, the disease process has transformed to a proliferative state—MDR-AML. A single observation of a high blast count in peripheral blood or marrow can be safely interpreted as progression to AML, despite myelodysplastic features or a history of MDS.

World Health Organization Classification

In 1976 and 1982 the FAB working group proposed that the previously chaotic nomenclature of MDS be standardized.[3,37,97,100] The resulting classification included five categories: refractory anemia (RA), RA with ring sideroblasts (RARS), RA with excess blasts (RAEB), RAEB in transformation (RAEB-T), and chronic myelomonocytic leukemia (CMML). This classification standardized the reporting of data related to

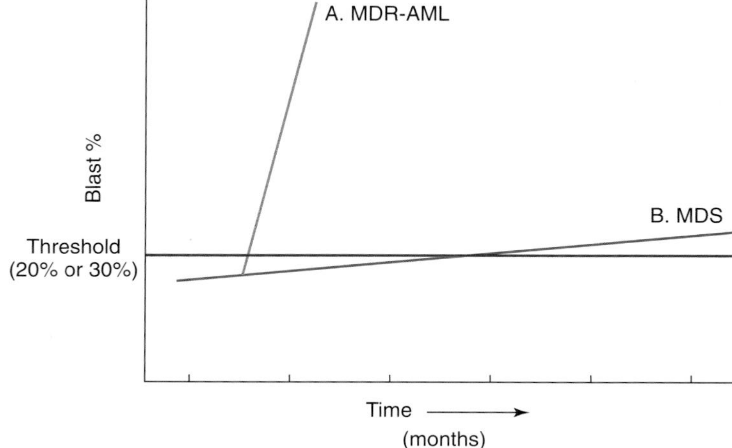

Figure 44-5. Blast progression over time in myelodysplastic syndrome (MDS). If the blast percentage in marrow rises rapidly (A), the case has transformed to MDS-related acute myeloid leukemia (MDR-AML). In contrast, if the blast percentage rises slowly over months (B) to exceed an artificial threshold (whether 20% or 30%), the case should be considered persistent MDS. A single observation of a high blast percentage in this setting may be interpreted as transformation to MDR-AML.[3,97]

these diseases and allowed the comparison of treatment regimens in standardized sets of patients. Subsequent revisions of this classification were incorporated in the WHO classification published in 2001.[2] These changes were retained with modest modifications in the edition of this classification published in 2008 (Table 44-2).[7-10,91-94,101] In the 2008 classification, CMML remains in the myelodysplastic/myeloproliferative subgroup. (In clinical practice, this group is frequently subdivided, and cases with low peripheral white blood cell counts are treated as a subset of MDS rather than as a proliferative disease.) The 5q− syndrome is still a discrete entity. The blast threshold for separating MDS from MDR-AML remains at 20% (see the previous discussion). The illogical FAB rule excluding erythroid precursors from the blast percentage calculation only when erythroid precursors exceed 50% of marrow cells is retained for the separation of MDR-AML from MDS but has been dropped for the subclassification of MDS. Use of this rule can lead to a misdiagnosis of AML despite a marrow blast percentage of less than 5% of total cells, and we strongly discourage its use. The distinction between MDS and de novo AML with a low blast count is appropriately retained. Emphasis on unilineage erythroid dysplasia and unilineage anemia in RARS is retained as well. The RA category in the 2001 WHO classification has been subsumed into a new category: refractory cytopenia with unilineage dysplasia (RCUD). RCUD includes cases with unilineage anemia, neutropenia, or thrombocytopenia or any combination of bicytopenia, all with unilineage dysplasia. Refractory cytopenia with multilineage dysplasia (RCMD), created in the 2001 WHO classification, is retained. The last major change in the 2008 WHO classification is the introduction of a separate category for childhood MDS with insufficient blasts for a diagnosis of RAEB; this new category is designated refractory cytopenia of childhood (RCC).

Refractory Cytopenia with Unilineage Dysplasia

In the 2008 WHO classification, RA is included in this new category,[91] along with refractory neutropenia and refractory

Table 44-2 Revised World Health Organization Classification of Myelodysplastic Syndrome (MDS)

Classification	Features
Refractory cytopenia with unilineage dysplasia (RCUD)	Uni- or bilineage cytopenia, unilineage dysplasia, <5% marrow blasts, <1% peripheral blasts
Refractory anemia with ring sideroblasts (RARS)	Anemia, unilineage erythroid dysplasia, <5% marrow blasts, ≥15% ring sideroblasts in marrow, no peripheral blasts
Refractory cytopenia with multilineage dysplasia (RCMD)	Cytopenias, multilineage dysplasia, <1% peripheral blasts, <5% marrow blasts, no Auer rods, no peripheral monocytosis (<1000/μL)*
Refractory anemia with excess blasts (RAEB-1, RAEB-2)	Cytopenias, no peripheral monocytosis (<1000/μL)*, uni- or multilineage dysplasia RAEB-1: <5% peripheral blasts, 5%-9% marrow blasts, no Auer rods RAEB-2: 5%-19% peripheral blasts, 10%-19% marrow blasts, ± Auer rods
MDS associated with isolated del(5q) chromosome abnormality (5q− syndrome)	Anemia, usually normal or increased platelets, <5% marrow blasts, <1% peripheral blasts, normal to increased and hypolobate or mononuclear megakaryocytes, isolated del(5q), no Auer rods
MDS, unclassifiable	Cytopenias, no Auer rods, ≤1% peripheral blasts, <10% dysplasia in any lineage, <5% marrow blasts, cytogenetic abnormality characteristic of MDS
Refractory cytopenia of childhood (RCC; provisional)	Cytopenias, multilineage dysplasia, <5% marrow blasts, <2% peripheral blasts
MDS, therapy related†	MDS of any morphologic subtype after therapy with agents that cause cross-link DNA damage (alkylating agents, platinum derivatives, nitrosoureas) or exposure to ionizing radiation

*≥1000 monocytes/μL suggests a diagnosis of chronic myelomonocytic leukemia, which may have similar features.
†Included under acute myeloid leukemia (AML), not under MDS, in the WHO classification, combined with AML, therapy related.[117]
See references 7-10, 91-94, and 101.
From Swerdlow SH, Campo E, Harris NL, et al, eds. *WHO Classification of Tumours of Haematopoietic and Lymphoid Tissues*. Lyon, France: IARC Press; 2008.

infancy and childhood MDS predominates in incidence over the CDAs and must be assiduously ruled out before CDA is diagnosed. In older patients, this caveat is even more important because CDA becomes progressively less frequent with advancing age. In the CDAs, dysplastic morphology and cytopenias are restricted to the erythroid lineage. If neutropenia, thrombocytopenia, or dysplasia of either lineage is present, a diagnosis of MDS should be strongly considered. Cytogenetics may be helpful, as is sequential observation; progressive disease over time is suggestive of MDS.

Non–Myelodysplastic Syndrome Sideroblastic Anemias

By far the most frequent cause of ring sideroblasts in bone marrow is MDS, but other diverse diseases are also associated with ring sideroblasts. The most common is alcoholism, although it is infrequently studied with bone marrow examination. Active alcohol abuse results in inhibition of multiple steps of heme synthesis, resulting in the accumulation of mitochondrial iron as ring sideroblasts. Dietary deficiencies associated with alcoholism may result in megaloblastoid hematopoiesis, and acute alcohol intoxication may cause vacuolization of erythroid precursors.[146,147] Thus, alcohol abuse may pose a difficult diagnostic problem. Fortunately, the diagnosis is usually easily resolved by the clinical history. Other reversible causes of ring sideroblasts are antituberculosis drugs (especially isoniazid),[148] severe copper deficiency (in premature infants, with prolonged parenteral hyperalimentation, or with copper chelation therapy),[149-151] zinc poisoning (which causes copper deficiency),[152] chloramphenicol,[153] and penicillamine therapy.[154] Copper deficiency and chloramphenicol also cause vacuolated erythroid precursors, and copper deficiency may cause vacuolated granulocyte precursors and neutropenia.

Congenital causes of sideroblastic anemia are diverse, including X-linked (most common), autosomal, and mitochondrial inheritance forms.[155,156] Anemia is microcytic hypochromic, variable in severity (may be severe), and may respond to exogenous pyridoxine; patients may have accompanying iron overload. Pearson's syndrome is a mitochondrial cytopathy characterized by refractory sideroblastic anemia, vacuolated marrow precursors, exocrine pancreatic dysfunction, mitochondrial inheritance pattern, and onset of disease symptoms in infancy. Variant mitochondrial cytopathies with ring sideroblasts have also been described. Ring sideroblasts may be seen with erythropoietic protoporphyria. All these congenital diseases are rare. In most of them, quantitative and morphologic abnormalities are restricted to the erythroid lineage.

Copper Deficiency and Zinc Toxicity

Copper deficiency, including that caused by zinc toxicity, deserves special comment. It can present with pancytopenia with dysplastic marrow morphology, closely mimicking MDS.[101,157] Vacuolization of precursors may be prominent. Patients typically are on total parenteral nutrition or enteral feedings, have undergone gastrectomy, or are malnourished, but exceptions have been described. Patients may experience progressive and irreversible wallerian degeneration of cervical and thoracic spinal cord tracts if the metal abnormality is not corrected.[101] Hematopoietic parameters may improve with folate and B_{12} treatment, but this does not prevent progression of the neurologic abnormalities. Accurate diagnosis and early treatment are essential to prevent irreversible neurologic damage and to avoid erroneous treatment for MDS.

Chronic Viral Infections

Epstein-Barr virus, herpesvirus, and cytomegalovirus infection may present with hypercellular marrow and dysplastic marrow morphology.[158,159] However, because of leukocytosis, the clinical differential diagnosis usually consists of the mixed myelodysplastic/myeloproliferative processes rather than MDS. Chronic parvovirus B19 infection has also been described as a mimic of MDS.[160] Abnormalities in parvovirus infection are restricted to the erythroid lineage.

Cytogenetic Abnormalities Mimicking Myelodysplastic Syndrome

The cytogenetic abnormalities of MDS appear to be secondary events. They may mark progression of the disease but seem to be unrelated to the underlying pathogenesis of MDS. They are not pathognomonic for MDS, occurring in other settings as well. For example, +8 is a common additional finding in the de novo AML subtype acute promyelocytic leukemia with t(15;17). MDS-like cytogenetic abnormalities may occur and then recede in aplastic anemia and in some of the congenital marrow failure syndromes, as well as in reversible megaloblastic processes.[86-89] Familial −7 is clinically heterogeneous, with some patients manifesting no symptoms of MDS.[161] Similarly, in rare pediatric patients with −7, the cytogenetic abnormality regresses spontaneously to a normal karyotype, with no subsequent evidence of MDS or hematologic disease.[162]

Reticulin Fibrosis in Myelodysplastic Syndrome versus Primary Myelofibrosis

Mild reticulin fibrosis in marrow is frequent in MDS, presumably secondary to the release of connective tissue growth factors from dysplastic precursors, similar to the pathogenesis of primary myelofibrosis (PMF).[132,133] Fibrosis in MDS may lead to confusion with PMF because neither entity has definitive diagnostic criteria. Although both diseases are clonal and involve an acquired genetic abnormality of a multipotential marrow progenitor, the distinction is of some consequence. High-grade MDS is a progressive disease with a mutator phenotype, a high incidence of progression to MDR-AML, and a relatively short survival. PMF has a considerably longer median survival (4 to 5 years), with prolonged survival possible, and it has a low propensity for progression to AML. Organomegaly, such as splenomegaly, is unusual in MDS. Marked extramedullary hematopoiesis supports a diagnosis of PMF. A striking leukoerythroblastic peripheral blood smear is suggestive of PMF. Teardrop RBCs may be found in either setting but are more common in PMF. PMF typically has clusters of dysplastic megakaryocytes in marrow; these megakaryocytes may mimic the large hyperchromic megakaryocytes sometimes seen in MDS, but not the more characteristic mononuclear or hypolobate megakaryocytes of MDS. Dysplasia of other lineages is typical of MDS but is sometimes present in cases that otherwise appear to be PMF. Moderate or marked reticulin fibrosis in marrow, mature collagen fibrosis (trichrome positive), and osteosclerosis all strongly suggest PMF. PMF frequently has clonal cytogenetic abnormalities (13q−, 20q−, +8, and abnormalities of chromosomes 1, 5, 7, 9, and 21), which may be helpful in the differential diagnosis but overlap partially with MDS.[163,164] The *JAK2* kinase mutation V617F is found in up to 50% of PMF patients, and analysis may help confirm the diagnosis.[165,166] However, this mutation has also been described in a subset of MDS patients with fibrosis.[167] This differential diagnosis is sometimes impossible to resolve with a single marrow examination and may require clinical follow-up and reexamination of the marrow at a later date. Fibrosis in MDS is found more frequently in secondary than primary disease.[120-122] Spent polycythemia vera and some cases of chronic myelogenous leukemia may also have marrow fibrosis, but history and routine studies usually suffice to separate these entities from MDS.

Reticulin Fibrosis in Myelodysplastic Syndrome versus Acute Megakaryoblastic Leukemia

Acute megakaryoblastic leukemia, regardless of genetic abnormalities, prior history, or classification as MDR-AML or de novo AML, is characterized by reticulin fibrosis and is frequently accompanied by dysplastic megakaryocytes and intermediate precursors.[6,31-33] In adults it frequently evolves from MDS or has dysplastic background hematopoiesis. Thus, acute megakaryoblastic leukemia may closely mimic MDS with reticulin fibrosis. The reticulin fibrosis in each is presumably secondary to dysplastic megakaryocytes and megakaryoblasts. Distinction of the two entities is based on the same principles used to distinguish MDS from MDR-AML—namely, blast percentages and, more important, the rate of progression of blasts (see the earlier discussion).

Leukemoid Reaction in Low-Grade Myelodysplastic Syndrome versus Chronic Myelomonocytic Leukemia

Superimposition of an inflammatory process on MDS may result in a leukemoid reaction, which may include monocytosis and thus mimic CMML.[168] It is important to recognize this possibility, because patients with MDS are prone to infectious complications (neutropenia, neutrophil dysfunction), and the treatment and prognosis of a leukemoid reaction in low-grade MDS differ substantially from those of CMML.

Aplastic Anemia versus Hypocellular Myelodysplastic Syndrome

Aplastic anemia may have dysplastic morphology in hematopoietic progenitors and may have transient cytogenetic abnormalities similar to those of MDS. Some cases of aplastic anemia progress to MDS, and some cases of MDS have hypocellular marrow biopsies.[86,88,123,124,126] This differential diagnostic problem was previously discussed in the section on hypocellular MDS.

Paroxysmal Nocturnal Hemoglobinuria

The interrelationship of paroxysmal nocturnal hemoglobinuria (PNH) and MDS is unclear. MDS patients may exhibit a positive Ham (acid serum hemolysis) test, similar to straightforward cases of PNH.[54,123,124] MDS patients may also have marrow hypocellularity, similar to those with PNH.[123,124] A subset of PNH patients progresses to MDS (up to 5%) or MDR-AML (1%).[169-171] It is possible that patients with mutator phenotype MDS, who acquire a variety of seemingly random DNA damage (discussed previously), could secondarily acquire homozygous loss of function of *PIGA*, the gene necessary for glycosyl-phosphatidylinositol anchoring of proteins to the cytoplasmic membrane in hematopoietic cells (the PNH anomaly).[172] An alternative explanation is that an abnormal clone with the PNH anomaly arises first through marrow damage and evolves over time to MDS. Neither a positive Ham test nor the diagnosis of PNH precludes a diagnosis of MDS if other criteria corroborate the diagnosis, even in the presence of overt clinical PNH. If a PNH patient develops significant marrow dysplasia or a clonal cytogenetic abnormality consistent with MDS, evolution to MDS should be strongly considered.

Arsenic Exposure

Arsenic trioxide—now used to treat acute promyelocytic leukemia and under investigation for use in other disorders, including MDS—causes striking dysplastic morphology in marrow, particularly in erythroid progenitors, mimicking the erythroid dysplasia of MDS.[32,173]

CAUSATIVE AGENTS

A variety of agents and diseases are associated with an increased incidence of MDS and are presumed to contribute to disease pathogenesis. Inherited abnormalities include Fanconi's anemia, severe congenital neutropenia (Kostmann's syndrome), Shwachman-Diamond syndrome, dyskeratosis congenita, amegakaryocytic thrombocytopenia, familial monosomy 7 or 5q−, other familial MDS, and Bloom syndrome.[113] Although these diseases may eventually provide insight into the pathogenesis of MDS, the clues have not yet been deciphered. The incidence of MDS and related leukemia in Down syndrome is also markedly increased, but the clinical behavior in Down syndrome differs so drastically from that in other clinical settings that the relationship is uncertain. Cytogenetic abnormalities found in MDS all appear to be secondary events; they may provide insight into the steps related to disease progression but probably not to the underlying pathogenesis of MDS. Indeed, in neither familial monosomy 7 nor familial 5q− does the causative defect appear to localize to the respective chromosomes.[174,175] The interrelationship of aplastic anemia and MDS is unclear, but a high percentage of aplastic anemia patients subsequently develop MDS or MDR-AML, and both aplastic anemia and MDS may respond to immunosuppressive therapy, suggesting an interrelated pathogenesis. A variety of exposures (ionizing radiation, agents that cause cross-link DNA damage, benzene, other solvents and petrochemicals, agricultural or farming chemicals, smoking, hair dyes) have been linked to an increased incidence of MDS and MDR-AML. With some (radiation, alkylating agents, benzene) the association is strong; with others it is less definite. In all cases, any specific contribution to pathogenesis, other than random DNA damage, remains unclear. Notably, some of these agents have also been linked to aplastic anemia. Genes known to be mutated in MDS, such as *NRAS* or *CSF1R* (*c-FMS*) mutations, appear to contribute to disease progression rather than to the underlying pathogenesis.

PATHOGENESIS

Understanding the pathogenesis of MDS appears to be the key to both refining classification systems and improving treatment results. However, the pathogenesis remains unknown. Many reports cite an apparent increase of both apoptosis and cell cycling in hematopoietic precursors in patients with MDS, leading to a model of MDS as a hyperproliferative disease with apoptotic destruction of maturing cells before their release from marrow.[64-66] The apoptosis is demonstrable by multiple ex vivo methods, and dying cells may exceed 50% of total nucleated cells. Observations include the rapid appearance of a DNA digestion ladder, suggesting synchronized degradation of a large number of cells triggered by removal of the marrow sample rather than the in vivo death of marrow precursors. Notably, although uric acid is a requisite by-product of cellular degradation in vivo, hyperuricemia is not a usual complication of MDS. The evidence for hyperproliferation in MDS is similarly problematic, being based on an increase in S and G_2 phase DNA content by flow cytometry and analyses of in vivo DNA incorporation of labeled nucleotides. The flow cytometric data could indicate cell cycle arrest rather than cell cycling, and the DNA synthesis data are difficult to interpret because of the absence of control data. Finally, this model lacks an explanation for the cause and apparent synchronization of these events, for the cause of genetic instability and leukemic progression, and for the various clinical and morphologic subgroups of MDS. These findings are not currently used for the diagnosis of MDS. An alternative hypothetical model is that MDS is characterized by a combination of unrepaired DNA damage (with cell cycle arrest mimicking proliferation and creating a mutator phenotype), failure of the damage to induce apoptosis in vivo (with accumulation of clonal arrested cells), and progression of damaged cells to apoptosis only upon the removal of marrow from its normal milieu.

CONCLUSION

MDS is an enigmatic set of diseases of unknown pathogenesis. We are required to diagnose it using secondary disease features, most of which are neither completely specific nor pathognomonic. It is important that MDS be diagnosed and subclassified accurately because of the prognostic and therapeutic implications of specific diagnoses. MDS has an extensive and difficult set of differential diagnoses, some of which can be ruled in or out only by clinical follow-up. It is hoped that discovery of the pathogenesis of MDS will result in improved diagnostic capabilities and clarification of important clinical and biologic subsets of disease.

Pearls and Pitfalls

- A good marrow sample (aspirate smear or touch preparation, biopsy section, iron stain on smear or touch preparation) and a full complement of related tests (peripheral smear, complete blood count with differential, flow cytometric characterization of increased blasts, cytogenetic and fluorescence in situ hybridization analysis) are essential for the correct diagnosis and classification of MDS.
- None of the features of MDS (morphology, cytogenetics, cytopenias, increased blasts) are pathognomonic or a sine qua non for diagnosis. At least two of these features are recommended to support the diagnosis.
- Low-grade MDS subtypes may be nonprogressive, with survival approaching that of age-matched peers.
- High-grade MDS subtypes, if not treated with stem cell transplantation, are typically progressive and fatal, regardless of transformation to AML. Only 10% to 40% actually progress to AML.
- The differential diagnosis of MDS is extensive, but given the significance of the diagnosis and the lack of definitive diagnostic tests, exclusion of other possible entities is imperative.
- Chemotherapy for MDR-AML often leads to reversion to high-grade MDS rather than a true complete remission with normal hematopoiesis.
- The important distinction in these diseases, from both a clinical and a biologic perspective, is separation of MDS-related disease from de novo AML, not separation of high-grade MDS from MDR-AML.

References can be found on Expert Consult @ www.expertconsult.com

Chapter 45

Acute Myeloid Leukemia

Daniel A. Arber and Amy Heerema-McKenney

CHAPTER OUTLINE

Acute myeloid leukemia (AML) is a heterogeneous group of diseases that represent clonal proliferations of immature, nonlymphoid, bone marrow–derived cells that most often involve the bone marrow and peripheral blood and may present in extramedullary tissues. If untreated, AML follows an aggressive clinical course. AML has traditionally been differentiated from other myeloid neoplasms based on a minimum blast cell count in bone marrow or peripheral blood. Although this remains the case for some disease types, several specific AML types are now defined without regard to blast cell count.

The French-American-British Cooperative Group (FAB) described a number of AML subtypes based originally on morphologic and cytochemical features; other studies, including immunophenotyping and electron microscopy, were added later as defining features of some subtypes.[1-4] The FAB classification defined all AML types as proliferations of 30% or more marrow blasts of either all bone marrow cells or all marrow nonerythroid progenitor cells. Although other classification systems were subsequently proposed to incorporate more comprehensive immunophenotyping studies, cytogenetic studies, and combinations of these two ancillary testing methods,[5-8] the FAB classification remained the primary system used by most pathologists and hematologists for many years. The terminology of the FAB classification continues to be used, but this system is now considered obsolete owing to

Box 45-4 *Key Features of Acute Promyelocytic Leukemia with t(15;17)(q22;q12) (PML-RARA)*

- Hypergranular type exhibits abundant cytoplasmic granules and bundles of Auer rods
- Characteristic myeloid-lineage immunophenotype, with weak or absent HLA-DR and absent CD34
- Hypogranular type exhibits indistinct granules and folded nuclei and is often CD34 positive
- Common association with disseminated intravascular coagulation
- Favorable prognosis in cases that are *FLT3* negative and treated with combination chemotherapy that includes all-*trans*-retinoic acid

cytosis, with numerous circulating abnormal promyelocytes.[41,42] Both forms have abnormal reniform or bilobed nuclei, and recognition of these characteristic nuclear features is an important element of the diagnosis. In hypergranular APL, the abnormal promyelocytes have numerous red to purple cytoplasmic granules (Fig. 45-3A). The granules are often larger and more darkly stained than normal neutrophil granules, and they may be so numerous that they obscure the nuclear borders. In some cases a high percentage of leukemic cells has deeply basophilic, granular cytoplasm. Cells containing multiple Auer rods are reportedly found in up to 90% of cases of the hypergranular form. The Auer rods may be numerous and intertwined. Large globular inclusions of Auer rod–like material are found in the cytoplasm of occasional cells. Typical myeloblasts are a minor component in most cases, rarely reaching 20%. The abnormal promyelocytes are considered comparable to blasts for the purpose of diagnosing APL. In the microgranular variant of APL, the leukemic cells have sparse or fine granulation and markedly irregular nuclei (see Fig. 45-3B). The bilobed or butterfly-shaped nuclei should raise suspicion of the microgranular variant. Cells containing multiple Auer rods are less abundant than in typical hypergranular APL. Myeloperoxidase and Sudan black B reactions are strong in both variants.

The immunophenotype of hypergranular APL displays increased side scatter, lack of expression of HLA-DR and CD34, bright CD33, bright cytoplasmic myeloperoxidase, and variable expression of CD13.[43,44] The microgranular variant shows similar CD13, CD33, and myeloperoxidase expression but may show dim HLA-DR and commonly demonstrates dim CD34. The $CD34^-$, $HLA\text{-}DR^-$ immunophenotype is not specific to APL[45]; it is also observed in some cases of cytogenetically normal AML without differentiation. Expression of CD15 is uncommon. CD117 is expressed in both morphologic variants. Many cases exhibit CD64 expression, and caution is warranted to avoid misdiagnosing microgranular APL as AML with monocytic differentiation. Aberrant expression of CD2 is more commonly observed in microgranular APL.[46] CD56 expression is described in 15% to 20% of patients with APL and has been associated with shorter complete remissions and poorer overall survival in some studies.[47]

Three breakpoint regions are described on the *PML* gene at band q22 of chromosome 15.[48] Two lead to long transcripts, and the third leads to the short transcript. The short transcript is more common in the microgranular variant. Cytogenetics, FISH, or RT-PCR is necessary for genetic confirmation of the *PML-RARA* fusion. FISH, RT-PCR, and immunofluorescence for the microspeckled nuclear distribution of PML protein may facilitate a rapid diagnosis.[49] RT-PCR is the only technique that can identify the *PML-RARA* isoform useful for the monitoring of minimal residual disease.[50] The PML-RARA fusion protein mediates a block in myeloid differentiation, which can be overcome using ATRA or arsenic trioxide therapy. ATRA targets the RARA component of the fusion protein, whereas arsenic trioxide targets PML, causing maturation and apoptosis. In most cases remission can be achieved with ATRA alone, but relapse invariably occurs. Therefore, standard induction chemotherapy with high-dose anthracyclines is generally given with or after ATRA. In adult patients who achieve complete remission, the prognosis is better than

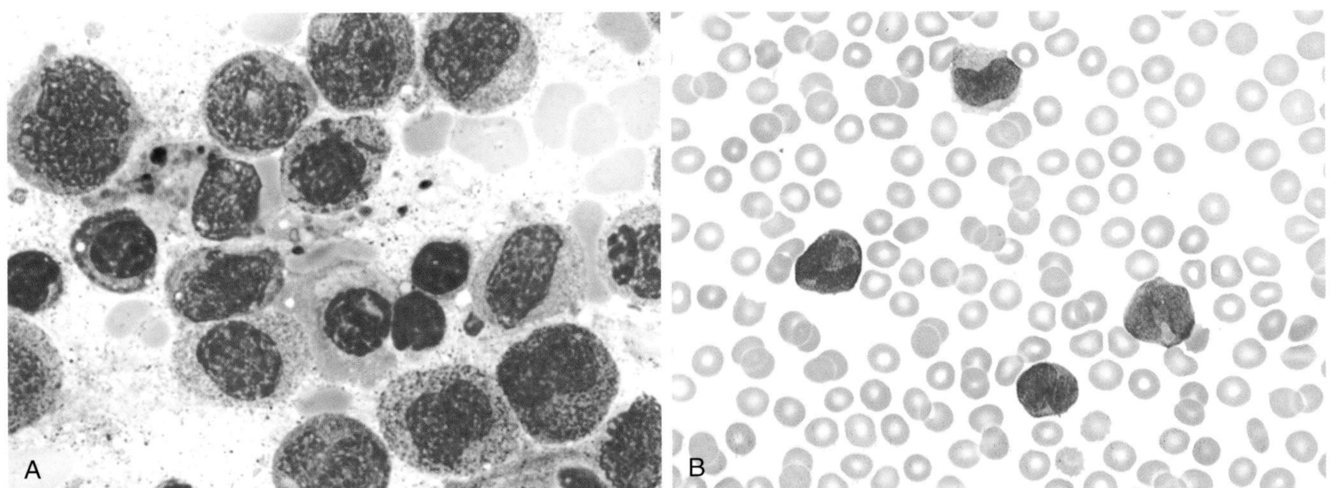

Figure 45-3. Acute promyelocytic leukemia with t(15;17)(q22;q12), *PML-RARA*. A, Bone marrow aspirate shows increased promyelocytes and blasts with folded nuclei and numerous cytoplasmic granules, characteristic of the hypergranular type of acute promyelocytic leukemia. Note one blast in the *upper center* of the panel exhibiting Auer rods. **B,** Peripheral blood from another case shows blasts with bilobed nuclei and less obvious cytoplasmic granules, characteristic of the microgranular variant of acute promyelocytic leukemia.

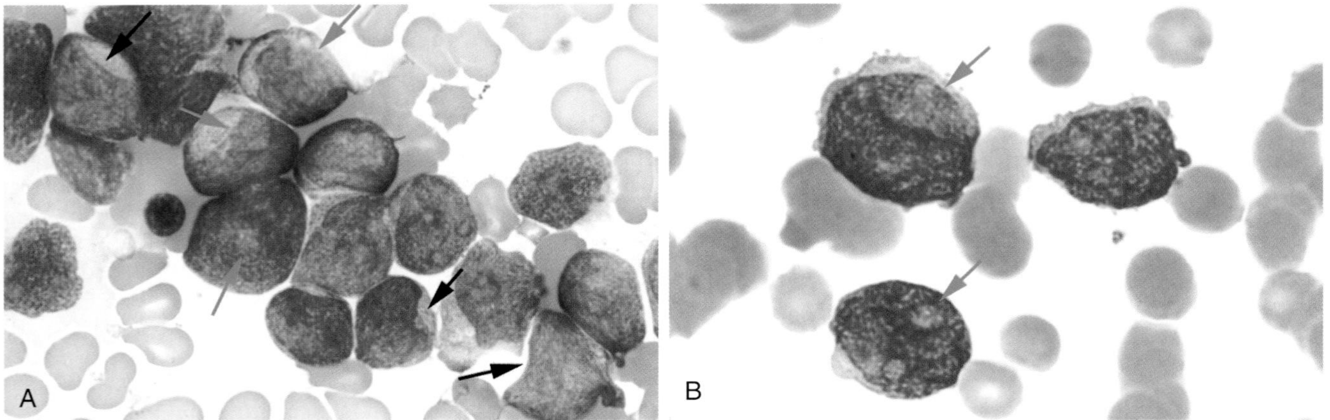

Figure 45-4. Acute myeloid leukemia with cup-like nuclear inclusions. A and **B**, Nuclear indentations from the side are most obvious (*black arrows*); from other angles, they may appear as large, pale nucleoli (*green arrows*). These features are reportedly associated with *FLT3* or *NPM1* mutations.

for any other category of AML. Rapid diagnosis and initiation of therapy are critical in APL. Because of the high risk of early death and the high potential for cure, initiation of therapy should not await genetic confirmation when clinical, morphologic, flow cytometric, and rapid molecular pathology results all suggest a diagnosis of APL.

FLT3 mutations are common in APL[51-53] and occur in approximately 40% of patients, with the majority being internal tandem duplication (ITD) mutations. *FLT3* ITD in APL is strongly associated with the microgranular subtype, high white blood cell counts in peripheral blood, and breakpoint region 3 (short form) in *PML*. In one retrospective study, patients with mutant *FLT3* had a higher rate of death during the induction of chemotherapy but no significant difference in relapse rate or 5-year overall survival.

Atypical promyelocytes may persist in the marrow for several weeks after induction chemotherapy, as may the detection of *PML-RARA* by karyotyping, FISH, or RT-PCR. These findings do not necessarily indicate resistant disease. The postinduction detection of *PML-RARA* by RT-PCR does not impact subsequent clinical outcome. However, detection of *PML-RARA* after complete remission is obtained strongly predicts the risk of relapse.

The differential diagnosis of the hypergranular variant of APL includes agranulocytosis with arrested maturation at the promyelocyte stage. With careful assessment, this distinction can usually be made quickly. In cases of agranulocytosis, the platelet count and hemoglobin are generally normal, the marrow is not hypercellular, the nuclear features of neoplastic promyelocytes are not present, and Auer rods are not observed. The immunophenotypic differential diagnosis includes cases of HLA-DR$^-$, CD34$^-$ AML, usually AML without differentiation. These cases can be distinguished by the abnormal "butterfly" nuclei and cytoplasmic granulation of APL. Cases of HLA-DR$^-$, CD34$^-$ AML without differentiation often show the "fish mouth" deformity or cup-like nuclear inclusions (Fig. 45-4). The microgranular variant of APL may mimic AML with monocytic differentiation, displaying folded nuclei. Strong myeloperoxidase reactivity by cytochemistry or flow cytometry can resolve this dilemma. In difficult cases, rapid FISH or RT-PCR assessment for the *PML-RARA* fusion can be requested, but in most cases, treatment should not be dealyed for molecular genetic confirmation.

Acute Promyelocytic Leukemia with Variant *RARA* Translocations

Uncommonly, a case with many of the morphologic, immunophenotypic, and clinical features of promyelocytic leukemia has a variant cytogenetic translocation that involves the *RARA* gene on chromosome 17 but not the *PML* gene on chromosome 15.[54-56] Table 45-1 shows the most common partner genes. The t(11;17)(q23;q12) (*ZBTB16-RARA*; formerly known as *PLZF-RARA*) is the best described translocation. The morphology differs from that of hypergranular or microgranular APL in that the majority of blast cell nuclei are round to oval (Fig. 45-5), Auer rods are usually absent, and pelgeroid neutrophils may be seen. Patients with variant *RARA* translocations often experience disseminated intravascular coagulation. These cases are important to recognize because although they have many of the features of typical APL, some variants, including those with *ZBTB16-RARA*, do not respond to ATRA therapy.

Acute Myeloid Leukemia with t(9;11)(p22;q23) (*MLLT3-MLL*)

Translocations involving the *MLL* gene on chromosome 11q23 are found in approximately 6% of cases of AML and are associated with more than 70 different partner genes.[57-59]

Table 45-1 Common Translocation Partners in Acute Promyelocytic Leukemia with Variant *RARA* Translocations

Chromosome Region	Involved Gene (Prior Name)	Expected ATRA Response
11q23	*ZBTB16* (*PLZF*)	Resistant
11q13	*NUMA1*	Probably responsive
5q35	*NPM1*	Probably responsive
17q11.2	*STAT5B*	Resistant

ATRA, all-*trans*-retinoic acid.

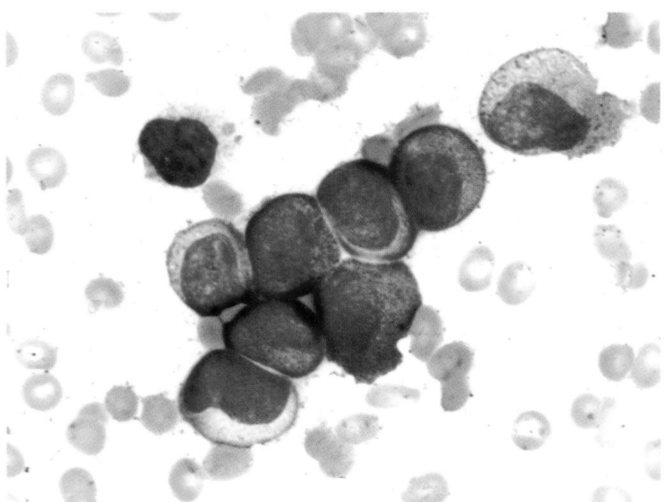

Figure 45-5. Acute promyelocytic leukemia with t(11;17)(q23;q12), *ZBTB16-RARA*. This rare type of acute promyelocytic leukemia is associated with abundant cytoplasmic granules, similar to the more common acute promyelocytic leukemia with t(15;17)(q22;q12). However, it has more round to oval blast cell nuclei, rather than the typical bilobed nuclei of the disease with t(15;17)(q22;q12).

In addition to de novo AML, *MLL* rearrangements are common in therapy-related myeloid proliferations, acute lymphoblastic leukemia, and acute leukemias of ambiguous lineage. The 2008 WHO category of AML with recurrent genetic abnormalities limits cases of 11q23 translocations specifically to AML with t(9;11)(p22;q23). AML with t(9;11)(p22;q23) typically occurs in children and has an intermediate prognosis (Box 45-5).[60] These patients may present with disseminated intravascular coagulation or extramedullary disease involving the gingiva and skin. The blasts typically have monocytic or myelomonocytic morphology, although occasionally they lack differentiation (Fig. 45-6). Cases composed morphologically of mostly monoblasts and promonocytes are typically myeloperoxidase negative by cytochemistry. In children, AML with t(9;11)(p22;q23) expresses CD33, CD4, CD65, and HLA-DR, with minimal to no CD13, CD14, and CD34 expression.[61] In adults, AML with 11q23 translocations often shows monocytic morphologic differentiation and may express multiple monocytic antigens, including CD14, CD64, CD11b, CD11c, and CD4. CD34 is often negative, with variable CD117 and CD56 reactivity.[62]

AML with balanced translocations of 11q23 other than t(9;11)(p22;q23) are diagnosed as AML, NOS, and the translocation is stated in the diagnosis line. The exceptions are those cases occurring after cytotoxic therapy, which are considered therapy-related AML, and those with the MDS-associated genetic abnormalities t(11;16)(q23;p13.3) and t(2;11)(p21;q23), which are considered AML with myelodysplasia-related changes. Another common translocation of *MLL* in de novo AML is t(11;19)(q23;p13) (*MLL-ELL*). Table 45-2 lists the more common *MLL* translocations in AML, with their

Box 45-5 *Key Features of Acute Myeloid Leukemia with t(9;11)(p22;q23) (MLLT3-MLL)*

- Typically occurs in childhood
- Monocytic morphology of blast cells most common
- Intermediate prognosis

Table 45-2 Most Common Translocation Partners with *MLL* in Acute Myeloid Leukemia (AML)

Chromosome Region	Involved Gene (Prior Name)	Frequency in *MLL*-Translocated AML (%)
9p22	*MLLT3* (*AF9*)	27-34
10p12	*MLLT10* (*AF10*)	13-18
19p13.1	*ELL*	11-18
6q27	*MLLT4* (*AF6*)	10-16
19p13.3	*MLLT1* (*ENL*)	5-8

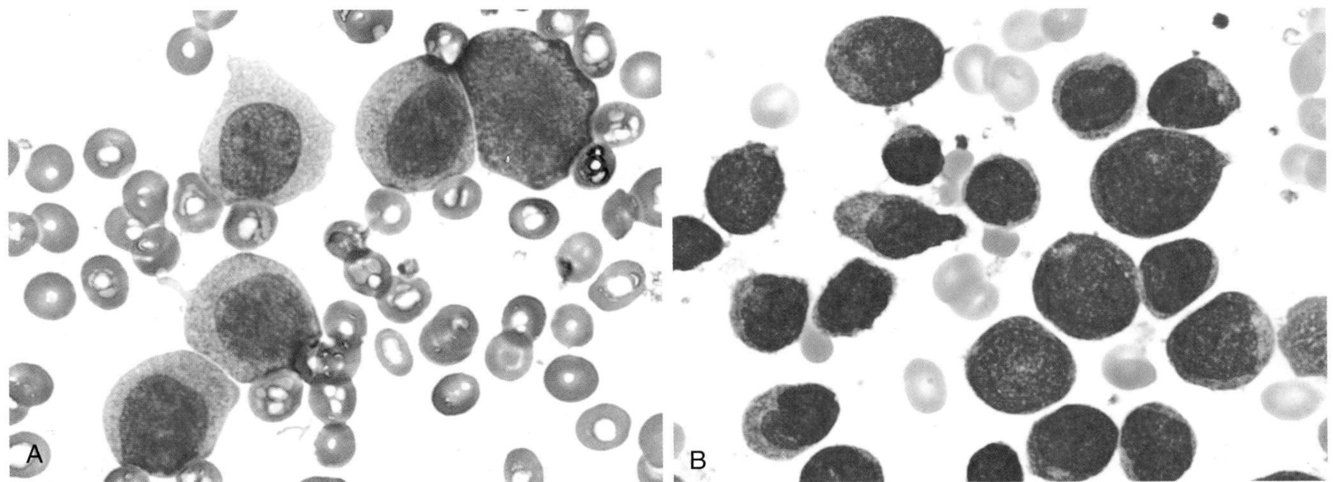

Figure 45-6. Acute myeloid leukemia with t(9;11)(p22;q23), *MLLT3-MLL*. The morphologic appearance is variable. **A,** This case shows abundant basophilic cytoplasm, suggestive of monocytic differentiation. **B,** This case shows blasts with a more myeloblastic appearance, including some cells with granules. Although myelomonocytic or monocytic features are most common, there are no specific morphologic features of this translocation.

relative frequencies and common morphologies. Translocation (4;11) is most common in acute lymphoblastic leukemia and acute leukemias of ambiguous lineage. Gene mutations in *KIT* or *FLT3* ITD are very uncommon in AML with 11q23 translocations. Approximately 20% of AML with t(9;11)(p22;q23) have activating loop domain point mutations in *FLT3*, but these are of uncertain prognostic significance. Pediatric AML with t(9;11)(p22;q23) has an intermediate prognosis, whereas leukemias with an 11q23 translocation involving a different partner chromosome generally have a poorer prognosis. Overexpression of the *EVI1* (ectopic virus integration-1) gene has been described in multiple variant translocations of 11q23 and is associated with a very poor prognosis.[63]

The differential diagnosis of AML with t(9;11)(p22;q23) includes various categories of AML, NOS; therapy-related AML; and mixed phenotype acute leukemia. The morphologic and immunophenotypic features cannot resolve the differential diagnosis with AML, NOS or therapy-related AML; proper classification depends on the cytogenetic findings and a clinical history of prior therapy. A history of prior cytotoxic therapy takes precedence over this de novo AML category. Cases that meet immunophenotypic criteria for mixed phenotype acute leukemia with *MLL* rearranged may be designated as such, but the presence of t(9;11)(p22;q23) should be clearly designated because this may be a more important prognostic finding than the mixed phenotype.

Acute Myeloid Leukemia with t(6;9)(p23;q34) (*DEK-NUP214*)

AML with t(6;9)(p23;q34) is a rare subtype accounting for approximately 1% of cases in both children and adults.[64-67] The median age in adults with this subtype of AML is 35 years. The translocation is reported in de novo AML, AML arising from MDS, and, less commonly, therapy-related AML. Most cases would have been classified as AML with multilineage dysplasia in the 2001 WHO classification and meet the criteria for a variety of FAB AML types, other than M3 (Box 45-6). Adults with AML with t(6;9)(p23;q34) tend to present with low white blood cell counts compared with other types of AML. Children may have more profound anemia. The blasts of AML with t(6;9)(p23;q34) may show occasional Auer rods and may exhibit monocytic features. Anisopoikilocytosis, circulating nucleated red blood cells, hypogranular neutrophils, and hypogranular platelets may be seen on the peripheral blood smear. Residual myeloid maturation is often present in the marrow, with dysplastic-appearing mature forms. Erythroid hyperplasia with dyserythropoiesis is also common, including ring sideroblasts in some cases. Small hypolobated megakaryocytes may be seen (Fig. 45-7). These dysplastic features are common to t(6;9) disease, but AML with t(6;9)(p23;q34)—now a distinct disease category—should be diagnosed rather than the less specific AML with myelodysplasia-related changes. Basophilia (>2% marrow or blood basophils) is present in roughly half of reported cases, a feature unique to this type of AML. By flow cytometry, blasts typically express CD45, CD13, CD33, HLA-DR, and intracytoplasmic myeloperoxidase, with variable expression of CD34, CD15 and CD11c. Terminal deoxynucleotidyl transferase (TdT) may be positive in some cases by flow cytometry or immunohistochemistry. *FLT3* ITD mutations are common in this type of AML,[65] with a reported frequency of 70%. Although the majority of patients with t(6;9) AML may achieve complete remission, survival rates are very poor with conventional chemotherapy. Like other high-risk categories of AML, patients may benefit from allogeneic stem cell transplantation. It is unclear whether the poor prognosis of AML with t(6;9) is independent of *FLT3* status. Some studies suggest a role for monitoring *DEK-NUP214* molecular status in patient manage-

Box 45-6 *Key Features of Acute Myeloid Leukemia with t(6;9)(p23;q34) (DEK-NUP214)*

- No specific blast cell morphology
- Often associated with erythroid hyperplasia and dysplasia
- Basophilia common
- Frequently associated with *FLT3* mutations
- Generally poor prognosis

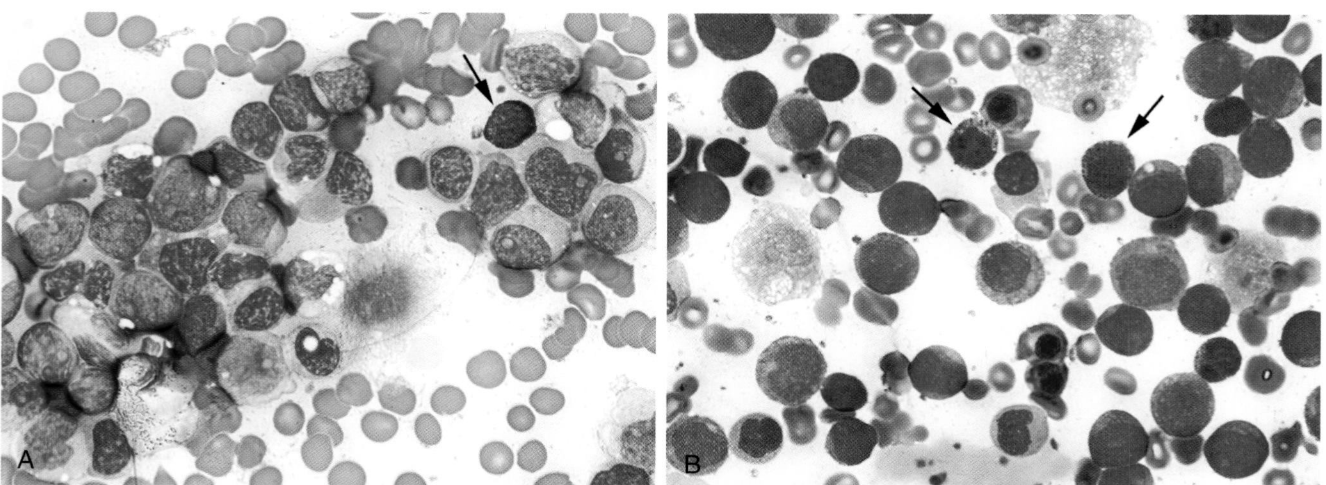

Figure 45-7. Acute myeloid leukemia with t(6;9)(p23;q34), *DEK-NUP214*. Blast cells exhibit variable morphology but are often associated with admixed basophils (*arrows*). **A,** Blasts with monocytic features. **B,** Myeloblasts without maturation and dysplastic erythroid precursors.

ribosome biogenesis, centrosomal duplication, and regulation of the *ARF-TP53* tumor suppressor pathway.[99,100] Mutations in exon 12 affect the amino acid composition of the nucleophosmin C-terminus; this creates a nuclear export motif, with resultant dislocation of nucleophosmin to the cytoplasm. *NPM1* is a chromosomal translocation partner in various types of leukemia and lymphoma in which the aberrantly regulated product appears to be oncogenic. The native product apparently has both oncogenic and tumor suppressor capabilities. *NPM1* is typically located in nucleoli. In patients with *NPM1* mutations, nucleophosmin becomes aberrantly localized to the cytoplasm, identifiable by immunohistochemistry. However, it should be stressed that the mutation status of both *NPM1* and *FLT3* needs to be assessed, and at present there are no immunophenotypic methods of detecting *FLT3* mutations. For this reason, many laboratories perform a multiplex PCR assay to evaluate the mutation status of both genes in new cases of AML, making immunohistochemical evaluation unnecessary.[101,102]

The frequency and prognostic significance of *NPM1* mutations in AML with myelodysplasia-related changes are not yet clear, although such mutations do not appear to be common in MDS. Because of this uncertainty, cases that meet the criteria for AML with myelodysplasia-related changes and have *NPM1* mutations should be classified as such, with the mutation results included in the diagnosis (i.e., AML with myelodysplasia-related changes [multilineage dysplasia] and mutated *NPM1*).[15]

Acute Myeloid Leukemia with Mutated *CEBPA*

CEBPA is a tumor suppressor gene located on chromosome 19q31.1 that encodes a differentiation-inducing transcription factor involved in granulocytic differentiation as well as diverse programs such as lung development, adipogenesis, and glucose metabolism.[103] *CEBPA* may be inactivated through multiple mechanisms, including transcriptional repression by the *RUNX1-RUNX1T1* fusion protein of t(8;21) AML and epigenetic modification. Point mutations of *CEBPA* are detected in 13% of cytogenetically normal AML in adults and in 17% to 20% of cytogenetically normal AML in children.[104-106] More than 100 different nonsilent mutations have been described. This range of mutation sites makes routine testing for this mutation more complicated, and the assay is not widely available at this time.[107] Mutations commonly lead to synthesis of a smaller dominant negative isoform that inhibits wild-type protein function. Unlike the common association between *NPM1* and *FLT3* ITD mutations, *FLT3* abnormalities are relatively uncommon in AML with *CEBPA* mutations. Recent studies suggest that the prognostic significance of *CEBPA* mutations in AML relates to the presence of double mutations of the gene and to the lack of *FLT3* mutations and poor prognostic cytogenetic abnormalities.[108-111] In the absence of these adverse prognostic factors, AML with *CEBPA* mutations has a favorable prognosis, and patients are unlikely to benefit from allogeneic stem cell transplantation; however, further study is needed to address optimal postremission therapy because the number of cases studied is too small to be definitive.

The morphologic subtypes of myeloblasts in AML with *CEBPA* mutations are most commonly AML with and without differentiation. AML with myelomonocytic or monocytic differentiation is less commonly seen, and erythroleukemia or megakaryoblastic leukemia has not been described. *CEBPA* mutations are rarely described in therapy-related AML, but when they occur, the diagnosis should be therapy-related AML, with a comment on the detection of a *CEBPA* mutation. Approximately 70% of AML with *CEBPA* mutations have a normal karyotype. Approximately 10% have a single karyotypic abnormality, and only rare cases have a complex karyotype. No specific immunophenotype of AML with *CEBPA* mutations has been described.

Box 45-9 ***Key Features of Acute Myeloid Leukemia with Myelodysplasia-Related Changes***

- More common in older patients
- May arise from myelodysplasia or de novo
- Dysplastic changes usually present in ≥50% of cells from two cell lines
- Generally poor prognosis

ACUTE MYELOID LEUKEMIA WITH MYELODYSPLASIA-RELATED CHANGES

The 2001 WHO category of AML with multilineage dysplasia was revised in 2008 in an effort to more accurately characterize this clinicobiologic entity.[15,112] AML with multilineage dysplasia was commonly associated with poor-risk cytogenetic abnormalities, and the significance of the morphologic changes independent of the cytogenetic findings was debated.[23,113-118] The 2008 WHO classification revised and expanded this category to AML with myelodysplasia-related changes (AML-MRC; Box 45-9). The category now includes patients with any of the following: (1) AML arising from a previous MDS or myelodysplastic/myeloproliferative neoplasm (MDS/MPN), (2) AML with a specific MDS-associated cytogenetic abnormality, and (3) AML with multilineage dysplasia (Box 45-10; Table 45-3).

AML-MRC is more common in elderly patients. Older literature suggested a frequency of 25% to 30% of all AML; however, given the new criteria, the diagnosis of AML-MRC may account for 50% of adult AML. Although it is reportedly rare in children, more children will likely be recognized as having AML-MRC, given the incorporation of cytogenetic criteria.

Box 45-10 ***Criteria for the Diagnosis of Acute Myeloid Leukemia with Myelodysplasia-Related Changes***

- ≥20% blood or marrow blasts
  AND
- Any one of the following:
  - Previous history of myelodysplastic syndrome
  - Myelodysplastic syndrome–related cytogenetic abnormality (see Table 45-3)
  - Multilineage dysplasia

  AND
- Absence of both of the following:
  - Prior cytotoxic therapy for an unrelated disease
  - Recurring cytogenetic abnormality as described for acute myeloid leukemia with recurrent genetic abnormalities

Table 45-3 Cytogenetic Abnormalities Sufficient to Diagnose Acute Myeloid Leukemia with Myelodysplasia-Related Changes When ≥20% Blood or Marrow Blasts Are Present

Complex Karyotype*	
Unbalanced Abnormalities:	**Balanced Abnormalities:**
	t(11;16)(q23;p13.3)†
−7/del(7q)	t(3;21)(q26.2;q22.1)†
−5/del(5q)	t(1;3)(p26.3;q21.1)
i(17q)/t(17p)	t(2;11)(p21;q23)
−13/del(13q)	t(5;12)(q33;p12)
del(11q)	t(5;7)(q33;q11.2)
del(12p)/t(12p)	t(5;17)(q33;p13)
del(9q)	t(5;10)(q33;q21)
idic(X)(q13)	t(3;5)(q25;q34)

*Three or more unrelated abnormalities, none of which is included in the acute myeloid leukemia (AML) with recurrent genetic abnormalities subgroup (such cases should be classified in the appropriate cytogenetic group).
†These abnormalities most commonly occur in therapy-related disease, and therapy-related AML should be excluded before using these abnormalities to diagnose AML with myelodysplasia-related changes.

The blast count is variable but must be 20% or more in the blood or marrow. To meet the morphologic criteria for AML-MRC, there must be evidence of dysplasia in 50% or more of developing cells in two or more lineages (Fig. 45-12). Cases of AML-MRC frequently have the features of AML with maturation or acute myelomonocytic leukemia, although cases with features of AML without maturation and erythroleukemia may also exhibit multilineage dysplasia. Many of the uncommon examples of hypocellular AML have multilineage dysplasia and may evolve from hypocellular MDS. Hypocellular AML and MDS are defined by a bone marrow cellularity of less than 30% (<20% in patients older than 60 years), although they are not considered distinct entities in the WHO classification.

There are no distinctive immunophenotypic findings in AML-MRC.[15,118] In general, the blasts are $CD34^+$ and $CD117^+$ and express the pan-myeloid markers CD13 and CD33. Aberrant expression of CD7, CD10, and CD56 may occur. Similar to the frequent morphologic suggestion of monocytic differentiation, this AML type often expresses CD4 and CD14. Cases with abnormalities of chromosomes 5 and 7 may show "aberrant" expression of TdT and CD7, along with CD34.

MDS-associated chromosomal abnormalities are commonly high-risk changes. Monosomy 7 has a particularly poor prognosis in pediatric AML.[119] Although trisomy 8, del(20q), and loss of chromosome Y are common in MDS, they are not considered sufficient in isolation for a diagnosis of AML-MRC. A complex karyotype, defined as three or more unrelated clonal abnormalities, is universally considered unfavorable.[120] Unbalanced structural abnormalities leading to a loss of genetic material are the most common aberrations.[121] The most common constituents of the complex karyotype are (in order of decreasing frequency) deletions of 5q, loss of 7q, loss of 17p, loss of 18q, and loss of 12p. Gains of chromosomal material are much less common and often involve chromosome 8q, 21q, or 11q.

Nine balanced abnormalities are included in the MDS-associated cytogenetic abnormalities diagnostic of AML-MRC. Almost all these rearrangements are also seen in therapy-related myeloid proliferations. If a history of cytotoxic therapy for another neoplasm is present, the case should be diagnosed as therapy-related AML, not AML-MRC. Four of the nine rearrangements involve 5q33, often with activation of the platelet-derived growth factor receptor-β (*PDGFRB*) at that locus. Imatinib is approved for the treatment of MDS and chronic myelomonocytic leukemia with translocations involving 5q33, but its efficacy in AML-MRC with this rearrangement is unclear. Two other rearrangements involve 3q26 (*EVI1* locus) and 3q21 (*RPN1* and *GATA2* loci), both involved in the recurrent genetic abnormality AML with inv(3)(q21q26.2) or t(3;3)(q21;q26.2) (see earlier). Two additional rearrangements involve the *MLL* locus at 11q23, and they should be diagnosed as AML-MRC (MDS-associated cytogenetic abnormality), not AML with 11q23 rearrangement (which is now restricted to t[9;11]). The final rearrangement, t(3;5)(q25;q35), may represent a unique genetic abnormality

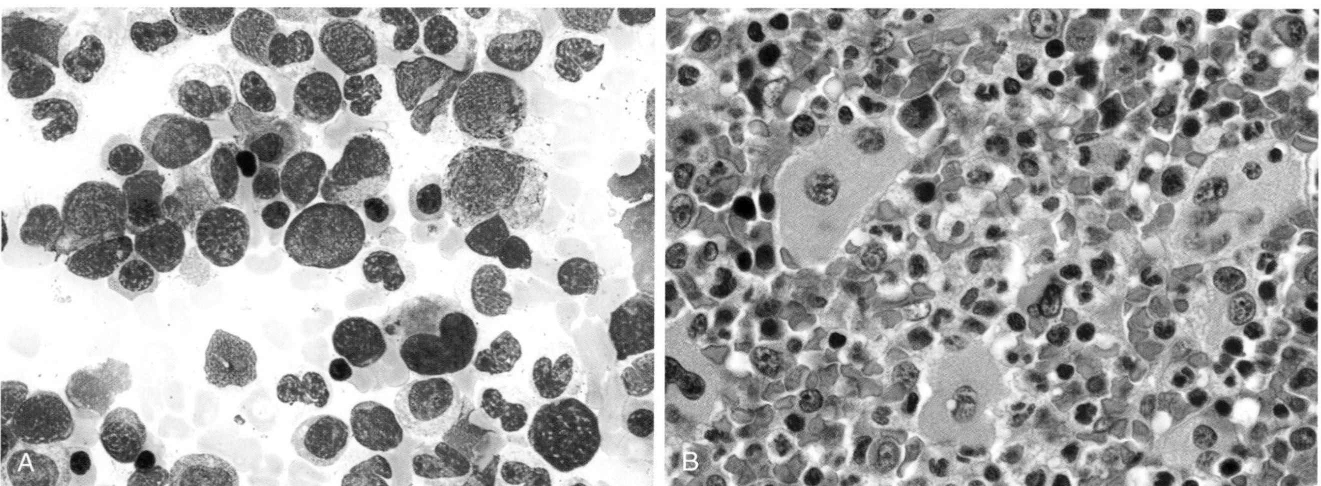

Figure 45-12. Acute myeloid leukemia with myelodysplasia-related changes. This proliferation requires 20% or more blood or bone marrow myeloblasts, as well as dysplastic changes in 50% or more of cells in at least two cell lines to diagnose this category by morphologic criteria. The dysplastic changes are best seen on aspirate smears (**A**), but dysplastic megakaryocytes are often apparent on biopsy sections (**B**). On the aspirate smear (**A**), note the hypogranular neutrophils with abnormal nuclear lobation, erythroid precursors with irregular nuclear contours, and small hypolobated megakaryocytes with admixed blasts cells.

in AML and has already been discussed. Patients with AML-MRC characterized by multilineage dysplasia and normal cytogenetics may have mutations of *FLT3* or *NPM1*, or both that affect their prognosis; however, the prognostic significance of these combinations of factors is unclear at this time. Therefore, the diagnosis should reflect the presence of these mutations in addition to the designation AML-MRC (multilineage dysplasia). *CEBPA* mutations are generally not found in this setting.

The prognosis of AML-MRC is typically unfavorable but is somewhat dependent on individual factors. In patients with lower blast counts and multilineage dysplasia (20% to 29% blasts), the disease may behave more like MDS, especially in children, with a slower disease progression. Patients with MDS-associated cytogenetic abnormalities have a more consistently poor prognosis. Multilineage dysplasia may not be detected in up to half of cases with MDS-associated cytogenetic abnormalities. It has been observed that patients with MDS-associated cytogenetic abnormalities have a worse prognosis than those with multilineage dysplasia lacking cytogenetic abnormalities.[115,117] The morphologic designation seems to be clinically useful, however, because patients with a normal or intermediate-risk karyotype and multilineage dysplasia have worse outcomes than those with AML, NOS.[118] The presence of a monosomal karyotype or overexpression of the *EVI1* gene may confer a particularly poor prognosis.[122,123]

The basis for categorization as AML-MRC should be stated in the diagnosis (e.g., AML-MRC [multilineage dysplasia and myelodysplasia-associated cytogenetic abnormality]), as should the presence of mutations in *NPM1*, *CEBPA*, or *FLT3*. The blast count should be clearly stated in the report so that patients with lower blast counts can be followed closely for progression.

The differential diagnosis of AML-MRC includes MDS, various categories of AML with recurrent genetic abnormalities, and AML, NOS. Differentiation between AML-MRC and MDS is resolved by the bone marrow blast cell count performed on aspirate smears; cases with 20% or more blasts are designated AML, and those with less than 20% are MDS. Blast cell counts based on flow cytometric immunophenotyping studies are not suitable owing to potential problems related to gating, cell lysis, and cell preservation that may lead to a different result than that obtained by a manual count. AML with recurrent cytogenetic abnormalities, especially inv(3)(q21q26.2) or t(3;3)(q21;q26.2) and t(6;9)(p23;q34), often meet the criteria for AML-MRC but should be diagnosed as the more specific cytogenetic disease type. In contrast, cases of AML-MRC with *NPM1* mutations and, much less commonly, *CEBPA* mutations should be diagnosed as AML-MRC with the specific mutation noted. The criteria for AML-MRC take precedence over all categories of AML, NOS, as long as the blast cell count is 20% or greater in the marrow.

Recent data suggest that autosomal monosomies are an even better marker of poor prognosis than complex cytogenetic abnormalities when there are either two autosomal monosomies in the karyotype or one autosomal monosomy in the presence of one or more structural chromosomal abnormalities (excluding core binding factor abnormalities).[122] Monosomy 7 appears to be most frequent, but the dismal prognosis seems to be independent of which particular autosomal chromosome is monosomic. AML-MRC criteria capture many of these cases in which monosomy 7 or 5 is involved, but this category does not capture all cases with this poor prognostic indicator.

THERAPY-RELATED MYELOID NEOPLASMS

Therapy-related myeloid neoplasms include cases of AML, MDS, and MDS/MPN that occur after cytotoxic chemotherapy or radiation therapy (Box 45-11).[16,124] They account for approximately 10% of AML and 20% of MDS and are among the deadliest late complications of chemotherapy. Although the various diseases can be subclassified based on marrow and blood blast cell counts, they are considered a single disease entity owing to their similar behavior, which appears to be somewhat independent of blast cell count. The recognition of therapy-related myeloid neoplasms in the late 1970s coincided with the first time patients treated with chemotherapy for cancer actually survived long enough to develop the disease. Alkylating agents were the first to be implicated, with latency periods of 5 to 7 years and a dose-dependent effect related to the number of cycles of chemotherapy received. Radiotherapy, alone or in combination with chemotherapy, also increases the risk of therapy-related myeloid neoplasms. The myelodysplastic phase can precede overt therapy-related AML and last for months to years. Use of topoisomerase II inhibitors is associated with a different syndrome in which overt therapy-related AML develops 1 to 3 years after exposure, commonly without a myelodysplastic phase. Other treatments now recognized to be associated with therapy-related disease include autologous bone marrow transplantation and fludarabine chemotherapy. Hematologic malignancies are the most common primary tumor, accounting for approximately half the cases. Breast and ovarian cancers are also common primary tumors. A minority of patients receive chemotoxic agents for nonneoplastic disease. Why some patients are susceptible but others treated with similar regimens are not is a matter of current investigation.

Cases with longer latency typically present with cytopenias and multilineage dysplasia (Fig. 45-13). Typical MDS-associated morphologic features, such as macrocytosis and poikilocytosis of erythrocytes and hypogranular neutrophils with abnormal nuclear lobation, are usually present. The bone marrow may be hypercellular, normocellular, or hypocellular and may have associated fibrosis. Dyspoiesis of all three lineages is common and often striking. Erythropoiesis may exhibit megaloblastic maturation with abnormal nuclear contours or multinucleation; ring sideroblasts are common. Megakaryocytes often display small, abnormal forms with hypolobation or widely separated nuclear lobes. Blast counts

Box 45-11 *Key Features of Therapy-Related Acute Myeloid Leukemia*

- Cases with short latency are usually associated with topoisomerase II inhibitor therapy, have abnormalities of *MLL* or *RUNX1*, and may not exhibit associated dysplastic changes
- Cases with longer latency are more commonly associated with alkylating chemotherapy, deletions of chromosomes 5 and 7, complex karyotypes, and a myelodysplastic phase
- Both types are generally associated with a poor prognosis

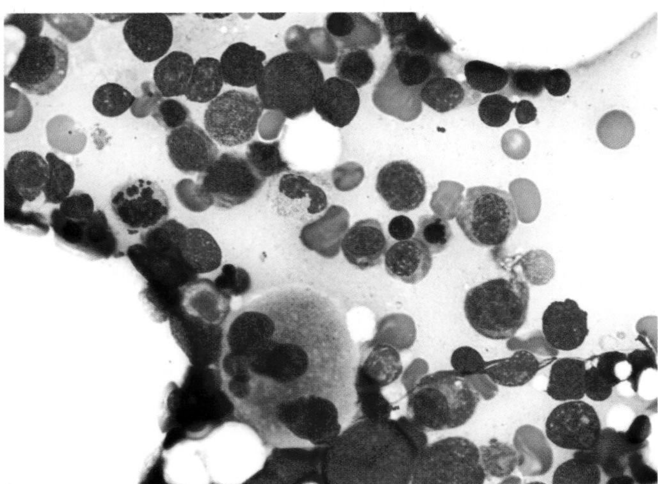

Figure 45-13. Therapy-related acute myeloid leukemia (AML) following alkylating agent chemotherapy. Multilineage dysplasia is characteristically present, similar to many cases of AML with myelodysplasia-related changes; however, the history of prior therapy places this case in the category of a therapy-related myeloid neoplasm.

are variable; approximately half the patients with therapy-related MDS have less than 5% blasts when initially diagnosed. Because of a similar poor outcome regardless of blast cell count, cases should not be classified as a specific subtype of MDS and should simply be diagnosed as therapy-related MDS.[125] Rare patients with therapy-related disease have features of MDS/MPN, and such cases are now included as therapy-related myeloid neoplasms. No specific immunophenotypic profile is associated with therapy-related disease, and there is immunophenotypic overlap with AML-MRC. Blasts are typically CD34^{+}, with expression of CD13 and CD33. CD7 and CD56 expression is not uncommon. Cytogenetic characterization of therapy-related myeloid neoplasms shows that cases with longer latency are similar to AML-MRC; are often associated with chromosomal losses, commonly of chromosomes 5 and 7; and often occur in the setting of a complex karyotype.[126]

A shorter latency period is seen in 20% to 30% of therapy-related myeloid neoplasms. Cases with shorter latency commonly have balanced chromosomal translocations that involve *MLL* at 11q23 or *RUNX1* at 21q22.[126-128] The morphologic features are similar to those of de novo AML without associated dysplastic changes (Fig. 45-14).[129] They usually exhibit morphologic features of AML with maturation, acute myelomonocytic leukemia, and acute monocytic leukemia. Some patients with short-latency therapy-related AML have karyotypic changes identical to those of de novo AML, including some good prognostic categories similar to those of the core binding factor leukemias or APL.[127,130] In contrast to the dismal prognosis of most therapy-related AML some reports suggest that cases with t(15;17) or inv(16) may have a prognosis more similar to their de novo counterparts. However, a recent study of therapy-related core binding factor AML showed a significantly worse survival rate when compared with de novo core binding factor AML.[131]

The prognosis of therapy-related myeloid neoplasms is generally poor, with reported overall survival less than 10%.[124] Treatment is impaired by dose-limiting toxicities of the prior chemotherapeutic agents, as well as by the expression of drug-resistance mechanisms in the neoplastic cells. Patients with monosomy 5 or 7 karyotypes have a particularly dismal prognosis, with a median survival of less than 1 year, regardless of the blast percentage. *FLT3* mutations have been observed in therapy-related AML, but their contribution to prognosis is unknown. There are few data on *NPM1* or *CEBPA* mutations in this disorder,[126,132,133] but a recent study found *NPM1* mutations in 7 of 51 patients with therapy-related AML. These cases were associated with *FLT3* mutations, and most had normal karyotypes, similar to more typical cases of AML with mutated *NPM1*. The prognostic significance of these mutations in therapy-related AML is not yet known. Therapeutic options for patients with therapy-related myeloid neoplasms are limited owing to the high rate of treatment-related mortality, high rate of treatment failure, and early disease recurrence for those patients who respond to therapy.

The differential diagnosis of the therapy-related myeloid neoplasms consists of their de novo counterparts, including the various categories of AML, NOS and MDS/MPNs, as well as various subtypes of non–therapy-related myelodysplasia and AML-MRC. A history of cytotoxic or radiation therapy for a prior neoplastic or nonneoplastic disorder takes precedence over these other categories, and all such cases should be considered therapy-related neoplasms, despite morphologic or cytogenetic similarities to these other disease categories. As mentioned previously, it is not appropriate to classify cases as specific subtypes of more traditional MDS when the disorder occurs as a therapy-related neoplasm.

ACUTE MYELOID LEUKEMIA, NOT OTHERWISE SPECIFIED

Cases of AML that do not fulfill the definition of AML with recurrent genetic abnormalities, AML-MRC, therapy-related myeloid neoplasm, or myeloid neoplasm of Down syndrome are considered AML, NOS.[13] There are a number of subtypes

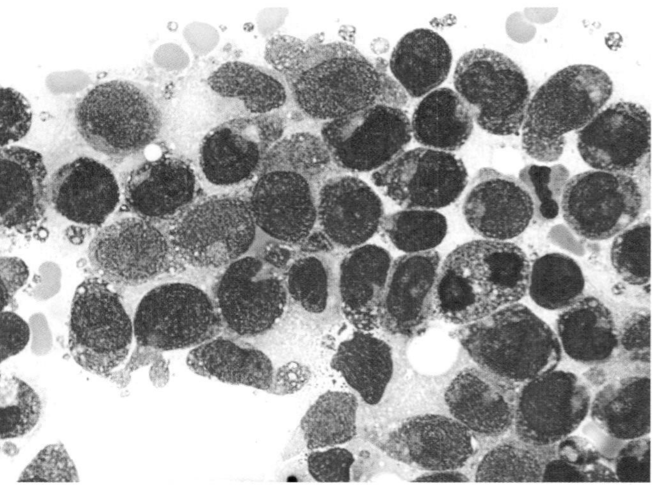

Figure 45-14. Therapy-related acute myeloid leukemia following topoisomerase II inhibitor therapy. This case, which has an 11q23 translocation involving *MLL*, shows blasts with monocytic features and no background dysplasia, typical of therapy-related disease with this cytogenetic abnormality.

of AML, NOS in the 2008 WHO classification, but most of these lack the cytogenetic or clinical features that would warrant calling them specific disease types, and they should be considered morphologic subtypes. Because these morphologic subtypes lack clinical or biologic significance,[23,134] subclassification of AML, NOS is not essential. The exceptions are the erythroid leukemias and acute panmyelosis with myelofibrosis, which are defined by different criteria. Most of the morphologic subtypes of AML, NOS are defined by previous FAB criteria,[2] with the exception of a 20% marrow blast cell count being sufficient for a diagnosis of acute leukemia (as opposed to a 30% cutoff by the FAB). Because flow cytometric immunophenotyping is routine in modern practice, cytochemical studies are not required for the subtyping of AML, NOS, although they may provide helpful information in selected cases.

There are few data on the clinical and genetic features of the AML, NOS subtypes. Prior studies of the epidemiology and clinical relevance of FAB subtypes are not useful because the various FAB types contained numerous other AML subtypes that are now considered separate entities. As a group, AML, NOS represents approximately 40% of adult AML, occurs at a younger age than AML-MRC, and has an intermediate prognosis.[118] This category includes many cases of AML with a normal karyotype, and mutation analysis is probably the most predictive marker of prognosis in this group. Cases with *NPM1* or *CEBPA* mutations should be classified as the provisional entities of AML with *NPM1* mutations or *CEBPA* mutations rather than as AML, NOS.

Acute Myeloid Leukemia with Minimal Differentiation

AML with minimal differentiation has 20% or more marrow blasts that lack definitive cytologic and cytochemical evidence of myeloid lineage but demonstrate immunophenotypic evidence of myeloid lineage. The blasts lack granules or Auer rods and may be confused with lymphoblasts. The blasts are cytochemically negative for myeloperoxidase or Sudan black B (<3% positive) and are nonspecific esterase negative (<20%), but they may show immunophenotypic evidence of myeloperoxidase expression. By flow cytometry, blasts express CD34, CD38, and HLA-DR. They commonly express CD13, CD33, or CD117. The blasts usually lack expression of monocytic or myeloid antigens such as CD15, CD11b, CD14, or CD64. Expression of CD7, CD19, and TdT may be present, but blasts are negative for the more definitive B- and T-lymphoid–associated cytoplasmic antigens CD79a, CD22, and CD3. Mutations of *RUNX1* (*AML1*) and mutations or deletions of *ETV6* are reported in a subset of cases based on older diagnostic criteria.[135,136]

Acute Myeloid Leukemia without Maturation

AML without maturation is defined as a bone marrow blast population of 20% or more that is cytochemically positive for myeloperoxidase or Sudan black B and negative (<20%) for nonspecific esterase. In addition, blasts must constitute 90% or more of the nonerythroid marrow cells. Blasts usually have sparse granules and infrequent Auer rods, although the identification of these features does not preclude this diagnosis. Cases may be mistaken for lymphoblastic proliferations without immunophenotyping or cytochemical studies. Blasts express myeloid-associated antigens, but there is no specific immunophenotypic profile.

Acute Myeloid Leukemia with Maturation

AML with maturation is probably the most common morphologic type of AML, NOS. It has cytochemical features identical to those of AML without maturation, with 20% or more marrow blasts; however, it differs by having more than 10% of nonerythroid marrow cells showing maturation to the promyelocyte or later stage of differentiation. Blasts more frequently contain cytoplasmic granules or Auer rods but exhibit no specific cytogenetic abnormalities or immunophenotypic profile.

Acute Myelomonocytic Leukemia

In acute myelomonocytic leukemia (AMML), the sum of myeloblasts, monoblasts, and promonocytes is 20% or more. Twenty percent to 79% of the bone marrow cells are of monocyte lineage, often demonstrated by reactivity with the nonspecific esterase stain; however, cytochemical studies are not necessary for diagnosis when the morphologic identity of the monocyte lineage is obvious. Numerous monocytes may be present in the peripheral blood and may mimic MDS/MPN, especially chronic myelomonocytic leukemia. Both granulocytic and monocytic differentiation are observed in varying proportions in the bone marrow. The major criterion distinguishing AMML from AML with maturation is the proportion of neoplastic cells with monocytic features, which collectively must equal 20% or more. The immunophenotype of AMML generally reflects the dual differentiation pattern of the leukemic cells, with some populations expressing fairly typical myeloid antigens and others expressing more monocytic antigens, including CD14 and CD64.

Careful distinction of promonocytes from abnormal monocytes in the bone marrow is essential to separate AMML from chronic myelomonocytic leukemia.[17] Promonocytes retain fine chromatin, indistinct nucleoli, and delicate nuclear folds, reflecting their immaturity. In contrast, abnormal immature-appearing monocytes of chronic myelomonocytic leukemia have more condensed chromatin and generally more folded or convoluted nuclear contours. In a new diagnosis, the distinction between chronic myelomonocytic leukemia from AMML may not be possible with a peripheral blood smear. Correlation with bone marrow findings is essential to resolve the diagnosis, because the immature populations of AMML are more readily identified in marrow. A reliable discriminating immunophenotype is not available because promonocytes typically lack CD34.

Acute Monoblastic and Monocytic Leukemias

Acute monoblastic and monocytic leukemias have 20% or more immature cells (blasts or promonocytes) in bone marrow, and 80% or more of the marrow cells have monocytic features by morphology (Fig. 45-15), cytochemistry, or immunophenotyping studies. Cases can be further

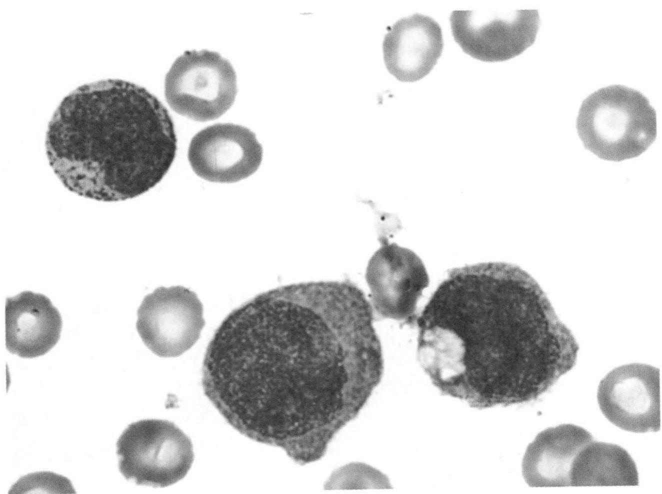

Figure 45-15. Acute monocytic leukemia. Blasts may have round or more monocytoid folded nuclei and cytoplasmic vacuoles. The leukemia in Figure 45-14 also has monocytic features, but the history of prior therapy takes precedence over the categories of acute myeloid leukemia, not otherwise specified.

subdivided by the maturity of the monocytic cells. If 80% or more of the monocytoid cells are immature (monoblasts), the case is considered acute monoblastic leukemia; if the cells show evidence of monocytic maturation and less than 80% are monoblasts, it is considered acute monocytic leukemia. Monoblasts are large and have moderately abundant, variably basophilic cytoplasm, which frequently contains delicate peroxidase-negative azurophilic granules or vacuoles. Auer rods are not observed. The nucleus is round, with reticular chromatin and one or more prominent nucleoli. Monoblasts are nonspecific esterase positive and myeloperoxidase negative. The leukemic cells in acute monocytic leukemia manifest more obvious cytologic evidence of monocytic differentiation and maturation. The nuclei have delicate chromatin and a characteristic folded or cerebriform appearance. The promonocyte cytoplasm is less basophilic than that of monoblasts and contains a variable number of azurophilic granules. The promonocytes are usually nonspecific esterase positive; some exhibit weak myeloperoxidase activity.

The immunophenotype of acute monoblastic and monocytic leukemia is characterized by the expression of monocytic differentiation antigens, but the patterns of expression vary. Both subtypes often lack CD34 but may express CD117. They commonly express HLA-DR, CD13, and bright CD33, with CD15 and CD65. Typically, at least two markers of monocytic differentiation are present, including CD14, CD4, CD11b, CD11c, CD64, CD68, CD36, lysozyme, and CD163. Aberrant expression of CD7 and CD56 is not unusual. Myeloperoxidase may be weakly positive in acute monocytic leukemia. Immunohistochemistry may show positivity for CD68 and lysozyme, but these are relatively nonspecific. CD163 appears to be a more specific marker for monocyte lineage, but it may be less sensitive.

Monoblastic and monocytic leukemias are associated with a high incidence of organomegaly, lymphadenopathy, and other tissue infiltration. In a significant number of cases, the first clinical manifestations of leukemia result from extramedullary tissue infiltrates. Despite these seemingly unique clinical features, a diagnosis of acute monoblastic or acute monocytic leukemia does not confer prognostic significance.[134]

Box 45-12 *Key Features of Acute Erythroid Leukemia*

- Erythroid/myeloid form must have >50% marrow erythroid precursors, with myeloblasts constituting ≥20% of nonerythroid marrow cells
- Pure erythroid leukemia does not have increased myeloblasts but has ≥80% pronormoblasts or early basophilic normoblasts
- Cases must be distinguished from therapy-related myeloid neoplasms and acute myeloid leukemia with myelodysplasia-related changes
- Both forms have an aggressive clinical course with a generally poor prognosis

Acute Erythroid Leukemia

Acute erythroid leukemias are composed predominantly of erythroid cells and are diagnosed using criteria that differ significantly from those of most other AML (Box 45-12). Two subtypes are included in the 2008 WHO classification, and these are distinguished by the presence or absence of an apparent myeloid blast component (erythroid/myeloid versus pure erythroid leukemia).

Erythroid/myeloid leukemia is the more common subtype. In this type, 50% or more of all nucleated bone marrow cells are erythroid precursors, and 20% or more of the remaining cells (nonerythroid) are myeloblasts (Fig. 45-16; see also Fig. 45-10). Most patients with erythroid/myeloid leukemia present with pancytopenia and nucleated red cells in the blood. The predominant leukemic cell in the marrow is the erythroblast. There is striking erythroid hyperplasia and dyserythropoiesis characterized by abnormalities of nuclear

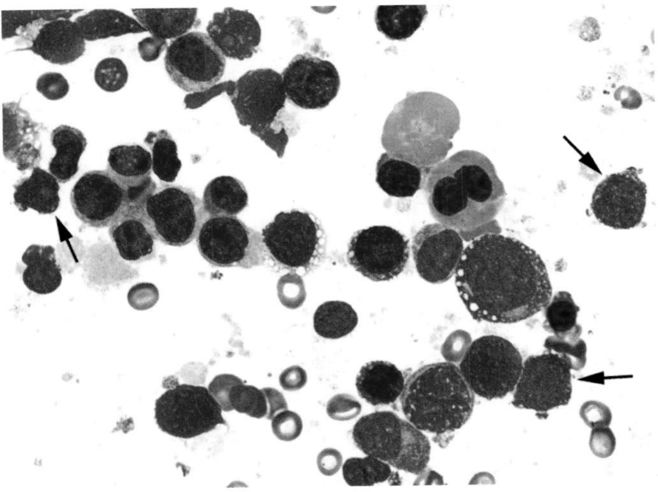

Figure 45-16. Acute erythroid leukemia (erythroid/myeloid). The majority of cells are dysplastic erythroid precursors, with scattered myeloblasts (*arrows*) present. Myeloblasts represent less than 20% of all marrow cells but more than 20% of nonerythroid cells, thus fulfilling the criteria for the erythroid/myeloid type of acute erythroid leukemia.

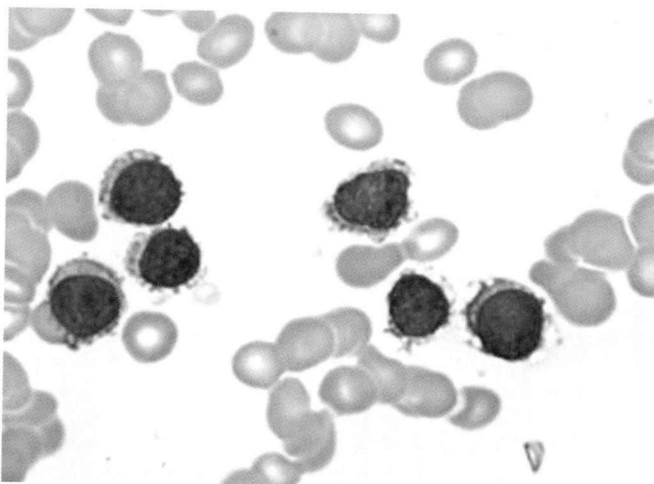

Figure 45-17. Pure erythroid leukemia. This rare leukemia exhibits a pure population of immature erythroid cells with cytoplasmic vacuoles and no myeloblast proliferation. These cells represent more than 80% of peripheral blood and marrow cells and express erythroid-associated markers of hemoglobin and glycophorin.

development, including megaloblastoid changes and karyorrhexis. The erythroblasts may contain cytoplasmic vacuoles that are periodic acid–Schiff positive. There is often evidence of a panmyelosis with striking megakaryocytic and platelet abnormalities. When more than 50% of the cells of two or more lineages are dysplastic and the myeloid blast cell percentage is 20% or more of all nucleated bone marrow cells, the case should be classified as AML-MRC on the basis of multilineage dysplasia. The erythroblasts are commonly $CD45^-$ by flow cytometry and lack expression of myeloid antigens. They may express detectable hemoglobin A or glycophorin, with aberrantly dim expression of CD71. The myeloid blasts are similar to those of AML without differentiation or AML with minimal differentiation. Auer rods may be present. Progression of the disease is frequently marked by an increase in myeloblasts and a decrease in erythroblasts.

In the rare cases of pure erythroid leukemia, the erythroid lineage is the only obvious component of acute leukemia; no myeloblast component is apparent. The neoplastic cells are predominantly or exclusively pronormoblasts and early basophilic normoblasts (Fig. 45-17). These cells must constitute 80% or more of the marrow elements. The erythroblasts are commonly $CD34^-$ and $HLA\text{-}DR^-$ by flow cytometry and lack expression of myeloid-associated antigens. The more mature forms express hemoglobin A and glycophorin. The more immature erythroid progenitors may be $CD36^+$. Some cases may also express megakaryocytic markers, such as CD41 and CD61, and it may not be possible to distinguish such cases as having an erythroid or a megakaryocytic lineage.[137]

There is often significant overlap among the erythroid leukemias, AML-MRC, and MDS. Myelodysplasia-related cytogenetic abnormalities and multilineage dysplasia are common in these disorders, and cases that fulfill the criteria for other disease categories, especially AML-MRC, should be diagnosed as such. A third type of erythroleukemia in which the marrow contains 30% or more myeloblasts and 30% or more erythroid precursors has been proposed,[138] but such case are best diagnosed in other categories, such as AML-MRC. The erythroid leukemias must also be distinguished from several nonneoplastic disorders that manifest marked dyserythropoiesis. These include megaloblastic anemia due to vitamin B_{12} or folate deficiency, heavy metal intoxication from arsenic, drug effects, and congenital dyserythropoiesis.

Acute Megakaryoblastic Leukemia

Acute megakaryoblastic leukemia is defined by the presence of 20% or more bone marrow blasts, at least 50% of which are megakaryoblasts, in patients who do not meet the criteria for a myeloid neoplasm of Down syndrome, AML with t(1;22)(p13;q13), AML with t(3;3)(q21;q26) or inv(3)(q21;q6), or AML-MRC.[13,79,139] Using these criteria, the acute megakaryoblastic leukemia type of AML, NOS is uncommon. In blood and bone marrow smears, megakaryoblasts are usually medium to large cells with a high nuclear-to-cytoplasmic ratio. Nuclear chromatin is dense and homogeneous. Nucleoli are variably prominent. There is scant to moderately abundant cytoplasm, which may be vacuolated. An irregular cytoplasmic border is often noted, and projections resembling budding platelets are occasionally present. Transitional forms between poorly differentiated blasts and recognizable micromegakaryocytes may be observed. In some cases the majority of the leukemic cells consist of small lymphoid-like blasts. A marrow aspirate may be difficult to obtain because of frequent myelofibrosis. Trephine biopsy sections may reveal morphologic evidence of megakaryocytic differentiation that is not appreciated in the marrow aspirate smears.

Identification of a megakaryocyte lineage cannot be made by morphologic features alone and requires immunophenotyping or electron microscopy and ultracytochemistry.[3] The more differentiated blasts are recognized by the presence of demarcation membranes and "bull's-eye" granules by electron microscopy. Ultrastructural peroxidase activity is found in the nuclear envelope and endoplasmic reticulum and absent from the granules and Golgi complexes of leukemic megakaryoblasts. This pattern of localization of the ultrastructural peroxidase reaction distinguishes megakaryoblasts from myeloblasts and is the earliest distinctive, recognizable characteristic of megakaryoblasts. By flow cytometry, the megakaryoblasts are myeloperoxidase negative and may be $CD45^-$, $CD34^-$, and $HLA\text{-}DR^-$, with variable expression of CD13 or CD33. Aberrant CD7 expression may be seen. Immunophenotyping by flow cytometry or immunohistochemistry using antibodies to megakaryocyte-restricted antigens, such as CD41 and CD61, is usually diagnostic. Bone marrow cytogenetics may be difficult to obtain owing to the presence of marrow fibrosis.

Acute Basophilic Leukemia

Acute basophilic leukemia is an extremely rare AML with 20% or more bone marrow blast cells and evidence of basophilic differentiation. Described cases have been defined by morphologic features of basophilic blast cell granules or solely by the ultrastructural detection of basophilic features (Fig. 45-18).[140-142] The latter criterion is problematic because electron microscopy studies are not routinely performed on acute leukemias. The blasts may resemble AML without differentiation, lacking myeloperoxidase or Sudan black B. By flow cytometry, they lack CD117 (excluding mast cell leukemia)

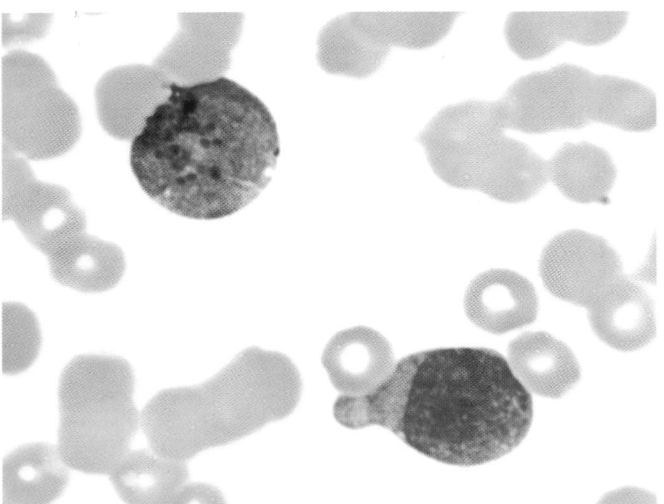

Figure 45-18. Acute basophilic leukemia. Blast cell proliferation in which many of the blasts contain basophilic granules. This patient had no history of chronic myelogenous leukemia and did not meet the criteria for another type of acute myeloid leukemia and was therefore diagnosed with acute basophilic leukemia.

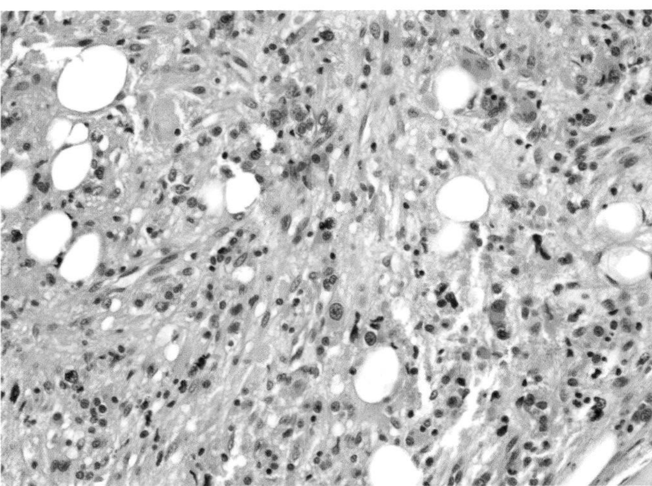

Figure 45-19. Acute panmyelosis with myelofibroisis. The marrow is replaced by fibrosis, with admixed immature cells that include myeloblasts, dysplastic and immature megakaryocytes, and erythroid precursors. The patient lacked splenomegaly and other features of a myeloproliferative neoplasm.

and show variable expression of CD34 and HLA-DR. CD13 and CD33 are usually detected, and blasts are usually positive for CD123 and CD11b.[143,144] Expression of CD203c in the absence of CD117 is considered fairly specific for a basophilic lineage.[143] Other leukemias with basophilia must be excluded, including AML with t(6;9)(p23;q34) and blast transformation of CML.

Acute Panmyelosis with Myelofibrosis

Acute panmyelosis with myelofibrosis (APMF) is a rare disorder that is included as a subtype of AML, NOS. It occurs most commonly in adults with pancytopenia and no splenomegaly (Box 45-13).[145-147] The marrow is fibrotic and shows panmyelosis, usually involving immature granulocytic, megakaryocytic, and erythroid cells (Fig. 45-19). Marrow myeloblast counts are usually difficult to perform owing to the inability to aspirate marrow as well as the panmyelosis, but most cases have 20% or more marrow blasts. The differential diagnosis of APMF includes primary myelofibrosis and other MPNs in their later stages, acute megakaryoblastic leukemia, AML-MRC, MDS with myelofibrosis, and other neoplasms with fibrosis in the marrow, including metastatic tumors. The lack of splenomegaly helps distinguish this disorder from many of the MPNs. Exclusion of AML-MRC may be difficult owing to poor aspirates for morphologic or cytogenetic analysis, but a diagnosis of AML-MRC takes precedence over APMF. APMF can be distinguished from acute megakaryoblastic leukemia by the frequent expression of CD34 on the blasts of APMF and the proliferation of immature cells from all three lineages, not just megakaryoblasts. APMF has an aggressive course and a more abrupt clinical onset, with fever and bone pain, than MDS with increased blasts and myelofibrosis; however, in some cases it may be impossible to distinguish APMF from myelodysplasia with fibrosis.[148]

Box 45-13 *Key Features of Acute Panmyelosis with Myelofibrosis*

- Occurs in adults with pancytopenia and no splenomegaly
- Fibrosed marrow with increased immature myeloid cells (blasts), erythroid precursors, and immature megakaryocytes (panmyelosis)
- Rapidly progressive clinical course

MYELOID PROLIFERATIONS OF DOWN SYNDROME

Patients with Down syndrome are at increased risk for both acute lymphoblastic leukemia and AML. Infants and children with Down syndrome often have myeloid proliferations in blood and bone marrow that in some cases would meet the criteria for AML.[149] Because of the unique nature of these myeloid proliferations, they were grouped in a separate category in the 2008 WHO classification.[150] Approximately 10% of neonates with Down syndrome manifest a transient myeloproliferative disorder indistinguishable from acute leukemia that is called *transient abnormal myelopoiesis* (TAM). This proliferation spontaneously resolves in most cases. In the first 4 years of life, children with Down syndrome are at high risk for developing acute megakaryoblastic leukemia. This AML most commonly follows TAM and is phenotypically and, in many respects, genetically identical to the blasts of TAM. After the age of 5 years, the ratio of AML to acute lymphoblastic leukemia normalizes to that of the general pediatric population, but children with Down syndrome remain at higher risk for developing acute leukemia. Both TAM and the myeloid leukemia of Down syndrome are associated with mutations in the megakaryocyte transcription factor *GATA1* acquired in utero.[151]

Transient Abnormal Myelopoiesis

TAM presents in the newborn period; the median age at diagnosis was 5 days in one study.[152] Most patients present

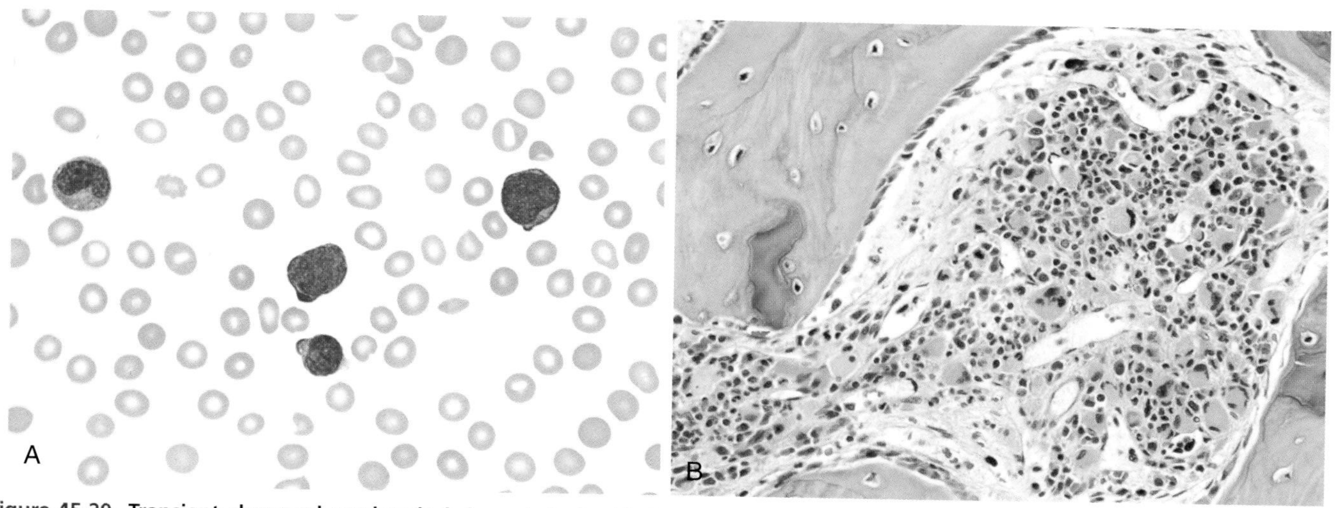

Figure 45-20. Transient abnormal myelopoiesis in an infant with Down syndrome. A, Peripheral blood from an infant with Down syndrome contains blasts with basophilic cytoplasm and shows cytoplasmic blebbing. These blasts mark with CD41 and CD61, consistent with megakaryoblasts. **B**, Bone marrow biopsy shows a predominance of immature cells and megakaryocytes.

with leukocytosis and increased peripheral blood blasts.[153] The blasts usually show morphologic features similar to megakaryoblasts in other settings, including basophilic cytoplasm with or without coarse basophilic granules and cytoplasmic projections (Fig. 45-20). Red blood cell and platelet indices are variable, with near-normal median values. Dysplastic changes of marrow elements may be present. By flow cytometry, the blasts of TAM commonly express moderate CD45 and HLA-DR, the myeloid antigen CD33 with or without CD13, as well as CD38, CD117, and CD34.[154,155] They frequently show aberrant CD7 and CD56 expression and evidence of megakaryocytic differentiation, with expression of CD41, CD61, and CD71. Clonal cytogenetic abnormalities are typically limited to trisomy 21, although nonclonal abnormalities are frequently observed. *GATA1* and *JAK3* mutations are both common in TAM.[156-158]

Hepatic dysfunction is a marker for poor outcome in TAM. Patients frequently demonstrate hepatomegaly. Clinically significant liver disease manifests as hyperbilirubinemia with or without elevated transaminases. Biopsy may demonstrate cholestasis, fibrosis (portal and perisinusoidal), a paucity of bile ducts, variable hepatocellular necrosis, and a variable amount of extramedullary hematopoiesis. Some cases show an abundance of megakaryocyte precursors; others may show only occasional mononuclear cells. This may be a function of their myeloproliferative state and whether the biopsy is performed during TAM, with elevated blast counts, or after the resolution of TAM. Patients with severe perinatal disease may have fibrosis of other organs, including the pancreas and kidneys. The exact cause of the fibrosis is not clear, but circulating proinflammatory cytokines such as interleukin-1β, tumor necrosis factor-α, interferon-γ, or possibly platelet-derived growth factor have been implicated.[159,160]

Only a subset of patients requires intervention for hyperviscosity, blast counts greater than 100,000/μL, organomegaly with respiratory compromise, renal dysfunction, or disseminated intravascular coagulation. Three risk groups have been described: low risk, with no palpable hepatomegaly or hepatic dysfunction (38% of patients, overall survival 92 ± 8%); intermediate risk, with hepatomegaly and non-life-threatening hepatic dysfunction (40% of patients, overall survival 82 ± 11%); and high risk, with a white blood cell count greater than 100,000/μL or life-threatening cardiorespiratory compromise due to TAM (21% of patients, overall survival 49 ± 20%). The reported median time to TAM resolution is 46 days. A later myeloid proliferation develops in 10% to 12% of patients, including some treated with low-dose chemotherapy.[152]

Myeloid Leukemia Associated with Down Syndrome

AML in Down syndrome typically presents in the first 3 years of life, often following a prolonged myelodysplasia-like phase.[161] Because cases with 5% to 20% blasts and cases of overt AML are biologically and clinically similar, they are often treated with similar protocols. Acute megakaryoblastic leukemia is the most common subtype of AML. Studies suggest that nearly all AML in children younger than 4 years with Down syndrome is megakaryoblastic leukemia.

Blasts in Down syndrome AML accumulate in the blood, bone marrow, liver, and spleen and exhibit features common to megakaryoblasts, as described earlier (Fig. 45-21). Dyserythropoiesis is usually evident in the blood (anisopoikilocytosis) and marrow (megaloblastic changes, nuclear contour abnormalities, multinucleate forms). By flow cytometry, the blasts show a similar immunophenotypic profile to that of TAM, with a few possible differences.[154,155] The blasts of AML may show more consistent expression of CD13 and CD11b, with less CD34 (93% of TAM cases, compared with 50% of AML) and possibly less HLA-DR. In addition, AML often demonstrates clonal karyotypic abnormalities as well as trisomy 21; these include complete or partial trisomies of chromosomes 1 and 8. Despite these clonal abnormalities, many of which are considered myelodysplasia related in non–Down syndrome patients, the prognosis of AML in Down syndrome is very good compared with that in non–Down syndrome patients, especially when treated with high-dose cytarabine. However, the prognosis in patients older than 5 years is similar to that in non–Down syndrome patients.[162] Age is a significant predictor of outcome even in younger

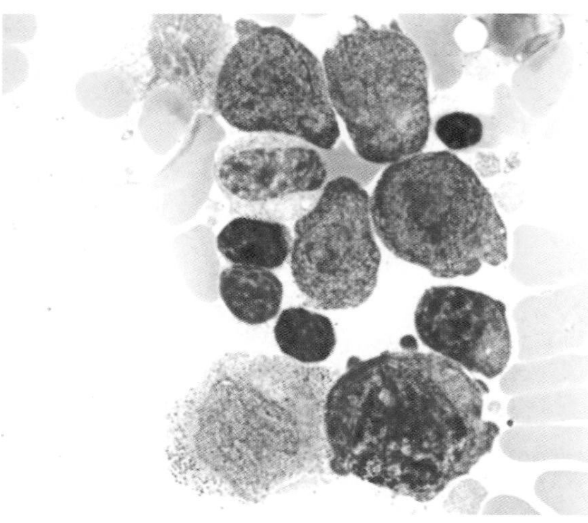

Figure 45-21. Acute myeloid leukemia (megakaryoblastic) of Down syndrome. Bone marrow shows abnormal erythroid precursors and blasts that mark as megakaryoblasts. Although the features are similar to those in Figure 45-20, the diagnosis of acute leukemia rather than transient abnormal myelopoiesis is dependent on the child's age and the clinical features.

children. The event-free survival for children aged 0 to 2 years is 86%; for those aged 2 to 4 years, it is 70%; and for those older than 4 years, it is 28%.[162] There is a trend toward more frequent monosomy 7 in older children, but it is not clear whether this significantly affects outcome. The frequency of tyrosine kinase activating mutations is unclear, with variable reports on the frequency of *JAK2*, *JAK3*, or *FLT* mutations in small studies.[163,164]

MYELOID SARCOMA

Myeloid sarcoma is an extramedullary proliferation of myeloid blasts that may be associated with a concurrent myeloid neoplasm involving the bone marrow, but such an association is not required.[165-169] In some cases, myeloid sarcoma may herald relapse in a patient with previously treated disease. In others, it may be the first indication of acute leukemia. In adults, roughly one third of myeloid sarcomas present with concurrent myeloid disease (including AML, MDS, MPN, or MDS/MPN), and one third have a history of a prior myeloid neoplasm. By definition, the infiltrates efface the underlying tissue architecture. Synonyms include *chloroma*, *granulocytic sarcoma*, and *extramedullary myeloid tumor*. The presence of myeloid sarcoma is diagnostic of AML, regardless of the bone marrow or blood status. The most common site of involvement is the skin, followed by mucous membranes, orbits, central nervous system, lymph nodes, bones, gonads, and other internal organs. Myeloid sarcoma is considered more common in pediatric AML, occurring in approximately 10% of cases,[170] although the true incidence in adults is unknown. The frequency in children may reflect associations with the t(8;21), inv(16), and 11q23 translocation subtypes, which are relatively more common in younger patients.

Previously, three subtypes of myeloid sarcoma were described based on the degree of maturation: blastic, immature, and differentiated.[169,171] Such subtyping is no longer considered relevant, but it may be useful in recognizing the morphologic variability of the myeloid blast infiltrate. Myeloid sarcoma should not be considered a type of AML but rather a type of presentation of AML. Every attempt should be made to classify myeloid sarcoma cytogenetically and immunophenotypically, in the same manner as if it were AML in the bone marrow. In patients with concurrent bone marrow or peripheral blood involvement, this classification is straightforward. In patients with de novo disease limited to myeloid sarcoma, precise classification may be difficult. Repeat biopsy or fine-needle aspiration may be necessary to obtain smears and fresh material for flow cytometric immunophenotyping and cytogenetic studies to properly classify the AML.

The myeloblasts of myeloid sarcoma usually form sheets of mononuclear cells, with an interfollicular pattern common in lymph nodes (Fig. 45-22). The blast cells may have admixed maturing granulocytes, erythroid precursors, or megakaryocytes, which are useful clues to the myeloid lineage of the immature cell population (see Fig. 45-22A). Eosinophilic myelocytes are the most easily recognized maturing cell population. Although they are present in only a subset of myeloid sarcomas, their presence is highly associated with a myeloblast cell population. The blasts themselves may have round to folded nuclei, usually with fine nuclear chromatin with a more stippled pattern than that typically seen in large B-cell lymphoma. Flow cytometric immunophenotyping usually demonstrates a lack of lineage-specific B- or T-cell markers and expression of myeloid or myelomonocytic markers such as CD13, CD33, myeloperoxidase, CD14, or CD64. However, as with AML in other sites, aberrant lymphoid antigen expression commonly occurs, and a relatively large panel of antibodies is useful to ensure accurate lineage determination. Fewer antibodies are available for characterization in paraffin sections, but lack of specific B- or T-lineage markers with expression of myeloperoxidase or the monocyte-specific marker CD163 is fairly specific for myeloid sarcoma. Other markers that are commonly positive but less lineage specific are CD43, lysozyme, and CD68. Only about half of cases are CD34$^+$, but CD117 expression is apparently more common. Recently, a paraffin antibody against CD33 was developed, which should prove useful in the detection of myeloid sarcoma.[172] Rare cases are of megakaryocytic lineage, especially extramedullary presentations of AML with t(1;22)(p13;q13) in infants (see earlier). Paraffin detection of CD41 and CD61 expression is useful in these cases, which are characteristically myeloperoxidase negative. Von Willebrand's factor and LAT (linker for activation of T cells) are less specific markers of megakaryocytic lineage. In addition to aberrant expression of B- and T-cell markers, rare cases may express CD30 or even cytokeratin.

Myeloid sarcoma shows some variability in presentation. Nearly one quarter of children with AML with t(8;21)(q22;q22) develop myeloid sarcoma.[173,174] Head and neck localization with orbital, skull, and central nervous system extramedullary involvement is most common in this group. A smaller percentage (approximately 10%) of adults with t(8;21) AML have myeloid sarcoma,[173] without the pattern of head and neck localization. Skin involvement in pediatric patients (leukemia cutis) tends to occur at a younger age (median, 2.6 years), and the skin lesions are most commonly associated with 11q23 translocations and with abnormalities of chromosome 16. Myelomonocytic morphology is most common in this setting. A unique and rare subset of skin

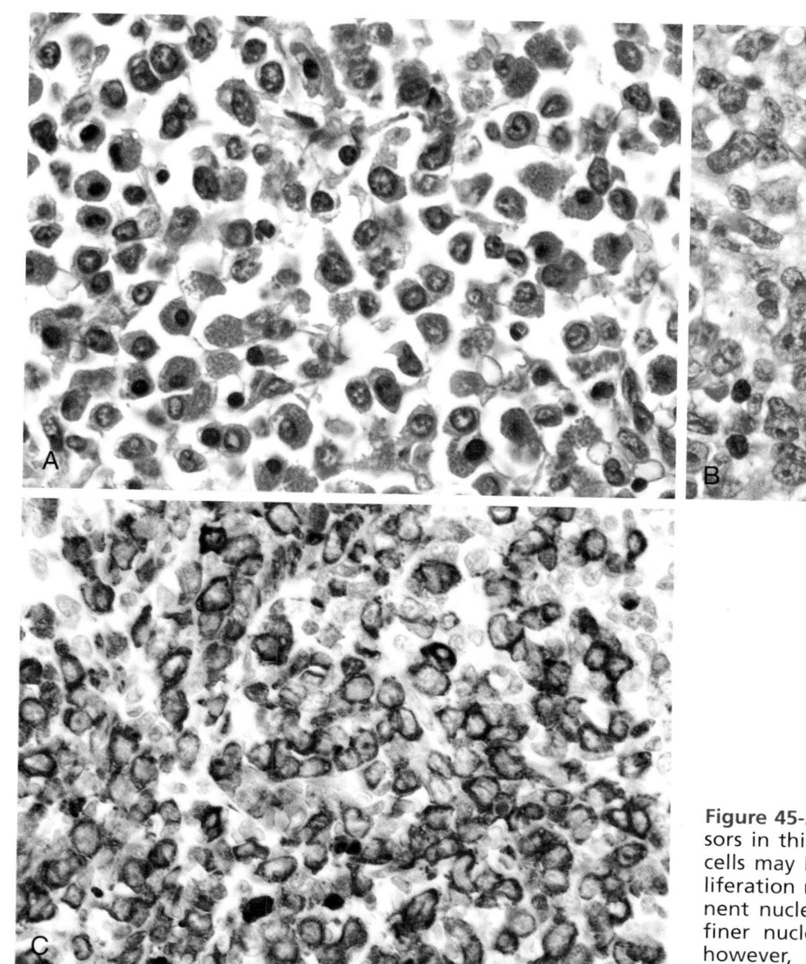
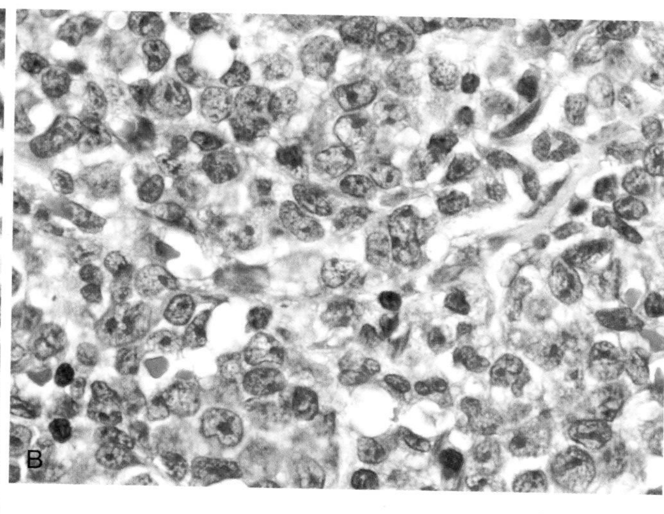

Figure 45-22. Myeloid sarcoma. A, Admixed eosinophil precursors in this myeloid sarcoma are a clue that the mononuclear cells may be myeloid cells. **B**, This more undifferentiated proliferation mimics a diffuse large B-cell lymphoma, with prominent nucleoli and some chromatin clearing. **C**, The cells have finer nuclear chromatin than most large B-cell lymphomas, however, and the cells are myeloperoxidase positive by immunohistochemistry.

tumors appears to represent a congenital leukemia, with multiple skin lesions of myeloid sarcoma presenting within the first week after birth (a form of "blueberry muffin" baby). In some of these babies, disease is limited to the skin. Such cases tend to have spontaneous remissions, sometimes over a period of days. The most common cytogenetic abnormality in this setting is t(8;16)(p11;q13) (*MYST3/CREBBP*),[86] which is frequently associated with erythrophagocytosis, therapy-related disease, and a poor prognosis in adults (see earlier). Because chemotherapy is very toxic to newborns, some reports recommend careful observation for patients with congenital myeloid sarcoma limited to the skin and no systemic manifestations, cytopenias, or lymph node involvement. Some spontaneously remitting cases with t(8;16) recur. Reserving chemotherapy for recurrences in spontaneously remitting cases may be an appropriate course of action,[175] sparing the infant excessive and possibly unnecessary toxicity. In contrast to babies with t(8;16) disease, those with 11q23 translocations tend to have a poor prognosis.

The clinical significance of myeloid sarcoma remains unclear. Other than the self-limited congenital forms, it is not clear whether myeloid sarcoma confers any specific prognosis in the era of high-dose cytarabine therapy, particularly when cases are classified according to known risk groups.[173,176] Low-dose radiation therapy may be useful for the emergent treatment of life-threatening or organ-threatening (e.g., orbital) myeloid sarcomas. The use of radiation therapy in the routine management of these patients does not appear to be indicated, however.

The differential diagnosis of myeloid sarcoma versus lymphoma, especially diffuse large B-cell lymphoma, lymphoblastic lymphoma, blastic mantle cell lymphoma, and Burkitt's lymphoma, is challenging on morphologic grounds alone. Fine nuclear chromatin with a high mitotic rate is often helpful in differentiating large B-cell lymphoma, which usually shows more distinct nucleoli and chromatin clearing. As mentioned, the presence of admixed erythroid cells, megakaryocytes, or eosinophilic myelocytes is a helpful clue to the possibility of a myeloid tumor. Immunophenotyping, however, is essential to the proper diagnosis of myeloid sarcoma. Cases of suspected lymphoma that lack B- or T-lineage–specific markers, including those with a CD43-only immunophenotype, should be further evaluated for evidence of myeloid sarcoma. Aberrant B-lineage marker expression, particularly CD19 and PAX5, in AML with t(8;21)(q22;q22) can lead to an incorrect diagnosis of B-cell lymphoma in a case of myeloid sarcoma. Subsets of APL and AML with inv(16)(p13.1q22) or t(16;16)(p13.1;q22) aberrantly express the T-lineage–associated marker CD2 and can be mistaken for T-cell lymphomas. CD7 and CD56 are also frequently expressed in myeloid sarcoma, and neither marker should be used alone to diagnose a T-cell or natural killer (NK) cell malignancy. Extramedullary tumors of AML (megakaryocytic) with t(1;22)(p13;q13) often show cell clustering in infants and may be mistaken for small blue round cell tumors of infancy. Without knowledge of this tumor and investigation with megakaryocytic markers, the diagnosis may be missed.

Other aspects of the differential diagnosis include the interpretation of sparse immature myeloid cell infiltrates in extramedullary sites. The diagnosis of myeloid sarcoma should be restricted to tumors that form space-occupying lesions. Patients with AML may have leukemic infiltrates in multiple sites that do not form masses that disrupt normal tissue architecture, and such cases should not be considered myeloid sarcoma. Patients receiving growth factors may have left-shifted granulocytes in various tissues that do not form masses, and these should not be overinterpreted as myeloid sarcoma. Similarly, maturing granulocyte proliferations of the skin must be distinguished from a dermal myeloid sarcoma. Sweet's syndrome,[177] also known as *acute febrile neutrophilic dermatosis*, may occur in patients with AML, but this does not represent an extramedullary leukemic infiltrate. Sweet's syndrome is associated with marked dermal edema with a marked mature neutrophilic infiltrate, in contrast to the more immature cell infiltrate of cutaneous myeloid sarcoma. Sweet's syndrome often resolves with treatment of the associated AML; the lesions also respond to systemic corticosteroid therapy.

INTEGRATED APPROACH TO THE DIAGNOSIS OF ACUTE MYELOID LEUKEMIA

A complex approach is necessary to diagnose and appropriately classify cases of AML. This requires an integration of morphologic, immunophenotypic, cytogenetic, and molecular genetic data. Such integration is best done in a single, final pathology report. Such reports need to be amended as genetic results become available, and diagnoses will be revised based on those data. Although morphologic and immunophenotypic clues can suggest specific cytogenetic abnormalities, cytogenetic or molecular genetic confirmation is essential. Diagnosis based on any single element of the workup of AML is fraught with difficulty and pitfalls. Some cases with less than 20% bone marrow blast cells on morphologic examination are now considered acute leukemia if they have specific recurring cytogenetic abnormalities. These cases might be missed if the appropriate cytogenetic studies are not available to the diagnosing pathologist. Similarly, samples with high numbers of marrow red blood cell precursors may result in falsely elevated blast cell counts when such counts are performed only by flow cytometry, and these cases may be overdiagnosed as AML. Cases of AML with specific recurring cytogenetic abnormalities, such as AML with t(8;21)(q22;q22), may be misdiagnosed as mixed phenotype acute leukemia if only flow cytometry methods are used for diagnosis.

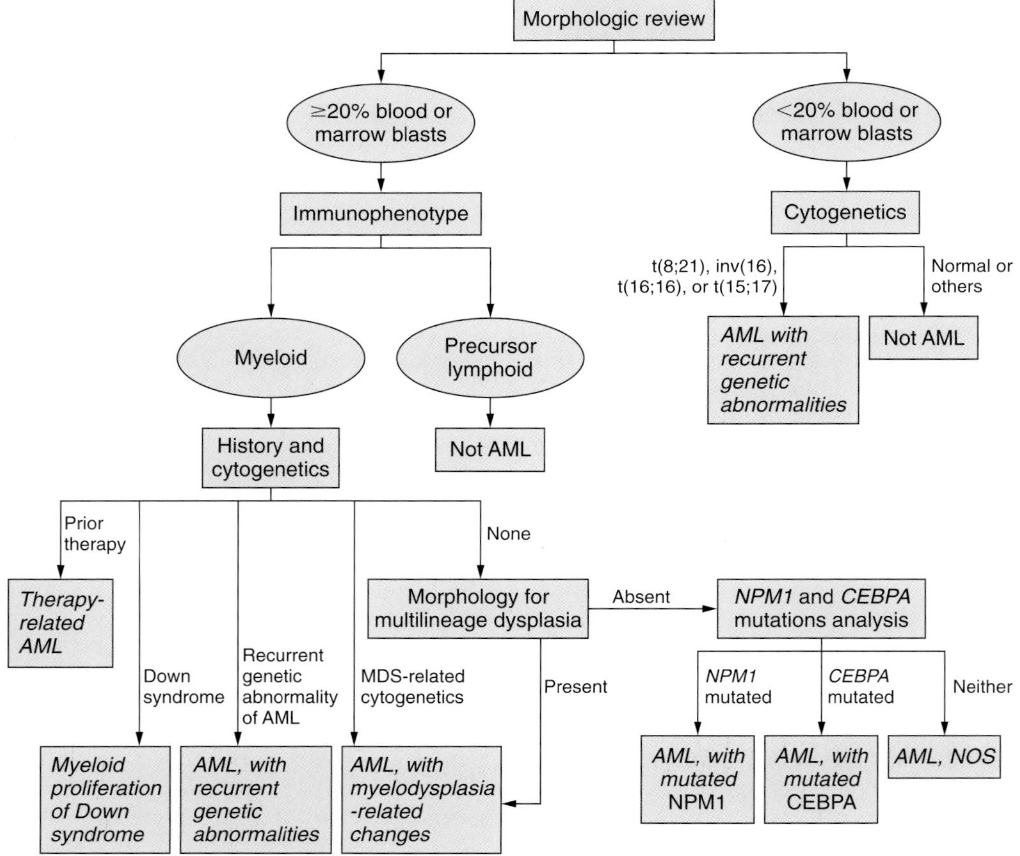

Figure 45-23. Algorithmic approach to the classification of acute myeloid leukemia (AML). MDS, myelodysplastic syndrome; NOS, not otherwise specified.

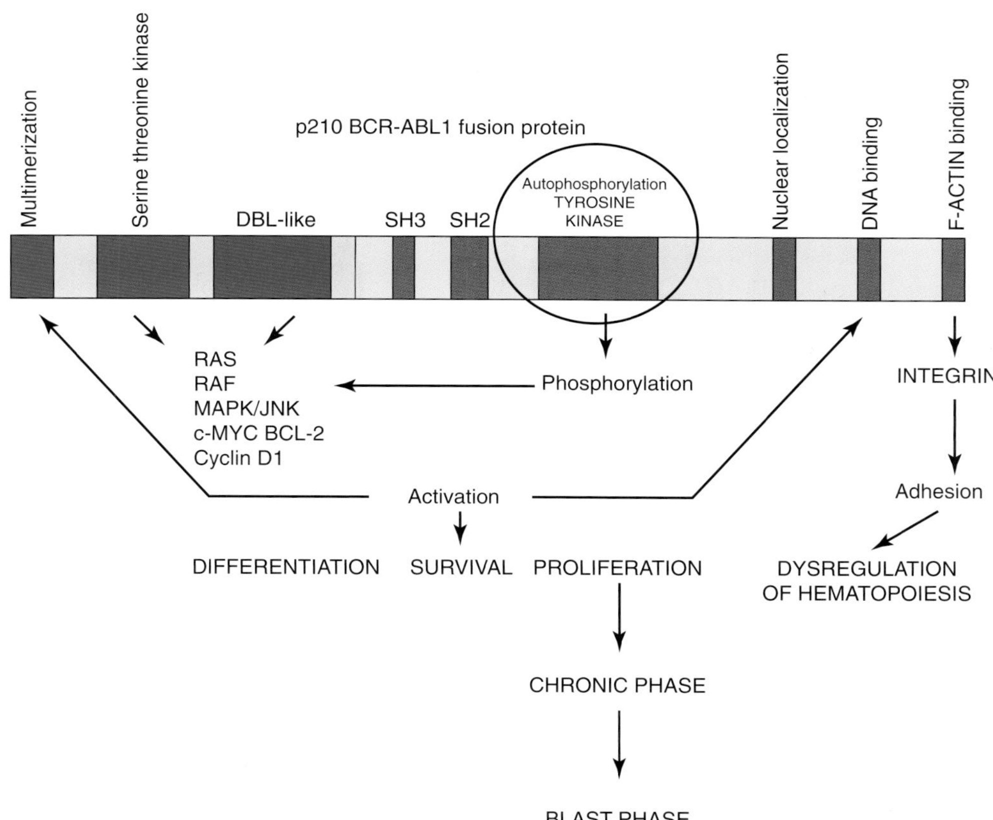

Figure 46-4. *BCR-ABL1* fusion on chromosome 22 leads to a BCR-ABL1 fusion protein with a constitutively activated tyrosine kinase in a domain of the protein encoded by *ABL1*. This tyrosine kinase plays a pivotal role in the pathogenesis of chronic myelogenous leukemia and leads to autophosphorylation of other sites on the oncoprotein. These serve as sites of phosphorylation of cellular proteins involved in pathways of differentiation, survival, proliferation, cellular adhesion, and regulation of hematopoiesis.

gene, located at chromosome 4q12, which encodes the tyrosine kinase receptor platelet-derived growth factor receptor-α (PDGFRA), and of the *PDGFRB* gene at 5q33, which encodes platelet-derived growth factor receptor-β (PDGFRB), have been reported in patients with myeloproliferative processes associated with marked eosinophilia. In these cases, the rearrangements lead to constitutive activation of PDGFRA or PDGFRB, respectively, resulting in proliferation.[41-47] Despite many similarities to the other MPNs, the neoplasms associated with these abnormalities have several unique features and have been placed in a separate category (see Chapter 49), yet they illustrate the role of constitutively activated signaling proteins in MPNs and closely related disorders. Furthermore, almost all cases of mastocytosis are associated with activating mutations of *KIT*, which encodes the surface tyrosine kinase receptor KIT. Mutations in *KIT* at codons 560 (V560G) and 816 (D816V) result in the ligand-independent activation of KIT, which is important in the pathogenesis of mast cell disease (see Chapter 48).[48-51]

In view of the accumulated data regarding CML, mastocytosis, and some cases of eosinophilic leukemia, it was not unexpected that a constitutively activated signaling protein would eventually be found in PV, ET, and PMF. What was surprising was that these three diseases, which have different clinical, laboratory, and morphologic features, share the same genetic defect. In 2005, four different groups of investigators working independently identified a mutation of the gene that encodes Janus kinase 2 (JAK2; a member of the Janus family of cytoplasmic nonreceptor tyrosine kinases) in most patients with PV and approximately 50% of those with ET and PMF.[52-55] The mutation, *JAK2* V617F, is a guanine-to-thymidine substitution that results in a substitution of valine for phenylalanine at codon 617 in the JAK2 protein. It is an acquired somatic mutation that occurs in hematopoietic cells of all myeloid lineages, as well as in some B and T lymphocytes in affected individuals.[56,57]

The JAK kinases are essential to cytokine signaling and signal transduction through their association with homodimeric type 1 cytokine receptors that lack intrinsic kinase activity (Fig. 46-5). The JAK2 protein is the sole JAK kinase that associates with the EPO receptor (EPOR), but it also associates with the thrombopoietin (TPO) receptor (MPL) and the granulocyte colony-stimulating factor receptor (GCSFR), among others.[55,58,59] Engagement of the cytokine receptor with its ligand normally results in receptor dimerization, followed by autophosphorylation and transphosphorylation of the receptor and of the JAK2 kinase. The activated JAK2 receptor complex leads to recruitment and phosphorylation of substrate molecules, including signal transducers and activators of transcription (STAT) proteins, and subsequently results in target gene transcription in the nucleus.[9,59]

The JAK2 protein has several domains, including a catalytic domain (JH1) and a pseudokinase domain (JH2). Normally, the latter domain is thought to play an inhibitory role in the catalytic domain.[60,61] The *JAK2* V617F mutation

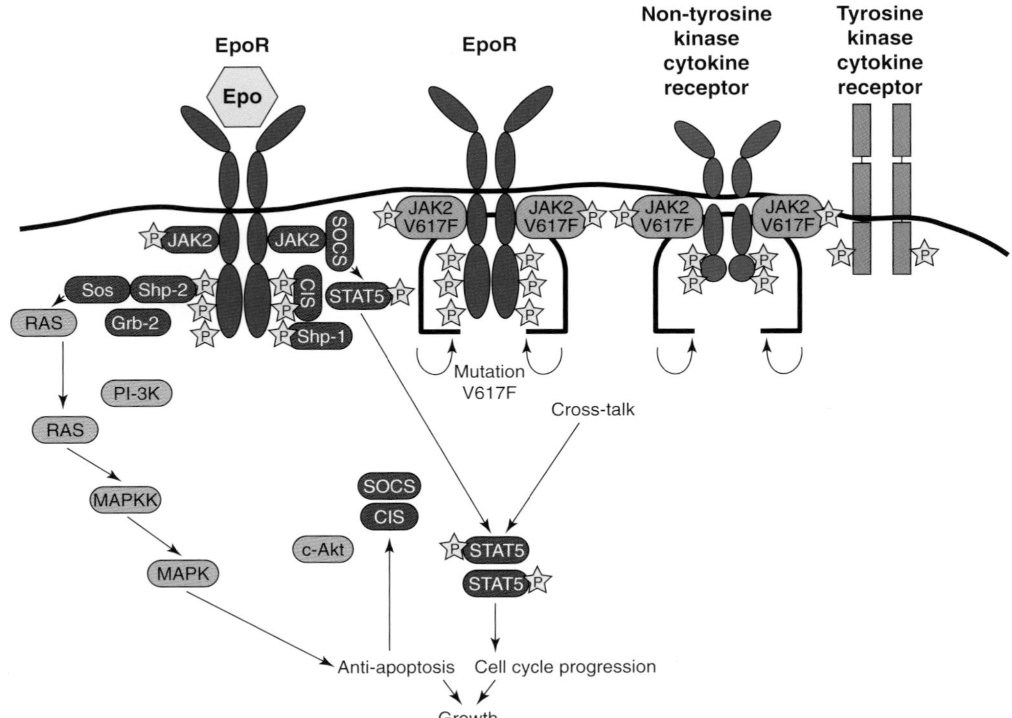

Figure 46-5. Interaction of JAK2 and cytokine receptors important in the pathogenesis of myeloproliferative neoplasms. **The homodimeric erythropoietin receptor EpoR (*green*); another JAK2-utilizing, homodimeric, non–tyrosine kinase cytokine receptor such as MPL or granulocyte colony-stimulating factor receptor (*blue*); and a tyrosine kinase cytokine receptor (*orange*) such as platelet-derived growth factor receptor are illustrated. In normal erythroid precursors, as illustrated on the left side of the diagram, activation of JAK2 occurs when there is binding of Epo to EpoR and an activated dimeric form of the receptor results. Various signaling proteins, including STAT5, are recruited by the phosphorylated sites and, in turn, are phosphorylated and activated, leading to a series of activated proteins that ultimately results in cellular proliferation and inhibition of apoptosis. Inhibitory proteins, such as suppressors of cytokine signaling (SOCS), are also recruited to the activated receptor and act to modulate the activation. In diseases in which the *JAK2* V617F mutation is present, JAK2 is constitutively activated (second *green* receptor to the right, activated JAK2 colored *orange*), which leads to phosphorylation of EpoR and activation of the downstream proteins, even without binding to Epo. Similar events occur in other cytokine receptors for which JAK2 serves as an activating kinase, such as MPL. JAK2 does not serve as the activation protein for tyrosine kinase cytokine receptors such as PDGFR, although there is likely cross-talk between the various activated receptors.** (Modified from Vainchenker W, Constantinescu SN. A unique activating mutation in JAK2 (V617F) is at the origin of polycythemia vera and allows a new classification of myeloproliferative diseases. *Hematology Am Soc Hematol Educ Program.* 2005:195-200.)

affects the JH2 region and leads to the loss of its inhibitory function, which essentially accounts for a gain of function of JAK2; JAK2 is constitutively activated.[55,62] Expression of *JAK2* V617F confers growth factor hypersensitivity and cytokine-independent growth to hematopoietic cells, which explains the finding of EECs in the bone marrow noted by earlier investigators. The association of abnormal JAK2 with various growth factor and cytokine receptors, particularly EPOR, GCSFR, and MPL, explains the proliferation of multiple lineages that is often observed in MPNs. Confirmation of the mutation's role in the pathogenesis of PV has come from animal models, in which retroviral transduction of *JAK2* V617F into murine hematopoietic stem cell lines led to PV and in some cases to myelofibrosis.[63-65]

Discovery of the *JAK2* mutation has revolutionized the diagnostic approach to the *BCR-ABL1*–negative MPNs, particularly PV, ET, and PMF. It is important to appreciate, however, that the mutation has also been reported, albeit with low frequency, in other myeloid neoplasms, including rare cases of acute myeloid leukemia (AML), myelodysplastic/myeloproliferative neoplasms (MDS/MPNs), and myelodysplastic syndrome (MDS).[66-68] Discovery of *JAK2* V617F in diseases with diverse clinical, laboratory, and morphologic features raises the obvious questions of how one mutation contributes to the pathogenesis of different MPN entities and whether other, yet to be discovered factors may be more important in determining disease characteristics. Because all myeloid lineages, as well as some B and T lymphocytes, carry the mutation in affected individuals, it seems unlikely that distribution of the mutation among the hematopoietic lineages accounts for the variable disease manifestations. Rather, data suggest that the genetic background of the host, the allele dosage of the mutation, a preceding acquired but unknown genetic abnormality, or any combination of these factors may determine the ultimate disease characteristics when the *JAK2* V617F mutation is present.[18,69-71]

Another question is the pathogenesis of cases of PV, ET, and PMF that lack *JAK2* V617F mutations. In the case of PV, further investigations revealed another recurring mutation of *JAK2* in exon 12 that is present in most PV patients who lack *JAK2* V617F.[72] A gain-of-function mutation of *MPL*, the gene that encodes the TPO receptor MPL, has also been reported in approximately 5% of cases of PMF and 1% of cases of ET.[73,74] Still, the molecular pathogenesis is currently unknown in 40% to 50% of cases of PMF and ET, in most cases of chronic neutrophilic leukemia (CNL), and in those cases of chronic eosinophilic leukemia that lack abnormalities of *PDGFRA*, *PDGFRB*, or *FGFR1*.

CHRONIC MYELOGENOUS LEUKEMIA, *BCR-ABL1* POSITIVE

Although CML is a rare disease with an annual incidence of only 1 or 2 cases per 100,000 people,[75] it is perhaps the most studied of all hematopoietic neoplasms. This leukemia originates in an abnormal pluripotent stem cell and is consistently associated with the Ph chromosome or the *BCR-ABL1* fusion gene, or both (see Fig. 46-1). The fusion gene encodes an abnormal oncoprotein with constitutively activated tyrosine kinase activity. Although the principal manifestation of CML is marked expansion of neutrophils and their precursors in the blood and bone marrow, *BCR-ABL1* is found in all the myeloid lineages; in B, T, and NK lymphoid cells; and in endothelial cells. The natural history of untreated CML is bi- or triphasic: an initially indolent chronic phase (CP) is followed by an accelerated phase (AP) or a blast phase (BP), or both. Agents that specifically inhibit the abnormal tyrosine kinase activity of the BCR-ABL1 protein have significantly altered the course of the disease and improved survival in most patients.[76]

Diagnosis

The National Comprehensive Cancer Network practice guidelines recommend that the initial evaluation of patients suspected of having CML include a complete clinical history and physical examination, complete blood cell count with platelet count and leukocyte differential, bone marrow aspiration and biopsy, complete karyotype analysis, FISH for the *BCR-ABL1* fusion gene, and baseline quantitative RT-PCR for the measurement of BCR-ABL1 transcripts.[77] The major features of CML at the time of presentation in CP are listed in Box 46-2.

Box 46-2 *Common Features of the Chronic Phase of Chronic Myelogenous Leukemia*, BCR-ABL1 *Positive*

Annual Incidence
- 1 to 2 per 100,000 individuals

Age
- Any, but pediatric cases are rare; median age about 65 years

Clinical Findings
- Fatigue
- Weight loss
- Fever
- Splenomegaly
- 20%-40% of patients are asymptomatic at initial diagnosis

Blood Findings
- Leukocytosis
- Platelets normal or increased
- Anemia often present
- Spectrum of maturing granulocytes; "myelocyte bulge"
- Blasts usually <2% of white blood cells
- Absolute basophilia
- No significant dysplasia

Bone Marrow Findings
- Hypercellularity
- Increased myeloid-to-erythroid ratio
- Blasts usually <5%, always <10%
- Megakaryocytes normal or increased in number, but with "dwarf" morphology
- Reticulin fibers normal to moderately increased

Genetics
- 100% have Philadelphia chromosome or *BCR-ABL1* fusion gene

Clinical Findings

Although CML can occur at any age, the median age at diagnosis is approximately 65 years, and there is a slight male predominance.[38,75,78,79] Rare cases of pediatric *BCR-ABL1*–positive CML occur[80] and should not be confused with juvenile myelomonocytic leukemia (JMML), a leukemia that lacks the *BCR-ABL1* fusion gene but was called *juvenile CML* in the older literature (see Chapter 47).

Most patients with CML are diagnosed in CP, which has an insidious onset. Nearly 20% to 40% of patients are asymptomatic and are diagnosed when blood collected during a routine medical examination reveals an abnormality.[81,82] Symptoms at presentation include those due to anemia or an enlarged spleen, or both, such as fatigue, lethargy, left upper abdominal pain, or early satiety. Symptoms related to a hypermetabolic condition, including fever, night sweats, and weight loss, also occur, and occasional patients present with bleeding manifestations. Splenomegaly is found in 30% to 50% of patients, and some also have enlarged livers. Significant lymphadenopathy is uncommon, but if the other findings are in keeping with CML, a lymph node biopsy should be considered to exclude a blastic proliferation (myeloid sarcoma).[38,81,82] Atypical presentations sometimes occur, including initial presentation in a transformed phase with no preceding detectable CP.

Laboratory Findings

Peripheral Blood

The most prominent finding in the peripheral blood is leukocytosis, with median white blood cell (WBC) counts of approximately 100 × 10^9/L. However, a wide range of values is reported—from normal WBC counts in rare patients to counts exceeding 500 × 10^9/L.[38,79,82] The increase in the WBC count is largely due to neutrophils in different stages of maturation, with peaks in the percentages of myelocytes and segmented neutrophils (Fig. 46-6).[81,83] The neutrophils are generally normal morphologically, and there is no significant dysplasia.[84] Typically, blasts account for less than 2% of WBCs at the time of diagnosis.[83,85,86] Absolute basophilia is virtually always seen. It is important to quantify basophils accurately because their percentage is commonly used to judge disease progression.[81,85] Eosinophils may be increased in number as well. Because of the very high WBC count, only a few monocytes may result in absolute monocytosis, but their percentage is usually 3% or less.[86] The platelet count is normal or elevated in almost all cases and exceeds 1000 × 10^9/L in up to 10% to 15% of patients at diagnosis.[82]

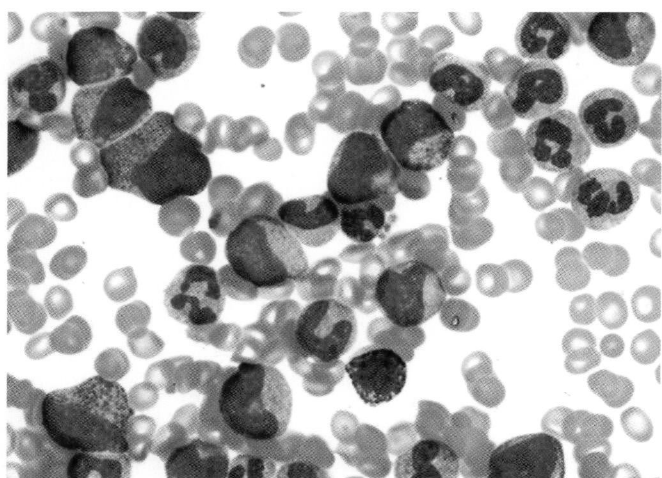

Figure 46-6. Peripheral blood smear of a patient with chronic myelogenous leukemia illustrates marked leukocytosis with a spectrum of neutrophil maturation, including a prominence of myelocytes and segmented neutrophils. Basophils are invariably increased in absolute numbers.

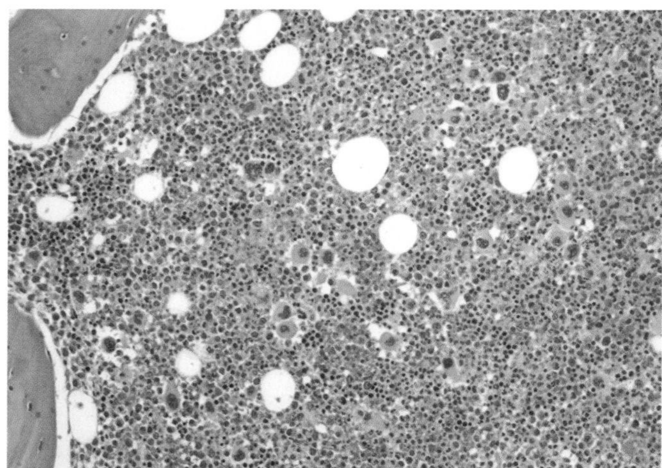

Figure 46-7. The bone marrow in the chronic phase of chronic myelogenous leukemia is hypercellular. It shows granulocytic proliferation, with small islands of erythroid precursors interspersed, and increased numbers of megakaryocytes, many of which are "dwarf" megakaryocytes.

Thrombocytopenia is uncommon and, if marked, should prompt consideration of a more advanced stage of disease or thrombocytopenia due to another cause. Platelet morphology is usually not remarkable at presentation, but occasional giant platelets may be seen. Abnormal platelet function studies are common, however, and contribute to the hemorrhagic episodes sometimes observed.[38] Although anemia is common, hemoglobin values less than 10 g/dL are initially observed in only 25% to 30% of patients.[82]

Bone Marrow

Although some might argue that the WBC count, leukocyte differential, and FISH study of peripheral blood cells that demonstrates *BCR-ABL1* fusion are sufficient for the diagnosis of CML, the value of the bone marrow biopsy and aspirate cannot be overstated. Bone marrow aspiration provides the best specimen for complete karyotype analysis, which should be done at the time of diagnosis in every case to detect the presence of chromosomal abnormalities in addition to the Ph chromosome. This initial study is essential because the detection of additional chromosomal abnormalities in a later cytogenetic study signifies disease evolution.[87,88] Furthermore, morphologic inspection of the aspirate and biopsy provides a baseline against which future changes, such as an increase in reticulin fibrosis, can be judged.

In CP of CML, the bone marrow biopsy and aspirate smears are hypercellular (Fig. 46-7) and nearly devoid of fat cells owing to proliferation of the neutrophil lineage, which shows a maturation pattern similar to that observed in the peripheral blood. There is a prominent increase of neutrophil myelocytes ("myelocyte bulge") and of segmented neutrophils. In the biopsy the cuff of immature granulocytes along the bony trabecula is increased from its normal two or three layers of immature cells to four or five layers or more, and abundant segmented neutrophils are found deeper in the intertrabecular regions (Fig. 46-8).[81,85,89] On aspirate smear preparations, the neutrophils lack evidence of significant dysplasia.[84] Blasts usually account for less than 5% of the nucleated bone marrow cells and are scattered throughout the marrow. The finding of 10% or more blasts or the finding of large clusters of blasts in the biopsy specimen indicates disease progression.[85] The myeloid-to-erythroid ratio is often elevated and is sometimes greater than 20 : 1.[38] In the biopsy, erythroid islands are reduced in size and number but show maturation.[89] Dyserythropoiesis is either absent or minimal. The number of megakaryocytes varies considerably. In nearly half of patients, megakaryocytes are normal or slightly decreased in number, but in a nearly equal number, there is moderate to marked megakaryocytic proliferation that is best appreciated in biopsy sections (Figs. 46-9 and 46-10). Although usually singly dispersed in the bone marrow in CP, the megakaryocytes may also occur in sizable clusters as the disease progresses.[89] The megakaryocytes in CML are notable for

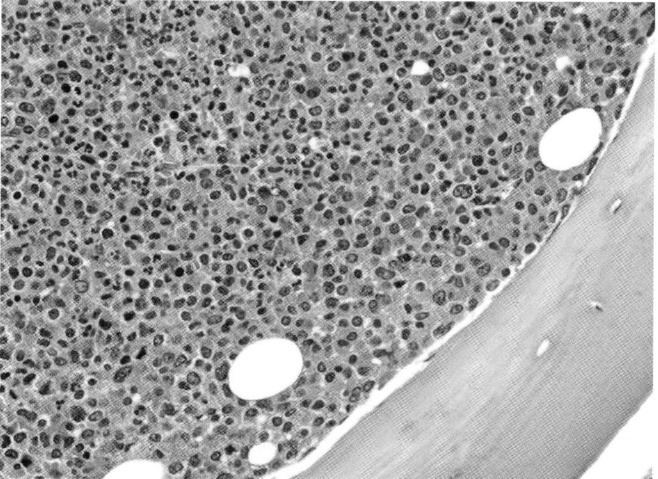

Figure 46-8. In chronic myelogenous leukemia, the peritrabecular rim of immature granulocytes thickened from the normal two to three cell layer to five or more cells, with mature cells farther from the bone in the intertrabecular region.

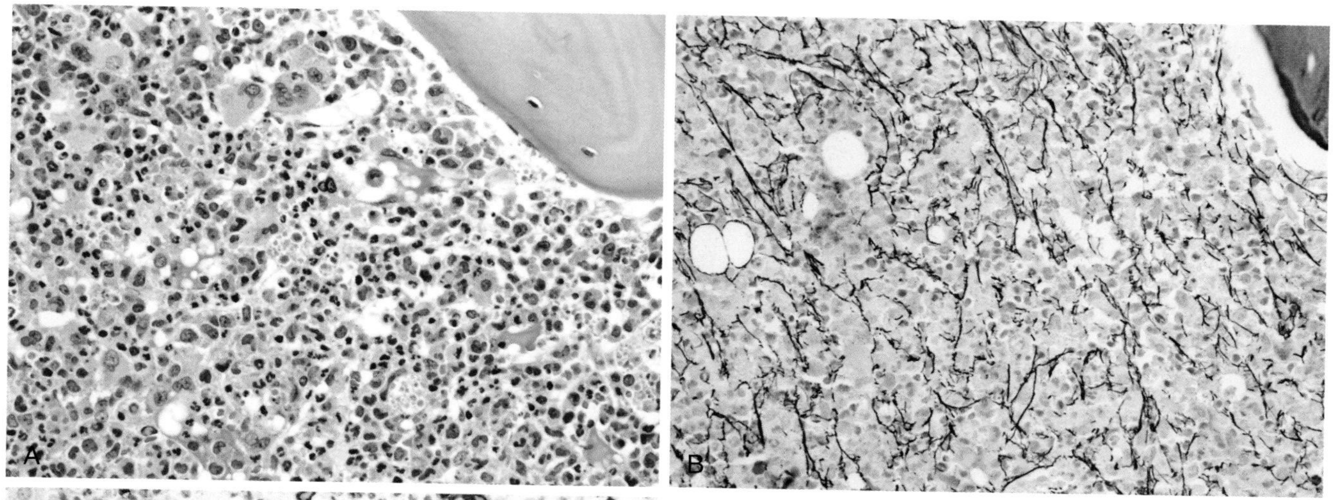

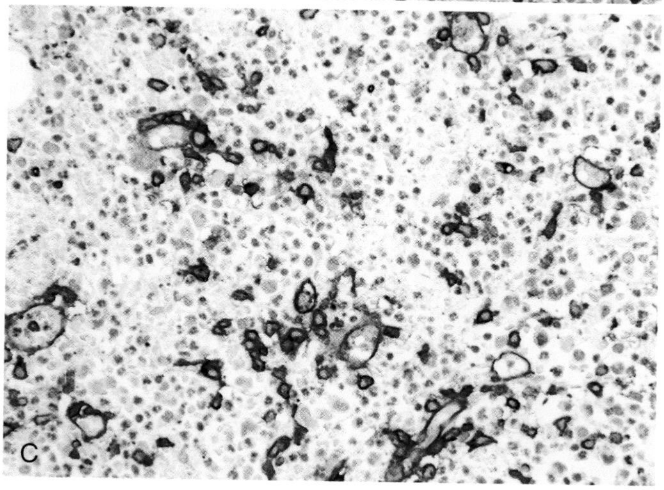

Figure 46-14. Chronic myelogenous leukemia, accelerated phase. This patient, who had Ph⁺ CML for 5 years, developed cytopenia in the blood, with 12% blasts. The bone marrow biopsy specimen is hypercellular (**A**), with reticulin fibrosis (**B**). An immunohistochemical stain for CD34 (**C**) reveals more blasts than were appreciated in the hematoxylin-eosin–stained section.

have no favorable impact when they are found in association with the Ph chromosome in CML, BP.[119] In myeloid BP, the blasts express myeloid-related antigens such as CD117, CD33, CD13, CD61, or myeloperoxidase, although it is not uncommon for the blasts to also express one or more lymphoid antigens. In 20% to 30% of BP, the blasts are lymphoblasts, most commonly with a precursor B-cell phenotype (Fig. 46-17), with expression of terminal deoxynucleotidyl transferase (TdT), CD19, CD10, and PAX5, although rare cases of T-cell origin have been reported as well.[115,117] Mixed

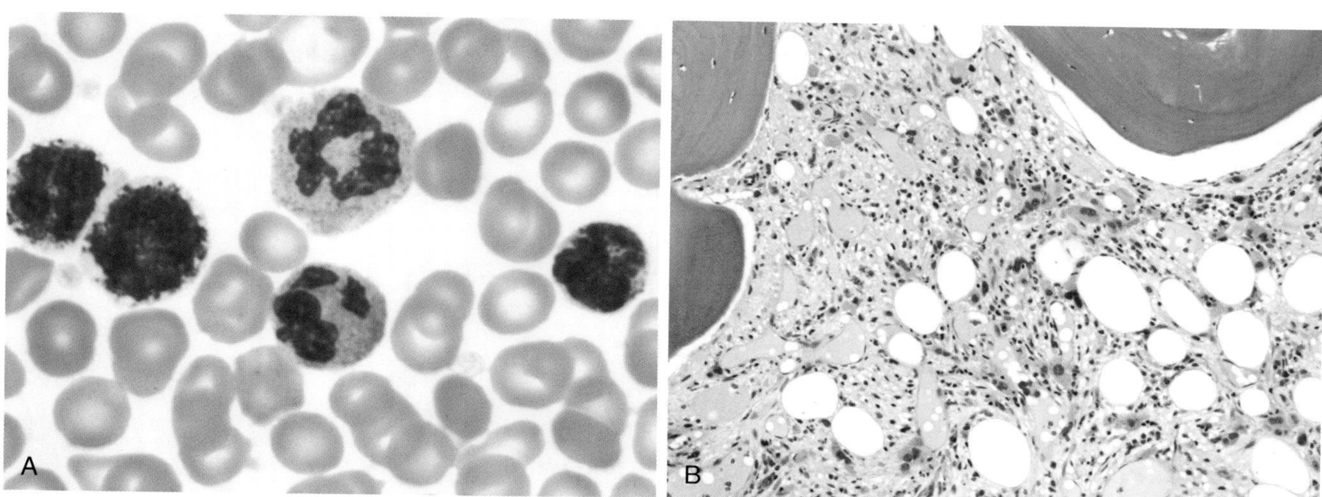

Figure 46-15. A, This patient with chronic myelogenous leukemia developed greater than 20% basophils in the blood. **B,** The bone marrow biopsy shows marked fibrosis and atypical megakaryocytic proliferation.

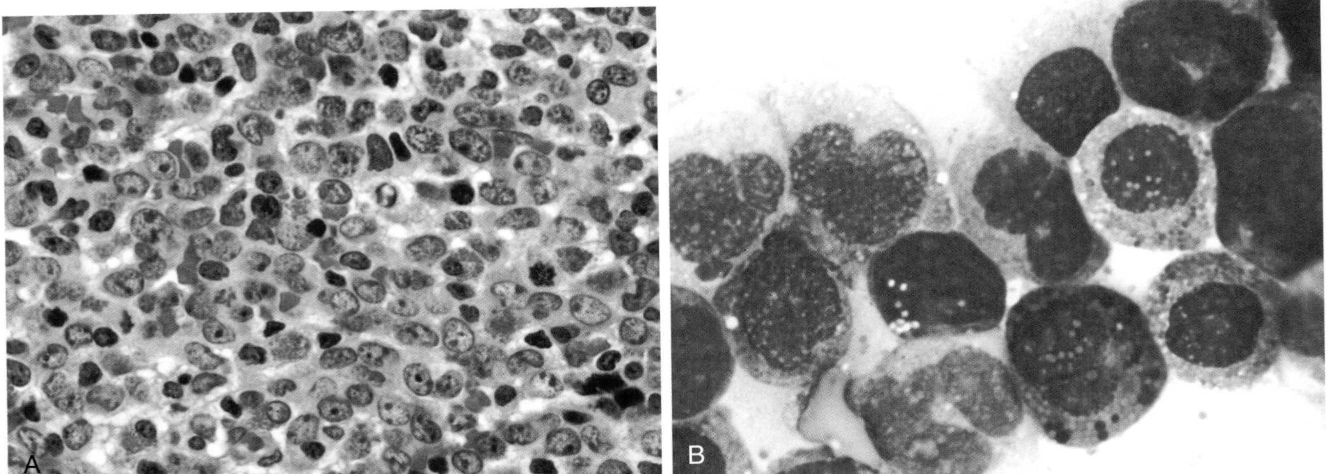

Figure 46-16. Chronic myelogenous leukemia, myeloid blast phase. A, Bone marrow biopsy shows sheets of blasts with some eosinophils intermixed. **B,** Marrow aspirate contains abnormal eosinophils and monocytic cells. This patient's leukemic cells showed t(9;22)(q34;q11.2) plus inv(16)(p13.1q22).

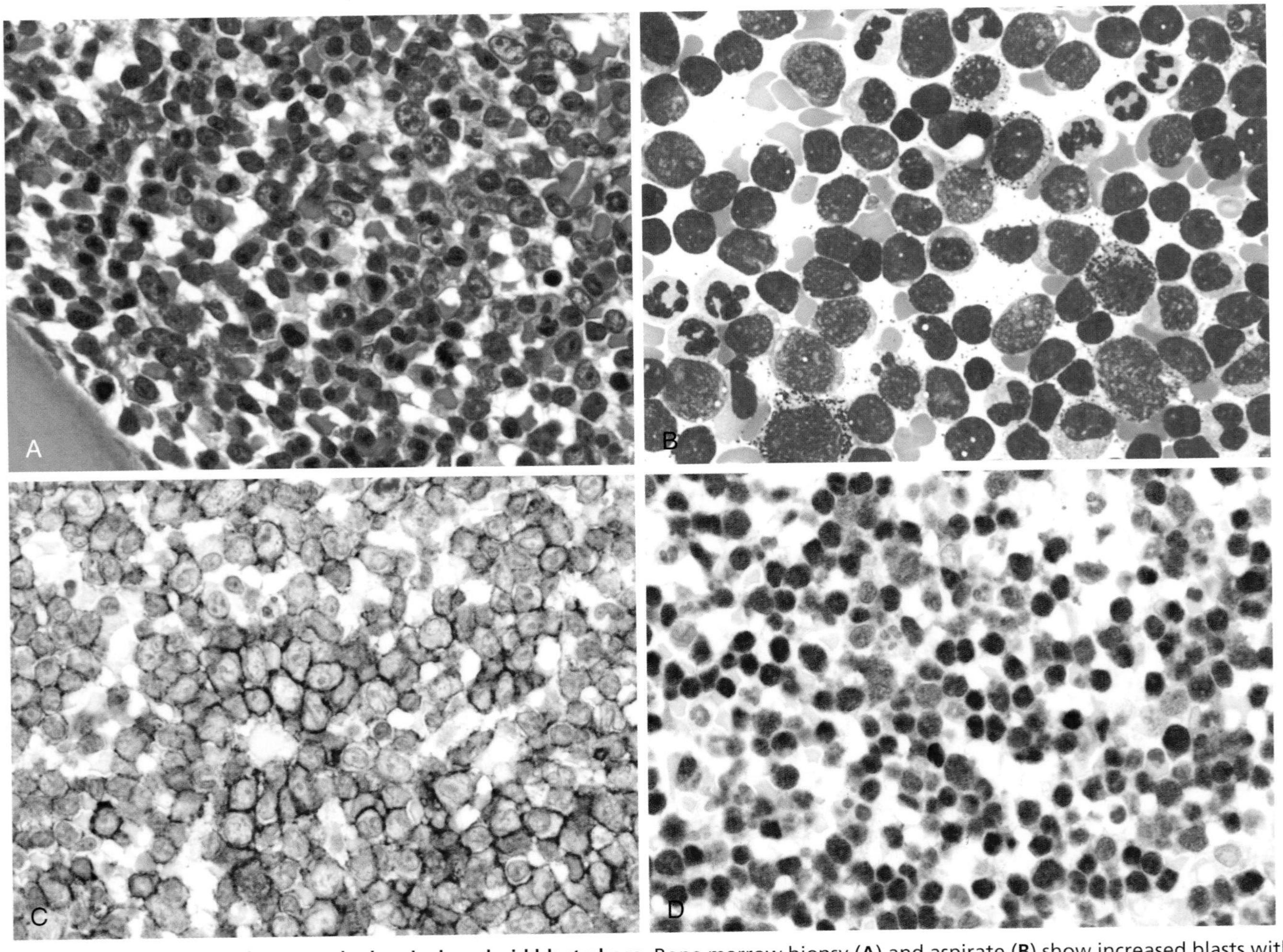

Figure 46-17. Chronic myelogenous leukemia, lymphoid blast phase. Bone marrow biopsy (**A**) and aspirate (**B**) show increased blasts with lymphoid morphology in a background of granulocytic cells. The blasts express CD19 (**C**) and terminal deoxynucleotidyl transferase (**D**), from a patient with *BCR-ABL1*–positive CML diagnosed 8 years previously.

phenotype blasts may also be found, manifesting as blasts with myeloid- and lymphoid-related antigens on the same cells or on separate and distinct myeloid and lymphoid populations present simultaneously or sequentially.[117,120] An extramedullary proliferation of blasts can precede or occur simultaneous with or subsequent to the recognition of BP in the bone marrow. This can occur at any site but is usually encountered in the skin, lymph nodes, spleen, or central nervous system[121] and may be comprised of myeloblasts, lymphoblasts, or mixed phenotype blasts. The diagnosis of an extramedullary blast proliferation is synonymous with CML, BP, regardless of the bone marrow findings.

Appearance of *BCR-ABL1*–Negative Clonal Myeloid Proliferations

As noted previously, in occasional patients with CML who have been treated and may be in cytogenetic or even molecular remission, a clonal population of myeloid cells is found that lacks the Ph chromosome or *BCR-ABL1* fusion gene. Most often the myeloid clones demonstrate clonal chromosomal abnormalities, such as +8 or del(20q). In some cases the clone may be transient, but in others there may be clinical and morphologic manifestations of an MDS or acute leukemia.[105,106] Such clones may be a new therapy-induced disorder, or they may represent evolution of a clone that preceded even the Ph chromosome. At present, their relation to the initial CML clone is unknown in most cases.[76]

Therapy and Disease Monitoring

Our understanding of the molecular pathogenesis of CML and the development of therapy to target the causative molecular defect have led to dramatic improvements in patient survival and quality of life. Before there was any effective therapy, median survival in patients with CML ranged from 2 to 3 years. Conventional chemotherapy, such as busulfan, improved median survival to about 4 years but did little to delay the onset of AP or BP, and with such therapy, less than 10% of patients were alive 10 years after diagnosis.[122] Currently, the first line of therapy is the TKI imatinib, which inhibits the abnormal tyrosine kinase activity associated with the BCR-ABL1 fusion protein. In a large cohort of more than 500 patients treated continuously with imatinib and followed for 6 years, 97% achieved and maintained a complete hematologic response; 82% achieved a complete cytogenetic response, with disappearance of the Ph chromosome at some time during the follow-up period; and 63% of patients still exhibited a complete cytogenetic response at the end of follow-up.[76] Measurement of BCR-ABL1 transcripts by quantitative RT-PCR in the same cohort showed a greater than 3-log reduction in 80% of the patients by 48 months after the start of therapy.[123] Astoundingly, for those who achieved a complete cytogenetic response, the annual rates of progression to AP or BP fell throughout the observation period, from 2.8% at 2 years to 0% at 6 years.[76] Imatinib is also effective in many patients in the transformed stages, although the response rate is not as high as in CP and is sometimes short-lived.

Despite the efficacy of imatinib, it is not curative, and transcripts of BCR-ABL1 remain detectable by quantitative RT-PCR in most patients. In addition, a number of mechanisms may lead to therapy resistance. These include amplification of the *BCR-ABL1* gene, point mutations in the tyrosine kinase domain that interfere with binding of TKIs, additional genetic evolution, and a number of pharmacokinetic considerations.[124] Therefore, patients with CML need to be monitored continually to detect the level of BCR-ABL1 transcripts in the blood or bone marrow, as well as to detect evidence of cytogenetic remission or cytogenetic evolution. A number of recommendations have been proposed for the assessment of patients on TKI therapy. Most include routine cytogenetic studies at diagnosis and at regular intervals thereafter until a complete cytogenetic remission is achieved, as well as quantitative RT-PCR at diagnosis to determine a baseline value for BCR-ABL1 transcripts and regular measurements thereafter. When a complete cytogenetic response is obtained, levels of BCR-ABL1 transcripts in the blood should be analyzed at regular (usually 3-month) intervals by quantitative RT-PCR.[79,124,125] A routine karyotype of bone marrow cells is recommended whenever the transcript level increases or there is any change in the clinical status. In the event of acquired resistance during therapy, the mechanism should be ascertained, including analysis for mutations in the tyrosine kinase domain.

Imatinib and other TKIs have predictable effects on the morphologic findings of CML in the blood and bone marrow. The most striking effect is normalization of the peripheral blood counts and of bone marrow cellularity (Fig. 46-18). In some patients, hypocellular bone marrow may be seen, depending on the duration of therapy. However, if marrow fibrosis was present initially, it may take months to resolve. Lymphoid aggregates are commonly observed in the biopsy during therapy with imatinib. Signs of failure of response include sustained hypercelluarity of the bone marrow or abnormal blood counts, persistence of an increased or increasing percentage of basophils or blasts, and increasing marrow fibrosis. Nevertheless, the findings should always be correlated with cytogenetic and quantitative assessment of BCR-ABL1 transcripts. Currently, the most important prognostic indicator is the response to treatment at the hematologic, cytogenetic, and molecular level.[126]

Differential Diagnosis

Chronic Phase

The differential diagnosis of CML in CP includes reactive leukocytosis; other MPNs, particularly CNL; chronic eosinophilic leukemia, not otherwise specified (CEL, NOS); the myeloid neoplasms associated with rearrangements of *PDGFRA*, *PDGFRB*, and *FGFR1*; the MDS/MPN subtypes of CMML; atypical chronic myeloid leukemia, *BCR-ABL1* negative; and, in the pediatric population, JMML. There is no Ph chromosome or *BCR-ABL1* fusion gene in any of these disorders, but they have to be considered as alternative diagnoses if a case thought to be CML turns out to have no Ph chromosome and no *BCR-ABL1* by FISH or by RT-PCR. Rare cases may be encountered that closely resemble CML but do not have a Ph chromosome or *BCR-ABL1* fusion gene and that do not meet the criteria for any other well-defined myeloid neoplasm. Such cases are best considered MPN, unclassifiable, until additional evolution of the disease leads to a better characterization. Each of the disorders considered in the differential diagnosis is described in detail elsewhere in

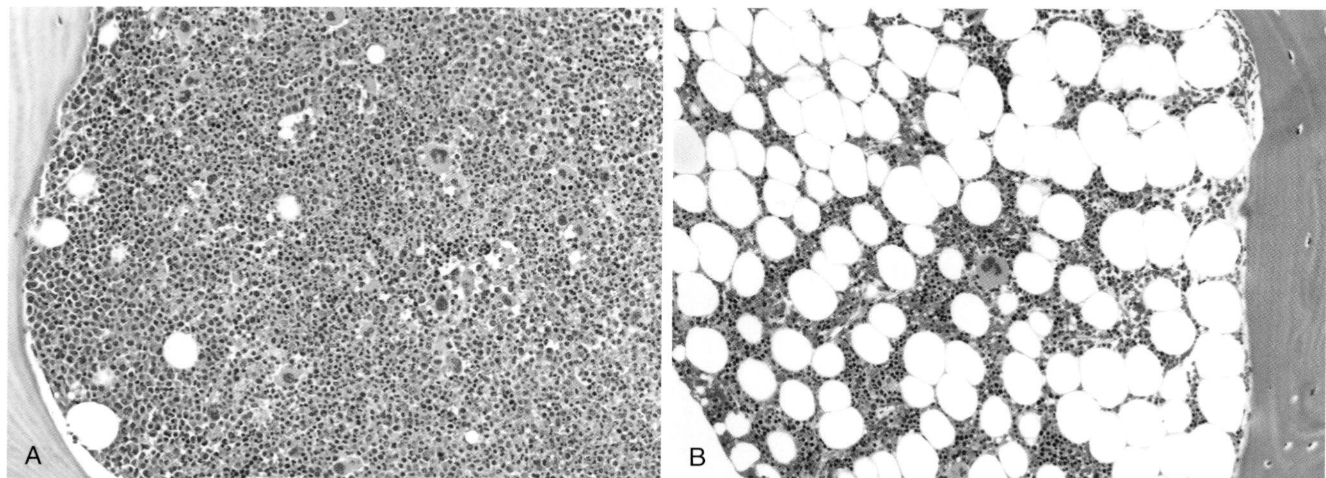

Figure 46-18. Initial bone marrow biopsy (**A**) of a patient with Ph⁺ chronic myelogenous leukemia and a repeat biopsy 12 months after the institution of imatinib therapy (**B**), at which time a complete hematologic and cytogenetic remission had been achieved. Notice the small megakaryocytes in the initial marrow and the normal-sized megakaryocytes in the remission marrow.

this book, but the major features that distinguish them from CML and from one another are briefly described here and in Table 46-1.

Reactive leukocytosis or leukemoid reactions can usually be distinguished from CML by the clinical history and a thorough search for an underlying infectious, inflammatory, or neoplastic process. In the peripheral blood, most cases of reactive leukocytosis lack basophilia and the myelocyte bulge that characterizes CML. In questionable cases, molecular or FISH studies performed on peripheral blood cells may be necessary and are advisable if no cause for persistent neutrophilia can be found. Bone marrow samples are usually not required to distinguish reactive leukocytosis from CML, but the bone marrow may occasionally provide a clue to the reason for the leukocytosis, such as a metastatic tumor or infectious process.

CNL is a rare, *BCR-ABL1*–negative, clonal myeloid leukemia characterized by sustained neutrophilia, hepatosplenomegaly, and bone marrow hypercellularity (see the later section for a more detailed description).[127-130] Briefly, peripheral blood smears in CNL lack the spectrum of immature and mature neutrophils typical of CML, exhibiting mainly segmented neutrophils, often with toxic granulation; basophilia is absent or minimal. In the bone marrow there is granulocytic proliferation, with a shift to mature forms; importantly, the "dwarf" megakaryocytes seen in CML are not observed. In *BCR-ABL1*–positive CML associated with the p230 BCR-ABL1 protein, segmented neutrophils predominate in the blood and may resemble CNL; in these cases, cytogenetic and, if necessary, molecular genetic studies are essential to exclude CML.[97]

Eosinophilic disorders—including myeloid neoplasms associated with abnormalities of *PDGFRA*, *PDGFRB*, and *FGFR1*; CEL, NOS; and hypereosinophilic syndrome—are characterized by a sustained eosinophil count of at least 1.5×10^9/L. However, occasionally in CML, eosinophils are

Table 46-1 Comparison of Major Features of Chronic Myelogenous Leukemia and Other Entities in the Differential Diagnosis

Feature	Chronic Phase CML, *BCR-ABL1* Positive	CNL	CMML-1, -2	aCML, *BCR-ABL1* Negative
Philadelphia chromosome	≈95%	0	0	0
BCR-ABL1 fusion gene	100%	0	0	0
Principal proliferating cells	Granulocytes, megakaryocytes	Granulocytes	Monocytes, granulocytes	Granulocytes
Monocytes	Usually <3%	$<1 \times 10^9$/L	$>1 \times 10^9$/L; >10%	$<1 \times 10^9$/L; <10%
Basophils	>2%	<2%	<2%	<2%
Dysplasia	Absent to minimal	Absent, "toxic" changes frequent	Usually in one or more lineages	Always dysgranulopoiesis, often trilineage dysplasia
Blasts (peripheral blood)	<10%	<1%	<20%	<20%
Immature granulocytes (peripheral blood)	Often >20%	<10%	Usually <20%	10%-20%
Megakaryocytes	Usually normal or increased numbers, with "dwarf" morphology; occasionally mildly decreased	Normal or increased numbers, with normal morphology	Decreased, normal, or occasionally increased numbers, with variable but often dysplastic morphology	Normal, decreased, or rarely increased numbers, often with dysplastic morphology

aCML, atypical chronic myeloid leukemia; CML, chronic myelogenous leukemia; CMML, chronic myelomonocytic leukemia; CNL, chronic neutrophilic leukemia.

markedly increased and may reach this quantity. No matter what the cause, sustained eosinophilia leads to tissue damage due to the release of eosinophil cationic proteins, and patients may suffer irreparable damage to cardiac, pulmonary, neurologic, or other tissues. Therefore, discovering the reason for the eosinophilia is essential. In CEL, NOS and in those cases associated with rearrangement of *PDGFRA*, *PDGFRB*, or *FGFR1*, the eosinophilia is due to clonal, autonomous proliferation of eosinophil precursors; in contrast, in hypereosinophilic syndrome, no underlying cause for the eosinophilia can be discovered, such as hypersensitivity pneumonia, parasitic infection, T-cell lymphoma, or Hodgkin's lymphoma, nor is there any evidence of eosinophil clonality.[131,132] Many of the disorders associated with eosinophilia have some granulocytic proliferation as well, so confusion with CML is possible. Although the bone marrow in any of these disorders, including CML, may show a marked increase in eosinophils, eosinophil precursors, and Charcot-Leyden crystals, the "dwarf" megakaryocytes typical of CML are not found in CEL, NOS; the disorders associated with *PDGFRA*, *PDGFRB*, or *FGFR1*; or hypereosinophilic syndrome. In a patient with marked eosinophilia and no apparent underlying inflammatory or nonmyeloid neoplastic disease, studies for the Ph chromosome and *BCR-ABL1* fusion and for rearrangements of *PDGFRA*, *PDGFRB*, and *FGFR1* should be performed, and the case categorized appropriately if any of these are found.[133] If the case does not fit into any of these categories but there is a myeloid-related clonal abnormality or an increase in blasts in the blood or bone marrow, the diagnosis is CEL, NOS. If there is no evidence of clonality, no increase in blasts, and no apparaent reason for the eosinophilia, the diagnosis is hypereosinophilic syndrome.[133]

CMML is characterized by monocytosis greater than 1000/μL and 10% or more monocytes in the peripheral blood, dysplasia in one or more of the myeloid lineages, and less than 20% blasts in the blood or bone marrow.[134] There is no Ph chromosome or *BCR-ABL1* fusion gene. The 10% or greater monocyte rule of thumb is important because in a patient with CML who presents with a WBC count of 100 × 10^9/L, only 1% monocytes in the leukocyte differential would result in absolute monocytosis. However, CML in CP rarely has 10% or more monocytes in the peripheral blood. Not uncommonly, blood and bone marrow specimens of patients with CMML have a significant granulocytic component, and there may also be small, dysplastic megakaryocytes. Further, splenomegaly is common, so confusion between CML and CMML is clinically and morphologically possible. In addition, the rare cases of CML that carry the shorter BCR-ABL1 fusion protein (p190) frequently have monocytosis and may initially be misdiagnosed as CMML.[96] Therefore, the leukemic cells of all patients in whom CMML is suspected should be analyzed by routine karyotyping and, if no Ph chromosome is present, by FISH or RT-PCR to exclude CML. See Chapter 47 for a detailed description of CMML.

Atypical chronic myeloid leukemia is not merely an atypical form of CML, as its name might imply (see Chapter 47). There is no *BCR-ABL1* fusion gene in atypical chronic myeloid leukemia. Furthermore, in contrast to *BCR-ABL1*–positive CML, the granulocytes demonstrate prominent dysplasia, there is no significant basophilia, and thrombocytopenia is common. In the bone marrow, there is often dysplasia of the erythroid and megakaryocytic lineages, as well as the granulocytic lineage.[86,135] Median survival times of less than 2 years are reported,[136] although relatively few patients have been studied.

JMML is a disorder of children; more than 90% of cases are diagnosed before the age of 4 years. There is no Ph chromosome or *BCR-ABL1* fusion gene, but nearly 80% of children demonstrate mutated *NRAS* or *KRAS*, *NF1*, or *PTNP11*. Monosomy 7 is found in 20% to 30% of cases. The peripheral blood shows leukocytosis with monocytosis greater than 1000 × 10^9/L, with variable numbers of immature granulocytes and nucleated RBCs.

Transformed Stages

The differential diagnosis of CML in AP or BP is not problematic if there is a history of CML. However, occasional patients with CML initially present in BP, and it may be nearly impossible to distinguish between BP CML and de novo Ph^+ ALL, Ph^+ mixed phenotype acute leukemia, or Ph^+ AML. If the blood shows blasts in a background of granulocytic proliferation with a left shift, a myelocyte bulge, and absolute basophilia and there are "dwarf" megakaryocytes in the bone marrow, the diagnosis of BP CML is most likely. However, if these features are absent and blasts constitute the majority of cells in the blood and bone marrow, the diagnosis is more difficult. If the breakpoint in *BCR* is in the minor breakpoint cluster region, with the production of p190, the diagnosis of de novo acute leukemia is supported but not proved. A breakpoint in the major breakpoint cluster region does not resolve the issue either, because in a minority of cases of de novo Ph^+ ALL, particularly in adults, the p210 protein is present. The issue of whether Ph^+ AML is a distinct entity is not yet settled. Although Ph^+ AML has been reported,[137-139] the criteria to distinguish it from BP CML are not entirely convincing, and for this reason, Ph^+ AML is not currently recognized in the WHO classification. The category of Ph^+ mixed phenotype acute leukemia is recognized, however, provided that BP CML can be excluded.[120]

CHRONIC NEUTROPHILIC LEUKEMIA

CNL is a clonal MPN characterized by a sustained proliferation of mature neutrophilic granulocytes in the bone marrow, with leukemic involvement of the peripheral blood and infiltration of the spleen and liver. There is no Ph chromosome or *BCR-ABL1* fusion gene and no rearrangements of *PDGFRA*, *PDGFRB*, or *FGFR1*. Although some data suggest that it is a clonal disorder that arises in a pluripotent stem cell, with involvement of lymphoid as well as myeloid lineages,[140] other data indicate that the lineage involvement in CNL is more limited, perhaps involving only the granulocytes.[141] Granulocyte-macrophage colony-stimulating factor and granulocyte colony-stimulating factor are reportedly low in CNL,[142] and mononuclear cells isolated from the blood and bone marrow reportedly give rise to colonies of maturing and mature granulocytes without added growth factors.[141] The abnormalities in signal transduction pathways that account for the endogenous colony formation are not known, although the *JAK2* V617F mutation has been reported in a few cases.[143-145] CNL is so rare, however, that not enough cases have been studied to reliably assess its cell of origin, its underlying biology, or even its incidence in the population. Fewer than 150 cases have been reported in the literature, and it is likely that less than 40% of those would meet the WHO criteria for the diagnosis of CNL.[129]

Diagnosis

When considering a diagnosis of CNL, the major challenge is to exclude reactive neutrophilia due to an underlying infection, inflammatory disorder, or nonhematopoietic or hematopoietic neoplasm, including other myeloid neoplasms. The clinical history and physical findings are of paramount importance, and it is often necessary to observe the patient for an appropriate period to ensure that the neutrophilia is sustained. Correlation of the hematologic data, morphologic findings in blood and bone marrow, and cytogenetic and molecular genetic information, including studies for *JAK2* V617F and *BCR-ABL1* fusion, is necessary to confidently make a diagnosis of CNL. Although studies for clonality using inactivation patterns of X-linked genes, such as the human androgen receptor gene assay, may support the diagnosis of CNL in some cases, such studies must be interpreted with caution and are rarely used in clinical practice.[146] The WHO criteria for CNL are listed in Box 46-4.

Clinical Findings

Although CNL usually affects adults in their 60s, it has been reported in adolescents as well. The sexes appear to be nearly equally affected. Many patients are asymptomatic, and a blood count performed during a routine medical examination reveals leukocytosis; other patients complain of fatigue, gout, or pruritus.[127,129] The most consistent physical finding is splenomegaly, which may be symptomatic.[127,129,147] Hepatomegaly may be present but is uncommon, as is lymphadenopathy. A tendency for bleeding from mucosal surfaces has been reported in 25% to 30% of patients with CNL.[127,148]

Laboratory Findings

Peripheral Blood

The WBC count is 25×10^9/L or greater (median, 50×10^9/L). Segmented neutrophils and bands account for 80% or more of the WBCs, whereas the sum of immature granulocytes (promyelocytes, myelocytes, and metamyelocytes) is usually less than 5% and always less than 10% of the WBCs (Fig. 46-19). Myeloblasts are almost never seen in the blood at diagnosis.[130] Toxic granulation in the neutrophils is commonly reported, but there is no significant dysplasia.[127,128,147] The neutrophil alkaline phosphatase score is often elevated,[127,130,147] but this is a nonspecific finding. Monocytes are not increased

Box 46-4 *World Health Organization Diagnostic Criteria for Chronic Neutrophilic Leukemia*

- Peripheral blood leukocytosis: white blood cell count ≥25×10^9/L
  - Segmented neutrophils and bands are >80% of white blood cells
  - Immature granulocytes (promyelocytes, myelocytes, metamyelocytes) are <10% of white blood cells
  - Myeloblasts are <1% of white blood cells
- Hypercellular bone marrow biopsy
  - Neutrophilic granulocytes increased in percentage
  - Myeloblasts are <5% of nucleated bone marrow cells
  - Neutrophilic maturation pattern normal or shifted to segmented forms
  - Megakaryocytes normal
- Hepatosplenomegaly
- No identifiable cause for physiologic neutrophilia or, if present, proof of clonality of myeloid cells
  - No infectious or inflammatory process
  - No underlying tumor
- No Philadelphia chromosome or *BCR-ABL1* fusion gene
- No rearrangement of *PDGFRA*, *PDGFRB*, or *FGFR1*
- No evidence of polycythemia vera, essential thrombocythemia, or primary myelofibrosis
- No evidence of myelodysplastic syndrome or myelodysplastic/myeloproliferative neoplasm
  - No granulocytic dysplasia
  - No myelodysplastic changes in other myeloid lineages
  - Monocytes <1×10^9/L

From Swerdlow SH, Campo E, Harris NL, et al, eds. *WHO Classification of Tumours of Haematopoietic and Lymphoid Tissues*. Lyon, France: IARC Press; 2008.

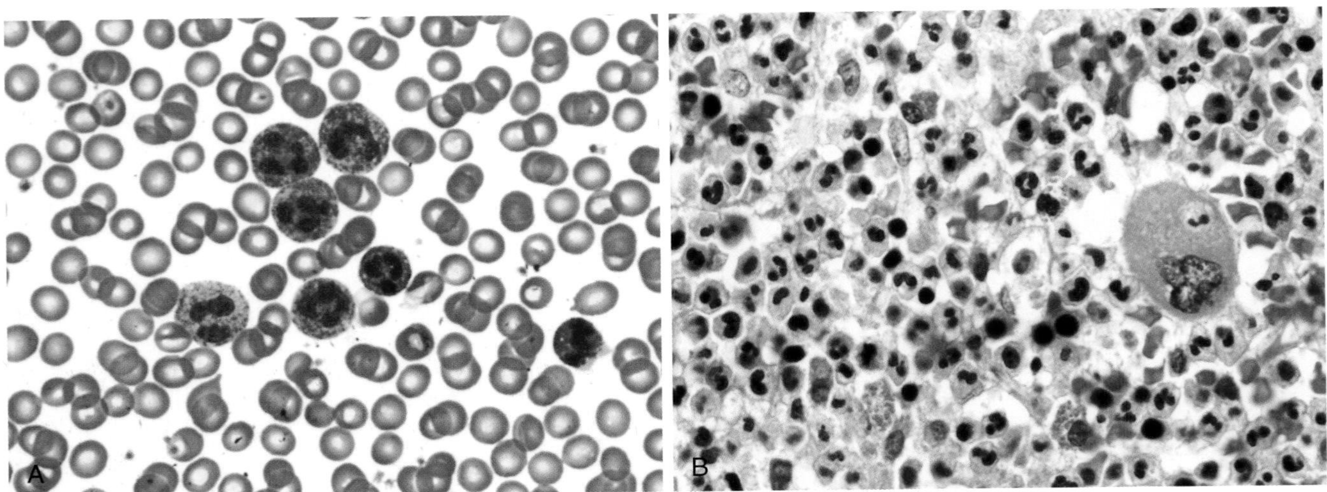

Figure 46-19. Chronic neutrophilic leukemia. A, Peripheral blood shows mainly segmented neutrophils with toxic granules. **B,** Biopsy shows a similar shift toward mature forms. No underlying disease could be found to explain the neutrophilia, and splenomegaly was present.

in absolute numbers ($<1 \times 10^9/L$), and basophilia and eosinophilia are not observed. Mild to moderate anemia is common, although RBC morphology is usually normal.[128,130] The platelet count is most often within the normal range or slightly reduced, but severe thrombocytopenia or thrombocytosis is uncommon.[129] Platelet function studies are reportedly abnormal in rare cases, but the vast majority of patients reported in the literature have not been evaluated for platelet defects.[148]

Bone Marrow

In CNL the bone marrow biopsy is markedly hypercellular due to neutrophil proliferation, with a myeloid-to-erythroid ratio of 20:1 or more (see Fig. 46-19). The percentages of blasts and promyelocytes are not increased at the time of diagnosis, but the percentages of myelocytes, metamyelocytes, bands, and segmented neutrophils are increased.[127,129,130] As in the blood, the neutrophils may show significant reactive changes, with toxic granules; however, there is no significant dysplasia, and basophilia and eosinophilia are not observed. In the bone marrow, erythroid precursors are reduced in percentage but are usually normoblastic. Megakaryocytes are morphologically normal, although mild megakaryocytic proliferation has been reported in some cases.[129,147] Reticulin fibrosis is uncommon.

In the older literature, nearly 30% of cases of CNL were associated with plasma cell myeloma or other plasma cell dyscrasias,[149-152] although in virtually none of the reported cases was neutrophil clonality documented. It is likely that the neutrophilia associated with plasma cell dyscrasia is reactive and driven by cytokines released from the plasma cells or other accessory cells. The WHO classification specifically recommends that CNL not be diagnosed when another neoplastic process, such as myeloma, is present, unless there is documentation of neutrophil clonality.[130] Because of the frequent association between neutrophilia and plasma cell myeloma, the bone marrow should be examined for evidence of excess plasma cells using morphologic and immunohistochemical studies when considering the diagnosis of CNL.

Extramedullary Tissues

Splenomegaly and hepatomegaly are caused by tissue infiltration by neutrophils. In the spleen the infiltration assumes the usual leukemic pattern, with infiltration in the red pulp cords and sinuses, whereas in the liver the sinuses or portal areas, or both, may be infiltrated.[127,130,147]

Genetics

Cytogenetic abnormalities are found in 20% to 25% of patients at diagnosis and are helpful in proving the clonal nature of the process, but none are specific.[129,130] Abnormalities reported include +8, +9, +21, del(20q), and del(11q). Additional abnormalities may occur with disease progression. By definition, there is no Ph chromosome or *BCR-ABL1* fusion gene and no rearrangement of *PDGFRA*, *PDGFRB*, or *FGFR1*. Although the *JAK2* V617F mutation has been reported in CNL, its incidence is unknown owing to the limited number of patients studied.[143-145]

Disease Progression and Prognosis

CNL follows a progressive disease course. Acceleration of the disease is often associated with increasing neutrophilia, worsening anemia, and thrombocytopenia. Transformation to a BP reportedly occurs in 10% to 15% of cases.[129] Intracranial hemorrhage as a cause of death has been reported in a disproportionate number of patients. Although this may be a manifestation of an underlying coagulation or platelet abnormality, it may also be related to thrombocytopenia related to progressive disease or to the therapy for progressive disease.[148]

Differential Diagnosis

The differential diagnosis of CNL includes reactive neutrophilia and other neoplastic myeloid proliferations. Chronic infection and inflammation and nonmyeloid hematopoietic or nonhematopoietic malignancies can lead to sustained reactive neutrophilia that mimics CNL. Toxic granulation is often seen in reactive neutrophilia and in CNL, so peripheral blood morphology is not a reliable means of distinguishing between these two disorders. Often the underlying cause is revealed by a thorough clinical history and additional clinical and laboratory studies. The bone marrow should always be carefully examined to exclude a plasma cell dyscrasia or another underlying neoplasm. Some epithelial tumors and sarcomas secrete cytokines that stimulate neutrophil production, so nonhematopoietic tumors must be excluded as well.[129,153,154] In the presence of either a plasma cell dyscrasia or another neoplastic condition, the diagnosis of CNL should be deferred unless there is convincing evidence of clonality of the neutrophil population or of their precursors or until it has been proved that the underlying tumor is not responsible for the neutrophilia and no other cause can be found. The other disorders to be considered in the differential diagnosis of CNL are *BCR-ABL1*–positive CML, particularly when associated with the variant p230 BCR-ABL1 fusion protein; CMML; and *BCR-ABL1*–negative atypical chronic myeloid leukemia. The distinguishing features of these entities are listed in Table 46-1. In a pediatric patient, JMML may also be considered, but the finding of monocytosis in the blood, which is required for the diagnosis of JMML, excludes CNL from further consideration.

POLYCYTHEMIA VERA

Erythropoiesis is fine-tuned to produce sufficient numbers of RBCs to carry oxygen to the tissues. Tissue hypoxia leads to an increase in the production of EPO, which is the primary regulator of erythropoiesis. When EPO binds to the EPOR on erythroid progenitors, there is homodimerization of EPOR and autophosphorylation of the associated JAK2 kinase, which in turn activates downstream effectors to culminate in the proliferation and reduced apoptosis of erythroid precursors (see Fig. 46-5).[155] Downregulation of EPOR and JAK2 signaling is mediated by protein tyrosine phosphatases such as SHP-1, by suppressors of cytokine signaling, and by other inhibitors of the activated downstream pathways.[156] The synthesis of EPO occurs in peritubular cells in the kidney and is regulated by a family of transcription factors produced in response to hypoxia, the hypoxia-inducible factors (HIFs).[157,158] The HIFs undergo degradation as normal oxygen levels are reached through an interaction among HIF, oxygen, prolyl hydroxylase domain (PHD)–containing enzymes, and the von Hippel-Lindau tumor suppressor protein (VHL). Under conditions of hypoxia, HIF degradation is slowed, leading to the

Box 46-5 *Causes of Polycythemia*

"True" Primary Polycythemia
- Congenital: primary familial congenital erythrocytosis, including *EPOR* mutations
- Acquired: polycythemia vera

"True" Secondary Polycythemia
- Congenital
  - *VHL* mutations, including Chuvash polycythemia
  - 2,3-bisphosphoglycerate mutase deficiency
  - High-oxygen-affinity hemoglobin
  - Congenital methemoglobinemia
  - Hypoxia-inducible factor-2α mutations
  - Prolyl hydoxylase domain-2 mutations
- Acquired
  - Physiologically appropriate response to hypoxia: cardiac, pulmonary, renal, and hepatic diseases; carbon monoxide poisoning; sleep apnea; renal artery stenosis; smoker's polycythemia; after renal transplant*
  - Inappropriate production of erythropoietin: cerebellar hemangioblastoma, uterine leiomyoma, pheochromocytoma, renal cell carcinoma, hepatocellular carcinoma, meningioma, parathyroid adenoma

Relative, "Spurious," or "False" Polycythemia
- Acute, transient hemoconcentration due to dehydration or other causes of contraction of plasma volume; red cell mass is not increased, so it is not true polycythemia

*The cause of post–renal transplant polycythemia is not clear; in some cases it is likely due to retained, chronically ischemic native kidney with endogenous erythropoietin production plus increased sensitivity of the erythroid precursors to EPO.

promotion of EPO synthesis.[159] Disturbances anywhere in the EPOR signaling pathway or in the production of EPO can lead to either too few or too many RBCs.

Polycythemia is an increase in the number of RBCs per unit volume of blood, usually defined as a greater than 2 standard deviation increase from the age-, sex- and race-adjusted normal value for hemoglobin (Hb), hematocrit, or red cell mass.[160,161] There are multiple causes of polycythemia (Box 46-5). Usually, polycythemia is a "true" increase in the red cell mass, but occasionally, diminished plasma volume may lead to hemoconcentration and to "relative" or "spurious" polycythemia. True polycythemia may be primary, in which an inherent abnormality of the erythroid progenitors renders them hypersensitive to (or independent of) factors that normally regulate their proliferation, or secondary, in which case the increase in RBCs is caused by an increase in serum EPO due to an appropriate physiologic response to tissue hypoxia or to the inappropriate secretion of EPO by various neoplasms. Primary and secondary polycythemia may be either acquired or congenital.

PV is an acquired primary polycythemia. It is a rare disease with an annual incidence of approximately 1 to 3 per 100,000 individuals in the Western world; the incidence is reportedly lower in Asia. It is a clonal proliferation not only of erythroid precursors but also of granulocytes and megakaryocytes in the bone marrow (i.e., panmyelosis), so in addition to polycythemia there are leukocytosis and thrombocytosis in the blood. The clinical manifestations are usually related to the vascular consequences of the increased red cell mass and consist mainly of thrombosis and hemorrhage. Three phases of PV have been described: (1) a prodromal, prepolycythemic phase with borderline to mild erythrocytosis, often with prominent thrombocytosis; (2) an overt polycythemic phase; and (3) a postpolycythemic phase, which is characterized by cytopenias (including anemia), bone marrow fibrosis, and EMH (post-PV myelofibrosis [post-PVMF]).[161] The natural history of PV also includes a low incidence of evolution to a BP (1% to 2%). In addition, a number of patients with PV may develop myelodysplasia or a BP related to cytotoxic therapy given to suppress the myeloproliferation.

More than 90% of cases of PV are associated with the acquired somatic mutation *JAK2* V617F, and most of the remainder have a similar *JAK2* exon 12 activating mutation. Families with a high incidence of MPNs, including PV, have been well described. In such cases *JAK2* V617F is an acquired somatic mutation.[16] Recent evidence gained from the study of single nucleotide polymorphisms in patients with PV suggests that variation in germline genes, including germline *JAK2*, may predispose to acquisition of the somatic *JAK2* mutation in a hematopoietic stem cell.[19]

Diagnosis

In the past a major diagnostic difficulty was the distinction of PV from secondary polycythemia. In the absence of any specific biologic marker, previous diagnostic criteria for PV, such as those suggested by the venerable Polycythemia Vera Study Group,[162] included nonspecific clinical and laboratory parameters intended to exclude secondary erythrocytosis and to support the presence of a primary MPN. There was virtually no role for histopathology in these criteria. Now, with the knowledge that virtually all cases of PV are associated with *JAK2* V617F or *JAK2* exon 12 mutations, it is much simpler to distinguish PV from causes of secondary polycythemia. However, because *JAK2* V617F is also found in ET and PMF, additional laboratory and histopathologic parameters are needed to distinguish PV from these MPNs. Box 46-6 lists the WHO criteria for the diagnosis of PV. Figure 46-20 provides a simple algorithm for the evaluation of patients with suspected PV.

Clinical Findings, Polycythemic Phase

PV is usually diagnosed in the polycythemic phase. It is most often encountered in patients in their 60s; patients younger than 20 years are only rarely reported.[163,164] Men are more likely to be affected than women. The principal symptoms of PV are related to thrombosis and hemorrhage, which are also the leading causes of morbidity and mortality.[165,166] The most common initial symptoms, including headache, dizziness, paresthesia, scotomata, and erythromelalgia (increased skin temperature, burning sensations, and redness in the lower extremities), are related to thrombotic events in the microvasculature.[165-169] Thrombosis involving the major arteries or veins occurs as well, and some patients initially have life-threatening events such as myocardial infarct or stroke.[165,166] In 10% to 15% of cases these manifestations occur up to 2 years before development of the abnormal blood parameters characteristic of PV.[165] Although uncommon, splanchnic vein thrombosis or Budd-Chiari syndrome should always raise suspicion of an MPN, including PV. In up to 35% to 40% of such cases, *JAK2* V617F may be present,

Box 46-6 *World Health Organization Diagnostic Criteria for Polycythemia Vera*

Diagnosis requires the presence of both major criteria and one minor criterion *or* the presence of the first major criterion together with two minor criteria:

Major Criteria

- Hemoglobin >18.5 g/dL in men and >16.5 g/dL in women, or other evidence of increased red cell volume*
- Presence of *JAK2* V617F or other functionally similar mutation, such as *JAK2* exon 12 mutation

Minor Criteria

- Bone marrow biopsy showing hypercellularity for age with trilineage growth (panmyelosis) and prominent erythroid, granulocytic, and megakaryocytic proliferation
- Serum erythropoietin level below the reference range for normal
- Endogenous erythroid colony formation in vitro

*Other evidence includes hemoglobin or hematocrit >99th percentile of method-specific reference range for age, sex, and altitude of residence; *or* hemoglobin >17 g/dL in men and >15 g/dL in women if associated with a documented and sustained increase of at least 2 g/dL from the individual's baseline value that cannot be attributed to correction of iron deficiency; *or* elevated red cell mass >25% above the mean normal predicted value.
From Swerdlow SH, Campo E, Harris NL, et al, eds. *WHO Classification of Tumours of Haematopoietic and Lymphoid Tissues*. Lyon, France: IARC Press; 2008.

even though there is no laboratory evidence of a hematologic disorder.[164,170] Overall, thrombotic events are more common in patients older than 65 than in younger patients.[168] Other symptoms include generalized fatigue, aquagenic pruritus, gout, and gastrointestinal complaints related to ulcers and hemorrhage.[165,166] The most prominent physical findings in the polycythemic phase include plethora in up to 80% of cases, splenomegaly in 70%, and hepatomegaly in 40% to 50%.[166]

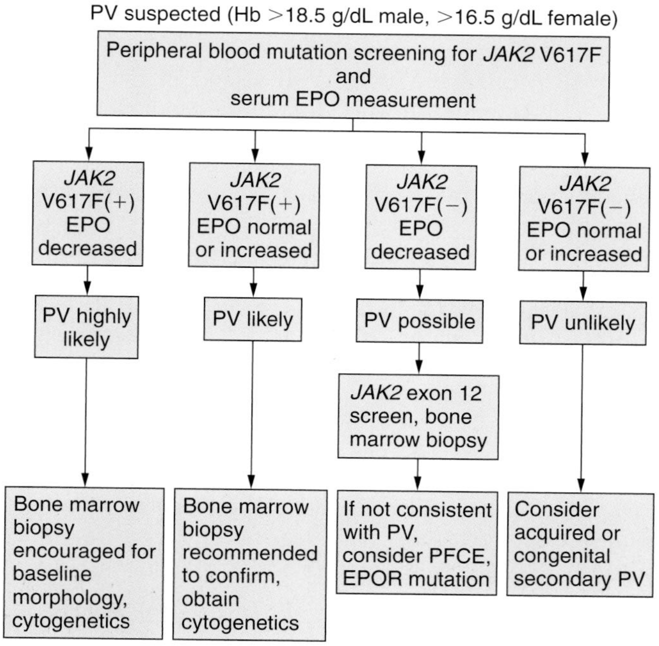

PV suspected (Hb >18.5 g/dL male, >16.5 g/dL female)

Peripheral blood mutation screening for *JAK2* V617F and serum EPO measurement

JAK2 V617F(+) EPO decreased	*JAK2* V617F(+) EPO normal or increased	*JAK2* V617F(−) EPO decreased	*JAK2* V617F(−) EPO normal or increased
PV highly likely	PV likely	PV possible	PV unlikely
		JAK2 exon 12 screen, bone marrow biopsy	
Bone marrow biopsy encouraged for baseline morphology, cytogenetics	Bone marrow biopsy recommended to confirm, obtain cytogenetics	If not consistent with PV, consider PFCE, EPOR mutation	Consider acquired or congenital secondary PV

Figure 46-20. Simplified approach to the diagnosis of polycythemia. EPO, erythropoietin; EPOR, erythropoietin receptor; Hb, hemoglobin; PFCE, primary familial congenital erythrocytosis; PV, polycythemia vera.

Some patients initially have clinical findings suggestive of PV but with Hb values and a red cell mass insufficient to meet the diagnostic criteria. In such "latent" or "prepolycythemic" cases, the diagnosis can be substantiated if *JAK2* V617F or a similar activating mutation is present, serum EPO levels are decreased, and the typical histologic features of PV are seen in a bone marrow specimen.

Laboratory Findings, Polycythemic Phase

Peripheral Blood

The major findings in the peripheral blood are increased Hb, hematocrit, and RBC count (see Box 46-6). The Hb level required for diagnosis is greater than 18.5 g/dL in men and greater than 16.5 g/dL in women; alternatively, it is greater than 17 g/dL in men and greater than 15 g/dL in women if the Hb value is associated with at least a 2 g/dL increase from an individual's baseline level that cannot be attributed to correction of iron deficiency. The RBC indices are usually normal, except in patients with iron deficiency, which is relatively common in PV[167]; in this case, the mean corpuscular volume and mean corpuscular Hb concentration may be low. More than 60% of patients have increased WBC counts due to neutrophilia, and thrombocytosis is found in 50%.[166,167]

The peripheral blood smear shows crowding of RBCs that are usually normochromic and normocytic; they may be microcytic and hypochromic if there is concomitant iron deficiency caused by gastrointestinal bleeding or phlebotomy (Fig. 46-21). A mild left shift in the neutrophils may be present, with occasional immature granulocytes; blasts are rarely seen. Modest basophilia is common, and eosinophils are sometimes slightly increased as well. Thrombocytosis may be marked.

Bone Marrow

Although some have argued that a bone marrow specimen is not necessary to make the diagnosis of PV,[171] others have suggested that a bone marrow specimen helps confirm the diagnosis, provides the best material for cytogenetic studies, and establishes a baseline against which future studies can be compared to assess progression or response to therapy.[167,172] The characteristic bone marrow findings of PV are best observed in a bone marrow biopsy.[89,161,173] The histopathology of latent or early-stage PV and of full-blown polycythemia is similar and is characterized by a proliferation of granulocytic, erythroid, and megakaryocytic lineages (see Fig. 46-21). The cellularity of the bone marrow reportedly ranges from 30% to 100% (median, 80%),[173] but it is characteristically hypercellular for the patient's age. The hypercellularity may be particularly noticeable in the subcortical bone marrow spaces, an area that is often hypocellular in normal, age-matched control patients.[161] Although a modest left shift in granulopoiesis may be observed, there is no increase in the percentage of myeloblasts. Erythropoiesis often occurs in expanded erythroid islands throughout the marrow and is normoblastic, except when iron deficiency leads to iron-deficient

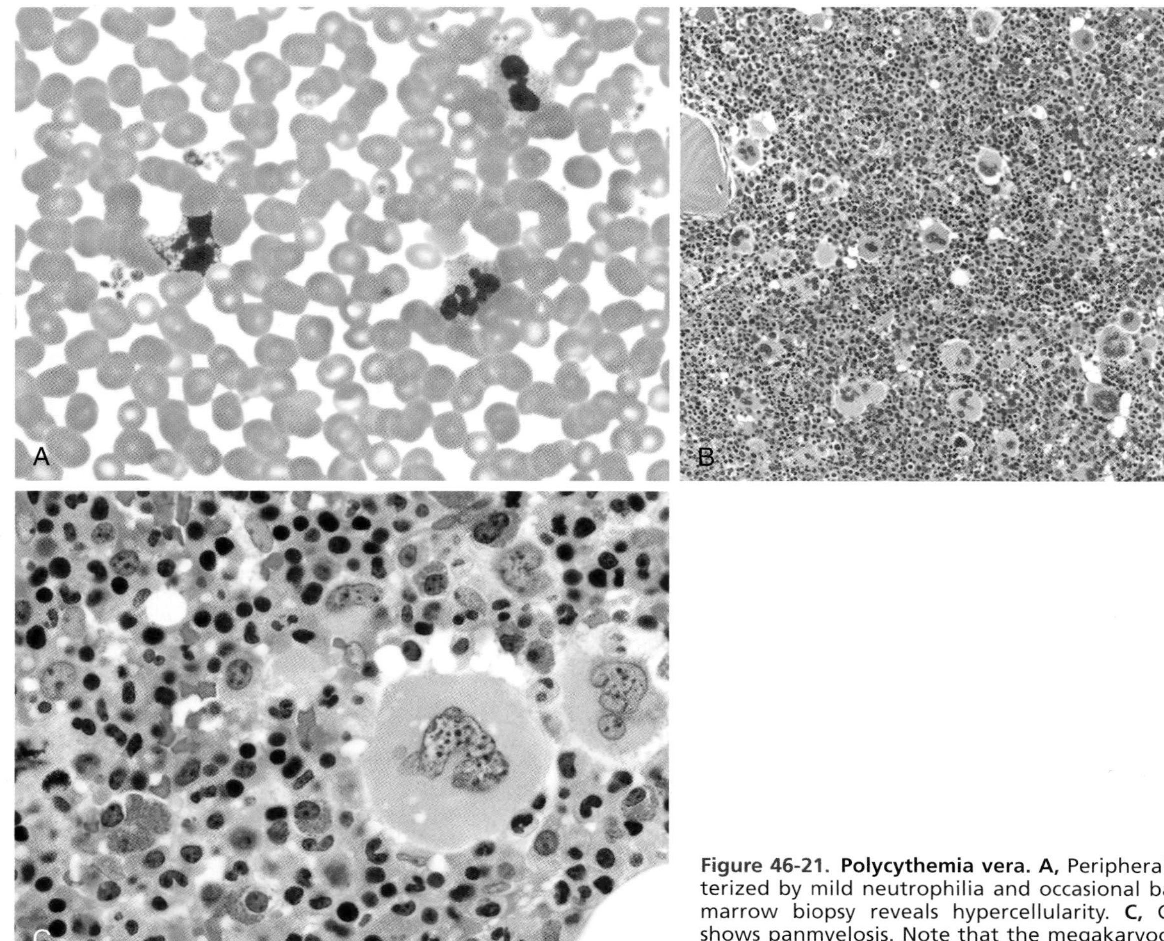

Figure 46-21. Polycythemia vera. A, Peripheral blood is characterized by mild neutrophilia and occasional basophils. **B,** Bone marrow biopsy reveals hypercellularity. **C,** Closer inspection shows panmyelosis. Note that the megakaryocytes are variable in size, but overall, they are not highly atypical or bizarre.

erythropoiesis.[89,161] The megakaryocytes in PV are increased in number. Small, medium, and large megakaryocytes may be dispersed throughout the bone marrow or may form loose clusters, often located abnormally next to bony trabeculae. Although some atypical megakaryocytes are found, they generally lack the marked cytologic atypia that characterizes the megakaryocytes seen in PMF.[89] Stainable iron is absent in the aspirate in more than 90% of cases.[173] In most cases, reticulin fibers are normal, but in about 20% of patients, reticulin and even borderline collagen fibrosis may be found at the time of diagnosis.[161,173] Lymphoid nodules are occasionally seen.

Patients with PV and *JAK2* exon 12 mutations have similar clinical features as those with *JAK2* V617F. In the bone marrow, however, there is mainly erythroid proliferation, with less granulocytic and megakaryocytic expansion than observed in patients with *JAK2* V617F.[174]

Extramedullary Tissues

The splenomegaly present in the polycythemic phase is due to engorgement of the cords and sinuses with RBCs, with minimal if any evidence of EMH.[175] Similar changes are seen in the hepatic sinuses.

Genetics

More than 95% of patients with PV have the *JAK2* V617F mutation, and a *JAK2* exon 12 mutation is found in most of the remaining patients. The *JAK2* V617 F mutation is not unique to PV and is present in nearly 50% of cases of ET and PMF, occasionally in MDS/MPN, and in rare cases of AML.[66,67] It is unknown what determines the disease phenotype in an individual patient with this mutation, but the genetic background of the host as well as the dosage of the mutant allele may be important factors (see the earlier discussion on pathogenesis). Homozygosity for *JAK2* V617F, which results from mitotic recombination, is more common in PV than in other MPNs.[66,176] In virtually all cases of PV, colony-forming cells homozygous for *JAK2* V617F are found, which is almost never the case in ET and uncommon in PMF. In addition to the mutations of *JAK2*, approximately 10% to 20% of patients have cytogenetic abnormalities at diagnosis.[167,177] The most common recurring abnormalities are +8, +9, del(20q), del(13q), and del(9p); sometimes trisomy 8 and trisomy 9 are found together. There is an increased incidence of cytogenetic abnormalities associated with disease progression.

Other Laboratory Findings

The serum EPO level is typically decreased in PV, in contrast to the elevated level often seen in secondary causes of polycythemia. Measurement of the EPO level is therefore an important study that should be performed early in the evaluation of polycythemia (see Fig. 46-20). However, a normal

EPO value does not exclude either PV or secondary erythrocytosis.[171] When grown in vitro in a semisolid medium, bone marrow cells from patients with PV form EECs without the addition of EPO.[22] In contrast, precursors from normal individuals and those with secondary erythrocytosis require EPO for in vitro colony formation and survival. However, EECs are not specific for PV and are seen in ET and PMF as well.[24] Although testing for EECs may provide information that supports the diagnosis of PV, it is rarely performed in most clinical laboratories.

Abnormal platelet function studies, such as decreased primary and secondary aggregation in response to epinephrine or adenosine diphosphate, or both, are frequently observed in patients with PV but correlate poorly with bleeding or thrombotic episodes.[178-180] Acquired storage pool deficiency is common and is likely a manifestation of platelet activation, although the mechanism of activation is not clear.[180] Patients with platelet counts of 1000×10^9/L or more may develop an acquired von Willebrand's syndrome that is associated with decreased functional activity of von Willebrand's factor as measured by collagen binding activity and ristocetin cofactor activity.[179] This defect in von Willebrand's factor activity predisposes to bleeding episodes and explains why patients with higher platelet counts are more prone to hemorrhage than those with lower counts, although there is no direct correlation between platelet count and thrombosis.[180] Usually, the prothrombin time and partial thromboplastin time are normal.

Most patients with PV have hyperuricemia and elevated histamine levels. Serum ferritin is usually low, but such a finding is not specific and may be seen in secondary erythrocytosis as well. Although elevated vitamin B_{12} levels resulting from transcobalamin release from the increased granulocyte mass is typical of PV, this information has little utility in the modern-day workup. In PV, arterial oxygen saturation is normal, as is P50 (the partial pressure of oxygen in blood at which 50% of the Hb is saturated with oxygen).[159]

Disease Progression and Prognosis

Untreated PV patients usually die within 1 to 2 years due to thrombosis or hemorrhage.[165] Currently, aggressive phlebotomy to keep the hematocrit below 45% is the most common therapy. If the patient is at increased risk for thrombosis, cytoreductive therapy with hydroxyurea or similar agents may be used. When patients are carefully managed, survival of 15 years or more is commonly reported, particularly in those who are younger than 70 years at diagnosis.[165]

Aside from thrombosis and hemorrhage, anemia, post-PVMF, and acute leukemia are possible complications. Whether they are part of the natural disease progression or related to previous therapy is not always clear. Further, there is some confusion regarding the terminology used to describe these events. The term *spent phase* is used by some to indicate a phase in which the polycythemia and panmyelosis in the bone marrow have given way to bone marrow failure with anemia. However, anemia in a previously polycythemic patient does not necessarily equate with bone marrow failure. It may be due to iron deficiency resulting from gastrointestinal hemorrhage or phlebotomy or to the volume expansion that often accompanies splenomegaly, even when splenic EMH is not prominent.[171] Nevertheless, two important patterns of disease progression are recognized by all investigators: post-PVMF and AML.

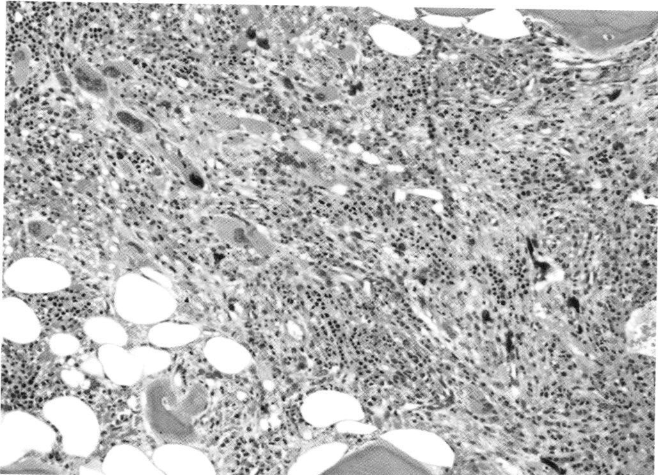

Figure 46-22. Post-polycythemic myelofibrosis. Bone marrow biopsy from a patient with polycythemia vera for nearly 15 years who then developed anemia, leukoerythroblastosis, and increasing splenomegaly. The bone marrow is somewhat depleted, with a background of reticulin fibrosis and atypical megakaryocytes.

Post-polycythemic Myeloid Metaplasia

This progressive and often terminal complication develops in approximately 15% to 20% of patients 10 to 15 years after the initial diagnosis of PV and in up to 50% who survive 20 years or more.[166,181] Post-PVMF is characterized by anemia, a leukoerythroblastic blood smear with red cell poikilocytosis and teardrop-shaped red cells, myelofibrosis of the bone marrow, and splenomegaly due to EMH.[161] Bone marrow specimens are variably cellular but demonstrate overt reticulin and often collagen fibrosis (Fig. 46-22). Osteosclerosis may be present as well. Granulopoiesis and particularly erythropoiesis are diminished in quantity, and clusters of abnormal megakaryocytes of variable sizes with hyperchromatic, bizarre nuclei are frequently the predominant marrow component. The marrow sinuses are often dilated and filled with hematopoietic precursors and megakaryocytes.[89,161] In the spleen, EMH in the cords and sinuses contributes to the leukoerythroblastosis in the blood. A similar pattern of EMH is seen in the liver. Overall, the findings are very similar to those seen in the fibrotic stages of PMF, from which post-PVMF cannot be readily distinguished without an appropriate clinical history. Nearly 80% to 90% of patients with post-PVMF exhibit an abnormal karyotype.[182]

Acute Leukemia/Myelodysplastic Phase

MDS and AML occur as rare and usually late events in PV. The incidence of MDS and AML in patients with PV who have been treated with phlebotomy alone is reportedly 1% to 2%,[182,183] which is often assumed to be the incidence of AML and MDS that would occur during the natural course of the disease. However, the incidence of AML and MDS in some series ranges from 5% to 15% of PV patients followed for 10 years or more.[182,184] The risk of developing a myelodysplastic or leukemic complication appears to be related to the patient's age (higher risk in older patients) and exposure to certain cytotoxic treatment modalities, such as alkylating agents and P32,[182-184] which are now being used less frequently. In virtually all cases the acute leukemia is of myeloid origin and is often preceded by a myelodysplastic phase. Sometimes the transformation to AML occurs in the setting of post-PVMF. In such cases the fibrosis may prevent aspiration, and the detection of blasts in the biopsy may be facilitated by staining for CD34. The finding of 10% or more blasts generally heralds transformation to an accelerated or myelodysplastic stage, and the finding of 20% or more blasts indicates a diagnosis of acute leukemia. Rare cases of lymphoblastic leukemia have been reported and may represent de novo disease.[185]

Almost all patients who develop MDS or AML show karyotypic evolution, often with the acquisition of complex chromosomal abnormalities. The karyotype may include loss of all or part of chromosome 5 or chromosome 7—abnormalities that are commonly associated with therapy-related myeloid neoplasms.[184] At the time of development of acute leukemia, the leukemic blasts may not carry the *JAK2* V617F mutation, giving rise to speculation that the transformation may occur in a clone that preceded the *JAK2* mutated clone.[185]

Differential Diagnosis

The different causes of polycythemia are listed in Box 46-5. Most cases encountered are either primary or secondary acquired polycythemia. Serum EPO levels and genetic testing for *JAK2* V617F should be considered "up-front" tests for the diagnosis of PV and its differentiation from other causes of erythrocytosis.

Primary Polycythemia, Acquired and Congenital

PV is the only acquired primary polycythemia. The only congenital primary polycythemia that has been well characterized is primary familial congenital polycythemia, a rare condition caused by mutations in *EPOR*, usually with an autosomal dominant inheritance pattern.[164,186] So far, 16 different mutations of the gene have been described that lead to truncation of the cytoplasmic portion of *EPOR* and loss of the binding site of SHP-1, which normally downregulates EPO-mediated activation of the JAK2/STAT5 pathway.[159,186] Loss of this domain is, in essence, an activating mutation that results in hypersensitivity of the erythroid precursors to EPO. As a consequence, serum EPO levels are low or normal. There is erythrocytosis but not granulocytosis or thrombocytosis. Patients are often asymptomatic, but there is reportedly a predisposition to develop cardiovascular disease.[186] *EPOR* mutations account for only a small number of cases of primary familial congenital polycythemia; for the majority, the defects are unknown.

In some families there is a predilection to develop PV or other MPNs owing to a genetic factor that predisposes them to acquire a somatic *JAK2* mutation. Such cases should not be considered congenital polycythemia but rather familial primary acquired PV.[15,16]

Secondary Polycythemia, Acquired and Congenital

Most cases of secondary polycythemia are acquired and induced by hypoxia (see Box 46-5). Chronic obstructive lung disease, right-to-left cardiopulmonary shunts, sleep apnea, and renal disease that compromises blood flow to the kidney are among the most frequent causes.[159,187,188] Individuals living at high altitudes compensate for the lower atmospheric oxygen by increasing their Hb levels as a consequence of tissue hypoxia. Chronic carbon monoxide poisoning causes tissue hypoxia and is responsible, in part, for "smoker's polycythemia"; nicotine also contributes by lowering plasma volume through its diuretic effect.

Inappropriate production of EPO is an important but often overlooked cause of secondary erythrocytosis. A number of tumors, including cerebellar hemangioblastoma, uterine leiomyoma, pheochromocytoma, hepatocellular adenoma, and meningioma, have been associated with inappropriate EPO production. Exogenous EPO administration to improve performance in competitive sports may also lead to polycythemia; administration of androgens has a similar effect. The pathogenesis of post–renal transplant polycythemia, which occurs in 10% to 15% of renal transplant recipients 6 to 24 months after transplantation, is thought to be multifactorial. Abnormal EPO production from retained native kidneys, as well as increased sensitivity of erythroid precursors to EPO stimulation, may contribute to the erythrocytosis.[187]

Congenital secondary polycythemia should be considered in young patients or in those with lifelong polycythemia in whom the serum EPO level is normal or elevated. Two broad groups of defects are found in this category—those associated with abnormal Hb affinity for oxygen, and those associated with mutations of genes in the oxygen-sensing–EPO synthesis pathway.

More than 90 Hb variants have been described that have abnormal Hb-oxygen dissociation curves. Those with increased affinity for oxygen (high-oxygen-affinity Hb) do not readily give up oxygen to tissues, and the oxygen dissociation curve is shifted to the left. This is associated with a reduced P50, and the resulting tissue hypoxia leads to increased EPO levels and secondary erythrocytosis. Although some of the high-oxygen-affinity Hb variants may be detected by electrophoretic techniques, a substantial number are not. Therefore, the P50 is an appropriate screening test when such a Hb variant is suspected.[159,187] A similar but very rare disease is that caused by 2,3-bisphosphoglycerate (2,3-BPG) mutase deficiency. The absence of mutase does not permit the conversion of 1,3-BPG to 2,3-BPG, which is necessary to convert Hb into a lower-oxygen-affinity state so that it can release its oxygen to the tissues. Therefore, the mutase deficiency results in a shift of the oxygen dissociation curve to the left, reduced P50, and secondary erythrocytosis.[189]

Mutations in genes encoding proteins in the oxygen-sensing pathway and in the regulation of EPO production do not result in abnormalities of the oxygen dissociation curve and thus have a normal P50. Chuvash polycythemia is the most frequent of these disorders. It is an inherited form of polycythemia that affects individuals in the Chuvash region of Russia and results from a mutation in the von Hippel-Lindau (*VHL*) gene.[190] Specifically, the alpha subunit of HIF (HIF-α), a transcription factor for EPO synthesis, is degraded by the collaborative effect of oxygen, PHD-containing enzymes, and VHL. The mutated *VHL* produces a VHL protein that does not bind with HIF-α, thus disrupting the degradation of this transcription factor and allowing increased EPO production. Mutations of the genes that encode the PHD-containing enzymes important in the degradation of HIF-α (*PHD2*) and of the genes that encode the HIF-α isoforms (*HIF-2α*) can lead to similar changes. Patients with mutations affecting these genes may have erythrocytosis and increased serum EPO.[159]

PRIMARY MYELOFIBROSIS

Myelofibrosis is an increase in the amount and density of the discontinuous linear network of delicate reticulin fibers that provides the structural framework on which hematopoiesis normally occurs. This increase can vary from a focal, loose, yet nearly continuous network of reticulin fibers to a diffuse, dense network of markedly thickened fibers associated with collagen fibrosis and osteosclerosis. Myelofibrosis is a nonspecific response to various injuries and diseases that involve the bone marrow and is mediated by a number of cytokines released from bone marrow hematopoietic cells, particularly megakaryocytes and cells of the monocyte-macrophage lineage, as well as from other bone marrow stromal cells.[13,191,192] Marrow fibrosis can be associated with infections and inflammatory conditions that involve the bone marrow, and it commonly accompanies neoplastic diseases such as carcinoma or lymphoma when they involve the marrow. However, almost half of all cases of myelofibrosis are associated with myeloid neoplasms and, in particular, with MPNs.[193] Although any MPN can be associated with marrow fibrosis—often as a manifestation of disease progression—PMF stands out because of the prominent role that marrow fibrosis plays in the disease process.

PMF is a clonal myeloid neoplasm characterized by a neoplastic proliferation of predominantly megakaryocytes and granulocytes, accompanied by an increase in bone marrow connective tissue and often by EMH. Two phases of the disease are recognized: a prefibrotic or early stage, in which the marrow is hypercellular, with absent or only slight reticulin fibrosis and minimal if any EMH, often accompanied by peripheral blood thrombocytosis; and a fibrotic stage, which is characterized by a usually hypocellular bone marrow with marked reticulin or collagen fibrosis and, often, osteosclerosis. This latter stage is commonly associated with a leukoerythroblastic peripheral blood smear and prominent hepatosplenomegaly due to EMH. There is a gradual, stepwise progression from the prefibrotic to the fibrotic stage.[194]

In PMF, the megakaryocytic and granulocytic lineages have the most proliferative and survival advantage, but as in the other MPNs, all the myeloid lineages and some B and T lymphocytes are derived from an abnormal bone marrow stem cell.[195] In contrast, the fibroblasts are not derived from the neoplastic clone; instead, they proliferate and deposit connective tissue in response to a number of cytokines that are abnormally produced and released.[13,196,197] Fibrogenic factors include, among others, platelet-derived growth factor and transforming growth factor-β, which are synthesized, packaged, and released by the neoplastic megakaryocytes and platelets. In addition to fibrosis, there is prominent neoangiogenesis in the bone marrow and spleen. Increased serum levels of vascular endothelial growth factor are found in patients with PMF, and an increase in the microvascular density in the bone marrow correlates with the degree of fibrosis and the extent of EMH in the spleen.[198,199] In addition to cytokines that promote vascular proliferation and connective tissue deposition, other cytokines are increased in PMF, including macrophage inflammatory protein 1-β, tissue inhibitor of metalloproteinase, insulin-like growth binding factor-2, and tumor necrosis factor-α1. Therefore, the findings in PMF are related to the hematologic effects of the neoplastic proliferation in the bone marrow and to the "cytokine storm" that occurs in PMF but not in other MPNs.[13,196,197]

Approximately 50% of patients with PMF exhibit the *JAK2* V617F mutation, which identifies the proliferation as neoplastic. Animal models have demonstrated that *JAK2* V617F leads to a phenotype in some strains of mice that includes myelofibrosis,[63,65,71] thus establishing that the mutation is important in the pathogenesis of PMF. In approximately 5% of cases of PMF, the gene encoding the TPO receptor, *MPL*, is mutated. The *MPL* W515L/K mutation, like *JAK2* V617F, is believed to result in cytokine-independent growth and TPO hypersensitivity. In animal models, mutated *MPL* bestows a more PMF-like phenotype than does *JAK2* V617F.[73]

Diagnosis

The diagnostic criteria for PMF are shown in Box 46-7. As with the other MPNs, PMF is a progressive disease, and the findings at diagnosis depend on the stage of disease when the patient's symptoms are first recognized. In contrast to the other MPNs, in which most patients are diagnosed during the early proliferative stage, nearly 70% of patients with PMF are first encountered in the fibrotic stage, when leukoerythroblastosis, myelofibrosis, and massive splenomegaly are evident.[89,194,200] For the 20% to 25% of patients who are recognized in the early prefibrotic stage of PMF, the marked thrombocytosis often present at that time may lead to misclassification as ET.[200] Thus, careful correlation of the clinical findings with laboratory data and a careful examination of the peripheral blood and bone marrow biopsy are required to reach a correct diagnosis in the early stage.

Clinical Findings

The annual incidence of PMF reportedly ranges from 0.5 to 1.5 per 100,000 people.[201,202] The median age at diagnosis is usually in the seventh decade, and less than 10% of cases are diagnosed before age 40 years. Although PMF reportedly occurs in children, it is uncommon, and every effort should be made to exclude other diseases that might mimic PMF in a child.[203,204]

The onset of PMF is usually insidious. Almost 25% of patients are asymptomatic when their illness is discovered by a routine blood count that shows anemia or marked thrombocytosis.[205] Nonspecific symptoms, such as fatigue, are noted by more than half of symptomatic patients. Hypercatabolic symptoms, including weight loss, night sweats, and low-grade fever, are common, as are symptoms related to hyperuricemia, such as gouty arthritis or renal stones.[202]

In the prefibrotic stage, symptoms such as fatigue, easy bruising, and weight loss are commonly reported, but palpable splenomegaly and hepatomegaly are usually absent or only minor to moderate in degree.[194] Patients in this phase may present with bleeding or thrombosis, and because the platelet count is often markedly elevated, the clinical picture may overlap that of ET.

During the fibrotic stage of PMF, symptoms related to anemia, which can be profound, are common. Splenomegaly may be massive, leading to early satiety, abdominal

Box 46-7 World Health Organization Diagnostic Criteria for Primary Myelofibrosis

(Diagnosis requires all 3 major and 2 minor criteria)

Major Criteria

- Presence of megakaryocyte proliferation and atypia,* usually accompanied by either reticulin or collagen fibrosis; ***OR***, in the absence of significant reticulin fibrosis, megakaryocyte changes must be accompanied by increased bone marrow cellularity characterized by granulocytic proliferation and often decreased erythropoiesis (i.e., prefibrotic cellular-phase disease)
- Failure to meet the WHO criteria for polycythemia vera,† *BCR-ABL1*-positive chronic myelogenous leukemia,‡ myelodysplastic syndrome,§ or other myeloid disorders
- Demonstration of *JAK2* V617F or another clonal marker (e.g., *MPL* W515K/L); ***OR***, in the absence of clonal markers, no evidence that bone marrow fibrosis is secondary to infection, autoimmune disorder or other chronic inflammatory condition, hairy cell leukemia or other lymphoid neoplasm, metastatic malignancy, or toxic (chronic) myelopathies‖

Minor Criteria

- Leukoerythroblastosis¶
- Increased serum lactate dehydrogenase level¶
- Anemia¶
- Palpable splenomegaly¶

*Small to large megakaryocytes with an aberrant nuclear-to-cytoplasmic ratio and hyperchromatic, bulbous, or irregularly folded nuclei and dense clustering.

†Requires the failure of iron replacement therapy to increase the hemoglobin level to the polycythemia vera range in the presence of decreased serum ferritin. Exclusion of polycythemia vera is based on hemoglobin and hematocrit levels; red cell mass measurement is not required.

‡Requires the absence of *BCR-ABL1*.

§Requires the absence of dyserythropoiesis and dysgranulopoiesis.

‖Patients with conditions associated with reactive myelofibrosis are not immune to primary myelofibrosis, and the diagnosis should be considered in such cases if other criteria are met.

¶Degree of abnormality can be borderline or marked.

From Swerdlow SH, Campo E, Harris NL, et al, eds. *WHO Classification of Tumours of Haematopoietic and Lymphoid Tissues*. Lyon, France: IARC Press; 2008.

discomfort, or acute abdominal pain due to splenic infarct.[202] The splenomegaly is caused by EMH. Hepatomegaly is found in up to 50% of patients in the fibrotic stage, caused in part by EMH but also by accompanying portal vein hypertension. Ascites and variceal bleeding are common complications. The clinical findings in the fibrotic stage of PMF mimic those seen in post-PVMF and post-ET myelofibrosis (post-ETMF), and currently, only documentation of the initial disease distinguishes among these entities.

Progression from the prefibrotic to the fibrotic stage of PMF is a gradual transition, and patients may have symptoms and physical findings at various times that range along a spectrum between the two extremes of this disease process.[194]

Laboratory Findings

Peripheral Blood

In one of the few studies in which hematologic parameters measured during the prefibrotic and fibrotic stages of PMF were reported separately, the prefibrotic stage was characterized by modest anemia (mean Hb 13 g/dL; range, 7.0 to 15.5), mild leukocytosis (mean WBC count 14×10^9/L ; range, 5.6 to 32.7), and moderate to marked thrombocytosis (mean platelet count 962×10^9/L; range, 104 to 3215).[194] The most striking finding on the peripheral blood smear in this early stage is usually marked thrombocytosis, often leading to an initial diagnostic impression of ET (Fig. 46-23). Mild neutrophilia and a left shift, with occasional myelocytes, may be present, but myeloblasts, nucleated RBCs, and teardrop-shaped RBCs are only rarely observed.

There is a gradual worsening of hematologic parameters as the disease progresses, and patients in the fibrotic stage are more anemic (mean Hb 11.5g/dL; range, 4.2 to 14.0) and have lower platelet counts (mean platelet count 520×10^9/L; range, 190 to 2496) than those in the prefibrotic stage. Although mild leukocytosis is common in the fibrotic period, severe leukopenia may also occur as bone marrow failure

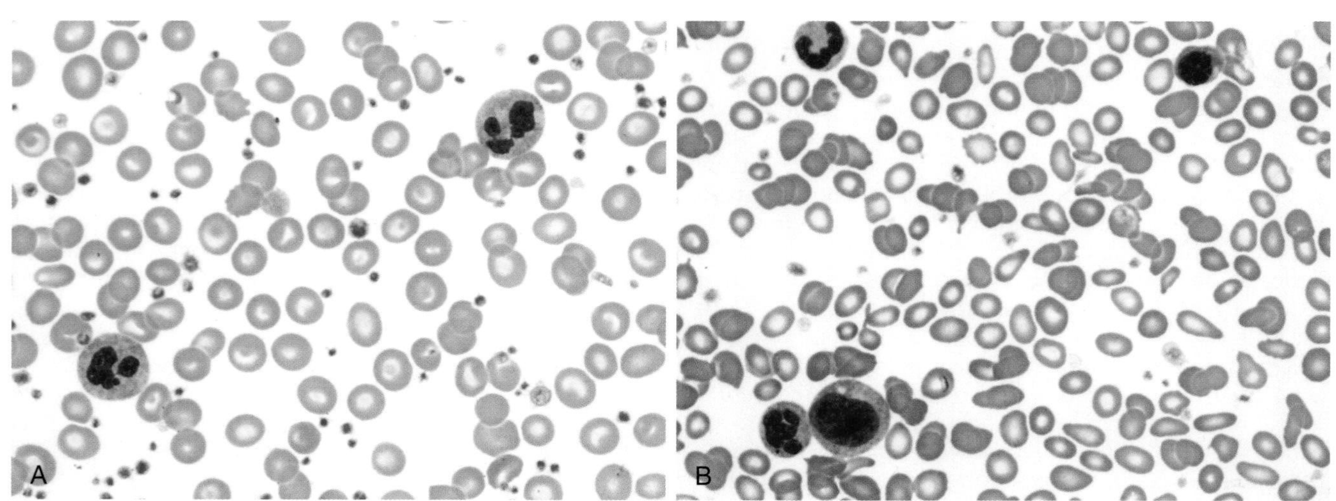

Figure 46-23. Blood smears from prefibrotic and fibrotic stages of primary myelofibrosis. A, This smear from the prefibrotic stage shows neutrophilia and thrombocytosis but minimal red cell changes (corresponding bone marrow is shown in Figure 46-25). **B,** This smear from the fibrotic stage shows leukoerythroblastosis with marked red cell abnormalities, including many teardrop forms (corresponding bone marrow is shown in Figure 46-27).

becomes more prominent due to increasing myelofibrosis (mean WBC count ≈14.0 × 10^9/L; range, 1.0 to 62.2).[194]

The classic findings on blood smears of patients with PMF—leukoerythroblastosis with numerous teardrop-shaped RBCs and large, abnormal platelets—are evident in the fibrotic stage of the disease and are due in large part to the abnormal release of immature and abnormal cells from sites of EMH (see Fig. 46-23). Circulating megakaryocyte nuclei and fragments are frequently observed. Blasts can be seen on the peripheral blood smear during the fibrotic stage of disease and occasionally account for 5% to 9% of the WBCs. When this is the case, the patient should be carefully monitored to determine whether there is progression to a more aggressive, accelerated stage of disease or to acute leukemia. However, in many patients, blast percentages of 5% to 9% may remain stable for long periods and do not indicate progression. In contrast, blast percentages of 10% to 19% in the peripheral blood should arouse concern for an AP or an impending transformation to AML, and a bone marrow specimen is warranted for further evaluation. If blasts account for 20% or more of the cells in the blood, the diagnosis of acute leukemia/acute transformation should be made.[206]

Bone Marrow

A bone marrow biopsy is essential for the diagnosis of PMF. The biopsy should be processed to allow the accurate assessment of cellularity, the relative number of cells in the various myeloid lineages and their degree of immaturity, the amount and grade of fibrosis, and the careful evaluation of megakaryocyte morphology—all of which are critical for making the diagnosis and following disease progression. The bone marrow biopsy specimen should always be stained for reticulin fibers, and every attempt should be made to perform this test using a standard, uniform protocol to avoid technical variation. The reticulin fiber content should be evaluated using a semiquantitative grading system that is reproducible (Table 46-2; Fig. 46-24).[207] An immunostain for CD34, CD105, or other endothelial markers may provide additional information regarding neoangiogenesis, and CD34 may highlight more blasts than suspected from routinely stained sections. When a bone marrow aspirate can be obtained, it can provide helpful information regarding blast percentages and maturation of the neoplastic populations.

In the prefibrotic stage the bone marrow is hypercellular and shows an increased number of neutrophils, but often a decrease in erythropoiesis that is shifted toward immaturity (Fig. 46-25). Although there may be a left shift in granulopoiesis, neutrophils at the band and segmented stage usually predominate.[161] The percentage of myeloblasts is not increased, which can be confirmed by immunohistochemical staining for CD34. The megakaryocytes are markedly abnormal in both topography and cytology and demonstrate features that are helpful in distinguishing PMF from other MPNs, particularly ET. The megakaryocytes vary from small to large forms, with an abnormal nuclear-to-cytoplasmic ratio and disorganized, plump, "cloud-like" or "balloon-like" nuclear lobation. Often the nuclei are hyperchromatic, and numerous bare megakaryocytic nuclei are seen. Overall, the megakaryocytes of PMF, even in the early stages, have a pleomorphic and bizarre appearance that, when combined with the background of exuberant neutrophil proliferation, can distinguish prefibrotic PMF from ET, with which it is frequently confused (Fig. 46-26). Reticulin fibers vary in quantity and thickness but are often not increased, except focally around blood vessels. A stain for CD34 demonstrates the increased vascularity evident at this stage, but clusters of blasts or a significant increase in blasts should not be observed. Lymphoid nodules are reportedly present in up to 25% of patients with PMF, most frequently in the prefibrotic stage.[208] In some cases the B and T lymphocytes have been shown to be derived from the neoplastic clone.[209]

As PMF progresses to the fibrotic stage, marrow cellularity gradually decreases, and reticulin or even collagen fibrosis of the marrow becomes more obvious. Islands of hematopoiesis are sometimes separated by loose connective tissue or fat; dilation of marrow sinuses may be prominent, and they may contain megakaryocytes and other immature hematopoietic cells. Atypical megakaryocytes are often the predominant cells in the marrow in the fibrotic stage and occur in sizable clusters or sheets. New bone formation and osteosclerosis may occur (Fig. 46-27). The fibrotic stage of PMF cannot be distinguished from post-PVMF or post-ETMF based on morphology alone.

The finding of 10% to 19% blasts in the bone marrow or blood should prompt the diagnosis of accelerated stage of PMF, and the finding of 20% or more blasts should be considered evidence of transformation to AML.[161,206] Occasionally, patients may present for the first time with overt AML and a background of fibrosis and enlarged, atypical megakaryocytes that resemble those of PMF. In such cases the best diagnosis is AML, with mention of its possible origin from PMF or another MPN.

Table 46-2 Semiquantitative Grading of Bone Marrow Fibrosis

Grade	Description
MF-0	Scattered linear reticulin fibers with no intersections (crossovers), corresponding to normal bone marrow
MF-1	Loose network of reticulin with many intersections, especially in perivascular areas
MF-2	Diffuse and dense increase in reticulin with extensive intersections, occasionally with focal bundles of collagen or focal osteosclerosis
MF-3	Diffuse and dense increase in reticulin with extensive intersections and coarse bundles of collagen, often associated with osteosclerosis

Extramedullary Tissues

Many of the abnormalities observed in the peripheral blood, such as teardrop-shaped RBCs and leukoerythroblastosis, are caused by the abnormal release of cells from sites of EMH. The most common sites of EMH in PMF are the spleen and liver,[210] but almost any organ can demonstrate EMH, including kidney, breast, adrenal gland, lymph node, and dura mater. In the spleen, the splenic trabeculae are widely separated by the red pulp, which is expanded by trilineage hematopoiesis in the sinuses (Fig. 46-28). Megakaryocytes are often the most prominent component and may exhibit cytologic atypia.[205] The red pulp cords may show fibrosis or contain a few developing granulocytes. Hepatic sinuses also demonstrate EMH, but fibrosis and cirrhosis of the liver are common; they, along with EMH, play a major role in the pathogenesis of the portal hypertension that can develop.

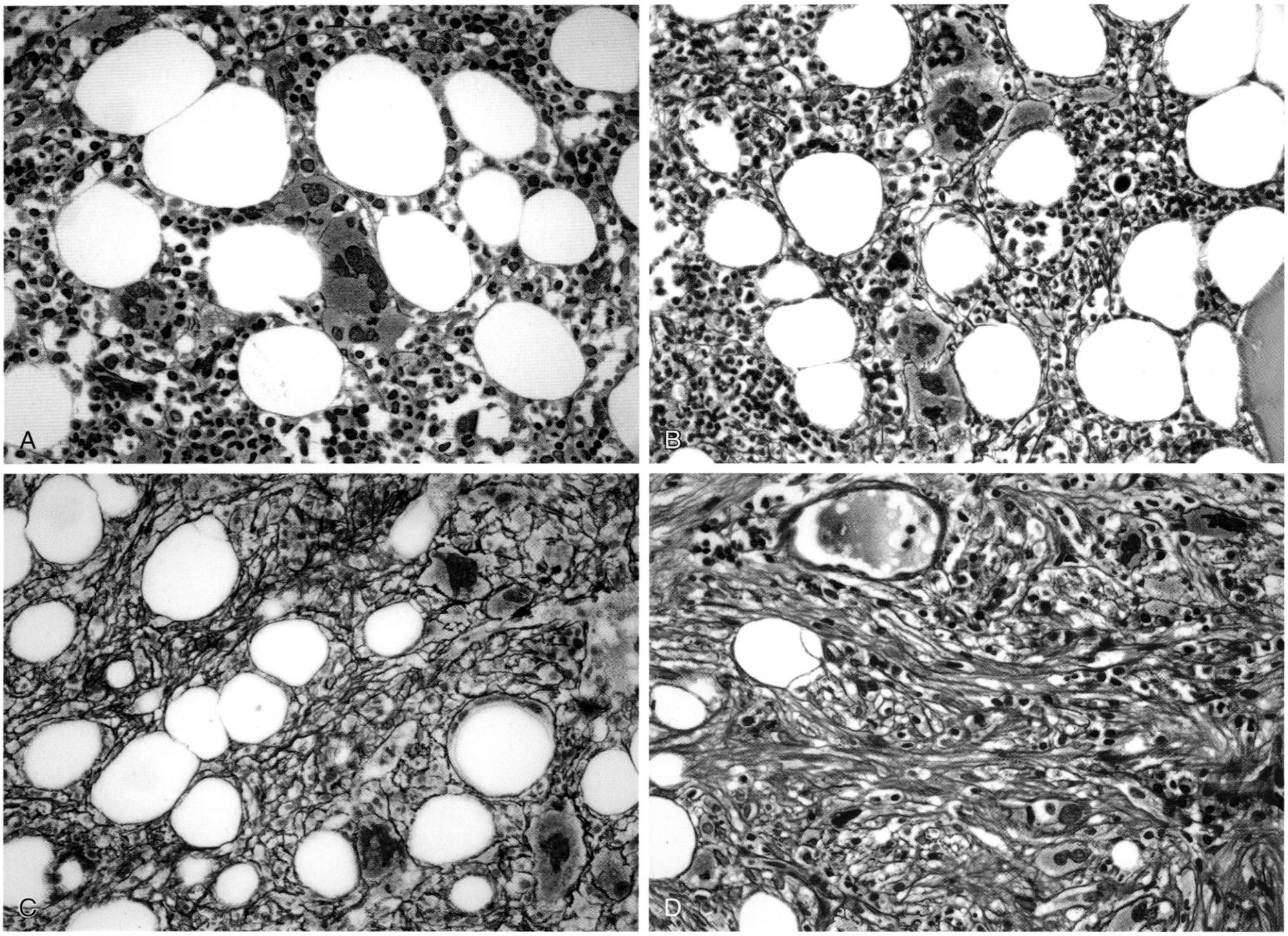

Figure 46-24. Semiquantitative grading of bone marrow fibrosis. A, Grade MF-0. **B,** Grade MF-1. **C,** Grade MF-2. **D,** Grade MF-3. See Table 46-2 for a description of the grades. (Courtesy of Drs. H. Kvasnicka and J. Thiele.)

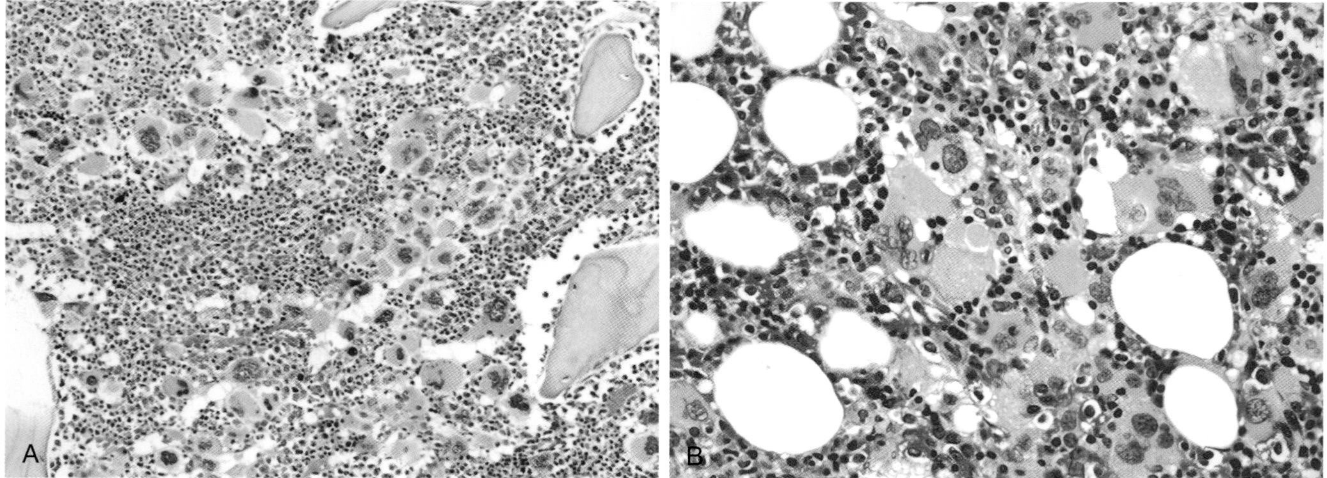

Figure 46-25. Prefibrotic primary myelofibrosis. A, Note the clusters of abnormal megakaryocytes in a background of neutrophils. This patient's peripheral blood is illustrated in Figure 46-23A. **B,** The neutrophil-rich background of the bone marrow in prefibrotic PMF can be better visualized with the naphthol-ASD-chloroacetate esterase reaction, as illustrated here. (**B,** Courtesy of Dr. H. Kvasnicka.)

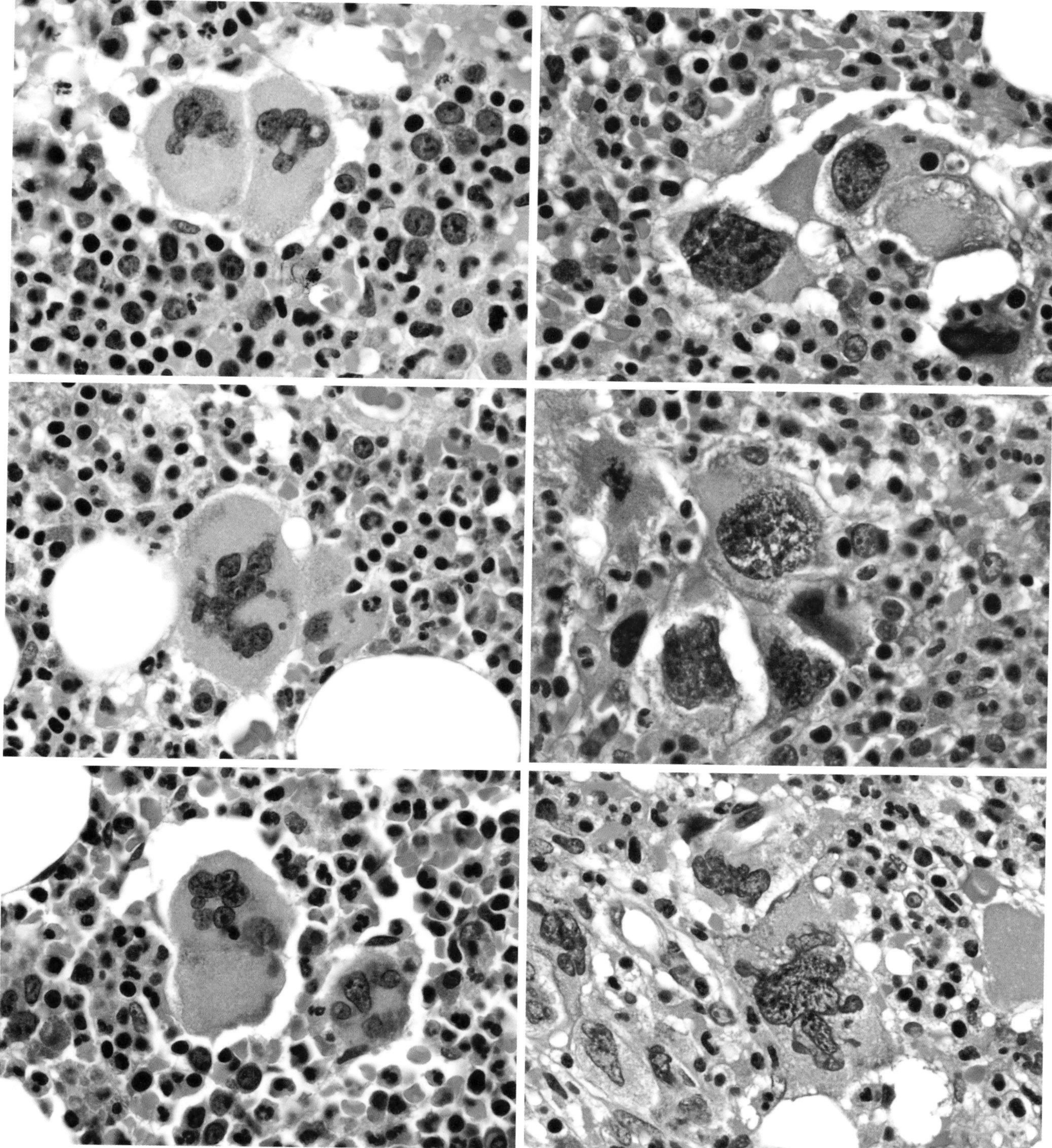

Figure 46-26. Megakaryocytes in essential thrombocythemia (ET) and prefibrotic primary myelofibrosis (prefibrotic-PMF). Although ET and prefibrotic-PMF may have overlapping clinical and laboratory features, the megakaryocytes differ morphologically between the two disorders, although megakaryocyte morphology is not the sole basis for diagnosis. **Images to the left,** Megakaryocytes from different cases of ET in which the majority (but not all) of the megakaryocytes have hyperlobulated nuclei and voluminous cytoplasm. **Images to the right,** In contrast, in these cases of prefibrotic PMF, the majority of megakaryocytes have an altered nuclear-to-cytoplasmic ratio; bulky, "cloud-like" nuclei; and an overall bizarre appearance. (From an unpublished study in which there was consensus with regard to the diagnosis among a group of experienced observers—Drs. C. Hanson, J. Thiele, A. Orazi, and J. Vardiman—correlated with clinical data.)

Continued

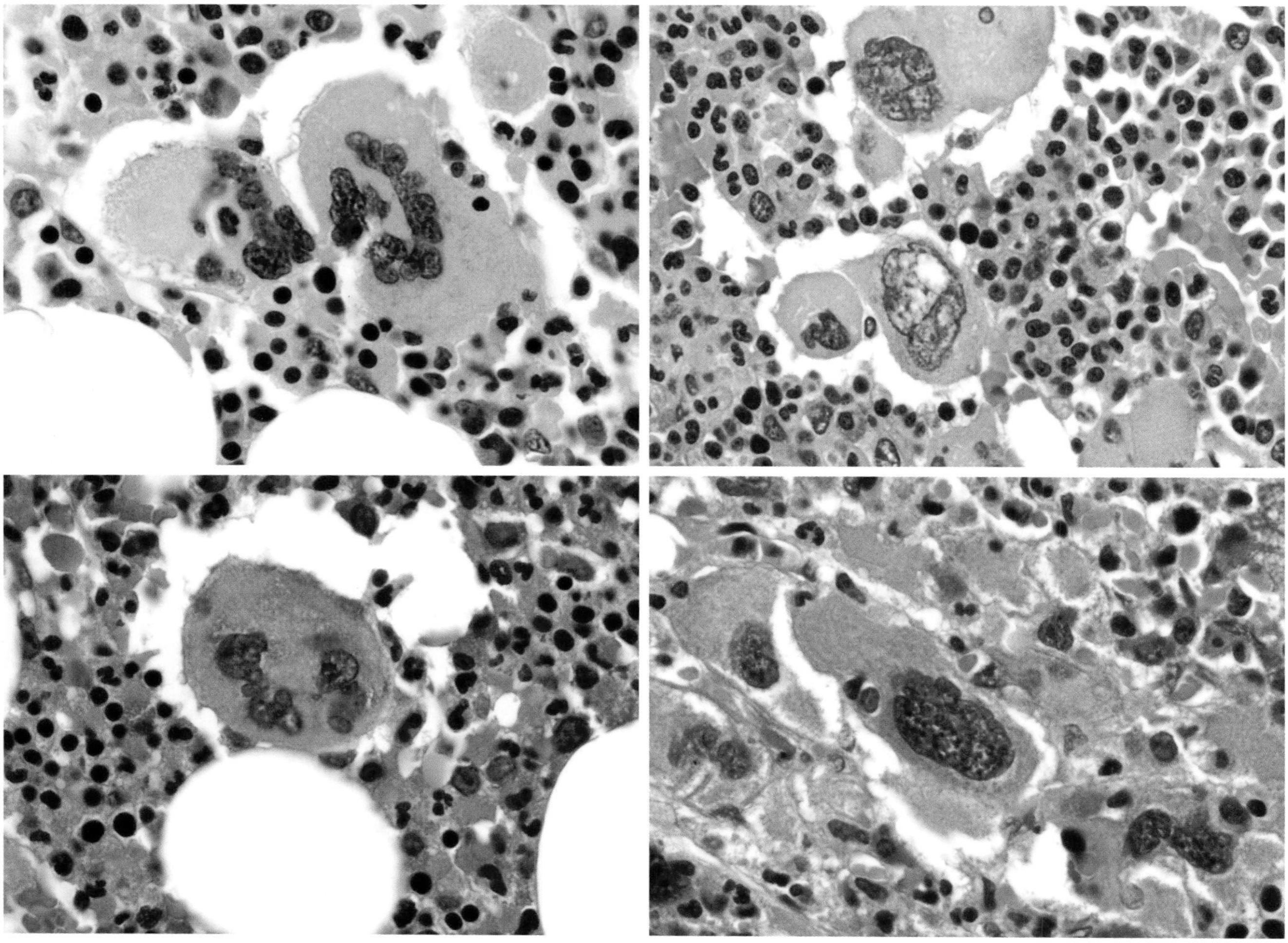

Figure 46-26, cont'd.

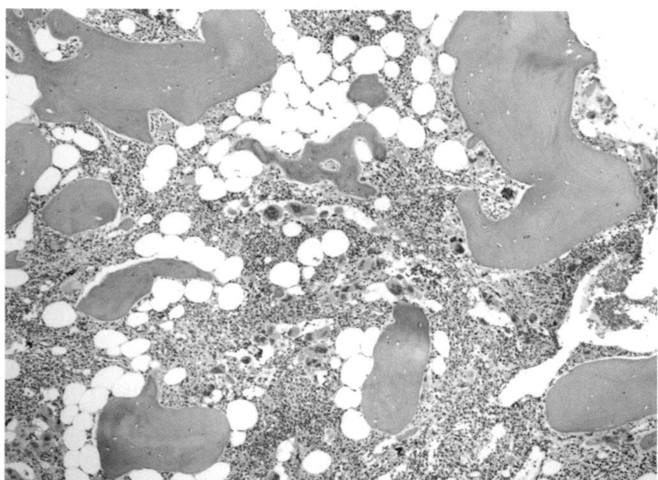

Figure 46-27. Primary myelofibrosis, fibrotic stage. Biopsy shows numerous clusters of atypical megakaryocytes, some of which occur in dilated sinuses, and osteosclerosis. This patient's peripheral blood is illustrated in Figure 46-23B.

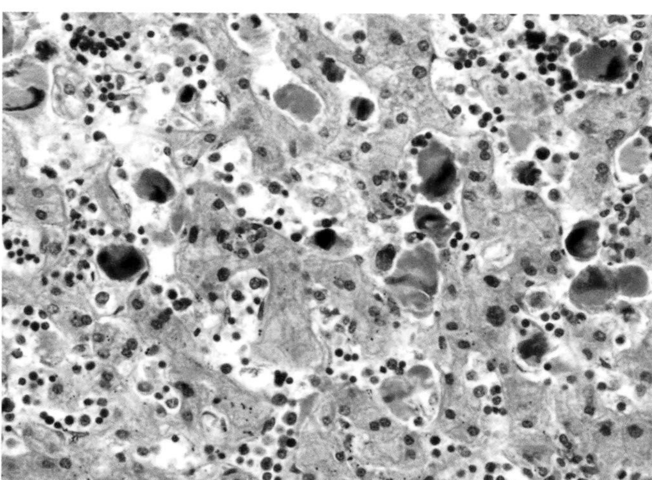

Figure 46-28. Extramedullary hematopoiesis in the liver of a patient with primary myelofibrosis. Note that the sinuses are filled with hematopoietic cells, and megakaryocytes are particularly prominent.

Extramedullary tissues may also be the site of transformation to a BP, and myeloid sarcoma should be considered in the differential diagnosis of any extramedullary lesion in a patient with PMF. Immunohistochemical stains for CD34 may be very helpful in excluding this possibility.

The EMH in PMF is composed of neoplastic cells and is likely derived from hematopoietic stem cells and precursor cells that arise in the bone marrow. The structure of the marrow sinuses is distorted and compromised by the surrounding connective tissue increase, and immature bone marrow cells more readily gain access to the marrow sinuses and hence the circulation in patients with PMF.[175] Whatever the mechanism, CD34$^+$ cells are markedly increased in the blood of patients with PMF, particularly in the fibrotic stage, compared with those with other MPNs and normal controls, and an increase in CD34$^+$ cells can also be demonstrated in the spleen.

Genetics

Approximately 50% of patients with PMF have the *JAK2* V617F mutation; mutations of *MPL*, such as *MPL* W515L/K, are found in an additional 5%.[73] These mutations are not specific for PMF. Clonal chromosomal abnormalities are reported in 30% to 50% of patients at the time of diagnosis, and the frequency gradually increases over time.[211,212] There are no abnormalities that are specific for PMF; del(13q), del(20q), +8, +9, and abnormalities of chromosome 1q are most frequently found, but −7/del(7q), −5/del(5q), and del(12p) are reported as well. When present as the sole abnormality, del(20q) and del(13q) are considered prognostically favorable abnormalities; all others, particularly +8, are unfavorable.[212] More than 90% of patients who experience transformation to MDS or AML have cytogenetic abnormalities that are often complex and often include abnormalities of chromosome 5 or 7. There is no Ph chromosome or *BCR-ABL1* fusion gene.

Other Laboratory Findings

Lactate dehydrogenase is increased in most patients with PMF, and the increase reportedly correlates directly with the degree of microvascular density in the bone marrow.[213] Nearly half of patients with PMF have some disturbance of the immune system. Circulating immune complexes, positive studies for antinuclear antibodies, and autoimmune hemolysis have been reported in some cases of PMF. Some authors have suggested that autoimmune abnormalities are more common in patients whose bone marrow demonstrates lymphoid aggregates.[208]

Disease Progression and Prognosis

The natural evolution of PMF is progressive bone marrow fibrosis accompanied by bone marrow failure. In addition to severe anemia, leukopenia, and thrombocytopenia, a number of other serious complications may develop. An increasing spleen size can be very problematic, leading not only to pain and discomfort but also to worsening of cytopenias, portal hypertension, and hypercatabolic symptoms.[13] Splenectomy may benefit occasional patients, but a significant number develop more prominent hepatomegaly following the procedure. Myeloid blast transformation occurs in about 5% to 20% of cases at a median of 3 years after the initial recognition of PMF; it usually responds poorly to therapy. Transformation is almost always accompanied by karyotypic evolution.[202]

In a number of reports, the most important adverse prognostic indicators at diagnosis include anemia (Hb <10 g/dL), advanced age (older than 64 years), circulating blasts (≥1%), leukopenia (<4.0 × 10^9/L), leukocytosis (>30 × 10^9/L), and various cytogenetic abnormalities, such as +8.[13,202,212] Length of survival depends on the stage of disease at diagnosis. The overall median survival of patients diagnosed in the fibrotic stage is approximately 5 years, whereas 10- and 15-year relative survival rates of 72% and 59%, respectively, have been reported in patients diagnosed in the prefibrotic stage.[202,214]

Differential Diagnosis

The differential diagnosis of the fibrotic stage of PMF includes post-PVMF and post-ETMF; however, without a history of preceding PV or ET, the distinction between these entities and fibrotic PMF is essentially impossible. The differentiation of other myeloid neoplasms, metastatic tumors, and even inflammatory diseases can also be problematic (Tables 46-3 and 46-4).

Prefibrotic PMF versus ET is a challenging diagnostic problem that has only recently been appreciated.[194,215] Thrombocytosis, sometimes in excess of 1000 × 10^9/L, is not uncommon in prefibrotic PMF and may prompt the erroneous diagnosis of ET. Because the overall survival times of ET and PMF differ, their distinction is important (see Table 46-3).[205,214] The peripheral blood smear may not be helpful in distinguishing these two entities, although the findings of neutrophilia, occasional immature granulocytes, basophilia, and even rare teardrop-shaped RBCs favor prefibrotic PMF. In bone marrow biopsy specimens, in contrast to the clustered, highly atypical, variably sized megakaryocytes of PMF, the megakaryocytes of ET are often more dispersed, are uniformly large or giant, and

Table 46-3 Comparison of Prefibrotic Primary Myelofibrosis and Essential Thrombocythemia

Feature	Prefibrotic PMF	Essential Thrombocythemia
White blood cell count	Variable, often increased	Usually normal, occasionally mildly increased
Platelet count	Often ≥450 × 10^9/L, sometimes normal or decreased	Always ≥450 × 10^9/L
Marrow cellularity	Increased	Normal to increased, rarely decreased
Major proliferating cells	Megakaryocytes, granulocytes	Megakaryocytes
Megakaryocyte morphology	Loose and tight clusters of ≥3 small to large megakaryocytes with altered nuclear-to-cytoplasmic ratio, "cloud-like" bulky nuclei, bare megakaryocytic nuclei; often bizarre forms	Dispersed or loose clusters of large to giant megakaryocytes with abundant cytoplasm, hyperlobulated nuclei; bizarre forms rarely seen
Genetic findings	*JAK2* V617F in ≈50%; *MPL* W515L/K in ≈5%	*JAK2* V617F in ≈50%; *MPL* W515L/K in ≈1%-2%

Table 46-4 Comparison of Myeloid Neoplasms Commonly Associated with Myelofibrosis

Feature	CML, *BCR-ABL1* Positive	Fibrotic PMF	MDS-F	APMF
BCR-ABL1 fusion gene	100%	0	0	0
WBC count	Increased	Increased, normal, or decreased	Decreased, rarely normal	Decreased
Bone marrow blasts	CP: <9% AP: 10%-19% BP: ≥20%	<20%	<20%	≥20%
Megakaryocyte morphology	Small "dwarf" megakaryocytes	Variable size, small to large; atypical morphology; bizarre; altered nuclear-to-cytoplasmic ratio; in clusters	Small, dysplastic megakaryocytes, dispersed or in clusters or sheets	Mainly small and dysplastic, but large abnormal forms also seen; megakaryoblasts may be frequent
Dysgranulopoiesis	CP: minimal AP/BP: may be present	Minimal, but may be present as disease transforms	Usually prominent	Usually prominent
Dyserythropoiesis	CP: minimal AP/BP: may be present	Minimal	Often prominent	Usually prominent

AP, accelerted phase; APMF, acute panmyelosis with myelofibrosis; BP, blast phase; CML, chronic myelogenous leukemia; CP, chronic phase; MDS-F, myelodysplastic syndrome with fibrosis; PMF, primary myelofibrosis; WBC, white blood cell.

have abundant, mature cytoplasm and deeply lobulated ("staghorn") nuclei (see Fig. 46-26). The neutrophilic proliferation that is commonly seen in the bone marrow in prefibrotic PMF is absent in ET. Any appreciable reticulin fibrosis is a strong argument in favor of PMF.

Acute panmyelosis with myelofibrosis is an uncommon subtype of AML, not otherwise specified. It is characterized in the peripheral blood by pancytopenia with minimal RBC poikilocytosis and an absence of teardrop-shaped RBCs. The granulocytes are dysplastic, and a few circulating blasts are common. There is minimal if any organomegaly (see Table 46-4). The bone marrow is variably cellular, with a proliferation of erythroid and granulocytic precursors and megakaryocytes in variable proportions. Blasts constitute 20% or more of the marrow cells, although often only barely so.[216] In most cases megakaryocytes are particularly conspicuous, but in contrast to the megakaryocytes of PMF, they are small and dysplastic, although large dystrophic forms may occasionally be seen. Immature megakaryocytes and megakaryoblasts may be present, and in most cases it is more difficult to distinguish acute panmyelosis with myelofibrosis from high-grade MDS or acute megakaryocytic leukemia than from PMF. However, differentiation from PMF in an AP or BP may be more problematic.[216]

MDS with myelofibrosis is not a distinct entity. Significant myelofibrosis may be found in 5% to 10% of cases of MDS, generally in those with excess blasts; these cases are collectively referred to as MDS with fibrosis.[217] In contrast to PMF, patients with MDS with fibrosis lack significant organomegaly, and the blood and marrow demonstrate prominent dysplastic features involving multiple lineages. In the bone marrow the megakaryocytes are small, dysplastic forms, in contrast to the pleomorphic, bizarre, and often enlarged forms of PMF. Often, cellular bone marrow aspirates are not obtained, but immunohistochemical staining of the bone marrow biopsy specimen for CD34 usually identifies an increased blast population.[217]

Autoimmune myelofibrosis may develop in patients with autoimmune disorders such as systemic lupus erythematosus. Recently, attention has been drawn to bone marrow fibrosis in patients who do not have lupus or any other well-characterized autoimmune disease but who consistently have autoantibody production and develop modest reticulin fibrosis in their bone marrow. These patients often present with peripheral blood cytopenia, particularly anemia, and may have mild RBC poikilocytosis with rare teardrop-shaped RBCs. The bone marrow varies from hypocellular to nearly 100% cellular, with increased numbers of megakaryocytes dispersed in the marrow with normal morphology. There is usually erythroid hyperplasia, sometimes with a shift toward immature forms; interstitial infiltrates or aggregates of lymphoid cells are also present, usually comprising a mixture of T and B cells. Modest plasmacytosis is often seen, and the plasma cells are frequently in a perivascular distribution. Significant splenomegaly is absent.[218,219]

ESSENTIAL THROMBOCYTHEMIA

Thrombocytosis is a common hematologic finding that can present a diagnostic challenge. It can accompany numerous hematopoietic and nonhematopoietic malignancies but is also found in iron deficiency anemia and in a variety of infectious and inflammatory disorders (Box 46-8). In the majority of patients, even those in whom the platelet count is greater than $1000 \times 10^9/L$, the thrombocytosis is due to reactive megakaryocytic proliferation that resolves when the underlying disease is adequately treated.[220] In a minority of cases, however, the thrombocytosis is caused by a clonal megakaryocytic proliferation that occurs independent of the mechanisms that normally control platelet production. Such a proliferation is usually associated with one of the MPNs but may also be seen in some cases of MDS, MDS/MPN, and rare subtypes of AML. Within the subgroup of MPNs, ET is the disorder that, in the minds of many clinicians and pathologists, is most characteristically associated with a markedly elevated platelet count; however, any MPN, including CML, PV, and PMF, can demonstrate marked thrombocytosis, with platelet counts exceeding $1000 \times 10^9/L$.

ET is an MPN that involves primarily the megakaryocytic lineage.[200,221] It is characterized by sustained thrombocytosis ($\geq 450 \times 10^9/L$) in the peripheral blood; increased numbers of large, mature megakaryocytes in the bone marrow; and episodes of thrombosis or hemorrhage. The *JAK2* V617F mutation is present in approximately 50% of cases, and *MPL*

Box 46-8 *Causes of Thrombocytosis**

Secondary (Reactive) Thrombocytosis
- Infection
- Inflammatory diseases
  - Collagen vascular disease
  - Chronic inflammatory bowel disease
- Blood loss, hemorrhage
- Chronic iron deficiency
- After splenectomy
- Hyposplenism
- Trauma (particularly brain)
- Postsurgical procedures
- Neoplasms (nonhematopoietic and nonmyeloid hematopoietic)
- Regeneration, rebound after chemotherapy

Myeloid Neoplasm Related
- Myeloproliferative neoplasms
  - Chronic myelogenous leukemia, *BCR-ABL1* positive
  - Polycythemia vera
  - Primary myelofibrosis
  - Essential thrombocythemia
- Acute myeloid leukemia with t(3;3)(q21;q26) or inv(3)(q21q26)
- Myelodysplastic syndrome with isolated del(5q) abnormality
- Myelodysplastic/myeloproliferative neoplasm
- Provisional entity: refractory anemia with ring sideroblasts and thrombocytosis

*Platelet count ≥450 × 10^9/L.

W515K/L is present in 1% to 2%. These mutations lead to constitutive activation of pathways that stimulate megakaryocyte proliferation and platelet production. The cause of the proliferation in the remaining cases is currently unknown. The finding of a *BCR-ABL1* fusion gene excludes the diagnosis.

The megakaryocyte originates from a hematopoietic stem cell that gives rise to early myeloid progenitors. The erythroid and megakaryocytic lineages share a common megakaryocyte-erythroid progenitor. Differentiation of the megakaryocyte-erythroid progenitor toward the megakaryocyte and erythroid lineages is driven in part by the transcription factor GATA1, whereas downregulation of the transcription factor PU.1 favors megakaryocytic development and suppresses erythroid maturation by the megakaryocyte-erythroid progenitor.[222,223] Megakaryocytic proliferation and maturation are complex and are characterized by DNA endoreduplication, cytoplasmic maturation and expansion, and release of megakaryocytic cytoplasmic fragments into the circulation as platelets.[222] TPO plays a central role in the maturation, survival, and proliferation of the megakaryocyte. It is produced in the liver and binds to MPL, its receptor on the megakaryocyte and platelet surface. Circulating levels of TPO are regulated by the extent of its binding to MPL. As the megakaryocyte and platelet mass increases, levels of TPO fall as it binds to MPL. The MPL-TPO complex is destroyed as platelets are removed from the circulation, and TPO levels increase to stimulate more platelet production.[222,223] The binding of TPO with MPL on the megakaryocyte normally initiates conformational changes of MPL and activation of the JAK kinase constitutively bound to the cytoplasmic domain of MPL. This initiates signaling through the STAT5, PI3K, and MAPK pathways to stimulate proliferation, endoreduplication, and expansion of the megakaryocytic mass.

In patients with ET and mutated *JAK2* V617F or *MPL* W515K/L, the normal pathway of stimulation by TPO is constitutively activated owing to the mutation, and megakaryocyte proliferation and platelet production are either independent of or hypersensitive to TPO. A similar but as yet unknown defect is presumably present in the remaining cases of ET. Why the *JAK2* V617F mutation leads to ET in some cases and to PV or PMF in others is not clear, although patients with ET tend to have lower allele burden of the mutated *JAK2* than patients with PV or PMF.[9,70]

Diagnosis

There is no unique genetic or biologic property that specifically identifies ET, so all other causes of thrombocytosis must be excluded before making the diagnosis. Although the *JAK2* V617F mutation is found in about half the cases of ET and the *MPL* W515K/L mutation in another 1% to 2%, neither is specific; both are seen in other MPNs. Still, when one of these mutations is present, it confirms the clonal nature of the process and eliminates further consideration of reactive thrombocytosis. This is important, because the distinction between reactive and clonally derived thrombocytosis is clinically relevant and can be a rather urgent matter. Patients with reactive thrombocytosis infrequently experience bleeding or thrombotic episodes, but patients with clonal megakaryocytic proliferations associated with thrombocytosis are at increased risk for these events. In cases of ET that lack a mutation or a clonal chromosomal marker, additional studies to exclude not only reactive but also neoplastic causes of thrombocytosis are necessary. The diagnostic criteria for ET are listed in Box 46-9.

Clinical Findings

ET is a rare disorder, with an estimated incidence of about 0.6 to 2.5 per 100,000 persons per year.[224] The disease can occur at any age, including in children, but most cases occur in patients in the sixth decade of life. A second peak, particularly in women, occurs at 30 years of age.[224-226]

Nearly 30% to 50% of patients with ET are asymptomatic at diagnosis and are identified when a blood count is obtained for routine screening or for the evaluation of another illness.[226] The remaining patients have symptoms related to microvascular occlusive events (headaches, transient ischemic attacks, dizziness, visual disturbances, erythromelalgia, seizures), major vascular occlusive events (stroke, myocardial infarction, deep venous thrombosis, Budd-Chiari syndrome), or, less commonly, hemorrhage from mucosal surfaces (epistaxis, gastrointestinal bleeding).[227-229] Splenomegaly or hepatomegaly is present in only a minority of patients and is usually not marked.[214,221]

Laboratory Findings

Peripheral Blood

Unfortunately, there are limited data regarding the laboratory findings in patients who meet the WHO criteria for ET, and the data presented here are based on only a few series.

Box 46-9 World Health Organization Diagnostic Criteria for Essential Thrombocythemia

Diagnosis requires that all of the following criteria be met:

- Sustained platelet count ≥450 × 10^9/L*
- Bone marrow biopsy specimen showing proliferation mainly of the megakaryocytic lineage, with increased numbers of enlarged, mature megakaryocytes; no significant increase or left shift of neutrophil granulopoiesis or erythropoiesis
- Failure to meet the WHO criteria for polycythemia vera,[†] primary myelofibrosis,[‡] *BCR-ABL1*–positive chronic myelogenous leukemia,[§] myelodysplastic syndrome,[‖] or other myeloid neoplasms
- Demonstration of *JAK2* V617F or other clonal marker; or, in the absence of *JAK2* V617F, no evidence of reactive thrombocytosis[¶]

*Sustained during the workup process.
[†]Requires the failure of iron replacement therapy to increase the hemoglobin level to the polycythemia vera range in the presence of decreased serum ferritin. Exclusion of polycythemia vera is based on hemoglobin and hematocrit levels; red cell mass measurement is not required.
[‡]Requires the absence of relevant reticulin fibrosis, collagen fibrosis, peripheral blood leukoerythroblastosis, or markedly hypercellular marrow accompanied by megakaryocyte morphology typical for primary myelofibrosis—small to large megakaryocytes with an aberrant nuclear-to-cytoplasmic ratio and hyperchromatic, bulbous, or irregularly folded nuclei and dense clustering.
[§]Requires the absence of *BCR-ABL1*.
[‖]Requires the absence of dyserythropoiesis and dysgranulopoiesis.
[¶]Causes of reactive thrombocytosis include iron deficiency, splenectomy, surgery, infection, inflammation, connective tissue disease, metastatic cancer, and lymphoproliferative disorders. However, the presence of a condition associated with reactive thrombocytosis does not exclude the possibility of essential thombocythemia if other criteria are met.
From Swerdlow SH, Campo E, Harris NL, et al, eds. *WHO Classification of Tumours of Haematopoietic and Lymphoid Tissues*. Lyon, France: IARC Press; 2008.

Regardless of the diagnostic criteria, thrombocytosis is the most striking abnormality found on the hemogram and may range from 450 to more than 2000 × 10^9/L.[200,229] On the blood smear, platelets often show anisocytosis, ranging from very small to large. Although highly atypical platelets—including giant, bizarre forms and hypogranular platelets—may be seen, they are not common (Fig. 46-29). In most cases there is minimal if any leukocytosis, with WBC counts usually in the range of 8 to 15 × 10^9/L,[200] although the WBC count may be elevated in patients who have experienced hemorrhage. Generally, the leukocyte differential is not remarkable, and basophilia and immature granulocytes are infrequent; leukoerythroblastosis is not observed at the time of diagnosis of ET. Mild anemia may be present, but the RBCs usually lack significant aniso- or poikilocytosis, and teardrop-shaped cells are not observed. Hypochromia and microcytosis may be present in patients with a history of bleeding.

Bone Marrow

A bone marrow biopsy is essential in distinguishing ET from the other MPNs, including the prefibrotic stage of PMF, and from reactive causes of thrombocytosis. In patients with ET, bone marrow cellularity is variable but is often normal or slightly hypercellular (see Fig. 46-29). The most striking abnormality is an increase in the number and size of megakaryocytes. They may occur in loose clusters or be singly dispersed in the marrow; the megakaryocytes are large to giant, with abundant, mature cytoplasm and deeply lobulated and hyperlobulated nuclei that have been likened to a "staghorn" (see Fig. 46-26).[89,221] A significant population of bizarre, highly atypical megakaryocytes with an increased nuclear-to-cytoplasmic ratio or marked pleomorphism is not observed in ET. If such forms are frequently encountered, the diagnosis of PMF should be considered rather than ET.[89,200,221] In most cases the myeloid-to-erythroid ratio is normal, but if there has been hemorrhage, there may be some erythroid proliferation. Granulocytic proliferation is uncommon and, if present, should raise doubts about the diagnosis of ET. Blasts are not increased in number, and there is no myelodysplasia. The network of reticulin fibers is either normal or only mildly increased.[221] On aspirate smears the megakaryocytes often appear as huge forms, often associated with large pools of platelets. Emperipolesis of bone marrow cells is sometimes seen, but this is not specific and can be found even in normal megakaryocytes from normal bone marrow.

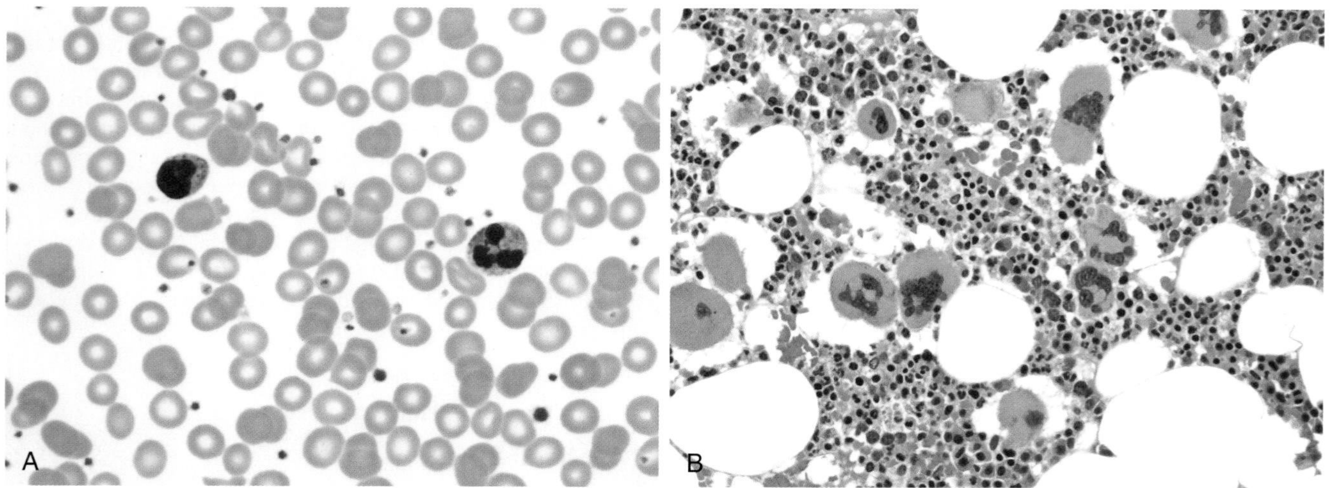

Figure 46-29. Essential thrombocythemia in a 42-year-old woman. A, Peripheral blood is largely unremarkable, except for thrombocytosis (800 × 10^9/L). **B,** Bone marrow biopsy exhibits normal cellularity but increased numbers of large megakaryocytes with hyperlobulated nuclei.

Extramedullary Tissues

Splenic enlargement is uncommon at the time of diagnosis; if present, it may be largely due to pooling and sequestration of platelets. EMH is absent or minimal.[221]

Genetics

Nearly 50% of cases of ET have the *JAK2* V617F mutation, and 1% to 2% have mutated *MPL*.[66,73] The finding of these mutations establishes the clonality of the process, but they are not specific for ET, nor does their absence exclude ET. Cytogenetic abnormalities are detected in less than 10% of cases at the time of diagnosis.[230,231] The abnormalities most frequently found, such as del(20q) and trisomy 8, are not specific and can be found in any myeloid neoplasm; however, they do establish that the megakaryocytic proliferation is clonal. Cytogenetic abnormalities are more common when ET evolves to acute leukemia, perhaps as a result of cytotoxic therapy. Cytogenetic studies may also be helpful in excluding ET as the reason for thrombocytosis in some cases. The discovery of del(5q) as a sole abnormality suggests the diagnosis of MDS associated with thrombocytosis rather than ET, whereas t(3;3)(q21;q26.2) or inv(3)(q21q26.2) indicates MDS or AML rather than ET. Detection of a Ph chromosome or the *BCR-ABL1* fusion gene indicates that the diagnosis is CML, not ET. Each of these disorders is associated with characteristic megakaryocyte morphology that differs from the large, hyperlobulated megakaryocytes seen in ET.

Other Laboratory Findings

Patients with ET usually demonstrate abnormal platelet function studies, with evidence of abnormal platelet activation by unknown mechanisms.[179,180] Correlation between an abnormal study and the ability to predict hemorrhagic or thrombotic episodes is not good. However, higher platelet counts tend to be associated with a greater probability of hemorrhage, most likely because of acquired von Willebrand's syndrome. This is associated with the loss of large von Willebrand's factor multimers and the loss of function of von Willebrand's factor.[178,180] Serum uric acid levels may be elevated in 25% to 30% of cases of ET, and pseudohyperkalemia may be present as well. Serum ferritin is almost always normal, and stainable iron is found in the marrow of the majority of patients at diagnosis.[221]

Disease Progression and Prognosis

The natural history of ET is that of an indolent disorder punctuated by episodes of thrombosis or hemorrhage and by long symptom-free intervals. Progression to post-ET myelofibrosis occurs in a minority of cases after years of follow-up.[200,232] Similarly, a small number of cases (<5%) show transformation to acute leukemia, and the majority of these patients have been treated previously with cytotoxic agents.[226,228] Overall, median survival times of 10 to 15 years have been reported, and in the large majority of patients, life expectancy is near normal.[214]

Differential Diagnosis

The first question to answer when a patient with marked thrombocytosis is encountered is whether the increase in the platelet count is reactive and caused by an underlying disease process or is due to a clonal myeloid neoplasm with excess platelet production. The clinical history, physical findings, and a few ancillary laboratory studies are often sufficient to distinguish between reactive and neoplastic causes of thrombocytosis. A history of chronic thrombocytosis, hemorrhagic or thrombotic episodes, and the finding of splenomegaly favor ET, whereas the lack of these findings plus evidence of an underlying inflammatory disease, such as elevated C-reactive protein, favors reactive thrombocytosis. Nevertheless, if an underlying cause for the thrombocytosis cannot be readily identified, studies for the *JAK2* V617F mutation should be performed and a bone marrow specimen obtained and examined for the characteristic features of ET or another myeloid neoplasm, as well as for marrow involvement by a disorder that might lead to reactive thrombocytosis (see Box 46-8).

The most commonly encountered myeloid neoplasms associated with thrombocytosis that might be confused with ET include the polycythemic stage of PV, the prefibrotic stage of PMF, and CML. Each of these diseases has been characterized in the preceding sections and tables in this chapter; the characteristic morphology that distinguishes prefibrotic PMF from ET, which is often a difficult issue, is illustrated in Figure 46-26. It should be remembered that some cases of CML, particularly those with the p230 oncoprotein, initially display marked thrombocytosis and minimal leukocytosis, so cytogenetic or molecular genetic studies should always be performed to exclude a *BCR-ABL1* fusion gene and CML as a cause of thrombocytosis.

A provisional entity, refractory anemia with ring sideroblasts and thrombocytosis (RARS-T), is yet another diagnostic consideration. It resembles ET, in that it is characterized by a platelet count of 450×10^9/L or greater and has a proliferation of megakaryocytes in the bone marrow that morphologically resemble those of ET or PMF.[233] However, RARS-T demonstrates ineffective erythroid proliferation, with dyserythropoiesis and ring sideroblasts that account for 15% or more of the erythroid precursors. There is marked anemia. Nearly half the cases of RARS-T have been demonstrated to carry the *JAK2* V617F mutation, but it is currently debatable whether this is a unique entity, an MPN that has evolved to acquire ring sideroblasts, or MDS that has secondarily acquired an additional genetic abnormality that links it to the MPNs.[234-236]

Other Myeloid Neoplasms Associated with Thrombocytosis

Elevated platelet counts are uncommon in MDS or AML, but in some specific instances, the platelet count may be markedly elevated. MDS associated with del(5q) as the sole abnormality and MDS or AML with t(3;3)(q21;q26.2) or inv (3)(q21q26.2) are frequently associated with thrombocytosis. In the case of MDS with del(5q), in contrast to the hyperlobulated nuclei of the megakaryocytes of ET, there is hypolobation of the megakaryocyte nucleus. MDS or AML cases associated with t(3;3) or inv(3) are characterized by the proliferation of micromegakaryocytes.

MYELOPROLIFERATIVE NEOPLASMS, UNCLASSIFIABLE

The designation MPN, unclassifiable should be applied only to cases that have definite clinical, laboratory, and morphologic features of an MPN but fail to meet the criteria for any of the specific MPN entities. Most cases fall into one of three categories: (1) early stages of PV, PMF, or ET in which the clinical, laboratory, and morphologic manifestations are not yet fully developed; (2) the myelofibrotic, accelerated, or blast phase of any MPN in which the underlying disease is not clear or was never previously recognized; and (3) patients with convincing evidence of an MPN in whom a coexisting inflammatory, metabolic, or neoplastic process obscures the diagnosis. The designation MPN, unclassifiable, should not be used if the laboratory data necessary for classification are incomplete or were never obtained, the size or quality of the bone marrow specimen is inadequate for complete evaluation, or the patient has received prior growth factor therapy or cytotoxic therapy. The finding of a *BCR-ABL1* fusion gene or rearrangements of *PDGFRA*, *PDGFRB*, or *FGFR1* preclude the diagnosis of MPN, unclassifiable. Although *JAK2* V617F is most commonly observed in MPNs, it has also been described in AML, MDS, and MDS/MPN[66] and cannot be used as the sole evidence to designate a case MPN, unclassifiable if other data are not supportive.

If a case does not have features of one of the well-defined MPN entities, the possibility (or probability) that it is not an MPN at all must be seriously considered. Reactive bone marrow responses to a number of inflammatory and infectious agents must be kept in mind, particularly when considering CNL and CEL. Marrow fibrosis with osteosclerosis may be found in a number of inflammatory and neoplastic conditions as well, including chronic osteomyelitis, Paget's disease, metabolic bone diseases, osteosclerotic myeloma, hairy cell leukemia, metastatic carcinoma, and malignant lymphoma.

When a diagnosis of MPN, unclassifiable is made, the report should indicate why a more definitive diagnosis is not possible. If one or more specific MPNs can be excluded on the basis of the laboratory, clinical, and morphologic data, that should be stated as well. Recommendations for additional studies to clarify the diagnosis should be given, even if only a suggestion to repeat the same studies after an appropriate time interval. Sharing the case with colleagues, particularly with the clinicians responsible for the patient's care, is important. Sending the case for an expert opinion may help reach a diagnostic conclusion or at least confirm that someone with more experience with MPNs could not classify the case either.

Pearls and Pitfalls

- Reliable clinical and laboratory information is essential for the diagnosis of MPNs. The clinician caring for the patient should be invited to review the slides and discuss the case.
- Well-prepared peripheral blood smears, bone marrow aspirate smears, or touch preparations and adequate biopsy specimens that are well processed are vital for diagnosing MPNs.
- Routine karyotypes, best performed from bone marrow specimens, should be done in all patients during the initial evaluation for a myeloid neoplasm. Molecular genetic studies can add important diagnostic and other information but should not be considered a substitute for an initial karyotype study.
- Although CML usually presents in a straightforward manner, it may have unusual manifestations. Keep this in mind when dealing with any unusual myeloid neoplasm, and obtain cytogenetic and molecular testing when even remotely suspicious.
- Do not get hung up on megakaryocyte morphology in the *BCR-ABL1*–negative MPNs. Although megakaryocyte morphology is important, the diagnosis of an MPN is made by also considering the background cells of the bone marrow in which the megakaryocytes occur, along with the clinical history and other laboratory data.
- The diagnosis of MPN, unclassifiable is not intended for cases in which there is insufficient material to evaluate or an inadequate clinical or laboratory workup. In such cases the report should indicate what additional material or studies are required to reach a conclusion.

References can be found on Expert Consult @ www.expertconsult.com

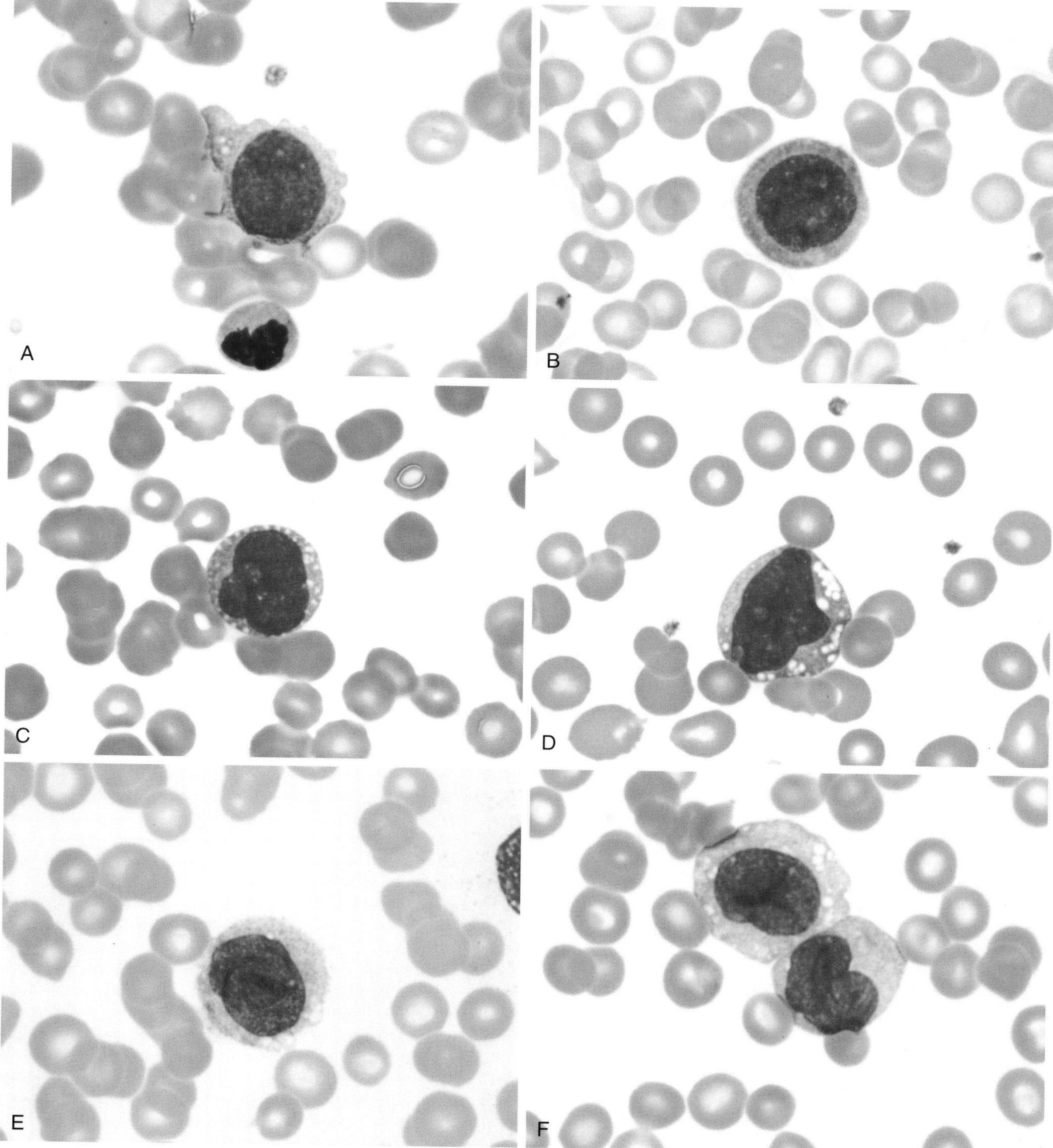

Figure 47-3. Monoblasts, promonocytes, and abnormal monocytes. A–D, Monoblasts are large, with round to oval nuclei that may be slightly irregular, lacy chromatin, one or more variably prominent nucleoli, and moderate to abundant cytoplasm that may contain a few vacuoles or fine granules. **E–H**, Promonocytes have more irregular and slightly folded nuclei with fine chromatin, indistinct nucleoli, and moderate to abundant finely granulated cytoplasm that may contain a few vacuoles.

Continued

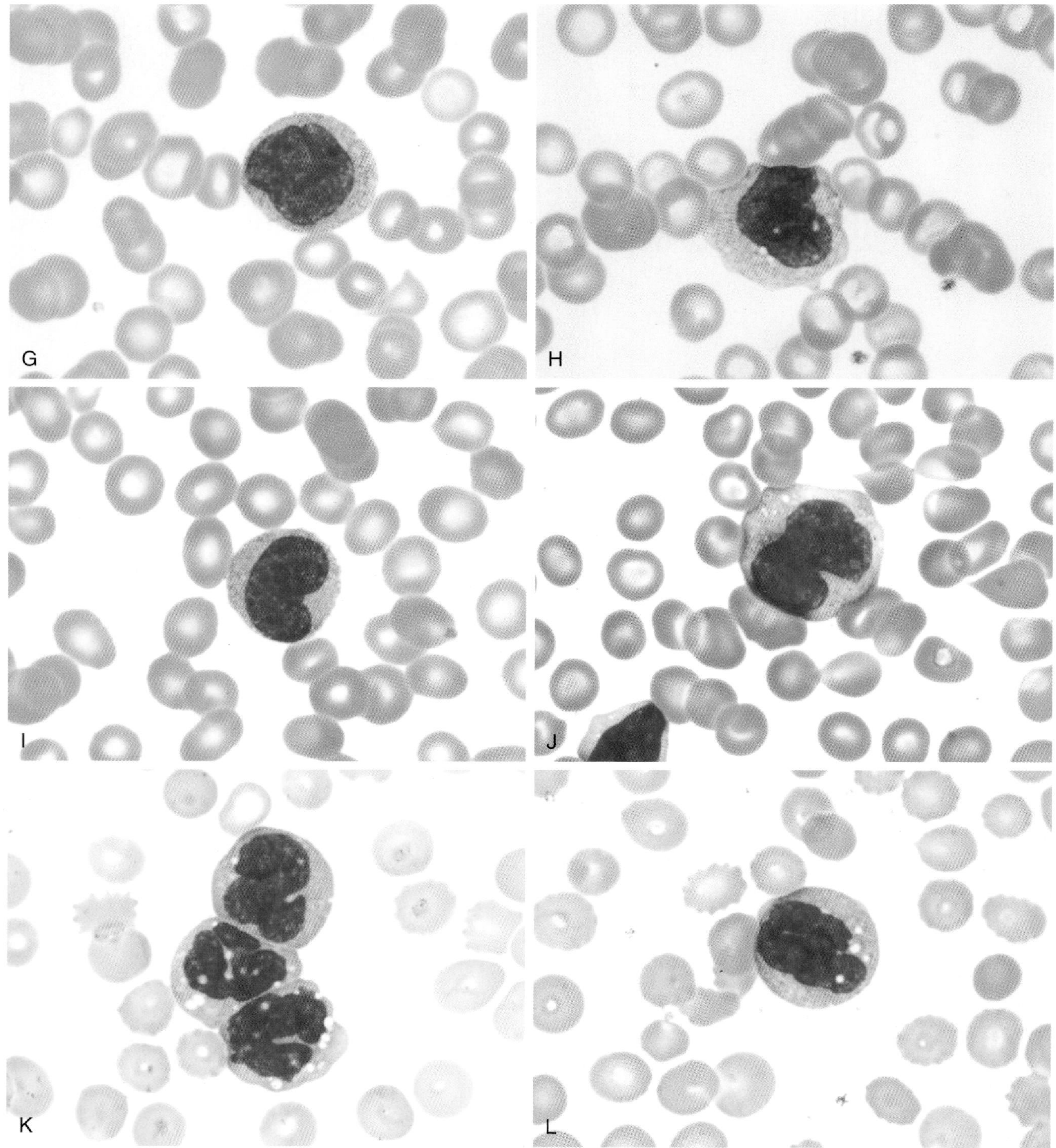

Figure 47-3, cont'd. I–L, Abnormal monocytes in chronic myelomonocytic leukemia appear immature. However, they have more condensed chromatin; abnormally shaped, irregular, or folded nuclei; and abundant grayish blue cytoplasm, with more cytoplasmic granules and, often, more cytoplasmic vacuoles.

Dysgranulopoiesis, including neutrophils with hypolobated or abnormally segmented nuclei or hypogranular cytoplasm, is usually present in the peripheral blood, but it may be minimal, if present at all, in a substantial minority of cases.[43] It is commonly believed that patients with higher WBC counts have less dyspoiesis than those with lower counts, but some authors have reported that there is no significant relationship between severity of dysplasia and the leukocyte count.[33]

Bone Marrow

The bone marrow biopsy is hypercellular in more than 75% of cases (Fig. 47-4), but normally cellular or even hypocellular specimens may be encountered.[40,44,45] Granulocytic proliferation is often the most prominent feature in the biopsy, with a significant increase in the myeloid-to-erythroid ratio (see Fig. 47-4); however, erythroid precursors are usually readily identified and, in some cases, even increased in number. The number of megakaryocytes may be increased, normal, or decreased. Up to 75% of patients are reported to have micromegakaryocytes or megakaryocytes with abnormal nuclear lobation,[43,44] although in some cases, enlarged megakaryocytes can be found as well. Clustering of megakaryocytes is unusual in CMML.

The number of monocytes required in the bone marrow for the diagnosis of CMML has never been established, and the percentages reported in the literature vary widely. When the biopsy has been well fixed, thinly sectioned, and nicely stained, a proliferation of monocytes may be appreciated (see Fig. 47-4B). Immunohistochemical stains performed on the biopsy, such as CD14 and CD68, may aid in their identification (Fig. 47-4),[43,44] although cytochemical stains for nonspecific esterase performed on blood and aspirate smears are, in our experience, more reliable (Figs. 47-5 and 47-6). An increase in blasts can often be appreciated in the biopsy. Staining the biopsy specimen for CD34 may be useful in estimating the blast percentage (Fig. 47-7), but CD34 may not be expressed by monoblasts or promonocytes; therefore, undue reliance should not be placed on the number of cells that express this antigen, and careful morphologic inspection is necessary. Reportedly, in up to 20% of cases (and an even greater percentage of cases of CMML-2), variably sized nodules of differentiated plasmacytoid dendritic cells can be found in the biopsy (see Fig. 47-4).[43] A mild increase in reticulin fibers has been reported in most cases of CMML, and 30% to 60% of cases (particularly CMML-2) can demonstrate a substantial increase.[44,46] Increased numbers of lymphocytes and lymphoid nodules may be observed as well.[44]

Cellular bone marrow aspirate smears provide the best material for assessing the number of myeloblasts, monoblasts, promonocytes, and monocytes and for appreciating dysplasia in the various lineages. Cytochemical staining for alpha naphthyl acetate esterase or alpha naphthyl butyrate esterase to detect monocytes—either alone or in combination with naphthol-ASD-chloroacetate esterase (CAE), which stains primarily neutrophils—is strongly recommended when the diagnosis of CMML is being considered (see Fig. 47-6). Dysgranulopoiesis, which is usually present, is more often appreciated in aspirate smears than in the peripheral blood. Dyserythropoiesis, particularly megaloblastoid changes or ring sideroblasts, is reported in about 25% of cases. The abnormal megakaryocyte morphology described in the biopsy can be appreciated in the aspirate as well.

Extramedullary Tissues

Splenic enlargement is frequent and is due to leukemic infiltration of primarily the red pulp by myelomonocytic cells (Fig. 47-8).[31] Trilineage extramedullary hematopoiesis has been reported in some splenectomy specimens from patients with CMML, and numerous foamy macrophages may be seen, particularly when the spleen has been removed as a therapeutic maneuver to relieve thrombocytopenia.[47] Some authors report high mortality and morbidity rates associated with splenectomy in patients with CMML.[47] Lymphadenopathy is seen in a minority of patients, and a biopsy is recommended in such cases because it may indicate extramedullary transformation to acute leukemia. In rare patients with CMML, tumoral proliferations of plasmacytoid dendritic cells, identical to those described in the bone marrow, may be seen in splenectomy or lymph node specimens.[48,49]

Immunophenotype

By flow cytometric analysis, the leukemic cells express myelomonocytic antigens such as CD33 and CD13, with variable expression of CD14, CD68, and CD64.[31] Often the monocytes in CMML exhibit aberrant expression of two or more antigens, including overexpression of CD56, aberrant expression of CD2, or decreased expression of HLA-DR, CD14, CD13, CD15, or CD64.[50-52] Some of these phenotypic abnormalities, such as decreased expression of CD14, may reflect immaturity of the monocytes. The maturing neutrophils may also show aberrant phenotypic features, such as asynchronous expression of maturation-associated antigens or aberrant light scatter properties. An increased number of $CD34^+$ cells or an emerging blast population with an aberrant immunophenotype may herald the onset of transformation to AML; however, as noted previously, CD34 does not always detect transformation to AML because the immature monocytic component may not express CD34.[52]

Immunohistochemistry on tissue sections of bone marrow biopsies may facilitate the assessment of cellular components in their architectural context and be helpful in distinguishing CMML from other MPNs and reactive conditions (see Fig. 47-7). Both granulocytes and monocytes, including immature forms and blasts, express CD33, which may be demonstrated in paraffin-embedded specimens.[53] Immunostaining for lysozyme may help highlight granulocytic and monocytic components, but neither CD33 nor lysozyme can discern between them. The combined use of CD33 or lysozyme immunohistochemistry and cytochemistry for CAE may facilitate the identification of monocytic cells, which are CD33 and lysozyme positive but CAE negative; in contrast, granulocytic cells are positive for CD33, lysozyme, and CAE. Other markers such as CD68 (KP1), CD68R (PG-M1), CD11b, CD11c, CD14, CD16, CD56, CD117, CD163, and HLA-DR are reportedly helpful in assessing the granulocytic and monocytic components of CMML, and some authors have suggested that when a number of these markers are used in combination, the staining pattern may be useful in the differential diagnosis of CMML, aCML, and CML.[43,44,54] Interestingly, Orazi and coworkers[43] reported that clusters of plasmacytoid dendritic cells, which could be identified with CD123, were restricted to cases of CMML (particularly

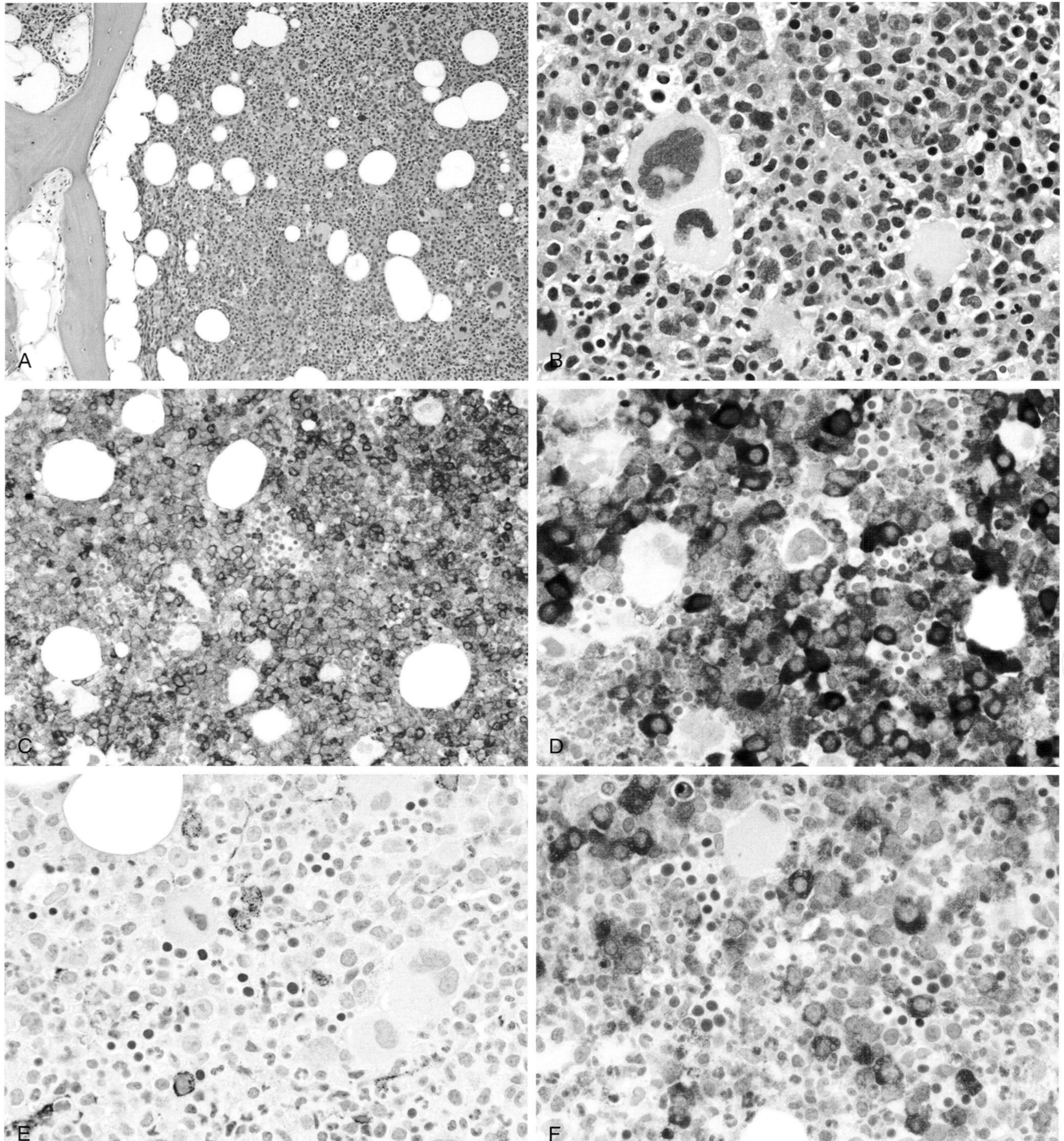

Figure 47-4. Bone marrow biopsy from a patient with chronic myelomonocytic leukemia-1. **A**, The bone marrow is hypercellular, with prominent granulocytic and monocytic components and variably sized megakaryocytes. **B**, On higher magnification, the folded nuclei of monocytes dispersed among granulocytes and large megakaryocytes can be better appreciated. There is also a distinct erythroid component present. **C** and **D**, Immunohistochemical stains for CD33 (**C**) and lysozyme (**D**) highlight granulocytic and monocytic components, respectively. **E**, Immunohistochemical stain for CD34 demonstrates only occasional immature $CD34^+$ mononuclear cells. **F**, Immunohistochemical stain for myeloperoxidase highlights numerous immature and maturing granulocytes.

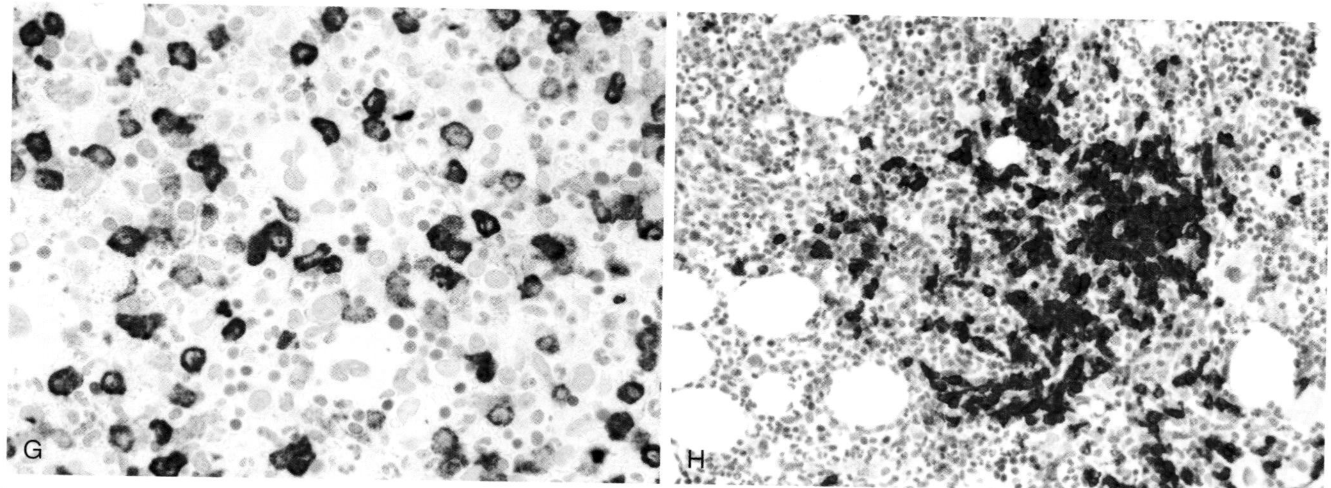

Figure 47-4, cont'd. **G**, CD14 demonstrates increased monocytes. **H**, Immunohistochemical stain for CD123 highlights a nodule of CD123^{+} plasmacytoid dendritic cells present in the biopsy specimen.

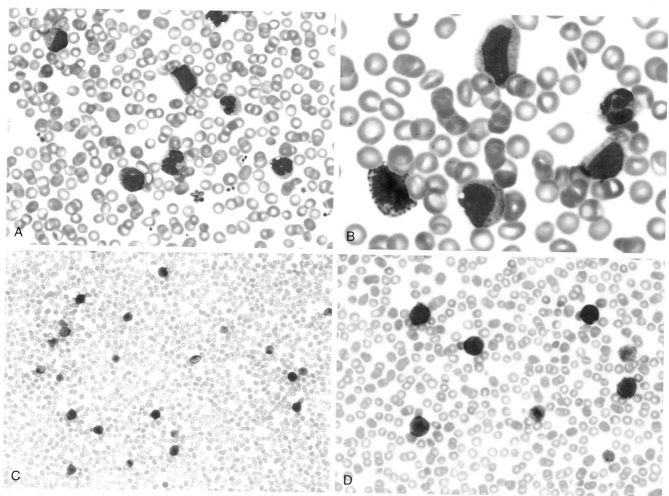

Figure 47-5. Chronic myelomonocytic leukemia-2. A and **B**, Peripheral blood smear demonstrates immature granulocytes, circulating blasts, and monocytes. **C** and **D**, The monocytic component can be better appreciated with the combined esterase stains: naphthol-ASD-chloroacetate esterase reaction combined with naphthyl butyrate esterase (monocytes are *brown*; neutrophils are *blue*).

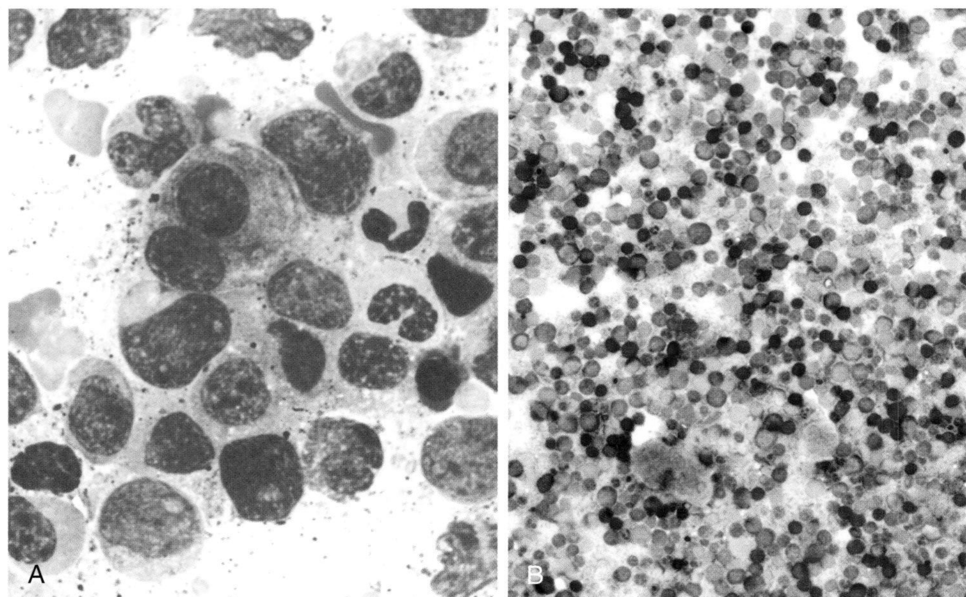

Figure 47-6. Chronic myelomonocytic leukemia-2. A, Bone marrow aspirate smear demonstrates monocytic and granulocytic components, scattered blasts, and a dysplastic megakaryocyte. **B**, Monocytic and granulocytic components in the bone marrow can be better appreciated with the combined esterase stains: naphthol-ASD-chloroacetate esterase reaction combined with naphthyl butyrate esterase (monocytes are *brown*; neutrophils are *blue*).

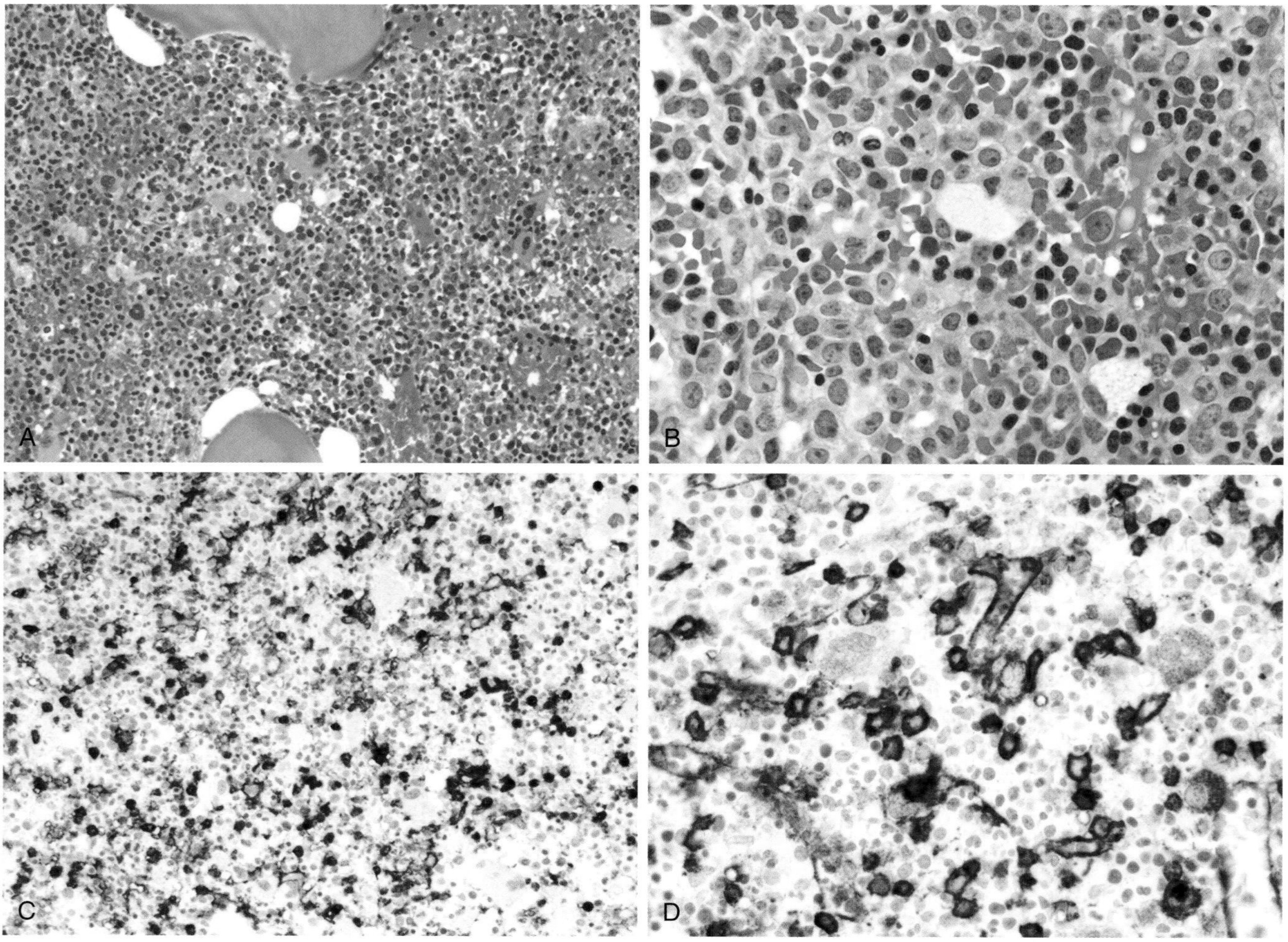

Figure 47-7. Chronic myelomonocytic leukemia-2. A, Bone marrow biopsy shows hypercellular bone marrow with prominent granulocytic and monocytic components, increased blasts, and numerous morphologically variable megakaryocytes, including dysplastic forms. **B**, On higher magnification, an increase in immature cells and blasts can be better appreciated, and there is a distinct erythroid component. **C**, Immunohistochemical stain for CD14 demonstrates increased monocytes scattered throughout the marrow. **D**, Immunohistochemical stain for CD34 demonstrates an increase in $CD34^+$ blasts.

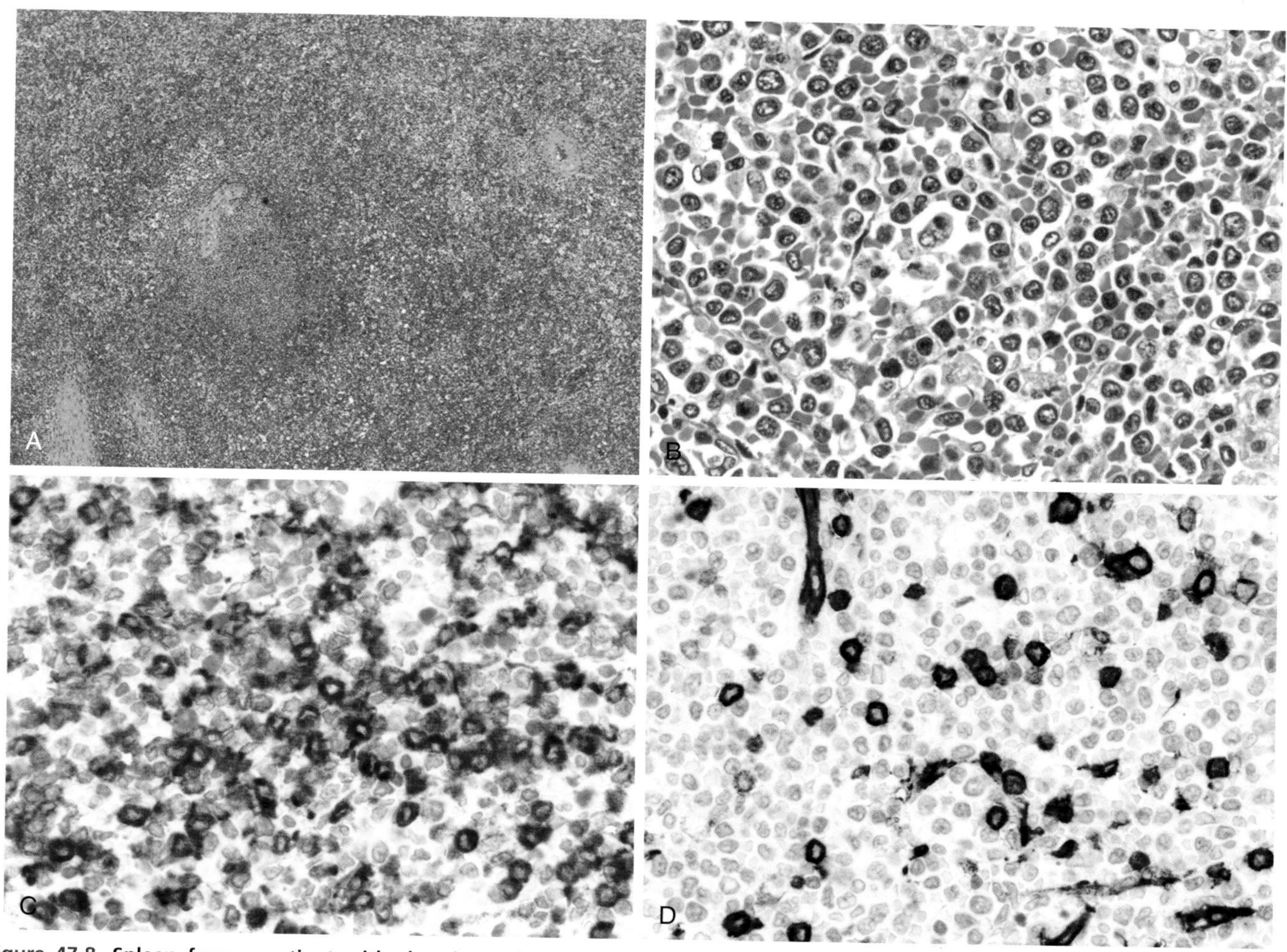

Figure 47-8. Spleen from a patient with chronic myelomonocytic leukemia-2. A, Leukemic infiltrate in the red pulp of the spleen encroaches on the white pulp. **B,** The infiltrate is comprised of blasts, immature granulocytes, and monocytes. **C,** Immunohistochemical stain for CD14 highlights the monocytic component of the infiltrate. **D,** Immunohistochemical stain for CD34 demonstrates increased $CD34^+$ blasts.

CMML-2) and were not found in cases of aCML or CML, *BCR-ABL1* positive. Immunoassaying for CD61 or CD42b highlights abnormal megakaryocytes.[43] Staining for glycophorin C by immunohistochemistry may also be helpful in demonstrating erythroid precursors.

Cytogenetics and Genetics

No specific cytogenetic or genetic abnormalities have been identified in CMML. Abnormal karyotypes are reported in only 20% to 40% of cases, and the recurring abnormalities most frequently reported include +8, −7, −5, del(12p), del(20q), and complex karyotypes.[33,34,55] Abnormalities involving *MLL* at 11q23 are unusual in CMML; if present, special care should be taken to rule out AML.

Some authors have suggested that patients whose leukemic cells carry an isochromosome 17q have a unique form of MDS/MPN characterized by marked Pelger-Huët–like nuclei and peripheral cytoplasmic vacuolization of neutrophils (Fig. 47-9), often associated with marrow fibrosis, dysmegakaryocytopoiesis, and usually a poor prognosis.[56] However, almost all patients have absolute monocytosis and meet the criteria for CMML, although rare patients may fit into the aCML or MDS/MPN, unclassifiable category.

As noted in the section on pathogenesis, SNP-A analysis has revealed somatic uniparental disomy in nearly 50% of cases of CMML.[4,5] The segments most commonly affected are chromosomes 1p, 4q, 7q, 21q, 6p, 13q , 14q, and 11q.[4] The significance of these cryptic chromosomal aberrations, which often lead to loss of heterozygosity, is currently unknown. Recently, investigation of genes in an area of chromosome 4q24 commonly affected by loss of heterozygosity and deletions in myeloid malignancies identified frequent mutations of *TET2* in patients with MDS/MPNs, including CMML, thus implicating a role for this putative tumor suppressor gene in the pathogenesis of CMML.[57]

As noted earlier, mutations of *NRAS* or *KRAS* occur in 20% to 60% of patients. Although some authors have linked mutated RAS proteins to higher WBC counts,[3] this has not been found in other studies.[6] Array comparative genomic hybridization profiling of CMML has found frequent alterations of *RUNX1*,[3] which often occur in conjunction with *RAS* mutations. In addition, it has been reported that *RUNX1* mutation in the C-terminal region may predict early AML transformation.[58] Other mutations in CMML have been reported that involve class I and class II genes and likely play a role in biology and disease progression.[59,60]

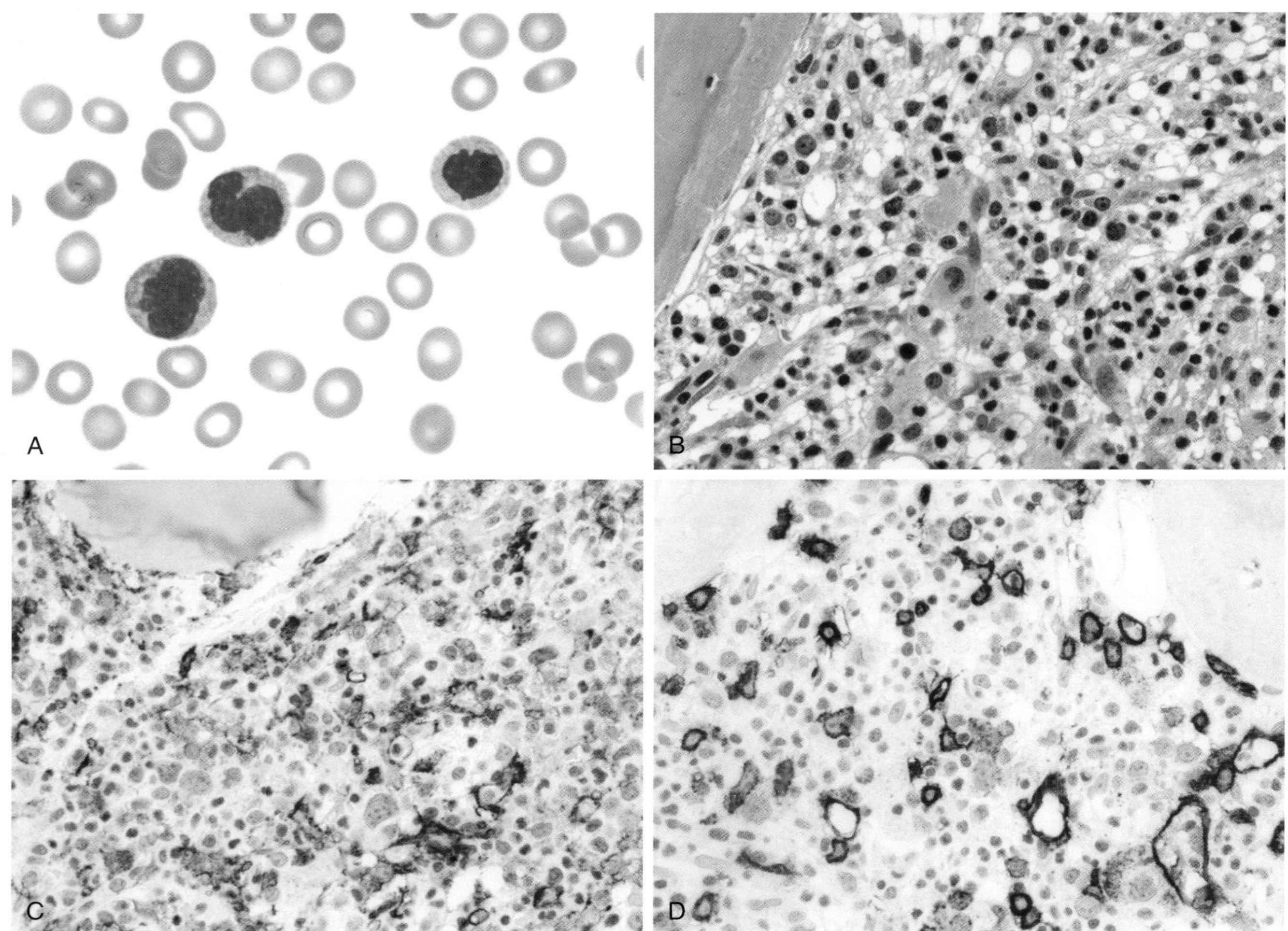

Figure 47-9. Isochromosome 17q. A, Many patients with i(17q) have an absolute monocytosis, with abnormal monocytes and dysplastic granulocytes showing Pelger-Huët–like nuclei with condensed chromatin and hypogranular cytoplasm. **B**, Bone marrow biopsy demonstrates granulocytic proliferation with marked dysplasia and dysmegakaryopoiesis. **C**, Immunohistochemical stain for CD14 highlights the increased monocytic component. **D**, Immunohistochemical stain for CD34 demonstrates increased CD34⁺ blasts.

Although there has been long-standing interest in epigenetic abnormalities of gene methylation in MDS and MDS/MPN, information regarding gene methylation in CMML is limited to a small number of cases that are usually included in MDS studies and to a limited number of specific genes.[61] Methylation of the promoter of the cell cycle regulatory gene *p15INK4* was reported in 58% of 33 CMML cases and correlated with reduced messenger RNA and protein expression and with increased expression of the DNA methyltransferase DNMT 3A.[62] Methylation of *RASSFIA* and *SHIP-1*, negative regulators of RTK/RAS signaling, is rare in CMML.[63] The data on *SOCS1* are conflicting, but *SOCS1* methylation is reportedly associated with a higher frequency of *NRAS* mutation, poor prognosis, and greater cumulative risk of transformation to acute leukemia but has no independent effect on survival.[63]

Recently, genome-wide DNA methylation microarray analysis combined with high-density SNP-A karyotyping in a large series of patients with AML, MDS, and MDS/MPNs, including CMML, has shown that aberrant methylation of tumor suppressor genes occurs frequently in all myeloid malignancies, including CMML, and can cooperate with chromosomal deletions to silence tumor suppressor genes and affect disease progression.[64] Furthermore, clinical trials with demethylating agents reported encouraging clinical responses in a fraction of CMML patients, thus underscoring the importance of this epigenetic mechanism to the pathogenesis and progression of CMML.[65-67]

Other Laboratory Findings

Serum lysozyme levels are usually elevated and parallel the degree of monocytosis in the blood. Polyclonal hypergammaglobulinemia has been reported in 50% to 60% of patients, and rarely, monoclonal proteins may be detected.[68,69] A positive Coombs test in the face of no prior transfusion history was reported in almost 20% of patients evaluated in one study.[69]

Differential Diagnosis

The diagnosis of CMML is sometimes difficult, particularly when dysplasia is minimal, the degree of monocytosis is slight, no cytogenetic abnormalities are present, and the dura-

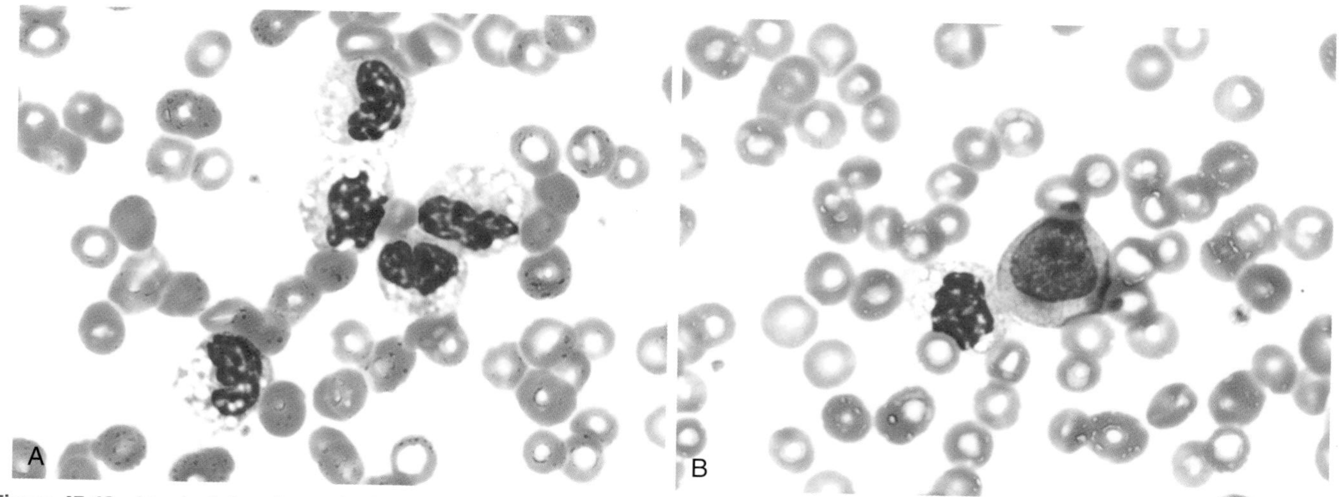

Figure 47-12. Atypical chronic myeloid leukemia, "syndrome of abnormal chromatin clumping" variant. A and **B**, Peripheral blood smear shows marked granulocytic dysplasia, with abnormally lobated nuclei, clumped chromatin, and immature neutrophils.

Most cases reported as the *syndrome of abnormal chromatin clumping* can be considered variants of aCML.[80-82] These are characterized in the blood and bone marrow by a high percentage of neutrophils and precursors, with exaggerated clumping of the nuclear chromatin (Fig. 47-12).

Extramedullary Tissues

Splenomegaly and hepatomegaly are frequently observed,[79] but there are no studies detailing the histologic findings in these organs in aCML. However, the pattern of involvement would be expected to be similar to that observed in other myeloid diseases—that is, mainly red pulp involvement of the spleen and sinus and periportal infiltrates in the liver.

Immunophenotype

No specific immunophenotypic characteristics have been reported. When studied by multiparameter flow cytometry, however, asynchronous expression of maturation antigens on the myeloblasts and maturing granulocytes, similar to that reported in MPNs, would be expected,[83] as would abnormal orthogonal light scatter properties due to the hypogranular cytoplasm of neutrophils and their precursors.

Cytogenetics and Genetics

Karyotypic abnormalities are reported in up to 80% of patients with aCML. The most common chromosome abnormalities include trisomy 8 and del(20q), but deletions involving chromosomes 12, 13, 14, and 17 are also seen.[2,78] Rarely, patients who have isochromosome 17q may have features resembling aCML, although most meet the diagnostic criteria for CMML. Some cases with the t(8;9)(p22;p24), *PCM1-JAK2* chromosomal rearrangement have been diagnosed as aCML, but because eosinophilia is usually present in these cases, they are better classified as chronic eosinophilic leukemia.[84] Patients with rearrangements of *PDGFR* or *FGFR1* are also excluded from this diagnostic category. Although there are reports of *JAK2* V617F mutation in aCML,[12] in one study in which the WHO diagnostic criteria for aCML were rigidly applied, there were no cases that demonstrated mutated *JAK2*.[15] Mutations of *NRAS* or *KRAS* are reported in 30% to 40% of cases.[6,8]

Differential Diagnosis

Chronic Myelomonocytic Leukemia

The major distinguishing features between CMML and aCML are the percentage of monocytes in the blood (≥10% in CMML and <10% in aCML) and the more severe dysplasia in most cases of aCML. Differences in the morphologic findings and in the reported median survival times argue that CMML and aCML are biologically separate entities, but in practice, occasional cases may arise in which the distinction is somewhat arbitrary and cannot be made with any degree of confidence.

Chronic Myelogenous Leukemia, *BCR-ABL1* Positive

As indicated by the nomenclature, CML, *BCR-ABL1* positive has the Ph chromosome or *BCR-ABL1* fusion gene, which is not present in aCML; appropriate cytogenetic or molecular genetic studies should always be performed when either diagnosis is suspected. Usually, morphology can readily distinguish between them; dysplasia is usually minimal in the chronic phase of CML but prominent in aCML. Basophilia may be present in both diseases, but it is usually less than 2% of the peripheral blood cells in aCML and greater than 2% in CML. Nevertheless, the accelerated phase of CML may be difficult to distinguish from aCML because dysplasia becomes more noticeable when CML progresses beyond the chronic phase. Cytogenetic studies are always required.

Myelodysplastic Syndrome

Although the dysplasia observed in aCML is similar to that in MDS, the leukocytosis observed in aCML would not be expected in MDS.

Prognosis and Prognostic Factors

The limited number of cases reported in the literature precludes any definitive statement regarding disease outcome, but most patients seem to fare poorly, with overall median survival of 11 to 25 months. Age older than 65 years, female sex, WBC counts greater than 50 × 10^9/L, severe anemia, and thrombocytopenia are generally considered unfavorable prognostic features. Patients who receive bone marrow transplants may have an improved outcome. In 15% to 40% of patients aCML evolves to AML, whereas the remainder succumb to bone marrow failure.[78,79]

JUVENILE MYELOMONOCYTIC LEUKEMIA

JMML is a clonal hematopoietic neoplasm of early childhood characterized by a proliferation of mainly the granulocytic and monocytic lineages. Nevertheless, because it originates in a pluripotent stem cell, abnormalities of erythroid and megakaryocytic lineages are often present as well. Blasts plus promonocytes are less than 20% of the peripheral blood WBCs and of the nucleated bone marrow cells. As noted previously, aberrations in the RAS signaling pathway contribute to the pathogenesis of JMML and account for the hallmark finding of hypersensitivity of the progenitor cells to GM-CSF.

Previously JMML was referred to as *juvenile chronic myeloid leukemia*. This nomenclature led to some confusion between JMML and CML, *BCR-ABL1* positive, which does occur in children, although rarely. In contrast to CML, the leukemic cells of JMML lack the Ph chromosome and the *BCR-ABL1* fusion gene. In addition, some children with monosomy of chromosome 7 were separately diagnosed as having *monosomy 7 syndrome*. The findings in many of these children overlap with those of JMML, and such cases should be classified as JMML if they meet the diagnostic criteria (Box 47-5).

Clinical Findings

The annual incidence of JMML is only 1.3 per million children between birth and 14 years of age.[85,86] More than 75% of cases of JMML are diagnosed in children younger than 3 years, and 95% are diagnosed before the age of 6, with a median age of 2 years at diagnosis. Boys are affected about twice as commonly as girls.[10] About 10% of cases occur in children with NF-1, and rarely, children with Noonan syndrome develop JMML.

Pallor, failure to thrive, and decreased appetite are common symptoms reported by the parents. Many patients have constitutional findings that resemble those of acute or subacute infection,[10,87-90] but these are usually related to infiltration of various tissues by leukemic cells. Fever, often in conjunction with symptoms of bronchitis or tonsillitis, is present in 50% or more of patients at the time of initial diagnosis. Maculopapular rashes due to leukemic infiltrates usually involve the face and occur in 40% to 50% of patients. Between 10% and 15% of patients with JMML also exhibit clinical manifestations of NF-1,[10,88] including café au lait spots and dermal neurofibromas. Hepatosplenomegaly is almost always present, and lymphadenopathy is seen in up to 80% of cases.[90] A few patients present with gastrointestinal symptoms, including intractable diarrhea, due to leukemic infiltration of the intestine.[91] When evaluating a patient for JMML, it is important to carefully search for features of the inherited diseases with which it may be associated—namely, NF-1 and Noonan's syndrome.

Box 47-5 World Health Organization Diagnostic Criteria for Juvenile Myelomonocytic Leukemia

- Peripheral blood monocytosis >1 × 10^9/L
- Blasts (including promonocytes) are <20% of leukocytes in the blood and <20% of nucleated bone marrow cells
- No Philadelphia chromosome or *BCR-ABL1* fusion gene
- Plus two or more of the following:
  - Hemoglobin F increased for age
  - Immature granulocytes in peripheral blood
  - WBC count >10 × 10^9/L
  - Clonal chromosomal abnormality (may be monosomy 7)
  - GM-CSF hypersensitivity

GM-CSF, granulocyte-macrophage colony-stimulating factor; WBC, white blood cell.

From Swerdlow SH, Campo E, Harris NL, et al, eds. *WHO Classification of Tumours of Haematopoietic and Lymphoid Tissues*. Lyon, France: IARC Press; 2008.

Laboratory Findings

Blood

Examination of the peripheral blood is necessary to reach the diagnosis of JMML and is often more revealing than the bone marrow (Fig. 47-13). Characteristic findings include moderate leukocytosis, monocytosis, occasional immature neutrophils, rare blasts, a few nucleated red blood cells, and thrombocytopenia.[10,87,88,90] However, there is considerable variation. The median reported WBC count is 25 to 35 × 10^9/L, but it may range from 10 to, rarely, more than 100 × 10^9/L. Neutrophils, including a few immature forms, often constitute the majority of the white cells, but monocytosis, which can vary from 1 to greater than 60 × 10^9/L, is invariably present; at least 1 × 10^9/L monocytes are required for the diagnosis of JMML.[86] Blasts plus promonocytes usually account for less than 5% of the WBCs at diagnosis and always for less than 20%. Normocytic red blood cells are usually seen, but some children, particularly those with monosomy 7, have macrocytic indices. Acquired thalassemia with microcytosis has been reported in some children.[92] Nucleated red blood cells are frequently observed. Platelet counts are decreased in at least 75% of patients, and the thrombocytopenia may be severe.

Bone Marrow

It is not always easy to determine whether a marrow specimen from a baby is hypercellular, yet most investigators report that bone marrow biopsy and aspirate specimens are hypercellular for the patient's age (see Fig. 47-13). In most cases the myeloid-to-erythroid ratio is increased, but it may vary from less than 1:1 to more than 50:1.[87] Blasts and promonocytes usually account for less than 5% of the marrow cells and are always less than 20%. Monocytes may be difficult to appreciate, particularly if only a Wright-stained aspirate smear or hematoxylin-eosin–stained bone marrow biopsy section is examined. Staining the bone marrow aspirate with nonspecific esterase or the bone marrow biopsy specimen for CD68 or CD14 may enhance the recognition of monocytes. Dyspla-

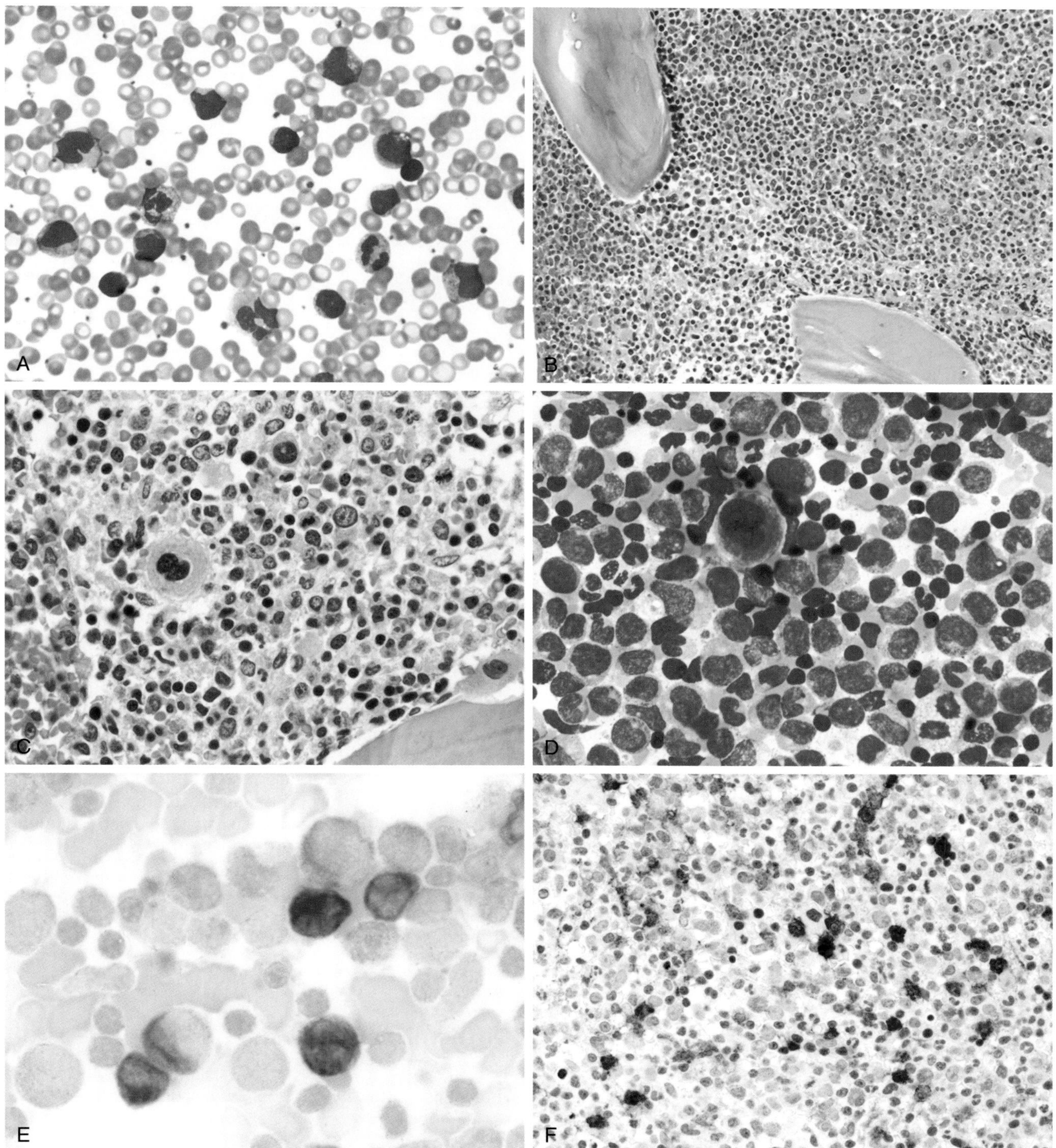

Figure 47-13. Juvenile myelomonocytic leukemia. A, Peripheral blood smear shows monocytosis, with abnormal monocytes and immature granulocytes. **B**, Bone marrow is hypercellular, with granulocytic proliferation and mildly reduced megakaryocytes. **C**, On higher magnification, scattered monocytes intermingled with granulocytes can be identified; however, the monocytic component is difficult to appreciate. Blasts are not significantly increased. **D**, Bone marrow aspirate reflects the findings in the bone marrow and demonstrates granulocytic proliferation and increased monocytes. **E**, Combined alpha naphthyl acetate esterase and naphthol-ASD-chloroacetate esterase reaction is helpful in identifying both the granulocytic component (*blue*) and the monocytic component (*brown*). **F**, The monocytic component can also be demonstrated by immunohistochemical stain for CD14.

Continued

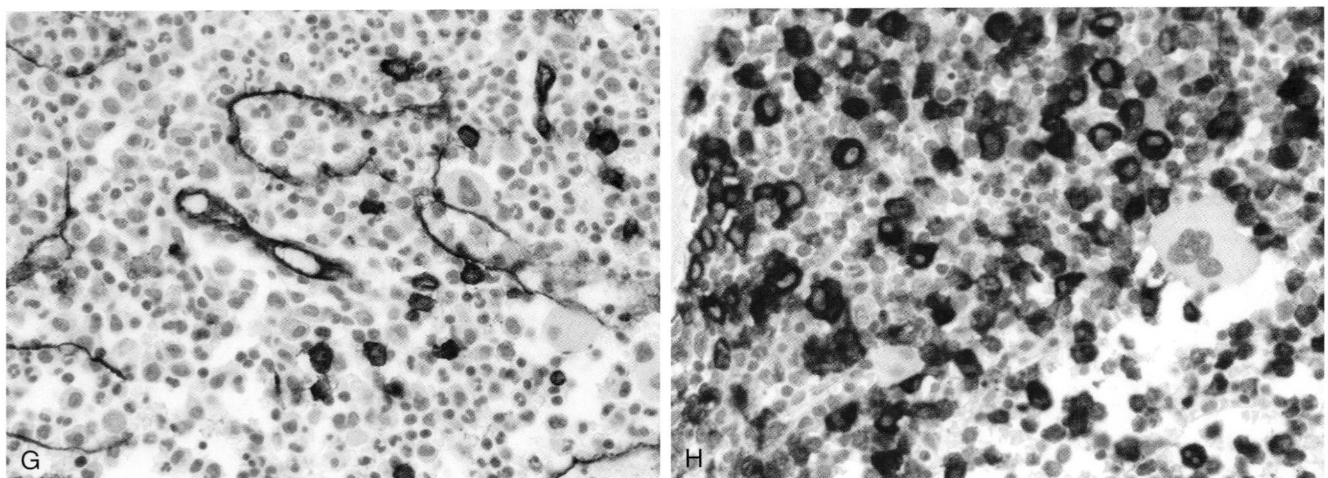

Figure 47-13, cont'd. G, Immunohistochemical stain for CD34 demonstrates a small number of $CD34^+$ blasts and highlights dilated marrow sinuses filled with leukemic cells that may go to extramedullary sites. **H,** Immunohistochemical stain for myeloperoxidase highlights the granulocytic component.

sia is minimal, if present at all, but pseudo–Pelger-Huët neutrophils and neutrophils with hypogranular cytoplasm have been reported.[88] Auer rods are not observed. Erythroid precursors may show megaloblastic changes. Megakaryocytes are often reduced in number, but megakaryocytic dysplasia is not usual.

Extramedullary Tissues

The hepatosplenomegaly observed clinically is due to leukemic infiltration. In the spleen, leukemic cells infiltrate the red pulp and compress and obliterate the white pulp (Fig. 47-14). Liver biopsies often show both portal tract and sinusoidal infiltration. The skin is often infiltrated with myelomonocytic cells in the upper and lower dermis. Myelomonocytic infiltration of the lungs accounts for the pulmonary symptoms at presentation—sometimes complicated by simultaneous infections—and contributes to the significant morbidity in JMML (see Fig. 47-14). The cells spread from the peribronchial lymphatics and alveolar capillaries into the alveolar septa and alveoli.[93]

Immunophenotype

No specific phenotypic abnormalities have been reported in JMML. In tissue sections the monocytic component may be detected by analysis for CD14, CD11b, CD68R, or lysozyme expression.

Cytogenetics and Genetics

There is no Ph chromosome or *BCR-ABL1* fusion gene. No consistently recurring cytogenetic abnormalities are reported in JMML, and normal karyotypes are found in 40% to 70% of patients.[10,90] Monosomy 7, del(7q), or other abnormalities of chromosome 7 have been reported in approximately 25% of cases.[10,94] Mutations of *NRAS* or *KRAS*, *NF1*, and *PTPN11* have each been reported in about 20% to 35% of JMML patients and are mutually exclusive; thus, overall, nearly 75% of patients with JMML have one of these abnormalities.[21] These mutations are not specific for JMML, however, and have been reported in AML, MDS, and other MDS/MPNs. Nevertheless, detection of one of these mutations can certainly help confirm the diagnosis; unfortunately, the tests to do so are not widely available for clinical use.

Other Laboratory Findings

Most patients with JMML have hemoglobin F levels that are increased for their age; however, patients with monosomy 7 are more likely to have normal or only modestly elevated hemoglobin F levels compared with children with JMML and normal karyotypes or other cytogenetic abnormalities.[87] More than half the patients with JMML have polyclonal hypergammaglobulinemia of uncertain significance. Autoantibodies and a positive direct Coombs test have also been reported in up to 25% of cases. Hypersensitivity of the myeloid progenitors to GM-CSF is characteristic for JMML. Unfortunately, analysis of progenitor cells' response to GM-CSF is not readily available, but every attempt should be made to do this study if the diagnosis of JMML cannot be readily substantiated by other clinical and laboratory findings.

Differential Diagnosis

The diagnosis of JMML can be challenging for the clinician and the pathologist. Although the neoplastic nature of the proliferation can be appreciated in most patients, in some cases the initial symptoms resemble those of an infection or a systemic inflammatory illness, and a careful examination of the peripheral blood smear is often the first clue to the diagnosis of JMML.

Infection

The clinical and morphologic findings of JMML can be imitated by a variety of infectious diseases, including those caused by Epstein-Barr virus, cytomegalovirus, and human herpesvirus 6.[89,95] However, the possibility that a patient with JMML may have a concomitant infection that obscures the diagnosis must also be considered. Serologic investigations

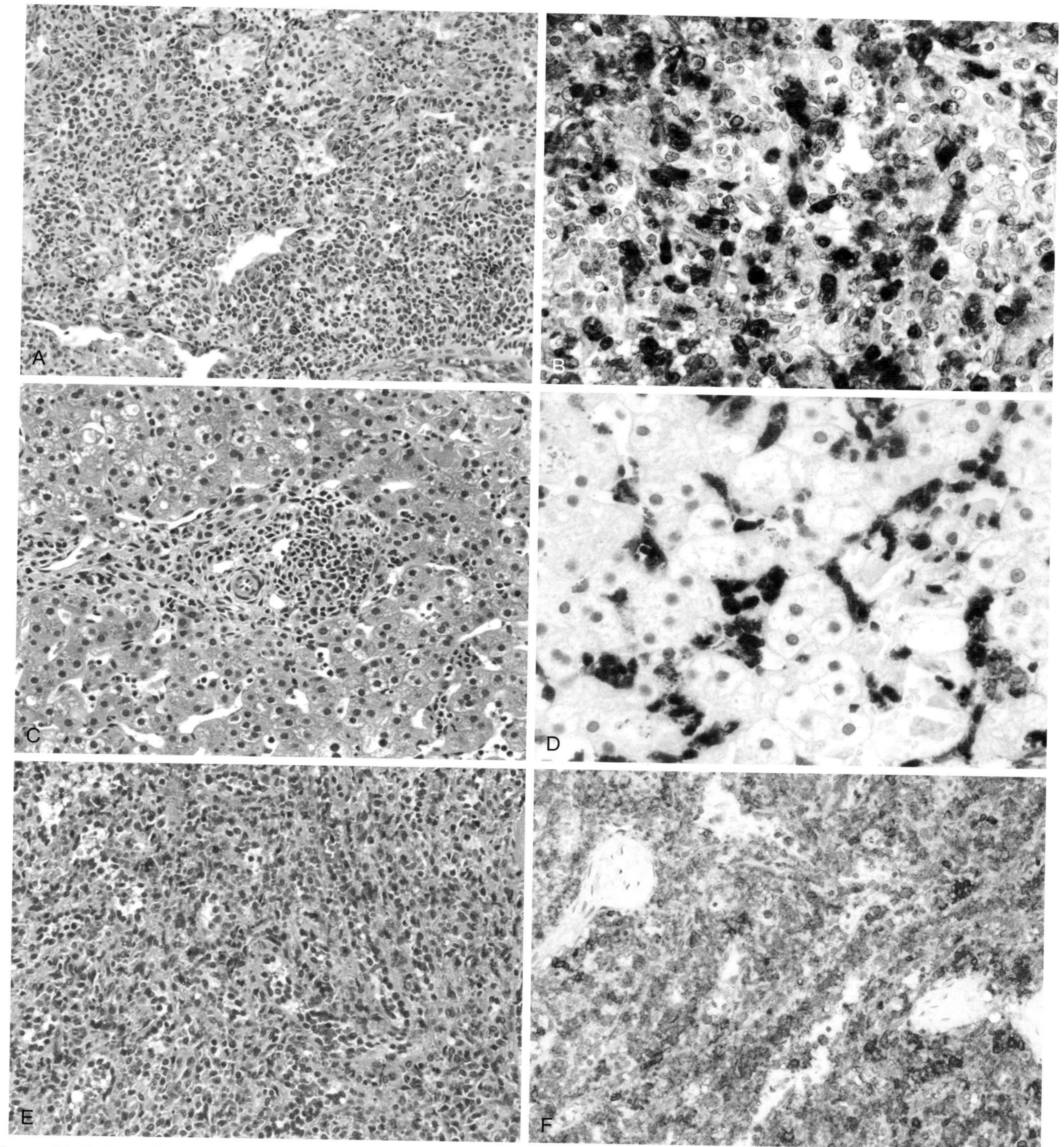

Figure 47-14. Juvenile myelomonocytic leukemia, extramedullary tissue. A, Interstitial leukemic infiltrate in the lung. **B**, Immunohistochemical stain for lysozyme highlights both the granulocytic and monocytic components of the infiltrate. **C**, Leukemic infiltrate in the portal region and sinuses of the liver. **D**, Immunohistochemical stain for lysozyme highlights leukemic cells in the liver sinuses. **E**, Leukemic infiltrate in the red pulp of the spleen. **F**, Immunohistochemical stain for CD33 highlights leukemic cells in the splenic cords and sinuses.

Continued

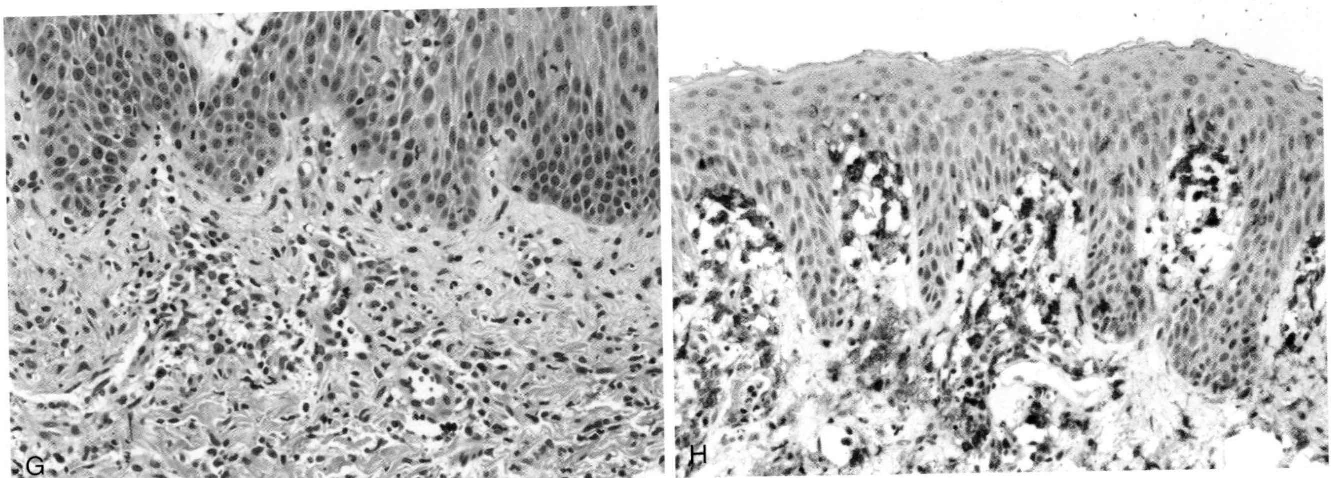

Figure 47-14, cont'd. G, Perivascular and subepidermal leukemic infiltrate in the skin. **H,** Immunohistochemical stain for CD33 highlights the leukemic infiltrate in the dermis, which focally extends into the epidermis.

have shown that children with JMML have a similar prevalence of antibodies for cytomegalovirus, Epstein-Barr virus, and herpesvirus type 1 as does the normal infant population. The finding of a clonal chromosomal abnormality or other genetic defect, such as *NRAS* mutation, would substantiate the neoplastic nature of the process.

Other Myeloid Diseases

Adult-type CML, *BCR-ABL1* positive, is even less common in children than is JMML, particularly in those younger than 5 years. Nevertheless, cytogenetic and molecular studies should always be performed to exclude this possibility whenever the diagnosis of JMML is considered. In contrast to JMML, adult-type MDS usually occurs in children older than 5 years and is generally associated with leukopenia rather than leukocytosis. Dysplasia that involves two or all three of the myeloid lineages is usually much more prominent in MDS, which also has a lower frequency of hepatosplenomegaly compared with JMML.[87,90] It has been reported that children with MDS have a higher incidence of cytogenetic abnormalities than do those with JMML. Monosomy 7 can be seen in childhood MDS and in AML but is also common in JMML; thus the diagnosis of a patient with monosomy 7 depends on clinical, laboratory, and morphologic findings rather than on karyotype alone.[96] The distinction between AML and JMML is based on the percentage of blasts including promonocytes in the blood and bone marrow. At the time of diagnosis, JMML has fewer than 20% whereas in acute leukemia, blasts including promonocytes account for 20% or more.[86]

Prognosis and Outcome

The prognosis of JMML is quite variable. Spontaneous improvement has been reported in some patients, particularly those with *PTPN11* mutations who are younger than 1 year; unfortunately, the majority of patients experience disease progression.[10] Standard chemotherapy regimens are usually ineffective, and allogeneic stem cell transplantation is the only curative treatment. Even then, a substantial number of patients, perhaps 30% to 40%, relapse after the transplant. Factors that predict a worse outcome include age older than 2 years, platelet counts less than $100 \times 10^9/L$, and fetal hemoglobin greater than 15%.[86,88] Transformation of JMML into overt AML occurs in only 10% to 15% of patients; rare cases with evolution to B-lymphoblastic leukemia have also been reported.[97]

MYELODYSPLASTIC/ MYELOPROLIFERATIVE NEOPLASM, UNCLASSIFIABLE

When patients exhibit features that do not easily fit into any existing subcategory of disease, the entity is unclassifiable. It should be emphasized, however, that the term *unclassifiable* is justified only when the appropriate and requisite clinical, morphologic, immunophenotypic, and genetic studies have been performed to determine that the disease truly does not fit a well-defined category. In the case of MDS/MPN, a case can be considered unclassifiable if the disorder in question meets the criteria for the MDS/MPN category—that is, at the time of initial diagnosis, there are clinical, morphologic, and laboratory features that overlap both MDS and MPN—but the case does not meet the criteria for CMML, aCML, or JMML. The finding of a *BCR-ABL1* fusion gene or rearrangements of *PDGFRA*, *PDGFRB*, or *FGFR1* excludes the diagnosis of MDS/MPN, unclassifiable. It is important that this designation not be applied to patients with previously well-defined MPNs who develop dyspoietic features in association with therapy or disease progression. The diagnosis may be appropriate, however, for some patients in whom the chronic phase of an MPN was not previously recognized and who present initially with what appears to be an MPN in transformation with dysplastic features. If the underlying MPN cannot be accurately identified, the designation MDS/MPN, unclassifiable may be appropriate. If the patient has received any growth factor or cytotoxic therapy before the initial diagnostic evaluation, additional clinical and laboratory studies are essential to prove that the dyspoietic or proliferative features are not related to the therapy.

Box 47-6 World Health Organization Diagnostic Criteria for Refractory Anemia with Ring Sideroblasts and Thrombocytosis

- Platelets ≥450 × 10^9/L
- No Philadelphia chromosome or *BCR-ABL1* fusion gene
- Case meets the criteria for refractory anemia with ring sideroblasts: refractory anemia; no blasts in the blood and <5% blasts in the bone marrow; and ineffective erythroid proliferation with dyspoietic features, including ring sideroblasts that account for ≥15% of marrow erythroid precursors
- Proliferation of abnormal megakaryocytes with morphology similar to those observed in the *BCR-ABL1* negative myeloproliferative neoplasms primary myelofibrosis and essential thrombocythemia

From Swerdlow SH, Campo E, Harris NL, et al, eds. *WHO Classification of Tumours of Haematopoietic and Lymphoid Tissues*. Lyon, France: IARC Press; 2008.

Refractory Anemia with Ring Sideroblasts Associated with Marked Thrombocytosis

In the WHO classification of myeloid neoplasms, this provisional entity is included in the MDS/MPN, unclassifiable category.[98] This may seem to be a strange situation for a disorder with such stringent diagnostic criteria (Box 47-6), but the controversy is whether RARS-T is an actual MDS/MPN entity, the evolution and progression of a previously unrecognized MPN, or two distinct disorders that occur simultaneously. Until some of these questions can be answered, it seems best to leave RARS-T exactly where it is, as a provisional entity.

Initially, RARS-T was proposed to encompass patients with the clinical and morphologic features of refractory anemia with ring sideroblasts (RARS) along with marked thrombocytosis associated with abnormal megakaryocytes, similar to those observed in *BCR-ABL1* negative MPNs. The myeloproliferative component of RARS-T is supported by the finding of the *JAK2* V617F mutation in up to 50% of the cases analyzed[25-29,99,100] or, much less commonly, abnormalities involving *MPL* W515K/L.[7,101] However, in the few cases of RARS-T with *JAK2* mutations that have been studied for in vivo endogenous colony formation, the growth pattern is more akin to that of MDS than MPN.[26,29] Furthermore, RARS and RARS-T share a high frequency of hemochromatosis-associated gene mutations.[102] Thus, it may be that the MDS/MPN designation is appropriate, and RARS-T will gain its place as the fourth MDS/MPN entity. The finding of the *BCR-ABL1* fusion gene or rearrangements of *PDGFRA*, *PDGFRB*, or *FGFR1* excludes this diagnosis, as does the presence of isolated del(5q), t(3;3)(q21;q26), or inv(3)(q21q26).

Clinical Findings

The incidence of RARS-T is unknown, but it appears to be a rare entity. In the cases reported to date, there appears to be no sex predilection. Patients may present with symptoms related to the refractory anemia, which is often quite severe, or to the excessive thrombocytosis, with bleeding or thrombosis; in many, the symptoms are related to both abnormalities. Organomegaly is usually absent or mild.

Laboratory Findings

Blood. The WBC count is usually normal to modestly elevated, and there are no blasts. Dysplasia is lacking in the neutrophils. Red blood cells often show the typical dimorphic pattern observed in RARS (Fig. 47-15). Platelets are at least 450 × 10^9/L.[98]

Bone Marrow. The bone marrow biopsy is hypercellular and shows increased numbers of megakaryocytes, many of which are enlarged and have features similar to those seen in essential thrombocythemia or primary myelofibrosis (see Fig. 47-15).[2,98] Erythropoiesis usually predominates and is dysplastic, a feature that can best be appreciated in aspirate smears. At least 15% of the erythroid precursors must be ring sideroblasts, demonstrated with an iron stain on the aspirate smear.

Immunophenotype. There are no specific immunophenotypic features reported with RARS-T.

Cytogenetics and Genetics. No karyotypic abnormality has been specifically associated with RARS-T. Most patients have normal cytogenetics, although trisomy 8, del(12p), and del(13q) have been mentioned in some cases. As noted earlier, nearly 50% of patients have the *JAK2* V617F mutation, and a smaller number have mutated *MPL* W515K/L. Recently, using SNP-A, a number of cryptic cytogenetic lesions were discovered in a cohort of 18 RARS-T patients who did not have mutated *JAK2*, including 4 patients with uniparental disomy for chromosome 1p (UPD1p)—an area that contains *MPL*.[7]

Differential Diagnosis

Refractory Anemia with Ring Sideroblasts. Slightly elevated platelet counts are common in RARS and can lead to diagnostic confusion with RARS-T.[103] It is important to adhere to all the WHO criteria in establishing the diagnosis, particularly the requirement that the megakaryocytes in RARS-T resemble those seen in essential thrombocythemia or primary myelofibrosis. Such megakaryocytes are not observed in RARS.

Myeloproliferative Neoplasm with Ring Sideroblasts. Although not commonly observed initially in MPNs, ring sideroblasts may appear as a result of disease evolution.[99] Thus, the finding of ring sideroblasts in association with thrombocytosis and atypical, large megakaryocytes is not sufficient for the diagnosis of RARS-T. In addition to these findings, the erythroid precursors must show morphologic dysplasia with evidence of ineffective erythropoiesis, and there cannot be a previous history of an MPN or other myeloid neoplasm.[98]

Prognosis and Prognostic Features

In general, the prognosis of the reported cases of RARS-T has been more favorable than that of the other MDS/MPN categories, with survival ranging from 5 to 233 months in one series[25] and a median survival of 88 months in another.[28] However, RARS-T patients do not fare as well as those with essential thrombocythemia, who may have a near-normal life span if appropriately managed.[2] Thus, the distinction between these disorders is important.

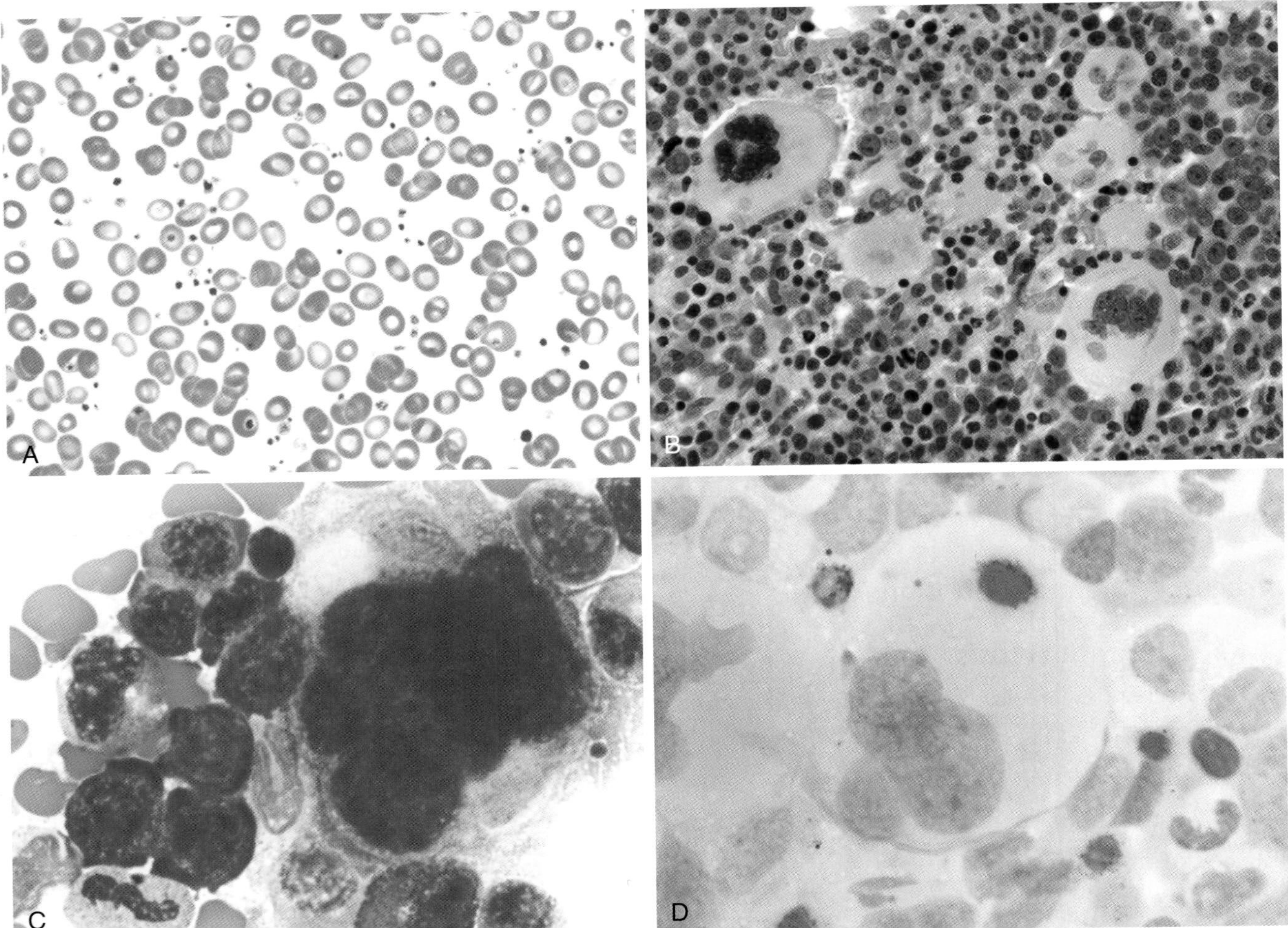

Figure 47-15. Refractory anemia with ring sideroblasts and thrombocytosis. A, Peripheral blood smear from an 83-year-old man with severe anemia and thrombocytosis of 1048 × 10^9/L demonstrates abnormal macrocytic hypochromic red cells and a marked increase in platelets showing anisocytosis. **B**, Bone marrow biopsy from the same patient demonstrates hypercellular bone marrow, with marked erythroid and megakaryocytic proliferation and dyserythropoiesis. The megakaryocytes are large and show clustering. Some of the megakaryocytes have hyperchromatic nuclei. **C**, Megaloblastoid erythroid precursors and atypical megakaryocytes are evident in the bone marrow aspirate smear from this patient. **D**, The majority of erythroid precursors are ring sideroblasts.

Pearls and Pitfalls

- Reactive monocytosis is much more common than CMML.
- If there is no significant myeloid dysplasia, no clonal myeloid-related cytogenetic abnormality, and no significant increase in blasts, and if the duration of the monocytosis is not known or is less than 3 months, it is best to wait to determine that the monocytosis is persistent and that no other cause of monocytosis is found before making the diagnosis of CMML.
- Eosinophilia in MDS/MPN should always prompt the consideration of rearrangement of *PDGFRA*, *PDGFRB*, or *FGFR1*.
- CML, *BCR-ABL1* positive with the p190 protein may exhibit monocytosis and resemble CMML; genetic studies are always necessary before diagnosing CMML.
- Atypical CML is not just an unusual form of CML.
- Some cases of RARS have high platelet counts; follow all the criteria for RARS-T, including abnormal essential thrombocythemia-like or primary myelofibrosis–like megakaryocyte morphology, before making the diagnosis of RARS-T.

References can be found on Expert Consult @ www.expertconsult.com

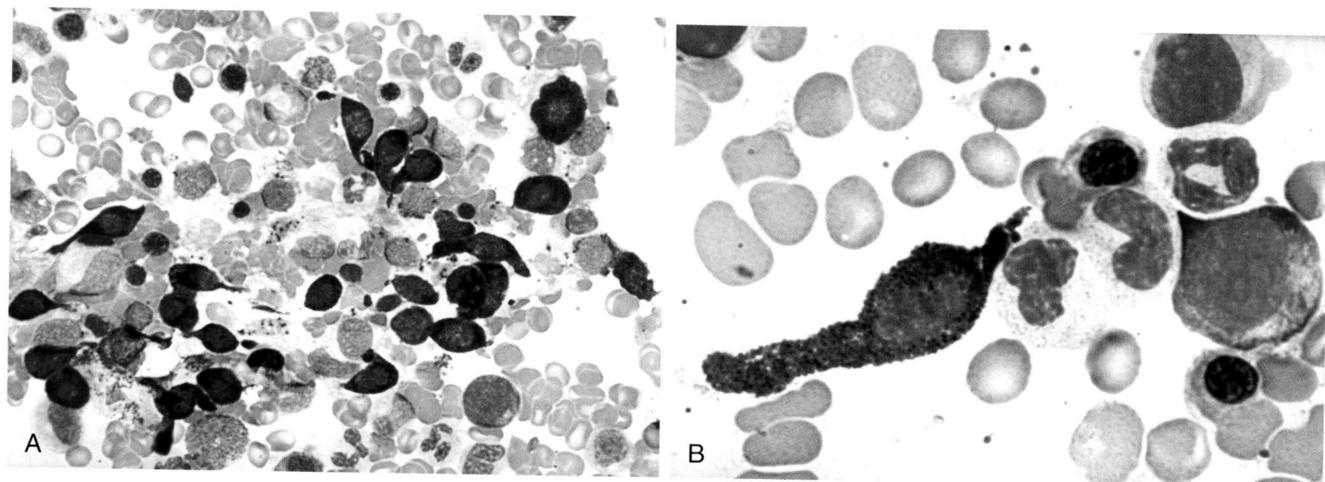

Figure 48-1. Indolent systemic mastocytosis: bone marrow smear. A, This case exhibits unusually large numbers of strongly metachromatic mast cells, which are round or spindle shaped and contain centrally located, slightly pleomorphic nuclei without prominent nucleoli. **B,** On higher magnification, note that the spindle-shaped mast cell is larger than the normal blood cell precursors.

patients, circulating MCs usually exhibit varying degrees of atypia. MCs may be strongly metachromatic and easily identifiable, or they may be very atypical, with scanty metachromatic granules and, occasionally, a blast-like appearance (Fig. 48-3). A definitive diagnosis of MCL can be made when MCs constitute greater than 20% of all nucleated cells in bone marrow smears and circulating MCs represent greater than 10% of blood leukocytes (Fig. 48-4). If MCs constitute more than 20% of nucleated bone marrow cells but less than 10% of leukocytes in the peripheral blood, the final diagnosis of an aleukemic variant of MCL must be established.[30] In both instances, the presence of an AHNMD has to be excluded by bone marrow examination.

Histology

Histologic investigation is imperative for the diagnosis and subtyping of mastocytosis.[30,76,77] Histologic evaluation of bone marrow trephine biopsies taken from the iliac crest provides the definitive diagnosis of SM in most cases.[78,79] This investigation should always include immunostaining with antibodies against tryptase, KIT/CD117, and CD25.[80] Staining for tryptase not only enables MC numbers to be assessed easily and reliably but also facilitates the assessment of MC infiltration patterns in the bone marrow, allowing the detection of compact MC infiltrates (which, by definition, are a histologic prerequisite for the diagnosis of mastocytosis), even if they are very small (Figs. 48-5 to 48-7). Expression of CD25 confirms the neoplastic state of an MC and enables the diagnosis of SM to be established, given that CD25 is not expressed on normal or reactive MCs. CD2 expression also defines an atypical immunophenotype of MC.[81]

Four major types of bone marrow infiltration patterns have been defined, based on the number and localization of tryptase-expressing MCs[82]:

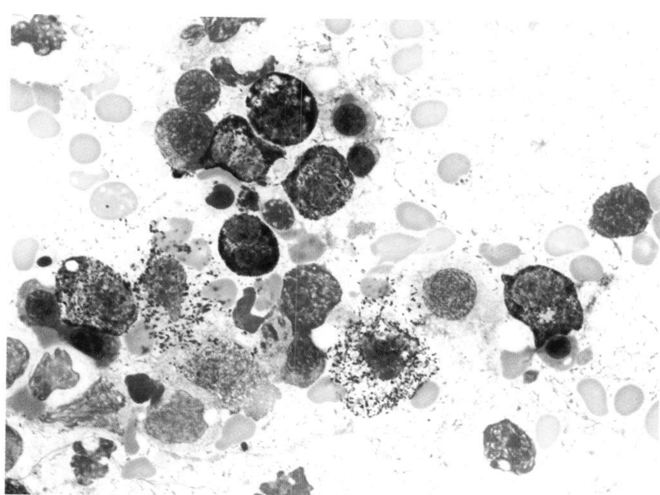

Figure 48-2. Aggressive systemic mastocytosis: bone marrow smear. In this case with an unusually large number of mast cells, note that the mast cells contain considerably fewer granules than those depicted in Figure 48-1.

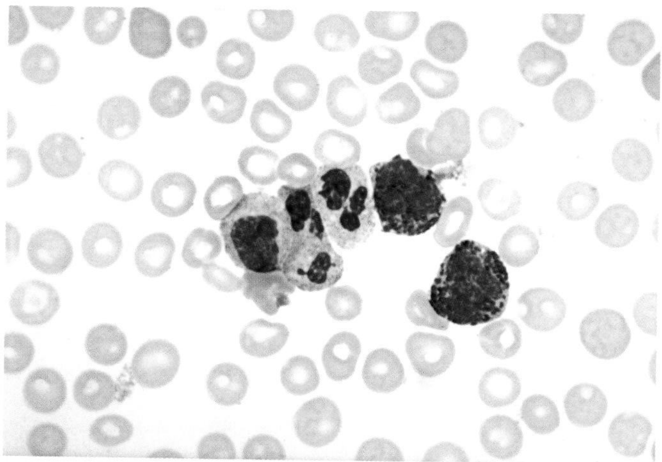

Figure 48-3. Myelomastocytic leukemia: blood smear. Two atypical medium-sized cells with metachromatic granules are shown. However, it is not possible to determine the nature of these cells (mast cells or basophils) on the basis of cytomorphology alone. Because bone marrow sections from this case showed a significant increase in tryptase-positive, $CD117^+$ mast cells (see Fig. 48-13), it can be assumed that these circulating cells are atypical mast cells.

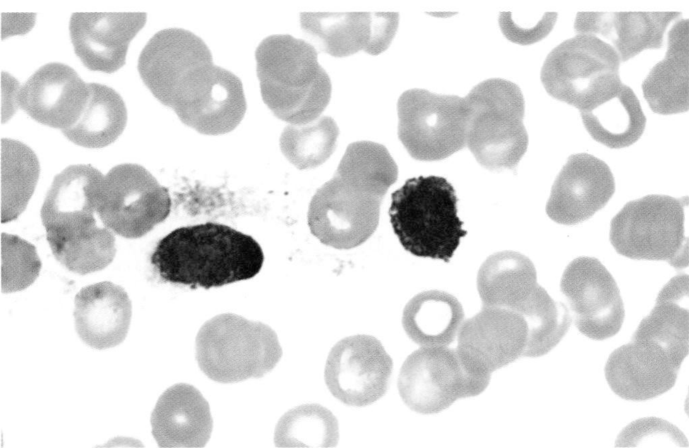

Figure 48-4. Mast cell leukemia: blood smear. Circulating pleomorphic mast cells with many metachromatic granules can be seen. Note the round nuclei, which distinguish these cells from basophils.

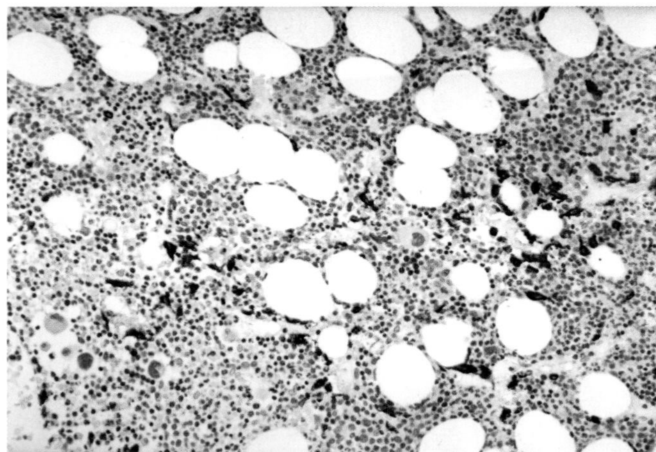

Figure 48-5. Bone marrow from a patient with cutaneous mastocytosis. Immunostaining for tryptase reveals an increase in loosely scattered mast cells within a slightly hypercellular bone marrow. Some small groups of mast cells can be seen, but there are no compact infiltrates. By definition, such findings should not be interpreted as bone marrow involvement by indolent systemic mastocytosis. This case illustrates the diffuse infiltration pattern (interstitial subtype) seen in reactive states (mast cell hyperplasia) and in bone marrow involvement by mastocytosis, especially the indolent variant of systemic mastocytosis. Note that this type of infiltration pattern is not diagnostic of mastocytosis.

1. Focal, with disseminated or multifocal compact MC infiltrates. This is the usual pattern in ISM and SM-AHNMD.
2. Diffuse-interstitial, with an increase in loosely scattered MCs. The exclusive occurrence of a diffuse-interstitial pattern generally indicates the reactive state of MC hyperplasia, but it may also be encountered in the bone marrow of patients with CM.
3. Diffuse-compact, with complete effacement of preexisting bone marrow. This type of infiltration pattern is usually seen in MCL, but it may also be encountered in advanced stages of smoldering SM and ASM.
4. Mixed (focal and diffuse-interstitial). This pattern is typically seen in ASM and MCL and is commonly associated with clinical signs of bone marrow failure, but it also occurs in a subgroup of patients with ISM, typically the so-called smoldering variant.

It has been shown by morphometry that the number of MCs in diffuse-interstitial infiltration patterns is usually significantly higher in cases of mastocytosis, irrespective of subtype, than in reactive states.[50] However, it cannot be overemphasized that the demonstration of at least one dense or compact MC infiltrate comprising more than 15 cells is the key finding for a definitive diagnosis of mastocytosis.[30] This holds true for the bone marrow as well as for extramedullary organs such as the spleen, lymph nodes, or gastrointestinal (GI) tract.

Immunophenotype

Virtually all reactive and neoplastic MCs express tryptase, for which staining is granular and intracytoplasmic, and KIT/CD117, for which staining is annular and membrane associ-

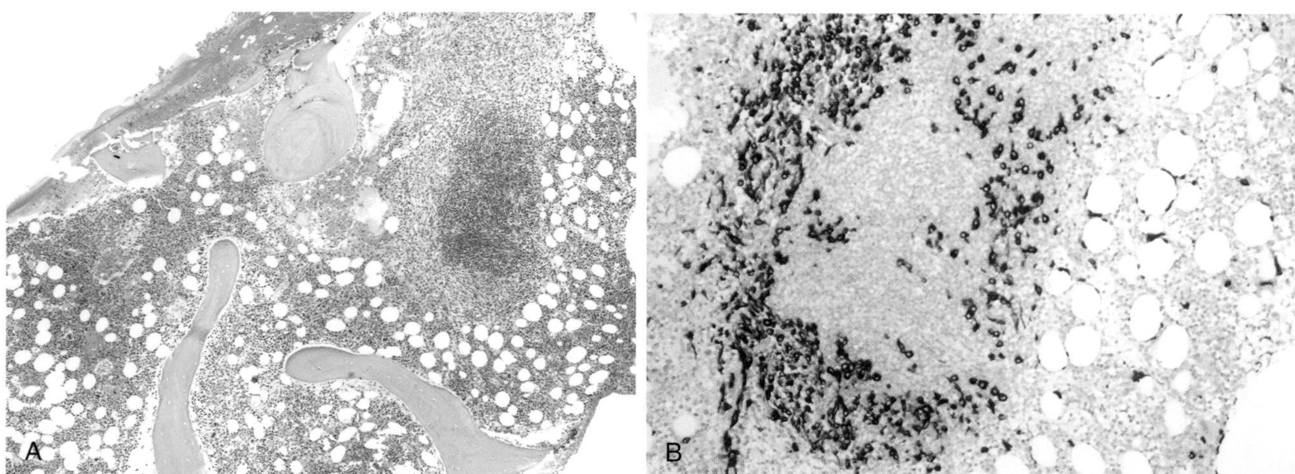

Figure 48-6. Indolent systemic mastocytosis: bone marrow findings. The marrow is slightly hypercellular and exhibits intact hematopoiesis and an aggregate of mast cells with admixed lymphocytes (**A**). The mast cells surrounding the lymphocytes show strong expression of tryptase (**B**). Note the spindle shape of most of the mast cells and the absence of increased mast cell numbers in the diffuse infiltrate (compare with Fig. 48-5). The patient has skin lesions of urticaria pigmentosa.

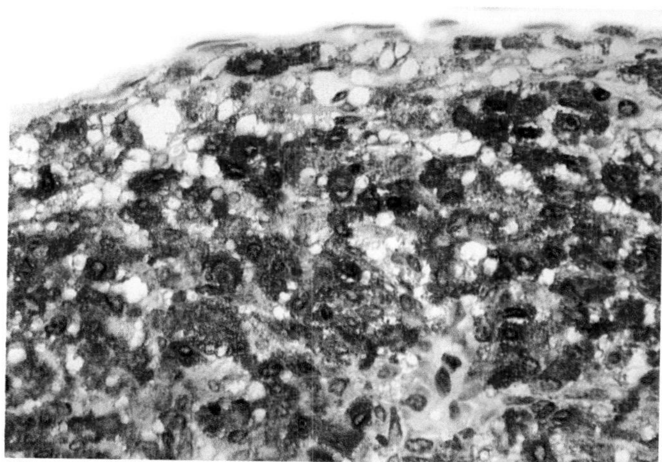

Figure 48-7. Mast cell leukemia: bone marrow findings. The diffuse-compact infiltration pattern on tryptase staining is found almost exclusively in mast cell leukemia (compare with Figs. 48-5 and 46-7). The mast cells exhibit strong expression of tryptase, reflected in the typical granular cytoplasmic staining. Note the absence of spindling of mast cells and the subtotal depletion of fat cells and normal blood cell precursors.

ated (Fig. 48-8).[48-50] The coexpression of tryptase and KIT enables MCs to be clearly distinguished from basophils. The latter may produce small amounts of tryptase in neoplastic states, usually CML, but they are always negative for KIT.[44] Flow cytometric studies have shown that neoplastic MCs in cases of mastocytosis react with antibodies against CD2 and CD25, whereas normal and reactive MCs are usually negative for CD2 and CD25.[26,27] CD2 is immunohistochemically detectable in MCs in a significant proportion of cases of proven SM. In about 50% of cases, tissue infiltrates of SM in the bone marrow are CD2$^+$, although the reactivity is often relatively weak; in contrast, the surrounding or intermingled T cells are strongly positive for CD2.[81] CD25 staining produces a positive and clearly diagnostic result in almost all patients with SM. However, there are also cases in which SM cannot be diagnosed but MCs still express CD25. Examples are chronic inflammatory reactions, MPN with eosinophilia (MPNEo), and chronic eosinophilic leukemia (CEL). In MPNEo, the presence of CD25$^+$ MCs is a pathognomonic finding; in some cases, MCs may also form focal infiltrates, leading to the final diagnosis of SM-MPNEo. In most cases of MPNEo, however, MCs do not form compact (diagnostic) infiltrates, so the diagnosis of SM cannot be made (MCs in these patients have been found to lack *KIT* D816V). Because lymphoid cells expressing CD25 are only rarely found in normal and reactive bone marrow, and because megakaryocytes, which are always CD25$^+$, can clearly be distinguished from MCs, the bone marrow is the ideal tissue to confirm or exclude the presence of CD25-expressing atypical MCs, even in cases with a predominantly mild diffuse-interstitial involvement.[26] However, identifying CD25$^+$ MCs is often very difficult in extramedullary tissues, especially in those containing large amounts of preexisting lymphatic cells such as mucosal layers, lymph nodes, and spleen. MCs also may react with some of the routinely used macrophage-associated antibodies, especially those against CD68.[83] Neoplastic MCs in more aggressive variants of SM have been found to react more often and more intensely than normal MCs with antibodies against CD30 (unpublished observation) and PG-M1/CD68r.[84] MCs also express a variety of other antigens, such as CD45, vascular endothelial growth factor, and chymase, which is another highly specific but less sensitive MC-associated protease; all these are of minor importance in the diagnosis of mastocytosis.[85,86] A summary of the markers relevant to the diagnosis of mastocytosis is provided in Table 48-3.

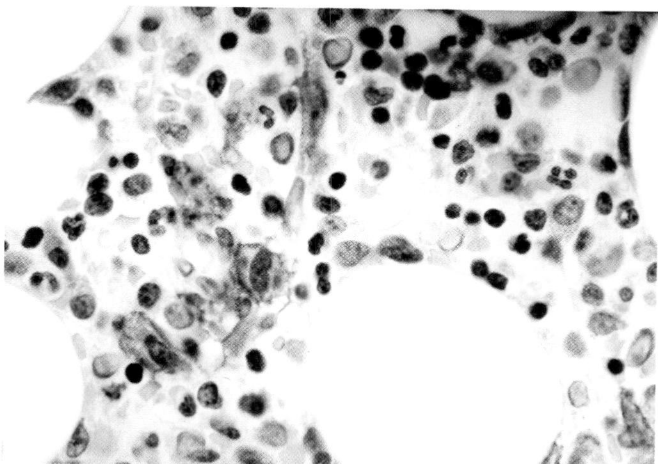

Figure 48-8. Indolent systemic mastocytosis: bone marrow findings. Slightly hypercellular marrow with a significant increase in mast cells that exhibit typical annular membrane-associated staining by an antibody against CD117.

Histopathologic Findings

In the following sections, the histopathologic findings commonly associated with tissue infiltration by mastocytosis in different organs are provided (Box 48-2).

Table 48-3 Sensitivity and Specificity of Antigens and Markers Used to Diagnose Mastocytosis*

Antigen/Marker	Specificity: For MCs	Specificity: For SM	Sensitivity
Metachromasia	++	–	++
CAE	++	–	++
Tryptase	+++	–	+++
Chymase	+++	–	++
CD2	–	+++†	+
CD9	+	–	+++
CD14	–	+	+
CD25	–	+++†	+++
CD30	–	+	+
CD45	–	–	++
CD68	–	–	+++
CD73	+	+	+
CD117 (KIT)	+	–	+++
HDC	+	–	++
VEGF	–	–	++

+++, high; ++, moderate; +, low; –, absent.
*In routinely processed tissues, including mildly decalcified bone marrow trephine biopsy specimens.
†High specificity for MCs in SM; not expressed in normal or reactive MCs.
CAE, naphthol AS-D chloroacetate esterase; HDC, histidine decarboxylase; MC, mast cell; SM, systemic mastocytosis; VEGF, vascular endothelial growth factor.

Box 48-2 *Histopathologic Findings Associated with Tissue Infiltrates of Mastocytosis**

- Reticulin fibrosis
- Angioneogenesis
- Collagen fibrosis
- Osteosclerosis (bone marrow)
- Eosinophilia
- Lymphocytosis
- Plasmacytosis

*Listed in decreasing order of frequency.

Bone Marrow

Because the bone marrow is involved in almost all patients with SM,[11,78,79,82,87,88] the definitive diagnosis of mastocytosis is usually based on the histopathologic findings in trephine specimens taken from the iliac crest. The typical histopathologic picture is a multifocal or disseminated, usually perivascular and peritrabecular, granulomatoid-appearing infiltrate of mixed cellularity. The cellular composition of these infiltrates varies greatly, but diagnostically, MCs are the most important component. They form cohesive groups of round or spindle-shaped cells that may be located centrally or peripherally. The reactive lymphocyte component may be so pronounced that a diagnosis of lymphocytic non-Hodgkin's lymphoma of low-grade malignancy may be suspected.[87] The fact that immunocytoma and the nodular infiltrates of chronic lymphocytic leukemia are usually associated with markedly increased numbers of reactive MCs may also cause diagnostic problems.[89,90] Recently, a case of SM associated with chronic lymphocytic leukemia mimicking a mixed SM infiltrate with a prominent (polyclonal) lymphocytic component was published.[91] Lymphocytic aggregates adjacent to compact MC infiltrates are commonly seen in bone marrow infiltrates of ISM but are rarely encountered in ASM and MCL. There is almost always an increase in eosinophils, plasma cells, histiocytes, and fibroblast-like cells within or around tissue infiltrates of mastocytosis. Compact MC infiltrates are the histologic hallmark of mastocytosis and contain a dense network of reticulin fibers. In long-standing SM, marked collagen fibrosis develops. A diagnosis of primary (idiopathic) myelofibrosis can be excluded in such cases by immunostaining for tryptase. Peritrabecular MC infiltrates almost always produce signs of osteosclerosis, which is predominantly focal. Finally, prominent angioneogenesis, with an increase in small blood vessels of the capillary type, is almost always seen in compact MC infiltrates. The highly specific microarchitecture of such compact MC infiltrates is related to certain MC mediators, such as fibroblast growth factor, tryptase, chymase, vascular endothelial growth factor, chemokines, and interleukins.[92] The number and size of MC infiltrates vary greatly and show no strong correlation with disease subtype. However, ASM usually exhibits far more MC infiltrates, which are also larger and sometimes confluent. Accordingly, hematopoiesis is largely intact in most cases of ISM but is markedly reduced and often associated with clinical signs of bone marrow failure and cytopenia in ASM. MCL can be easily recognized by the extreme hypercellularity of the marrow due to diffuse-compact infiltration, which leads to pronounced depletion of fat cells and normal blood cell precursors. Usually there is only a slight to moderate increase in reticulin fibers. SM-AHNMD represents a particular diagnostic challenge because small, compact MC infiltrates may be obscured by the associated hematologic malignancy and can be detected only in tryptase immunostains.[93] It is also important to note that in some cases of SM-AHNMD, the AHNMD component is a primary myelofibrosis exhibiting the activating point mutation *JAK2* V617F. In most of these patients, both activating point mutations (i.e., *KIT* D816V and *JAK2* V617F) have been detected through microdissection of single cells of both disease compartments.[71]

Spleen

Normal and reactive splenic tissue (except the fibrous capsule) is virtually devoid of MCs; therefore, an increase in metachromatic cells, especially cohesive groups or larger infiltrates of MCs, is almost pathognomonic of mastocytosis.[94-96] The degree of infiltration varies greatly; it may be very pronounced and associated with marked splenomegaly (>1000 g). MC infiltrates may be found predominantly in the red pulp or the white pulp, but they are more often evenly distributed between the two compartments (Fig. 48-9). As in the bone marrow, MC infiltrates often have a granulomatoid appearance so that a histiocytic or reticulum cell tumor may initially be suspected, especially if the MCs are atypical and metachromatic granules are virtually absent. The correct diagnosis is easily missed in cases of SM with an associated hematologic disorder and may be almost impossible to identify without immunostaining for tryptase. Staining for CD25 leads to the diagnosis of SM in such cases, even if other organs are not affected. Isolated splenic mastocytosis is a rare diagnosis, although a few cases of mastocytosis with predominant involvement of the spleen associated with splenomegaly and clinical signs of hypersplenism have been reported.[97] In such cases, the degree of bone marrow involvement may be very small and can be assessed definitively only by tryptase immunohistochemistry. This underlines the fact that in mastocytosis, as in other malignancies, the extent of infiltration of one organ does not allow one to draw definitive conclusions about other tissues. As in the bone marrow, MC infiltrates in the spleen are always accompanied by an increase in recticulin and, in later stages of the disease, collagen fibers. A reactive increase in eosinophils and plasma cells is often seen as well.

Liver

It is likely that involvement of the liver is more frequent in SM than would be supposed from clinical findings alone.[98-102] Even in patients with no significant hepatomegaly and normal liver enzyme levels, microscopy may reveal small periportal or intrasinusoidal MC infiltrates. Because intrasinusoidal MCs are never encountered in normal or reactive states, such findings can be regarded as proof of involvement by mastocytosis (Fig. 48-10). In almost all cases, the portal triads are the main site of infiltration and show fibrotic enlargement. Accordingly, liver fibrosis is a frequent finding in mastocytosis and may even be associated with clinical signs of portal hypertension, especially in ASM and MCL. Cirrhosis does not develop and therefore should not be regarded as a consequence of MC infiltration. As in other tissues, immunohistochemical staining for tryptase and CD25 must always be performed to evaluate the number of infiltrating MCs and establish a definitive diagnosis. Periportal MC infiltrates may be accompanied

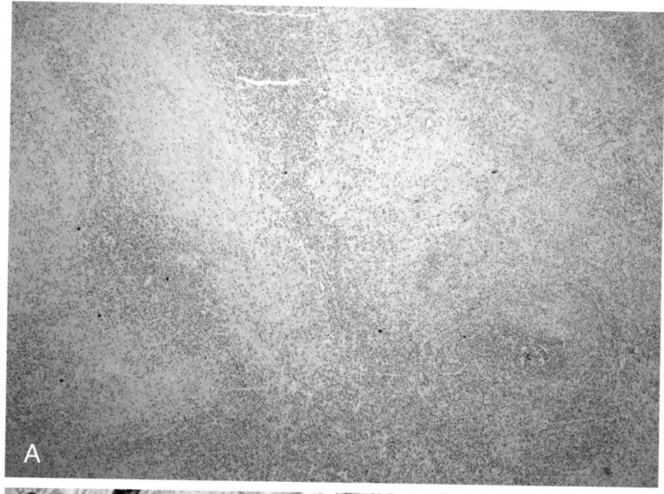

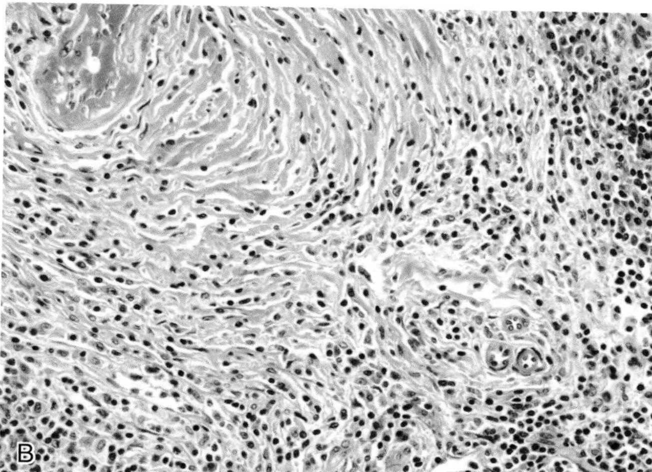

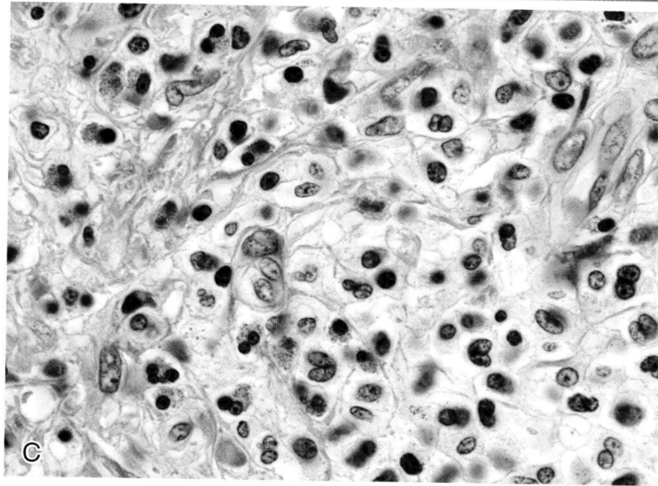

Figure 48-9. Spleen findings in systemic mastocytosis. A, The spleen shows patchy areas of fibrosis and mast cell aggregates in the red pulp and adjacent to the white pulp. **B,** Fibrotic areas show an infiltration of spindled and round mast cells with admixed eosinophils. **C,** Red pulp aggregates of round mast cells with abundant cytoplasm and admixed eosinophils are also present. The mast cell infiltrate stained for c-Kit, tryptase, and CD25 (not shown).

by large numbers of lymphocytes, so a low-grade malignant lymphoma with liver involvement may initially be suspected in a small number of cases.

Lymph Nodes

Lymph node infiltration is seen in about half the patients with SM, making it less frequent than involvement of the bone marrow, spleen, and liver.[96,100,103] The peripheral lymph nodes in patients with long-standing CM may be enlarged. Histologically, these nodes almost always exhibit MC infiltration, which may be minimal and therefore difficult to detect. However, generalized lymphadenopathy is a rare finding in SM and is usually associated with a smoldering or aggressive clinical course. This rare subtype of ASM has been described as *lymphadenopathic mastocytosis with eosinophilia*.[104] Because lymph nodes in normal and reactive states (nonspecific lymphadenitis) often contain large numbers of MCs located predominantly in the sinuses, it can be difficult to confirm or exclude involvement by mastocytosis. The most relevant findings concern the number and distribution of MCs. Compact MC infiltrates within the paracortical regions or the pulp can be regarded as evidence of nodal involvement by mastocytosis (Fig. 48-11). These infiltrates are often small and are visible only when immunostaining with an antibody against tryptase is performed. Again, CD25 staining may be helpful to confirm the presence of neoplastic MCs and thus the diagnosis of SM. Loosely scattered intrasinusoidal MCs may be numerous in reactive states (e.g., in a node draining an invasive cancer), as well as in mastocytosis. In patients with known mastocytosis, a significant increase in intrasinusoidal MCs should be regarded as specific involvement, even if there are no compact infiltrates. As in other tissues involved by mastocytosis, reticulin or even collagen fibrosis is a consistent finding, but eosinophilia, plasmacytosis, and germinal center hyperplasia are not present in all cases.

Gastrointestinal Tract

An increase in loosely distributed reactive MCs (MC hyperplasia) is a common finding in inflammatory processes involving the GI tract mucosa, and GI symptoms are very frequent in patients with SM. Thus, it may be difficult to determine whether the GI tract is directly involved by mastocytosis, even if immunostaining for tryptase is performed.[105-107] In these cases, immunohistochemical staining with antibodies against tryptase and CD117 should be performed to determine the number of MCs and also to detect small groups or compact infiltrates of MCs. Anti-CD25 may be a useful additional marker to determine the atypical immunophenotype in the setting of mastocytosis. However, special care must be taken to ensure the proper recognition of CD25$^+$ MCs, because

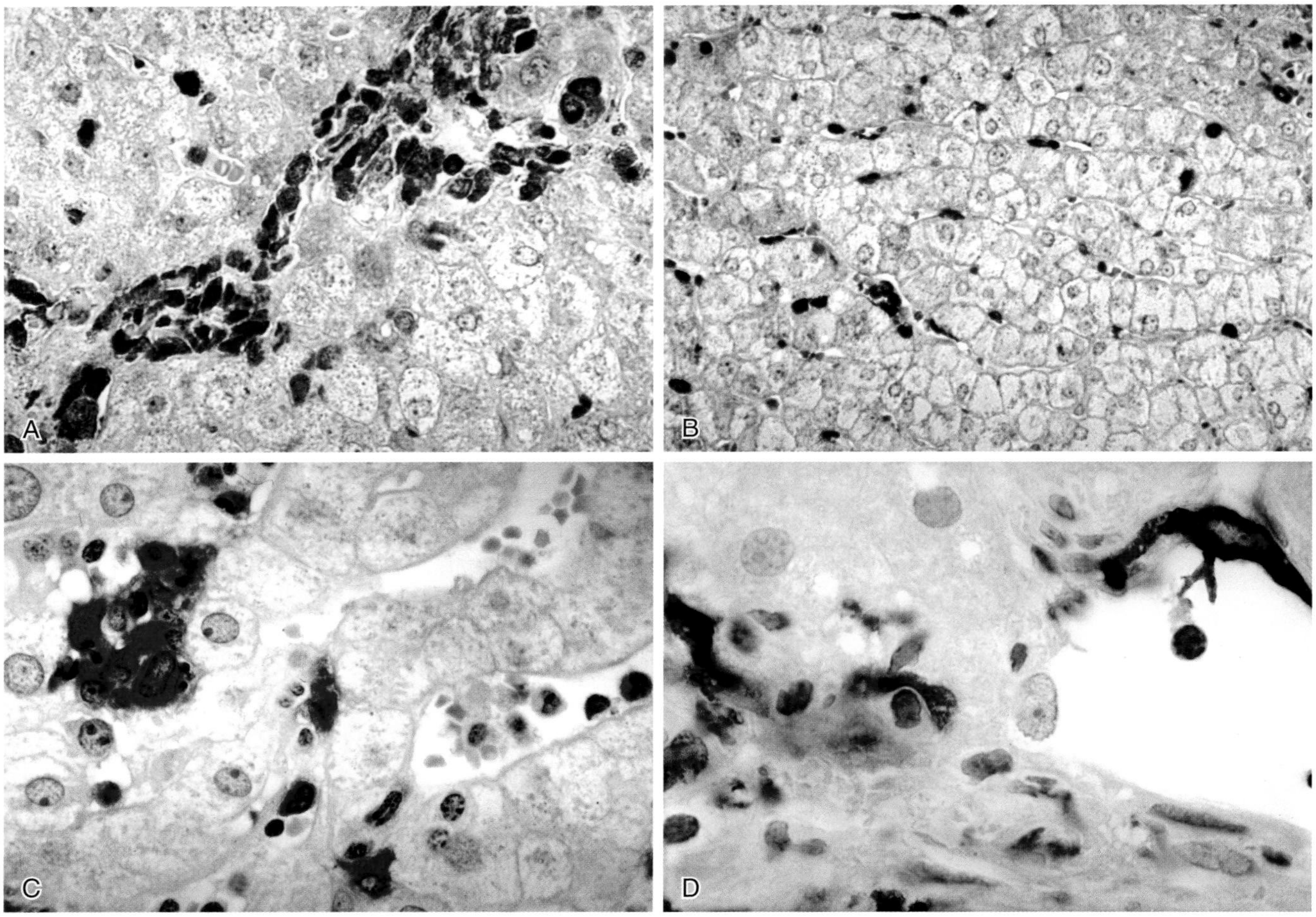

Figure 48-10. Liver findings in systemic mastocytosis. A, On Giemsa stain, the portal triads are infiltrated by strongly metachromatic mast cells in a case of indolent systemic mastocytosis. **B,** In the same case, there are loosely scattered intrasinusoidal mast cells in otherwise normal liver tissue. Although there are no compact infiltrates, such findings must be interpreted as involvement by mastocytosis. **C,** At higher magnification, the same case shows pleomorphic mast cells strongly reactive with chloroacetate esterase but negative for myeloperoxidase (not depicted). This marker constellation proves that the disease is mastocytosis and rules out myeloid leukemia. **D,** Immunostaining for tryptase reveals some unusual stellate mast cells resembling endothelial cells.

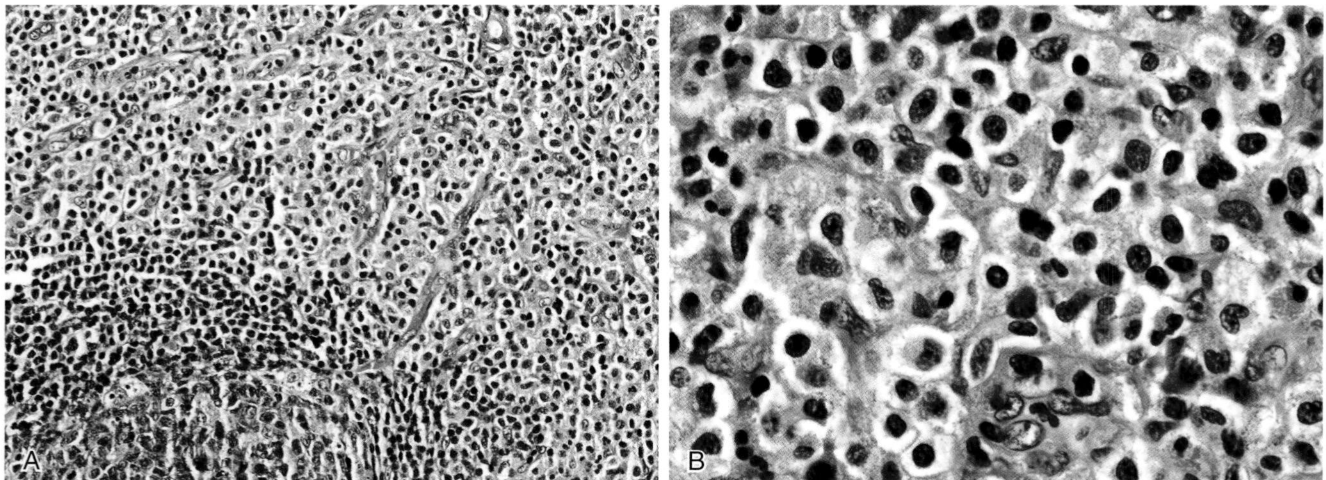

Figure 48-11. Lymph node findings in systemic mastocytosis. A, Diffuse infiltration and partial destruction of the paracortical lymph node architecture by metachromatic mast cells. Such histologic findings are typical in enlarged peripheral lymph nodes in patients with long-standing cutaneous mastocytosis (urticaria pigmentosa) and signify a diagnosis of indolent systemic mastocytosis. **B,** At higher magnification (same case), the mast cells have abundant granular or clear cytoplasm with admixed eosinophils.

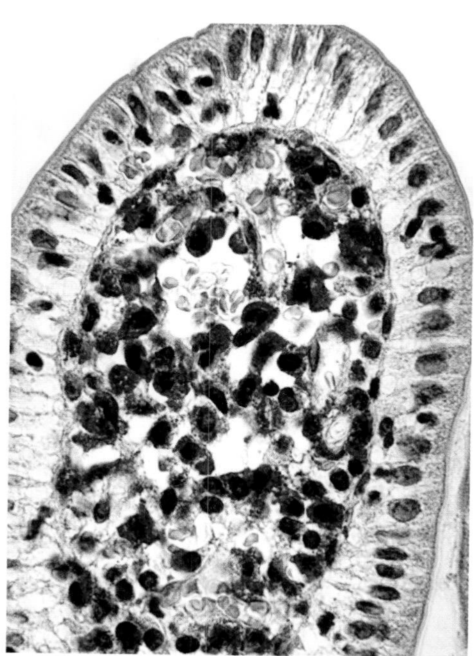

Figure 48-12. Systemic mastocytosis involving the duodenum. The lamina propria of the duodenal mucosa is densely infiltrated by slightly pleomorphic mast cells exhibiting strong reactivity for chloroacetate esterase. The patient had complained of diarrhea. Because there was also mild focal involvement of the bone marrow, this case could be classified as indolent systemic mastocytosis. Note that the epithelium is completely intact and contains no mast cells.

some lymphocytes also express this antigen. Overall, mucosal biopsies are much more difficult to interpret than the bone marrow with respect to CD25 immunohistochemistry. Compact intramucosal MC infiltrates are relatively rare, but as in the bone marrow and other tissues, these are the histologic hallmark of involvement by mastocytosis (Fig. 48-12). Such dense MC infiltrates are often located in the deeper layers of the lamina propria, often in the immediate vicinity of the muscularis mucosae. The small and large bowel are more often involved than the stomach. Surprisingly, one study detected a decrease of intramucosal MCs in patients with SM, compared with patients exhibiting pure UP and normal controls, and expression of CD25 by intramucosal MCs was not seen.[108] However, CD25 expression by intramucosal MCs was found in a case of SM associated with chronic lymphocytic leukemia with focal involvement of the duodenum; gastric mucosa of the same patient showed a reactive increase in MCs, without CD25 expression and without the formation of compact infiltrates.[91] Evaluation of 200 cases of eosinophilic mucositis (mostly eosinophilic enteritis and colitis) using antibodies against tryptase, CD25, and CD117 and molecular studies for the presence of *KIT* D816V revealed five cases of mastocytosis (authors' unpublished observations). Accordingly, it can be stated that a small number of patients diagnosed with eosinophilic mucositis in fact have mastocytosis. There are several different forms of involvement of the GI tract by SM when comparing histomorphologic features and infiltration patterns:

- Loosely scattered MCs expressing CD25 or carrying the *KIT* D816V mutation (usually seen in patients with known SM). However, diagnostic criteria of mastocytosis involving the mucosa are not fulfilled, and a preliminary diagnosis of monoclonal MC activation syndrome can be established.
- Disseminated nodular (granulomatoid) compact MC infiltrates (comparable to findings in other organs, especially the bone marrow). If MCs express CD25 or carry the mutation *KIT* D816V, the diagnostic criteria of mastocytosis involving the mucosa are fulfilled.
- Band-like, subepithelial, compact MC infiltrates (detectable only in GI tract mucosa). If MCs express CD25 or carry the mutation *KIT* D816V, the diagnostic criteria of mastocytosis are fulfilled.
- Diffuse-compact MC infiltrates distorting preexisting cryptal structures and mimicking inflammatory bowel disease. Expression of CD25 by MCs or demonstration of *KIT* D816V allows the diagnosis of mastocytosis.
- Sarcomatous destructive growth (one case report). SM should be excluded by proper recognition of its diagnostic criteria.

Skin

The histopathologic findings in patients with CM vary greatly, irrespective of the age of onset, but there is generally good correlation with the macroscopic appearance of the lesions.[45,109,110] Disseminated perivascular and periadnexal MC infiltrates throughout the dermis are the most common cutaneous lesions and are associated with the maculopapular subtype, the most frequent form of UP. MCs usually show an abundance of intracytoplasmic granules and are therefore strongly metachromatic. In more long-standing lesions, the basal layers of the epidermis show marked hyperpigmentation due to an increase in melanin, producing the lesions' red-brown color. Only rarely is the number of melanophages in the dermis also increased. An increase in reticulin and collagen fibers is almost always seen in CM. The number of eosinophils and lymphocytes is slightly or moderately increased in most cases. Although solitary mastocytoma and the rare nodular or plaque-like variants of UP exhibit strands and sheets of strongly metachromatic round MCs within a thickened fibrotic dermis, the increase in MCs in patients with the telangiectatic subtype of CM (telangiectasia macularis eruptiva perstans) may be minimal and detectable only by immunostaining for tryptase. As in the common macular and maculopapular UP subtypes, MCs in telangiectatic lesions tend to accumulate in the upper third of the dermis and often assume a spindle shape. A band-like infiltrate consisting almost exclusively of MCs is seen in the subepidermal connective tissue in the rare erythrodermic subtype of CM. In contrast to other involved tissues, expression of CD2 or CD25 is variable in cases of clinically and histologically diagnosed UP; therefore, CD2 and CD25 negativity is not as useful as in other (extracutaneous) tissues (authors' unpublished observations).

DIFFERENTIAL DIAGNOSIS

Tables 48-4 and 48-5 summarize the major conditions that must be considered in the differential diagnosis of mastocytosis on the basis of cytologic or, more often, histologic findings. The main problem is the recognition of MC hyperplasia, which can be very pronounced in solid tumors of neurogenic origin and in hematologic malignancies, especially

Table 48-4 Differential Diagnosis of Mastocytosis

Diagnosis	Definition
Mast cell hyperplasia	Nonneoplastic, local or systemic increase in mast cells
Myelogenous/myeloid tumor with mast cell differentiation but lacking SM criteria	MDS, MPD, or AML with focal increase in neoplastic atypical mast cells, especially myelomastocytic leukemia
Tryptase-positive AML or AML with *KIT* D816V	AML with aberrant expression of tryptase but without compact infiltrates or other criteria for SM
Mastocytosis (mast cell disease)	Typical skin lesions of cutaneous mastocytosis, fulfilled SM criteria, or localized mast cell tumor

AML, acute myeloid leukemia; MDS, myelodysplastic syndrome; MPD, myeloproliferative disorder; SM, systemic mastocytosis.

lymphoplasmacytic lymphoma and chronic lymphocytic leukemia.[109-111] However, even if the reactive increase in MCs is massive, compact infiltrates are virtually absent; they have been detected only in a unique case of stem cell factor–induced extreme MC hyperplasia.[112] It is therefore crucial to look carefully for compact or dense MC infiltrates, which should consist of at least 10 to 15 cells. The compact infiltrates in many cases of ISM are typically intermingled with many small lymphocytes, which sometimes form follicle-like structures, making it very difficult to distinguish this disorder from low-grade non-Hodgkin's lymphoma involving the bone marrow.[90,91] Myeloid neoplasms, especially myelodysplastic and myelodysplastic/myeloproliferative syndromes, occasionally show a marked increase in atypical, sometimes blast-like MCs in the bone marrow and peripheral blood. Such phenomena are best considered signs of MC differentiation and must be distinguished from "true" mastocytosis. If the number of circulating atypical metachromatic cells is greater than 10%, the designation *myelomastocytic leukemia* is appropriate (Fig. 48-13).[113] The existence of tryptase-expressing blast cells in cases of AML can be designated *tryptase-positive AML*, which often belongs to the M0 and M1 subtypes of the French-American-British classification (Fig. 48-14). This immunohistochemical finding is reflected in an elevation of the serum tryptase level, which is sometimes extremely high and can exceed levels found in patients with aggressive mastocytosis.[114] However, such cases should not be classified as mastocytosis. When tryptase immunostainings are routinely used in the workup of bone marrow trephine biopsy specimens, the recently described phenomenon preliminarily termed *tryptase-positive compact round cell infiltrate of the bone marrow* (TROCI-bm) should be considered. By definition, TROCI-bm may be focal or diffuse and consists exclusively of round (not spindle-shaped) cells forming compact (dense) tissue infiltrates.[115] The differential diagnosis of TROCI-bm comprises six distinct but rare hematologic neoplasias that can be separated only by using a panel of antibodies mainly directed against MC- and basophil-related antigens such as KIT (CD117), CD25, 2D7, and BB1. Because the BB1 and 2D7 antigens are expressed exclusively on basophilic granulocytes, focal TROCI-bm in the setting of CML indicates secondary basophilic leukemia and therefore disease progression.[39,40] TROCI-bm with coexpression of KIT and CD25 indicates SM, whereas lack of CD25 in this setting is typical for WDSM.[59] Finally, coexpression of CD34 by tryptase-positive cells in diffuse TROCI-bm indicates either myelomastocytic leukemia or tryptase-positive AML.

If the diagnostically relevant antibodies against tryptase and KIT are not applied, the differential diagnosis includes a much broader range of reactive and neoplastic disorders. When hematoxylin-eosin– or Giemsa-stained sections are evaluated, systemic granulomatoses, histiocytoses, myelofibrosis, and Hodgkin's disease represent the most important considerations. In cases of SM-AHNMD, the associated hematologic malignancy often dominates the histologic picture and may obscure small MCs.[93] The principal clue to the diagnosis of mastocytosis is to be aware that clusters of fibroblast-like spindle cells in the bone marrow are almost always the primary histologic sign of SM. Spindle cells are extremely rare in other hematopoietic neoplasms but may be seen in reticulum cell sarcoma and exceedingly rare cases of multiple myeloma. Infiltrates or metastases of solid spindle cell tumors (sarcoma or GIST) are also exceedingly rare. GIST with expression of KIT might be the only difficult differential diagnosis; however, GIST involving the bone marrow has not been reported.

Table 48-5 Differential Diagnosis of Subtypes of Mastocytosis

Subtype	Differential Diagnosis
CM	ISM
ISM	MCH, MMAS, BMM, SSM, WDSM
SM-AHNMD	Tryptase-positive AML, MML, SSM, ASM
ASM	SSM, aleukemic MCL, malignant lymphoma*
MCL	MML, ASM, chronic basophilic leukemia
MCS	High-grade sarcoma, myelosarcoma, mastocytoma

*Only lymphadenopathic mastocytosis with eosinophilia.

AML, acute myeloid leukemia; ASM, aggressive systemic mastocytosis; BMM, isolated bone marrow mastocytosis; CM, cutaneous mastocytosis; ISM, indolent systemic mastocytosis, MCH, mast cell hyperplasia; MCL, mast cell leukemia; MCS, mast cell sarcoma; MMAS, mast cell activation syndrome; MML, myelomastocytic leukemia; SM-AHNMD, systemic mastocytosis with associated clonal hematologic non–mast cell lineage disorder; SSM, smoldering systemic mastocytosis; WDSM, well-differentiated systemic mastocytosis.

CLASSIFICATION

The following sections describe each of the variants of mastocytosis defined in the 2008 WHO classification (Box 48-3).[30,31] It should be emphasized that transitions between disease categories may occur, and the exact diagnosis may depend on the accuracy of the investigatory procedures.[116] The incidence of transition to a higher disease category (e.g., from ISM to ASM) is unknown. In patients with CM, ISM always has to be excluded by careful histologic investigation of the bone marrow, which should include immunohistochemical staining for tryptase and CD25. In a minority of patients with ASM, the bone marrow infiltrates may be so extensive that both aleukemic MCL and SM-AHNMD with an obscured AHNMD should be included in the differential diagnosis. Table 48-5 summarizes the defined disease categories and the main diseases and conditions to consider in the differential diagnosis. Because most pediatric cases are pure CM, bone marrow biopsy is not of major importance and is not recommended unless there are clinical or laboratory signs of systemic or aggressive disease.

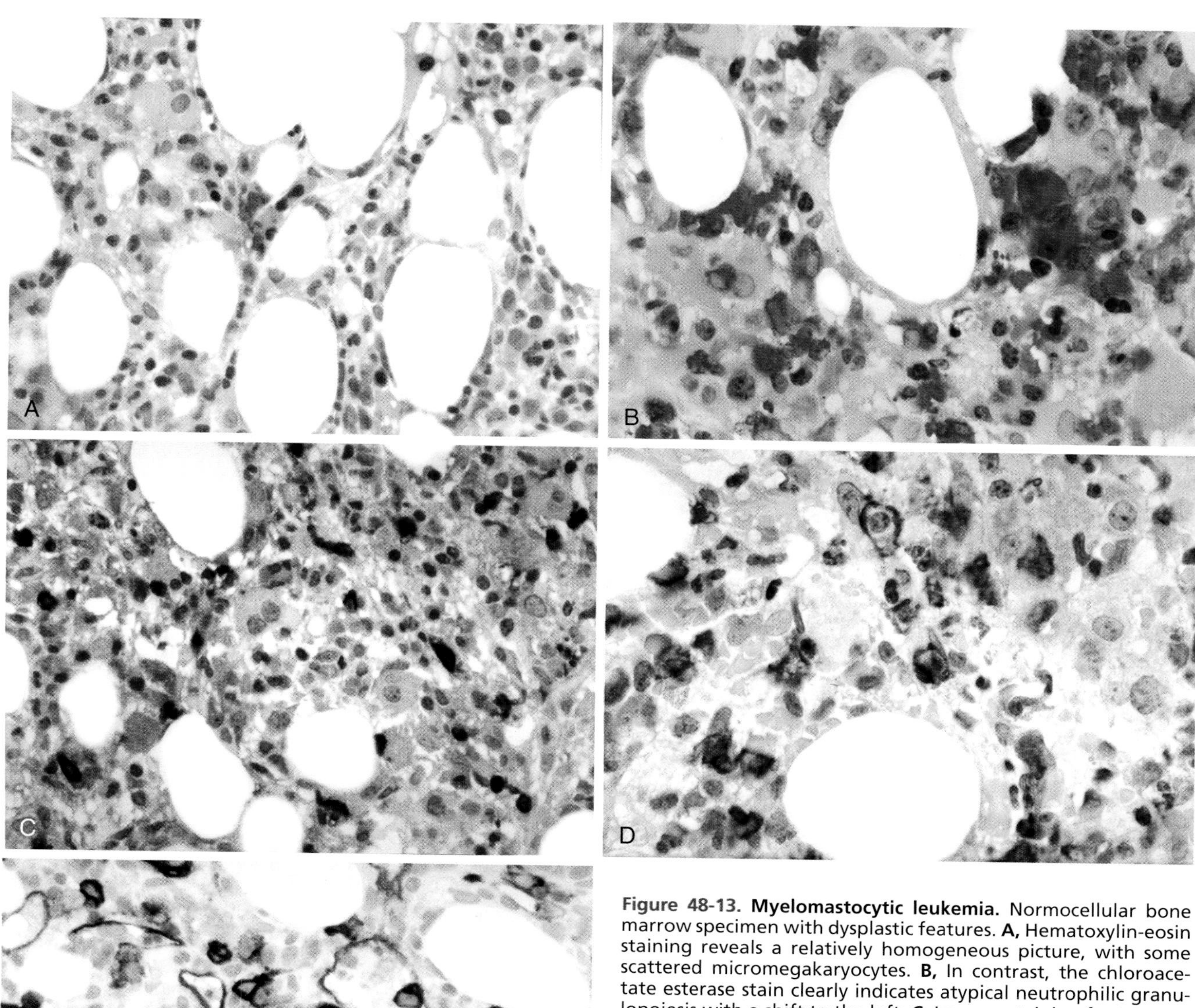

Figure 48-13. Myelomastocytic leukemia. Normocellular bone marrow specimen with dysplastic features. **A,** Hematoxylin-eosin staining reveals a relatively homogeneous picture, with some scattered micromegakaryocytes. **B,** In contrast, the chloroacetate esterase stain clearly indicates atypical neutrophilic granulopoiesis with a shift to the left. **C,** Immunostaining for tryptase reveals a significant increase in round and spindle-shaped mast cells, which are strongly stained but do not form dense infiltrates. **D,** These cells are confirmed to be mast cells and not atypical basophils by immunostaining with an antibody against CD117. **E,** The number of CD34^{+} progenitor or blast cells is also significantly increased, but compact infiltrates cannot be detected. Altogether, the CD34^{+} cells constitute 5% to 10% of all nucleated bone marrow cells, which, by definition, signifies a diagnosis of the myelodysplastic syndrome refractory anemia with excess blasts-1. Because a small number of circulating mast cells was also detected, this case shows the typical features of so-called myelomastocytic leukemia and cannot be diagnosed as mastocytosis or mast cell leukemia (compare with Fig. 48-3).

Cutaneous Mastocytosis

Definition

CM is an accumulation of MCs within the dermis associated with typical clinical findings, usually disseminated maculopapular lesions of UP. CM can be diagnosed only if there are no signs of systemic disease, especially no elevated serum tryptase, hematologic abnormalities, hepatosplenomegaly, or lymphadenopathy. Compact MC infiltrates should not be found on histologic evaluation of the bone marrow or other extracutaneous tissues. The skin lesions in the majority of patients with ISM are clinically and histologically indistinguishable from pure CM.

Epidemiology

CM is the most common variant of MC disease, especially in children (juvenile CM), and it reportedly accounts for more than 80% of cases. However, if patients with mastocytosis are staged—especially with an appropriate investigation of bone marrow trephine specimens, including immunostaining (e.g.,

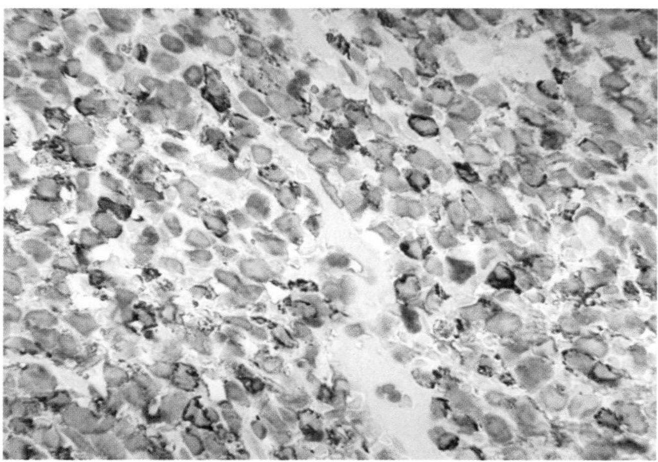

Figure 48-14. Secondary acute myeloid leukemia expressing tryptase. Extremely hypercellular bone marrow with subtotal depletion of normal blood cell precursors and fat cells in a patient with a blast crisis of Ph1⁺ chronic myelogenous leukemia (CML). Immunostaining for tryptase reveals strong focal cytoplasmic reactivity in most of the blast cells. These findings can be interpreted as indicative of (secondary) tryptase-positive acute myeloid leukemia. The blast cells also express c-Kit (CD117), further strong evidence of mast cell differentiation and not of a so-called basophilic crisis, which is more common in CML.

tryptase and CD25), and molecular analyses for *KIT* codon 816 mutations—the incidence of SM markedly increases.

Clinical Features

Three major clinical types of CM are recognized.

1. UP is the most common subtype, exhibiting disseminated red-brown macules or papules.
2. Diffuse or erythrodermic CM is very rare and is almost always seen in young children.
3. Solitary mastocytoma of the skin is also rare, occurs almost exclusively in children, and has a tendency to regress spontaneously.

Box 48-3 *World Health Organization Classification of Mastocytosis*

- Cutaneous mastocytosis (CM)
  - Variants: urticaria pigmentosa (UP), diffuse (erythrodermic) CM, solitary mastocytoma of the skin
- Indolent systemic mastocytosis (ISM)
  - Provisionally defined variants: isolated bone marrow mastocytosis, smoldering systemic mastocytosis, well-differentiated (round cell) mastocytosis
- Systemic mastocytosis with an associated clonal hematologic non–mast cell lineage disorder (SM-AHNMD)
- Aggressive systemic mastocytosis (ASM)
  - Variant: lymphadenopathic mastocytosis with eosinophilia
- Mast cell leukemia (MCL)
  - Variant: aleukemic MCL
- Mast cell sarcoma (MCS)
- Extracutaneous mastocytoma (ECM)

From Swerdlow SH, Campo E, Harris NL, et al, eds. *WHO Classification of Tumours of Haematopoietic and Lymphoid Tissues*. Lyon, France: IARC Press; 2008.

Whether telangiectasia macularis eruptiva perstans should be regarded as a special type of CM is debatable because the number of MCs in most cases is not significantly increased.[117] Primary mast cell sarcoma (MCS) of the skin has been observed; the tumor occurred in the scalp, relapsed several times, and showed minor infiltration of the bone marrow without overt MCL (authors' unpublished observations).

Morphology

The histologic picture in typical cases of UP is one of disseminated aggregates of mature-appearing, strongly metachromatic, mostly round to ovoid MCs found mainly around small blood vessels and adnexal structures within the dermis (Fig. 48-15). Prominent signs of epidermotropism are not seen. Confluent clusters of MCs are rarely found. Erythrodermic CM can be recognized by a diffuse, band-like, subepider-

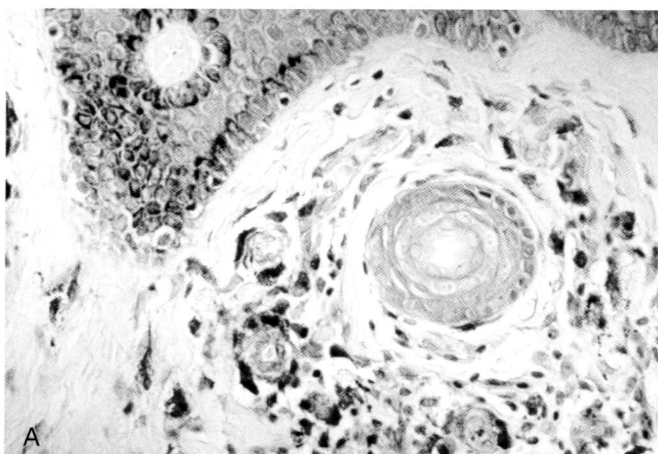

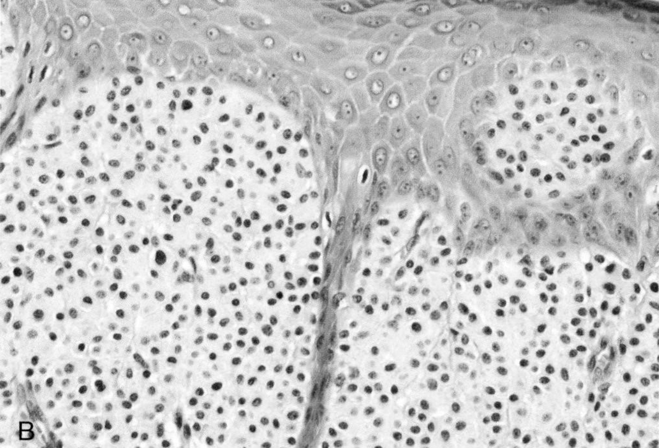

Figure 48-15. Cutaneous mastocytosis. A, Giemsa stain of a skin biopsy specimen from a patient with long-standing urticaria pigmentosa. Note the preferential perivascular and periadnexal localization of the metachromatic mast cells, without the formation of larger infiltrates. Hyperpigmentation of the basal layer of the epidermis is responsible for the typical red-brown macroscopic appearance of the lesions. **B,** Hematoxylin-eosin section of a skin biopsy from a child with solitary mastocytoma. Note the sheets of slightly pleomorphic mast cells within the dermis.

mal infiltrate of MCs, whereas mastocytoma shows nodular compact infiltrates, often elevating the overlying intact epidermis.

Immunophenotype

Virtually all MCs in all cases of CM express tryptase and KIT (CD117), whereas coexpression of CD25 varies considerably. The MCs in CM, unlike those in SM, usually also express chymase, although this is of little diagnostic relevance. The frequency of expression of the T-cell–associated antigen CD2 in CM is not known.

Postulated Cell of Origin

The postulated cell of origin is a committed (circulating) MC precursor.

Clinical Course

The clinical course of CM is usually that of a benign dermatologic disorder, and spontaneous regression occurs in a significant proportion of juvenile cases. Solitary mastocytoma is often resected under suspicion of a nevus. In patients with diffuse CM, severe mediator syndrome and shock resulting from massive degranulation of MCs may occur, leading to a fatal outcome.

Differential Diagnosis

Because of the typical dermatologic findings, including Darier's sign, the diagnosis of UP is rarely missed. Histopathologic features are nearly pathognomonic. In patients with CD25-expressing MCs, the presence of *KIT* D816V, and persistently elevated serum tryptase, ISM is much more likely than pure CM. These findings in an adult require appropriate staging procedures, including histologic investigation of a bone marrow biopsy specimen. Solitary mastocytoma may be misinterpreted as a cellular neoplasm or even a malignancy unless appropriate stains (e.g., Giemsa, toluidine blue, tryptase) are performed.

Indolent Systemic Mastocytosis

Definition

ISM is defined by multifocal MC infiltrates in at least one extracutaneous organ, usually the bone marrow. Most patients have the typical skin lesions of UP. Involvement of lymph nodes, liver, spleen, or GI tract mucosa is less frequent than in aggressive or leukemic SM. By definition, signs of aggressive disease (organomegaly with signs of organ failure, or C findings), MCL (circulating MCs), or AHNMD are not present.

Epidemiology

ISM is the most common subtype of SM and is probably much more frequent than all the other defined variants of systemic MC disease put together.

Clinical Features

Because cutaneous involvement is present in almost all cases of ISM, the clinical picture is usually dominated by the typical lesions of UP, but it may also include a significant mediator syndrome due to MC activation. The serum tryptase level exceeds 20 ng/mL in almost all patients. Organomegaly (hepatosplenomegaly or lymphadenopathy) is usually not found.

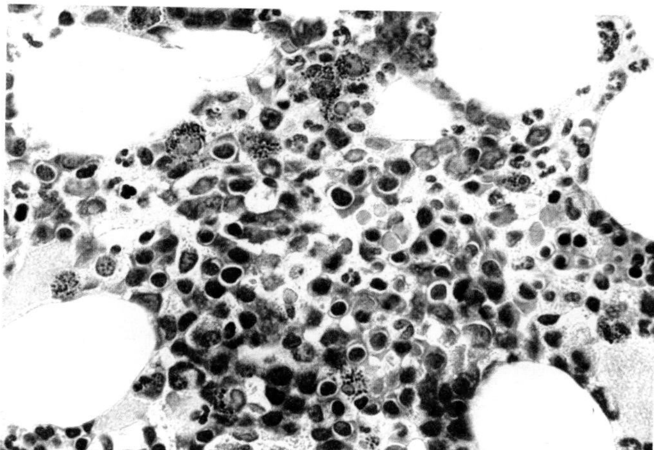

Figure 48-16. Mast cell hyperplasia. Slightly hypercellular bone marrow specimen with prominent erythropoiesis and an increase in loosely scattered metachromatic mast cells. This finding alone does not establish a diagnosis of indolent systemic mastocytosis, even in patients with known cutaneous mastocytosis and elevated serum tryptase levels. Note that the mast cells do not form clusters or compact infiltrates. This case illustrates the interstitial type of diffuse infiltration, which is typically seen in hyperplastic states (mast cell hyperplasia).

Morphology

ISM is characterized by a multifocal, often peritrabecular, compact MC infiltrate in the bone marrow (Figs. 48-16 and 48-17). The MCs may be round or, especially in later stages of the disease, spindle shaped. In most cases the degree of infiltration is low and does not exceed 10% of the section area. There is a normal distribution of fat cells. Hematopoiesis is intact. Mild reactive bone marrow changes, including hemosiderosis, eosinophilia, lymphocytosis, and plasmacytosis, are frequently seen. An increase in reticulin or collagen fibers is confined to the compact MC infiltrates. Slight

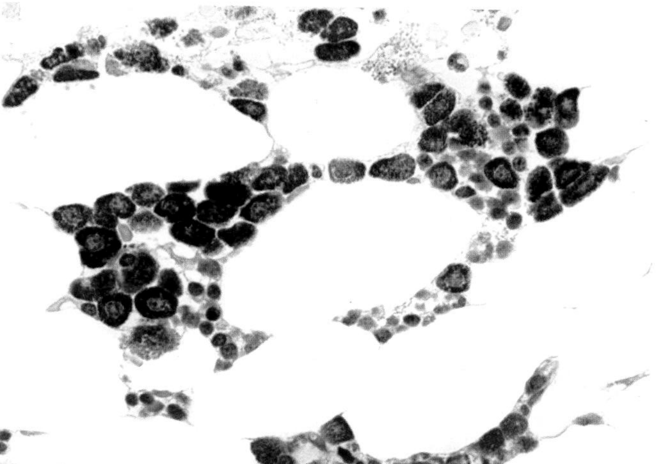

Figure 48-17. Indolent systemic mastocytosis (ISM). Hypocellular bone marrow specimen with a focal increase in strongly metachromatic mast cells. Because the patient was known to have urticaria pigmentosa, a diagnosis of ISM was established (compare with Fig. 48-16). The finding of mast cell infiltrates in a hypocellular marrow specimen is uncommon.

osteosclerosis in the immediate vicinity of compact MCs may occur.

Immunophenotype

Immunostaining for tryptase is crucial for the diagnosis of ISM to identify even very small compact MC infiltrates. The neoplastic MCs almost always coexpress KIT and CD25; in a significant subset of cases, CD2 is also present. In the rare cases of WDSM, however, expression of both CD25 and CD2 is absent. Focal accumulations of lymphocytes, composed of almost equal proportions of $CD20^+$ B cells and $CD3^+$ T cells, are found relatively often in the immediate vicinity of the compact MC infiltrates in ISM, but they are rarely seen in other variants of SM. MCs coexpressing tryptase and chymase (MC_{TC}) are seen relatively frequently in ISM and CM but are relatively rare in ASM and MCL. The latter entities exhibit a majority of MCs belonging to the MC_T type.

Postulated Cell of Origin

The postulated cell of origin is an MC-committed $CD34^+$ hematopoietic progenitor cell.

Clinical Course

The course of the disease is usually benign. Patients apparently have a slightly increased risk of developing an associated myeloid neoplasm compared with the general population.

Provisional Subvariants and Differential Diagnosis

Isolated bone marrow mastocytosis represents a subtype of SM exhibiting a histologic picture indistinguishable from that of ISM but lacking skin involvement and clinical signs of SM; in particular, an increased serum tryptase level is missing. Isolated bone marrow mastocytosis accounts for the majority of cases formerly designated *eosinophilic fibrohistiocytic bone marrow lesion*.[9] It is nearly impossible to make a definitive diagnosis of isolated bone marrow mastocytosis during life.

Smoldering SM assumes an intermediate position between ISM and ASM, exhibiting B findings but no C findings and no AHNMD. The degree of bone marrow infiltration is higher than that seen in typical ISM, exceeding 30% of the section area; there are sometimes signs of mild cellular dysplasia of hematopoiesis. A markedly elevated serum tryptase level is seen in almost all patients with smoldering SM.[118-119]

WDSM is characterized by the presence of round, hypergranulated MCs forming multifocal infiltrates; CD25 is not expressed, and the *KIT* D816V mutation is lacking. A published case of this rare subvariant of SM was found to have a transmembrane point mutation of *KIT* F522P not associated with imatinib resistance.[59]

Systemic Mastocytosis with an Associated Clonal Hematologic Non–Mast Cell Lineage Disorder

Definition

The diagnosis of SM-AHNMD can be made only when there is clear morphologic evidence of both SM with multifocal tissue infiltrates and an AHNMD. The diagnosis of SM-AHNMD can be extremely difficult to establish because the histologic and cytologic features of SM may be obscured by the associated malignancy. In some patients, diagnosis and subtyping of the AHNMD is possible only in the blood owing to an extensive compact infiltration of the bone marrow, mimicking pure ASM or MCL at first glance. In some patients the initial bone marrow biopsy specimen enables establishment of a diagnosis of SM-AHNMD, whereas in the second biopsy some years later progression of SM with extensive infiltration of the bone marrow now obscures the AHNMD. The following diseases (classified according to WHO criteria) have been identified within the setting of SM-AHNMD: SM–myelodysplastic syndrome, SM-AML, SM-CML, SM–myelodysplastic/myeloproliferative neoplasm (almost always chronic myelomonocytic leukemia), SM–MPN, SM–non-Hodgkin's lymphoma, and SM–multiple myeloma.

Epidemiology

SM-AHNMD is the second most common subtype of SM. However, its true incidence is probably underestimated because the SM component is often missed owing to the dominance of the associated hematologic malignancy. Cases have been recognized in which the presence of SM was disclosed after therapy for AML, enabling the diagnosis of SM-AML only retrospectively.[120] Such cases can also be termed *occult mastocytosis*, but they must be separated from other variants of occult mastocytosis. We use this term primarily to designate rare cases of histologically proven SM in which the patient underwent operations before the SM diagnosis and the initially removed tissues (e.g., lymph nodes) were found to contain the activating point mutation of *KIT* without morphologic evidence of mastocytosis at the time.[121]

Clinical Features

The clinical features are generally dominated by the non-MC hematologic neoplasm, usually leading to the diagnosis of suspected myeloid or lymphatic malignancy. The skin lesions of UP that are seen in ISM are absent in the vast majority of patients.[122-124]

Morphology

The histologic picture of SM-AHNMD in the bone marrow is heterogeneous and largely dependent on the type of AHMND (Fig. 48-18). Except for cases of associated non-Hodgkin's lymphoma or plasma cell myeloma, the bone marrow almost always exhibits marked hypercellularity, with subtotal depletion of fat cells. It must be emphasized that both multifocal compact MC infiltrates and the typical morphologic findings of a myelodysplastic or myeloproliferative neoplasm, acute leukemia, or, very rarely, malignant lymphoma, lymphoblastic leukemia, or plasma cell myeloma must be detectable.[125-130] Remarkably, despite the rarity of lymphoproliferative disorders in the setting of AHNMD, two cases of plasma cell myeloma have been reported.[131,132] Another case of autopsy-proven isolated bone marrow mastocytosis was found to be associated with an extramedullary sarcomatous tumor of myeloid origin; however, the definitive diagnosis of MCS could not be established.[133] A few cases of pure CM with associated hematologic malignancies have also been reported.[134] We believe that such cases should not be termed *SM* (or *SM-AHNMD*) and represent coincidental findings. An association between hairy cell leukemia and SM represents a particular histopathologic challenge because the strong

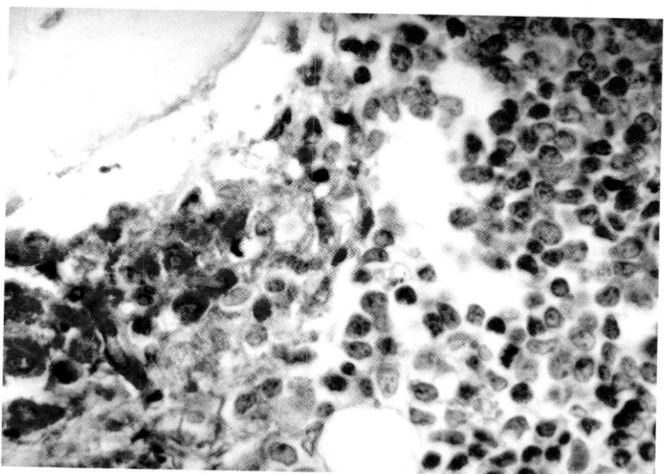

Figure 48-18. Systemic mastocytosis with an associated clonal hematologic non–mast cell lineage disorder. Immunostaining for tryptase in this case of acute myeloid leukemia reveals a focal peritrabecular infiltrate of strongly reactive mast cells, clearly indicating the presence of an associated systemic mastocytosis. Note that such clear differentiation between the two tumor cell populations can be achieved only by immunohistochemistry.

expression of CD25 by the neoplastic B cells can obscure the neoplastic phenotype of the MCs (authors' unpublished observations).[135]

It is especially important to emphasize that an association between SM and hypereosinophilic syndrome (HES); CEL, not otherwise specified; and MPNEo exhibiting *PDGFRA* or *PDGFRB* fusion genes does exist. In the setting of MPNEo, the occurrence of CD25-expressing, loosely scattered MCs does not allow the diagnosis of SM-AHNMD unless compact MC infiltrates or two other minor criteria of SM are detected.[136-140] In other words, WHO criteria for both SM and HES, CEL, or MPNEo have to be fulfilled to establish the diagnosis of SM-HES, SM-CEL, or SM-MPNEo. In the case of HES, it is also important to demonstrate the specific organopathy (lung, heart, skin, other), because SM can be associated with eosinophilia that is mild to moderate in most cases and is not associated with HES- or CEL-associated organopathy. Unlike most other subtypes of SM-AHNMD, cases of MPNEo (based on the detection of platelet-derived growth factor receptor [PDGFR] anomalies) do not carry the *KIT* D816V mutation; in contrast, in cases with an associated primary myelofibrosis, both *KIT* D816V and *JAK2* V617F mutations (the latter highly characteristic for MPN) have been demonstrated, including some cases in which MCs carried both activating point mutations.[71]

Immunophenotype

Immunostaining with antitryptase and anti-CD25 antibodies is usually sufficient to establish the diagnosis of SM within the setting of SM-AHNMD. Because chymase is not always expressed by the MCs in SM-AHNMD, the major MC subtype involved can be defined as MC_T.

Postulated Cell of Origin

The postulated cell of origin is a pluripotent $CD34^+$ hematopoietic progenitor cell.

Clinical Course

In most patients the clinical course and prognosis are dominated by the AHNMD, not by the SM.

Differential Diagnosis

SM-AHNMD must be distinguished from non-MC myelogenous tumors with signs of MC differentiation (e.g., tryptase-positive AML) and from myelodysplastic sydrome–AML with prominent involvement of the MC lineage, which is seen in so-called myelomastocytic leukemia.[141,142] MC differentiation in AML is associated with tryptase expression in otherwise morphologically unremarkable blast cells, which sometimes form clusters, without the typical focal MC infiltrates of SM. In myelomastocytic leukemia there is a diffuse but variable increase in tryptase-expressing metachromatic cells (metachromatic blasts) that are often highly atypical and may express CD34, an antigen never expressed by MCs. As in tryptase-positive AML, focal compact MC infiltrates are not seen in myelomastocytic leukemia.

Aggressive Systemic Mastocytosis

Definition

ASM is a very rare subtype of SM that exhibits the clinical characteristics of a high-grade hematologic neoplasm and signs of severe organ damage caused by MC infiltration, usually involving the bone marrow and liver (C findings).

Epidemiology

ASM is much less common than ISM and SM-AHNMD, but its exact incidence is unknown. It is therefore a rare but distinct subtype of SM accounting for about 5% of all cases.

Clinical Features

ASM is characterized by an aggressive clinical course due to marked MC infiltration of various organs and tissues, including bone marrow, liver, spleen, GI tract mucosa, and skeleton. The typical skin lesions of UP are usually absent. The total MC burden is high, with corresponding organomegaly (usually hepatomegaly) and signs of impaired organ function (e.g., cytopenias, ascites, malabsorption, osteolysis).[143-145] Serum tryptase levels are almost always markedly elevated.

Morphology

The bone marrow is markedly hypercellular, with focal and diffuse infiltration by atypical, hypogranular, nonmetachromatic MCs that usually show prominent spindling. There may be slight atypia of blood cell precursors or signs of myeloproliferation. However, criteria for an associated myeloid neoplasm must not be fulfilled, excluding SM-AHNMD. A distinct variant of ASM with clinical features mimicking generalized malignant lymphoma has been termed *lymphadenopathic mastocytosis with eosinophilia*. In contrast to classic ASM, this condition is associated with generalized lymphadenopathy and marked blood eosinophilia.[104]

Immunophenotype

The MCs in ASM are always tryptase positive and coexpress CD25 and KIT (CD117). In a significant proportion of cases the MCs also express CD2, whereas chymase is relatively rarely detected and is usually not expressed by all MCs in a given case. Accordingly, the major immunophenotype of MC in ASM is MC_T.

Postulated Cell of Origin

The postulated cell of origin is a $CD34^+$ hematopoietic MC-committed precursor cell.

Clinical Course

The prognosis of ASM is much worse than that of ISM. However, it is almost impossible to predict survival in individual patients. Many patients die within a few years of diagnosis with signs of severe bone marrow or hepatic insufficiency. The serum tryptase levels are usually markedly increased.

Differential Diagnosis

ASM must be differentiated from the smoldering variant of ISM (C findings are missing), SM-AHNMD, and aleukemic MCL (MC count <20% in bone marrow smears favors ASM). When bone marrow MCs are 20% or greater, it is impossible to distinguish ASM from aleukemic MCL on the basis of bone marrow histology alone.

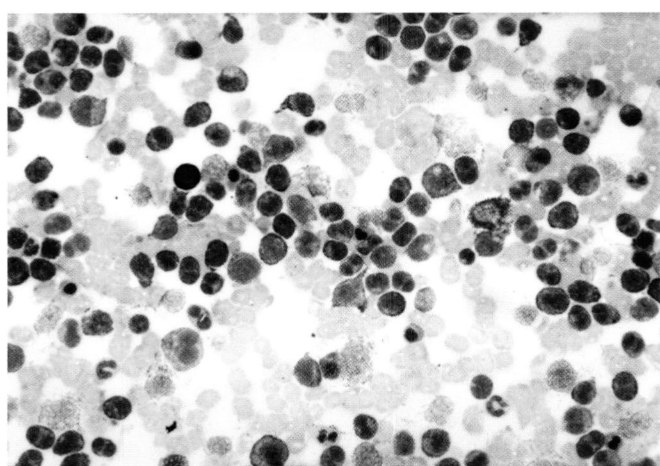

Figure 48-19. Mast cell leukemia (MCL). This bone marrow smear shows an extremely pronounced increase in atypical mast cells containing varying amounts of metachromatic granules. The mast cells constitute more than 90% of all the nucleated cells. Because a large number of circulating mast cells was also present, this case was diagnosed as MCL (compare with Fig. 48-4).

Mast Cell Leukemia

Definition

MCL is a highly malignant neoplasm with a significant increase in atypical MCs in the bone marrow (>20% of all nucleated cells in bone marrow smears) and in the blood (in typical cases, >10% of leukocytes). If circulating MCs constitute less than 10% of all leukocytes, a diagnosis of aleukemic MCL should be made. The latter disease was formerly designated *malignant mastocytosis with circulating MCs*. It should be emphasized that the term *malignant mastocytosis* is not used in the current classification system of mastocytosis and should therefore not be applied in any case.

Epidemiology

MCL is extremely uncommon and probably represents the rarest form of leukemia in humans. Fewer than 50 well-documented cases have been reported.[35,51-55,146,147]

Clinical Features

Patients with MCL present with signs of acute leukemia, including prominent cytopenia. The typical skin lesions of UP are usually absent, but disseminated leukemic skin infiltrates have occasionally been described. Owing to the large MC burden, serum tryptase levels may be markedly elevated, and mediator-related symptoms, including episodes of flushing, may occur. Most patients with MCL die within 1 year of diagnosis. More prolonged survival (i.e., "chronic" MCL) may be observed in a few exceptional cases.

Morphology

As in most cases of acute leukemia, the bone marrow in MCL usually shows a dense, diffuse-compact infiltration pattern, with subtotal depletion of fat cells and normal blood cell precursors (Fig. 48-19). Abundant, highly atypical, often round MCs are seen in bone marrow and blood smears in most cases. These MCs are often hypogranular and exhibit immature blast-like morphology, with monocytoid or even lobulated nuclei (metachromatic blasts). In rare cases the MCs exhibit a mature phenotype, with round nuclei and an abundance of metachromatic granules.

Immunophenotype

The tumor cells of MCL express tryptase, CD25, and KIT.[148] Like the neoplastic MCs in all other types of SM, they may also coexpress CD2.

Postulated Cell of Origin

The postulated cell of origin is a $CD34^+$ MC-committed hematopoietic progenitor cell.

Clinical Course

MCL almost always behaves very aggressively. The median survival time is only about 6 months. However, in a few exceptional patients, complete remission and long-term survival after poly-chemotherapy and bone marrow transplantation have been reported.

Differential Diagnosis

The differential diagnosis includes basophilic leukemia, SM-AHNMD, and myelomastocytic leukemia. The aleukemic variant of MCL has to be discriminated from ASM on the basis of bone marrow smears.

Mast Cell Sarcoma

Definition

MCS is even rarer than MCL. There is local, sarcomatous, destructive growth of highly atypical MCs, initially without clinical signs of dissemination or generalization.

Epidemiology

Only a few well-documented cases of MCS have been described.[149-151] Interestingly, involved sites were not the

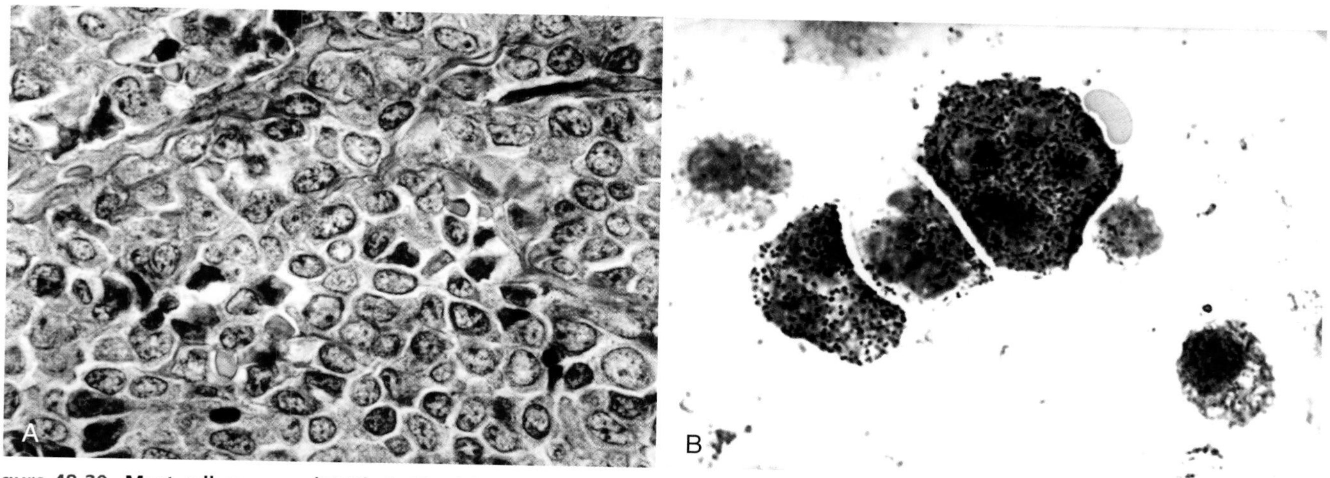

Figure 48-20. Mast cell sarcoma (MCS). A, The histopathologic picture is that of a cellular pleomorphic tumor with only a mild desmoplastic reaction. Even with the meticulous evaluation of Giemsa-stained sections, no metachromatic granules could be detected. Because most of the tumor cells strongly expressed chloroacetate esterase, CD117, and tryptase, a diagnosis of MCS was established. **B,** The simple technique of imprint cytology also provides the correct diagnosis. Using this technique, the pleomorphic, sometimes multinucleated tumor cells can be seen to contain an abundance of metachromatic granules; these were not detectable in routinely processed specimens, presumably because of water solubility. The granules of normal basophils are water soluble, as may be the case for highly malignant mast cell tumors (mast cell leukemia and MCS).

lymphoreticular tissues commonly affected by mastocytosis but the larynx, colon, and dura. However, a case of MCS involving the capillitium has been recognized in which minimal bone marrow infiltration could be detected after immunohistochemical analysis (authors' unpublished observations).

Clinical Features

MCS presents with signs of local tumor growth that are largely nonspecific. Based on the small number of cases described, it appears that MCS shows secondary dissemination and leukemic transformation indistinguishable from MCL.

Morphology

MCS is one of the most aggressive neoplasms within the spectrum of MC disorders and is characterized by atypical hypogranular tumor cells that often exhibit bizarre nuclei and prominent nucleoli, mimicking a high-grade sarcoma at first glance (Fig. 48-20). The morphology of these cells only vaguely resembles that seen in the other subvariants of mastocytosis.

Immunophenotype

The tumor cells must express tryptase and KIT (CD117) for a definitive diagnosis of MCS to be made.

Postulated Cell of Origin

The postulated cell of origin is an MC-committed precursor cell.

Clinical Course

The disease followed a highly aggressive course in all three published cases. The terminal phase resembled MCL. Survival time was short. However, one female patient with primary MCS of the larynx treated by radiotherapy and chemotherapy survived for more than 3 years.

Differential Diagnosis

The differential diagnosis includes all highly malignant (grade 3) round cell soft tissue sarcomas, granulocytic sarcoma/myelosarcoma, and extracutaneous (benign) mastocytoma. The main difficulty lies in the fact that granulocytic sarcoma, which is much more common than MCS, expresses chloroacetate esterase, a feature shared with the tumor cells of MCS. However, the expression of tryptase by MCS clearly distinguishes it from granulocytic sarcoma. A diagnosis of extracutaneous mastocytoma, which exhibits monomorphic, round, well-differentiated, strongly metachromatic tumor cells, is easy to exclude. Fibromastocytic tumor, which is extremely rare, should also be considered in the differential diagnosis.[152]

Extracutaneous Mastocytoma

Definition

Extracutaneous mastocytoma (ECM) is a benign localized tumor consisting of mature-appearing MCs, with no signs of systemic involvement.

Epidemiology

Unlike cutaneous mastocytoma, ECM is extremely rare and has been found almost exclusively in the lung.[153-156]

Clinical Features

In pulmonary ECM, the clinical features are those of an intrathoracic tumor, with no specific macroscopic or clinical signs.

Morphology

In contrast to MCS, ECM exhibits relatively monomorphic, strongly metachromatic, round MCs that are easily recognizable when basic dyes such as Giemsa or toluidine blue are applied.

Immunophenotype

No information concerning the immunophenotype has been published, but it can be expected that the tumor cells express tryptase and KIT (CD117).

Postulated Cell of Origin

The postulated cell of origin is an MC-committed precursor.

Clinical Course

The clinical course is that of a benign tumor, with complete remission after resection. Progression to an aggressive disease with generalization has not been reported.

Differential Diagnosis

The major differential diagnosis of ECM is SM, which is much more frequent. Therefore, the diagnosis of ECM should be established only after a careful and thorough investigation of the adjacent tissue and definitive exclusion of all other SM criteria. In some instances, the hematopathologist may ask for another organ biopsy (to detect a second infiltrate) before making the final diagnosis of ECM. Because ECM consists of sheets of well-differentiated metachromatic MCs, it can be easily distinguished from MCS and soft tissue sarcomas. In hematoxylin-eosin stains, the MCs may have a plasmacytoid appearance, initially suggesting a diagnosis of plasma cell granuloma.

Pearls and Pitfalls

Pearls

- A multifocal, compact mast cell infiltrate in tissues such as bone marrow or spleen is the only major diagnostic criterion for mastocytosis.
- Mast cells exhibiting a spindle-shaped appearance, an atypical immunophenotype with expression of CD25, and an activating point mutation of *KIT* at exon 17 (*KIT* D816V) are strongly indicative of mastocytosis.
- The most common variants of mastocytosis—cutaneous mastocytosis and indolent systemic mastocytosis—usually have a benign clinical course.
- Systemic mastocytosis with an associated clonal non–mast cell hematologic disorder is distinctive among hematologic neoplasms.

Pitfalls

- Mastocytosis must be distinguished from a variety of rare hematologic disorders, especially the myelomastocytic overlap syndromes (tryptase-positive AML, myelomastocytic leukemia, eosinophilic and chronic basophilic leukemias).
- Mast cells in reactive and neoplastic states coexpress tryptase and CD117 (KIT); cells expressing only tryptase (neoplastic basophils) or CD117 (hematopoietic progenitor cells) must not be termed *mast cells*.
- Tryptase immunohistochemistry in mucosal layers can easily lead to false-positive results and the misdiagnosis of mastocytosis; therefore, application of tryptase, CD117, and CD25 is strongly recommended in all cases of suspected mastocytosis with mucosal infiltration.

Acknowledgment

The authors wish to thank Dr. M. Ruck for his help in preparing this chapter.

References can be found on Expert Consult @ www.expertconsult.com

Chapter 49

Eosinophilia and Chronic Eosinophilic Leukemia, Including Myeloid/Lymphoid Neoplasms with Eosinophilia and Abnormalities of *PDGFRA*, *PDGFRB*, and *FGFR1*

Barbara J. Bain

CHAPTER OUTLINE

Eosinophilia is an increase in the number of circulating eosinophils accompanied by an increase of eosinophils and precursors in the bone marrow and often in other tissues as well. The upper limit of normal for the eosinophil count, if subjects with trivial allergic conditions are excluded, is about $0.46 \times 10^9/L$; however, $0.5 \times 10^9/L$ is a practical working limit. The eosinophilia may vary from mild to marked, but patients with prolonged eosinophilia, particularly when the eosinophilia is marked ($\geq 1.0 \times 10^9/L$), are at risk of suffering serious organ damage due to release of the contents of eosinophilic granules. Cardiac damage is most common, with congestive cardiac failure and arrhythmias being common manifestations. Essentially any organ can be involved, however, and symptoms related to damage to the central nervous system, lungs, gastrointestinal tract, and skin are also observed. It is therefore essential to recognize and treat the underlying cause of the eosinophilia as quickly as possible.

Recognizing the cause can be challenging at times. Eosinophilia may be reactive, due to an underlying infection or an immune response that results in increased interleukin (IL)-5, IL-3, or other cytokines produced by activated T cells or by the cells of a neoplastic process such as Hodgkin's or non-Hodgkin's lymphoma. In other cases, the eosinophils themselves are part of a clonal neoplastic hematopoietic neoplasm, such as chronic myelogenous leukemia, acute myeloid leukemia (AML), or myelodysplastic syndrome. When the eosinophils are clonal and are the dominant component and they number $1.5 \times 10^9/L$ or greater in the peripheral blood, the possibility of chronic eosinophilic leukemia (CEL) should also be considered. Sometimes the underlying pathology remains elusive and unknown. In these cases, the diagnosis of idiopathic eosinophilia is the last diagnostic option, as long as the reason for the eosinophilia has been fully investigated.

This chapter focuses on the evaluation of eosinophilia and on the various reactive and neoplastic conditions in which it can be found (Box 49-1).

EVALUATION OF EOSINOPHILIA

The differential diagnosis and definitive diagnosis of hypereosinophilic conditions cannot be based solely on laboratory data. An initial clinical history and physical examination are required to orient the diagnostic process. Questioning should specifically seek any history of atopy (eczema, asthma, hay

Box 49-1 *Classification of Eosinophilia by Cause*

Reactive
- Allergy
  - Asthma
  - Atopic eczema
  - Urticaria
  - Allergic rhinitis
  - Allergic bronchopulmonary aspergillosis
  - Adverse drug reaction
- Skin disease
  - Pemphigus vulgaris
  - Bullous pemphigoid
  - Dermatitis herpetiformis
- Parasitic infection
  - Nematodes (e.g., ascariasis, hookworm infection, strongyloidiasis, filariasis)
  - Trematodes (e.g., fascioliasis, fasciolopsiasis, schistosomiasis)
  - Cestodes (e.g., cysticercosis, echinococcosis)
- Fungal infection
  - Coccidioidomycosis
- Neoplasia
  - Carcinoma
  - Sarcoma
  - Hodgkin's lymphoma
  - Non-Hodgkin's lymphoma
  - Acute lymphoblastic leukemia
  - Systemic mastocytosis*
- Vasculitis
  - Churg-Strauss syndrome
  - Systemic necrotizing vasculitis
- Endocrine disorder
  - Addison's disease
  - Hypopituitarism
- Administration of cytokines
  - Interleukin-3
  - Interleukin-5

Neoplastic
- Acute myeloid leukemia (occasionally)
- Lymphoid and myeloid neoplasms with *PDGFRA* rearrangement
- Myeloid neoplasms with *PDGFRB* rearrangement
- Lymphoid and myeloid neoplasms with *FGFR1* rearrangement
- Chronic eosinophilic leukemia, not otherwise specified
- Eosinophilic transformation of myeloproliferative neoplasms (e.g., chronic myelogenous leukemia, primary myelofibrosis)
- Systemic mastocytosis*

Unknown
- Idiopathic hypereosinophilic syndrome

*Eosinophilia can be reactive or neoplastic.

fever), cyclic angioedema, drug intake (particularly any recent changes, and including alternative medicines), and travel (particularly to the tropics, remote in time as well as recent, and any illness while there). The physical examination should be thorough and systematic; of particular note are abnormalities that might provide a clue to the cause of eosinophilia, such as lymphadenopathy, hepatomegaly, splenomegaly, and cutaneous lesions (erythema, eczematous rash, edema, and more specific lesions such as urticaria pigmentosa or lymphomatous infiltration). The examination should also be directed at abnormalities that might indicate tissue damage by eosinophils or their secreted products, such as cardiac valvular lesion, cardiac failure, bronchospasm, peripheral neuropathy, and vasculitis.

How the investigation proceeds depends on the degree of eosinophilia, the differential diagnosis based on the history and examination, and whether the situation appears to be clinically urgent. Clinical urgency is indicated by any cardiac signs or symptoms, a seriously ill appearance, a very high eosinophil count ($>100 \times 10^9/L$), a high proportion of degranulated eosinophils, or suspicion of a hematopoietic or nonhematopoietic malignancy. If there is clinical urgency, it is important to identify any readily treatable conditions rapidly, so it may be necessary to do multiple unrelated investigations within a short time. If the situation is not urgent, a logical sequence can be followed, as suggested by the clinical features. In fact, most causes of hypereosinophilia are amenable to treatment, but ideally, treatment should be targeted correctly by first establishing the diagnosis. Mild eosinophilia that can be explained by the history and physical examination (e.g., due to atopy or skin disease) does not necessarily require any further investigation. Eosinophilia that is more than trivial ($>1.5 \times 10^9/L$) and unexplained should generally be investigated. In the absence of clinical urgency, the initial investigation should focus on the diagnoses that seem most probable (Table 49-1). Flow charts for diagnostic pathways are provided in Figures 49-1 to 49-3.

CAUSES OF EOSINOPHILIA

Parasitic Infection

This diagnosis requires a detailed history of previous residence and travel.[1-3] It is important to be aware that strongy-

Table 49-1 Investigations Indicated for Unexplained Persistent Hypereosinophilia

Investigation	Possible Diagnostic Yield
Blood film	Lymphoblasts, myeloblasts, or lymphoma cells indicating hematologic neoplasm
Investigation of stool, urine, or blood for parasites; serology for parasitic infection	Parasitic infection
Immunoglobulin E and tests for allergy	Allergic disease
Bone marrow aspiration and trephine biopsy	Eosinophilic leukemia, Hodgkin's or non-Hodgkin's lymphoma, or systemic mastocytosis
Cytogenetic analysis of bone marrow aspirate	Eosinophilic leukemia
Molecular analysis of peripheral blood cells for *F1P1L1-PDGFRA* fusion gene	Eosinophilic leukemia
Molecular analysis of bone marrow cells for *KIT* mutation	Systemic mastocytosis
Serum tryptase	Eosinophilic leukemia or systemic mastocytosis
Immunophenotyping of peripheral blood T cells	Cytokine-driven eosinophilia
Computed tomography scan of chest and abdomen	Underlying lymphoma or other neoplasm

Modified from Fletcher S, Bain B. Eosinophilic leukaemia. *Br Med Bull.* 2007;81:115-127.

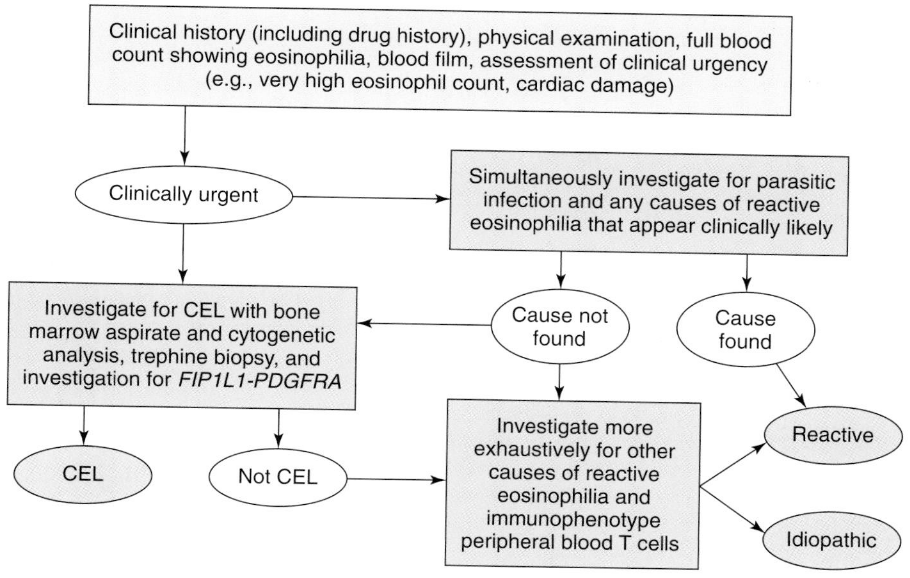

Figure 49-1. Flow chart of the suggested diagnostic process in a patient with hypereosinophilia when there is clinical urgency. CEL, chronic eosinophilic leukemia.

loidiasis can present clinically as long as 50 years after exposure, and schistosomiasis can also present a considerable time after leaving an endemic area. Parasitic infection is particularly prevalent among refugees from endemic areas who have lived in overcrowded, unsanitary conditions, as well as in immigrants from rural areas of relevant countries. Examination of the stool for ova, cysts, and parasites and examination of blood films for microfilaria (when indicated) should be carried out whenever there is a possibility of exposure. Three separate stool specimens should be examined. Serology is more sensitive than stool examination in the diagnosis of strongyloidiasis and schistosomiasis, and it is also applicable to the diagnosis of fascioliasis and clonorchiasis. It is the primary diagnostic method for gnathostomiasis, opisthorchiasis, trichinosis, and toxocariasis. Urine should be examined for parasite ova when *Schistosoma japonicum* infection is suspected.

The only parasitic infection in which the hematologist often has a diagnostic role is filariasis. However, other patients with unexplained eosinophilia may be referred to a clinical hematologist for investigation. The hematologist must also be aware of the possibility of occult parasitic infection, particularly strongyloidiasis, in patients with actual or predicted immune deficiency, including those with adult T-cell leukemia/lymphoma and those who are about to undergo combination chemotherapy or stem cell transplantation; in such

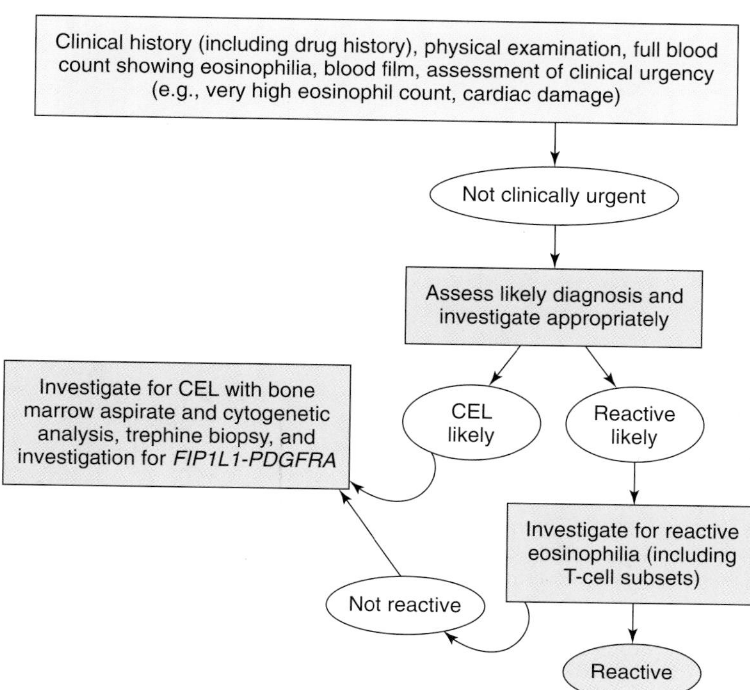

Figure 49-2. Flow chart of the suggested diagnostic process in a patient with hypereosinophilia when there is no clinical urgency. CEL, chronic eosinophilic leukemia.

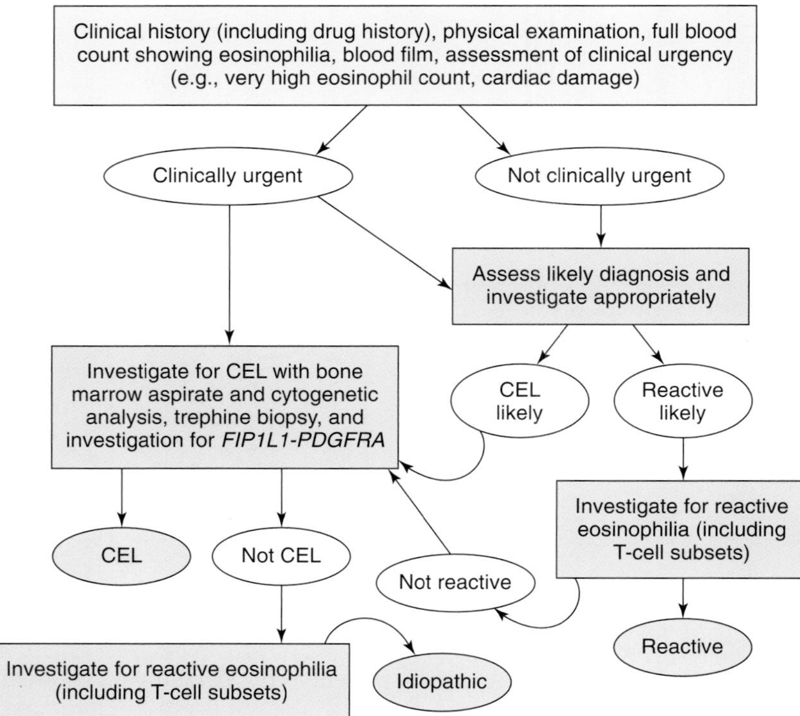

Figure 49-3. Flow chart of various diagnostic pathways in patients with hypereosinophilia. CEL, chronic eosinophilic leukemia.

patients, investigation (including serology) should not be confined to those with eosinophilia.

Coccidioidomycosis

A history of residence and travel is critical to determine the need to suspect and investigate for coccidioidomycosis. Endemic areas include the southwestern United States (California, Arizona, New Mexico, Texas), northern Mexico, and some parts of Central and South America. Blood and bone marrow examinations are not relevant.

Other Reactive Eosinophilias

A history of atopy and recently added or altered medications may be relevant (Fig. 49-4). Physical examination may disclose evidence of the primary disease. Causes of reactive eosinophilia include drug reactions, lymphomas (Hodgkin's and non-Hodgkin's), acute lymphoblastic leukemia, solid tumors, and autoimmune diseases. A blood film, bone marrow aspiration, computed tomography and other imaging studies, and tissue biopsy may be needed to investigate these possibilities. Information is available online on drugs known to cause pulmonary hypereosinophilia.[4] Causes of reactive eosinophilia that are sometimes diagnosed by examination of the peripheral blood and bone marrow include Hodgkin's and non-Hodgkin's lymphoma and acute lymphoblastic leukemia (Fig. 49-5). Bone marrow aspiration and particularly trephine biopsy can lead to a diagnosis of Hodgkin's lymphoma or metastatic nonhematopoietic malignancy underlying eosinophilia. Increased serum immunoglobulin (Ig) E is seen not only in atopy but also in T-cell–driven hypereosinophilia (lymphocytic variant of hypereosinophilic syndrome) and even occasionally in eosinophilic leukemia. Serum IL-5 may be elevated in reactive and T-cell–driven hypereosinophilia. The diagnosis of cyclic angioedema with eosinophilia rests on the clinical history and observation of cycling of both the eosinophil count and the body weight; pathologic investigation is not particularly useful. Likewise, Churg-Strauss syndrome generally cannot be diagnosed by examination of the peripheral blood and bone marrow; tissue biopsy and serology are needed. The

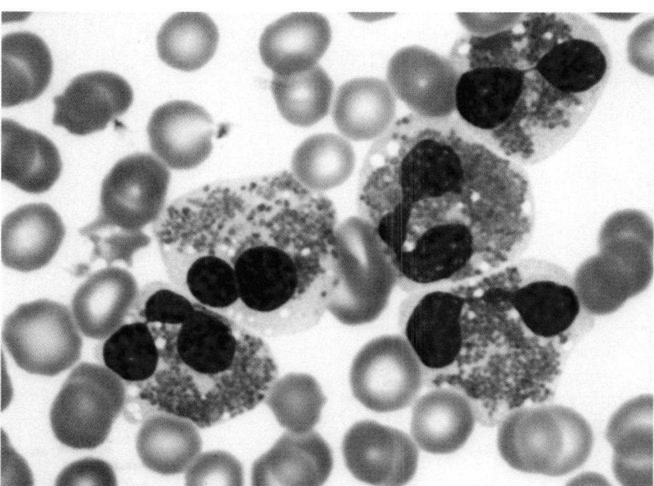

Figure 49-4. Reactive eosinophilia. Peripheral blood film from a 9-year-old asthmatic boy who developed pruritus within hours of receiving antibiotic therapy for a presumed pulmonary infection. The white blood cell count was 64.5×10^9/L, with more than 90% eosinophils. Note that some eosinophils have vacuoles, and others are partially degranulated. The eosinophilia resolved within 3 days of withdrawal of the antibiotic.

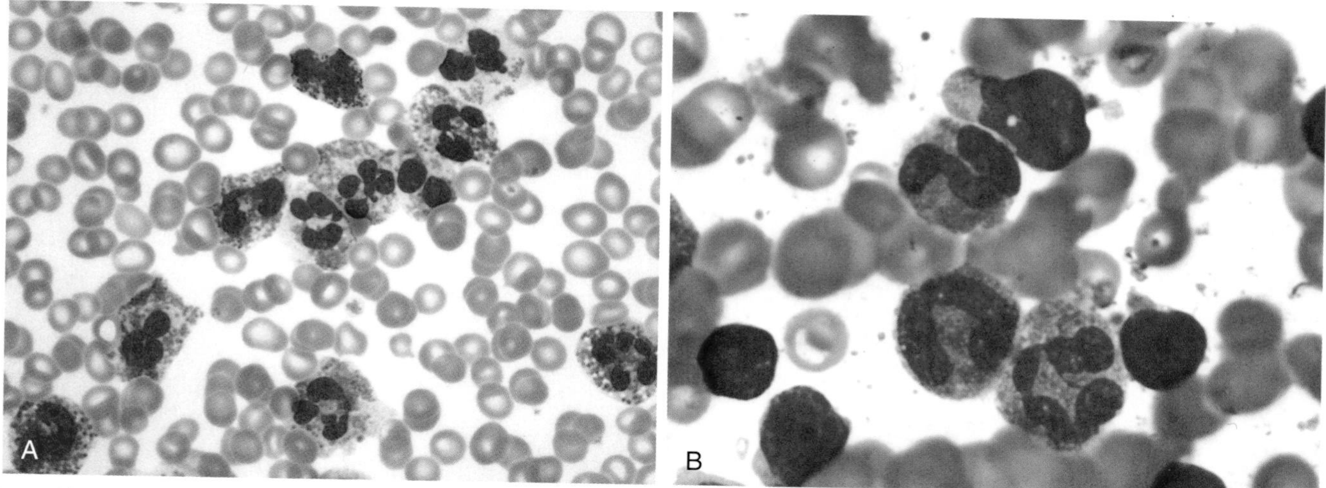

Figure 49-5. Reactive eosinophilia and acute lymphoblastic leukemia. A, Peripheral blood film from a 16-year-old girl referred for persistent eosinophilia of unknown cause. The white blood cell count was 40.0×10^9/L, with 85% eosinophils and occasional basophils; note the hypersegmented nuclei of the eosinophils. **B,** Bone marrow aspirate shows lymphoblasts of precursor B-cell origin, and the t(5;14)(q31;q32), *IL3-IGH* abnormality was found by karyotypic analysis. This rearrangement in the leukemic lymphoid blasts leads to constitutive activation of *IL3*, which in turn leads to reactive eosinophilia.

American College of Rheumatology has provided diagnostic criteria.[5]

Acute Myeloid Leukemia

Eosinophilia is uncommon as the predominant manifestation of AML. It has been reported in rare patients with AML associated with t(8;21)(q22;q22)[6,7] and in one patient leading to hypereosinophilic syndrome.[7] In AML associated with inv(16)(p13.1q22) or t(16;16)(p13.1;q22), peripheral blood eosinophilia is usually minor but is occasionally marked. In the rare patients in whom eosinophilia is a feature of AML, other peripheral blood features suggestive of acute leukemia are usually present, and bone marrow examination and cytogenetic analysis give the diagnosis.

Systemic Mastocytosis

Eosinophilia can be a feature of systemic mastocytosis. The eosinophils may be part of the neoplastic clone, but there may also be reactive eosinophilia as a result of the release of cytokines by the neoplastic mast cells. The bone marrow is usually infiltrated, so a bone marrow aspirate and particularly a trephine biopsy are indicated if systemic mastocytosis is suspected. Elevated serum mast cell tryptase may provide a clue, although this can also occur in CEL and other myeloproliferative neoplasms. Serum tryptase levels are higher in systemic mastocytosis, but there is some overlap. In the bone marrow the infiltrating mast cells are cohesive, are often spindle shaped, and may be preferentially located in a periarteriolar or paratrabecular position. There may be an associated increase of eosinophils and lymphocytes (Fig. 49-6). Immunohistochemistry for mast cell tryptase is very useful to confirm the nature of a suspected mast cell infiltrate. Eosinophilia as a result of mastocytosis must be distinguished from CEL (see later), which can also exhibit bone marrow infiltration by neoplastic mast cells. The former condition is characterized by a *KIT* mutation, usually *KIT* D816V, whereas the latter often has rearrangement of *PDGFRA* or *PDGFRB*.

Lymphocytic Variant of Hypereosinophilic Syndrome

An aberrant cytokine-secreting lymphocyte population can lead to eosinophilia, sometimes designated the *lymphocytic variant of hypereosinophilic syndrome*.[8] Clinical features are mainly cutaneous and include pruritus, eczema, erythroderma, urticaria, and angioedema.[9] There may be lymphadenopathy or a history of atopy. In contrast to CEL (see later), cardiac involvement is very uncommon, and the sex incidence is equal. The blood count shows eosinophilia and a normal

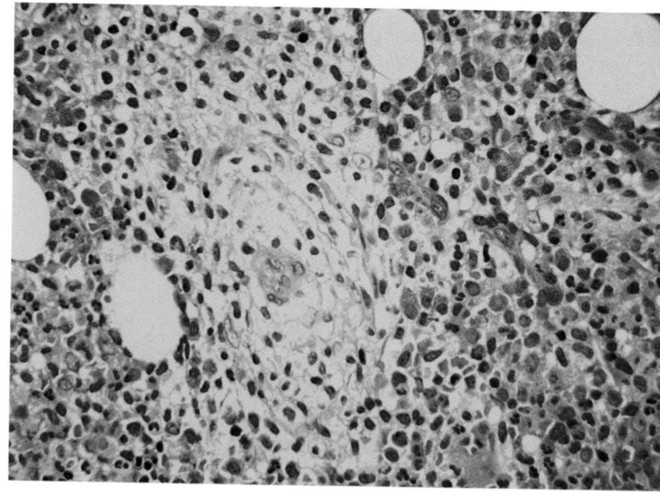

Figure 49-6. Eosinophilia and mast cell disease. Bone marrow trephine biopsy section from a patient with systemic mastocytosis shows a small blood vessel encircled by mast cells. The surrounding marrow exhibits a marked increase in eosinophils. The patient had peripheral blood eosinophilia.

or slightly elevated lymphocyte count but is otherwise normal. The bone marrow shows increased eosinophils and precursors. The lymphocytes are abnormal on flow cytometry. They usually lack CD3 but do express CD4, often with expression of CD2, overexpression of CD5, and loss of CD7 expression. Other cases have shown a range of different aberrant phenotypes, such as $CD3^+/CD4^-/CD8^-$ or $CD3^+/CD4^+/CD7^-$ (weak). In patients whose lymphocytes express CD3, there is restricted use of T-cell receptor-β gene variable regions (but specialized immunophenotyping to detect this is not widely available). The lymphocytes can express markers of activation such as CD25 and HLA-DR. It may be possible to demonstrate clonality by the analysis of T-cell receptor genes (*TCRB*, *TCRG*). Serum IL-5 is often increased, and sometimes there is a polyclonal increase of serum immunoglobulins (IgG and IgM). Serum vitamin B_{12} is not increased. It is important to distinguish the lymphocytic variant of hypereosinophilic syndrome from overt T-cell lymphoma with reactive eosinophilia; skin infiltration and marked lymphadenopathy suggest the latter diagnosis. Some patients who present with the lymphocytic variant of hypereosinophilic syndrome subsequently develop T-cell lymphoma, with reported intervals ranging from 3 to 20 years.[8] In addition to corticosteroids, the lymphocytic variant of hypereosinophilic syndrome responds to mepolizumab, an anti–IL-5 monoclonal antibody.

Chronic Eosinophilic Leukemia and Other Myeloid and Lymphoid Neoplasms Associated with *PDGFRA* Rearrangement

Definition

Many patients who would have been regarded as having idiopathic hypereosinophilic syndrome in the past are now known to have CEL as a result of a cryptic deletion of part of chromosome 4q that leads to the *FIP1L1-PDGFRA* fusion gene.[10] These leukemias are defined by the presence of the fusion gene, and because they can manifest initially as AML or T-lineage acute lymphoblastic leukemia or transform into either one, they have been designated *lymphoid and myeloid neoplasms associated with PDGFRA rearrangement* in the 2008 World Health Organization classification of tumors of hematopoietic and lymphoid tissues.[11]

Epidemiology

There is a remarkable male predominance and a wide age range.

Etiology

No etiologic factors have been identified.

Clinical Features

Clinical features include fever, weight loss, malaise, cardiac signs and symptoms (dyspnea, chest pain, palpitations), cough, diarrhea, skin lesions (angioedema, urticaria), mucosal and genital ulceration,[9] and peripheral neuropathy. There may be embolic phenomena, including splinter hemorrhages of the nail beds. Serum IgE is usually normal, but an increase does not exclude the diagnosis.[12] Increased serum IL-5 does not exclude the diagnosis either.[12]

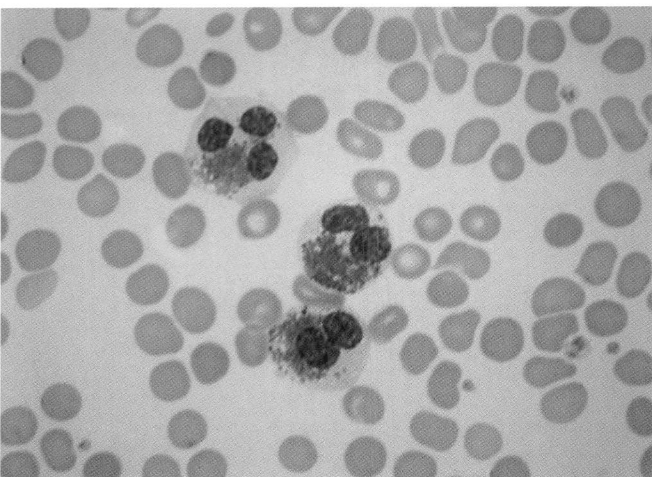

Figure 49-7. Peripheral blood film from a patient with chronic eosinophilic leukemia associated with the *FIP1L1-PDGFRA* fusion gene. There is eosinophilia, and the eosinophils show extensive degranulation and some vacuolation.

Morphology

The blood film shows eosinophilia (Fig. 49-7); based on current knowledge, this appears to be invariable. Eosinophils may be cytologically abnormal (degranulation, vacuolation, hyperlobation), but such features can also be seen in reactive eosinophilia. Sometimes there is neutrophilia. The bone marrow shows increased eosinophils and precursors (Fig. 49-8). On trephine biopsy sections there is an increase of eosinophils and precursors and often of mast cells as well, which may be spindle shaped (Fig. 49-9). Usually the mast cells do not form the cohesive infiltrates seen in systemic mastocytosis, but sometimes a histologic distinction from

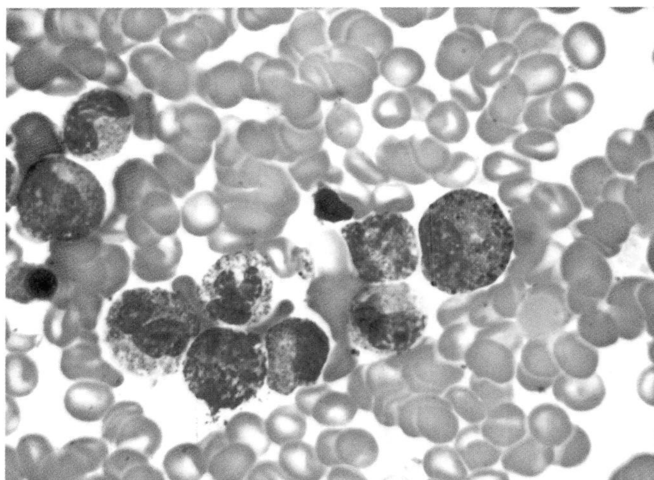

Figure 49-8. Bone marrow aspirate film from another patient with chronic eosinophilic leukemia associated with the *FIP1L1-PDGFRA* fusion gene shows eosinophils and precursors. An eosinophil promyelocyte has a mixture of eosinophilic and proeosinophilic (purple-staining) granules; this feature can also be seen in reactive eosinophilia.

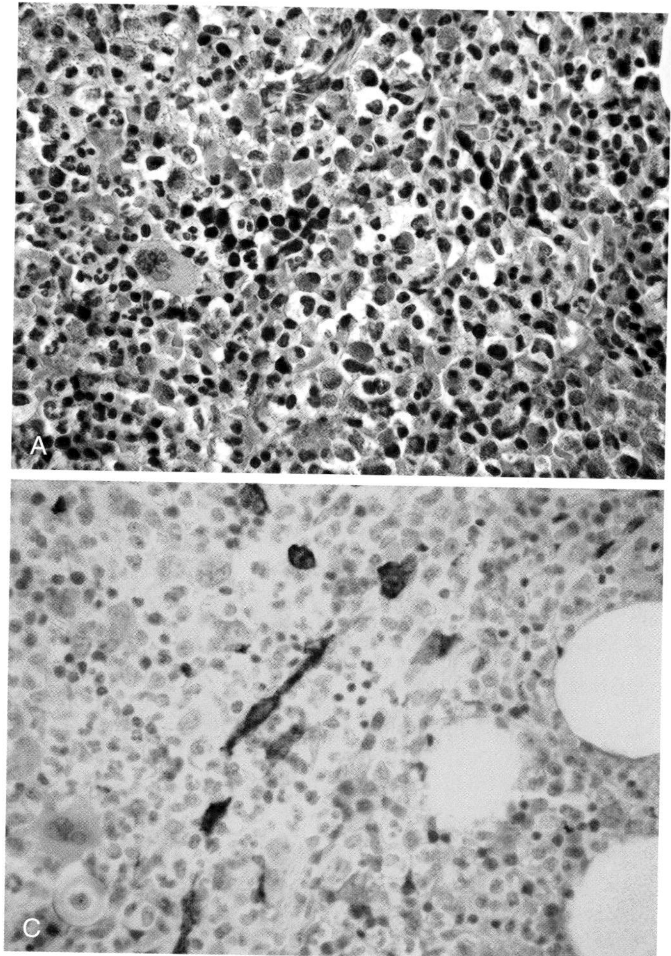
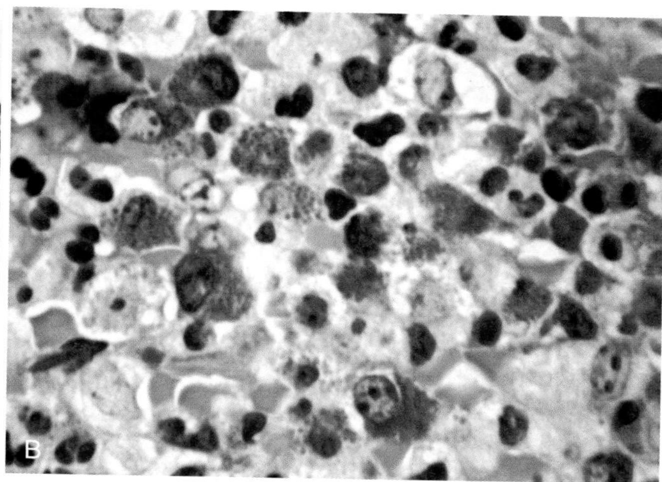

Figure 49-9. Bone marrow trephine biopsy sections from a patient with chronic eosinophilic leukemia associated with the *FIP1L1-PDGFRA* fusion (same patient as in Fig. 49-8). **A,** Hypercellular, disorganized marrow with increased eosinophils and precursors. **B,** Giemsa stain shows hypercellular marrow with increased eosinophil precursors. **C,** Scattered spindle-shaped mast cells and several cells with a high nuclear-to-cytoplasmic ratio that are likely to be hematopoietic precursors (immunoperoxidase for CD117).

systemic mastocytosis is not possible. Reticulin may be increased.

Immunophenotype

Eosinophils may show immunophenotypic features of activation, but this is not diagnostically helpful.

Genetics and Molecular Findings

Usually cytogenetic analysis is normal, but occasionally there is a related chromosomal rearrangement with a 4q12 breakpoint or, more often, an unrelated chromosomal abnormality (e.g., trisomy 8, del(20q), del(17p)). The *FIP1L1-PDGFRA* fusion gene encodes a constitutively activated tyrosine kinase that is pathogenetic. A minority of patients have a different chromosomal rearrangement that also leads to rearrangement of *PDGFRA* but involves a different partner gene.[13] Diagnosis is by polymerase chain reaction (PCR; nested PCR is often needed) or fluorescence in situ hybridization (FISH), or both. A combination of the two is recommended.[13] FISH techniques often rely on detecting deletion of the *CHIC2* gene, which is located between *FIP1L1* and *PDGFRA* and is lost when this deletion occurs.

Postulated Cell of Origin

The cell of origin is a pluripotent lymphoid/myeloid stem cell.

Clinical Course

The clinical course may be chronic, but some patients die of cardiac or other complications; in some, there is transformation to AML. The prognosis is likely to be much improved since identification of the fusion gene and discovery of the marked sensitivity of this condition to imatinib therapy. Even patients who present in the acute phase may respond. Sensitivity to imatinib is greater than in chronic myelogenous leukemia, and if molecular monitoring is available, treatment can start at the low dose of 100 mg daily.

Differential Diagnosis

The differential diagnosis includes other causes of hypereosinophilia, but as long as a sensitive technique for detecting the cryptic deletion or fusion gene is used, there is no diagnostic difficulty. The presence of abnormal bone marrow mast cells should not be misinterpreted as indicating systemic mastocytosis.

Myeloid Neoplasms Associated with *PDGFRB* Rearrangement

Definition

Myeloid neoplasms in this group result from a translocation that leads to rearrangement of *PDGFRB* and formation of a fusion gene to which *PDGFRB* contributes.[14-16] The most frequently observed translocation is t(5;12)(q31-q33;p12), with formation of an *ETV6-PDGFRB* fusion, but more than a dozen different translocations and fusion genes have been recognized, most of which have been reported in only single patients.[15] The hematologic features are heterogeneous, even in patients with *ETV6-PDGFRB*.

Epidemiology

There is a wide age range, from childhood to old age. The incidence in males is twice that in females.

Etiology

No etiologic factors have been identified.

Clinical Features

Splenomegaly is common. Sometimes there is skin infiltration or cardiac damage. Serum vitamin B_{12} and serum tryptase may be increased.

Morphology

There is leukocytosis and sometimes anemia or thrombocytopenia. The great majority of patients, but not all, have eosinophilia (Fig. 49-10). Hematologic features may be those of CEL, atypical chronic myeloid leukemia (usually with eosinophilia), or chronic myelomonocytic leukemia (usually with eosinophilia). Some patients have presented with AML (with or without eosinophilia). Occasional patients have had chronic basophilic leukemia (associated with t(4;5;5)(q23;q31;q33) or t(4;5)(q21.2;q31.3) and a *PRKG2-PDGFRB* fusion gene), and one child presented with juvenile myelomonocytic leukemia with eosinophilia (associated with t(5;17)(q33;p11.2) and a *SPECC1-PDGFRB* fusion gene). The bone marrow is hypercellular, with a variable increase of eosinophils, neutrophils, monocytes, and their precursors. Trephine biopsy may show increased mast cells, increased reticulin, and, less often, increased collagen.

Immunophenotype

Immunophenotyping is not diagnostically helpful.

Genetics and Molecular Findings

All patients show a translocation or, rarely, another chromosomal rearrangement with a 5q31-q33 breakpoint.

Postulated Cell of Origin

The cell of origin appears to be a multipotent myeloid stem cell.

Clinical Course

In the past, median survival was only about 2 years; however, with the early institution of imatinib therapy, it is greatly improved.

Differential Diagnosis

The differential diagnosis includes other causes of hypereosinophilia, and particularly other myeloproliferative or myelodysplastic/myeloproliferative neoplasms. To date, all cases diagnosed have had a relevant abnormality on conventional cytogenetic analysis.

Lymphoid and Myeloid Neoplasms Associated with *FGFR1* Rearrangement

Definition

This group of lymphoid and myeloid neoplasms is hematologically heterogeneous, but the entities are linked by rearrangement of *FGFR1* and formation of a fusion gene to which it contributes.[15,16]

Epidemiology

There are no specific epidemiologic features.

Etiology

No etiologic factors have been identified.

Clinical Features

Common presenting features include lymphadenopathy and splenomegaly. The prognosis is poor because of early acute transformation.

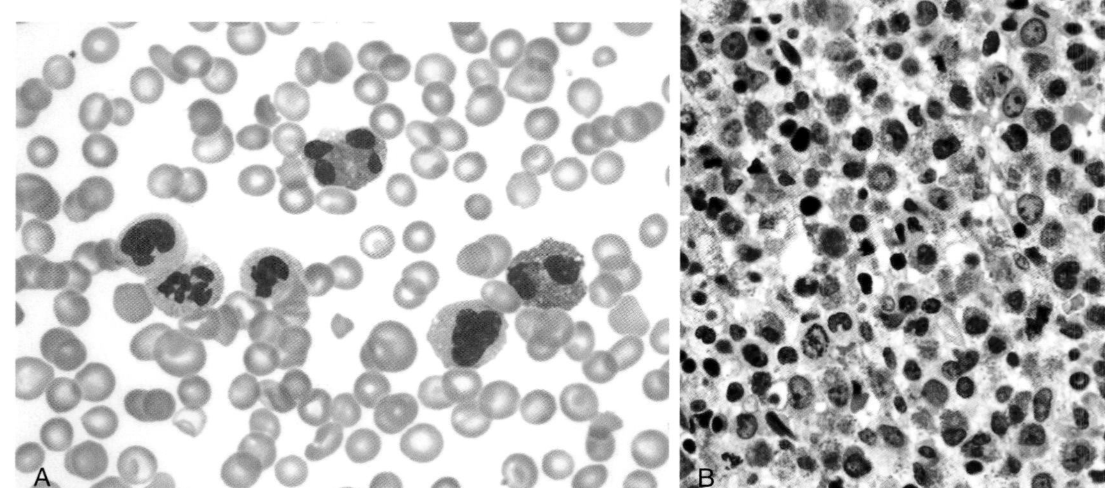

Figure 49-10. Peripheral blood film (**A**) and bone marrow biopsy (**B**) showing marked eosinophilia in a patient with monocytosis, resembling chronic myelomonocytic leukemia. Cytogenetic analysis revealed t(5;12)(q31;p12), *ETV6-PDGFRB*.

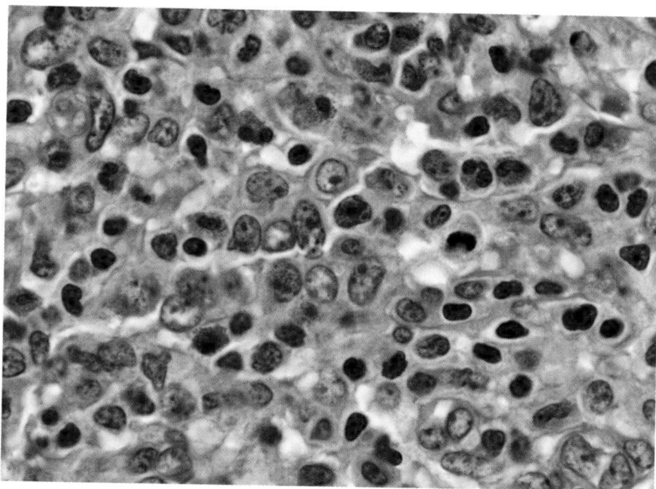

Figure 49-11. Lymph node biopsy from a patient with T-lymphoblastic lymphoma and t(8;13)(p11;q12), *ZNF198-FGFR1*. Lymphoblasts are admixed with mature eosinophils. The patient later developed acute myeloid leukemia with eosinophilia. (Courtesy of Dr. Elaine Jaffe.)

Morphology

Presentation may be CEL (with subsequent acute myeloid or lymphoblastic transformation), AML, or T-lineage or B-lineage lymphoblastic lymphoma or acute lymphoblastic leukemia (Fig. 49-11).[17] Patients who present in the acute phase have eosinophilia. The disease phenotype differs somewhat in cases with *BCR-FGFR1* fusion, which tend to have hematologic features resembling those of chronic myelogenous leukemia with eosinophilia rather than CEL; both T-lymphoblastic and B-lymphoblastic transformations have been reported in this subgroup. An unusual feature of patients with *FGFR1OP1-FGFR1* is four cases of associated polycythemia vera.

Immunophenotype

Immunophenotyping is informative for phenotypic analysis of blasts when blast cells are increased but is not otherwise useful.

Genetics and Molecular Findings

A variety of cytogenetic and molecular genetic abnormalities have been described. The four most often observed are t(8;13)(p11;q12) with a *ZNF198-FGFR1* fusion gene, t(8;9)(p11;q33) with a *CEP110-FGFR1* fusion gene, t(6;8)(q27;p11-12) with an *FGFR1OP1-FGFR1* fusion gene, and t(8;22)(p11;q11) with a *BCR-FGFR1* fusion gene. Other rearrangements have generally been observed only in single cases. Trisomy 21 is the secondary chromosomal abnormality most often seen.

Postulated Cell of Origin

The postulated cell of origin is a pluripotent lymphoid/myeloid hematopoietic stem cell.

Clinical Course

Patients usually present in the acute phase or experience acute transformation within 1 to 2 years. Remissions may occur with chemotherapy but are not sustained.

Differential Diagnosis

Other lymphoid and myeloid neoplasms may be considered, including lymphoid neoplasms with reactive eosinophilia. Cytogenetic analysis clarifies the diagnosis.

Chronic Eosinophilic Leukemia, Not Otherwise Specified

Definition

This heterogeneous group of disorders is recognized as leukemic in nature by an increase in blast cells in the blood or bone marrow (>2% in blood or >5% in bone marrow) or by the demonstration of clonality of the myeloid cells.[16] Clinical features such as splenomegaly may also indicate the likelihood of leukemia.

Epidemiology

CEL, not otherwise specified, occurs mainly in adults. No specific epidemiologic features are recognized, although patients with t(8;9)(p22;p24) are usually male.

Etiology

No etiologic factors have been recognized.

Clinical Features

Clinical features can relate to either the leukemic nature of the condition (e.g., splenomegaly, hepatomegaly) or tissue damage by eosinophils (e.g., cardiac damage).

Morphology

The eosinophil count is increased—by convention, to at least 1.5×10^9/L—but without a sufficient increase of monocytes or dysplastic neutrophil precursors to suggest that a diagnosis of chronic myelomonocytic leukemia or atypical chronic myeloid leukemia would be more appropriate. Blast cells may be increased in the peripheral blood and bone marrow, and cells of eosinophil lineage may be cytologically abnormal (Fig. 49-12). Patients with t(8;9)(p22;p24) and *PCM1-JAK2* may have increased bone marrow mast cells.[18]

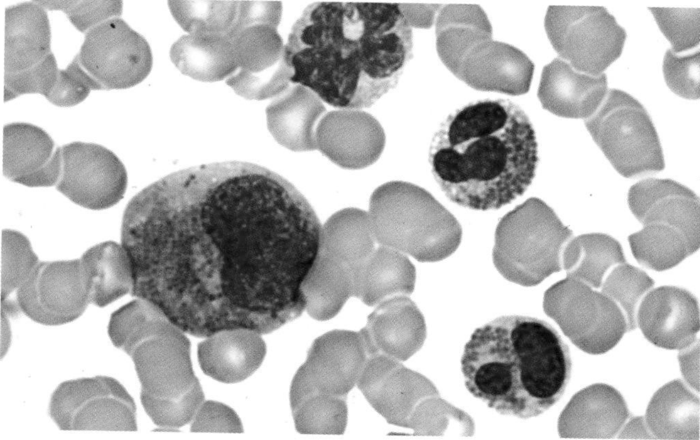

Figure 49-12. Peripheral blood film from a patient with chronic eosinophilic leukemia, not otherwise specified, associated with trisomy 10 and increased bone marrow and peripheral blood blast cells. There are two abnormal eosinophils and an eosinophil precursor.

Immunophenotype

Immunophenotyping is indicated only if there is an increase of blast cells and it is necessary to demonstrate that they are myeloid rather than lymphoid.

Genetics and Molecular Findings

Clonality may be demonstrable by the presence of skewed expression of X chromosome genes, mutation of an oncogene (e.g., *RAS* or *JAK2*),[19] or demonstration of a clonal cytogenetic abnormality with or without a demonstrable fusion gene. By definition, cases with rearrangement of *PDGFRA*, *PDGFRB*, or *FGFR1* are excluded from this diagnostic category. However, other recurrent translocations and fusion genes, such as t(8;9)(p22;p24) with *PCM1-JAK2* fusion, may be found.[20] Other cytogenetic abnormalities that have been described include trisomy 8, i(17p), and a complex karyotype.

Postulated Cell of Origin

The postulated cell of origin is a multipotent myeloid stem cell.

Clinical Course

The clinical course may be chronic, with death sometimes resulting from cardiac damage. Acute transformation can occur.

Differential Diagnosis

This condition is distinguished from both specific molecular subtypes of eosinophilic leukemia and idiopathic hypereosinophilic syndrome by the results of cytogenetic and molecular genetic analysis.

Idiopathic Hypereosinophilic Syndrome

Definition

By definition, this is a diagnosis of exclusion. No cause for a reactive eosinophilia is found, and there is no evidence of a myeloid neoplasm. Presence of the *FIP1L1-PDGFRA* fusion gene must be specifically excluded. Diagnosis requires the presence of unexplained eosinophilia of at least 1.5×10^9/L persisting for at least 6 months and leading to tissue damage. In some patients there is abnormal cytokine release from immunophenotypically aberrant, sometimes clonal, T cells, but an overt T-cell neoplasm excludes the diagnosis.

Epidemiology

This disorder occurs mainly in adults. The marked male predominance previously observed is no longer present when patients with *FIP1L1-PDGFRA* fusion are excluded.

Etiology

By definition, the cause is unknown, although the disorder is sometimes T-cell and cytokine driven.

Clinical Features

Splenomegaly is present in a minority of patients, and a small minority have lymphadenopathy.[18] Cutaneous manifestations and cardiac damage are common.[18] Liver, central nervous system, muscle, pulmonary, and nasal sinus involvement are more common than in eosinophilic leukemia.[18] IgE is increased in about half of patients. Serum vitamin B_{12} is usually normal. Serum tryptase is sometimes elevated.[18]

Morphology

By definition, the eosinophil count is at least 1.5×10^9/L. Otherwise, the differential count is usually normal. There may be anemia. The platelet count is usually normal. The bone marrow is normocellular or hypercellular, with increased eosinophils and precursors and no increase in blast cells. Mast cells are increased in the bone marrow in more than half the patients, and these cells may show aberrant expression of CD2 and CD25.[18]

Immunophenotype

Immunophenotyping of the eosinophils is not useful, but immunophenotyping of peripheral blood lymphocytes is indicated and may show an aberrant population.

Genetics and Molecular Findings

By definition, no abnormality is detected, and clonality of myeloid cells is not shown.

Postulated Cell of Origin

There is no postulated cell of origin. It can be hypothesized that some cases represent a myeloid stem cell disorder, whereas others are a lymphoid disorder. A minority of patients exhibit a sustained hematologic response to imatinib, inviting speculation that there is an undiscovered point mutation or fusion gene involving a tyrosine kinase gene. In one study, five of six patients with idiopathic hypereosinophilic syndrome who responded to imatinib came from a group of eight patients with increased bone marrow mast cells.[18]

Clinical Course

The clinical course is one of slow progression, with death sometimes occurring as a result of cardiac damage.

Differential Diagnosis

The differential diagnosis includes all known causes of hypereosinophilia.

CONCLUSION

The differential diagnosis of eosinophilia is very wide. The clinical history is of great importance and may point to a specific diagnosis. In other cases there are no diagnostic clues, and extensive investigation is needed. Eosinophils may have striking cytologic abnormalities in both eosinophilic leukemias and reactive conditions. Conversely, cytologic abnormalities are sometimes quite minor in CEL. Eosinophil morphology is therefore not useful in terms of diagnosis; however, other features in blood films, bone marrow aspirates, and trephine biopsy sections may be diagnostic or at least suggest a limited range of diagnoses. These include the presence of blast cells, lymphoma cells, and even parasites. One pitfall to be avoided is the misdiagnosis of CEL as systemic mastocytosis. A second is diagnosing idiopathic hypereosinophilic syndrome before exhaustive investigations have been performed. As increasingly specific treatments become available, detecting the cause of eosinophilia is becoming increasingly important, and thorough investigation is justified.

Pearls and Pitfalls

- There are hundreds of different causes of eosinophilia.
- The integration of clinical features and laboratory results is essential for identifying clonal and reactive eosinophilia and determining the cause of reactive eosinophilia.
- Some cases of eosinophilic leukemia cannot be recognized with current techniques and are identified only in retrospect, when disease evolution occurs.
- Reactive eosinophilia and eosinophilic leukemia can lead to life-threatening tissue damage mediated by eosinophil products.
- Because of the therapeutic implications, it is important not to misdiagnose eosinophilic leukemia as systemic mastocytosis.
- Cytologic abnormalities are not reliable indicators of neoplastic eosinophils; reactive eosinophils may have abnormal morphologic features, and neoplastic eosinophils may appear morphologically normal.

References can be found on Expert Consult @ www.expertconsult.com

Chapter 50

Blastic Plasmacytoid Dendritic Cell Neoplasm

Fabio Facchetti

DEFINITION

Blastic plasmacytoid dendritic cell neoplasm (BPDCN) is a rare hematologic malignancy characterized by the clonal proliferation of immature plasmacytoid dendritic cells (PDCs), also known as *professional type I interferon-producing cells,*[1] or their precursors. This neoplasm was originally recognized in 1994,[2] and the uncertainty about its histogenesis was reflected by several name changes, including *agranular CD4⁺ natural killer (NK) cell leukemia,*[3] *blastic NK cell leukemia/lymphoma,*[4] and *agranular CD4⁺, CD56⁺ hematodermic neoplasm*[5] or *tumor.*[6] In 2001 the World Health Organization (WHO) classification of tumors of hematopoietic and lymphoid tissues coined the term *blastic NK-cell lymphoma* on the basis of the blastic cytology and the expression of CD56 in the absence of other lineage-specific markers. A relationship to PDCs was hypothesized first by Lucio and colleagues[7] in 1999 and subsequently confirmed by several other studies.[5,8-13] The term *blastic plasmacytoid dendritic cell neoplasm* was introduced in 2008 in the updated WHO classification.[14]

The clinical hallmarks of BPDCN are predominant cutaneous involvement, with subsequent or simultaneous extension to bone marrow and peripheral blood (Box 50-1). Systemic dissemination and short survival are characteristic. Morphologically, the tumor cells show an immature "blastic" appearance; the diagnosis rests on the demonstration of CD4 and CD56, along with markers that are more restricted to PDCs (e.g., BDCA-2, CD123, TCL1, CD2AP, BCL11a), and negativity for lymphoid, NK, and myeloid lineage–associated antigens.

BPDCN must be distinguished from other tumoral conditions of PDCs. In these conditions, massive nodal or extranodal localizations of mature PDCs develop in association with another myeloid neoplasm, in most cases, chronic myelomonocytic leukemia.[15]

EPIDEMIOLOGY

This is a rare hematologic tumor with no racial or ethnic predominance.[8] It represents less than 1% of acute leukemias,[8] and in two series of lymphomas it accounted for 0.27% to 0.7 %.[16,17]

Data from 207 cases collected from several Western series or single reports (including 11 unpublished cases) indicate that the male-to-female ratio is 3.5:1 (Fig. 50-1). Most patients are older adults, with a mean age at diagnosis of 57.5 years and a median age of 66.0 years; women with BPDCN are generally younger than men (mean age, 51.6 versus 59.2 years; median age, 55.5 versus 67.0 years). In an additional series from Japan (47 cases; 33 males, 14 females), the total mean age was 52.9 years.[18] Infrequent cases in children have been reported, and these must be distinguished from lymphoblastic malignancies.

ETIOLOGY

There are currently no clues to the etiology of BPDCN. Rare (questionable) cases positive for Epstein-Barr virus (EBV) have been reported, but EBV as well as other lymphotropic viruses (human immunodeficiency virus, hepatitis C virus, human herpesvirus 6 and 8, cytomegalovirus, human T-lymphotropic virus 1 and 2) are generally negative.[8]

CLINICAL FEATURES

The clinical features and evolution of BPDCN are rather homogeneous from series to series[3,4,6,8,9,17-21] and consist of two main patterns. One (90% of cases) is characterized by an indolent onset dominated by cutaneous lesions followed by tumor dissemination; the other (10%) has features of an acute leukemia with systemic involvement from the beginning.

Box 50-1 ***Major Diagnostic Features of Blastic Plasmacytoid Dendritic Cell Neoplasm***

- Diffuse dermal skin infiltrate composed of medium-sized immature cells, resembling lymphoblasts or myeloblasts
- Absence of necrosis and angioinvasion
- Positive for CD4, CD56, and PDC-associated antigens (BDCA-2, CD123, TCL1, CD2AP, BCL11a)
- CD2, CD7, CD33, and TdT can be expressed; CD34 is negative
- Negative for lineage-associated antigens for T cells (CD3, CD5, LAT, TCR-AB, TCR-GD), B cells (CD19, CD20, PAX5), NK cells (CD16, TIA-1, perforin), and myelomonocytic cells (myeloperoxidase, lysozyme, CD11c, CD14, CD163, esterases)
- Germline configuration of B-cell and T-cell receptor genes
- Negative for Epstein-Barr virus–associated antigen (LMP-1) and RNA (EBER)
- No specific chromosomal aberrations, but frequent complex abnormalities in the same cells

LAT, linker for activation of T cells; NK, natural killer; PDC, plasmacytoid dendritic cell; TCR, T-cell receptor; TdT, terminal deoxynucleotidyl transferase.

Patients usually present with asymptomatic skin lesions (sometimes lasting for months) and are in good general health without systemic symptoms, concealing the aggressive nature of the underlying disease. Skin lesions can be nodules, plaques, or bruise-like areas; in several cases one cutaneous lesion was described, but more often they are multiple and can occur in any body site. The lesions can be erythematous, reddish or bluish in color; the size varies from a few millimeters to several centimeters (Fig. 50-2).[8] In about half the cases, skin lesions are the only detectable clinical manifestation.[6,17] Localized or disseminated lymphadenopathy at presentation is common (20% of cases), as well as spleen enlargement (40% to 60% of

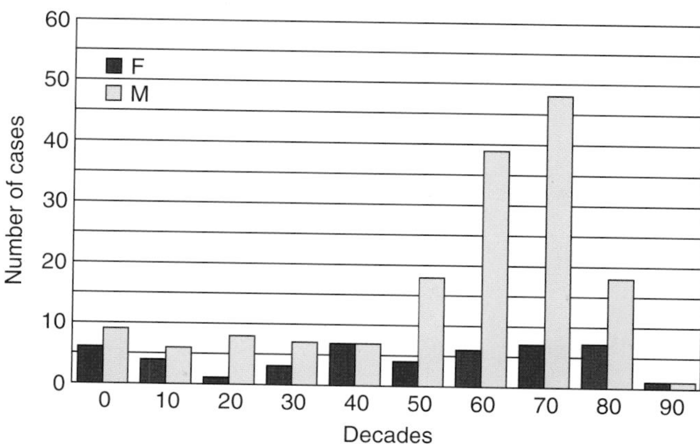

Figure 50-1. Distribution of blastic plasmacytoid dendritic cell neoplasm according to age and sex (data from 207 cases). F, female; M, male.

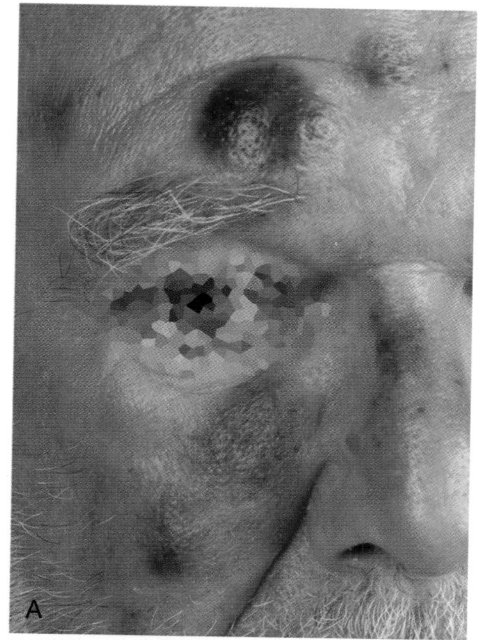

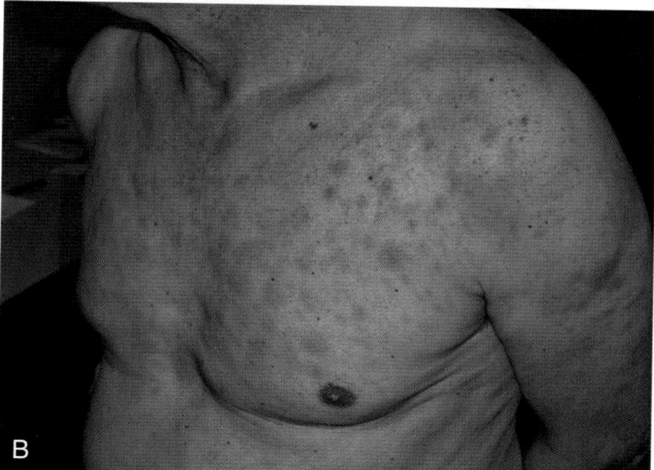

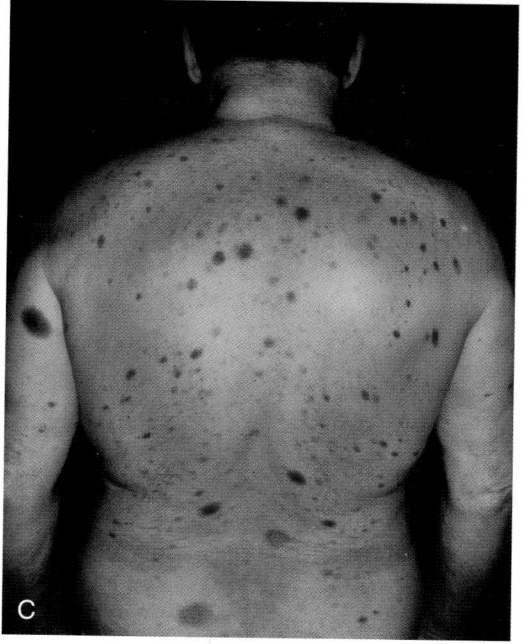

Figure 50-2. A–C, Examples of skin lesions in blastic plasmacytoid dendritic cell neoplasm. Lesions may consist of nodules, plaques, or bruise-like areas; they can be erythematous and reddish or bluish. (Courtesy of Prof. Lorenzo Cerroni, Graz, Austria; Dr. Stefano Corsico, Brescia, Italy; and Prof. Piergiacomo Calzavara, Brescia, Italy.)

cases). Bone marrow involvement at disease onset has been reported in 40% to 90% of cases; it may be minimal and demonstrable only with immunohistochemistry but invariably increases with progression. Anemia and thrombocytopenia frequently occur at diagnosis, and in a minority of cases they are severe, indicating bone marrow failure.[6,22] Circulating tumor cells are found in about half the patients, but counts are generally low (median, 2%; range, 0% to 94%).[18,22]

The acute leukemic variant is characterized by an elevated white blood cell count, circulating blasts, and massive bone marrow infiltration. Multiple skin nodules are frequently present.[18]

The noteworthy cutaneous tropism of BPDCN tumor cells in all clinical presentations contrasts with the absence of normal PDCs in the skin and might depend on the expression of antigens that favor skin migration, such as CLA and CD56,[23] as well as on the production of ligands of chemokines expressed by tumor cells (CXCR3, CXCR4, CCR6, CCR7) by the invaded organs.[24]

In about 15% to 20% of cases, BPDCN is associated with or develops into a chronic myelomonocytic leukemia or acute myeloid leukemia.[6,9,17,20,22,25-27] Marked marrow or blood monocytosis at diagnosis can reveal the associated leukemic proliferation, even if myelodysplasia or blasts are absent.[6] Myeloid leukemic cells are phenotypically distinct from BPDCN tumor cells but can express CD4 and CD56 as well as TCL1 and CD123, suggesting that the two diseases are more than coincidental and may have a common cellular origin. BPDCN with associated myeloid leuekmia should be distinguished from the tumoral proliferation of mature PDCs regularly associated with other myeloid neoplasms (see Differential Diagnosis); the pathogenesis may be analogous, however, with a common clonal origin in both settings.[15,28,29]

MORPHOLOGY

BPDCN is characterized by a diffuse, dense, monomorphic infiltrate of medium-sized cells with an obvious blastic morphology, suggesting either lymphoblasts or myeloblasts. The nuclei are single, with a variably irregular contour; the chromatin is fine; and the nucleoli, when present, are eosinophilic, single or multiple. The cytoplasm is usually scant and appears gray-blue, devoid of cytoplasmic azurophilic granules on Giemsa stain. Mitotic activity is markedly variable, and Ki-67 antigen labeling is generally moderate to high (20% to 80%)[25,30,31] (Fig. 50-3).

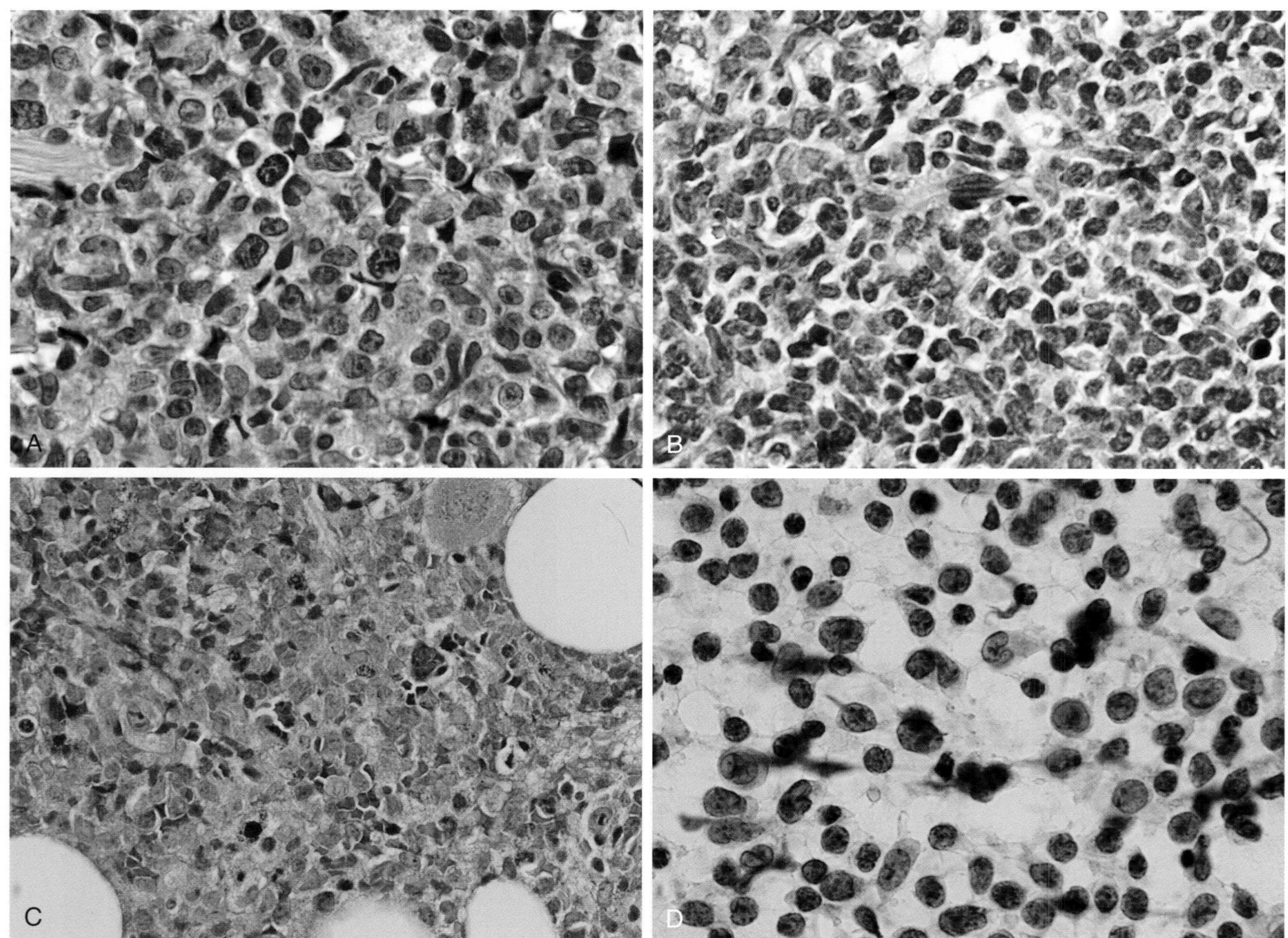

Figure 50-3. The cytomorphology of the immature tumor cells in blastic plasmacytoid dendritic cell neoplasm varies from myeloblast-like (**A**) to lymphoblast-like (**B** and **C**) cells (hematoxylin-eosin; Giemsa). Fine-needle aspiration from a lymph node (**D**) shows medium-size immature cells with variable amounts of cytoplasm (Papanicolaou).

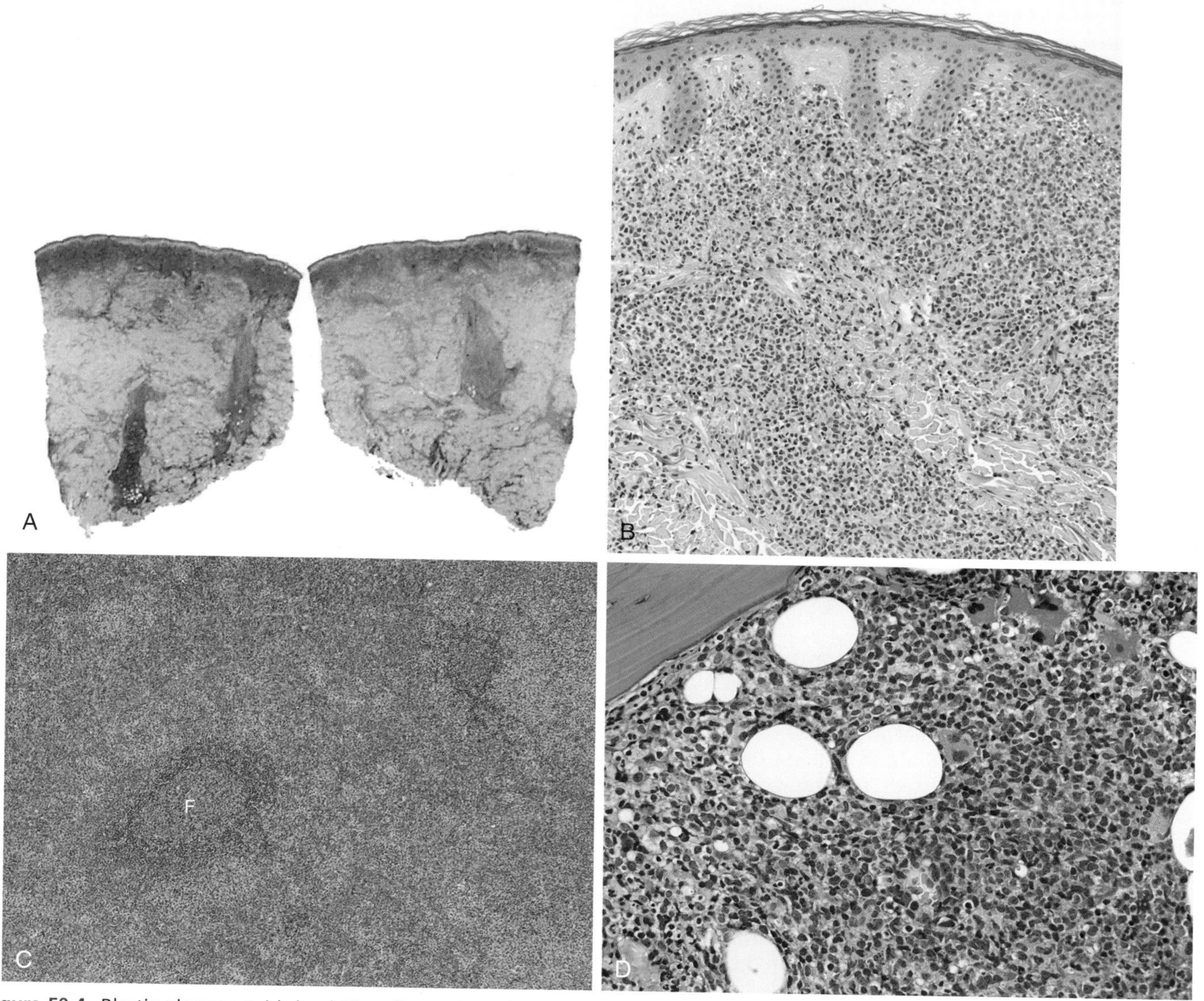

Figure 50-4. Blastic plasmacytoid dendritic cell neoplasm (BPDCN) involving the skin (**A** and **B**), lymph node (**C**), and bone marrow (**D**). In the skin (**A** and **B**) the infiltrate is diffuse and extends from the superficial to the deep dermis, sparing the papillary dermis. In the lymph node (**C**), BPDCN obliterates the interfollicular and paracortical areas; residual follicles (F) may be present. Bone marrow (**D**) can show extensive replacement of the bone lacuna, with residual hyperchromatic megakaryocytes.

In skin biopsies, tumor cells occupy predominantly the dermis but may extend to the subcutaneous fat; they spare the epidermis. Their density and distribution largely depend on the lesion selected for biopsy; low-density infiltrates from flat lesions are generally superficially located. Lymph nodes are involved in the interfollicular areas and medulla, with a leukemic pattern of infiltration that frequently spares B follicles. Bone marrow contains either a subtle interstitial infiltrate or a massive localization; dysplastic megakaryocytes are frequently found in residual hematopoietic tissue.[17] Angioinvasion and coagulative necrosis are regularly absent (Fig. 50-4).

On fine-needle aspirate preparations stained with Papanicolaou or hematoxylin-eosin, the medium-sized cells exhibit blastic features but may also resemble mature lymphomatous cells (e.g., marginal zone B-cell lymphoma) or atypical monocytes (see Fig. 50-3). On blood and bone marrow smears, tumor cells may show cytoplasmic microvacuoles localized along the cell membrane and pseudopodia.[22]

IMMUNOPHENOTYPE

At present, the diagnosis of BPDCN is based primarily on immunohistochemistry and relies on the expression of CD4 and CD56, along with other antigens more specific for PDCs (Table 50-1). Lineage markers for B cells, T cells, myeloid or monocytic cells, and NK cells are generally absent, with the exception of CD33 and CD7. Cytoplasmic but not surface CD3 has been reported rarely, generally with the use of polyclonal anti–CD3ε antibodies.

By definition, BPDCN is positive for CD4 and CD56,[5,8,19,20,22,32-34] but rare cases lacking CD4 or CD56 have been reported[30,35-39]; this negativity might be the result

Table 50-1 Comparison of Immunohistochemical Markers Expressed in Paraffin Sections by Normal Cells and Tumor Cells

Expression	Markers
Positive in normal PDCs and BPDCN	CD4, CD43, CD45RA, CD68,* CD123, BDCA-2/CD303, CD2AP, TCL1, BCL11a, CLA, granzyme B,† MxA
Positive in BPDCN	CD56, CD2, CD7, CD33, CD38, CD117, TdT‡
Negative in normal PDCs and BPDCN	CD1a, CD3, CD5, CD8, CD10, CD11c, CD13, CD14, CD16, CD19, CD20, CD21, CD23, CD25, CD30, CD34, CD45RO, CD57, CD138, FOXP3, immunoglobulin (surface and cytoplasmic), langerin/CD207, LAT, lysozyme, myeloperoxidase, neutrophil elastase, perforin, T-bet, TCR-AB and -GD, TIA-1, ZAP-70

*In normal PDCs, CD68 expression is constantly diffuse; in neoplastic PDCs, it is variable, punctate, and limited to the Golgi region.
†Granzyme B is rarely found in BPDCN on tissue sections.
‡The expression of all these markers, except for CD56, is inconstant; CD33 was found in normal circulating PDCs in a single study.[54]
BPDCN, blastic plasmacytoid dendritic cell neoplasm; CLA, cutaneous lymphocyte antigen; PDC, plasmacytoid dendritic cell; LAT, linker for activation of T cells; TCR, T-cell receptor; TdT, terminal deoxynucleotidyl transferase.

of low sensitivity of the technique or poor preservation of the antigen.[6,35,39a] Nevertheless, the diagnosis is supported by the demonstration of antigens typically labeling PDCs, such as CD123, TCL1, BDCA-2/CD303, CD2AP, and BCL11a.[5,6,9,10,17,19,20,26,38,40,41] Notably, all these antigens can be demonstrated on formalin-fixed, paraffin-embedded tissue sections (Fig. 50-5). At present, there is no consensus on the minimal phenotype to establish the diagnosis of BPDCN immunohistochemically,[6] but it is prudent to identify at least one of the PDC-associated antigens, especially when CD4 or CD56 is not found. CD123 represents the interleukin-3 receptor alpha chain, a cytokine receptor fundamental for PDC survival and function[42,43]; it is positive in the majority of BPDCNs.[5,38,44] CD123 can also be strongly expressed in various myeloid leukemias and leukemic stem cells,[45-47] as well as in Langerhans cell histiocytosis.[48] The oncogene *TCL1*, a coactivator for Akt, is regularly expressed in BPDCN.[26,38,40] However, its specificity is low; TCL1 is also positive in about 20% of acute myeloid leukemias,[20,26,40] in a broad variety of B-cell lymphoproliferative disorders, and in T-cell prolymphocytic leukemia. In the appropriate context, this marker can be a very useful tool for BPDCN diagnosis.

BDCA-2 (CD303), a C-type lectin transmembrane glycoprotein involved in antigen uptake and regulation of interferon production by PDCs, currently represents the most specific marker for these cells.[49,50] Using an antibody reactive on frozen sections, BDCA-2 has been regularly demonstrated in small series of BPDCN.[8,10,31,51] Using their own reagent for paraffin sections, Jaye and coworkers[52] reported that only 10 of 19 cases (55%) were positive for BDCA-2. Because the BDCA-2 antigen is downregulated upon PDC activation,[49] it is possible that its expression may depend on the degree of tumor cell differentiation or activation. Preliminary results using the anti–BDCA-2 monoclonal antibody that reacts on paraffin sections (clone 124B3.13) indicate that it is an excellent marker for normal and neoplastic PDCs.

In a recent immunohistologic screening, the adapter protein CD2AP (CD2-associated protein) emerged as a selective marker of normal PDCs and BPDCN.[38] It recognized 35 of 37 cases (95%) of BPDCN but only 1 of 24 cases (4%) of acute myeloid leukemia and none of 12 cases of precursor or lymphoblastic B- and T-cell leukemia. It should be noted that CD2AP also weakly stains subsets of normal B lymphocytes, and reactivity with peripheral B-cell lymphomas can be found (T. Marafioti, personal communication).

CD68 is positive in about half the cases of BPDCN in the form of small cytoplasmic dots,[5,17,19] an expression pattern that markedly differs from the strong and diffuse reactivity regularly observed in normal PDCs or macrophages.[53] Among lymphoid- and myeloid-associated antigens, CD7 and CD33 are relatively common,[54] and some cases have shown expression of CD2, CD10, and CD38. The cytotoxic molecules perforin and TIA-1 are negative. Interestingly, granzyme B is generally undetectable in tissue sections, despite positive results with flow cytometry and evidence of expression at the messenger RNA level in BPDCN[11,55]; additionally, it is normally found in reactive PDCs.[56]

The results of staining for terminal deoxynucleotidyl transferase (TdT) have been quite variable in different series.[4,5,19,20,34,38] Overall, TdT is expressed in about one third of cases, with positivity ranging between 10% and 80% of cells. Other hematopoietic precursor cell markers such as CD34 and CD117 are negative. EBV antigens and EBV-encoded small nuclear RNA (EBER) are not found.

On flow cytometry, the lack of lineage-associated antigens, together with the expression of CD4, CD45RA, CD56, and CD123, is considered to represent a unique and virtually pathognomonic phenotype.[33] Other immunophenotypic characteristics useful in flow cytometric analysis include both negative (CD45RO, CD57, CD117, myeloperoxidase, CD116 [granulocyte-macrophage colony-stimulating factor receptor]) and positive (CD36, CD38, BDCA-2, HLA-DR) markers.[12,22,55]

CYTOCHEMISTRY

BPDCN tumor cells are nonreactive for alpha-naphthyl butyrate esterase, naphthol AS-D chloroacetate esterase, and peroxidase cytochemical reactions.[9,22,25,30]

GENETICS AND MOLECULAR FINDINGS

T-cell and B-cell receptor genes are usually germline.[9,17,20] Only a few cases have been reported with T-cell receptor gamma chain gene rearrangement,[6,17,57,58] but the presence of clonal bystander T cells cannot be ruled out. In addition, lineage promiscuity at the molecular level is sometimes observed in immature hematolymphoid neoplasms.[59] Sixty-six percent of patients with BPDCN have an abnormal karyotype; no specific chromosomal aberrations have been identified, but complex abnormalities in the same cells are a distinctive feature, with an average of six to eight abnormalities. Genetic changes are characterized by gross genomic imbalances (mostly losses), including both lymphoid and myeloid lineage–associated rearrangements. The most frequent chromosomal targets are 5q (5q21 or 5q34; 72%), 12p (12p13; 64%), 13q (13q13-21; 64%), 6q (6q23-qter; 50%), monosomy 15 (43%), and monosomy 9 (28%).[9,19,30,60]

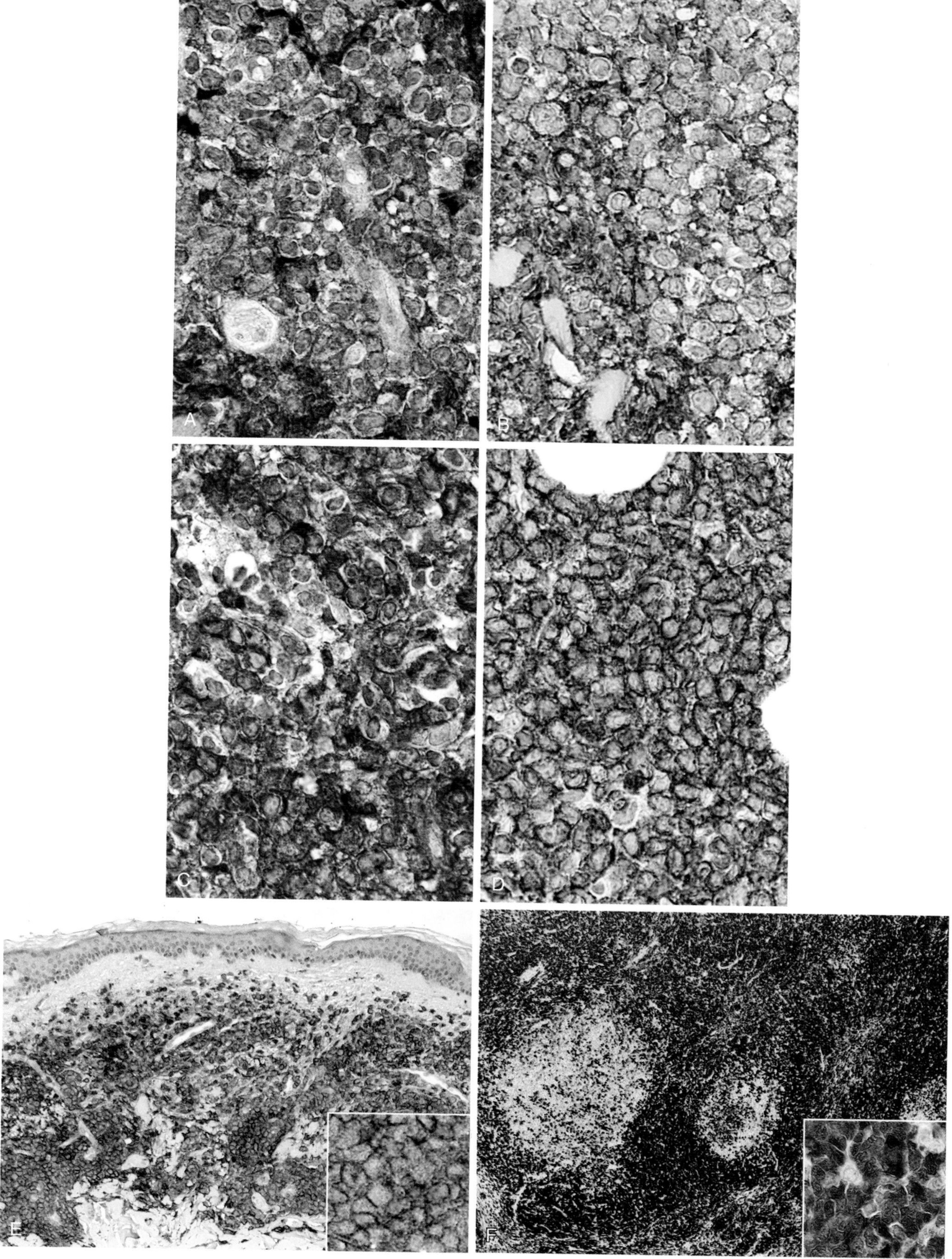

Figure 50-5. For legend see p. 794.

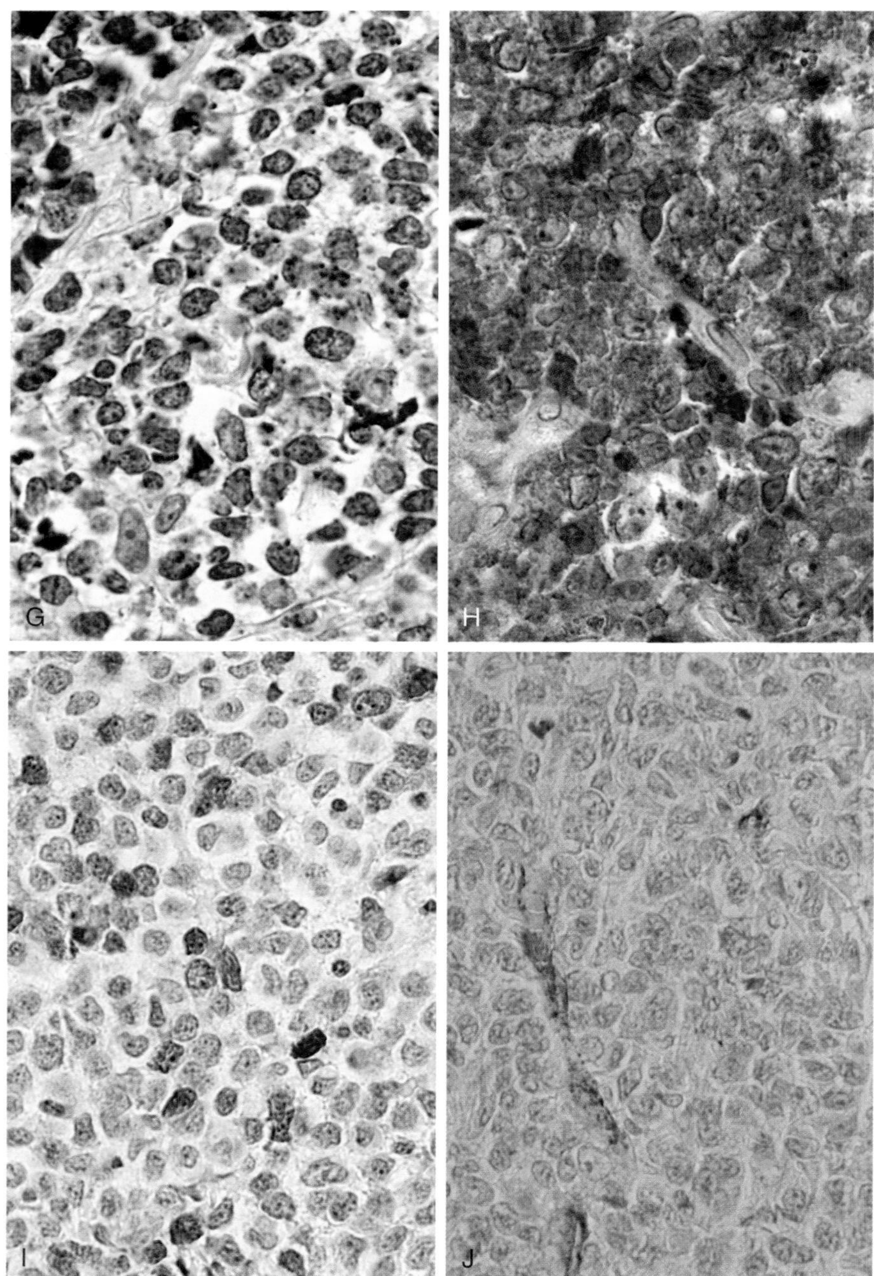

Figure 50-5, cont'd. Immunohistochemical features of blastic plasmacytoid dendritic cell neoplasm. A–F, Positive tumor markers are represented by CD4, CD56, CD123, CD2AP, BDCA-2, and TCL1, respectively. In the lymph node **(F)**, there is massive involvement of the interfollicular area; note also some reactivity on germinal center B cells. **G,** CD68 is typically expressed in the form of dot-like positivity. **H,** CD33 can be positive. **I,** Terminal deoxynucleotidyl transferase is variably expressed. **J,** CD34 is regularly negative.

Gene expression profiling and array-based comparative genomic hybridization have shown that BPDCN is genetically distinct from cutaneous myelomonocytic leukemia.[61] It is characterized by recurrent deletion of regions on chromosomes 4 (4q34), 9 (9p13-p11 and 9q12-q34), and 13 (13q12-q31) that contain several tumor suppressor genes, with consequent diminished expression (*Rb1*, *LATS2*). In addition, there is overexpression of the oncogenes *HES6*, *RUNX2*, and *FLT3* that is not coupled with genomic amplification. BPDCN does not show cytoplasmic expression of nucleophosmin, the immunohistochemical surrogate for *NPM1* mutations, indicating that the gene is wild type.[62]

POSTULATED CELL OF ORIGIN AND NORMAL COUNTERPART

There is a large series of data indicating that PDCs (previously known as *plasmacytoid T cells*,[28] *plasmacytoid T-zone cells*,[29] or *plasmacytoid monocytes*[33]) are the normal counterpart of BPDCN (Fig. 50-6). Identifying the cell of origin of BPDCN was hampered by several factors, including the blastic appearance of the tumor cells, which is nonspecific and lacks any morphologic clue that might suggest a PDC origin. Moreover, CD56, one of the BPDCN-defining molecules, is absent from PDCs in normal tissues,[56] although Petrella and associ-

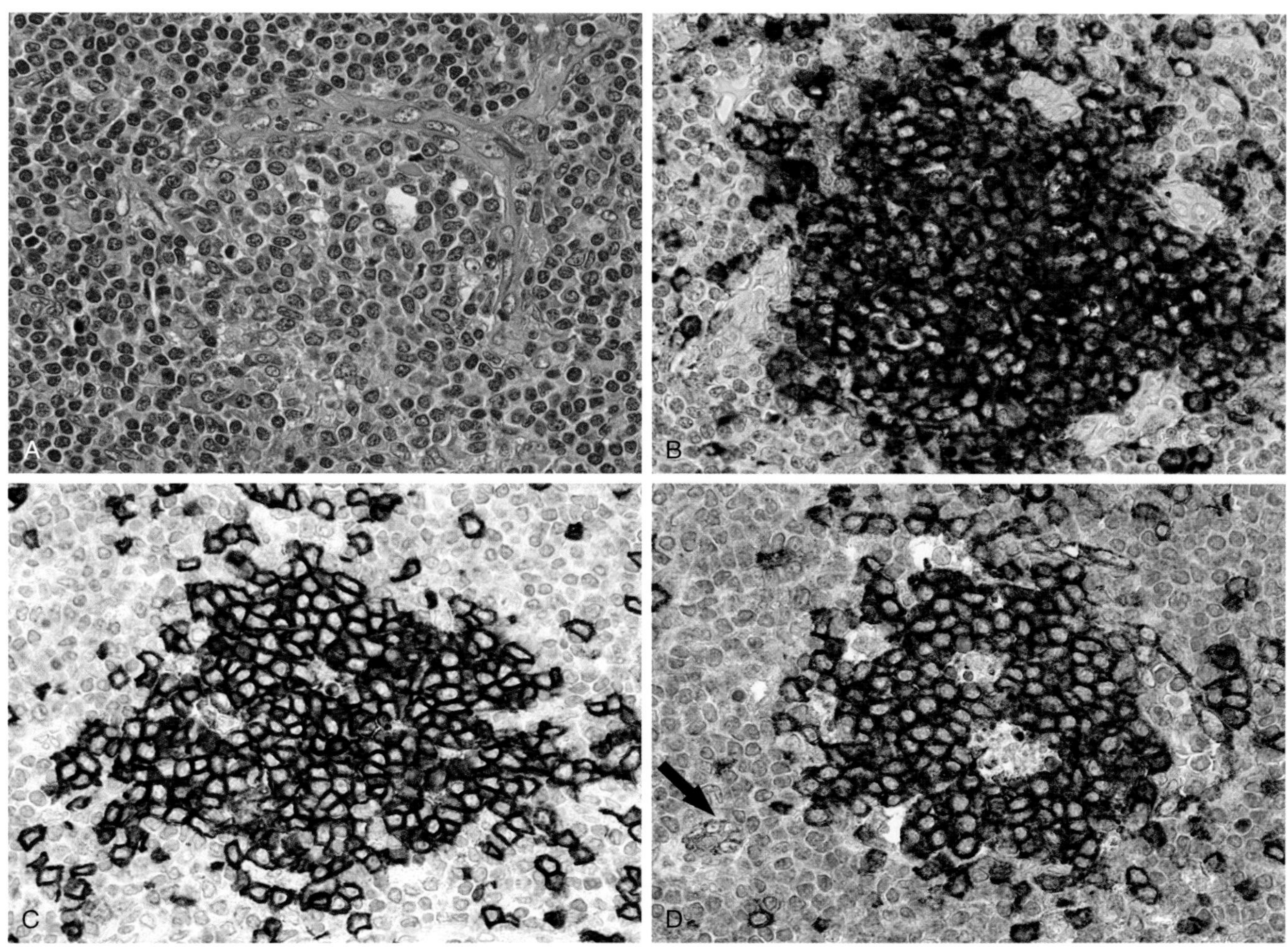

Figure 50-6. Plasmacytoid dendritic cell (PDC) clusters in a reactive lymph node. The cytomorphology (**A**) and three markers typically strongly expressed on PDCs are illustrated: CD68 (**B**), BDCA-2 (**C**), and CD123 (**D**). Note that CD123 also stains high endothelial venules (*arrow*).

ates[5] demonstrated that it can occur in a small subset of peripheral blood PDCs upon treatment with FLT3 ligand. The unique features of normal PDCs were discovered only in the late 1990s,[42,43,63-65] so only recently have the tools to define this hematopoietic neoplasm become available. These features include the expression of PDC-restricted antigens[5,6,8,10-12,26,31,40,52,55] and chemokine receptors,[24] the production of type I interferon,[10,12,31,54] and the maturation into dendritic cells with an antigen-presenting capacity upon appropriate stimuli.[12,24] Box 50-2 lists the main morphologic and functional features of normal PDCs.

CLINICAL COURSE AND PROGNOSIS

Despite the apparently indolent clinical presentation, the course is aggressive. Median survival is approximately 12 to 14 months, based on several series.[6,8,17,21,22] The tumor cells are very sensitive to cytotoxic drugs and to steroids, and several remissions can be induced in most cases (80% to 90%); however, early relapses occur, and chemoresistance eventually develops. Sites of relapse are the skin, where disseminated lesions usually develop at the terminal stage of the disease, as well as the bone marrow, lymph nodes, spleen, soft tissues, nasopharynx, gums, and bronchial mucosa. The central nervous system represents a frequent site of tumor recurrence, suggesting that it may be a reservoir of neoplastic cells requiring intrathecal prophylaxis.[22,66] In most cases a fulminant leukemic phase ultimately develops.[22]

Meta-analysis of large series[18,21,66] has shown that better survival may be related to age, tumor stage, clinical presentation, or tumor cell phenotype. Younger patients have a better prognosis than older ones, but this might be related to the option of using more aggressive therapy in young as compared with elderly individuals.[66] Patients with disease restricted to the skin showed slightly better survival than those with advanced disease (17 and 12 months,[66] 21 and 12 months,[21] and 25 and 14 months,[18] respectively). The presentation as isolated skin nodules versus skin plus extracutaneous involvement was a favorable factor in one series[66] but did not influence survival in another.[21] Nevertheless, the single reported patient with extended survival (>15 years) presented with isolated skin lesions.[3] High blast counts in the marrow or peripheral blood are unfavorable factors.[18] The expression of TdT seems to correlate with longer survival,[18,21,52] suggesting a heterogeneous response based on maturational stage.

At present, there is no consensus on the optimal treatment of BPDCN. Local chemotherapy or radiotherapy is inefficient

Box 50-2 *Features of Normal Plasmacytoid Dendritic Cells*

Occurrence

- Especially in lymph nodes and tonsils, more rare in the thymus (medulla) and other lymphoid tissues
- 0.1% to 0.05% of total peripheral blood leukocytes
- Tissue and circulating PDC numbers decline significantly with age

Morphology

- Typically occur in the vicinity of high endothelial venules, as scattered elements or aggregates; the latter typically contain apoptotic bodies
- Medium-sized cell with a single round-oval or indented nucleus, finely dispersed chromatin, and one or two small nucleoli; moderately abundant eosinophilic cytoplasm, basophilic on Giemsa stain
- No mitotic activity

Immunohistochemical Recognition*

- Best markers for PDC identification on paraffin sections: CD68, BDCA-2, CD123, CD2AP, TCL1, BCL11a

In Vitro/Ex Vivo Functional Properties

- Production of high amounts of IFN-I
- Differentiation into dendritic cells; compared with other dendritic cells, PDCs are less efficient in antigen presentation and T-cell expansion
- Main activating and differentiating factors are viruses, CpG, IL-3, and CD40L; TLR-7 and TLR-9 are the main PDC sensors for pathogen recognition

PDCs in Human Diseases

- Marked PDC increase in lymph nodes in Kikuchi-Fujimoto disease and the hyaline-vascular subtype of Castleman's disease; can be numerous in infectious and noninfectious granulomatous lymphadenitis and metastatic lymph nodes
- PDCs play a pivotal role (by secreting high amounts of IFN-I and interacting with other immune cells) in autoimmune diseases, especially SLE and psoriasis
- In SLE, PDCs are reduced in peripheral blood but accumulate in tissues (e.g., skin)
- PDCs strongly suppress HIV replication in $CD4^+$ T cells; PDC numbers in peripheral blood are severely reduced in HIV-infected patients and correlate with HIV load and decrease of $CD4^+$ lymphocytes
- PDC function is defective in human neoplasms (e.g., melanoma, ovarian carcinoma, head and neck squamous cell carcinoma)
- PDCs are associated with the local antitumoral and antiviral response to imiquimod, a potent stimulator of TLR-7

*See also Table 50-1.
CpG, Cytidine-phosphate-Guanosine oligodeoxynucleotides; HIV, human immunodeficiency virus; IFN, interferon; IL, interleukin; PDC, plasmacytoid dendritic cell; SLE, systemic lupus erythematosus; TLR, Toll-like receptor.

in BPDCN, and only patients receiving systemic polychemotherapy regimens are likely to achieve complete remission. Different protocols have been applied,[66] including chemotherapy less intensive than CHOP (cyclophosphamide, hydroxydaunomycin [doxorubicin], Oncovin [vincristine], and prednisone), CHOP and CHOP-like regimens, therapy for acute leukemia, and allogeneic or autologous stem cell transplantation. A CHOP or CHOP-like regimen induces complete remission in most cases, but relapse is nearly constant, and evolution is rapidly fatal.[66] With intensive therapy for acute leukemia, the rate of sustained complete remission increases, but only myeloablative treatment with allogeneic bone marrow transplantation during the first remission results in the chance of long-term survival.[22,66]

DIFFERENTIAL DIAGNOSIS

In the vast majority of cases, a skin biopsy represents the first diagnostic procedure in BPDCN. Thus, the differential diagnosis includes primarily cutaneous infiltrates composed of immature hematopoietic cells, some mature T/NK-cell lymphomas with predominant dermal involvement, and primary or metastatic undifferentiated neoplasms (e.g., Merkel cell neuroendocrine carcinoma) (Box 50-3). The expression of markers for myeloblasts (CD13, myeloperoxidase), monoblasts (CD14, lysozyme), and B and T lymphoblasts (CD19,

Box 50-3 *Differential Diagnosis of Blastic Plasmacytoid Dendritic Cell Neoplasm*

Precursor Lymphoblastic Leukemia/Lymphoma

- Positive for B- and T-cell–associated antigens (e.g., CD19, PAX5, CD3, LAT, ZAP-70)
- Clonal configuration of B-cell and T-cell receptor genes
- Caveats
  - TdT can be positive in BPDCN, but rarely diffuse and intense
  - PDC markers CD56, CD2AP, or TCL1 can be positive in T- and B-cell precursor lymphoblastic lymphomas

Acute Myeloid Leukemia* and Chronic Myelomonocytic Leukemia

- Occurrence of granulated myeloid cells (in the more differentiated forms)
- Positive for myeloperoxidase, lysozyme, CD11c, CD13, CD14, and esterase reactions
- Caveats
  - CD4 and CD56 can be positive in acute myeloid and monocytic leukemia
  - CD7 and CD33 are commonly expressed by BPDCN
  - CD123 and TCL1 can occur in acute myeloid leukemia

Cutaneous T/NK-Cell Nasal-Type Lymphoma

- Pleomorphic tumor cells
- Angioinvasion and necrosis frequent
- Positive for T/NK-cell markers (cCD3, CD2, LAT, ZAP-70)
- Positive for cytotoxic molecules (granzyme B, perforin, TIA-1)
- Positive for Epstein-Barr virus RNA (EBER)
- Caveat: CD56 (and occasionally CD4) can be positive

Cutaneous Mature T-Cell Lymphoma (Unspecified)

- Pleomorphic tumor cells
- Positive for T-cell markers (CD2, CD3, LAT, ZAP-70)
- Positive for cytotoxic molecules (TIA-1)
- Caveat: CD56 (and occasionally CD4) can be positive

Langerhans Cell Histiocytosis

- Nuclei more irregular, abundant eosinophilic cytoplasm
- Eosinophils usually present (sometimes rare)
- Positive for CD1a, langerin, S-100
- Caveat: CD4, CD56, and CD123 frequently positive

*Especially minimally differentiated, undifferentiated, and monocytic subtypes.
BPDCN, blastic plasmacytoid dendritic cell neoplasm; LAT, linker for activation of T cells; NK, natural killer; PDC, plasmacytoid dendritic cell; TdT, terminal deoxynucleotidyl transferase.

PAX5, CD3) excludes BPDCN. It should be taken into consideration that the CD4$^+$, CD56$^+$ phenotype can be observed in cases of acute myeloid leukemia, especially those with monocytic differentiation,[20,21,40,61,67,68] whereas it is very infrequent in lymphoblastic leukemia.[69] Cases of Langerhans cell histiocytosis exhibiting an immature morphology and few associated eosinophils should also be excluded using appropriate markers (S-100, CD1a, langerin). Notably, tumoral Langerhans cells regularly express CD4 and CD56[70] and can be positive for CLA and CD123.[48,71]

Cutaneous T-cell or NK/T-cell lymphomas expressing CD4 or CD56, or both (with marked variability from series to series) include nasal-type extranodal NK/T-cell lymphoma and primary cutaneous T-cell lymphomas, unspecified.[20,21,34,72,73] None of these tumors display a blastic morphology; rather, they are composed of a pleomorphic cell population and may exhibit necrosis and angiotropism. These features, associated with the expression of T-cell markers (CD3, LAT, ZAP-70), cytotoxic molecules (TIA-1, perforin), and EBV (in nasal-type NK/T-cell lymphoma), unquestionably exclude BPDCN.

Merkel cell carcinoma is an uncommon, aggressive primary cutaneous neuroendocrine carcinoma that may mimic BPDCN owing to the "blastic" appearance of tumor cells; another potential pitfall is its expression of CD56 and TdT.[74]

The tumoral proliferations of PDCs occurring in association with another myeloid neoplasm, usually chronic myelomonocytic leukemia, differ from BPDCN by their clinical, morphologic, and phenotypic features. The bone marrow in these cases may contain PDC aggregates.[75,76] More rarely, patients with chronic myelomonocytic leukemia may develop systemic lymphadenopathy due to extensive "tumor-forming" localizations of PDC nodules.[15,28,29,77] Finally, foci of PDCs are occasionally observed within myeloid sarcomas.[78]

In all these circumstances, the PDCs exhibit mature morphology and appear as well-defined clusters containing apoptotic bodies, as typically found in reactive PDC foci.[79] Moreover, CD56 is mostly negative or only weakly expressed on a minority of cells,[15,56] and CD68 and granzyme B are consistently positive, as in normal PDCs (Fig. 50-7).[15] Finally, although extranodal lesions may occur, skin involvement is

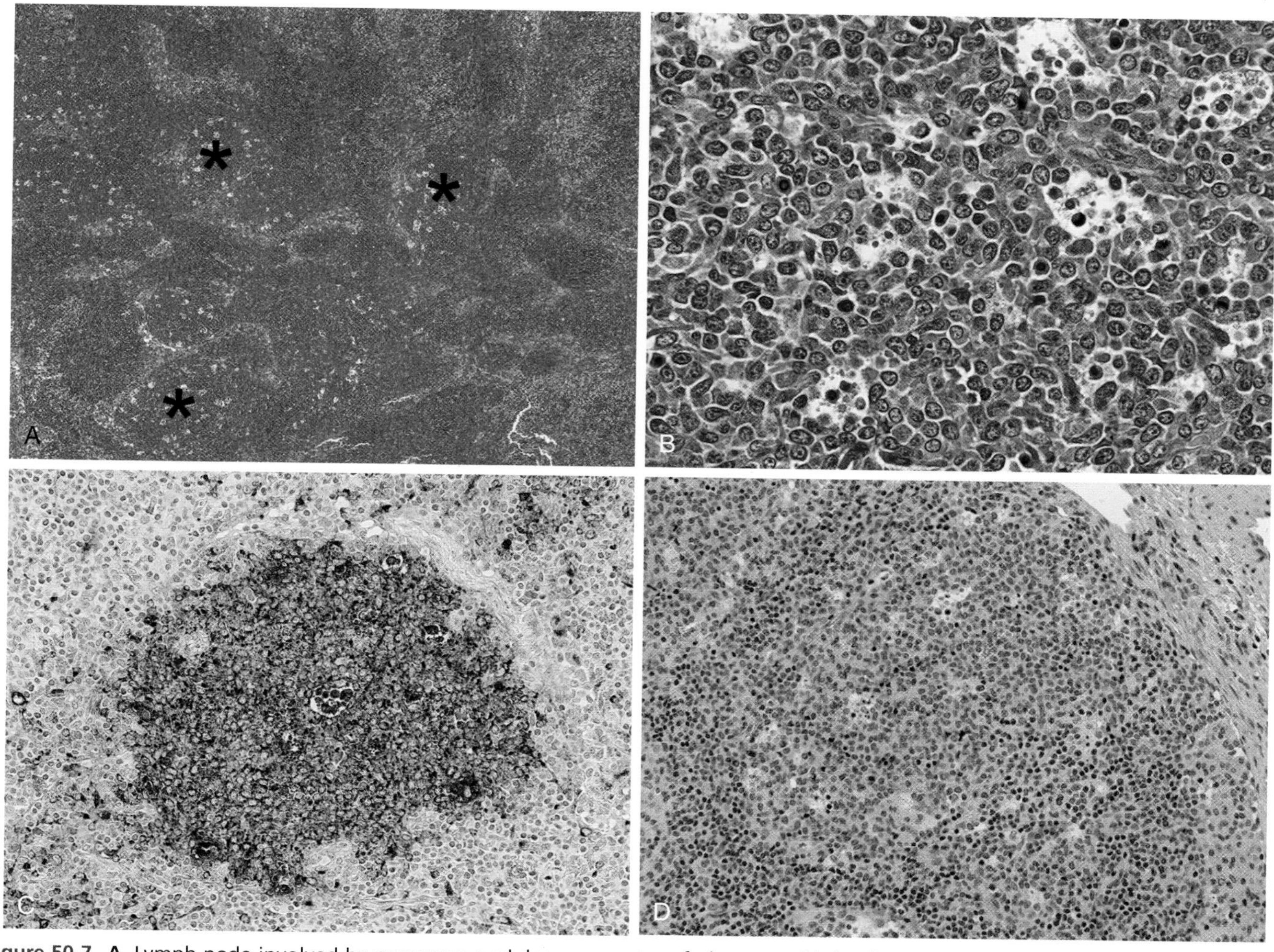

Figure 50-7. A, Lymph node involved by numerous nodular aggregates of plasmacytoid dendritic cells (PDCs; *asterisks*) in a patient with chronic myelomonocytic leukemia. **B,** Note the mature morphology of the PDCs and the numerous apoptotic bodies. **C,** There is strong expression of CD68. **D,** CD56 is negative.

uncommon and never represents an overwhelming clinical feature.[15,28,80] It should be noted that this condition shares with BPDCN a dismal prognosis, and patients usually die from rapid progression of the associated myeloid leukemia.[15] It has been questioned whether these PDC nodules may simply represent a reactive phenomenon.[29,77,80] Fluorescence in situ hybridization analysis, however, demonstrated identical chromosomal abnormalities in PDCs and the associated myeloid neoplasm,[15,78,81] indicating that the PDCs are clonal, neoplastic in nature, and closely related to the leukemic clone.

Pearls and Pitfalls

- There is no single morphologic feature absolutely distinctive for BPDCN.
- Consider BPDCN in any infiltrate composed of monotonous medium-sized immature cells, especially involving the skin or lymph nodes.
- Skin infiltrates do not involve the epidermis and lack obvious necrosis; angiotropism is absent.
- Expression of CD4 and CD56 strongly suggests the diagnosis of BPDCN but cannot be used as the only diagnostic marker; moreover, CD4 or CD56 can be negative.
- Specific markers for PDCs (e.g., BDCA-2, CD123, TCL1, CD2AP, BCL11a) are very useful for making a definitive diagnosis.
- The indolent clinical presentation contrasts with the systemic character of the infiltrate and should not divert one from the correct diagnosis, which leads to aggressive treatment.

References can be found on Expert Consult @ www.expertconsult.com

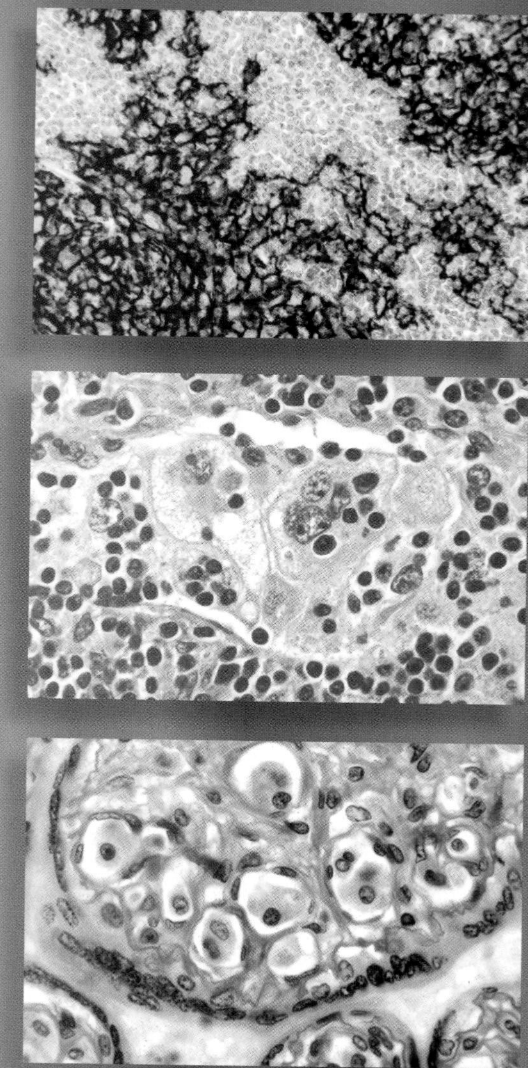

PART V

Histiocytic Proliferations

Chapter 51

Nonneoplastic Histiocytic Proliferations of Lymph Nodes and Bone Marrow

Sherif A. Rezk, John L. Sullivan, and Bruce A. Woda

CHAPTER OUTLINE

The histiocytoses are a group of disorders characterized by the proliferation of macrophages and dendritic cells. The contemporary classification of histiocytic disorders divides them into three groups: dendritic cell–related disorders, macrophage-related disorders, and malignant disorders.[1] The World Health Organization classifies neoplasms of histiocytes and dendritic cells according to their putative normal counterparts.[2] These entities are covered in Chapter 53. In this chapter, we discuss the nonneoplastic proliferations of histiocytes and their differential diagnosis. Box 51-1 lists the disorders discussed in this chapter.

SINUS HISTIOCYTOSIS WITH MASSIVE LYMPHADENOPATHY (ROSAI-DORFMAN DISEASE)

Definition

Sinus histiocytosis with massive lymphadenopathy (SHML), also known as *Rosai-Dorfman disease,* is a rare, self-limited histiocytic disorder of unknown cause. It is typically characterized by massive bilateral enlargement of the cervical lymph nodes, often accompanied by fever and weight loss; extranodal presentations can occur, and lymph nodes in other sites may be involved (see Pearls and Pitfalls).

Epidemiology

SHML can occur at any age but is most common in the first and second decades of life (median age, 20 years); there is a slight male preponderance.[3,4] The disease has been found worldwide, with a slightly higher prevalence in Africans.[3] It is generally regarded as a nonfamilial hematopoietic disorder, although one report described the presence of the disease in three brothers.[5] Moreover, histologic features closely resembling SHML have been reported in lymph nodes of patients with autoimmune lymphoproliferative syndrome.[6]

Etiology

The cause and pathogenesis of SHML remain unclear. The indolent clinical course suggests a reactive disorder rather than a neoplasm. Studies of clonality indicate that it is a polyclonal process.[1,7] It has been hypothesized that SHML is a lymphoreticular reaction to an infectious agent such as human herpesvirus 6 or Epstein-Barr virus (EBV); however, an infectious agent has not been identified.[8,9]

Clinical Features

Patients with SHML usually present with painless, massive bilateral cervical lymphadenopathy accompanied by low-

Box 51-1 *Nonneoplastic Histiocytic Proliferations*

- Reactive sinus histiocytosis
- Sinus histiocytosis with massive lymphadenopathy
- Hemophagocytic syndromes
  - Familial hemophagocytic lymphohistiocytosis
  - Secondary hemophagocytic syndromes
- Storage disorders
  - Neimann-Pick disease
  - Gaucher's disease
  - Tangier disease

grade fever, weight loss, leukocytosis, polyclonal gammopathy, and elevated erythrocyte sedimentation rate.[10] A mild normochromic, normocytic anemia may also be present.[10] Extranodal involvement occurs in 25% to 40% of patients and may be the initial manifestation of SHML in rare cases.[8,10-12] The most common extranodal sites, in order of frequency, are the skin,[13] upper respiratory tract,[11] soft tissue,[10] orbit,[14] bone,[15] salivary gland,[16] central nervous system,[4] breast,[17] and pancreas.[18]

Morphology

SHML is characterized by the expansion of lymph node sinuses by large histiocytes accompanied by lymphocytes and plasma cells, causing pronounced dilation (Fig. 51-1). Total effacement of the normal lymph node architecture occurs as the disease progresses. The histiocytes have large, round or oval nuclei with dispersed chromatin, often prominent nucleoli, and abundant pale cytoplasm. Within the histiocytes, the presence of lymphocytes and plasma cells in intracytoplasmic vacuoles that protect them from degradation by cytolytic enzymes—a process called *emperipolesis*—is characteristic of SHML but not specific (Fig. 51-2). Erythrophagocytosis may also be observed.[8] Plasma cells are typically numerous in the medullary cords. Granulomas may be seen in rare cases. In extranodal sites, where there are no sinuses, the histiocytes form aggregates that resemble dilated sinuses. Emperipolesis may be less conspicuous in extranodal sites.

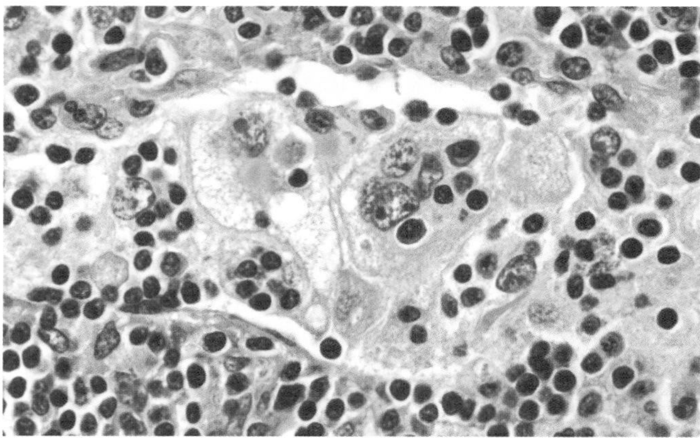

Figure 51-2. Rosai-Dorfman disease (sinus histiocytosis with massive lymphadenopathy). Higher magnification shows emperipolesis of lymphocytes. Note the plasma cells within and around the sinus. (Courtesy of Dr. Bharat Nathwani.)

Immunophenotype

The histiocytes in SHML express S-100 (Fig. 51-3) and other macrophage-associated markers such as CD4, CD11c, CD14, CD33, and CD68. Variable numbers of cells express the macrophage-associated enzymes lysozyme, α_1-antitrypsin, and α_1-antichymotrypsin.[19,20] CD30 is reportedly positive in half the cases.[3] In contrast to Langerhans cell histiocytosis, CD1a is reactive in less than 10% of patients with SHML; cathepsin D and E are positive in both disorders.[1,8]

Clinical Course

SHML patients typically have an indolent, protracted course and an excellent prognosis. The disease usually lasts between 3 and 9 months, followed by spontaneous remission. However, a few cases with persistent disease lasting more than 5 years have been described.[3,8] Occasionally, the disease is fatal.[21,22] Patients with an aggressive course and recurrences after com-

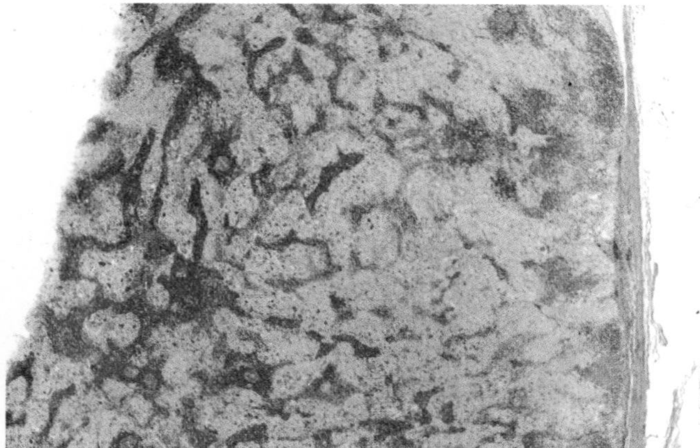

Figure 51-1. Rosai-Dorfman disease (sinus histiocytosis with massive lymphadenopathy). Lymph node almost entirely occupied by benign-appearing histiocytes in association with marked dilation of the sinuses. Note the fibrotic capsule of the node. (Courtesy of Dr. Bharat Nathwani.)

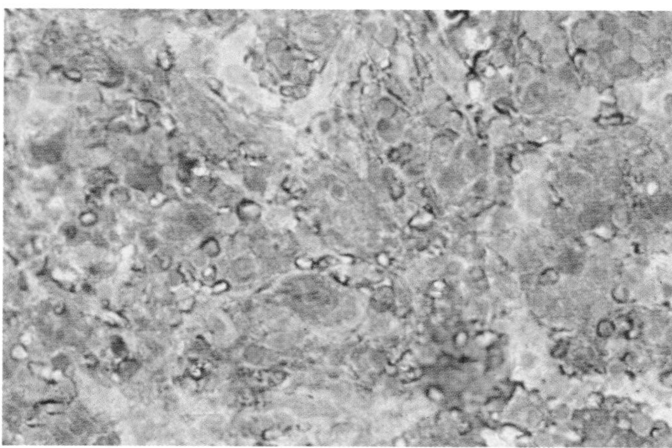

Figure 51-3. Rosai-Dorfman disease (sinus histiocytosis with massive lymphadenopathy). Proliferating histiocytes express S-100. (Courtesy of Dr. Bharat Nathwani.)

plete remission tend to have multiple sites of lymph node involvement or involvement of multiple extranodal sites.[3,8] Development of lymphoma in patients with SHML has been reported rarely, as has focal SHML in lymph nodes involved by lymphoma, but an increased risk of lymphoma has not been documented.[12,21]

Differential Diagnosis

It is important to differentiate SHML from Langerhans cell histiocytosis. In contrast to the histiocytes of SHML, the characteristic cytologic features of Langerhans cells include elongated, grooved nuclei; inconspicuous nucleoli; and a smaller amount of pale cytoplasm. Eosinophils are typically numerous, plasma cells are absent, and emperipolesis does not occur in Langerhans cell histiocytosis. Other disorders in the differential diagnosis are reactive sinus histiocytosis and sinusoidal malignancies. Both disorders lack the massive expansion of sinuses by histiocytes and lymphophagocytosis emperipolesis that occur in SHML. Although the prominent nucleoli of the histiocytes in SHML can give them an atypical appearance, the absence of mitotic activity is useful in ruling out malignancy. Hemophagocytic syndromes, especially the familial form that occurs in early life, can mimic SHML; however, these syndromes are characterized by disseminated disease and an aggressive clinical course, so the clinical presentation aids in the diagnosis. Infectious processes inducing the proliferation of histiocytes, such as tuberculosis, should also be considered in the differential diagnosis, but true granulomas and necrosis are uncommon in SHML.

HEMOPHAGOCYTIC SYNDROMES

A classification of histiocytic disorders, including the hemophagocytic syndromes, has been presented by the Reclassification Working Group of the Histiocyte Society and the World Health Organization Committee on Histiocytic/Reticulum Cell Proliferations.[1] They divided the hemophagocytic syndromes into *primary (familial)* and *secondary hemophagocytic lymphohistiocytoses*. In some reports the term *infection-associated hemophagocytic syndrome* is used for the latter. The clinical, laboratory, and pathologic features of the hemophagocytic syndromes are listed in Box 51-2.

Box 51-2 *Diagnostic Criteria for Hemophagocytic Syndromes*

- Fever >38.5°C lasting ≥7 days
- Splenomegaly
- The following hematologic abnormalities
  - Anemia (hemoglobin <9 g/dL)
  - Thrombocytopenia (<100,000 cells/μL)
- One of the following abnormalities
  - Hypertriglyceridemia (>2 nmol/L)
  - Hypofibrinogenemia (<150 mg/dL)
- Hemophagocytosis in bone marrow, spleen, or lymph node

Adapted from McMahon HE, Bedizel M, Ellis CA. Familial erythrophagocytic lymphohistiocytosis. *Pediatrics*. 1963;32:868; and Henter JI, Samuelsson-Horne A, Arico M, et al. Treatment of hemophagocytic lymphohistiocytosis with HLH-94 immunochemotherapy and bone marrow transplantation. *Blood*. 2002;100:2367.

Familial (Primary) Hemophagoctyic Lymphohistiocytosis

Definition

Familial hemophagocytic lymphohistiocytosis (FHLH) is a systemic syndrome of histiocyte activation manifested by the widespread proliferation of benign macrophages throughout the reticuloendothelial system and extranodal sites; this is associated with florid hemophagocytosis, various systemic symptoms, and peripheral blood cytopenias. This disorder encompasses familial erythrophagocytic lymphohistiocytosis, which was described by McMahon and colleagues[23] in 1963.

Epidemiology

FHLH has an incidence of approximately 1 to 2 per 1 million children.[24] The onset of the disease is before 1 year of age in the majority of cases; however, a few cases have been reported in adolescence or early adulthood.[24,25] The disease occurs in a known familial setting in about 50% of cases and as a sporadic event in about 50%.[24]

Etiology

It is hypothesized that all hemophagocytic syndromes are a manifestation of an immune defect that results in immunologic dysregulation and persistent hypercytokinemia, which triggers T-cell and macrophage activation and the resultant clinical syndrome. In healthy individuals, agents that trigger the immune system, such as infectious organisms or toxins, stimulate the activation of cytotoxic T cells, natural killer (NK) cells, and macrophages, resulting in elimination of the infected cell and termination of the immune response. Cytotoxic T lymphocytes and NK cells eliminate their target by the release of cytolytic granules containing perforin and granzyme. In FHLH, certain gene mutations have been identified that are thought to impair the production, release, or intracellular trafficking of these granules, thereby causing impaired removal of the inciting antigen, sustained immune activation, and high cytokine levels.[25] Mutations in *PFR1* lead to impaired perforin production and are the most common reported mutations in FHLH (30% to 50%).[25] *Munc13D* mutations impair the release of granules and have been reported in up to 30% of cases.[26] A third mutation in *STX11*, which plays a role in intracellular trafficking, was recently identified in a minority of patients mostly of Turkish descent.[25,27] Other mutations that have yet to be identified are also thought to be involved in the pathogenesis of FHLH.

Immunologic studies have illustrated a variety of cellular immune defects in patients with FHLH. These include depressed lymphocyte proliferation, antigenic and mitogenic anergy, and a loss of delayed cutaneous hypersensitivity.[28-30] Plasma from patients with FHLH inhibits the in vitro antigen-induced proliferation of lymphocytes from normal individuals; this inhibitory factor is reduced after plasma exchange. Patients with FHLH may exhibit elevated interferon gamma and tumor necrosis factor levels.[28,31] In patients with perforin deficiency, T- and NK-cell–mediated cytotoxicity is decreased.[32]

Clinical Features

The clinical presentation is characterized by fever, failure to thrive, hepatosplenomegaly, rash, anemia, and thrombocytopenia

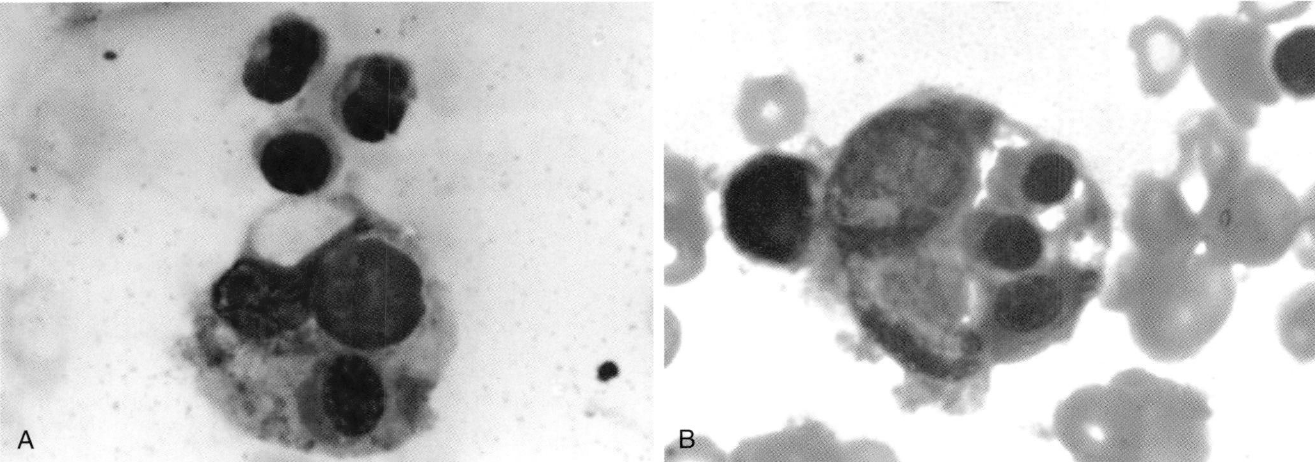

Figure 51-4. Familial hemophagocytic lymphohistiocytosis due to a mutation in the perforin gene. A and B, Bone marrow aspirate smear shows a macrophage demonstrating phagocytosis of a plasma cell and nuclear debris in a patient with primary (familial) hemophagocytic syndrome. (Courtesy of Dr. Nancy Lee Harris; from Lipton JM, Westra S, Haverty CE, et al. Case records of the Massachusetts General Hospital. Weekly clinicopathological exercises. Case 28-2004. *N Engl J Med.* 2004;351:1120.)

(see Box 51-2). Patients may have lymphadenopathy, hepatosplenomegaly and pulmonary, central nervous system, pericardial, and gastrointestinal involvement. Leukopenia and a coagulopathy may be present. Circulating atypical or bizarre-appearing mononuclear cells are often recognized. Liver dysfunction is common, with jaundice and elevated transaminase levels. A common laboratory finding is elevated plasma triglyceride and cholesterol levels. Recently, hyperferritinemia (>500 mcg/L) has been added as a criterion,[32a] and levels >10,000 have been reported to be highly sensitive and specific for the diagnosis of HPS/HLH.[32b] The onset of the syndrome often coincides with the occurrence of a viral infection.[33]

Morphology

Pathologic examination of affected organs shows an infiltration of benign-appearing histiocytes with hemophagocytosis—predominantly red blood cells and neutrophils. Virtually all organs of the reticuloendothelial system are affected, and central nervous system involvement is common.[34] Bone marrow is the tissue most widely used for diagnostic examination, and bone marrow smears may best demonstrate hemophagocytosis (Fig. 51-4). Examination of lymph nodes and spleen may reveal profound generalized lymphoid depletion, with sinusoidal infiltration by hemophagocytic histiocytes.[34] In some patients, a massive infiltration of histiocytes into the lymph node and spleen involves virtually the entire organ.[34] Liver biopsy shows hemophagocytic histiocytes in sinusoids (Fig. 51-5).

Immunophenotype

One study of a small number of cases suggested that the histiocytes of FHLH express a characteristic phenotype exhibiting CD11b, CD21, CD25, CD30, CD35, CD36, and S-100 positivity.[35] A CD14 dim, CD16 bright monocytic population was described in one case—a phenotype associated with macrophages that secrete interleukin (IL)-1β, IL-6, and tumor necrosis factor-α.[36] In individuals with the perforin gene mutation, the perforin protein is absent in $CD8^+$ T cells.[37] Recently, three cases were described in which a small number of circulating and bone marrow $CD8^+$ T cells with an abnormal immunophenotype (reduced CD7 and absent CD5) was revealed by flow cytometry.[38,39]

Genetics

Chromosomal linkage analysis has shown that FHLH is genetically heterogeneous[32,40,41]; in up to 40% of patients, it has been linked to a chromosomal locus and is inherited in an autosomal recessive fashion. A linkage to chromosome 10q21-22 leading to *PFR1* gene mutation is seen in up to 50% of cases.[32,41] *Munc13D* mutations on chromosome 17q25 have been reported in up to 30% of cases.[26] *STX11* gene mutations located on chromosome 6q24 are very rare and so far have been found only in patients of Turkish descent.[27] A linkage to chromosome 9q21.3-22, leading to an unknown gene mutation, has been found in about 10% of cases.[25,32] In indi-

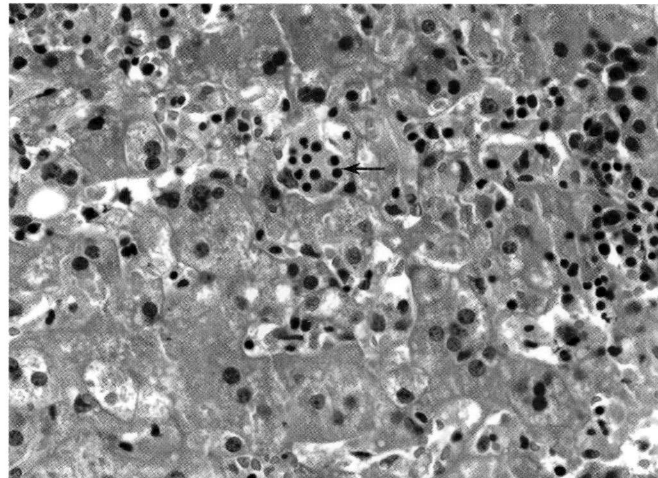

Figure 51-5. Familial hemophagocytic lymphohistiocytosis due to a mutation in the perforin gene. Hemophagocytosis is evident in the liver sinusoids (*arrow*) of a patient with primary (familial) hemophagocytic syndrome. (Courtesy of Dr. Nancy Lee Harris; from Lipton JM, Westra S, Haverty CE, et al. Case records of the Massachusetts General Hospital. Weekly clinicopathological exercises. Case 28-2004. *N Engl J Med.* 2004;351:1120.)

viduals from consanguineous families, the mutations are homozygous, whereas those with sporadic disease may be compound heterozygotes. True heterozygous cases are rare but have been reported.[38,42]

Clinical Course

Most patients with FHLH have a rapid downhill course, and death may occur in weeks to months. Clinical deterioration is characterized by hemorrhage, sepsis, and neurologic impairment.[43] Patients have been treated with chemotherapeutic agents such as etoposide and cyclosporine, the intention being to decrease the number and function of monocytes and lymphocytes.[44] Some patients have responded with reduction in fever, normalization of hematologic indices, and return of the lipid profile to normal.[43-45] The treatment of choice, when feasible, is allogeneic bone marrow transplantation, which may be curative.[46,47]

Secondary Hemophagocytic Syndromes

Definition

Secondary hemophagocytic syndromes (HPSs) are characterized by a systemic proliferation of benign histiocytes with hemophagocytosis. By definition, FHLH is excluded. Owing to its similar clinical and pathologic features, macrophage activation syndrome (MAS) has been integrated into the family of secondary HPSs in the contemporary classification of histiocytic disorders.[48,49] Any MAS that is secondary to malignancy, infection, or rheumatic disease is designated a secondary HPS.[48,49] Synonyms of secondary HPS include *virus-associated hemophagocytic syndrome* and *infection-associated hemophagocytic syndrome*.

Epidemiology

Secondary HPS, although infrequent, is more common than the familial form and can occur at any age. It is often associated with immunodeficiency, immunosuppressive therapy, infection, or underlying malignancy. This syndrome has been observed most often in individuals with underlying immunosuppression, including allograft recipients, patients with leukemia or lymphoma, and those with severe collagen vascular diseases.[8] HPS is often seen in patients with X-linked lymphoproliferative syndrome; about 75% of such patients exhibit the pathologic features of infection-associated HPS.[8] In some cases HPS occurs as an evolution of Chediak-Higashi disease.[50]

Secondary HPS was first recognized in association with primary EBV infection.[51] It can occur with carcinoma, graft-versus-host disease,[52] and virtually any infection. The infectious agents most commonly associated with HPS are viral and include cytomegalovirus,[53] human immunodeficiency virus (HIV),[54] parvovirus,[55] and adenovirus[56]; however, other nonviral agents have been reported, such as clostridial infection,[57] salmonellosis,[58] *Escherichia coli* infection,[59] tuberculosis,[60] malaria,[61] histoplasmosis,[62] and leishmaniasis.[63] Hematologic malignancies, particularly T-cell and NK-cell lymphomas and those that are EBV$^+$, have also been associated with HPS.[64-66]

MAS was originally reported as a rare complication of rheumatic diseases in children. It results in high morbidity and mortality owing to the excessive activation and proliferation of T cells and macrophages. It was first described in 1985 in seven patients with juvenile rheumatoid arthritis who presented with serious systemic complications during the course of their disease.[67] MAS has also been reported in systemic lupus erythematosus,[68] juvenile dermatomyositis,[69] Kawasaki's syndrome,[70] systemic-onset juvenile rheumatoid arthritis,[71,72] and children with Langerhans cell histiocytosis (see Chapter 52).[73]

Etiology

It is thought that immunodeficiency or underlying immunosuppression plays a role in the pathogenesis of HPS. Many of the infectious agents associated with hemophagocytic lymphohistiocytosis (HLH) are potent stimulators of the immune system and require complex interactions of immunoregulatory cells for host recovery. Underlying immunoregulatory disturbances may predispose to an inappropriate antiviral response. As this response progresses, cytokines secreted by activated T lymphocytes elicit the proliferation and activation of histiocytes. It is likely that the activated histiocytes in association with the high cytokine levels are responsible for this syndrome.[62,74]

Clinical Features

HPSs are characterized by fever, myalgias, and malaise. Physical examination reveals hepatosplenomegaly with generalized lymphadenopathy. Laboratory studies commonly demonstrate pancytopenia, abnormal liver function tests, and coagulopathy. The disease course is morbid, and the mortality rate is high.

Morphology

The pathologic features of secondary HPS vary according to the stage of disease when the biopsies are performed.[75,76] Early after the onset of the clinical syndrome, lymph nodes may exhibit an intense immunoblastic proliferative response, resulting in partial effacement of the lymph node architecture, and the number of histiocytes may be low. At this stage, the lymph node histology may be consistent with a viral lymphadenopathy. Later in the disease, lymphoid depletion occurs, and there may be massive sinusoidal infiltration by benign histiocytes, many of them exhibiting erythrophagocytosis (Figs. 51-6 and 51-7). The liver reveals portal infiltrates of lymphocytes, immunoblasts, and histiocytes. Histiocytes, many of which exhibit erythrophagocytosis, are seen in liver sinusoids. The spleen shows atrophy of the white pulp and extensive infiltration by histiocytes, many of which exhibit erythrophagocytosis. The bone marrow biopsy shows variable degrees of histiocytic infiltration, typically with hemophagocytosis. Hemophagocytic histiocytes may be best seen on marrow aspirate smears. Careful evaluation for an associated lymphoma should be performed.[77]

Immunophenotype

Immunologic studies have been reported in only a few patients.[35,75,78] In the majority of studies, EBV was found to be the infectious agent. Atypical lymphocytes, which are the hallmark of acute EBV infection, are absent or diminished, reflecting a decrease in the number of activated CD8$^+$ T cells normally seen in response to EBV. In EBV-associated HPS, CD8$^+$ T cells are infected with EBV; in contrast, CD4$^+$ T cells are infected in chronic EBV infection, and B cells are infected in acute infectious mononucleosis.[79,80]

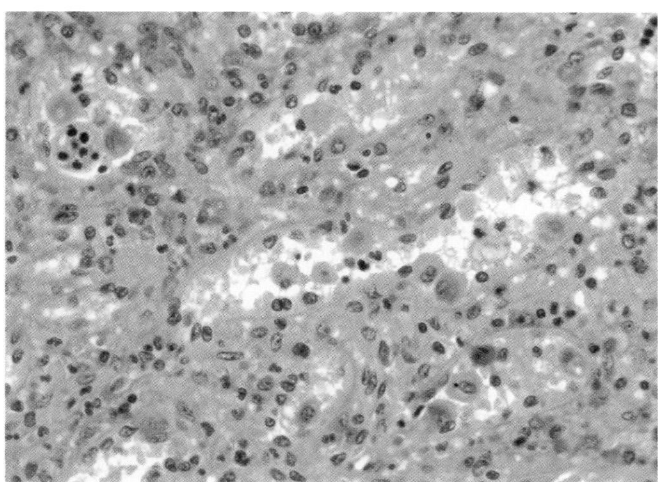

Figure 51-6. Hemophagocytic syndrome. Erythrophagocytosis and lymphophagocytosis are readily apparent in the dilated splenic sinuses of a patient with malignancy-associated hemophagocytic syndrome.

Genetics

There is no known genetic association in the vast majority of cases of secondary HPS. It may be associated with congenital or acquired immunodeficiency, especially the X-linked lymphoproliferative (XLP) syndrome. It has been shown that the genetic defect in XLP maps to chromosome Xq25.[81] The gene (*SH2DIA*) responsible for XLP syndrome has recently been identified and encodes a 128–amino acid protein thought to play a role in signal transduction and activation of T lymphocytes.[81-83] The XLP protein may be involved in regulation of the intense CD8⁺ T-cell cytotoxicity stimulated by acute EBV infection.

Clinical Course

At present, there is no specific treatment for secondary HPS. Immunosuppressive therapy has been used to treat infection-associated HPS that was confused with malignant histiocytosis, with apparently deleterious results.[84] Therefore, patients with symptoms compatible with infection-associated HPS should be thoroughly studied for evidence of infection with EBV, cytomegalovirus, adenovirus, or other viral infections before immunosuppressive therapy is initiated. It has been suggested that in HLH associated with EBV infection, permissive infection may take place in the lymphoreticular tissues. In such cases, a trial of the antiviral agent acyclovir may be beneficial. Treatment of the underlying lymphoma is essential for patients with lymphoma-associated HPS. For individuals without underlying immunodeficiency or lymphoma who survive the acute syndrome, the prognosis is excellent.[85]

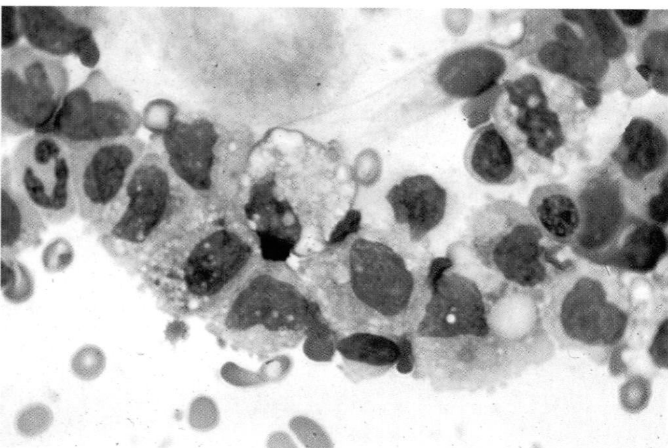

Figure 51-7. Hemophagocytic syndrome. Bone marrow aspirate smear shows histiocytes demonstrating phagocytosis of red blood cells and nuclear debris in a patient with virus-associated hemophagocytic syndrome.

Differential Diagnosis

In patients who exhibit a clinical syndrome consistent with HPS, the preferred diagnostic method is bone marrow biopsy and aspirate. If the marrow is hypocellular and exhibits infiltration by histiocytes, a diagnosis of HPS can be rendered. In patients with lymphadenopathy, a biopsy that exhibits the features of lymphoid depletion associated with histiocytic infiltration and hemophagocytosis is indicative of HPS. It should be noted that increased histiocytes in the bone marrow may be associated with hypercellularity, such as a chronic myeloproliferative disorder or myelodysplastic syndrome, and do not represent HPS. Similarly, reactive lymph nodes may show sinus histiocytosis, with occasional histiocytes exhibiting hemophagocytosis. In the absence of the clinical features of HLH, such a diagnosis should not be proposed.

An important distinction in HPS is that between primary and secondary syndromes. Patients with FHLH typically present in infancy, whereas secondary HPS is recognized in all age groups (Table 51-1). However, approximately 50% of patients with FHLH present as the first proband, and its onset is often associated with a viral infection, making it difficult to distinguish the two types. When a diagnosis of HPS is established, it is essential that a complete genetic history be elicited and a thorough investigation for a viral infection be performed. Analysis of perforin expression and NK-cell function should be undertaken if an acute viral infection is not identified or if the syndrome persists. If perforin expression by T cells is absent or decreased, analysis for the perforin gene mutation or other less common mutations such as *Munc13D* and *STX11* should be performed. If perforin expression is normal, NK-cell function can be used to distinguish FHLH from secondary HPS. NK cells are normal in number, but NK-cell function is absent in familial cases. NK-cell function may be decreased in patients with secondary HPS, but this is associated with a decrease in the number of NK cells and an increase in the number of CD8⁺ T cells.[86] Definitive diagnosis of XLP syndrome can now be accomplished by sequencing of the *SH2DIA* gene.

Because secondary HPS may be associated with an underlying lymphoma or leukemia, a search for a concurrent neoplasm should be conducted. The presence of secondary HPS associated with a T-cell lymphoma may obscure recognition of the lymphoma. Moreover, the identification of hemophagocytosis in a node involved by T-cell lymphoma may suggest a histiocytic neoplasm or malignant histiocytosis. Most cases of the latter reported in the literature are in fact examples of T-cell lymphoma associated with HPS; thus, this diagnosis should be made with great caution, and only after T-cell lymphoma has been excluded.[64] Immunophenotypic analysis,

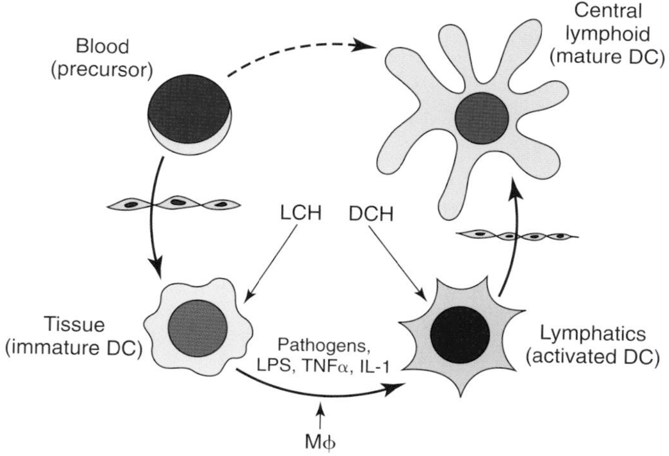

Figure 52-2. Dendritic cell (DC) cycle. Bone marrow precursors circulate in the blood, reaching peripheral sentinel sites. Immature dendritic cells can be activated by a number of stimuli; the stimulated cells migrate centrally to cluster with T cells in central lymphoid paracortex as mature dendritic cells. Langerhans cell histiocytosis (LCH) has the phenotype of the immature tissue DC but retains the capacity to mature to some degree. DCH, dendritic cell histiocytosis (non-Langerhans type, maturing phenotype); IL-1, interleukin-1; LPS, lipopolysaccharide; TNFα, tumor necrosis factor-α.

lesions are the most common manifestation in the newborn, and these may ulcerate. These lesions have been referred to as *congenital* or *self-healing reticulohistiocytosis* or *Hashimoto-Pritzker disease*, but neither term is satisfactory. Hashimoto and Pritzker[31] described solitary congenital reticulohistiocytoma, which is a different condition, and some infants with congenital disease progress or even die of their disease.[32,33] Skin lesions may be unusual, in that the deep dermis is involved but the epidermis is spared, whereas classic LCH has epidermotropism and exocytosis. Congenital Langerhans cell disease of the skin has $CD1a^+$, langerin-positive Langerhans cells with Birbeck granules on electron microscopy. Lesions involute slowly over a few months,[21,34] although recurrent skin or bone involvement and progression to multisystem disease can occur.[12,32,35] Congenital reticulohistiocytoma is included in the differential diagnosis.

Sites Involved in Localized Disease

The sites most commonly involved with single or a few discrete, localized Langerhans cell lesions (single or multiple eosinophilic granulomas) are the bones and adjacent soft tissues, lymph nodes, lungs, thymus, and, rarely, thyroid. Skin is occasionally a solitary site, but it is such an integral part of multisystem disease that it is considered later. Basic

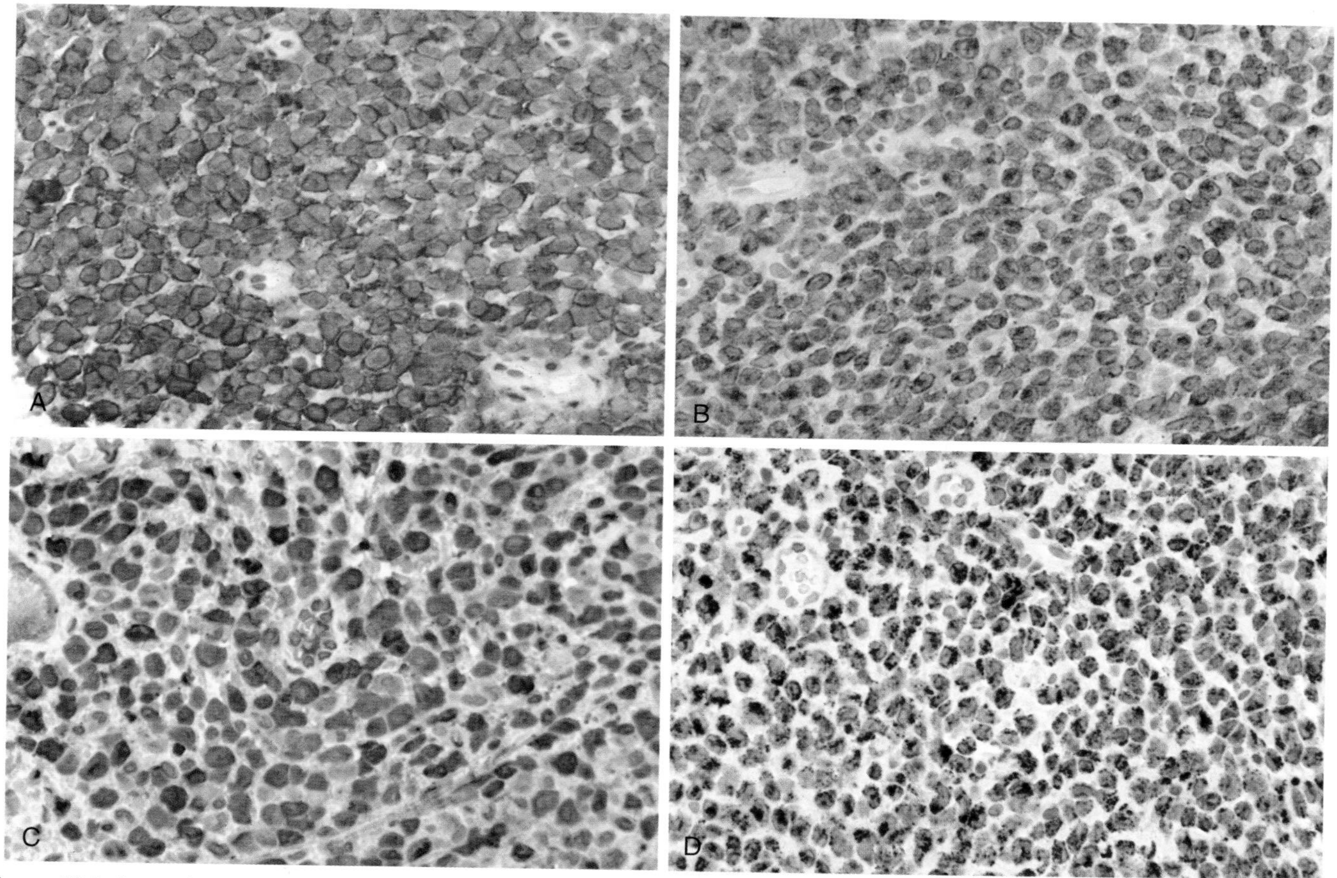

Figure 52-3. Langerhans cell histiocytosis demonstrated in an immature dendritic cell. **A,** Strong surface staining for CD1a (010). **B,** Granular and paranuclear staining for langerin (12D6). **C,** Strong but variable expression of S-100 (polyclonal). **D,** Paranuclear intracytoplasmic dot of HLA-II (LN3).

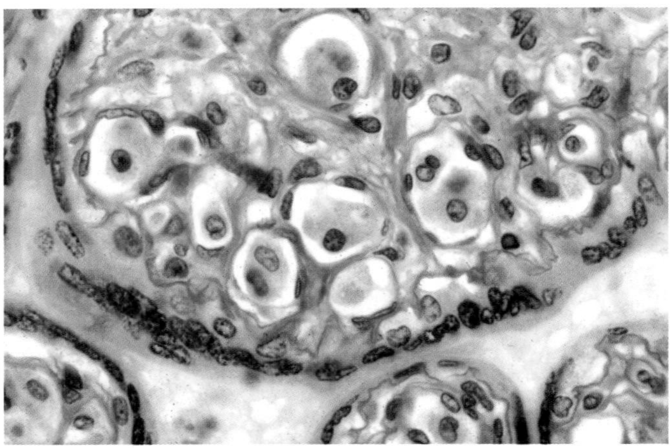

Figure 52-4. Placenta from a stillborn fetus is filled with cells that have features of Langerhans cell histiocytosis. The fetus had foci of autolytic histiocytic cells (periodic acid–Schiff).

diagnostic criteria do not vary by site, although local features can complicate the diagnosis; therefore, these confounders are stressed.

Bone

The skull, especially the calvaria and temporal bones, is the most distinctive site. The vertebrae, jaws, ribs, pelvic bones, and proximal long bones are also typical sites of involvement, but the small bones of the hands and feet are not.[36] Pain at the site is the most common clinical presentation; however, orbital involvement may present with proptosis, and temporal bone lesions may present as chronic otitis or mastoiditis. Vertebral collapse may produce its own clinical presentation, and loose teeth herald jaw involvement.[17]

Plain-film radiographs remain the basic imaging modality for the construction of a differential diagnosis of bone lesions. The lesions are typically lytic and rapidly growing, with poorly defined margins; later or regressing lesions have a more sclerotic rim (Fig. 52-5).[36] Involuting lesions undergo

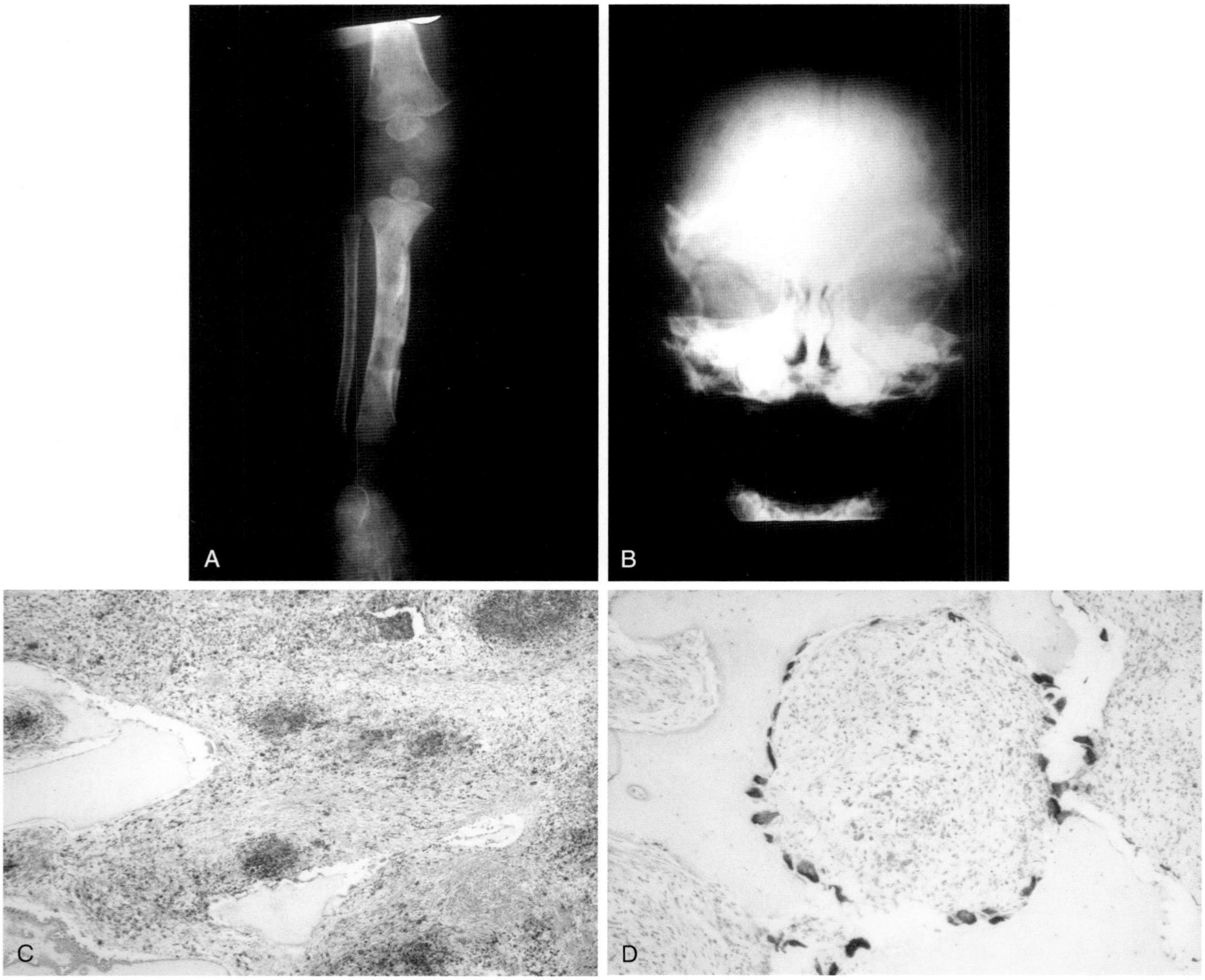

Figure 52-5. Langerhans cell histiocytosis (LCH) in bone. A and **B,** Bones of the lower limb (**A**) and skull (**B**) have numerous osteolytic lesions. **C,** Low-power view reveals the nodular aggregates of LCH cells that do not directly abut the bone (S-100). **D,** Exaggerated osteoclastic activity is most likely responsible for the bone resorption (CD68).

sclerosis and loss of margins and eventually reconstitute completely. Early lesions may raise the possibility of a more aggressive process because the margins may be permeative, and cortical rupture with soft tissue extension is the rule. Later lesions, because of their sclerosis, raise the possibility of lower-grade lesions, most notably chronic osteomyelitis. Specific recommendations for imaging at various sites are given by Meyer and DeCamargo.[36] Whole-body imaging is part of the clinical staging of patients with LCH.

The diagnosis can be made on fine-needle aspiration cytology or biopsy; needle or trephine biopsy; or open biopsy. The classic eosinophilic granuloma has a dominant population of oval cells that are positive for CD1a, langerin, and S-100, with an interspersed population of osteoclast-type giant cells, eosinophils that can vary from sparse to overwhelming, phagocytic macrophages, and T lymphocytes. Necrosis, hemorrhage, or eosinophilic "abscesses" can dominate the picture. CD1a is demonstrable on lesional cells by immunocytology or immunohistology, and care must be taken to ensure that the staining pattern is membranous. S-100 stains the same cells, and S-100$^+$ chondroid elements in the tissue should be no impediment to interpretation. The clinical differential diagnosis in sites such as the skull, long bones, or vertebrae in the early phase includes high-grade lesions, the Ewing's sarcoma family, osteosarcoma, neuroblastoma, tuberculosis, and, rarely and only in children, myofibromatosis. In late and involuting lesions, untangling the differential diagnosis may be more complicated. The LCH cells disappear as lesions involute and may not be demonstrable on biopsy, resulting in failure to confirm the clinical and imaging suspicion. Bone lesions subjected to pathologic fracture, necrosis, or hemorrhage can heal with an extensive xanthomatous macrophage component in which the LCH cells may not be demonstrable, and they may be confused with fibrohistiocytic lesions. Plasma cells, which are rare in uncomplicated LCH, may be seen in late complicated lesions, making the distinction from chronic recurrent multifocal osteomyelitis difficult or impossible. Rosai-Dorfman disease of bone is a rare mimicker, compounded by the fact that the cells are also S-100$^+$ but morphologically distinct. Juvenile xanthogranuloma and the adult counterpart, Erdheim-Chester disease, can affect bone, making the phenotypic differences from LCH important.

Single bone lesions may require only biopsy and pain management, although curettage is widely practiced. Nonsteroidal anti-inflammatory agents are thought to accelerate healing. Symptomatic lesions or those in vulnerable sites have been given low-dose irradiation or intralesional steroid injections.[5,37]

Lymph Node

Lymph nodes can be the only site involved in LCH, or they can be part of a more systemic involvement associated with adjacent bone or skin lesions.[38] The clinical presentation is usually asymptomatic swelling of the nodes, most commonly cervical, inguinal, axillary, mediastinal, or retroperitoneal.[21] Computed tomography or magnetic resonance imaging (MRI) defines the extent of lymph node enlargement, and plain radiographs are used to screen for bone involvement as part of the staging workup.[36]

The diagnosis is established by identifying Langerhans cell histiocytes in the lesions, but lymph nodes provide their own set of confounders. Resected lymph nodes reveal a primarily sinus pattern of involvement in LCH, which is an important diagnostic feature.[38,39] As the disease progresses, there is spillover into the paracortex, sparing the follicles. Complete node replacement effaces most landmarks, although the sinus pattern is still discernible in the nodal medulla. The lesions consist of an almost pure population of LCH cells, but the phenotypic variation mimics the normal maturation, differentiation, and migration of peripheral Langerhans cells. Sinus cells have the phenotypic characteristics of the classic LCH cell, with high expression of surface CD1a and langerin. Paracortical cells, by contrast, lose some of their langerin and CD1a expression, are larger, and acquire high expression of surface HLA-II molecules (Fig. 52-6). A range of intermediate forms between these two can be found. Caution should be exercised when using langerin in place of CD1a because there is an endogenous population of langerin-positive, CD1a$^-$ cells in medullary sinuses.[23]

Eosinophils, macrophages, giant cells, areas of necrosis, and hemosiderin can be present in varying amounts. An occasional lymph node may be so heavily filled with hemosiderin that the underlying LCH involvement is not readily apparent (Fig. 52-7).

There are no histologic features that can predict outcome. The proliferative index of the LCH cells can be very high and ranges from 2% to 48%.[21]

An unusual pattern is replacement of a node by an epithelioid granulomatous process, in which the histiocytes exhibit strong surface expression of CD1a (see Fig. 52-7). This phenomenon has been encountered only in abdominal sites in the absence of LCH elsewhere in the body, and it is not clear whether it actually represents LCH.[38] In multifocal or disseminated LCH there can be an element of macrophage activation or hemophagocytosis, and this macrophage histiocytosis can obscure the LCH.[40]

Diagnosis is made by lymph node biopsy in most instances, and the architectural context permitted by an examination of the entire node is informative. Confirmation is achieved by demonstrating the sinus pattern and LCH cell profile of the lesional cells. The apparent presence of two populations—CD1a$^+$ sinus cells and CD1a$^-$ paracortical cells—has led to some diagnostic confusion. Notably, S-100 stains all LCH cells. Fine-needle aspiration is an acceptable mode of diagnosis if the immunophenotype and cytology of the aspirated cells are typical. Cytology is complicated by the fact that CD1a positivity is present not in all LCH cells but in a varying population, depending on the site, age of the lesion, and possibly other factors. Similarly, langerin is seen in only some lesional cells (Fig. 52-8). Aspiration immunocytology should be interpreted with this in mind, and typical cytology with immunocytologic confirmation is diagnostic if dermatopathic lymphadenopathy is excluded.

Although the differential diagnosis is wide (Table 52-1), in practical terms, it resides between LCH and other histiocyte-rich lesions such as dermatopathic lymphadenopathy (Fig. 52-9), Kikuchi's disease, granulomatous lymphadenopathies (cat-scratch disease and toxoplasmosis in particular), and histiocyte-rich malignant disorders such as the histiocyte-rich variant of anaplastic large cell lymphoma and some T-cell leukemias. The architectural cues provided by lymph node biopsy dispense with most of the confounders. Aspiration cytology requires greater caution.

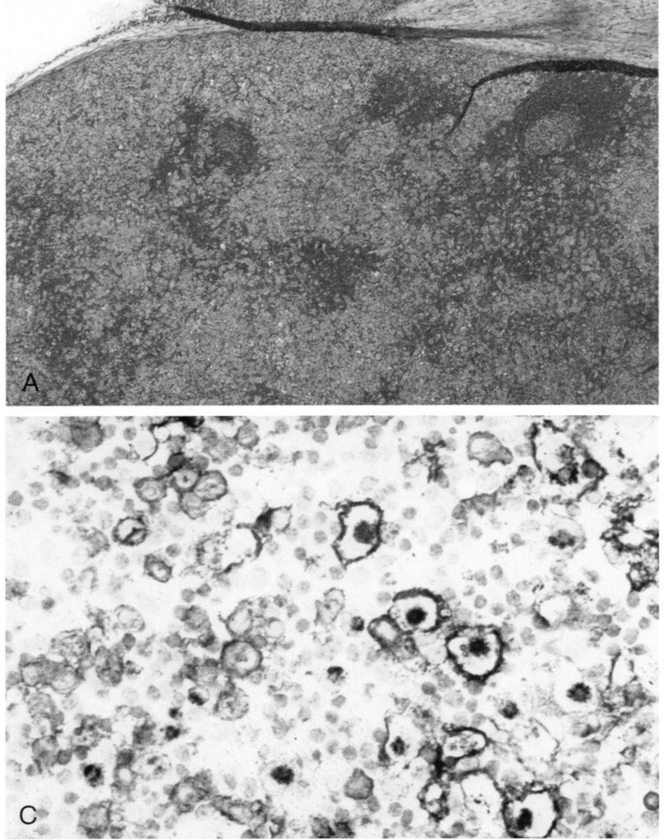

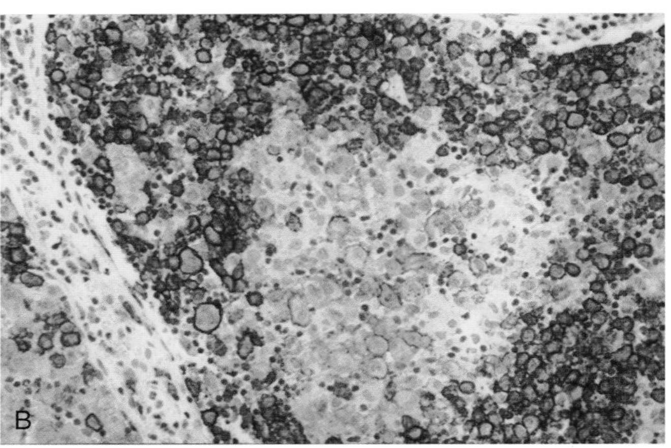

Figure 52-6. Langerhans cell histiocytosis (LCH) in a lymph node. A, The node is largely replaced by LCH cells, sparing the follicles. **B,** The sinus pattern has cells that are strongly $CD1a^+$, and the paracortical LCH involvement exhibits low to absent CD1a. **C,** HLA-II expression on the cell surface of the larger paracortical cell is increased. The cells also have prominent juxtanuclear staining. This mimics the normal migration and maturation of epidermal Langerhans cells, although no dendrites are present and no lymphocyte clustering occurs (LN3).

There are occasional reports of LCH occurring in the same node as a lymphoma. Because none of these patients have LCH elsewhere, either at presentation or at follow-up, the phenomenon is best regarded as focal Langerhans cell hyperplasia rather than LCH.[41,42] Microdissection has shown these lesions to be polyclonal, reinforcing the suggestion that they represent an exaggerated local hyperplasia.[43] Reactive dendritic cell hyperplasia can mimic LCH (see Fig. 52-9). Isolated lymph node involvement with LCH, like isolated disease elsewhere, is self-limited or responds to gentle therapy and regresses without consequence.

Thymus

The thymus can be partially or totally involved with LCH as an isolated site,[44] and it is commonly enlarged in systemic LCH.[45] In common with other thymic infiltrates, such as Hodgkin's disease (its prime differential diagnosis), LCH involvement of the thymus leads to cystic transformation of the organ. Diagnosis is established by identifying LCH cells, mostly medullary, and confirming the phenotype. $CD1a^+$ cortical thymocytes do not present a diagnostic difficulty, given their small size and lack of cytoplasm. Extensive hemorrhage, cystic transformation, necrosis, and xanthomatous response may mask the lesional cells, a point to remember when needle aspiration cytology is the diagnostic procedure. Small clusters of $CD1a^+$ cells in myasthenia gravis and other conditions are not LCH[46] and are best considered further examples of focal Langerhans cell hyperplasia.

Thyroid

The thyroid is not an unusual site of localized LCH.[47] The diagnosis, by aspiration cytology or biopsy, requires the recognition of LCH cells and confirmation of their immunophenotype.[48] The main differential diagnoses are other granulomatous processes that involve the thyroid, none of which should meet the criteria for the diagnosis of LCH. Increased numbers of reactive (dendritic) Langerhans cells are reported in papillary carcinomas of the thyroid, and this should be borne in mind when attempting a cytologic diagnosis.

Lung

The lung can be involved in disseminated multivisceral LCH in young children, but adult-type pulmonary LCH is far more common and is usually a single-organ phenomenon. Most patients with pulmonary LCH (>90%) are smokers,[49] and smoking is known to increase the number of Langerhans cells in the lungs of normal subjects.[50] Smoking can rapidly reinduce LCH in adults who had LCH in childhood.[51]

The incidence of LCH in the lung is unknown but rare, and no genetic associations are known. Supporting the suggestion that Langerhans cell proliferation is a reactive phenomenon in smokers is evidence that the lesions appear to be largely nonclonal.[28]

Clinical presentation can include a nonproductive cough or dyspnea, although many patients are asymptomatic; one third or less present with constitutional symptoms.[49] A chest radiograph reveals micronodular or reticulonodular

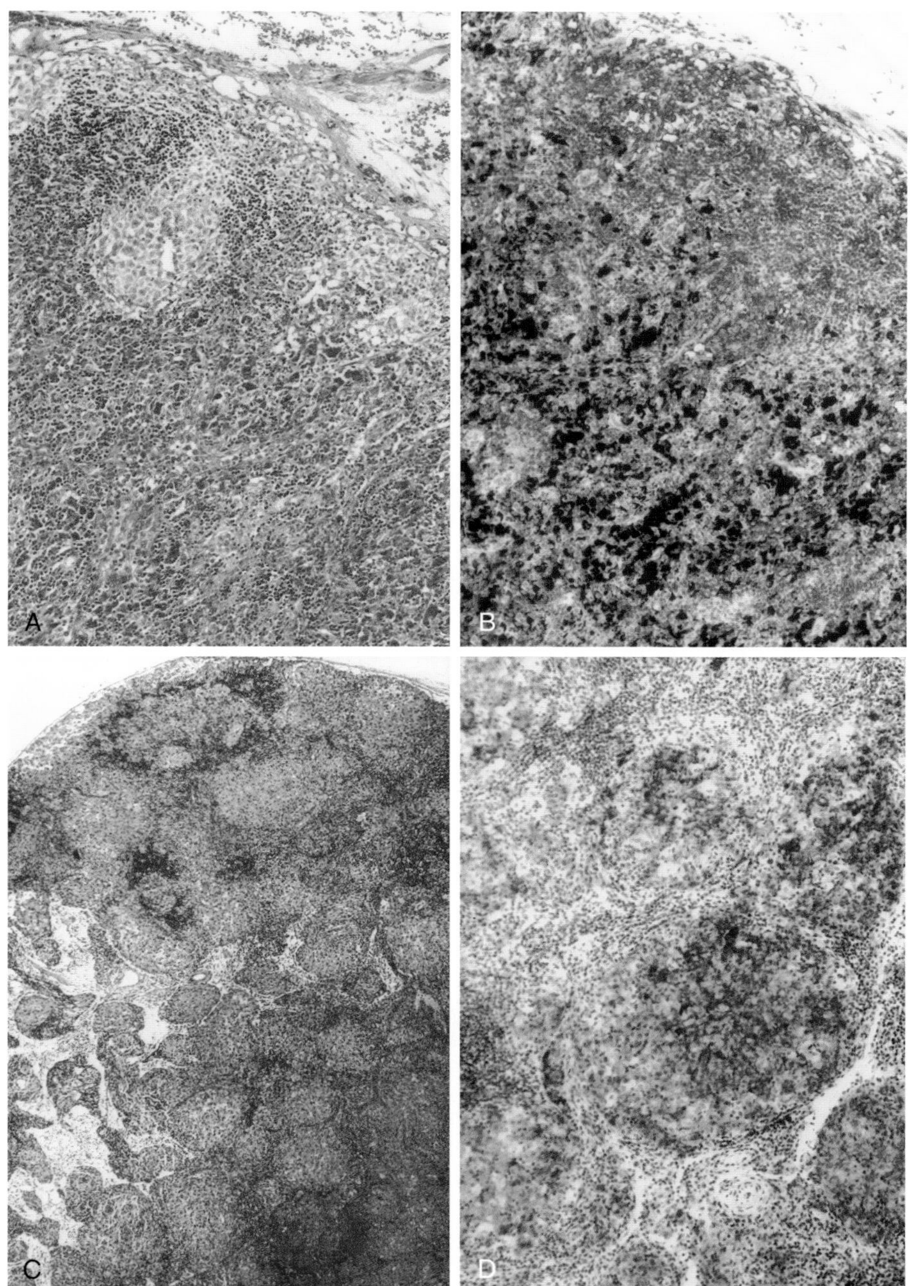

Figure 52-7. Langerhans cell histiocytosis (LCH) in a lymph node. A, Massive hemosiderosis obscures the LCH. **B**, CD1a staining of the sinusoidal LCH cells can still be demonstrated, however (CD1a, amino ethyl-carbazole (AEC) with hemosiderin counterstain). **C**, An unusual epithelioid granulomatous pattern is occasionally noted in abdominal lymph nodes. This probably does not represent LCH. **D**, Histiocytes stain intensely for CD1a.

interstitial infiltrates, mostly in the middle and upper lobes, that are bilateral and symmetric. Cystic changes may supervene or even dominate.[48] High-resolution computed tomography is very sensitive in demonstrating the nodular and cystic changes.[52]

Staging may reveal lung involvement to be the sole site; however, other lesions, especially bone lesions, may be present in adults. In children, pulmonary involvement is seen almost exclusively as part of disseminated disease. In patients with documented disease at other sites, the diagnosis can be inferred from the typical findings on high-resolution computed tomography.[52]

Immunocytology of a bronchoalveolar lavage specimen can be used in conjunction with typical radiographic features. Although Langerhans cells are a prominent component of many interstitial and some neoplastic pulmonary processes, a bronchoalveolar lavage specimen with greater than 5% CD1a$^+$ large cells is strongly suggestive of LCH in the appropriate setting in children[53] but not in adults, in whom the sensitivity is low.[54]

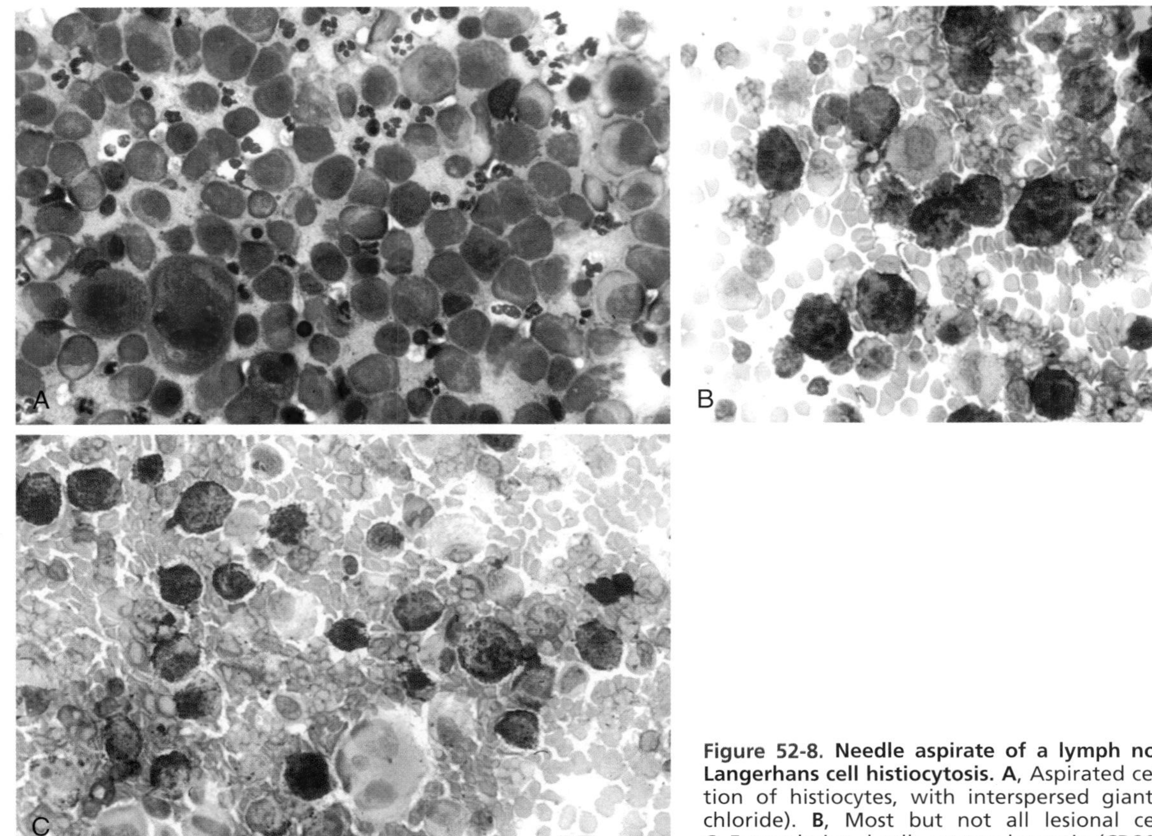

Figure 52-8. Needle aspirate of a lymph node involved with Langerhans cell histiocytosis. A, Aspirated cells show a population of histiocytes, with interspersed giant cells (pinacyanol chloride). **B**, Most but not all lesional cells express CD1a. **C**, Fewer lesional cells express langerin (CD207).

Table 52-1 Differential Diagnosis of Langerhans Cell Histiocytosis

Site	Conditions	Distinguishing Features
Skin	Langerhans cell hyperplasia, many dermatologic conditions	Perivascular distribution of dendritic-shaped cells, CD1a$^+$, langerin negative
	Non-Langerhans dendritic cell lesions (indeterminate cell, immature dendritic cell)	CD1a$^+$, lacks Birbeck granules
	Dendritic cell histioma (mature)	CD1a$^-$, CD68$^+$, MHC class II high, fascin high, S-100$^+$
	Juvenile xanthogranuloma family	S-100$^-$, factor XIIIa positive, fascin high
	Reticulohistiocytoma	Large cells, PAS$^+$, CD68$^+$, CD1a$^-$, S-100$^-$
	Rosai-Dorfman disease	Large cells, emperipolesis CD1a$^-$, S-100$^+$, fascin high, CD68$^+$
Lymph node	Dendritic cell hyperplasias Dermatopathic lymphadenopathy	No sinus involvement, fascin high, patchy CD1a$^+$
	Macrophage histiocytosis Sinus histiocytosis	CD1a$^-$, fascin positive, CD68$^+$
	Histiocyte-rich lymphomas T-cell and anaplastic large cell lymphomas	CD68$^+$ (vacuolar), S-100$^-$, no CD1a, identification of a specific lymphoma
Bone and soft tissue	Chronic relapsing osteomyelitis, benign fibroxanthomatous lesions	Plasma cells, CD1a$^-$, lack of other LCH lesions
Brain	Cytoplasm-rich space-occupying lesions, including rhabdoid tumors	CD1a$^-$, no Birbeck granules, other neural or stromal proteins

LCH, Langerhans cell histiocytosis; MHC, major histocompatibility complex; PAS, periodic acid–Schiff.

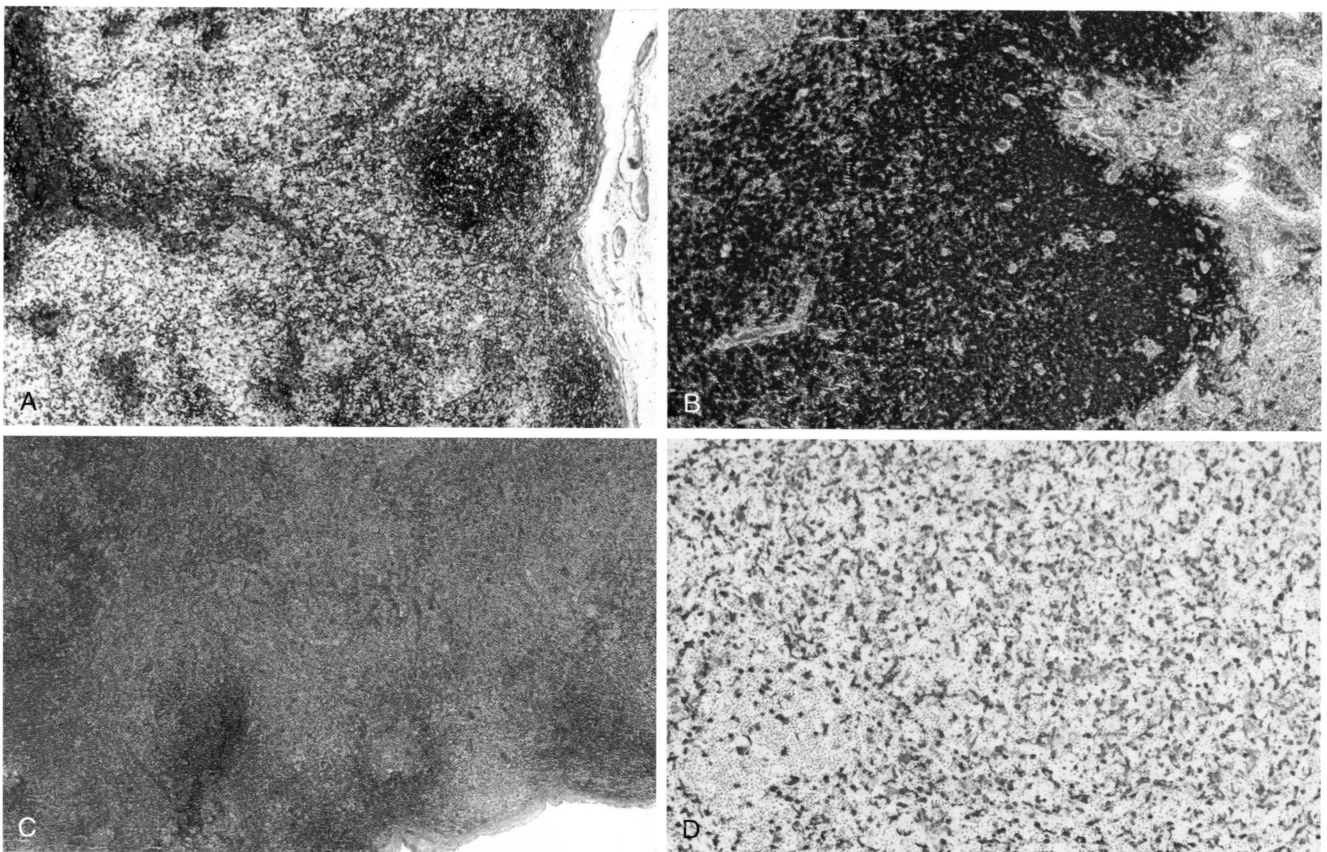

Figure 52-9. Lymph nodes simulating Langerhans cell histiocytosis (LCH). A, Paracortical expansion in a lymph node draining an area of dermal LCH raises the possibility of dermatopathic lymphadenopathy versus LCH involvement. **B,** Fascin staining and the lack of a sinus component indicate that this is dermatopathic lymphadenopathy, not LCH. **C,** Lymph node with striking dendritic cell hyperplasia. The node was found to harbor a T-cell leukemia. **D,** S-100 highlights the massive dendritic cell hyperplasia, simulating LCH.

Transbronchial biopsy is of limited value owing to the patchy nature of the condition; thoracoscopic or open biopsy is more likely to yield diagnostic tissue.[49] CD1a and langerin staining of the lesional oval cells is sensitive and specific at this site, given that reactive Langerhans cells in the airways are smaller and dendritic. Sholl and colleagues[24] documented 6 CDla$^+$, langerin-positive cells per high-power field (HPF) in the adult lung, 14 per HPF in interstitial pneumonia, and more than 30 per HPF in adult lungs with LCH, with more than 100 from intralesional sites. The major differential diagnostic considerations once the clinical and radiographic features have been determined are sarcoidosis and hypersensitivity pneumonitis in adults, which do not have an accumulation of CD1a$^+$ cells.

Pulmonary lesions are strictly bronchocentric, with intervening normal lung (Fig. 52-10). Macrophages, especially alveolar macrophages, can accumulate and obscure the Langerhans cells. Eosinophils, lymphocytes, and, rarely, plasma cells may contribute to the nodules. Centrifugal fibrosis produces a stellate nodule with cystic changes peripheral to the nodule as the disease progresses. Once the disease is advanced, with fibrosis and honeycombing, Langerhans cells may no longer be visible, and the distinction from other causes of honeycombing may be lost.[55]

Pneumothorax from ruptured bullae can occur and provoke an eosinophilic response, regardless of the cause of the pneumothorax; thus, documentation of LCH cells is still required for confirmation, unless they have been previously demonstrated.[56]

Cessation of smoking is the mainstay of treatment in adults, with corticosteroids and then chemotherapeutic agents for progressive disease.[49] Lung transplantation has been used for advanced disease, and recurrence has been reported.[57]

Sites Involved in Disseminated Disease

Skin

Skin may be the only site of Langerhans cell disease, or it may be part of more widespread involvement; skin involvement is present in half of all patients with LCH.[34] An earlier suggestion that loss of E-cadherin on LCH cells could distinguish between systemic and localized disease has not been confirmed prospectively.[58] However, it has been suggested that the LCH cells of congenital self-limited disease and of isolated cutaneous disease have a more mature dendritic cell phenotype, being CD83$^+$ and CD86$^+$, in contrast to other forms of LCH.[29]

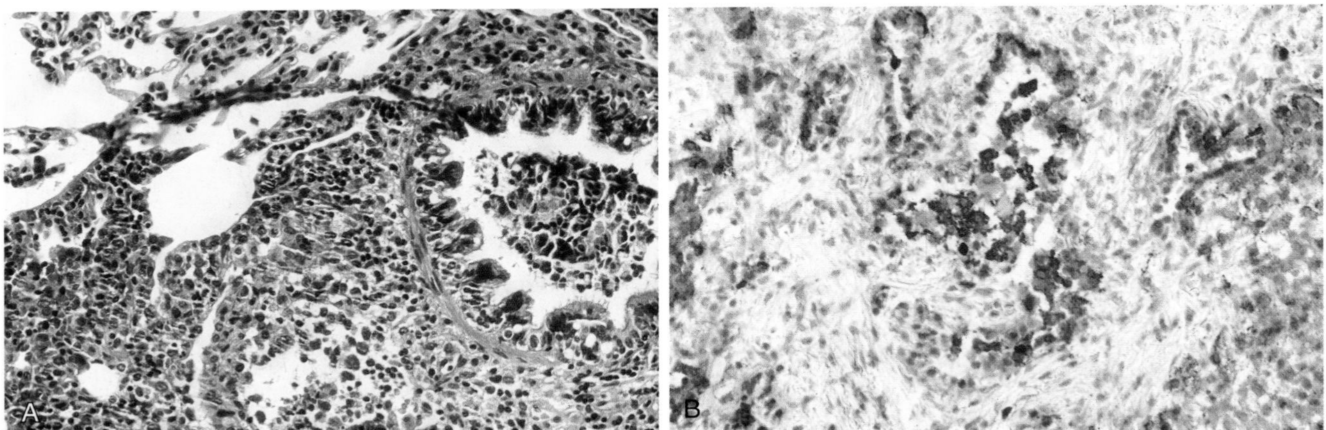

Figure 52-10. Langerhans cell histiocytosis (LCH) in the lung. A, LCH cells aggregate around and infiltrate the bronchi. **B,** CD1a staining reveals the LCH accumulation (frozen tissue).

In children the common sites of involvement are the scalp, flexural folds, and diaper area; petechiae are characteristic. Seborrheic dermatitis, dermatophytes, and diaper rash are the usual differential diagnoses. Lesions may ulcerate.

An overriding consideration in the differential diagnosis is that Langerhans cells normally reside in the epidermis, and large numbers of CD1a^{+} but langerin-negative cells may be present in the perivascular superficial dermis as a reactive phenomenon in many dermatitides (see Table 52-1).[59] Histiocyte-rich lesions in some patients with immune deficiencies such as Omenn's syndrome may be especially rich in CD1a^{+} but langerin-negative dendritic cells. These normal CD1a^{+} cells are dendritic in shape; the cells of LCH are not. If ultrastructural demonstration of a Langerhans cell granule is the method used to confirm the diagnosis, the Birbeck granule must be in a lesional cell, not in an intervening normal Langerhans cell. The disorder is epidermotropic, with cells filling the upper dermis, especially the papillary dermis, and infiltrating the epidermis. Parakeratosis, accumulation of neutrophils in the epidermis, ulceration, and secondary infection can complicate the diagnosis. LCH cells are seen in active lesions; they are large cells occurring in the context of a mixed infiltrate of T lymphocytes, eosinophils, and macrophages, but multinucleated cells are unusual. The density of the mixed infiltrate may mask the LCH cells. The diagnosis is confirmed by demonstrating staining for CD1a in a membrane pattern in the population of large oval cells (Fig. 52-11). S-100 stains the same cells but in the skin the presence of nevus cells can

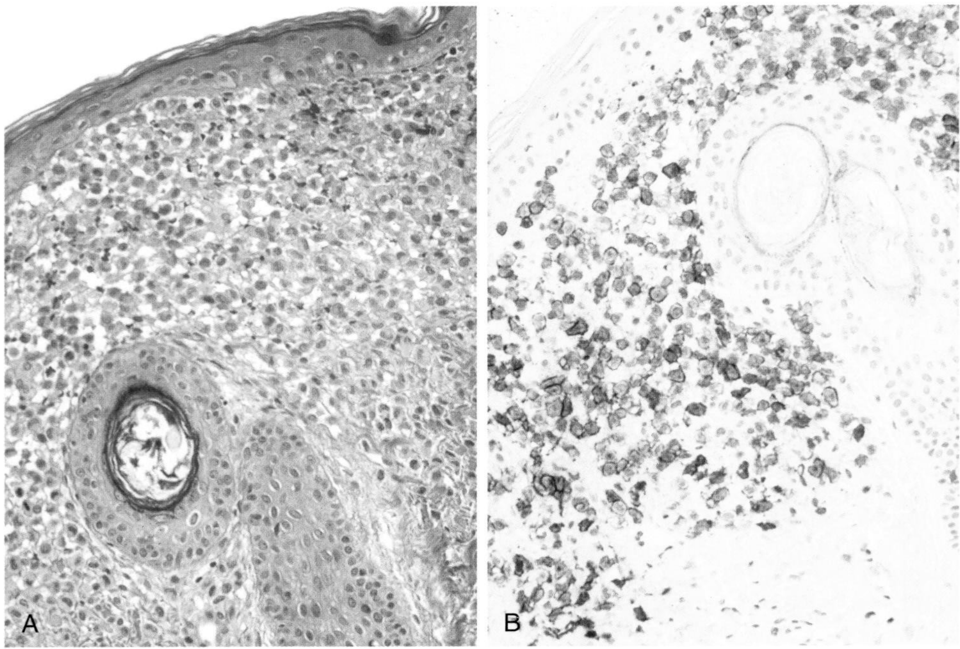

Figure 52-11. Langerhans cell histiocytosis in the skin. A, Skin involvement is epidermotropic, filling the papillary dermis. **B,** CD1a immunostain confirms the diagnosis.

be a confounding finding. Staining for langerin carries the same diagnostic specificity as demonstration of CD1a or the Birbeck granule. By convention, dendritic cell infiltrates that are CD1a⁺ but lack Birbeck granules (and, presumably, langerin) have been called *indeterminate cell lesions*, but sampling may contribute to their indeterminate nature, and more detailed phenotyping is required.

As later lesions resolve, they have more macrophages, some of which are xanthomatous, and the diagnostic LCH cells may be sparse or even absent. In these circumstances, distinction from other inflammatory lesions or juvenile xanthogranuloma may be difficult or impossible.

Liver

It is rare for the liver to be the sole site of involvement in LCH, but it is involved in an undetermined number of children with multivisceral LCH.[60] In early cases of disseminated disease there may be transient hepatomegaly and hypoalbuminemia, but biopsy at this stage may yield only a picture of macrophage activation.[61]

Liver involvement with LCH presents as silent progression to cholestasis.[62] LCH has a peculiar tropism for the larger bile ducts, and this can be demonstrated on imaging, where biliary stenoses and dilations are accompanied by peribiliary changes (Fig. 52-12). Enlarged hilar nodes may also be demonstrable.[36] Features of sclerosing cholangitis appear and commonly progress to biliary cirrhosis. Intrahepatic involvement is usually portal and associated with bile duct involvement, but in advanced disease, lobular infiltration may occur.[21] Because the disease is focal in nature, biopsy often highlights only the upstream effects of sclerosing cholangitis without revealing the LCH, but the features of small duct involvement are subtle and require immunostaining for S-100, CD1a, or langerin. In cases of isolated hepatic disease, the diagnosis must be made by demonstrating LCH and confirming the phenotype of the LCH cell using CD1a. In disseminated disease, hepatomegaly should not be assumed to be liver involvement; however, if features of sclerosing cholangitis are present, along with raised levels of γ-glutamyltransferase or bilirubin, LCH involvement can be inferred. As at other sites, Langerhans cell disease involutes to leave scar, and in the cirrhotic phase of sclerosing cholangitis, LCH cells may no longer be demonstrable.[60] Recurrence after liver transplantation has been documented,[63] as has a case of systemic LCH after living donor transplantation.[64]

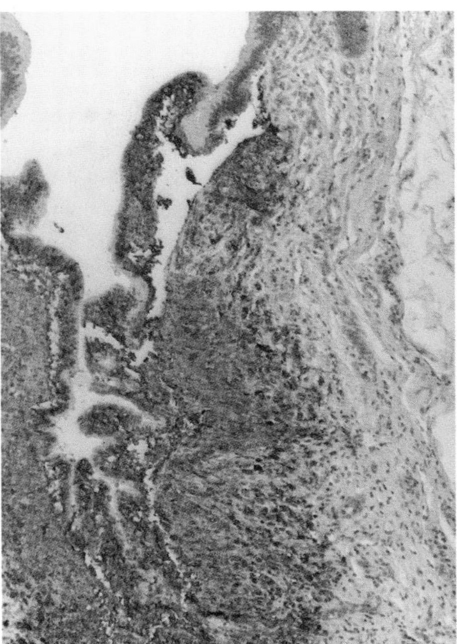

Figure 52-12. Langerhans cell histiocytosis in the bile duct. The infiltrate destroys the biliary epithelium and the bile duct, resulting in sclerosing cholangiopathy (CD1a).

Bone Marrow

Patients with disseminated LCH may be anemic or even pancytopenic, and this has been attributed to marrow involvement. Pancytopenia is not due to massive LCH infiltration or myelofibrosis; rather, examination of aspirates using immunocytochemistry for CD1a and CD68 reveals that only some patients with cytopenia have demonstrable LCH infiltration.[65] When present, LCH cells are oval and occur in groups or clusters in the marrow[66]; they can be stained after decalcification or fixation in B5-type fixatives (e.g., B-plus) using the O10 antibody to CD1a (Fig. 52-13) and langerin. CD1a is not demonstrable by immunohistochemistry in the normal marrow, although a few cells (<0.5%) are detected by flow cytometry.[65] S-100 staining alone is not acceptable in the marrow because reactive S-100⁺ spindle and dendritic cells and activated macrophages may also stain.[21] Macrophage activation syndrome and frank hemophagocytic syndrome are not uncommon in children who have disseminated LCH, and the marrow can be filled with CD68⁺ and CD163⁺ macrophages, even in the absence of LCH cell infiltration.[40] The same features can be seen in the marrow after treatment for LCH. Treated and untreated marrow can be replaced by sheets of foamy macrophages and disrupted by stromal fibrosis. Hemosiderosis may be overwhelming, obscuring any residual LCH cells.

Central Nervous System

Central nervous system (CNS) involvement is dominated by the endocrine effects of hypothalamic and posterior pituitary involvement, but a wide variety of signs and symptoms can be due to mass or degenerative effects. The advent of MRI has led to a major reevaluation of the incidence and type of CNS lesions.[67-69] The incidence of CNS involvement is 1% to 3% of all patients with LCH, but the incidence of diabetes insipidus with posterior pituitary disease can be as high as 12%.[70,71] Risk factors have been identified for CNS disease. There are no age or sex differences in patients with or without CNS involvement, but the presence of multisystem disease elsewhere and skull lesions of the temporal and orbital bones with intracranial extension are associated with a higher risk of CNS disease.[71]

Three broad types of CNS involvement are described: hypothalamic-pituitary, space occupying, and neurodegenerative.[68,69] Hypothalamic-pituitary involvement is most common, but MRI reveals an unexpectedly high incidence of involvement of the pineal gland as well. Diabetes insipidus can precede or follow other manifestations of LCH,[70] and once established, it is rarely reversible.[72] Other hypothalamic or pituitary effects, such as growth hormone and thyroid-stimulating hormone deficiency, can occur.[73] Damage to the

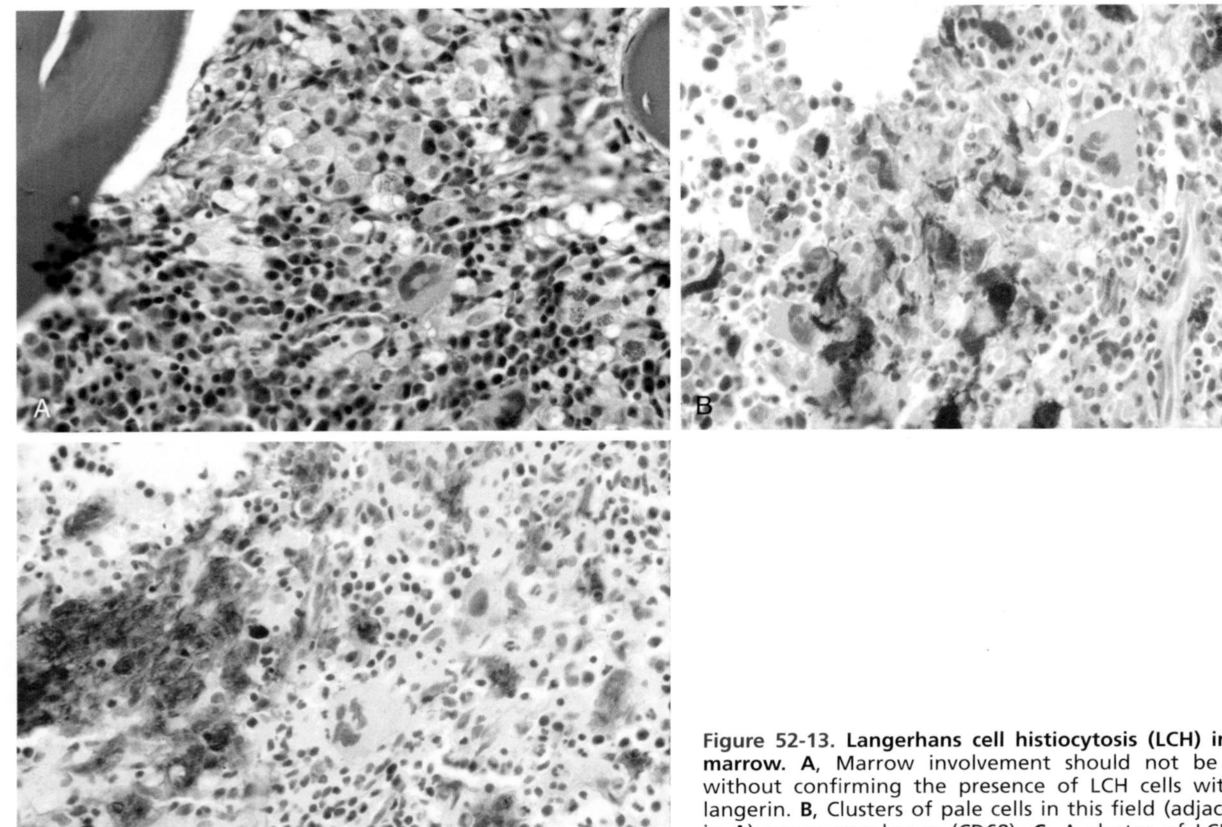

Figure 52-13. Langerhans cell histiocytosis (LCH) in the bone marrow. A, Marrow involvement should not be diagnosed without confirming the presence of LCH cells with CD1a or langerin. **B,** Clusters of pale cells in this field (adjacent to that in **A**) are macrophages (CD68). **C,** A cluster of LCH cells was found elsewhere in the marrow (CD1a).

area is due to direct infiltration with LCH cells that are CD1a reactive and S-100⁺, although there may be an inflammatory component rich in T cells as well.

Space-occupying lesions can be intracerebral, in the meninges, or in the choroid plexus.[68] Disease confined to the brain is unusual, and isolated brain involvement is frontal or temporal.[74] Intracerebral lesions may be difficult to diagnose because of the paucity of classic LCH cells and the relative exuberance of the inflammatory, macrophage, and astroglial component.[21] Early, fresh lesions are more likely to contain CD1a⁺ LCH cells. Space-occupying lesions that involve the meninges or choroid plexus are characterized by a striking xanthomatous macrophage response, and at the time of surgery or biopsy, a fibroxanthoma or juvenile xanthogranuloma may be suspected (Fig. 52-14). In contrast to juvenile xanthogranuloma, the xanthomatous cells do not demonstrate factor XIIIa staining. LCH cells may not be detectable, and LCH involvement may have to be inferred from the presence of documented disease elsewhere.[21]

The third type of CNS involvement is the occurrence of neurodegenerative lesions, often years after the diagnosis of LCH. About 2% to 3% of LCH patients develop cerebellar symptoms. MRI shows signal alterations that simulate multisystem atrophy and involve the cerebellum bilaterally, including dentate nuclei and basal ganglia. These lesions do not contain LCH cells but exhibit demyelination, neuronal and axonal degeneration, edema, and an inflammatory component rich in T cells like those seen in paraneoplastic lesions (see Fig. 52-14).[69] There is thus no merit in trying to biopsy lesions of this kind to document LCH involvement.

Gastrointestinal Tract

The gastrointestinal tract is most commonly involved as part of disseminated disease, but it may also be a presenting site.[75,76] Usually the lamina propria is involved, with only minor changes in glandular structure; characteristically, the superficial lamina propria, under the surface epithelium, is loaded with LCH cells (Fig. 52-15). Depending on the major site of involvement, symptoms may vary, but mass lesions in the stomach may cause obstruction.[77] Diffuse large and small bowel disease can lead to diarrhea and protein-losing enteropathy.[78] Diagnosis is by demonstrating the LCH cell nature of the pale histiocytes, which are CD1a⁺ and S-100⁺.[21,79]

Spleen

The spleen is involved in disseminated LCH, but splenomegaly alone is not sufficient grounds for diagnosis because it may be due to macrophage activation with hemophagocytosis, even in the absence of LCH. Documentation of LCH in the spleen requires the demonstration of LCH cells (CD1a⁺) by splenectomy or splenic puncture-aspiration. Phenotypic confirmation is absolutely required because both LCH and

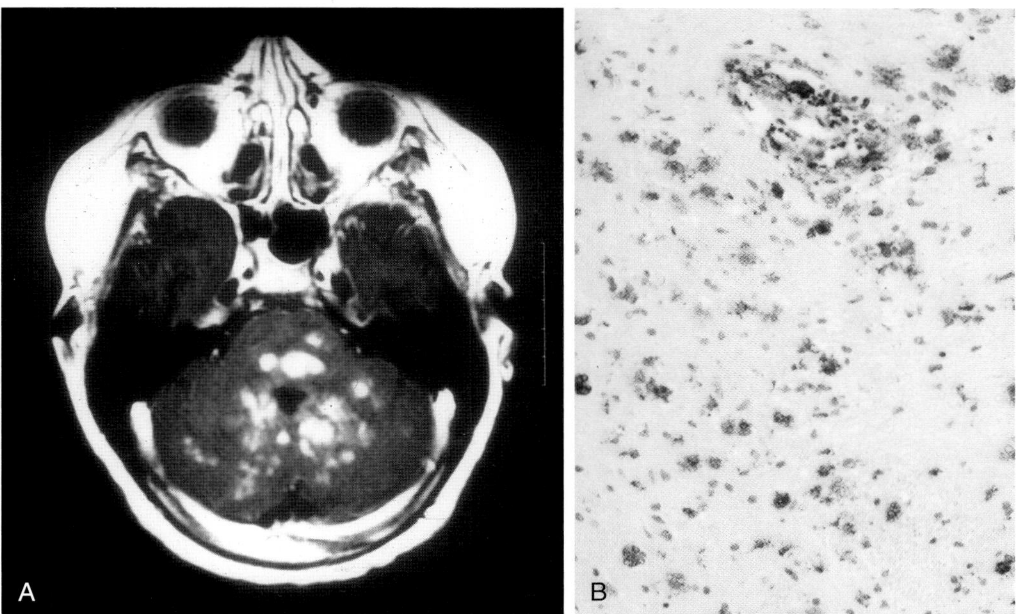

Figure 52-14. Langerhans cell histiocytosis (LCH) in the brain. A, Computed tomography scan of a child with LCH and cerebellar lesions. The lesions are inflammatory, with T cells and destruction of white matter, but LCH cells are not present. **B**, The phagocytic macrophage response is highlighted (CD68).

macrophage histiocytoses coexist and cannot be reliably distinguished without it (Fig. 52-16).

Langerhans Cell Disease and Macrophage Activation

As already noted with respect to LCH involvement of the bone marrow and spleen, a vigorous macrophage response occurs at some sites. Langerhans cell disease, especially multifocal and disseminated disease, can be accompanied by varying degrees of macrophage activation.[40] The extreme form is a full-blown secondary hemophagocytic syndrome. In its milder manifestations, a generalized increase in the size and state of activation of macrophages may be seen throughout the body. Hepatomegaly that is subjected to biopsy may show enlarged, prominent, even phagocytic Kupffer cells. The

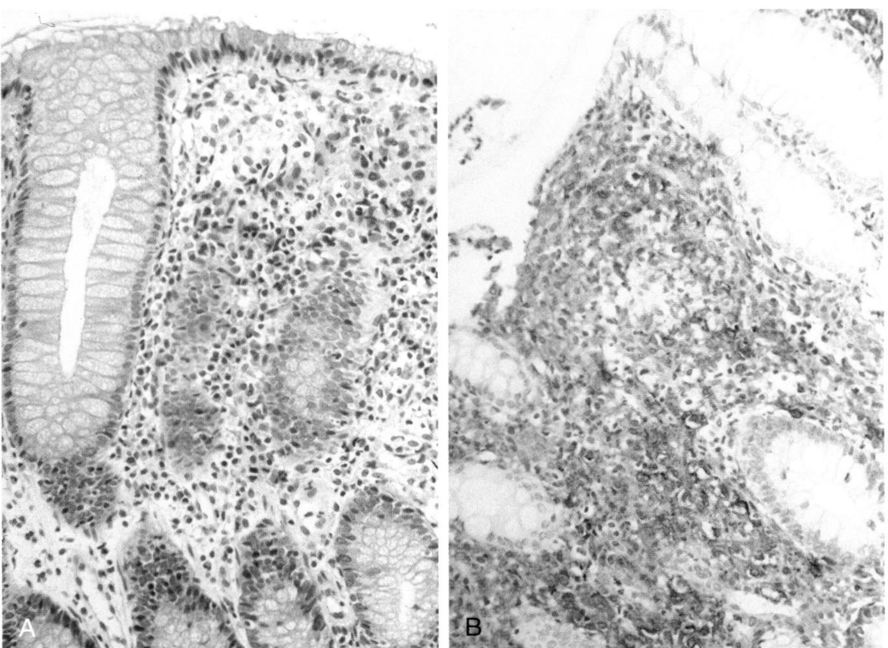

Figure 52-15. Langerhans cell histiocytosis in the gastrointestinal tract. A, The colonic lamina propria contains pale histiocytes in a child with widespread disease. **B**, S-100 immunostain confirms the identity of the histiocytes.

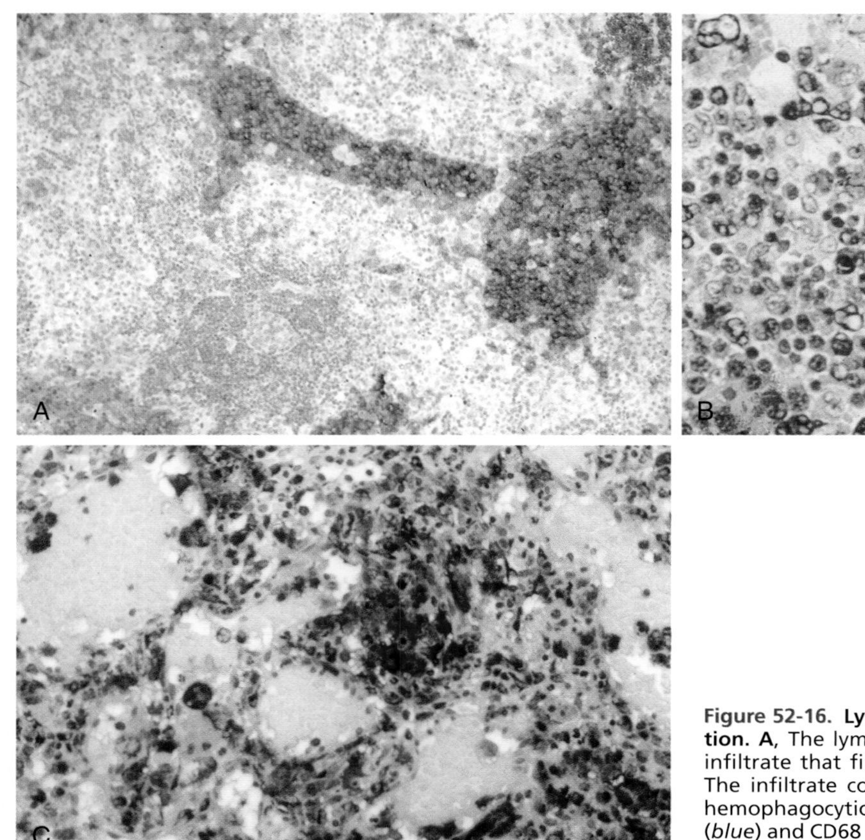

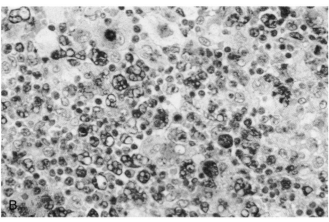

Figure 52-16. Lymph node and spleen with macrophage activation. A, The lymph node has CD1a+ cells in the sinuses, but an infiltrate that fills the rest of the node is unstained (CD1a). **B,** The infiltrate consists mostly of macrophages, phagocytic and hemophagocytic (CD68). **C,** Spleen, double stained for CD1a (*blue*) and CD68 (*brown*), reveals clusters of LCH cells and phagocytic macrophage histiocytes.

spleen, lymph nodes, and especially bone marrow may exhibit a prominent increase in the number of macrophages that obscures LCH, when present, or leads to misdiagnosis when LCH cells are absent. In the hemophagocytic syndrome associated with disseminated LCH, organomegaly and pancytopenia may be due to infiltration of hemophagocytic macrophages in the presence or absence of LCH cells at that site (see Fig. 52-16).[38] It is not clear whether the macrophages are reacting to cytokines produced by the LCH or whether some of them actually derive from the same precursors as the LCH cells.

MALIGNANT LANGERHANS CELL DISEASE AND LANGERHANS CELL SARCOMA

There appear to be three forms of malignant disease characterized by cells with a Langerhans cell phenotype:

1. Transition from LCH to sarcoma. Only rare examples exist, almost all in adults. The clinical and histopathologic onset of LCH is followed by recurrences with increasingly bizarre or anaplastic cells (which retain the CD1a phenotype) and atypical mitoses, eventuating in a frank sarcoma that may retain or lose CD1a positivity (Fig. 52-17).[80]
2. Langerhans cell disease with atypical (aggressive) clinical behavior. This has been described after acute T-cell lymphoblastic leukemia, and both the leukemia and the subsequent LCH showed evidence of clonality by virtue of an identical T-cell receptor gamma gene rearrangement.[81] CD56 positivity has been recorded in some cases,[82] and this may help identify LCH with aggressive clinical behavior.
3. Primary Langerhans cell sarcoma. Confined almost entirely to adults, this malignant and metastasizing tumor is not preceded or accompanied by LCH. Widespread tumefaction, metastases, and poor outcome in 50% of patients have been documented.[80-86] The lesions are cytologically malignant, with pleomorphism and atypical mitoses, but retain their Langerhans cell phenotype of CD1a, S-100, and langerin positivity, although staining may be less uniform than for LCH (see Fig. 52-17).

Dermal and soft tissue sarcomas with Langerhans cell features may occur in patients with monocytic leukemias or myeloproliferative syndromes. Rarely, a deep dermal or subcutaneous nodular mass occurs in adults; histiocytes are present, sometimes around a zone of central necrosis, as well as CD1a+ cells. This is not LCH but appears to be a cutaneous manifestation of a monocytic leukemia or myelodysplastic syndrome, with Langerhans cell maturation in the dermal deposits (see Fig. 52-17). This is different from the well-described occurrence of leukemia following etoposide therapy for LCH.[87-90]

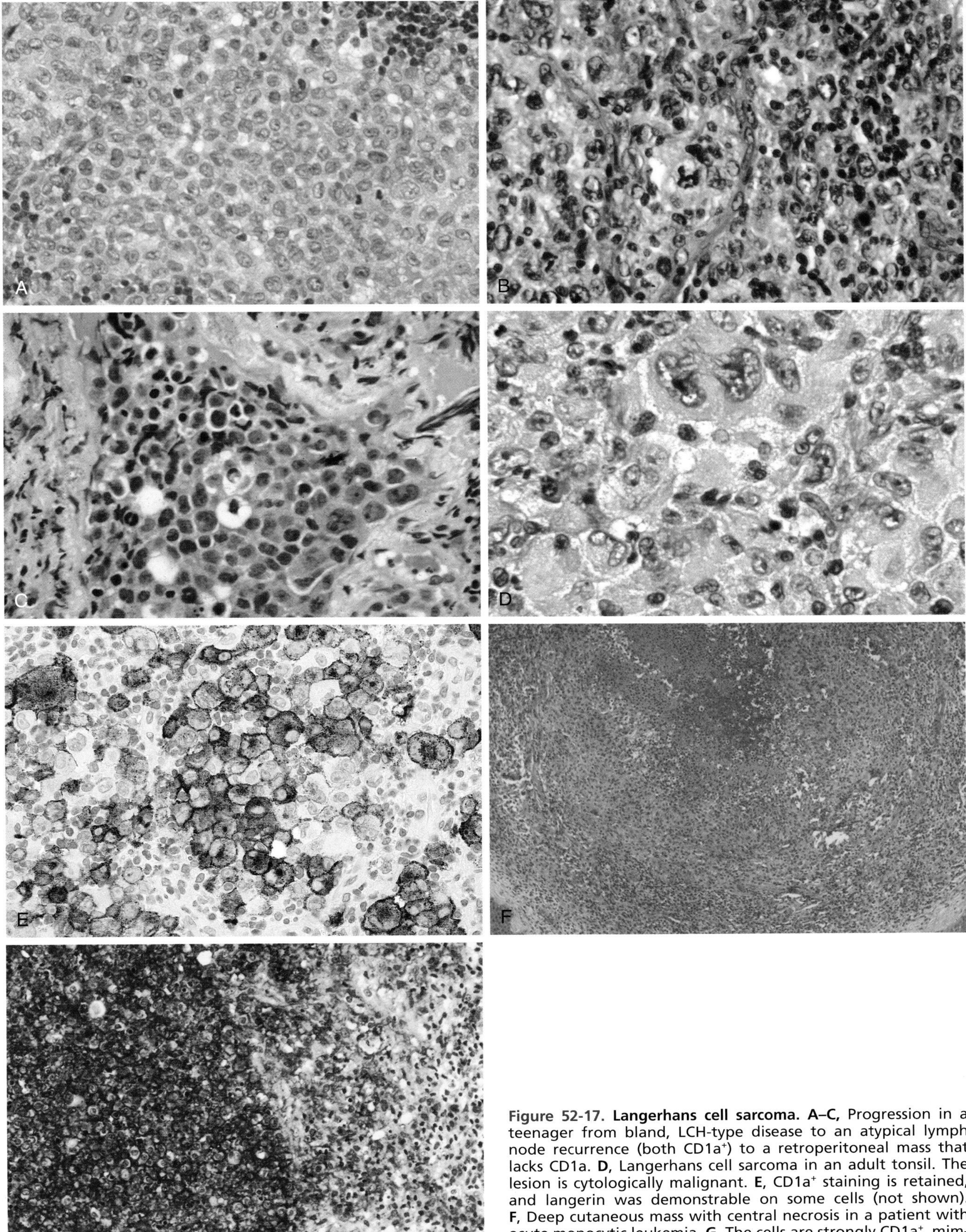

Figure 52-17. Langerhans cell sarcoma. A–C, Progression in a teenager from bland, LCH-type disease to an atypical lymph node recurrence (both CD1a⁺) to a retroperitoneal mass that lacks CD1a. **D,** Langerhans cell sarcoma in an adult tonsil. The lesion is cytologically malignant. **E,** CD1a⁺ staining is retained, and langerin was demonstrable on some cells (not shown). **F,** Deep cutaneous mass with central necrosis in a patient with acute monocytic leukemia. **G,** The cells are strongly CD1a⁺, mimicking LCH.

Pearls and Pitfalls

Pearl

- Typical hematoxylin-eosin cytomorphology and demonstration of CD1a and langerin is powerful at all sites.

Pitfalls

- $CD1a^+$ dendritic cells are part of the inflammatory response at many sites: skin, lung, some tumors. These may be confused with LCH cells (false positive).
- Macrophage activation and hemophagocytic syndrome can obscure LCH or cause confusion in bone marrow, lymph node, and spleen.
- LCH-related disease, such as degenerative cerebellar disease, does not have LCH cells.
- Major bile duct involvement in the liver can lead to false-negative needle or wedge biopsies.
- Natural regression of LCH can lead to false-negative biopsies in bona fide LCH disease.

References can be found on Expert Consult @ www.expertconsult.com

Chapter 53

Other Histiocytic and Dendritic Cell Neoplasms

Karen L. Chang and Lawrence M. Weiss

CHAPTER OUTLINE

The four major functional compartments of a lymph node (and the corresponding predominant immunologic cell components) are, simplistically, the (1) lymphoid follicle (follicular dendritic cells, lymphoid cells, tingible body macrophages), (2) medullary cords (plasma cells, lymphoid cells, macrophages, mast cells), (3) paracortex (interdigitating cells, epithelioid venules, T lymphocytes), and (4) sinuses (macrophages, B cells). One of the primary functions of lymph nodes is to process antigens.

Normal histiocytes are defined as having a high lysosomal enzyme content and phagocytosing capabilities and deriving from bone marrow monocytes (which in turn derive from myeloid stem cells). Histiocytes are freely mobile and are found circulating in the sinuses of the lymph nodes, tonsils, and spleen. Fixed tissue histiocytes are called *macrophages*. Whether freely mobile or fixed, histiocytes have large oval nuclei with a bland nuclear chromatin pattern and a moderate to abundant amount of cytoplasm, depending on their functional state.

Unlike histiocytes, for which phagocytosis (antigen processing) is a major component, dendritic cells are primarily antigen-presenting cells. Some dendritic cells, such as Langerhans cells, interdigitating dendritic (interdigitating reticulum) cells, and plasmacytoid dendritic cells, also arise from marrow myeloid stem cells. The follicular dendritic (or dendritic reticulum) cells, a specialized type of dendritic cell, are thought to arise from a mesenchymal stem cell.

In this chapter we discuss tumors derived from the histiocytic and dendritic cells, with the exception of Langerhans cell–derived tumors (Langerhans cell histiocytosis and Langerhans cell sarcoma), which are covered in Chapter 52. Box 53-1 provides the World Health Organization (WHO) classification of histiocytic and dendritic cell neoplasms.[1]

HISTIOCYTIC SARCOMA

Definition

Histiocytic sarcoma is defined in the WHO classification as a malignant proliferation of cells with morphologic and immunophenotypic features of mature tissue histiocytes.[1-4] Extramedullary myeloid tumors with monocytic differentiation (e.g., acute monoblastic leukemias) and dendritic cell neoplasms are specifically excluded. Histiocytic sarcoma was

Box 53-1 *World Health Organization Classification of Histiocytic and Dendritic Cell Neoplasms*

- Macrophage/histiocytic neoplasm
  - Histiocytic sarcoma
- Dendritic cell neoplasms
  - Langerhans cell histiocytosis
  - Langerhans cell sarcoma
  - Interdigitating dendritic cell sarcoma
  - Follicular dendritic cell sarcoma
  - Fibroblastic reticular cell tumor
  - Indeterminate dendritic cell tumor
- Disseminated juvenile xanthogranuloma

From Swerdlow SH, Campo E, Harris NL, et al, eds. *WHO Classification of Tumours of Haematopoietic and Lymphoid Tissues*. Lyon, France: IARC Press; 2008.

previously called *true histiocytic lymphoma* and, even more remotely and less accurately, *malignant histiocytosis*. The latter term is no longer used because most reported cases of that entity were subsequently shown to be lymphomas, generally of T-cell origin, including many cases of anaplastic large cell lymphoma, which was later recognized as a distinct entity.[5-8]

Other entities historically associated with so-called malignant histiocytosis include *histiocytic medullary reticulosis* and *regressing atypical histiocytosis*. Histiocytic medullary reticulosis, an entity first described in 1939, is now regarded in most cases as a hemophagocytic syndrome that may occur in association with a T-cell or natural killer (NK)–cell lymphoma or in association with a variety of infections, most commonly Epstein-Barr virus (EBV) but also other viral infections.[9-14] Some cases of histiocytic medullary reticulosis were subsequently shown to be Hodgkin's lymphoma, anaplastic large cell lymphoma, peripheral T-cell lymphoma with or without hemophagocytosis, or Lennert's lymphoma, as well as hyperimmune reactions. Cases of regressing atypical histiocytosis have been reclassified as lymphomatoid papulosis/anaplastic large cell lymphoma, cutaneous type, not histiocytic sarcoma.[15]

Epidemiology

Histiocytic sarcoma accounts for less than 1% of all hematolymphoid neoplasms and occurs most commonly in adults, with an equal distribution between men and women.[16] Infants and children may also be affected. Some cases of histiocytic sarcoma are associated with or occur subsequent to a non-Hodgkin's lymphoma, such as lymphoblastic lymphoma/leukemia, follicular lymphoma, and low-grade B-cell neoplasms.[17,18] A subset of histiocytic sarcomas is associated with primary mediastinal nonseminomatous germ cell tumors, particularly malignant teratoma with or without yolk sac differentiation.[19-21] In addition to mediastinal neoplasms, rare cases of malignant histiocytosis have been described in patients with primary gonadal germ cell tumors.[22,23] Interestingly, in patients with primary mediastinal nonseminomatous germ cell tumors, the risk of developing a hematologic disorder is statistically significantly higher than in the general population. The hematologic malignancies often occur within 1 year of diagnosis of the germ cell tumor and adversely affect prognosis. Many of the hematologic neoplasms exhibit a megakaryocytic lineage (acute megakaryoblastic leukemia, myelodysplasia with abnormal megakaryocytes, idiopathic or essential thrombocytosis), but cases of lymphoblastic leukemia or other acute myeloid leukemias, systemic mastocytosis, and histiocytic sarcoma have also been described.[21,24-26] Investigators hypothesize that the association results from the divergent differentiation of a shared multipotential progenitor cell into both a hematologic malignancy and a germ cell tumor.[21,24,25]

Etiology

No etiologic agents have been uncovered. A subset of cases occurs in patients with mediastinal germ cell tumors (previously discussed) or B-cell lymphomas (discussed later).

Clinical Features

Patients generally present with fever, fatigue, weight loss, and weakness. Physical findings usually include lymphadenopathy and may include hepatosplenomegaly, splenomegaly alone, or skin lesions (ranging from solitary tumors to innumerable lesions on the trunk and extremities).[4,27-29] Some patients may present with intestinal obstruction. Bones may show lytic lesions. Rare cases may occur as primary tumors in the central nervous system.[30]

Morphology

Lymph nodes involved by histiocytic sarcoma may show partial or complete effacement by a proliferation of cytologically malignant cells resembling histiocytes.[4] Visceral organ involvement may exhibit a sinusoidal pattern. The extent of mitotic activity closely parallels the degree of cellular pleomorphism, which is quite variable. A variable number of host cells is present, including small lymphocytes, plasma cells, benign histiocytes, and eosinophils. The malignant cells have large, eccentrically placed, oval nuclei with vesicular chromatin and a prominent single, irregular nucleolus (Fig. 53-1).

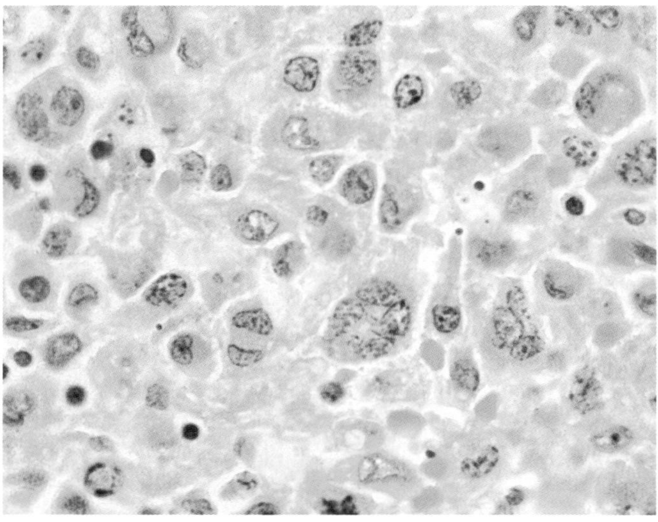

Figure 53-1. Histiocytic sarcoma, high power. Tumor cells have large pleomorphic nuclei. Hemophagocytosis is present.

The nucleus may appear grooved. Cytoplasm is abundant and eosinophilic, and it may be foamy or vacuolated. Large multinucleated tumor cells and multiple nucleoli may also be seen. Hemophagocytosis of tumor cells is extremely rare. Spindle cell sarcoma-like areas are present in some tumors. The tumor cytology and architecture are not particularly distinctive; thus, immunophenotypic and molecular studies are absolutely essential for diagnosis.

Ultrastructure

Ultrastructural features of the neoplastic cells include abundant cytoplasm with numerous lysosomes. Birbeck granules and cellular junctions are not seen (Table 53-1).

Immunophenotype

There should be immunophenotypic evidence of a histiocytic lineage, including expression of CD68, CD163, CD14, CD4, CD11c, lysozyme, and α_1-antitrypsin (Table 53-2). CD163 is a more specific marker of histiocytic lineage than CD68, which may be expressed in a variety of nonhematolymphoid tumors.[31-33] The granular staining pattern of lysozyme, with Golgi region accentuation, may offer a clue that one is dealing with histiocytic sarcoma and not some other neoplasms, which usually show more diffuse staining. CD45, CD45RO, CD4, and HLA-DR are usually positive in histiocytic sarcoma. S-100 may also be positive, and rare cases are CD56$^+$.[4,34,35] Weak CD15 staining may be seen.[34] By definition, markers of B lineage and T lineage are negative, as are markers of dendritic cells (CD21, CD23, CD35) and Langerhans cells (langerin, CD1a), CD34, CD30, HMB45, myeloperoxidase, epithelial membrane antigen (EMA), and keratins.[16,27,34,36] The Ki-67 index varies from 10% to 90% of tumor cells.

Genetics and Molecular Findings

In many cases, immunohistochemistry cannot definitively identify the lineage of the neoplasm, and one must resort to molecular studies (see Table 53-1). Most pathologists (including the authors) require the absence of clonal immunoglobulin (Ig) and T-cell receptor antigen genes for the diagnosis of histiocytic sarcoma.[4,5,37,38] Rare bona fide cases have been reported that show IgH gene rearrangements, and t(14;18) has been detected by polymerase chain reaction and fluorescence in situ hybridization in cases of histocytic sarcoma occurring synchronously with or subsequent to a diagnosis of follicular lymphoma.[39] This phenomenon suggests the possibility of "lineage plasticity" or transdifferentiation in these tumors. No consistent cytogenetic abnormalities have been found in studies of cases that fulfill the modern immunophenotypic criteria for the diagnosis of histiocytic sarcoma. However, an isochromosome 12p was detected in both neoplastic components of histiocytic sarcomas associated with mediastinal germ cell tumor.[21] Rare cases have been reported with deletion of the long arm of chromosome 5, trisomy 8, or trisomy 9.[40,41]

Postulated Cell of Origin

Histiocytic sarcoma cells have morphologic and immunophenotypic features similar to those of mature tissue histiocytes.

Clinical Course

Many cases of histiocytic sarcoma have an aggressive clinical course, with most patients dying from progressive disease within the first year.[28,34,42] However, in a subset of patients presenting with clinically localized, resectable disease treated with surgery alone, a favorable long-term outcome has been reported, with follow-up times ranging from 13 to 92 months.[28] Although there are no well-established prognostic markers, tumor size may correlate with prognosis.[28]

Differential Diagnosis

The differential diagnosis of histiocytic sarcoma includes anaplastic large cell lymphoma, B- or T-cell large cell lymphomas (particularly those associated with benign erythrophagocytosis), anaplastic carcinomas with hemophagocytosis, follicular dendritic cell neoplasms, hepatosplenic T-cell lymphoma, and malignant melanoma (Table 53-3; see Pearls and Pitfalls). By adhering to strict clinical, immunophenotypic, and molecular criteria for histiocytic sarcoma, one can exclude these other anaplastic tumors.[4,14,43,44] Myeloid sarcomas (particularly those with monoblastic differentiation) also may be confused with histiocytic sarcoma, but the former has smaller, more monomorphic tumor cells and may be CD34$^+$.[34] Benign entities with a proliferation of histiocytes, such as infection-associated hemophagocytic syndrome, familial hemophagocytic lymphohistiocytosis, and storage diseases such as Gaucher's or Niemann-Pick disease, can generally be excluded because of a lack of malignant cytologic features.[43,44]

DENDRITIC CELL NEOPLASMS

Follicular Dendritic Cell Sarcoma

Definition

Follicular dendritic cell sarcoma is a neoplastic proliferation with morphologic and immunophenotypic features similar to those of normal follicular dendritic cells. In the past, this tumor was also termed *reticulum cell sarcoma/tumor* or *dendritic reticulum cell sarcoma/tumor*.

Epidemiology

This is a rare tumor. Most studies consist of single case reports or small series.[34,45-49] The tumors occur primarily in young or middle-aged adults, with median age of occurrence in the fifth decade. Rare cases have been reported in childhood. There is no gender preference.[50]

Approximately 10% to 20% of cases of follicular dendritic cell sarcoma are associated with antecedent or concurrent Castleman's disease, mostly the hyaline vascular type and rarely the plasma cell variant.[47,49,51,52] In some cases, the antecedent Castleman's disease harbors areas of follicular dendritic cell proliferation, and the follicular dendritic cell sarcomas are hypothesized to arise in this hyperplastic setting.[53] Some patients with both follicular dendritic cell sarcoma and Castleman's disease also have paraneoplastic pemphigus.[54] Some patients have a history of long-standing schizophrenia.[34]

Etiology

Human herpesvirus 8 is negative. There is no association with EBV in most nodal cases.[50,55,56] However, a monoclonal

Table 53-1 Ultrastructural, Enzyme Immunohistochemical, and Molecular Characteristics of Histiocytic and Dendritic Cell Neoplasms

	Ultrastructure				*Enzyme Immunohistochemistry*				*Molecular Features*			
Neoplasm	Desmosomes	Birbeck Granules	Lysosomes	Cytoplasmic Processes	α-Naphthyl Acetate Esterase	Naphthol AS-D Chloroacetate Esterase	Lysozyme	α_1-Antitrypsin	Recurring Cytogenetic Abnormalities	IgH	TCR	EBV
Langerhans cell histiocytosis	–	+	–	–	+	–	–	–	–	–	–	–
Histiocytic sarcoma	–	–	Numerous	–	+	–	+	+	–	–	–	–
Follicular dendritic cell sarcoma	Numerous	–	Rare	Numerous	–	–	–	–	–	–	–	–
Interdigitating dendritic cell sarcoma	Not well formed; numerous complex, interdigitating cell processes seen instead	–	Scattered	–	+	–	+	–	–	–	–	–

EBV, Epstein-Barr virus; IgH, immunoglobulin H; TCR, T-cell receptor.

Table 53-2 Immunohistochemical Characteristics of Histiocytic and Dendritic Cell Neoplasms

Neoplasm	CD1a	CD3	CD20	CD21	CD23	CD30	CD34	CD35	CD45	CD56	CD68	CD163	S-100	Langerin	Lysozyme
Langerhans cell histiocytosis	+	–	–	–	–	–	–	–	–	–	+	+	+	+	+/–
Histiocytic sarcoma	–	–	–	–	–	–	–	–	Usually +	Rarely +	+	+	+/–	–	+ (granular)
Follicular dendritic cell sarcoma	–	–	Rarely +	+	+	–	–	+	Weakly +	–	+/–	+/–	Rarely +	–	–
Interdigitating dendritic cell sarcoma	–	–	–	–	–	–	–	–	+	?	+/–	+	+	–	+

Table 53-3 Differential Diagnosis of Histiocytic and Dendritic Cell Neoplasms

Neoplasm	Differential Diagnosis	Useful Morphologic Features	Useful Ancillary Test Results
Histiocytic sarcoma	Anaplastic large cell lymphoma	Sinusoidal pattern of involvement, "hallmark" cells	Immunohistochemistry: $CD30^+$, $ALK^{+/-}$ FISH or molecular studies: t(2;5)
	T-cell lymphoma with erythrophagocytosis	Large histiocytes with emperipolesis	Immunohistochemistry: tumor cells $CD68^-$ Molecular studies: T-cell gene rearrangements present
	Myeloid sarcoma	Monomorphic tumor cells with fine blastic chromatin	Immunohistochemistry: strong myeloperoxidase positivity
	Malignant melanoma	Fine brown pigment in cytoplasm	Immunohistochemistry: $HMB45^+$, melan A positive
Follicular dendritic cell sarcoma	Interdigitating dendritic cell sarcoma	Cells form a whorled or storiform pattern	Immunohistochemistry: lacks CD21, CD35, and CD1a expression Electron microscopy: lacks desmosomes
	Thymoma	Hassall's corpuscles	Immunohistochemistry: keratin positive
	Spindle cell carcinoma	Tight clustering of tumor cells	Immunohistochemistry: keratin positive
	Melanoma	Fine brown pigment in cytoplasm	Immunohistochemistry: $HMB45^+$, melan A positive
Interdigitating dendritic cell sarcoma	Follicular dendritic cell sarcoma	Small reactive lymphocytes interspersed throughout neoplasm	Immunohistochemistry: $CD21^+$, $CD35^+$, may be EMA^+; small reactive lymphocytes may be B lineage Electron microscopy: numerous desmosomes
	Langerhans cell sarcoma	Oval indented nuclei	Immunohistochemistry: $S\text{-}100^+$, $CD1a^+$ Electron microscopy: Birbeck granules
	Pleomorphic large cell lymphoma	Small reactive lymphocytes interspersed throughout neoplasm	Immunohistochemistry: B- or T-lineage markers present; small reactive lymphocytes are T lineage Molecular studies: IgH or TCR gene rearrangements
	Fibroblastic reticular cell tumor	May have fine collagen fibers throughout tumor	Immunohistochemistry: $S\text{-}100^-$, positive for smooth muscle actin and desmin

ALK, anaplastic lymphoma kinase; EMA, epithelial membrane antigen; FISH, fluorescence in situ hybridization; IgH, immunoglobulin H; TCR, T-cell receptor.

proliferation of EBV has been found in a subset of follicular dendritic cell sarcomas occurring in the liver and spleen (discussed later).[57]

Clinical Features

Most patients present with a painless, slow-growing lymphadenopathy that typically involves the cervical neck nodes. Axillary, mediastinal, mesenteric, retroperitoneal, and supraclavicular lymph node involvement is also common. Approximately 30% of cases present in extranodal sites, which include the tonsil, oral cavity, gastrointestinal tract, intra-abdominal soft tissue, and breast. Patients with abdominal disease may present with abdominal pain. Systemic symptoms are unusual, except in a subset of patients with the inflammatory pseudotumor–like variant of follicular dendritic cell sarcoma.[58]

Gross Description

Follicular dendritic cell sarcomas have a median size of approximately 5 cm. The largest tumors are found in the retroperitoneum or mediastinum and measure up to 20 cm; the smallest tumors (1 cm) are usually found in the cervical neck lymph nodes or tonsils. Most of the tumors are well circumscribed, with cut sections showing solid pink or tan-gray masses. Necrosis or gross hemorrhage may be seen on occasion, particularly in larger tumors.

Morphology

Microscopic sections of the tumor show storiform or whorled bundles of spindle cells with ovoid to elongated bland nuclei, sometimes resembling the whorled pattern of meningiomas (Fig. 53-2). Rarely, the tumor has a dense, fibroblast-like appearance. The tumor cell nuclei have vesicular or granular chromatin, thin nuclear membranes, and a small but distinct nucleolus (Fig. 53-3). Cytoplasm is eosinophilic, moderate in amount, and somewhat fibrillar. The tumor cells have indistinct borders. Rare cases have tumor cells with nuclear pseudoinclusions or multinucleated giant cells, occasionally resembling Warthin-Finkeldey giant cells. A distinctive characteristic of these tumors is the admixture of small lymphocytes (or, more rarely, plasma cells) between the individual tumor cells and in perivascular spaces (Fig. 53-4). Uncommonly, there may be fluid-filled cystic spaces, some in a perivascular location, or myxoid change. Necrosis is not prominent. The mitotic rate is usually 0 to 10 per 10 high-power fields. Recurrent or metastatic tumors may show

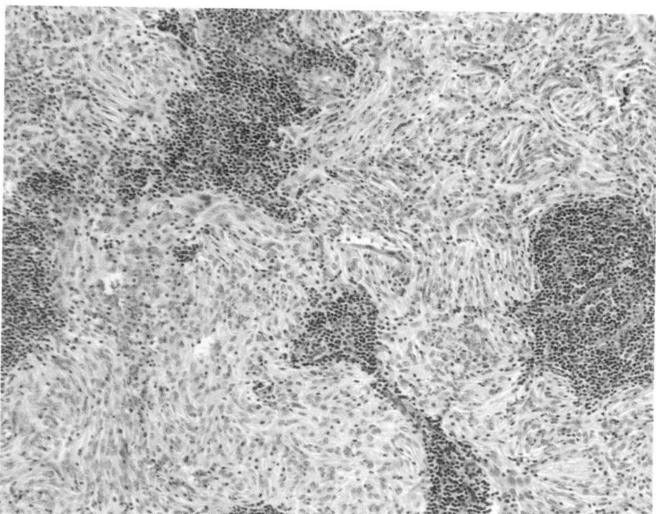

Figure 53-2. Follicular dendritic cell sarcoma. Whorling bundles and fascicles of tumor cells are admixed with adjacent lymphoid infiltrates.

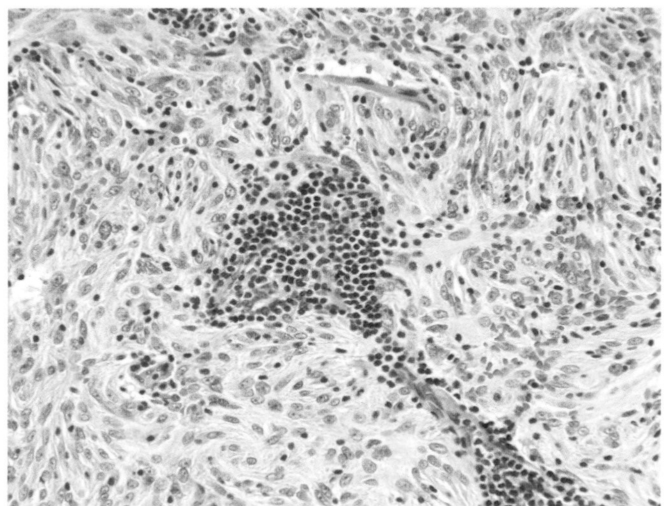

Figure 53-3. Follicular dendritic cell sarcoma. Spindled tumor cells are admixed with numerous small lymphocytes.

increased cytologic atypia, nuclear pleomorphism, and mitotic activity when compared with the original tumor.[45,47]

Rare cases show histologic changes following chemotherapy or radiotherapy, including squamous metaplasia of the tumor cells, increased nuclear atypia, and sheets of foamy histiocytes.[59] Other rare cases resembling thymoma or thymic carcinoma may have perivascular spaces filled with proteinaceous fluid and blood and prominent fibrous septa surrounding rounded and angulated tumor nodules, imparting a jigsaw puzzle–like appearance.[60]

Some hepatic and splenic proliferations show histologic features of inflammatory pseudotumor and focal markers of follicular dendritic cell differentiation; these may represent a subset of follicular dendritic cell sarcoma. These tumors are not as cellular as typical cases of follicular dendritic cell sarcoma. The spindled proliferation is often obscured by a prominent lymphoplasmacytic reaction. The spindle cell nuclei usually have a vesicular chromatin pattern, with varying degrees of nuclear atypia, and they may possess prominent nucleoli, occasionally resembling Hodgkin or Reed-Sternberg cells. By morphology, they may be easily confused with inflammatory pseudotumor. Some pathologists use the presence of well-formed fascicles, concentric whorls, cellular atypia, and decreased numbers of plasma cells to make the diagnosis of follicular dendritic cell tumor over inflammatory pseudotumor.[57]

Grading

Most of these tumors are considered low-grade sarcomas. However, significant cytologic atypia may be found in a small subset of cases (but not in the inflammatory pseudotumor variant) and may be associated with a much higher mitotic rate, as well as easily identified atypical mitotic figures. High-grade morphologic features, including nuclear pleomorphism, high mitotic activity, abnormal mitoses, and necrosis, are associated with deep-seated lesions.

Ultrastructure

The most distinctive ultrastructural feature of the neoplastic cells of follicular dendritic cell sarcoma is the numerous long, thin cytoplasmic processes connected by numerous cell junctions and mature desmosomes. The nuclei are elongated and may show cytoplasmic invaginations. The cytoplasm often contains numerous polysomes. No Birbeck granules are seen, and lysosomes are rare (see Table 53-1).

Immunophenotype

Immunohistochemical studies are essential for diagnosing follicular dendritic cell sarcoma (see Table 53-2). The neoplastic cells retain the immunophenotype of nonneoplastic follicular dendritic cells.[61,62] Thus, they are positive for one or more of the follicular dendritic cell markers, including CD21 (C3b complement receptor), CD23, CD35 (C3d complement receptor), and R4/23 (a nonclustered follicular dendritic cell–specific marker) (Figs. 53-5 to 53-7).[50] The staining is usually focal, but it may be diffuse and strong. Both normal and neoplastic follicular dendritic cells are also positive for clusterin, vimentin, fascin, epidermal growth factor receptor, and

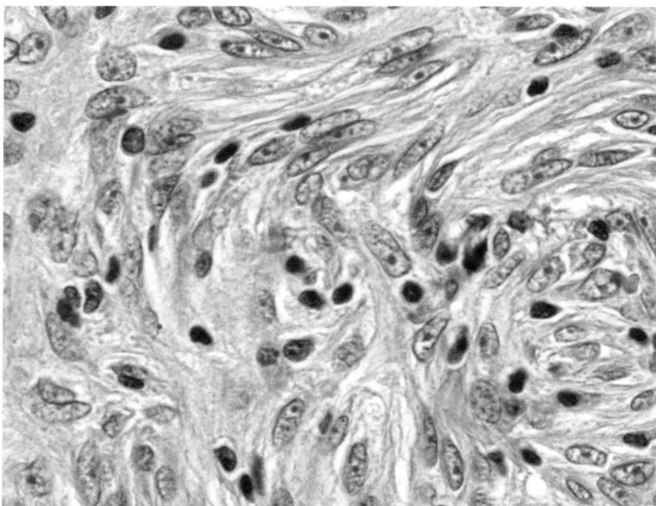

Figure 53-4. Follicular dendritic cell sarcoma, high power. The neoplastic cells have bland nuclei with indistinct cytoplasmic borders.

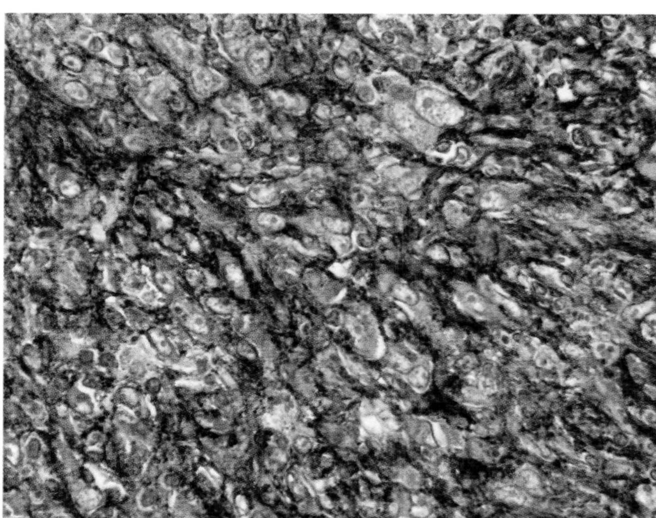

Figure 53-5. Follicular dendritic cell sarcoma. Tumor cells show strong membrane reactivity for CD21.

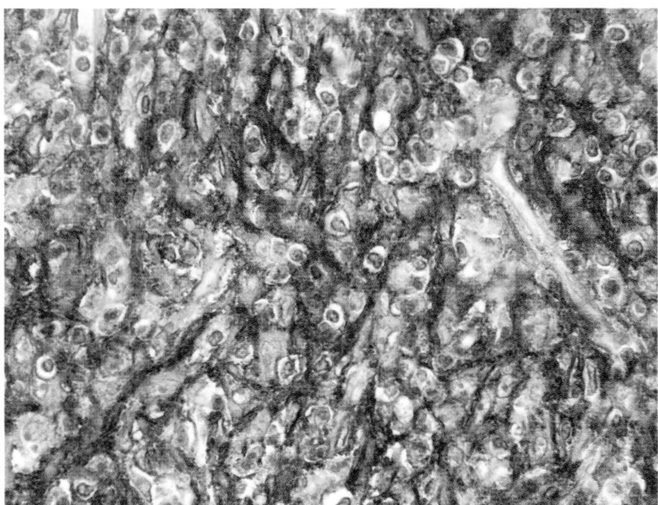

Figure 53-6. Follicular dendritic cell sarcoma. CD35 immunohistochemistry shows dense membrane staining of nearly all tumor cells.

HLA-DR.[63,64] EMA often stains the tumor cells but usually does not stain normal follicular dendritic cells. The tumor cells are variably and weakly positive for CD68 and desmoplakin. CD45/45RB and CD20 are almost invariably negative, but adjacent lymphoid cells may lead to the appearance of positive staining. Muscle-specific actin, EMA, and S-100 are rarely positive. Staining for CD1a, lysozyme, myeloperoxidase, CD34, CD3, CD79a, CD30, HMB45, desmin, and high-molecular-weight cytokeratins is not seen. Ki-67 labeling ranges from 1% to 25%. The admixed small lymphocytes have a variable phenotype; in some cases there is a B-cell predominance, and in other cases T cells predominate. The inflammatory pseudotumor variant of follicular dendritic cell sarcoma involving the liver and spleen shows a similar immunophenotype, but the expression of follicular dendritic cell immunohistochemical markers is often weak and focal.

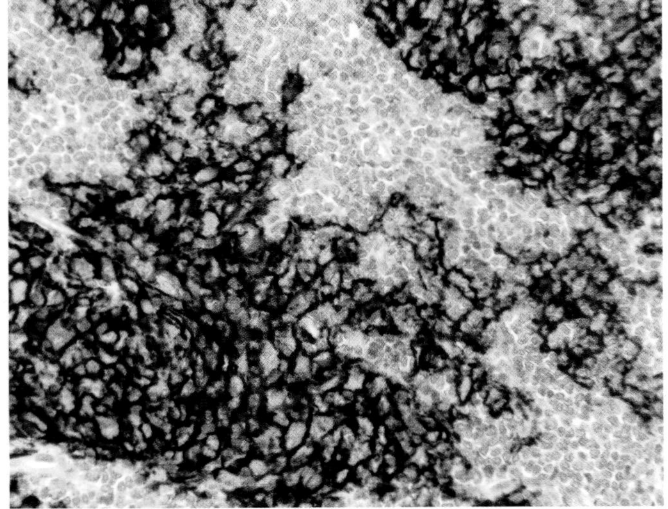

Figure 53-7. Follicular dendritic cell sarcoma. CD23 stains all the tumor cells, highlighting the tight dendritic network of these cells.

Genetics and Molecular Findings

Follicular dendritic cell sarcomas have no B-cell or T-cell gene rearrangements. No recurring cytogenetic abnormalities have been described. EBV-encoded RNA (EBER) has been detected in most of the proliferating spindle cells in cases of hepatic and splenic follicular dendritic cell sarcoma with inflammatory pseudotumor–like features, and the EBV is present in a monoclonal episomal form (see Table 53-1).[57]

Postulated Cell of Origin

The presumed normal counterpart is the antigen-presenting follicular dendritic cell of the lymph node follicle. This cell is not thought to be of hematolymphoid origin.

Clinical Course

The behavior of follicular dendritic cell sarcoma resembles that of low-grade soft tissue sarcoma rather than malignant lymphoma.[59] Complete surgical excision, with or without adjuvant radiotherapy or chemotherapy, is the usual treatment. Local recurrences are common (40% to 50% of cases), and metastases occur in approximately 25% of patients, often after local recurrence.[50,59] Indicators of a poorer prognosis include an intra-abdominal presentation, significant cytologic atypia, extensive coagulative necrosis, high proliferative index, tumor size greater than 6 cm, and lack of adjuvant therapy. Approximately 20% of patients ultimately die of their disease, often after a protracted course.

Differential Diagnosis

The differential diagnosis of follicular dendritic cell sarcoma includes interdigitating dendritic cell sarcoma, dendritic cell sarcoma (not otherwise specified), thymoma, spindle cell carcinoma, malignant melanoma, and sarcoma (see Table 53-3). All the dendritic cell neoplasms require immunohistochemistry for diagnosis. CD21 and CD35 staining has high specificity for follicular dendritic cell sarcomas. Keratin positivity is seen in thymomas and spindle cell carcinomas and in a moderate number of epithelioid leiomyosarcomas, but not in follicular dendritic cell sarcomas.

These tumors often have an immunohistochemical profile of follicular dendritic cells when involving the liver and spleen and, interestingly, are often EBV$^+$.[57] In these cases, EBER has been found in nearly all the proliferating spindle cells, and Southern blot studies have demonstrated that the virus is present in a monoclonal proliferation.[57] The expression of follicular dendritic cell immunohistochemical markers is often weak and focal. Thus, these cases may be considered a variant of follicular dendritic cell sarcoma associated with EBV.

Interdigitating Dendritic Cell Sarcoma

Definition

Interdigitating dendritic cell sarcoma has a lineage phenotype consistent with interdigitating dendritic cells, which normally reside in the paracortical areas of a lymph node. This tumor has also been called *interdigitating dendritic cell tumor* and *interdigitating reticulum cell tumor/sarcoma*.[65-68]

Epidemiology

Interdigitating dendritic cell sarcomas are rare and have been reported in adults and teenagers.[68] Slightly more men than

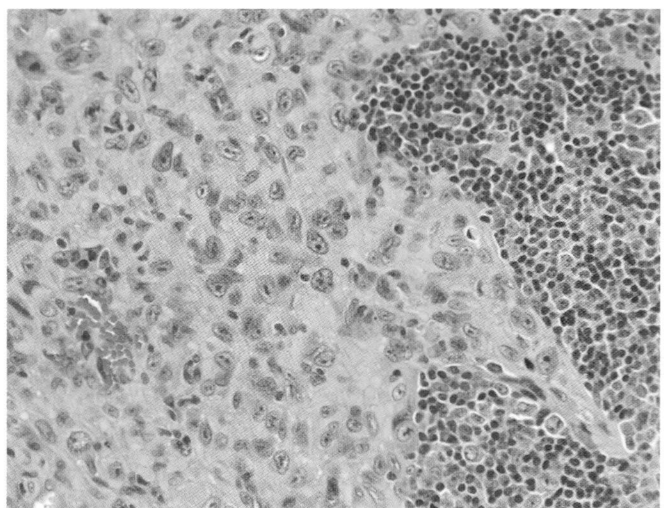

Figure 53-8. Interdigitating dendritic cell sarcoma, low power. Residual reactive lymphoid follicles are often sharply demarcated from the tumor cells.

women have been reported with the disease, but the paucity of cases precludes a definitive assessment of gender preference.

Etiology

No specific etiology has been discerned, although occasional cases have been reported in patients with a low-grade B-cell lymphoproliferation or T-cell lymphoma.[69,70]

Clinical Features

Most patients have an asymptomatic mass. Some patients present with fatigue, fever, and night sweats. Patients may present with solitary lymph node enlargement or involvement of extranodal sites such as the skin, soft tissue, small intestine, liver, kidney, lung, and spleen.

Morphology

The usual histologic appearance of interdigitating dendritic cell sarcoma is that of a paracortical proliferation of indistinct fascicles (sometimes with a storiform or whorled pattern) of ovoid to spindle cells. Sometimes there is no specific fascicle formation and instead there are just diffuse sheets of spindle or round cells. One reported case consisted of a spindled neoplasm in the initial biopsy and a more pleomorphic and less spindled neoplasm in a recurrence.[59] At low magnification one often sees residual lymphoid follicles as well as small lymphocytes scattered throughout the neoplasm (Fig. 53-8). Plasma cells may be admixed with tumor cells. Necrosis is usually not present, although in rare cases, particularly those with atypical nuclear features, there may be large foci of coagulative necrosis. The neoplastic cell nuclei range in shape from round to ovoid to markedly spindled (Fig. 53-9). The nuclear chromatin may be bland but is often vesicular, with a single medium-sized nucleolus. Delicate nuclear folds, occasional nuclear grooves, and rare intranuclear cytoplasmic invaginations have all been described in some cases. The cytoplasm is usually abundant and lightly eosinophilic and often has poorly defined borders.

Grading

The degree of cytologic atypia varies from case to case. The mitotic rate is usually low: less than 5 per 10 high-power fields. The cytologic grade does not appear to correlate with clinical outcome.

Enzyme Cytochemistry

The neoplastic cells in most of the studied cases stain for adenosine triphosphatase, α-naphthyl esterase, acid phosphatase, and 5′-nucleotidase.[65,66,71,72] The tumor cells do not show staining for alkaline phosphatase, peroxidase, β-glucuronidase, or chloroacetate esterase (see Table 53-1).

Ultrastructure

Electron microscopic features of the neoplastic cells and normal interdigitating cells are similar.[72-74] The neoplastic cells show complex, elongated interdigitating cell processes and scattered lysosomes. However, one does not observe well-formed desmosomes, such as those seen in follicular dendritic cell sarcoma, or Birbeck granules, such as those seen in Langerhans cell histiocytosis. Basal lamina, tonofilaments, dense-core secretory granules, and melanosomes are not seen (see Table 53-1).

Immunophenotype

The diagnosis of interdigitating dendritic cell sarcoma rests on immunohistochemical studies (see Table 53-2). The immunohistochemical features of neoplastic and nonneoplastic interdigitating dendritic cells are similar.[34] The cells consistently express S-100 protein and vimentin and are usually negative for histiocytic antigens (CD68, CD163, lysozyme, CD45). They are consistently negative for markers of follicular dendritic cells (CD21, CD23, CD35), langerin, CD1a, complement markers, myeloperoxidase, CD34, specific B- and T-cell markers, CD30, EMA, desmin, HMB45, and cytokeratins. Ki-67 usually stains 10% to 20% of tumor nuclei. The admixed small lymphocytes are almost always of T-cell lineage, with a paucity of B cells. Some reports of interdigitating tumors include CD1a$^+$ tumors; however, we consider these to be indeterminate cell tumors (discussed later).

Genetics and Molecular Findings

In the rare cases analyzed by molecular methods, the immunoglobulin heavy-chain gene and the alpha, beta, and delta

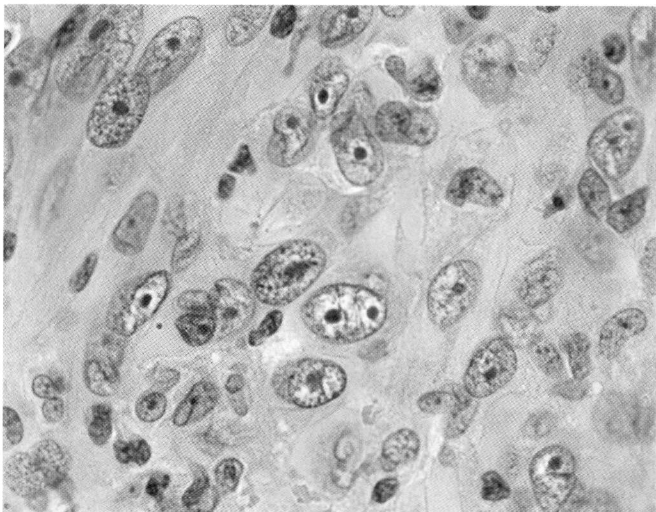

Figure 53-9. Interdigitating dendritic cell sarcoma, high power. Hematoxylin-eosin stain shows numerous spindle and plump ovoid cells with vesicular chromatin.

chains of the T-cell receptor are in a germline configuration (see Table 53-1).[48]

Postulated Cell of Origin

The presumed normal counterpart of these tumor cells is the interdigitating dendritic cell of the paracortical region of the lymph node. Interdigitating dendritic cells derive in part from Langerhans cells.

Clinical Course

The disease usually has an aggressive clinical course. The reported therapies for interdigitating dendritic cell sarcoma are varied. Most patients have been treated with local excision, usually with adjuvant radiotherapy or chemotherapy, or both. One patient underwent bone marrow transplantation. Local recurrence may be seen. Approximately half the patients die of their disease, generally within 1 year of diagnosis. To date, prognosis does not correlate with any clinical, histologic, or treatment variables.

Differential Diagnosis

The differential diagnosis of interdigitating dendritic cell sarcoma is similar to that of follicular dendritic cell sarcoma (see Table 53-3). In contrast to these tumors, interdigitating dendritic cell sarcomas do not have ultrastructural evidence of desmosomes and do not show immunohistochemical reactivity with monoclonal antibodies against complement receptors (CD21, CD35) and the DRC1 antigen. Interdigitating dendritic cell sarcomas may also be confused with large cell lymphomas, including pleomorphic large cell lymphoma with convoluted nuclei. CD20 or CD3 positivity excludes the diagnosis of interdigitating dendritic cell sarcoma.

Other Dendritic Cell Tumors

Rare dendritic cell neoplasms that do not meet the criteria for follicular dendritic cell sarcoma, interdigitating dendritic cell sarcoma, Langerhans cell histiocytosis, or Langerhans cell sarcoma include the indeterminate dendritic cell tumor (or indeterminate cell histiocytosis)[69,75-78] and the fibroblastic reticular cell tumor (or cytokeratin-positive interstitial reticulum cell tumor).[49]

Indeterminate dendritic cell tumors were previously thought to derive from a cell with overlapping features between Langerhans cells and interdigitating cells (morphologic and immunologic similarities to normal Langerhans cells, but without Birbeck granules by electron microscopy). These tumors are extremely rare and are a diagnosis of exclusion. Some cases are associated with prior low-grade B-cell malignancy, and one patient subsequently developed acute myeloid leukemia.[69,79]

Fibroblastic reticular cell tumors are very rare and are considered to be derived from fibroblastic reticular cells. These cells constitute a complex cellular network in the paracortex of lymph nodes. They ensheathe the high endothelial venules and are believed to play a role in the transport of soluble mediators (cytokines, chemokines) within the lymph node.[80] These cells are positive for vimentin and smooth muscle actin and may be positive for desmin. They also may stain for factor XIII but do not stain for CD21, CD23, or CD35.[81] The neoplasms, which arise in lymph nodes, have a similar phenotype to their normal cellular counterpart. Rare tumors have been reported to arise in the spleen.[82] These lesions are in the morphologic differential diagnosis of follicular dendritic cell sarcomas, interdigitating dendritic cell sarcomas, and inflammatory pseudotumors of the spleen.

DISSEMINATED JUVENILE XANTHOGRANULOMA

Definition

Disseminated juvenile xanthogranuloma is a rare systemic and clinically aggressive proliferation of histiocytes similar to those seen in dermal juvenile xanthogranuloma.[83-86] In its usual form, juvenile xanthogranuloma is a benign dermal histiocytic disorder that occurs as single or multiple yellowish nodules that usually involve primarily the head and neck, trunk, or upper extremities. Solitary extracutaneous lesions are rare and have been reported in the orbital and periorbital areas, as well as in the lung and liver. Rarely (<5% of cases), the disorder may present systemically and cause significant morbidity and sometimes death.

This rare entity has also been called *systemic or deep juvenile xanthogranuloma*, *progressive nodular histiocytosis*, *benign cephalic histiocytosis*, or *generalized eruptive histiocytosis*. Some cases of Erdheim-Chester disease (polyostotic sclerosing histiocytosis) and xanthoma disseminatum, a rare condition in which xanthomas involve the skin of flexor areas and the eyelids, may represent disseminated juvenile xanthogranuloma.

Epidemiology

Disseminated juvenile xanthogranuloma most often affects children from infancy to 10 years of age, but it has been reported in older children and adults (Erdheim-Chester type).[87]

Etiology

The etiology of disseminated juvenile xanthogranuloma is not known. Rare patients with disseminated xanthogranuloma have coexistent neurofibromatosis type 1; however, patients with neurofibromatosis type 1 have a higher incidence of the usual type of juvenile xanthogranuloma.[88] The true incidence of the latter is not known because the skin lesions are often not biopsied (because of the patient's young age, lesion location, and strong clinical suspicion of café au lait spots), but it has been reported to be between 0.7% and 18%. Although patients with both entities have a slightly increased risk of developing juvenile myelomonocytic leukemia (JMML),[89] screening of such patients for JMML is not recommeded.[90] Patients with neurofibromatosis type 1 alone have an increased risk of developing JMML over the general population.[91] Rare juvenile xanthogranuloma patients without neurofibromatosis have also been reported to develop JMML.

Sites of Involvement

Disseminated xanthogranuloma involves the skin in only 50% of cases, unlike the usual solitary type, which is predominantly cutaneous (although it may involve other sites, as noted earlier). Sites involved in systemic disease include the kidney, lung, soft tissue, central nervous system, aerodigestive tract, and, rarely, bone (all usually with the skin as well). Unusual sites are the myocardium, pericardium, retroperitoneum, and spleen.[85,92]

Clinical Features

The disseminated form of juvenile xanthogranuloma usually occurs in children, but it has been described in adults (Erdheim-Chester disease).[85,92] Patients may have a preexisting or prior malignancy, such as Langerhans cell histiocytosis. Some of the disseminated cases may be associated with JMML or, rarely, lymphoblastic leukemia.[84,85,93-95] Clinical presentations include anemia, thrombocytopenia, and massive hepatosplenomegaly.[92,96] Liver or bone marrow failure may ensue from involvement. Serum lipid levels are normal and remain normal.

Morphology

The histologic appearance of juvenile xanthogranuloma is varied. There is no histologic difference between the usual type and the systemic type of juvenile xanthogranuloma. Early lesions show a dense, monomorphic, histiocytic infiltrate in the affected organ. Dermal lesions are predominantly in the dermis, with some extension into the subcutaneous tissues and muscle. Older lesions contain large to pale foamy histiocytes, Touton giant cells, and foreign body giant cells, as well as a mixed cellular infiltrate of neutrophils, lymphocytes, eosinophils, and (rarely) mast cells. The histiocytes may contain pleomorphic nuclei, particularly in disseminated cases. Fibrosis may be prominent in older lesions. Touton giant cells may not be present in every case of juvenile xanthogranuloma. Mitotic figures are few or absent. Deep lesions tend to be more cellular and monotonous, with fewer Touton cells.[97]

Ultrastructure

Electron microscopy examination of the lesions shows features of histiocytes.[96] The cells have short cell processes and abundant cytoplasm containing mitochondria, rough endoplasmic reticulum, ribosomes, lysosomes, and phagolysosomes, with occasional comma-shaped dense bodies. Birbeck bodies are not seen.

Immunophenotype

Use of special stains is important to differentiate juvenile xanthogranuloma from Langerhans and non–Langerhans cell histiocytoses. In disseminated juvenile xanthogranuloma, the histiocytic cells are usually positive to antibodies against factor XIIIa, CD68, CD163, lysozyme, and vimentin.[83-85,90,98] Fascin, CD4, and S-100 are variably positive. The histiocytic cells are generally negative for CD1a and langerin. One case of possible disseminated juvenile xanthogranuloma reportedly exhibited membranous and cytoplasmic anaplastic lymphoma kinase (ALK) positivity, although it is not clear whether that case represented a distinct clinicopathologic entity of ALK$^+$ histiocytosis of infancy.[99]

Genetics and Molecular Findings

No consistent cytogenetic or molecular genetic abnormalities have been identified. Rare cases are associated with neurofibromatosis type 1. No detectable T- or B-cell gene rearrangements have been detected. In a limited study, clonality was detected by X-linked androgen receptor gene assay.[100]

Postulated Cell of Origin

The cell of origin is not definitively known, but dermal dendrocytes have been proposed, based on immunoreactivity to fascin, CD4, and factor XIIIa. However, this is a nonspecific immunophenotype.[84,98]

Clinical Course

The lesions are considered benign. However, disseminated xanthogranuloma may result in significant morbidity, particularly when it involves the central nervous system or deep-seated vital organs, and it may even lead to death.[101]

Differential Diagnosis

The differential diagnosis of disseminated juvenile xanthogranuloma includes the xanthomatous variant of Langerhans cell histiocytosis. The latter entity shows immunohistochemical reactivity for CD1a and langerin, which are never positive in disseminated juvenile xanthogranuloma. Also, the presence of Birbeck granules in Langerhans cell histiocytosis is a distinguishing feature.

CONCLUSION

Histiocytic and dendritic neoplasms are extremely rare entities and may be difficult to diagnose (see Pearls and Pitfalls). Furthermore, their rarity has hindered our ability to study their clinical and biologic properties. However, the WHO classification for this category of tumors offers highly reproducible and reliable diagnostic criteria, providing a framework for further study.

Pearls and Pitfalls

- Histiocytic and dendritic cell neoplasms are extremely uncommon.
- If an S-100$^+$ lesion is identified in the lymph node, be sure to exclude metastatic malignant melanoma first, because melanoma is far more common than histiocytic lesions.
- If melanoma has been excluded in an S-100$^+$ lesion, consider Langerhans cell histiocytosis next, because that is more common than the other histiocytic or dendritic lesions.
- When a limited amount of tissue is available, immunohistochemistry is far more useful than molecular, flow, or cytogenetic studies in the classification of these lesions.
- The five most discriminatory immunohistochemical stains are S-100, CD1a, CD163, CD21, and CD35. Lysozyme, CD68, and EMA are also very useful.
- Langerin (CD207) is more specific for Langerhans cells than is CD1a; CD163 is more specific for histiocytes than is CD68 or lysozyme.

References can be found on Expert Consult @ www.expertconsult.com

Table 54-1 Major Categories of Primary Immunodeficiency Conditions

Designation	Pathogenesis/Defect	Inheritance	Associated Features
B-cell Immunodeficiencies			
X-linked agammaglobulinaemia	Mutations in *btk*	XL	—
Hyper IgM syndrome	Mutation in CD40 ligand	Variable	Neutropenia; thrombocytopenia; hemolytic anemia; gastrointestinal and liver involvement
Common variable immunodeficiency	Variable; ICOS, TACI, BAFFR	Variable	See text
IgA deficiency	Failure of terminal differentiation in IgA + B cells	Variable	Autoimmune and allergic disorders
Selective IgG subclass deficiency	Defects of isotype differentiation	Unknown	—
T-Cell Immunodeficiencies			
Purine nucleoside phosphorylase (PNP) deficiency	Deficiency of PNP		Small lymph nodes
ZAP-70 deficiency		AR	CD8 lymphopenia
Nezelof syndrome	Unknown	AR, XL	Absent or abnormal differentiation of thymus
CD3g and CD3e deficiency	Defect in TCR signaling	AR	Poor response to T-cell mitogens
Severe Combined Immunodeficiencies			
T-B-SCID			
RAG1/2 deficiency and Omenn syndrome	Mutation in RAG1/2 genes	AR	
Reticular dysgenesis	Defective maturation of T- and B-cells and myeloid cells (stem cell defect)	AR	Granulocytopenia; thrombocytopenia
Adenosine deaminase (ADA) deficiency	T- and B-cell defects from toxic metabolites (e.g., dATP, S-adenosyl homocysteine)	AR	
T-B+SCID			
X-linked severe combined immunodeficiency	Mutations in common cytokine receptor gamma chain gene	XL	Lymphadenopathy; hematosplenomegaly
JAK3 Deficiency	Mutation in JAK3	AR	
Other SCID		AR	
Bare lymphocyte syndrome Type I	Mutations in TAP1 and TAP2 genes	AR	Defect in NK cell cytotoxicity
Bare lymphocyte syndrome Type II	Mutation in transcription factors (CIITA bare lymphocyte syndrome, or RFX5, RFXAP, RFXANK genes) for MHC class II molecules	AR	Decrease in CD4 + T-cells
CD45 deficiency	Mutation in CD45	Unknown	Poor response to T-cell mitogens
Other Immunodeficiencies			
Wiskott-Aldrich syndrome	Mutations in WAS gene; cytoskeletal defect affecting hematopoietic stem cell derivatives	XL	Thrombocytopenia; small defective platelets; eczema; lymphomas; autoimmune disease
DiGeorge/velocardiofacial syndrome	Deletion of 22q11.2	De novo defect or AD	Hypoparathyroidism; conotruncal malformation; abnormal facies; partial monosomy of 22q11-pter or 10p in some patients
Ataxia-telangiectasia	Mutation in ATM gene	AR	Increase in sensitivity to x-rays
Immunodeficiency with albinism			
Chédiak-Higashi syndrome	Defect in *Lyst*	AR	Albinism; acute phase reaction; low NK and CTL activities; giant lysosomes
Griscelli syndrome	Defect in *myosin 5a*; defect in *RAB27A*	AR	Albinism; acute phase reaction; low NK and CTL activities; progressive encephalopathy in severe cases

Continued on following page

Table 54-1 Major Categories of Primary Immunodeficiency Conditions (Continued)

Designation	Pathogenesis/Defect	Inheritance	Associated Features
X-linked lymphoproliferative syndrome	Defect in *SAP*	XL	Clinical and immunological manifestations induced by EBV infection; hepatitis; aplastic anaemia; lymphomas
ICF syndrome	*DNMT3B* mutation (20q11.2)	AR	Developmental delay; facial abnormalities; reduction of at least two Ig classes +/–; defective cell-mediated immunity
Nijmegen breakage syndrome	Defect in *NBS1* (*Nibrin*); disorder of cell cycle checkpoint and DNA double-strand break repair	AR	Microcephaly; lymphomas; ionizing radiation sensitivity; chromosomal instability
Job's syndrome	Unknown	AD	Elevated serum IgE rash; bone abnormalities
Autoimmune LPS	Defects in Fas-Fas ligand system	AR	Lymphadenopathy; autoimmunity

AD, autosomal dominant; AR, autosomal recessive; CTL, cytotoxic lymphocyte; EBV, Epstein-Barr virus; ICF, immunodeficiency, centromeric instability, facial anomaly; Ig, immunoglobulin; IL, interleukein; MHC, major histocompatibility complex; NK, natural killer; SCID, severe combined immunodeficiency; TAP, transport associated with antigen processing protein; TCR, T-cell receptor; XL, X-linked; ZAP, zeta-associated polypeptide.

The histopathologic spectrum of lymphoid lesions ranges from mild, nonspecific, reactive or follicular hyperplasia[15,17,25] to atypical lymphoid hyperplasia and overt lymphoma. Compared with lymphomas occurring in immunocompetent individuals, these neoplasms show a predilection for extranodal sites, such as the central nervous system and gastrointestinal tract. They are frequently diffuse large B-cell lymphomas. Burkitt's lymphoma, low-grade B-cell lymphomas, peripheral T-cell lymphomas, and Hodgkin's lymphoma are rare.[16,17] More recent studies show that the molecular genetic detection of clonality and the degree of immunosuppression are better predictors of clinical outcome than is clinical stage.[17]

PATHOGENESIS OF LYMPHOPROLIFERATIVE DISORDERS

The pathogenetic mechanisms underlying the development of lymphoproliferative disorders in primary immunodeficiencies generally involve the interplay of one or more of the following factors: (1) polyclonal lymphocyte activation, (2) abnormal regulation of lymphoid proliferation by the dysfunctional immune system, and (3) development of somatic genetic abnormalities in the proliferating lymphoid cells.

Table 54-2 Prevalence of Primary Immunodeficiencies

Disease	Prevalence
X-linked agammaglobulinemia	1/200,000
X-linked lymphoproliferative syndrome	<1/1 million live births in males
X-linked immunodeficiency with hyper-IgM	<1/1 million live births in males
X-linked SCID	1/50,000 to 100,000
JAK3-deficient SCID (autosomal recessive T^-, B^+ SCID)	<1/500,000 live births
Adenosine deaminase deficiency	1 to 2/100,000
B-cell–negative SCID; Omenn's syndrome	≈1/100,000
Ataxia-telangiectasia	≈1/100,000

IgM, immunoglobulin M; SCID, severe combined immunodeficiency.

Polyclonal Activation of Lymphoid Proliferation

Viruses are the agents most often implicated in the polyclonal activation of lymphoid cells in the primary immunodeficiencies. Among these, Epstein-Barr virus (EBV) is most common.[26-29] Much less frequently, human herpesvirus 6 (human B-lymphotropic virus) has been identified.[30] Polyclonal activation of B cells can also occur due to stimulation of a T-helper 2 (Th2) cytokine response, as seen in autoimmune lymphoproliferative syndrome.[31]

Abnormal Regulation of Lymphoid Proliferation by the Dysfunctional Immune System

The immunologic defect that allows uncontrolled lymphocyte proliferation varies among the immunodeficiency syndromes. For example, in WAS, defects of the surface glycoprotein sialophorin/leukosialin (CD43), which is involved in T-cell proliferation, may result in impaired regulation of B-cell activity.[32] In contrast, in adenosine deaminase (ADA)–deficient severe combined immunodeficiency (SCID), EBV-reactive cytotoxic T cells are selectively sensitive to the toxic conditions of absent ADA activity.[33] In different forms of hypogammaglobulinemia, persistently elevated levels of interleukin (IL)-6[34] or impaired NK-cell activity[35] may contribute to abnormal lymphoid proliferation.

Genetic Abnormalities

Somatic genetic abnormalities may result in the emergence of a malignant clone in the lymphoproliferative disorders occurring in some congenital immunodeficiencies, principally AT and Nijmegen breakage syndrome (NBS). In AT and NBS, most of the chromosomal aberrations involve chromosome 14q11 (the T-cell receptor alpha chain gene locus), which on occasion may be juxtaposed to band 14q32 (the immunoglobulin heavy-chain gene locus). The accumulation of several genetic aberrations may then result in the development of malignant lymphoma.[36,37] DNA hypomethylation due to mutations of the DNA methyltransferase 3B results in aberrant expression of key growth regulatory genes, leading to lymphoproliferation.[38]

PREDOMINANTLY ANTIBODY DEFICIENCIES

The B-cell immunodeficiencies are predominantly antibody defects.

X-Linked Agammaglobulinemia

Clinical Features

The prevalence of X-linked agammaglobulinemia is about 1 in 200,000 live births. Serum concentrations of IgG, IgA, and IgM are markedly reduced. Levels of circulating B lymphocytes are significantly decreased, and plasma cells are absent from lymph nodes and bone marrow; however, the number of T cells is normal or even increased. The clinical phenotype is variable, and members of the same family can have different symptoms. Nonetheless, the majority of affected boys present with recurrent bacterial infections from the age of 4 to 12 months, after the disappearance of maternal immunoglobulin.[39] Patients with X-linked agammaglobulinemia have a normal response to viral infections and normal VDJ rearrangement. Infections caused by pyogenic bacteria are the most common clinical manifestations.

Genetic and Cellular Defects

X-linked agammaglobulinemia, the first genetic immunodeficiency to be specifically identified, was described by Bruton.[40] It is caused by a block in B-cell differentiation due to mutations involving the Bruton tyrosine kinase gene (BTK), which encodes a tyrosine kinase that regulates the activity of signaling pathways by phosphorylation.[41,42] Flow cytometric methods to detect Btk protein expression[43] and molecular diagnostic tests allow identification of the carrier state and enable prenatal diagnosis of the disorder.[44] However, approximately one third to one half of X-linked agammaglobulinemia cases are sporadic.

Pathology

Patients have markedly hypoplastic or absent tonsils, adenoids, and lymph nodes. The germinal centers are severely atretic, with decreased numbers of B lymphocytes. Immunophenotypic studies demonstrate the presence of B cells in the bone marrow; however, few if any are seen in the peripheral blood.[45] Plasma cells are not present in either the bone marrow or the peripheral blood.

Hyper-IgM Syndrome

Clinical Features

Hyper-IgM syndrome is a group of distinct entities characterized by defective normal or elevated IgM in the presence of diminished IgG and IgA levels.[46] Seventy percent of cases are X-linked,[47] and others are autosomal recessive.[48] Affected individuals have recurrent pyogenic infections and are particularly susceptible to *Pneumocystis carinii*. They may have profound neutropenia, autoimmune hemolytic anemia, and thrombocytopenic purpura. Liver disease, including sclerosing cholangitis, viral hepatitis, and hepatic lymphoma, is common, and its frequency increases with age.[49] The long-term survival for patients with X-linked hyper-IgM syndrome is poor, despite the regular use of intravenous immunoglobulin. Less than 30% of patients are alive at 25 years of age. Levy and colleagues[50] estimated that only 20% of patients reach the third decade of life, and 75% of those have liver complications. Major causes of death include *Pneumocystis carinii* pneumonia early in life and liver disease and malignancies later in life.[50] Allogeneic bone marrow transplantation[51] or nonmyeloablative bone marrow transplantation from matched unrelated donors[52] has been successful in the treatment of hyper-IgM syndrome.

Genetic and Cellular Defects

The genetic abnormality in X-linked hyper-IgM syndrome has been mapped to Xq26 and involves mutations of the CD40 ligand (CD40L) gene, now known as CD154.[53] Interaction between the CD40 ligand present on activated T cells and CD40 on B cells is required for productive isotype switching in B cells.[54] Studies of CD40L (CD154) knockout mice that are also susceptible to *Pneumocystis carinii* infections show that the defect in CD40L expression prevents CD40-mediated upregulation of CD80/CD86 expression in B lymphocytes and other antigen-presenting cells, ultimately resulting in poor T-cell priming and a defective type I immune response.[55]

Pathology

The blood in patients with X-linked hyper-IgM syndrome contains normal numbers of B lymphocytes that bear surface IgM and IgD. There are no germinal centers in lymph nodes or the spleen, despite the presence of normal numbers of B cells and T cells.[3] Lymphoid tissue shows disorganization of the follicular architecture and periodic acid–Schiff–positive plasmacytoid cells containing IgM. Tonsillar hypertrophy due to infiltration with these cells may occur. In addition, extensive proliferation of IgM-producing polyclonal plasma cells may involve the gastrointestinal tract, liver, and gallbladder and cause death.[3]

In 16 tumors in patients with hyper-IgM syndrome, the Immune Deficiency–Cancer Registry reported 9 cases of non-Hodgkin's lymphoma (56.3%) and 4 cases of Hodgkin's lymphoma (25%). The lymphomas showed a predilection for extranodal sites, particularly the gastrointestinal tract and brain. No leukemias were recorded, but other tumors accounted for 18.8% of cases. The median age at diagnosis of lymphoma was 7.8 years, and the male-to-female ratio was 7:2.[14] Hayward and coworkers[49] described various gastrointestinal cancers, including cholangiocarcinoma, hepatocellular carcinoma, and adenocarcinoma, in a cohort of boys with hyper-IgM syndrome and cholangiopathy.

Common Variable Immunodeficiency

Clinical Features

CVID is a heterogeneous group of disorders characterized by defective antibody formation.[4] It is also known as *late-onset hypogammaglobulinemia*, *adult-onset hypogammaglobulinemia*, and *acquired immunodeficiency*. The diagnosis is based on the exclusion of other known causes of humoral immune defects. The feature common to all patients is hypogammaglobulinemia, generally affecting all antibody classes, but sometimes only IgG. Several modes of inheritance (autosomal recessive, autosomal dominant, and X-linked) have been reported; however, most cases are sporadic. CVID is the most frequent primary immunodeficiency disease among populations of European descent, and it affects both sexes equally.[56] The usual age at presentation is in the second or third decade. CVID is the most common clinically significant primary immunodeficiency disease that can present initially in adulthood.[5] The typical clinical manifestations of CVID are recurrent pyogenic sinopulmonary infections. Recurrent attacks of herpes simplex virus infection are common, and herpes zoster develops in about 20% of patients.[3] In addition, CVID patients are prone to persistent episodes of diarrhea caused by *Giardia lamblia*. A high frequency of autoimmune diseases, including rheumatoid arthritis, pernicious anemia, and autoimmune hemolytic anemia, thrombocytopenia, and neutropenia, is seen.[3] A syndrome resembling sarcoidosis can also affect some patients; the granulomas tend to involve the lung, liver, spleen, and conjunctiva. Patients are also at risk for Crohn's disease, celiac disease, and nodular lymphoid hyperplasia of the intestine.

Genetic and Cellular Defects

Mutations in four genes have been identified as being associated with CVID: inducible T-cell costimulator (ICOS)[57]; tumor necrosis factor receptor superfamily member 13B (TNFRSF13B), also known as TACI[58]; tumor necrosis factor receptor superfamily member 13C (TNFRSF13C), also known as BAFFR[59]; and CD19.[60]

Pathology

A reduction in $CD4^+$ T cells is often seen in CVID, predominantly in the $CD45RA^+$ population. There is a correlation between disease severity and reduction of $CD4^+$ T cells and B cells.[61]

Reactive lymphoid hyperplasia is more common than lymphoma in CVID patients.[18,23,24] Extranodal sites such as the gastrointestinal tract, lung, skin, spleen, and other viscera may be involved. Figure 54-1 demonstrates the histopathologic findings in the enlarged spleen of an elderly woman with a long history of CVID. Organisms were not identified by periodic acid–Schiff, acid-fast, or Gram stains. There was polytypic immunoglobulin kappa and lambda light-chain

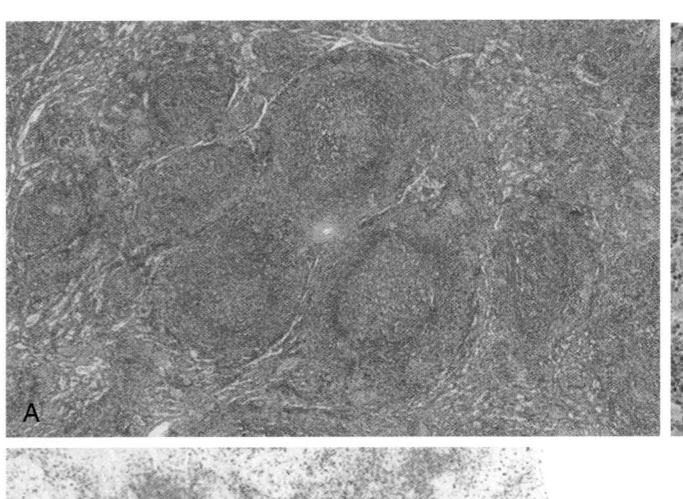

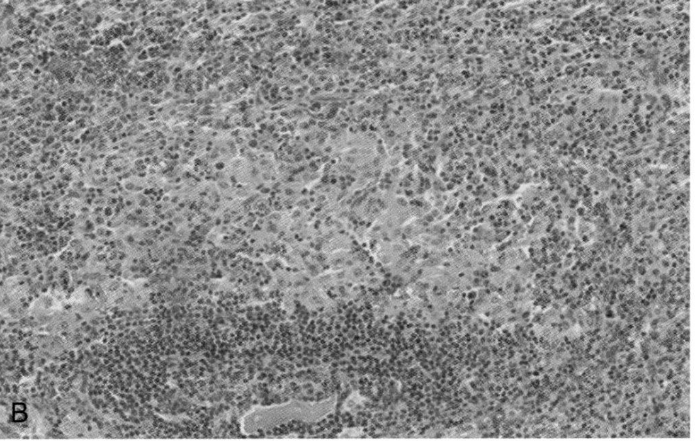

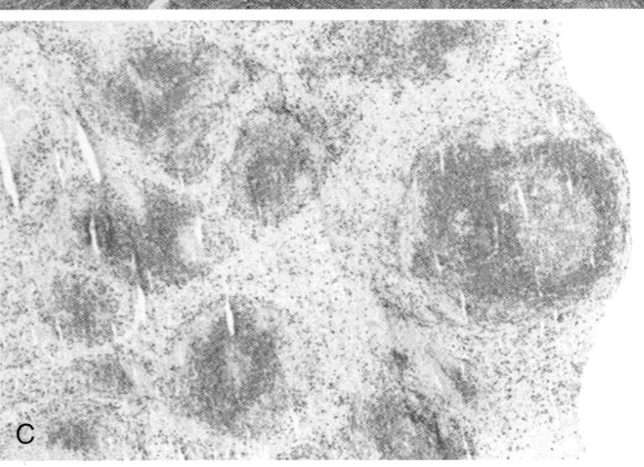

Figure 54-1. Atypical lymphoid hyperplasia involving the spleen. This 61-year-old woman had a 20-year history of common variable immunodeficiency with chronic diarrhea, bronchiectasis, and immune hemolytic anemia treated with intravenous gammaglobulin. She was evaluated for a 2-year history of asymptomatic splenomegaly, retroperitoneal lymphadenopathy, and bilateral lung nodules. **A,** Sections of enlarged spleen (540 g) show expanded white pulp, with prominent marginal zones and maintenance of follicular germinal centers. **B,** Granulomas composed of plump epithelioid histiocytes are present. **C,** The expanded lymphocyte population is highlighted by CD20 (avidin-biotin immunoperoxidase stain).

expression, and immunoglobuin gene rearrangement studies revealed a polyclonal population of B cells. In situ hybridization studies for EBV-encoded RNA (EBER1) were negative.

Sander and associates[18] studied 30 biopsies of nodal and extranodal lesions from 17 CVID patients. Reactive lymphoid hyperplasia was diagnosed in 14 cases (47%), atypical lymphoid hyperplasia in 8 cases (27%), chronic granulomatous inflammation in 6 cases (20%), and malignant lymphoma in 2 cases (6.7%). The atypical hyperplasia seen in CVID patients may show architectural effacement, raising the suspicion of malignant lymphoma; however, immunohistochemistry reveals preserved architecture with florid expansion of the B- and T-cell compartments. In situ hybridization studies for EBV are positive in about 25% of cases of atypical lymphoid hyperplasia in CVID patients. Gene rearrangement studies have also supported the benign nature of these histologically atypical lesions. Figure 54-2 illustrates a case of polyclonal T-cell infiltration of the bone marrow in a patient with CVID.

Clonal expansions of B or T lymphocytes may also occur in the absence of malignancy in CVID patients.[25] Similarly, clonal T-cell receptor (TCR) gene rearrangement has been demonstrated in a clinically benign case of reactive lymphoid proliferation demonstrating paracortical hyperplasia in a CVID patient.[15]

Lymphomas occur in 1% to 7% of CVID patients[24] and are 300 times more common in women than in men. Lymphomas in CVID patients occur most frequently in the fifth to seventh decades of life.[24,62] They are usually extranodal, aggressive B-cell non-Hodgkin's lymphomas,[17,63] and many are associated with EBV.[17,18] Rare cases have monoclonal immunoglobulins in the blood.[24] Rare cases of T-cell lymphomas in CVID patients have been reported.[62,64,65]

CVID patients are also at increased risk for other malignancies; there is an estimated 47-fold increased risk of gastric cancer in CVID patients compared with the normal population.[66] Acute and chronic myelogenous leukemias have been reported in CVID.[62]

IgA Deficiency

Clinical Features

Selective IgA deficiency is the most common form of immunodeficiency in the Western world, affecting approximately 1 in 600 individuals. Most patients have IgA levels less than 5 mg/dL; those with levels between 5 and 10 mg/dL are diagnosed as having partial IgA deficiency. Serum concentrations of the other immunoglobulins are usually normal, but patients have a high incidence of autoantibodies, and many have allergies, including autoimmune gastrointestinal disorders, allergic conjunctivitis, rhinitis, urticaria, atopic eczema, and bronchial asthma.[67] In about one third of cases there is an increased occurrence of bacterial infections in both the upper and lower respiratory tracts.

Genetic and Cellular Defects

The major role of IgA is to facilitate the presentation of antigen to mucosal T cells. The pathogenesis of IgA deficiency involves

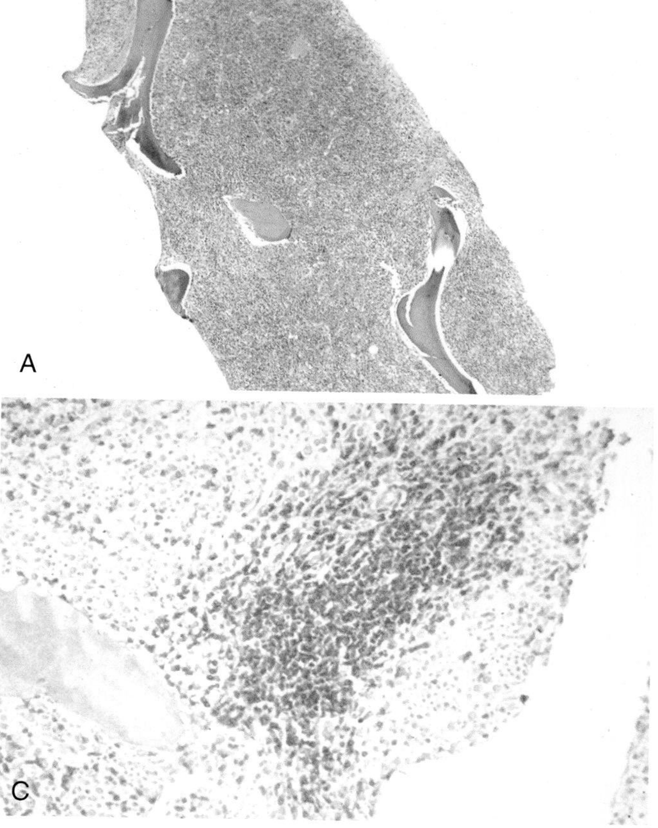

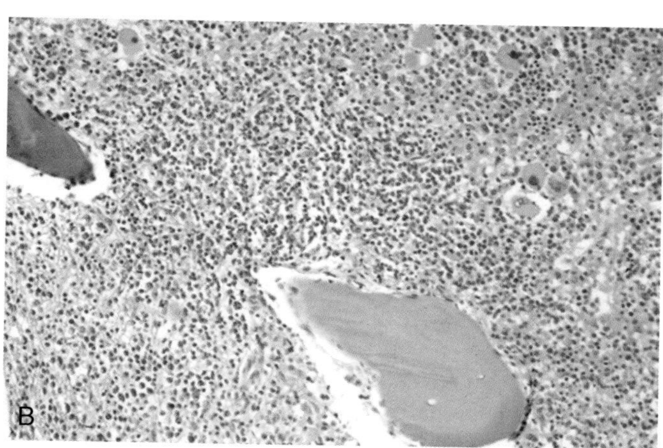

Figure 54-2. Atypical lymphocytic infiltrate in the bone marrow. This 22-year-old woman with common variable immunodeficiency presented with fever, sore throat, and intermittent diarrhea. **A,** Sections of bone marrow core biopsy are hypercellular and show numerous loosely cohesive aggregates of small lymphocytes diffusely scattered throughout the interstitium. **B,** At higher magnification, the paratrabecular aggregate contains small lymphoid cells that exhibit angulated nuclei with scant cytoplasm. **C,** The atypical lymphocytes are highlighted by CD3 (avidin-biotin immunoperoxidase stain). B cells were few in number but were polyclonal by immunohistochemical studies and flow cytometry. There was no evidence of T-cell receptor gene rearrangement by polymerase chain reaction.

a block in B-cell differentiation, which may be due to defective interaction between T and B cells. This is suggested by the observation that IL-12 treatment can overcome IgA deficiency by providing adequate T-cell priming in mice.[68] Susceptibility genes within the major histocompatibility complex (MHC), such as HLA-B8, SC01, and DR3, have been associated with IgA deficiency.[69] Other studies have implicated genomic polymorphisms in the tumor necrosis factor gene as a protective factor in IgA deficiency.[70]

Pathology

Lymphoid hyperplasia can occur in IgA deficiency.[71] In most cases the lymph node architecture and histology are normal, with the changes related mostly to infection. Enteropathy-associated reactive T-cell infiltration progressing to a clonal T-cell non-Hodgkin's lymphoma of gamma-delta type has been described in a patient with IgA deficiency.[72]

Selective IgG Subclass Deficiencies

Selective deficiencies of IgG subclasses, with or without IgA deficiency, are caused by defects in several genes. IgG2 deficiency is most common in children, whereas adults more often have low levels of IgG3. Patients with IgG2 deficiency have recurrent sinopulmonary infections caused by *Pneumococcus* and *Haemophilus*.[4]

T-CELL IMMUNODEFICIENCIES

Purine Nucleoside Phosphorylase Deficiency

Clinical Features

Purine nucleoside phosphorylase deficiency leads to dysfunction of the purine salvage pathway and accumulation of deoxyguanosine triphosphate (dGTP). Patients have defective T-cell immunity with variable abnormalities in humoral immunity,[73] often accompanied by a neurologic disorder and developmental retardation.[74]

Genetic and Cellular Defects

Mutations of purine nucleoside phosphorylase lead to the accumulation of dGTP, which is more toxic to T cells than to B cells.[75] Recent mouse models of purine nucleoside phosphorylase deficiency suggest that the accumulation of dGTP in the mitochondria results in impaired mitochondrial DNA repair with enhanced T-cell sensitivity to spontaneous DNA damage, leading to T-cell apoptosis.[76]

Pathology

Lymph nodes are generally small and lack paracortical regions because of depressed T-cell development. The thymus is small to absent and contains poorly formed Hassall's corpuscles. Other lymphoid tissues show marked depletion, with few T cells. Development of malignant lymphoma of the B-immunoblastic type has been reported in some patients.[77]

ZAP-70 Deficiency

ZAP-70 deficiency is an autosomal recessive disorder characterized by recurrent opportunistic infections within the first year of life.[4] ZAP-70 (zeta-associated polypeptide of 70 kDa) is a tyrosine kinase that binds to the TCR's phosphorylated immunoreceptor tyrosine-based activation motif sequences, a key molecule in TCR signaling. ZAP-70 deficiency results in CD8 lymphopenia.[78] In ZAP-70 deficiency, signaling through the TCR is defective, influencing T-cell development with a selective block in the positive selection of $CD8^+$ cells. There is failure of the peripheral $CD4^+$ T-cell proliferative response to mitogens or anti-CD3 antibody. By contrast, the activity of NK cells and B cells and serum immunoglobulin levels are normal.

Nezelof Syndrome

Nezelof syndrome is generally inherited in an autosomal recessive manner, although some report an X-linked inheritance pattern.[4] It is largely a T-cell deficiency, with little or no abnormality of gammaglobulins. The defect may be limited to the thymus, leading to abnormal thymocyte differentiation.[79] The thymus may be absent, with subsequent T-lymphocyte deficiency, impaired delayed hypersensitivity, and poor skin graft rejection. Lymphoid tissues are usually depleted, although plasma cells are normal in number.

CD3γ and CD3ε Deficiencies

Rare congenital immunodeficiencies are caused by mutations in the gamma[80] and epsilon[81] subunits of CD3. They are inherited in an autosomal recessive (11q23) manner and result in moderate to severe immunodeficiency due to decreased circulating $CD3^+$ T cells and poor responses to T-cell mitogens. They show decreased lymphocyte membrane expression of TCR/CD3.

SEVERE COMBINED IMMUNODEFICIENCIES (SCID)

SCID syndrome is characterized by impairment of both humoral and cell-mediated immunity and by susceptibility to fungal, bacterial, and viral infections. The syndrome is associated with various defects of the immune system involving T, B, and sometimes NK cells.

T-Cell–Negative, B-Cell–Negative Severe Combined Immunodeficiency

RAG1/RAG2 Deficiency and Omenn's Syndrome

Two related autosomal recessive deficiencies of the recombination-activating genes *RAG1* and *RAG2* result in a spectrum of SCIDs, called *RAG1/RAG2 deficiency* and *Omenn's syndrome*. RAGs are crucial proteins for VDJ recombination in B- and T-cell receptor genes. An absence of or defect in the VDJ recombination results in the arrest of B- and T-cell development, such that most of the circulating lymphocytes in affected patients are NK cells. Mutations that result in the total absence of *RAG1* or *RAG2* gene products lead to SCID without mature lymphoid cells,[82] whereas mutations that result in partial VDJ recombination activity lead to Omenn's syndrome.[83]

Clinical Features. Omenn's syndrome is characterized by the absence of circulating B cells and the infiltration of many organs by activated oligoclonal T lymphocytes. Most patients present with infantile diffuse erythroderma, alopecia, diarrhea, lymphadenopathy, hepatosplenomegaly, fever, hypereosinophilia, elevated serum IgE levels, and failure to thrive unless the condition is corrected by bone marrow transplantation.

Genetic and Cellular Defects. Patients with Omenn's syndrome have missense mutations of the *RAG1* and *RAG2* genes that decrease the efficiency of VDJ recombination.[83]

Pathology. There is massive infiltration of the skin and gut mucosa by activated CD45RO$^+$, HLA-DR$^+$ T cells, associated with marked eosinophilia. The T cells produce Th2-type cytokines and cause a disorder similar to graft-versus-host disease.[84] Peripheral lymphoid organs and the thymus are devoid of lymphocytes, with increased numbers of interdigitating reticulum cells and eosinophils.[85] The thymus is hypoplastic and often lacks Hassall's corpuscles.

Reticular Dysgenesis

Reticular dysgenesis is a rare and severe form of combined immunodeficiency.[86] It is characterized by congenital agranulocytosis, lymphopenia, and thymic hypoplasia. The red blood cells and platelets are usually normal in number. Cellular and humoral immune functions are absent owing to the failed maturation of both lymphoid and myeloid precursor cells, with maturation arrest at the promyelocyte stage,[87] and the absence of Langerhans cells within the skin.[88] Reticular dysgenesis can be corrected by bone marrow transplantation.

Adenosine Deaminase Deficiency

Clinical Features. ADA deficiency is the second most prevalent form of SCID, accounting for approximately 20% of cases. It is associated with the severe depletion of B cells, T cells, and NK cells. Affected individuals die from overwhelming opportunistic infections within the first few months of life if untreated. In addition to immunologic defects, most patients with ADA deficiency have skeletal abnormalities.

Genetic and Cellular Defects. ADA catalyzes the deamination of adenosine and deoxyadenosine; in its absence, these molecules as well as dGTP accumulate in the cells and inhibit cell division, resulting in a profound decrease in the maturation of lymphocyte precursors.[89] Some mutations result in partial ADA activity, allowing some lymphocyte differentiation to occur; these patients present as adults with infections and autoimmunity.[89] Allogeneic bone marrow transplantation or enzyme replacement may restore sufficient T-cell immunity to prevent infectious sequelae. Treatment of ADA deficiency by gene transfer has also been attempted.[90]

T-Cell–Negative, B-Cell–Positive Severe Combined Immunodeficiency

X-Linked Severe Combined Immunodeficiency

Clinical Features. Approximately 50% of patients with SCID have an X-linked recessive pattern of inheritance. Affected infants have infections caused by a wide range of pathogens, including *Candida albicans, Pneumocystis carinii, Pseudomonas,* cytomegalovirus, and varicella. Fatal giant cell pneumonia has been described as a result of measles infection or the live measles vaccine, and progressive vaccinia has occurred after smallpox vaccination. Infants have profound lymphopenia.[3] The number of NK cells may be normal or high. In contrast to the autosomal recessive forms of SCID, in which both T and B lymphocytes are profoundly deficient, X-linked SCID is characterized by the presence of a normal number of peripheral blood B cells.

Genetic and Cellular Defects. The disease results from a defect in the common cytokine receptor gamma chain gene that encodes a shared, essential component of the receptors for IL-2, IL-4, IL-7, IL-9, and IL-15.[91] Thus, the early lymphoid progenitor cells that lack intact interleukin receptors fail to be stimulated by these growth factors, which are vital to the normal development of T and B cells.

Pathology. There is thymic involution, with a marked paucity of lymphoid cells. Remnants of the thymus may be found in the neck owing to its failure to descend into the anterior mediastinum.[92] The thymus is composed of tightly packed lobules of undifferentiated thymic epithelium, with characteristic rosette formation. No vestiges of Hassall's corpuscles are present. Lymph nodes are few in number and very small; they often show only a marginal sinus and reticular framework devoid of lymphocytes. Mucosa-associated lymphoid tissues are atrophic. The spleen shows marked lymphoid depletion; B cells may localize around the central arteriole, where T cells are normally present.[93]

Lymphomas occur in about 1% to 5% of cases; approximately 74% are non-Hodgkin's lymphomas and 9.5% are Hodgkin's lymphomas. The median age at diagnosis of non-Hodgkin's lymphoma is 1.6 years, and it is usually extranodal.[13] When three SCID patients with non-Hodgkin's lymphoma were examined for the presence of EBV, it was detected in only one case by in situ hybridization. Other malignancies such as carcinomas occur much less frequently than lymphomas.[13,14]

JAK3 Deficiency

Mutations of the *JAK3* kinase gene lead to a non–X-linked form (autosomal recessive) of SCID. Clinically, patients resemble infants with X-linked SCID, with elevated levels of B cells and very low levels of T cells and NK cells in the blood.[91] The JAK3 protein, an intracellular tyrosine kinase, is crucial for signal transmission of cytokine receptors to signal transducers and activators of transcription, which drive gene expression in the nucleus. The mutations result in almost complete absence of JAK3 kinase activity with impairment of IL-2 and IL-4 signaling.[94,95]

Other Severe Combined Immunodeficiencies

Bare Lymphocyte Syndrome Type I (TAP1 and TAP2 Deficiency)

Clinical Features. Bare lymphocyte syndrome is characterized by a severe decrease of human leukocyte antigen (HLA) class I or class II molecules. It manifests within the first 6 years of life with recurrent bacterial infections of the upper respiratory tract.

Genetic and Cellular Defects. Transport associated with antigen processing (TAP) proteins encoded by genes within the MHC play a role in the presentation of antigenic peptides to T cells. The TAP complex is composed of TAP1 and TAP2, which, via the adenosine triphosphate–binding cassette transporter, translocate peptides from the cytosol to MHC class I molecules in the endoplasmic reticulum. TAP1 and TAP2 deficiencies have identical clinical manifestations. Mutations of both *TAP1* and *TAP2* genes result in deficient expression of HLA class I proteins on the cell surface, with defects in NK cell cytotoxicity.[96,97]

Pathology. Histologic examination reveals a necrotizing granulomatous inflammation similar to that of Wegener's granulomatosis.[98]

Bare Lymphocyte Syndrome Type II (MHC Class II Deficiency)

Children with hereditary MHC class II deficiency are susceptible to bacterial, viral, and fungal infections beginning in the first year of life. Most children die from infection by age 4 years.[99] Three forms occur, caused by impaired transcription of MHC class II genes. Regulatory factor X, a complex binding to the X-box of MHC II promoters in the nucleus, is mutated in one form; mutations of the class II transcription activator, a positive regulator of MHC class II gene transcription and regulatory factor X–associated protein, occur in the others.[100] $CD4^+$ T cells are decreased in all three forms, although circulating lymphocyte numbers are normal, and immunoglobulin levels can be decreased.[101-103]

CD45 Deficiency

A molecular defect of CD45 is a rare cause of SCID.[104,105] CD45 is an abundant transmembrane tyrosine phosphatase expressed on all leukocytes, and it is required for efficient lymphocyte signaling, integrin-mediated adhesion, and migration of immune cells. Mutations leading to loss of a component of the extracellular domain of CD45 result in very low numbers of circulating T cells but a normal number of B cells. The T cells are unresponsive to mitogens, and serum immunoglobulin levels usually decrease with age.

OTHER IMMUNODEFICIENCIES

Wiskott-Aldrich Syndrome (WAS)

Clinical Features

WAS is an X-linked recessive disease characterized by immune dysregulation and thrombocytopenia. The estimated incidence in the United States is 4 per million male live births, accounting for six new cases per year.[4] Affected males have eczema, recurrent bacterial infections, and profound thrombocytopenia with small, dysfunctional platelets.[106] Serum IgM concentrations are reduced, IgA and IgE concentrations are elevated, and IgG is normal. Antibody formation, especially to encapsulated bacteria, is defective, as is the response to protein antigens. The number of B cells increases with time, whereas the number of T cells decreases.[107] There is a poor in vitro T-cell response to the mitogenic effects of anti-CD3.[108] Food allergy and autoimmune disease, including hemolytic anemia, vasculitides, and inflammatory bowel disease, may occur.[11] In the less severe form, known as *X-linked thrombocytopenia*, mutations in the same gene produce characteristic platelet abnormalities but minimal immunologic disturbances; the immune defects appear later and are variable and progressive.[109,110] In the past, WAS patients generally died within the first decade from infection, hemorrhage, or malignancy. However, improved management, including intravenous immune globulin therapy and splenectomy, has improved the life expectancy of WAS patients, with a median survival of 15 years.

Genetic and Cellular Defects

Several mutations of the WAS gene (Xp11.22) have been identified.[111,112] The normal gene encodes the WAS protein,[111] a member of a family of proteins responsible for the transduction of signals from the cell membrane to the actin cytoskeleton.[113] The interaction among WAS protein, the rho family GTPase CDC42, and the cytoskeletal organizing complex Arp2/3 is disturbed and leads to defects in cell signaling, polarization, motility, and phagocytosis.[114] The cell surface sialoglycoproteins, most notably CD43 (sialophorin/leukosialin), are unstable, with reduced expression.[111] Although the neutrophils and macrophages in WAS patients have been shown to exhibit impaired chemotactic responses,[115] other functional properties of these cells appear to be intact.[113] Deficiency of WAS protein can be detected in peripheral blood mononuclear cells by flow cytometry.[116]

Pathology

The lymph nodes and spleen frequently show depletion of lymphocytes from the T-cell zones, prominence of the stroma, atypical plasma cells, plasmacytosis, and extramedullary hematopoiesis.[117] Tissue eosinophilia may be seen. Less frequent features include hemophagocytosis and depletion of germinal centers.

The risk of malignancy in WAS patients is estimated to be 100 times greater than normal.[14] Approximately 10% to 20% of WAS patients develop lymphoma.[118] The risk increases with age,[22] with a median age of 6 years at the time of diagnosis of lymphoma. Non-Hodgkin's lymphomas, most commonly large B-cell lymphomas, account for 75% of the malignancies; Hodgkin's lymphoma and leukemias account for approximately 4% and 10%, respectively.[14] Extranodal sites such as the brain, skin, small bowel, and mediastinum are commonly involved. EBV-associated Hodgkin's lymphoma also has been reported (Fig. 54-3).[119] Fatal EBV^+ lymphoproliferative disorders can also occur.[120] Monoclonal expansions of B lymphocytes with monoclonal gammopathy have also been described,[121] although some have been documented to undergo spontaneous regression.

Nonlymphoid tumors such as Kaposi's sarcoma have rarely been described.[122] Of interest is the complete absence of the usual childhood malignancies such as Burkitt's lymphoma, lymphoblastic lymphoma, and other common pediatric tumors such as neuroblastoma, Wilms' tumor, Ewing's sarcoma, and rhabdomyosarcoma.

DiGeorge/Velocardiofacial Syndrome

Clinical Features

DiGeorge/velocardiofacial syndrome is characterized by lack of development or underdevelopment of the thymus and sur-

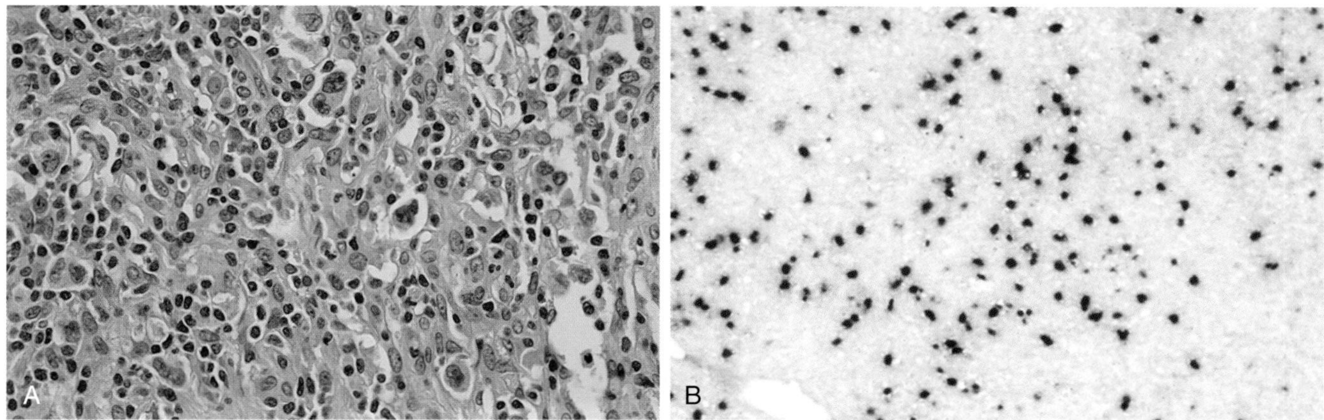

Figure 54-3. Hodgkin's lymphoma in a patient with Wiscott-Aldrich syndrome. An enlarged cervical lymph node in a 6-year-old patient with Wiskott-Aldrich syndrome was biopsied. **A,** The lymph node architecture is effaced by a polymorphic population of small reactive lymphocytes with admixed Reed-Sternberg cells. **B,** In situ hybridization demonstrates numerous EBER1+ Reed-Sternberg cells.

rounding organs and other associated defects, including cardiac outflow tract anomalies, abnormal facies, thymic hypoplasia, cleft palate, and hypocalcemia.[123] The degree of immunodeficiency varies, and only about 20% of patients have decreased T-cell numbers and function. Autoimmune diseases and recurrent infections are common.[124]

Genetic and Cellular Defects

The DiGeorge anomaly is one of a group of disorders that share a deletion involving chromosome 22q11.2 (the DiGeorge syndrome chromosome region), which includes 24 contiguous genes.[123] No causative gene or combination of genes has been demonstrated. Knockout studies have shown that mice heterozygous for a transcription factor of the T-box gene (*Tbx1*) display developmental anomalies encompassing almost all the common features of DiGeorge syndrome.[125] Standard karyotyping, polymerase chain reaction, and fluorescence in situ hybridization using probes from within the deletion segment are available for prenatal diagnosis of the 22q11.2 deletion.[126]

Pathology

There is depletion of thymic tissue, with no corticomedullary differentiation, and ill-defined Hassall's corpuscles in some patients; in others, thymic tissue is totally absent (Fig. 54-4). Lymph nodes also show depletion of lymphoid cells.

Ataxia-Telangiectasia

Clinical Features

AT is an autosomal recessive disorder characterized by neurologic deficits, including cerebellar degeneration with ataxia, oculocutaneous telangiectasia, and immunodeficiency.[4] Most patients develop recurrent bacterial sinopulmonary infections and have increased susceptibility to cancer.[127,128] The immunologic defects are of variable severity and may affect both T and B cells. Other important features include thymic hypoplasia, growth retardation, hypogonadism, and elevated levels of alpha fetoprotein, which may be useful in establishing the diagnosis.[127] Eighty percent of patients are IgA deficient, and serum levels of IgG4 and IgG2 may also be decreased. AT patients exhibit increased susceptibility to the effects of ionizing radiation because of defective DNA repair and chromosomal instability.[129]

Genetic and Cellular Defects

The *ATM* gene, on chromosome 11q22-23,[130] encodes a polypeptide with a phosphatidyl inositol-3′ kinase domain[131] and similarities to the catalytic subunit of DNA-dependent protein kinase[132]; this polypeptide can bind directly to and phosphorylate c-abl and p53. *ATM* is involved in mitogenic signal transduction, meiotic recombination, response to DNA damage, cell cycle control, and apoptosis.[133] The *ATM* gene is mutated in all AT patients.[131] Approximately 10% of all T lymphocytes in AT patients show the presence of translocations and inversions, mainly involving chromosomes 7 and 14 at specific breakpoints, the chromosomal location of T-cell antigen receptor genes, and immunoglobulin gene loci.[127]

Pathology

There is a progressive loss of Purkinje cells and the granular cell layer of the cerebellum.[134] Congenital hypoplasia of the ovaries and incomplete spermatogenesis have been reported.[135] Lymphoid tissues show nodal hypoplasia, with depletion of B cells within the follicles,[136] and thymic atrophy, with the absence of Hassall's corpuscles.

Approximately 10% of all AT homozygotes develop a malignancy, with a 70-fold and 250-fold excess risk for leukemias and lymphomas, respectively.[21] Both B- and T-cell tumors occur, with a four- to fivefold increase in the frequency of T-cell tumors compared with B-cell tumors (Fig. 54-5).[14] AT patients have an increased incidence of acute lymphoblastic leukemia[137] with a high proportion of unfavorable prognostic characteristics, including older age at presentation (median, 9 years), high initial white blood cell count, male gender, and mediastinal mass. Hodgkin's lymphoma accounts for approximately 10% of the neoplasms in AT patients.[138]

Young adult patients may develop a variety of T-cell lymphomas, including T-cell prolymphocytic leukemia[127,139] and

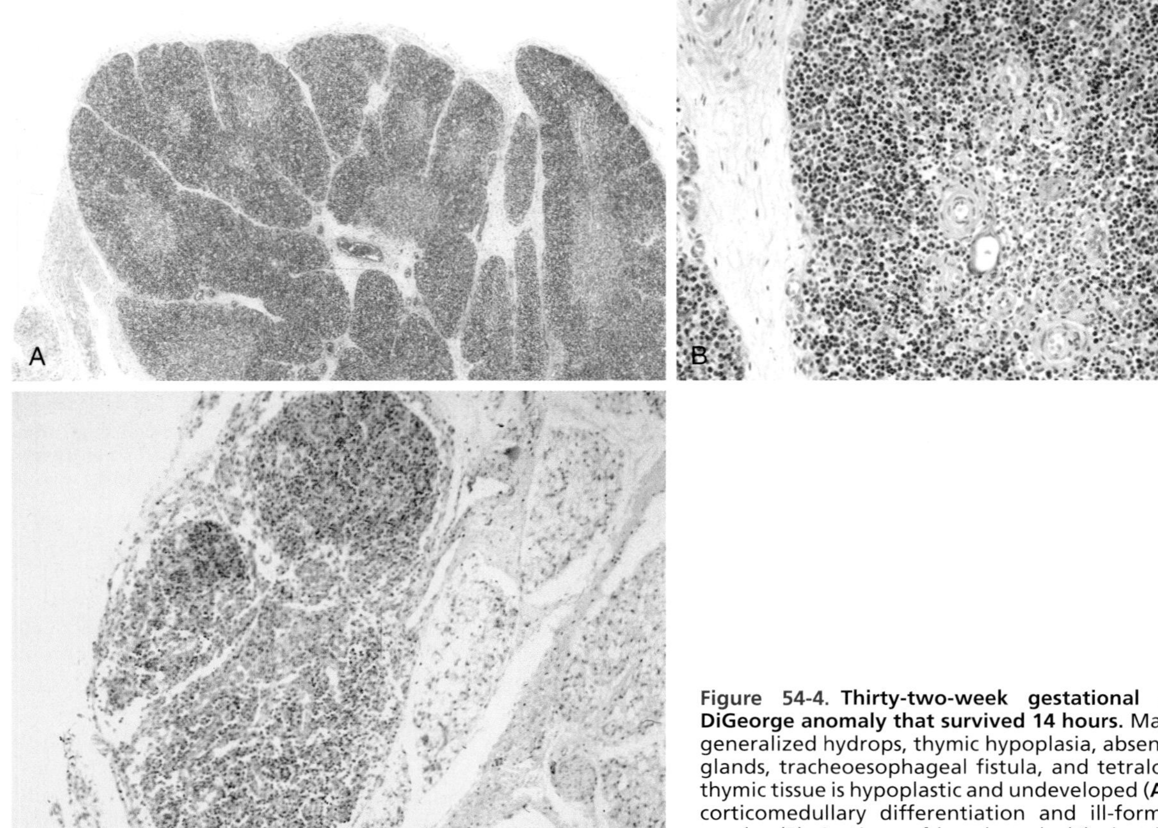

Figure 54-4. Thirty-two-week gestational age fetus with DiGeorge anomaly that survived 14 hours. Major findings were generalized hydrops, thymic hypoplasia, absence of parathyroid glands, tracheoesophageal fistula, and tetralogy of Fallot. The thymic tissue is hypoplastic and undeveloped **(A)**, with decreased corticomedullary differentiation and ill-formed Hassall's corpuscles **(B)**. Sections of lymph node **(C)** also show depletion of lymphoid cells.

T-lymphoblastic lymphoma.[140] Nonlymphoid tumors (mostly carcinomas) account for 13% to 22% of all malignancies in AT patients and occur in older patients, with a median age of 17 years.[21]

Immunodeficiency with Albinism

Chédiak-Higashi Syndrome

Clinical Features. Chédiak-Higashi syndrome is characterized by partial skin and ocular albinism, increased susceptibility to infection, and progressive neuropathy.[141] Most patients with Chédiak-Higashi syndrome develop lethal complications, called the *accelerated phase,* during which T cells and macrophages undergo overwhelming activation involving multiple organs.[142]

Genetic and Cellular Defects. Mutations of the gene encoding a cytoplasmic protein that controls lysosome traffic, called *LYST* (lysosomal trafficking regulator) in humans or *Beige* in mice, are thought to cause Chédiak-Higashi syndrome.[143] Many cell types have large intracytoplasmic granulations,[144] and there is deficient cytotoxic lymphocyte activity as a result of defective vesicular trafficking of the endosome-lysosome compartment. Defective T-cell and NK-cell cytotoxic function develops due to defective exocytosis and delivery of lytic proteins.[145]

Pathology. Peripheral blood films show abnormal granules in the leukocytes. Large lysosomal granules are also seen within melanocytes and gastric mucosal epithelial cells, among others.[144]

Griscelli Syndrome

Clinical Features. Griscelli syndrome is a rare autosomal recessive disorder that results in hypopigmentation of hair and skin, the presence of large clumps of pigment in hair shafts, and an accumulation of melanosomes in melanocytes.[146] Most patients develop an uncontrolled T-lymphocyte and macrophage activation process with hemophagocytosis, leading to death in the absence of bone marrow transplantation.[147] However, some Griscelli syndrome patients exhibit severe neurologic impairment without apparent immune abnormalities. Patients present with frequent pyogenic infections and acute episodes of fever, neutropenia, and thrombocytopenia. Despite an adequate number of T and B lymphocytes, the patients are hypogammaglobulinemic, deficient in antibody production, and incapable of delayed skin hypersensitivity and skin graft rejection. Griscelli syndrome resembles Chédiak-Higashi syndrome, but the characteristic giant granules of the latter are not present, and the polymorphonuclear leukocytes in Griscelli syndrome are morphologically normal.

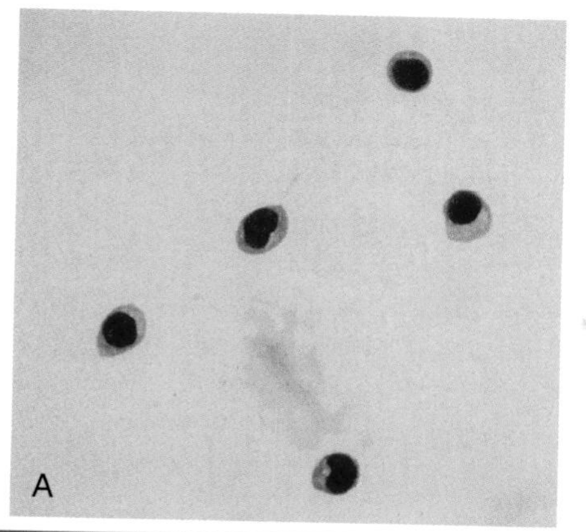

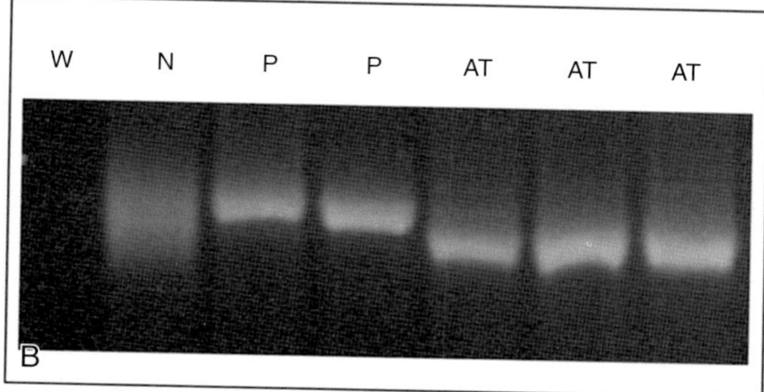

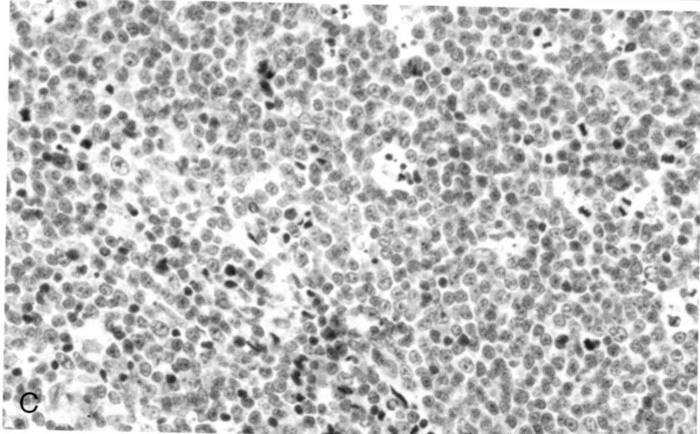

Figure 54-5. Lymphoid neoplasms in patients with ataxia-telangiectasia. A, Cytospin of cerebrospinal fluid from a 7-year-old girl with ataxia-telangiectasia shows predominantly lymphocytes with slight nuclear enlargement and ample, lightly basophilic cytoplasm. Nuclear chromatin shows variable maturity, and occasional cells show nucleoli (Wright stain). **B,** Subsequent analysis of pleural fluid demonstrates a clonal population of T cells by T-cell receptor gene polymerase chain reaction. *Lane W*, template-free control (H_2O), shows no product. *Lane N*, negative (polyclonal) DNA control from a hyperplastic tonsil, shows a polyclonal smear pattern. *Lanes P*, positive (monoclonal) DNA controls from the MOLT 4 and Karpas 299 cell lines, respectively. *Lanes AT*, DNA from lymphoma in a patient with ataxia-telangiectasia. **C,** Pelvic mass in a 13-year-old white girl with ataxia-telangiectasia exhibits the morphologic features of Burkitt's lymphoma.

Genetic and Cellular Defects. Nucleotide substitutions of the myosin-5A gene (*MYO5A*) have been reported in two affected patients with neurologic impairment but without susceptibility to infection or hemophagocytic syndrome.[148] Myosin-5A, a member of the unconventional myosin family thought to participate in organelle transport, is important for lymphocyte cytotoxic function.[147] A second locus involves the *RAB27A* gene on chromosome 15q21, which encodes a RAB guanosine triphosphate binding protein that is important for regulating intracellular protein trafficking.[147] Patients lack neurologic features but have hemophagocytic syndrome. T cells of RAB27A-deficient individuals have a normal granule content of perforin and granzymes but defective granule release.

Pathology. The liver, spleen, lymph nodes, and lungs may show reactive histiocytic proliferations.[149]

X-Linked Lymphoproliferative Syndrome

Clinical Features

XLP syndrome, or Duncan's disease, is a rare inherited immunodeficiency characterized by lymphohistiocytosis, hypogammaglobulinemia, and lymphoma that usually develops in response to EBV,[150,151] leading to uncontrolled expansion of EBV-infected B cells and cytotoxic T cells. The average age of onset is 2.5 years, with 100% mortality by age 40 years.[152] Patients are totally asymptomatic before EBV infection; following infection with EBV, a vigorous, uncontrolled polyclonal expansion of T and B cells occurs. Fever, pharyngitis, lymphadenopathy, hepatosplenomegaly, and atypical lymphocytosis develop; serum immunoglobulins may be reduced or absent, or there may be a polyclonal hypergammaglobulinemia. The primary cause of death is hepatic necrosis and bone marrow failure.

Genetic and Cellular Defects

XLP syndrome is caused by mutations in SH2 domain protein-1A,[151] also called signaling lymphocyte activation molecule (SLAM)–associated protein (SAP), and in X-linked inhibitor of apoptosis (XIAP; also termed BIRC4).[153] SLAM (also known as CDw150) on the surface of T cells has a crucial function in cell stimulation. Mutations in SAP affect the interaction between T cells and B cells and lead to uncontrolled B-cell proliferation during EBV infection.[150] Mutations in XIAP lead to a heightened apoptotic response to a variety of stimuli, including TCR-CD3 complex, the death receptor CD95, and tumor necrosis factor–associated apoptosis-inducing ligand receptor. Patients have reduced numbers of NK/T lymphocytes (NKT cells).[153,154]

Pathology

The extent of lymphoid proliferation in response to EBV can vary from a reactive lymphocytic vasculitis[155] to extensive involvement of hematopoietic organs, viscera, and central nervous system by lymphocytes, plasma cells, and histiocytes. The extensive tissue destruction of the liver and bone marrow appears to stem from the uncontrolled cytotoxic T-cell response.[150] Hemophagocytic lymphohistiocytosis occurs in a subset of patients.[156] The phenotype is that of severe or fatal infectious mononucleosis in approximately 50% of cases, acquired hypogammaglobulinemia in about 30%, and malignant lymphoma in about 25%, alone or in combination.

Most of the malignant lymphomas are extranodal non-Hodgkin's lymphomas, usually diffuse large B-cell lymphoma or Burkitt's lymphoma, involving the ileocecal region. In a registry study of 100 patients, 35 developed B-cell lymphoma, and the terminal ileum was involved in 26.[157] Of 17 cases of lymphoma occurring in XLP syndrome patients, 41% were classified as small noncleaved cell, 18% as immunoblastic, and 12% as small cleaved cell or mixed lymphomas; 6% were unclassifiable.[158]

Immunodeficiency, Centromeric Instability, Facial Anomaly (ICF) Syndrome

Clinical Features

Variable immunodeficiency in association with centromeric instability of chromosomes 1, 9, 16, and, rarely, 2, with an increased frequency of somatic recombination of the arms of these chromosomes and a marked tendency to form multibranched configurations, has been reported.[159] Affected children have variable immunodeficiency, mild developmental delay, and facial abnormalities consisting of hypertelorism, a flat nasal bridge, epicanthal folds, protrusion of the tongue, and mild micrognathia. Most patients exhibit the absence or severe reduction of at least two immunoglobulin classes, with or without a defective cell-mediated immunity, and most patients die during childhood.

Genetic and Cellular Defects

Patients with immunodeficiency, centromeric instability, facial anomaly syndrome have marked hypomethylation of their DNA. Mutations involving the DNA methyltransferase 3B gene were identified in four patients from three families.[160,161] Genomic methylation is critical for the maintenance of structure and expression, and undermethylation of certain chromosomal segments is associated with centromere instability and abnormal expression of key immunoregulatory genes.

Nijmegen Breakage Syndrome

Clinical Features

NBS is a rare autosomal disorder characterized by microcephaly, stunted growth, mental retardation, café au lait spots, and immunodeficiency, with impaired DNA repair and hypersensitivity to ionizing radiation.[162,163] The disease has similarities to AT; recurrent infections, chromosomal instability, hypersensitivity to ionizing radiation and bleomycin, and radioresistance of DNA replication are common features of both. NBS patients lack the classic signs and symptoms of AT such as cerebellar ataxia, oculocutaneous telangiectasia, and increased alpha fetoprotein. Patients suffer from recurrent respiratory tract or urinary tract infections. Hypogammaglobulinemia is typically present; IgA, IgG2, IgG4, and IgE levels are low.[163] There is high predisposition to malignancy.

Genetic and Cellular Defects

Most patients have a truncating deletion of the *NBS-1* gene on chromosome 8q21. The *NBS-1* gene encodes the protein nibrin, involved in DNA double-strand break repair.[164] The defect is thought to result in defective immunoglobulin class switching and decreased immunoglobulin production.[165] There is a functional link between AT and NBS gene products, in that the phosphorylation and function of NBS-1 protein induced by ionizing radiation requires the kinase function of *ATM*.[166]

Pathology

NBS patients have thymic hypoplasia,[167,168] with fatty replacement, predominant thymic epithelial cells, and absent Hassall's corpuscles. The lymph nodes and spleen are normal but have small lymphoid follicles with sparse germinal centers, sinus histiocytosis, and medullary plasmacytosis. Peyer's patches are atrophic.[167]

Nine of the 30 documented NBS patients have developed malignancies, eight of which were lymphomas.[163,169] The average age of NBS patients with lymphoid malignancy is 10.25 years, with a male-to-female ratio of 1:1. Most lymphomas are of the diffuse large B-cell type.[167,170]

Job's Syndrome

Clinical Features

Job's syndrome is characterized by markedly elevated serum IgE levels and recurrent cutaneous and sinopulmonary infections.[171] Many patients have eczematoid rashes, mucocutaneous candidiasis, subcutaneous abscesses, bony abnormalities, and osteoporotic fractures.[172]

Genetic and Cellular Defects

The genetic basis is not known, and the immunologic defect is largely undefined. Reduced neutrophil chemotaxis and variable T-cell defects have been demonstrated in some patients. It has been hypothesized that hyper-IgE is associated with a Th1-Th2 imbalance.[173] Job's syndrome is inherited as a single-locus, autosomal dominant trait with variable penetrance.[174]

Pathology

Lymphomas have been reported in patients with Job's syndrome.[175-177] Of the five reported to date, three were diffuse large B-cell lymphomas, one was Burkitt's lymphoma, and one was Hodgkin's lymphoma. Immunohistochemistry for EBV latent membrane protein was negative in one case studied.[15]

Autoimmune Lymphoproliferative Syndrome

Clinical Features

Children with autoimmune lymphoproliferative syndrome (ALPS) present with peripheral lymphocytosis, diffuse lymphadenopathy, hepatosplenomegaly, hypergammaglobulinemia, autoimmune cytopenias, and, rarely, autoimmune glomerulonephritis and hepatitis.[178] The peripheral blood contains $CD5^+$ B cells; NK cells; and TCRαβ $CD4^-$, $CD8^-$ (double negative), HLA-DR^+ naïve T cells[179] constituting between 15% and 70% of the peripheral blood T cells. These cells have impaired proliferative and cytokine responses to activation. Patients with ALPS have a predilection for developing malig-

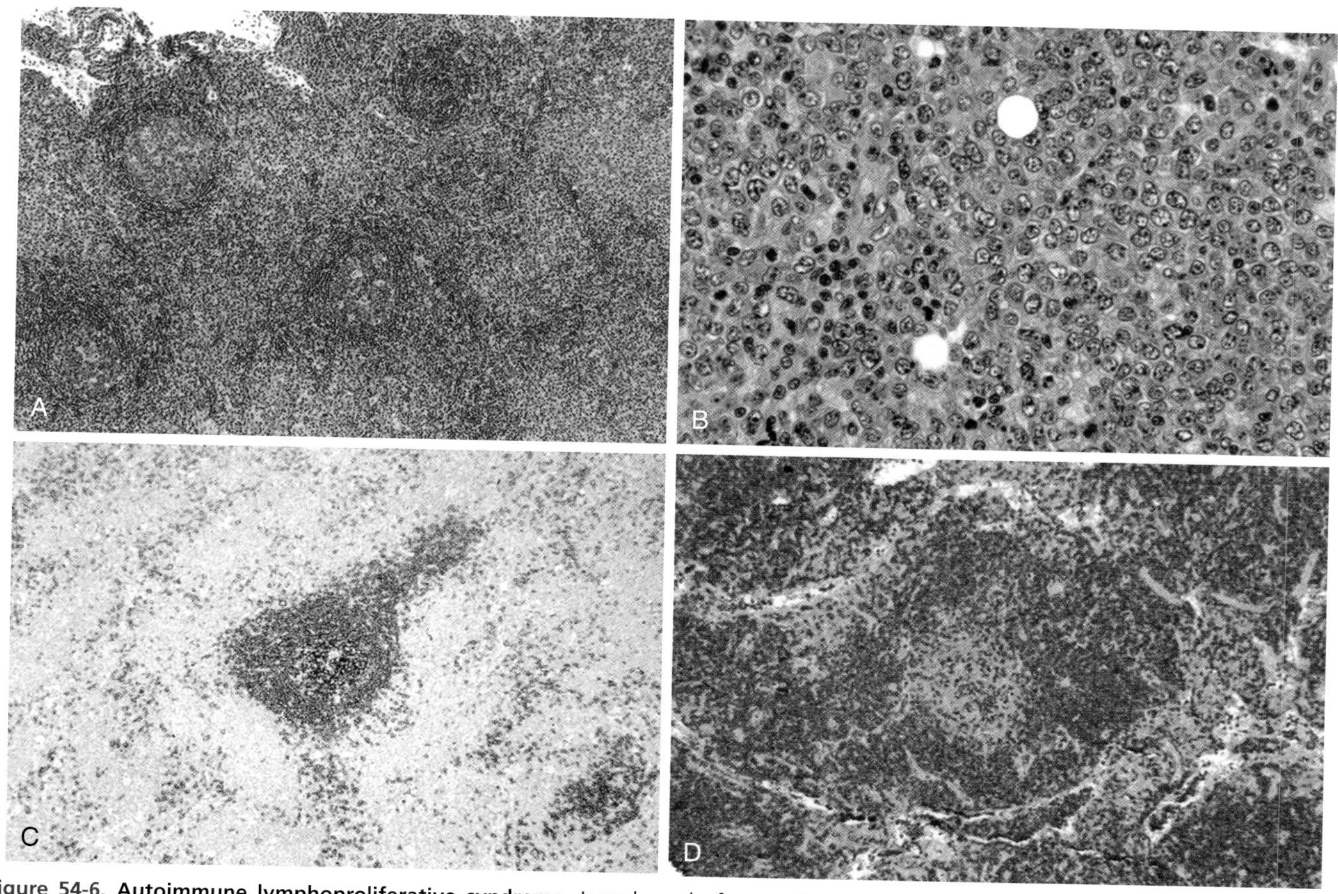

Figure 54-6. Autoimmune lymphoproliferative syndrome. Lymph node from a 4-year-old boy with autoimmune lymphoproliferative syndrome shows follicular hyperplasia and expansion of the paracortical zone (**A**) by small to intermediate-sized lymphocytes (**B**). The atypical lymphocytes are negative for CD20 (**C**) but express CD3 (**D**). (**C** and **D**, avidin-biotin immunoperoxidase stain.)

nant lymphomas of both non-Hodgkin's and Hodgkin's types.[180,181]

Genetic and Cellular Defects

ALPS result from mutations in several genes in the apoptosis pathway, including Fas,[182] Fas ligand, and caspases 8 and 10.[183] The disease is inherited as an autosomal dominant trait, but development of the full phenotype depends on additional factors, suggesting that other host factors or genes play a role in modulating the disease phenotype. The observation of ALPS in individuals without mutations of the above-mentioned genes suggests a role for other apoptosis pathway genes.

Pathology

Lymph nodes are characteristically enlarged and demonstrate a spectrum of appearances, from follicular hyperplasia with numerous follicles showing hyperplastic germinal centers to others showing atrophic features.[184] There is expansion of the paracortex by the proliferation of small to medium-sized T cells that are $CD4^-$, $CD8^-$, and $CD3^+$ and have a naïve ($CD45RA^+$) phenotype. They may appear cytologically atypical and must be recognized to avoid the misdiagnosis of lymphoma (Fig. 54-6).

Pearls and Pitfalls

- Although the majority of patients with primary immunodeficiencies present during early childhood, a subset (CVID) can present in adulthood.
- The abnormal lymphoid proliferations that occur in primary immunodeficiences represent a biologic continuum of reactive and atypical to clonal populations, requiring the integration of clinical, immunophenotypic, and molecular analyses.
- Serial biopsies or other analyses may be required to determine the nature of lymphoid proliferations in patients with primary immunodeficiencies.
- Common histologic findings in tissues obtained from patients with primary immunodeficiencies include eosinophilia, histiocytic proliferation, and hemophagocytosis.
- Lymphoid tissues from patients with primary immunodeficiencies commonly exhibit underdeveloped germinal centers.
- Lymphomas that arise in patients with primary immunodeficiencies occur in extranodal sites and are usually associated with EBV.

References can be found on Expert Consult @ www.expertconsult.com

Chapter 55

Iatrogenic Immunodeficiency-Associated Lymphoproliferative Disorders

Steven H. Swerdlow and Fiona E. Craig

CHAPTER OUTLINE

DEFINITION

Lymphoproliferative disorders (LPDs) associated with iatrogenic immunodeficiency constitute a spectrum of lymphoid or plasmacytic proliferations, including a major subset that occurs following solid organ, stem cell, or bone marrow transplantation (posttransplant lymphoproliferative disorders, or PTLDs). A smaller number of cases (other iatrogenic immunodeficiency-associated LPDs) occur in other situations, such as in patients with rheumatoid arthritis treated with methotrexate or in young patients with Crohn's disease treated with tumor necrosis factor-α (TNF-α) antagonists. Many but not all LPDs are associated with Epstein-Barr virus (EBV). They require further classification because of the great variation in their cytologic composition, degree of destructiveness, immunophenotype, cytogenetic and molecular findings, clinical behavior, and therapeutic approach.[1-7] Cases range from hyperplastic-appearing lesions to others that are indistinguishable from non-Hodgkin's or Hodgkin's lymphomas in immunocompetent hosts. Even the latter cases, however, are separately designated, because reducing or discontinuing immunosuppression, when possible, or administering therapy that would be considered inadequate in immunocompetent hosts may lead to resolution.

POSTTRANSPLANT LYMPHOPROLIFERATIVE DISORDERS

The World Health Organization (WHO) classification recognizes four major categories of PTLD (Box 55-1).[5] Which of these disorders is truly neoplastic is debatable, and such a determination is not necessarily of clinical utility. Biopsies performed when there is a question of PTLD should be handled using a standard "rule out lymphoma" protocol that includes all the necessary ancillary techniques required for a complete diagnosis (Box 55-2). Although cytologic and fine-needle aspiration biopsy specimens can be useful in some circumstances, excisional biopsy is preferred because of the importance of assessing architectural features, the need for sufficient material for ancillary studies, and the intralesional heterogeneity present in a moderate number of PTLDs.

Epidemiology

PTLD develops in approximately 2% of all transplant recipients, but there is a significant variation in incidence based on the type of organ transplanted. As recently reported, the incidence in adults after kidney transplantation is less than 1%; after liver, heart, marrow, or stem cell transplantation, it is

Box 55-1 *World Health Organization Classification of Posttransplant Lymphoproliferative Disorders (PTLDs)*

Early Lesions*
- Plasmacytic hyperplasia
- Infectious mononucleosis–like PTLD

Polymorphic PTLDs

Monomorphic PTLDs
Classify according to the lymphoma they resemble.
- B-cell neoplasms
  - Diffuse large B-cell lymphoma, not otherwise specified
  - Burkitt's lymphoma
  - Plasma cell myeloma
  - Plasmacytoma-like lesion
  - Other[†]
- T-cell neoplasms
  - Peripheral T-cell lymphoma, not otherwise specified
  - Hepatosplenic T-cell lymphoma
  - Other

Classical Hodgkin's Lymphoma–Type PTLD

*Some posttransplant mass lesions may have the appearance of florid follicular hyperplasia or other marked but non–infectious mononucleosis–like lymphoid hyperplasia.
[†]Small B-cell lymphomas arising in transplant patients are not considered PTLD.
From Swerdlow SH, Campo E, Harris NL, et al, eds. *WHO Classification of Tumours of Haematopoietic and Lymphoid Tissues*. Lyon, France: IARC Press; 2008.

generally 1% to 2%; the incidence is higher after lung, heart-lung, and intestinal transplants, particularly multivisceral transplants.[5] Multivisceral transplantation has been associated with an incidence of 33% to 47%.[8,9] Many other factors impact the incidence of PTLD. EBV seronegativity at the time of organ transplantation is an extremely important risk factor and explains in part the much higher incidence of PTLD in children than in adults.[5] Transplanting an organ from an EBV-seropositive donor into an EBV-seronegative recipient (EBV mismatch) increases the incidence of PTLD 10- to 75-fold.[10] Lack of previous exposure to cytomegalovirus (CMV) is also associated with an increased incidence of PTLD if the recipient is CMV$^-$ and either the donor is CMV$^+$ (CMV mismatch) or the recipient experiences a symptomatic primary CMV infection.[10] The effects of EBV mismatch and CMV mismatch appear to be synergistic. Patients who are transplanted for hepatitis C–induced cirrhosis reportedly have an increased incidence of PTLD, suggesting that hepatitis C may potentiate the oncogenicity of EBV.[11,12] Host factors, such as polymorphisms leading to lower expression of proinflammatory cytokines or greater expression of anti-inflammatory cytokines, may also influence the risk of selected PTLDs.[13-15]

Another important risk factor is the immunosuppressive regimen required to maintain the transplant or to treat graft-versus-host disease. The cumulative intensity of immunosuppressive therapy and the agents used are associated with the risk of developing early PTLD in the first year after transplantation, whereas the overall duration of immunosuppression is associated with the risk of developing later PTLD.[10,16] Some of the newer immunosuppressive strategies may be associated with a lower risk for PTLD.[17] Anti–T-cell antibody preparations, such as OKT3 and antithymocyte globulin (ATG), have been associated with an increased risk of PTLD, as has the use of these agents to remove T cells from bone marrow or stem cell products before transplantation.[10,16-19] However, depletion of both T cells and B cells is not associated with as great a risk.[18]

Etiology

The majority of PTLDs are caused by EBV-infected lymphoid or plasmacytic cells that are not adequately controlled because of an impaired cytotoxic T-cell response related to immunosuppression and, in the case of stem cell and bone marrow transplants, myeloablative regimens.[16,20,21] Specifically, patients with PTLD have decreased EBV-specific CD8$^+$ T cells

Box 55-2 *Major Diagnostic Features of and Recommended Diagnostic Testing for Posttransplant Lymphoproliferative Disorders (PTLDs)*

Morphology
- Required for diagnosis and best accomplished with histologic sections
- Findings are extremely variable, ranging from lymphoplasmacytic proliferations with underlying architectural preservation to destructive polymorphic lymphoplasmacytic proliferations with moderately numerous transformed cells or immunoblasts to lesions fulfilling the criteria for one of the non–small cell B-cell lymphomas, a plasma cell neoplasm, one of the T-cell lymphomas, or occasionally classical Hodgkin's lymphoma

Immunophenotype
- Required for diagnosis
- Findings are extremely variable, including polyclonal lesions, often with many admixed B and T cells, or lesions with the classic immunophenotypic features of one of the lymphoid or plasmacytic neoplasms
- Stains for EBV should be performed, with the majority of (but not all) cases positive using EBER in situ hybridization or, in a somewhat smaller proportion of cases, using an EBV LMP-1 immunohistochemical stain

Genetics
- Variably required
- Clonal B cells are demonstrable in the vast majority of cases, except in plasmacytic hyperplasia, some IM-like PTLDs, and T-cell PTLDs
- Clonal T cells are demonstrable in T-cell monomorphic PTLD
- Various additional cytogenetic and karyotypic findings are related to the type of PTLD, such as *MYC* rearrangements and *TP53* mutations
- These studies are most important in recognizing T-cell PTLD and classifying some of the B-cell monomorphic PTLDs

Clinical Features
- Assessment required for patient care
- PTLDs can present with an IM-type illness, like conventional lymphoid or plasmacytic neoplasms, or sometimes with vague or absent symptoms
- PTLDs are sometimes discovered only because of routine EBV monitoring or at autopsy; overall mortality is up to 50% to 80%, with many different factors affecting outcome

EBER, EBV-encoded small RNA; EBV, Epstein-Barr virus; IM, infectious mononucleosis; LMP-1, latent membrane protein-1.

and decreased numbers of CD4+ T cells.[22] EBV may be acquired from the donor or other sources as a primary infection, superinfection by a second strain of EBV in a seropositive recipient, or, especially in adults, reactivation of recipient EBV. Humoral responses to EBV are also diminished after transplantation, but whether this plays a role in the development of PTLD is not known.[23] EBV-associated PTLD shows variable latency patterns, and individual cells can express different sets of latency proteins[24,25]; however, many cases have a type III latency pattern, similar to that seen in EBV+ lymphoblastoid cell lines.[16,26] Some monomorphic PTLDs, including plasmacytoma-like cases, and occasional polymorphic cases are associated with latency pattern type I, as seen in Burkitt's lymphoma, and Hodgkin-type PTLD may demonstrate pattern type II.[25,27,28] Most PTLDs also have at least some replicative EBV activity.[24] Patients with PTLD reportedly demonstrate a T-helper (Th)-2 serum cytokine profile that promotes EBV-induced B-cell proliferation.[10,29] In fact, monitoring interleukin-10 levels has been proposed as a way to follow patients at risk for PTLD and as a diagnostic tool.[30] Related to these observations, it is of interest that ATG not only causes an overall decrease in lymphocyte counts (predominantly due to decreased CD4+ cells) but also affects Th1 (but not Th2) CD4+ T-cell responses.[31]

EBV cannot be demonstrated in up to 30% of PTLDs; some report an even higher percentage, and the proportion of EBV− cases is greater now than in the past.[32-37] The cause of EBV− PTLD is uncertain, but at least some cases may represent EBV-related proliferations that have lost the virus following transformation (hit-and-run theory)[38]; others may reflect technical difficulties in the detection of EBV, represent lymphoid proliferations driven by other viral or other infectious agents, or be related to chronic antigenic stimulation, possibly by the transplant itself. Rare cases of human herpesvirus 8–positive PTLD have been reported, including polymorphic lesions, a Castleman-like lesion, and primary effusion lymphoma.[39-41] Rare reports have described other viral associations that remain to be established. A recent gene expression profiling study demonstrated distinct differences between EBV− and EBV+ monomorphic B-cell PTLDs.[42] The EBV− PTLDs lacked some viral-associated changes present in the EBV+ group, suggesting a possible nonviral etiology for these cases; however, another gene profiling study that included a broader spectrum of PTLDs failed to distinguish EBV+ from EBV− PTLDs.[43]

Most PTLDs following solid organ transplantation are derived from recipient lymphoid cells, whereas those occurring following bone marrow transplantation are most often donor derived.[44,45] PTLDs limited to the allograft following solid organ transplantation are more frequently of donor origin.[46,47]

Although very few patients demonstrate a sequential development of the disorder, PTLDs are thought to begin as polyclonal proliferations related to EBV or other stimuli, with the development over time of oligoclonal and then monoclonal B-cell or, much less frequently, T-cell proliferations (Fig. 55-1).[4,35,48,49] Antigenic selection may be important in the development and progression of the B-cell clonal proliferations in PTLDs.[43,50] Cytogenetic or genotypic abnormalities of the types seen in conventional lymphoid or plasmacytic neoplasms (described later) also occur as the lesions progress, making them less responsive to immune regulation.[4,6,43,51,52]

Clinical Features

Most cases of PTLD present within 1 year of transplantation. A relatively short interval has been reported for younger patients, those presenting with an infectious mononucleosis (IM)-like syndrome, and PTLD following bone marrow, lung, and heart-lung transplants.[18,53,54] Although there are conflicting data, patients presenting after a longer interval are reportedly older and have localized extranodal disease, a higher frequency of EBV− PTLD, and a worse prognosis.[34,55] T-cell and Hodgkin-type PTLDs are also more common among the PTLDs that occur later.

Patients with PTLD may present with tumorous masses, often at extranodal sites; widely disseminated disease; an IM-like illness; vague, nonlocalized symptoms, such as fever; or no symptoms at all.[56] The most common sites of involvement include the gastrointestinal tract, lymph nodes, lung, and liver. Gastrointestinal tract involvement is often multifocal and may present with hemorrhage, obstruction, or perforation.[57] PTLD may involve the central nervous system; however, the incidence appears to have decreased following the introduction of cyclosporin A. Early lesions often present with tonsil or adenoid enlargement, and IM-like presentations are particularly common in younger patients. Approximately 20% of PTLDs occurring following solid organ transplantation are localized to the allograft; the highest incidence is in lung transplant patients, and it is very rare in the heart.[58] Disease involving the allograft is often associated with allograft dysfunction and may be difficult to distinguish clinically from transplant rejection. Some PTLDs present with widely disseminated disease, including the plasma cell myeloma type, which usually occurs in older patients and following bone marrow transplantation.

EBV viral load often increases in the blood in association with PTLD, before the development of overt disease, and this has been proposed as a surveillance tool for high-risk patients.[15,59-63] However, there are no agreed-on methodologic or interpretive standards for viral load testing, nor is it clear how these results should be used in combination with other markers, such as monitors of EBV-specific T-cell response.[60] EBV viral load has also been used together with cytokine genotyping to predict PTLD.[15] It should be recognized that even EBV+ PTLD can develop in the setting of low viral loads; persistent high levels predict an increased risk of PTLD only in selected settings and may resolve spontaneously; and at least in some series, EBV loads relate to the type of immunosuppressive regimen or the degree of iatrogenic immunosuppression.[63-68]

Morphology

The PTLDs form a morphologic spectrum from early, nondestructive polymorphic lesions to more infiltrative and destructive polymorphic or monomorphic proliferations (see Boxes 55-1 and 55-2).[5] PTLDs are classified based largely on their morphologic appearance, but doing so can be difficult and very subjective, in part because of frequent intralesional variability or variation among different sites of disease. Vascular wall and, at extranodal sites, neural infiltration, as well as areas of geographic necrosis, are characteristic but not required features. Extranodal involvement may be mass-like or more infiltrative, and parenchymal necrosis is sometimes present.

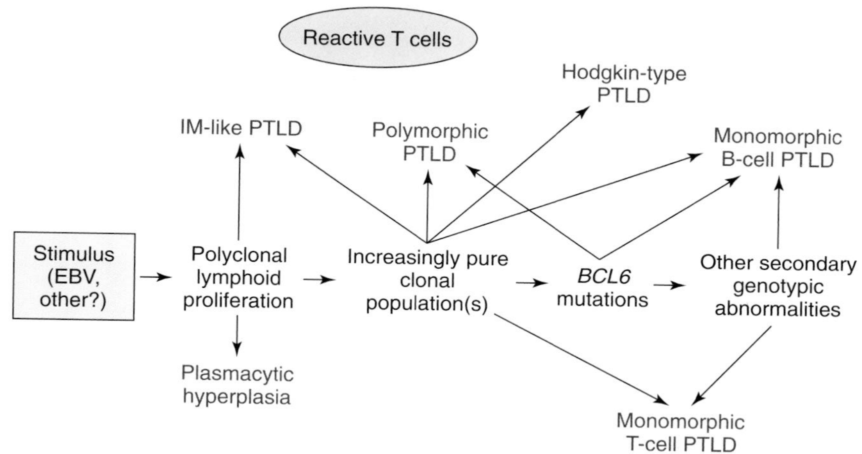

Figure 55-1. Model of posttransplant lymphoproliferative disorder (PTLD) development and correlation with clinicopathologic categories. Epstein-Barr virus (EBV) infection or, in a minority of cases, other stimuli (possibly including chronic antigenic stimulation), in the presence of iatrogenic immunosuppression and an insufficient cellular immune response, lead to a polyclonal lymphoid proliferation without causing significant destruction of the underlying tissue structures. Cases with few transformed cells fulfill the criteria for plasmacytic hyperplasia; those with a more florid proliferation, including moderate numbers of transformed cells, are infectious mononucleosis (IM) like. Increasingly pure clonal populations develop over time that are often but not always of B-cell origin. These may still be plasmacytic hyperplasia or IM like but often fulfill the criteria for a polymorphic or monomorphic PTLD. If there is a pure plasma cell proliferation, a plasmacytoma or myeloma-type PTLD is diagnosed; if there are clonal T cells, one of the T-cell PTLDs is diagnosed. Occasional cases are T-cell rich, sometimes resembling either a T-cell–rich diffuse large B-cell lymphoma or Hodgkin's lymphoma. Cytokine production by the PTLD and other cells may help foster the proliferation. Additional genotypic or karyotypic abnormalities may accumulate, with *BCL6* mutations seen in polymorphic PTLDs, and other secondary abnormalities such as *MYC* translocations seen in some types of monomorphic PTLD. Documentation of progression through these varied stages is lacking in the vast majority of cases, and the possibility that many lesions do not progress through all stages must be considered.

Areas adjacent to a main lesion may show more focal involvement, such as involvement of hepatic portal tracts involvement or preservation of nodal sinuses.

Overt bone marrow involvement occurs only in a minority of patients with PTLD, and occasional patients may demonstrate peripheral blood involvement as well.[69,70] The marrow lesions, which can be either extensive or small and focal, are morphologically similar to those seen at other sites.[69,71] Not uncommonly, children with PTLD may demonstrate an EBV+ polyclonal-appearing plasmacytosis or small lymphoid or plasmacytic aggregates in the marrow that are of uncertain significance.[69]

Early Lesions

Plasmacytic hyperplasia (PH) is usually diagnosed in biopsies of lymph nodes or sometimes tonsils in which the underlying architectural features are intact and there is a proliferation of small lymphocytes and plasma cells, with few transformed cells (Fig. 55-2).[6,7] These cases are not considered PTLD by all pathologists, and particularly when EBV is lacking, they are indistinguishable from nonspecific lymphoid hyperplasia.

IM-like PTLD is also usually diagnosed in biopsies of lymph nodes or tonsils (Fig. 55-3).[4,48] The specimens demonstrate changes associated with IM in the normal host, with a florid proliferation of small lymphocytes, plasma cells, and often very prominent transformed cells and immunoblasts. Although nodal sinuses may be obscured and hyperplastic follicles may appear indistinct, the basic architecture of the lymph node or tonsil is intact. In florid cases it may be impossible to distinguish IM-like PTLD from a polymorphic PTLD in tonsils. As long as the changes are acceptable for IM in the normal host, the former diagnosis is preferred. IM-like changes have also been identified in other extranodal sites such as the liver; these are often considered to be more like IM or simple EBV infection than PTLD; however, these changes may precede overt PTLD.[72] It is also important to rule out the possibility of partial nodal involvement by a monomorphic PTLD. More recently, it has been suggested that some early lesions may have the morphologic appearance of florid follicular hyperplasia, without the interfollicular changes that characterize the other early lesions.[5,43]

Polymorphic Posttransplant Lymphoproliferative Disorder

Polymorphic PTLD, the most morphologically characteristic type of PTLD, is a diffuse and destructive proliferation of variably sized and variably shaped lymphocytes, plasma cells, transformed cells, and immunoblasts (Fig. 55-4).[7] Many of the small lymphocytes may have angulated or cleft-appearing nuclei. The immunoblasts may be multinucleated, with very prominent nucleoli resembling Reed-Sternberg cells. Many cases previously diagnosed as Hodgkin-like PTLD (a category that is no longer recognized) undoubtedly represent polymorphic PTLD and require immunohistologic studies to distinguish them from classical Hodgkin's lymphoma (CHL)-type PTLD. Some cases demonstrate large geographic areas of necrosis that are often associated with neutrophils and histiocytes and are surrounded by increased numbers of transformed cells or immunoblasts. Apoptosis may also be present. Pulmonary cases with prominent angioinvasion and geographic necrosis resemble lymphomatoid granulomatosis (see

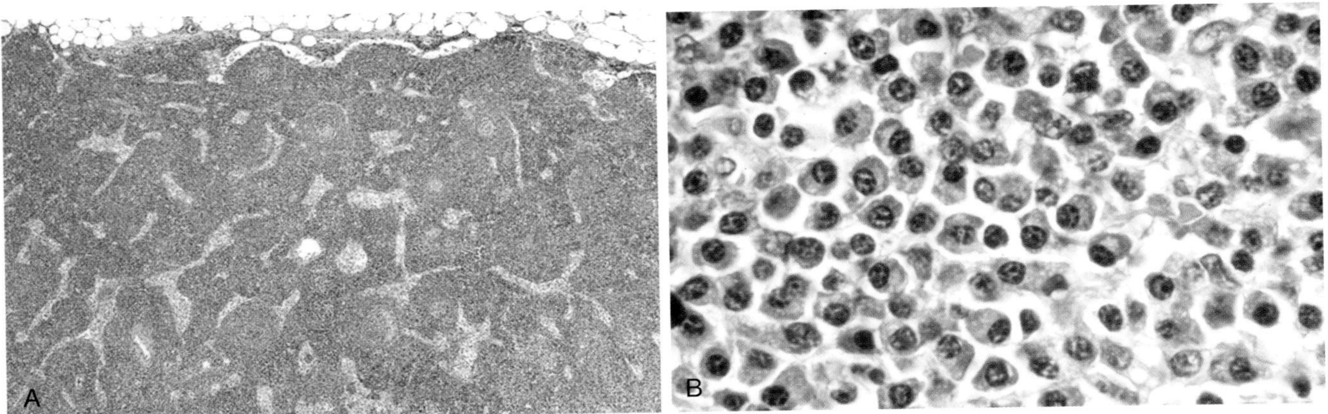

Figure 55-2. Plasmacytic hyperplasia in a perigastric lymph node. A, Normal architecture of the lymph node is preserved, with intact sinuses and occasional small follicles. **B**, Note the numerous plasma cells, which were shown to be polyclonal using in situ hybridization stains for kappa and lambda. EBER in situ hybridization stain for Epstein-Barr virus showed scattered positive cells.

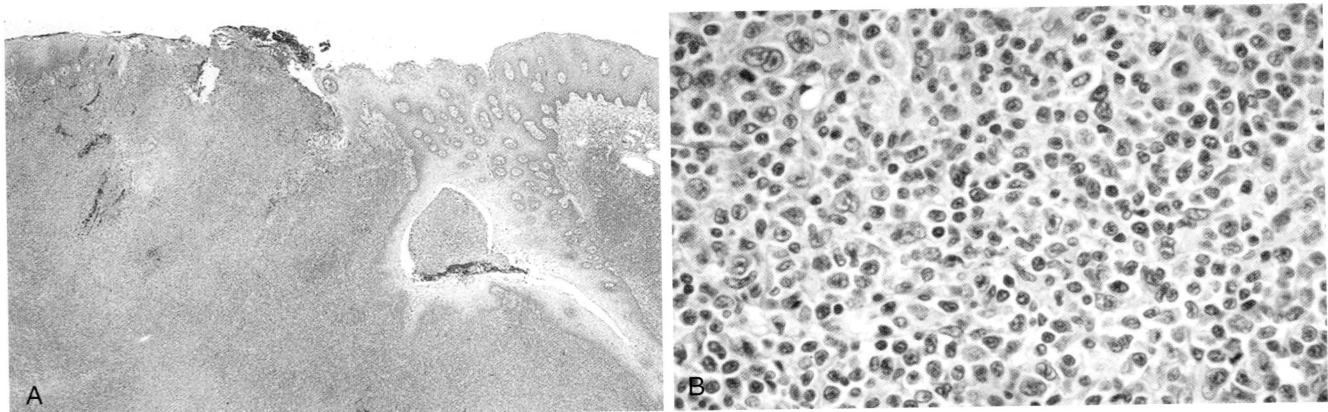

Figure 55-3. Infectious mononucleosis–like posttransplant lymphoproliferative disorder. Tonsil from an adolescent male who presented with enlarged tonsils and adenoids and a sore throat several months after liver transplantation. The patient did well following reduction of tacrolimus immunosuppressive therapy and acyclovir treatment. **A**, Although the normal architecture of the tonsil is difficult to see, intact crypts are present. There is some superficial necrosis. **B**, The very polymorphic proliferation would be consistent with infectious mononucleosis in a normal host. Southern blot analysis of this lesion did not demonstrate a monoclonal B-cell population.

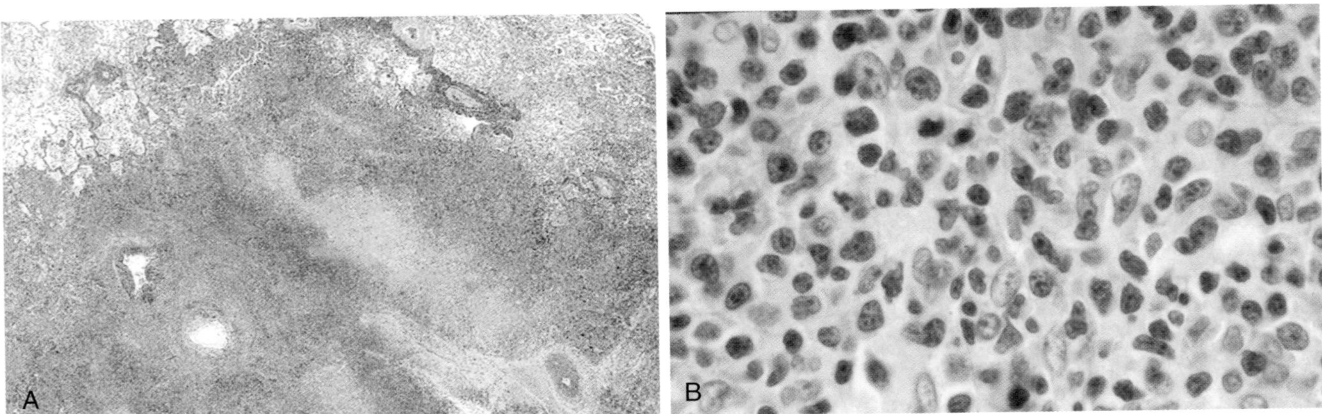

Figure 55-4. Polymorphic posttransplant lymphoproliferative disorder with numerous transformed cells focally. Lung from an adult male who presented with multiple pulmonary nodules 6 months after liver transplantation. **A**, Note the mass lesion, with infiltration of vascular and bronchial structures as well as a large area of geographic necrosis. **B**, Most areas demonstrate a very polymorphic infiltrate composed of transformed cells and smaller lymphoid cells, including some with angulated or cleaved nuclear contours.

Fig. 55-4). Cases that demonstrate a predominance of transformed cells or immunoblasts are classified as monomorphic PTLD according to the WHO criteria, even if the cells are pleomorphic or demonstrate differentiation to mature plasma cells.

Monomorphic Posttransplant Lymphoproliferative Disorder

Monomorphic PTLDs are lymphoid or plasmacytic proliferations that fulfill the criteria for one of the non-Hodgkin's lymphomas (not the small B-cell type) or plasma cell neoplasms that arise in immunocompetent hosts. They must be further categorized based on the type of neoplasm they most closely resemble.

Monomorphic B-Cell Posttransplant Lymphoproliferative Disorder

Many monomorphic PTLDs are composed of numerous transformed B cells that most commonly resemble diffuse large B-cell lymphoma (DLBCL), not otherwise specified (Fig. 55-5); less commonly Burkitt's lymphoma (Fig. 55-6); or occasionally one of the DLBCL subtypes. As with other DLBCLs, the transformed B cells may be very pleomorphic, and plasmacytic differentiation may create a variable degree of pleomorphism. Some cases are T-cell rich and therefore demonstrate only a minority of large transformed B cells.

Distinguishing polymorphic PTLD from DLBCL-type monomorphic PTLD can be extremely difficult, and there are no absolute guidelines for dealing with borderline lesions. Some cases exhibit a definite polymorphic background but either focal or extensive areas of numerous transformed B cells or immunoblasts. These cases are considered at least focally monomorphic in the WHO classification, but others have considered them polymorphic PTLD or polymorphic PTLD with numerous transformed cells.[4] Cases with admixed monoclonal plasma cells and transformed cells or immunoblasts can also be problematic when the latter are not the dominant population; like polymorphic PTLD, there is a complete spectrum of B-cell maturation, but like monomorphic PTLD, these cases fulfill the criteria for malignant lymphoma in a nonimmunocompromised host.

The other major (but much less common) types of B-lineage monomorphic PTLDs include plasma cell myeloma and plasmacytoma-like lesions (Fig. 55-7). The former should fulfill all the criteria for plasma cell myeloma in a normal host. The latter occur most commonly in the gastrointestinal tract but also at nodal and other extranodal sites; they contain sheets of plasma cells, sometimes with occasional foci of small lymphoid cells.

Mucosa-associated lymphoid tissue (MALT) lymphomas in the stomach and, rarely, in the salivary glands have been specifically recognized in the posttransplant setting.[73,74] However, like the other types of small B-cell lymphomas

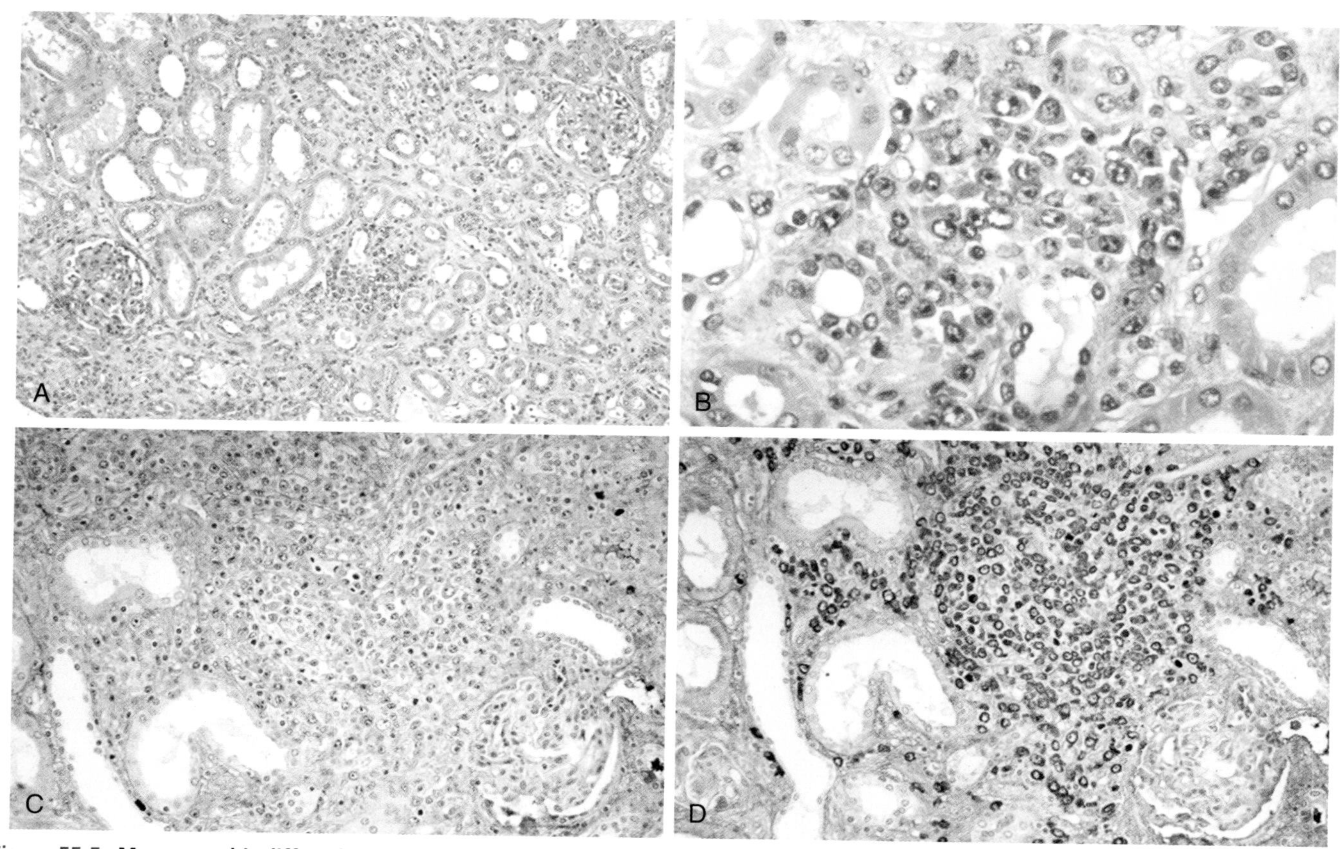

Figure 55-5. Monomorphic diffuse large B-cell lymphoma–type posttransplant lymphoproliferative disorder. A, Note the patchy infiltrate in the renal parenchyma of an adult male 4 months after renal transplantation. **B,** The infiltrate is composed predominantly of transformed and plasmacytoid-appearing large cells. In other areas there was a prominent intravascular component. **C,** Kappa immunostain is essentially negative. **D,** Lambda immunostain is positive, supporting the monoclonality of this lesion.

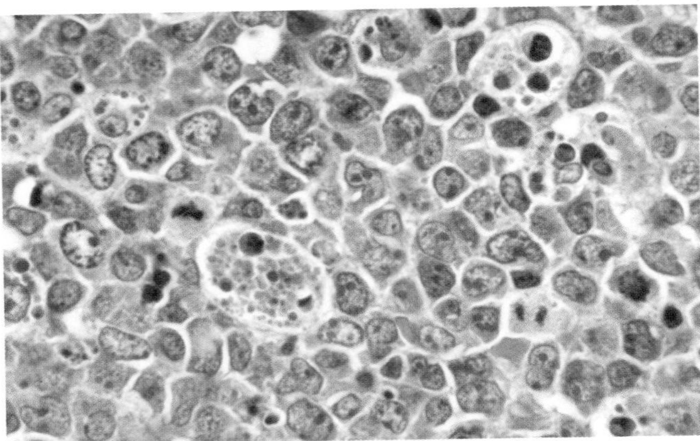

Figure 55-6. Monomorphic B-cell posttransplant lymphoproliferative disorder (PTLD) with *MYC* rearrangement. This example of PTLD in an adult woman after kidney transplantation is composed of intermediate-sized to large transformed cells. It has some Burkitt-type features, with a high mitotic rate and tingible body macrophages, creating a "starry sky" appearance.

that can occur in these patients, they are currently not considered PTLD.

Monomorphic T/NK-Cell Posttransplant Lymphoproliferative Disorder

T-cell or the rare natural killer (NK)-cell PTLDs account for less than 15% of PTLDs and, by definition, are monomorphic.[5,75] In contrast to most monomorphic B-cell PTLDs, the T-cell cases are not necessarily composed of predominantly large transformed cells. Most fulfill the criteria for a peripheral T-cell lymphoma, not otherwise specified; others represent a variety of specific types of mature T-cell lymphomas (Fig. 55-8).[75] Approximately 15% of all hepatosplenic T-cell lymphomas occur in the posttransplant setting (Fig. 55-9).[76] Very rare, aggressive true NK-cell neoplasms also occur in this setting[77,78] and must be distinguished from indolent posttransplant T-cell large granular lymphocytic leukemia. The latter cases should not be grouped with the other T-cell monomorphic PTLDs. Nonneoplastic oligoclonal increases in $CD8^+$, $CD57^+$ T cells have been described following bone marrow transplantation,[79] and clonal $CD8^+$ T cells can also be seen in IM.[80] Rare cases of T-lymphoblastic leukemia/lymphoma have been reported, including some cases that could be clonally related to prior non–T-cell blastic neoplasms. The varied T-cell PTLDs are morphologically similar to their counterparts in the normal host. Particularly because some of these cases appear morphologically indistinguishable from polymorphic PTLDs, phenotypic and genotypic studies are critical whenever the possibility of a T-cell PTLD is raised.

Classical Hodgkin's Lymphoma–Type Posttransplant Lymphoproliferative Disorder

CHL-type PTLD, the least common type, often resembles mixed cellularity CHL.[2,27,81,82] These cases should fulfill both the morphologic and the immunophenotypic criteria for CHL because atypical immunoblasts or Reed-Sternberg–like cells are commonly found in many PTLDs, and Hodgkin-like cases are no longer included in this category (Figs. 55-10 and 55-11). Some cases have occurred following non-Hodgkin–type PTLD.[48]

Immunophenotype

The immunophenotype of PTLDs is very variable, as would be expected for a spectrum of disorders that can resemble hyperplastic proliferations; B-, T-, or NK-cell neoplasms; Hodgkin's lymphoma; or plasma cell neoplasms. In PH or IM-like PTLD, immunophenotypic studies do not demonstrate B-cell clonality, plasma cell clonality, or aberrant B- or T-cell phenotypes.

Polymorphic PTLDs demonstrate admixtures of B cells with variable pan–B-cell marker expression and heterogeneous T cells. Paraffin section immunostains may demonstrate B-cell clonality; however, often only polyclonal plasma cells are identified. In addition, they may demonstrate intra- or interlesional clonal heterogeneity with polyclonal and monoclonal areas or both kappa monoclonal and lambda monoclonal regions.[7] Flow cytometric studies also show variable results, with polyclonal, monoclonal, or surface immunoglobulin-negative B cells.[83] T cells may predominate.

Monomorphic PTLDs have an immunophenotype consistent with that of the lymphomas they resemble. Those of the DLBCL type usually express pan–B-cell antigens, and if immunoglobulin staining is present and can be demonstrated, they have clonal surface or cytoplasmic immunoglobulin. Most monomorphic B-cell PTLDs have a late germinal center or post–germinal center phenotype ($CD10^-$, $BCL6^{+/-}$, IRF4/$MUM\text{-}1^+$, $CD138^{+/-}$); a minority, especially EBV^- cases, have a germinal center phenotype ($CD10^{+/-}$, $BCL6^+$, IRF4/$MUM\text{-}1^-$, $CD138^-$).[43,84-86] Burkitt-type cases should have a typical $CD10^+$ monoclonal B-cell phenotype. Plasma cell myeloma–like and plasmacytoma-like PTLDs should demonstrate monoclonal plasma cell populations with few if any admixed lymphoid cells. T-cell–type monomorphic PTLDs have the phenotypic characteristics of one of the T-cell lymphomas. A moderate number of T-cell PTLDs are composed of $CD8^+$ cytotoxic T cells that express TIA-1 and sometimes other cytotoxic granule proteins.[75,87] Some PTLDs include both B-cell and T-cell components.[88]

CHL-type PTLD can be diagnosed with the greatest degree of confidence when $CD15^+$, $CD30^+$, $CD45^-$ Reed-Sternberg cells are present in an appropriate T-cell–rich background; however, as with CHL in an immunocompetent host, some $CD15^-$ cases can be expected. The Reed-Sternberg–like cells in other non-Hodgkin's lymphoma–type PTLDs are expected to be $CD20^+$, $CD45^+$, and $CD15^-$. CD30 positivity cannot help in the distinction between these two entities; however a $CD30^-$ phenotype makes CHL-type PTLD extremely unlikely.

All types of PTLDs demonstrate variable numbers of admixed T cells; the IM, polymorphic, and CHL types are most likely to have the most numerous T cells.[89] Some cases not of clonal T-cell origin have greater than 80% T cells.[90] Some series report a predominance of $CD8^+$ T cells, whereas others have found a predominance of $CD4^+$ T cells.[90-92] In one of the latter series, 24% to 47% of T cells expressed the TIA-1 cytotoxic marker.[91] In contrast to lymph nodes involved with

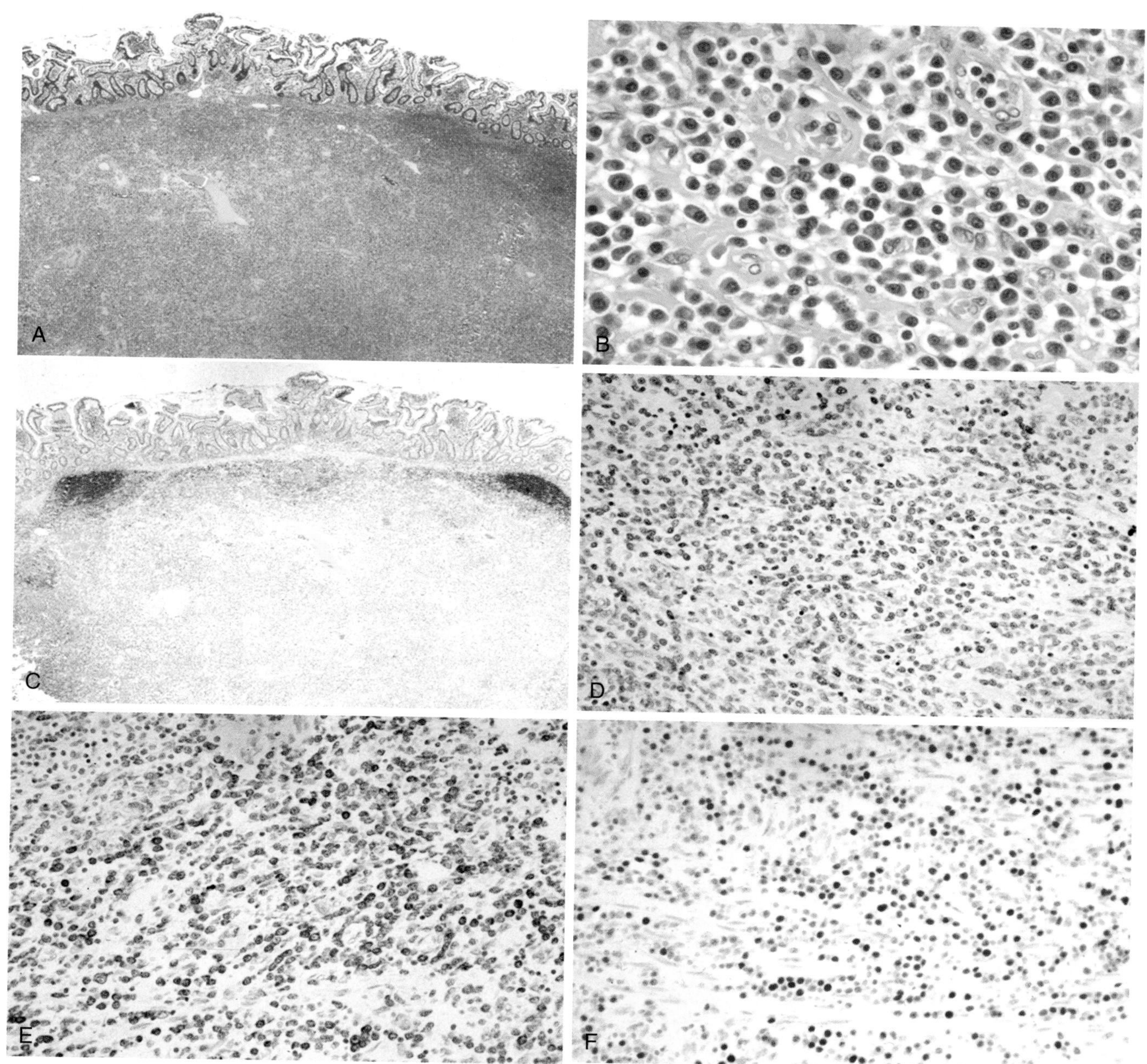

Figure 55-7. Monomorphic plasmacytoma-type posttransplant lymphoproliferative disorder in the small intestine. A, The mass lesion includes occasional lymphoid aggregates but otherwise demonstrates numerous plasma cells. **B,** There is a relatively homogeneous population of plasma cells. **C,** CD20 immunostain highlights the occasional lymphoid aggregates but is otherwise essentially negative. **D,** Kappa in situ hybridization stain is negative. **E,** Lambda in situ hybridization stain shows numerous positive cells, supporting the monoclonality of the plasma cells. **F,** EBER in situ hybridization stain for Epstein-Barr virus shows numerous positive nuclei.

IM, CD56+ cells were reported to be absent in at least one series.[93] Some cases have many CD57+ T cells.[90] Studies of cytokine and chemokine expression are complex and have been reviewed elsewhere.[94] Consistent with reported serum findings, at least some PTLDs have a Th2-like cytokine microenvironment in the involved tissues.[10,29,95] Differences from IM have been reported.[93,96]

About 70% to 85% of PTLDs are associated with EBV; this is best demonstrated by in situ hybridization for EBV-encoded small RNAs (EBER).[32-36,97] EBER in situ hybridization is somewhat more sensitive than the immunohistochemical stain for EBV latent membrane protein-1 (LMP-1), but it is also somewhat more likely to be positive in the absence of a diagnosable PTLD. EBV− PTLDs are more often monomorphic compared with EBV+ cases.[33,34] Cases of EBV− PH are completely indistinguishable from nonspecific hyperplasia. EBV is described in all other types of PTLDs, although plasma cell myeloma cases are often negative, and CHL-type cases are almost invariably positive. About one third of T-cell PTLDs are EBV+, as are at least some of the rare NK-cell neoplasms.[75,78]

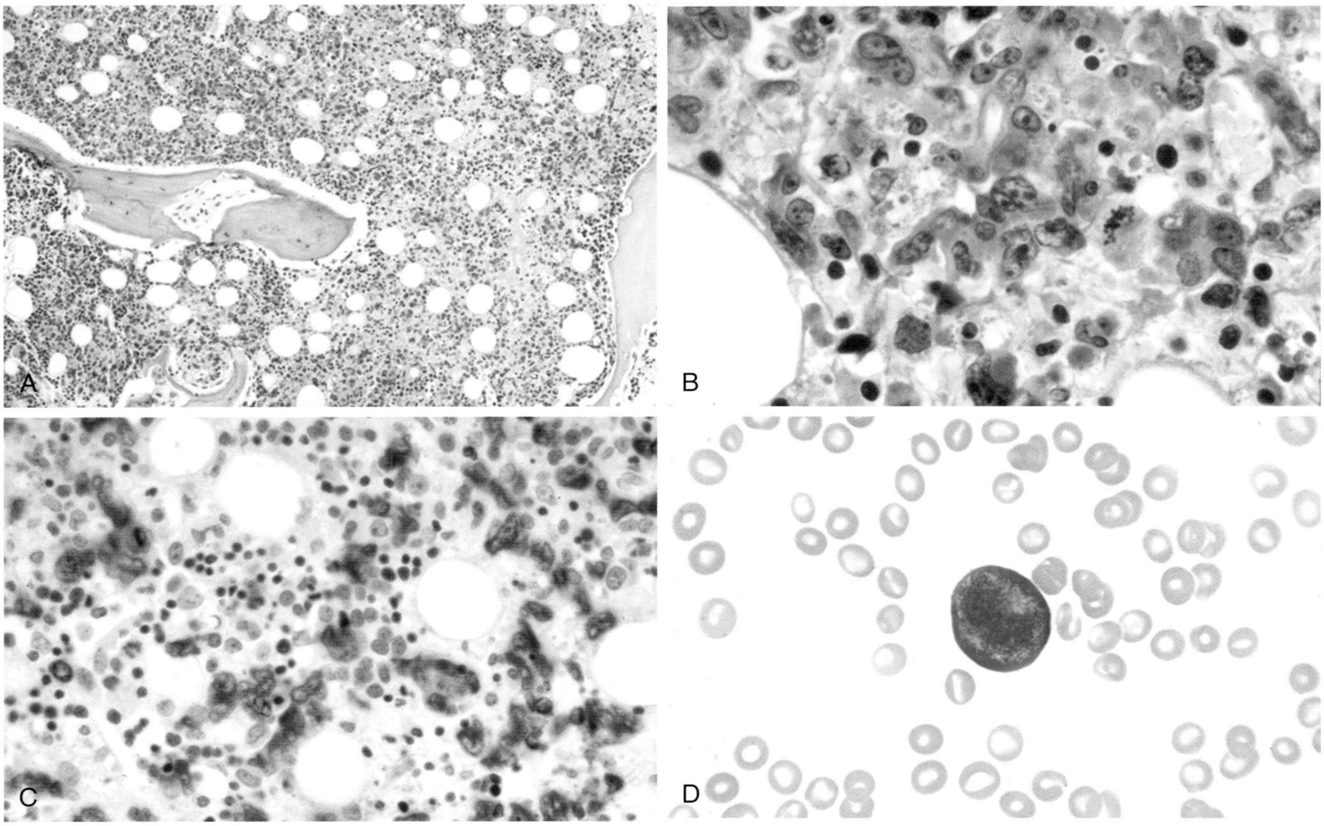

Figure 55-8. **Monomorphic peripheral T-cell lymphoma–type posttransplant lymphoproliferative disorder. A**, Bone marrow biopsy in a 39-year-old woman with pancytopenia, 4 years after kidney transplantation, shows a mostly interstitial large cell infiltrate admixed with hematopoietic elements, including an increased proportion of immature myeloid cells. There are also bony changes, consistent with hyperparathyroidism. **B**, The large abnormal cells have nucleoli and often irregular nuclear contours. Admixed hematopoietic elements are also seen. **C**, CD3 immunostain highlights the interstitial and scattered nature of the abnormal cells in many areas. The cells were also positive for TIA-1, indicating their cytotoxic nature, although CD4 and CD8 immunostains were both negative. The cells were negative for CD30 but positive for epithelial membrane antigen. Genotypic studies demonstrated a clonal T-cell population. **D**, Peripheral blood demonstrates a small proportion of very large abnormal lymphoid cells, some of which have cytoplasmic granules.

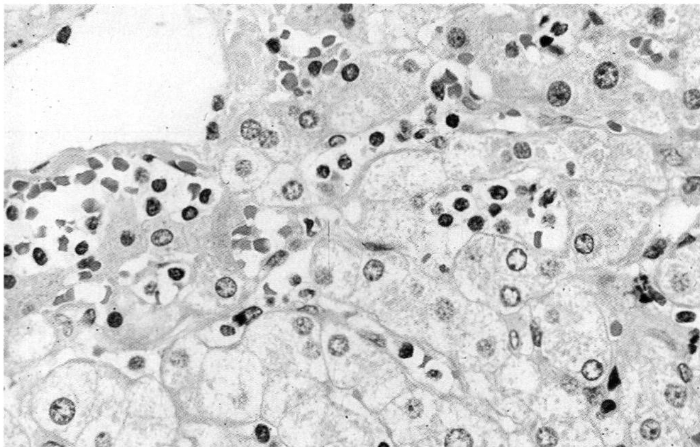

Figure 55-9. **Hepatosplenic T-cell lymphoma–type posttransplant lymphoproliferative disorder.** Note the lymphoid cells infiltrating the hepatic sinuses. (Courtesy of Dr. Nancy Lee Harris.)

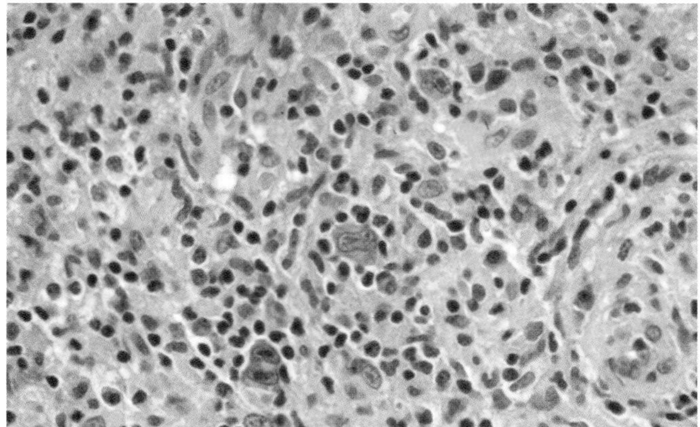

Figure 55-10. **Mixed cellularity classical Hodgkin's lymphoma–type posttransplant lmphoproliferative disorder in an adult male after kidney transplantation.** Note the Reed-Sternberg and Reed-Sternberg variant cells admixed with numerous small lymphocytes, plasma cells, and histiocytes.

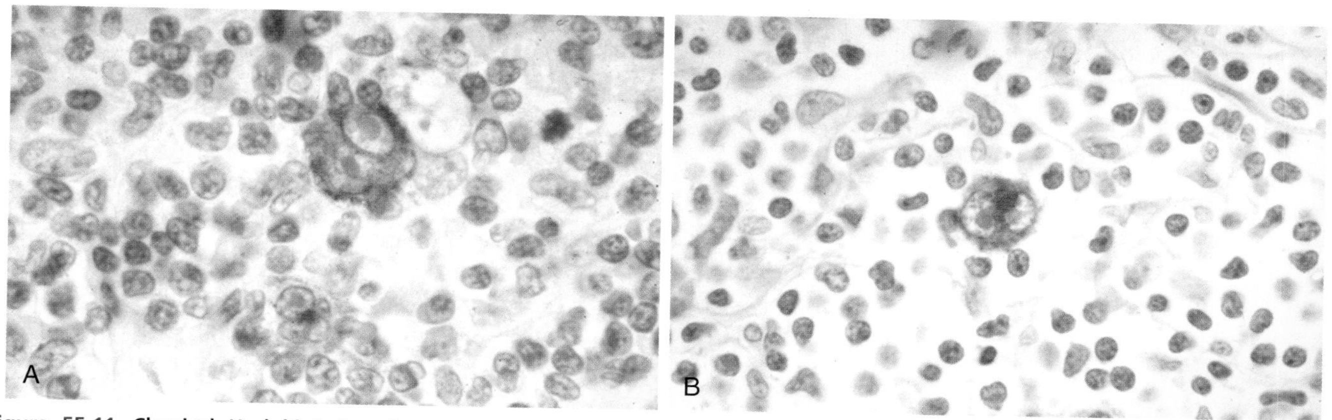

Figure 55-11. Classical Hodgkin's lymphoma–type posttransplant lymphoproliferative disorder. A, CD30 stain highlights a Reed-Sternberg cell. **B,** Reed-Sternberg cells are also highlighted by Epstein-Barr virus latent membrane protein-1 immunostain.

Genetics

Clonality Studies

In contrast to the results of immunophenotypic studies, virtually all polymorphic PTLDs and B-cell monomorphic PTLDs can be shown to be monoclonal by Southern blot analysis of immunoglobulin heavy-chain rearrangements or EBV terminal repeat analysis.[6,41,98] With the very sensitive latter technique, many IM-like PTLDs are demonstrably clonal, as are some cases of PH and even occasional hyperplastic lymph nodes in a nontransplant setting.[99] Genotypic studies demonstrate occasional cases with more than one clone or with an oligoclonal B-cell proliferation. Monomorphic PTLDs usually have more dominant clones than do polymorphic PTLDs.[100,101] Polymerase chain reaction studies have largely replaced Southern blot analysis, although depending on the primers used, the occurrence of false-negative results can be problematic.

It is important to recognize that distinct simultaneous or subsequent lesions in the same patient may show different B-cell clones or a monoclonal population at one site and a polyclonal population elsewhere.[6,7,100] The presence of numerous clonally distinct PTLD lesions is particularly well recognized in the gastrointestinal tract.[102] Recurrent PTLD may represent the same or different clones.[48] Southern blot analysis using *IGH@* probes demonstrates clonal B cells in some CHL-type PTLDs; in others, clonality is demonstrated using EBV terminal repeat analysis.[3] Studies of *IGH@ V* gene usage and mutational patterns suggest that antigen selection may be important in the development or progression of PTLDs.[43,48,50] A minority of cases show crippling *IGH@* mutations.[43] T-cell clonality is documented in the vast majority of monomorphic T-cell lymphoma–type PTLDs using genotypic studies. Occasional cases can be shown to have both clonal B cells and T cells either simultaneously or in different lesions.[88]

Epstein-Barr Virus Studies

Genotypic studies can be used to demonstrate the presence of EBV in PTLDs; however, Southern blot EBV terminal repeat analysis is not as sensitive as EBER stains, and EBV polymerase chain reaction studies are so sensitive that they simply indicate prior EBV infection, with a significant minority of hyperplastic lymph nodes positive in a nontransplant setting.[99] In addition, EBV terminal repeat analysis can distinguish latent from replicative infections. Evidence of lytic EBV infection in PTLD can also be documented with immunostains to certain EBV-associated proteins, such as ZEBRA.[24]

Additional Genotypic Abnormalities

In addition to increasing clonal dominance, progression in PTLDs is associated with other genotypic abnormalities. *BCL6* mutations are reported to be absent in PH and present in 43% of polymorphic PTLDs and 90% of monomorphic PTLDs.[52] Others have found similar proportions of *BCL6* mutations in polymorphic and monomorphic PTLDs.[43] Aberrant somatic hypermutation involving other genes is more common in monomorphic than polymorphic PTLDs.[43] Other abnormalities reported in B-cell monomorphic PTLDs include *MYC* rearrangements and *NRAS* and *TP53* mutations.[6,100] Those with *MYC* rearrangements do not necessarily resemble Burkitt's lymphoma. Overall, the frequency of these genotypic abnormalities in PTLDs is quite low. The proportion in WHO-defined monomorphic PTLDs remains uncertain. Alpha-interferon gene deletion has been reported in 44% of monomorphic PTLDs but in only 1.7% of other intermediate- to high-grade non-Hodgkin's lymphomas.[103] *BCL2* and *BCL6* but not *CCND1* gene rearrangements are described in rare PTLDs.[6,88,104,105] Lack of expression of the cyclin-dependent kinase inhibitor p16/INK4a has also been identified in almost half of PTLDs and is associated with predominantly monomorphic or EBV$^-$ cases and those with a higher proliferative fraction.[106] *TP53* and other oncogene mutations are also reported in a high proportion of T-cell PTLDs.[107] Characteristic isochrome 7q and trisomy 8 are found in posttransplant hepatosplenic T-cell lymphoma.[76]

Classic Cytogenetic Studies

Classic cytogenetic studies have been used less extensively but show recurrent clonal abnormalities in a variable proportion of PTLDs; these recurrent abnormalities were not consistent, however, among the limited studies in which they were reported.[2,71,108,109] Abnormalities are most commonly found in monomorphic PTLDs but are also reported in some polymorphic PTLDs and even occasional early lesions. Some of the more commonly reported abnormalities include trisomy 9, trisomy 11, 8q24 rearrangements, 14q32 rearrangements, and breaks at 1q11-21. Comparative genomic hybridization studies demonstrate a variety of recurring chromosomal gains and losses, as well as some high-level amplifications.[110]

Postulated Normal Counterparts

The postulated normal counterparts are mature follicular or postfollicular B cells and postthymic T cells.

Clinical Course

PTLD is a serious complication of transplantation and is associated with significant morbidity and mortality. Reported mortality rates are as high as 50% to 80%, but they vary widely.[111] A uniform PTLD treatment strategy does not exist, and it is an area with many controversies, in part because of the protean nature of these LPDs.[57,111-115] In general, most patients are treated with a decrease in their immunosuppressive regimens whenever possible, keeping in mind that the patient's well-being is dependent on the status of the graft. The ability to reconstitute many patients' immune systems is one of the major features that distinguish PTLD from other LPDs. The reported response rate is extremely variable.[112,115] Surgical excision and sometimes radiation therapy for localized lesions are other important and frequently successful therapeutic strategies in appropriate cases. More recently, the addition of rituximab in CD20$^+$ cases has become an important component of therapy. There is controversy over the point at which combination chemotherapy is appropriate; it is used initially by some, and after other therapies have failed by others. Patients with PTLD reportedly have greater morbidity and mortality from chemotherapeutic regimens than other patients with non-Hodgkin's lymphomas, although newer strategies may be more effective.[112,113] As with all the therapies discussed, the timing and exact nature of chemotherapeutic regimens depend on the type of PTLD and other clinical findings. For example, many patients with CHL-type PTLD receive conventional Hodgkin's lymphoma therapy, and patients with Burkitt's lymphoma type–PTLD start an appropriate chemotherapeutic regimen without a waiting period to see whether reduced immunosuppression leads to remission. Antiviral agents have been widely used, but with the possible exception of some newer strategies, they have not been very effective in PTLD; this is because most antiviral agents target the lytic phase of EBV infection, which is (at most) a minor component of the EBV infection in PTLD.[112] Cytokine therapy with interferon-α has been used, as well as treatment with an anti–interleukin-6 antibody. Finally, varied strategies involving cellular immunotherapy have been implemented in a much smaller group of bone marrow, stem cell, and solid organ transplant patients, using either nonselected cytotoxic T cells or EBV-specific cytotoxic T cells.[112,116] In addition to all the uncertainties about the best treatment for PTLD, another issue (not covered here) relates to prophylaxis and preemptive therapies for high-risk patients.[10,112]

Prognostic factors are another problematic area; the literature is inconsistent, and one must take into account the specific type of PTLD and the clinical setting. Nevertheless, several prognostic factors that are probably applicable in many PTLDs have been reported, although rigorous proof does not exist, and it is unknown which factors are independent prognostic indicators. One important predictor of outcome is response to a trial of decreased immunosuppression; however, the proportion of responding patients is very variable, and those who fail to respond may still be cured of their disease.[57,112,115] PTLD following bone marrow transplantation has a very poor prognosis, with reported survival rates of only 8% to 12.5%.[45,117] Many solid organ transplantation patients fare better, and those with PTLD of donor origin reportedly have better outcomes than those with the much more common PTLD of recipient origin.[46,47] PTLD localized to the allograft is usually associated with a good prognosis, with about three quarters of patients surviving.[47,57,118] Although many patients who present with an IM-like syndrome have a good outcome, with a course typical of IM, some go on to develop rapidly progressive PTLD that may be fatal.[119-121] Central nervous system, bone marrow, and serous effusion involvement are all adverse prognostic indicators.[122-124] PTLD presenting as disseminated disease is associated with a survival rate of less than 10%.[118] There appears to be a worse prognosis for patients who present with PTLD several years after the transplant, and perhaps because of the duration of prior immunosuppressive therapy, they are often less responsive to decreased immunosuppression.[10,105] Elevated lactate dehydrogenase, organ dysfunction, central nervous system involvement, and multiorgan involvement adversely affect the likelihood of responding to decreased immunosuppression.[112,122]

Data allowing prognostication based on pathologic subtype are limited; however, some generalizations can be made. Patients with PH generally do well, whereas those with monomorphic PTLD appear to be less likely to respond to decreased immunosuppression and have a worse prognosis.[120,125,126] The degree to which patients with polymorphic PTLD do better than those with monomorphic PTLD, if at all, is controversial; some investigators report major differences, and others report excellent survival among those with monomorphic disease.[10,70,125,127-133] Patients with PTLD resembling plasma cell myeloma have a very bad prognosis.[6] Plasmacytoma-like PTLD appears to have a more variable outcome.[134] Except for cases of indolent T-cell large granular lymphocytic leukemia, PTLDs of T- and NK-cell phenotype are often but not invariably associated with a poor prognosis[75]; occasional patients respond to a decrease in immunosuppression. Absence of detectable EBV is also associated with a worse prognosis in some studies but not in others.[33,37]

Although PTLDs with B-cell clonality demonstrated principally by immunophenotyping are more frequently resistant to decreased immunosuppression than are polyclonal-appearing PTLDs, a significant number of the former patients respond to this therapeutic strategy.[7,70] It has also been reported that PTLDs with the most dominant B-cell clones are among those least likely to respond to decreased immunosuppression.[101] Secondary *NRAS* and *TP53* mutations and *MYC* translocations are associated with a poor prognosis.[6,100] *BCL6* mutation is reportedly associated with a shorter survival and refractoriness to therapy with decreased immunosuppression; however, an association with outcome is not uniformly found.[43,52] Absence of comparative genomic hybridization abnormalities in monomorphic PTLD was associated with a better outcome in one study.[110]

Differential Diagnosis

The possibility of specific infectious or other inflammatory processes must always be ruled out when lymphoplasmacytic infiltrates are seen in posttransplant patients. These diagnoses may be based on the presence of viral inclusions or other organisms, the assessment of pathologic findings that suggest another specific diagnosis, and even the clinical situation, to some extent. Extensive EBV positivity or findings associated with any of the B- or T-cell lymphomas support the diagnosis of PTLD. Transplant patients may also have lymph node biopsies that show a completely nonspecific hyperplasia, with architectural preservation and an absence of EBV. It is important to question whether such lymph nodes are representative of whatever is causing the clinical concern in the patient. Lymphadenopathy may also occur as an apparent allergic reaction to the therapeutic use of OKT3 and ATG.[135]

When allograft biopsies are being evaluated, the distinction from florid rejection can be difficult. The presence of expansile nodules or a mass lesion, numerous transformed cells, lymphoid atypia, a very B-cell–rich infiltrate, extensive serpiginous necrosis within the infiltrate, a high proportion of frank plasma cells, and evidence of many EBV⁺ cells are among the features that support the diagnosis of PTLD rather than rejection.[36,136-138] Necrosis by itself and venous wall infiltration are not helpful findings. Significant arterial infiltration and variable numbers of eosinophils are among the features favoring rejection. Caution is advised, however, because PTLD can infiltrate arterial walls, have numerous T cells, and lack atypia. Conversely, some inflammatory processes, including in transplant patients, may have scattered (≤10%) EBV⁺ cells.[9,137,139] Lesions not diagnostic of PTLD but with scattered EBV⁺ cells may be associated with PTLD at another site or with an increased risk of developing PTLD.[9,72] Some allografts demonstrate evidence of both PTLD and rejection.

IATROGENIC IMMUNODEFICIENCY-ASSOCIATED LYMPHOPROLIFERATIVE DISORDERS IN NONTRANSPLANT SETTINGS

Outside the transplant setting, iatrogenic LPDs have been described in patients receiving a number of immunosuppressive agents.[140,141] Some of the implicated agents are the same as those used following transplantation, such as azathioprine and tacrolimus.[142,143] Others are immunosuppressive agents used in the therapy of autoimmune disorders or lymphoid neoplasms. Assessment of whether an immunosuppressive agent is responsible for an LPD is complicated by the fact that the patient's underlying disorder may be associated with an increased incidence of lymphoma or the patient may be taking multiple immunosuppressive medications.

The best recognized iatrogenic LPDs in the nontransplant setting are those associated with methotrexate in patients being treated for rheumatoid arthritis, dermatomyositis, and, rarely, psoriasis.[140,144-150] These patients usually have long-standing rheumatic disease (often as long as 15 years), are receiving methotrexate at the time of diagnosis, and have been taking methotrexate for a median of 3 years. About half the cases involve one or more extranodal sites.[144,146,148]

Methotrexate-associated LPDs form a morphologic spectrum similar to that of the PTLDs, but with a different distribution among the morphologic subtypes.[141,144] Most commonly, cases fulfill the criteria for DLBCL or, less commonly, Burkitt's lymphoma (Fig. 55-12). Areas of geographic necrosis may contribute to the resemblance to a PTLD. Only a small proportion of cases resemble a polymorphic PTLD or are described as a lymphoplasmacytic infiltrate (Fig. 55-13). Although an infrequent type of PTLD, up to 25% of cases reportedly fulfill the criteria for CHL of mixed cellularity or another type. Caution is advised, because many Hodgkin-like lesions are also described in this setting. As with the PTLDs, progression from a polymorphic proliferation to a monomorphic or Hodgkin-type lesion can occur. A small proportion of the monomorphic cases represent peripheral T-cell lymphomas, with rare cases described as large granular lymphocytic lymphoma reported as well. Finally, some cases included in series of iatrogenic LPDs are small B-cell neoplasms of varied types. Although series vary, about 40% of the methotrexate-associated LPDs are EBV⁺, including some follicular lymphomas; the Hodgkin-type cases have the highest proportion.[140,141,144,148,149] Very few data exist about molecular diagnostic studies in methotrexate-associated LPDs;

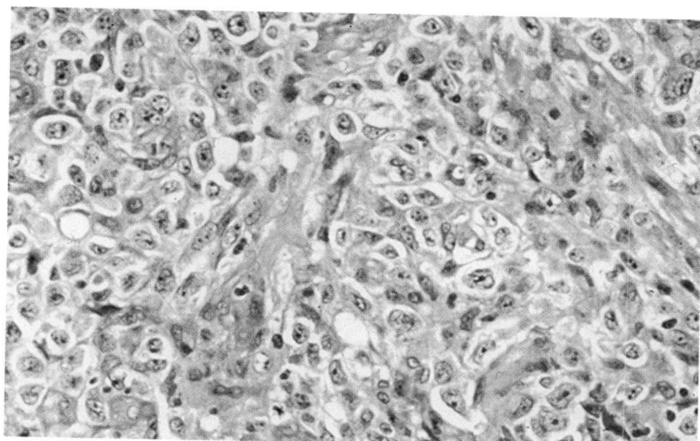

Figure 55-12. Diffuse large B-cell lymphoma–type methotrexate-associated lymphoproliferative disorder (EBV⁺) in a patient with rheumatoid arthritis. This relatively monomorphic proliferation of large transformed B cells is indistinguishable from many diffuse large B-cell lymphomas in normal hosts. (Courtesy of Dr. Nancy Lee Harris.)

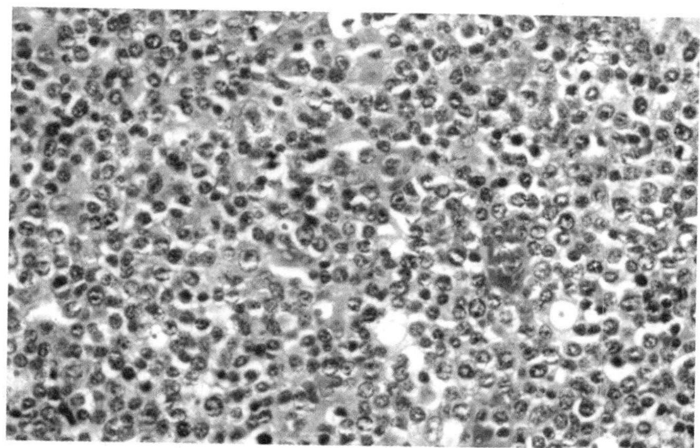

Figure 55-13. Polymorphic methotrexate-associated lymphoproliferative disorder (EBV⁺) that regressed following cessation of methotrexate therapy. There is a diffuse proliferation of very heterogeneous lymphoid cells. (Courtesy of Dr. Nancy Lee Harris.)

however, the vast majority appear to be clonal, including polymorphic cases.

Recognition of methotrexate-associated LPD is important, because about one third of patients respond to withdrawal of methotrexate therapy.[141] The reported frequency of response varies widely, and about half the reported cases that regress eventually recur and require chemotherapy. Responses to discontinuation of methotrexate can occur even in monoclonal lesions.[148] EBV$^+$ methotrexate-associated LPDs are most likely to respond; however, some responses are seen with EBV$^-$ lesions.[144,148] Hodgkin-type cases have also responded in some but not all reports. In the absence of a response or following relapse, conventional lymphoma therapies are required.

Fludarabine has been associated with the development of EBV-associated LPD, most frequently in the treatment of low-grade lymphoma.[151] Fludarabine is a purine analogue that has a well-recognized side effect of long-lasting T-cell lymphopenia. The association between fludarabine therapy and LPD is more difficult to prove than that with methotrexate because of the presence of a preexisting LPD and the difficulty encountered in reversing the immune defect.[152,153] Evidence of the association includes increased serum EBV DNA viral load seen in a few patients receiving fludarabine, development of an EBV-associated LPD that is morphologically and clonally distinct from the lymphoid neoplasm that was being treated, and, most important, regression described in a few patients without antineoplastic therapy. The cases of EBV-associated LPD following fludarabine therapy include polymorphic PTLD–like, monomorphic PTLD–like, and CHL-like clonal B-cell proliferations.[151] It is important in these cases to rule out a Richter-like transformation of the original neoplasm. EBV$^+$ LPD may also follow the use of other chemotherapeutic regimens, such as the LPD resembling lymphomatoid granulomatosis reported in a small number of children and rare adults following therapy for acute lymphoblastic leukemia.[154,155]

Infliximab and other TNF-α antagonists have been associated with LPDs of varied types in patients with autoimmune diseases; infliximab, used with azathioprine or mercaptopurine, has also been associated with hepatosplenic T-cell lymphomas in young patients with Crohn's disease.[141,156] As with the other immunosuppressive medications discussed, it is very difficult to determine the role of any given agent. TNF-α inhibitors have a profound effect on the immune system, including decreased T-cell–mediated responses, and infliximab has been associated with EBV reactivation and an increased EBV viral load that reverses following discontinuation of the drug.[157] The hepatosplenic T-cell lymphomas in patients receiving infliximab have been completely typical of that entity and almost uniformly fatal.

Pearls and Pitfalls

- Diagnosis of a PTLD rests heavily on the history of a prior transplant; however, not every lymphoid proliferation in a transplant patient is a PTLD.
- Recognition of a PTLD is extremely important for clinical purposes, even if categorization is problematic. Absolute distinction between a "benign" and a "malignant" PTLD can be more of a philosophical problem than a practical one; the WHO classification should be used as much as possible. Early lesions can be fatal, and lymphoma-like lesions may regress with decreased immunosuppression. Small tissue biopsies may preclude a precise classification.
- Presence of a clonal lymphoid population does not indicate that a PTLD is a "lymphoma" type and should not be considered pathognomonic of PTLDs.
- Patients with polymorphic or monomorphic PTLDs may have an "early-type" PTLD seen in regional lymph nodes, at other more distant sites, or immediately adjacent to the involved tissues.
- Before diagnosing a polymorphic PTLD, exclude a possible T-cell monomorphic PTLD, because morphologically, the latter may be very polymorphic.
- Even if not required for the diagnosis, the finding of numerous EBV$^+$ cells is very helpful in making the diagnosis of an iatrogenic immunodeficiency-associated LPD; however, their absence does not rule out the diagnosis, and the presence of small numbers of positive cells is not pathognomonic. EBV$^+$ cases should be distinguished from EBV$^-$ cases.
- Transplant patients can show both allograft rejection and PTLD at the same time.
- Iatrogenic immunodeficiency-associated LPDs are best described in patients following solid organ, stem cell, or bone marrow transplantation; in patients with rheumatoid arthritis following methotrexate therapy; and most recently in young males with Crohn's disease treated with infliximab (and azathioprine or mercaptopurine); however, they can occur following immunosuppression or immunosuppressive chemotherapeutic regimens in many other circumstances as well.

References can be found on Expert Consult @ www.expertconsult.com

Chapter 56

Hematopathology of Human Immunodeficiency Virus (HIV) Infection

Jonathan Said

CHAPTER OUTLINE

HIV infection is associated with a diverse group of lymphoid proliferations with varied clinical and pathologic features. Despite the control of HIV in industrialized countries, lymphoma remains the most common HIV-related malignancy.[1] Entities reviewed in this chapter are listed in Box 56-1.

HIV-RELATED LYMPHOID HYPERPLASIA

Immunopathogenesis

Primary HIV infection may be associated with an acute mononucleosis-like syndrome 3 to 6 weeks after infection, characterized by a burst of viremia and a drop in $CD4^+$ T cells. The viremia disappears within 1 week to 3 months, in association with the advent of a detectable immune response. Although the viral burden in peripheral blood mononuclear cells is low during this clinically latent period, there is dissemination throughout the body and propagation in lymphoid tissue.[2] Viral replication continues at these sites and, if untreated, is associated with the progressive depletion of $CD4^+$ T cells.

In the early phases of viral infection, the lymph node germinal centers remain intact but contain numerous extracellular HIV virions associated with follicular dendritic cells and their processes. HIV stimulates oligoclonal proliferation of follicular B lymphocytes. Dendritic cells trap the virus, and although viremia is temporarily curtailed, viral replication continues in the lymphoid tissue. HIV is present in the lymphoid tissue throughout the period of so-called clinical latency, even when minimal viral activity is demonstrated in the blood.[3] Without specific antiretroviral therapy, dendritic cell processes eventually degenerate, and HIV particles are released from the constraints of lymph node entrapment and recirculate.[2] Morphologically, this manifests as loss of follicular dendritic cells and the appearance of follicular lysis.

Persistent Generalized Lymphadenopathy

Persistent generalized lymphadenopathy (PGL) is part of an HIV-related symptom complex and is defined as lymphadenopathy of at least 3 months' duration involving two or more noncontiguous sites, in the absence of intercurrent illness or the use of drugs associated with lymphadenopathy. Associated constitutional symptoms include fever, headache, photophobia, night sweats, weight loss, and severe malaise. There may be hepatosplenomegaly, anemia, leukopenia, and

Box 56-1 ***HIV/AIDS-Related Lymphoid Proliferations***

- Nonneoplastic conditions involving lymph nodes and extranodal sites, including salivary gland, thymus, and bone marrow
  - HIV-related lymphoid hyperplasia and progressive generalized lymphadenopathy
  - Salivary lymphoid hyperplasia
  - Multicentric Castleman's disease
  - Kaposi's sarcoma–associated lymphadenopathy
  - Mycobacterial spindle cell tumor
  - *Pneumocystis* lymphadenopathy
- Bacillary angiomatosis

AIDS-Related Lymphomas

- Lymphomas also occurring in immunocompetent patients
  - Diffuse large B-cell lymphoma: immunoblastic or centroblastic
  - Burkitt's lymphoma: classic or with plasmacytoid differentiation
  - Classical Hodgkin's lymphoma
  - Extranodal marginal zone B-cell lymphoma (MALT lymphoma)
  - Peripheral T/NK-cell lymphoma
  - Mycosis fungoides
- Lymphomas occurring more specifically in HIV$^+$ patients
  - Primary effusion lymphoma
  - HHV8$^+$ solid lymphoma
  - Lymphoma associated with HHV8-associated multicentric Castleman's disease
  - Plasmablastic lymphoma (oral cavity type)
- Lymphomas occurring in other immunodeficient states
- Polymorphic B-cell lymphoma (PTLD like)

HHV8, human herpesvirus 8; MALT, mucosa-associated lymphoid tissue; NK, natural killer; PTLD, posttransplant lymphoproliferative disorder.

hypergammaglobulinemia. Lymphoid hyperplasia often affects the nasopharynx and Waldeyer's ring.[4]

The progressive stages of PGL and their histologic and immunohistochemical features are summarized in Boxes 56-2 and 56-3. In the early stage of PGL there is explosive follicular hyperplasia; expanded follicles, frequently without well-defined follicular mantles ("naked" follicles; Fig. 56-1A); and infiltration of follicles by CD8$^+$ T cells. Follicular lysis with hemorrhage and islands of mantle cells and T cells within follicular centers occur in the early phase (see Fig. 56-1B). Paracortical hyperplasia is also seen, with increased immunoblasts and plasma cells, as well as arborizing postcapillary venules with activated endothelial cells (high endothelial venules). Multinucleated giant cells, representing infected syncytia of T lymphocytes[5] or histiocytes,[4] may be present (see Fig. 56-1C). In addition to hyperplasia of sinus histiocytes, there are often aggregates of monocytoid B lymphocytes, similar to those seen in toxoplasmosis, often accompanied by neutrophils. Lymphoid hyperplasia also occurs in extranodal sites such as Waldeyer's ring and the paranasal sinuses and may be associated with multinucleated giant cells adjacent to crypt or surface epithelium.[4]

As the disease progresses, and in association with falling CD4$^+$ cell counts, follicular dissolution and disruption of germinal centers ensue. In the late stages there is lymphoid depletion, absence of follicles or residual "burnt out" follicles, and increased vasculature associated with immunoblasts and plasma cells (see Fig. 56-1D). Although none of these features is specific for HIV infection, the constellation of clinical features and histologic findings is highly characteristic of HIV-related lymphadenopathy.

Using monoclonal antibodies or in situ hybridization, HIV can be localized to the processes of follicular dendritic cells, and extracellular viral particles can be identified in extracellular locations by electron microscopy. Commercial antibodies useful to localize HIV in routinely processed tissue sections include antibodies to p24, p17, gp41, and gp120. Tubuloreticular inclusions similar to those found in systemic lupus erythematosus and other abnormal immune states are frequently present in vascular endothelium. Epstein-Barr virus (EBV) can be found in interfollicular B lymphocytes and rare T lymphocytes in cases of PGL.

Box 56-2 ***Stages of Lymphoid Hyperplasia in Persistent Generalized Lymphadenopathy***

Early

- Cortical hyperplasia
  - Enlarged irregular follicles
  - Follicles extending through cortex and medulla
  - Aggregates of small lymphocytes within follicles
  - Hemorrhage in germinal centers
- Paracortical hyperplasia
  - Small lymphocytes, immunoblasts, plasma cells
  - Polykaryocytes (multinucleated giant cells)
  - Arborizing postcapillary venules with high endothelium
  - Monocytoid B lymphocytes
  - Sinus reticular hyperplasia

Intermediate

- Follicular fragmentation and lysis
- Follicular involution
- Focal necrosis
- Vascular transformation of sinuses

Late

- Follicular depletion
- "Burnt out" follicles
- Hyaline vascular follicles
- Hypocellularity and lymphoid depletion
- Increased vascularity
- Fibrosis

Box 56-3 ***Immunohistochemical Findings in HIV-Related Lymphoid Hyperplasia (Persistent Generalized Lymphadenopathy)***

- Polyclonal immunoglobulins in germinal centers (dendritic pattern)
- Aggregates of small lymphocytes (CD8$^+$) in germinal centers
- CD4$^+$ polykaryocytes
- Increased Ki-67 staining in germinal centers
- Antibody to dendritic cells (CD21, CD23, DRC-1) reveals fragmentation of follicular framework (follicular lysis)
- Antibodies to HIV-1 localized in dendritic cell meshwork
- Inversion of normal CD4/CD8 cell ratio in paracortex
- Eventual depletion of CD4$^+$ cells
- Increased polyclonal plasma cells

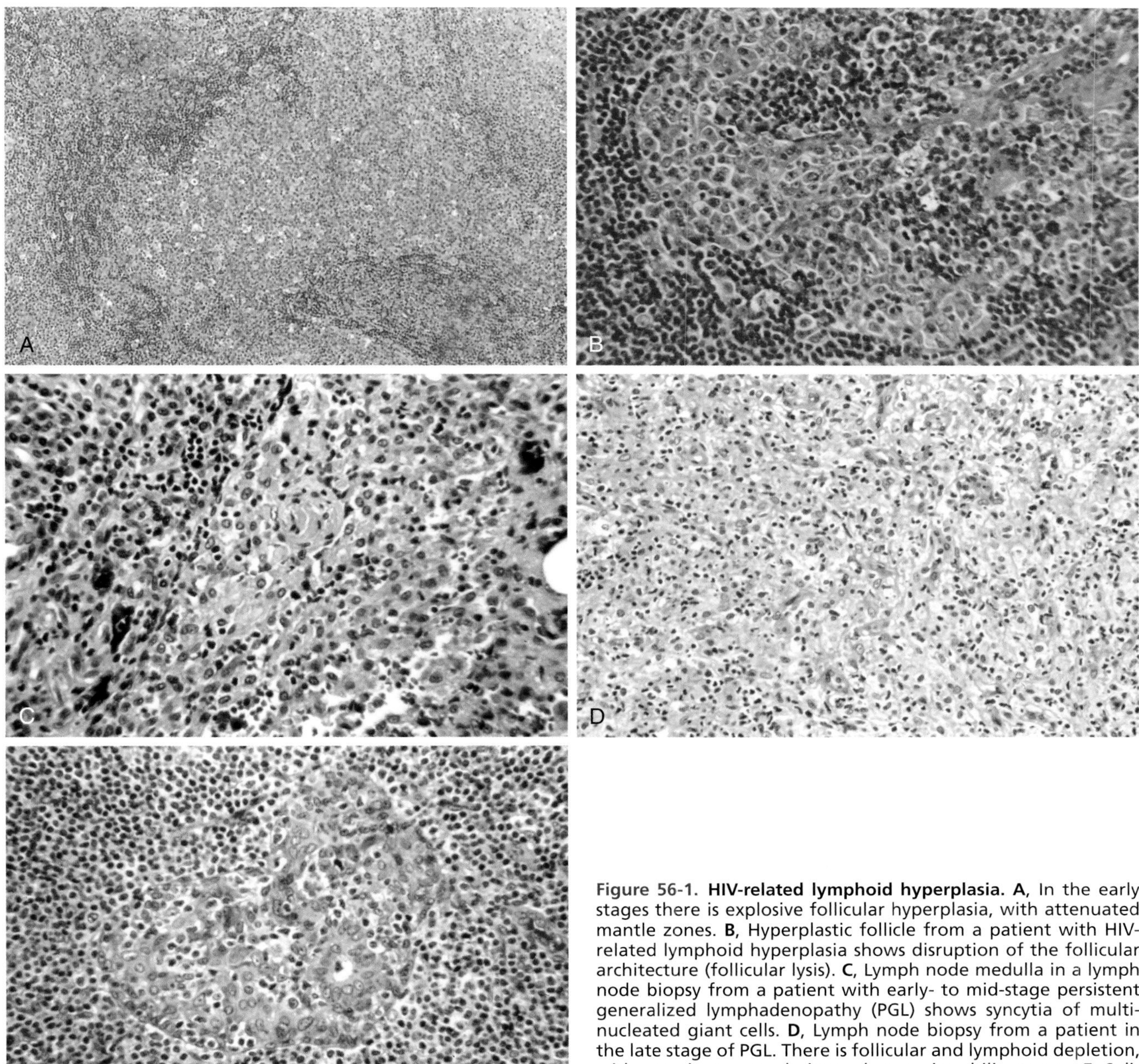

Figure 56-1. **HIV-related lymphoid hyperplasia. A,** In the early stages there is explosive follicular hyperplasia, with attenuated mantle zones. **B,** Hyperplastic follicle from a patient with HIV-related lymphoid hyperplasia shows disruption of the follicular architecture (follicular lysis). **C,** Lymph node medulla in a lymph node biopsy from a patient with early- to mid-stage persistent generalized lymphadenopathy (PGL) shows syncytia of multinucleated giant cells. **D,** Lymph node biopsy from a patient in the late stage of PGL. There is follicular and lymphoid depletion, with prominent vascularity and an eosinophilic stroma. **E,** Salivary lymphoid hyperplasia in the parotid gland. Salivary duct shows myoepithelial proliferation and lymphoid infiltration.

Salivary Lymphoid Hyperplasia and Salivary Duct Cysts

Lymphoid hyperplasia is common in the parotid gland (and, less frequently, the submandibular gland) and surrounding lymph nodes and is associated with ductal epithelial proliferations that resemble the lymphoepithelial lesions seen in Sjögren's syndrome (see Fig. 56-1E).[6] Other features of Sjögren's syndrome, including rheumatoid antibodies and the sicca syndrome, are absent. Salivary ducts may dilate to form gross fluid-filled cysts. Follicular dendritic cells within the hyperplastic follicles are a site of active replication of HIV-1. These lesions may give rise to a differential diagnosis of lymphoma of mucosa-associated lymphoid tissue (MALT lymphoma). However, the follicles in HIV-related lymphoid hyperplasia are prominent, often with follicular lysis; broad strands of extrafollicular monocytoid B cells are not seen. Plasma cells are polyclonal, and there is no clonal rearrangement of immunoglobulin genes or c-*MYC*.

HIV-Related Multicentric Castleman's Disease

Human herpesvirus 8 (HHV8), also known as Kaposi's sarcoma herpesvirus (KSHV), has been linked to multicentric Castleman's disease in both HIV-positive and -negative patients[7,8] and is present in most cases of multicentric Castleman's disease in the setting of acquired immunodeficiency syndrome (AIDS). The disease most commonly presents in the lymph nodes or spleen. In HIV-infected patients with Castleman's disease, there is a strong association between HHV8 and sexual transmission, as well as the development of KS.[9] The pathogenesis may be related to the production of viral interleukin (IL)-6.[10] Multicentric Castleman's disease occurs most often in older patients, predominantly men, and is associated with lymphadenopathy and constitutional symptoms. HHV8$^+$ large B-cell lymphoma may develop in patients with multicentric Castleman's disease (see later).

Small, hyaline vascular germinal centers are characteristic of Castleman's disease. Mantle zone lymphocytes are arranged in concentric rings ("onion skinning"), and mantle zones may intrude into the germinal centers (Fig. 56-2). Interfollicular vascular proliferation and prominent plasmacytic infiltrates are present. The mature plasma cells in the interfollicular region are polytypic.

Large cells with vesicular nuclei and amphophilic cytoplasm, resembling immunoblasts or plasmablasts, can be located in the mantle zones of the follicles and in the interfollicular regions (see Fig. 56-2B).[11,12] The plasmablasts are thought to proliferate in response to activation of the IL-6 signaling pathway.[12] Plasmablasts can form clusters of cells that encroach on the germinal centers, forming so-called microlymphomas (see Fig. 56-2C). HHV8 is present in the plasmablasts and can be detected by in situ hybridization or by immunohistochemistry using antibody against latency-associated nuclear antigen (LANA; see Fig. 56-2D). Plasmablasts variably express CD20 and are positive for CD138 and monotypic immunoglobulin (Ig) Mλ, although in the early stages, they are polyclonal. They do not harbor somatic mutations in the rearranged immunoglobulin genes, however, and appear to originate from naïve B cells.[12] Unlike the solid variant of primary effusion lymphoma (PEL), another HHV8+ lymphoma, they are negative for EBV-encoded small RNA (EBER). With disease progression, frank plasmablastic lymphomas develop, which efface the nodal or splenic architecture and may involve other sites, including the lung and liver. These lymphomas are monoclonal, although the immunoglobulin genes remain unmutated.

Kaposi's Sarcoma–Associated Lymphadenopathy

In some patients KS involves the lymph nodes in the absence of skin lesions. This lymphoma-like presentation of KS is frequently associated with hyaline vascular follicular hyperplasia, similar to Castleman's disease.[9] Nodal involvement is

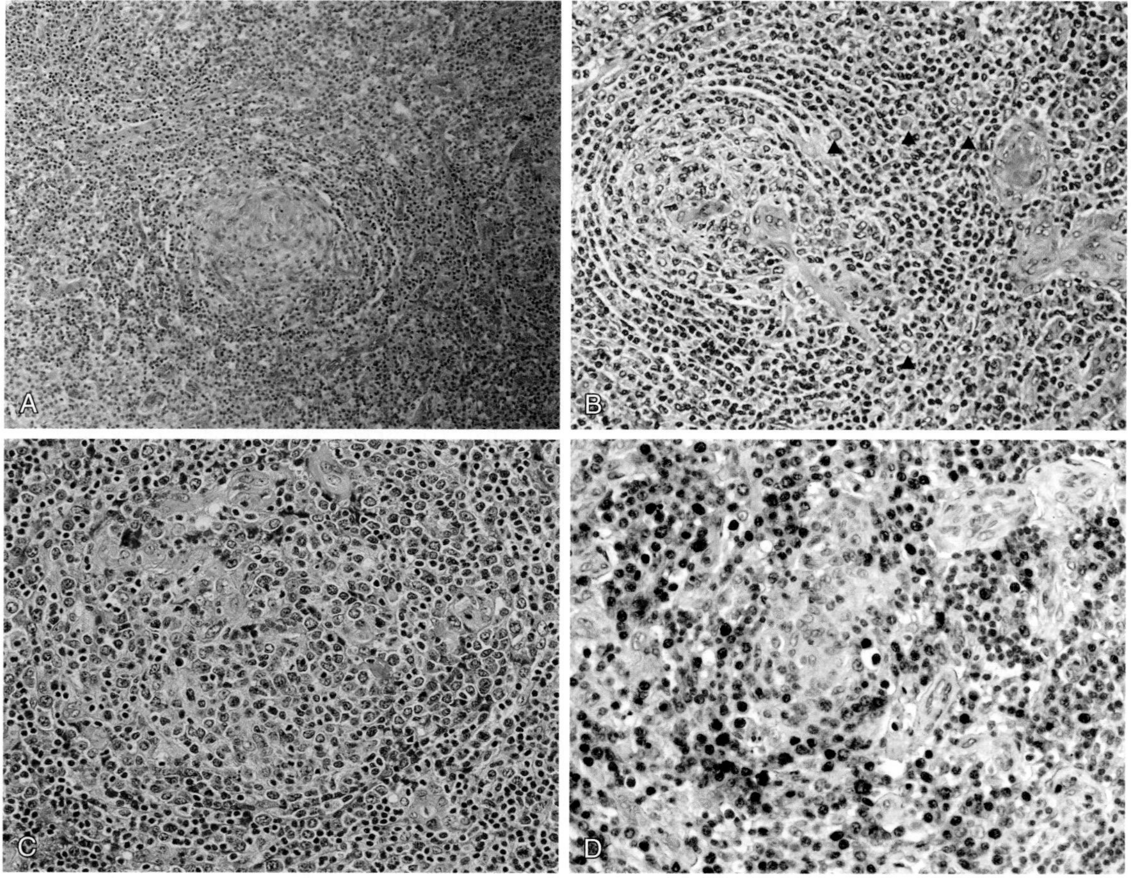

Figure 56-2. HIV-related multicentric Castleman's disease. A, Typical hyaline vascular follicle with a penetrating venule. **B,** Castleman's disease shows a follicle with a penetrating venule and an expanded mantle zone with single large lymphoid cells or plasmablasts (*arrowheads*). **C,** Multicentric Castleman's disease with numerous plasmablasts, including clusters. **D,** Plasmablasts are positive for human herpesvirus 8 latency-associated nuclear antigen (LANA) (immunoperoxidase stain for LANA; hematoxylin counterstain).

characterized by peripheral and subcapsular dilated lymphatic and vascular channels and spindle cell nodules (Fig. 56-3). HHV8 can be demonstrated with immunohistochemistry and antibodies to LANA within spindle and endothelial cells.[13]

Mycobacterial Spindle Cell Pseudotumor

Mycobacterial spindle cell pseudotumor occurs in lymph nodes in which the parenchyma is replaced by spindled macrophages containing numerous mycobacterial organisms, usually *Mycobacterium avium-intracellulare* (Fig. 56-4).[14] In addition to lymph nodes, mycobacterial spindle cell tumors may occur in the skin, bone marrow, spleen, lung, retroperitoneum, and central nervous system (CNS).[15]

Pneumocystis Lymphadenopathy

Pneumocystis infection may involve the lymph nodes, bone marrow, or spleen and can be recognized by the

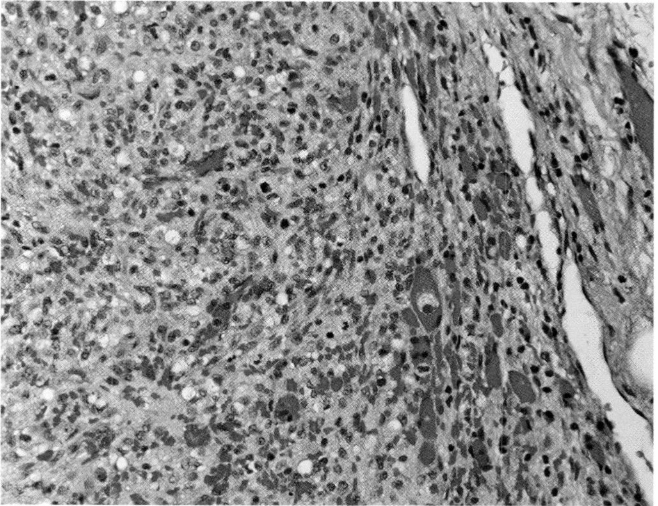

Figure 56-3. **Kaposi's sarcoma of lymph node.** Kaposi's sarcoma involves the lymph node sinus and extends into the capsule and lymph node parenchyma.

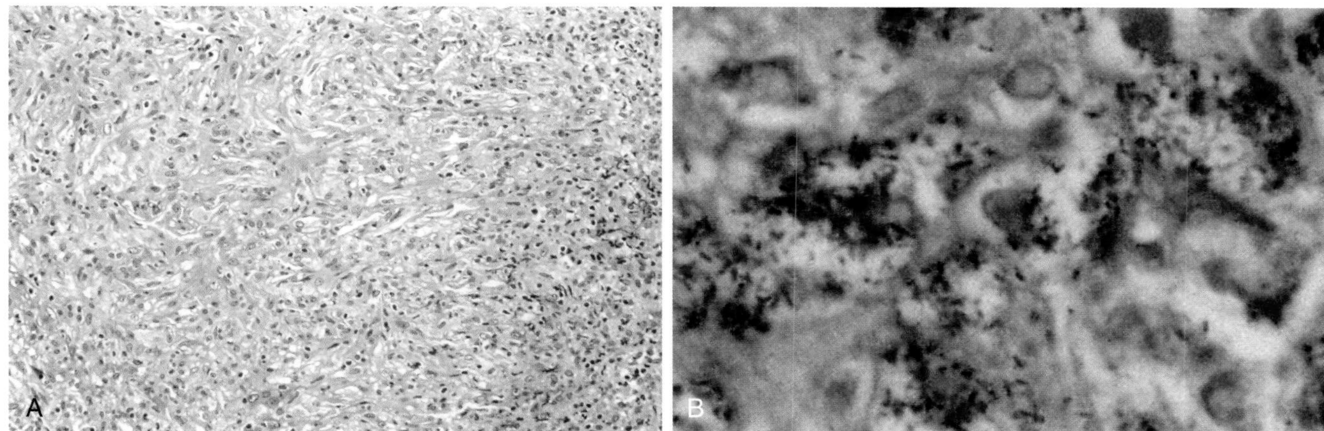

Figure 56-4. **Mycobacterial spindle cell pseudotumor of lymph node. A,** Histologic appearance of mycobacterial spindle cell pseudotumor. The lymph node is replaced by spindled histiocytes containing mycobacteria. **B,** Acid-fast stain shows innumerable bacteria (Ziehl-Neelsen stain).

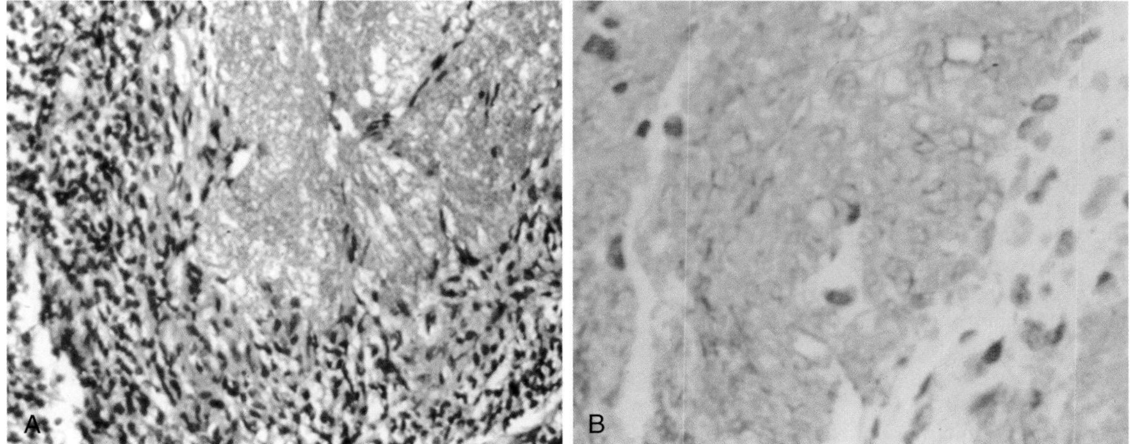

Figure 56-5. ***Pneumocystis* infection in lymph node. A,** Lymph node biopsy from a patient with *Pneumocystis* infection shows foamy material replacing the lymph node architecture. **B,** Immunostain for *Pneumocystis* on a lymph node from a patient with *Pneumocystis* lymphadenitis (immunoperoxidase stain; hematoxylin counterstain).

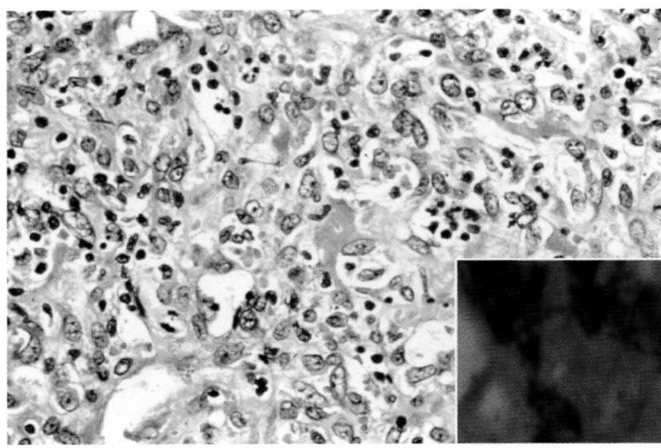

Figure 56-6. Bacillary angiomatosis of lymph node. The lymph node is replaced by a vascular proliferation with an edematous stroma, numerous neutrophils, and purple clumps of bacteria. *Inset*, Warthin-Starry stain of a lymph node in a patient with bacillary angiomatosis shows clumps of bacteria stained black.

characteristic foamy exudate similar to that seen in the lung (Fig. 56-5A). Organisms are readily identified by silver stains or immunohistochemistry (see Fig. 56-5B).

Bacillary Angiomatosis

Bacillary angiomatosis is a vascular proliferation caused by *Bartonella henselae* or *Bartonella quintana*.[16] It is most commonly seen in the skin but may occur in the lymph nodes, where it must be differentiated from KS. In bacillary angiomatosis, vascular proliferation is associated with eosinophilic interstitial edema and neutrophils with leukocytoclasis (Fig. 56-6).[17] Numerous organisms are typically seen with Warthin-Starry or Steiner stains.

HEMATOLOGIC AND BONE MARROW MANIFESTATIONS OF HIV INFECTION

Peripheral Blood

Most often, HIV infection is characterized hematologically by anemia, granulocytopenia, and lymphopenia. Anemia is usually normochromic and normocytic, consistent with anemia of chronic disease. Iron stores are typically increased, but there is low serum iron, low or normal total iron-binding capacity, and increased ferritin. Circulating atypical lymphocytes and vacuolated monocytes can be seen at all stages of HIV infection.

Thrombocytopenia occurs in asymptomatic HIV-infected individuals and is a common manifestation of AIDS. Thrombocytopenic purpura is not associated with a short-term risk of progression to AIDS and is not one of the case surveillance criteria of the Centers for Disease Control and Prevention (CDC). Causes of thrombocytopenia following HIV infection include immune-mediated destruction of platelets; impaired thrombopoiesis, including the effects of medication; and syndromes resembling hemolytic uremic syndrome and thrombotic thrombocytopenic purpura. Immune platelet destruction in HIV infection most often results from platelet-bound immunoglobulin and complement and immune complex formation. Antiplatelet antibodies have also been implicated. $CD34^+$ stem cells are susceptible to HIV infection and exhibit a reduced capacity to give rise to megakaryocyte colonies, a finding that has been linked to increased viral replication in the bone marrow microenvironment. Clinically significant bleeding is rarely seen with HIV-related thrombocytopenia, and patients seldom require splenectomy. Hemostatic abnormalities in HIV-infected individuals may also be due to circulating anticoagulant factors, particularly lupus anticoagulant.[18]

Bone Marrow

The bone marrow of patients infected with HIV is often hypercellular in the early stages. As the disease progresses, cellularity tends to decrease as a result of impaired production, leading to worsening cytopenias. Core biopsies frequently exhibit foci of serous atrophy, which is characterized by marrow hypoplasia and fat atrophy with gelatinous transformation of the stroma, suggesting a damaged hematopoietic microenvironment. Macrocytic erythroid maturation may be prominent, particularly after antiretroviral therapy (Fig. 56-7A). Megakaryocytes are usually increased and include dysplastic forms with "naked" nuclei (see Fig. 56-7B).[19] Lymphoid aggregates with or without germinal centers are common in the bone marrow and should not be confused with malignant lymphoma. Granulomas are common, but opportunistic organisms (e.g., mycobacteria, fungi) may be detected with special stains and cultured from the marrow even when granulomas are not identified (see Fig. 56-7C). For this reason, stains for acid-fast bacilli and fungi should routinely be performed on bone marrow biopsies from HIV-infected patients, even when no granulomas are seen (see Fig. 56-7D). The presence of granulomas correlates with opportunistic infection in about 80% of cases.[20] Parvovirus infection may be associated with red cell aplasia and may also suppress other lineage progenitors (see Fig. 56-7E).[21]

Bone marrow involvement is reported in about 25% of patients with newly diagnosed AIDS-related lymphoma.[22] Patients with marrow involvement have a higher incidence of lymphomatous meningitis and positive cerebrospinal fluid.[22] Impaired survival is correlated with extensive marrow infiltration (>50%). Patterns of lymphomatous infiltration in specific lymphoma types are discussed later.

THYMIC CHANGES IN HIV INFECTION

Thymic involvement may be particularly important in the pediatric population, because HIV infection of the thymus may prevent the regeneration of depleted T lymphocytes, contributing to profound early immune impairment. T-cell precursors at multiple stages of intrathymic maturation are susceptible to HIV infection via the CD4 molecule, and the T-cell pool is unable to regenerate in the setting of progressive HIV infection. Thymic epithelial cells may also be directly infected with HIV.

Pathologic examination of the thymus can help distinguish AIDS from other congenital deficiency syndromes. In almost all cases of AIDS the thymus is markedly reduced in size.[23,24] A spectrum of histologic changes is observed, including sclerosis and scarring. Thymic dysplasia is characterized by lymphoid depletion, profound reduction in Hassall's corpuscles, and sclerosis of the septa. Precocious involution is characterized by depletion of the thymus parenchyma and fatty replacement. Hassall's corpuscles may be microcystically dilated but are not markedly reduced. Thymitis is character-

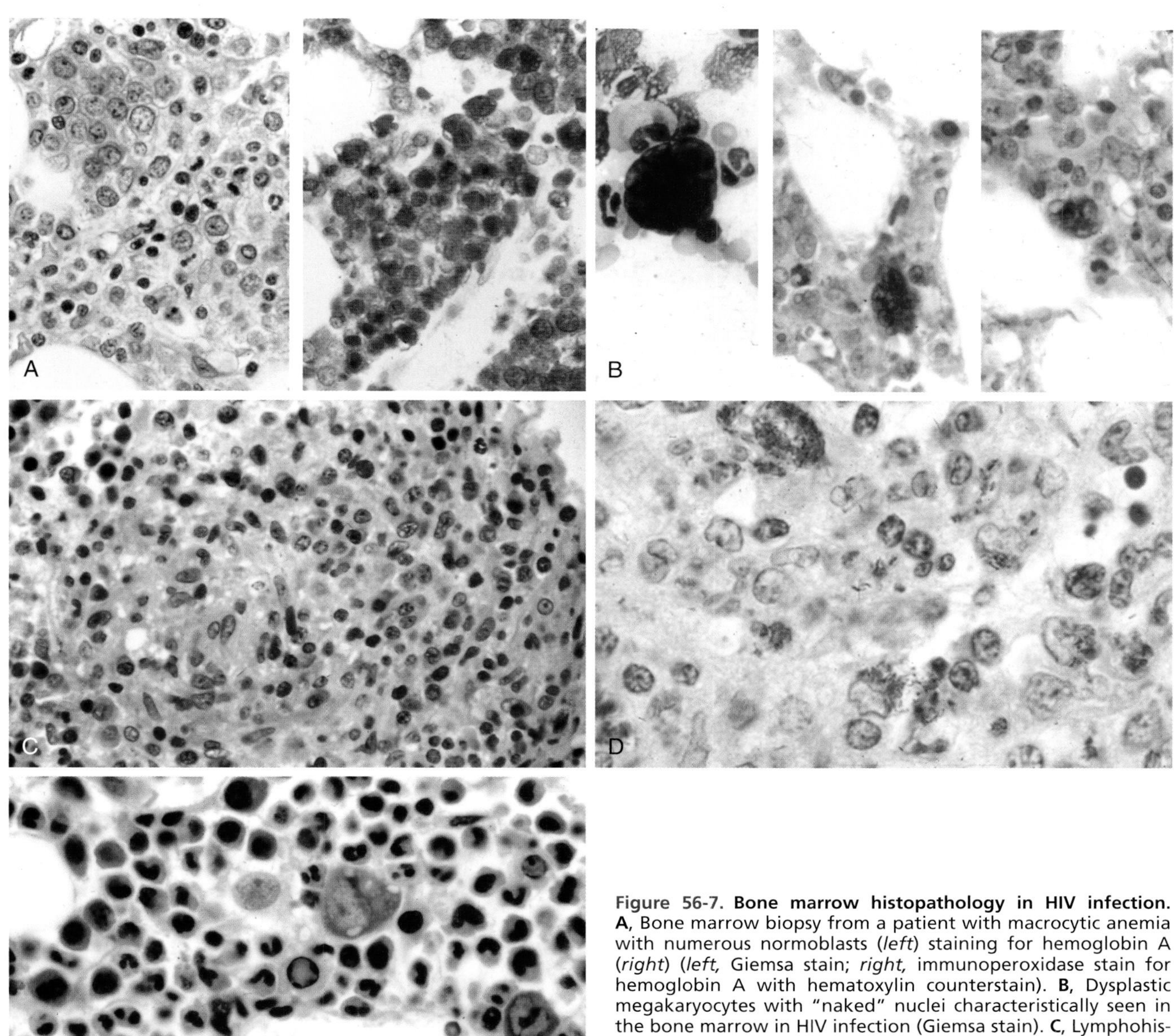

Figure 56-7. Bone marrow histopathology in HIV infection. **A,** Bone marrow biopsy from a patient with macrocytic anemia with numerous normoblasts (*left*) staining for hemoglobin A (*right*) (*left,* Giemsa stain; *right,* immunoperoxidase stain for hemoglobin A with hematoxylin counterstain). **B,** Dysplastic megakaryocytes with "naked" nuclei characteristically seen in the bone marrow in HIV infection (Giemsa stain). **C,** Lymphohistiocytic aggregate with poorly formed granuloma, a common feature in the bone marrow of patients with HIV. **D,** Acid-fast stain reveals macrophages containing large numbers of beaded acid-fast organisms, consistent with *Mycobacterium avium* complex infection. **E,** Giant normoblasts with characteristic parvovirus inclusions.

ized by medullary lymphoid follicles with germinal centers, multinucleated giant cells, and diffuse lymphoplasmacytic infiltrates. Thymitis can be followed by precocious involution and is thought to result from injury late in fetal life or after birth. Thymic lymphoid hyperplasia may result in significant thymic enlargement and can be associated with thymic cysts.[25]

AIDS-RELATED LYMPHOMAS

Epidemiology

Since the advent of highly active antiretroviral therapy (HAART), there has been a change in the incidence of HIV-related lymphomas.[26,27] In one cooperative study the incidence of non-Hodgkin's lymphoma per 100,000 decreased from 1.99 to 0.30.[26] This decline was most apparent in cases of primary CNS lymphoma, which decreased from 27.8 to 9.7 per 10,000 person-years.[28] There has also been a change in lymphoma subtypes, with a decreased incidence of Burkitt's lymphoma (BL) and a relative increase in diffuse large B-cell lymphoma (DLBCL).[29] Other changes include a higher prevalence of lymphoma in women infected with HIV and a longer history of HIV seropositivity before the onset of lymphoma.[28] In a population-based study comparing the cancer experiences of AIDS patients with those of the general population, incidence rates in the former were increased 113-fold for non-Hodgkin's lymphoma, 7.6-fold for Hodgkin's lymphoma, and 4.5-fold for myeloma.[27]

Lymphomas are a relatively late complication of HIV infection,[30] often preceded by low CD4+ cell counts and increased viral loads in plasma.[22,29] Unlike KS, which affects predominantly homosexual and bisexual males, lymphomas affect all sections of the HIV+ population, and the clinical and pathologic characteristics are the same in all groups, regardless of gender or mechanism of HIV transmission. Most HIV-related non-Hodgkin's lymphomas are derived from B cells and share clinical features, including an extranodal presentation and aggressive behavior.[31] AIDS lymphomas associated with EBV or HHV8 commonly exhibit plasmablastic differentiation. Prognosis can be improved with better combined chemotherapy regimens and antiretroviral drugs.[32]

Classification

Lymphomas associated with HIV have been classified by the World Health Organization (WHO) in three groups: those that also arise in immunocompetent patients, those occurring specifically in HIV+ patients, and those also occurring in other immunodeficiency states (see Box 56-1).[33]

Clinical Features

Systemic (B) symptoms are usually present and include weight loss, fever, and night sweats. Disease is usually widespread at presentation and may involve multiple extranodal sites, most commonly the CNS, gastrointestinal tract, bone marrow, and liver. Multiple tumor masses may be present in the gastrointestinal tract, which may represent separate clonal neoplasms. Lymphomas may present at unusual sites, including the myocardium, bile duct, soft tissue, gingiva and oral cavity, appendix, anorectum, kidney, and lung. There may be extensive organ infiltration leading to organ failure, particularly in the bone marrow and liver.

BL constitutes 30% to 40% of AIDS-related non-Hodgkin's lymphomas and is generally seen at a younger age than DLBCL.[34,35] Most cases of BL present in the abdomen or bone marrow. Primary CNS lymphomas are predominantly immunoblastic DLBCL.[36,37] The usual presentation consists of one or more mass lesions in the brain, which may be deep seated (Fig. 56-8A).[38] Computed tomography of the brain may lead to confusion with cerebral toxoplasmosis, although in the latter condition, the lesions are usually multiple and smaller. In children with AIDS, primary lymphoma is the most common cause of focal or multifocal mass lesions in the brain.[39]

Pathogenesis

Although the pathogenesis of lymphoma in AIDS patients is not completely understood, evidence suggests that chronic antigenic stimulation, as evidenced by PGL and polyclonal hypergammaglobulinemia, frequently precedes lymphoma.[40] EBV infection in association with impaired immune surveillance leads to B-cell overproduction and an increased risk of genetic alterations that lead to malignant lymphoma.[41,42] Polyclonal and oligoclonal B-cell expansion frequently precedes the development of lymphoma in HIV-infected individuals, and lymphomas may contain multiple copies of monomorphic EBV genomes, indicating that infection occurred before the clonal expansion in these tumors. Unlike lymphomas in the transplant setting, lymphomas in HIV+ patients have been associated with both A- and B-type EBV.[43-47] Viral infection (EBV and HHV8) may be associated with cytokine production, including IL-6, IL-10, and IL-13, which may contribute to lymphomagenesis.[31,48]

Table 56-1 Epstein-Barr Virus and AIDS-Related Lymphomas

Lymphoma Type	Cases Positive for EBV (%)
BL, classic type	30-40
BL, plasmacytoid type	50-75
B-cell lymphoma with features intermediate between DLBCL and BL (formerly atypical BL or Burkitt-like lymphoma)	30-50
Large cell lymphoma, centroblastic	20-30
Large cell lymphoma, immunoblastic	80
Large cell immunoblastic lymphoma of the CNS	100
Primary effusion lymphoma	100
Plasmablastic lymphoma of the oral cavity and other sites	100
Plasmablastic lymphoma associated with MCD	0

BL, Burkitt's lymphoma; CNS, central nervous system; DLBCL, diffuse large B-cell lymphoma; EBV, Epstein-Barr virus; MCD, multicentric Castleman's disease.

EBV infection of neoplastic cells has been demonstrated in about 40% of cases of HIV-related lymphomas (Table 56-1).[49,50] EBV is identified in a higher percentage of CNS lymphomas and those with immunoblastic morphology (80% to 100%) compared with BL, in which the incidence of tumor cell infection with EBV resembles that of sporadic rather than endemic cases (approximately 40%).[51,52] Latent EBV nuclear antigen (EBNA-1) transcripts detected in HIV-related lymphomas resemble the pattern seen in sporadic BL, but HIV-related lymphomas may also express transcripts for EBV latent membrane protein (LMP-1).[53]

Chromosomal translocations may result in the activation of oncogenes in about 40% of cases; these oncogenes include c-*MYC* and, less commonly, *RAS*, *BCL2*, and *p53*. *MYC* activation and *p53* inactivation occur more often in BL.[54] Molecular mechanisms of *MYC* activation resemble those found in sporadic rather than endemic BL.[52] Most HIV-related lymphomas contain at least one genetic abnormality, and three or four different lesions have been described in the same neoplasm. DLBCL with centroblastic morphology is associated with the expression of BCL6 protein, suggesting germinal center derivation.[55,56]

AIDS-Related Lymphomas Occurring in Immunocompetent Hosts

Diffuse Large B-Cell Lymphoma

DLBCL accounts for about 30% of lymphoma cases in HIV+ patients. The incidence of EBV infection in DLBCL is variable, ranging from about 30% in the centroblastic lymphomas to 80% or higher in cases with immunoblastic morphology; it is highest in immunoblastic lymphomas arising in the CNS. DLBCL often presents at extranodal sites and may form multiple tumor masses (see Fig. 56-8B).

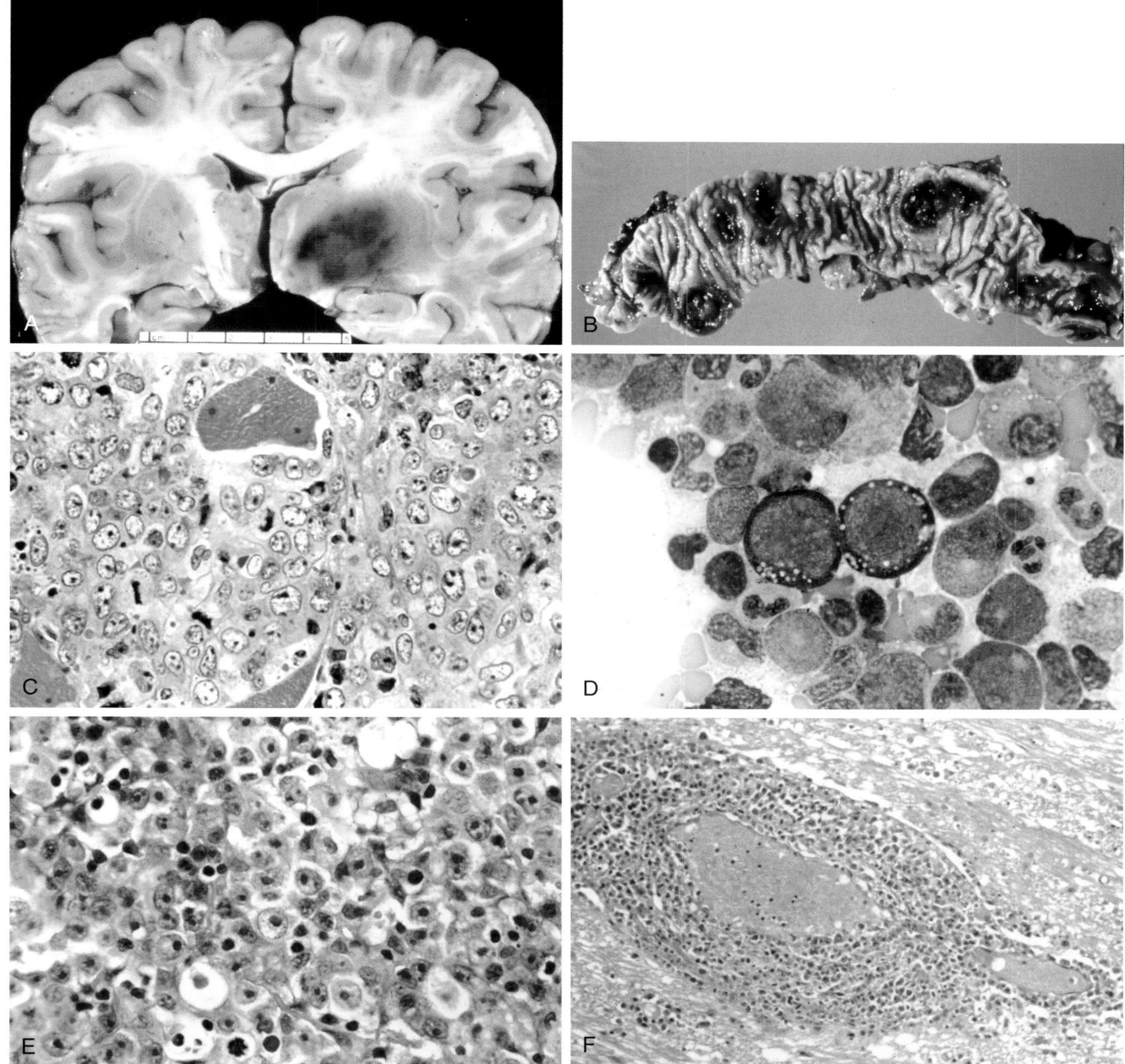

Figure 56-8. Diffuse large B-cell lymphoma (DLBCL) in HIV infection. A, Coronal section of the brain shows a deep-seated lymphoma mass, characteristic of immunoblastic DLBCL in the central nervous system. **B,** Large bowel contains multiple ulcerating tumor nodules of DLBCL. **C,** Soft tissue mass in the flank exhibits DLBCL, with neoplastic centroblasts infiltrating muscle fibers. **D,** DLBCL with single malignant cells with prominent nucleoli and vacuolated cytoplasm infiltrating the bone marrow (Giemsa stain). **E,** Immunoblastic DLBCL. The cells have large central nucleoli and abundant cytoplasm. **F,** DLBCL in the brain exhibits neoplastic immunoblasts clustered around blood vessels. (A and **B,** From Hsi ED. *Hematopathology*. Philadelphia: Churchill-Livingstone, 2007:321, 319.)

Morphology. There is a morphologic spectrum in DLBCL, ranging from cases with a diffuse proliferation of large centroblastic cells to those comprising predominantly immunoblasts. Cases made up almost entirely of centroblasts have a similar morphology to DLBCL in the general population. The neoplastic cells have round, oval, or irregular nuclei; vesicular chromatin; and two or more nucleoli, often evenly spaced at the nuclear membrane (see Fig. 56-8C). The pattern of marrow infiltration by DLBCL is variable; tumor aggregates may be present, but DLBCL can also infiltrate the marrow as single cells (see Fig. 56-8D).

The immunoblastic variant accounts for about 20% of cases of AIDS lymphomas and is composed almost entirely of immunoblasts (>90% of the cell population). The neoplastic lymphoid cells are large, with single central macronucleoli and amphophilic or plasmacytoid cytoplasm (see Fig. 56-8E). In some cases the cells are more pleomorphic and may contain polyploid Reed-Sternberg–like cells. In CNS lymphomas, the lymphoma cells are often clustered around vessels (see Fig. 56-8F).[38]

Molecular Genetics and Clonality. Immunoglobulin gene rearrangement studies reveal monoclonal patterns using Southern blot or polymerase chain reaction techniques.[57] Rearrangements of the *BCL6* gene are found in DLBCL with centroblastic morphology.[58] CNS lymphomas are homogeneous, monoclonal B-cell neoplasms, positive for EBV, and lack *MYC* rearrangements.[59] *RAS* mutations and *p53* point mutations are found in 40% of DLBCLs.[51,52,54] Translocations involving the *MYC* locus also occur in about 20% of DLBCLs.

Burkitt's Lymphoma

Epidemiology. BL constitutes 30% to 40% of AIDS-related non-Hodgkin's lymphomas. It is generally seen at a younger age than DLBCL and in patients with $CD4^+$ cell counts exceeding 200/μL[34,35,60]; it is often the first AIDS-defining illness. Most cases of BL present with advanced disease involving the abdomen or bone marrow. Symptoms can include abdominal pain, bowel obstruction, gastrointestinal bleeding, or syndromes mimicking appendicitis or intussusception.[60] Cases of extensive bone marrow infiltration may present as acute leukemia. Although uncommon, AIDS-related BL can present with localized stage I/Ie disease, resembling the endemic form.[61]

Morphology. Although similar in appearance to BL in non-immunosuppressed patients, a number of variants are described in association with HIV infection.[62] In the classic variant the cells are medium sized, with basophilic cytoplasm, monomorphic round or oval nuclei, and often multiple nucleoli (Fig. 56-9A). In patients with AIDS, BL cells more often appear plasmacytoid, with eccentric nuclei and amphophilic cytoplasm that is positive for immunoglobulin (see Fig. 56-9B). EBV is more likely to be positive in these cases (up to 75%). BL with plasmacytoid differentiation is characteristically associated with HIV infection. Occasional cases have greater pleomorphism in both nuclear size and shape compared with classic BL, and the nuclei may contain more prominent nucleoli (see Fig. 56-9C).[63]

BL commonly involves the marrow in patients with AIDS[64] and may present with extensive marrow infiltration or replacement of normal marrow in a pattern resembling acute lymphoblastic leukemia (see Fig. 56-9D).

Immunophenotype and Genetics. The immunophenotype and genetic features of AIDS-related BL are similar to those

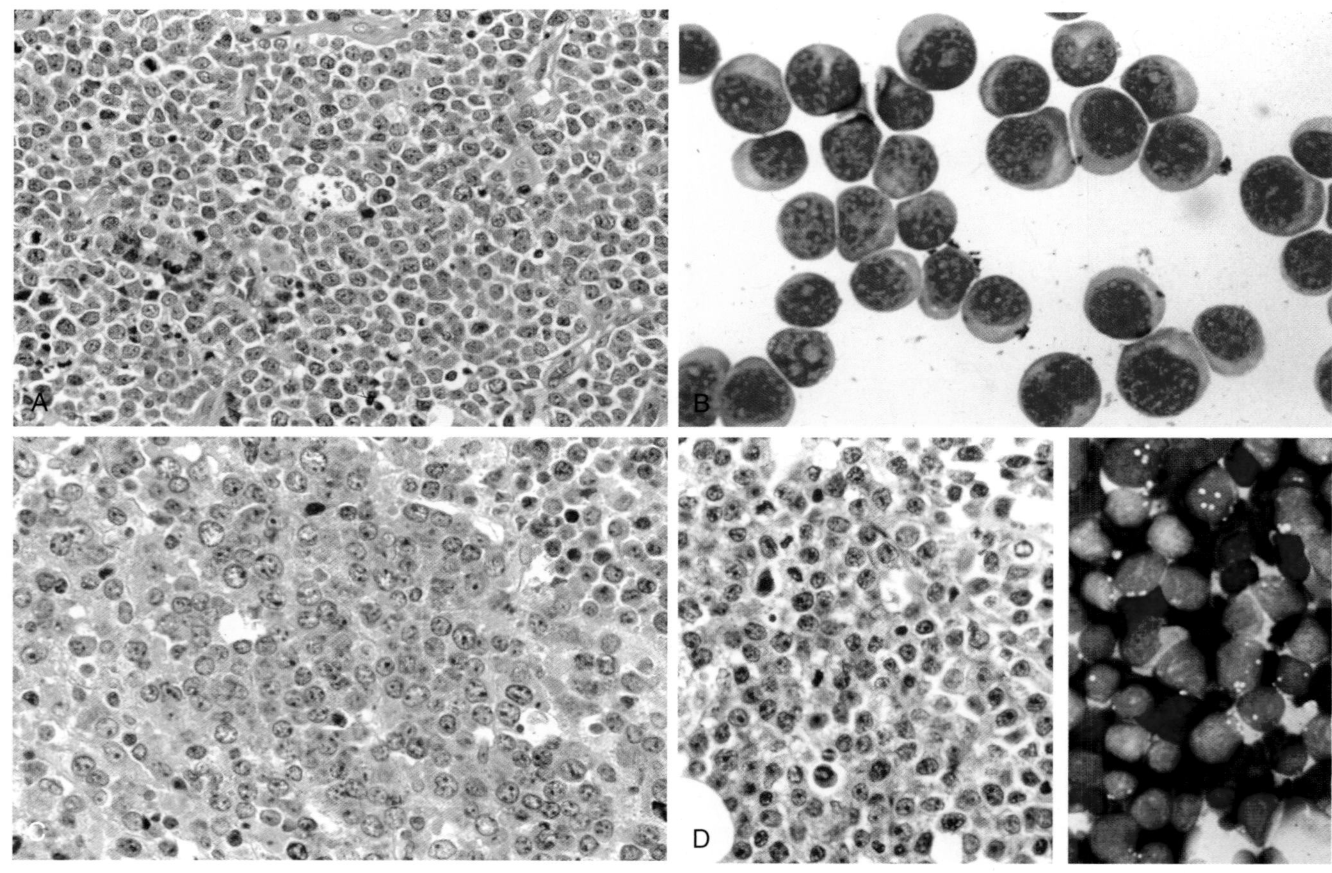

Figure 56-9. Burkitt's lymphoma in HIV infection. A, Classic Burkitt's lymphoma, with a diffuse proliferation of blastic cells with round nuclei and "starry sky" macrophages. **B,** Plasmacytoid variant of Burkitt's lymphoma. Imprint preparation shows blastic cells with round nuclei and basophilic or plasmacytoid cytoplasm (Giemsa stain). **C,** HIV-related Burkitt's lymphoma with cohesive clusters of medium-sized cells showing greater nuclear variability than in the classic type. **D,** Burkitt's lymphoma presenting with marrow packed with medium-sized blastic cells with round nuclei, abundant cytoplasm, and cytoplasmic vacuoles evident on the smear (*left*, biopsy; *right*, aspirate, Giemsa stain).

of sporadic BL. Cells express CD22, CD20, CD19, CD10, BCL6, and CD79a and are negative for CD5, CD23, BCL2, and terminal deoxynucleotidyl transferase (TdT). The cells express bright surface IgM with monoclonal light-chain restriction. The immunophenotypic evidence of somatic hypermutation[65] indicates that the cells of BL arise from germinal center B cells.

BL in HIV$^+$ patients has translocations involving the *MYC* gene on chromosome 8q24 and the heavy-chain locus on chromosome 14 (t[8;14]) or the light-chain loci on chromosomes 2 or 22.[63,66] Deregulation of *MYC* may also arise from point mutations in the first intron–first exon regulatory regions and amino acid substitution in the second exon. Point mutations of *p53* are also relatively common in BL (about 60% of cases).[54] EBV infection is present in about 30% to 40% of BLs with the classic morphology and in up to 75% of the atypical and plasmacytoid variants.

Extranodal Marginal Zone B-Cell Lymphoma of Mucosa-Associated Lymphoid Tissue (MALT Lymphoma)

MALT lymphomas have been associated with HIV, particularly in the lungs of children with a history of lymphocytic interstitial pneumonitis.[67] Cases have also been described in adults and at common MALT sites, including the stomach and conjunctiva.[68] These resemble MALT lymphomas in the general population and are characterized by marginal zone B cells forming multiple pulmonary nodules, associated with lymphoepithelial lesions involving the bronchiolar epithelium (Fig. 56-10).

Plasma Cell Myeloma

Epidemiologic studies indicate that AIDS leads to a significantly increased risk of myeloma.[69] However, many of these cases may actually be examples of plasmablastic lymphoma (see later) because they are aggressive, with an anaplastic appearance and involvement of ascitic and other fluids.[70]

Other Lymphoma Types

Single cases of other B-cell lymphoma types, including primary mediastinal large B-cell lymphoma,[71] have been reported in patients with HIV, but it is unclear whether these are related to HIV infection. Similarly, there are rare cases of T-lymphoblastic lymphoma/leukemia in patients with HIV.[72]

Mature T/NK-Cell Lymphoma

T-cell/natural killer (NK)–cell lymphomas are relatively uncommon, but the incidence appears to be increasing in HIV-infected individuals.[73-76] T-cell lymphomas tend to involve the skin and other extranodal sites. Morphologically they resemble peripheral T-cell lymphomas in the general population, with diffuse infiltration by a spectrum of small and large T cells with irregular nuclei and clear cytoplasm. In most tumors, large cells predominate (Fig. 56-11A). Peripheral T-cell lymphomas associated with HIV may have a cytotoxic phenotype.[75] In the skin, T-cell lymphomas characteristically form one or more tumor masses in the dermis, without epidermotropism. The lymphomatous infiltrates may demonstrate angiotropism and may be associated with necrosis.

Mycosis fungoides can occur in the setting of HIV,[74] and it may be difficult to diagnose because it must be differentiated from other forms of lymphocytic interface dermatitis commonly associated with HIV. Cases of mycosis fungoides have a characteristic appearance, with convoluted or cerebriform Sézary-type cells infiltrating the epidermis and forming Pautrier's microabscesses. Patients with advanced HIV infection and CD4 depletion may have a cutaneous eruption characterized by a dense infiltrate of mycosis-like cells that are CD8$^+$.[77] These cells may also infiltrate lymph nodes and bone marrow, and the prognosis is poor.[74]

Anaplastic large cell lymphoma, including expression of anaplastic lymphoma kinase (ALK) protein, may occur in AIDS patients; it usually presents in extranodal sites, and the histology may mimic that of carcinoma (see Fig. 56-11B and C). Cases of neutrophil-rich anaplastic large cell lymphoma have also been described.[78] There is one report of nasal-type NK/T-cell lymphoma, EBV$^+$, in a patient with AIDS.[79]

Immunophenotype and genetic features are similar to those of T-cell lymphomas in nonimmunocompromised persons. Many large T/NK-cell lymphomas in the skin of HIV patients express CD30 but are negative for ALK protein. In one study, monoclonally integrated HIV-1 was demonstrated within the T-cell lymphoma cell genome.[80]

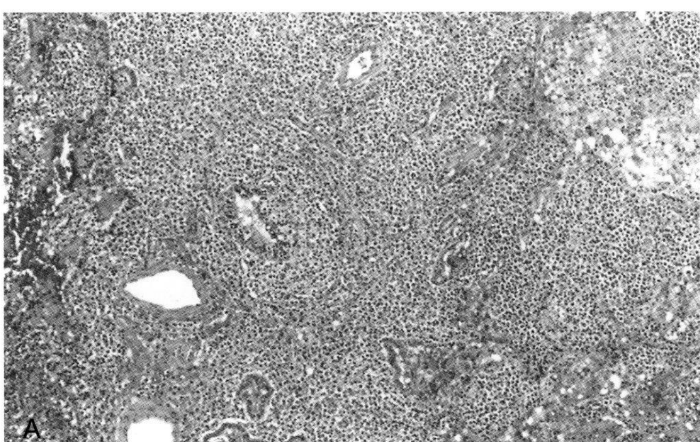

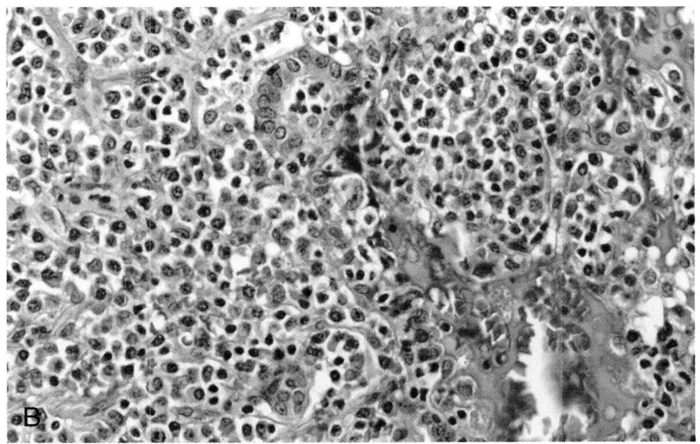

Figure 56-10. Marginal zone lymphoma in HIV infection. A (low magnification) and **B** (high magnification), Extranodal marginal zone (MALT) lymphoma in a child with HIV infiltration of a bronchiole forming a lymphoepithelial lesion.

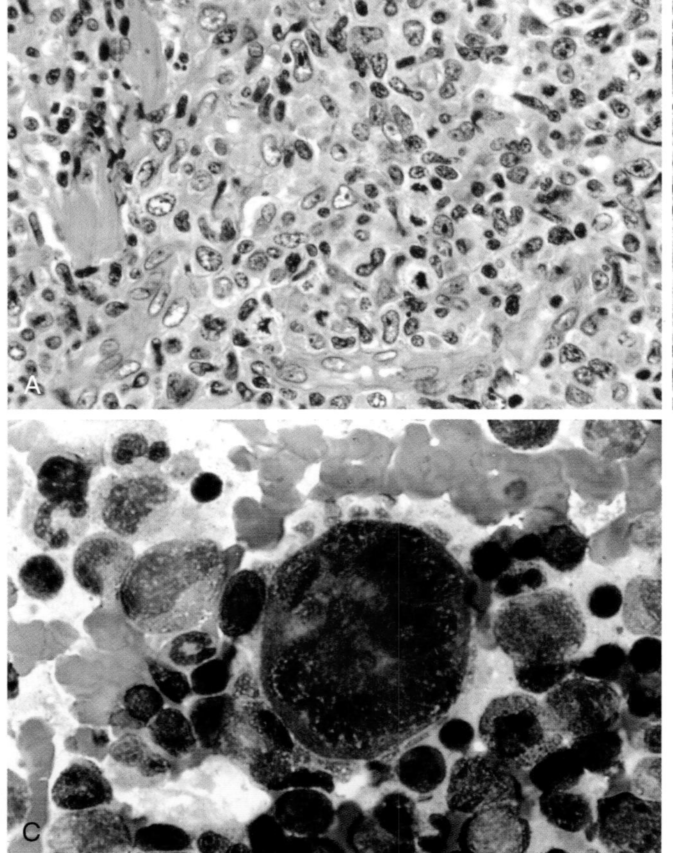
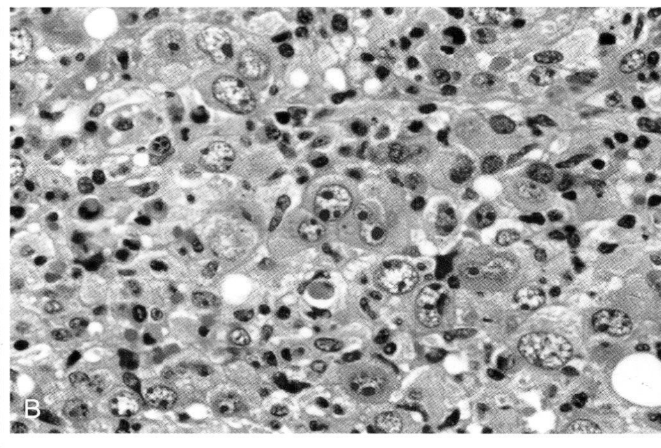

Figure 56-11. **AIDS-related peripheral T-cell lymphoma. A**, Peripheral T-cell lymphoma in a patient presenting with a skin mass. The dermal collagen is infiltrated by mainly large pleomorphic T cells. **B** and **C**, Anaplastic large cell lymphoma (anaplastic lymphoma kinase negative) involving the nasal sinus (**B**) and bone marrow (**C**) of an AIDS patient. The bizarre appearance and cytoplasmic nature of the cells can cause confusion with carcinoma (**C**, Giemsa stain).

Classical Hodgkin's Lymphoma

Clinical Features. Although not considered an AIDS-defining cancer by the CDC, an excess incidence of classical Hodgkin's lymphoma (CHL) has been found in HIV-infected homosexual men, and recent epidemiologic studies indicate a significantly increased risk of Hodgkin's lymphoma in patients with AIDS.[69] Paradoxically, the incidence of CHL has increased in the era of HAART for patients with HIV.[81]

Hodgkin's lymphoma is the most common type of non–AIDS-defining tumor that occurs in the HIV$^+$ population.[82] The mean interval between the diagnosis of HIV and the diagnosis of Hodgkin's lymphoma is about 5 years.[83] Development of CHL in a patient at risk for AIDS is a potent predictor of HIV positivity.[84] HIV-associated CHL and NHL occur in patients of similar age and gender with similar HIV risk factors, degree of immunodeficiency, and incidence of previous AIDS.[85] CD4$^+$ cell counts are relatively high at presentation compared with those in non-Hodgkin's lymphomas. The clinical presentation of HIV-associated CHL is atypical, and the disease is more aggressive than in HIV$^-$ patients. About 11% of HIV$^+$ patients with Hodgkin's lymphoma have mediastinal involvement, and more than 80% present in stage III or IV with B symptoms.[85] The bone marrow is involved at presentation in about 50% of patients and may be the only site involved.[86] Patients may respond to conventional CHL chemotherapy but are at risk for opportunistic infections and other complications of AIDS. The overall 5-year survival in one series was estimated at 24%.[85]

Pathogenesis. The pathogenesis of CHL in the HIV$^+$ population may be related to EBV infection because there is increased expression of EBV DNA in HIV$^+$ patients with CHL compared with the HIV$^-$ population.[80,87-90] Composite Hodgkin's and non-Hodgkin's lymphoma has been reported in AIDS patients, in which both neoplasms express the EBV genome.[91] Moreover, the same EBV$^+$ clone has been identified in multiple locations and at different times in the same patient, supporting a causal role for EBV in the pathogenesis of CHL.[92] CHL in HIV-infected patients is associated with morphologic features of aggressiveness, higher frequency of neoplastic cells, and constant LMP-1 expression.[93] Since HAART was introduced, the incidence of CHL has increased in patients with HIV, and this likely relates to improvements in CD4$^+$ cell counts. One explanation for this phenomenon is that background CD4$^+$ cells are required for the pathogenesis of CHL (particularly nodular sclerosis CHL), so patients with advanced immunosuppression do not develop CHL.[81,94]

Morphology. Although the full spectrum of CHL is seen, including nodular sclerosis, the more aggressive subtypes (mixed cellularity and lymphocyte depletion) are more common (Fig. 56-12A). Neoplastic cell–rich cases with increased Reed-Sternberg cells are frequent.

Immunophenotype. In contrast to the general population, HIV$^+$ patients with CHL often exhibit a depletion of CD4$^+$ cells and a predominance of CD8$^+$ T cells in the background proliferation. Reed-Sternberg cells consistently express EBV anti-

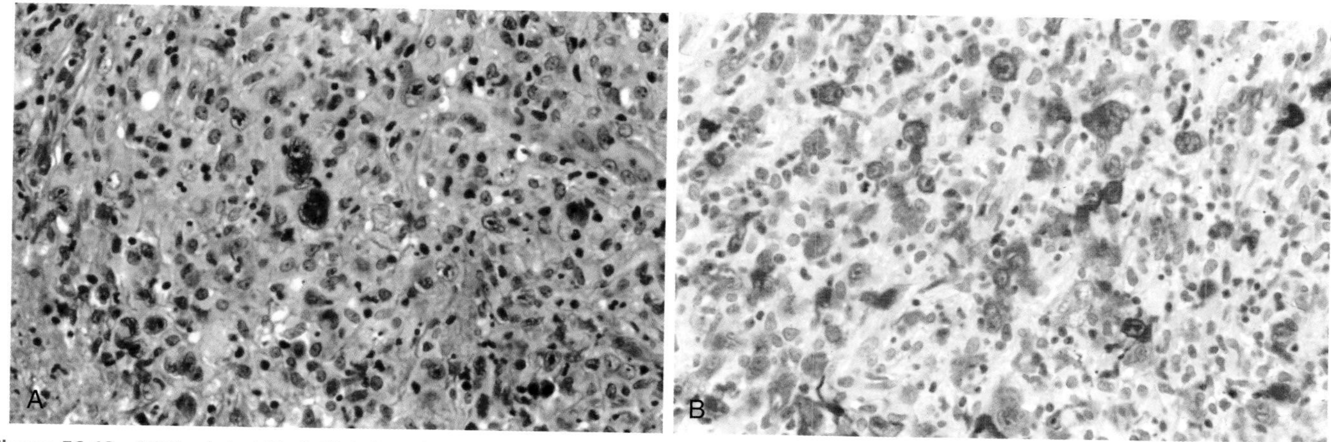

Figure 56-12. AIDS-related Hodgkin's lymphoma. A, Pleomorphic Reed-Sternberg cells are seen in a mixed inflammatory background. **B,** Numerous Reed-Sternberg cells stain for Epstein-Barr virus latent membrane protein-1.

gens, including LMP-1 (see Fig. 56-12B).[93] Reed-Sternberg cells in HIV-related Hodgkin's lymphoma have the phenotype of post–germinal center B cells.[95] Although the Reed-Sternberg cells express CD40 and EBV, they are not surrounded by CD40 ligand–positive reactive T cells, as in the general population with Hodgkin's lymphoma.[95]

Lymphomas Occurring Specifically in HIV Infection and Other Immune-Deficient States

Primary Effusion Lymphoma

Definition. PEL is a distinct clinicopathologic entity defined in the WHO classification as a neoplasm of large B cells usually presenting as a malignant effusion involving the pleural, peritoneal, or pericardial cavities, without a detectable tumor mass.[96] PEL is universally associated with KS-associated HHV8.

Epidemiology. Most cases of PEL occur in HIV$^+$ homosexual or bisexual men, but it can also occur in other immunodeficiency settings and in females.[97,98] Infection with HHV8 has been documented following bone marrow transplantation,[99] and cases of PEL have been reported following solid organ allografts.[100] PEL also occurs in elderly patients, mostly in areas with a high prevalence of HHV8, such as the Mediterranean, but not in Africa.

Pathogenesis. HHV8 was first identified in KS lesions by representational sequence analysis, which identified two DNA sequences (KS330 Bam and KS631 Bam) unique to HHV8.[101] The association between HHV8 and PEL was first demonstrated by molecular genetic techniques used to screen a large group of HIV-related lymphomas.[102] HHV8 sequences are present in much greater copy numbers in PEL compared with KS. Viral particles consisting of 100- to 115-nm capsids with central cores can be readily identified within the nucleus and cytoplasm of the neoplastic cells with electron microscopy (Fig. 56-13A).[103-105] Virus can also be demonstrated by immunohistochemistry in fixed tissue sections using an antibody to LANA (ORF-73) or other viral antigens (see Fig. 56-13B).

The risk group for HIV-related PEL is similar to that for KS, and KS lesions can be identified in approximately one third of patients with PEL.[106] Seropositivity rates for HHV8 are far higher than the incidence of HHV8-related disorders (including PEL), indicating that other factors, including immunosuppression, are involved in the pathogenesis.[107] PELs occurring in the setting of HIV are invariably associated with EBV, which is usually monoclonal, but EBV has restricted gene expression and is not required for pathogenesis.[106,108-110]

Clinical Features. HIV-related PELs tend to occur in older patients (mostly in the fourth decade of life) and at a somewhat later stage of the disease than BL. Patients are usually severely immunosuppressed (T cell counts $<100/mm^3$), and most have prior manifestations of AIDS, including opportunistic infections. Patients present with lymphomatous effusions (pleural, pericardial, or ascitic), without a contiguous tumor mass.[31,97,106,111-113] Although the majority of patients have disease localized to body cavities, there may be extension to adjacent organs such as the lung, soft tissues, regional nodes, and bone marrow, either at presentation or with advanced disease. The prognosis is poor, and the majority of patients die within 1 year of diagnosis. Improved survival has been reported with chemotherapy and immune reconstitution, as well as interferon-α in combination with azidothymidine.[114]

Morphology. Neoplastic cells in PEL have similarities with both B-cell immunoblastic lymphoma and anaplastic large cell lymphoma, including large cells with polyploid and lobated nuclei, prominent nucleoli, and abundant amphophilic or plasmacytoid cytoplasm (see Fig. 56-13C to E). Occasional multinucleated Reed-Sternberg–like cells may be seen (see Fig. 56-13F). Cells in the associated solid tumor masses are similar to those in malignant effusions but may appear less anaplastic.

Immunophenotype. The immunophenotype of PEL is distinctive, with neoplastic cells expressing common leukocyte antigen (CD45) in the absence of most B-lineage antigens, including CD20, CD19, CD79a, and surface immunoglobulin (Table 56-2). The lack of B-cell antigen expression may reflect a preterminal stage of B-cell differentiation, as exemplified by the lack of expression of PAX5 and the expression of

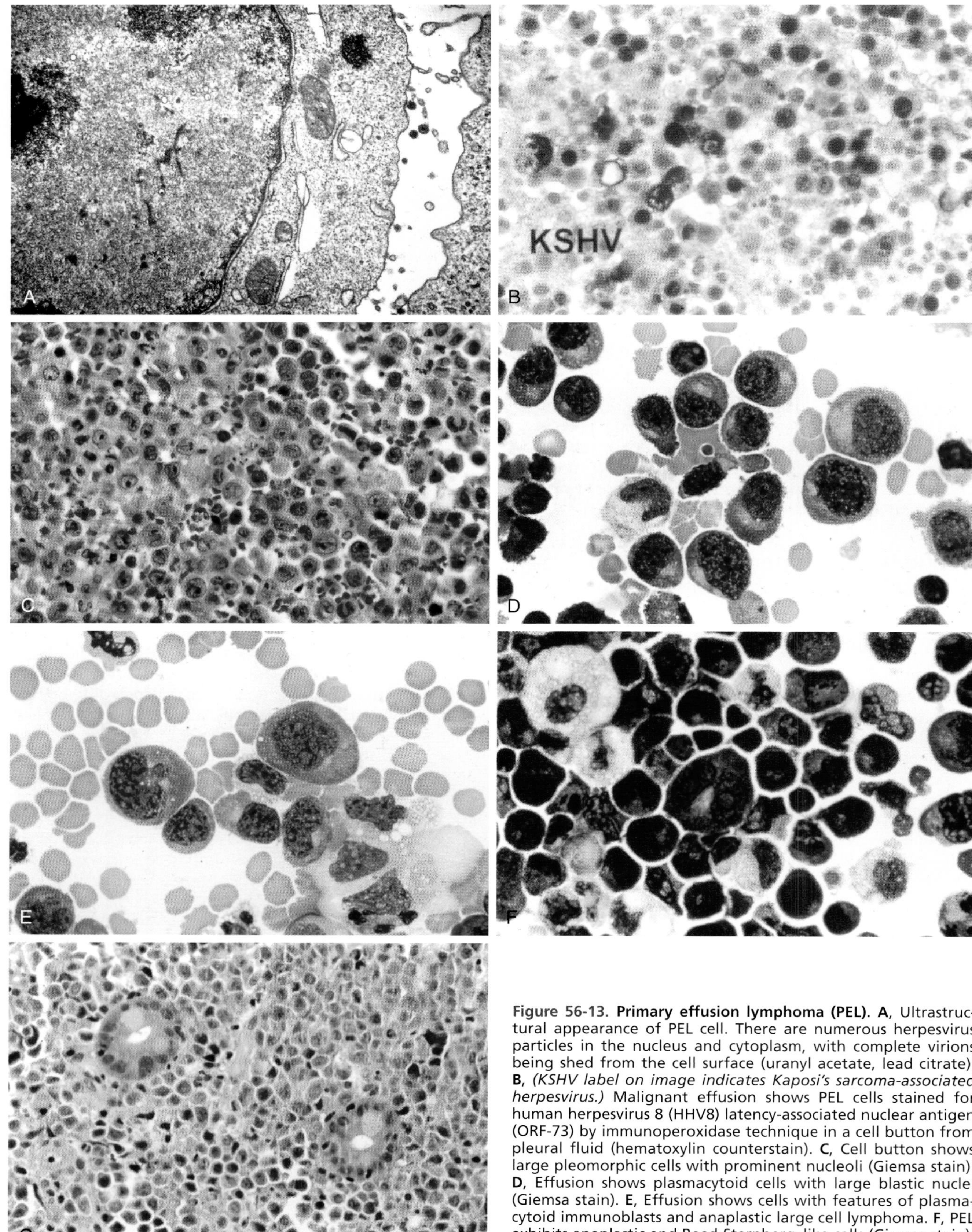

Figure 56-13. **Primary effusion lymphoma (PEL).** **A**, Ultrastructural appearance of PEL cell. There are numerous herpesvirus particles in the nucleus and cytoplasm, with complete virions being shed from the cell surface (uranyl acetate, lead citrate). **B**, *(KSHV label on image indicates Kaposi's sarcoma-associated herpesvirus.)* Malignant effusion shows PEL cells stained for human herpesvirus 8 (HHV8) latency-associated nuclear antigen (ORF-73) by immunoperoxidase technique in a cell button from pleural fluid (hematoxylin counterstain). **C**, Cell button shows large pleomorphic cells with prominent nucleoli (Giemsa stain). **D**, Effusion shows plasmacytoid cells with large blastic nuclei (Giemsa stain). **E**, Effusion shows cells with features of plasmacytoid immunoblasts and anaplastic large cell lymphoma. **F**, PEL exhibits anaplastic and Reed-Sternberg–like cells (Giemsa stain). **G**, HHV8^{+} solid lymphoma of the bowel.

Table 56-2 **Immunophenotype of Primary Effusion Lymphoma**

Antigen	Expression
TdT (precursor stages of T- and B-cell differentiation)	–
CD45 (leukocyte common antigen)	+ (95% cases)
B-cell antigens (CD19, CD20, CD22)	–
PAX5	–
Immunoglobulins	– (80% cases)
T-cell antigens (CD2, CD3, CD5, CD7)	–/+*
Reed-Sternberg cell–associated antigen (CD15)	–
Activation antigens (EMA, CD30, CD38, CD138, CD77)	+

*Rare cases express T- and B-cell antigens.
EMA, epithelial membrane antigen; TdT, terminal deoxynucleotidyl transferase.

activation and plasma cell–related markers. A variety of activation and nonlineage-associated antigens may be found, including CD30, CD38, CD138 (syndecan-1), and epithelial membrane antigen (EMA).[115] Cases of HHV8⁺ lymphoma have been identified with aberrant expression of T-cell antigens, including CD3, CD2, CD5, and CD7.[105,116] Cases of T-cell PEL, with a T-cell phenotype and genotype, are extremely rare. Because of the aberrant antigen expression, PELs may be difficult to phenotype, and nuclear staining for HHV8-associated LANA (ORF-73) may be invaluable in making the diagnosis.

Genetics. Immunoglobulin heavy-chain genes are rearranged, and occasional cases have rearrangements of both immunoglobulin and T-cell receptor genes.[105] There is no involvement of *MYC* or *BCL6* gene rearrangements or *RAS* oncogene or *TP53* tumor suppressor gene mutations.[106] Cytogenetic studies reveal multiple chromosomal abnormalities (most commonly gains in chromosomes 12 and X),[117] suggesting that secondary genetic events may contribute to neoplastic transformation. The HHV8 genome contains potential oncogenes, including a viral cyclin homologue, viral IL-6, and a gene homologous to the cellular G protein–coupled receptor family of proteins.[118] EBV genomes, but not latency-associated antigens, are detected in the majority of cases in HIV⁺ patients. The cells are positive for EBER but negative for latent membrane proteins. Rare cases have been reported with both a T-cell phenotype and gene rearrangement, and these appear to be cases of T-cell PEL.[119] Gene expression profiling indicates that PELs have features of both plasma cells and EBV transformed cell lines.[120]

Differential Diagnosis. Lymphomas presenting as effusions in the absence of a tumor mass are unusual, but not all are associated with HHV8.[121] Pyothorax-associated lymphomas occur in the pleural cavity following long-standing inflammation in mine workers, artificial pneumothorax, or tuberculous pleuritis.[122,123] There is no association with HHV8, but like PEL, they consist of B cells with plasmacytoid differentiation and are associated with EBV.[124]

Other high-grade lymphomas, including BL and atypical BL, may involve body cavities in patients with HIV, but these are morphologically and immunophenotypically distinctive, have the c-*MYC* gene rearrangement, and are not associated with HHV8. To make the diagnosis of PEL, a combination of clinical, morphologic, and phenotypic studies is required, and the association with HHV8 should be confirmed with polymerase chain reaction or by immunohistochemical staining for HHV8.

Plasmablastic lymphomas may arise in patients with HHV8 and multicentric Castleman's disease and usually involve the spleen or lymph nodes. They are negative for EBV, and unlike PEL, they often express CD20 and cytoplasmic immunoglobulin, which is always IgMλ restricted.

Rare cases of HHV8⁻ effusion-based lymphomas similar to PEL have been described in patients with liver disease.[125-127]

Extracavitary Human Herpesvirus 8–Positive Lymphoma

HHV8⁺ lymphomas with a morphology and immunophenotype similar to those of PEL can present as solid tumor masses in the absence of an effusion; they have been called *extracavitary PEL*[115] or *solid immunoblastic/plasmablastic lymphoma*.[128] These may occur in the gastrointestinal tract and other extranodal sites, including the lung, CNS, and skin, as well as in lymph nodes (see Fig. 56-13G).[129] Solid lymphomas may express B-cell antigens or immunoglobulin in up to 25% of cases (more often than the neoplastic cells in PEL).[115] HIV⁺ patients who develop HHV8⁺ solid lymphomas may be less immunosuppressed and have a better survival than those who develop PEL.[115,129]

The solid lymphomas may have an anaplastic or immunoblastic-plasmacytoid appearance, similar to that of the malignant cells in PEL; they may also resemble anaplastic large cell lymphoma[130] or plasmablastic lymphoma.[129] As with PEL, the lack of B-cell antigens may relate to the preterminal stage of B-cell differentiation, as exemplified by the lack of expression of PAX5.[115] There are no abnormalities in c-*MYC*, *BCL2*, *BCL1*, or *BCL6*, and the solid lymphomas are positive for EBV. Unlike plasmablastic lymphomas of the usual type (see later), they contain both EBV and HHV8.

Plasmablastic Lymphoma

Definition and Clinical Features. Plasmablastic lymphoma is an aggressive B-cell lymphoma first described in the oral cavity of HIV⁺ patients.[131] Since then it has become apparent that large cell lymphomas with plasmablastic features, including a CD20⁻, CD138⁺ phenotype, are clinically heterogeneous and may be seen in both HIV⁺ and HIV⁻ patients.[132] Although there is a predilection for the oropharyngeal region in patients with HIV, plasmablastic lymphomas can occur at other sites, including the sinus, gastrointestinal tract, soft tissue, lung, bone, and even skin.[129,133,134] These cases must be differentiated from HHV8⁺ plasmablastic lymphomas associated with multicentric Castleman's disease and solid PEL, as discussed previously.

Morphology. Plasmablastic lymphomas vary in morphology from typical plasmablastic to immunoblastic cells.[132] The cells characteristically have large blastic nuclei, prominent central nucleoli, and amphophilic cytoplasm (Fig. 56-14). Mature plasma cells are few or absent.

Immunophenotype. Despite their resemblance to DLBCL, plasmablastic lymphomas lack B-cell antigens, including CD20, PAX5, CD45, and CD10, and they have a plasma cell signature, staining for MUM-1/IRF4, CD38, CD138, EMA, and cytoplasmic immunoglobulin (Table 56-3). Some cases

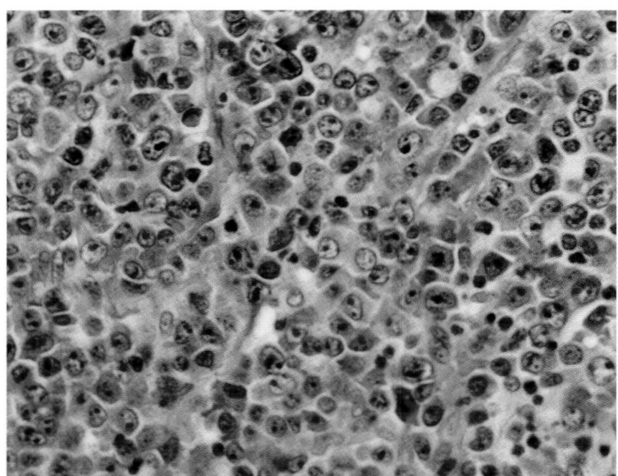

Figure 56-14. Plasmablastic lymphoma from the jaw. Note the large lymphoid cells with one or more nucleoli and plasmacytoid cytoplasm.

Table 56-3 Immunophenotype of Plasmablastic Lymphoma

Antigen	Expression
CD45	– to –/+
CD20	– to –/+
CD79a	– to +
Surface immunoglobulin	–/+
J-chain	+
Cytoplasmic immunoglobulin	+
PAX5	–
CD138	+
MUM-1 (IRF4)	+
BCL6	–/+
EBV EBER	+
EBV LMP-1	+/–
EBNA2	–
HHV8	–

EBER, EBV-encoded small RNA; EBNA, EBV nuclear antigen; EBV, Epstein-Barr virus; HHV8, human herpesvirus 8; LMP, latent membrane protein.

are positive for CD79a. BCL6 expression is negative to weak. Although most are EBER$^+$ and HHV8$^-$, they are negative for EBNA-2 and variably positive for EBV LMP-1.[135] Table 56-4 summarizes the immunohistochemical features helpful in the differential diagnosis of lymphomas that are similar to plasmablastic lymphoma.

Genetics. The immunoglobulin genes are clonally rearranged. Most cases are positive for EBER and negative for HHV8, although HHV8$^+$ cases have been described.[136]

Polymorphic B-Cell Lymphoma

Definition. Lymphoid proliferations following organ transplantation (posttransplant lymphoproliferative disorders [PTLDs]) include polymorphic B-cell proliferations related to EBV infection, which may be either polyclonal or monoclonal. Although rare, similar proliferations occur in the setting of HIV and have been termed *AIDS-related polymorphic lymphoproliferative disorders*.[57,137]

Clinical Features. These proliferations affect men, women, and children,[138] and the incidence does not correlate with the means of acquiring the viral infection. They may involve lymph nodes or extranodal sites, including the lungs, salivary glands, and skin.

Morphology. The histologic appearance mimics the polymorphic spectrum displayed by PTLDs, with a diffuse proliferation of small lymphocytes, plasma cells, histiocytes, and variable numbers of immunoblasts (Fig. 56-15). Cytologic atypia and necrosis are variable.

Immunophenotype. The proliferations comprise mainly CD20$^+$ B cells admixed with smaller populations of T cells. In most cases kappa or lambda light-chain restriction can be demonstrated.

Genetics. Monoclonality, as evidenced by gene rearrangement studies, can be demonstrated in about 80% of cases.[57] The rearranged bands are mostly faint, however, and may be superimposed on a polyclonal background. EBV sequences can be demonstrated in about 60% of cases, and the cases studied have been type A, analogous to the transplant population.[57]

Prognosis and Predictive Factors

The presence of an AIDS diagnosis before the diagnosis of lymphoma and a low CD4$^+$ cell count (<100/mm^3) correlate

Table 56-4 Differential Diagnosis of AIDS-Related Lymphomas with Overlapping Morphology*

	DLBCL—Centro-blastic	DLBCL—Immunoblastic	Plasmablastic Lymphoma	PEL	Burkitt's Lymphoma
Cell size	Large	Large	Large	Large	Intermediate
CD20	+	+/–	–/+	–	+
Leukocyte common antigen	+	+/–	–	+/–	+
Plasma cell antigens, including CD138	–	–/+	+	+	–
BCL6	+	–	–/+	–	+
EBV	–	+/–	+	+	–/+
HHV8	–	–	–	+	–
CD30	–	–/+	–/+	+/–	–

*Immunohistochemical findings refer to the most common patterns. In this group of neoplasms, aberrant phenotypic patterns are commonly observed.
DLBCL, diffuse large B-cell lymphoma; EBV, Epstein-Barr virus; HHV8, human herpesvirus 8; PEL, primary effusion lymphoma.

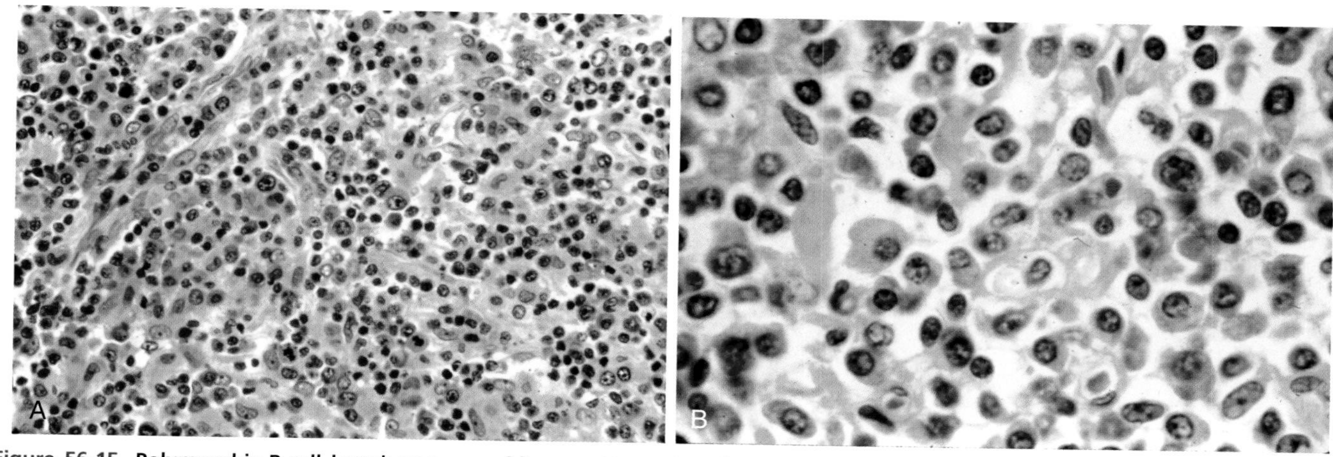

Figure 56-15. Polymorphic B-cell lymphoma resembling posttransplant lymphoproliferative disorder (PTLD). A, There is a mixture of small lymphocytes, plasma cells, and immunoblasts, resembling polymorphic PTLD. **B,** Focally, there are sheets of plasma cells.

with poor survival, as do advanced-stage disease and extensive bone marrow involvement. The degree of immunodeficiency correlates with an increasing International Prognostic Index score, suggesting that immunodeficiency may be an important factor in the aggressive clinical presentation of lymphoma.[139] Survival rates are lower in patients with DLBCL than BL, possibly because of a greater degree of immunodeficiency in the former group.[85] Survival rates in patients with AIDS-related Hodgkin's and non-Hodgkin's lymphomas appear to be similar, with less than 25% 5-year survival overall.[85] In addition to chemotherapy and radiation therapy, improved results may be obtained with antiretroviral therapy and hematopoietic growth factor support, including granulocyte-macrophage colony-stimulating factor and erythropoietin. Autologous stem cell transplantation has also been used successfully in patients on antiretroviral therapy.[140] Survival of patients has improved in the era of HAART, increasing in one series from 6 to 20 months.[28] An immunologic response to HAART (development of a higher $CD4^+$ cell count), receipt of a higher relative dose of chemotherapeutic agents, and attainment of complete remission are associated with longer survival.[27,141] Clinical outcomes for patients with DLBCL are now approaching those of patients with de novo lymphoma.[142]

Pearls and Pitfalls

Benign Lymphoid Proliferations

- Most HIV-related lymphoid hyperplasias are not specific but have characteristic features that suggest an immunodeficiency-related condition and infection with HIV.
- Lymphoid hyperplasias are commonly associated with HIV, may have atypical histologic features, and must be differentiated from neoplastic conditions. Indications for biopsy include a suspected treatable infection or neoplasm.
- Plasmacytic infiltrates are often prominent and should not be confused with the plasma cell variant of Castleman's disease or plasma cell dyscrasias.
- HHV8 LANA staining is useful for ruling out HHV8-related disease.

Infectious Conditions

- A high index of suspicion is required to rule out specific infections because HIV patients may not mount the characteristic immune reaction to infectious organisms.
- The presence of granulomas, irrespective of necrosis, indicates the need for special stains for organisms.
- Multiple infections are common.
- The presence of spindled macrophages is an indication of mycobacterial infection (*Mycobacterium avium-intracellulare*) and requires acid-fast stains for diagnosis.
- Parvovirus is a common cause of marrow failure, and characteristic cells with inclusions can be missed if they are not specifically looked for and confirmed with immunohistochemistry.

AIDS-Related Lymphomas

- Lymphomas often present at unusual sites and can mimic other neoplastic processes.
- Lymphomas may involve multiple sites and present with organ failure.
- Central nervous system lymphomas may have multiple infiltrates and mimic infections such as toxoplasmosis.
- Burkitt's lymphomas often present with marrow involvement and have atypical histologic features, particularly plasmacytoid morphology.
- Classical Hodgkin's lymphoma may have unusual clinical features (e.g., bone marrow involvement, advanced stage at presentation). Reed-Sternberg cells are invariably positive for EBV.
- Primary effusion lymphomas have overlapping cytologic features with carcinomas in body fluids. The HHV8 LANA stain is useful for the specific identification of effusion-based or solid $HHV8^+$ lymphomas.

References can be found on Expert Consult @ www.expertconsult.com

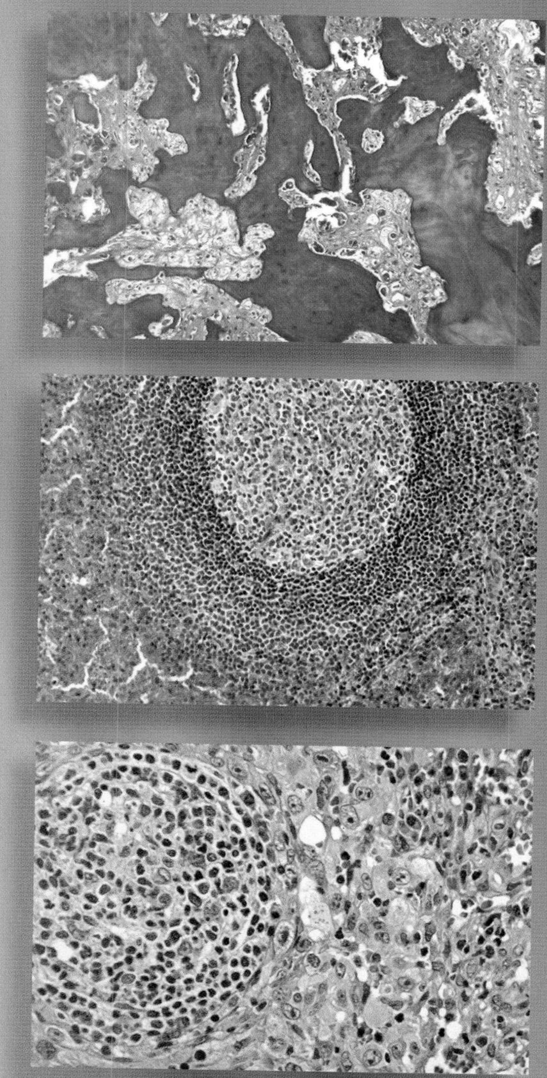

PART VII

Site-Specific Issues in the Diagnosis of Lymphoma and Leukemia

Chapter 57

Bone Marrow Evaluation for Lymphoma

Beverly P. Nelson and LoAnn C. Peterson

CHAPTER OUTLINE

One of the most common indications for bone marrow biopsy is to detect involvement of the bone marrow by malignant lymphoma. Bone marrow biopsies are routinely performed after patients have been diagnosed with lymphoma to determine the stage and extent of disease,[1,2] and they are frequently performed during the course of the disease to evaluate response to therapy or possible progression. Occasionally an initial diagnosis of lymphoma is made from a bone marrow specimen[3]; in some of these cases, lymphoma may not have been suspected clinically.

Even though pathologists commonly evaluate bone marrow biopsies for lymphoma, this task is often challenging. For example, benign lymphoid aggregates are frequently encountered in trephine biopsies, especially in older patients, and they can be exceedingly difficult to distinguish from malignant lymphoma, even with the help of ancillary techniques.[4,5] In patients with a prior diagnosis of lymphoma, assessment is complicated by the fact that lymphoma in the bone marrow may differ from the original extramedullary lesion; that is, the bone marrow frequently exhibits a more indolent or low-grade morphology.[6,7] When a lymphoid lesion is determined to be malignant, the lymphoma must be classified. Although this is usually straightforward in patients already diagnosed with lymphoma, determining the lymphoma subtype in a patient without a prior diagnosis may be difficult and requires not only knowledge of the diagnostic features of the various types of lymphoma but also appropriate use of ancillary techniques.

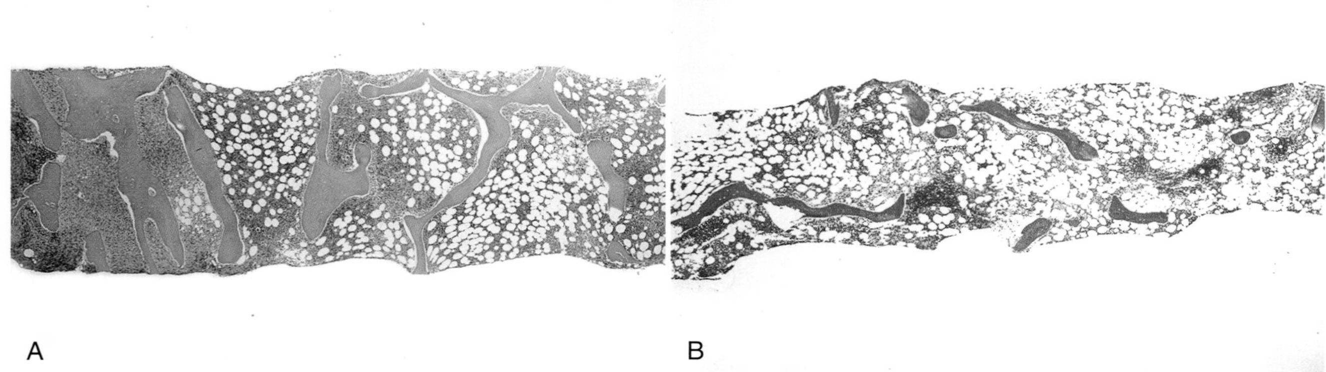

Figure 57-1. Bilateral bone marrow trephine biopsy sections obtained for staging purposes from a patient with diffuse large B-cell lymphoma. A, Only the left trephine biopsy specimen is involved by lymphoma. The lymphomatous infiltrate is focal but exhibits a diffuse growth pattern. **B,** The right trephine biopsy specimen is uninvolved.

The trephine biopsy is usually the most informative when evaluating the bone marrow for lymphoma. However, peripheral blood smears, aspirate smears, particle clot sections, and touch imprints also provide valuable complementary information and may be diagnostic in themselves. Therefore, all these preparations should be examined together and the findings correlated. Because adequate sampling of the bone marrow is important to ensure the detection of focal lymphomatous infiltrates, bilateral iliac crest trephine biopsies are recommended. The yield of lymphoma detection is significantly higher with bilateral versus unilateral posterior iliac crest trephine biopsies (Fig. 57-1).[8,9] Because the size of trephine biopsy specimens also correlates with the frequency with which lymphoma is identified, each biopsy should be at least 2 cm long.[10] In addition, sections obtained from multiple levels representative of each paraffin block should be examined.

Ancillary techniques, including immunophenotyping by flow cytometry, paraffin section immunohistochemistry, cytogenetic analysis, and molecular diagnostic tests, are becoming increasingly important in evaluating bone marrow specimens for lymphoma. The most effective technique varies with the clinical setting and morphologic findings. For instance, anaplastic large cell lymphoma can infiltrate the bone marrow as scattered single cells that may not be aspirated and are difficult to identify on hematoxylin-eosin (H&E)–stained sections. Immunohistochemical studies of the biopsy section for CD30 or anaplastic lymphoma kinase (ALK)-1 may be required to detect and distinguish these neoplastic cells from normal hematopoietic elements. Whenever ancillary techniques are employed, the resulting data should be correlated with one another and with the morphologic findings. It is also worth noting that although ancillary techniques are essential to adequately evaluate many bone marrow lymphoid lesions, knowledge of each technique, including its limitations, is required before it can be used as an effective diagnostic aid.

This chapter focuses on the distinction between benign lymphoid aggregates and lymphoma, including the role of morphology and ancillary techniques such as flow cytometry, immunohistochemistry, and molecular testing. Characteristic features of non-Hodgkin's and Hodgkin's lymphoma involving the bone marrow are discussed. Also addressed are issues pertinent to the evaluation of bone marrow biopsies when there is an established diagnosis of lymphoma and when a primary diagnosis of lymphoma is made based on the bone marrow biopsy. In addition, nonlymphoid lesions that may mimic lymphoma in the bone marrow are covered.

DISTINCTION BETWEEN BENIGN LYMPHOID INFILTRATES AND LYMPHOMA

Benign Lymphoid Aggregates

Benign lymphoid aggregates are common in older individuals, increase in frequency after age 50 years, and are of unknown clinical significance. They are often identified in bone marrow biopsies from patients with autoimmune disorders such as rheumatoid arthritis, systemic lupus erythematosus, autoimmune hemolytic anemia, and idiopathic thrombocytopenic purpura.[4,10] Patients with either chronic myeloproliferative neoplasms or myelodysplastic syndromes may also exhibit lymphoid aggregates in the bone marrow.[4,11]

The assessment of lymphoid infiltrates in the bone marrow is often based on histopathology alone; however, sometimes other studies such as immunohistochemistry, flow cytometric immunophenotyping, or molecular analysis are required to determine their biologic potential. Although these techniques are often informative, in some cases the nature of the lymphoid infiltrate remains unknown. The extent of testing to analyze a lymphoid infiltrate in the bone marrow depends on the clinical setting and the degree of suspicion for lymphoma. Table 57-1 summarizes the major features that aid in the distinction between benign lymphoid aggregates and non-Hodgkin's lymphoma. They are discussed in the following sections on morphology, immunohistochemistry, flow cytometry, and molecular genetics.

Morphology

Several morphologic features can be used to distinguish benign lymphoid aggregates from lymphomatous infiltrates.[4,5] Benign aggregates are usually single or few in number in the biopsy specimen. They are distributed randomly, away from

Table 57-1 Features That Distinguish Benign Lymphoid Aggregates from Non-Hodgkin's Lymphoma in Bone Marrow Biopsies

Benign	Malignant
Aggregates are few in number	Aggregates are variable in number and may be numerous
Random distribution of aggregates	Aggregates are frequently paratrabecular
Aggregates are usually round, well circumscribed	Aggregates are often irregularly shaped, with infiltration into adjacent marrow
Polymorphic cellular composition	Usually homogeneous cellular composition (except some peripheral T-cell lymphomas); atypical cytologic features may be present
Intrasinusoidal infiltrates absent (except in polyclonal B-cell lymphocytosis)	Intrasinusoidal infiltration may be present
Vascularity is often prominent	Vascularity is usually not prominent (except in peripheral T-cell lymphomas)
Germinal centers are occasionally present	Germinal centers are not present (except in splenic marginal zone lymphoma)
No lymphoma cells in smears or imprints	Lymphoma cells may be present in smears or imprints
Immunostains show a mixture of B and T cells (exceptions occur)	Immunostains that show a predominance of B cells, aberrant phenotype, or monoclonal plasma cells suggest B-cell lymphoma; an aberrant T-cell phenotype suggests T-cell lymphoma
No monoclonal B-cell population or T-cell abnormalities by flow cytometry	Immunoglobulin light-chain restriction or T-cell abnormalities by flow cytometry
No monoclonal B- or T-cell receptor gene rearrangement by molecular analysis	Monoclonal B- or T-cell receptor gene rearrangement by molecular analysis

the bony trabeculae, and are typically round and well circumscribed (Fig. 57-2). The lymphocytes within the aggregates are usually small and mature appearing, with round nuclei, condensed chromatin patterns, and absent or inconspicuous nucleoli. The aggregates are frequently polymorphic and may contain histiocytes and plasma cells. Often a vessel is visible within the aggregate. Germinal centers are rare, but when they are present, they usually indicate that the lymphoid aggregate is benign (Fig. 57-3); they are more common in lymphoid aggregates associated with autoimmune diseases. However, germinal centers are not specific for benign infiltrates. Rarely, non-Hodgkin's lymphoma, particularly splenic marginal zone lymphoma, may exhibit reactive germinal centers in the bone marrow in association with the lymphomatous infiltrate.[12]

Malignant infiltrates, in contrast to benign lymphoid aggregates, are frequently multiple, are often large, and may exhibit irregular infiltrative borders. Paratrabecular infiltrates that touch and grow along the surface of the bone and conform to the bony contour are malignant in the vast majority of cases.[4] The presence of distinct intrasinusoidal infiltrates is usually an indication of a neoplastic process. An exception is polyclonal B-cell lymphocytosis, in which intrasinusoidal infiltrates have been described.[13-17]

Cytologically, indolent lymphomas are difficult to distinguish from benign lymphoid lesions because they tend to be composed of small lymphocytes with condensed chromatin. More aggressive lymphomas, especially those with clearly abnormal morphologic features such as medium to large cell size, irregular nuclear outlines, partially condensed chromatin, prominent nucleoli, and abundant mitotic figures, are often easily distinguished from benign aggregates, even if the lymphomatous infiltrate is small. Malignant lymphomas generally exhibit a more homogeneous cellular composition than do benign lymphoid aggregates. However, it should be noted that a polymorphic cellular population also characterizes some lymphomas, most notably peripheral T-cell lymphoma and Hodgkin's lymphoma.[10,18] Importantly, the presence of atypical cells, frequent mitoses, and architectural features such as infiltrative borders should raise the suspicion of a malignant proliferation. The aspirate smear, touch imprint, or

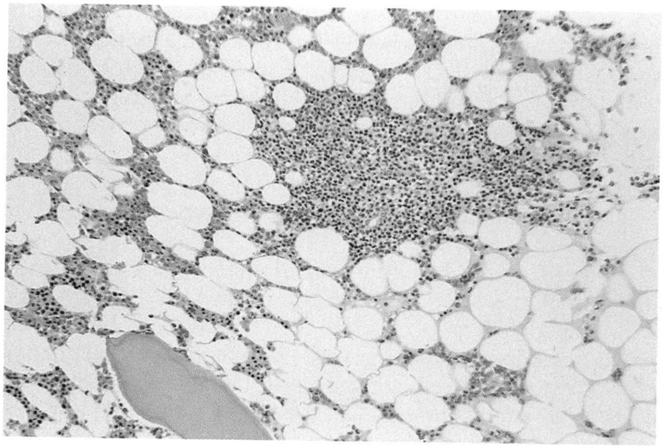

Figure 57-2. Benign lymphoid aggregate in a bone marrow trephine biopsy section. The single lymphoid aggregate is small, well circumscribed, and located between bony trabeculae. A small blood vessel is present in the lymphoid aggregate, which consists of predominantly small, mature-appearing lymphocytes.

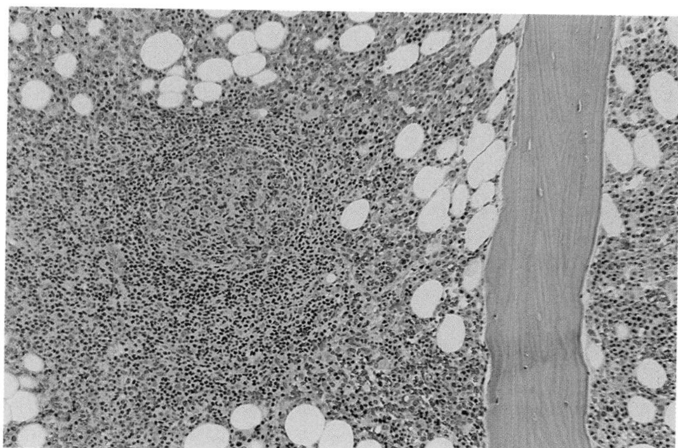

Figure 57-3. Benign lymphoid aggregate containing a reactive follicle. Note the discrete germinal center with an attenuated mantle zone within the lymphoid aggregate.

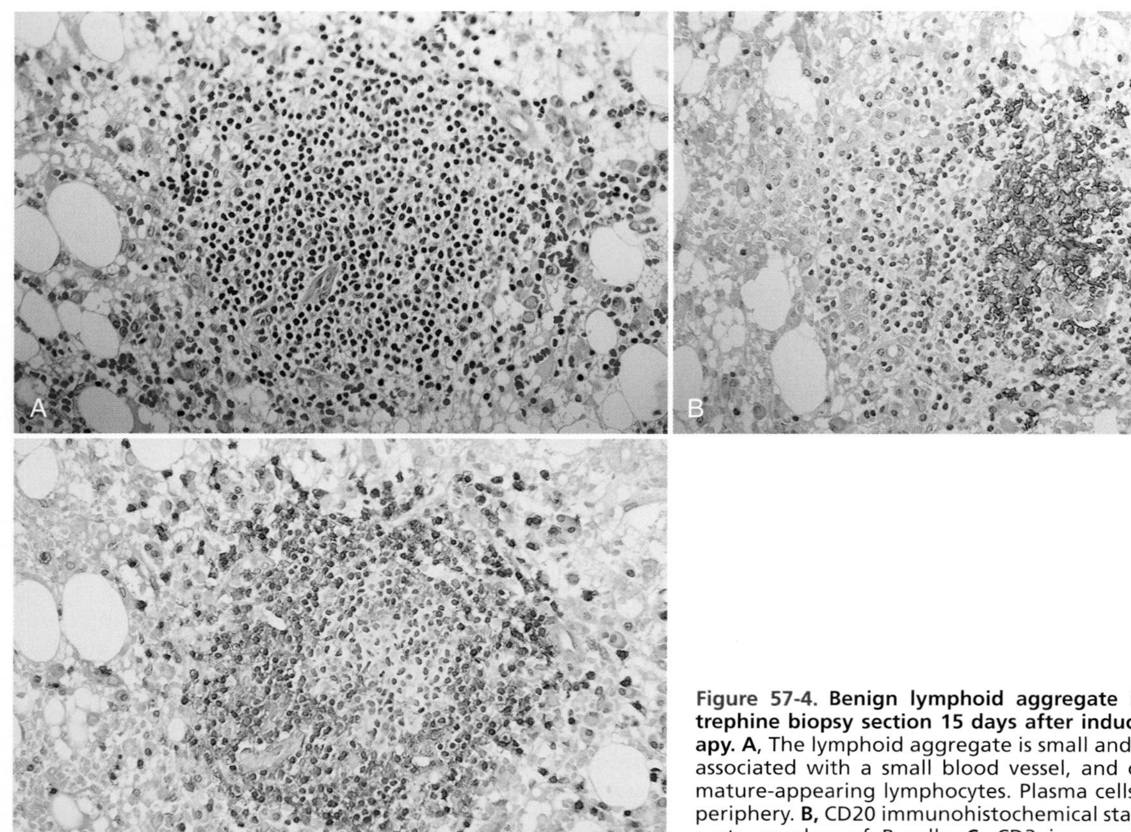

Figure 57-4. Benign lymphoid aggregate in a bone marrow trephine biopsy section 15 days after induction of chemotherapy. A, The lymphoid aggregate is small and well circumscribed, associated with a small blood vessel, and composed of small, mature-appearing lymphocytes. Plasma cells are present at the periphery. **B,** CD20 immunohistochemical stain illustrates a moderate number of B cells. **C,** CD3 immunohistochemical stain shows a moderate number of T cells.

peripheral blood film often contains lymphoma cells; their presence also helps confirm that a lymphoid lesion in bone marrow biopsy sections is malignant.

Immunohistochemistry

Despite the preceding guidelines, it is not always possible to distinguish between benign and malignant lymphoid infiltrates by morphology alone. In problematic cases, a panel of immunohistochemical stains performed on the bone marrow trephine biopsy or particle section can assist in this distinction. Immunhistochemical stains with B-cell–associated antibodies (CD20, CD79a, PAX5) and T-cell–associated antibodies (CD3) are often used to determine the proportions of B cells and T cells within the aggregates. Benign lymphoid aggregates usually have a mixture of B and T cells; frequently T cells predominate (Fig. 57-4). Lymphoid infiltrates composed of primarily B cells, especially if multiple, are often neoplastic (Fig. 57-5). However, these studies must be interpreted cautiously because a wide variety of reaction patterns can occur with both benign lymphoid aggregates and lymphoma. For instance, B-cell lymphomas may be accompanied by large numbers of reactive T lymphocytes. Therefore, a mixture of B cells and T cells or a predominance of T cells does not rule out a B-cell lymphoma.[19]

Immunohistochemical stains for BCL2 protein are reported to be negative or only weakly positive in the majority of benign lymphoid aggregates, whereas malignant infiltrates are usually moderately to intensely positive.[20] However, in our experience, the BCL2 stain is almost always positive in bone marrow lymphoid aggregates, and the determination of staining intensity is inconsistent between individual observers. Others have reported considerable overlap of BCL2 staining in benign and malignant lymphoid infiltrates in the bone marrow.[21,22] Small lymphocytic lymphoma, chronic lymphocytic leukemia, follicle center cell lymphoma, and mantle cell lymphoma are BCL2$^+$; normal T cells and normal mantle zone cells are positive as well. However, when germinal centers are present in the bone marrow, an immunostain for BCL2 is helpful in establishing whether the germinal centers are reactive or neoplastic. CD10 and BCL6 have also been evaluated to determine their utility in differentiating benign aggregates from follicular lymphoma involving the bone marrow. CD10 was more commonly positive in infiltrates of follicular lymphoma than in benign lesions, but the staining pattern for BCL6 was similar among the different types of lymphoid aggregates.[21]

Demonstrating an aberrant B-cell phenotype within a lymphoid infiltrate strongly supports a diagnosis of malignant lymphoma. CD5, a T-cell–associated antigen, can be used in paraffin sections to demonstrate an aberrant B-cell phenotype.[23] Another T-cell antigen, preferably CD3, should be assessed in parallel to establish the number of T cells present in the lymphoid infiltrate. If the B cells aberrantly express CD5, virtually all the lymphocytes in the aggregate will show positive staining with CD5, whereas if there is no aberrant expression of CD5, their staining pattern will parallel that of CD3.

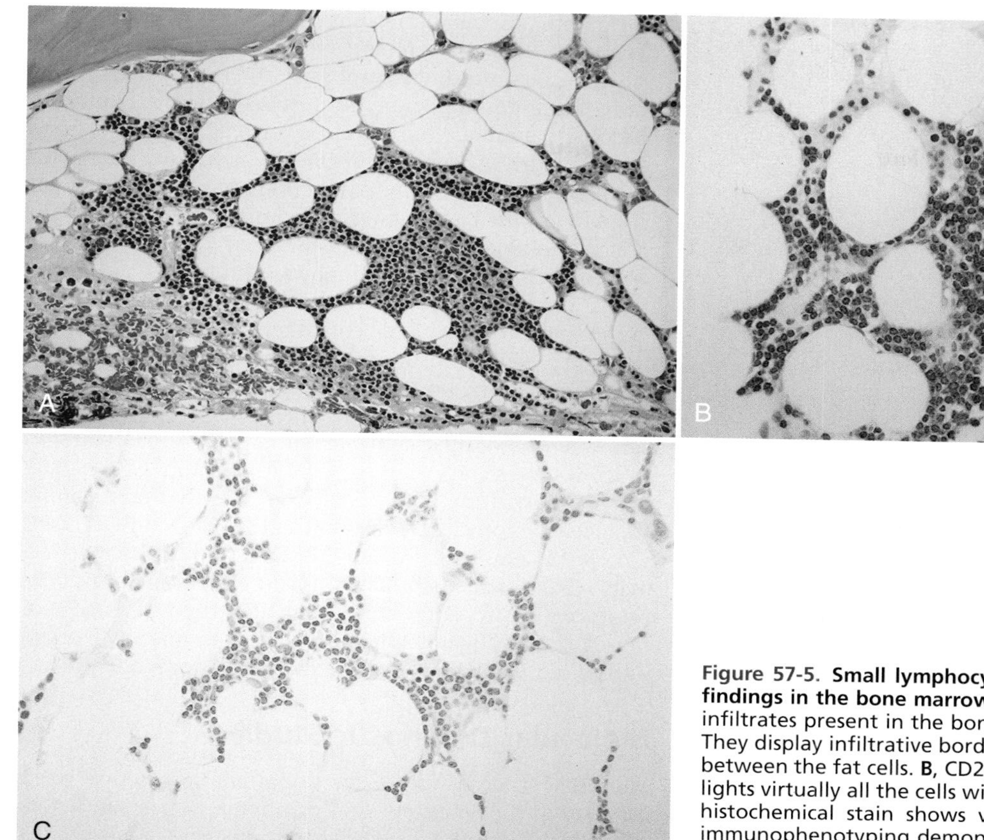

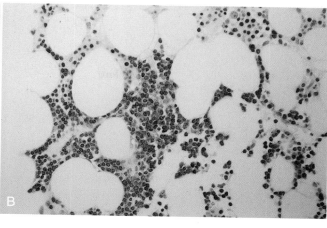

Figure 57-5. Small lymphocytic lymphoma (SLL) diagnosed by findings in the bone marrow. A, One of the multiple lymphoid infiltrates present in the bone marrow trephine biopsy section. They display infiltrative borders, with lymphocytes that migrate between the fat cells. **B,** CD20 immunohistochemical stain highlights virtually all the cells within the infiltrate. **C,** CD3 immunohistochemical stain shows very rare T cells. Flow cytometric immunophenotyping demonstrated monotypic B cells with the phenotype of SLL ($CD19^+$, dim $CD20^+$, $CD5^+$, $CD23^+$, $CD10^-$, $FMC7^-$).

Immunohistochemical or in situ hybridization studies for kappa and lambda immunoglobulin light chains are also valuable when the lymphoid lesion contains significant numbers of plasma cells; demonstration of cytoplasmic immunoglobulin light-chain restriction supports a malignant B-cell population. Detecting surface immunoglobulin in paraffin-embedded bone marrow sections is not consistently reliable for evaluating immunoglobulin light-chain restriction in many laboratories.

A T-cell infiltrate that exhibits absent or dim staining with one or more of the pan–T-cell antigens (CD2, CD3, CD5, CD7) displays an abnormal phenotype. The presence of an aberrant T-cell phenotype raises the possibility of a T-cell lymphoma. However, care should be taken when interpreting $CD7^-$ T cells in an infiltrate because small numbers of $CD7^-$ T cells may be found in reactive conditions.

Flow Cytometric Immunophenotyping

Immunophenotyping by flow cytometry performed on a fresh bone marrow aspirate or peripheral blood is helpful in distinguishing between reactive and malignant lymphoid infiltrates.[24-26] Excellent correlation exists between morphologic and immunophenotypic findings when bone marrow specimens are evaluated for B-cell lymphomas. Hanson and colleagues[25] reported flow cytometric immunophenotyping results of 175 patients with B-cell lymphomas who had staging bone marrow biopsies. A monoclonal lymphoid population was found in 83% of patients with morphologically positive bone marrow biopsies. No monoclonal population was identified in 96% of morphologically negative biopsies. A similar study that evaluated 39 B-cell non-Hodgkin's lymphomas found a 56% concordance rate between flow cytometric immunophenotyping and the morphology of bone marrow aspirate and trephine biopsy sections.[27] Because flow cytometry does not identify monoclonal lymphocytes in every patient with bone marrow involvement by lymphoma, this technique should always be used in conjunction with morphologic evaluation. Flow cytometry is most useful when bone marrow biopsy specimens contain morphologically equivocal lymphoid infiltrates; if flow cytometry demonstrates a monoclonal B-cell population, the lesions are likely malignant. Discrepancy between the trephine biopsy and the aspirate can occur because small, focal lesions may be missed during aspiration or bone marrow fibrosis prevents the aspiration of bone marrow cells. Thus, the demonstration of polyclonal B cells by flow cytometry does not ensure that the bone marrow is negative for lymphoma.

Flow cytometric immunophenotyping can be performed on a peripheral blood specimen when a bone marrow aspirate is not available, especially if the patient is known to have a lymphoma associated with a high incidence of peripheral blood involvement, such as follicular lymphoma, small lymphocytic lymphoma, mantle cell lymphoma, lymphoplasmacytic lymphoma, and splenic marginal zone lymphoma. Hanson and colleagues[25] identified monoclonal B cells in the peripheral blood in the majority of patients whose bone marrow biopsies showed involvement by these types of

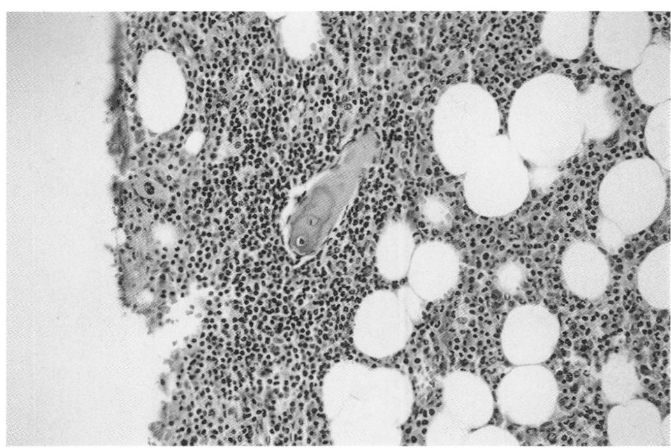

Figure 57-6. Mantle cell lymphoma demonstrated in the bone marrow trephine biopsy from a 37-year-old man with mantle cell lymphoma involving a lymph node. Deeper sections of the paraffin block were obtained because flow cytometric immunophenotyping of the bone marrow demonstrated monoclonal B cells, and the initial histologic sections were negative for lymphoma. The deeper section demonstrates small lymphoma cells that partially surround a bony trabecula and migrate between fat cells.

lymphomas. However, a negative result does not exclude the presence of lymphoma in the bone marrow.

Occasionally, flow cytometry documents a population of monoclonal B cells when no morphologic evidence of lymphoma is present. It is likely that many of these discrepancies are due to sampling. Whenever monoclonal B cells are identified without morphologic evidence of lymphoma, it is prudent to examine multiple histologic sections, even if the block must be cut through (Fig. 57-6); it may also be appropriate to perform immunohistochemical stains to ensure that an abnormal infiltrate is not missed. If lymphoma is not identified in the histologic sections, the report should note the presence of the monoclonal B cells identified by flow cytometry and the absence of morphologic evidence of lymphoma. Most therapeutic regimens are based on the morphologic findings in the bone marrow; thus, the clinical significance of monoclonal B cells identified only by flow cytometry is not clear. If the patient does not have an established diagnosis of lymphoma, another bone marrow biopsy or biopsy of any lesion suspicious for lymphoma can be considered and follow-up studies recommended.

It is also important to recognize that low levels of monoclonal B cells can be identified in individuals who are otherwise healthy and without clinical or morphologic evidence of lymphoma, most frequently in older individuals.[28,29] In most cases the monoclonal B cells represent a very small number of cells, usually less than 1% of the total cellular events analyzed.[28,29] Rawstron and associates[30] identified low levels of monoclonal B cells with a non–chronic lymphocytic leukemia phenotype in 1% of individuals with normal complete blood counts and no hematopoietic malignancy; in addition, 3.5% of subjects in the same study had low levels of monoclonal B cells with a chronic lymphocytic leukemia phenotype. The significance of these small populations of monoclonal B cells is unknown, and some authors have used the term *monoclonal B cells of undetermined significance* to emphasize this point. Although follow-up studies are warranted, most individuals who exhibit a small monoclonal population of B cells will not develop malignant lymphoma (see also Chapter 14).[28,29] Nevertheless, these findings emphasize the importance of correlating the immunophenotypic results with the clinical and pathologic findings. Furthermore, in patients with a history of lymphoma, it is important to compare any monoclonal population with the immunophenotypic profile of the prior lymphoma when evaluating the clinical significance of the monoclonal B cells.

Flow cytometric immunophenotyping also aids in the evaluation of bone marrow involvement by peripheral T-cell lymphomas. Crotty and coworkers[26] reported that flow cytometry has a sensitivity of 28.6% for identifying T-cell lymphomas in the bone marrow based on the detection of an abnormal phenotype, such as the absence of one or more pan–T-cell–associated antigens or an abnormal pattern of antigen expression, such as $CD4^+/CD8^+$ and $CD4^-/CD8^-$ T cells. Although the absence of CD7 was the most common abnormality noted, CD7 deletion can also be found in reactive T cells.[31] A more recent study reported a much higher sensitivity (92%) for identifying T-cell lymphomas with flow cytometry.[32] This latter study evaluated the abnormal intensity of T-cell antigen expression relative to normal T cells, as well as the parameters evaluated in the prior study.

Molecular Diagnostic Studies

Molecular analysis plays an important adjunctive role in evaluating bone marrow for lymphoma, especially in cases with focal lymphoid lesions that are suspicious but not diagnostic for lymphoma. Molecular diagnostic studies are usually performed on paraffin-embedded tissues using polymerase chain reaction (PCR), but fresh bone marrow aspirate or peripheral blood can also be used. Because formalin fixation is the least damaging to DNA, bone marrow processed in formalin is better suited for PCR analysis; however, in some studies B5-fixed bone marrow tissues have been analyzed successfully.[33,34]

The sensitivity of PCR for detecting bone marrow lymphoma depends on case selection, specimen type, and molecular technique used, including the number of primers used. Results obtained from gene rearrangement studies of bone marrow lymphoid aggregates correlate with the morphologic interpretations in the majority of cases. Coad and associates[35] tested 225 staging or posttherapy bone marrow aspirates from patients with B-cell lymphoma using consensus immunoglobulin heavy-chain gene (*IGH@*) and *IGH@/BCL2* gene PCR primers. In this study, 57% of bone marrow specimens positive for lymphoma by morphologic examination of the trephine biopsy showed monoclonally rearranged *IGH@* genes; this value was 25% for morphologically suspicious lesions, 5% for indeterminate lesions, and 11% for morphologically negative biopsies. DNA was also extracted from 11 B5-fixed, morphologically positive trephine core biopsy sections and analyzed by PCR in the Coad study; monoclonal bands were detected in 10 cases (91%), suggesting that similar analyses can be performed successfully on B5-fixed, paraffin-embedded trephine biopsy sections and on bone marrow aspirates. Using 83 bone marrow trephine biopsy sections obtained from 26 patients, Braunschweig and colleagues[36] were able to amplify DNA from nearly all cases (80 of 83; 96%) that were fixed in formaldehyde sublimate (73) or alcoholic Bouin (10);

a monoclonal B-cell population was detected in 63% (50 of 80), providing further evidence of the effectiveness of PCR analysis of paraffin-embedded bone marrow trephine biopsy sections. Interestingly, the bone marrow had a different monoclonal B-cell population than lymphoma at an extramedullary site in 4 of the 26 patients, and the different monoclonal *IGH@* population recurred in subsequent bone marrow specimens in 3 patients. Careful analysis, including sequencing, indicated that a different monoclonally rearranged *IGH@* gene appeared during tumor evolution in 3 patients, and that one human immunodeficiency virus (HIV)–positive patient had an oligoclonal B-cell lymphoma at the extramedullary site with one clone preferentially involving the bone marrow. Therefore, PCR results may be complex and may require a more detailed analysis, such as sequencing, for accurate interpretation. These reports and others show that PCR detects the majority of both T-cell and B-cell lymphomas and may be particularly useful in morphologically equivocal cases.[26] However, because a substantial number of false-negative PCR results occur, it is necessary to use molecular techniques in collaboration with morphology. Possible causes of false-negative findings include the following: (1) lymphoma cells may not be aspirated owing to reticulin fibrosis, (2) the lesion of interest may be absent from the paraffin block used for analysis, (3) the fixation technique may render the sample unsuitable for PCR analysis, (4) DNA quality in the specimen analyzed may be poor, and (5) nonbinding of the primers to rearranged genes may occur due to somatic DNA mutations in the primer binding regions.

The sensitivity of gene rearrangement studies is particularly high when focal lymphoid lesions are microdissected from the bone marrow and the cells of interest are analyzed, rather than analyzing the entire bone marrow section. In one study using microdissection technique and probes for *IGH@*, all lymphoid lesions that were categorized as benign based on their morphology had a polyclonal *IGH@* gene rearrangement pattern; all the lymphoid infiltrates classified as malignant based on their morphology had monoclonal *IGH@* gene rearrangement.[37] In addition, most cases (four of five) in which the lymphoid infiltrates were classified as suspicious for lymphoma also had a monoclonally rearranged *IGH@* gene. Although the sensitivity of microdissection is high, this technique is not routinely used for clinical samples.

Occasionally PCR demonstrates monoclonal lymphoid populations in the absence of morphologic evidence of lymphoma. Although this finding may represent lymphoma, such results must be interpreted with caution. Monoclonality is not synonymous with malignancy, and PCR can detect monoclonal lymphoid populations that are not clinically significant. PCR products obtained from the bone marrow and from the primary lymphoma (if available) can be compared to avoid the detection of biologically irrelevant monoclonal populations.[38]

Unique gene rearrangements of *BCL2* or c-*MYC* can also be identified with PCR; when present, they not only support a diagnosis of malignant lymphoma but also facilitate subclassification.[39,40] Currently, molecular diagnostic tests are not routinely used to identify bone marrow involvement by Hodgkin's lymphoma, although microdissected Hodgkin's lymphoma cells have been shown to harbor monoclonally rearranged *IGH@* genes.[41,42]

Unusual Reactive Lymphoid Infiltrates

Compared with the more typical benign lymphoid aggregates, differentiating other reactive lymphoid proliferations from malignant lymphoma is frequently more problematic.

Systemic Polyclonal Immunoblastic Proliferations

Systemic polyclonal immunoblastic proliferations are rare and unusual reactive lymphoplasmacytic proliferations that are often encountered in the setting of an acute immune disorder.[43] This disorder involves the peripheral blood, bone marrow, and lymph nodes; other organs, such as the liver and spleen, are often involved as well. The leukocyte count is usually elevated, with an absolute lymphocytosis that includes reactive lymphocytes, immunoblasts, and plasma cells; a neutrophilia with a shift toward immaturity may be present (Fig. 57-7). Anemia and thrombocytopenia are almost always present; the anemia is frequently immune mediated, with a positive antiglobulin test. Affected patients have polyclonal hypergammaglobulinemia.

Bone marrow aspirate smears and core biopsy sections show numerous lymphocytes, immunoblasts, and plasma cells. Focal lymphocytic aggregates are characteristically present in the biopsy sections; they may be inconspicuous or large and extensive (see Fig. 57-7). The plasma cells and immunoblasts in the infiltrate show a polyclonal immunoglobulin light-chain staining pattern. Flow cytometry reveals polyclonal B cells. Molecular analysis shows germline immunoglobulin heavy-chain and T-cell receptor genes or, rarely, oligoclonal B- and T-cell populations. Although the cause of this disorder is unknown, clonal cytogenetic abnormalities have been found in a subset of patients, raising the possibility of a cryptic neoplastic proliferation. Underlying peripheral T-cell lymphoma should be excluded since they exhibit clinical and pathologic features that overlap with systemic polyclonal immunoblastic proliferation.

The clinical behavior is variable. Many patients respond to steroid therapy, but others require chemotherapy. In the small number of reported cases, the mortality rate during the acute phase of the illness was high, about 50%. The majority of patients who recover do not experience recurrence or relapse.[43]

Reactive Polymorphic Lymphohistiocytic Proliferations

Reactive polymorphic lymphohistiocytic lesions are composed of heterogeneous cellular infiltrates of lymphocytes, including small, mature-appearing forms and large transformed lymphocytes with irregular nuclei and nucleoli. Admixed plasma cells, eosinophils, mast cells, and epithelioid histiocytes, some arranged in poorly formed granulomas, are frequently present in these lesions. These infiltrates are variably sized and are often larger than typical benign lymphoid aggregates. They may be multiple, situated adjacent to bony trabeculae, and have irregular borders (Fig. 57-8). They are particularly difficult to differentiate from malignant lymphomas. Most commonly, polymorphic lymphohistiocytic proliferations are found in patients with immunodeficiency disorders, including acquired immunodeficiency syndrome (AIDS).[44,45] However, they may also be seen in patients with connective tissue disorders such as rheumatoid arthritis. Malignant lymphoma should be diagnosed with caution in

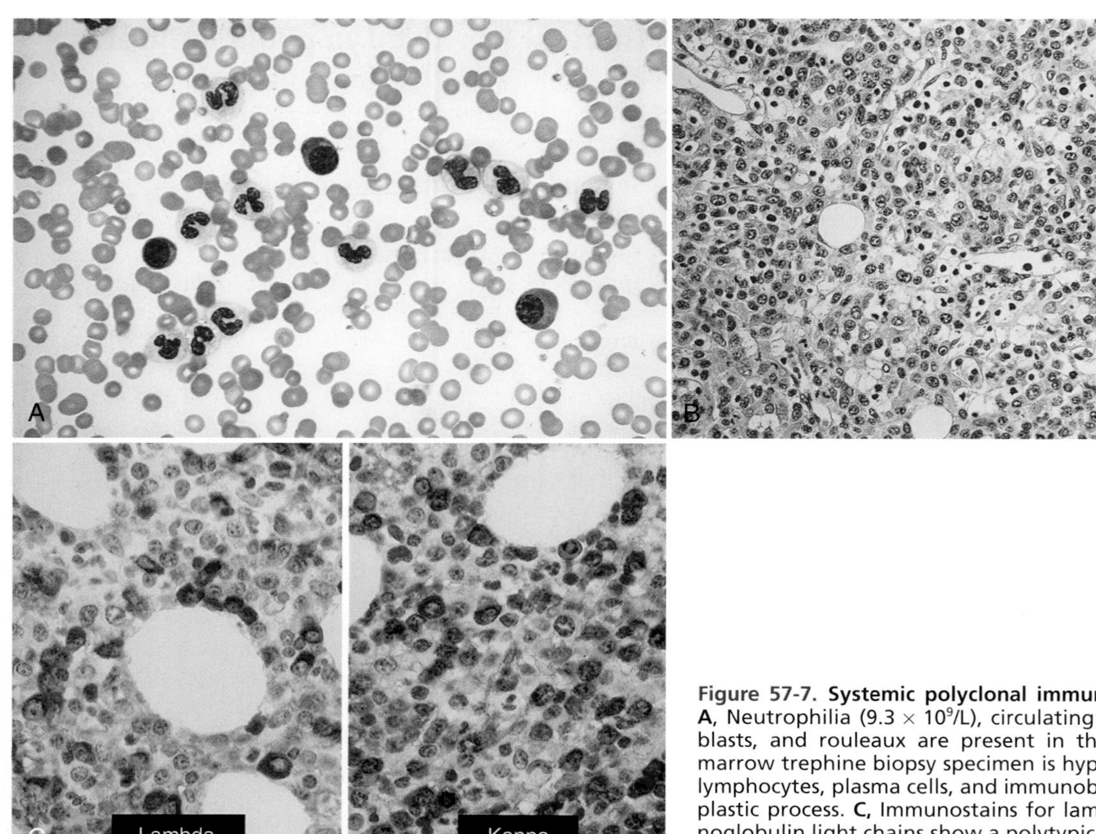

Figure 57-7. Systemic polyclonal immunoblastic proliferation. A, Neutrophilia (9.3×10^9/L), circulating plasma cells, immunoblasts, and rouleaux are present in the blood. **B**, The bone marrow trephine biopsy specimen is hypercellular and contains lymphocytes, plasma cells, and immunoblasts, mimicking a neoplastic process. **C**, Immunostains for lambda and kappa immunoglobulin light chains show a polytypic staining pattern in the plasma cells.

immunodeficient patients in the absence of histologic confirmation from another extramedullary site or in whom there is no supporting evidence from ancillary studies such as flow cytometric immunophenotyping, immunohistochemical stains, or molecular studies.

NON-HODGKIN'S LYMPHOMA

Incidence of Bone Marrow Involvement

The presence of lymphoma within the bone marrow is regarded as dissemination and represents stage IV disease.[46,47] The overall incidence of bone marrow involvement by lymphoma is 35% to 50%.[10] However, there is considerable variability in the frequency with which specific types of lymphoma involve the bone marrow (Table 57-2). In general, indolent lymphomas, aggressive lymphomas, and most peripheral T-cell lymphomas have the highest incidence of bone marrow involvement. For example, follicular lymphoma and small lymphocytic lymphoma involve the bone marrow in up to 60% and 85% of cases, respectively.[10,48] The mere presence of indolent lymphoma in the bone marrow does not always indicate a poor clinical outcome. Rather, the extent of marrow involvement has a more direct impact on patient survival.[49] Mantle cell lymphoma, which is an aggressive lymphoma, involves the bone marrow in the majority of cases (up to 95%).[50] Burkitt's lymphoma involves the bone marrow in 35% to 60% of cases.[10,51] In contrast, diffuse large B-cell lymphomas infiltrate the bone marrow in only about 15% to 30% of cases.[51-53] The incidence of bone marrow involvement by the specific subtypes of peripheral T-cell lymphomas has a wide range, but overall, these lymphomas involve the bone marrow in up to 80% of cases.[54] Some types, such as hepatosplenic T-cell lymphoma, infiltrate the bone marrow in virtually all cases.[14,15,55] The bone marrow is less frequently involved in mycosis fungoides,[56] anaplastic large cell lymphoma,[57] and nasal-type natural killer (NK)/T-cell lymphoma.[58]

Histologic Patterns of Bone Marrow Involvement

Non-Hodgkin's lymphomas infiltrate the bone marrow in a variety of architectural patterns (see Table 57-2), and more than one pattern is often seen in an individual patient.[7] Knowledge of these features is helpful in identifying malignant lymphoid infiltrates and in some cases facilitates lymphoma classification.

Lymphomatous infiltrates in the bone marrow can occur in five different patterns: focal random (nodular), focal paratrabecular, interstitial, diffuse, and intrasinusoidal (Fig. 57-9). Focal infiltrates are the most common and are characterized by discrete collections of malignant cells. Even though they focally displace bone marrow and fat cells, they are usually associated with considerable sparing of normal hematopoietic tissue. Focal infiltrates are present in either random or paratrabecular locations. Focal random lymphoid infiltrates occupy space away from the bony trabeculae. Focal paratrabecular infiltrates preferentially grow along the bone surface and conform to the bony contour. Paratrabecular infiltrates may expand out from the bony trabeculae, but one portion remains adjacent to the bone, often giving the infiltrate an asymmetric appearance. Random infiltrates that expand to

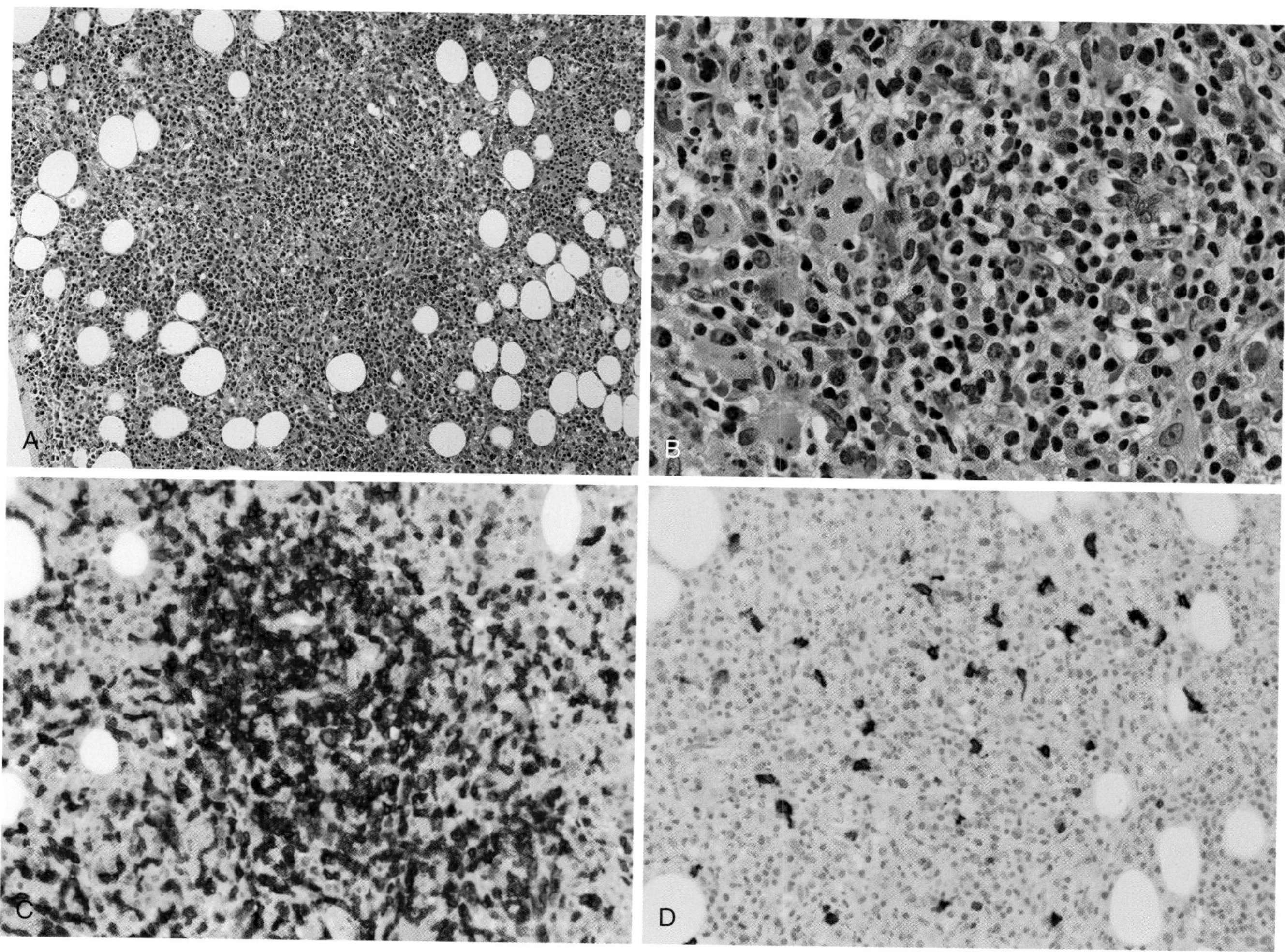

Figure 57-8. Reactive polymorphic lymphohistiocytic infiltrate in a bone marrow trephine biopsy section. A, The infiltrate blends imperceptibly with the normal bone marrow cells. **B,** Small, medium, and large lymphocytes, plasma cells, eosinophils, and histiocytes are present in the infiltrate. **C,** CD3 stain shows that virtually all the lymphocytes are T cells. **D,** CD20 stain shows only rare B cells in the infiltrate.

touch the bone focally are not considered paratrabecular. In interstitial infiltrates, the malignant cells infiltrate between normal hematopoietic cells without significantly disrupting the bone marrow architecture. They usually do not replace large amounts of bone marrow tissue, even though there is generally widespread bone marrow involvement. Diffuse infiltrates completely replace the hematopoietic elements between the bony trabeculae in a portion or all of the trephine biopsy section. Intrasinusoidal infiltration is characterized by collections of malignant cells within the bone marrow sinuses; these infiltrates are typically subtle and difficult to appreciate on routinely stained H&E sections but can be highlighted with immunohistochemical stains.

CHARACTERISTIC FEATURES OF B-CELL LYMPHOMAS INVOLVING BONE MARROW

This section describes the characteristics of each type of B-cell lymphoma when it involves the bone marrow; the next section does the same for T-cell lymphomas. The morphologic characteristics specific to bone marrow are emphasized. Other features such as immunophenotype and genetic characteristics are discussed in detail in the chapters covering each type of lymphoma.

Small Lymphocytic Lymphoma/Chronic Lymphocytic Leukemia

Small lymphocytic lymphoma (SLL) and chronic lymphocytic leukemia (CLL) are regarded as the same disease process with different tissue expressions. SLL is diagnosed when the neoplasm involves primarily lymph nodes or extranodal sites, without overt leukemia. About 85% of SLL cases have bone marrow involvement at diagnosis; rarely, patients with SLL have isolated bone marrow involvement.[10,48] Although, by definition, an absolute lymphocytosis is absent, a small population of circulating monoclonal B cells can frequently be detected by flow cytometry.[25,59,60] Approximately 15% of patients who present with SLL later develop overt lymphocytosis identical to CLL.[60,61] The patterns in which SLL/CLL infiltrates the bone marrow are focal random (Fig. 57-10), diffuse, interstitial, and mixed. Although focal random infiltrates can expand to touch bone, distinctly paratrabecular

Table 57-2 Histologic Features of Non-Hodgkin's Lymphomas Involving Bone Marrow

Type of Lymphoma	Incidence of Involvement (%)	Pattern of Involvement*	Cytology	Comments
Small lymphocytic	85	FR, I, D	Small, mature lymphocytes; proliferation centers may be present	Paratrabecular infiltrates essentially rule out this diagnosis
Lymphoplasmacytic	80-100	FR, I, D, FP	Spectrum of cells from lymphocytes to plasma cells; immunoblasts may be present; Dutcher bodies common	Unlike SLL/CLL, occasional paratrabecular infiltrates may be present
Mantle cell	55-95	FR, I, D, FP	Small irregular lymphocytes; may be blastoid; rare cells with prominent nucleoli	Cyclin D1 positive; paratrabecular infiltrates may be present
Follicular	50-60	FP, D, FR, I	Small cleaved lymphocytes usually predominate; large cleaved or noncleaved cells may be present	Characteristically paratrabecular; neoplastic follicles may be apparent
Splenic marginal zone	73-100	FR, I, D, IS	Small lymphocytes with slightly irregular nuclei, condensed chromatin, and abundant cytoplasm	Intrasinusoidal infiltrates often prominent; reactive germinal centers may be present
Low-grade extranodal marginal zone	44	FR, P, I, IS	Small cells with condensed chromatin and scant to moderate amounts of cytoplasm; rare large cells may be admixed	Extent of bone marrow infiltration usually minimal
Nodal marginal zone	30-40	FR, I, P, D	Small cells with condensed chromatin and scant to moderate amounts of cytoplasm	
Diffuse large B-cell	15-30	FR, D	Large cells with prominent nucleoli	Prominent component of T lymphocytes with or without histiocytes may be present; immunohistochemistry for B-cell antigens and other markers is essential in these cases; rare cases of large cell lymphoma are intravascular
Burkitt's	35-60	I, D	Medium-sized cells with reticular chromatin, multiple small nucleoli, and basophilic cytoplasm; cytoplasmic vacuoles common	Necrosis common; "starry sky" pattern may be seen
Peripheral T-cell (unspecified)	80	FR, D	Polymorphic lymphoid population—nuclei often hyperchromatic and irregular; large cells with nucleoli may be present; prominent reactive cell component often intermixed with lymphoma cells	Vascularity and reticulin fibrosis frequently prominent
Anaplastic large cell	4-40	FR, I (scattered cells), D	Large cells with lobulated nuclei, prominent nucleoli, and abundant cytoplasm	Detection rate is higher with immunostaining for CD30 or ALK-1
Hepatosplenic T-cell	100	IS	Medium-sized lymphocytes with dispersed chromatin	Lesions may be subtle; immunohistochemistry is often helpful
Lymphoblastic	50-60	I, D	Blastic cells with high mitotic rate	Identical to acute lymphoblastic leukemia
NK/T-cell	0-25	I (scattered cells)	Variable size with pleomorphic nuclei	Immunostains or in situ hybridization (EBER) may be necessary to identify lymphoma cells in bone marrow sections

*Patterns may be mixed; the most common patterns are listed.
D, diffuse; EBER, Epstein-Barr virus–encoded RNA; FP, focal paratrabecular; FR, focal random; I, interstitial; IS, intrasinusoidal; NK, natural killer; P, paratrabecular.

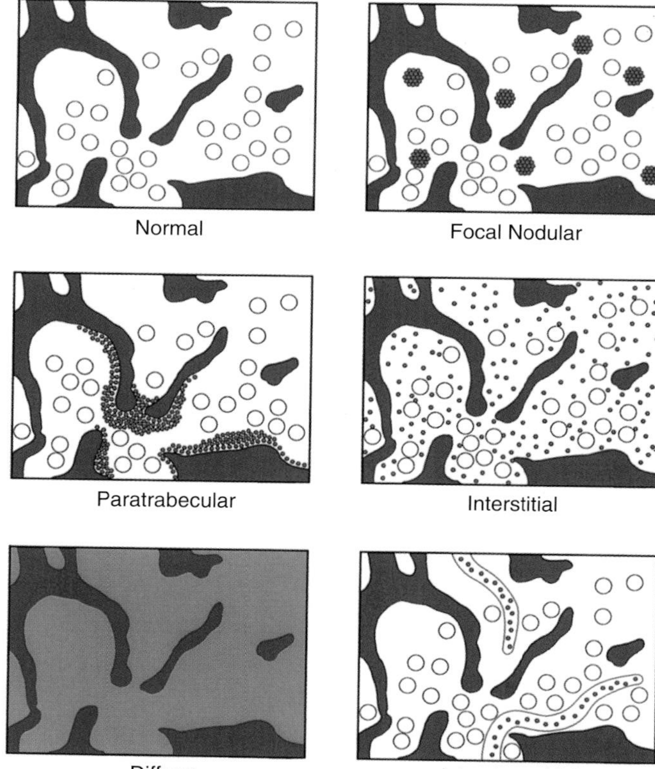

Figure 57-9. Diagram illustrating normal bone marrow and the five different patterns of infiltration by lymphoma.

infiltrates are absent; when paratrabecular infiltrates are observed, the diagnosis of SLL/CLL can be excluded, and other types of lymphoma should be considered. The malignant lymphocytes show similar morphology in the peripheral blood and bone marrow aspirate smears; they are small and mature appearing, with round nuclei, condensed chromatin, and scant cytoplasm. Although occasional cells may have slightly irregular nuclei, deep clefts are not common. Prolymphocytes are present in low numbers. Proliferation centers

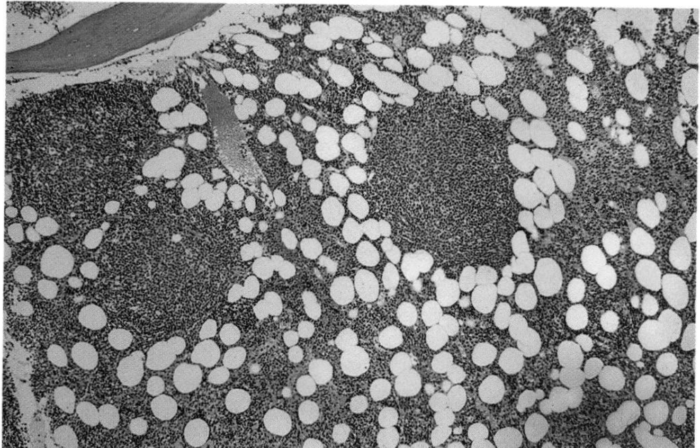

Figure 57-10. Small lymphocytic lymphoma. Three focal nodular lymphoid infiltrates and interstitial infiltrates composed of small lymphocytes with condensed chromatin and round nuclei are demonstrated in this hematoxylin-eosin–stained section.

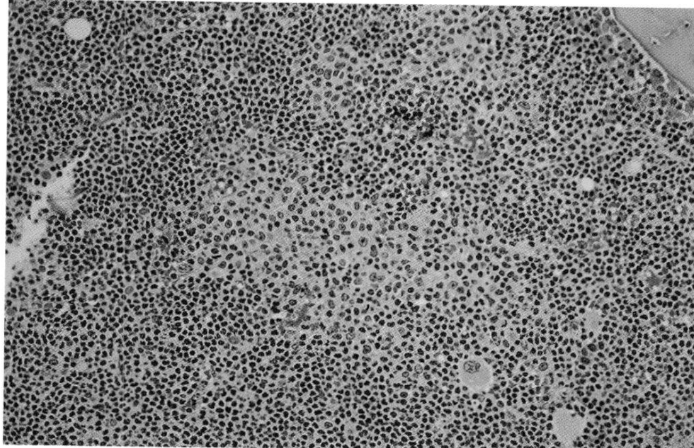

Figure 57-11. Proliferation centers of small lymphocytic lymphoma in a bone marrow trephine biopsy section. Pale-staining prolymphocytes with an ample amount of cytoplasm, slightly dispersed chromatin, and visible central nucleoli are present within the proliferation centers. Small, mature-appearing lymphocytes surround the proliferation centers.

identical to those commonly observed in lymph node biopsies in SLL/CLL are occasionally encountered in bone marrow trephine biopsy sections (Fig. 57-11; see also Chapter 14).

Lymphoplasmacytic Lymphoma and Waldenström's Macroglobulinemia

Lymphoplasmacytic lymphoma (LPL) is a rare neoplasm of small B lymphocytes, plasmacytoid lymphocytes, and plasma cells. Waldenström's macroglobulinemia (WM) is found in most patients with LPL.[62,63] WM is currently defined as LPL with bone marrow involvement and a serum immunoglobulin (Ig) M monoclonal protein of any concentration. LPL infiltrates in the bone marrow are usually intertrabecular, but paratrabecular infiltrates may be present in up to one third of cases. The characteristic immunophenotype of LPL is $CD19^+$, $CD20^+$, $CD22^+$, $CD25^+$, $FMC7^+$, and surface IgM^+. Although CD5, CD10, and CD23 are usually negative, heterogeneous expression of one these antigens may be observed in up to 10% of cases and does not necessarily exclude the diagnosis of LPL/WM, as long as appropriate measures to exclude mantle cell lymphoma, SLL/CLL, and follicular lymphoma have been taken.[64] In practice, the infiltrate of LPL/WM in the bone marrow includes a wide spectrum of cells, including small lymphocytes similar to those of SLL/CLL, a variable number of plasmacytoid lymphocytes, and plasma cells with monoclonal cytoplasmic immunoglobulin light chain. The number of plasma cells varies considerably, ranging from occasional to numerous; their chromatin may be condensed or immature, with visible nucleoli. Intranuclear inclusions (Dutcher bodies) are often identified in plasma cells (Fig. 57-12) but are not specific for LPL; they can also be seen in plasma cell myeloma, other lymphomas with plasmacytic differentiation, and occasionally reactive lymphoid infiltrates. Transformed lymphocytes with distinct nucleoli may be present in LPL, but they are usually in the minority. Mast cells and histiocytes are often increased in the bone marrow infiltrates of LPL. The bone marrow aspirate contains lymphoma cells similar to those in the trephine biopsy section. An

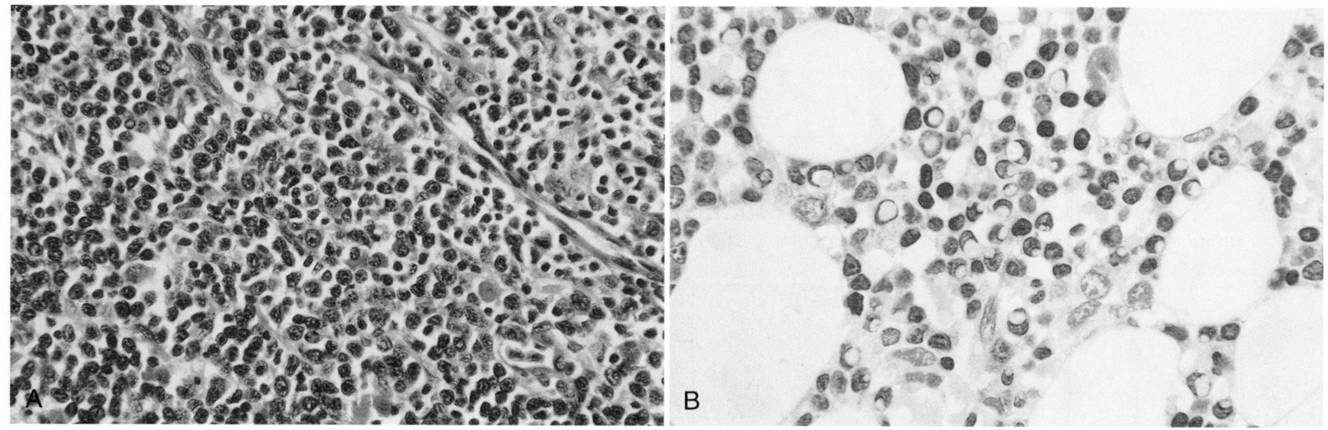

Figure 57-12. Lymphoplasmacytic lymphoma in a bone marrow trephine biopsy section. A, The infiltrate is dense and contains numerous plasma cells and small lymphocytes. **B,** Intranuclear inclusions (Dutcher bodies) are present within some plasma cells.

absolute lymphocytosis is present in the peripheral blood in 10% to 30% of cases.[65,66] The circulating lymphoma cells are small, with condensed chromatin and round nuclei, similar to those present in SLL/CLL; plasmacytoid lymphocytes may also be present.

LPL/WM should be distinguished from other B-cell neoplasms that frequently involve the bone marrow and show plasmacytic differentiation. These include splenic marginal zone lymphoma, B-cell lymphoma of mucosa-associated lymphoid tissue (MALT lymphoma), and plasma cell myeloma.[67] Although clinical and laboratory features such as IgM serum paraprotein with hyperviscosity, lack of lytic bone lesions, and presence of lymphadenopathy help distinguish LPL from multiple myeloma, the distinction from some other indolent B-cell lymphomas can be problematic.[63] This is especially true for marginal zone lymphoma because the lymphoma cells in both malignancies can exhibit similar morphology, be associated with IgM serum paraprotein, and commonly involve the spleen.[67] Careful attention to the affected anatomic sites can help exclude extranodal MALT lymphoma, which typically originates at mucosal sites and tends to spread to other MALT sites when it disseminates; in contrast, LPL/WM is rarely localized to extranodal sites and tends to involve lymph nodes or spleen in addition to bone marrow. Splenic marginal zone lymphomas exhibit splenomegaly and almost always involve the bone marrow, but peripheral lymph nodes are typically not involved, in contrast to LPL. Cytogenetic studies may also be helpful; several aneuploidies such as trisomy 3, 7, 12, or 18 and structural chromosomal rearrangements such as t(1;14)(p22;q32), t(11;18)(q21;q21), and t(14;18)(q32;q21) are associated with marginal zone lymphoma.[68-72] Although t(9;14)(q13;q32), which fuses *PAX5* with *IGH@*, has been associated with LPL/WM, more recent reports with a larger number of cases have not verified that association and have found that the *PAX5/IGH@* fusion is more commonly observed in large B-cell lymphoma.[73-75]

Splenic Marginal Zone Lymphoma

Splenic marginal zone lymphoma is an indolent B-cell lymphoma that includes the disorder previously known as *splenic lymphoma with villous lymphocytes*. It involves the bone marrow at presentation in nearly all cases.[12,69] Infiltration of the bone marrow by splenic marginal zone lymphoma may occur in one or more of the following patterns: intrasinusoidal (Fig. 57-13),[12] interstitial, focal random, and focal paratrabecular.

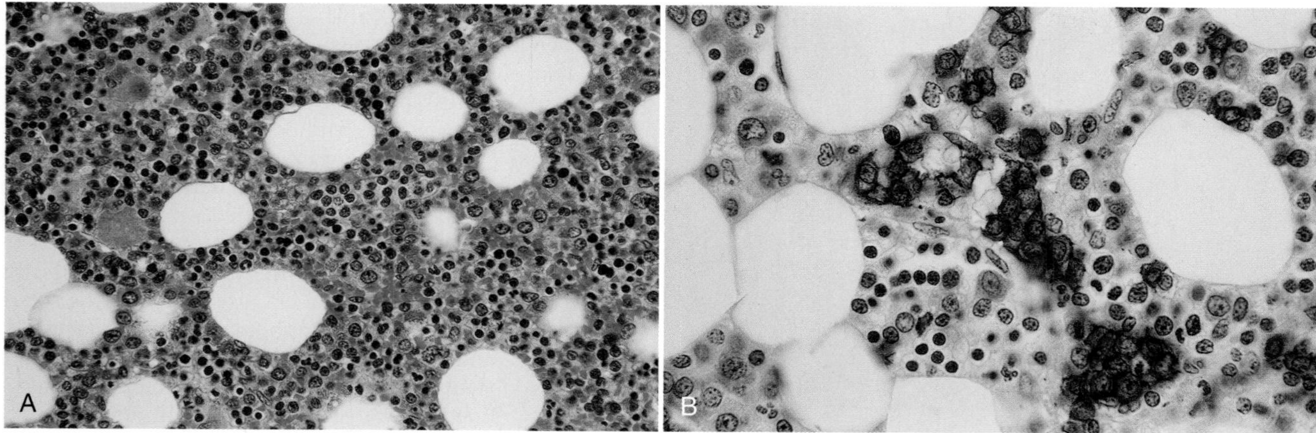

Figure 57-13. Splenic marginal zone lymphoma in a bone marrow trephine biopsy section. A, The infiltrate blends in with the normal hematopoietic elements and is difficult to identify on the hematoxylin-eosin–stained section. **B,** CD20 immunohistochemical stain highlights lymphoma cells within a bone marrow sinus.

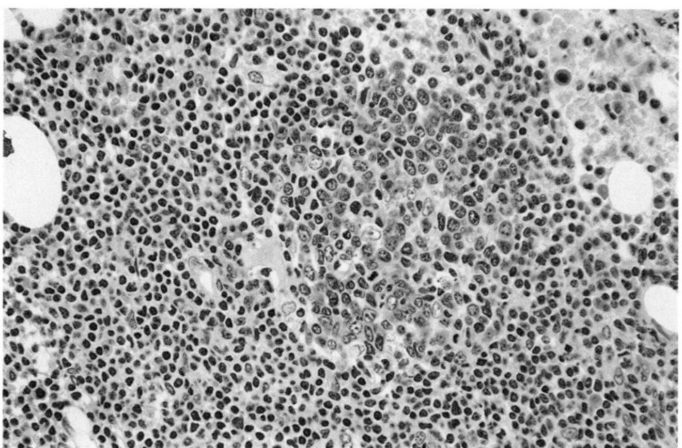

Figure 57-14. Splenic marginal zone lymphoma in a bone marrow trephine biopsy section. Most of the lymphoma cells are small, with slightly irregular nuclei, and they surround a reactive germinal center.

Diffuse involvement is rare. Intrasinusoidal infiltration may be prominent in splenic marginal zone lymphoma but is not specific for this disorder; a similar pattern occurs in other lymphomas.[12] Intrasinusoidal infiltrates are often difficult to appreciate in H&E-stained sections but can be highlighted by immunostains that mark the infiltrating cells. Another important finding is the presence of reactive germinal centers in the lymphomatous infiltrate, reported in about 30% of cases (Fig. 57-14).[12] Identification of cytologically abnormal cells outside the reactive germinal centers may be a clue that these lesions are malignant infiltrates, although the distinction is often difficult based on morphology alone. Immunostaining for CD21 or CD23 can be used to highlight follicular dendritic meshwork within the germinal centers, making the germinal centers stand out as discrete structures within the infiltrate. These reactive germinal centers should not be confused with foci of large cell lymphoma within the marginal zone lymphomatous infiltrate or with malignant germinal centers in follicular lymphoma, which are typically $BCL2^+$, unlike the $BCL2^-$ reactive germinal centers.[76]

The lymphoma cells in trephine biopsy sections are small to medium sized, with round to slightly irregular nuclei, condensed chromatin, and moderate amounts of pale, gray-blue cytoplasm. Rare large lymphocytes with vesicular nuclei and visible nucleoli, as well as plasmacytoid cells with or without Dutcher bodies, may be admixed among the smaller lymphoma cells but are absent in most cases.[77] Neoplastic cells are present in the peripheral blood in virtually all cases of splenic marginal zone lymphoma, although an absolute lymphocytosis is not a constant feature.[16] The circulating malignant lymphocytes are small to medium sized, with round or ovoid nuclei, condensed chromatin, and small to abundant amounts of lightly basophilic cytoplasm. Thin, short, polar villi may be present on the cytoplasmic surfaces in some cells.[78]

Extranodal Marginal Zone Lymphoma of Mucosa-Associated Lymphoid Tissue

Low-grade extranodal marginal zone lymphoma of the MALT type typically involves the gastrointestinal tract and is usually localized at diagnosis. Salivary gland, lung, thyroid, and conjunctiva are other commonly involved sites. When dissemination occurs, low-grade extranodal marginal zone lymphoma preferentially spreads to other mucosal sites; however, up to 44% of low-grade cases involve the bone marrow.[79] Most bone marrow infiltrates are focal random, although they may be paratrabecular, interstitial, or intrasinusoidal.[12,80,81] The extent of bone marrow involvement is variable,[12,82] and dissemination does not appear to affect prognosis.[79] Infiltrates of extranodal marginal zone lymphoma include a spectrum of lymphoma cells, ranging from small cells with condensed chromatin resembling mature lymphocytes to slightly larger cells with irregular nuclei, ample cytoplasm, and distinct cell borders. There may be admixed plasma cells. The absolute lymphocyte count is normal in most patients; circulating lymphoma cells are identified morphologically in only a minority of patients.

Nodal Marginal Zone Lymphoma

Nodal marginal zone lymphoma (formerly called *monocytoid B-cell lymphoma*) is a primary lymphoma of the lymph node that is distinct from low-grade extranodal MALT-type lymphoma.[83] Nodal marginal zone and MALT-type lymphomas share some features, such as the propensity to colonize reactive germinal centers. The malignant cells closely resemble nodal monocytoid B cells, which are frequently encountered in reactive lymphadenitis. Bone marrow involvement has been observed in 32% to 54% of cases, with mostly focal random or interstitial infiltrates; paratrabecular infiltrates occur less frequently.[82,84,85] Diffuse infiltrates occur in patients in the leukemic phase of nodal marginal zone lymphoma, but both are rare.[86] The infiltrates include small centrocyte-like cells with irregular nuclei, condensed chromatin, and scant cytoplasm, as well as medium to large monocytoid-like cells with ample cytoplasm; plasma cells may be intermixed. Nodal marginal zone lymphoma only rarely involves the peripheral blood and bone marrow aspirate; however, the cytology of the circulating lymphoma cells is similar to that observed in bone marrow core biopsy sections.[86]

Follicular Lymphoma

Follicular lymphoma involves the bone marrow in a high percentage of cases, approximately 50% to 60%, at initial diagnosis.[87] The infiltrates are often distinctly paratrabecular and may be exclusively paratrabecular (Fig. 57-15). However, other patterns, including focal random and diffuse, also occur.[10] The bone marrow infiltrates are most frequently composed of small lymphocytes with condensed chromatin and cleaved or irregularly shaped nuclei. Large lymphocytes with prominent single nucleoli may be present, but they are usually few in number. A follicular growth pattern can occur in the bone marrow but is not common, accounting for only 5% of cases (12 of 260) in one study (Fig. 57-16).[88] Interestingly, $CD3^+$ pseudo–mantle zones were noted in five of the cases (42%) with a follicular growth pattern, and the malignant follicles were distributed in a focal random pattern in all but one case. The lack of paratrabecular localization of the malignant follicles may cause confusion with benign infiltrates. However, as with follicular lymphoma that occurs at extramedullary sites, immunohistochemical stains demonstrate an

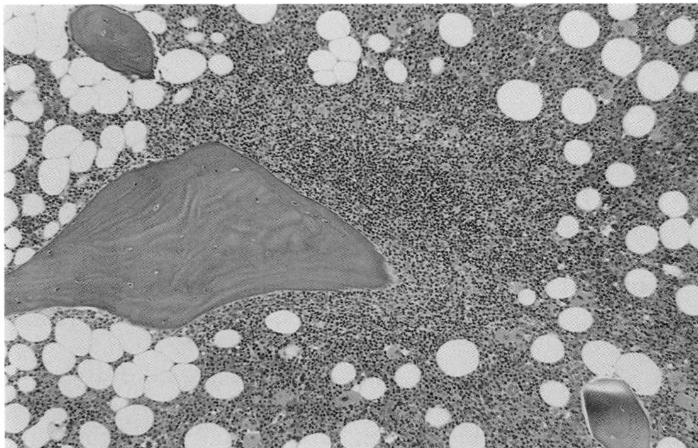

Figure 57-15. Follicular lymphoma. Paratrabecular lymphoid infiltrates hug the bone and conform to its contour.

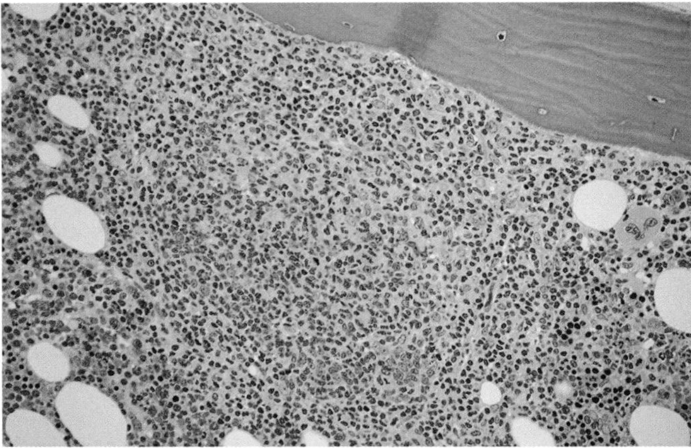

Figure 57-16. Follicular lymphoma with a follicular growth pattern. In this bone marrow trephine biopsy section, the infiltrate is paratrabecular, and the neoplastic germinal center is homogeneous and contains mostly small cleaved cells.

abnormal phenotype of the malignant germinal centers ($CD20^+$ B cells that are also $CD10^+$, $BCL6^+$, and $BCL2^+$, associated with a meshwork of dendritic cells that can be highlighted by CD21, CD23, or CD35).

Discordant morphology between the lymphoma at nodal or extranodal sites and the lymphoma in the bone marrow occurs in approximately 20% of cases; in the majority of cases, the bone marrow contains a more indolent infiltrate.[7,10,52,89,90] Discordant morphology also occurs between bilateral trephine biopsy sections in rare cases (Fig. 57-17). Circulating lymphoma cells are occasionally identified in the peripheral blood smear but are usually few in number. In a minority of cases, follicular lymphoma presents with an absolute lymphocytosis; rarely, the lymphocytosis is marked.[91] The lymphoma cells are typically slightly larger than mature lymphocytes and have deep nuclear clefts, smooth condensed chromatin, and scant cytoplasm (Fig. 57-18). In rare cases the lymphoma cells resemble blasts, there is marked leukocytosis, and the trephine biopsy specimen exhibits a diffuse infiltrate.[92,93] In these latter cases, ancillary studies such as immunophenotyping and genetic studies are essential to exclude acute leukemia and to identify follicular lymphoma in the leukemic phase.

Mantle Cell Lymphoma

Mantle cell lymphoma (MCL) involves the bone marrow in 55% to 95% of cases.[50] The infiltrates are typically focal and randomly distributed, but paratrabecular infiltrates are seen in up to 45% of cases; in occasional patients the lymphoma is exclusively paratrabecular (Fig. 57-19). Interstitial or diffuse patterns of infiltration may also occur.[50,94,95] The lymphocytes in MCL can exhibit a heterogeneous morphology, but in most cases there is a uniform population of small to medium-sized lymphocytes with condensed chromatin and irregularly shaped nuclei. Scattered larger cells with visible nucleoli may be admixed.[96] Occasionally the lymphoma cells are predominantly small, with condensed chromatin and round nuclei, resembling those present in SLL/CLL. There is also a blastoid variant in which the cells possess dispersed chromatin and scant cytoplasm, resembling acute leukemia (Fig. 57-20); the lymphoma cells can also be pleomorphic with lobated nuclei.[97] Bone marrow infiltrates tend to be interstitial or diffuse in the blastoid variant.[95]

Circulating lymphoma cells are common even when lymphocytosis is not present. If lymphoma cells are numerous,

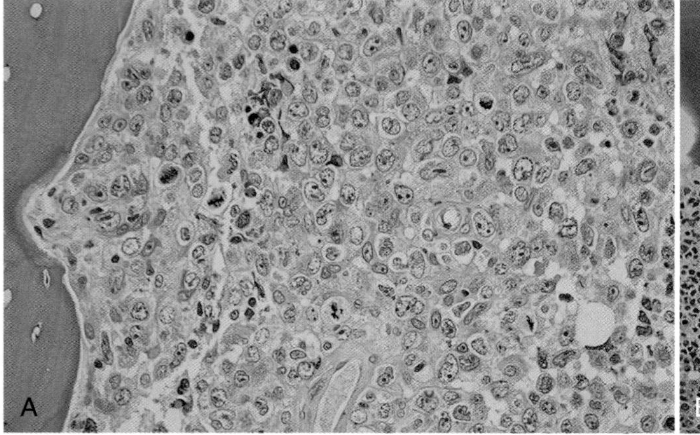

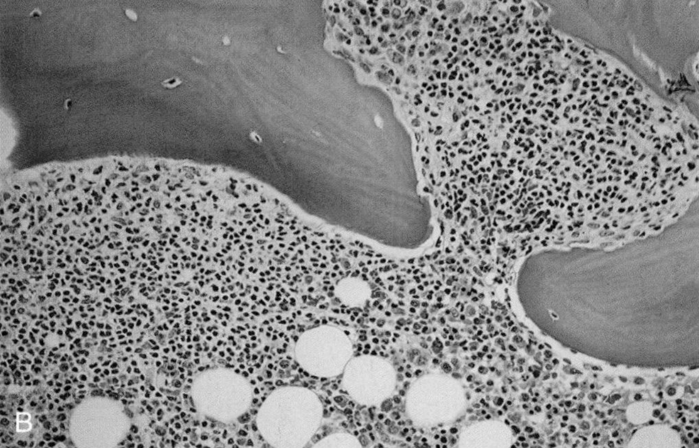

Figure 57-17. Lymphoma with discordant morphology in bilateral trephine biopsy sections. A, Large cell lymphoma involves the right trephine biopsy section. Necrosis (not shown) was also present. **B,** Small cleaved cell lymphoma in the left trephine biopsy section. Predominantly grade 1 follicular lymphoma with focal, diffuse large cell lymphoma was present in a lymph node.

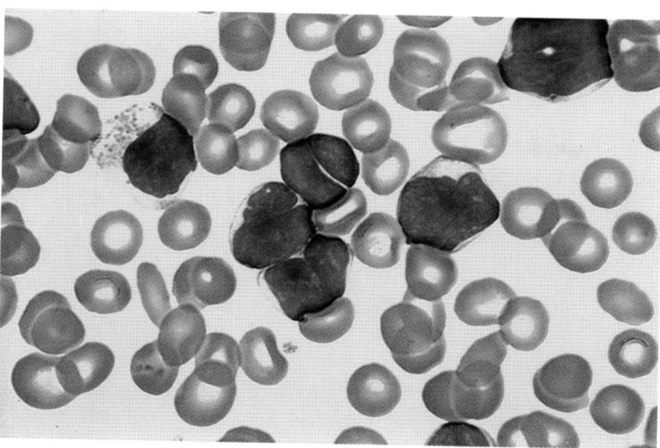

Figure 57-18. Follicular lymphoma cells in peripheral blood. The lymphoma cells are slightly larger than small, mature lymphocytes; they have a smooth chromatin pattern and deeply cleaved nuclei. A benign large granular lymphocyte is also present.

an absolute lymphocytosis may occur and has been reported in up to 28% of cases.[50,98] When a peripheral blood lymphocytosis is present and the lymphocytes are small and round, the morphologic appearance of MCL can closely resemble that of SLL/CLL (Fig. 57-21).[99] Other features similar to CLL, such as an absence of lymphadenopathy and an indolent disease course, may also be present. In addition, the MCL cells that resemble CLL often have a mutated immunoglobulin variable heavy-chain gene (56%) and are frequently $CD38^-$ (52%).[100] Immunophenotyping by flow cytometry may help distinguish between CLL and MCL. In contrast to CLL, MCL cells typically display strong-intensity surface immunoglobulin light chain and are usually $CD79b^+$, $FMC7^+$, and $CD23^-$, although they can be weakly $CD23^+$ in up to 50% of cases.[101,102] If bone marrow biopsies from these cases show paratrabecular infiltrates, a diagnosis of SLL/CLL can be excluded and the possibility of other disorders, including MCL, should be considered. MCL may also exhibit a morphology indistinguishable from that of prolymphocytic leukemia or CLL/prolymphocytic leukemia.[96,103] Therefore, a primary diagnosis

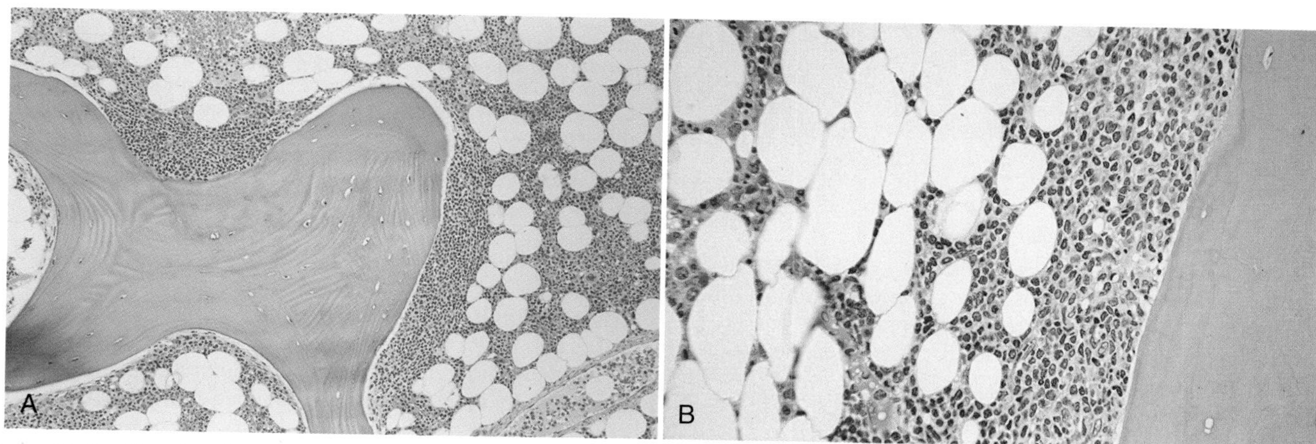

Figure 57-19. Mantle cell lymphoma in a bone marrow trephine biopsy section. A, The lymphomatous infiltrates are exclusively paratrabecular. **B,** The lymphoma cells are small to medium sized, with condensed chromatin and round to irregular nuclei.

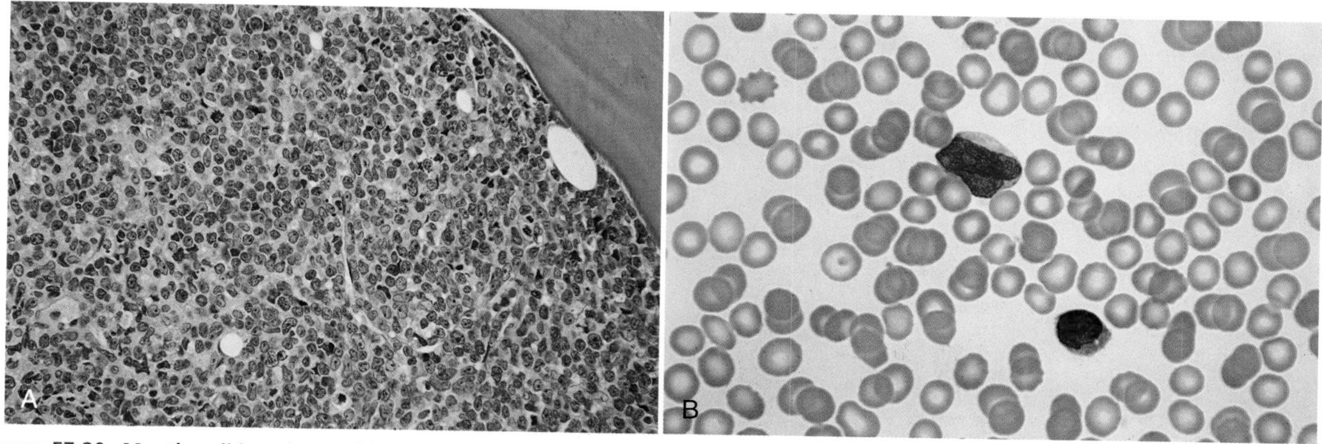

Figure 57-20. Mantle cell lymphoma, blastoid variant, in the bone marrow and peripheral blood. A, The infiltrate in the trephine biopsy section displays a diffuse growth pattern and contains medium to large cells with dispersed chromatin and one or more visible nucleoli. **B,** A lymphoma cell with a folded nucleus, slightly dispersed chromatin, and scant cytoplasm is present in the peripheral blood.

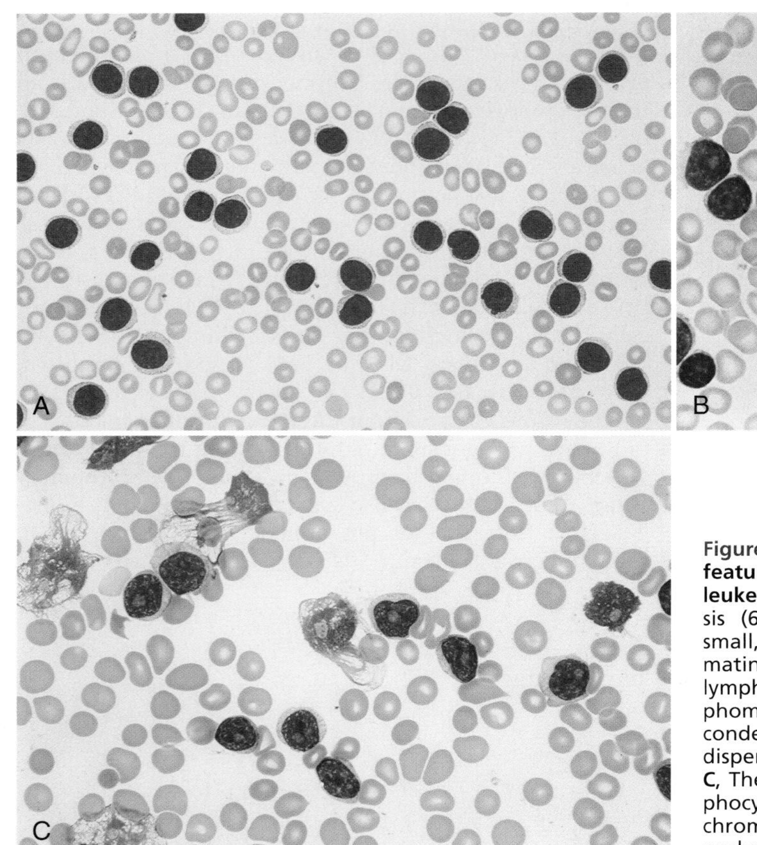

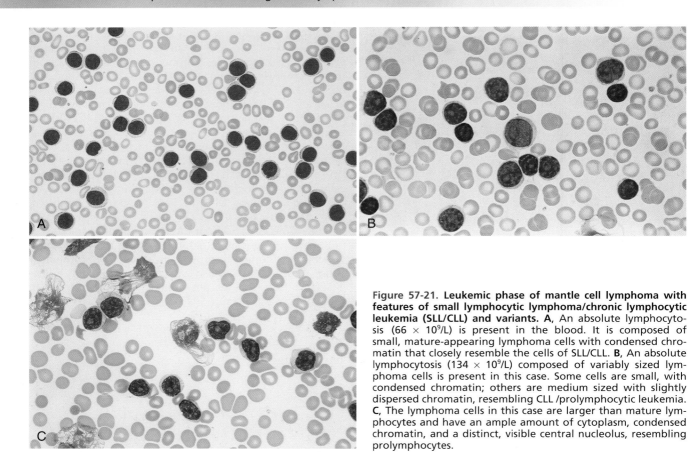

Figure 57-21. Leukemic phase of mantle cell lymphoma with features of small lymphocytic lymphoma/chronic lymphocytic leukemia (SLL/CLL) and variants. A, An absolute lymphocytosis (66×10^9/L) is present in the blood. It is composed of small, mature-appearing lymphoma cells with condensed chromatin that closely resemble the cells of SLL/CLL. **B**, An absolute lymphocytosis (134×10^9/L) composed of variably sized lymphoma cells is present in this case. Some cells are small, with condensed chromatin; others are medium sized with slightly dispersed chromatin, resembling CLL /prolymphocytic leukemia. **C**, The lymphoma cells in this case are larger than mature lymphocytes and have an ample amount of cytoplasm, condensed chromatin, and a distinct, visible central nucleolus, resembling prolymphocytes.

of MCL based on a bone marrow biopsy requires correlation with ancillary studies, such as flow cytometric immunophenotyping that shows the characteristic phenotype for MCL, immunostains showing BCL1 positivity, or genetic studies documenting t(11;14)(q13;q32).

Diffuse Large B-Cell Lymphoma

At diagnosis, diffuse large B-cell lymphoma (DLBCL) infiltrates the bone marrow in about 15% to 25% of cases.[52,53] Focal random, diffuse, and mixed patterns of infiltration occur most frequently, followed by paratrabecular infiltrates; interstitial infiltrates are rare.[104] The lymphoma cells are large and have one or more prominent nucleoli and scant to medium amounts of cytoplasm. Lymphomatous infiltrates are usually easily identified in H&E-stained bone marrow biopsy sections (Fig. 57-22). Bone marrow aspirates or touch imprints occasionally show lymphoma cells with one or more nucleoli and scant to ample basophilic cytoplasm (see Fig. 57-22). Peripheral blood involvement is uncommon but does occur.

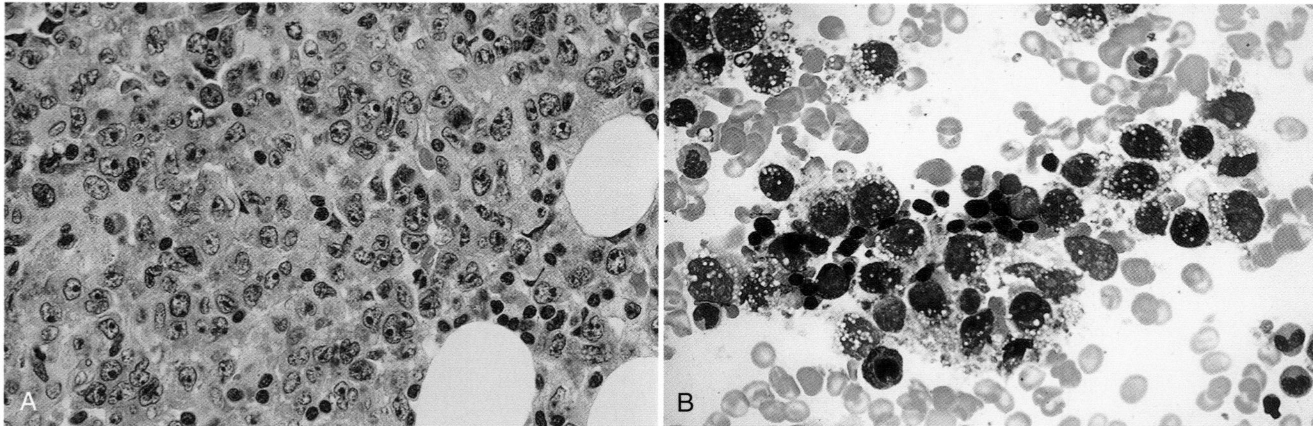

Figure 57-22. Diffuse large B-cell lymphoma in a bone marrow trephine biopsy and aspirate smear. A, Lymphoma cells in the trephine biopsy section are large, with dispersed chromatin; many have distinct nucleoli. **B**, The cytoplasm of the large lymphoma cells contains vacuoles.

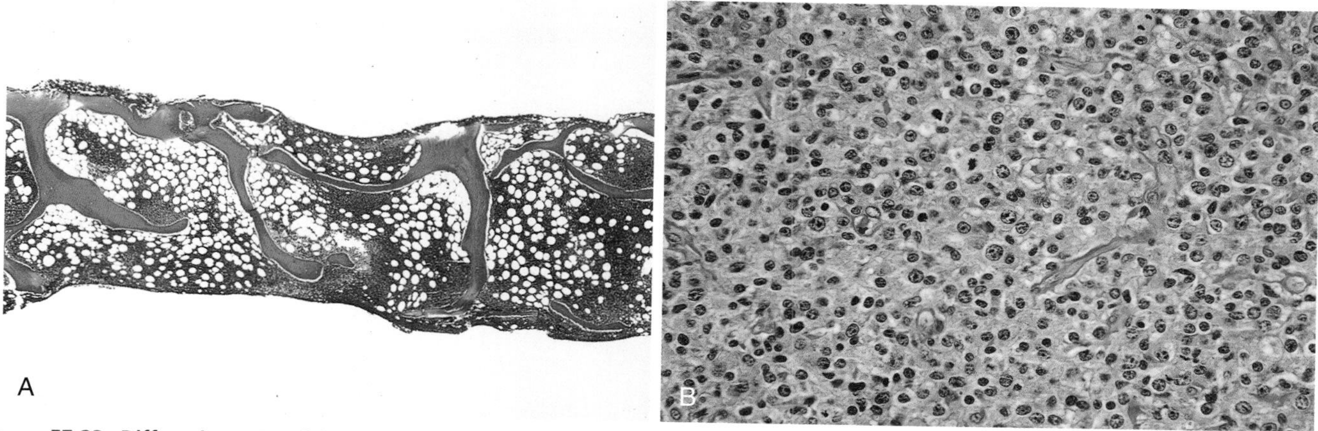

Figure 57-23. Diffuse large B-cell lymphoma with discordant morphology between lymph node and bone marrow. A, Trephine biopsy section contains several paratrabecular lymphoid infiltrates composed of small cells. **B,** Lymph node contains diffuse large B-cell lymphoma.

In a significant percentage of cases (up to 40%), DLBCL in a lymph node or extranodal tissue may exhibit discordant morphology from the lymphoma observed in the bone marrow.[6,52,53] In these cases the bone marrow usually exhibits a less aggressive histology, with the lymphoma composed entirely of small cells with condensed chromatin or a mixture of small and large cells (Fig. 57-23).[53,104] Two thirds of these discordant lymphomas exhibit identical monoclonal *IGH@* or *BCL2* gene rearrangements in the bone marrow infiltrates and the extramedullary large B-cell lymphoma, supporting the origin of both lymphomas from a single B-cell clone. About one third of these discordant, indolent bone marrow lymphomas are unrelated to the extramedullary DLBCL, as evidenced by the presence of distinct *IGH@* or *BCL2* gene rearrangements and gene sequences in both lymphomas.[105] In up to 40% of cases the infiltrates are paratrabecular, a histologic feature that helps support the conclusion that the more indolent-appearing lesions are lymphoma,[48] particularly because reactive lymphoid infiltrates may also occur in the bone marrow of patients with lymphoma at extramedullary sites.[105] Patients with discordant (indolent) lymphoma in the bone marrow have better overall survival rates than those with large cell lymphoma in the marrow. Extensive bone marrow infiltration by lymphoma (>70% infiltrate) or a diffuse infiltrative pattern composed of more than 50% large cells is also associated with a poor prognosis.[52,104]

A subset of DLBCL, T-cell/histiocyte-rich lymphoma, exhibits relatively few large neoplastic B cells admixed with numerous small T cells with or without histiocytes[106]; these lymphomas occasionally involve the bone marrow and may be difficult to distinguish from other lymphomas, especially peripheral T-cell lymphoma (Fig. 57-24) and Hodgkin's lymphoma. Immunostains showing that the large abnormal cells are B cells ($CD20^+$, $CD79a^+$, or $PAX5^+$ and $CD3^-$) that are $CD45^+$, $CD30^-$, and $CD15^-$ are useful to exclude both peripheral T-cell lymphoma and classical Hodgkin's lymphoma.

Mediastinal large B-cell lymphoma is a subset of DLBCL that arises in the mediastinum and has a female predominance.[107] Bone marrow involvement has been reported (3% to 9%), but the characteristics of marrow infiltration have not been described in detail.[108]

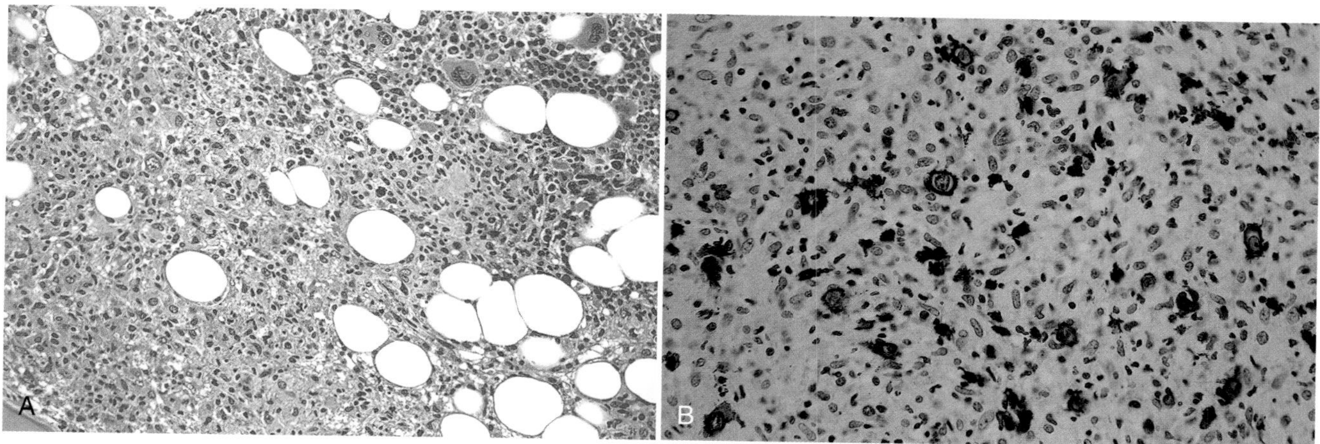

Figure 57-24. Diffuse large B-cell lymphoma, T-cell/histiocyte-rich subtype, involving the bone marrow. A, The infiltrate has poorly defined borders and contains histiocytes, many small lymphocytes, and scattered large, abnormal lymphocytes. **B,** CD20 immunostain highlights the scattered large lymphoma cells that constitute only a small part of the infiltrate. The majority of the cells are $CD3^+$ T cells (not shown).

Intravascular Large B-Cell Lymphoma

Intravascular large B-cell lymphoma is an uncommon variant of extranodal large B-cell lymphoma. The lymphoma cells preferentially localize within the lumens of small blood vessels and are usually widely disseminated, including to the bone marrow.[109] Rarely, bone marrow may be the initial diagnostic site.[110,111] Involved bone marrow sections exhibit intrasinusoidal lymphoma cells that can be highlighted by immunostains to B-cell–associated markers such as CD20 and CD79a.[17] In general, intravascular large B-cell lymphoma cells do not form extravascular tumor masses. Rarely, lymphoma cells are identified in peripheral blood or bone marrow aspirate smears; they are large lymphocytes with irregular nuclei and basophilic cytoplasm that is occasionally vacuolated (Fig. 57-25).

Analysis of intravascular large B-cell lymphoma using conventional G-banding combined with multicolor karyotyping has identified a complex abnormal karyotype characterized by structural rearrangements involving additions, deletions, duplications, inversions, and cryptic translocations.[112] Common recurring alterations include monosomy 6/6q– (59%) and trisomy 18/duplication (18q) (41%); the deleted region of chromosome 6 is often 6q21-q23, similar to findings in other DLBCLs.

Primary Effusion Lymphoma

Primary effusion lymphoma (also known as *body cavity–based lymphoma*) is a large B-cell lymphoma that most commonly occurs in the setting of immunodeficiency. Tumor masses do not occur outside body cavities. Bone marrow involvement has not been reported.

Burkitt's Lymphoma

Burkitt's lymphoma involves the bone marrow in 30% to 60% of cases, most often with a diffuse or interstitial pattern of infiltration.[10,87] Burkitt's lymphoma may also present with a leukemic picture. The cells are medium sized, with reticular chromatin, multiple small nucleoli, and moderate amounts of basophilic cytoplasm. Intracytoplasmic vacuoles, representing dissolved lipid, are often present and are best appreciated in aspirate smears (Fig. 57-26), touch preparations, or peripheral blood. Mitoses are abundant, and bone marrow necrosis is common; the "starry sky" pattern typically seen at extramedullary sites can also be present.

B-Lymphoblastic Leukemia/Lymphoma

B-lymphoblastic lymphoma has an identical morphology and phenotype to precursor B-cell acute lymphoblastic leukemia; the distinction between the two is arbitrary. The designation *lymphoblastic lymphoma* is used when the patient presents with an extramedullary mass, commonly in the skin, soft tissues, or lymph nodes; bone marrow involvement is absent, or the blasts account for less than 25% of the hematopoietic cells in the bone marrow.[113-115] B-lymphoblastic lymphoma usually infiltrates the bone marrow in a focal random pattern. The

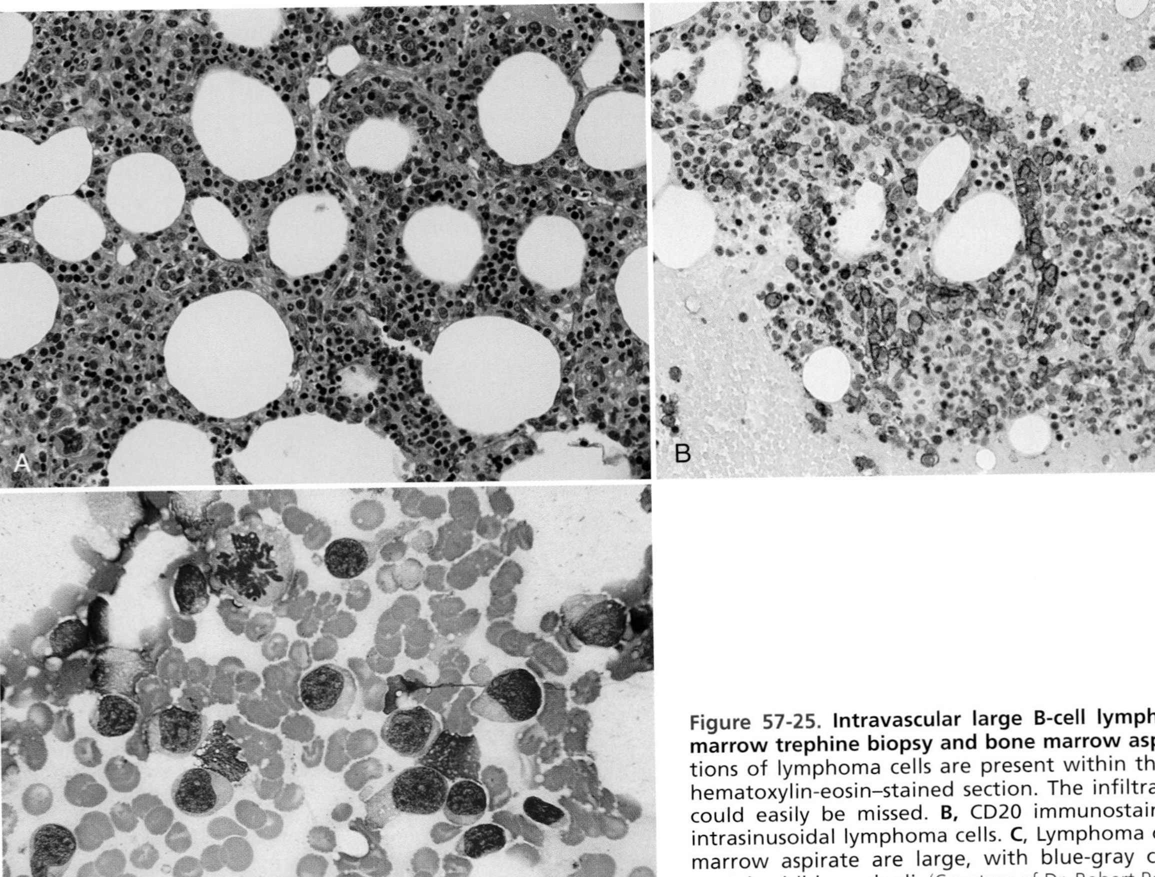

Figure 57-25. Intravascular large B-cell lymphoma in a bone marrow trephine biopsy and bone marrow aspirate. A, Collections of lymphoma cells are present within the sinuses of the hematoxylin-eosin–stained section. The infiltrate is subtle and could easily be missed. **B,** CD20 immunostain highlights the intrasinusoidal lymphoma cells. **C,** Lymphoma cells in the bone marrow aspirate are large, with blue-gray cytoplasm; many contain visible nucleoli. (Courtesy of Dr. Robert Pooley, Department of Pathology, Little Company of Mary Hospital, Evergreen Park, IL.)

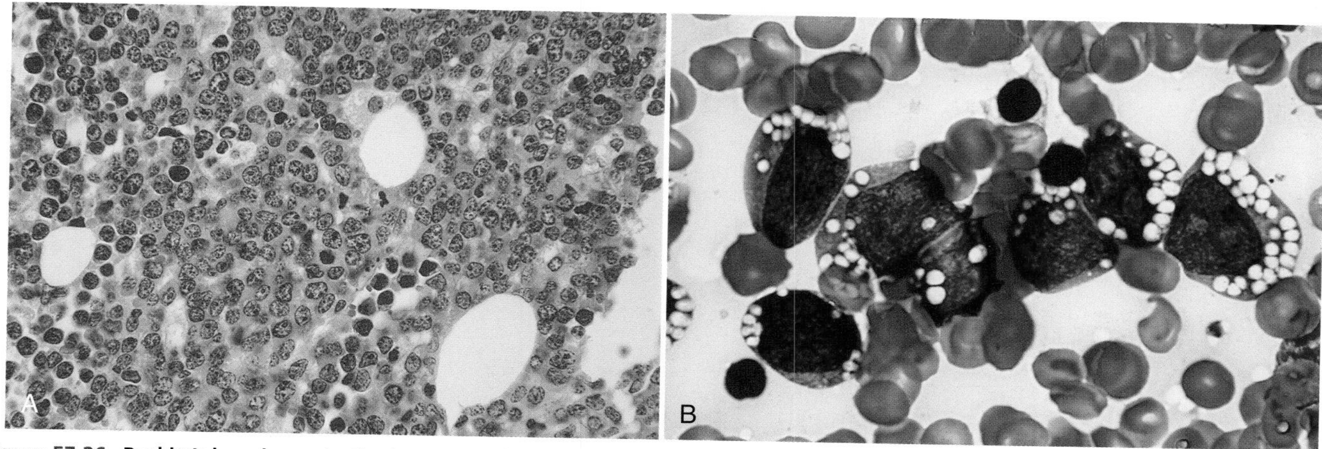

Figure 57-26. Burkitt's lymphoma in the bone marrow. A, Bone marrow trephine biopsy section contains a diffuse infiltrate of medium-sized cells with several small visible nucleoli, round nuclei, and an ample amount of cytoplasm. Note the mitoses. **B,** Bone marrow aspirate contains lymphoma cells with multiple vacuoles in their cytoplasm.

malignant cells are small to medium sized, with fine chromatin patterns, scant cytoplasm, absent to several small nucleoli, and frequent mitoses. When patients with acute leukemia are excluded, malignant cells are rarely detected in the peripheral blood and bone marrow aspirate at diagnosis, but they may be numerous if more extensive bone marrow involvement develops during the course of the disease.[116] B-lymphoblastic lymphoma can be difficult to distinguish from more mature B-cell neoplasms that involve the marrow extensively, such as the blastic variant of MCL. Immunophenotypic analysis is crucial in making this distinction; the demonstration of terminal deoxynucleotidyl transferase (TdT) or CD34 can exclude a more mature B-cell neoplasm.

CHARACTERISTIC FEATURES OF T-CELL LYMPHOMAS INVOLVING BONE MARROW

T-Lymphoblastic Leukemia/Lymphoma

The cells of T-lymphoblastic lymphoma are virtually identical to those of T-cell acute lymphoblastic leukemia. Overall, lymphoblastic lymphoma more commonly has a T-cell than a B-cell phenotype.[117,118] The designation *lymphoblastic lymphoma* is used when bone marrow involvement is absent or there is minimal involvement, with less than 25% blasts. When bone marrow is involved, the bone marrow biopsy shows focal random infiltrates of blasts with scant cytoplasm. Blasts range from small to large cells with dispersed or condensed chromatin and may have convoluted nuclei (Fig. 57-27).

Extranodal NK/T-Cell Lymphoma

Extranodal NK/T-cell lymphoma frequently arises in the nasal cavity and is called *nasal NK/T-cell lymphoma*.[119] *Nasal-type NK/T-cell lymphoma* refers to a similar lymphoma that presents outside the nasal cavity—commonly in the skin, nasopharynx, or testis. The cytology of the tumor cells varies from case to case; they can be small, medium sized, large, or a combination of sizes. The nuclei are irregular and pleomorphic. The cytoplasm is pale and moderately abundant; azurophilic granules are apparent in some cases. Epstein-Barr virus is demonstrable in almost all cases of both nasal and nasal-type NK/T-cell lymphomas.[120] Both nasal and nasal-type NK/T-cell tumors are surface $CD3^-$ but are positive for intracytoplasmic CD3ε in paraffin sections. Hemophagocytic syndrome manifesting as fever, pancytopenia, abnormal liver function tests, and bone marrow hemophagocytosis has been described in both nasal and nasal-type NK/T-cell lymphomas.[121,122]

Bone marrow involvement by nasal NK/T-cell lymphoma is subtle and uncommon (up to 8% of cases).[58] However, it is important to recognize marrow involvement because it is associated with early death. Typically, single lymphoma cells are found scattered in interstitial areas among the normal bone marrow elements.[58] They may be difficult to identify on H&E-stained sections, but in situ hybridization for Epstein-Barr virus–encoded RNA (EBER) or immunostains for CD56 can be used to demonstrate these isolated cells (Fig. 57-28). Although neither EBER in situ hybridization nor CD56 is specific for lymphoma cells, the normal bone marrow contains only a few NK cells and rarely contains $EBER^+$ cells. CD3 is less helpful because T cells are common in the bone marrow;

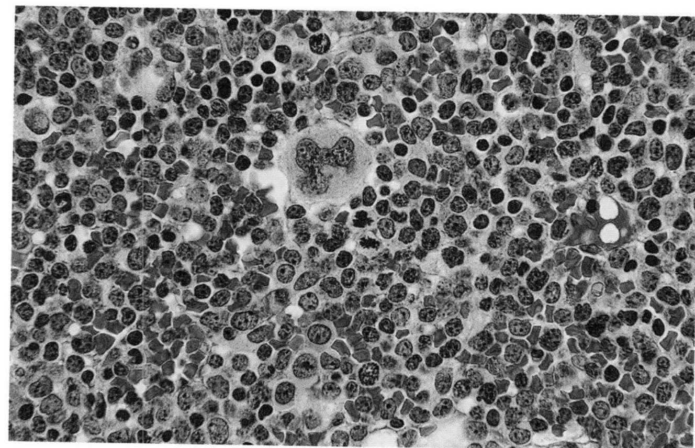

Figure 57-27. T-lymphoblastic leukemia/lymphoma involving the bone marrow. Bone marrow trephine biopsy demonstrates that the infiltrate has a diffuse growth pattern, replaces nearly all the normal hematopoietic elements, and is composed of variably sized lymphoma cells with dispersed chromatin. Note the mitoses within the infiltrate. A megakaryocyte is present in the infiltrate.

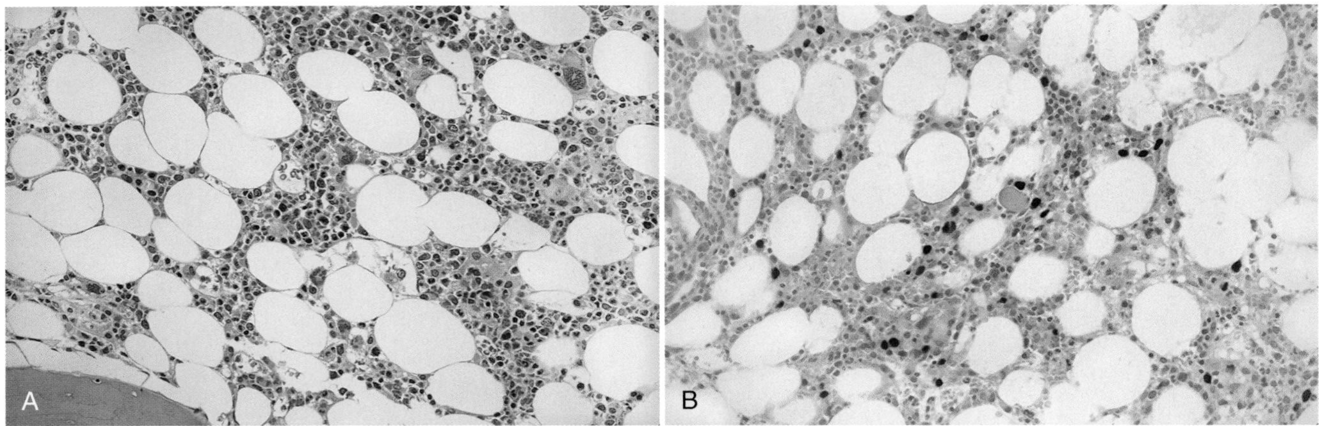

Figure 57-28. Nasal NK/T-cell lymphoma involving the bone marrow. A, The tumor cells are difficult to appreciate in hematoxylin-eosin–stained trephine biopsy sections. **B,** In situ hybridization for Epstein-Barr virus–encoded RNA (EBER) highlights the scattered tumor cells.

however, it may be helpful when morphologically abnormal $CD3^+$ tumor cells are identified.

In contrast to nasal NK/T-cell lymphoma, which is usually localized to the upper aerodigestive tract at presentation, most patients (80%) with nasal-type NK/T-cell lymphoma occurring outside the nasal cavity present with advanced disease involving multiple anatomic sites. In 15% to 25% of cases the bone marrow is involved by lymphoma.[58,121-123] The pattern of bone marrow infiltration has not been described in detail; however, we have observed bone marrow involvement by testicular nasal-type NK/T-cell lymphoma. The bone marrow contained scattered lymphoma cells in the interstitial areas among the normal hematopoietic elements, a pattern similar to that reported with nasal NK/T-cell lymphoma.

Enteropathy-Type T-Cell Lymphoma

Enteropathy-type T-cell lymphoma typically arises in the small intestine as a complication of long-standing celiac disease.[124] Bone marrow involvement has not been described.

Hepatosplenic T-Cell Lymphoma

Hepatosplenic T-cell lymphoma is a rare, aggressive peripheral T-cell lymphoma that occurs primarily in young adult males who present with marked splenomegaly and the absence of lymphadenopathy.[55] Affected patients often have anemia and thrombocytopenia.[14,15,55,125] The bone marrow and peripheral blood are almost always involved, although the number of circulating lymphoma cells is usually insufficient to cause an absolute lymphocytosis in the blood.[125] Bone marrow trephine biopsy sections are often hypercellular, with a subtle and predominantly intrasinusoidal infiltrate that is difficult to appreciate without immunohistochemical stains; interstitial infiltrates may also occur. The cytology of hepatosplenic T-cell lymphoma cells is similar in the blood and aspirate smears; they vary from medium-sized cells with moderately dispersed chromatin and conspicuous nucleoli, resembling blasts, to small lymphocytes with condensed chromatin and irregular nuclei.[55,125] Immunophenotyping shows that hepatosplenic T-cell lymphoma cells are mature, cytotoxic T cells that are $CD4^-$, $CD8^{+/-}$, and TIA-1^+ and express CD56, one of the NK-cell–associated markers. Most cases are positive for T-cell receptor gamma-delta, but cases positive for T-cell receptor alpha-beta also occur.[14,15] Isochromosome 7q is identified in 66% to 100% of evaluated cases.[125,126]

Subcutaneous Panniculitis-Like T-Cell Lymphoma

Subcutaneous panniculitis-like T-cell lymphoma is a rare neoplasm of cytotoxic ($CD8^+$) T cells that has a predilection for subcutaneous tissue.[127] The tumor remains localized and does not involve the bone marrow. Frequently, cases are complicated by pancytopenia related to hemophagocytic syndrome; in these cases the bone marrow exhibits features of hemophagocytic syndrome, including abundant histiocytes with hemophagocytosis.[128]

Mycosis Fungoides and Sézary Syndrome

Mycosis fungoides is a primary cutaneous T-cell lymphoma that generally remains localized for years.[129] Sézary syndrome is a rare disorder characterized by diffuse erythroderma, lymphadenopathy, and circulating lymphoma cells (Sézary cells).[130] An early report indicated that mycosis fungoides involves the bone marrow in up to 25% of patients at initial diagnosis,[56] but in a more recent study, only 1 in 60 patients (<2%)—53 with mycosis fungoides and 7 with Sézary syndrome—had bone marrow involvement at initial staging.[131] Borderline or atypical lesions not diagnostic of lymphoma were common in both studies (19 of 50 [38%] and 8 of 60 [13%]). With these borderline lesions, it was difficult to obtain a consistent neoplastic classification among different observers.[131] The extent of bone marrow infiltration is usually minimal to mild in patients with disseminated disease.[56,132] The infiltrates are focal random or interstitial, or both. Paratrabecular and diffuse infiltrates are rare.[133] The infiltrates are composed primarily of variably sized abnormal lymphocytes with convoluted nuclei, and they are often subtle and difficult to recognize on H&E-stained sections. Immunohistochemical stains for T-cell–associated markers, such as CD3, aid in the recognition of lymphoma cells (Fig. 57-29), but even with immunostains, in some studies there is poor agreement between histologic-immunophenotypic detection

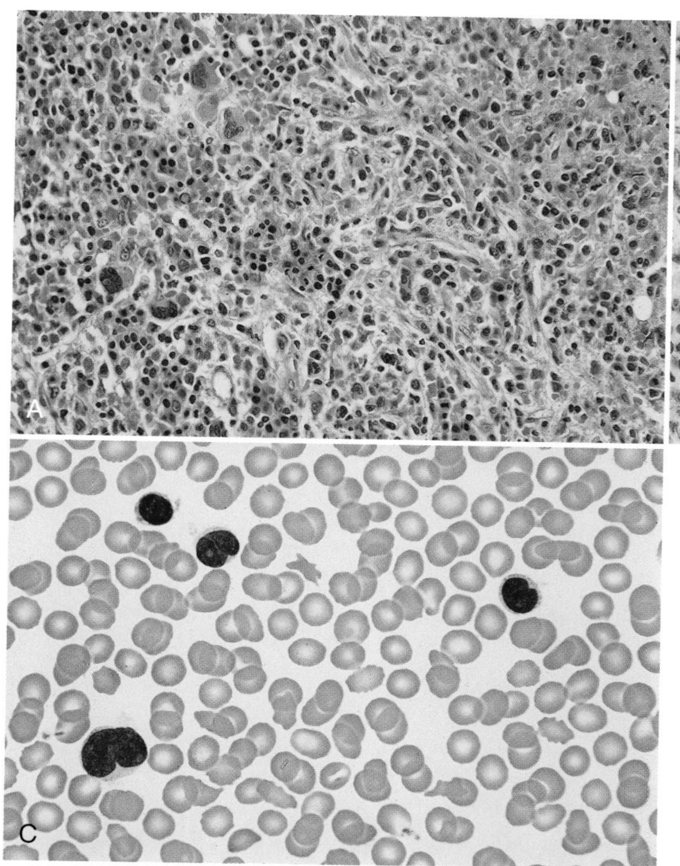

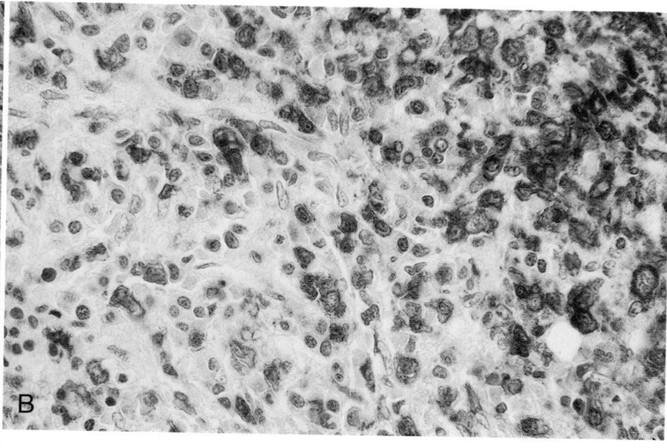

Figure 57-29. Cutaneous T-cell lymphoma (Sézary syndrome) in the bone marrow and peripheral blood. A, Hematoxylin-eosin–stained section show a focal lymphomatous infiltrate in loose stroma, with poorly demarcated margins. **B,** CD3 immunohistochemical stain accentuates the variably sized T cells within the infiltrate. **C,** Lymphoma cells in the peripheral blood vary in size but are larger than small, mature lymphocytes; they have less condensed chromatin, with cerebriform nuclei and indistinct nucleoli.

of disease and molecular studies for T-cell clonality.[134] Eosinophilia isolated to the bone marrow is present in some patients.

The number of circulating lymphoma cells in Sézary syndrome is highly variable, ranging from occasional cells to a frankly leukemic picture with an elevated white blood cell count. The malignant lymphocytes may be small or large with variable amounts of cytoplasm. The nuclei are characterized by striking convolutions that may give them a cerebriform appearance; nucleoli are absent or inconspicuous (see Fig. 57-29). Occasionally Sézary cells exhibit cytoplasmic vacuoles encircling the nuclei; the vacuoles are periodic acid–Schiff positive. The lymphoma cells have a characteristic immunophenotype and are typically $CD3^+$, may show a lack of staining with one of the pan–T-cell antigens (often CD7), and are $CD4^+$, $CD8^-$, and $CD26^-$ (Fig. 57-30).

Angioimmunoblastic T-Cell Lymphoma

Angioimmunoblastic T-cell lymphoma involves the bone marrow in 50% to 80% of cases.[18] The bone marrow infiltrates have a morphologic appearance similar to that of involved lymph nodes. The infiltrates are typically focal random, with infiltrative margins, and are less cellular than the surrounding uninvolved marrow. Paratrabecular infiltrates have been reported but are less common; diffuse infiltrates are exceedingly rare.[18,135] Reticulin fibrosis is usually prominent.[135] The cellular composition of the infiltrate is heterogeneous and consists of lymphocytes, immunoblasts, plasma cells, a variable number of histiocytes, eosinophils, and numerous small blood vessels (Fig. 57-31).

The peripheral blood findings in angioimmunoblastic T-cell lymphoma vary,[135,136] but anemia is found in the majority of patients (85%), neutrophilia in up to 50%, and eosinophilia in nearly 25%; thrombocytopenia is occasionally present. Circulating plasma cells, lymphocytes with plasmacytoid features, and immunoblasts are present in one third of patients. Bone marrow aspirate smears are usually cellular, with increased numbers of myeloid or erythroid elements as well as plasma cells and plasmacytoid lymphocytes. Small mature lymphocytes are usually decreased, and eosinophils are occasionally increased.

Peripheral T-Cell Lymphoma, Not Otherwise Specified

Peripheral T-cell lymphomas generally have a high incidence (80%) of bone marrow involvement at diagnosis.[54] The bone marrow infiltrates are diffuse in slightly more than 50% of cases and are focal, nonparatrabecular in about 40%; they are typically associated with prominent vascularity and reticulin fibrosis.[135,137,138] As with many other peripheral T-cell lymphomas, the lesions tend to be less sharply demarcated than B-cell lymphomas and intercalate into the surrounding normal marrow (Fig. 57-32). The lymphoma cells are variably sized, often with convoluted or irregular nuclei and usually indistinct nucleoli; they are frequently present in a polymorphic infiltrate that includes immunoblasts, many histiocytes,

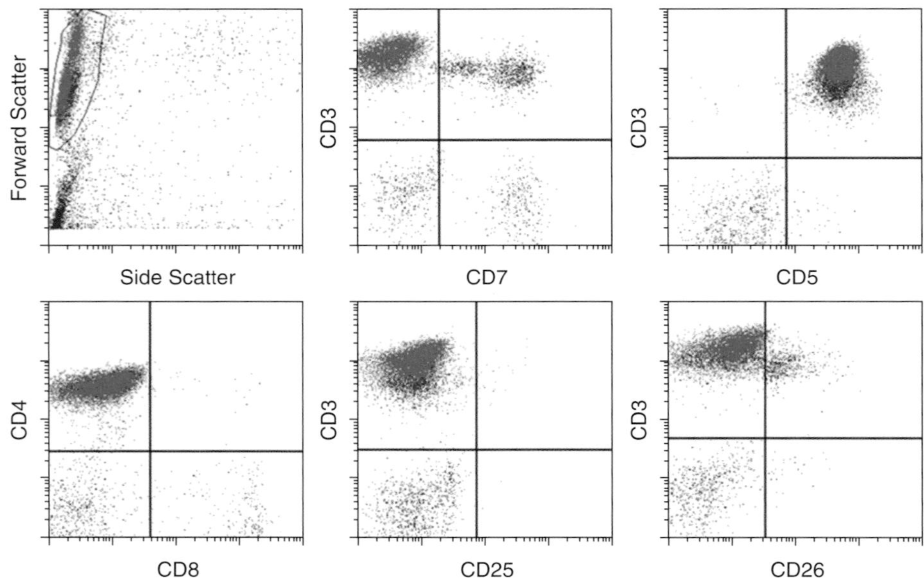

Figure 57-30. Sézary syndrome. Flow cytometric immunophenotyping histograms demonstrate a population of lymphoma cells (*red*) with an aberrant T-cell phenotype. The cells display high forward scatter, indicating that they are large. They are CD3^{+}, CD5^{+}, CD7^{-}, CD4^{+}, CD8^{-}, CD25^{-}, and CD26^{-}.

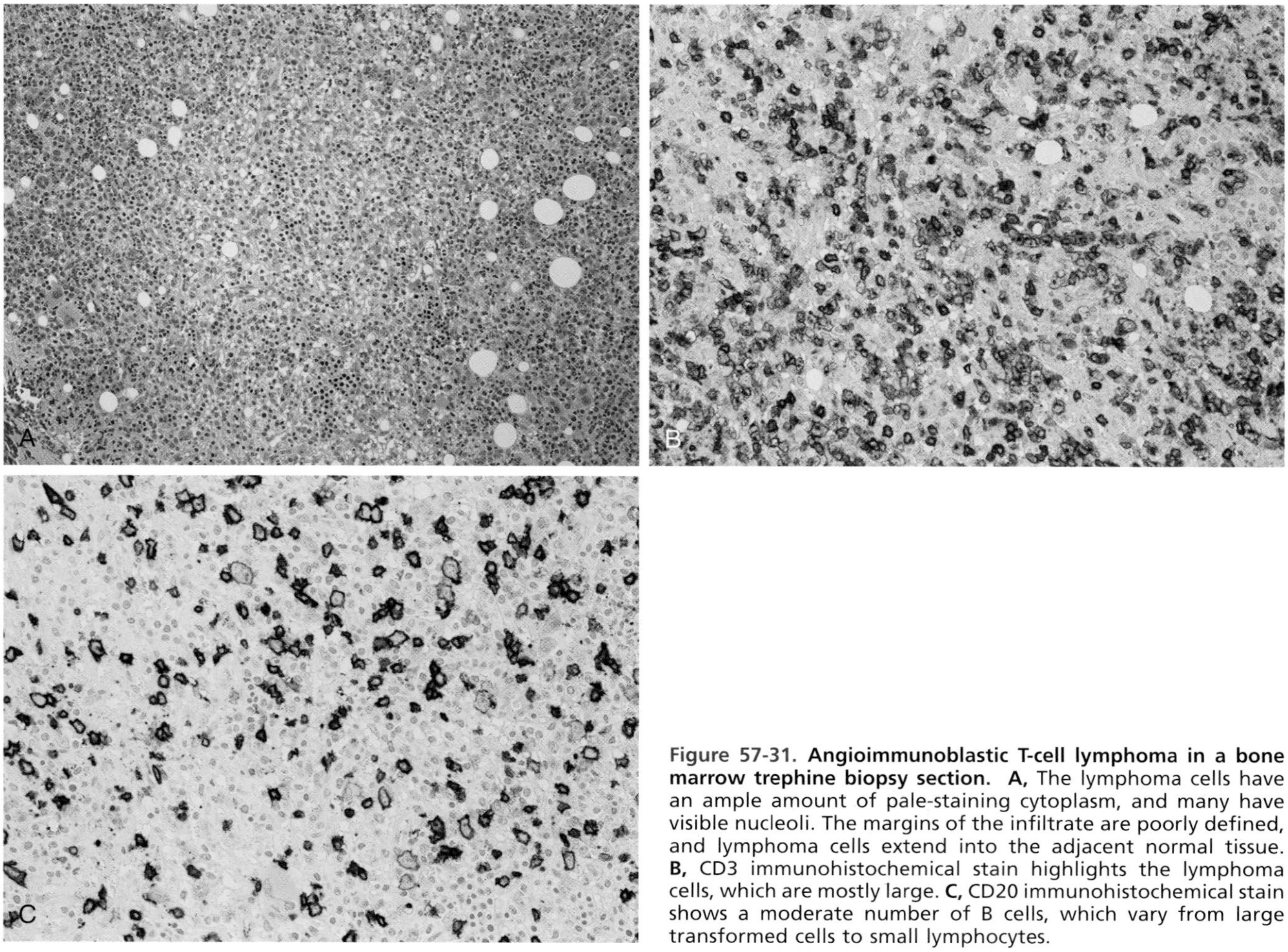

Figure 57-31. Angioimmunoblastic T-cell lymphoma in a bone marrow trephine biopsy section. A, The lymphoma cells have an ample amount of pale-staining cytoplasm, and many have visible nucleoli. The margins of the infiltrate are poorly defined, and lymphoma cells extend into the adjacent normal tissue. **B,** CD3 immunohistochemical stain highlights the lymphoma cells, which are mostly large. **C,** CD20 immunohistochemical stain shows a moderate number of B cells, which vary from large transformed cells to small lymphocytes.

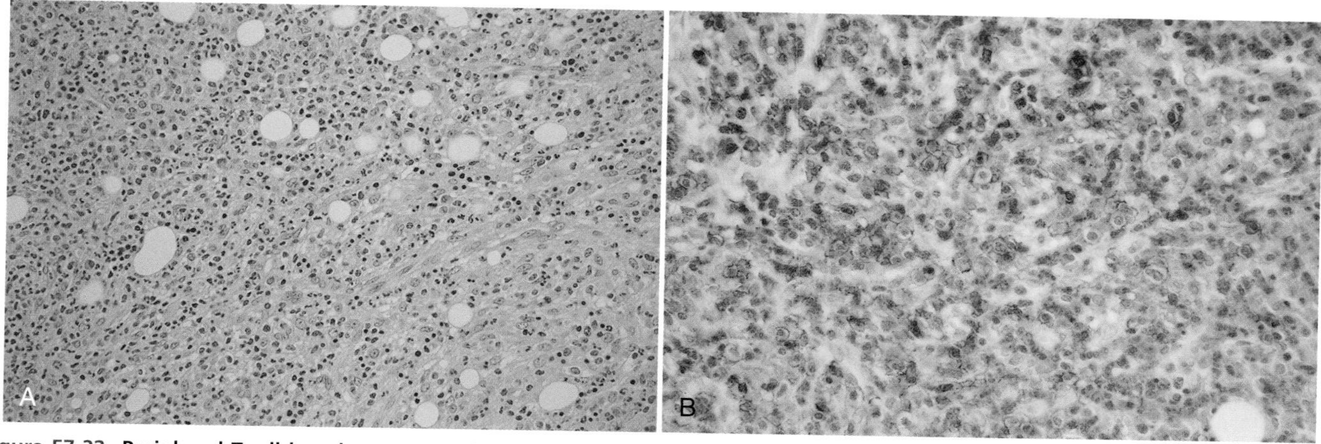

Figure 57-32. Peripheral T-cell lymphoma, not otherwise specified, in the bone marrow. A, Hematoxylin-eosin–stained section demonstrates an infiltrate with poorly circumscribed margins, many small blood vessels, and less intense staining than the adjacent normal bone marrow. **B,** CD3 immunohistochemical stain highlights the majority of lymphocytes within the infiltrate.

eosinophils, and plasma cells. The extent of disease within the bone marrow can be difficult to determine from H&E-stained sections, although immunostains with antibodies directed against T-cell antigens can aid in the assessment.

Lymphoma cells are present in the aspirate smears in most cases (70%) with bone marrow involvement; they vary from occasional to numerous (>90%) and are morphologically similar to those in trephine biopsy sections, with the exception that large lymphoma cells are usually rare in the aspirate.[54] Circulating lymphoma cells are present in about 30% of cases; rarely, a marked leukocytosis is present.[54] Eosinophilia may be present. Circulating lymphoma cells are similar to those in the bone marrow and are small, medium sized, or large, with convoluted and nonconvoluted nuclei; nucleoli are generally indistinct in the small lymphoma cells but may be visible in medium-sized and large cells.

Anaplastic Large Cell Lymphoma

Anaplastic large cell lymphoma involves the bone marrow in about 40% of cases.[57,139] The infiltrates are focal random or diffuse, or they may occur as small clusters of cells or isolated single cells. Isolated lymphoma cells are often difficult to identify among the normal immature hematopoietic elements when only routine H&E-stained sections are examined, but they can be highlighted by immunostains using antibodies to ALK-1, CD30, or epithelial membrane antigen (EMA) (Fig. 57-33). In one study using immunostains, lymphoma cells were found in 23% of patients with negative bone marrow by routine histology.[57] It is important to identify bone marrow involvement by anaplastic large cell lymphoma, even when subtle, because it is associated with a poor prognosis. The lymphoma cells are large but variably sized (ranging from the size of a promyelocyte to that of a megakaryocyte); they have irregular nuclei with dispersed chromatin, multiple prominent nucleoli, and abundant basophilic, occasionally vacuolated cytoplasm. In occasional cases tumor cells can be found in the peripheral blood (see Fig. 57-33) and bone marrow aspirate smears; rarely, the peripheral blood exhibits numerous circulating lymphoma cells.[140-142] The circulating lymphoma cells have a similar morphology to those in the core biopsy section.[141]

CHARACTERISTICS OF HODGKIN'S LYMPHOMA INVOLVING BONE MARROW

The overall incidence of Hodgkin's lymphoma (HL) involving the bone marrow at diagnosis is 5% to 15%.[10,47,48] The frequency of bone marrow involvement varies according to the HL subtype. Mixed cellularity HL involves the bone marrow in approximately 22% of cases at diagnosis,[143] nodular sclerosis HL involves the bone marrow at diagnosis in slightly less than 10% of cases, and lymphocyte-predominant HL almost never involves the bone marrow at diagnosis.[47,144] Lymphocyte-depleted HL reportedly has the highest incidence of bone marrow involvement. However, both the overall incidence of lymphocyte-depleted HL and the incidence of bone marrow involvement are lower than previously thought, owing to the recognition and exclusion of some carcinomas and non-Hodgkin's lymphomas that were diagnosed as lymphocyte-depleted HL before the routine use of immunohistochemical studies.[143]

Patients with HL who present with constitutional symptoms such as weight loss and fever are more likely to have bone marrow disease. Bone marrow involvement by HL represents stage IV disease. The value of routine bone marrow staging of all patients is controversial because the incidence of bone marrow involvement is less than 1% in patients with clinical stage IA or IIA disease. The bone marrow is more likely to be involved in patients with higher-stage disease, and biopsies in this group may provide additional prognostic information.[145]

In rare cases bone marrow is the primary diagnostic tissue in HL; this occurs most often in patients with AIDS.[146-148] HIV$^+$ patients who are diagnosed with HL in the bone marrow often present with peripheral blood cytopenias. HL is isolated to the bone marrow at diagnosis in approximately 14% of cases[148]; these patients lack lymphadenopathy and usually do not develop HL at extramedullary sites during the course of the disease.

Trephine biopsy is the procedure of choice for the diagnosis or staging of HL. The aspirate is insensitive for the detection of HL.[145] Reed-Sternberg cells are usually absent in aspirate smears, although they can be identified in rare cases

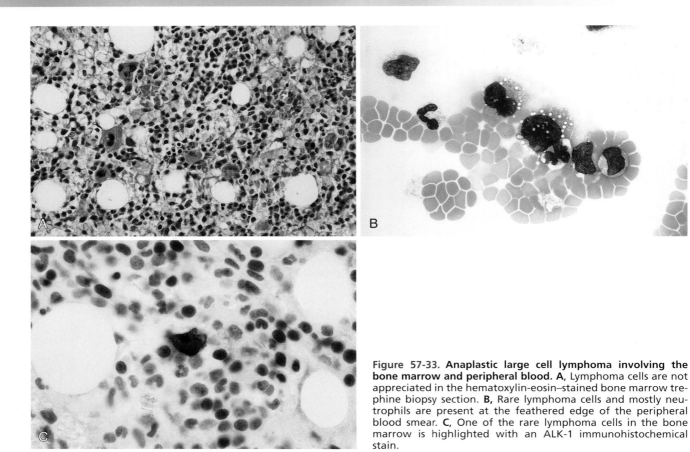

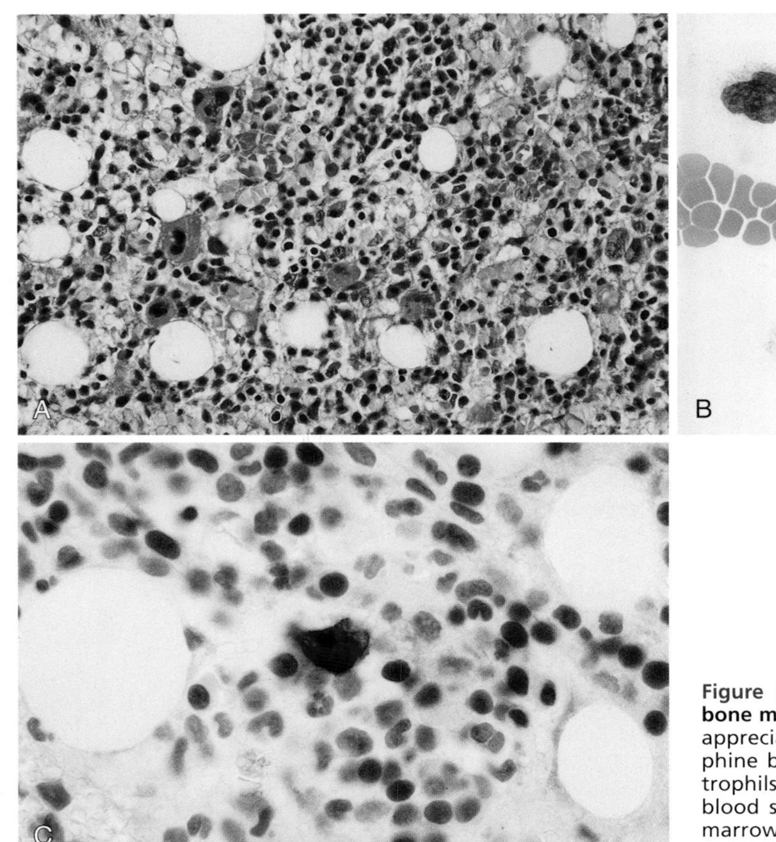

Figure 57-33. **Anaplastic large cell lymphoma involving the bone marrow and peripheral blood. A,** Lymphoma cells are not appreciated in the hematoxylin-eosin–stained bone marrow trephine biopsy section. **B,** Rare lymphoma cells and mostly neutrophils are present at the feathered edge of the peripheral blood smear. **C,** One of the rare lymphoma cells in the bone marrow is highlighted with an ALK-1 immunohistochemical stain.

with extensive bone marrow involvement. HL in the bone marrow is characterized by discrete, space-occupying lesions that are usually clearly demarcated from normal bone marrow tissue. Focal involvement is present in about 30% of cases; the infiltrates may be single or multiple, random or paratrabecular. Diffuse bone marrow involvement is present in about 70% of cases (Fig. 57-34).[10] The infiltrates are polymorphic and frequently contain a prominent component of small lymphocytes, histiocytes, plasma cells, and eosinophils (Fig. 57-35). Reed-Sternberg cells or variants are almost always present, although in some cases, multiple sections must be examined to find diagnostic neoplastic cells. Fibrosis is almost always present in the infiltrate and may be prominent, especially in diffuse lesions. Necrosis may be present and is more common in treated patients.

Historically, the criteria for diagnosing HL in the bone marrow varied, depending on whether the bone marrow was the initial diagnostic site.[149,150] HL can be diagnosed in the

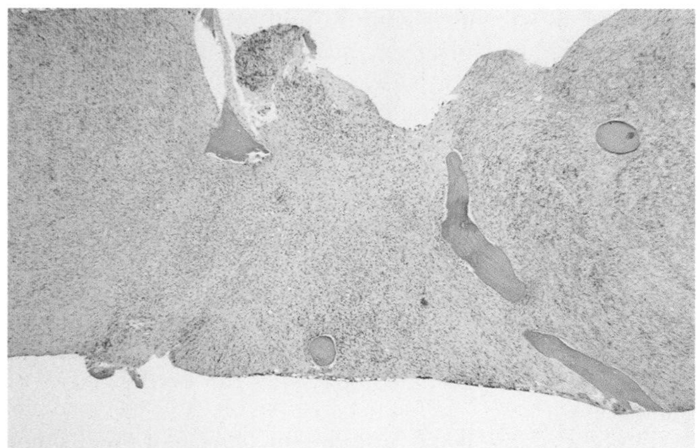

Figure 57-34. **Hodgkin's lymphoma in the bone marrow.** The diffuse infiltrate completely replaces the normal hematopoietic elements in the bone marrow.

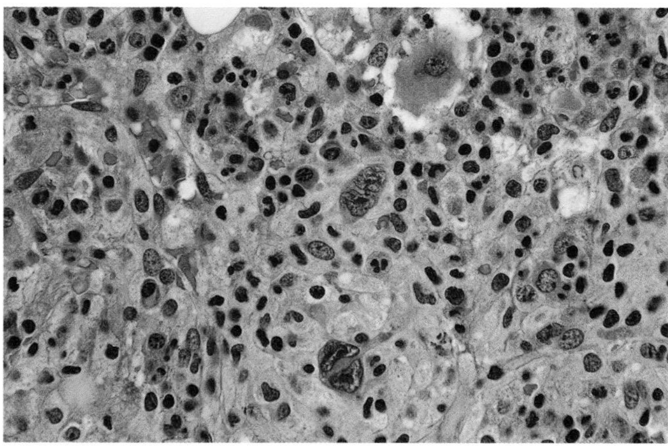

Figure 57-35. **Hodgkin's lymphoma in the bone marrow.** The lymphomatous infiltrate is polymorphic and contains Reed-Sternberg cells, small lymphocytes, histiocytes, plasma cells, and neutrophils.

bone marrow when Reed-Sternberg cells are found in a cellular environment characteristic of HL. When classic Reed-Sternberg cells are identified at another anatomic site, mononuclear Reed-Sternberg variants in an environment characteristic of HL is sufficient for diagnosis, even if classic Reed-Sternberg cells are not present in the bone marrow. Atypical cells (i.e., not classic Reed-Sternberg cells or mononuclear variants) in a patient with histologically proven HL elsewhere are suspicious for bone marrow involvement. Foci of fibrosis without Reed-Sternberg cells or mononuclear variants are suspicious for HL in patients with HL diagnosed at another site. In current practice, when abnormal cells with the characteristic immunophenotype of Hodgkin cells are identified in the bone marrow in the correct cellular background, detection of morphologically classic Reed-Sternberg cells is not always necessary for a primary diagnosis of HL.

HL in the bone marrow is not subclassified. The small sample size and variability of histopathology between lymph node and bone marrow make subclassification unreliable.[149] Patients with HL occasionally have granulomas in one or more organs, including the bone marrow, but granulomas are not sufficient to diagnose HL. Areas of bone marrow that are not involved by HL frequently exhibit other nonspecific changes, including granulocytic hyperplasia, eosinophilia, plasmacytosis, and increased numbers of megakaryocytes. Areas of bone marrow not involved by HL in AIDS-related cases may show pronounced fibrosis.

Non-Hodgkin's lymphomas such as anaplastic large cell lymphoma, T-cell–rich DLBCL, and peripheral T-cell lymphoma may mimic HL in the bone marrow. In addition, HL infiltrates may exhibit a granulomatous appearance and be mistaken for a benign infiltrative process. HL must be differentiated from reactive polymorphic lymphohistiocytic lesions, which are commonly encountered in the bone marrow of patients with immunodeficiency disorders such as AIDS.[44,45] Appropriate immunohistochemical stains allow this distinction. The demonstration of "atypical" cells that are negative for B-cell– and T-cell–associated markers, as well as $CD45^-$, EMA^-, and ALK-1^- but $CD30^+$ and $CD15^+$, supports the diagnosis of HL. In equivocal cases, biopsy of the lymph node or other tissue may be necessary.

EVALUATION OF BONE MARROW SPECIMENS FROM PATIENTS WITH AN ESTABLISHED DIAGNOSIS OF LYMPHOMA

Bone marrow biopsies are commonly performed in patients who have been diagnosed with lymphoma to determine the stage of disease and extent of bone marrow involvement; they may be repeated to evaluate response to therapy or disease progression.

Lymphoid infiltrates encountered in the bone marrow of patients with an established diagnosis of lymphoma at an extramedullary site are determined to be benign or malignant using the criteria discussed earlier (see the section on distinguishing benign lymphoid infiltrates from malignant lymphoma). As noted previously, this morphologic distinction is not always straightforward and may require the use of ancillary techniques such as immunohistochemistry, flow cytometric immunophenotyping, and molecular analysis. When a bone marrow specimen is examined for staging purposes, it is important to know the specific type of lymphoma present in the lymph node or other extramedullary sites; this may influence which ancillary techniques, if any, are required to evaluate the bone marrow. For instance, immunostains may be necessary to detect the lymphoma cells of anaplastic large cell lymphoma and NK/T-cell lymphoma because single lymphoma cells can infiltrate the bone marrow, making them difficult to appreciate in routine H&E-stained sections. Intrasinusoidal infiltrates commonly associated with splenic marginal zone lymphoma and hepatosplenic T-cell lymphoma are also best appreciated with immunostains that are capable of highlighting the malignant cells or endothelial cells.

When lymphoma is identified, the extent of bone marrow involvement should be noted by estimating the percentage of hematopoietic elements the lymphomatous infiltrate constitutes. In addition, morphologic concordance or discordance with the initial diagnostic specimen should be noted. In most cases both sites have similar morphology. However, 20% to 40% of cases show discordant morphology between the lymphoma in the bone marrow and that in the extramedullary site.[6,52] Follicular lymphomas and large B-cell lymphomas most commonly exhibit discordant morphology (see Fig. 57-23), with the less aggressive component usually present in the bone marrow.[52] The reasons for this discrepant morphology are not well understood, but postulated mechanisms include the presence of two or more unrelated tumors, preferential recirculation of the less aggressive lymphoma, tumor evolution from one histologic subtype to another, and differences in the microenvironment of the bone marrow and extramedullary sites.[6,53,105] Better remission rates and longer survival have been demonstrated for patients with diffuse large cell lymphoma at an extramedullary site and discordant bone marrow involvement than for those with concordant disease.[53]

Special consideration is needed for bone marrow specimens obtained following therapy. Posttherapy bone marrow biopsies should be compared with prior specimens to determine whether the extent of bone marrow involvement by lymphoma has changed. Some therapies such as colony-stimulating factor can impact interpretation. For example, early in the course of granulocyte colony-stimulating factor therapy, the bone marrow frequently exhibits a marked myeloid shift to immaturity, with a predominance of promyelocytes.[151] Trephine biopsy sections may contain sheets of promyelocytes, often in a paratrabecular location, that can closely mimic lymphoma, particularly large cell lymphoma (Fig. 57-36). Knowledge of the history of growth factor therapy can aid in the distinction from lymphoma. If the history is not provided, characteristic changes associated with growth factor therapy, such as severe toxic changes in peripheral blood neutrophils and a shift to immaturity in the blood and aspirate, can also alert one to this possibility. Evaluating the aspirate and touch preparation for lymphoma cells may also be helpful. Well-prepared histologic sections that allow observation of the morphologic features of promyelocytes, including granules, are essential. Immunostains for myeloperoxidase, CD20, or CD3 performed on the trephine biopsy specimen may be required to make the distinction.

Special consideration should also be given to patients who have been treated with anti-CD20 monoclonal antibody

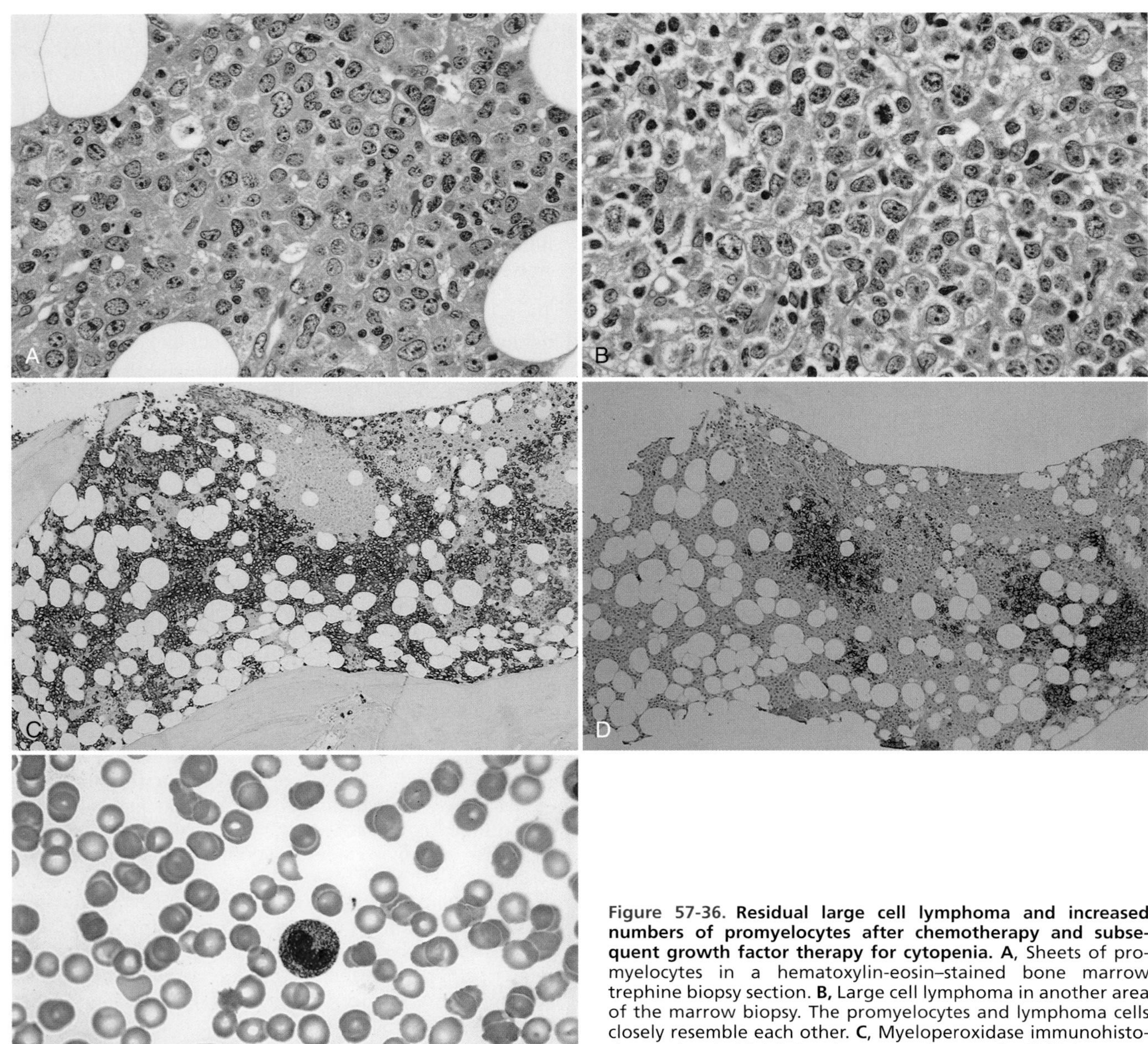

Figure 57-36. Residual large cell lymphoma and increased numbers of promyelocytes after chemotherapy and subsequent growth factor therapy for cytopenia. A, Sheets of promyelocytes in a hematoxylin-eosin–stained bone marrow trephine biopsy section. **B,** Large cell lymphoma in another area of the marrow biopsy. The promyelocytes and lymphoma cells closely resemble each other. **C,** Myeloperoxidase immunohistochemical stain highlights the promyelocytes. **D,** CD20 immunohistochemical stain highlights the lymphoma cells. **E,** Neutrophil with prominent toxic granules and Döhle's body due to colony-stimulating factor therapy.

(rituximab) and continue to exhibit lymphoid infiltrates in the bone marrow. In some cases, the lesions represent residual lymphoma.[152] In others, the lymphoma has been eliminated by anti-CD20 therapy, and lymphoma cells are no longer present; the lymphoid infiltrates are composed entirely of $CD3^{+}$ T cells, histiocytes, and stromal cells localized to the same area as the initial lymphoma. These aggregates may mimic residual lymphoma because they can be large, multiple, or even paratrabecular (Fig. 57-37). Even when residual B-cell lymphoma remains in the bone marrow of patients treated with anti-CD20 therapy, the lymphoma cells may be $CD20^{-}$. For all these reasons, immunostains or flow cytometric immunophenotyping using B-cell antigens other than CD20 (e.g., CD79a, PAX5) is often necessary to differentiate T-cell aggregates from residual B-cell lymphoma.

PRIMARY DIAGNOSIS OF LYMPHOMA IN BONE MARROW

A primary diagnosis of lymphoma is occasionally made on the basis of a bone marrow biopsy. This may occur when a biopsy is obtained for unexplained cytopenia or fever or when organomegaly and extramedullary masses are absent or inaccessible for biopsy. Classification of lymphomas from the bone marrow is clinically important because therapy is increasingly stratified according to specific lymphoma sub-

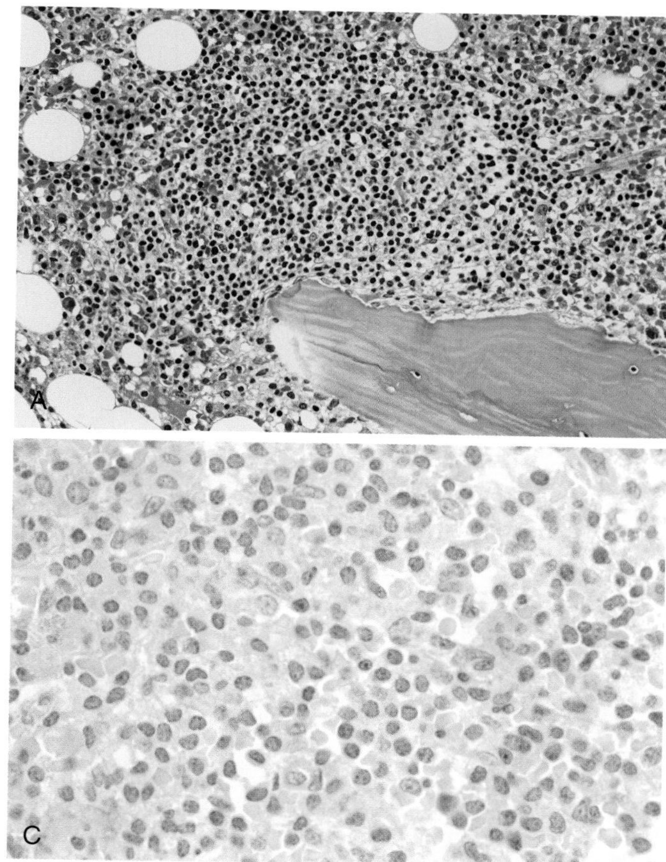
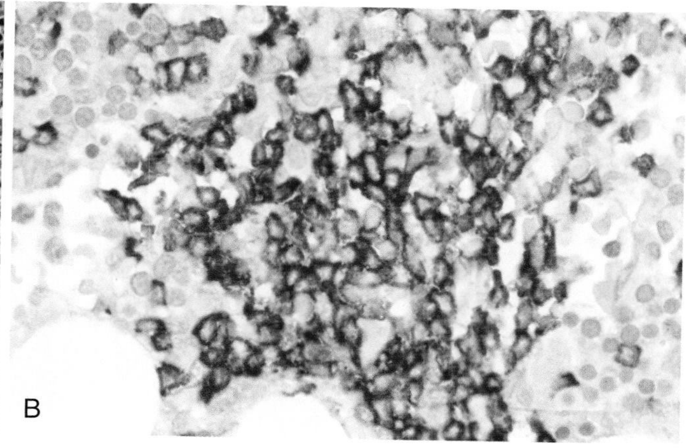

Figure 57-37. Lymphoid infiltrate in bone marrow following rituximab therapy. A, This paratrabecular lymphoid aggregate in the bone marrow, following rituximab therapy for low-grade follicular lymphoma, is composed of mostly small lymphocytes, with rare histiocytes and stromal cells, mimicking lymphoma. **B,** CD3 immunohistochemical stain shows that the lymphocytes are virtually all $CD3^+$ T cells. **C,** PAX5 immunohistochemical stain, which detects B cells, is completely negative, indicating that no B cells are present in the infiltrate. Therefore, the lymphoid aggregate does not represent residual lymphoma.

types. Although morphologic features are of paramount importance in making a primary diagnosis of lymphoma in the bone marrow and may also provide critical information indicating the lymphoma subtype, flow cytometric immunophenotyping or immunohistochemistry is essential for classification. Molecular genetic or cytogenetic studies may also be required. When all this information is integrated, the majority of lymphomas can be classified on the basis of a bone marrow biopsy alone. One study achieved an 85% concordance rate between lymphomas classified in the bone marrow and those independently classified at extramedullary sites.[89]

The small B-cell lymphomas, such as SLL, follicular lymphoma, MCL, and splenic marginal zone B-cell lymphoma, involve the bone marrow frequently and are therefore likely to be initially encountered there. Although the morphologic features of these small B-cell lymphomas overlap, some findings indicate or exclude specific types. For example, proliferation centers indicate SLL. Distinct paratrabecular infiltrates are not encountered in SLL and, when present, exclude this diagnosis.

Paratrabecular infiltrates, although not specific, are characteristic of follicular lymphoma; infiltrates of follicular lymphoma may be entirely paratrabecular. However, other patterns of involvement can also be observed in follicular lymphoma, and in some cases paratrabecular infiltrates are absent. The finding of a lymphomatous lesion in the bone marrow composed of cells with cleaved nuclei that are documented to be B cells with surface immunoglobulin light-chain restriction and that are $CD5^-$, $CD10^+$, and $FMC7^+$ supports the diagnosis of follicular lymphoma. Malignant follicles, although not common, may be present within the infiltrate; the neoplastic follicle center cells are $CD10^+$ and $BCL2^+$ in the majority of cases, and BCL6 is positive in slightly less than 50% of cases.[21] Documenting a t(14;18) further supports the diagnosis of follicular lymphoma.[153] The cytologic appearance (size and chromatin pattern) of the lymphoma cells should be described; however, grading of follicular lymphoma based on bone marrow histology alone should be avoided or done with the knowledge that the nodal counterpart may have discordant morphology.[5,90] An enlarged lymph node or an extranodal mass can be biopsied for grading purposes.

MCL, similar to follicular lymphoma, has a high incidence of bone marrow involvement and may be encountered for the first time in the marrow (Fig. 57-38). MCL can also manifest as an exclusively paratrabecular infiltrate in the bone marrow, similar to follicular lymphoma (see Fig. 57-19).[94] Its morphologic appearance may also closely mimic SLL/CLL, CLL/prolymphocytic leukemia, or prolymphocytic leukemia (see Fig. 57-21).[99] An accurate diagnosis of MCL encountered initially in the bone marrow is possible when a lymphomatous infiltrate with an MCL growth pattern and cytomorphology is present and an immunophenotype characteristic of MCL is documented—that is, a B-cell population with surface immunoglobulin light-chain restriction that is $CD5^+$, $CD10^-$, $CD23^-$ or dimly $CD23^+$, $FMC7^+$, and $CD79b^+$ (see Fig. 57-38).[98,99,101]

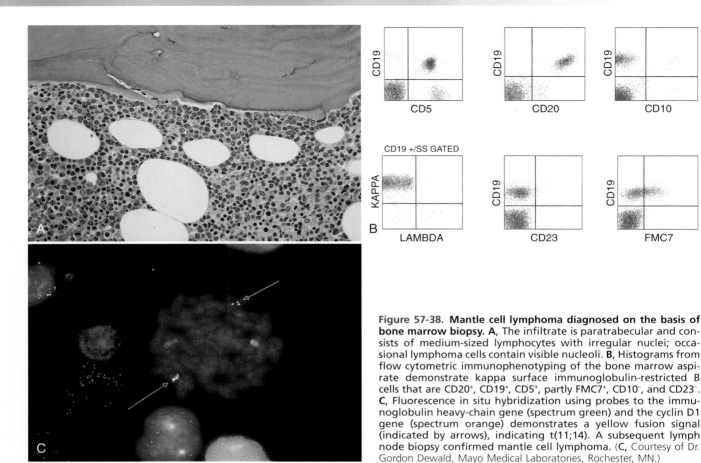

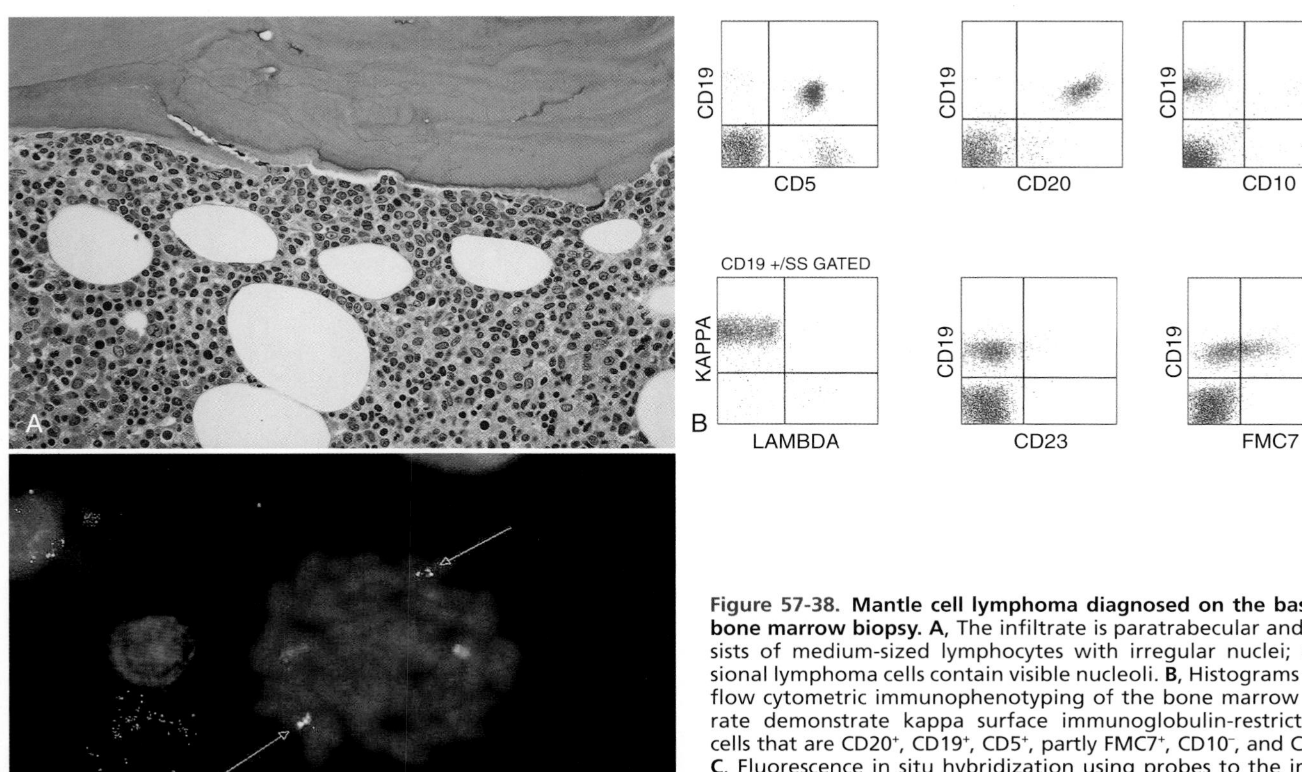

Figure 57-38. Mantle cell lymphoma diagnosed on the basis of bone marrow biopsy. A, The infiltrate is paratrabecular and consists of medium-sized lymphocytes with irregular nuclei; occasional lymphoma cells contain visible nucleoli. **B,** Histograms from flow cytometric immunophenotyping of the bone marrow aspirate demonstrate kappa surface immunoglobulin-restricted B cells that are CD20$^+$, CD19$^+$, CD5$^+$, partly FMC7$^+$, CD10$^-$, and CD23$^-$. **C,** Fluorescence in situ hybridization using probes to the immunoglobulin heavy-chain gene (spectrum green) and the cyclin D1 gene (spectrum orange) demonstrates a yellow fusion signal (indicated by arrows), indicating t(11;14). A subsequent lymph node biopsy confirmed mantle cell lymphoma. (**C,** Courtesy of Dr. Gordon Dewald, Mayo Medical Laboratories, Rochester, MN.)

The diagnosis should be confirmed by immunohistochemistry showing cyclin D1 positivity or by molecular or genetic studies that demonstrate t(11;14) (see Fig. 57-38).[98,99,154] Confirmation of MCL can also be obtained from a lymph node biopsy in cases with accessible lymphadenopathy.

Diagnosis of splenic marginal zone lymphoma in the bone marrow is more difficult; it requires the exclusion of other small B-cell lymphomas because the phenotype of the lymphoma cells is less distinctive, and the morphology overlaps considerably with that of the other small B-cell lymphomas. However, when intrasinusoidal infiltrates are noted within a lymphomatous infiltrate composed of small cells that exhibit an immunophenotype compatible with splenic marginal zone lymphoma—CD5$^-$, CD10$^-$, CD23$^-$, FMC7$^+$, CD79b$^+$, CD43$^-$, and cyclin D1$^-$—splenic marginal zone lymphoma is suggested.[12] Documenting the absence of t(11;14)(q13;q32) or t(14;18)(q32;q21) helps exclude MCL and follicular lymphoma. The clinical findings are also helpful because affected patients typically demonstrate splenomegaly without peripheral lymphadenopathy. Splenectomy allows definitive diagnosis but is not always performed.

Large cell lymphoma infiltrates can usually be easily recognized in bone marrow sections, and scattered lymphoma cells may also be present in aspirate smears or touch preparations. Intravascular large B-cell lymphoma involving the bone marrow can be difficult to recognize on routine H&E-stained sections. Ancillary studies such as immunostains or flow cytometric immunophenotyping are needed to verify that the infiltrate is lymphoid and to determine the lineage (B, T, or NK) of the lymphoma cells.

Aggressive lymphomas such as Burkitt's and precursor lymphoblastic lymphomas are occasionally diagnosed initially in the bone marrow; in these cases peripheral blood involvement may be minimal or absent. The morphologic features of the aggressive lymphomas overlap. Flow cytometric immunophenotyping or immunohistochemistry is essential not only to confirm the diagnosis of lymphoma but also to distinguish among the precursor types. The morphologic features of Burkitt's lymphoma are more distinctive, but immunophenotyping is required to document its mature B-cell phenotype. As in lymph node or extranodal tissue, distinguishing between Burkitt-like lymphoma and large B-cell lymphoma based on bone marrow morphology alone is often difficult. However, genetic studies demonstrating translocation between the c-*MYC* gene on chromosome 8 and the immunoglobulin heavy-chain gene on chromosome 14 (t[8;14][q24; q32]) or the immunoglobulin kappa (t[2;8][p12;q24]) or lambda (t[8;22][q24;q11]) light-chain genes on chromosomes 2 and 22, respectively, in the lymphoma cells supports the diagnosis of Burkitt's lymphoma.

Peripheral T-cell lymphomas are encountered in the bone marrow less frequently. They can be difficult to distinguish from reactive lesions or HL because they are often composed of a polymorphic infiltrate. Immunophenotyping is necessary to identify the infiltrates of T-cell lymphomas, and it may suggest that the infiltrate is malignant when an aberrant T-cell

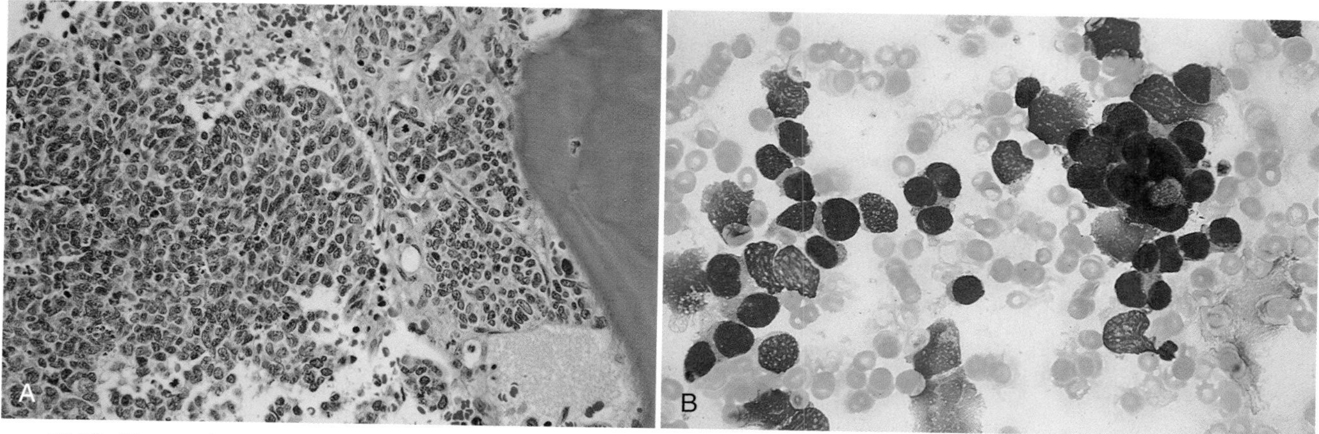

Figure 57-39. Metastatic neuroendocrine carcinoma involving the bone marrow. A, Cohesive tumor cells completely replace normal bone marrow cells in the trephine biopsy section. **B,** Discohesive, small carcinoma cells that resemble lymphoma cells in the bone marrow aspirate smear. A cohesive cluster of tumor cells, which is more typical of carcinoma, is also present.

phenotype is detected (see Fig. 57-30). It may also be necessary to establish T-cell monoclonality with molecular diagnostic studies. It should be noted that large B-cell lymphomas that are rich in T cells can mimic T-cell lymphomas based on the results of immunohistochemical stains. However, the large abnormal cells are highlighted with B-cell stains such as CD20, and the majority of the remaining cells are small, mature-appearing T cells. Thus, when data from different sources such as clinical, morphologic, phenotypic, molecular, and genetic studies are combined, peripheral T-cell lymphoma can usually be diagnosed. However, subtypes are often difficult to specify based on the bone marrow findings. For instance, distinguishing angioimmunoblastic T-cell lymphoma from peripheral T-cell lymphoma, not otherwise specified, may not be possible. Hepatosplenic T-cell lymphoma can usually be diagnosed when the characteristic morphologic, clinical, and immunophenotypic findings are present; cytogenetic or fluorescence in situ hybridization analysis may help confirm the diagnosis. In many cases only the broad category of peripheral T-cell lymphoma can be diagnosed, and biopsy of a tumor at an extramedullary site is needed for more specific classification.

The bone marrow is rarely the primary diagnostic site for HL, occurring most often in patients with acquired immunodeficiency disease.[146,147] As discussed earlier, Reed-Sternberg cells in an environment characteristic of HL must be present for a primary diagnosis of HL in the bone marrow. It is advisable to confirm the phenotype of the Reed-Sternberg cells with appropriate immunostains (i.e., $CD45^-$, $CD20^-$, $CD15^+$, $CD30^+$, EMA^-, $ALK\text{-}1^-$) because Reed-Sternberg–like cells can also be present in non-Hodgkin's lymphomas, including peripheral T-cell lymphomas. As noted previously, HL should not be subclassified in the bone marrow because the small sample size and variability of morphology between lymph node and bone marrow make subclassification unreliable.

In some cases subclassification of the lymphoma is not possible even with the use of ancillary techniques; diagnosis in these cases is often limited to broad categories such as small B-cell lymphoma or peripheral T-cell lymphoma, not otherwise specified. Biopsy of a lymph node or extranodal mass is needed for accurate classification.

NONLYMPHOID MALIGNANCIES THAT MIMIC LYMPHOMAS

Metastatic Tumors

Metastatic tumors in the bone marrow are usually easily distinguished from lymphoma because the malignant cells occur as cohesive clusters of cells (Fig. 57-39). However, tumor cells from small cell carcinoma and other small round blue cell tumors such as embryonal rhabdomyosarcoma, neuroblastoma, retinoblastoma, and Ewing's sarcoma are occasionally aspirated as single cells and mimic lymphoma cells in the aspirate smears (Fig. 57-40).[66,155] Scanning the aspirate smear at low magnification (10×) is useful to identify cohesive nests of tumor cells, even when they are rare. In the trephine biopsy section, foci of metastatic tumor are almost always sharply demarcated from normal hematopoietic cells and occur as clusters of morphologically neoplastic cells that are readily identified as metastatic tumor. Rarely, they focally infiltrate as groups of cells between hematopoietic tissue and resemble a large cell lymphoma (Fig. 57-41). In other cases the metastatic tumor may be extensive and diffusely replace virtually all the normal cellular elements of the bone marrow. When the infiltrating cells are diffuse, with no differentiation into glands or other epithelial structures, they can resemble a large cell lymphoma or HL (see Fig. 57-40). Immunostains appropriate for the tumor (e.g., cytokeratin, EMA, chromogranin, CD45, CD3, CD20) performed on the trephine biopsy or clot section can confirm the diagnosis of a metastatic tumor and exclude lymphoma.

Systemic Mastocytosis

Systemic mastocytosis involves the bone marrow in at least 90% of cases and shows similar patterns of infiltration as lymphoma, including paratrabecular, perivascular, random, or, rarely, diffuse infiltrates.[156] In most cases the mast cell lesions in the bone marrow are polymorphic, and the mast cells are admixed with lymphocytes, eosinophils, neutrophils, histiocytes, endothelial cells, and fibroblasts in varying proportions. The polymorphic mast cell lesions can mimic lymphoma, particularly peripheral T-cell lymphoma or HL.

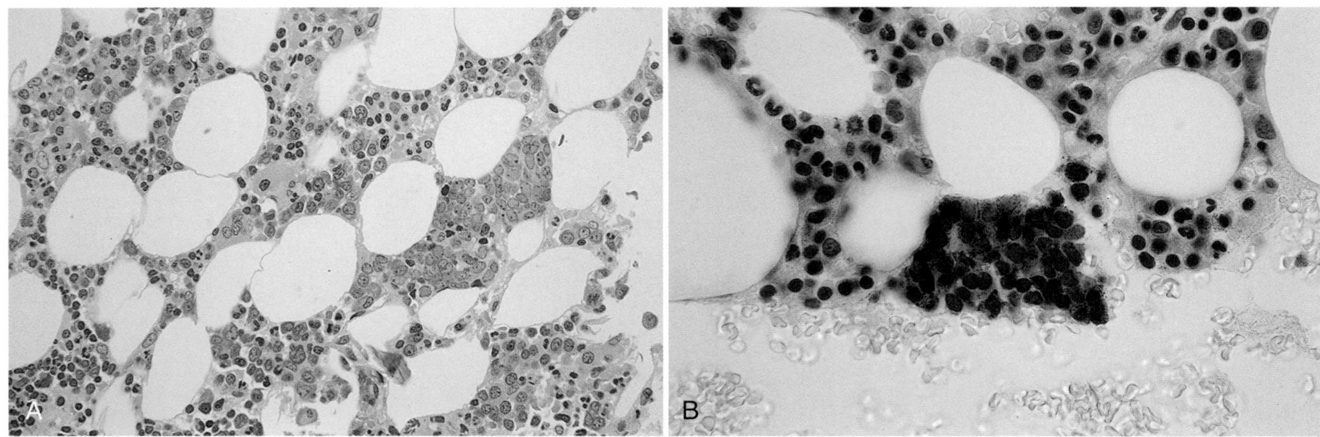

Figure 57-40. Neuroendocrine carcinoma (simulating a large cell lymphoma) in the bone marrow. A, Focal clusters of carcinoma cells with dispersed chromatin and lacking gland formation are nestled among the normal hematopoietic elements. The carcinoma cells superficially resemble a large cell lymphoma. **B,** Carcinoma cells in the clot section; immunohistochemstry demonstrates chromogranin-positive tumor cells.

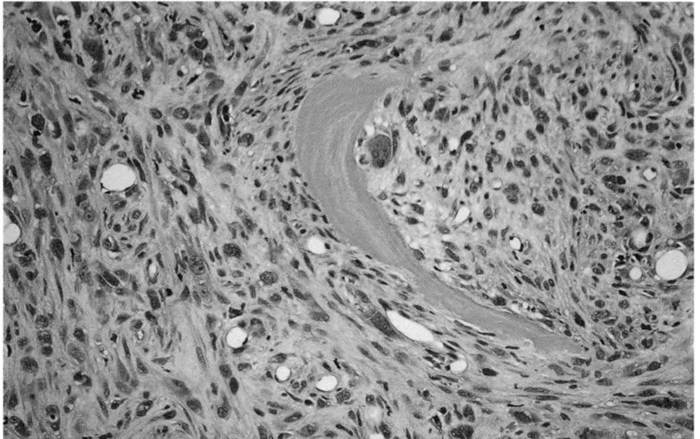

Figure 57-41. Metastatic carcinoma involving the bone marrow. The carcinoma is associated with marked bone marrow fibrosis; contains large, anaplastic tumor cells; and resembles Hodgkin's lymphoma. A cytokeratin immunohistochemical stain (not shown) was positive.

Occasionally, lymphocytes predominate; these lesions can closely resemble non-Hodgkin's lymphoma (Fig. 57-42). Recognition of mast cells in the bone marrow sections is critical to arrive at a diagnosis of systemic mastocytosis. They show variable morphology and may have round, oval, spindle-shaped, or monocytoid nuclei with abundant, slightly eosinophilic cytoplasm. One helpful morphologic clue to recognizing systemic mast cell disease in the bone marrow is the frequent compartmentalization of cells, with clusters of small lymphocytes surrounded by mast cells, creating the classic "bull's-eye" lesion. The most specific immunostain for identifying mast cells is tryptase (see Fig. 57-42). In addition, mast cells express CD45, CD33, CD68, and CD117 but are negative for CD3, CD20, CD15, and CD30.[157] Neoplastic mast cells also express CD25 or CD2, which can help distinguish them from reactive mast cell hyperplasia.[157,158] Somatic mutations of *KIT*, a proto-oncogene that encodes the tyrosine receptor for stem cell factor (CD117), is found in the mast cells from patients with systemic mastocytosis (see also Chapter 48).[159]

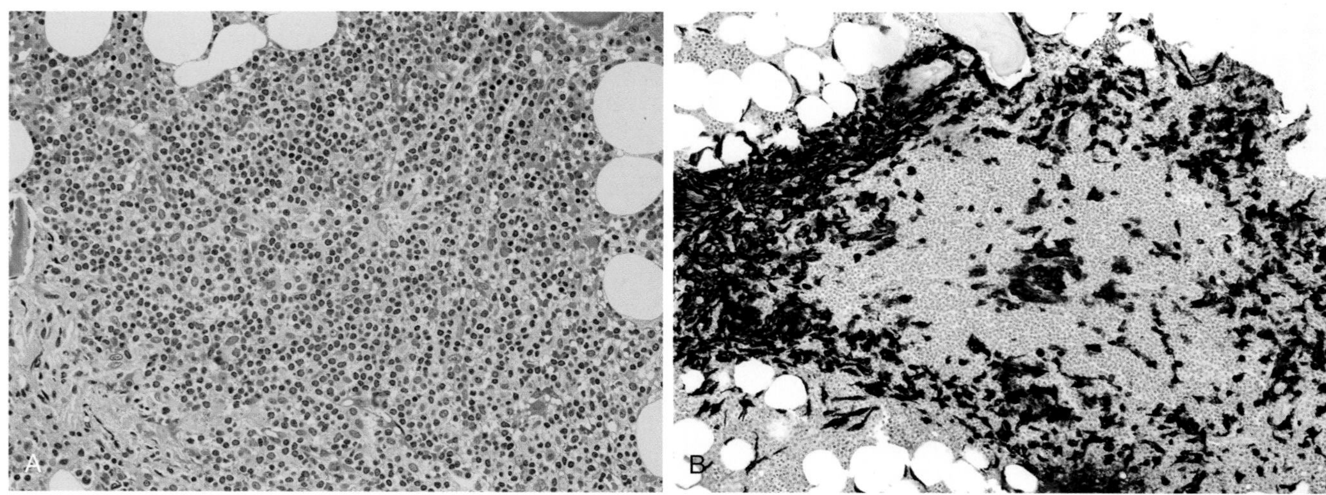

Figure 57-42. Systemic mastocytosis involving the bone marrow. A, The polymorphic mast cell infiltrate contains numerous small lymphocytes, occasional eosinophils, and small vessels, resembling a non-Hodgkin's lymphoma. The mast cells are difficult to appreciate on the hematoxylin-eosin–stained section, but they have elongated nuclei, more dispersed chromatin, and more cytoplasm than the small lymphocytes. **B,** Tryptase immunohistochemical stain highlights the mast cells.

Pearls and Pitfalls

Pearls

- Benign lymphoid aggregates can occur in patients with lymphoma.
- Distinct paratrabecular lymphoid infiltrates essentially exclude the diagnosis of SLL/CLL.
- Intravascular localization of lymphoid infiltrates usually indicates a malignant proliferation.
- Benign lymphoid aggregates are usually morphologically heterogeneous.
- Germinal centers usually indicate benign lymphoid infiltrates and are most commonly seen in patients with autoimmune disorders.
- Lymphoid infiltrates associated with lipogranulomas are benign.
- Paratrabecular lymphoid infiltrates almost always indicate lymphoma.
- Immunostains aid in identifying intrasinusoidal infiltrates, which are common in intravascular large B-cell lymphoma, splenic marginal zone B-cell lymphoma, and hepatosplenic T-cell lymphoma in the bone marrow.
- Immunostains also help identify anaplastic large cell lymphoma and NK/T-cell lymphoma, which can infiltrate the bone marrow as single cells.
- Monoclonal B cells identified by ancillary techniques usually support bone marrow involvement by a B-cell neoplasm.

Pitfalls

- Small, focal random lymphoid aggregates may represent lymphoma.
- Exclusively paratrabecular lymphoid infiltrates are most common in follicular lymphoma but can also be present in the majority of other lymphomas, including mantle cell lymphoma.
- Intrasinusoidal infiltrates have been reported in polyclonal B-cell lymphocytosis.
- Lymphoma, particularly T-cell types, can be morphologically heterogeneous.
- Splenic marginal zone lymphoma involving the bone marrow is associated with germinal centers in about 30% of cases.
- Noninfectious granulomas can accompany many lymphomas, including indolent B-cell lymphomas, T-cell lymphomas, and Hodgkin's lymphoma.
- Paratrabecular, multiple, or large lymphoid infiltrates that mimic lymphoma but are T-cell rich and benign (lack B cells) can persist after rituximab (anti-CD20) therapy for B-cell lymphoma.
- Immunostains are not diagnostic as stand-alone tests and must be correlated with clinical and other laboratory findings. Immunostains that are not specific for lymphoma (e.g., CD30) do not always indicate marrow involvement by lymphoma when they are positive.
- Low-level monoclonal B-cell populations may be identified by flow cytometry in "healthy" individuals with no evidence of lymphoma.

References can be found on Expert Consult @ www.expertconsult.com

Chapter 58

Evaluation of the Bone Marrow After Therapy

Yasodha Natkunam and Daniel A. Arber

CHAPTER OUTLINE

GENERAL APPROACH

A great number of changes occur in the bone marrow during and after therapy for malignancy. Although the proper interpretation of these changes requires knowledge of the patient's original disease process, some general features are common to all cases. It may be assumed that the purpose of bone marrow studies performed during or after therapy is to evaluate disease involvement; however, other important information can be obtained from these specimens. With effective high-dose chemotherapy, the marrow is completely ablated, and bone marrow studies may be performed to confirm obliteration of the neoplastic process. Later in the patient's disease course, a bone marrow examination may be performed to confirm the presence of regenerating hematopoiesis. In these cases a comment on bone marrow cellularity and the presence of maturing trilineage marrow elements (granulocytes, erythroid precursors, megakaryocytes) is important. Following hematopoietic stem cell transplantation (which includes bone marrow transplantation or peripheral blood stem cell transplantation), an examination may be performed to confirm engraftment, and descriptions of marrow cellularity and trilineage hematopoiesis are of primary importance. Therefore, complete clinical information—including information about the primary disease process, type of treatment, and time interval since treatment—should be submitted with the bone marrow specimen.

Several studies have evaluated marrow changes after high-dose chemotherapy or chemotherapy with radiation, including regimens used for hematopoietic stem cell transplantation,[1-8] and there are many similarities in the findings (Box 58-1; Fig. 58-1). These changes are also similar to the toxic changes resulting from drug injury of the marrow.[9] The changes expected in the first week after treatment are those of complete marrow aplasia. The marrow cellularity is often nearly zero, with an absence of normal marrow fat. There is prominent edema, with dilated marrow sinuses; scattered stromal cells, histiocytes, plasma cells, and lymphocytes may be present. Normal hematopoietic cells such as maturing granulocytes, nucleated red blood cells, and megakaryocytes, are often not identifiable. Histiocytes containing cellular debris are often present, and acellular areas of pink-staining fibrinoid necrosis often predominate. Rare cases may also show zonal areas of tumor cell necrosis. The development of mild reticulin fibrosis and the reappearance of fat cells follow these changes. The early fat in regenerating marrow is often loculated. Although the marrow remains markedly hypocellular, the fat is associated with focal areas of early hematopoiesis in the second week after treatment. This may be represented by islands of erythroid cells, alone or in combination with areas of left-shifted granulocytes. Both elements are usually present after 2 weeks. Megakaryocytes, often occurring in clusters with atypical or hypolobated nuclei, occur later in this process but are usually easily identified by the third week. In some patients, particularly children, early regeneration may be accompanied by an increase in precursor B cells, or hematogones. The features of these cells are discussed later in this chapter.

Box 58-1 *Bone Marrow Changes in the Three to Four Weeks Following Myeloablative Therapy*

Initial Changes
- Marrow aplasia
- Absence of fat cells
- Edema
- Fibrinoid necrosis
- Dilated sinuses
- Rare stromal cells, histiocytes, lymphocytes, and plasma cells

Intermediate Changes
- Reappearance of fat, often lobulated
- Mild reticulin fibrosis
- Foci of left-shifted erythroid and granulocyte islands
- Increase in precursor B cells on smears

Late Changes
- Resolution of reticulin fibrosis
- Appearance of small megakaryocytes in clusters
- Normal or slightly increased marrow cellularity

The expected later changes usually include a loss of the mild reticulin fibrosis of early regeneration and a return to normal or even slightly increased marrow cellularity. All three normal marrow cell lines are present, although a left shift of granulocytes and erythroid cells and atypical megakaryocyte clustering may persist for some time.

Some additional marrow changes may be observed in patients who have undergone high-dose therapy followed by hematopoietic stem cell transplantation (Box 58-2). Foci of regeneration may occur earlier in patients treated with stem cell infusion. Although clusters of regenerating marrow elements usually show a spectrum of maturation, these islands of cells may have a more monotonous appearance, without obvious maturation, after transplantation. This is most commonly seen with erythroid precursors. In addition, the topographic pattern of regenerating cells may differ after transplantation. In the normal bone marrow and in normally regenerating marrow after cytotoxic therapy, immature granulocyte islands of blast cells and promyelocytes usually occur adjacent to bony trabeculae. The presence of such islands away from the bone is considered an abnormal feature, referred to as *abnormal localization of immature precursors*, and is described as a feature of myelodysplasia on biopsy sections. After hematopoietic stem cell transplantation, these immature cell islands often occur away from the bone, and this feature should not be considered evidence of recurrent or impending myelodysplasia (Fig. 58-2).

Increases in marrow iron storage or siderotic iron incorporation are also common findings following hematopoietic stem cell transplantation. This is usually apparent by an

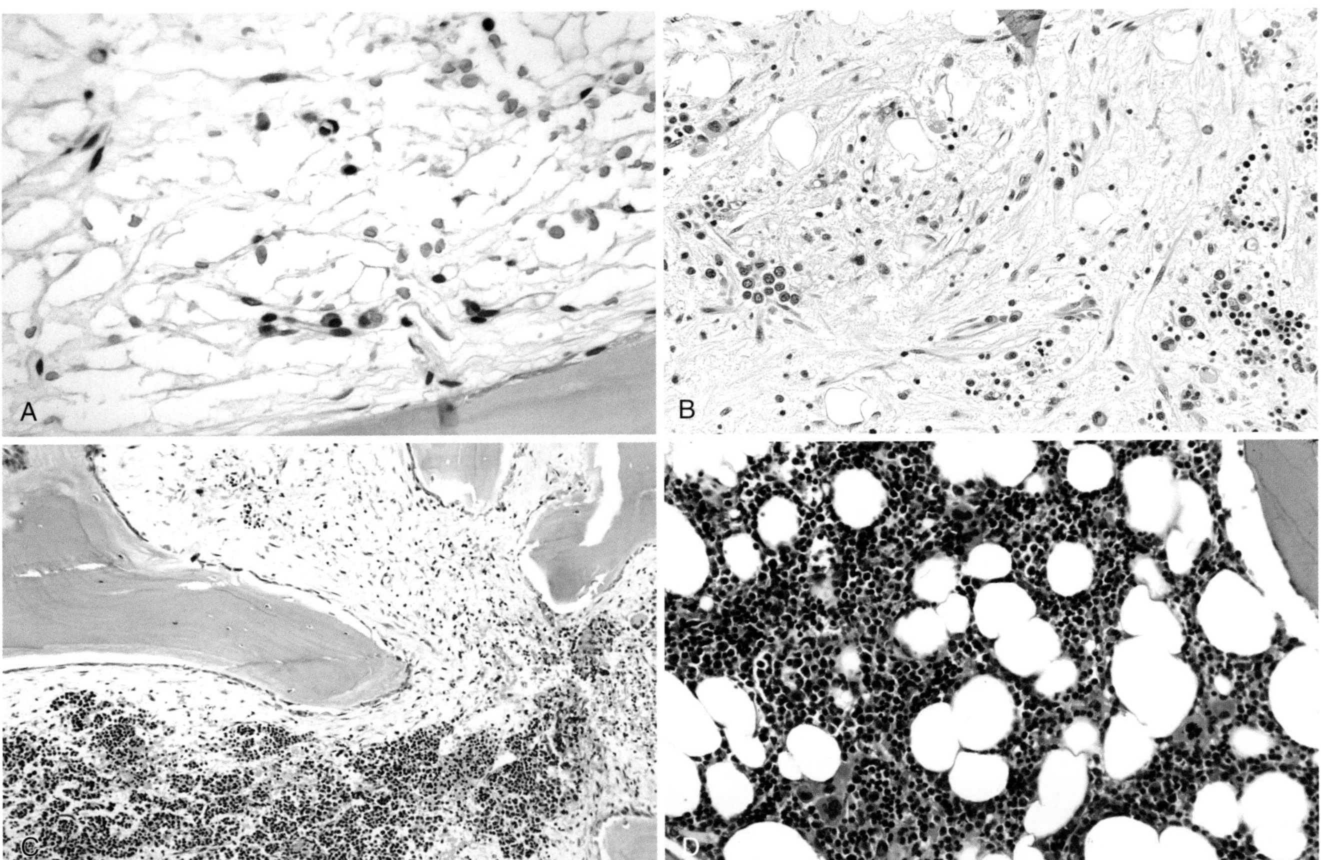

Figure 58-1. Bone marrow changes of myeloablative therapy. A, The marrow is initially acellular, with loss of fat cells. **B,** Islands of erythroid and granulocyte precursors then appear. **C,** The cellularity is often patchy, with acellular areas and areas of left-shifted cells. The hypocellular areas of this marrow still show mild fibrosis, which resolves as hematopoiesis returns. **D,** At 3 to 4 weeks, marrow cellularity returns.

Box 58-2 *Posttherapy Bone Marrow Changes Unique to Hematopoietic Stem Cell Transplantation*

- Regenerative islands with a monotonous, immature appearance
- Localization of immature cell precursors away from bony trabeculae
- Increased storage iron and siderotic iron with or without ring sideroblasts
- Prolonged variable cellularity with or without cytopenias
- Prolonged aplasia due to engraftment failure

increase in hemosiderin-laden macrophages on both aspirate smears and trephine biopsy sections. Although the increase in siderotic iron is usually less uniform than that seen in refractory anemia with ring sideroblasts, in some cases the pattern of iron staining may be similar or identical to that of sideroblastic anemia; therefore, iron stains must be interpreted with caution in post–marrow transplant patients.[10] Finally, after hematopoietic stem cell transplantation, marrow cellularity may never return to the normal range. These patients frequently exhibit variability in marrow cellularity and often have a persistently hypocellular marrow that may be accompanied by mild peripheral blood cytopenias for many years. Prolonged impairment of hematopoiesis has been demonstrated following standard as well as high-dose chemotherapy followed by bone marrow transplantation,[11,12] and this may explain the differences in cellularity in posttransplantation marrows.

A hypocellular posttreatment marrow may result from bone marrow failure after solid organ or hematopoietic stem cell transplantation, failure to engraft after stem cell transplantation, or delayed engraftment after stem cell transplantation. The marrow in these patients is similar and shows signs of aplasia even after several weeks. Histiocytes, stromal cells, lymphocytes, and plasma cells predominate.[13] Delayed engraftment may occur in patients with marked marrow fibrosis before transplantation,[14] and diffuse histiocytic proliferations have been reported with delayed engraftment.[13] Graft failure after hematopoietic stem cell transplantation or bone marrow failure after solid organ transplantation may occur secondary to viral infection, reactivation of virus, or hemophagocytic syndrome.[15-17] Late marrow failure may also occur as a terminal event of posttherapy myelodysplasia.

The immunodeficiency associated with chemotherapy also increases these patients' risk for infectious diseases. Examination of the bone marrow is one means of identifying infection. If an infectious disease is suspected, fresh bone marrow aspirate material should be sent for microbiology studies. Histochemical stains for acid-fast and fungal organisms should be performed on all biopsy specimens containing granulomas.

The optimal materials for evaluating posttherapy changes include the peripheral blood smear, bone marrow aspirate, and touch preparations (imprints), as well as trephine biopsy sections. Clot biopsy sections may also be useful, but focal lesions that cannot be aspirated may not be present on such sections. Aspirates and imprints generally offer the best cytologic detail and are helpful in evaluating residual blast cells after therapy. Biopsy material is useful for showing the pattern of blast cells, once they are identified on the aspirate material, as well as the presence and pattern of residual lymphoma or solid tumor involvement.

Ancillary studies are of increasing importance in the evaluation of posttherapy bone marrow specimens, particularly in the assessment of residual disease. These studies include flow cytometry, immunohistochemistry, and cytogenetic and molecular genetic studies. With the exception of immunohistochemistry and some molecular genetic tests, these ancillary methods require additional fresh bone marrow aspirate, and material must be saved at the time of specimen submission for these studies. The utility of each of these methods is discussed in the sections on the specific disease processes.

ACUTE LEUKEMIA OR MYELODYSPLASIA

Once the marrow has begun to regain its cellularity with normal hematopoietic cells, the pathologist is faced with the challenge of evaluating for residual or recurrent disease. It is well established that the presence of minimal residual disease (MRD) that is undetectable by morphologic methods is a

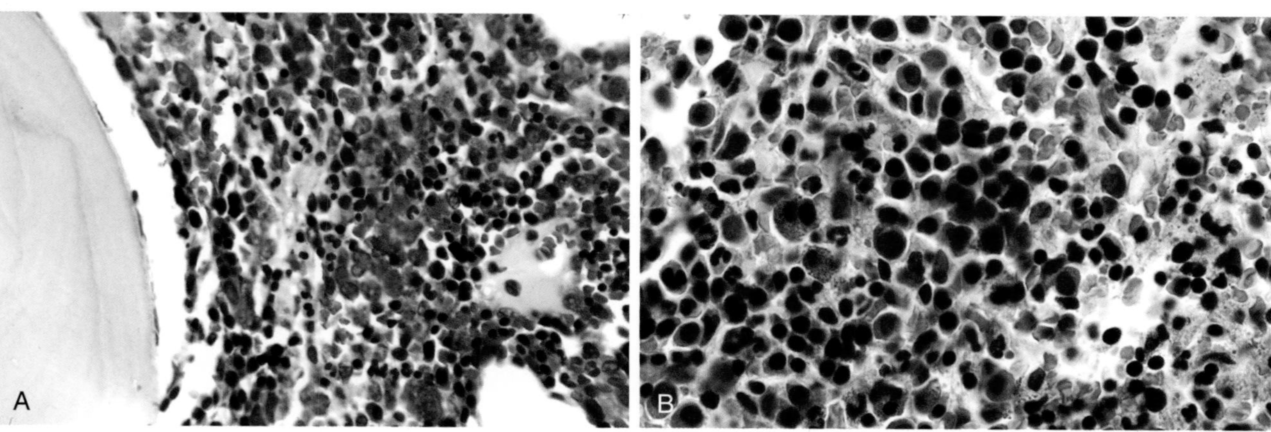

Figure 58-2. After bone marrow transplantation **(A)**, aggregates of immature-appearing cells may be present away from the bone. This is in contrast to regeneration in nontransplant patients, which usually occurs adjacent to bony trabeculae. Although this abnormal localization of immature precursors is a common feature of myelodysplasia **(B)**, it should not be overinterpreted as evidence of myelodysplasia in a post–hematopoietic stem cell transplant patient.

Table 58-1 Sensitivity of Methods for Detecting Residual Disease

Method	Sensitivity (%)
Morphology	1-5
Cytogenetic karyotype analysis	3-5
FISH	1-5
Immunohistochemistry	0.1-5
Consensus primer PCR for gene rearrangements	0.1-1
Flow cytometry	0.01-1
PCR and RT-PCR for specific translocations	0.001-0.01
Patient-specific PCR and RT-PCR	0.001

FISH, fluorescence in situ hybridization; PCR, polymerase chain reaction; RT-PCR, reverse transcriptase polymerase chain reaction.

powerful predictor of recurrence. Although different types of acute leukemia offer their own unique problems, some general features are common to all cases. A blast cell count of 5% in the bone marrow is the historic cutoff for delineating the presence of residual or recurrent leukemia. However, this cutoff is arbitrary, and the current goal is to detect the presence of neoplastic clones as early as possible. The use of multiparameter flow cytometry and molecular genetic techniques to detect MRD are redefining remission in many diseases.[18-20] A general overview of the sensitivity of the methods used to detect MRD is given in Table 58-1.

The common use of growth factors (discussed in more detail later) creates the problem of regenerative blast cell increases above 5% in some cases. Therefore, decisions regarding relapse or remission should not be based on blast cell counts alone. When the blast cell population in posttherapy bone marrow is suspicious for residual disease, comparison to the original acute leukemia is often helpful, and the presence of unique morphologic features such as Auer rods, distinctive cytoplasmic granules, prominent nucleoli, or nuclear irregularities that were identified in the original disease can be useful. In addition, the detection of an aberrant immunophenotype by flow cytometry is helpful, although this requires knowledge of the original immunophenotype of the tumor. The immunohistochemical detection of immature $CD34^+$ or terminal deoxynucleotidyl transferase (TdT)–positive cells in clusters in a bone marrow biopsy is also helpful, because immature cells in regenerating marrow do not normally show the clustering seen in recurrent leukemia specimens.

The detection of clonal cytogenetic abnormalities that were present in the patient's original leukemia can also be helpful in the evaluation of residual disease. Routine karyotype analysis or fluorescence in situ hybridization (FISH) studies are the most commonly performed genetic tests, but specific molecular genetic tests using polymerase chain reaction (PCR) may be useful as well.

To optimally assess a specimen for residual or recurrent disease, it is important that the original disease process be diagnosed and evaluated appropriately. Immunophenotyping for residual disease is more expensive owing to the larger panel of antibodies needed, and it is often less rewarding when information about the original leukemia is not available. Molecular genetic testing is usually not justified when the original karyotypic abnormality is not known. Ancillary testing is not necessary on all follow-up specimens. If residual or recurrent disease is suspected in the absence of material for these tests, such suspicion should be relayed to the treating physician. A repeat bone marrow evaluation after 1 or 2 weeks is often helpful to determine a change in the number of blasts, which would be expected to increase with recurrent disease, and appropriate ancillary tests can be performed on the second specimen. In contrast, increased immature cells in an early phase of marrow regeneration would be expected to show more mature precursors in the second bone marrow study.

Acute Myeloid Leukemia and Myelodysplasia

Morphologic Features

Published guidelines for the morphologic definition of remission in patients treated for acute myeloid leukemia (AML) require peripheral blood neutrophil counts of greater than 1.0 $\times 10^9$/L, platelet counts of at least 100 $\times 10^9$/L, and less than 5% blast cells without Auer rods.[21] Prior criteria requiring greater than 20% cellularity or stable counts for at least 4 weeks are no longer included. Before these changes are demonstrated, however, several morphologic features of the peripheral blood and bone marrow have prognostic significance. Failure to demonstrate a reduction in blast cells and cellularity at day 6 of induction chemotherapy usually results in a change in or augmentation of induction chemotherapy.[22] Not surprisingly, the presence of residual leukemic cells at the end of induction chemotherapy is a poor prognostic indicator.[23] Even after meeting the criteria for remission, patients with bone marrow hypercellularity, anemia, bone marrow blast cell counts of 1% or more, or peripheral blood blast cell counts exceeding 3% have a shortened duration of remission and shortened survival.[24,25] Therefore, more detailed evaluation of bone marrow and peripheral blood samples is needed than is suggested by the remission criteria.

The presence of an increased number of blast cells with features similar to the original AML or myelodysplasia should be regarded with suspicion. Auer rods (rod-shaped cytoplasmic aggregates of granules) are not a feature of regenerating or nonneoplastic myeloblasts and should be considered evidence of residual disease. Auer rods may rarely be encountered in maturing granulocytes but are nevertheless considered abnormal. Regenerating blast cells are usually admixed with promyelocytes and maturing granulocytes, and the presence of sheets of blasts on a smear is a sign of recurrent disease. In contrast, specimens with equal or fewer numbers of blast cells compared with promyelocytes usually represent regeneration.[26] Clustering of blast cells is often difficult to interpret on hematoxylin-eosin (H&E)–stained biopsy specimens, and aggregates of regeneration may be difficult to differentiate from leukemic blast cell aggregates. Regeneration usually occurs adjacent to bony trabeculae, and the presence of immature cell aggregates away from the bone is considered abnormal. This abnormal localization of immature cell precursors has been used as a feature of myelodysplasia, but caution should be applied when using these criteria in patients who have received hematopoietic stem cell transplants. After transplantation, the normal bone marrow architecture may change, and regenerating immature precursors may be present away from the bone on H&E-stained sections.

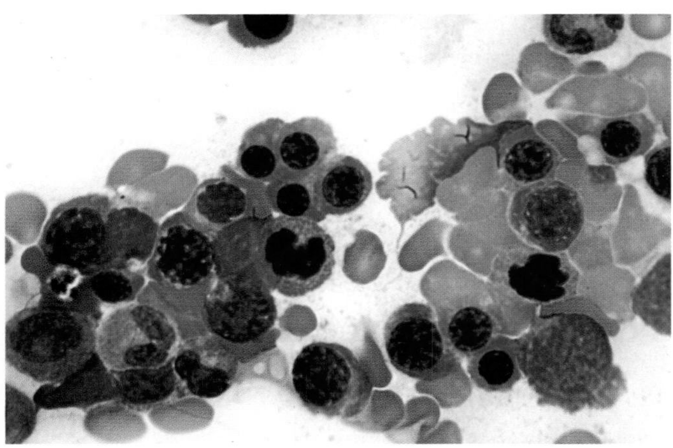

Figure 58-3. Posttherapy dyserythropoiesis associated with erythroid hyperplasia is common and should not be interpreted as myelodysplasia, which should exhibit dysplastic changes of other cell lines.

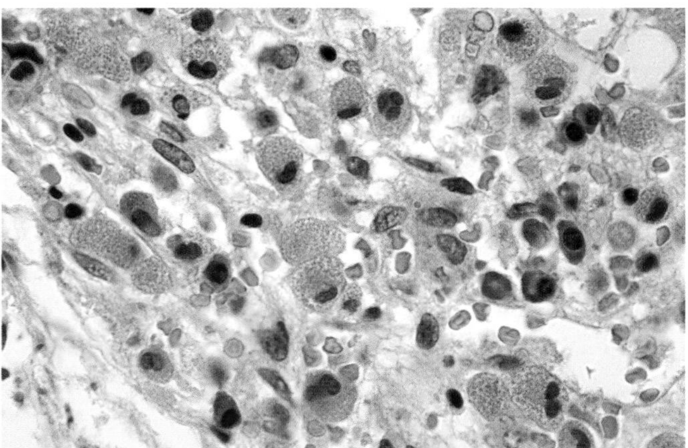

Figure 58-5. Residual promyelocytes during therapy for acute promyelocytic leukemia treated with all-*trans*-retinoic acid. Follow-up marrow examination showed continued maturation of granulocytes without a change in therapy.

AML with myelodysplasia-related changes and myelodysplasia may exhibit multilineage dysplasia before an increase in blast cells at relapse. Again, the features of the original multilineage dysplasia should be reviewed, and care should be taken not to overestimate multilineage dysplasia during or immediately after therapy. Dyserythropoietic changes are common during chemotherapy and often include a left shift of erythroid precursors and multinucleation of erythroid cells (Fig. 58-3). In addition, regenerating megakaryocytes are small and often cluster during or immediately after chemotherapy. Granulocyte changes after therapy are usually restricted to a left shift without hypogranulation or nuclear abnormalities commonly seen in association with myelodysplasia. Therefore, dysplastic changes of maturing granulocytes are probably more reliable in identifying recurrent AML with multilineage dysplasia during or immediately after chemotherapy than are erythroid abnormalities alone (Fig. 58-4).

Currently, most patients with acute promyelocytic leukemia are treated with both standard chemotherapy and all-*trans*-retinoic acid (ATRA), and their bone marrow changes are usually similar those seen in other AML samples. However, some patients treated with ATRA or combination chemotherapy without ATRA[27] may not show an initial marrow aplasia. The bone marrow in these patients may remain hypercellular, with markedly elevated numbers of promyelocytes (Fig. 58-5). These cells usually undergo slow maturation secondary to the therapy, with loss of the t(15;17) cytogenetic abnormality associated with acute promyelocytic leukemia. In this subgroup of patients, it should be understood that the presence of sheets of promyelocytes may not indicate treatment failure, and they should be followed closely with additional marrow examinations to confirm that maturational changes are occurring.

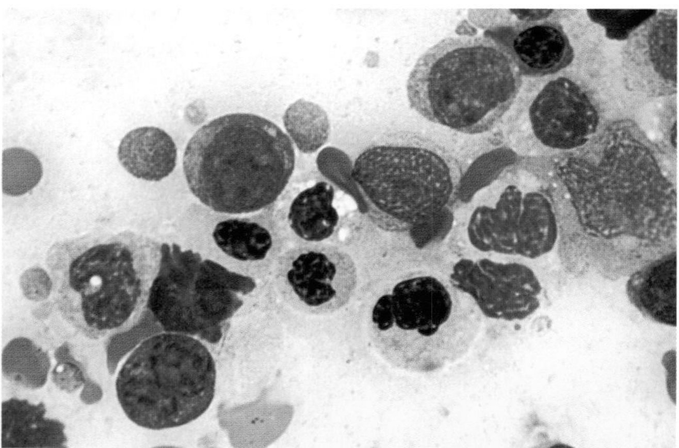

Figure 58-4. Relapse in a patient with previous acute myeloid leukemia with myelodysplasia-related changes. Although blasts are only slightly increased, dyspoietic changes are present in both neutrophils and erythroid precursors.

Immunophenotyping

Immunophenotyping studies in AML are often useful because a significant percentage of cases show aberrant expression of lymphoid-associated antigens, which can be used as an immunophenotypic "fingerprint" for residual disease testing. Lymphoid antigen expression is the most easily detected immunophenotypic abnormality, occurring in up to 48% of adult cases of AML.[28] Some aberrant immunophenotypes are commonly associated with a specific disease, such as the high frequency of CD2 expression in acute promyelocytic leukemia and in AML with inv(16)(p13.1q22) or t(16;16)(p13.1;q22), loss of HLA-DR in acute promyelocytic leukemia,[29,30] and aberrant expression of CD19 in AML with t(8;21)(q22;q22).[31,32] However, one of the most common aberrant immunophenotypes in AML is expression of CD7 on myeloblasts (Fig. 58-6),[28] which does not correlate with a specific disease type. More complex aberrant immunophenotypes have also been described, including overexpression of CD33 and CD34 on blast cells, abnormal light scatter of blast cells on flow cytometry, and asynchronous expression of mature markers on blast cells (Box 58-3).[28,33-36]

Knowledge of these aberrant immunophenotypes in the original leukemia specimen allows the use of a relatively small flow cytometry panel to evaluate for a residual population of blast cells. Detection of aberrant immunophenotypes after therapy for AML has prognostic significance, even in the absence of an increase in blast cells. Patients with only 1 aberrant cell in 100 to 1000 cells had a cumulative relapse rate of

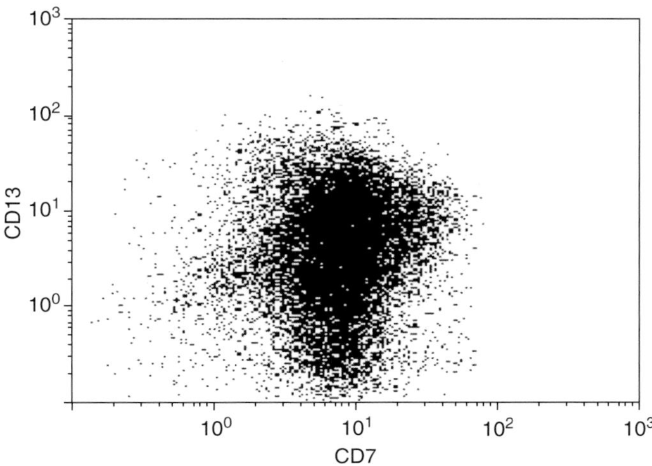

Figure 58-6. Flow cytometric scatter plot of the CD45-weak blast cell area in a patient with residual acute myeloid leukemia. The patient's original leukemia demonstrated aberrant coexpression of CD7 on $CD13^+$ myeloblasts, which are still detectable in the posttherapy sample.

50% in one study,[34] and detecting residual disease at a level of 3.5×10^{-4} or higher at the end of consolidation chemotherapy is reportedly a significant predictor of relapse.[35] The evaluation of CD117 and CD11b expression on promyelocytes can be useful in the detection of residual acute promyelocytic leukemia versus regenerating promyelocytes.[37] The leukemic promyelocytes express CD117 but not CD11b, whereas regenerating cells are $CD11b^+$ and $CD117^-$.

Paraffin section immunohistochemistry may be of value in selected cases, particularly in the presence of left-shifted cell aggregates on H&E-stained sections. Immunophenotyping can show that the immature cell aggregates of regeneration represent a spectrum of left-shifted cells that are not exclusively blast cells, whereas recurrent leukemia blast cell aggregates are a more uniform population of neoplastic cells. Therefore, the identification of clusters of cells expressing the immature cell antigen CD34 or an aberrant combination of markers that were present in the original leukemia favors residual or recurrent disease.

Box 58-3 *Aberrant Immunophenotypes in Acute Myeloid Leukemia Useful for Detecting Residual Disease*

Aberrant Lymphoid Antigen Expression on Myeloid Cells
- $CD7^+$
- $CD2^+$
- $CD4^+$
- $CD19^+$

Antigen Overexpression on Blast Cells
- $CD33^{++}$
- $CD34^{++}$

Asynchronous Antigen Expression on Blast Cells
- $CD33^{++}/CD34^+$
- $CD33^{++}/HLA\text{-}DR^-/CD34^-/CD14^-/CD15^-$
- $CD33^+/CD34^+/HLA\text{-}DR^-$
- $CD33^+/CD13^-$
- $CD33^+/CD117^+/CD34^-/CD15^-$
- $CD33^+/CD117^+/HLA\text{-}DR^-$
- $CD33^-/CD13^+$
- $CD33^-/CD14^+/HLA\text{-}DR^+$
- $CD33^-/CD15^+/HLA\text{-}DR^+$
- $CD34^+/CD11b^+$
- $CD34^+/CD69^+$
- $CD34^+/CD15^+/HLA\text{-}DR^+$
- $CD117^+/CD34^-/CD15^-$
- $CD117^+/CD11b^+$

Cytogenetics and Molecular Studies

Cytogenetic studies are not performed on all posttherapy samples but may be of value in some situations. Although some cases of AML are associated with normal karyotypes, most show a clonal cytogenetic abnormality.[38,39] Identification of that abnormality in a follow-up sample is highly supportive of relapsed disease. Karyotype analysis routinely includes the study of 20 cells; therefore, this method is not optimal for the detection of MRD when blast cells are below 5%. Most cytogenetic laboratories also perform FISH, which allows the screening of several hundred cells for a specific abnormality. This method may increase the detection rate of residual disease over karyotype analysis alone, but it requires knowledge of the karyotypic abnormality of the original disease, as well as probes specific for that abnormality. FISH probes are useful in identifying monosomies, trisomies, and masked 11q23 abnormalities, in addition to balanced chromosomal translocations. The detection of numerical chromosomal abnormalities by FISH during clinical remission has been shown to correlate with an increased risk of disease recurrence.[40] Another use of karyotype analysis and FISH is to evaluate for XX/XY chimerism.[41] If a patient receives an allogeneic transplant from a donor of the opposite sex, karyotype and FISH studies can reveal the presence of residual host cells in the marrow, even if they are of a normal karyotype. More recently, human leukocyte antigen (HLA)–based chimerism studies have been used in a similar fashion.[42] However, the detection of nondonor cells in the marrow is less predictive of recurrent disease than is the detection of a leukemia-specific abnormality.

The use of other molecular studies in the evaluation of residual disease is more controversial.[43] These methods generally employ PCR and can potentially detect 1 abnormal cell in 100,000 cells. Efforts have been made to standardize these procedures,[44] but there are still great differences in methodology and targets of study among laboratories. Similar to FISH analysis, PCR testing requires knowledge of the original karyotypic abnormality, as well as primers and probes for that abnormality. Because PCR tests are generally directed against balanced cytogenetic abnormalities, they cannot be used to detect the addition (trisomy) or deletion (monosomy) of chromosomes. However, because most de novo AML karyotypic abnormalities involve balanced translocations, PCR tests appear to be ideal for the identification of very low levels of disease. The PCR tests most often offered for AML are those for *RUNX1-RUNX1T1* (also known as *AML1-MTG8* or *AML1-ETO*) of t(8;21)(q22;q22), *PML-RARA* of t(15;17)(q22;q12), *CBFB-MYH11* of inv(16)(p13.1q22)-t(16;16)(p13.1q22), *MLL* translocations involving 11q23, and mutated *NPM1*, *FLT3*, and *CEBPA*. The *PML-RARA* PCR test is useful in the early detection of residual disease in acute promyelocytic leukemia and as a predictor of relapse of that disease.[45] Most assays for *PML-RARA* detect 1 translocated cell in 10,000 to

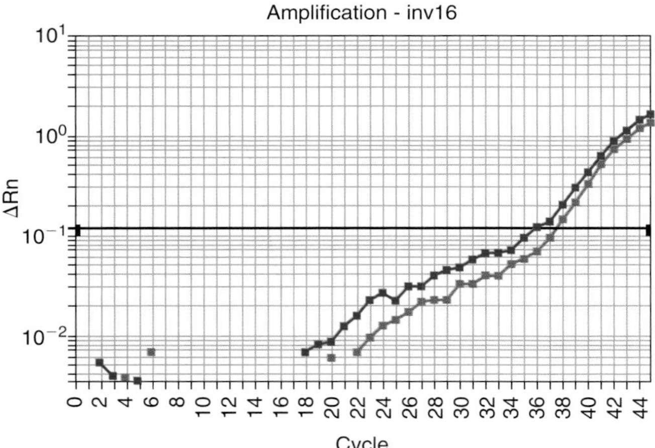

Figure 58-7. Real-time quantitative reverse transcriptase polymerase chain reaction (RT-PCR) for inv(16) detects a low level of the transcript following therapy for acute myeloid leukemia with inv(16) after normalization of the value against an internal control gene. This finding alone is not sufficient for a diagnosis of relapse because RT-PCR often continues to be positive for this abnormality at low levels, even in patients in remission. Follow-up samples showing an increase in the level of inv(16) would be needed before relapse could be suggested.

100,000 cells. However, this test appears to be less useful when more sensitive assays that detect 1 abnormal cell in 1 million are used. This ultrasensitive test is positive in patients who are in long-term remission and does not appear to be clinically relevant.[46] The *RUNX1-RUNX1T1* and *CBFB-MYH11* tests are even more problematic. It appears that other genetic aberrations, which may not be detectable by karyotype analysis, are necessary for these types of leukemia to develop.[47] In patients treated for AML with t(8;21)(q22;q22) or AML with inv(16)-(p13.1q22) or t(16;16)(p13.1;q22), standard qualitative PCR testing may detect low levels of these fusions during remission that often do not correlate with relapse of the disease (Fig. 58-7).[48,49] These PCR tests suggest that clonal cells with these fusions may persist indefinitely and that qualitative PCR for *RUNX1-RUNX1T1* and *CBFB-MYH11* is not clinically useful for residual disease testing. It is generally assumed, however, that quantitative PCR has clinical significance by showing that an increasing number of cells with *RUNX1-RUNX1T1* or *CBFB-MYH11* over time correlates with relapse of disease. Early studies appear to confirm this assumption.[50-52] Quantitative assays for *FLT3* gene mutations and Wilms' tumor gene (*WT1*) expression have also been used to detect residual disease in AML.[53] Mutations occurring in exon 12 of the nucleophosmin gene (*NPM1*) are the most frequent abnormality (60%) of normal-karyotype AML.[54] PCR and reverse transcriptase PCR (RT-PCR) assays for the detection of *NPM1* mutations have been successful in detecting MRD with good sensitivity,[55] although clonal evolution with loss of the mutation at relapse occurs in a small subset of patients.[56]

Acute Lymphoblastic Leukemia

Morphologic Features

Because of the morphologic overlap with myeloblasts, many of the features that are useful in distinguishing leukemic myeloblasts from regenerating myeloblasts also apply to lymphoblasts. Comparison to the original leukemia blasts is useful to identify distinctive features, such as variation in blast cell size and cytoplasm, cytoplasmic vacuoles, nucleoli, and nuclear convolutions. Some lymphoblasts may contain cytoplasmic granules, but Auer rods are not seen. Distinguishing lymphoblasts from normal precursor B cells or hematogones may create diagnostic difficulties and is discussed in detail later. Not surprisingly, the early clearance of blast cells from peripheral blood (by day 7) and bone marrow (by day 14 or 15) in acute lymphoblastic leukemia (ALL) is associated with an improved prognosis in both adults and children.[57-60] Even the detection of very low levels of bone marrow lymphoblasts by morphologic evaluation is significant. Sandlund and colleagues[61] demonstrated a significantly worse 5-year survival in children with 1% to 4% lymphoblasts by morphology on day 15 and by bone marrow aspirate examination on days 22 to 25 compared with children having less than 1% blast cells. Therefore, the morphologic examination for residual blast cells, even at low levels, is of clinical importance.

Bone marrow biopsy morphology can also help detect residual leukemia in ALL. As with leukemic myeloblasts, residual or recurrent lymphoblasts tend to cluster and form aggregates on biopsy material. Such suspicious aggregates can be evaluated by immunohistochemistry, as described later.

Immunophenotyping

Detection of aberrant immunophenotypes can be extremely helpful in the evaluation for residual ALL. Up to 46% of ALL cases show aberrant expression of myeloid-associated markers (Fig. 58-8).[62] The most common aberrant immunophenotypes are CD13, CD33, and CD38 expression in precursor B-cell ALL with t(9;22)(q34;q11.2)[63] and CD15 and CD65 expression but lack of CD10 expression in pro-B-cell ALL with *MLL* translocations, particularly t(4;11)(q21;q23)[64]; however, aberrant expression of myeloid antigens may occur in other ALL types. Other immunophenotypic abnormalities, such as dyssynchronous expression of B- or T-cell antigens for the stage of lymphocyte development, may be used for the evaluation of residual disease (Box 58-4).[62,65-69] Because of the presence of normal precursor B cells in the marrow, the detection of a small population of $CD19^+$, $CD10^+$, and TdT^+ cells in the marrow without other abnormalities is not sufficient for an interpretation of residual precursor B-cell ALL. However, precursor T cells should not be identified in the marrow, and the detection of any cytoplasmic $CD3^+$ and TdT^+ population is evidence of residual T-cell ALL.

The use of flow cytometry to detect aberrant immunophenotypes after treatment for ALL allows the detection of as few as 0.01% residual leukemic cells, and recent studies have demonstrated a significantly higher risk of relapse in children with 0.01% or higher leukemic cells by this method.[70-72]

Immunohistochemical studies are also useful in the evaluation of immature cell aggregates in the marrow of patients treated for ALL. Leukemic lymphoblasts tend to form clusters in the marrow, and the detection of clusters of TdT^+ or $CD34^+$ cells on biopsy material is strong evidence of residual disease (Fig. 58-9).[73] The immunophenotypic differences between leukemic cells and normal bone marrow progenitor cells are described in more detail in the section on hematogones.

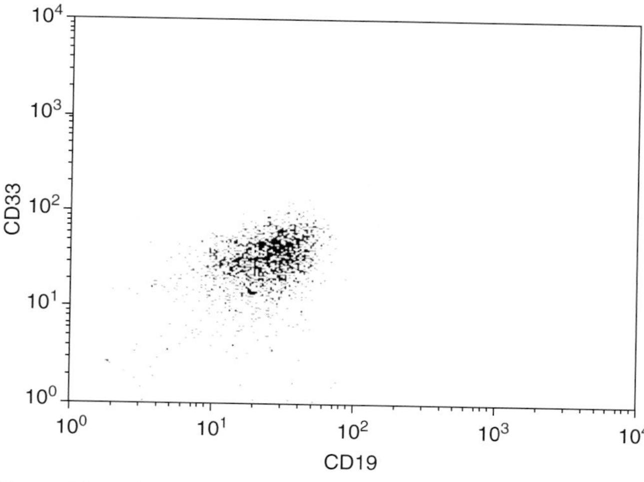

Figure 58-8. Flow cytometric scatter plot of the CD45-weak blast cell area in a patient with residual acute lymphoblastic leukemia. The patient's original leukemia demonstrated aberrant coexpression of CD19 and CD33, which are still detectable in the posttherapy sample.

Cytogenetics and Molecular Studies

Karyotype and FISH analyses offer results similar to those described for AML. Karyotype abnormalities are often detected at presentation with ALL, but a significant number of patients have normal karyotypes or abnormalities that are not easily followed by molecular methods. The specific abnormalities most often followed in patients with ALL are *BCR-ABL1* of t(9;22)(q34;q11.2), *TCF3-PBX1* of t(1;19)(q23;p13.3), *ETV6-RUNX1* of t(12;21)(p13;q22), and *MLL* translocations, particularly t(4;11).[74,75] ALL cells also demonstrate T- and B-cell receptor gene rearrangements.[76] Such rearrangements are not entirely lineage specific (dual immunoglobulin heavy-chain and T-cell receptor chain rearrangements are common in precursor B-cell ALL), but they can be used for residual disease testing. Most PCR tests for T- and B-cell gene rearrangements use consensus primers that can detect only 1 translocated cell in 100 to 1000 cells. Low levels of monoclonal cells are easily obscured by admixed polyclonal lymphocytes. In contrast, PCR testing directed to a specific balanced cytogenetic translocation is very sensitive and can detect abnormal cells at a level of 1 translocated cell in 100,000 cells. Therefore, specific PCR testing against balanced translocations is the easiest and most sensitive method of identifying molecular genetic evidence of residual disease.[77] Unfortunately, most patients with ALL do not have balanced translocations to target for these tests. To overcome this problem, several studies have used patient-specific gene rearrangement testing,[78,79] but this type of testing is labor intensive and is not routinely offered by most laboratories at this time. It requires the demonstration of a T- or B-cell gene rearrangement in the original acute leukemia specimen. The rearrangement is then sequenced, and PCR primers and probes are made specifically for the individual patient's abnormality. The follow-up samples are then tested with the patient-specific primers and probes for residual disease. This methodology can detect residual disease at the level of the specific translocation (usually 1 abnormal cell in 100,000 cells) and is useful for predicting relapse in childhood ALL.[78,80,81] This test appears to be even more powerful when quantitative assays are performed.

Molecular testing is reportedly useful when residual disease levels of 1 in 1000 (10^{-3}) cells are detectable at the end of induction chemotherapy and before the start of consolidation therapy.[80,82] Intensification of treatment based on MRD-directed risk groups was shown to benefit patients with ALL in a recent international multicenter trial.[83] The prognostic value of molecular MRD testing may be most significant for T-cell ALL.[80] Although most of the studies of MRD in ALL using gene rearrangements employ patient-specific primers, alternative approaches may also be effective. Using consensus primers and probes designed specifically for the quantitative monitoring of childhood ALL patients, a detection sensitivity of 1 clonal cell in 50,000 cells was described.[84] This appears to be sensitive enough to detect clinically significant disease. This method might be applicable to all childhood ALL cases and could become available in diagnostic laboratories in the near future.

Box 58-4 *Aberrant Immunophenotypes in Acute Lymphoblastic Leukemia Useful for Detecting Residual Disease*

Aberrant Myeloid Antigen Expression on Lymphoblasts
- CD13
- CD15
- CD33
- CD36
- CD65

Uniform Antigen Expression on Immature Cells
- CD34
- TdT

Antigen Overexpression on Blast Cells
- CD9
- CD10

Antigen Underexpression on Blast Cells
- CD19
- CD20
- CD38
- CD45
- HLA-DR

Other Asynchronous Antigen Expression on Blast Cells
- Cytoplasmic $CD3^+/TdT^+$
- $CD20^+/CD34^+$

Others Blast Cell Abnormalities
- Increased forward scatter
- Aberrant CD58 expression

Distinguishing Hematogones

One of the most challenging problems in the evaluation of posttherapy ALL specimens is distinguishing residual or recurrent disease from nonneoplastic precursor B cells, or hematogones. Hematogones are more frequent in children and may be the predominant cell type in bone marrow aspirates in some cases, such as in children with idiopathic thrombocytopenic purpura. They may also occur in children with other cytopenias, malignancies at other sites, or regenerating marrow after treatment for leukemia.[85-87] These cells also occur in adults, particularly after hematopoietic stem cell transplantation, but they may be seen in adults with lymphoma, autoimmune diseases, or acquired immunodeficiency

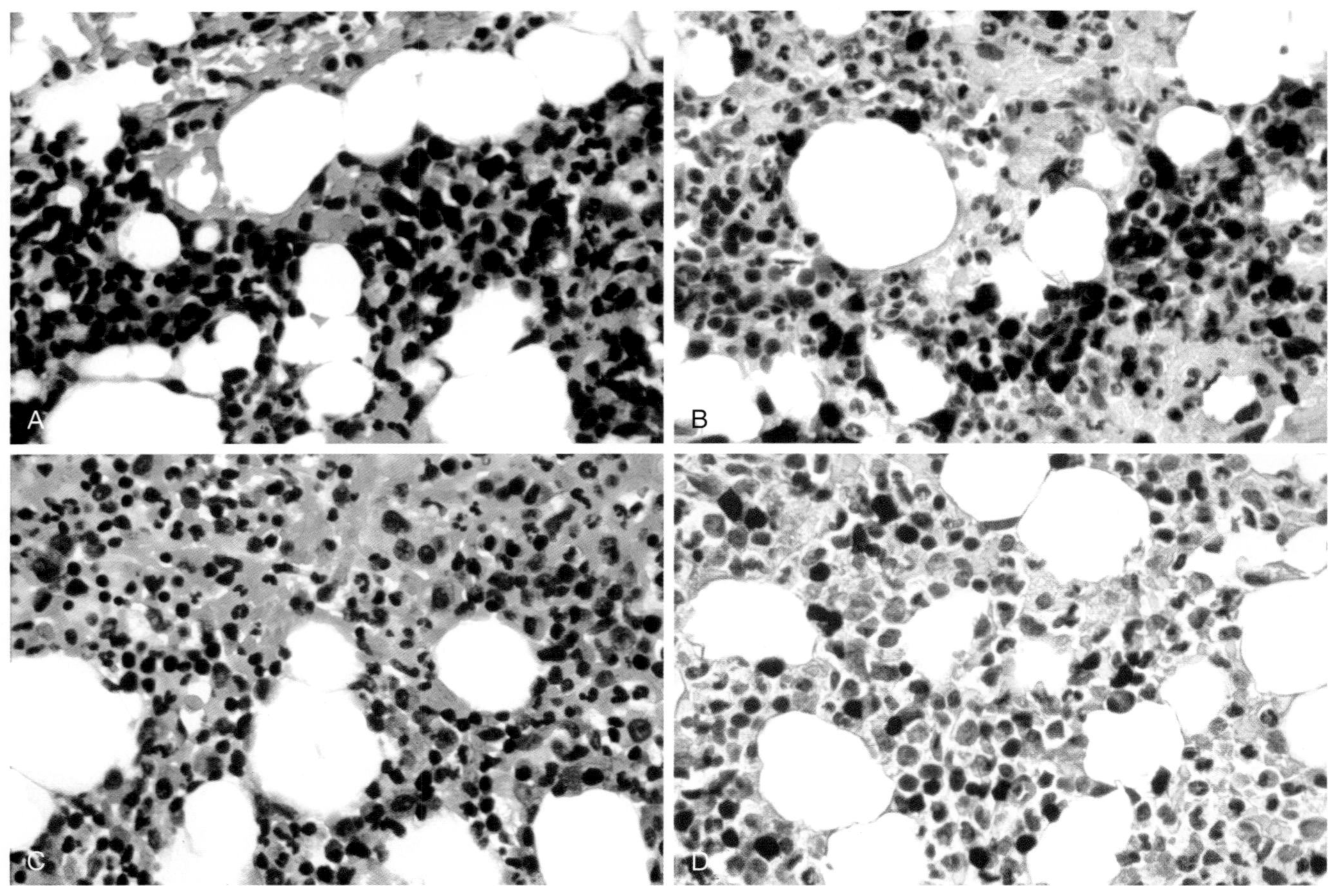

Figure 58-9. Immunohistochemical features of residual precursor B-cell acute lymphoblastic leukemia and normal precursor B cells (hematogones). **A** and **B,** This case of residual leukemia shows aggregates of terminal deoxynucleotidyl transferase (TdT)–positive cells. **C** and **D,** In this case there is an increase in hematogones, which do not form distinct aggregates on the biopsy material, and only scattered individual TdT^+ cells.

syndrome (AIDS) as well.[88,89] Because of their monotonous lymphoid appearance and precursor B-cell lineage, they are easily misinterpreted as leukemic cells. Hematogones are predominantly small cells with scant cytoplasm, with smaller numbers of admixed large cells (Fig. 58-10). The small cells are uniform in size but exhibit a spectrum of nuclear features, ranging from homogeneous, bland chromatin without nucleoli to mature, clumped chromatin. These cells differ from most lymphoblasts, which are usually larger and have more cytoplasm, more variation in size, distinct nucleoli, and no evidence of maturation. Although hematogones may be numerous in aspirate material, they are usually inconspicuous in biopsy material. Hematogones are usually found as interstitial infiltrates, whereas leukemic blasts often form aggregates in bone marrow biopsy specimens. Some adult patients with hematogones have been reported to have coexisting lymphoid aggregates, but in our experience, the cells in the lymphoid aggregates are not immature B cells by immunophenotyping. They are usually a mixture of T cells and mature B cells with surrounding interstitial precursor B cells.

Hematogones express CD19, CD10, and TdT; CD34 expression is variable; and CD20 expression is usually weak or absent. These cells exhibit the antigen expression profiles that are expected for developing B cells, in contrast to the aberrant immunophenotypes of ALL cells. Review of flow cytometric scatter plots usually reveals a spectrum of cells with varying degrees of CD10 and TdT expression, in contrast to the more uniform expression of these antigens in leukemic cells (Fig. 58-11). Several studies have now shown significant differences in antigen expression between hematogones and leukemic lymphoblasts.[65,67,90-92] Leukemic cells most often exhibit decreased expression of CD45 and increased expression of CD9, CD10, and CD34, with fairly uniform expression of these antigens in the blast cell population (see Box 58-4). Hematogones, in contrast, have a wider spectrum of antigen expression. For example, they usually show a spectrum of cells that vary from weak to bright CD10 positivity. This antigen expression profile follows normal B-cell development patterns and exhibits a high degree of immunophenotypic stability, regardless of therapy.[93] Aberrant myeloid antigen expression, which is common in ALL, is not seen in hematogones, and karyotypic and molecular genetic abnormalities should not be seen with proliferations of these cells. The interstitial pattern of hematogones seen in the biopsy specimen is easily confirmed by immunohistochemistry, whereas aggregates of precursor B cells in the biopsy specimen are strong evidence of leukemic cells. Although hematogones may be numerous in the bone marrow, they are usually not seen in the peripheral blood; therefore, circulating immature cells are a good indication of persistent or recurrent leukemia.

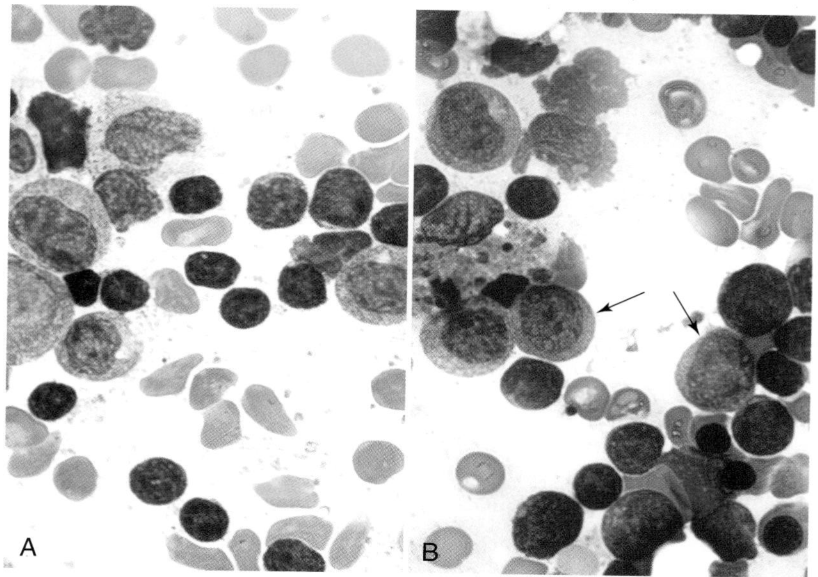

Figure 58-10. Hematogones after therapy. A, There is an increase in precursor cells, which are generally small and uniform in size and lack nucleoli. **B,** This similar population of cells also has larger blast cells (*arrows*) with nucleoli, in a specimen from an 8-month-old treated for *MLL*-positive pro-B acute lymphoblastic leukemia. This sample showed an immunoglobulin kappa gene rearrangement by polymerase chain reaction analysis and a small population of *MLL* rearranged cells by fluorescence in situ hybridization, consistent with minimal residual disease.

Table 58-2 summarizes the most useful features for distinguishing hematogones from residual or recurrent ALL.

CHRONIC MYELOGENOUS LEUKEMIA

The chronic myeloproliferative neoplasms have overlapping morphologic features and are generally diagnosed by a combination of morphologic, clinical, and genetic findings (see Chapter 46). Chronic myelogenous leukemia (CML) is the most common chronic myeloproliferative neoplasm and the one that most often requires posttherapy evaluation. A variety of therapies are now available for CML, including bone marrow transplantation, α-interferon therapy, and, most recently, tyrosine kinase inhibitor (TKI) therapy.

Morphologic Features

With treatment of the chronic phase of CML, the bone marrow becomes less cellular; with some therapies, it may become normocellular or even slightly hypocellular. The myeloid-to-erythroid (M/E) ratio, which is usually markedly elevated before treatment, usually returns to normal or may become decreased. In these cases it is often difficult to determine by morphologic features alone whether leukemic cells persist in the marrow. The most common clues to residual disease are hypercellularity, the presence of clusters of atypical "dwarf" megakaryocytes, prominent basophilia, and, in some cases, the continued presence of clusters of Gaucher-like histiocytes. Despite these clues, cytogenetic or molecular genetic studies to detect t(9;22)(q34;q11) *BCR-ABL1* are needed to definitively identify the continued presence of leukemia.

In the past, busulfan, hydroxyurea, and α-interferon therapies were used to treat CML, with some variation in the degree of bone marrow response. Some patients achieved clinical features of remission, with improvement of peripheral blood counts.[94,95] With busulfan, the bone marrow usually remains hypercellular, with an elevated M/E ratio. Megakaryocytes tend to be increased with therapy, and this increase is

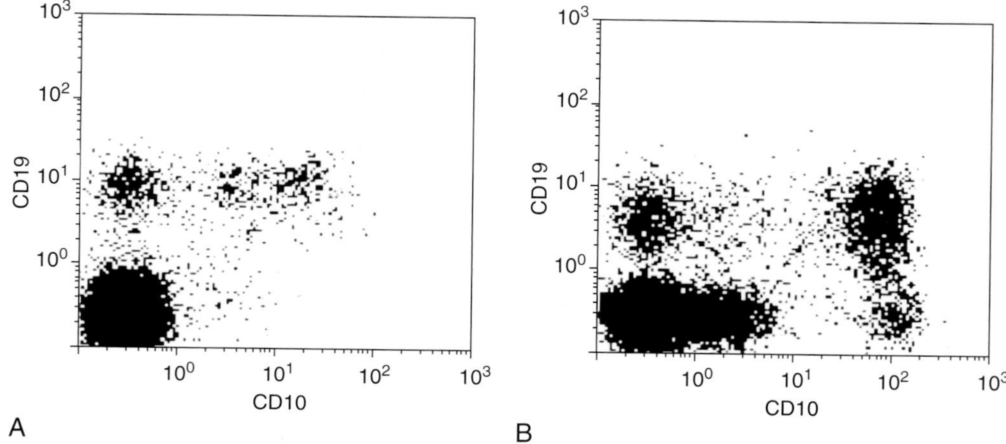

Figure 58-11. Flow cytometric features of hematogones (**A**) and residual precursor B-cell acute lymphoblastic leukemia (**B**). The hematogones show an immunophenotypic spectrum of CD10 expression among CD19⁺ cells, whereas the leukemia sample has a more distinct population of strongly CD10⁺ cells. Other immunophenotypic changes useful in this differential diagnosis are listed in Box 58-4.

Table 58-2 **Useful Features for Distinguishing Hematogones from Residual or Recurrent B Lymphoblastic Leukemia**

Feature	Hematogone	Leukemia
Homogeneous nuclear chromatin	+	–
Maturation spectrum	+	–
Most cells smaller than a maturing granulocyte	+	–
Nucleoli	–	+
Precursor B-cell clusters on biopsy	–	+
Aberrant antigen expression	–	+/–
Peripheral blood involvement	–	+/–

associated with an increase in marrow fibrosis. With hydroxyurea, the marrow cellularity decreases somewhat but usually remains above normal, with only a moderate correction in the M/E ratio. The number of megakaryocytes and degree of marrow fibrosis, however, tend to decrease with hydroxyurea. With α-interferon, complete normalization of peripheral blood counts may occur. The bone marrow remains slightly hypercellular in most patients, but approximately one quarter of patients develop normal bone marrow features on α-interferon.[95] Marrow megakaryocytes remain elevated, with associated fibrosis; bone marrow macrophages are reportedly increased in the marrow. Despite the improvement in marrow cellularity, most patients continue to show cytogenetic evidence of clonal marrow disease.

Bone marrow transplantation was the standard treatment for CML in the past and is still considered the only totally curative thrapy.[96] After transplantation the marrow undergoes the expected changes of aplasia, followed by regeneration. The majority of CML patients treated with transplantation are cured and show normocellular or hypocellular marrow without specific abnormalities. Relapse specimens from patients treated with transplantation show changes similar to de novo disease, with granulocytic hyperplasia, basophilia, and hypercellularity, and are usually not diagnostic dilemmas.

Currently, most patients with all phases of CML are treated with a TKI that directly blocks the effects of the *BCR-ABL1* fusion gene.[97] The TKI most commonly used is imatinib, although second-generation *BCR-ABL1* inhibitors are available for patients who fail to respond, relapse, or experience intolerance to imatinib. Imatinib therapy results in a clinical, morphologic, and at least partial or complete cytogenetic remission in many patients, with a reduction in marrow cellularity, normalization of the M/E ratio, and normalization of megakaryocyte number and morphology.[98-100] The peripheral blood is the first to respond to imatinib therapy; the white blood cell count returns to normal, basophils decrease, and the platelet count normalizes, with normal-appearing platelets occurring after about 2 months of therapy. The hemoglobin level tends to decrease slightly during therapy. A subset of patients may develop neutropenia or thrombocytopenia while receiving the drug. The bone marrow hypercellularity gradually decreases, and by 8 to 11 months the marrow is normocellular or hypocellular, with a normal or decreased M/E ratio in most patients. Even in the chronic phase, bone marrow blast cells and megakaryocytes decrease, the number of hypolobated megakaryocytes decreases, and megakaryocyte clustering becomes less common as the marrow cellularity decreases (Fig. 58-12). This therapy can also gradually eliminate the marrow fibrosis that is prominent is some cases of CML,[98,100,101] although progression of myelofibrosis has also been reported, mostly in cases with acceleration or blast phase.[99] Patients with accelerated or blast-phase CML, however, also show rapid decreases in peripheral blood and bone marrow blast cell counts.[98] After long-term treatment with imatinib, some patients may have increased pseudo-Gaucher cells and reactive lymphoid nodules.[99]

Relapse of CML may take the form of chronic or blast-phase disease and may result from natural evolution of the disease, with cytogenetic evolution; from loss of responsiveness to imatinib therapy through the acquisition of mutations

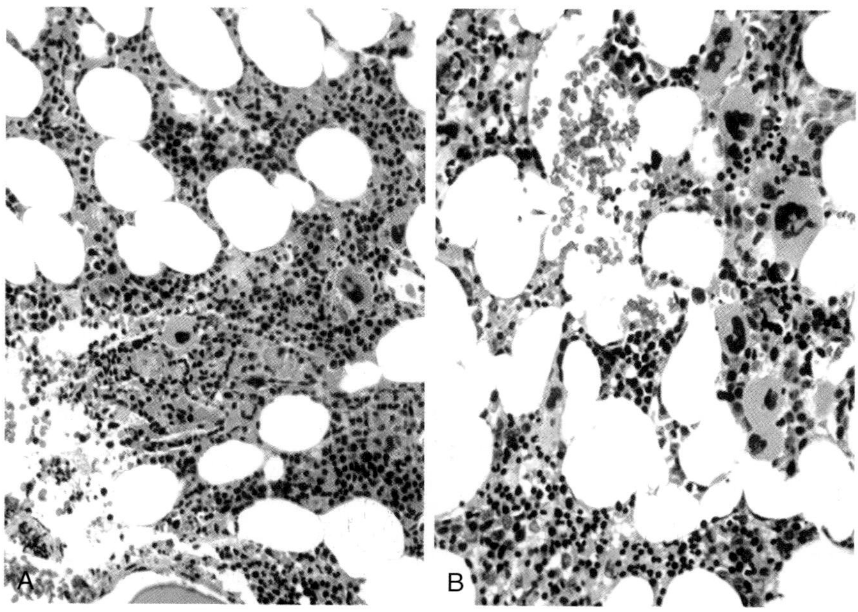

Figure 58-12. Posttherapy changes in chronic myelogenous leukemia. After tyrosine kinase inhibitor therapy, samples may be morphologically normal **(A)** or show residual clusters of atypical megakaryocytes **(B)**. Both samples remained positive for *BCR-ABL1* by reverse transcriptase polymerase chain reaction.

within the kinase domain of *BCR-ABL1* or amplification of the fusion gene; or through other mechanisms that are not yet clearly understood. Occasionally patients develop a myelodysplastic or blastic process in cells that are negative for the Philadelphia chromosome.[102] If the patient had a previous blast phase, comparison to the original material may be useful, similar to the evaluation of posttherapy acute leukemia specimens. Morphologic evaluation is of limited utility in predicting the type of blast crisis in CML, and immunophenotyping studies are required for accurate classification of the blast cell lineage.[103]

Immunophenotyping

Immunophenotyping studies generally are not useful in the evaluation of patients treated for CML. These studies may be of use in the follow-up of blast transformation, similar to that described for the acute leukemias. The majority of blast transformations in CML are of myeloid lineage,[103] with many showing expression of megakaryocyte-associated markers such as CD41, CD42, and CD61. Approximately one third of blast transformations are of precursor B-cell lineage with TdT expression, and only rare cases are of immature T-cell lineage. The lymphoblast proliferations are generally TdT$^+$ but also frequently express aberrant myeloid-associated antigens such as CD13 and CD33.

Cytogenetics and Molecular Studies

The majority of patients treated with busulfan, hydroxyurea, and α-interferon have karyotypic evidence of disease during and after treatment. However, approximately 13% of patients treated with α-interferon, 63% or more of patients on imatinib therapy for 60 months or longer, and most patients treated with hematopoietic stem cell transplantation have no karyotypic evidence of disease.[100,104,105] More sophisticated, ultrasensitive methods, however, reveal the continued presence of very low levels of the Philadelphia chromosome in the stem cells of patients treated with imatinib.[106] Many other patients receiving these therapies develop partial cytogenetic responses.[97] The reversion to normal bone marrow morphology does not correlate with loss of t(9;22) in all cases, and molecular or cytogenetic confirmation is needed. Patients treated with imatinib may develop a cytogenetic remission after only 2 months of therapy, but the time to achieve a cytogenetic response is variable. Patients who develop early normalization of bone marrow cellularity by 2 to 5 months are reportedly more likely to develop a complete cytogenetic response.

Various guidelines have been suggested for monitoring patients on therapy, particularly those receiving imatinib.[107-109] Most recommend that routine karyotyping and quantitative RT-PCR to measure *BCR-ABL1* transcripts be performed at regular intervals. FISH studies are generally not recommended for long-term follow-up, mainly because most FISH assays have background levels of up to 6%, limiting the ability to detect very low levels of disease. However, a highly sensitive interphase double-fusion assay, sometimes termed *D-FISH*, can detect very low levels of *BCR-ABL1* fusion and is much more sensitive than conventional karyotype analysis, although it does not allow the detection of additional chromosomal abnormalities.[110,111]

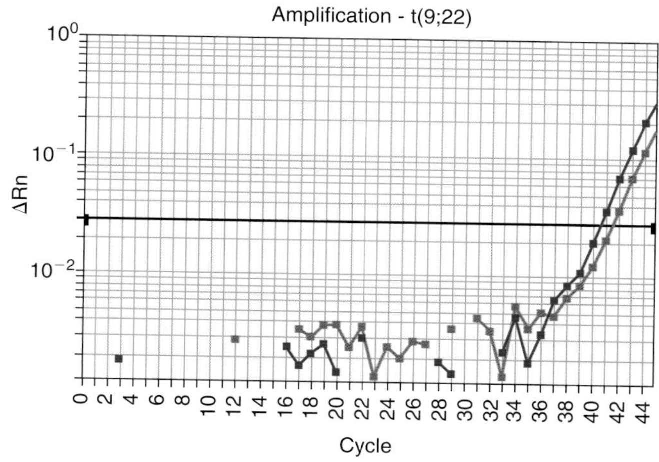

Figure 58-13. Low-level detection of residual *BCR-ABL1* fusion after therapy for chronic myelogenous leukemia, despite the presence of morphologic and cytogenetic karyotypic remission. These levels may continue to decline in the months immediately after bone marrow transplantation, but serial monitoring for an increase may allow early intervention and treatment of relapsed disease.

Following transplantation, patients frequently remain *BCR-ABL1* positive by PCR for several months, with no clinical evidence of relapse with long-term clinical follow-up.[112] In part, the cause of these presumably false-positive PCR results is the presence of the fusion product in terminally differentiated cells, such as Gaucher-like histiocytes.[113] With time these cells disappear, and the PCR test becomes negative. Therefore, PCR testing in the months immediately after transplantation may not have clinical relevance. Use of serial quantitative PCR methods may be one means of avoiding overinterpretation of a positive PCR result, with an interval increase in the amount of *BCR-ABL1* transcripts presumably indicating residual or recurrent disease (Fig. 58-13).[114] Performing quantitative PCR tests 18 months and longer after transplantation is useful in predicting relapse.[115] This type of testing is also useful in monitoring patients receiving imatinib mesylate so that molecular genetic relapses, with rising levels of *BCR-ABL1* fusion, can be treated before the development of morphologic evidence of disease recurrence.

CHRONIC LYMPHOPROLIFERATIVE AND PLASMA CELL DISORDERS

Morphologic Features

Most malignant lymphomas involve the bone marrow focally, forming aggregates of neoplastic cells. Because of the focal nature of the disease, it may be missed on a review of aspirate smears alone, and bone marrow trephine and clot biopsies are essential for a complete evaluation. Bilateral bone marrow biopsies increase the yield of detecting the focal lesions.[116] The finding of focal aggregates of atypical large lymphoid cells usually presents no diagnostic dilemma, but aggregates of small lymphoid cells of residual lymphoma must be distinguished from reactive lymphoid aggregates, which are common in older adults.[117,118] Even when the patient has a history of a large cell lymphoma, discordant lymphoma morphology may occur, with only low-grade lymphoma present in the bone marrow aggregates.[119-121]

Reactive lymphoid aggregates are usually composed of predominantly small lymphocytes with admixed large cells; they may contain histiocytes and plasma cells as well. These aggregates are usually small and well circumscribed and may contain intervening small vessels. The reactive aggregates are nonparatrabecular in location.[118] The pattern of neoplastic aggregates of residual or recurrent lymphoma in the marrow varies by the lymphoma type.[122,123] Follicular lymphoma characteristically involves the marrow in a paratrabecular pattern, with associated fibrosis and no fat spaces present between the lymphoid aggregate and the bone. This pattern of infiltrate is diagnostic of bone marrow involvement in a patient with a history of follicular lymphoma, and ancillary studies are not needed to confirm the diagnosis. After therapy, these aggregates may be less cellular, but they continue to exhibit lymphoid cells and fibrosis adjacent to bone.[124] Mantle cell lymphoma may show a mixed paratrabecular and nonparatrabecular pattern. An interstitial pattern of disease predominates in hairy cell leukemia and in some cases of chronic lymphocytic leukemia. Most other lymphomas show a predominantly nonparatrabecular pattern. Splenic marginal zone lymphoma may show an intrasinusoidal pattern of disease,[125,126] but this pattern does not appear to be specific for this disease, and patients who have undergone splenectomy for splenic marginal zone lymphoma may develop nodular bone marrow involvement.[127] The most helpful morphologic clues for identifying bone marrow involvement by lymphoma are a paratrabecular pattern of involvement, the presence of a monotonous cell population within the aggregates, and large, irregularly shaped aggregates that show infiltration into the surrounding normal hematopoietic marrow. Small nonparatrabecular lymphoid aggregates in patients with a history of lymphoma usually require ancillary immunohistologic studies to determine the nature of the aggregates.[120,128]

Residual or early recurrence of multiple myeloma is often most easily suspected based on bone marrow aspirate smears. In the absence of an absolute increase in marrow plasma cells, the presence of atypical plasma cells characterized by variably enlarged cells, immature chromatin, and prominent nucleoli should raise suspicion for involvement by disease. On biopsy material, only small clusters of atypical cells may be identified, or only individual cells may be present. In the absence of an increase in plasma cells or aggregates of atypical plasma cells, ancillary studies are usually needed.

Immunophenotyping

Immunophenotyping is the most common method of detecting residual disease in the marrow of patients with a history of lymphoma. Flow cytometry is often used, but several studies have failed to show a significant increase in disease detection over morphology when routine forward versus side scatter or CD45 gating is performed.[116,129,130] Other studies, however, have found flow cytometry to be superior to morphology in detecting residual disease,[131,132] and more recent four-color (or more) methods of analysis, with gating on $CD19^+$ or $CD20^+$ populations, increase the detection rate of this methodology. Sampling differences between bone marrow aspirate and biopsy material also decrease the yield of flow cytometry. When a suspicious lymphoid aggregate is present on the biopsy, immunohistochemical methods are useful. Because most malignant lymphomas are of B-cell lineage, and because most bone marrow lymphocytes are T cells, the detection of aggregates or sheets of B cells in lymphoid aggregates is often good evidence of involvement by lymphoma (Fig. 58-14).[118,123] The primary exception to the correlation between an increase in aggregate B cells and lymphoma is when reactive germinal centers are present in the marrow. Bone marrow germinal centers are most common in patients with autoimmune diseases,[133] and these types of aggregates should not automatically be considered evidence of marrow involvement by lymphoma. Bone marrow evaluation can usually be accomplished with a relatively small panel of antibodies, including CD3 and CD20, but more antibodies can be used if subclassification is needed. Aberrant expression of CD5 or CD43 in B cells is common in many lymphomas of small B cells in the marrow, and this finding is also useful to confirm bone marrow involvement by disease.[134]

Paraffin section immunophenotyping may cause confusion in cases of bone marrow involvement by follicular lymphoma. Follicular lymphoma at almost any site is usually accompanied by a relatively large number of T cells, and T cells may predominate in marrow involved by this type of lymphoma. Although CD10 expression is commonly seen with follicular lymphoma, this antigen is often lost in bone marrow lymphoma aggregates, and such antigen expression may be seen in nonneoplastic lymphocytes. Detection of BCL6 protein by immunohistochemistry may be useful in detecting follicular lymphoma, but this antigen is not restricted to germinal center cells. For this reason, the morphologic feature of paratrabecular aggregates is considered the most reliable means of detecting follicular lymphoma in the marrow.[128] A possible exception is in the setting of anti-CD20 therapy, in which paratrabecular aggregates devoid of B cells may persist after therapy.[135]

Many lymphoma patients are now treated with monoclonal antibodies directed against CD20. The most common of these is rituximab (Rituxan, IDEC Pharmaceutical, San Diego, CA). Patients treated with these antibodies may relapse with $CD20^-$ disease. In one study, 37% of lymphoma patients who relapsed after treatment with rituximab had $CD20^-$ relapsed disease.[136] This should be suspected when a subpopulation of cells does not appear to mark with either T-cell markers (e.g., CD3) or CD20. In such cases, or in patients with a known history of treatment with these antibodies, alternative B-cell markers, such as CD79a or PAX5, should be used to evaluate for possible lymphoma recurrence. Bone marrow lymphoid aggregates composed entirely of T cells, morphologically mimicking recurrent lymphoma, have also been described in patients who received rituximab therapy.[135]

Antibodies directed against annexin A1, tartrate-resistant acid phosphatase (TRAP), and DBA.44 are reportedly useful in the detection of hairy cell leukemia, but this tumor is almost always $CD20^+$, and additional markers are usually not needed to identify residual disease. In addition, annexin A1 is positive in myeloid-lineage cells, and although it is a robust marker of hairy cells, is difficult to interpret when small numbers of cells are present in a regenerating marrow.

For plasma cell disorders, cytoplasmic flow cytometric studies directed against $CD38^+$ or $CD138^+$ plasma cells may detect populations of residual clonal cells with kappa or lambda light chains.[137] However, these methods are not per-

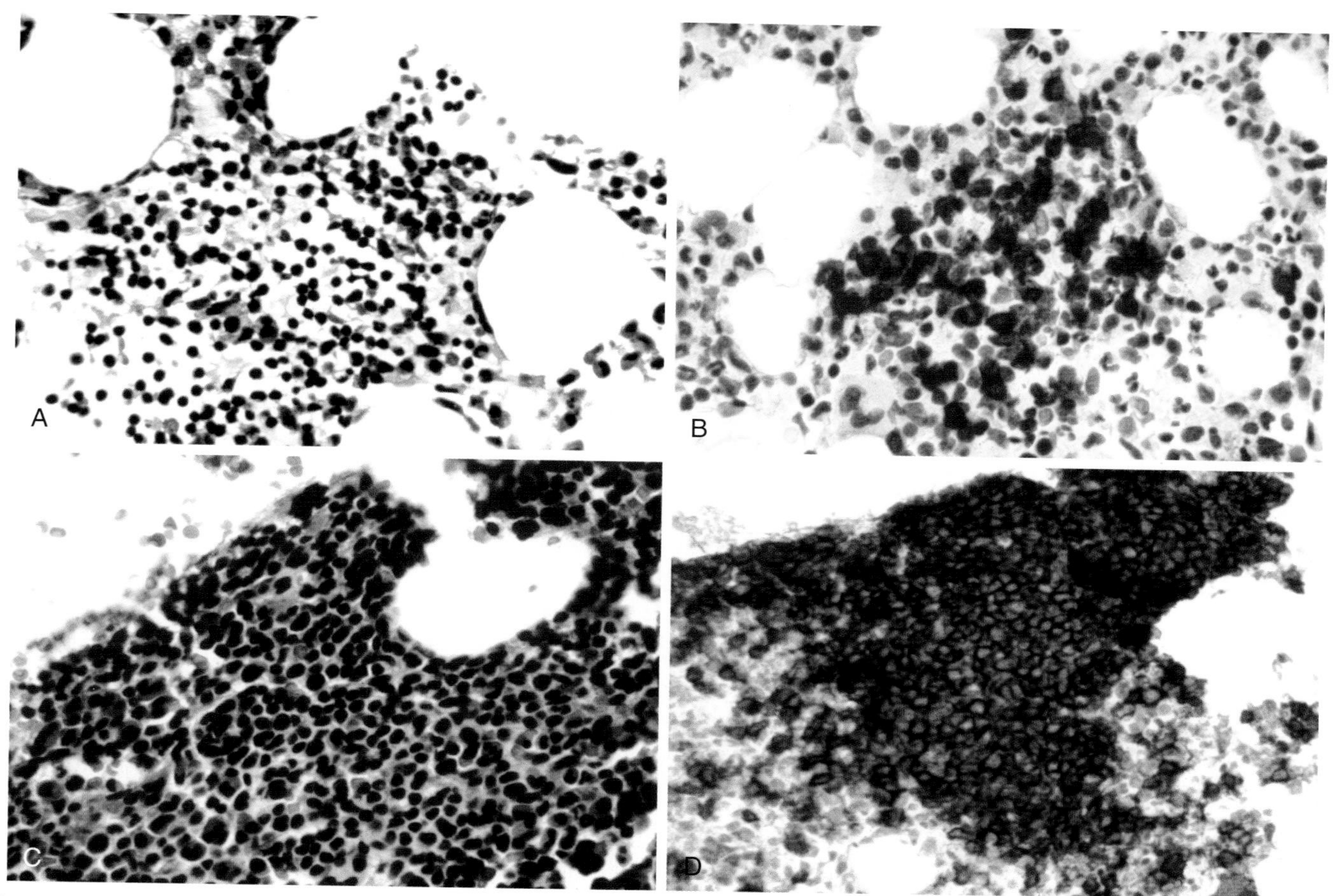

Figure 58-14. Morphologic and immunohistochemical features of reactive and neoplastic lymphoid aggregates. The reactive lymphoid aggregate (**A** and **B**) is small and well circumscribed, compared with the larger, infiltrating aggregate of lymphoma (**C** and **D**). The reactive aggregate is only partially composed of $CD20^+$ B cells (**B**), whereas sheets of B cells are present in the lymphoma aggregate (**D**). These B cells also showed aberrant expression of CD5 and CD43 and were positive for cyclin D1, consistent with recurrent mantle cell lymphoma.

formed in all laboratories, and immunohistochemical studies are more widely available. Paraffin section antibody panels that include CD138, kappa, and lambda are usually sufficient for the evaluation of residual myeloma cells (Fig. 58-15). CD138 staining is helpful in quantifying the plasma cell infiltrate and identifying the presence of plasma cell aggregates or clusters. Staining for immunoglobulin light chains may detect residual monotypic plasma cells at a level of 1% or less. Expression of CD31 or CD56 on neoplastic plasma cells has also been reported,[138,139] but these markers are usually not needed to evaluate residual disease. Autologous bone marrow and peripheral blood stem cell transplantation appear to significantly reduce the number of monotypic bone marrow plasma cells and result in improved survival.[137,140] In a recent study, multiparametric flow cytometric detection of monotypic plasma cells on day 100 was the most relevant independent prognostic factor in progression-free and overall survival among myeloma patients undergoing autologous stem cell transplantation.[141]

Cytogenetics and Molecular Studies

Karyotype analysis of the bone marrow is useful when a clonal population similar to the patient's original neoplastic clone is identified, but the low mitotic rate of many low-grade lymphomas results in many false-negative results. The addition of interphase FISH is one method of overcoming this problem and is useful in detecting lymphoma-associated translocations. Neither karyotype nor FISH analysis can detect T- or B-cell–associated gene rearrangements that are not associated with translocations or other clonal abnormalities.

Molecular methods are now being used more often to evaluate for residual disease in lymphoid and plasma cell disorders. Although Southern blot analysis is considered the "gold standard" for the detection of gene rearrangements, it is time-consuming, requires a relatively large amount of material, and does not routinely detect a clonal population that involves less than 5% of the marrow. Therefore, amplification methods are employed.[76] PCR and RT-PCR are the methods most commonly used to detect gene rearrangements and lymphoma-associated translocations. Gene rearrangement studies are usually directed against the immunoglobulin heavy-chain gene (*IGH@*; Fig. 58-16), immunoglobulin kappa light-chain gene (*IGK@*), T-cell receptor gamma gene (*TCRG*), and T-cell receptor beta gene (*TCRB*). These genes are fairly complex, so to achieve the highest rate of detection, the primers are fairly nonspecific (termed *degenerate* or *consensus primers*). With consensus primers, a relatively high

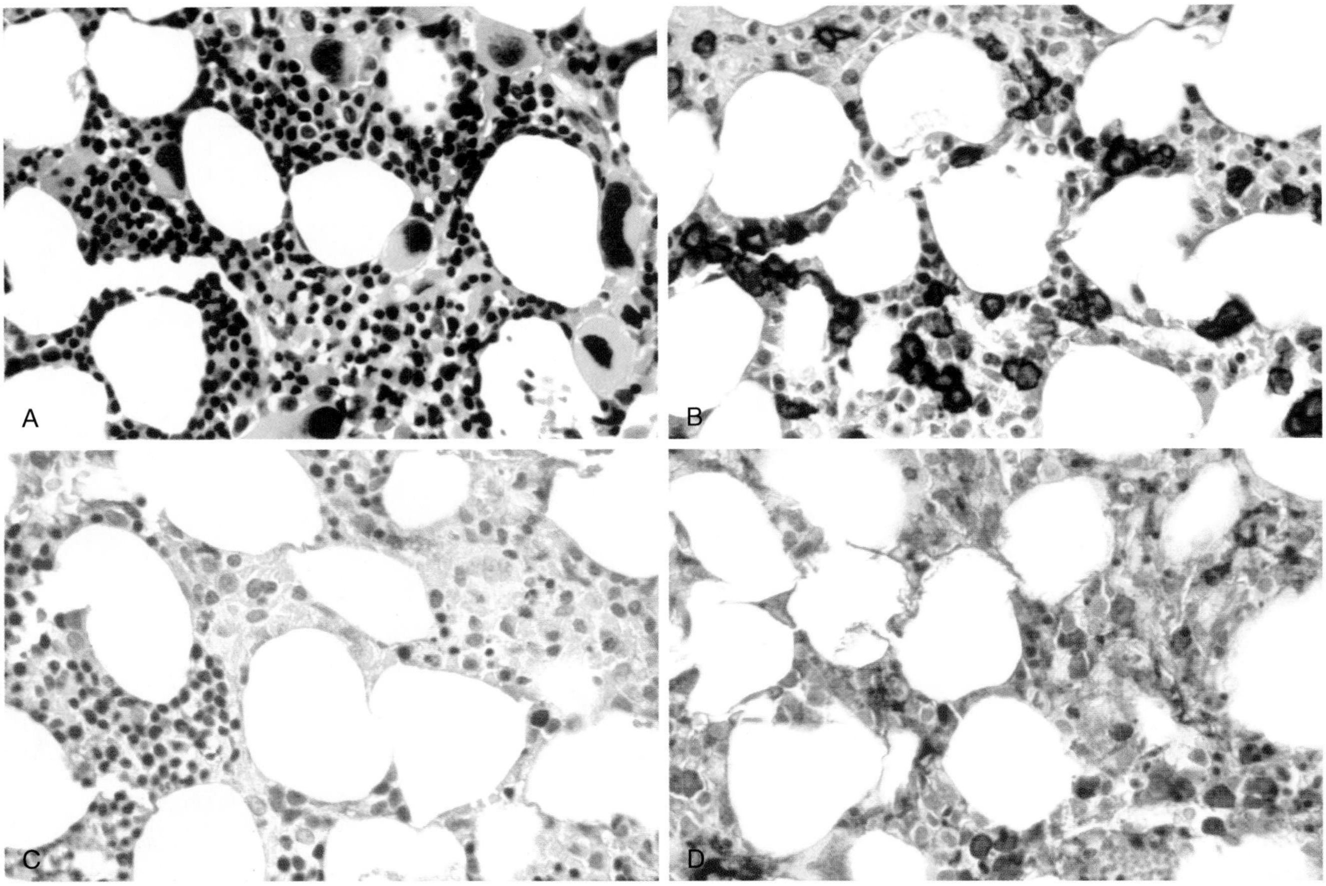

Figure 58-15. Residual plasma cell myeloma and therapy-related myelodysplasia after hematopoietic stem cell transplantation. Although plasma cell aggregates are not obvious on the hematoxylin-eosin–stained bone marrow biopsy section (**A**), an increase in $CD138^+$ plasma cells is identified (**B**). These plasma cells show lambda light-chain restriction, similar to the patient's original multiple myeloma (kappa, **C**; lambda, **D**). The bone marrow biopsy also shows atypical megakaryocytes (**A**). Multilineage dysplasia was present on the aspirate smears, and complex cytogenetic abnormalities were noted, consistent with therapy-related myelodysplasia.

false-negative rate occurs, especially for *IGH@* and *IGK@*.[142-144] Another major problem is that consensus primers do not detect very low levels of gene rearrangements, whereas tests directed against more specific targets, such as specific translocations, can detect them. Depending on the consensus primer set, the gene rearrangement test can detect 1 in 10 to 1000 cells. Not surprisingly, the utility of consensus primers to detect bone marrow involvement by lymphoma, compared with morphologic evaluation, has been variable in the literature.[131,145]

Laboratories have cloned and sequenced the specific gene rearrangements and created primers that are specific for an individual patient's disease,[146,147] similar to studies in ALL. Although this approach is very time-consuming and expensive, it allows the detection of very low levels of disease (in the range of 1 abnormal cell in 100,000 cells), which presumably results in earlier treatment. Even this approach has limitations, however, because patient-specific primers cannot be developed in all cases; in addition, some tumors have more than one clone, and all clones may not be detectable by the specific primers developed.

A subset of lymphomas has recurring cytogenetic abnormalities that make them ideal for evaluating residual disease by PCR.[76] These are discussed in more detail in other chapters. PCR tests directed against specific translocations offer a sensitivity similar to that of patient-specific gene rearrangement testing but do not require the development of primers specific for an individual patient. One of the most commonly studied translocations is the major breakpoint region of

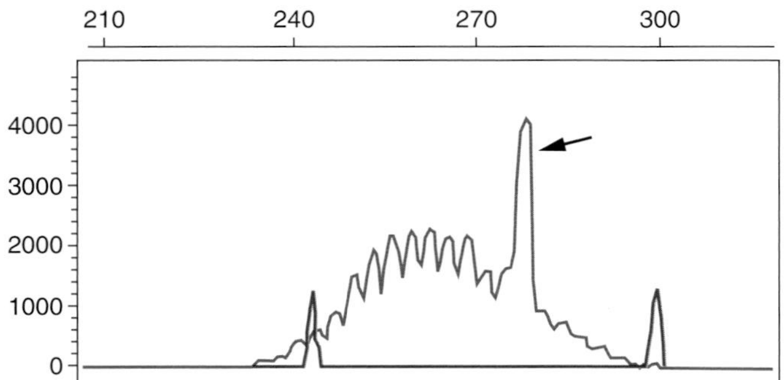

Figure 58-16. Detection of a residual clonal B-cell population in the bone marrow by immunoglobulin heavy-chain polymerase chain reaction. Multiple peaks (*blue*) of polyclonal B cells are detected with an admixed dominant clonal B-cell population (*arrow*). This population was the same size as the patient's original clonal lymphoma population, consistent with residual disease. *Red* peaks indicate molecular weight standards.

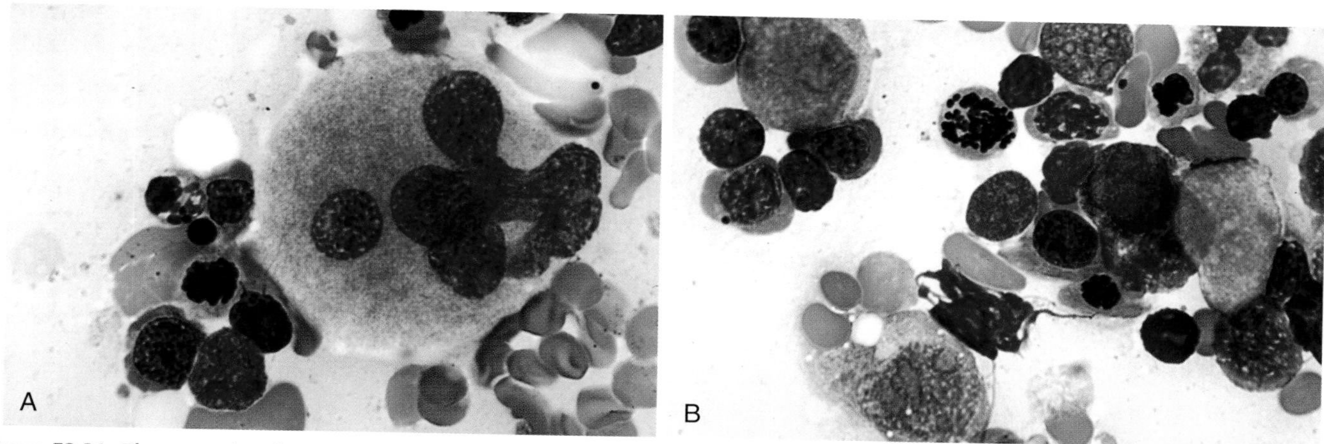

Figure 58-21. Therapy-related myelodysplasia. A and **B** are examples of cases that often show pronounced dyspoietic changes, including abnormal nuclear lobation of megakaryocytes and bizarre nuclear changes of erythroid precursors.

Secondary malignancies following solid organ transplantation, radiation therapy, or high-dose chemotherapy with hematopoietic stem cell transplantation are becoming increasingly common.[205,213-219] Although radiation-induced sarcomas may secondarily involve the bone marrow, such involvement is uncommon. However, therapy-related myelodysplasia, acute leukemia, and lymphoproliferative disorders may first be diagnosed on bone marrow examination.

Therapy-related myeloid neoplasms are fairly common in patients who have survived high-dose chemotherapy with hematopoietic stem cell transplantation (Fig. 58-21). These are aggressive diseases,[220] even in the case of therapy-related myelodysplasia without an increase in blast cells. Two main classes of drugs used to treat the primary disease have been implicated in therapy-related leukemia and myelodysplasia: alkylating agents and topoisomerase II inhibitors.[215,221,222] Disease associated with alkylating agents usually has a long latency period of 7 years or more and may be associated with the development of myelodysplasia or AML with multilineage dysplasia. These cases are usually associated with deletions of chromosome 5 or 7 or other unbalanced translocations. These chromosomal abnormalities may be detectable before the development of morphologic features of dysplasia, and cytogenetic studies should be performed on all cases of suspected therapy-related disease to detect this morphologically subtle presentation. Leukemias following topoisomerase II inhibitor therapy usually do not show changes of multilineage dysplasia and present as AML with monocytic or myelomonocytic features. These leukemias usually have a shorter latency period of 2 to 3 years and are associated with balanced cytogenetic translocations involving 11q23 and the *MLL* gene or 21q22 and the *AML1* gene. A variety of other cytogenetic abnormalities may occur in therapy-related leukemia and myelodysplasia, including many different balanced translocations.[223] Although the prognosis for therapy-related leukemia is generally poor, it may vary based on the different cytogenetic abnormalities.

Other therapy-related leukemias are less common but include myelodysplasia or AML associated with 17p deletions and *p53* mutations, which most often occur following hydroxyurea therapy for essential thrombocythemia.[224,225] There are prominent dysplastic changes of the neutrophil series, with pseudo–Pelger-Hüet cells, monolobated neutrophils, and prominent vacuolated cytoplasm. Similar morphologic and cytogenetic changes have been described in a subgroup of lymphoma patients with alkylating agent–related myelodysplasia and AML. Therapy-related ALL is also rare (Fig. 58-22),[226] but it occurs most often in patients treated with topoisomerase II inhibitors.[227] These leukemias are almost always of a pro-B ($CD10^-$) immunophenotype, with aberrant expression of the myeloid-associated antigens CD15 and CD65, and they are usually associated with balanced translocations of the *MLL* gene, particularly t(4;11).[64]

Donor-derived second malignancies after allogeneic transplantation have also been described but are extremely rare.[228,229] Reported cases have included acute leukemia and T-cell lymphoma.

Posttransplant lymphoproliferative disorders (PTLDs), which are covered in detail in Chapter 55, may involve the bone marrow. Over half of patients who develop PTLDs after solid organ transplantation have bone marrow involvement, and bone marrow changes are more common in children than in adults with PTLDs.[230] Bone marrow involvement is associated with a worse outcome. Aspirate smears tend to show an increased number of plasma cells. On the biopsy, the changes

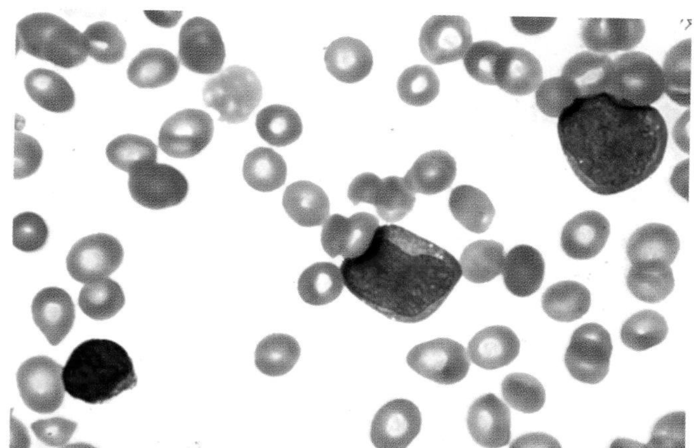

Figure 58-22. Therapy-related acute lymphoblastic leukemia. Blasts often show aberrant expression of the myeloid-associated antigens CD15 and CD65 and rearrangements of the *MLL* gene.

may range from aggregates of small lymphocytes or plasma cells without obvious atypia to aggregates of large atypical cells, usually with plasmacytoid features. Atypical cell infiltrates may be associated with fibrosis. The cellular infiltrate is usually of B lineage, but plasmacytoid cells may be underrecognized owing to their lack of immunoreactivity with antibodies directed against CD20. In situ hybridization studies for Epstein-Barr virus–encoded RNA (EBER) are positive in most cases. Although less common, PTLDs that occur after bone marrow transplantation are highly aggressive B-cell proliferations associated with Epstein-Barr virus and usually have a large cell or immunoblastic morphology.[231] These proliferations are associated with T-cell–depleted transplantation, unrelated donor transplantation, or HLA-mismatched related donor transplantation, and they usually occur within the first year after transplantation.[214]

Pearls and Pitfalls

- Bone marrow specimens must always be interpreted in the context of the clinical setting.
  - Slight increases in blast cells do not always mean residual disease.
  - Residual disease can be present in patients with less than 5% blast cells.
- Residual or recurrent leukemia is favored over regeneration when sheets of blasts are present on smear or when blasts outnumber promyelocytes.
- Growth factor therapy may be a factor in patients with numerous promyelocytes with distinct perinuclear hofs.
- Aggregates of $CD34^+$ or TdT^+ cells on bone marrow biopsy material favor leukemia over regeneration or hematogones.
- Dyserythropoietic changes, including ring sideroblasts, during or shortly after chemotherapy are not sufficient for an interpretation of myelodysplasia.
- Hematogones should be considered when a small lymphoid cell proliferation is present in children.
  - A spectrum of lymphoid cells that, by morphology or antigen expression, resemble precursor B-cell development is more characteristic of hematogones than leukemic cells.
  - Hematogones do not show cytogenetic abnormalities or aberrant immunophenotypes.
- Never rely on a single feature to exclude the presence of disease. False-negative results of ancillary studies are common.
- Consider the sensitivity and pitfalls of any test used, especially ancillary studies.
- Morphologically normal bone marrow may continue to show the Philadelphia chromosome in patients treated for chronic myelogenous leukemia.
- The molecular detection of very low levels of t(15;17), inv(16), and t(8;21) fusion transcripts after therapy do not necessarily predict relapse.
- Patients treated for multiple myeloma or chronic myelogenous leukemia may have small, decreasing but detectable populations of residual clonal disease for several months after transplantation, which may convert to molecular remission without additional therapy.

References can be found on Expert Consult @ www.expertconsult.com

Chapter 59

Nonhematopoietic Neoplasms of the Bone Marrow

Robert E. Hutchison

CHAPTER OUTLINE

The bone marrow acts principally as the site of hematopoiesis, and the majority of lesions arising in it are of hematopoietic origin. However, a wide variety of nonhematopoietic neoplasms and stromal abnormalities are encountered when evaluating bone marrow specimens, including metastatic tumors. Although metastases are usually best characterized from the primary site of involvement, sometimes the primary site is not obvious or is difficult to access; in these cases characterization may be performed or attempted from the bone marrow. Symptoms of nonhematopoietic neoplasms of the bone marrow are often related to cytopenias, metabolic disturbances, and the occupation of space (e.g., bone pain) and may mimic leukemias and lymphomas. Imaging studies are often helpful, but a bone marrow examination is usually required to directly visualize the process and to determine appropriate laboratory studies for its further characterization. Nonhematopoietic neoplasms are also found incidentally.

Bone marrow involvement by metastatic tumor is often referred to as *myelophthisis* and is sometimes first suspected when the peripheral blood smear shows leukoerythroblastic anemia with microangiopathic features, although the changes are usually subtle (Fig. 59-1). Circulating tumor cells are seen rarely.

Serum chemistry is often abnormal in metastatic disease as well as in metabolic diseases simulating metastasis, such as primary hyperparathyroidism and renal osteodystrophy. Elevated calcium, uric acid (>10 mg/dL), blood urea nitrogen (>25 mg/dL), and lactate dehydrogenase (>500 IU/L) combined with platelets less than 100,000/μL are helpful indicators of bone marrow metastasis, and elevation of lactate dehydrogenase and serum glutamic-oxaloacetic transaminase is often seen in bone marrow necrosis.[1] Bone pain is often present when the bone marrow is involved with tumor.

Bone marrow examination should include both aspiration and biopsy, and sampling at multiple sites may be necessary owing to the often focal and spotty nature of metastatic and some hematopoietic tumors. When the biopsy is negative, aspirates must be extensively scrutinized, particularly for tumors such as neuroblastoma and small cell carcinoma.

The nature of a metastatic tumor may be apparent from its morphology, but further evaluation is often required to determine a probable primary site or to confirm it, because multiple concurrent tumors can occur. This usually involves immunohistochemistry, but special histochemical stains and molecular assays are also used in some instances. Most immunohistochemical antibody stains work well in bone marrow biopsy and clot sections, although the detection parameters may vary with decalcification and fixation and should be optimized for the laboratory and, when possible, performed with controls that have been identically fixed and decalcified. Molecular assays such as fluorescence in situ hybridization (FISH) and polymerase chain reaction (PCR) techniques are often impaired by fixation involving metals (e.g., B5, Zenker's, zinc-formol fixatives), which results in nucleic acid fragmentation. Molecular assays often work best with fresh blood or bone marrow aspirates.

The selection of immunohistochemical assays follows the basic tenets of a diagnostic approach to a metastatic tumor with an unknown primary, guided by morphology and clinical findings. Immunohistochemical techniques can screen for a broad range of tumors in paraffin sections (Table 59-1), whereas molecular assays are typically more disease specific. It is particularly important to identify tumors that are responsive to therapy.[2] The basic approach is to determine the line of differentiation and then cell-specific products.

Virtually all carcinomas contain keratins that are composed of various keratin intermediate filament polypeptides, of which there are 20 types: 8 type II (basic), designated CK1 through CK8; and 12 type I (acidic), designated CK9 through CK20. Different carcinomas show characteristic cytokeratin expression, and a variety of monoclonal antibodies are available to detect them, along with strategies to simplify testing and interpretation.[2]

Antibody CAM5.2, recognizing CK8, and antibody 35βH11, recognizing CK18, identify simple keratins in most carcinomas, except for squamous cell types; they are often used for initial carcinoma screening, as are the

Table 59-1 Immunohistochemical Screening

Tumor Type	CK8 and CK18 (CAM5.2 and 35βH11), Pan-Keratin (AE1, AE3) CK19	CK7	CK20	CK5, CK6	EMA	CEA	p63	TTF-1	CDX2	PSA, PSAP	Villin	GCDFP-5, Mammaglobulin	Synaptophysin, CD56, NSE	NB84	HMB45, MART-1	Desmin	Myogenin, Myo-D1	CD99	FLI-1	CD117
Breast	+	+	–	Variable	+	–	–	–	–	–	–	+	–	–	–	–	–	–	–	–
Lung small cell	+	+	–	–	–	Variable	–	+	–	–	–	–	+	–	–	–	–	–	–	–
Lung squamous	+	+	–	+	+	–	+	–	–	–	–	–	–	–	–	–	–	–	–	–
Lung adenocarcinoma	+	+	Variable	–	+	+	–	+	–	–	–	–	–	–	–	–	–	–	–	–
Prostate	+	–	–	–	+	–	–	–	–	+	–	–	–	–	–	–	–	–	–	–
Gastroduodenal	+	+	Variable	–	+	+	–	–	+	–	Variable	–	–	–	–	–	–	–	–	–
Colorectal	+	–	+	–	+	+	–	–	+	–	+	–	–	–	–	–	–	–	–	–
Renal cell	+	–	–	–	+	–	–	–	–	–	–	–	–	–	–	–	–	–	–	–
Melanoma	Variable	–	–	–	–	–	–	–	–	–	–	–	–	–	+	–	–	–	–	Variable
Rhabdomyosarcoma	–	–	–	–	–	–	–	–	–	–	–	–	–	–	–	+	+	–	–	–
Neuroblastoma	–	–	–	–	–	–	–	–	–	–	–	–	+	+	–	–	–	–	–	–
Medulloblastoma	–	–	–	–	–	–	–	–	–	–	–	–	+	+	–	–	–	–	–	–
Ewing's family	–	–	–	–	–	–	–	–	+	–	–	–	Variable	Variable	–	–	–	+	+	–

CEA, carcinoembryonic antigen; EMA, epithelial membrane antigen; GCDFP, gross cystic disease fluid protein; NSE, neuron-specific enolase; PSA, prostate-specific antigen; PSAP, prostate-specific acid phosphatase.

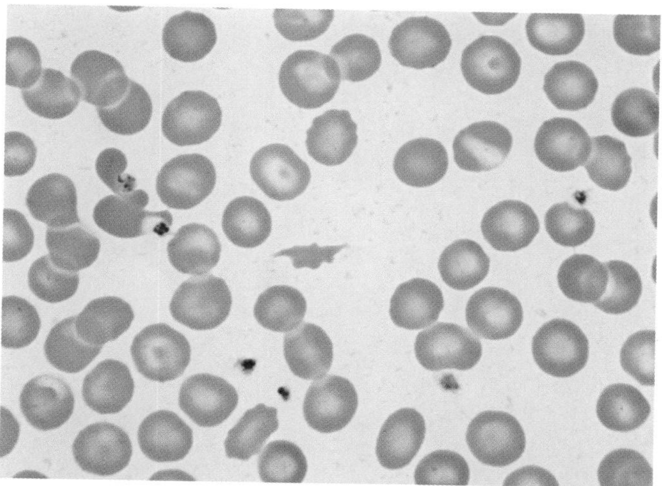

Figure 59-1. Normocytic anemia with schistocytes due to metastatic lung carcinoma.

cytokeratin antibodies AE1 and AE3. CK7 is more restricted and labels breast, lung, ovarian, endometrial, pancreaticobiliary, neuroendocrine, and transitional cell carcinomas but not colorectal, renal, or prostate carcinomas. CK20 expression is restricted to colorectal, pancreatic, gallbladder, Merkel cell, transitional cell, and pulmonary mucinous carcinomas. CK5 and CK6 identify squamous differentiation.

The most common tumors metastatic to the marrow are breast carcinoma in women and lung and prostate carcinomas in men. Marrow metastasis is present in up to 20% of patients with these primary tumors. Other tumors seen at lower frequency are adenocarcinoma of the stomach and colon, melanoma, renal cell carcinoma, ovarian and testicular carcinomas, transitional cell carcinoma, rhabdomyosarcoma, Ewing's sarcoma, and vascular tumors; many others are seen occasionally. Childhood tumors that frequently involve the marrow are neuroblastoma and variants, rhabdomyosarcoma, Ewing's sarcoma, retinoblastoma, and medulloblastoma.[1]

METASTATIC TUMORS IN ADULTS

In patients with skeletal metastatic breast cancer, the pelvis is the most common site of metastasis, followed by the lumbar spine, ribs, long bones, skull, and cervical spine.[3] Imaging techniques usually identify the disease with osteoblastic or osteoclastic activity, although purely intertrabecular disease also occurs. Ductal and lobular carcinomas of the breast most often metastasize, whereas papillary carcinomas typically do not.[4] Invasive ductal carcinoma grows in sheets, nests, cords, or individual cells, with variable gland differentiation (Fig. 59-2). Nuclei are usually large, with prominent nucleoli and

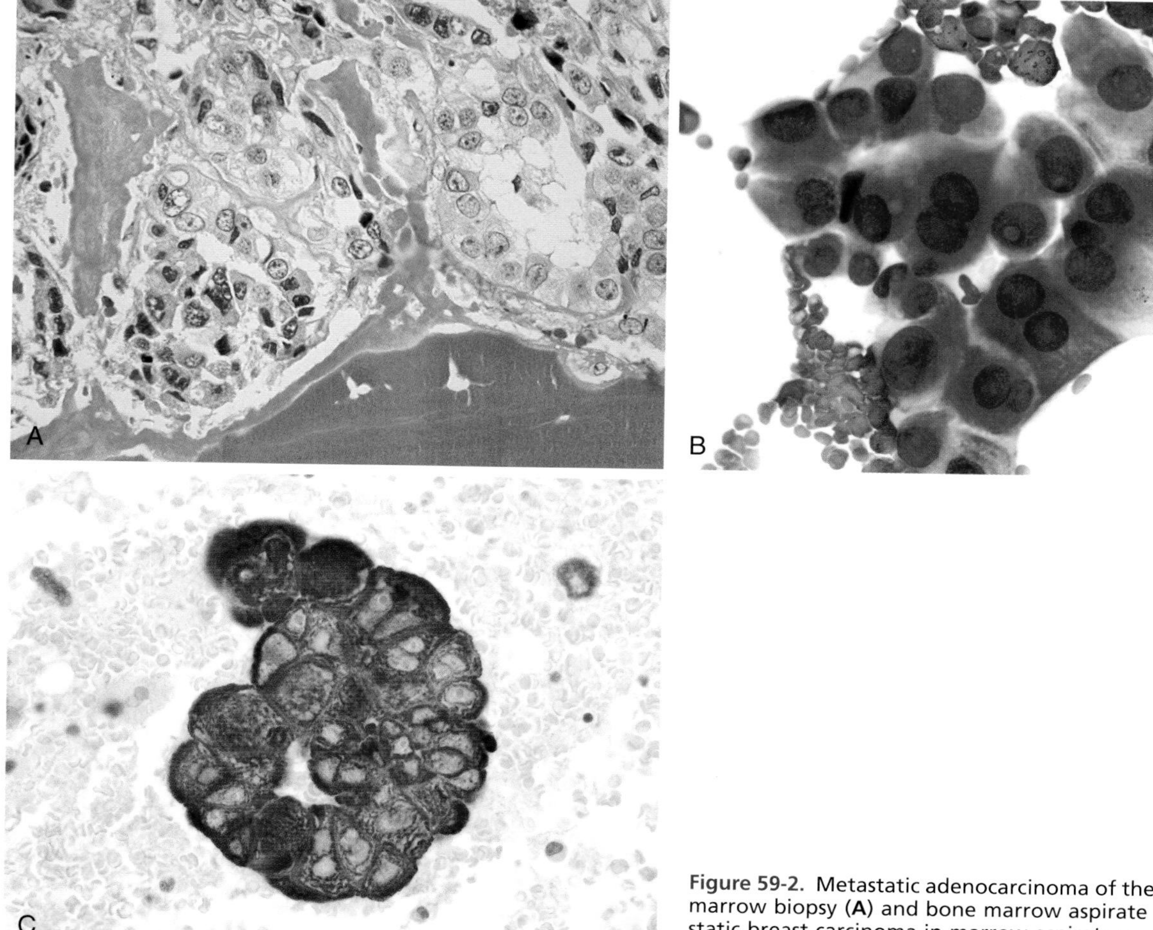

Figure 59-2. Metastatic adenocarcinoma of the breast in a bone marrow biopsy (**A**) and bone marrow aspirate smear (**B**). Metastatic breast carcinoma in marrow aspirate expressing the cytokeratin CK7 (**C**).

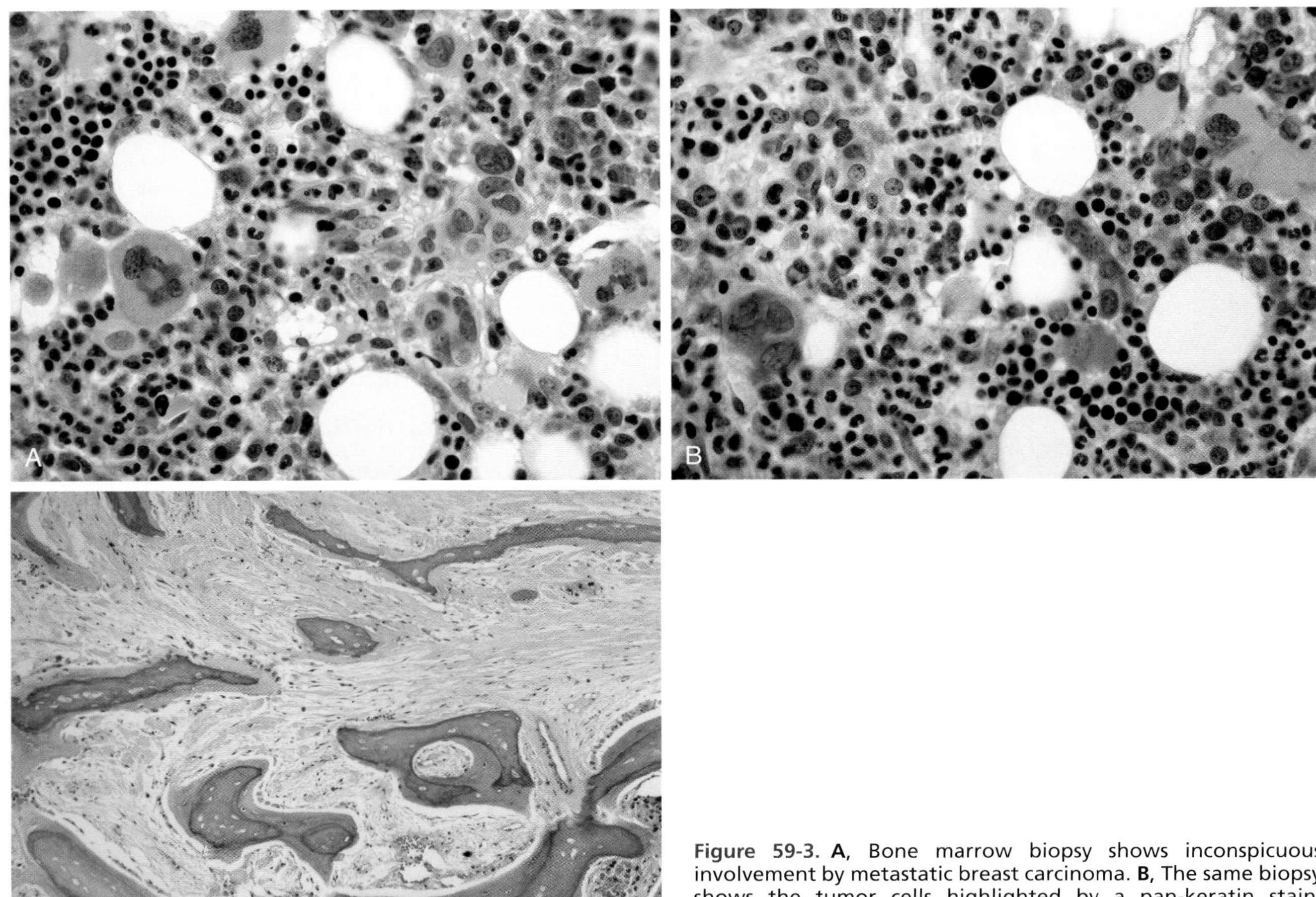

Figure 59-3. A, Bone marrow biopsy shows inconspicuous involvement by metastatic breast carcinoma. **B,** The same biopsy shows the tumor cells highlighted by a pan-keratin stain. **C,** Marrow fibrosis in a different specimen due to metastatic breast carcinoma.

frequent mitoses, and there is frequent fibrosis, desmoplasia, or necrosis. Mucin staining is present in about half of cases. Mucinous carcinoma shows nests of tumor floating in a mucinous background. Marrow involved by breast carcinoma may show abundant tumor nests, but areas of inconspicuous clusters or extensive fibrosis are also frequent (Fig. 59-3). Invasive lobular carcinoma, although derived from nest-like in situ lobular neoplasia, is characterized by small, uniform cells growing singly and in Indian files in dense, fibrous stroma.

Metastatic breast carcinoma is detected by antibodies for CK7 and CK19. The presence of diffuse CK20 is strong evidence against a breast primary tumor. Carcinoembryonic antigen (CEA) and estrogen receptor or progesterone receptor antibodies are often positive but nonspecific. More specific antibodies indicating breast carcinoma include gross cystic disease fluid protein (GCDFP-15), which also reacts with apocrine gland tumors, and mammaglobin A.[5]

The sensitivity of detecting marrow involvement by breast carcinoma is increased by immunohistochemistry using antibodies against CK19 and PCR for CK19 messenger RNA. Real-time quantitative PCR techniques have also been applied to peripheral blood. Semiautomated immunocytochemical screening of blood is available, as are other techniques, including expression array analysis and immunospot profiling of residual viable cells after CD45 depletion. Immunocytochemical screening is usually coupled with enrichment techniques, including density gradients, magnetic beads, or size filtration.[6] The identification of micrometastatic tumor cells in the marrow using sensitive techniques has been associated with an increased risk of relapse.[7] The clinical utility of detecting micrometastases has not been fully realized, but it may direct adjuvant therapy, particularly the use of bisphosphonates, which may limit the occurrence of bone metastases and improve long-term outcome.[8]

Carcinoma of the lung involves the bone marrow with a frequency that varies by histologic type. Small cell carcinoma most frequently metastasizes to the marrow (≈20%), followed by squamous cell carcinoma (3% to 15%) and adenocarcinoma (5% to 10%).[1] Tumor cells in the marrow resemble those in the primary site.

Small cell carcinoma (Fig. 59-4) is composed of small round or oval to elongated cells with hyperchromatic, finely granular chromatin, resembling blast cells but with frequent clustering and nuclear molding. Cells label for simple keratins (CK7, CAM5.2, AE1, AE3) and usually the neuroendocrine markers synaptophysin, CD56, and neuron-specific enolase (NSE), as well as CEA, TTF-1, and often CD117.[9] Patients frequently exhibit neuroendocrine syndromes, such as the syndrome of inappropriate antidiuretic hormone secretion, Cushing's syndrome, myasthenic-like syndrome (Eaton-Lambert syndrome), or carcinoid syndrome.[10] Large cell neuroendocrine and carcinoid tumors may also metastasize to the

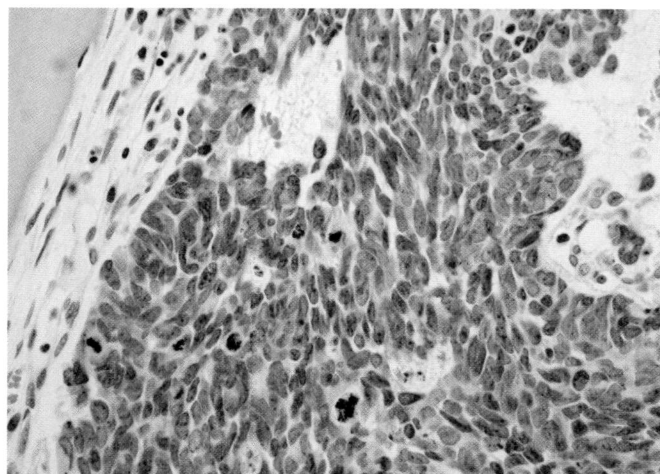

Figure 59-4. Small cell carcinoma of the lung, metastatic to the marrow.

marrow (Fig. 59-5). Marrow fibrosis and osteosclerosis may be striking (Fig. 59-6).

Squamous cell carcinoma, most common in males and smokers, is distinctive in the marrow biopsy but usually does not appear in aspirates, which may be acellular. Nests of cohesive tumor cells are often embedded in a fibrous background. Cells are usually strongly reactive for cytokeratins as detected by AE1 or AE3, 34βE12, and CK5/6; they also frequently label for epithelial membrane antigen (EMA), CEA, and p63, the last being a member of the p53 family.[9]

Adenocarcinomas are increasingly common and constitute about half of lung cancers. The histology is one of variable differentiation with acinar, papillary, or solid growth or, rarely, with signet ring, mucinous, or other morphology. There is usually some intracellular mucin production, as well as immunoreactivity for low-molecular-weight keratins (AE1 or AE3, 35βH11, CK7) and for CEA, Leu-M1, and TTF-1 (Fig. 59-7). Tumors with dual differentiation (adenosquamous) or with little differentiation (poorly differentiated large cell) also occur, as well as some tumors with an uncommon but distinctive histology (giant cell, spindle cell, lymphoepithelial-like, pseudoangiomatous, and large cell neuroendocrine types). Detection of marrow involvement is increased by imaging studies,[11,12] monoclonal antibody immunochemistry,[13] and PCR-based assays,[14,15] but the utility of detecting micrometastases is not proved.[16]

Prostate carcinoma frequently metastasizes to the skeletal system and lymph nodes, and this disease represents one of the most common sources of metastatic bone marrow disease in adult males.[1] This may be related to prostatic epithelial cells' increased affinity for bone marrow endothelium.[17] Most primary prostate tumors are well-differentiated adenocarcinomas with small acinar formation, but it is the less well differentiated types that tend to metastasize, particularly moderately differentiated forms with fused glands, cribriform or papillary formations, or the absence of apparent gland formation (Fig. 59-8).[18] Immunohistochemistry is usually positive for simple keratins (AE1 or AE3, CAM5.2) but not for CK5, CK7, or CK20. Prostate-specific antigen (PSA), prostatic acid phosphatase (PAP), and prostate-specific membrane antigen (PSMA) are, when combined with simple cytokeratins, specific for prostate carcinoma. PSMA has the advantage of increased expression in poorly differentiated tumors, and pro-PSA provides an additional marker of high-grade tumors.[2] Acid mucins are detected with alcian blue staining.[19] Neuroendocrine differentiation may also be detected. Micrometastases have been evaluated in the marrow using antibodies to cytokeratins and PSA and by reverse transcriptase PCR (RT-PCR) for PSA expression.[20,21]

Most upper gastrointestinal carcinomas are mucin-producing adenocarcinomas. Signet ring adenocarcinomas exhibit single cells with fibrosis and intracellular mucin. Immunohistochemistry of upper gastrointestinal tumors shows low-molecular-weight keratins, including CK7, as well as frequent CEA, CDX2, and villin. CDX2 is an intestinal cell transcription factor that labels all duodenal and most gastric and esophageal tumors. Antibodies to villin label a majority of esophageal and duodenal tumors, as well as colorectal carcinoma and almost half of gastric tumors. Neuroendocrine differentiation may be present, and small cell neuroendocrine carcinomas similar to those in the lung may arise in the stomach, as well as adenosquamous, mucinous, hepatoid, lymphoepithelioma-like, sarcomatoid, and other variants.[22]

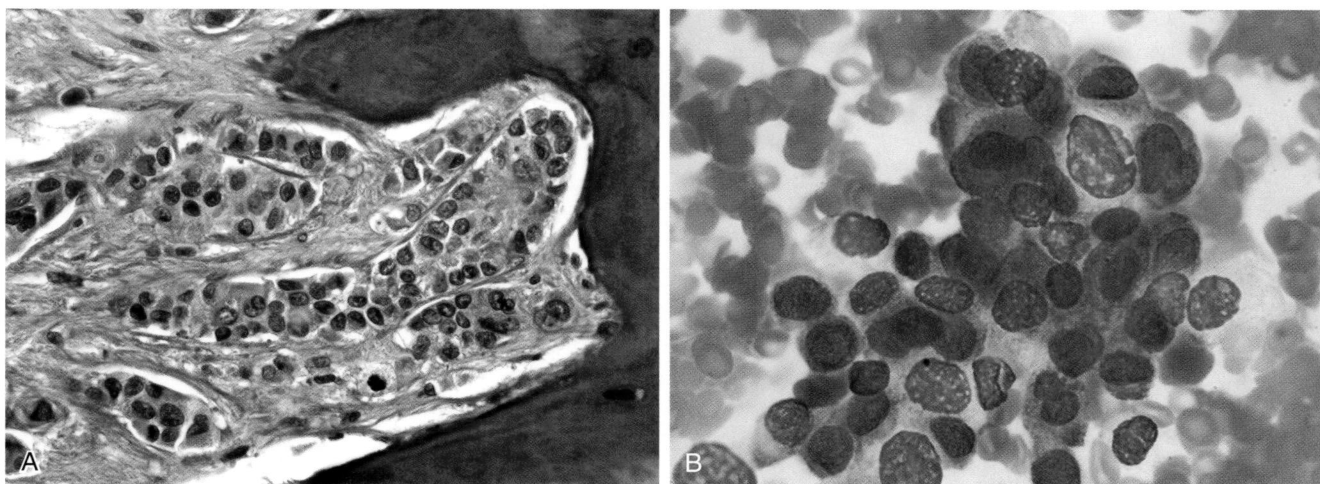

Figure 59-5. Metastatic malignant carcinoid tumor in a biopsy **(A)** and bone marrow aspirate smear **(B)**.

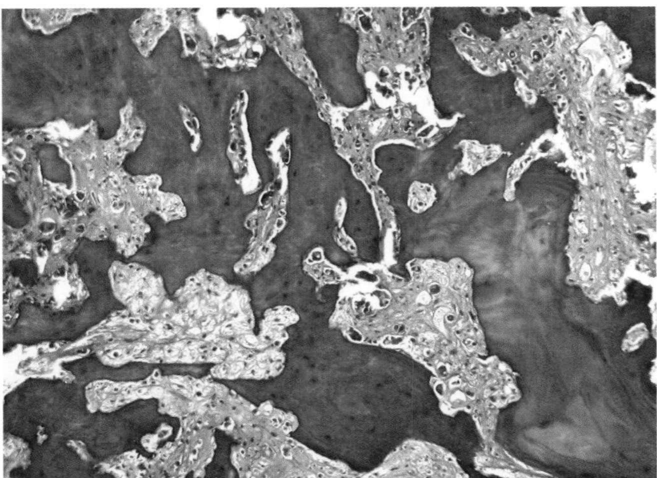

Figure 59-6. Osteosclerosis due to metastatic lung carcinoma.

Disseminated tumor cells in the marrow can be detected, as for many other tumors, but this is not routine practice.[23]

Most colorectal carcinomas are moderately differentiated adenocarcinomas with glandular formation and mucin production (Fig. 59-9). These tumors label with cytokeratins (typically positive for CK18, CK19, CAM5.2, and AE1 or AE3, with variable CK7 and CK20), villin, and CDX2. Most cases are strongly CK20^{+} and CDX-2^{+}, but CK7^{-}. Immunohistochemical detection of cytokeratins, EMA, and CEA, and PCR for CEA and other markers, can help detect micrometastases and minimal residual disease.[24,25]

Carcinomas of other primary sites may also involve the marrow; some, such as head and neck squamous cell carcinoma, may occur in an occult fashion more often than suspected.[26] We have rarely seen adenoid cystic carcinoma of the parotid involving the marrow (Fig. 59-10). Renal cell carcinoma can be detected with antibody RCC, CD10 and vimentin, adrenal neoplasms with A103 and Ad4BP, and urothelial carcinomas with uroplakin. CCR and A103 label other carcinomas as well; Ad4BP is specific for adrenal tumors.[2]

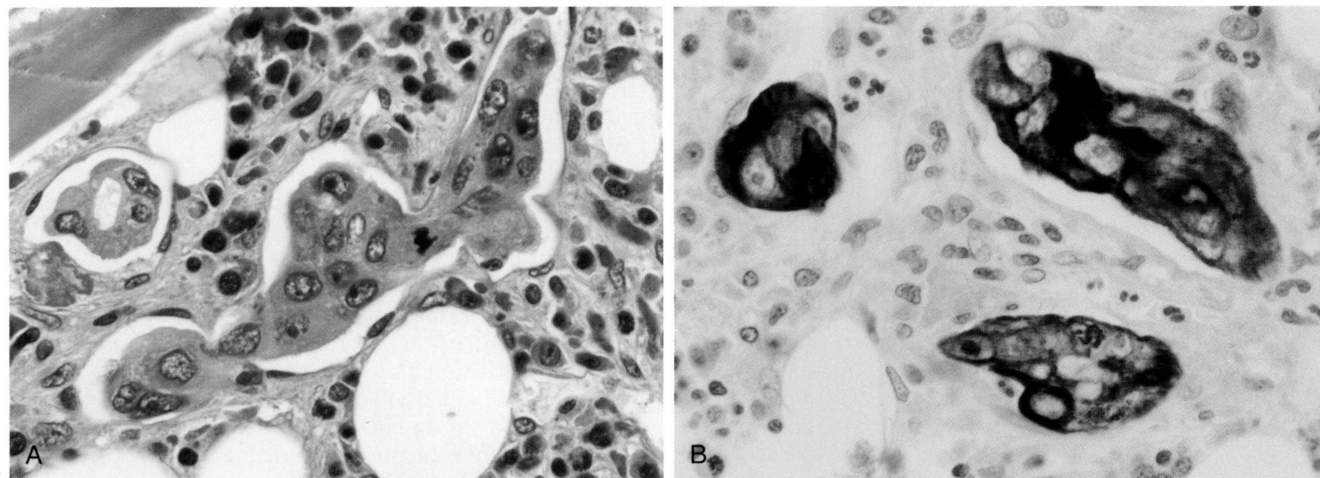

Figure 59-7. Metastatic adenocarcinoma of lung in a bone marrow biopsy (**A**) and expressing the cytokeratin CK7 (**B**).

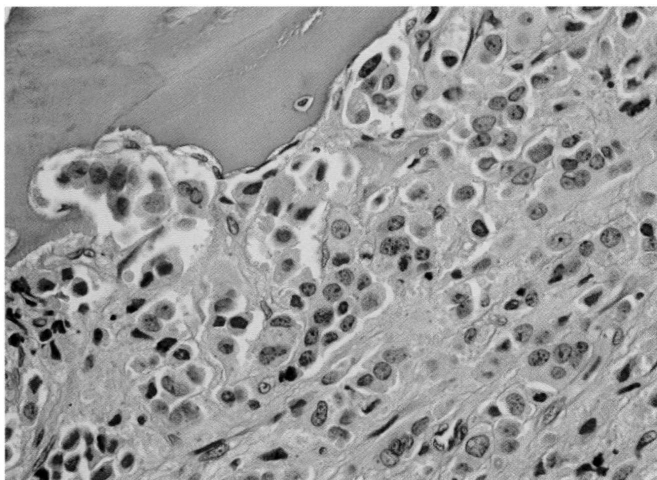

Figure 59-8. Metastatic prostate cancer in a bone marrow biopsy.

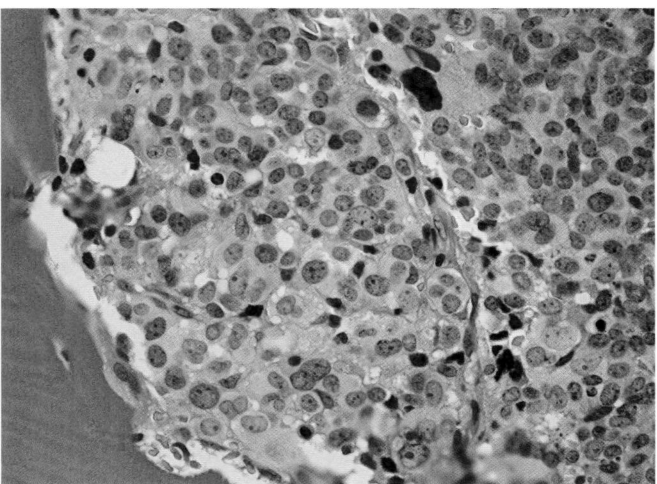

Figure 59-9. Bone marrow biopsy specimen extensively involved with metastatic colon carcinoma.

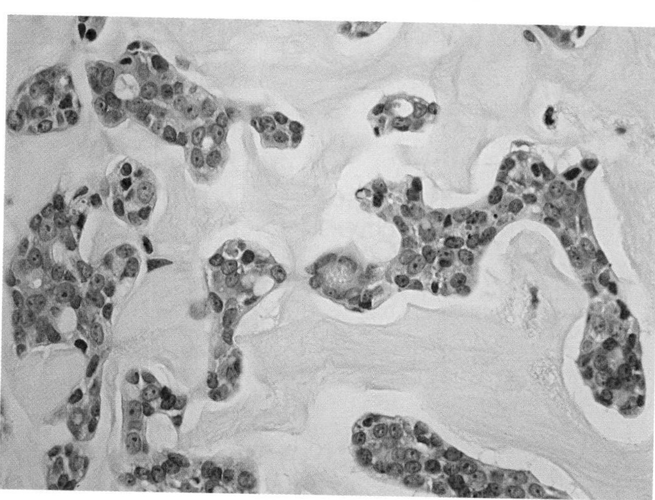

Figure 59-10. Bone marrow biopsy shows involvement by metastatic adenoid cystic carcinoma of the parotid gland.

Malignant melanoma is a great mimic of other tumors, and although melanin production is a helpful feature, it is not usual in marrow metastases. Tumor cells may be sarcomatoid or resemble diffuse or anaplastic lymphomas, myelomas, or other tumors. Melanoma should be considered in the differential diagnosis of any anaplastic or poorly differentiated tumor. Immunohistochemical staining (S-100 protein, HMB45, and MART-1/melan A) is usually diagnostic, although HMB45 is negative in desmoplastic and some other melanomas.[27] Melanoma also mimics other tumors in antigen expression and may express low-molecular-weight keratins, CEA, EMA, and the hematopoietic markers CD10, CD56, CD57, CD68, CD74, CD99, CD117, and others.[28] Sensitive assays may prove helpful in diagnosing occult metastases in the future.[29,30]

METASTATIC TUMORS IN CHILDREN AND ADOLESCENTS

Pediatric cancers, so-called small blue cell tumors of childhood, generally require bone marrow examination for staging purposes, and the results have a significant impact on treatment and prognosis. Most of these tumors show highly variable patterns of involvement, sometimes with extensive disease at one site but undetectable involvement nearby. Rhabdomyosarcomas are the most common soft tissue malignancies in children. They are derived from skeletal muscle cells and bear myogenic proteins. The primary histologic types are botryoid, in which solid tumor nests of small cells under an epithelium may have a grape-like appearance; embryonal, with solid growth of rhabdomyoblasts at different stages of myogenic maturation and loose myxoid stromal areas; and alveolar, with primitive round myoblasts often floating in alveoli-like spaces lined by tumor cells against fibrous trabeculae or forming a solid tumor, and usually with the cytogenetic abnormality t(2;13)(q35;q14) *PAX3-FKHR* or t(1;13)(p36;q14) *PAX7-FKHR*. Anaplastic rhabdomyosarcoma with pleomorphic nuclei occurs in adults, as do spindle cell tumors resembling smooth muscle.[31] Treatment and prognosis are based on age, stage, histology, and molecular or cytogenetic features, with the alveolar type being the most aggressive and the most likely to have discernible genetic abnormalities. Marrow involvement is seen in 25% to 30% of cases,[32] with an increased frequency in those with alveolar histology (50%).[33,34] Tumor cells in the marrow often occur as clusters of singly dispersed small, blast-like cells that may have eosinophilic granular cytoplasm, although their morphology can vary (Fig. 59-11). Hemophagocytosis has been described,[35] and presentation resembling acute leukemia is not rare.[36-41] These tumors typically label for vimentin, desmin, muscle-specific actin, myo-D1, and myogenin.[42] Similar to other tumors, molecular techniques appear to increase the sensitivity of detecting rhabdomyosarcoma and include RT-PCR for *PAX3-FKHR* of t(2;13)(q35;q14), *PAX7-FKHR* of t(1;13)(p36;q14),[43-45] myo-D transcripts,[46] and acetylcholine receptor.[47]

Neuroblastoma and related differentiated tumors (ganglioneuroblastoma and ganglioneuroma) occur primarily in young children. The natural history is variable, depending on age, histology, and biologic features, and complicated to predict. It is important, however, because some cases regress or mature to differentiated forms, whereas others are highly aggressive and refractory. Children younger than 18 months with histologic differentiation and a lower mitoses-to-karyorrhexis index have the best prognosis. Histologic classification systems have been reviewed.[48,49] *N-MYC* amplification is likely the most negative prognostic factor, whereas hyperdiploidy and *TRAK-A* gene expression are favorable.[50] Other biologic prognostic factors include ploidy, cytogenetics, serum ferritin, and a variety of others.[51] Neuroblastomas are derived from neural crest ectoderm and are most common in the adrenal cortex and abdomen, followed by the thoracic sympathetic ganglia, neck, pelvis, and other areas; they may be multifocal. Catecholamines, including dopamine, vanillylmandelic acid, and homovanillic acid, are elevated in serum and urine, and detection assists in diagnosis. Metastatic spread is both lymphatic and hematogenous, and bone marrow involvement is common. More than 50% of cases in some series have marrow involvement at diagnosis.[52] Bilateral biopsy of the bone marrow as well as aspiration is recommended for staging.[48,51-53] Better understanding of bone involvement in neuroblastoma may lead to specific treatment or prevention of metastases, such as with the use of bisphosphonates in breast cancer.[54]

Primary tumors (and metastases) contain combinations of primitive-appearing neuroblasts (undifferentiated small round cells with stippled chromatin), Schwann cells (spindle-shaped cells with elongated nuclei), and ganglion cells. Homer Wright rosettes may be present and consist of neuroblasts surrounding a tangle of neuropil (Fig. 59-12). Fibrillary stroma is present in most cases, and Schwann cells with organized fascicles of neuritic processes and fibrosis are present in cases with ganglioneuromatous components.

Immunohistochemical labeling is helpful but overlaps with other small blue cell tumors of childhood, particularly primitive neuroectodermal tumor (PNET) and Ewing's sarcoma. NSE, CD56 (Leu-7, HNK-1), NB84, and peripherin are usually positive.[48] S-100 labels Schwann cells, synaptophysin labels differentiated neuroblasts and ganglion cells, and chromogranin A labels ganglion cells. All these may be performed on paraffin blocks, but decalcified bone marrow fixed in B5 may produce variable results. An adequate bone marrow specimen in a child consists of at least 1 cm of biopsy past the

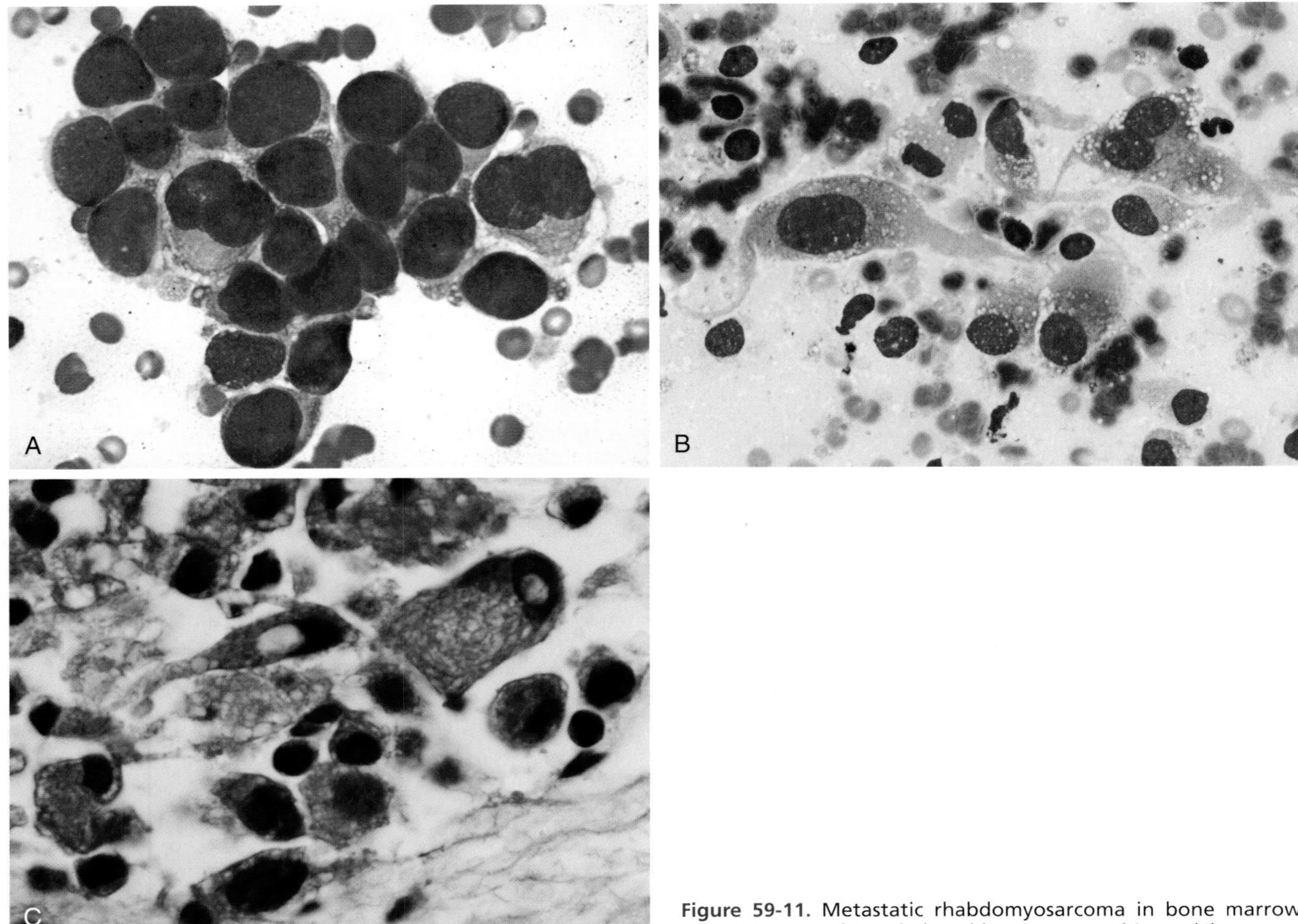

Figure 59-11. Metastatic rhabdomyosarcoma in bone marrow aspirate smears (**A** and **B**) and bone marrow biopsy (**C**).

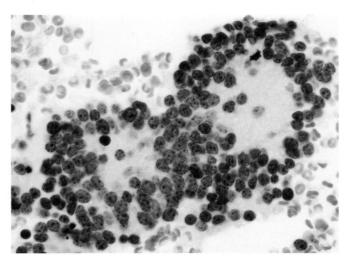

Figure 59-12. Rosettes of metastatic neuroblastoma in a clot section of bone marrow.

cortical bone and an aspirate containing particles. A low degree of marrow involvement (<10%) indicates a special favorable category (stage 4S) in infants with metastatic spread limited to liver, skin, and (localized) bone.[51] Morphologically, neuroblastoma may resemble acute leukemia (Fig. 59-13), and myelofibrosis may be present at diagnosis.[55] Similar to other diseases, there is an extensive body of literature that addresses the detection of minimal marrow involvement.[56-59] *N-MYC* amplification for prognostication can be determined from marrow and other samples by FISH techniques.[60]

Retinoblastoma is a prototypical aggressive childhood tumor of the eye.[61] It is one of the most common eye tumors (the most common in children, occurring in 1 in 14,000 births) and is associated with mutations of the tumor suppressor retinoblastoma gene on chromosome 13q14. It usually presents clinically before age 5 years as a white light reflex and is treated by surgery as well as chemotherapy and radiotherapy. Disseminated disease usually presents in the bone marrow or central nervous system, but the actual incidence of marrow involvement is less than 10%, and the value of routine marrow examination is controversial.[62-65] The histology varies from undifferentiated small blue cell tumor to more differentiated forms with rosette formation, including Homer Wright rosettes and Flexner-Wintersteiner rosettes, a circle of nuclei away from a central membrane-defined lumen contain-

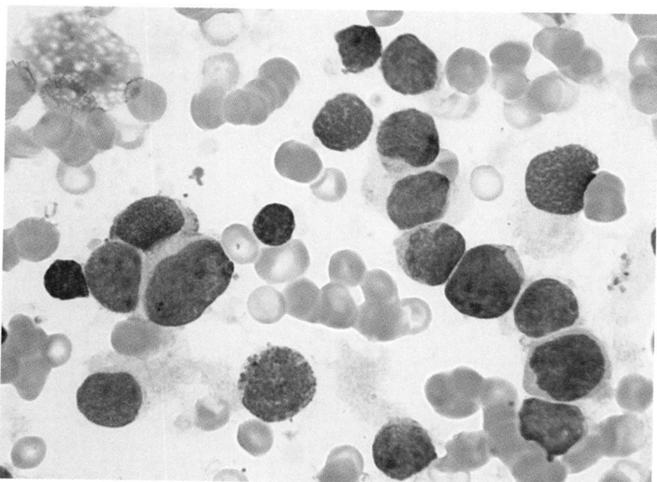

Figure 59-13. Neuroblastoma mimicking acute leukemia in the bone marrow aspirate; note the rare tumor cluster.

ing acid mucopolysaccharide similar to that around normal rods and cones.[58] Rare leukemic involvement late in the course of the disease has been described,[66] and disease in marrow and blood detected by RT-PCR (for expression of PGP9.5) has been treated successfully.[67] Immunohistochemical features include expression of the photoreceptor cell–associated proteins rhodopsin, rhodopsin kinase, transducin, and S antigen; often the glial marker glial fibrillary acidic protein (GFAP); S-100; vimentin; or Leu-7 (CD56).[61]

Medulloblastoma is a PNET of the cerebellum that occurs in children and sometimes metastasizes to the bone marrow. Metastatic cases require chemotherapy, and localized disease is treated with radiation.[68] The histology is that of a small blue cell tumor (blast-like cells) in sheets, often forming Homer Wright rosettes, and sometimes with features resembling neuroblastoma (neurofibrillary stroma or ganglionic differentiation). Tumors often are positive for synaptophysin and GFAP. Leukemic involvement has been reported.[69]

BONE TUMORS

Ewing's sarcoma is usually a primary bone tumor, although extraskeletal disease also occurs. It is one of the most undifferentiated tumors and occurs early in life, with a median age of 13 years.[70,71] The morphology is that of a small blue cell tumor, with sheets or nests of medium-sized blast-like cells with dispersed chromatin, high nuclear-to-cytoplasmic ratios, and interspersed small hyperchromatic cells resembling lymphocytes (Fig. 59-14). Mitoses are variable, and necrosis is often present. Pseudorosettes of tumor cells surrounding necrotic centers occur, and perivascular tumor cuffing is often present in necrotic areas. Tumor cells are characteristically periodic acid–Schiff positive owing to glycogen.

Neuroectodermal tumor of bone (PNET or primitive neuroepithelioma) is a similar tumor but demonstrates neuroectodermal differentiation. Along with small cell tumor of the thoracopulmonary region (Askin's tumor), these tumors belong to the Ewing's sarcoma family of tumors.

Immunohistochemical markers of Ewing's family tumors include vimentin, CD99, and FLI-1.[71] Neural markers, NSE, synaptophysin, and CD56 are expressed in PNET and sometimes in Ewing's sarcoma. CD99 must be interpreted with caution because lymphoblasts and occasionally myeloblasts also label with this marker (CD99 was raised against T lymphoblasts).[72] Ewing's sarcoma is characterized by the cytogenetic abnormality t(11;22)(q24;q12) involving the *EWS* gene on 22q12 and *FLI-1* or *ERG* on 11q24. Antibodies to the FLI-1 protein react in more than 70% of cases.[73] The fusion transcript can be detected by PCR, which provides a method of detecting occult marrow and blood involvement.[44,45,74,75] The fusion may also be detected by FISH from paraffin sections as well as from aspirated cells (Fig. 59-15).[76,77]

Desmoplastic small round cell tumor can be identified by antibody WT-1, as well as by the expression of simple keratins, desmin, and NSE. It only rarely metastasizes to the marrow, however.[78]

The bone-forming tumors (osteoma, osteoid osteoma, osteoblastoma, osteosarcoma) are characterized by the presence of osteoid. Osteosarcoma is the most common primary

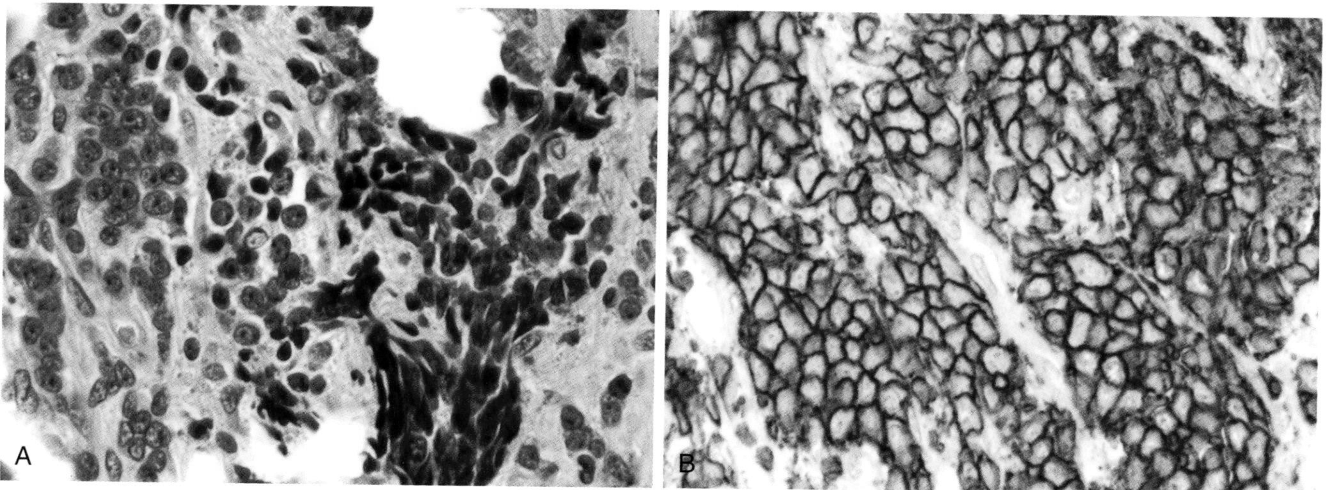

Figure 59-14. A, Appearance of Ewing's sarcoma in a hematoxylin-eosin–stained bone marrow section. **B,** The same tumor expresses CD99, which is not specific for Ewing's sarcoma.

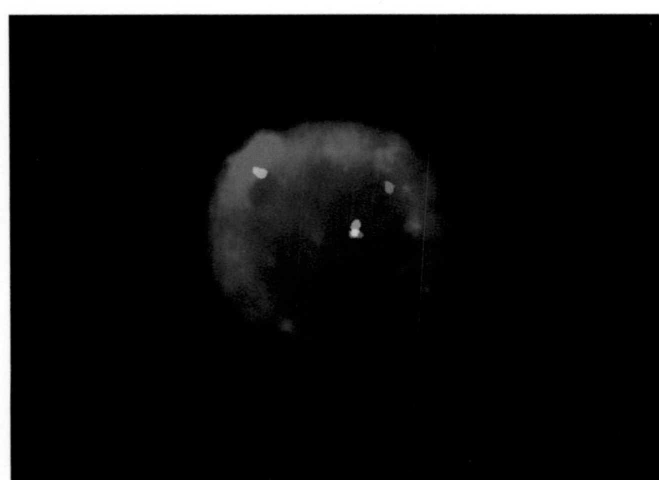

Figure 59-15. Break-apart fluorescence in situ hybridization probe demonstrating the t(11;22)(q24;q12) fusion in a cell from the bone marrow aspirate of a patient with Ewing's sarcoma.

bone tumor, usually occurring in individuals between 10 and 25 years of age or those older than 40 years. The incidence is increased in older patients with Paget's disease, following radiation or alkylating agent chemotherapy, and in the setting of preexisting bone lesions, including fibrous dysplasia, osteochondromatosis, and chondromatosis. These sarcomas present with a variety of appearances, including fibroblastic and chondroblastic, but they are diagnosed by the presence of malignant osteoid formation somewhere in the tumor.[79] Occasionally, multifocal osteosarcoma can masquerade as undifferentiated sarcoma in a bone marrow biopsy (Fig. 59-16).

Cartilage-forming tumors include benign chondromas (those originating in the diaphyses are termed *enchondromas*) composed of mature lobules of hyaline cartilage, often with myxoid degeneration, calcification, and ossification; osteochondromas, which are the most common benign bone tumors and have a characteristic radiologic appearance; chondroblastomas, which are cellular and may contain giant cells; and chondromyxoid fibromas, which are cellular benign cartilaginous tumors. Chondrosarcomas, similar to osteosarcomas, show a wide variation in differentiation; they may contain bone but lack malignant osteoid. Giant cell tumors (osteoclastoma) are usually low-grade malignancies occurring in the long bones or skull.

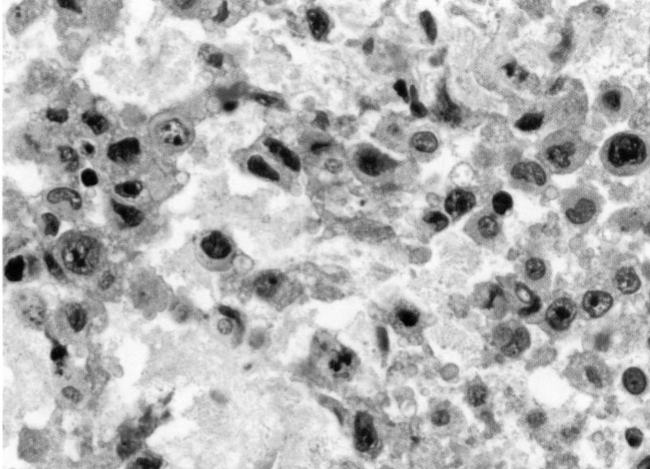

Figure 59-16. Multifocal osteosarcoma presenting as an undifferentiated sarcoma in a bone marrow aspirate smear.

VASCULAR AND MISCELLANEOUS TUMORS

Hemangiomas of bone occur principally in flat bones of the skull and jaw and in vertebrae. They are benign vascular malformations consisting of lattice-like formations of endothelium-lined cavernous spaces containing blood. Lymphangiomas occur less commonly. Massive osteolysis (Gorham's disease) appears similar to hemangioma but is destructive, leading to resorption of bone and replacement by heavily vascularized fibrous tissue.

Epithelioid hemangioendothelioma consists of vessels lined by plump eosinophilic epithelioid or histiocyte-like endothelial cells with large vesicular nuclei and often an inflammatory infiltrate rich in eosinophils. A range of cytologic atypia exists, from hemangioma to angiosarcoma. Endothelial cells express CD31, CD34, and von Willebrand's factor antigen. This disorder may simulate Langerhans cell histiocytosis.

A wide variety of other soft tissue tumors may present in bone, including desmoplastic fibroma, fibrosarcoma, malignant fibrous histiocytoma, leiomyoma, leiomyosarcoma, lipoma, liposarcoma, chordoma, and adamantinoma. For these, refer to texts on the surgical pathology of bone tumors.[79-82]

BENIGN TUMOR-LIKE LESIONS

Benign tumor-like lesions of the bone include solitary and aneurysmal bone cysts and ganglion cysts of bone. Radiographic changes are often characteristic. Solitary bone cysts occur most often in the proximal metaphysis of the humerus or femur of males younger than 20 years and consist of a membrane of well-vascularized fibrous tissue around a fluid-filled cyst; the surrounding bone is dense. Aneurysmal bone cysts occur mostly in the vertebrae and flat bones of adolescents. They expand eccentrically and erode the cortex. A grossly hemorrhagic mass consists of blood-filled spaces separated by fibroblasts, myofibroblasts, and histiocytes. Septa between cystic spaces contain these cells, blood vessels, osteoid, bone, degenerative calcifying fibromyxoid stroma, and rows of osteoclasts. Ganglion cysts occur near a joint space and contain gelatinous material lined by a thin fibrous membrane and surrounded by condensed bone.[79]

Metaphyseal fibrous defect (nonossifying fibroma) is a storiform fibrous lesion with scattered osteoclasts and hemosiderin-laden macrophages near the epiphyses of long bones in adolescents. Fibrous dysplasia is a benign lesion that consists of fusiform expansion of the medullary space, thinning of the cortex of long or flat bones, often highly cellular fibrous tissue, and irregular bone formation lined by abnormal fibroblast-like osteoblasts.

Paget's disease of the bone is a relatively common disorder of older adults. It usually involves multiple sites (polyostotic), most often the lumbosacral spine, pelvis, and skull. Pelvic involvement is likely to be seen in an iliac crest bone marrow biopsy. It is initially an osteoclastic lytic lesion in which irregular repair leads to thickened bony trabeculae with irregular cement lines demarcating areas of resorption and repair. More orderly cement lines are seen around reactive repair, such as near metastatic tumor, osteomyelitis, radiation damage, and chronic osteomyelitis. There may be an increase in primary bone tumors in Paget's disease, but this is controversial.

Chronic osteomyelitis is characterized by increased inflammatory neutrophils, lymphocytes, and plasma cells; often fibrosis; and the presence of sequestrum (infected dead bone) and involucrum (a surrounding formation of new bone). In acute osteomyelitis, pus often perforates the periosteum and forms a sinus tract to the skin. With healing, the epithelium of the sinus tract may become entrapped within the bone and form inclusion cysts or even, eventually, squamous carcinoma.

Epithelial inclusions are often seen as artifacts of bone marrow biopsies. If the central trocar of a biopsy needle is not firmly in place when the needle is pushed through skin overlying the biopsy site, fragments of skin can end up adjacent to or appear to be within the bone marrow space in histologic sections. Other dermal and subcutaneous structures can similarly be pushed into the biopsy. Other artifacts can occur during histologic processing, such as when "floaters" from other biopsies altogether appear in sections. This can usually, but not always, be suspected when there is space between unexpected tissue and the bone marrow biopsy. If this is suspected, it may be wise to repeat the procedure.

METABOLIC BONE DISEASE

Patients with a history of normal skeletal development but skeletal pain or fracture and radiologic evidence of osteopenia may suffer from a metabolic bone disease such as osteoporosis or osteomalacia or from an endocrine disorder, particularly hyperparathyroidism. Active osteoporosis (with accelerated bone turnover) exhibits increased osteoid formation, with an increased proportion (>20%) of trabeculae having osteoid seams of normal width. Greater than four collagen layers of lamellae are present, and bone surfaces contain plump osteoblasts. Increased osteoclasts (>1 or 2 per histologic section) or clustered osteoclasts are also present. Peritrabecular fibrous tissue (osteitis fibrosa), similar to that of hyperparathyroidism, may be seen. Inactive osteoporosis (with reduced turnover) exhibits thin osteoid seams, flattened osteoblasts, and reduced osteoclasts, with a reduction of both bone formation and bone resorption but an overall decreased loss of bone tissue.[83]

Hyperparathyroidism, due to parathyroid adenoma or secondary to renal failure, results in increased osteoclastic and osteoblastic activity with peritrabecular fibrosis, known as osteitis fibrosa (Fig. 59-17). This is not an uncommon finding in bone marrow biopsies and resembles mast cell disease, except for its characteristic pattern. It is one of the few disorders causing focal fibrosis in the marrow. Review of serum chemistries usually shows evidence of chronic renal failure.

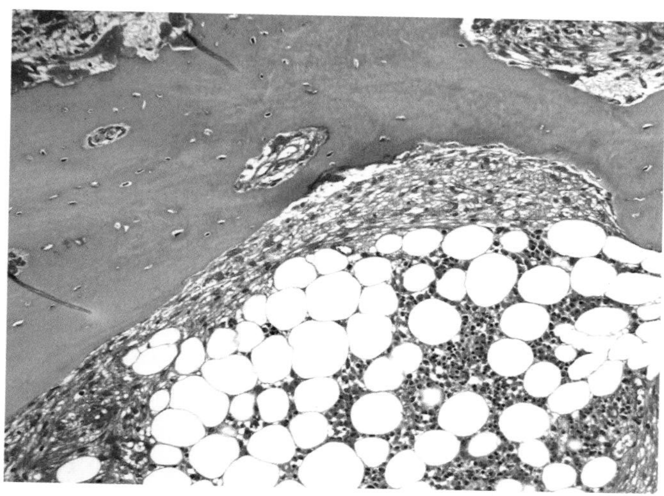

Figure 59-17. Osteitis fibrosa cystica due to hyperparathyroidism.

Osteomalacia and rickets (vitamin D deficiency) are abnormalities of calcification. Osteomalacia is histologically difficult to identify and may require fluorescence examination following tetracycline administration, with decreased deposition of fluorescence. Rickets results in uncalcified masses of cartilage in the growth plate of a child. Scurvy, or vitamin C deficiency, results in an inability to form osteoid due to abnormal collagen transformation. Calcified cartilage is seen, with radiologic evidence of increased density at the growth plate.[83]

CONCLUSION

Bone marrow is the primary site of hematopoiesis, and it must be examined when evaluating hematopoietic abnormalities. It may also provide information about diseases occurring in other organs, such as metastatic tumors, and about generalized metabolic disturbances. The underlying biology of bone marrow metastases from neoplasms of other organs is not yet well understood, but it likely involves both tumor-specific and stromal factors.[84] There is new evidence, in fact, that metastases of neoplasms to nonhematopoietic organs requires the establishment of vascular endothelial growth factor–expressing bone marrow–derived hematopoietic precursors at that site.[85]

The evaluation of nonhematopoietic disorders in the bone marrow requires careful correlation with clinical, imaging, and laboratory findings and communication with the patient's physician. Metastases are best characterized at the primary site whenever possible, and it is important to know that although modern immunohistochemical techniques are very powerful, few markers are entirely lineage specific. Many immunologic markers, including EMA, CD38, CD56, CD99, CD117, anaplastic lymphoma kinase, p63, and others, may be seen in both hematopoietic and nonhematopoietic neoplasms.[28,86,87] No single marker should be used to assign the lineage of a tumor found in the marrow; rather, targeted panels based on histology should be used and interpreted in light of clinical findings. When evaluated properly, the bone marrow examination is a powerful diagnostic tool for both hematopoietic and nonhematopoietic disorders.

Pearls and Pitfalls

- Nonhematopoietic neoplasms in the marrow are often focal. Sample adequately and examine each slide.
- Both the biopsy and the aspirate are important in the evaluation of metastatic disease. Some tumors, such as neuroblastomas, may show only rare clusters on aspirates even when there is extensive involvement. Request biopsies, even in pediatric patients, when looking for metastatic disease.
- Bare megakaryocyte nuclei frequently mimic metastatic tumor clusters on aspirates.
- Bilateral bone marrow biopsies increase the likelihood of finding metastases.
- Biopsy of radiologically suspicious sites may be necessary to identify focal marrow (or bone) involvement.
- Plan ahead. When a tumor is suspected, save appropriate material for genetic studies.
- When possible, use immunohistochemical controls that have been fixed and processed (e.g., decalcified) in the same way as the specimen being tested.
- Tumors are best classified from the primary site, even though the marrow may be more accessible.
- Always correlate findings with the clinical history and radiologic findings.
- Talk to clinicians.
- Hesitate before making an unlikely diagnosis, but realize that anything is possible.

References can be found on Expert Consult @ www.expertconsult.com

Chapter 60

Nonlymphoid Lesions of the Lymph Nodes

Dan Jones and L. Jeffrey Medeiros

CHAPTER OUTLINE

Nonlymphoid elements are frequently present in surgically excised lymph nodes. This chapter reviews the most commonly encountered tumors and nonneoplastic lesions. We begin with lymph node metastases because they can present the most diagnostic difficulty. We then summarize the use of sentinel lymph node biopsy for the staging of metastatic tumors and discuss the range of nonneoplastic inclusions included in the differential diagnosis of metastatic tumors. We also consider mesenchymal and vascular tumors, including those that are intrinsic to the lymph node.

METASTATIC TUMORS IN LYMPH NODES

The identification of metastatic solid tumors in lymph nodes is one of the most important tasks in diagnostic surgical pathology. Up to 5% of cancer patients present with lymph node metastasis from an occult primary tumor. Most of these neoplasms are carcinomas; however, 2% of patients with melanoma and a smaller percentage of patients with germ cell tumors and sarcomas may initially present with lymph node metastasis. In this section we review the histologic features and ancillary tests that can be performed on a metastatic tumor to identify its site of origin.

Histologic Features of Metastatic Tumors

Most solid tumors metastasize to regional lymph nodes following invasion of peritumoral lymphatics, with sequential progression down the lymphatic chain. As a result, metastatic deposits in lymph nodes are initially located preferentially in the extranodal vessels and subcapsular sinuses. This localization pattern is diagnostically useful because it is uncommon in lymphoma, with the exception of anaplastic large cell lymphoma. More extensive metastatic involvement is usually multifocal or geographic, but there is often a discrete boundary separating the tumor from uninvolved areas of lymph node. Metastatic solid tumors usually have a cohesive appearance, forming sheets, nests, or islands; undifferentiated carcinoma and melanoma may have a discohesive appearance, mimicking lymphoma.

Histologic clues to the site of origin of a metastatic tumor include keratinization or mucin production in carcinomas, rosette formation in neuroendocrine tumors, melanin pigment in melanomas, and abundant extracellular matrix or a fibrillary-filamentous cytoplasmic appearance in sarcomas. Metastatic papillary tumors of the thyroid, kidney, ovary, or lung can show nuclear pseudoinclusions and psammoma

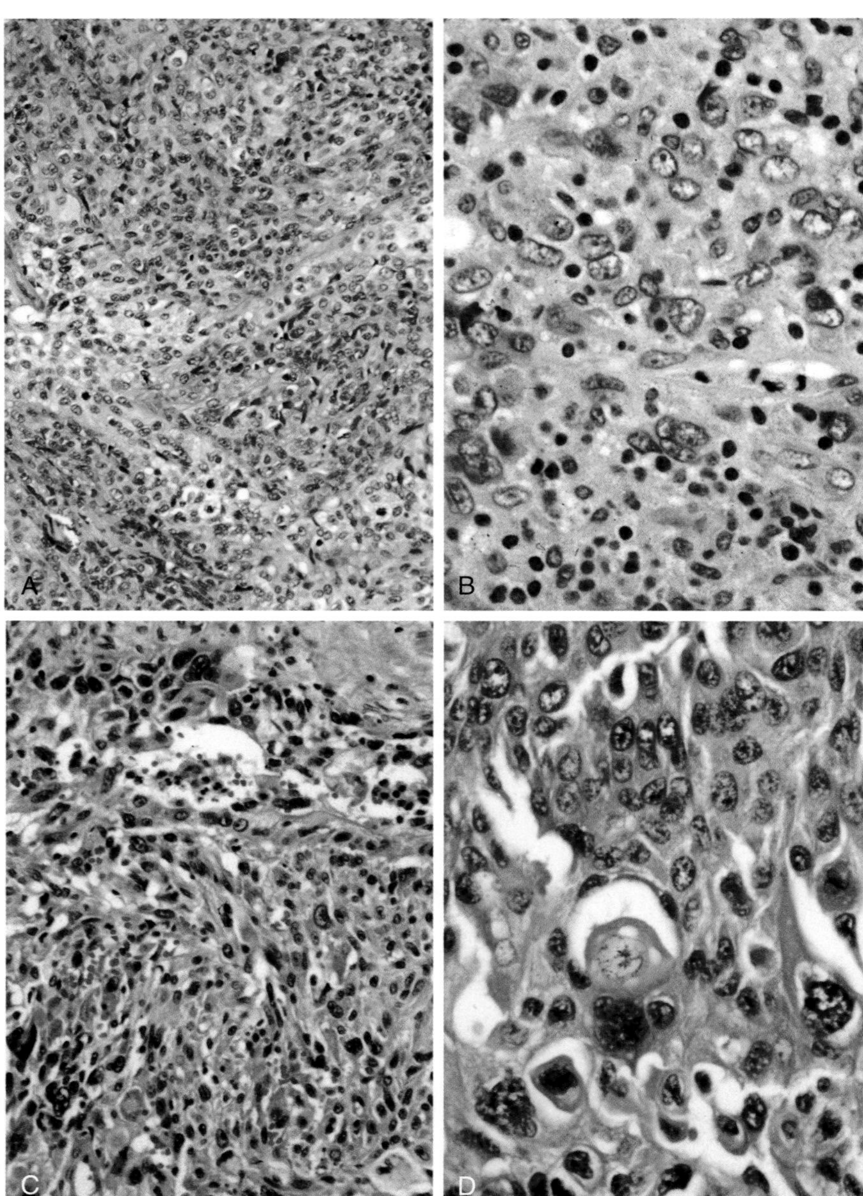

Figure 60-1. Histologic categories of metastatic tumor in lymph node. To simplify the differential diagnosis, metastatic tumors can be divided into those that have an epithelioid (**A**), anaplastic (**B**), or spindled (**C**) appearance. Areas of keratinization (**D**) can be useful in identifying carcinoma. All four cases shown are metastatic carcinoma.

bodies; carcinomas of lung and prostate origin often show evidence of partial neuroendocrine differentiation; and foci of necrosis are common in colon adenocarcinoma. Although still useful, cytochemical stains for mucin, neurosecretory granules (e.g., Grimelius and Fontana), or extracellular matrix proteins (e.g., reticulin and Masson trichrome) have largely been replaced by immunohistochemistry in routine diagnosis.

Poorly differentiated metastatic tumors are common and can be classified preliminarily as epithelioid, anaplastic, spindled, or small cell (Fig. 60-1). Table 60-1 outlines the differential diagnosis of metastatic tumors in each of these morphologic categories. Because of their relatively small cell size and discohesive growth, small cell tumors are among the most difficult to detect and distinguish from lymphoma; in some instances, immunohistochemistry is required for diagnosis. Lobular carcinoma of the breast (Fig. 60-2), carcinoid tumor, small cell carcinoma, Merkel cell carcinoma, and neuroblastoma can all show subtle infiltration of the interfollicular nodal areas. Colonization of lymphoid follicles is also occasionally observed. In the mediastinum, occult lung metastasis of small cell carcinoma can mimic lymphoblastic lymphoma but typically shows more prominent nuclear molding. Small cell carcinomas of the lung also commonly have abundant coagulative necrosis and basophilic deposition of DNA within blood vessels (known as nuclear encrustation or the Azzopardi phenomenon). Zonal areas of necrosis may also be seen in neuroblastoma. Although rare, rhabdomyosarcoma (Fig. 60-3) and primitive neuroectodermal tumor/Ewing's sarcoma (Fig. 60-4) can both show subtle interfollicular infiltration of the lymph node and should be considered in younger patients.

Table 60-1 Differential Diagnosis of Poorly Differentiated Metastatic Tumors

Histologic Pattern	Tumor Types	Useful Diagnostic Tests and Clues
Small cell tumors	Carcinoma (lobular breast, prostate)	Keratin
	Small cell, Merkel cell carcinoma	Chromogranin; keratin can be focal
	Neuroendocrine, carcinoid tumors	Chromogranin, synaptophysin, CD56
	Neuroblastoma	NSE, neurofilament, NB84, EM
	Lymphoblastic lymphoma	TdT, cytogenetics
	Ewing's sarcoma, other primitive sarcomas	PAS stain, CD99, cytogenetics
	Rhabdomyosarcoma	Desmin, EM, cytogenetics
Epithelioid tumors	Carcinoma (especially renal cell, prostate, breast)	Multiple keratin stains/cocktails often helpful
	Melanoma	S-100, HMB45, tyrosinase, MART-1
	Large cell lymphoma	CD45/LCA, CD3, CD20
	Seminoma (especially retroperitoneum, mediastinum)	PLAP, PAS stain, Oct-4
	Extramedullary myeloid cell tumor	Myeloperoxidase, lysozyme, CD34, CD43, CD68, CD117/c-KIT
	Plasma cell myeloma	CD138, CD38, immunoglobulins
Anaplastic tumors	Carcinoma (lung, bladder, breast, thyroid)	Focal keratinization or mucin
	Nasopharyngeal carcinoma	Epstein-Barr virus in situ hybridization
	Melanoma	S-100, HMB45, melan A, tyrosinase
	Anaplastic large cell lymphoma	CD30, EMA, ALK, CD43 (often CD3$^-$)
	Hodgkin's lymphoma	CD15, CD30 (CD45/LCA$^-$)
	Dendritic cell neoplasms	CD21 (FDC), S-100 (IDC), EM
	Angiosarcoma	CD31, CD34, factor VIII–related antigen
	Leiomyosarcoma	Desmin (actins are less specific), EM
Spindle cell tumors	Sarcomatoid carcinoma	Keratins (often only focally positive)
	Desmoplastic melanoma	S-100 (HMB45 and MART-1 often negative)
	Kaposi's sarcoma	PAS, CD34, HHV8 LNA-1, podoplanin
	Large cell lymphoma with fibrosis (especially mediastinal)	CD20 (works in necrotic tumor areas as well), PAX5
	Syncytial variant of Hodgkin's disease	CD15, CD30 (CD43$^-$, CD45/LCA$^-$)
	FDC neoplasms	CD21, CD35 (CD23 can be negative)
	Metastatic sarcoma (especially angiosarcoma, nerve sheath tumors, or myofibroblastic sarcoma)	EM and cytogenetics helpful
	Inflammatory pseudotumor	Admixed acute inflammatory cells, smooth muscle actin
	Infectious pseudotumor	AFB, fungal, and Gram stains

AFB, acid-fast bacillus; ALK, anaplastic lymphoma kinase; EM, electron microscopy; EMA, epithelial membrane antigen; FDC, follicular dendritic cell; HHV8 LNA-1, human herpesvirus 8 latent nuclear antigen-1; IDC, interdigitating dendritic cell; LCA, leukocyte common antigen; NSE, neuron-specific enolase; PAS, periodic acid–Schiff; PLAP, placental alkaline phosphatase; TdT, terminal deoxynucleotidyl transferase.

Among epithelioid tumors, metastatic carcinoma and melanoma are the most common nonhematopoietic tumors encountered. Metastatic seminoma (Fig. 60-5) should be considered, particularly in retroperitoneal lymph nodes. Large cell lymphomas can also appear cohesive and need to be excluded. Anaplastic tumors presenting in a lymph node have a broad differential diagnosis and can show abnormal antigen expression patterns. Thus, careful attention to cytoplasmic features is helpful. For example, focal mucin droplets can be present in poorly differentiated adenocarcinoma, intracellular lumens can be seen in vascular tumors, and so-called hallmark cells may suggest anaplastic large cell lymphoma.

Characteristic Biologic Patterns of Metastasis

In addition to histologic features and patient demographic data, the location of an involved lymph node can narrow the possible sources of a metastatic tumor. In cervical lymph nodes, the most commonly encountered occult tumor is squamous cell carcinoma or undifferentiated carcinoma from a head or neck primary tumor.[1] The primary site can be located in approximately 40% of these cases by subsequent clinical examination and is usually at the base of the tongue or tonsillar fossa. Survival is determined by the extent of lymph node involvement at presentation. Occult carcinomas originating in the lung and esophagus are the next most commonly encountered metastatic tumors in cervical lymph nodes.[2]

In patients with supraclavicular lymphadenopathy as a result of metastasis, carcinoma is the most common pathologic finding.[3] Tumors of abdominal origin preferentially result in left supraclavicular (Virchow's) lymph node enlargement, whereas tumors of the head and neck, lung, and breast (as well as lymphomas) can involve either side.[4] Metastatic tumors in axillary lymph nodes most often originate in the breast in women,[5,6] followed in frequency by melanoma, cutaneous squamous cell carcinoma, and lung cancers. In inguinal lymph nodes, the most common metastatic tumors are melanoma and prostate carcinoma in men and gynecologic malignancies in women.[7] Germ cell tumors, mostly seminoma, can present as metastases involving retroperitoneal lymph nodes and are frequently extensively necrotic.[8]

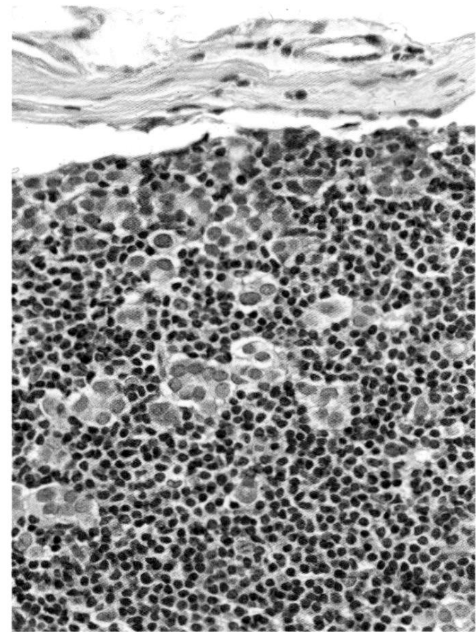

Figure 60-2. Metastatic lobular carcinoma of the breast. Subtle infiltration of the lymph node subcapsular sinus and paracortex by tumor cells in small nests is often observed.

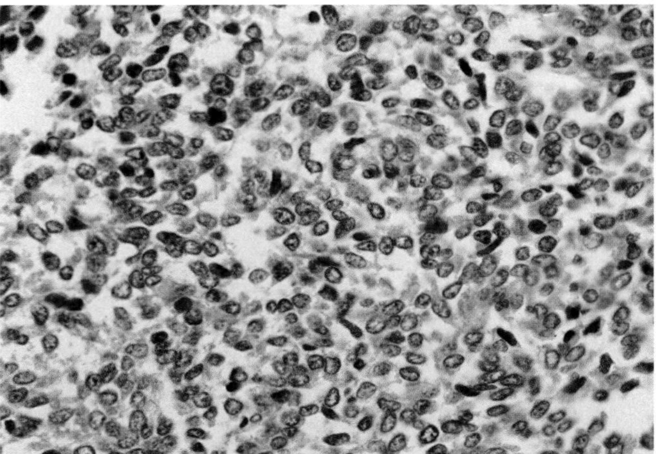

Figure 60-4. Metastatic Ewing's sarcoma/primitive neuroectodermal tumor. The fine nuclear chromatin (described as "smoky" or "dusty") of these small cell tumors may mimic blastic hematopoietic malignancies, but they usually have more abundant cytoplasm with indistinct borders, as well as large areas of necrosis (not shown). Pseudorosette formation is usually focal or absent in lymph node metastases.

Role of Immunohistochemistry in the Diagnosis of Metastatic Tumors

Immunohistochemical stains for metastatic tumors are divided into those used for diagnosis and those used for prognostic or treatment purposes. A review of the prognostic markers is beyond the scope of this chapter, and they are constantly evolving. Suggested diagnostic immunohistochemistry panels for different tumor categories are shown in Table 60-2.

In general, the commonly used first-tier diagnostic antibodies are highly specific but variably sensitive for the detection of particular tumor types.[9] However, aberrant or unrecognized patterns of staining with routine antibodies must always be considered. Most hematopoietic markers in common use are specific for hematopoietic cells, but some hematopoietic markers, such as CD5, CD7, CD10, CD43, and CD56, are commonly expressed in neuroendocrine tumors or carcinomas from certain sites.[10-12] Also, CD30 is strongly expressed by embryonal germ cell tumors and sometimes by mesotheliomas,[13] and CD45 (leukocyte common antigen [LCA]) may be positive in the cytoplasm of breast carcinoma, for example, with rare membranous positivity in poorly differentiated carcinomas.[14] Conversely, S-100 protein and the vascular marker CD31 are variably expressed by monocytes and macrophages. VS38, CD138/syndecan-1, and CD38 are plasma cell markers. However, VS38 and CD138/syndecan-1 are expressed by many solid tumors,[12] whereas CD38 is more restricted to plasma cells and some lymphocytes and histio-

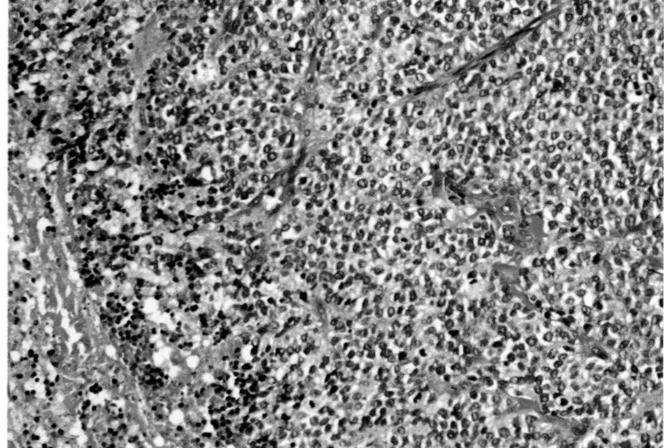

Figure 60-3. Metastatic rhabdomyosarcoma. Diffuse replacement of the lymph node by this small cell neoplasm may be difficult to distinguish histologically from lymphoblastic lymphoma, because diagnostic rhabdomyoblasts may be rare. A predominantly nested growth pattern can be a clue to the diagnosis.

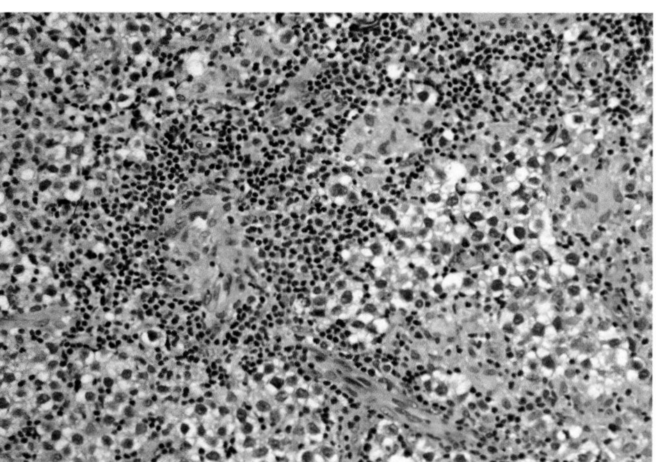

Figure 60-5. Seminoma metastatic to lymph node. The lymph node is infiltrated by large germ cells with abundant clear cytoplasm and distinct cell borders. A helpful feature in distinguishing metastatic seminoma from large cell lymphoma is the admixed granulomatous reaction and small lymphocytes.

Table 60-2 Routine Immunohistochemistry Panels for Diagnosis

Histologic Group	First Round of Staining	Second and Third Rounds of Staining
Small cell tumors	Pan-keratin, TdT, LCA, desmin	Chromogranin, synaptophysin, CD56, CD34, CD99, lymphoid markers, myogenin, myo-D1, myf-4, calcitonin
Anaplastic and epithelioid tumors	Pan-keratin, S-100, CD30, LCA	EMA, PLAP, immunoglobulins, HMB45, melan A, CD68, myeloperoxidase
Spindle cell tumors	Smooth muscle actin, desmin, S-100, pan-keratin	HHF35 actin, CD117/c-KIT, LCA, caldesmon, CD21 or CD35 (FDC sarcoma)

EMA, epithelial membrane antigen; FDC, follicular dendritic cell; LCA, leukocyte common antigen; PLAP, placental alkaline phosphatase; TdT, terminal deoxynucleotidyl transferase.

cytes. Finally, plasmacytomas are notorious for aberrant and false-positive immunoreactivity and can stain for cytokeratin, myeloperoxidase, and T-cell markers, among others.[15]

In metastatic carcinoma of unknown origin, a second group of immunostains can complement the histologic appearance and clinical data, suggesting a possible primary site.[16] Currently, the most broadly useful antibodies are those that detect the cytokeratin expression pattern, particularly keratin types 7 and 20 (Fig. 60-6).[17,18] The overall patterns of these markers are summarized in Table 60-3, but it is important to note that variations can be seen among the more poorly differentiated tumors. Other markers can be helpful in identifying metastasis from less common primary sites.[19] For example, hepatocellular carcinoma is typically negative for keratin 19 (in contrast to cholangiocarcinoma) but positive for low-molecular-weight keratin, as detected by CAM5.2.[20]

The pattern of keratin positivity can also be helpful. A punctate or dot-like cytoplasmic staining pattern observed in Merkel cell carcinoma and small cell carcinoma is characteristic but not completely specific for these tumor types. It should be noted that some lymphomas (approximately 2%) of both mature and lymphoblastic types can show some keratin positivity, most commonly cytokeratin 8.[21,22]

The complex pattern of immunohistochemical expression of the classic serum tumor markers, including carcinoembryonic antigen (CEA), CA19-9, CA15-3, CA125, epithelial membrane antigen/MUC1, β-human chorionic gonadotropin, and alpha fetoprotein, limits their role as diagnostic markers, except in particular cases (e.g., canalicular CEA staining detected by polyclonal antiserum in hepatocellular carcinoma).[10,23] Similarly, polypeptide hormones and their receptors, such as testosterone, estrogen, and progesterone receptors, can be expressed by a wide variety of carcinomas and should be used cautiously as evidence of a particular cell lineage.

Molecular profiling using a limited array of transcripts of lineage-associated genes has recently shown great promise in accurate classification[24-26] and the selection of appropriate therapies.[27] Cytogenetic analysis, although technically demanding, can be highly useful in evaluating the poorly differentiated blastoid tumors; there are characteristic translocations that support the diagnosis of lymphoblastic lymphoma, neuroblastoma, rhabdomyosarcoma, Ewing's sarcoma, and other sarcoma types. Targeted fluorescence in situ hybridization (FISH) analysis for specific chromosomal translocations can routinely be performed on cytologic smears and touch imprints, with high sensitivity. Although less sensitive, FISH is frequently done on fixed, paraffin-embedded tissue sections as well. Electron microscopy has a limited role in the differential diagnosis but can be helpful in the definitive diagnosis of poorly differentiated tumors, for example, by detecting melanosomes in poorly differentiated melanoma or cell junctions that would suggest a carcinoma or dendritic cell neoplasm. In small cell tumors, electron microscopy is especially useful in detecting muscle filaments in rhabdomyosarcoma.

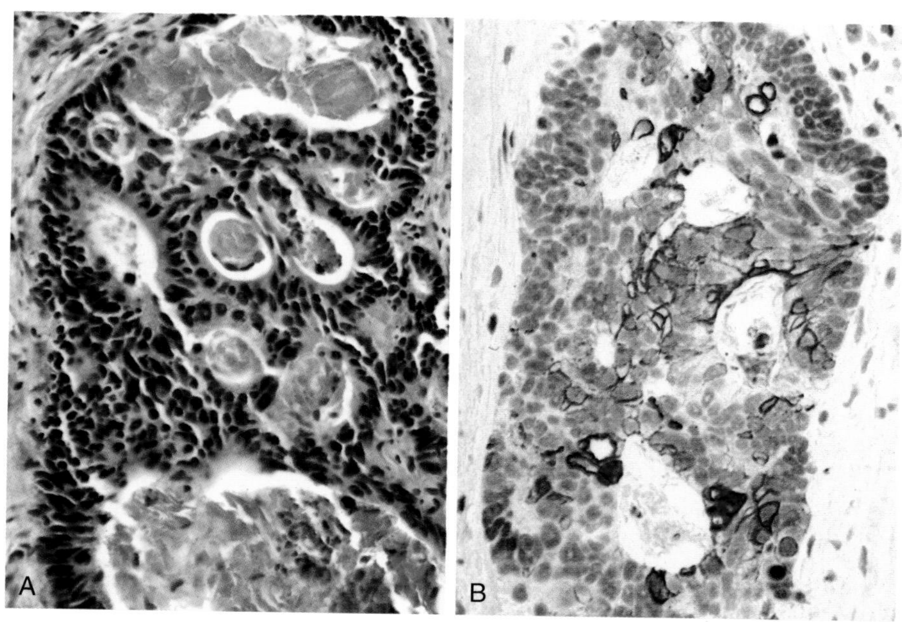

Figure 60-6. Keratin immunostaining of colon adenocarcinoma metastatic to lymph node. A, Columnar tumor cells that replace the nodal parenchyma exhibit gland formation with central necrosis, typical of colon adenocarcinoma. **B,** Tumor cells are positive for cytokeratin 20 but negative for cytokeratin 7 (not shown).

Table 60-3 **Immunostains Used to Identify the Site of Origin of Metastatic Carcinoma**

Marker	Specificity
Beta-catenin	GI tract, ovarian
CDX2	GI tract
Calcitonin	Medullary thyroid carcinoma; rarely, other neuroendocrine tumors
Chromogranin	Neuroendocrine differentiation, including small cell and Merkel cell carcinomas
Cytokeratin 7^+, 20^-	Lung, breast, transitional cell, ovarian, some neuroendocrine and squamous cell carcinomas; endometrioid ovarian
Cytokeratin 7^-, 20^+	GI tract, mucinous ovarian, Merkel cell
Cytokeratin 7^+, 20^+	Transitional cell (bladder), cholangiocarcinoma
Cytokeratin 7^-, 20^-	Adrenocortical, hepatocellular, prostate, renal cell, small cell carcinoma, squamous cell (esophageal), carcinoid, germ cell tumor
Gross cystic disease fluid protein (GCDFP)-15	Breast, salivary gland, some prostate tumors
HepPar1	Hepatocellular carcinoma, small subset (≈5%) of other adenocarcinomas and neuroendocrine tumors
HMB45	Melanoma, lymphangiomyomatosis
MART-1/melan A	Melanoma, adrenocortical carcinoma, other steroid-producing tumors
Napsin A	Lung adenocarcinoma
Oct-4	Seminoma and embryonal carcinomas of testis
Placental alkaline phosphatase (PLAP)	Germ cell tumors; occasional carcinomas of lung, GI, and müllerian origin; some histiocytes
Podoplanin/D2-40	Kaposi's sarcoma, some angiosarcomas, lymphangioma
Prostatic acid phosphatase (PAP)	Prostate, some carcinoids, apocrine breast and salivary tumors
Prostate-specific antigen (PSA)	Prostate carcinoma (decreased in poorly differentiated tumors), some breast carcinomas
RCC	Renal cell carcinomas
Surfactant A	Lung adenocarcinoma
Synaptophysin	Neuroendocrine differentiation, including small cell and Merkel cell carcinomas
Thyroglobulin	Thyroid tumors (not anaplastic or mucoepidermoid)
Thyroid transcription factor-1 (TTF-1)	Lung and thyroid carcinomas and neuroendocrine tumors at these sites
Villin	GI tumors (brush border–type staining)
Vimentin	Negative in endometrial and low-grade renal carcinomas, positive in most other carcinomas

GI, gastrointestinal

Nonlymphoid Tumors with Prominent Reactive Lymphoid Components

In several neoplasms the density of tumor-associated reactive lymphocytes can obscure the tumor cells. This is particularly common in seminoma, melanoma, and medullary carcinoma of the breast. In mediastinal biopsy specimens, thymoma should always be a diagnostic consideration when numerous small lymphocytes are associated with a spindle or epithelioid cell proliferation. The diagnosis of thymoma can be further complicated by the immature thymic immunophenotype of the reactive T-cell component, which can be indistinguishable from lymphoblastic lymphoma by flow cytometric analysis. In such cases, immunostains can easily detect the extensive cytokeratin-positive tumor meshwork.

Undifferentiated nasopharyngeal carcinoma (or undifferentiated carcinoma arising at other sites) is probably the solid tumor most frequently misdiagnosed as lymphoma.[28] This is due to its occasionally prominent inflammatory component and the fact that occult nodal presentations of nasopharyngeal carcinoma are common, occurring in up to 50% of cases. The keratinizing and nonkeratinizing squamous cell variants of nasopharyngeal carcinoma usually present few diagnostic difficulties (Fig. 60-7). However, in the lymphoepithelioma variant of undifferentiated nasopharyngeal carcinoma (also known as the Schmincke type), the neoplastic cells are often obscured by a dense lymphocyte infiltrate (Fig. 60-8). Other cases can be associated with numerous neutrophils and eosinophils and may mimic Hodgkin's lymphoma (Fig. 60-9). Tumor cell cohesiveness and central necrosis within tumor cell aggregates are helpful clues. The most useful ancillary tests for the diagnosis of nasopharyngeal and undifferentiated carcinoma are keratin immunostains and in situ hybridization

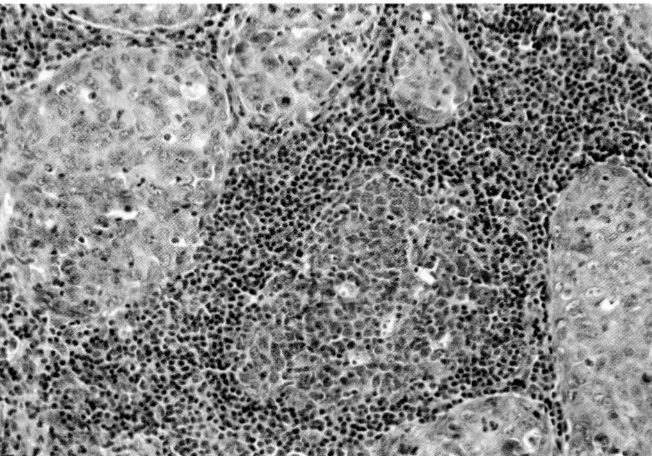

Figure 60-7. Metastatic nonkeratinizing squamous cell carcinoma of nasopharyngeal origin. Large nests of cohesive tumor cells are outlined by collagen bands and show multifocal nodal infiltration. In this field, a central reactive lymphoid follicle is surrounded by tumor.

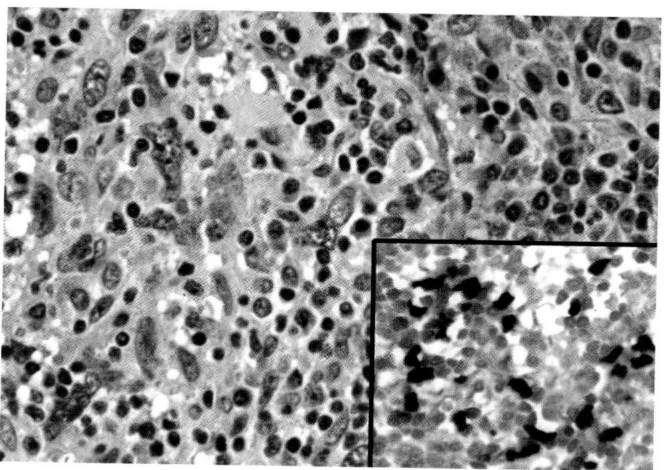

Figure 60-8. Metastatic undifferentiated nasopharyngeal carcinoma —Schmincke or lymphoepithelioma type. Anaplastic tumor cells are interspersed between numerous small lymphocytes. Keratin immunostain and Epstein-Barr virus in situ hybridization (*inset*) were positive in tumor cells.

for Epstein-Barr virus sequences using Epstein-Barr virus–encoded small RNA (EBER) probes.

STAGING AND PROGNOSTIC FACTORS IN LYMPH NODE METASTASIS

As tumor staging procedures have become more sophisticated, the surgical pathologist has been asked to record an increasing and ever-changing number of histologic parameters for metastatic tumors. The handling of sentinel and staging lymph node dissection specimens varies greatly at different institutions and for different tumor types. However, there have been recent efforts to codify such procedures.

Sentinel Lymph Node Biopsy for Carcinoma

Sentinel lymph node biopsy is now widely used for staging regional lymph node fields in patients with breast carcinoma[29] and Merkel cell tumor.[30] In contrast, the use of sentinel lymph node biopsy for colon[31] and prostate carcinoma has proved less useful in predicting metastasis, perhaps due to their unpredictable lymphatic drainage patterns. Sentinel lymph node biopsy involves the use of preoperative lymphoscintigraphy, followed by selective excision of the radioactively "hot" lymph node by the surgeon. This is usually guided by preoperative blue dye injection into the tumor field. Excision is followed by histologic examination using serial sections and sometimes immunohistochemical stains. Identification of a positive lymph node may be followed by immediate or delayed complete axillary dissection or by axillary irradiation. Full-body in vivo imaging studies using lymph node scintigraphy[32] or positron emission tomography[33] may be used in the future to localize sites of occult metastasis for selective biopsy.

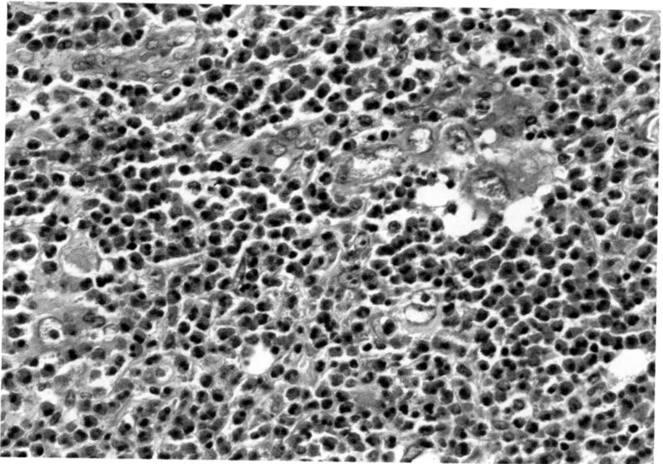

Figure 60-9. Metastatic undifferentiated nasopharyngeal carcinoma —eosinophil-rich variant. Large neoplastic tumor cells are interspersed between numerous eosinophils.

Lymph Node Dissection for Carcinoma

The Association of Directors of Anatomic and Surgical Pathology has promulgated guidelines for the handling of staging lymph node dissection specimens.[34] Data recorded in the report should include the number of lymph nodes positive for metastatic disease (out of the total number examined), the size of the largest metastatic deposit (greatest dimension, as measured on the slide), and whether the tumor is limited to extranodal lymphatic vessels. A separate accounting of tumor deposits not associated with a recognizable lymph node is also recommended.

In some centers the presence of extracapsular tumor extension is recorded for breast and prostate carcinomas, but overall, this finding has not been an independent prognostic factor in most studies. Extracapsular tumor extension has been associated with an increased rate of local recurrence in head and neck carcinomas.[35] The clinical significance of micrometastases remains controversial, and reporting probably varies according to specific tumor types. Carcinoma micrometastases are typically subcapsular and may resemble benign epithelial inclusions, as discussed later.

Sentinel Lymph Node Biopsy for Melanoma

Sentinel lymph node biopsy is now widely used for the staging of malignant melanoma,[36] and this is reflected in the newest American Joint Committee on Cancer (AJCC) classification scheme for melanoma.[37] Identification of any metastatic deposit in a sentinel lymph node is usually followed by complete lymph node dissection, both for further staging and as debulking treatment to reduce the chance of local recurrence.[38] The relevance of complete dissection of the nodal basin to overall disease-specific survival is controversial and the subject of ongoing study.[39,40] In such dissections, the number of lymph nodes involved, the presence of extracapsular extension of tumor, the diameter of the largest tumor focus, and its nodal sublocation (subcapsular versus medullary) are usually recorded and have a significant bearing on prognosis.[40-42] The presence of extracapsular extension has been associated with an increased frequency of local recurrence in melanoma.[43]

The use of immunohistochemistry or molecular analysis[44,45] to detect lymph node micrometastases in sentinel lymph node biopsy and staging lymphadenectomy specimens for melanoma is controversial,[46] but it has been shown that immunohistochemistry using antibodies such as anti–S-100 protein, antityrosinase, HMB45, or MART-1/melan A can detect melanoma micrometastases missed by routine histology.[47-49] However, staining of melanophages or nevus cells must be considered when these antibodies highlight only single cells or small benign-appearing aggregates of cells.[50] False-negative sentinel node biopsies can occur for a variety of reasons.[51]

BENIGN LYMPH NODE INCLUSIONS

Epithelial and Mesothelial Inclusions in Lymph Nodes Adjacent to Solid Organs

Müllerian inclusion cysts (MICs) are by far the most commonly encountered benign glandular inclusions, identified in up to 20% of lymph nodes excised from women. Such cysts may rarely be seen in males. Rare cases of florid MICs causing significant lymph node enlargement or ureteric obstruction have been reported.[52] MICs are most frequently located in the para-aortic lymph nodes and, less frequently, in the iliac lymph nodes. MICs are usually simple cysts lined by serous-type (müllerian) cuboidal to columnar epithelium that is cytologically bland (Fig. 60-10).[53] Histologic features distinguishing benign MICs from metastatic tumor deposits include an intertrabecular location in a lymph node, the presence of multiple types of benign lining cells, and the lack of mitoses or cellular atypia. The presence of a periglandular basement membrane and the absence of a desmoplastic stromal reaction are additional characteristics of MICs. The increased incidence of MICs in patients with borderline ovarian tumors suggests a neoplastic potential for benign-appearing MICs in rare cases.[54] Immunohistochemical stains may be helpful in cases that architecturally resemble metastatic gynecologic cancers, in that MICs are usually negative for CEA.[53]

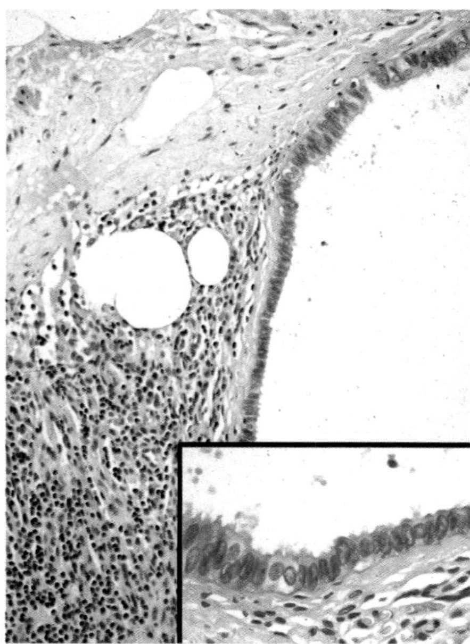

Figure 60-10. Endosalpingiosis of lymph node. A simple cyst in a subcapsular location, lined by cytologically bland cuboid and ciliated columnar epithelium (*inset*).

Endometriosis in lymph nodes is usually seen only in patients with extensive peritoneal deposits; it shows benign-appearing glands with columnar epithelium, edematous endometrial-type stroma, and hemosiderin-laden macrophages (siderophages), as at other sites.[55] Estrogen and progesterone receptors can be detected by immunohistochemistry. Endosalpingiosis with associated psammoma bodies has been rarely reported in lymph nodes.

Benign epithelial inclusions resembling glands from nearly all solid organs have been reported in adjacent lymph nodes. Apparent neoplastic transformation of such benign inclusions has also been rarely reported.[56] Given the close proximity of many lymph nodes to the salivary glands, it is not surprising that these nodal groups often contain numerous salivary ducts and glands. In dense lymphoepithelial lesions of the salivary gland (e.g., lymphoepithelial cysts, acquired immunodeficiency syndrome [AIDS]–associated sialoadenitis, Sjögren's syndrome), it may be difficult to distinguish salivary gland tissue from adjacent lymph node. Salivary gland neoplasms, including Warthin's tumor and pleomorphic adenoma, have been reported to arise from heterotopic salivary gland ducts within lymph nodes. Similar collections of benign ducts and glands can be observed in perithyroidal, axillary, and perirenal lymph nodes.

Bland but occasionally enlarged mesothelial cells can occur as detached groups within the lymph node sinuses, usually in the mediastinum and rarely at other sites.[57] These keratin-positive mesothelial inclusions are most problematic in crushed and fragmented mediastinal lymph node biopsy specimens obtained for the diagnosis of suspected malignancy. Immunohistochemical positivity for mesothelial cell markers (e.g., calretinin, HMBE-1) and the absence of staining for pan-epithelial markers (e.g., Ber-EP4) can be helpful in problematic cases.

Keratin-Positive Fibroblastic Reticular Cells

In interpreting immunostains of lymph nodes, it is important to recognize that the fibroblastic reticular cell network can be variably positive for keratin. Fibroblastic reticular cells, usually identified by antibodies that detect keratins 8 and 18 (e.g., CAM5.2), have a spindled or dendritic morphology and usually present few diagnostic difficulties in tissue sections. However, their presence in cytologic preparations may be more confusing. In some reactive lymph node expansions, keratin-positive fibroblastic reticular cells may be quite numerous but still maintain their dispersed pattern of infiltration (Fig. 60-11).

Nevus Cell Aggregates

Nevus cell aggregates are most commonly seen in axillary lymph node dissection specimens, where they may be mistaken for carcinoma or melanoma. Other common sites include cervical and inguinal lymph nodes; nevus cell aggregates are rare in deep lymph nodes.[58] Nevus cells are present much more frequently in staging lymph nodes from patients with melanoma (up to 25%) than in lymph nodes excised for other reasons.[58] This finding, as well as the increased frequency of nodal nevus aggregates in patients with congenital nevi, suggests aberrant developmental migration patterns of

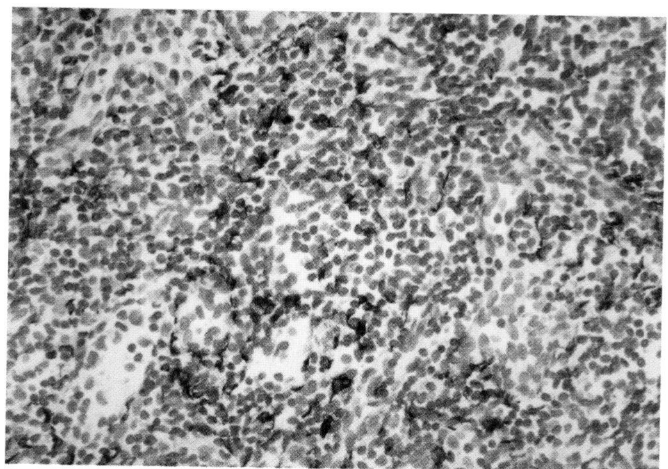

Figure 60-11. Keratin-positive fibroblastic reticular cells in lymph node. Cytologically benign nodal reticular cells with fine cytoplasmic cell processes are interspersed between lymphocytes (pankeratin immunostain). Keratin-positive stromal cells are more commonly detected with low-molecular-weight keratin immunostains (e.g., CAM5.2) but may be seen with any cytokeratin antibody.

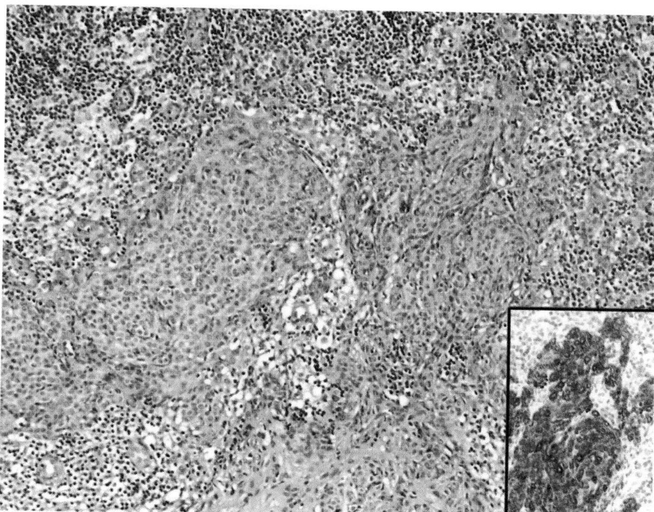

Figure 60-12. Nevus aggregates in lymph node. Variably pigmented nevus cells extend from lymph node trabeculae. MART-1 immunostain is diffusely positive (*inset*). (Courtesy Dr. Victor Prieto.)

melanocytes in patients who subsequently develop melanocytic neoplasms.[59]

Nevus cell aggregates are most commonly embedded in the collagen of the lymph node capsule or trabeculae but can also be found within the subcapsular sinus or rarely in the lymphatics or surrounding small intranodal vessels.[58] These aggregates are usually composed of small, uniform melanocytes that resemble those seen in intradermal melanocytic nevi (Fig. 60-12). When melanin pigment is inconspicuous, immunostaining for S-100 protein or MART-1 can be used to confirm their identity; these aggregates are often negative for HMB45, a useful marker in the differential diagnosis.[60]

Lymph node metastasis from blue nevi and other cytologically bland melanocytic proliferations has been reported.[61] Clues to this occurrence would be more widespread intranodal distribution of nevus cells than commonly seen in benign nevus cell aggregates. Correlation with the presence of a large nevus in the area of the draining lymph node can help provide a definitive diagnosis. The rarely reported primary nodal blue nevus usually represents similar capsular collections of spindle cells with abundant melanin pigment.[62]

MESENCHYMAL PROLIFERATIONS IN LYMPH NODES

A helpful and sensible approach to diagnosing stromal proliferations in lymph nodes is to identify the primary proliferating cell types. Benign proliferations of stroma intrinsic to the lymph node can arise from lymphatic vessels, blood vessels, fibroblastic stroma, dendritic cell types (covered in Chapter 53), or a combination of these types. In addition, the lymph node proliferation can be part of a (syndromic or sporadic) systemic mesenchymal disorder such as leiolymphangiomatosis or angiomatosis. Finally, both primary nodal sarcomas and metastatic sarcomas of all types must be considered.

Vascular Transformation of Lymph Node Sinuses and Lymphatic Proliferations

Vascular transformation of lymph node sinuses is probably the most commonly encountered reactive stromal lesion of lymph nodes. The overall architecture is preserved, but the lymph node sinuses are prominent and show complex anastomosing channels that may contain blood cells or fibrin or have a fibrotic appearance (Fig. 60-13). Some cases also show solid areas that resemble hemangiomas (Fig. 60-14); others show mixed solid and sinusoidal, multinodular, and even plexiform patterns. Rare cases may involve the obliteration of sinuses by a proliferation of cytologically bland, plump fibroblasts and histiocytoid cells.[63]

Vascular transformation of lymph node sinuses likely results from the effects of altered lymph flow due to pressure

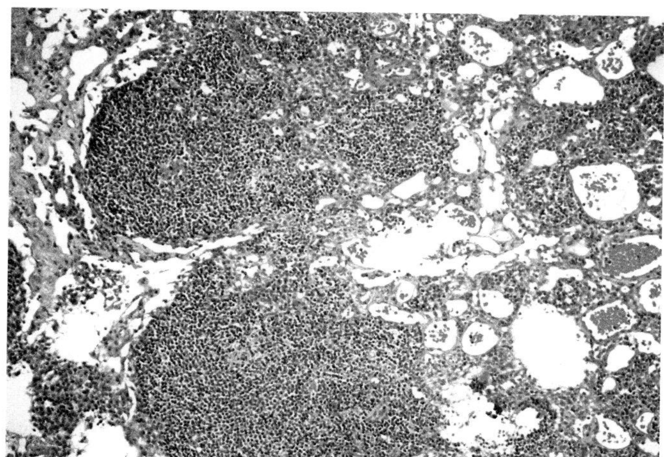

Figure 60-13. Vascular transformation of lymph node sinuses. Dilated sinuses show intraluminal fibrin deposition and red blood cells.

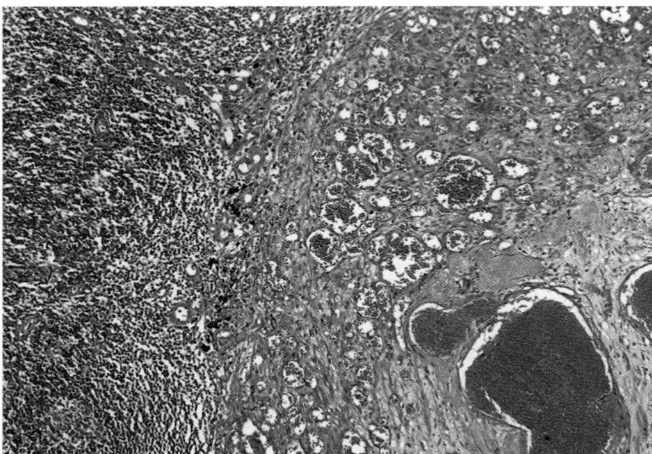

Figure 60-14. Solid hemangioma-like area in vascular transformation of lymph node sinuses. A hypervascular nodule of dilated blood vessels displaces nodal parenchyma. Elsewhere in the lymph node, typical changes of vascular transformation of lymph node sinuses were noted.

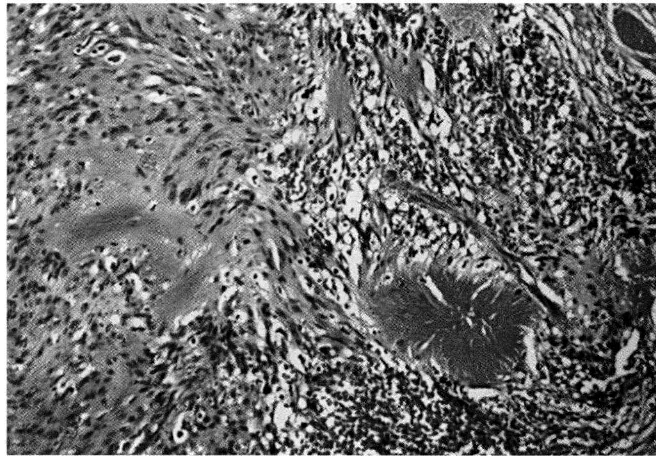

Figure 60-15. Palisaded myofibroblastoma. Stellate spindle cell proliferations radiate out from dense eosinophilic, sclerotic amianthoid collagen. (Courtesy of Dr. Mario Luna.)

changes or stasis secondary to venous or sinus obstruction.[64] Thus, it is common in lymph nodes compressed by adjacent solid tumors or in damaged lymphatic beds following surgery. The association of vascular transformation of lymph node sinuses and concurrent hemangiomas also suggests a role for angiogenic factors in inducing lymphatic proliferation or expansion. Similarly, vascular transformation–like changes can be seen in lymph nodes draining lymphomas or inflammatory conditions that produce abundant cytokines.

In contrast, lymphangioma of lymph nodes is a proliferation of greatly distended, thin-walled lymphatic vessels with dense fibrotic stroma, resembling the cystic hygroma of infancy. In these benign proliferations, variably sized lymphatic spaces, filled with proteinaceous fluid and occasional lymphocytes, displace the normal nodal architecture and extend outside the lymph node.[65]

Mixed Smooth Muscle–Vascular Proliferations

Benign smooth muscle proliferations in lymph nodes are common and appear to be related to extrinsic effects; they occur most often in pelvic, inguinal, and abdominal sites, where gravitational effects on vascular or lymphatic drainage may contribute to their development. These cytologically bland lesions, which radiate out from the lymph node hilum, have been diagnosed as *angiomyomatous hamartoma* in cases with a mixed proliferation of smooth muscle and blood vessels in sclerotic stroma[65,66] or as *leiomyomatous hamartoma* when the smooth muscle component is more prominent.[67] Stromal cells in both these lesions are variably positive for smooth muscle actin, desmin, and vimentin but are negative for HMB45.

Palisaded myofibroblastoma (also known as *hemorrhagic spindle cell tumor with amianthoid fibers*) is a similar benign fibromuscular proliferation largely restricted to the pelvic lymph nodes.[68,69] These tumors are well demarcated and composed of a fascicular proliferation of spindle cells with focal nuclear palisading and acellular stellate, occasionally calcified or ossified, amianthoid collagen fibers (Fig. 60-15). Thick-walled blood vessels and peripherally located hemorrhagic areas are admixed. Immunoreactivity for vimentin, α–smooth muscle actin (Fig. 60-16), and muscle-specific actin (detected by the HHF35 antibody) and electron microscopic studies showing intracytoplasmic bundles of microfilaments support smooth muscle cell differentiation.[70] The differential diagnosis of this tumor includes schwannoma, which may contain similar amianthoid collagen but shows more prominent nuclear palisading and is positive for S-100.

Lymphangiomyomatosis (also known as *leiolymphangiomatosis*) is a systemic proliferation of abnormal smooth muscle and malformed blood vessels and lymphatics occurring in young women. This lesion, which is linked to inactivation of the *TSC2* gene, can occur in association with tuberous sclerosis or sporadically in patients who may also have angiomyolipomas of the kidney. The primary site of disease is usually the lung, but lymph nodes are typically involved as well. Diagnosis is aided by the presence of HMB45$^+$ plump smooth muscle proliferations underlying the anastomosing lymphovascular spaces.[71]

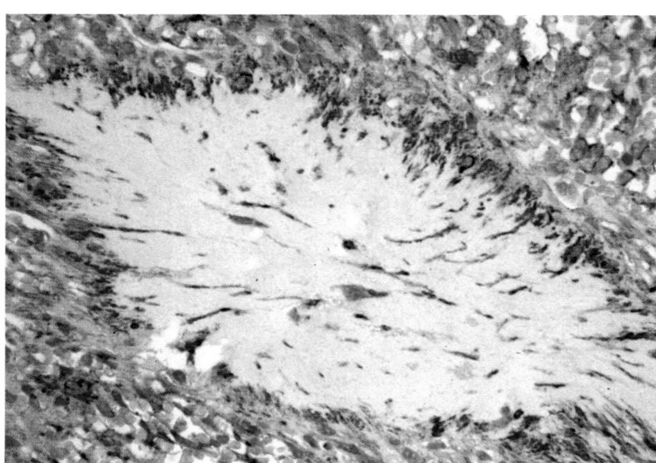

Figure 60-16. Palisaded myofibroblastoma. Smooth muscle actin expression. (Courtesy of Dr. Mario Luna.)

Inflammatory Pseudotumor of Lymph Nodes

Dense fibroblastic or myofibroblastic proliferations in lymph nodes are usually diagnosed as inflammatory pseudotumor. The pathologic spectrum and cause of this entity have not been firmly established. Patients with inflammatory pseudotumor can have marked lymph node enlargement and prominent constitutional symptoms, and surgical resection usually leads to a dramatic resolution of symptoms.[72]

Inflammatory pseudotumor initially involves the paracortical areas and often the fibrous trabeculae of the lymph node, secondarily spreading into follicles and perinodal adipose tissue. Some cases are composed of a polymorphic infiltrate of acute or chronic inflammatory cells embedded in collagen-rich fibroblastic stroma (Fig. 60-17A). Other cases are composed of a dense, storiform proliferation of myofibroblasts (see Fig. 60-17B). Unlike inflammatory pseudotumors of the liver, nodal cases are usually negative for Epstein-Barr virus.[73]

The differential diagnosis of inflammatory pseudotumor is broad and includes inflammatory myofibroblastic tumor; follicular dendritic cell sarcoma; lymphoproliferative disorders associated with a fibrohistiocytic response, including Hodgkin's disease and T-cell lymphomas; and infectious lymphadenitis caused by mycobacteria or fungi. In contrast to some cases of inflammatory myofibroblastic tumor, inflammatory pseudotumors are negative for anaplastic lymphoma kinase.[73]

Kaposi's Sarcoma

Kaposi's sarcoma (KS) is a virally induced tumor characterized by a proliferation of vascular elements and stromal cells with variable myofibroblastic differentiation. KS occurs in a variety of clinical settings, including immunosuppression (solid organ transplantation, human immunodeficiency virus [HIV] infection) and old age, particularly elderly patients of Mediterranean or African heritage. An endemic version of the disease occurs in those geographic areas. In Africa, epidemic variants of KS also occur, with a much younger age of onset.

KS often extends from the lymph node capsule along the fibrous trabeculae before completely replacing the nodal parenchyma. KS exhibits curvilinear fascicles of bland-appearing spindle cells with characteristic cytoplasmic periodic acid–Schiff–positive hyaline globules (Fig. 60-18) and admixed plasma cells, hemosiderin, and extravasated erythrocytes. In the less cellular areas, sieve-like vasoformative structures are easier to appreciate. Rare cases may show sinusoidal infiltration extending throughout the interfollicular areas, in a pattern resembling vascular transformation of lymph node sinuses.

The pathogenetic role of human herpesvirus 8 (HHV8) in KS is now well established. Immunostains for HHV8, particularly latency-associated antigen-1, are useful in confirming the diagnosis of KS (Fig. 60-19). Furthermore, KS changes in lymph nodes are often noted adjacent to the regressed follicles of multicentric Castleman's disease, another lesion related to HHV8 infection.

Vascular Tumors

Benign hemangiomas of lymph nodes can exhibit the full range of histologic variants seen at other anatomic sites. They are often centered in the hilum or medulla but can also completely efface the parenchyma. The most common types in lymph nodes are lobulated capillary hemangioma with myxoid stroma and cavernous hemangioma (Fig. 60-20). Cases of nodal cellular hemangioma have also been described. Rarely, lesions resembling epithelioid hemangioma or angiolymphoid hyperplasia with eosinophilia can be seen in lymph nodes.

Epithelioid hemangioendothelioma, which usually occurs in lymph nodes as a metastatic tumor, is characterized by sheets, nodules, or cords of plump, eosinophilic, vacuolated cells with small intracytoplasmic lumens that sometimes contain red blood cells, with abundant extracellular hyaline matrix (Fig. 60-21). The tumor cells are positive for vascular markers, including CD31 and factor VIII–associated protein. In nodal lesions of epithelioid hemangioendothelioma, central necrosis and dense fibrosis are frequently seen. Spindle cell

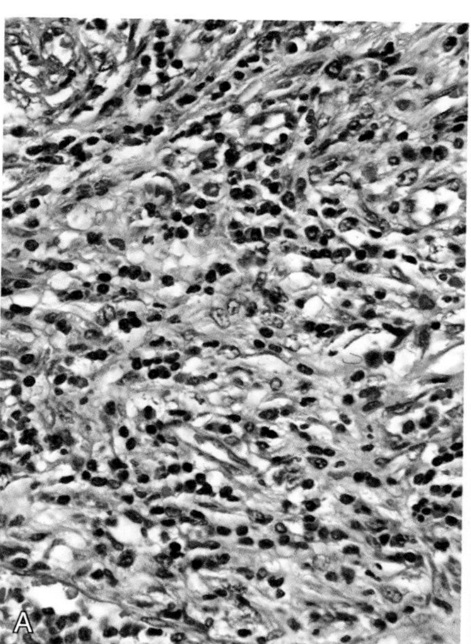

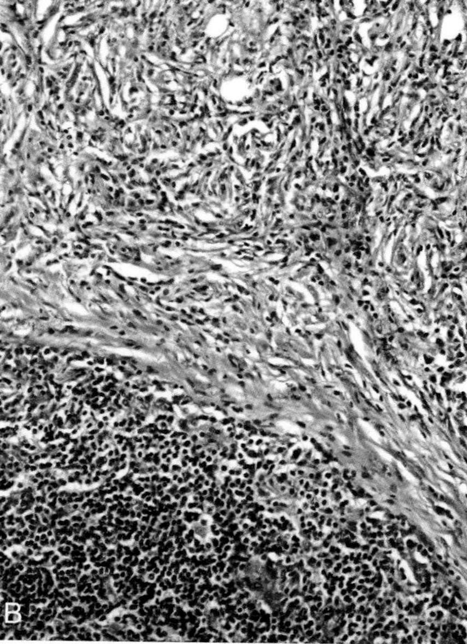

Figure 60-17. Inflammatory pseudotumor of lymph node. Various patterns have been described, including lesions rich in inflammatory cells **(A)** and other cellular or spindled lesions **(B)**. Differential diagnosis of the more cellular lesions includes myofibroblastic sarcoma.

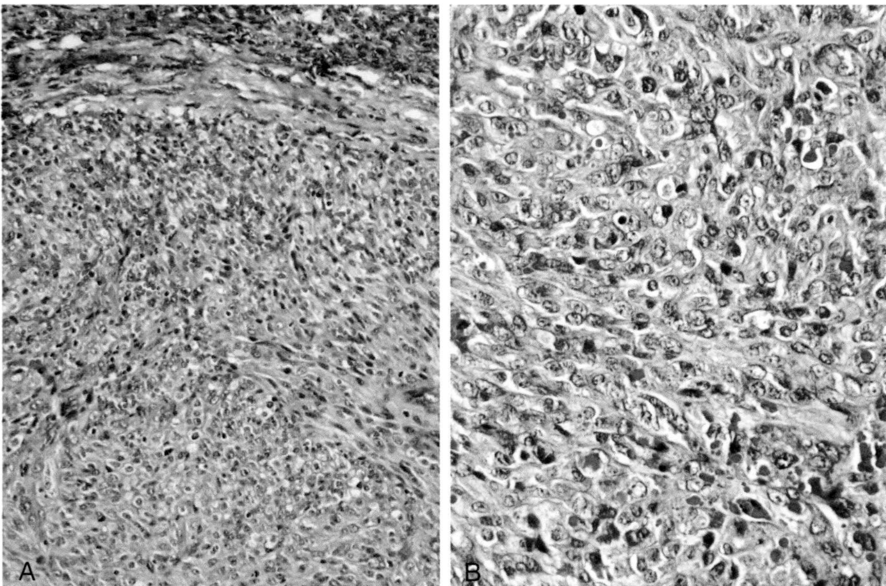

Figure 60-18. Kaposi's sarcoma of lymph node. A, Hypervascular spindle and epithelioid cell proliferation centered on the lymph node capsule. **B,** Entrapped red blood cells and extracellular hyaline globules are diagnostic clues.

hemangioendothelioma can be the sole histologic pattern but is more commonly a minor component of epithelioid hemangioendothelioma (Fig. 60-22).[74]

Nodal angiosarcoma appears to be an exceedingly rare primary neoplasm, but metastasis to lymph nodes from an occult tumor can occur. Angiosarcoma is distinguished from the lower-grade vascular tumors by marked atypia, an increased mitotic rate, and multilayering of tumor cells in the vasoformative areas. Tumors can have a spindled, epithelioid, or anastomosing pattern or a mixture of all patterns (Fig. 60-23). Epithelioid angiosarcoma is more common in retroperitoneal lymph nodes (Fig. 60-24).

Metastatic Sarcomas of Other Types

Primary nodal sarcomas of follicular dendritic cell, interdigitating dendritic cell, and fibroblastic reticular cell origin are described in Chapter 53 and are not discussed here.

Although any histologic type of sarcoma can metastasize to lymph nodes, different sarcomas have different frequencies of lymph node metastasis. Among adult soft tissue sarcomas, lymph node metastases are most common with rhabdomyosarcoma, angiosarcoma, and hemangioendothelioma.[75,76] Liposarcomas rarely metastasize to lymph nodes. Among childhood sarcomas, rhabdomyosarcoma and Ewing's sarcoma most frequently metastasize to lymph nodes, with a 10% to 15% incidence over the course of the disease.[77] Ganglioneuroblastoma may metastasize to lymph nodes, particularly in the mediastinum (Fig. 60-25). Among bone tumors, both chrondrosarcoma and osteosarcoma can metastasize to regional lymph nodes.

Bone Marrow Hematopoietic Elements and Tumors Involving Lymph Nodes

Bone marrow hematopoietic elements can appear in lymph nodes in a variety of settings. The most common is in asso-

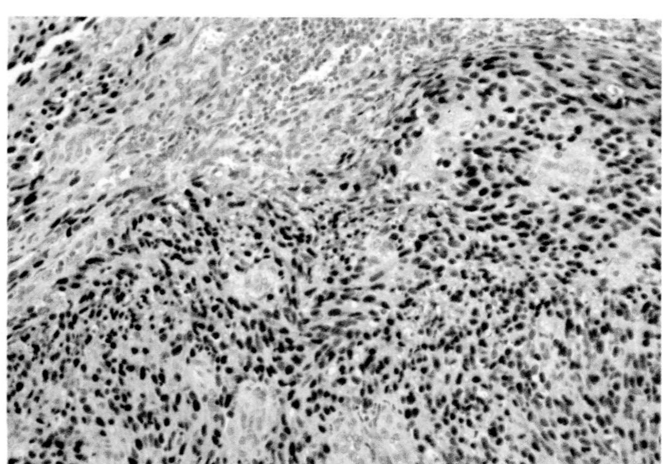

Figure 60-19. Human herpesvirus 8 (HHV8) infection in Kaposi's sarcoma. Immunostain for HHV8 latency-associated antigen-1 viral product is diffusely positive in proliferating spindle cells.

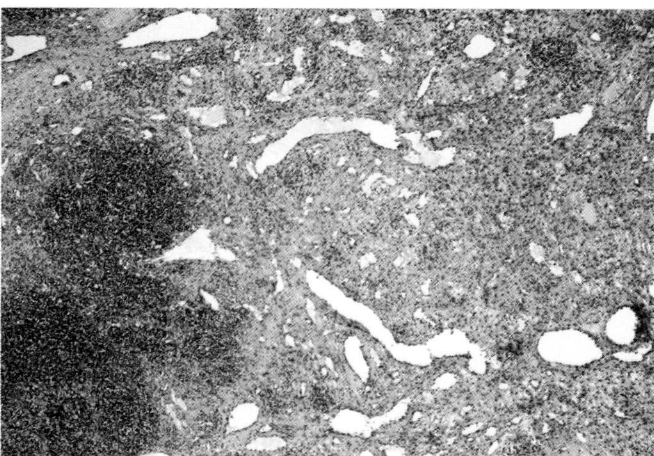

Figure 60-20. Hemangioma of lymph node. The nodal parenchyma is displaced by a proliferation of benign-appearing blood vessels of various sizes and dense sclerosis.

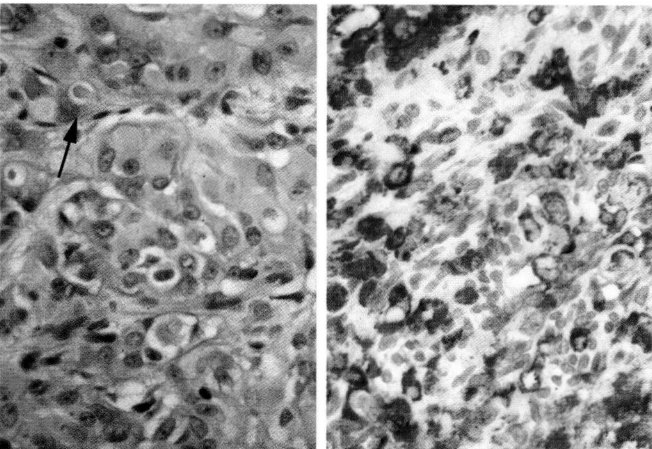

Figure 60-21. Epithelioid hemangioendothelioma involving lymph node. Large epithelioid cells with abundant pink cytoplasm show intracytoplasmic vacuolation (*left, arrow*). Factor VIII–associated protein immunostain is positive (*right*).

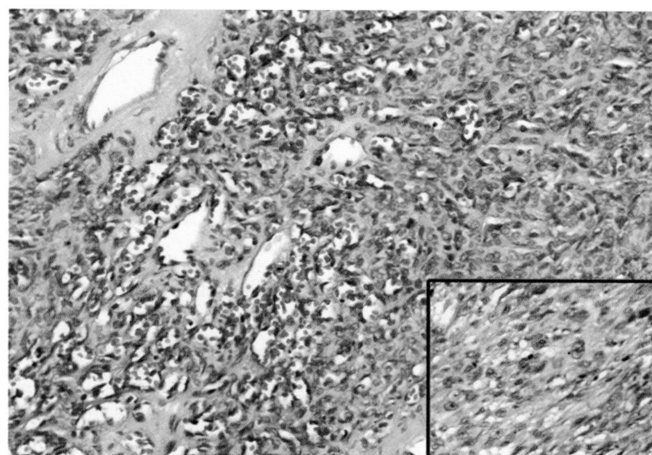

Figure 60-23. Angiosarcoma metastatic to lymph node. Tumor can have a wide variety of appearances, often with vasoformative areas mixed with cellular spindle cell areas (*inset*).

ciation with fibrotic myeloproliferative syndromes, where the bone marrow environment is no longer optimal. In such cases, megakaryocytes and other bone marrow elements appear in great numbers in the interfollicular areas of lymph nodes (Fig. 60-26). This is also known as *extramedullary hematopoiesis*.

Lymph nodes may be secondarily involved by acute leukemias and may be the first site of disease detection. Acute lymphoblastic leukemia involving lymph nodes resembles lymphoblastic lymphoma, as discussed in Chapter 41. An interfollicular pattern can be observed in lymphomas with early spread. Acute myeloid leukemia involving lymph nodes (also known as *granulocytic sarcoma*, *extramedullary myeloid cell tumor*, and *myeloid sarcoma*) is discussed in Chapter 45. The interfollicular pattern of infiltration in acute myeloid leukemia (Fig. 60-27) and the cytologic features, especially as seen on touch preparations (Fig. 60-28), are clues to the

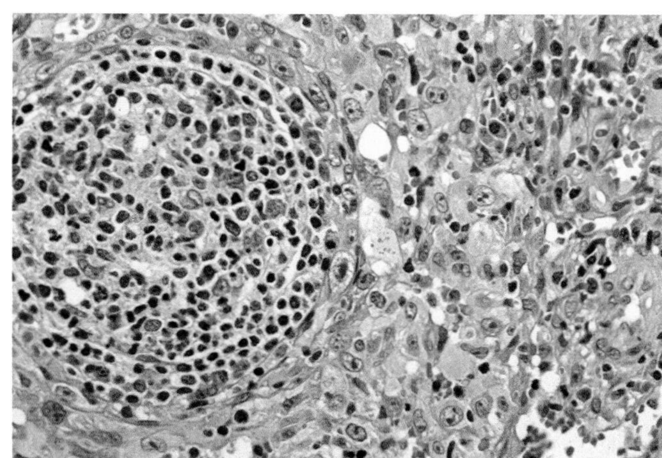

Figure 60-24. Epithelioid angiosarcoma metastatic to lymph node. An interfollicular pattern of tumor invasion is noted.

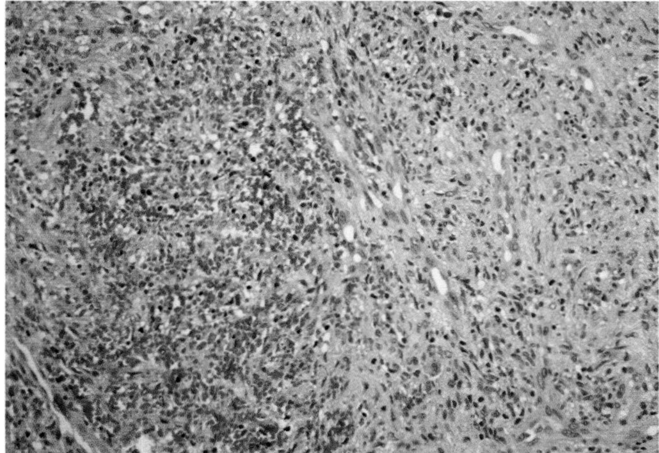

Figure 60-22. Hemangioendothelioma in lymph node with spindled and retiform growth patterns. A mixed pattern of solid collagenous areas and anastomosing vasoformative areas is common. The degree of atypia and number of mitoses are typically lower in epithelioid hemangioendothelioma than in angiosarcoma.

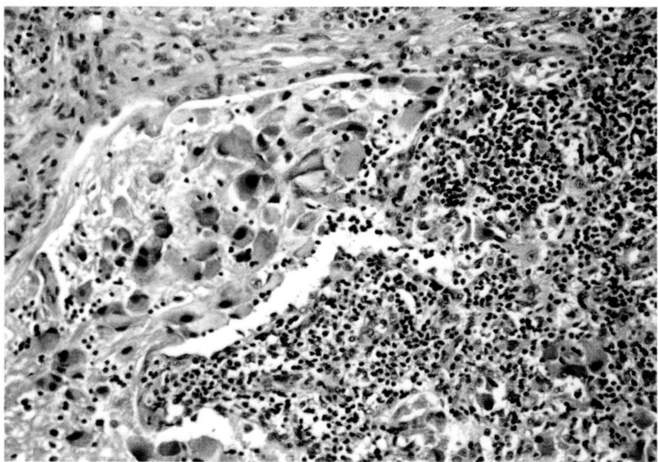

Figure 60-25. Metastatic ganglioneuroblastoma. Sinusoidal infiltration by spindled tumor cells with granular cytoplasm is noted. This patient had a history of a large posterior mediastinal mass.

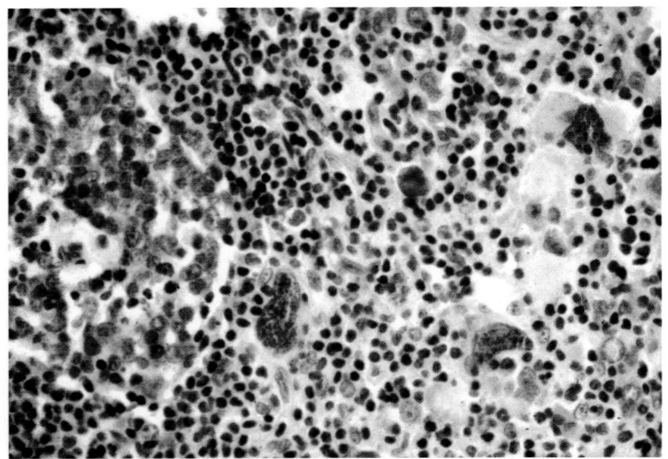

Figure 60-26. Extramedullary hematopoiesis in lymph node. Megakaryocytes and immature myeloid forms are scattered throughout the interfollicular areas in this patient with a chronic myeloproliferative disorder.

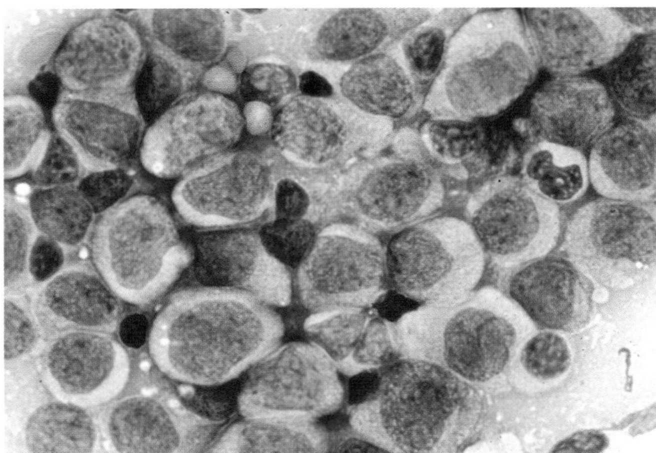

Figure 60-28. Acute myeloid leukemia in lymph node. Touch preparation reveals immature myelomonocytic forms.

correct diagnosis. The inclusion of CD45/LCA in routine immunohistochemical panels should detect most of these tumors, but the antibody is negative in a small subset of cases. Other stains, such as myeloperoxidase, lysozyme, CD43, CD68, and CD117, are very helpful for diagnosis.

Nodal involvement by mast cell disease is discussed in Chapter 48. Mast cell tumors in lymph node are often associated with perivascular fibrosis and eosinophils—two clues to the correct diagnosis. Low-grade tumors can have abundant pale cytoplasm, resembling nodal marginal zone B-cell lymphoma. High-grade tumors can be difficult to distinguish from other poorly differentiated neoplasms. Metachromatic staining with Giemsa or toluidine blue stains and immunohistochemical stains (e.g., tryptase, CD117) are helpful in establishing the diagnosis.

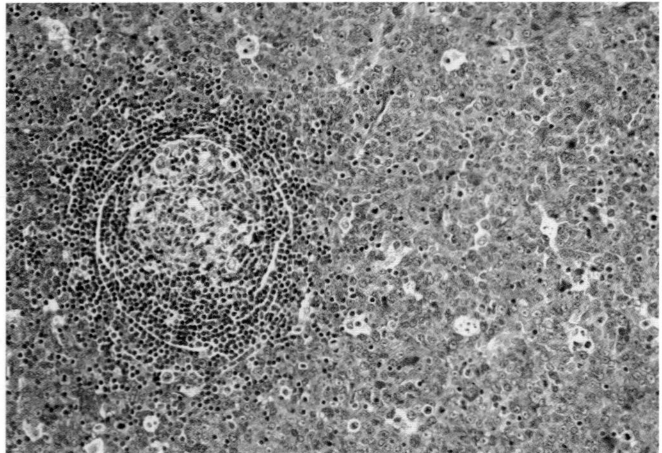

Figure 60-27. Acute myeloid leukemia in lymph node. The interfollicular areas are expanded by a neoplastic proliferation of immature myeloid forms.

Langerhans cell histiocytosis is a relatively common finding in lymph nodes and is discussed in Chapter 52. Rarely, these tumors can resemble poorly differentiated nonhematopoietic tumors and should be considered when the first round of immunostaining is negative. The strong, uniform immunoreactivity of tumor cells for CD1a and S-100 protein distinguishes these tumors from other histiocytic proliferations, which are negative or only focally positive.

Pearls and Pitfalls

- Lymph node location is often the most helpful clue to the primary site of origin of metastatic carcinoma. For instance, occult nasopharyngeal carcinoma commonly presents in neck lymph nodes.
- Sarcomatoid carcinoma should always be considered when a poorly differentiated spindle cell nodal metastasis is encountered.
- Anaplastic large cell lymphoma can have a variety of appearances and exhibit the loss of nearly all lymphoid-associated markers. Perform a CD30 immunostain before ruling out a nodal large cell malignancy.
- Follicular dendritic cell (FDC) neoplasms often have an epithelioid or anaplastic morphology that mimics other tumors. A panel of FDC markers (CD21, CD23, CD35) is recommended because partial FDC differentiation is common. Residual nodal tissue may show colonization of lymphoid follicles by dysplastic FDCs.

References can be found on Expert Consult @ www.expertconsult.com

Chapter **61**

Spleen: Normal Architecture and Neoplastic and Nonneoplastic Lesions

Attilio Orazi and Dennis P. O'Malley

CHAPTER OUTLINE

Few hematologic malignancies arise primarily in the spleen; most conditions occurring at this site represent secondary involvement by diseases originating elsewhere in the body. The role of the pathologist in most cases is to confirm the known or suspected diagnosis and to exclude unsuspected pathology. The keys to the successful interpretation of splenic pathology are careful gross evaluation of the organ and optimal tissue fixation. Because of the amount of blood in the spleen, thin sections are particularly important. In addition, care must be exercised in isolating lymph nodes of the splenic hilum. Their examination can provide valuable additional information, particularly in the diagnosis of low-grade B-cell lymphomas. Obtaining adequate clinical information is often critical for the diagnostic characterization of disorders that involve the spleen; this need cannot be overemphasized.

In this chapter we present a comprehensive account of those aspects of splenic pathology likely to be encountered by diagnostic hematopathologists. We outline principles for a systematic histopathologic analysis that can be applied to achieve a specific diagnosis after the recognition of broad categories of abnormalities affecting individual splenic compartments. To avoid the repetition of material covered elsewhere in this text, immunohistochemistry, cytogenetics, and molecular genetics are only briefly described where appropriate.

THE NORMAL SPLEEN

The characterization of disorders that involve the spleen can best be understood in light of the structure and function of that organ.[1-9] The spleen is composed of two anatomically and functionally distinct regions (Table 61-1). The lymphoid tissue of the spleen, called the *white pulp*, appears grossly as uniformly distributed white nodules. The white pulp is intimately associated with the splenic arterial circulation. The central arteries, which arise from trabecular arteries within the fibrous trabeculae, are surrounded by cylindrical cuffs of lymphocytes called *periarteriolar lymphoid sheaths*. The periarteriolar lymphoid sheaths contain an admixture of B and T cells, with a predominance of $CD4^+$ T lymphocytes. Periodically, splenic lymphoid follicles (malpighian corpuscles) occur as outgrowths of the periarteriolar lymphoid sheaths.[5,6] The morphology of the splenic white pulp varies with age and with its functional activity (e.g., presence of antigenic stimulation). Inactive or hypoplastic white pulp, in which no germinal centers are seen, is characteristic of infancy, senescence, and the immunologically unstimulated adult spleen. In the immunologically activated state, the splenic lymphoid follicle shows three distinct zones.[7-9] The *germinal center*, structurally similar to germinal centers in other lymphoid organs, is surrounded by a *mantle zone*. The mantle zone is encased by the outer *marginal zone*, a cellular layer at the interface between the white and red pulp. The marginal zone, composed of both B and T cells,[4] is the site of initial antigen trapping and processing (Fig. 61-1).

The *red pulp* of the spleen is composed of splenic vascular sinuses and the cords of Billroth, which are made up of splenic macrophages, scattered cord capillaries, venules, and stromal cells. All these cellular elements linked together, along with a relatively scanty amount of extracellular matrix, are responsible for the peculiar architecture of the red pulp.[10-12] The splenic vascular sinuses provide the mechanism for filtration of the peripheral blood, one of the important functions of the spleen. The sinus lining cells, also known as *littoral cells*, have long cytoplasmic processes that overlap and are closely opposed. However, because no tight junctions are present, circulating blood cells are able to squeeze through the interendothelial spaces and percolate through the cords of Billroth before entering the splenic sinuses and the venous system, thus returning to the systemic circulation. The ability of circulating blood cells to enter the splenic sinuses and subsequently percolate through the cords depends on their deformability. Cells without the ability to deform cannot enter the sinuses and are destroyed in the acidotic, hypoxic environment of the cords of Billroth.[2,13]

The T cells found in the red pulp are predominantly $CD8^+$ small lymphocytes, which are rarely found in the periarteriolar lymphoid sheaths and are virtually absent in the germinal centers. Gamma-delta T cells also reside normally in the red pulp. The distribution of immunoglobulin-containing B cells is comparable to that seen in the lymph nodes. The mantle zone B cells bear surface immunoglobulin, with coexpression of immunoglobulin (Ig) M and IgD. The marginal zone B cells express predominantly IgM, with only a small minority expressing IgD. IgG expression is lacking in these areas and is limited to scattered cells in the red pulp, where rare IgA-containing cells are also found. The red pulp contains numerous cells of monocyte-macrophage lineage, only a few of

Table 61-1 Normal Morphologic Compartments of the Spleen

Compartment	Elements	Description
White pulp	Follicles	
	Primary	Composed of small nodules of mantle-type B lymphocytes (see below)
	Secondary	Composed of a mixture of small, irregular B lymphocytes and large transformed cells, with intermixed dendritic cells and macrophages
	Mantle zone	Surrounds the germinal center; composed predominantly of small B lymphocytes with round to irregular nuclei, condensed chromatin, and scant cytoplasm
	Periarteriolar lymphoid sheaths	Sheaths of predominantly small T lymphocytes that surround arterioles and arteries; other cells include larger transformed lymphocytes, NK cells, plasma cells, B cells
Red pulp	Sinusoids	Lined by specialized endothelial cells with macrophage capacity; lack a continuous basal membrane
	Cords	Lie between the sinusoids; composed of extracellular space and cordal macrophages
Supporting stroma	Capsule and trabecular septa	Paucicellular dense fibrous tissue; thickened in reactive or chronic conditions

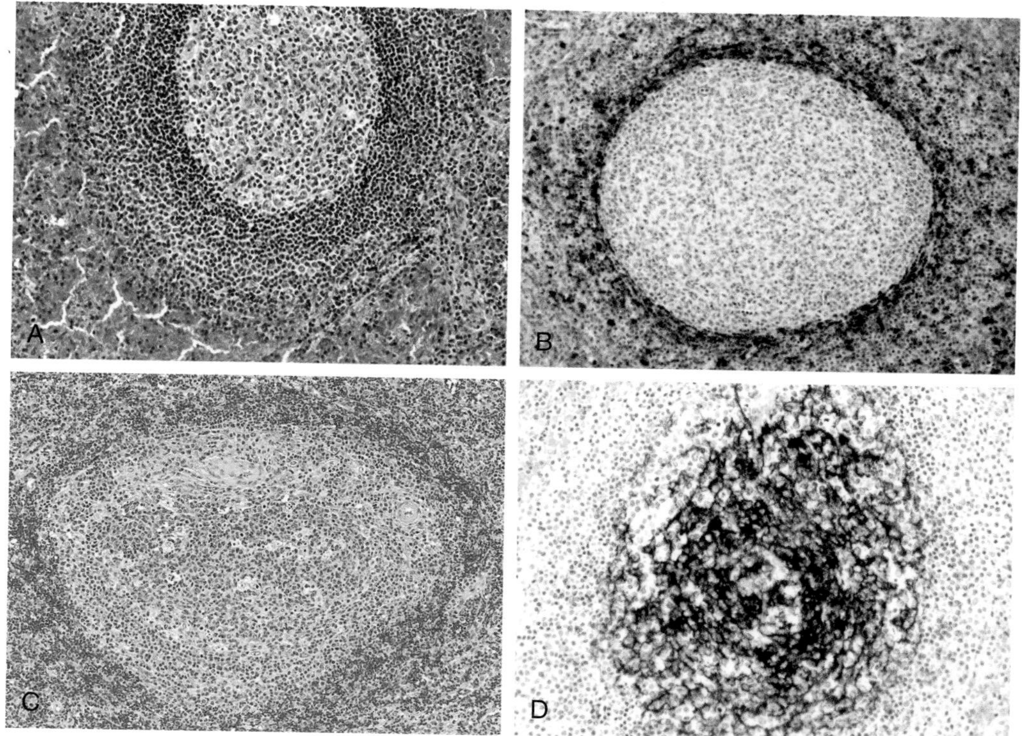

Figure 61-1. **A**, Splenic lymphoid follicle displaying its characteristic tripartite nature: germinal center, mantle zone, and well-defined marginal zone. **B**, DBA.44 immunohistochemical stain highlights mantle zone cells. Note negative staining in the follicle germinal center and rare positive cells within the predominantly negative marginal zone. **C**, Hyperplastic follicle, with less distinct mantle and marginal zones. **D**, CD21 immunohistochemical stain highlights the follicular dendritic cell network within a germinal center.

which are found in the white pulp. Natural killer (NK) cells are found scattered throughout the red pulp. The red pulp also contains granulocytes, monocytes, and lymphocytes that pass transiently through the red pulp circulation.

GROSS EXAMINATION

The initial evaluation of the spleen should consist of a gross examination of the organ. Three major patterns are recognized, based on involvement of the white pulp, red pulp, or more focal lesions (Table 61-2).

Diffuse Splenic Enlargement

White Pulp Involvement

Most proliferative disorders of the splenic lymphoid tissue produce a micronodular pattern owing to the abnormal expansion of preexisting splenic lymphoid structures (follicles and periarteriolar lymphoid sheaths). Grossly, multiple small, whitish nodules are noticeable on the cut surface, an appearance that is occasionally referred to as a *miliary* pattern. This pattern is most often seen in small B-cell lymphoid neoplasms involving the spleen. The nodules occasionally become confluent or present as larger, dominant masses. Lymphoid malignancies that affect the white pulp are largely the same as those that affect lymph nodes. These disorders include both classical and nodular lymphocyte-predominant Hodgkin's lymphoma and non-Hodgkin's lymphomas, primarily of B-cell lineage.

Red Pulp Involvement

Red pulp involvement has a different gross appearance. Typically, expansion of the red pulp gives the spleen a more homogeneous red or "beefy" appearance. The normal nodularity of the white pulp is typically diminished or not seen. Microscopically, the white pulp is often atrophic or compressed by the expanded red pulp. Neoplastic proliferations that involve the red pulp include myeloid and lymphoid leukemias, myeloproliferative disorders, and a variety of nonhematopoietic tumors. In general, disorders with a large component of circulating cells (e.g., chronic lymphocytic leukemia, large granular lymphocytic leukemia, hairy cell leukemia, acute leukemia) have significant red pulp involvement. However, some lymphomas (e.g., hepatosplenic T-cell lymphoma, intravascular large B-cell lymphoma, as well as other less well defined lymphoid malignancies) also involve the red pulp.

Focal Splenic Pathology

Some benign and malignant proliferations produce focal lesions rather than more diffuse involvement of the red or white pulp. These include lesions that involve vascular, stromal, and hematolymphoid elements.

Splenic Rupture

Pathologic rupture of the spleen can be seen in a variety of hematologic disorders, both benign and malignant.[5]

Table 61-2 Patterns of Involvement in Splenic Pathology

	Predominantly Red Pulp Based		Predominantly White Pulp Based	
Pattern	Neoplastic	Nonneoplastic	Neoplastic	Nonneoplastic
Diffuse	HCL and HCL variant Splenic diffuse red pulp small B-cell lymphoma Hepatosplenic T-cell lymphoma LGLL Acute leukemias MPN, other myeloid neoplasms CLL/SLL (rare) LPL (rare)	Hemolytic anemias Nonspecific congestion Extramedullary hematopoiesis Storage diseases Cytokine effects HPS	Small B-cell lymphomas (CLL/SLL, LPL, SMZL, MCL) PTCL	Hyperplasia
Focal* or variable	Hodgkin's lymphoma DLBCL T-PLL FDCT Other dendritic cell tumors Mast cell disease Vascular tumors[†] Metastases	—	—	Inflammatory pseudotumor Hamartoma Cyst Peliosis

*Focal lesions may have considerable overlap, with both red and white pulp involvement. At times, this division is arbitrary.
†Diffuse involvement is seen in systemic angiomatosis as well as in some cases of littoral cell angioma.
CLL/SLL, chronic lymphocytic leukemia/small lymphocytic lymphoma; DLBCL, diffuse large B-cell lymphoma; FDCT, follicular dendritic cell tumor; HCL, hairy cell leukemia; HPS, hemophagocytic syndrome; LGLL, large granular lymphocytic leukemia/lymphoma; LPL, lymphoplasmacytic leukemia/lymphoma; MCL, mantle cell lymphoma; MPN, myeloproliferative neoplasm; PTCL, peripheral T-cell lymphoma; SMZL, splenic marginal zone lymphoma; T-PLL, T-cell prolymphocytic leukemia.

Spontaneous rupture of the spleen should always prompt a pathologic evaluation of the splenic tissue because various infectious causes (particularly infectious mononucleosis) have pathologic findings that are distinctive enough to make a presumptive diagnosis or suggest additional serologic studies. Other causes, such as storage diseases, present with characteristic findings as well. Splenic rupture as a primary presentation of hematologic malignancy is rare, but it has been reported with both low-grade and high-grade lymphoid malignancies. Acute and chronic myeloproliferative disorders and, rarely, acute lymphoblastic leukemia can present as splenic rupture. Nonhematopoietic lesions associated with splenic rupture include cysts, infarctions, vascular lesions or neoplasms, and metastatic malignancies.

LYMPHOID HYPERPLASIA

Various reactive conditions that affect the splenic white or red pulp can simulate hematopoietic malignancies (Box 61-1). Reactive follicular hyperplasia, with the formation of germinal centers, is usually easily recognized as benign (see Fig. 61-1).[2] However, follicular hyperplasia must occasionally be distinguished from follicular lymphoma. The finding of tingible body macrophages and a polymorphic lymphoid cell population within polarized splenic follicles points to the diagnosis of a reactive hyperplasia. A rare entity that may grossly simulate lymphoma is localized (nodular) reactive lymphoid hyperplasia. The area of nodular hyperplasia appears quite distinct from adjacent normal spleen and may raise the suspicion of lymphoma (Fig. 61-2). Histologically, this area is composed of a focal aggregation of hyperplastic follicles that have typical, benign features.[14]

The marginal zones may become widely expanded, a phenomenon referred to as *splenic marginal zone hyperplasia*.[2,5,15-18] This usually occurs in association with follicular hyperplasia. It may be impossible to distinguish these reactive changes from cases of early marginal zone lymphoma on morphologic grounds alone.[15,19] Some autoimmune disorders can lead to this picture, including systemic lupus erythematosus or idiopathic thrombocytopenic purpura.

Reactive lymphoid hyperplasia without germinal center formation, which is characteristic of infectious mononucleosis as well as herpes simplex and other viral infections, can simulate both Hodgkin's and non-Hodgkin's lymphoma.[2,20-22] The white pulp in these conditions lacks expanded follicles and, on low-power examination, resembles the immunologically unstimulated spleen.[2,5,7,23,24] This is the splenic equivalent of paracortical hyperplasia and is primarily a reaction of T cells. High-power examination reveals morphologic evidence of antigenic stimulation, characterized by the presence of lymphocytes in varying stages of transformation, including small and large lymphocytes and immunoblasts. Transformed lymphocytes and immunoblasts also proliferate around splenic arterioles and may infiltrate the subendothelial zones

Box 61-1 *Benign Lesions of the Spleen That Simulate Hematopoietic Malignancies*

- Immune reactions
  - Florid follicular hyperplasia
  - Marginal zone hyperplasia
- Congenital immunodeficiencies
- Autoimmune conditions
- Disorders of the reticuloendothelial system
  - Storage diseases
  - Hemophagocytic syndrome
  - Langerhans cell histiocytosis
- Castleman's disease
- Reactive myeloid proliferations due to cytokine treatment
- Nonhematopoietic lesions
  - Cyst
  - Hamartoma
  - Inflammatory pseudotumor

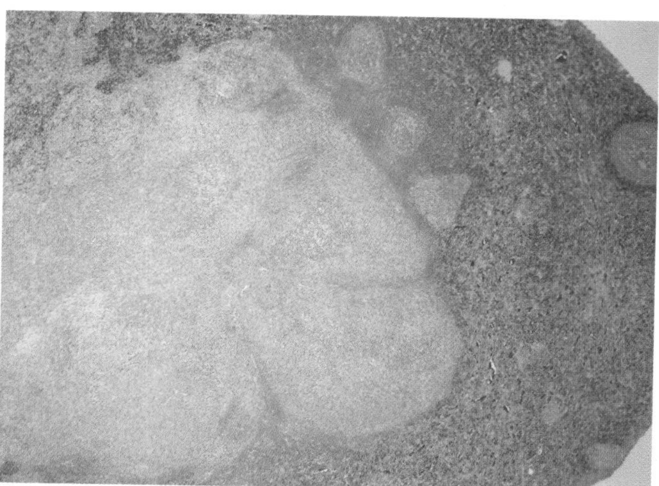

Figure 61-2. Nodular lymphoid hyperplasia of the spleen. Note the confluence of several hyperplastic follicles, which form a tumor-like lesion. This is surrounded by normal red pulp and other hyperplastic-appearing follicles. Although cytologically benign, this entity can mimic lymphoma or other focal splenic lesions.

of the trabecular veins and the connective tissue framework, resulting in splenic rupture in extreme cases.[25] This pattern of lymphoid hyperplasia can be seen in immunocompromised individuals, such as patients treated with steroids or other immunosuppressive therapies for conditions such as immune thrombocytopenic purpura or autoimmune hemolytic anemia.[26,27] Some peripheral T-cell lymphomas may produce a similar pattern of white pulp expansion. Nodular T-cell hyperplasia, simulating a peripheral T-cell lymphoma, can rarely be observed in patients with hypersensitivity reactions to phenytoin.[28] Abnormalities of the white pulp that may be worrisome for lymphoma can also be seen in patients with congenital conditions characterized by immunodeficiency or by abnormalities causing deregulated lymphoid production (e.g., autoimmune lymphoproliferative syndrome).

CASTLEMAN'S DISEASE

Occasional cases of Castleman's disease of both the unicentric hyaline-vascular type and the multicentric type associated with human herpesvirus 8 (HHV8) or Kaposi's sarcoma–associated herpesvirus (KSHV) reportedly occur in the spleen.[29-31] Multicentric Castleman's disease represents the majority of cases reported. Splenic involvement is rare in the unicentric form, and most such reports are from the older literature, before cases were evaluated for HHV8/KSHV; thus, the nature of these proliferations is not clearly established.[31-33] More recently, cases of human immunodeficiency virus (HIV)–related multicentric Castleman's disease involving the spleen have been described. The white pulp is expanded, with hypervascular germinal centers; the red pulp shows marked plasmacytosis. As seen in lymph nodes, immunoblastic cells expressing IgMλ are distributed in the perifollicular areas of the white pulp.[34,35] Multicentric Castleman's disease is generally negative for Epstein-Barr virus (EBV), but rare cases resembling germinotropic lymphoma have been described. These tumors are coinfected with EBV and HHV8/KSHV.[36]

AUTOIMMUNE LYMPHOPROLIFERATIVE SYNDROME

Autoimmune lymphoproliferative syndrome is a rare disorder that can mimic lymphoma in the spleen. It is a hereditary disorder, usually due to mutations of the CD95 (Fas) gene,[37,38] that presents in early childhood (younger than 2 years of age). Autoimmune lymphoproliferative syndrome is characterized by lymphoid hyperplasia, autoimmunity, and splenomegaly; the spleen frequently enlarges to more than 10 times its age-normal size. Histologically, the white pulp shows variable degrees of follicular hyperplasia, often with enlarged marginal zones. The periarteriolar lymphoid sheaths and red pulp are also expanded, owing to a markedly increased number of T cells (Fig. 61-3). These cells consist of a mixture of small lymphocytes and immunoblasts. As in lymph nodes in this disorder, many of these T cells are negative for both CD4 and CD8. The pathologic picture of the spleen is complicated by the frequent association with immune cytopenias affecting red cells, granulocytes, and platelets, contributing to splenomegaly.[39,40] Patients with this disorder have an increased risk of developing both Hodgkin's and non-Hodgkin's lymphomas.[41]

HODGKIN'S LYMPHOMA

Although the spleen is the most common extranodal organ involved by Hodgkin's lymphoma,[42,43] primary Hodgkin's lymphoma of the spleen is extremely rare.[44-48] The documentation of splenic involvement has therapeutic and prognostic implications, although these implications now appear to be less critical in light of the high rates of remission and cure obtained with current regimens of combination chemotherapy.[49,50] Involvement of the liver and bone marrow is rarely found in the absence of splenic involvement.[42] All histologic subtypes of Hodgkin's lymphoma can involve the spleen; nodular sclerosis and mixed cellularity are the most common,[42] and involvement by nodular lymphocyte-predominant Hodgkin's lymphoma is less common.[51] Lymphocyte-depleted Hodgkin's lymphoma characteristically presents with subdiaphragmatic disease and splenic involvement.[52]

Hodgkin's lymphoma produces either small miliary nodules or, more frequently, solitary or multiple tumor masses in the spleen (Fig. 61-4).[5,53] Splenic involvement is generally detectable grossly but may be subtle (Fig. 61-5). Foci of involvement may be only a few millimeters in size.[54,55] For this reason, the gross examination of the spleen must be meticulous in patients with Hodgkin's lymphoma so that small foci of involvement are not missed. The early lesions of Hodgkin's lymphoma in the spleen are found microscopically in the periarteriolar lymphoid sheaths or in the marginal zones.[5] As the disease progresses, the nodules expand to efface the lymphoid follicles and may involve the red pulp.

Sarcoid granulomas may be found in the spleens of patients with Hodgkin's lymphoma, in addition to various other disorders associated with abnormal T-cell function.[56,57] The granulomas are not related to prior lymphangiography, and their origin is unknown.[53] Several studies have suggested that granulomas occur more frequently in spleens uninvolved by Hodgkin's lymphoma than in those involved by the disease.[58,59] Grossly, the granulomas may be so large as to mimic involvement by Hodgkin's lymphoma. Microscopically, the granulomas are composed of clusters of epithelioid histiocytes that

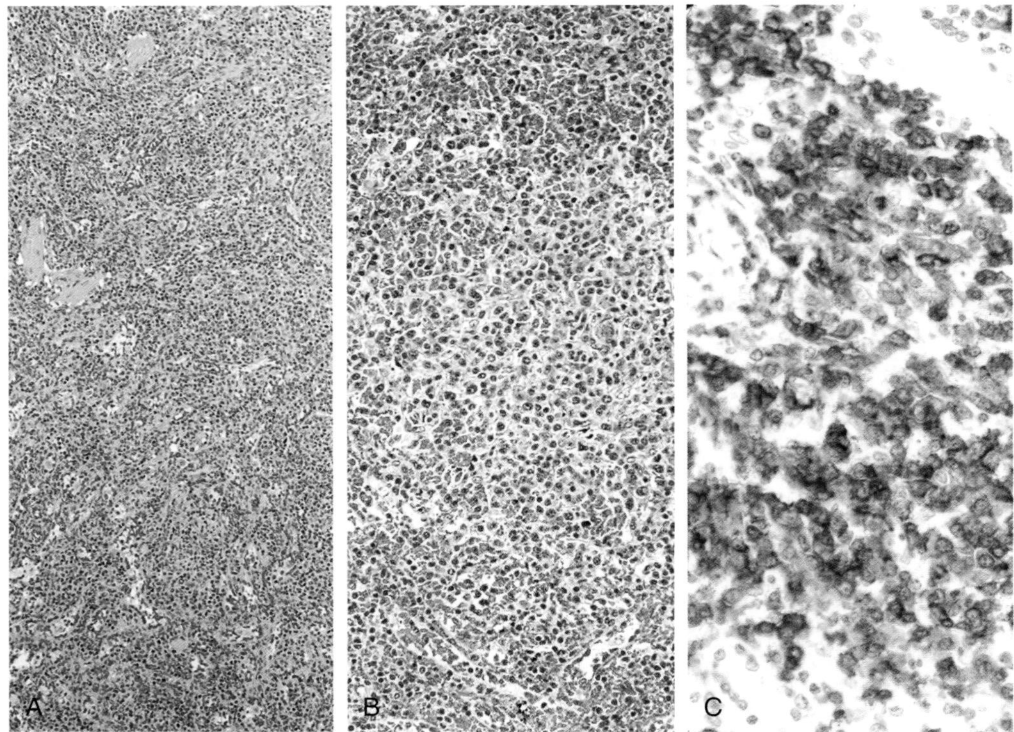

Figure 61-3. Splenic involvement in autoimmune lymphoproliferative syndrome. A, Low power shows atypical lymphoid hyperplasia that could easily be confused with lymphoma. Note the absence of reactive germinal centers due to prolonged steroid treatment. **B,** Higher magnification shows hyperplastic periarteriolar lymphoid sheaths and surrounding red pulp containing an increased number of atypical-appearing lymphocytes. **C,** CD3 stain demonstrates the T-cell nature of the proliferating lymphocytes.

occur in the white pulp in close association with the arterial circulation. It has been suggested that patients with splenic sarcoid granulomas have a better prognosis.[60]

The criteria for the diagnosis of Hodgkin's lymphoma in the spleen are the same as those for other nonnodal sites. In a patient with a previous nodal diagnosis, classical Hodgkin's lymphoma in the spleen can be documented if abnormally nucleolated large cells (mononuclear variant of Reed-Sternberg cells) are seen in a typical, mixed inflammatory background. A classic Reed-Sternberg cell is not necessary for the diagnosis in this setting. Immunohistochemical studies can be helpful in confirming the diagnosis of Hodgkin's lymphoma by showing that cytologically atypical cells have a phenotype appropriate for a given Hodgkin's lymphoma subtype.

The subclassification of Hodgkin's lymphoma in the spleen is sometimes difficult and is unnecessary in cases with a previous nodal diagnosis.[50] However, the unique morphologic and immunophenotypic characteristics of nodular lymphocyte-predominant Hodgkin's lymphoma allow its distinction from the classical Hodgkin's lymphoma subtypes (see Chapter 26).

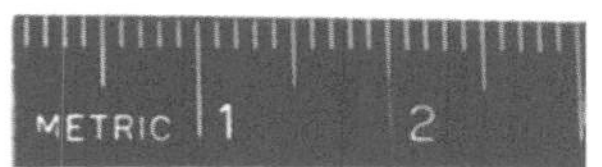

Figure 61-4. Gross photograph of Hodgkin's lymphoma involving the spleen. Hodgkin's lymphoma can present with a single mass or multiple discrete nodules. Thin sections after fixation are particularly valuable in detecting subtle involvement.

NON-HODGKIN'S LYMPHOMAS

Non-Hodgkin's lymphomas may involve the spleen in three clinical settings. In the first and rarest setting, termed *true primary splenic lymphoma*, the tumor is confined to the spleen or splenic hilar lymph nodes, without evidence of involvement of other sites. In the second and most common setting, the organ is involved as part of generalized, systemic lymphomatous spread. In the third setting, the lymphomatous process is characterized by prominent or predominant splenomegaly and often distinctive clinicopathologic features.

Primary Splenic Lymphoma

Primary splenic lymphoma is rare, accounting for less than 1% of all lymphomas. Excluding lymphomas thought to arise in the spleen, such as splenic marginal zone lymphoma, most of these cases were described in the older literature and are

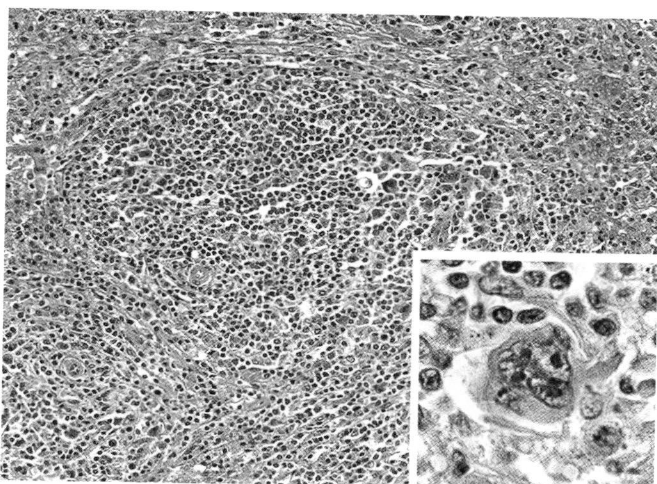

Figure 61-5. Early involvement of the spleen by Hodgkin's lymphoma. Reed-Sternberg cells are seen within a polymorphic cellular background in perifollicular areas. *Inset,* Higher magnification shows classic Reed-Sternberg cells.

not well defined.[61-71] Two cases occurred in HIV$^+$ patients,[62,63] and rare cases have been associated with hepatitis C infection.[70] Warnke and coworkers[61] were able to identify 47 cases of primary splenic lymphomas fulfilling the most stringent diagnostic criteria (i.e., tumor confined to the spleen and splenic hilar lymph nodes).[61] The patients were all adults; a slight male preponderance was noted. The most common presenting symptoms included left-sided abdominal pain and systemic symptoms such as fever, malaise, and weight loss. The gross findings and the histologic characteristics were similar to those observed in spleens secondarily involved by malignant lymphoma. Nearly all cases were of B-cell lineage. The most common subtype (30 of 47 cases) was diffuse large B-cell lymphoma (DLBCL), with the remainder being mostly low-grade B-cell malignancies. Kroft and associates[69] reported a CD5$^+$ form of DLBCL of the spleen, and a series of eight cases of DLBCL were reported by Grosskreutz and colleagues.[68] Of the 17 splenic lymphomas reported by Falk and Stutte[71] (which included cases with minimal extrasplenic involvement), three cases showed T-cell lineage. A recent report identified 32 patients presenting with follicular lymphoma first diagnosed in the spleen. There were two variants: one with the t(14;18), high BCL2, and CD10 expression, similar to nodal follicular lymphoma; and a second subset that lacked t(14;18) and was of a higher histologic grade.[72] The majority of patients relapsed with systemic disease.

Secondary Splenic Involvement by Lymphoma

Clinical assessment of the likelihood of splenic involvement by malignant lymphomas may be difficult. The weights of involved spleens vary widely.[73] Although tumor involvement usually results in palpable splenomegaly, Goffinet and coworkers[74] found that approximately one third of nonpalpable spleens were involved by lymphoma at staging laparotomy. Staging laparotomy has been replaced by imaging studies; positron emission tomography, in particular, provides an accurate determination.[75]

Non-Hodgkin's lymphomas of different types involve the spleen with variable frequency. Splenic involvement is particularly frequent in low-grade B-cell lymphomas. As mentioned earlier, evaluation of splenic hilar lymph nodes is very important. Histologic findings of lymphoma that are ambiguous or incompletely diagnostic in splenic sections may be more distinctive in splenic hilar lymph nodes. Liver involvement by lymphoma is rare in the absence of splenic disease.

PRECURSOR LYMPHOID NEOPLASMS

Although enlargement of the spleen often occurs during the course of either B- or T- lymphoblastic malignancies, it rarely approaches clinical significance. The histopathologic features are similar to those of other leukemic disorders, with diffuse infiltration of the red pulp by blastic-appearing cells.[5]

MATURE B-CELL LYMPHOMAS AND LEUKEMIAS

Most B-cell lymphomas involve the spleen in one of two main patterns: with uniform nodular expansion of the white pulp, as seen in small B-cell lymphomas such as chronic lymphocytic leukemia/small lymphocytic lymphoma (CLL/SLL), splenic marginal zone lymphoma, mantle cell lymphoma, and follicular lymphoma (Fig. 61-6); or with the formation of single or multiple tumor masses, as seen in most cases of DLBCL (Fig. 61-7; Table 61-3).[5,24] Occasionally, the spleen is the site of large cell transformation of a low-grade B-cell lymphoma (Fig. 61-8).

Chronic Lymphocytic Leukemia/Small Lymphocytic Lymphoma

Splenic involvement is common in CLL/SLL[76] (Fig. 61-9) and may be a presenting feature.[77] CLL/SLL often produces grossly visible nodules in a miliary pattern or, in more advanced stages of the disease, has a more homogeneous diffuse appearance, reflecting infiltration of both the red and white pulp.[5]

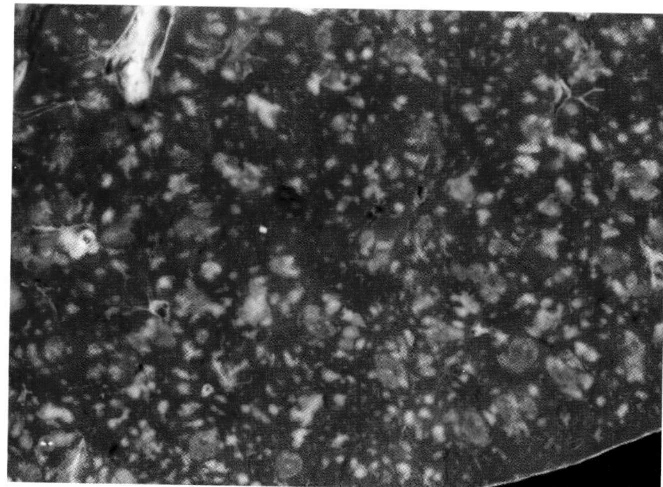

Figure 61-6. Gross photograph of miliary involvement of the spleen by low-grade B-cell lymphoma. This is an exaggeration of the normal white pulp appearance and is seen in lymphomas that preferentially involve the white pulp.

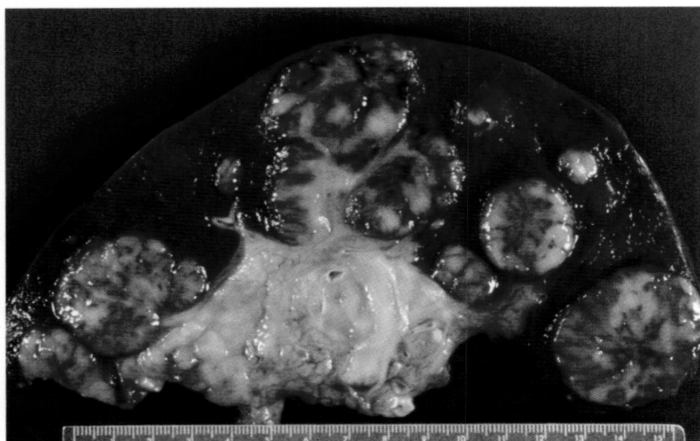

Figure 61-7. Gross photograph of diffuse large B-cell lymphoma involving the spleen. Large single or multiple tumor masses are not typically seen in low-grade lymphomas; they are more common in more aggressive lymphomas.

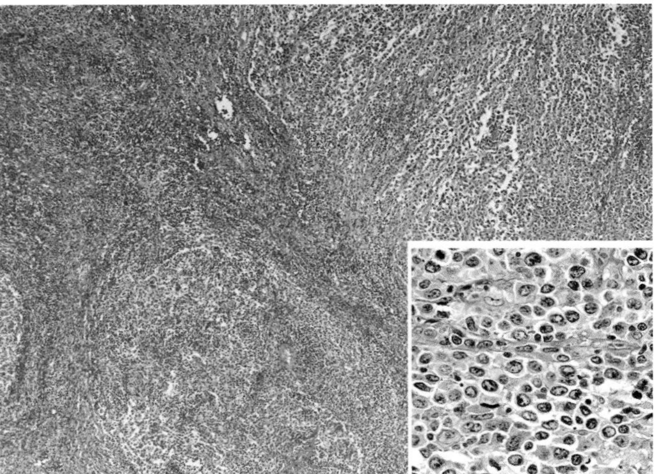

Figure 61-8. Low-power photomicrograph of follicular lymphoma (*lower left*) transforming to diffuse large B-cell lymphoma (*upper right*). *Inset,* Higher magnification of the large cell lymphoid component shows cytologic features consistent with a centroblastic subtype.

Infiltration of large vessels or trabeculae may be prominent (see Fig. 61-9). Prolymphocytes and paraimmunoblasts are identified, both intermingled with the small lymphoid cells and in proliferation centers. The spleen may be the site of large cell transformation (Richter's syndrome) in some cases. Early splenic involvement by CLL/SLL may be difficult to detect because the white pulp nodules resemble those of the immunologically unstimulated spleen.[5] The presence of scattered prolymphocytes and paraimmunoblasts and focal infiltration of the red pulp are useful clues. In some cases, however, the diagnosis rests on an examination of splenic hilar lymph nodes and flow cytometric or immunohistochemical confirmation.

B-Cell Prolymphocytic Leukemia

Prominent splenomegaly is one of the hallmarks of B-cell prolymphocytic leukemia, with the associated features of hypersplenism, peripheral cytopenias, and the absence of significant lymphadenopathy.[78-80] The white blood cell count is markedly elevated (often >100 × 10^9/L), with a predominance of prolymphocytes that have large vesicular nuclei and single prominent nucleoli. Both the red and white pulp are prominently involved (Fig. 61-10).[78]

Lymphoplasmacytic Lymphoma

Splenomegaly is a common feature of lymphoplasmacytic lymphoma and may be associated with hypersplenism. Patients with lymphoplasmacytic lymphoma often have immune-mediated cytopenias, and trapping of red cells and platelets may lead to further splenic enlargement. The most common pattern is a polymorphic infiltrate of lymphocytes, plasmacytoid lymphocytes, and plasma cells. Dutcher and Russell bodies may be prominent (Fig. 61-11). The infiltrate preferentially involves the red pulp, but expansion of the white pulp may be present. Because other lymphomas in the spleen, including CLL/SLL and marginal zone lymphoma,

Table 61-3 Features of B-Cell Lymphoproliferative Disorders in the Spleen

Disorder	White Pulp	Red Pulp	Critical Immunohistochemistry
CLL/SLL PLL	Homogeneous nodules of small, round lymphocytes; variable proportions of prolymphocytes	Frequent infiltration with intravascular involvement	CD5⁺,* cyclin D1⁻
MCL, classic type	Follicles with expanded mantle zones	Frequent infiltration	Cyclin D1⁺
MCL, blastoid/pleomorphic type	Blastoid cells in white pulp	Frequent infiltration with prominent intravascular involvement	Cyclin D1⁺
FL	Expansion of white pulp by neoplastic follicles	Rare, subtle	BCL2⁺ follicles
SMZL LPL	Homogeneous nodules with dimorphic cytology: small, round lymphocytes with occasional larger cells (more numerous at periphery)	Frequent infiltration, often with small nodules	IgD⁺
HCL HCL variant	Involvement very rare	Diffuse, with formation of pseudosinuses and blood lakes	TRAP⁺, DBA.44⁺ CD103⁺, Annexin A1⁺ (Annexin is negative in HCL variant)
Splenic diffuse red pulp small B-cell lymphoma		Diffuse, with infiltration of cords and sinuses	CD20⁺, DBA44⁺, Annexin A1⁻, CD25⁻, CD103⁻

*CD5 is less frequently positive in PLL than in CLL/SLL.
CLL/SLL, chronic lymphocytic leukemia/small lymphocytic lymhoma; FL, follicular lymphoma; HCL, hairy cell leukemia; Ig, immunoglobulin; LPL, lymphoplasmacytic leukemia/lymphoma; MCL, mantle cell lymphoma; PLL, prolymphocytic leukemia; SMZL, splenic marginal zone lymphoma; TRAP, tartrate-resistant acid phosphatase.

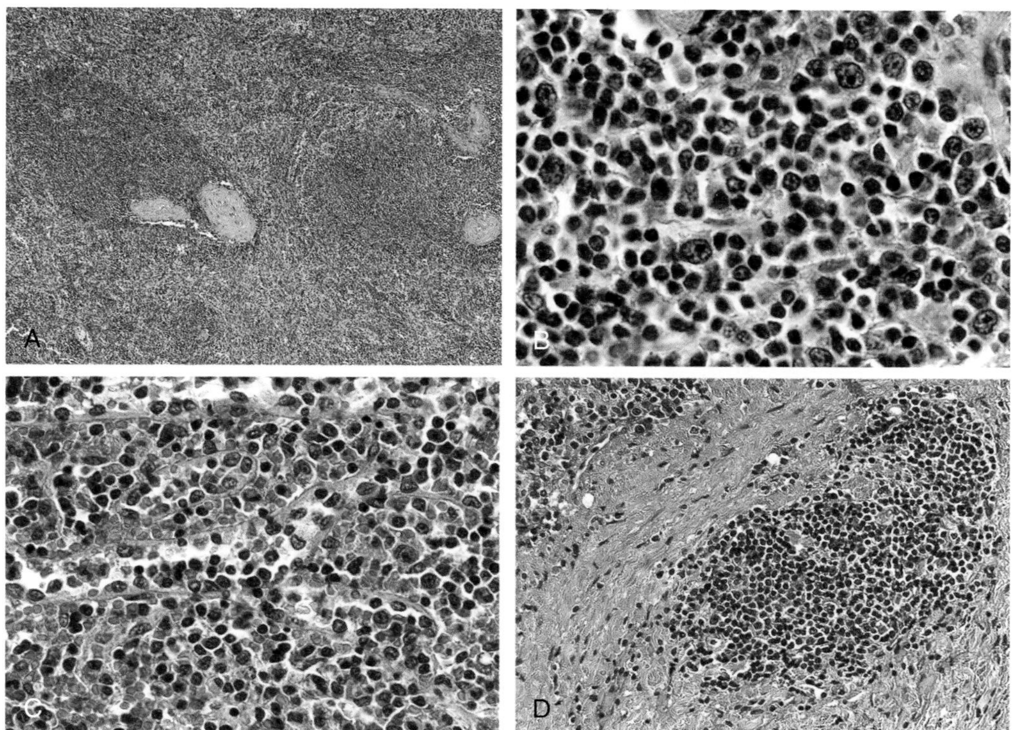

Figure 61-9. **A,** Low-power photomicrograph of chronic lymphocytic leukemia/small lymphocytic lymphoma (CLL/SLL) in the spleen. Note the homogeneous expansion of the white pulp. **B,** Higher power shows the cytomorphology of CLL/SLL; note the presence of scattered prolymphocytes and paraimmunoblasts. **C,** Photomicrograph highlights the pronounced lymphoid infiltration of the red pulp (both intravascular and cordal infiltration). **D,** Trabecular infiltration by CLL/SLL.

may show plasmacytoid differentiation, a primary diagnosis of lymphoplasmacytic lymphoma/Waldenström's macroglobulinemia should be made with caution.

Mantle Cell Lymphoma

Mantle cell lymphoma (MCL) frequently involves the spleen.[77,81,82] Although MCL may present initially with clinically isolated splenomegaly, workup of these patients reveals that most are actually stage IV at the time of diagnosis, with bone marrow or liver involvement or both.[77] The morphology of the disorder in the spleen is similar to that in involved lymph nodes. The white pulp is uniformly expanded, with neoplastic cells proliferating in widened mantle zones around benign, atrophic-appearing germinal centers. This pattern may superficially mimic reactive secondary splenic follicles. The latter are tripartite, however, with central follicles and

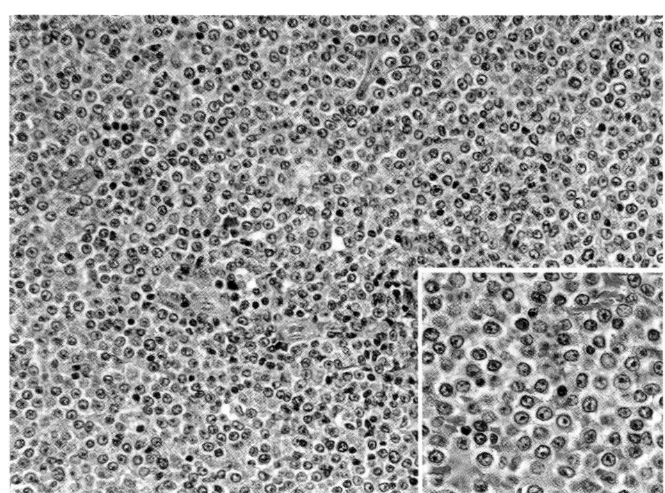

Figure 61-10. Intermediate-power appearance of B-cell prolymphocytic leukemia in the spleen. *Inset,* High power shows the prominent central nucleoli of prolymphocytes.

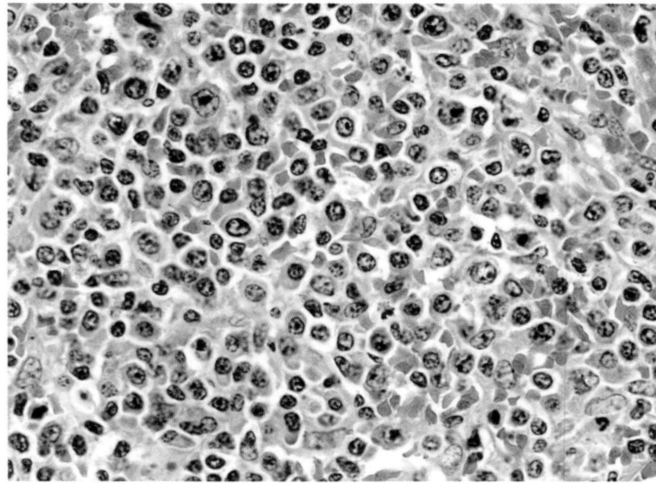

Figure 61-11. Lymphoplasmacytic lymphoma involving the spleen in a patient with Waldenström's macroglobulinemia. Note the obvious plasma cell differentiation and the presence of occasional plasmacytoid immunoblasts.

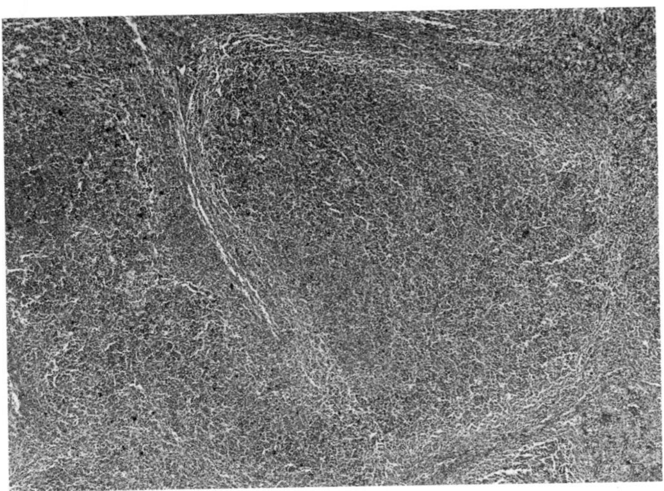

Figure 61-12. Small cell (nonblastoid) mantle cell lymphoma involving the spleen. Note the homogeneous expansion of the white pulp (similar to Fig. 61-9**A**) and the spillover of lymphocytes into the red pulp. Red pulp involvement is common in mantle cell lymphoma, although it can be subtle.

mantle and marginal zones. The spillage of lymphoma cells into the red pulp aids in the diagnosis of malignancy. Eventually, the neoplastic cells invade and replace the germinal centers (Figs. 61-12 and 61-13). Rarely, a marginal zone–like differentiation can be observed. Such cases must be distinguished from splenic marginal zone lymphoma. The immunophenotype is comparable to that of MCL in other sites, with cyclin D1 being a key diagnostic immunostain.

The blastoid and pleomorphic variants of MCL involve different diagnostic considerations. The blastoid variant may have more extensive red pulp involvement than typical MCL, and the cells may resemble lymphoblasts in tissue sections; immunohistochemical documentation of cyclin D1 positivity and lack of terminal deoxynucleotidyl transferase (TdT) expression is particularly useful in such cases. The pleomorphic variant of MCL may mimic DLBCL.

In a subset of cases presenting with leukemic involvement, there may be prominent splenomegaly without any peripheral lymphadenopathy.[83] Most of these cases exhibit blastoid morphology and aggressive clinical behavior. There has been controversy regarding the distinction of leukemic blastoid MCL from B-cell prolymphocytic leukemia associated with 14q32 rearrangements. The current view is that such cases should be regarded as leukemic MCL rather than B-cell prolymphocytic leukemia.

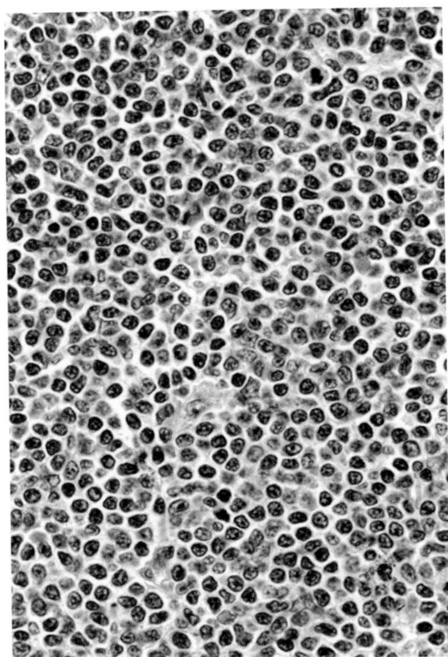

Figure 61-13. Cytology of mantle cell lymphoma at high power. Lymphoid cells are small and slightly irregular, with condensed chromatin.

Follicular Lymphoma

Secondary splenic involvement is common in follicular lymphoma, a disease that, like CLL/SLL and MCL, is often disseminated at initial presentation (Fig. 61-14). Rarely, cases of follicular lymphoma may present as isolated splenomegaly.[72] Grossly, the spleen shows a miliary pattern of involvement due to the expansion of abnormal white pulp follicles; occasionally, the neoplastic nodules coalesce to form larger tumor masses.[5,24] In follicular lymphoma grades 1 and 2, high-power examination typically reveals a monotonous population of centrocytes with coarse chromatin and inconspicuous nucleoli. In some cases admixed centroblasts may superficially resemble reactive germinal centers. The neoplastic follicles seen in follicular lymphoma usually lack tingible body macrophages, and the margin between the follicle center and mantle or marginal zone is indistinct. In addition, the red pulp does not display the plasmacytosis usually seen in reactive lymphoid hyperplasia and may contain satellite nodules composed of lymphoma cells. Immunohistochemistry or flow cytometry can aid in identifying monoclonality or aberrant expression of CD10. As with other lymphomas, the spleen may represent the initial site of high-grade transformation of follicular lymphoma to DLBCL (see Fig. 61-8).

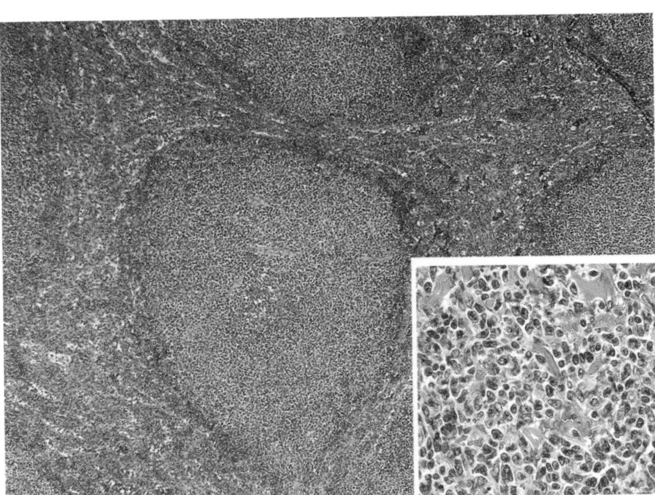

Figure 61-14. Low-power photomicrograph of follicular lymphoma involving the spleen. *Inset,* Higher power shows the characteristic mixture of small cleaved cells and larger noncleaved cells.

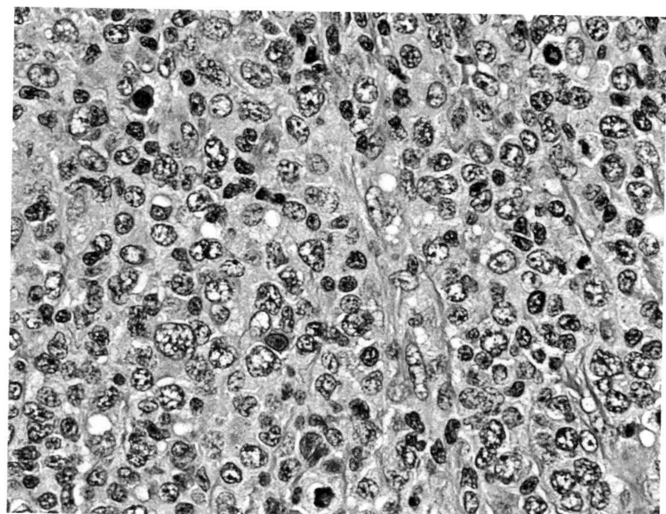

Figure 61-15. Diffuse large B-cell lymphoma involving the spleen.

Nodal and Extranodal Marginal Zone Lymphoma

Splenic involvement by nodal marginal zone lymphoma (MZL) has been reported in the older literature.[84-88] However, most of these reports predated the description of other B-cell lymphomas that more commonly involve the spleen, such as splenic MZL, splenic lymphoma with villous lymphocytes, and the newly recognized splenic diffuse red pulp small B-cell lymphoma (see later and Chapter 16). Thus, these cases are not well documented. Extranodal MZL usually does not involve the spleen unless the disease is widely disseminated.

Diffuse Large B-Cell Lymphoma

DLBCL in the spleen characteristically produces solitary or multiple tumor masses that are usually well demarcated and may show areas of necrosis (Fig. 61-15). Prominent splenomegaly may be a presenting feature.[5,61,74,77] Predominant red pulp involvement may be observed in some cases.[65,89-92] T-cell/histiocyte-rich large B-cell lymphoma, a variant of DLBCL, is associated with a micronodular pattern of infiltration that may be difficult to diagnose and often mimics a reactive process. The spleen in these cases is markedly enlarged, but without distinct nodules. Small aggregates of lymphocytes and histiocytes are distributed in the red and white pulp. The histiocytes are especially abundant, and neoplastic large B cells may be difficult to identify without the use of immunohistochemical studies.[90] In cases of DLBCL limited to the red pulp, the possibility of transformation from splenic diffuse red pulp small B-cell lymphoma or from red pulp–predominant splenic MZL (see later) should also be considered.

Burkitt's Lymphoma

Involvement of the spleen, lymph nodes, or liver is uncommon in Burkitt's lymphoma. Grogan and associates[93] reported splenic involvement in two patients, one of whom was leukemic; Banks and colleagues[94] found splenic involvement in 10 of 17 cases of sporadic Burkitt's lymphoma. Both the red and white pulp are involved in most cases, although more selective involvement of the white pulp, in either the malpighian corpuscles or the marginal zones, is occasionally seen.[95] Immunohistochemistry for TdT and CD99 can be used to separate Burkitt's lymphoma from lymphoblastic malignancies.[96-98] Demonstration of *MYC* rearrangement as well as additional genetic analysis (e.g., for *BCL2* and *BCL6* gene rearrangements) may be essential for the correct diagnosis.

B-CELL LYMPHOID NEOPLASMS PRESENTING WITH PROMINENT SPLENOMEGALY

Several types of B-cell lymphoma/leukemia, such as splenic marginal zone lymphoma (SMZL), present with splenomegaly. The histopathology is briefly discussed here; see Chapter 16 for a complete discussion of SMZL and related conditions.

Splenic Marginal Zone Lymphoma

The cut surface of the spleen in SMZL shows a characteristic miliary expansion of the white pulp.[99,100] Histologically, nodular involvement of the white pulp is centered on preexisting follicles (Fig. 61-16). The mantle zones are usually lost. Germinal centers are rarely identifiable, often being surrounded and occupied by small lymphocytes. This central zone merges at the periphery with a zone of medium-sized cells with more dispersed chromatin, less regular nuclei, and relatively abundant pale cytoplasm, resembling marginal zone cells.[101] Toward the periphery of the neoplastic nodules, a variable number of large, atypical lymphoid cells is usually seen (Fig. 61-17). When residual germinal centers are identified, the neoplastic cells are arranged in broad concentric bands around the germinal center (reactive or hyalinized), a pattern that may superficially resemble reactive marginal zone hyperplasia, particularly in cases with minimal or no splenomegaly.[16-19] However, in marginal zone hyperplasia, mantle

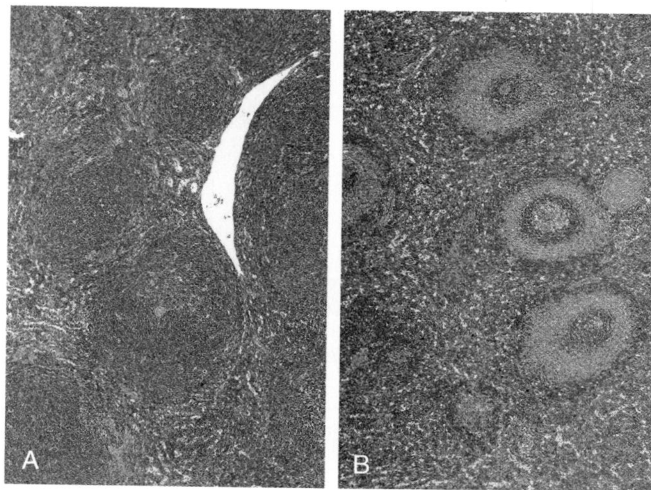

Figure 61-16. A, Low-power appearance of splenic marginal zone lymphoma. A proliferation of small lymphoid cells replaces the normal white pulp. **B,** An example of so-called indolent splenic marginal zone lymphoma, which retains the normal-appearing tripartite nature of the white pulp. Although difficult to distinguish from reactive marginal zone hyperplasia, this case was proved to be monoclonal.

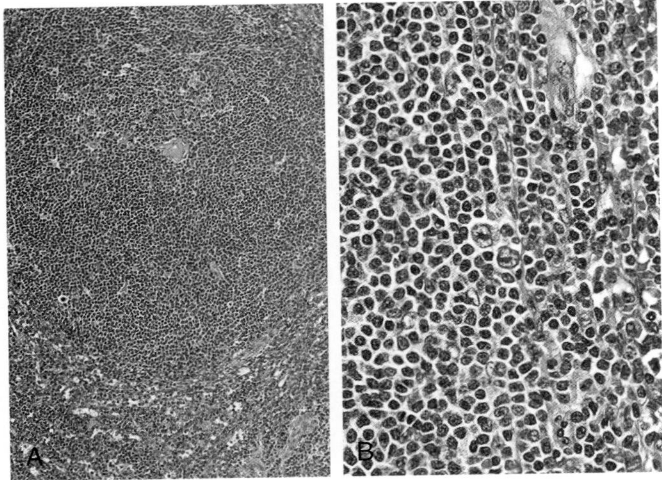

Figure 61-17. A, Intermediate magnification of splenic marginal zone lymphoma, with small lymphocytes constituting the majority of cells. Note the presence of larger pale marginal zone–like cells at the periphery of the neoplastic nodules, as wells as the subtle red pulp involvement. **B,** Higher magnification shows rare large transformed cells. Note the spillover of lymphocytes into the surrounding red pulp (*upper right*).

zones are preserved, and lymphoid infiltration of the germinal center is not observed. In addition, red pulp infiltration, which is a common feature of SMZL, is absent in reactive hyperplasia (Table 61-4). Transformation of SMZL to large B-cell lymphoma is seen in a proportion of cases; p53 overexpression may be detected in some of these cases.[102,103]

The differential diagnosis of SMZL includes other small B-cell lymphomas (Table 61-5). Both a micronodular pattern and marginal zone differentiation can be seen in follicular lymphoma, MCL, and, with less frequency, CLL/SLL. SMZL is distinguished by its characteristic dimorphic cytology, different from the monomorphic cytology of MCL, and by the distinctive mixture of centroblasts and small cleaved cells seen in follicular lymphoma. CLL/SLL may be identified on the basis of its monotonous small lymphocytic cytology in conjunction with the presence of scattered prolymphocytes and paraimmunoblasts. Lymphoplasmacytic lymphoma shows predominant red pulp involvement with prominent plasmacytic differentiation.

Hairy Cell Leukemia

Most patients with hairy cell leukemia (HCL) present with prominent splenomegaly associated with pancytopenia, lack of lymphadenopathy, and characteristic hairy cells in the peripheral blood.[104,105] The gross appearance of the spleen is homogeneous and dark red, with variably sized hemorrhagic areas (blood lakes). The white pulp is inconspicuous. The hairy cells appear in splenic touch smears as medium-sized atypical lymphoid cells with homogeneous chromatin, inconspicuous nucleoli, moderate amounts of clear to pink cytoplasm, and typical surface projections. A pericellular clear halo is often seen in histology sections. Tumor cells infiltrate both the splenic cords and the red pulp sinuses (Fig. 61-18), and subendothelial invasion of the trabecular veins may be prominent.[104] Blood lakes lacking an endothelial lining and lined by hairy cells are often seen (see Fig. 61-18).[106] The infiltrate in HCL may resemble T-cell large granular lymphocytic leukemia (T-LGLL) or T-cell lymphomas (hepatosplenic T-cell lymphoma in particular). Mastocytosis in the spleen occasionally resembles HCL; however, the characteristic trabecular distribution and associated fibrosis of mastocytosis are not seen in HCL. In HCL, characteristic tartrate-resistant acid phosphatase (TRAP) positivity can be demonstrated on touch imprints of the spleen and in tissue sections by immunohistochemistry (see Fig. 61-18). Other useful markers include annexin A1 (the most specific), DBA.44, CD25, and CD123. In addition, hairy cells characteristically express CD103 and CD11c by flow cytometry.

Splenic Lymphoma/Leukemia, Unclassifiable

The World Health Organization (WHO) classification provides for other small B-cell neoplasms that present in the spleen but do not correspond to any of the more well-defined entities already discussed. The two best defined of these relatively rare provisional entities are splenic diffuse red pulp small B-cell lymphoma and hairy cell leukemia variant (see Chapter 16). Other splenic small B-cell lymphomas not fulfilling the criteria for either of these provisional entities or for other better established B-cell lymphomas should be diagnosed as splenic B-cell lymphoma/leukemia, unclassifiable.

Table 61-4 Bone Marrow and Peripheral Blood Findings in Lymphomas with Prominent Splenic Involvement

Lymphoma	Blood	Bone Marrow
SMZL*	Atypical lymphoid cells with condensed chromatin and moderate amounts of cytoplasm; cytoplasmic projections, if present, are often polar and coarser than those in HCL	Nodular, interstitial aggregates of atypical lymphoid cells with abundant pale cytoplasm; residual follicles variably colonized or surrounded by atypical lymphoid cells; intrasinusoidal spread can be seen
HCL	Round nuclei with partially condensed chromatin and abundant cytoplasm; numerous hairy projections; monocytopenia common	Interstitial, diffuse infiltrates of small lymphocytes with abundant cytoplasm ("fried egg" appearance); spindle cell morphology can also be seen; typically associated with reticulin fibrosis
HSTCL	Occasional leukemic cases may show small to medium-sized lymphocytes, or blastoid-appearing forms	Hypercellular marrow with often subtle intrasinusoidal infiltrate of T cells

*Cytologic findings in the peripheral blood and bone marrow histology are similar to those seen in splenic diffuse red pulp small B-cell lymphoma, a provisional entity in the World Health Organization's 2008 classification that may correspond to cases previously diagnosed as the diffuse variant of SMZL. Splenic diffuse red pulp small B-cell lymphoma also overlaps with HCL variant.

HCL, hairy cell leukemia; HSTCL, hepatosplenic T-cell lymphoma; SMZL, splenic marginal zone lymphoma.

Table 61-5 Differential Diagnosis of Splenic Marginal Zone Lymphoma and Small B-Cell Lymphomas in the Spleen

Lymphoma	Pattern of Splenic Involvement	Cytology	Useful Immunophenotypic Markers	Cytogenetics
SMZL	Expansion of marginal zones, often with sparing of follicles; frequent red pulp and intrasinusoidal involvement (also in BM)	Small lymphocytes; occasional monocytoid morphology; biphasic cytology with rare large cells; mitoses rare; may have circulating villous lymphocytes	IgM/IgD$^+$, CD5$^-$, CD23$^-$, CD10$^-$, BCL6$^-$, CD43$^-$, cyclin D1$^-$, annexin A1$^-$	del(7q), +3, others Absent: t(11;18), t(14;18), t(11;14) Overrepresentation of VH1-2
CLL/SLL	Diffuse replacement of white pulp with neoplastic cells; proliferation centers occasionally seen; frequent red pulp and intravascular involvement	Small round lymphocytes with condensed chromatin; prolymphocytes present; mitoses rare	CD5$^+$, CD23$^+$, CD43$^+$, CD10$^-$	del(13q14), +12, del(11q), del(17p)
FL	Neoplastic follicles replacing normal white pulp	Mixture of small, irregular cleaved lymphocytes and larger centroblasts; mitoses dependent on grade	CD10$^+$, CD5$^-$, CD23$^-$, CD43$^-$	t(14;18)
MCL, conventional type	Diffuse replacement of white pulp with neoplastic cells, occasionally surrounding atrophic germinal centers; frequent red pulp and intravascular involvement	Small irregular lymphocytes with dense chromatin; mitoses common	Cyclin D1$^+$, CD5$^+$, CD43$^+$, CD23$^-$, CD10$^-$	t(11;14)
LPL	Expansion of marginal zone and other white pulp areas; frequent red pulp involvement	Mixture of small round lymphocytes, plasma cells, and plasmacytoid lymphocytes; mitoses rare; Dutcher bodies seen occasionally	IgM$^+$, IgG$^{+/-}$, CD25$^{+/-}$, CD38$^{+/-}$, CD43$^{+/-}$, CD5$^{-/+}$, CD23$^-$, CD10$^-$, IgD$^-$	del(6q), +4
Splenic diffuse red pulp small B-cell lymphoma*	Diffuse infiltration of red pulp sinuses and cords; atrophic or absent follicles; intrasinusoidal BM involvement	Small B cells with round nuclei, condensed chromatin, occasional distinct small nucleoli; mitoses rare; circulating villous lymphocytes	DBA.44$^+$, IgG$^+$, IgD$^-$, annexin A1$^-$, CD25$^-$, CD103$^-$, CD123$^-$, CD11c$^-$, CD10$^-$, CD23$^-$, CD5$^-$	t(9;14) Alterations of *TP53* Overrepresentation of VH3-23 and VH4-34, as in HCL

*This is a provisional entity in the World Health Organization's 2008 classification that may correspond to what was previously referred to as the diffuse variant of SMZL; it also overlaps with HCL variant.

BM, bone marrow; CLL/SLL, chronic lymphocytic leukemia/small lymphocytic lymphoma; FL, follicular lymphoma; HCL, hairy cell leukemia; Ig, immunoglobulin; LPL, lymphoplasmacytic leukemia/lymphoma; MCL, mantle cell lymphoma; SMZL, splenic marginal zone lymphoma.

Splenic Diffuse Red Pulp Small B-Cell Lymphoma

Splenic diffuse red pulp small B-cell lymphoma is an uncommon lymphoma with a diffuse pattern of involvement of the splenic red pulp by small monomorphic B lymphocytes.[107] The neoplasm also involves bone marrow sinusoids and peripheral blood, commonly with a villous cytology. Some of these cases may represent what has been termed in the bone marrow and peripheral blood *splenic lymphoma with villous lymphocytes*.[108,109]

Hairy Cell Leukemia Variant

HCL variant is a splenomegalic malignancy characterized by a high leukemic count without associated cytopenias.[110-112] The bone marrow is usually aspiratable. The tumor cells of HCL variant have a higher nuclear-to-cytoplasmic ratio than typical hairy cells, more condensed chromatin, and a prominent nucleolus, and they often lack TRAP, CD25, and CD103. The prognosis is generally worse than for typical HCL.[112] The cells resemble prolymphocytes, and this process may be related to B-cell prolymphocytic leukemia.

PLASMA CELL NEOPLASMS

Plasma cell neoplasms are a heterogeneous group of neoplastic conditions associated with monoclonal immunoglobulin production. These conditions can affect both the red and white pulp of the spleen. A common finding is evidence of immunoglobulin production, manifested by the presence of plasma cells or plasmacytoid lymphocytes with periodic acid–Schiff (PAS)–positive cytoplasmic globules (Mott cells) and intranuclear and cytoplasmic immunoglobulin inclusions (Dutcher and Russell bodies, respectively).

Plasma Cell Myeloma

Splenomegaly is rarely clinically significant in patients with plasma cell myeloma. However, the organ may be extensively involved, particularly in the presence of plasma cell leukemia.[113] Although rare, splenic rupture may be associated with myelomatous involvement of the spleen.[114] Splenomegaly in plasma cell myeloma can also result from amyloid deposition. In rare cases, light-chain deposition only (and not amyloid)

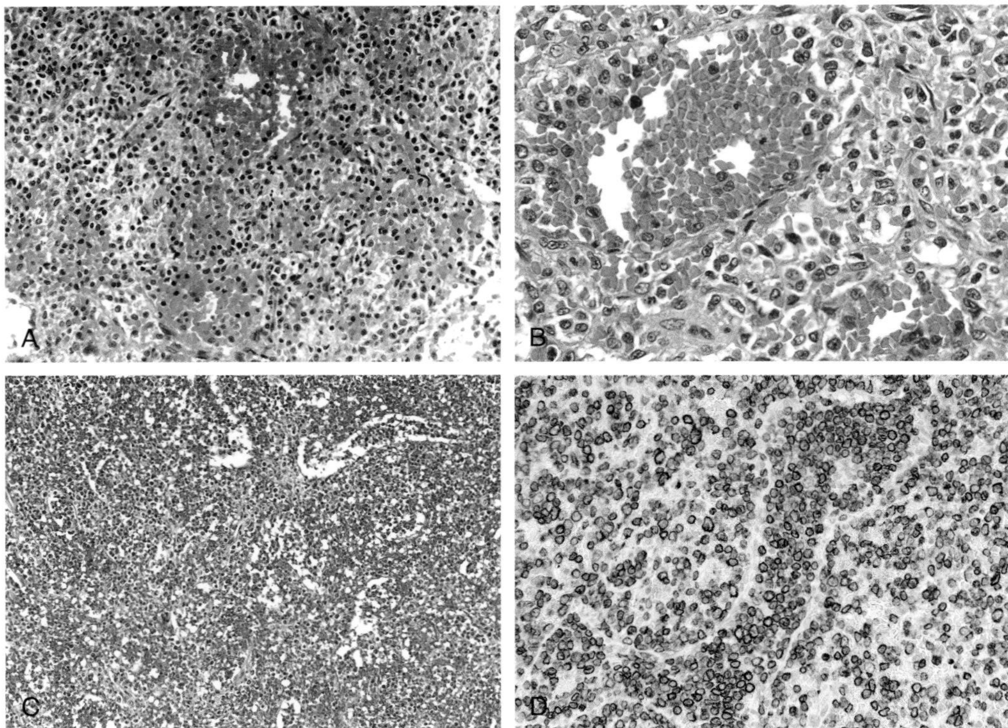

Figure 61-18. Hairy cell leukemia in the spleen. A, Note the obliteration of the white pulp. **B,** Red pulp infiltration by hairy cells with blood lakes. **C,** Hairy cell leukemia with marked intrasinusoidal spread. **D,** Strong positivity for tartrate-resistant acid phosphatase (TRAP) immunostaining in hairy cells.

has been described in myeloma patients. Rarely, excess light chain is taken up by histiocytes, causing so-called crystal-storing histiocytosis.[115] Masses of crystals produce engorged histiocytes, which morphologically may resemble Gaucher cells. These crystals are often only weakly positive with immunohistochemical stains for light chains, possibly owing to partial lysosomal degradation or masking of epitopes in the crystal structure. This can be accompanied by a foreign body type of granulomatous reaction. Although exceedingly rare, this phenomenon needs to be distinguished from coexistent multiple myeloma and Gaucher's disease, which has been reported several times in the literature.[116] The neoplastic plasma cells either infiltrate the red pulp diffusely or, rarely, produce grossly visible nodules.

Hepatosplenomegaly is a common feature of POEMS syndrome,[117] in which an osteosclerotic variant of myeloma occurs in association with polyneuropathy, organomegaly, endocrinopathy, the presence of a monoclonal paraprotein, and hyperpigmentation of the skin.[118]

The pattern of splenic involvement in plasma cell leukemia resembles that in other leukemic processes. Cytopenias resulting from hypersplenism[119,120] and splenic rupture have occasionally been reported in patients with plasma cell leukemia.[121,122]

Primary Amyloidosis

Although splenic involvement is possible in both primary and secondary amyloidosis, it is more common in the latter. Early in the disease, amyloid is deposited in the walls of small blood vessels. A nodular deposition of amyloid in the white pulp produces the miliary, or "sago," pattern, whereas the "lardaceous" spleen results from larger, more expansive sheets of amyloid in the sinuses of the red pulp. The white pulp in primary amyloidosis often contains numerous mature plasma cells and less numerous plasmacytoid lymphocytes. In a large percentage of these cases, monoclonal plasma cells with lambda light-chain restriction can be demonstrated. Functional hyposplenism may occur with extensive amyloid deposition.[122] Splenic rupture has also been reported in association with splenic amyloidosis.[123-125]

Heavy-Chain Diseases

Splenic involvement may be a feature of both gamma (Franklin's) and mu heavy-chain diseases; it has not been reported in alpha heavy-chain disease. Patients with these disorders usually have a serum paraprotein that consists of an intact but structurally abnormal heavy chain. Heavy-chain disease is not associated with amyloid deposition. Gamma heavy-chain disease most often has the histologic features of lymphoplasmacytic lymphoma.[126,127] The lymphoplasmacytoid infiltrates may also contain eosinophils and immunoblasts. Mu heavy-chain disease is a B-cell lymphoproliferative disorder resembling chronic lymphocytic leukemia.[128,129] The spleen is infiltrated by small lymphocytes and plasma cells that typically have vacuolated cytoplasm and Russell bodies.

MATURE T- AND NK-CELL NEOPLASMS

Mature T-cell and NK-cell malignancies are relatively uncommon, and few studies have focused on the splenic pathology. Among the nonleukemic forms, splenic involvement is relatively common in cases of advanced-stage mycosis fungoides/Sézary syndrome. Splenic involvement in mycosis fungoides usually affects the white and red pulp alike.[130] The marginal zones and the periarteriolar lymphoid sheaths are infiltrated by large atypical cells, associated with both diffuse and patchy nodular involvement of the red pulp.[130,131] Not all cells have cerebriform nuclear contours, and a variable proportion of the tumor cells may appear blastic.

The node-based peripheral T-cell lymphomas (PTCLs) are perhaps the least-studied group of T-cell neoplasms that occur in the spleen. The pattern of splenic involvement in these diseases is different from that in B-cell lymphomas and is centered more on the red pulp (Fig. 61-19).[23,132-134] We have seen a variety of patterns of involvement—some expanding the periarteriolar lymphoid sheath, some producing discrete masses, and one mimicking the pattern seen in mycosis fungoides. The lymphoepithelioid cell (Lennert's) variant,[135] a cytologic subtype of PTCL unspecified, is characterized by a high content of epithelioid histiocytes. Early involvement usually occurs in the peripheral zones of follicles and the periarteriolar lymphoid sheaths, consistent with the T-cell origin of this lymphoma. The epithelioid histiocytes tend to localize in a ring-like arrangement at the periphery of the white pulp, but they occasionally form clusters.[23] Although originally thought to be characteristic of this type of lymphoma, the ring-like arrangement of epithelioid cells may be seen in other forms of both B-cell and T-cell lymphoma. The epithelioid cells may be difficult to differentiate from the sarcoid type of granulomas sometimes seen in the spleens of patients with Hodgkin's lymphoma.[135] Some cases of PTCL with marked splenomegaly have been associated with hemophagocytic syndrome.[136,137] In these cases, expansion of the red pulp predominates, and the erythrophagocytic histiocytes may overshadow the neoplastic T cells. A hemophagocytic syndrome may be seen with both T-cell and NK-cell malignancies, many of which are associated with EBV (see later).

Angioimmunoblastic T-Cell Lymphoma

In addition to generalized lymphadenopathy, fever, weight loss, and a pruritic rash, hepatosplenomegaly is often a presenting feature in patients with angioimmunoblastic T-cell lymphoma.[138-144] Most descriptions of the morphology of the spleen have come from autopsy series. Splenectomy is occasionally performed in cases associated with severe hemolytic anemia.[143] A variety of patterns of involvement have been described. In some, a polymorphic infiltrate predominates in the marginal zones (see Fig. 61-19). Focal aggregates of large lymphoid cells are seen in the surrounding red pulp.[143] There may be an increased reticulin content in the marginal zone, which produces a characteristic perifollicular fibrosis. Other authors have described nonspecific reactive follicular hyperplasia.[143] Other cases show a more extensive pattern of involvement, with large nodules involving both the white and red pulp.[144] The arborizing vascular network typically seen in lymph nodes has not been reported in the spleen. The majority of reports in the older literature were based on autopsy series, and the findings may reflect end-stage disease or therapeutic effects; these include lymphoid depletion and diffuse fibrosis.

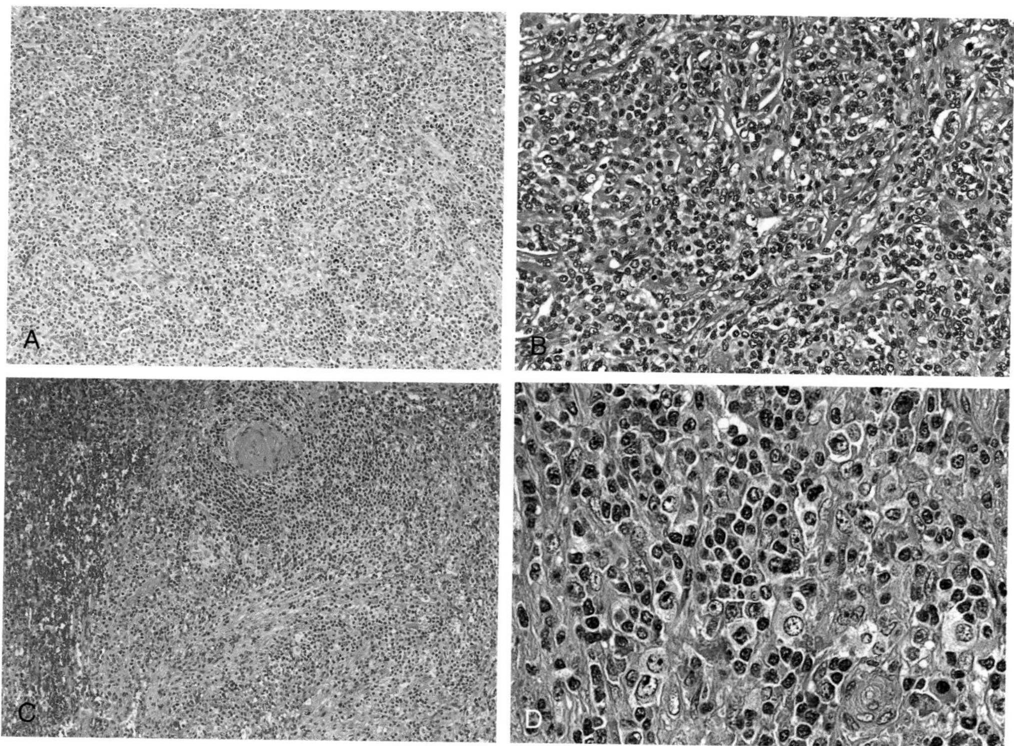

Figure 61-19. **A**, Peripheral T-cell lymphoma, unspecified, involving the spleen. Note the absence of follicles and the polymorphic cell proliferation within the red pulp. **B**, Higher magnification of the same case shows pleomorphic atypical lymphoid cells within red pulp areas. **C**, Peripheral T-cell lymphoma, angioimmunoblastic type, involving the spleen. Note the perifollicular distribution, with sclerosis and a relatively abundant vascular network. **D**, High magnification of the same case shows several large, pale, atypical lymphoid cells.

Anaplastic Large Cell Lymphoma

Anaplastic large cell lymphoma consists of anaplastic lymphoma kinase (ALK)–positive and –negative cases, which are distinguished in the WHO classification. Both types can have splenic involvement[145-147] and may present with a splenic mass. Rare cases may present with splenic rupture. In older reports the differentiation from aggressive variants of classical Hodgkin's lymphoma may be problematic.

T-CELL LYMPHOID NEOPLASMS PRESENTING WITH PROMINENT SPLENOMEGALY

Several types of lymphomas and leukemias present with splenomegaly and distinct clinicopathologic characteristics.

Hepatosplenic T-Cell Lymphoma

Hepatosplenic T-cell lymphoma is a distinct clinical entity within the spectrum of PTCLs. It is characterized by hepatosplenomegaly, sinusoidal tropism, and, in most cases, a T-cell receptor gamma-delta (TCRγδ) phenotype of malignant cells.[148-150] It typically occurs in young adults, more frequently males, and has a poor prognosis. The presenting symptoms include fever, weight loss, hepatosplenomegaly, and variable cytopenias. Some cases of hepatosplenic T-cell lymphoma are associated with a hemophagocytic syndrome, a condition that once was termed *erythrophagocytic T-gamma lymphoma*.[151] Macroscopically, the spleen is enlarged (usually weighing ≥3000 g), with a homogeneous cut surface and loss of white pulp markings. Histologically, the neoplastic cells infiltrate the red pulp cords and sinuses (Fig. 61-20). The lymphoid cells are usually medium sized and have oval or folded nuclei, with chromatin less condensed than that of small lymphocytes and a moderate amount of pale cytoplasm. Occasional cases have larger, more blastic-appearing cells. The histologic appearance of the spleen may mimic that of HCL[150]; however, in hepatosplenic T-cell lymphoma, blood lakes are not seen, and the immunophenotypic differences are distinctive. The main histologic feature of liver as well as bone marrow involvement is an intrasinusoidal distribution of neoplastic cells (see Table 61-4). The neoplastic cells stain with various pan–T-cell markers but are often double negative for CD4 and CD8. Most cases express TCRγδ,[148,150] although some cases also express TCRαβ.[148,149,151-153] There is a strong association with isochromosome 7q10 in both gamma-delta and alpha-beta variants.[150,154]

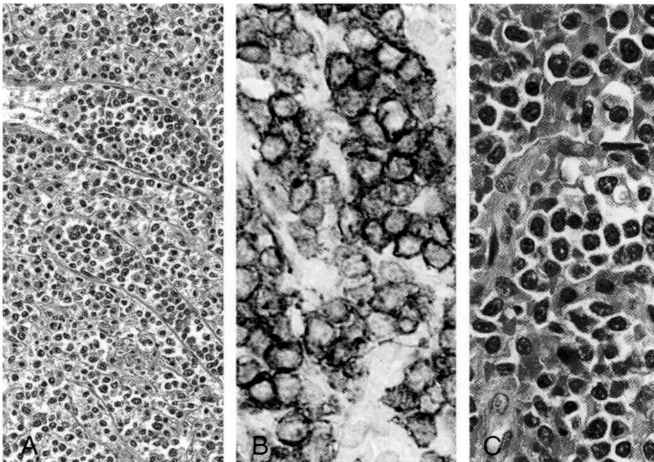

Figure 61-20. Hepatosplenic T-cell lymphoma. A, Intermediate magnification of hepatosplenic T-cell lymphoma. Note the prominent degree of intravascular infiltration observed throughout the red pulp. **B,** CD3 stain highlights the intravascular distribution of the atypical lymphoid cells. **C,** Higher magnification shows intermediate-sized atypical lymphoid cells within vascular sinuses and red pulp cords.

The differential diagnosis includes both B-cell and T-cell lymphomas. A careful review of the morphology and immunohistochemical stains allows separation from B-cell lymphomas. Rarely, T-cell prolymphocytic leukemia (T-PLL) can present with predominant splenic involvement in the absence of prominent leukocytosis. In these cases, histology of the spleen shows predominant involvement of the red pulp, similar to that seen in hepatosplenic T-cell lymphoma.[80] However, a variable degree of white pulp involvement is always present in T-PLL.[5,155] This important characteristic, which is also useful to separate T-PLL from T-LGLL, can be better appreciated by immunohistochemistry.[155] There are additional differences in the immunophenotypes of these disorders. T-PLL may show coexpression of CD4 and CD8, whereas both antigens may be absent in hepatosplenic T-cell lymphoma.

T-Cell Prolymphocytic Leukemia

T-PLL is a rare leukemic condition that presents with a high lymphocyte count and generalized lymphadenopathy and hepatosplenomegaly.[80] The circulating lymphocytes may be small, but in many cases they show nuclear irregularity and visible nucleoli. As opposed to T-LGLL, the cells of T-PLL do not have cytoplasmic granules. In addition to bone marrow involvement, infiltration of splenic red pulp and hepatic sinusoids is common. T-PLL involves both the red and white pulp. The presence of double positivity for CD4 and CD8 (25% of cases) may be helpful in the differential diagnosis. Surface CD3 expression is often weak. CD52 is usually highly expressed in T-PLL and can be used as a therapeutic target. *TCL1* expression by immunohistochemistry and cytogenetic abnormalities (e.g., abnormalities of chromosome 14q11) can also be demonstrated and may be useful in confirming the diagnosis.

T-Cell Large Granular Lymphocytic Leukemia

T-LGLL is a proliferation of CD3⁺, CD8⁺, and TCRαβ⁺ T lymphocytes.[156,157] Some patients with T-LGLL have only a moderate lymphocytosis with neutropenia and minimal splenomegaly. Others have progressive disease with marked blood and bone marrow lymphocytosis and prominent splenomegaly (see Chapter 30).[158,159]

Splenic involvement in T-LGLL is confined to the red pulp, where large granular lymphocytic cells infiltrate both cords and sinuses (Fig. 61-21).[160] T-LGLL may mimic HCL and T-PLL; however, the blood lakes characteristic of HCL are not present. As previously mentioned, in contrast to T-LGLL, T-PLL shows infiltration of the white pulp as well.[5,155] In addi-

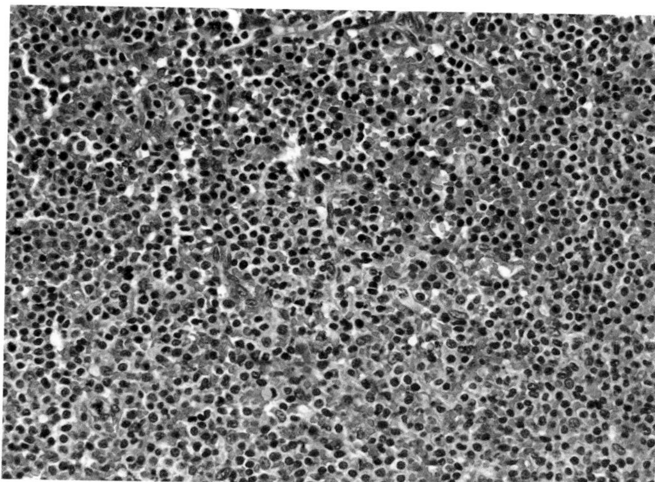

Figure 61-21 Large granular lymphocytic leukemia exhibits diffuse involvement of the red pulp by small lymphocytes.

tion, immunophenotypic findings are distinctively different in the three disorders (see Chapters 15 and 30).

MYELOID NEOPLASMS

Red pulp disease is characteristic of splenic involvement in leukemic processes (Fig. 61-22).[5,161] The leukemic cells usually appear localized to the cords of Billroth, with secondary involvement of the sinuses. Peritrabecular and subendothelial deposits may be seen early in the course of leukemic infiltration. Although splenic involvement is invariable in leukemic disorders, the degree of splenomegaly depends on the type of leukemia and the duration of the disease. The acute leukemias usually result in only mild to moderate splenic enlargement, but the chronic leukemias may produce prominent splenomegaly that often results in hypersplenism. Peripheral cytopenias may necessitate splenectomy, which may be effective in ameliorating the cytopenias but usually does not affect the course of the underlying disease. Splenic rupture is an occasional complication of leukemia. This is believed to result from tumor cells infiltrating the trabecular framework and vascular structure of the organ or from infarction within the spleen.[162-164] Rupture of the spleen is far more common in the chronic leukemias (particularly chronic myeloid leukemia) than in the acute forms.[163,164]

Acute Myeloid Leukemias

Acute myeloid leukemias include forms that may be derived from granulocytic, erythroid, monocytic, or megakaryocytic lineages. Distinguishing among these forms is often difficult based on examination of the spleen alone, although touch imprints supplemented by cytochemical stains are often helpful. Immunohistologic studies and immunophenotypic analysis by flow cytometry may be required to adequately characterize the leukemia. Splenic involvement with acute myeloid leukemia may precede or occur concurrently with systemic evidence of leukemia, or it may be a manifestation of relapse. It may also occur as part of the blast transformation process of a chronic myeloproliferative neoplasm (MPN), myelodysplastic syndrome (MDS), or myelodysplastic/myeloproliferative neoplasm (MDS/MPN). The existence of an underlying MPN may be suggested by the concomitant presence of background hematopoietic cells of different myeloid cell lines (extramedullary hematopoiesis). All the various subtypes of myeloid leukemias involve the spleen in a similar topographic manner (Fig. 61-23), with the exception of erythroleukemia, in which the leukemic cells tend to cluster preferentially in the red pulp sinuses.[5] In some cases focal proliferation of blasts may result in identifiable tumor-like masses, usually referred to as *myeloid sarcomas*.

Chronic Myeloid Neoplasms

The chronic MPNs are a group of interrelated clonal disorders of the hematopoietic stem cell.[165-167] These disorders include polycythemia vera, primary myelofibrosis, essential thrombocythemia, and chronic myelogenous leukemia. A variable degree of splenomegaly occurs in all these disorders. Although

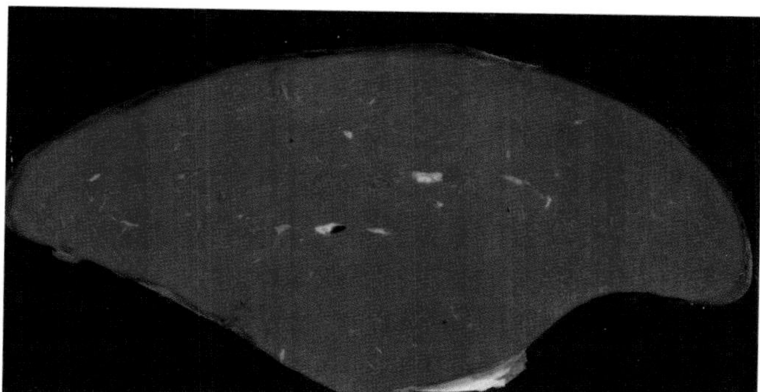

Figure 61-22. Leukemic involvement of the spleen. Disorders characterized by red pulp involvement, such as acute and chronic leukemias, produce a uniform red to purple appearance. The normal white pulp nodularity is typically absent.

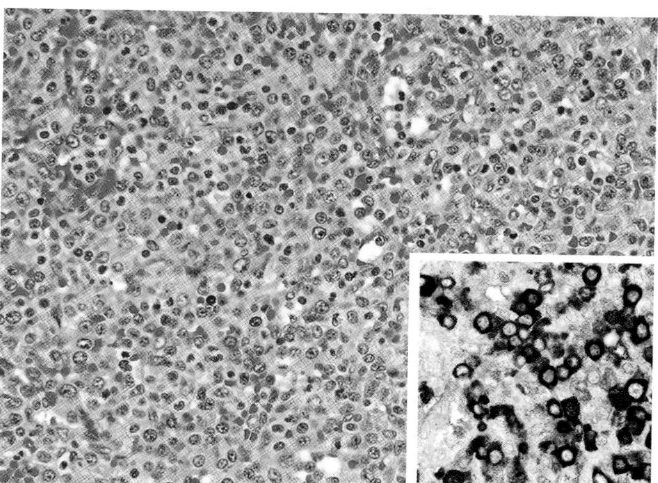

Figure 61-23. Acute myeloid leukemia in the spleen. Note the numerous blasts throughout the red pulp. This case represents transformation of a long-standing chronic myelomonocytic leukemia. The spleen can be the initial site of acute transformation in myeloproliferative and myelodysplastic disorders. *Inset,* Myeloperoxidase immunostain confirms the myeloid nature of the blasts.

each has its own somewhat distinctive characteristics, a precise diagnostic subtyping of the MPNs cannot be based on a morphologic examination of the spleen alone; this requires relevant clinical and laboratory data, as well as an examination of bone marrow and peripheral blood smears.[167-169]

Chronic Myelogenous Leukemia

Chronic myelogenous leukemia (CML) is frequently associated with massive splenomegaly. The cut surface of the spleen is deep red, without visible white pulp, because CML generally obliterates the lymphoid follicles, although small remnants of white pulp are occasionally seen.[5] Infarcts are common because of subendothelial invasion of the splenic trabecular veins, and fibrosis of the cords may be prominent. Histologic examination reveals a polymorphic cellular infiltrate in the red pulp, which includes myeloid cells at all stages of maturation.[5] The identification of immature myeloid cells (i.e., promyelocytes, myelocytes) can be facilitated by using immunohistologic stains for CD34, CD117, CD68 (or CD68R), and myeloperoxidase (or lysozyme) in combination with the enzymatic chloroacetate esterase reaction (Leder stain); the latter is particularly strongly expressed in promyelocytes. Localized collections of ceroid-containing histiocytes (pseudo–Gaucher cells), similar to those seen in the bone marrow, may also be observed in the spleens of CML patients.

The majority of CMLs terminate with the development of an accelerated or blastic phase that resembles de novo acute leukemia.[170,171] Approximately one third of cases of blast crisis arise in an extramedullary site, most commonly the spleen. Blast crisis in CML may result in a dramatic increase in spleen size.[172] Several studies have indicated that the myeloid cells in the spleen develop additional cytogenetic abnormalities before this occurs in such cells at other sites,[173-180] and they may proliferate in the spleen more rapidly than at other sites of blastic transformation.[181,182] Gross examination may reveal a homogeneous cut surface or, in some cases, discrete nodules that represent discrete collections of blasts.[5] Most often the blasts are myeloblasts, although they are lymphoblasts in approximately 25% of cases and megakaryoblasts or erythroblasts in rare cases. Immunohistochemistry with a panel of antibodies that includes both myeloid- and lymphoid-associated antigens (e.g., CD34, CD117, CD68, myeloperoxidase, CD42b [or CD61], TdT, CD79a [or PAX5], CD10, CD3) may be helpful in confirming the presence of an increased number of blasts and in identifying their lineage.

Therapy with colony-stimulating factors (e.g., granulocyte colony-stimulating factor) may simulate splenic involvement with CML or another myeloid neoplasm (Fig. 61-24) or, occasionally, may even mimic extramedullary acute myeloid leukemia.[183] Rarely the administration of this cytokine has been associated with splenic rupture.[183]

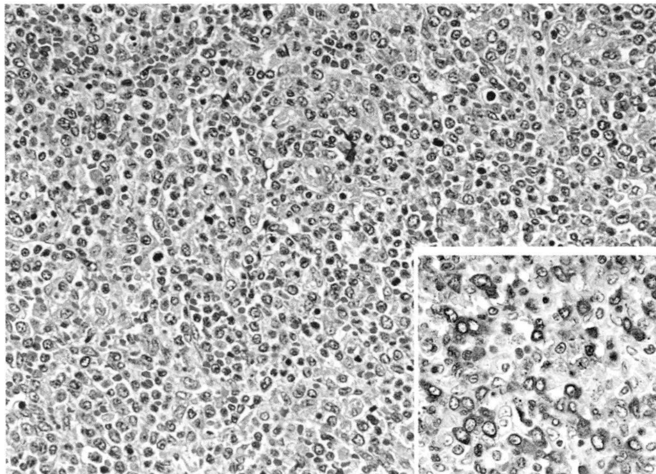

Figure 61-24. Left-shifted granulocytic hyperplasia in the spleen induced by granulocyte colony-stimulating factor. The red pulp is diffusely occupied by promyelocytes and other immature granulocytic forms, a finding that could be interpreted as evidence of acute myeloid leukemia. *Inset,* Myeloperoxidase immunostain highlights the myeloid cells.

Polycythemia Vera

Splenomegaly occurs in the majority of patients with polycythemia vera.[169] The degree of splenomegaly in the erythrocytotic phase of polycythemia vera is usually mild or moderate; the size of the spleen roughly correlates with the duration of the disease.[184-187] In approximately 15% of cases, however, polycythemia vera evolves to a spent phase, also called *postpolycythemic myeloid metaplasia*, in which the development of reticulin fibrosis in the bone marrow is accompanied by leukoerythroblastosis in the peripheral blood and marked splenomegaly.[186,188]

Although it was previously believed that splenic enlargement in polycythemia vera results from myeloid metaplasia, it has been demonstrated that extramedullary hematopoiesis is not a feature of this disease before the development of reticulin fibrosis in the bone marrow.[186] Spleens in the erythrocytotic phase show intense congestion of the cords of Billroth and the sinuses of the red pulp, accompanied by a proliferation of cordal macrophages without significant myeloid metaplasia. In contrast, spleens obtained from patients whose disease has evolved to postpolycythemic myeloid metaplasia show prominent myeloid metaplasia indistinguishable from that observed in cases of de novo primary myelofibrosis (see next section).[189,190]

Primary Myelofibrosis

The degree of splenomegaly seen in cases of primary myelofibrosis (PMF) characterized by myeloid metaplasia (also termed *agnogenic myeloid metaplasia* or *idiopathic myelofibrosis with myeloid metaplasia*) is most striking among the MPNs. In PMF, splenomegaly is associated with reticulin fibrosis in the bone marrow and the presence of leukoerythroblastosis (circulating erythroblasts in association with immature myeloid cells—usually myelocytes or metamyelocytes) and teardrop erythrocytes in the peripheral blood.[169,190] Symptoms related to massive enlargement of the organ may be the presenting feature of this disorder. The degree of splenomegaly correlates with disease duration.[185,186,190] Increasing splenomegaly may be arrested, but only transiently, by splenic irradiation or chemotherapy.

Splenomegaly in PMF results from the presence of extramedullary hematopoiesis in the red pulp, also known as *myeloid metaplasia*. On gross examination, the spleen is enlarged and purple-red, with indistinct white pulp markings. Infarcts are common. In some cases, however, focal proliferations with grossly recognizable nodules, usually composed predominantly of one cell type, are observed.[5] Microscopic

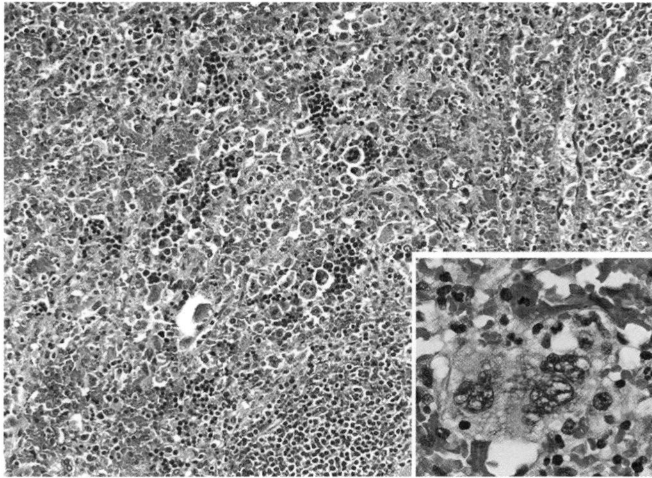

Figure 61-25. Extramedullary hematopoiesis in the spleen in a case of primary myelofibrosis. *Inset,* High-power photograph shows atypical megakaryocytes with cloud-like nuclear morphology and abnormally clumped chromatin. When comparing reactive versus hematopoietic neoplasm–associated extramedullary hematopoiesis, the presence of atypical megakaryocytes favors a clonal hematopoietic process.

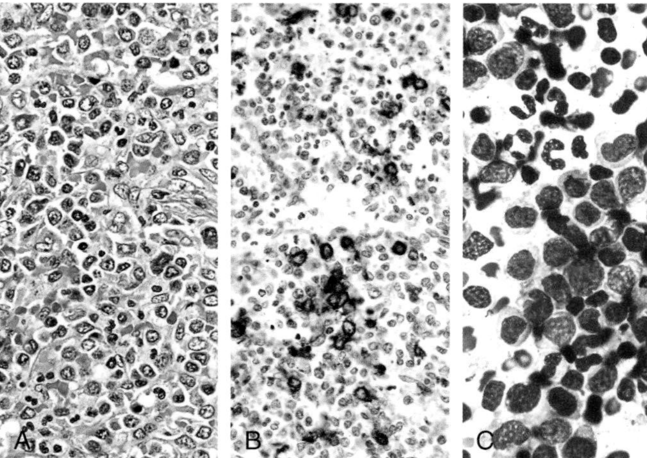

Figure 61-26. Juvenile myelomonocytic leukemia involving the spleen. A, The red pulp contains a polymorphic cellular population that includes blasts, other immature myeloid cells, monocytes, neutrophils, and eosinophils. **B,** CD34 stain highlights the presence of a variable proportion of blasts. **C,** Touch preparation of the spleen (Wright-Giemsa stain) shows immature and mature granulocytic and monocytic cells.

examination usually reveals multiple foci of extramedullary hematopoiesis distributed throughout the red pulp sinuses and in the splenic cords (Fig. 61-25; Table 61-6). Extramedullary hematopoiesis may be accompanied by a variable degree of fibrosis.

Histologically, although the hematopoiesis is always trilinear, one cell line may predominate in a given case. Erythroid precursors occur in easily recognizable clusters, frequently in the sinuses. Megakaryocytes show the same dysplastic features as those in the bone marrow, with clusters of large, often bizarre forms. Although granulocytic precursors may be difficult to distinguish from cordal macrophages, they can be recognized in touch imprints or in tissue sections by using the immunoperoxidase technique with antibodies to myeloperoxidase or lysozyme.[191] Extramedullary hematopoiesis is accompanied by a proliferation of cordal macrophages, and phagocytosis of hematopoietic precursors may be seen.[5] The trilinear nature of the hematopoiesis seen in PMF aids in distinguishing this disorder from other types of myeloid neoplasms (e.g., CML). Blastic transformation in PMF may be heralded by an increase in immature cells. In these cases the identification of an increased proportion of blasts can be facilitated by the use of appropriate immunohistochemical stains, as previously described. In addition to CML, the differential diagnosis of myeloid metaplasia in the spleen includes various disorders associated with bone marrow fibrosis and peripheral blood leukoerythroblastosis. Metastatic carcinoma and infectious disorders that involve the bone marrow are well-known causes of bone marrow fibrosis that may mimic PMF to a certain extent. Others that are much less frequent include MDS[192] and MDS/MPNs such as chronic myelomonocytic leukemia[191,193] and juvenile myelomonocytic leukemia (Fig. 61-26).[194]

Essential Thrombocythemia

Essential thrombocythemia is characterized by a marked megakaryocytic proliferation in the bone marrow associated with thrombocytosis.[169,195-197] Clinical manifestations include hemorrhagic or, less commonly, thrombotic phenomena.[169,195] The degree of splenomegaly in essential thrombocythemia is

Table 61-6 Evaluation of Myeloid Metaplasia in the Spleen

	Etiology	Hematopoiesis
Benign	Hypersplenism due to nonneoplastic causes	Typically trilineage
	"Hematopoietic" hemolytic anemias and other anemias	Predominantly erythroid, with occasional megakaryocytes
	Cytokine induced (e.g., G-CSF)	Predominantly myeloid; may simulate acute myeloid leukemia (M2 or M3 types in particular)
	Lymphoma, other malignancies (carcinoma, sarcoma)	Variable degrees of trilineage, without atypia
Clonal	MPN	Usually trilineage—occasionally one lineage predominant; atypia seen in megakaryocytes; may represent initial site of blast transformation
	MDS/MPN	Overlapping findings of both MPN and MDS
	MDS	Usually trilineage, occasionally with increased monocytes-macrophages; dysplasia seen in megakaryocytes; increased immature myeloid blasts may herald blast transformation

G-CSF, granulocyte colony-stimulating factor; MDS, myelodysplastic syndrome; MPN, myeloproliferative neoplasm.

usually less marked than that seen in the other chronic myeloproliferative disorders, and hypersplenism is not a common clinical manifestation. Because of the scarcity of splenectomy specimens, there are no large studies of the splenic pathology in essential thrombocythemia. In the few cases studied, the most notable finding was widening of the cords of Billroth, which may appear hypocellular at low power because of the presence of large masses of platelets, which may also be seen in the sinuses. Touch preparations of the spleen may be useful for demonstrating the sequestration of platelets. Although mild to moderate, splenomegaly is characteristic of most cases of essential thrombocythemia. In advanced cases, the spleen may become atrophic and nonfunctional, with atrophy probably resulting from infarction caused by the pooling of platelets.[198] The presence of fibrosis and microinfarcts (Gamna-Gandy bodies) may mimic the morphology of the spleen in advanced sickle cell disease. In our experience, no significant extramedullary hematopoiesis is seen. Occasionally, however, in the rare cases of essential thrombocythemia evolving to myelofibrosis, significant myeloid metaplasia reportedly occurs in the spleen.

Other Chronic Myeloid Neoplasms

Other types of myeloid neoplasms may produce splenomegaly. This complication is more likely to be associated with MDS/MPNs such as chronic myelomonocytic leukemia or juvenile myelomonocytic leukemia.[191-194] In these cases, the splenic red pulp contains an increased number of myelomonocytic cells (see Fig. 61-26). An increased number of blasts can be seen in cases undergoing acute transformation. Immunohistochemistry may be helpful to confirm the diagnosis and is necessary to confirm acute transformation. Aggregates of mature plasmacytoid dendritic cells (plasmacytoid monocytes) can also be observed in cases of chronic myelomonocytic leukemia,[199,200] as well as in other types of myeloid neoplasms.

SYSTEMIC MASTOCYTOSIS

The spleen is usually involved in systemic mastocytosis, although the degree of splenomegaly is frequently only mild to moderate.[201-203] The pattern of involvement of the spleen in mast cell disease is variable.[201-204] Early involvement may preferentially localize to paratrabecular areas or to the marginal zones of the white pulp. A characteristic fibroblastic reaction resulting in a concentric rimming of the lymphoid follicles may be observed (Fig. 61-27). Some investigators have reported a diffuse infiltration of the red pulp, and multinodular perivascular infiltrates have also been described.[204] Increased eosinophils are associated with the mast cell aggregates. Mast cells typically appear cuboid or spindle shaped, with pale nuclei and grayish cytoplasm. Mast cell granules can be demonstrated with chloroacetate esterase stain and are metachromatic with toluidine blue and Giemsa stains, although neoplastic mast cells are often hypogranular. Tryptase and CD117 positivity may be helpful in confirming splenic involvement, particularly in cases associated with a marked fibroblastic reaction and relatively rare mast cells. Systemic mast cell disease may be associated with other clonal hematologic non–mast cell disorders, most notably chronic myelomonocytic leukemia, MPN, MDS, or acute myeloid leukemia,[205,206] which may be present concurrently in the spleen. Their identification within the splenic red pulp may be facilitated by immunohistology for myeloid-associated antigens.

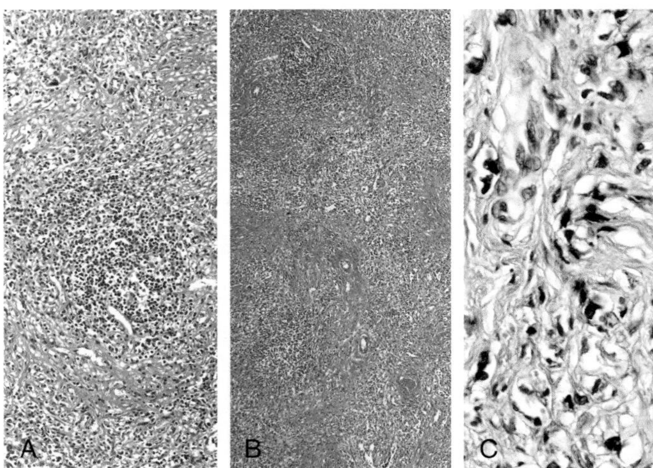

Figure 61-27. Systemic mastocytosis. A, Marked perifollicular fibrosis, with mast cells embedded in the fibrotic stroma. **B,** Perivascular, perifollicular, and trabecular fibrosis is often seen in mast cell disease in the spleen. **C,** Tryptase immunohistochemical stain highlights the mast cells entrapped in the sclerotic matrix.

PROLIFERATIONS OF THE MONOCYTE-MACROPHAGE SYSTEM

See also Chapters 51-53.

Hemophagocytic Syndromes

The hemophagocytic syndromes (HPSs) are a group of systemic disorders characterized by acute-onset pancytopenia caused by a proliferation of macrophages in lymphoreticular organs associated with prominent phagocytosis of hematopoietic elements (Box 61-2).[207] A familial (primary) form of HPS affecting infants and young children is termed *familial hemophagocytic lymphohistiocytosis*.[208-211] It is inherited in an autosomal recessive manner and is caused by the overwhelming activation of T lymphocytes and macrophages associated with defective triggering of apoptosis and reduced cytotoxic activ-

Box 61-2 *Disorders Associated with Hemophagocytosis in the Spleen*

Benign
- Storage diseases
- Congenital hemophagocytic syndromes
- Viral infections (Epstein-Barr, other viruses)
- Other infections (bacterial, fungal, rickettsial, parasitic)
- Autoimmune hemolytic anemia
- Drug induced (e.g., fludarabine)

Malignant
- Histiocytic sarcoma (malignant histiocytosis)
- Hepatosplenic T-cell lymphoma
- Other peripheral T-cell lymphomas
- B-cell lymphomas

ity. Mutations in the perforin gene have been found in patients with familial hemophagocytic lymphohistiocytosis.[210] Most secondary cases of HPS are related to either infection or an NK- or T-cell neoplasm, most often EBV⁺. Because of the acute clinical course, culminating in death in many cases; the systemic distribution; and the striking proliferation of cells in all lymphoreticular organs, these cases were once thought to represent malignant histiocytosis. They are characterized by a proliferation of benign histiocytes demonstrating prominent hemophagocytosis. Patients exhibit fever and varying cytopenias in a clinical context of underlying viral infection or malignancy.[136,212] Cases associated with infection have been referred to as either *viral-associated* or, later, *infection-associated HPS*. Numerous subsequent studies have revealed that HPS may be preciptated by a wide variety of microorganisms, as well as by a variety of tumors.[5,136,212]

The spleen in infection-associated HPS is moderately to markedly enlarged. The red pulp shows a proliferation of macrophages that display prominent hemophagocytosis, most characteristically of erythrocytes, but also of granulocytes, lymphocytes, and platelets. Fibrosis, focal infarctions, and gradual obliteration of the white pulp with B-cell depletion may occur.[5]

HPS-associated malignancies of the hematopoietic system differ morphologically because the spleen usually but not always contains a component of malignant cells. Lymphomas associated with HPS are most often of peripheral T-cell or NK-cell type.[213] Association with EBV is a major risk factor, and HPS is a common complication of extranodal NK/T-cell lymphoma, aggressive NK-cell leukemia, and systemic EBV⁺ lymphoproliferative disease of childhood associated with chronic active EBV infection. When only rare neoplastic T cells are found admixed with the numerous histiocytes, the resemblance to malignant histiocytosis may be marked (Fig. 61-28). The diagnosis of T-cell lymphoma in these cases usually requires molecular confirmation.

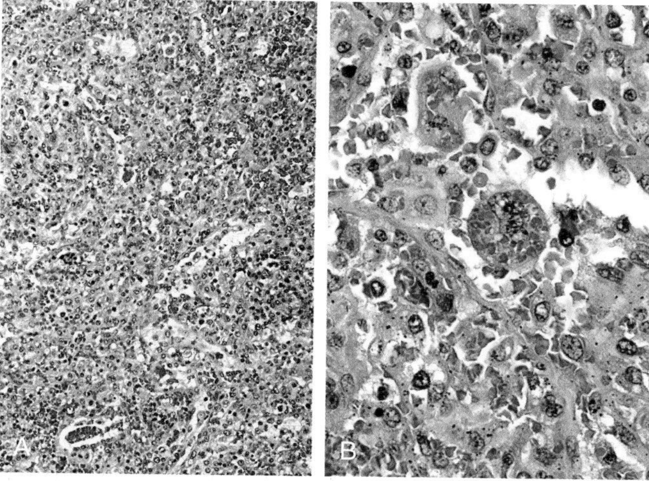

Figure 61-28. Peripheral T-cell lymphoma in the spleen associated with hemophagocytic syndrome. A, At low magnification, the findings are subtle. A variety of other disorders can be associated with hemophagocytosis in the spleen, most notably those with infectious or viral causes. **B,** Macrophage with ingested red blood cells (*center*). Also note the atypical-appearing lymphocytes, which proved to be T-cell lymphoma.

Histiocytic Sarcoma

Histiocytic sarcoma is a malignant proliferation of cells showing morphologic and immunophenotypic features similar to those of mature tissue histiocytes. Historically, cases characterized by a systemic presentation, with multiple sites of involvement, were referred to as *malignant histiocytosis*.[214] The pattern of splenic involvement resembles that of leukemia, with diffuse infiltration of the red pulp, sometimes obliterating the white pulp. The infiltrate is pleomorphic, with the proliferating cells showing a variable degree of differentiation and cytologic atypia. Occasional hemophagocytosis may be present, but it is usually seen in only a small fraction of the tumor cells; in contrast, the majority of cells show evidence of phagocytosis in HPS. Immunohistology with CD68, CD68R, CD163, and lysozyme is helpful to confirm the diagnosis. S-100 (but not CD1a) is frequently positive. Histiocytic sarcoma was reported in the spleen as a "secondary" malignancy following B-lymphoblastic leukemia/lymphoma; however, it was shown to be clonally related to the initial tumor, bearing both *IGH@* and *TCR* gene rearrangements. Possible mechanisms include transdifferentiation from the original B-lymphoblastic malignancy or a common stem cell.[215]

The differential diagnosis of histiocytic sarcoma in the spleen includes DLBCL with prominent red pulp involvement, anaplastic large cell lymphoma,[216,217] hepatosplenic T-cell lymphoma, and HPS associated with other lymphoid malignancies, previously mistakenly diagnosed as malignant histiocytosis in many cases.[136,218-220] Cases of acute monoblastic leukemia with histiocytic differentiation overlap morphologically with disseminated histiocytic sarcoma.[221]

"Malignant Histiocytosis" Associated with Mediastinal Germ Cell Tumor

An unusual association occurs between mediastinal nonseminomatous germ cell tumors and hematologic malignancies.[222] Approximately half these hematologic malignancies have been characterized as malignant histiocytosis.[222-225] These proliferations of histiocytes may occur either diffusely or in the form of ill-defined nodules within the red pulp of the spleen.[226] They are thought to represent an unusual form of metastasis from hematologic elements originating within the germ cell tumor through the aberrant differentiation of malignant germ cells.[224]

DENDRITIC CELL NEOPLASMS

See also Chapters 52-53.

Follicular Dendritic Cell Sarcoma

Follicular dendritic cell sarcoma is a rare neoplasm derived from follicular dendritic cells of the germinal center; it has been described rarely in the spleen.[227-230] Follicular dendritic cells are mesenchymal cells that are not of hematopoietic origin, in contrast to myeloid dendritic cells, including Langerhans cells. Follicular dendritic cell sarcoma is characterized grossly by fleshy or solid nodules and histologically by oval or spindle cells usually growing in bundles and whorls. Nuclei are bland in appearance and have a low mitotic rate. The neoplastic cells are typically CD21⁺ and CD35⁺. The clinical behavior of these tumors appears to be more aggressive than the relatively bland cytology would suggest.[230] A rare EBV+ variant of follicular dendritic cell sarcoma shares morphologic features with splenic inflammatory pseudotumor, from which it should be distinguished.[231]

Interdigitating Dendritic Cell Sarcoma

Interdigitating dendritic cell sarcoma is a rare tumor that is thought to arise from interdigitating dendritic cells.[229] The disease usually involves lymph nodes, but splenic involvement may occur, particularly in cases of disseminated disease with involvement of the bone marrow, skin, liver, kidney, and lung, as well as the spleen.[232,233] The gross and histologic features of interdigitating dendritic cell sarcoma are similar to those described for follicular dendritic cell sarcoma. In paraffin sections, the cells are positive for S-100 and variably positive for CD68; they lack CD1a, langerin, B-cell, T-cell, and specific follicular dendritic cell antigen expression.

Langerhans Cell Histiocytosis

Langerhans cell histiocytosis, a clonal proliferation of CD1a+, S-100+, langerin-positive Langerhans cells, has multiple clinical presentations, ranging from an isolated lytic lesion of bone to a fulminating, disseminated disorder mimicking leukemia. This latter presentation, historically termed *Letterer-Siwe disease*,[234] is most common in young children and is the form of disease in which splenic involvement may occur.[235-238] The abnormalities observed in the spleen include hemorrhage and areas of necrosis and infarction. Red pulp involvement is predominant and may take the form of a diffuse infiltrate or ill-defined tumor aggregates resembling loosely formed granulomas. The characteristic cell in Langerhans cell histiocytosis is a large macrophage-like cell with abundant pale, sometimes vacuolated cytoplasm.[239] Nuclei are frequently deeply indented or grooved, with fine chromatin and one or two small nucleoli. Electron microscopy usually reveals characteristic structures, termed *Birbeck granules,* within the cytoplasm.[240,241] The cells of Langerhans cell histiocytosis are typically S-100, CD1a, and langerin positive. As in other involved sites, eosinophils and histiocytes may be found intermixed with the Langerhans cells.

Rare cases of Langerhans cell sarcoma, the malignant counterpart of Langerhans cell histiocytosis, have been reported.[242,243] There is a male predominance, patients are older, and there is disseminated involvement, frequently including the spleen. In these cases the Langerhans cells appear cytologically malignant, with marked atypia.

TUMOR-LIKE AND NONHEMATOPOIETIC NEOPLASTIC LESIONS

Several benign lesions involving the spleen can grossly mimic malignant lymphoma by virtue of the production of mass lesions that may be associated with hypersplenism, although their benign nature is usually readily apparent microscopically.

Splenic Cyst

Splenic cysts are most commonly single and unilocular. The majority of these are so-called false cysts that lack epithelial linings.[244] Approximately 20% of splenic cysts have an epithelial lining, which is usually of a stratified squamous type.[245-249] These are termed *true cysts* or *epidermoid cysts.* Rarely, true cysts can result in hypersplenism.

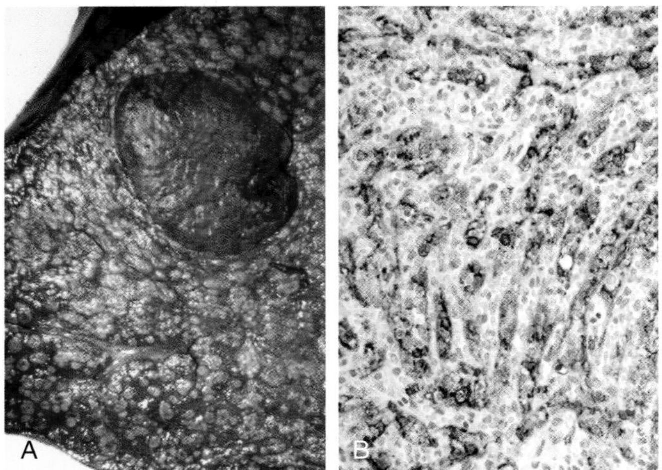

Figure 61-29. A, Gross photograph of a splenic hamartoma. Note the well-circumscribed mass. The lesion consists of red pulp only and lacks white pulp. **B,** CD8 immunohistochemical stain highlights the splenic sinuses.

Splenic Hamartoma

Similarly, splenic hamartomas occasionally result in hypersplenism,[250] although they are more commonly an incidental finding at autopsy or in spleens removed for unrelated causes.[5,251] Splenic hamartomas are well-circumscribed nodules that resemble normal red pulp histologically, with slit-like vascular spaces lined by plump endothelial cells of littoral cell derivation (i.e., CD8+) (Fig. 61-29). Splenic trabecular architecture and white pulp structures are only rarely seen in hamartomas, although scattered lymphocytes are often found. The typical splenic hamartoma can be easily distinguished from capillary hemangioma by virtue of its immunohistochemical reactivity with CD8 and CD68 and lack of CD34 expression. More problematic, however, is the distinction between hamartoma and rare entities such as cordal capillary hemangioma[252] and splenic myoid angioendothelioma.[253] The extensive morphologic overlap between these entities is well acknowledged, and their separation may be at least partially arbitrary.[252]

Inflammatory Pseudotumor

Splenic inflammatory pseudotumor (IPT) is a distinctive lesion that differs from most other neoplastic and nonneoplastic lesions bearing this name in other organ systems. It presents as an isolated mass, mimicking a tumor, but is composed of a mixture of inflammatory cells and stromal cells (Fig. 61-30).[231,254-257] The stromal component appears to be the proliferative component of IPT, but clonality has not been established. IPTs that occur in the spleen are most commonly of either myofibroblastic or follicular dendritic cell origin. Both are typically associated with EBV and have similar clinical and histologic features, differing mainly in the phenotype

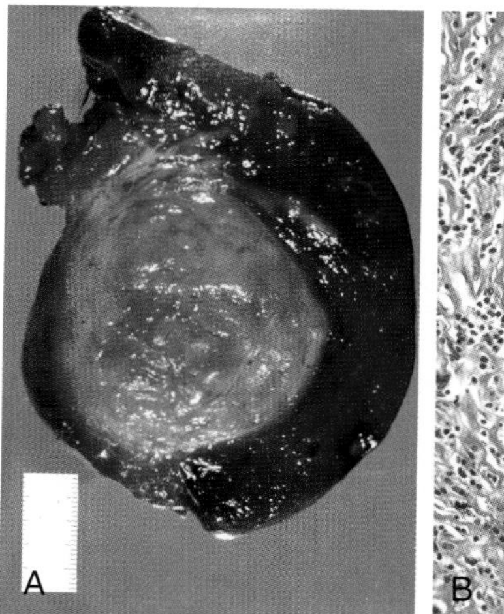

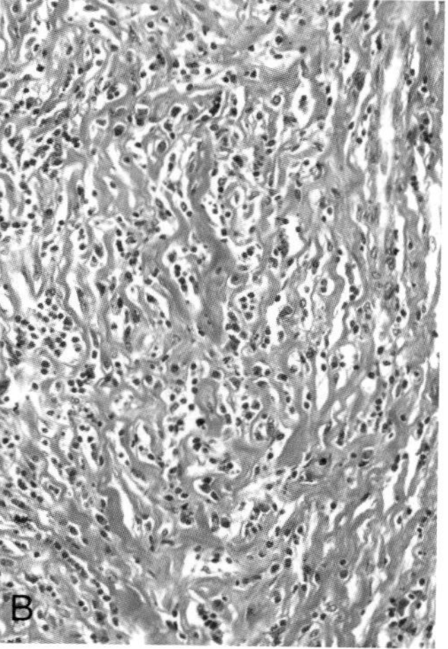

Figure 61-30. A, Gross photograph of a sclerotic splenic inflammatory pseudotumor. The mass may mimic splenic involvement by a variety of malignancies, including Hodgkin's and non-Hodgkin's lymphomas. **B**, Microscopic appearance. This inflammatory pseudotumor has a predominance of fibrous bands, with a few spindle-shaped cells. Mixed inflammatory cells and spindle cells may be more prominent in other cases.

of the proliferating spindle cells. The clinical outcome is typically benign, without recurrences following splenectomy. IPT is often asymptomatic; occasional patients have abdominal pain or a sense of fullness. Splenic IPT usually presents as a solitary, circumscribed, firm nodule, often with central necrosis. The borders are usually well circumscribed. Histologically, common findings include a proliferation of bland-looking spindle-shaped cells within a polymorphic background that contains variable numbers of monocytes, lymphocytes, and polyclonal plasma cells.

In IPT of myofibroblastic origin, immunohistochemical staining for smooth muscle markers (smooth muscle actin) is positive in the spindle cell population. EBV-encoded small RNA (EBER) is usually positive, whereas latent membrane protein-1 (LMP-1) is more uncommonly expressed.[255,258] A possibly related entity is the IPT-like follicular dendritic cell tumor.[231] Unlike conventional follicular dendritic cell tumors (see the eariler section), the IPT-like variant has a marked female predominance. IPT-like follicular dendritic cell tumors have been reported to occur in the spleen or liver. As the name implies, there is a mixed inflammatory background associated with bland spindle cells. The spindle cells are positive for dendritic cell markers (CD21, CD23, CD35), and essentially all cases are positive for EBV.[231] In rare cases of IPT the patient has a history of infection, but the relationship between IPT and infection may be coincidental, with only EBV being found on a consistent basis.[254,259]

IPT should be distinguished from inflammatory myofibroblastic tumor, a neoplasm common in children and associated with the expression of ALK.[256] This is not problematic, because involvement of the spleen and lymph nodes has not been reported with ALK$^+$ inflammatory myofibroblastic tumor. In addition to splenic lymphoma, the differential diagnosis of splenic IPT includes various benign or tumor-like splenic lesions, such as hamartoma and hemangioma. Splenic hamartomas are typically surrounded by a rim of compressed red pulp, usually without associated fibrosis. In addition, the sinus or cord-like spaces characteristically observed in splenic harmartoma are not observed in IPT.

Sclerosing Angiomatoid Nodular Transformation

Sclerosing angiomatoid nodular transformation of the spleen is a poorly understood condition that presents as a tumor-like nodule or mass lesion in the spleen (Fig. 61-31).[260-262] It may be related to splenic hamartoma because the components are those of the splenic red pulp. Grossly, it resembles IPT. The lesions of sclerosing angiomatoid nodular transformation can be large, up to 17 cm in diameter. Histologically, it has a multinodular appearance. The individual nodules have an angiomatoid appearance, being composed of slit-like vascular channels with interspersed spindle cells and dense sclerosis. The vessels have a phenotype that is intermediate between that of true vascular channels (sometimes CD34$^+$ or CD31$^+$) and splenic sinusoidal lining cells (CD8$^+$). It has been postulated that the lesion is nonneoplastic and represents altered red pulp entrapped by a stromal proliferation. The clinical outcome has been benign in all reported cases.

Peliosis

Peliosis is a rare condition of unknown cause in which ectatic sinusoids and blood-filled cysts are present throughout the spleen.[263,264] Peliotic cysts are lined by sinusoidal endothelium, but in larger lesions this is often absent. The cysts are often located adjacent to the periarteriolar lymphoid sheaths and in the perifollicular zones. Its clinical importance lies in its association with spontaneous splenic rupture,[263,264] caused by a combination of splenic enlargement and fragility of the dilated, cystic sinusoids. Peliosis also affects the liver.

Splenic Vascular Tumor

Capillary and cavernous angiomas can occur in the spleen. Their morphologic features are similar to those observed elsewhere. Problems in the differential diagnosis may be encountered, however, in cases of diffuse angiomatosis and littoral cell angiomas, benign conditions that must be distinguished from the highly malignant angiosarcoma of the spleen. In littoral cell angiomas,[265] the endothelial cells are usually plump and cuboid (Fig. 61-32). They may express CD8, typical of splenic sinusoidal endothelium. Papillary projections of endothelial cells may protrude into the vascular spaces. Vascular lumens also contain abundant desquamated littoral cells and macrophages (sometimes exhibiting erythrophagocytosis). Mild cytologic atypia may be present, and the distinction between littoral cell angioma and low-grade angiosarcoma can be difficult in individual cases.[265,266]

Angiosarcomas of the spleen are rare multifocal proliferations, heterogeneous in morphology and clinical behavior (Fig. 61-33).[267] In some areas they may appear benign, resembling littoral cell angiomas (see Fig. 61-33); elsewhere, they may contain areas of unequivocal malignancy resembling high-grade angiosarcoma at other sites. Expression of CD8 is weak or absent in the areas that appear most malignant. The presence of CD8 positivity in some of these tumors supports the concept that a subset of angiosarcomas may arise from sinusoidal endothelium.[266]

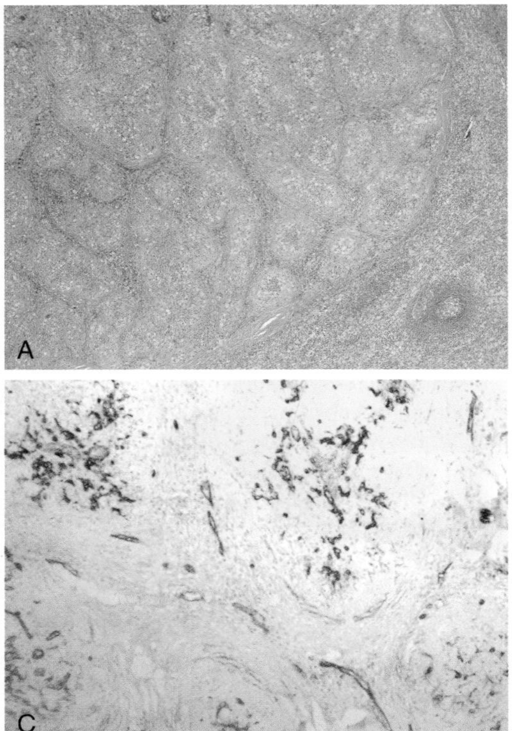

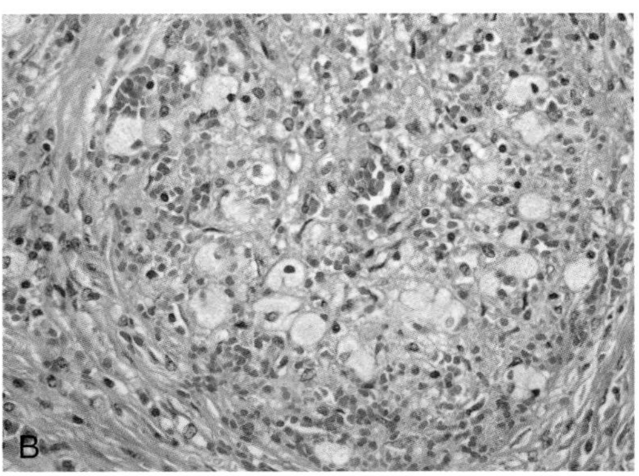

Figure 61-31. Sclerosing angiomatoid nodular transformation. A, The lesion is multinodular, with slit-like spacing surrounded by dense sclerosis. The gross appearance mimics inflammatory pseudotumor, but histologically, the distinction is usually not difficult. The lesion is sharply demarcated from adjacent spleen. **B**, Foam cells may be present in the nodules. **C**, The vascular slits within the nodules stain with CD34 and varibly with CD31 and CD8 (not shown).

High-grade angiosarcomas in the spleen usually contain areas with spindle cell morphology and little evidence of vascular differentiation (Fig. 61-34). Occasional malignant neoplasms of the spleen have been described with a pure spindle cell composition; these have variously been regarded as malignant fibrous histiocytoma or solid angiosarcoma.[268] Solid malignant tumors with the characteristics of Kaposi's sarcoma have also been described in the spleen, not always in patients with HIV infection or other immunodeficient states.[269] Lymphangiomas are thin-walled cysts of various size lined by flat endothelial cells; they contain watery, pink proteinaceous material but not blood.[270] Single cases of primary splenic nonvascular mesenchymal tumors, including rhabdomyosarcoma and fibroblastic reticular cell tumor, have also been reported.[271,272]

Metastatic Tumors

Metastatic tumors are uncommon in the spleen, perhaps because of the absence of afferent lymphatics. Many types of carcinoma, as well as melanoma and, more rarely,

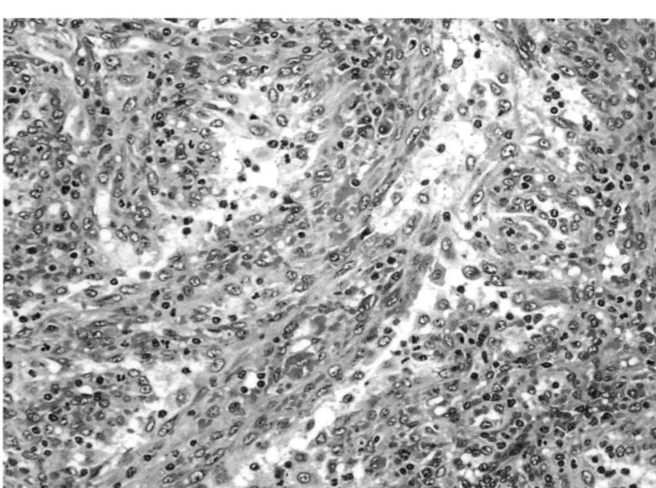

Figure 61-32. Littoral cell angioma with vascular spaces lined by plump endothelial cells lacking cytologic atypia. Sinus lining cells desquamate into the vascular lumens.

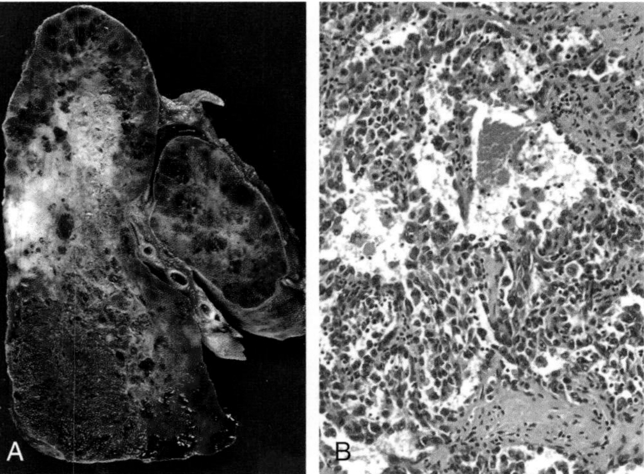

Figure 61-33. A, Gross photograph of littoral cell angiosarcoma of the spleen. Note the mixture of spongy, dark red cystic areas and more malignant-looking solid areas. **B**, Note the presence of significant nuclear pleomorphism and the arborizing vascular pattern.

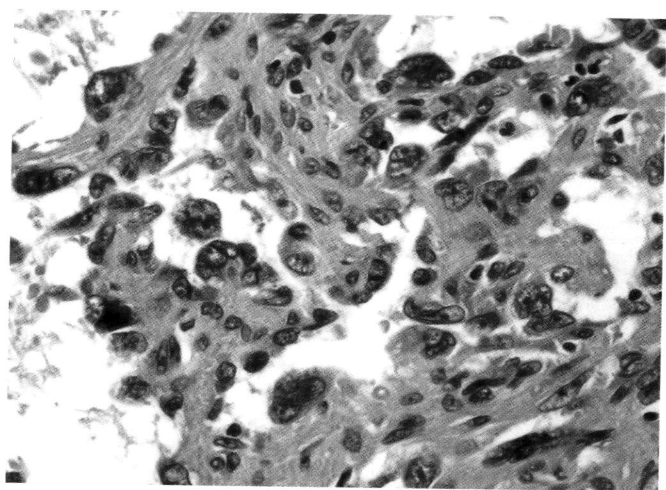

Figure 61-34. Photomicrograph of splenic angiosarcoma. The marked cellular pleomorphism is consistent with a diagnosis of angiosarcoma. Note the irregular, anastomosing appearance of the vascular channels.

sarcoma, have been reported in the spleen. Most cause tumor masses, but some may infiltrate the organ diffusely (Fig. 61-35).

STORAGE DISEASES

The spleen is involved in many of the lysosomal storage diseases. These are predominantly autosomal recessive conditions whose diagnosis and classification are based on the enzymatic defect characteristic of each disease, often in combination with specific genetic testing. Although most of these conditions are rare, three of the lipid storage diseases are encountered (uncommonly) in surgical pathology practice. Gaucher's and Niemann-Pick diseases, particularly in their nonneuronopathic forms, are the most common storage diseases encountered in removed spleens.[5,273,274] The significant splenomegaly observed in these cases may cause hypersplenism. Not uncommonly in these cases, the spleen is removed to confirm the diagnosis or to ameliorate cytopenias. Ceroid histiocytosis (sea-blue histiocytosis) can also be observed. Accumulation of sea-blue histiocytes may be seen in association with lipid disorders, infectious diseases, red blood cell disorders, and myeloproliferative disorders. However, it is also a prominent feature in spleens removed from patients with Hermansky-Pudlak syndrome, a rare, often fatal autosomal recessive condition that is currently classified among the disorders of lysosome-related organelle biogenesis.[275]

In most storage disorders, affected spleens are usually pale and homogeneous in appearance. Rarely, areas of fibrosis are noted.[5] Microscopically, the red pulp is expanded because of the accumulation of numerous histiocytes in the splenic cords.[5]

Gaucher's disease is the most common of the storage disorders. Gaucher cells range in size from 20 to 100 μm in diameter and have fibrillar cytoplasm that appears brownish in hematoxylin-eosin–stained preparations. Multinucleated cells may occur. The cytoplasm is intensely PAS positive, and this positivity is resistant to diastase digestion. The glucocerebroside in Gaucher cells is autofluorescent. Because Gaucher cells are macrophages and ingest red blood cells, they frequently stain positively for iron. Lipid stains are only weakly positive. Ultrastructural studies reveal numerous lysosomes containing characteristic lipid bilayers. Pseudo–Gaucher cells are often seen in the spleens of patients with CML.

Niemann-Pick cells are large, ranging from 20 to 100 μm in diameter, and appear foamy or bubbly owing to numerous small vacuoles. They are clearer than Gaucher cells and usually stain only faintly with PAS, but they contain neutral fat, as demonstrated by Sudan black B and oil red O stains. The lipid deposits are birefringent and, under ultraviolet light, display yellow-green fluorescence. Electron microscopy reveals lamellated structures resembling myelin figures within lysosomes.

In cases of ceroid histiocytosis, smaller histiocytes with more basophilic cytoplasm and vacuoles are characteristically seen. These cells can also be seen in Niemann-Pick disease. Ceroid-containing histiocytes measure up to 20 μm and contain cytoplasmic granules that measure 3 to 4 μm. The histiocytes show a variable degree of granulation. Foamy histiocytes with smaller, darker granules may also occur. Ceroid is composed of phospholipids and glycosphingolipids and is similar to lipofuscin in its physical and chemical properties. Histiocytes containing ceroid appear faintly yellow-brown in hematoxylin-eosin–stained sections but blue-green with Romanowsky stains, resulting in the term *sea-blue histiocyte*. Ceroid is PAS-positive and resistant to diastase digestion and stains positively with lipid stains. It shows a strong affinity for basic dyes such as fuchsin and methylene blue. Ceroid is acid-fast and becomes autofluorescent with aging of the pigment. Ultrastructural studies reveal inclusions of lamellated membranous material with 4.5- to 5-nanometer periodicity.

None of the cell types identified in storage disorders is specific for a given disease, and their actual diagnosis should be based on biochemical or molecular genetic testing specific for these diseases.

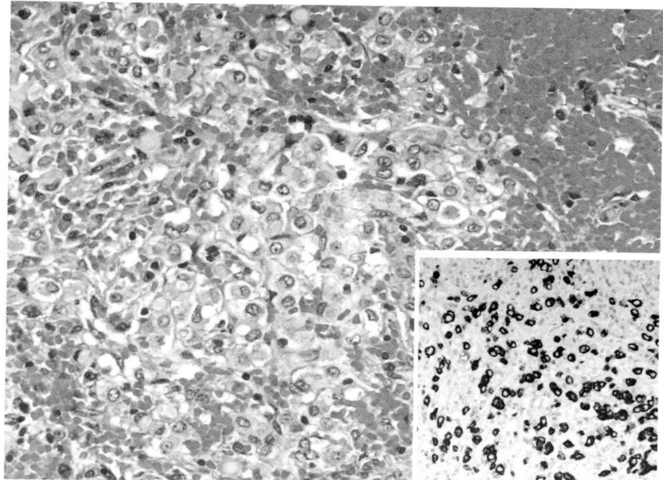

Figure 61-35. Signet ring carcinoma metastatic to the spleen. *Inset,* The malignant cells are strongly positive with a pancytokeratin immunostain.

Pearls and Pitfalls

Benign

- Infectious mononucleosis may be misdiagnosed as DLBCL or PTCL, not otherwise specified. A polymorphic infiltrate of lymphocytes with large cells that seems malignant but is unusual for a specific type of lymphoma should be evaluated for possible EBV infection, especially in a young person.
- Immunodeficiency-associated lymphoproliferative disorders can be confused with malignant lymphoma in the spleen. The clinical history is critical. In adults, common variable immunodeficiency and related disorders can be particularly difficult to distinguish from lymphomas.
- Myeloid hyperplasia in the red pulp, which can mimic acute myeloid leukemia, may be caused by cytokines, particularly granulocyte colony-stimulating factor.
- True IPT, inflammatory myofibroblastic tumor, and IPT-like follicular dendritic cell tumor are difficult to distinguish—extensive immunohistologic panels are usually necessary.
- Careful interpretation of CD8, CD31, and CD34 stains is useful in assessing splenic vascular lesions (e.g., endothelial cells in hamartoma are $CD8^+$).

Malignant

- Many types of small B-cell lymphomas (CLL/SLL, MZL, MCL) involve the white pulp with a miliary pattern and thus display considerable morphologic overlap. Immunohistology in conjunction with careful attention to cellular composition is critical. Splenic hilar lymph node examination may be valuable.
- Small B-cell lymphoma with exclusive involvement of the red pulp must be distinguished from classic HCL. Preponderant red pulp involvement can be seen in rare cases of MZL.
- Large granular lymphocytic leukemia and other PTCLs (e.g., mycosis fungoides/Sézary syndrome) often have subtle splenic involvement. In these cases, immunohistology may be of great value.
- Autoimmune lymphoproliferative syndrome may be confused with splenic lymphoma. Autoimmune lymphoproliferative syndrome typically presents in pediatric patients. A family history of "congenital splenomegaly" may be a clue.
- Hepatosplenic T-cell lymphoma has distinctive clinical and morphologic features and is usually gamma-delta type but may also be alpha-beta. An important diagnostic clue is that most cases are double negative for CD4 and CD8.
- In both myeloid and lymphoid leukemic disorders, as well as in low-grade lymphomas, the spleen may be the initial site of high-grade transformation.

References can be found on Expert Consult @ www.expertconsult.com

found in only HIV+ patients.[8] Many cases coexpress BCL6 and IRF4/MUM-1. Loss of human leukocyte antigen (HLA) class I and II molecules is reportedly frequent.[19,20]

Genetic Features

Molecular genetic analysis shows monoclonal immunoglobulin gene rearrangements in DLBCL.[7,8] Virtually all cases of PCNS DLBCL in immunosuppressed patients are positive for EBV-encoded small RNA (EBER) by in situ hybridization, whereas such tumors in immunocompetent patients are EBER−.[3,8] About half of cases (less often in HIV− than HIV+ cases) show mutations of the *BCL6* gene, consistent with transition through the germinal center.[8] There appears to be preferential use of certain VH families, as well as a high load of somatic mutations, in some cases accompanied by intraclonal diversity. The pattern suggests that the neoplastic cells are derived from antigen-selected B cells of the germinal center.[7,18]

Postulated Normal Counterpart

Immunophenotypic and genetic features suggest that primary CNS DLBCL is derived from a post–germinal center B cell. Some investigators have suggested that the cell of origin is a B cell in peripheral lymphoid tissue that crosses the blood-brain barrier and then proliferates to form a tumor in this immunologically protected environment. In such a scenario, it is unclear whether neoplastic transformation takes place before or after entry into the CNS or whether the immunoglobulin genes of tumor cells can continue to mutate outside the germinal center.[7,8,15] The loss of HLA molecules may be related in some way to the survivial of lymphomas in immune-privileged sites such as the CNS and testis.[19,20]

Staging, Treatment, and Outcome

Staging should be performed to exclude systemic lymphoma with secondary involvement of the CNS, but staging is usually negative in patients presenting with the findings described earlier.[2] PCNS DLBCL is an aggressive neoplasm requiring prompt diagnosis and therapy.[18] Survival is only a few months without therapy. In the past, traditional therapy was whole-brain radiation combined with steroids. This resulted in complete remission in 90% of cases, but the lymphoma usually relapsed within a year, with a median survival of 12 to 18 months and a 5-year survival rate of only 3% to 4%.[4,5,15] More recently, survival has improved with the addition of high-dose methotrexate, an agent that can penetrate the blood-brain barrier, to radiation. Unfortunately, long-term survivors who have received radiation therapy are at high risk for the development of leukoencephalopathy, manifested by severe progressive dementia, ataxia, and urinary incontinence.[15] To avoid this complication, regimens without radiation are being tested. Relatively good outcomes without cognitive loss have been achieved using intensive chemotherapy-based regimens.[5]

When patients with PCNS DLBCL relapse, the CNS is involved in the vast majority of cases. In a small proportion of cases, lymphoma spreads outside the CNS; sites of spread are usually extranodal, with frequent testicular involvement.[5] The prognosis is better for patients who are younger than 60 years[4,5] and immunocompetent.[6] The low-grade B-cell lymphomas appear to have a relatively favorable prognosis, although this topic has not been well studied.[3,11]

Differential Diagnosis

Sampling artifact or prior steroid therapy can result in a biopsy that shows a predominance of small reactive T cells, mimicking a chronic inflammatory process.[2] Avoiding prebiopsy steroids and obtaining intraoperative frozen sections to ensure that the tissue is representative in any case of suspected PCNSL are helpful in establishing a diagnosis. There may be a surrounding glial reaction that mimics astrocytoma. Other neoplasms, including primitive neuroectodermal tumor, undifferentiated carcinoma, melanoma, anaplastic oligodendroglioma, and small cell astrocytoma, can grow in sheets and mimic lymphoma.[11] Arteritis can mimic areas of lymphoma with perivascular growth.[11]

Eye

Clinical Features

Ocular lymphoma or intraocular lymphoma—lymphoma involving the eye itself—is uncommon, but its frequency has increased in recent years.[10,21-23] Ocular DLBCL is considered part of the spectrum of PCNS DLBCL. It occurs predominantly in older adults,[23-25] although occasionally young adults[26] and rarely children[27] are affected. There is a female preponderance.[10,23,28] Most patients have no known predisposing conditions, but cases have been described in HIV-infected patients[22] and in iatrogenically immunosuppressed allograft recipients.[21,27]

Patients typically complain of blurred vision or floating spots, or both.[23] Although symptoms are often unilateral, ophthalmologic examination reveals involvement of both eyes in about 80% of cases.[10] Translucent gray cells appear in sheets and clumps suspended in the vitreous. In the majority of cases the vitreous, retina or uveal tract (choroid, iris, and ciliary body), or a combination are affected. Whitish, yellow-white, or gray-white infiltrates; plaque-like lesions; or large masses may be seen beneath the retinal pigment epithelium, in the uvea, or invading the optic nerve, sometimes with edema, hemorrhage, necrosis, or retinal detachment. The posterior uvea (choroid) is more often involved than the anterior uvea (iris and ciliary body). Other manifestations include increased intraocular pressure, keratic precipitates (deposits of cells on the posterior surface of the cornea), and anterior chamber cells and flare (the presence of increased protein causes the normally clear fluid of the anterior chamber to become cloudy [flare] with tiny particles [cells] suspended in the fluid).[10,23,24,29]

Ocular lymphoma can mimic nonneoplastic conditions, including chronic idiopathic uveitis, retinal vasculitis,[23] optic neuritis, amyloidosis, sarcoidosis, and infections such as toxoplasmosis, syphilis, tuberculosis, Whipple's disease, and cytomegalovirus infection.[10] The possibility of lymphoma may be raised when there is a poor response to steroids or antimicrobial therapy or the onset of neurologic symptoms due to CNS involvement.[10,23]

Techniques used to establish a diagnosis include vitreous aspirate, vitrectomy, biopsy, or, in patients with a blind, painful eye, ocular enucleation. The most common method is microscopic examination of the vitreous, but the sensitivity of this procedure may be limited by admixed inflammatory cells or by prior steroid therapy, which may eliminate many of the tumor cells.[23] Diagnostic yield may be improved by combining routine light microscopy with flow cytometry and molecular genetic analysis.[30] An elevated interleukin-10 level in the vitreous is strongly associated with ocular lymphoma and may prompt repeat biopsy if the initial specimen is nondiagnostic.[10]

Pathologic Features

Nearly all ocular lymphomas are DLBCL.[22,23] The pathologic features are identical to PCNS DLBCL presenting in the brain. Rare cases of peripheral T-cell lymphoma presenting with ocular involvement have also been described.[26,28,31]

Staging, Treatment, and Outcome

The majority of cases of ocular DLBCL are associated with CNS DLBCL either at presentation or, without treatment, during follow-up; a minority are associated with systemic lymphoma or remain confined to the eye. Aggressive treatment of isolated ocular lymphoma can decrease the risk of progression.[10,23,24,32]

Ocular DLBCL frequently responds well to radiation therapy,[24] but restoration of sight is not guaranteed because the retina may already be irreversibly damaged, and radiation may be associated with retinopathy and cataracts. Patients treated with ocular radiation alone often develop ocular recurrence or progress to CNS or, less often, systemic involvement. Other types of therapy have been suggested, including combined chemotherapy and radiation, chemotherapy alone, intensive chemotherapy with autologous stem cell transplantation, and intravitreal methotrexate.[10,29]

Peripheral Nerves

Lymphomas can affect the peripheral nervous system in several ways. The most common is a paraneoplastic syndrome, most often in association with Waldenström's macroglobulinemia. Less often there is direct extension into nerves from lymphoma in adjacent tissues. Lymphoma arising in other sites can relapse in peripheral nerves.[33] Patients may present with symptoms related to neural involvement, but staging usually reveals more widespread disease involving the CNS or sites outside the nervous system.[34,35] Primary lymphoma confined to peripheral nerves is exceedingly rare. Involvement of multiple nerves with or without involvement of spinal nerve roots, dorsal root ganglia, and meninges (neurolymphomatosis) is more common than involvement of a single nerve.[33,34,36]

Clinical Features

Patients are usually adults; males and females are equally affected. They typically present with a subacute onset of neuritic pain, often accompanied by sensory and motor deficits. Physical examination or magnetic resonance imaging reveals a tumor expanding the nerves, sometimes imparting a fusiform contour.[33,35] When a single nerve is involved, it is usually the sciatic nerve.[33] Lymphoma infiltrates the nerve, resulting in segmental demyelination and axonal degeneration.[34,36] Patients may respond to chemotherapy, but most develop relapses in other nerves, the CNS, or a variety of extranodal sites, and the majority succumb to their lymphoma.[33]

Pathologic Features

The lymphomas are most often DLBCL, but low grade B-cell lymphomas and T-cell lymphomas have been described.

Differential Diagnosis

On clinical grounds, the differential diagnosis includes paraneoplastic syndrome, degenerative disease, Guillain-Barré syndrome, and schwannoma.[33,36] On histologic examination, early involvement by low-grade lymphoma can be difficult to distinguish from an inflammatory process.

Dura Mater

Clinical Features

Lymphoma arising in the dura mater is uncommon, but well-documented cases have been described. Patients are mostly middle-aged and older adults. There are no known risk factors. They present with seizures, headaches, cranial nerve abnormalities, radicular pain, syncope, or a combination of these findings.[37-41] Radiologic evaluation usually reveals a localized, expansile mass or plaque-like thickening of the dura over the brain[40,42,43]; preoperatively, this is most often thought to be a meningioma or, less often, a nerve sheath tumor or subdural hematoma.[39,40]

Pathologic Features

Approximately half of cases are diffuse large cell lymphomas (B lineage when immunophenotyped). The remainder are a variety of types in older classifications, but recent publications suggest that many are extranodal marginal zone B-cell lymphomas.[40,41] The marginal zone lymphomas have histologic and immunohistologic features similar to those seen in other sites. They are composed of small lymphocytes and marginal zone cells, usually with plasmacytic differentiation and admixed reactive follicles (Fig. 62-2). Entrapped meningothelial cells may be seen.[39-41] Dural marginal zone lymphomas may arise in association with meningothelium, just as marginal zone lymphomas arise in association with epithelium in other sites.[39,40] Dural lymphomas are localized (stage IE) tumors. Therapy varies from case to case, but almost all recently reported patients (undergoing thorough staging and optimal therapy) have done well.[39-41]

Differential Diagnosis

Other low-grade B-cell lymphomas, such as lymphoplasmacytic lymphoma and chronic lymphocytic leukemia, can have histologic features mimicking those of marginal zone lymphoma, but the immunophenotype and localized nature can be used to exclude other low-grade lymphomas. Some cases previously interpreted as dural plasmacytoma may actually represent marginal zone lymphoma with marked plasmacytic differentiation.[39,40] Some cases may raise the question of inflammatory pseudotumor, a chronic inflammatory process, or lymphoplasmacyte-rich meningioma, but immunophenotyping or genotyping can help establish the diagnosis.

OCULAR ADNEXA

Clinical Features

Primary ocular adnexal lymphomas are defined as lymphomas arising in the orbit (including the lacrimal gland), conjunctiva, or eyelids. The orbit is the most common site, followed by the conjunctiva and then the eyelids.[44] One percent to 2% of all lymphomas[45] and approximately 8% of all extranodal lymphomas[46] arise in the ocular adnexa. Lymphoid tumors

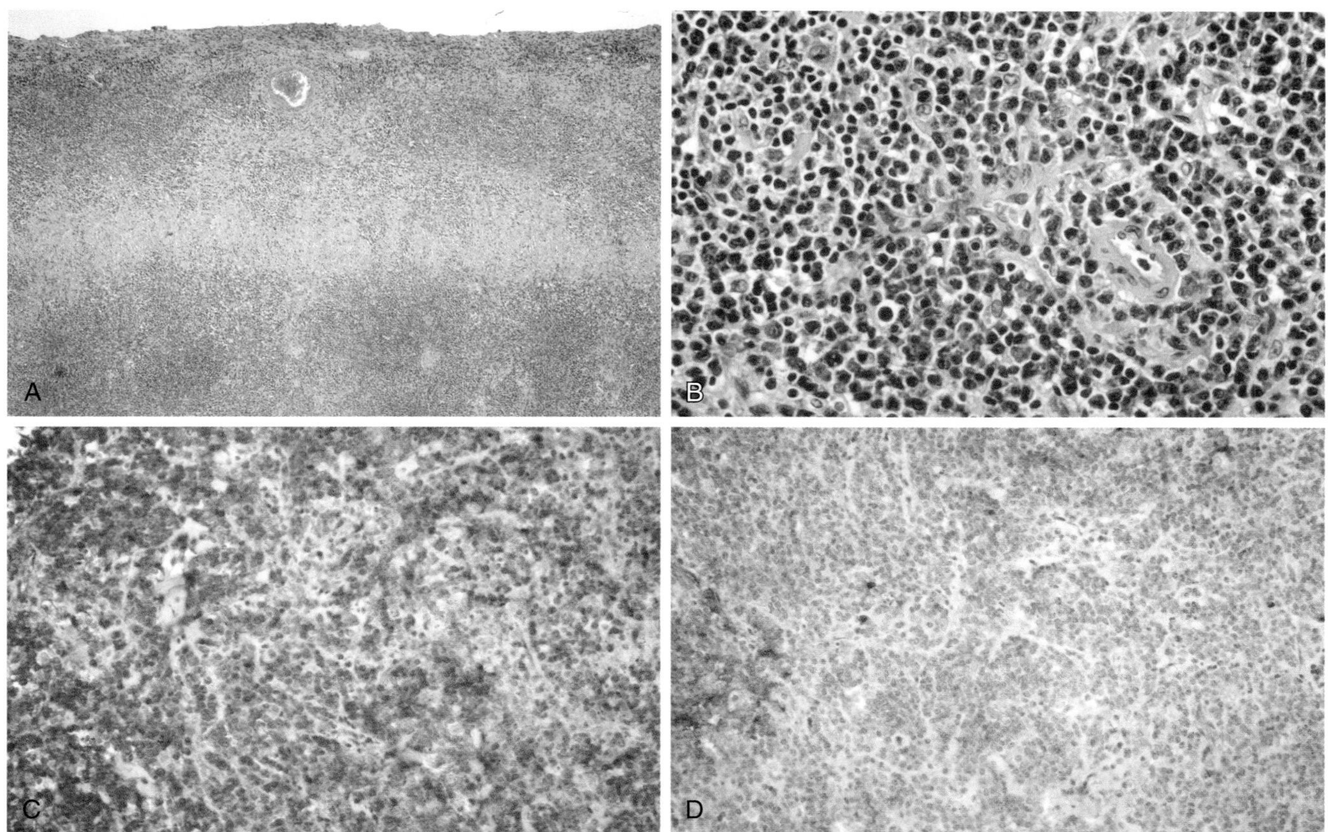

Figure 62-2. Marginal zone lymphoma in the dura mater. A, The dura shows a dense lymphoid infiltrate. **B,** Higher power shows small lymphoid cells and aggregates of plasma cells. **C,** Plasma cells express monotypic cytoplasmic kappa light chain. **D,** Staining for cytoplasmic lambda light chain is negative (**C** and **D**, immunoperoxidase technique on paraffin sections).

constitute 10% of orbital mass lesions, and lymphoma is the most common orbital malignancy.[45] Lymphomas in this site affect predominantly older women (male-to-female ratio of 3:4), with a median age in the 60s.[47] Children are only rarely affected.[47] Occasionally patients have a history of an autoimmune disorder,[47] another malignancy,[48] HIV infection,[49] or contact lens wear.[50] Recently, an association between some ocular adnexal lymphomas and *Chlamydia psittaci* infection has been identified; in a subset of patients harboring *C. psittaci*, their lymphomas responded to antibiotic therapy.[51]

Patients present with proptosis, ptosis, a palpable or visible mass, diplopia, tearing, or discomfort.[47] Systemic symptoms are rare. Conjunctival lymphoma usually produces a salmon-colored plaque that is mobile over the surface of the eye. The orbital soft tissue is involved in the majority of cases, sometimes accompanied by lacrimal gland involvement; the conjunctiva is involved in up to approximately one third of cases.[47] In 10% to 25% of cases there is bilateral involvement.[47,52,53]

Pathologic Features

Lymphomas of all types can present with ocular adnexal involvement, but most (60% to 75%) are marginal zone B-cell lymphoma.[47,54] Most of the remainder are follicular lymphoma, followed by DLBCL. Rare cases of chronic lymphocytic leukemia, mantle cell lymphoma, Burkitt's lymphoma, and precursor B-lymphoblastic lymphoma present with ocular adnexal involvement.[47] The few primary ocular adnexal lymphomas encountered in children or in HIV$^+$ patients are usually high-grade B-cell lymphomas, either DLBCL or Burkitt's lymphoma.[55,56] Rare cases of T-cell lymphoma and natural killer (NK)–cell lymphoma[47] have ocular adnexal involvement at presentation.

The immunophenotypic and genetic features are generally similar to those of the same lymphomas arising elsewhere, although ocular adnexal lymphomas show a tendency for site-specific genetic changes. Approximately one quarter of ocular adnexal marginal zone lymphomas harbor t(14;18)(q32;q21), a translocation involving the immunoglobulin heavy-chain gene and the *MALT1* gene; this translocation has also been found in marginal zone lymphomas arising in the liver, skin, and salivary glands but is rare in marginal zone lymphomas at other sites. Conversely, t(11;18)(q21;q21), a translocation involving the *API2* and *MALT1* genes, is relatively common in gastric and pulmonary marginal zone lymphoma but is only rarely encountered in the ocular adnexa.[57] In patients with bilateral ocular adnexal lymphoma, the morphologic, immunophenotypic, and molecular genetic features are reportedly identical, consistent with a single neoplastic clone involving both sites, rather than two distinct, unrelated primary tumors.[49,50]

Staging, Treatment, and Outcome

Approximately 80% of patients have disease confined to the ocular adnexa, unilaterally or bilaterally.[48,53,58] In some studies marginal zone lymphoma was more likely than other lymphoma types to present with stage I disease.[59] Localized low-grade lymphomas are usually treated with radiation. Cases of high-grade lymphomas, whether localized or widespread, are usually treated more aggressively.[53] Radiation therapy achieves excellent local control of disease, and freedom from local recurrence is close to 100%.[59] The overall prognosis of ocular adnexal lymphoma is good. Overall survival at 5 years is approximately 90%, and the 5-year disease-free survival is approximately 70%.[53,58,59] When relapses occur, they may be in lymph nodes, the opposite orbit, or other extranodal sites.[53]

Patients who present with disease localized to the ocular adnexa have a much better prognosis than those with more widespread disease.[44,49,60] However, isolated bilateral ocular adnexal disease does not have a worse prognosis than unilateral disease.[53,61] The histologic type of lymphoma is also important in defining outcome. In most reports, patients with high-grade lymphoma have a worse outcome.[58,60,62,63]

Differential Diagnosis

Because most ocular adnexal lymphomas are low-grade lymphomas, the main differential diagnosis is a reactive process, including inflammatory pseudotumor and reactive lymphoid hyperplasia. Inflammatory pseudotumor is a lesion, although relapses may occur at sites other than the eye, with a variably cellular, polymorphic infiltrate of small lymphocytes, plasma cells, immunoblasts, histiocytes, and sometimes eosinophils or neutrophils, in a stroma with areas that are hyalinized or edematous, or both. Vascularity can be prominent, and endothelial cells may appear hyperplastic. Immunohistochemical studies in such cases show a mixture of T cells, B cells, and polytypic plasma cells. In some cases the plasma cells are predominantly IgG4$^+$, suggesting that some inflammatory pseudotumors may be part of the spectrum of IgG4$^+$ sclerosing disease. Rare cases of lymphoma arising in a background of IgG4$^+$ inflammatory pseudotumor have been described, emphasizing the importance of careful histologic and immunophenotypic study of orbital inflammatory pseudotumors.[64] Reactive lymphoid hyperplasia usually consists of follicular hyperplasia without a prominent diffuse lymphoid proliferation and without cytologic atypia. A dense, diffuse infiltrate composed predominantly of B cells favors a diagnosis of lymphoma. Such lesions usually express monotypic immunoglobulin and contain clonal B cells on molecular genetic analysis.

WALDEYER'S RING

Waldeyer's ring is the circle of lymphoid tissue guarding the entrance to the alimentary and respiratory tracts. It consists of the faucial or palatine tonsils, the nasopharynx, and the base of the tongue. Waldeyer's ring is the primary site for 5% to 10% of all non-Hodgkin's lymphomas. More than half of all non-Hodgkin's lymphomas primary in the head and neck arise in Waldeyer's ring.[65]

Clinical Features

Most patients are adults, with a median age in the 50s and a male-to-female ratio of 1:1 to 1:1.5.[65-67] Children may also develop lymphomas in this site.[68] A few patients are HIV$^+$ or iatrogenically immunosuppressed. Patients present with dysphagia, dyspnea, snoring, or a neck mass due to cervical lymphadenopathy. A minority of patients have systemic symptoms.[66,68,69]

The tonsil is the most frequently involved site, accounting for more than half of Waldeyer's ring lymphomas, followed by the nasopharynx and base of the tongue.[65-67,70] Physical examination reveals a mass that is unilateral and exophytic in most cases and may be polypoid, fungating, or ulcerated. The lymphoma is localized (stage I or II) in approximately three quarters of cases; stage II disease, with cervical lymph node involvement, is more common than stage I.[66,67]

Pathologic Features

Sixty percent to 84% of cases are DLBCL (Fig. 62-3). Other types are uncommon; they include follicular lymphoma, Burkitt's lymphoma, mantle cell lymphoma, marginal zone B-cell lymphoma, and peripheral T-cell lymphoma.[65-67,70] Mantle cell lymphoma can present with involvement of Waldeyer's ring, but in contrast to DLBCL, mantle cell lymphoma is usually widespread at the time of diagnosis. Among children with Waldeyer's ring lymphoma, Burkitt's lymphoma is much more frequent than it is among adults (Fig. 62-4).[68] The lymphoepithelioid cell type of peripheral T-cell lymphoma, not otherwise specified (Lennert's lymphoma), has a

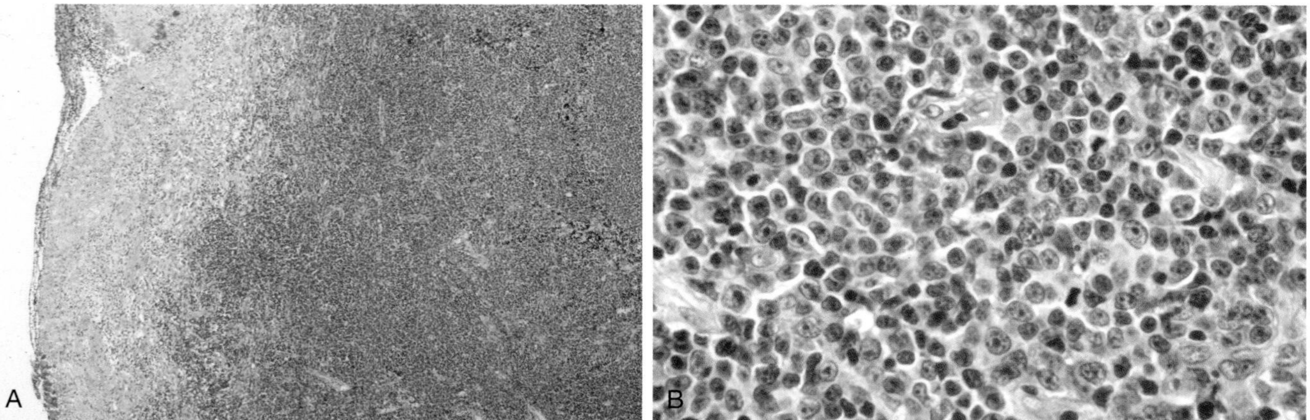

Figure 62-3. Diffuse large B-cell lymphoma in the nasopharynx. A, The surface of the tissue is necrotic. The rest of the tissue is replaced by a dense lymphoid infiltrate. **B,** Higher power reveals a predominance of immunoblasts.

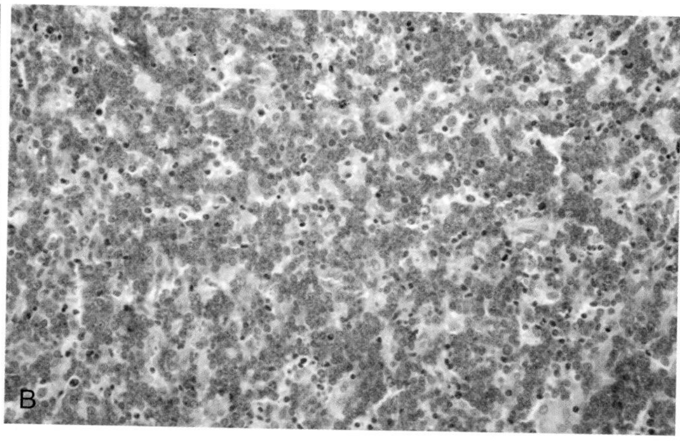

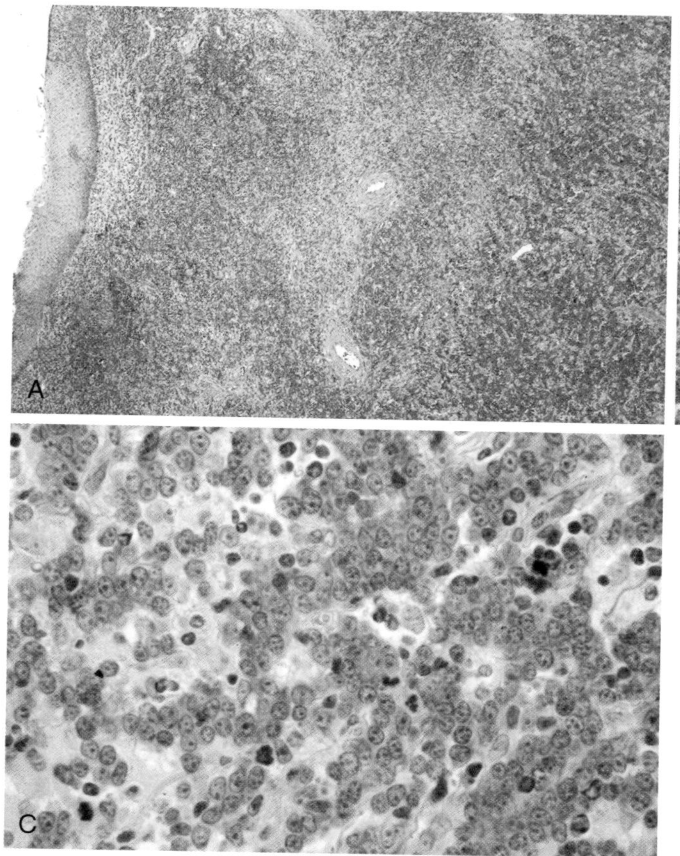

Figure 62-4. Burkitt's lymphoma in the tonsil of a child. A, A dense lymphoid infiltrate is seen beneath intact squamous epithelium. Normal crypt architecture has been obliterated. **B,** Medium power shows a striking "starry sky" pattern. **C,** High power shows uniform medium-sized round cells with finely stippled chromatin and small nucleoli, numerous mitotic figures, and many admixed tingible body macrophages.

predilection for Waldeyer's ring. These lymphomas have pathologic features similar to those seen in other sites.

Hodgkin's lymphoma, almost always of the classical type, occasionally presents with involvement of Waldeyer's ring. In most cases staging reveals Hodgkin's lymphoma involving other sites as well. In one study, among those cases confined to Waldeyer's ring, lymphocyte-rich classical Hodgkin's lymphoma was the most common type.[71] The presence of EBV may be more prevalent in Hodgkin's disease in this anatomic site than elsewhere, possibly because Waldeyer's ring is a reservoir for EBV.[71,72]

Treatment and Outcome

Patients respond well to therapy, with a high proportion achieving complete remission. However, there is a high rate of distant relapse, particularly in those treated with radiation alone. Although relapses may occur in any lymph node and in a variety of extranodal sites, there is a predilection for spread to the gastrointestinal tract. A better prognosis is associated with a tonsillar primary tumor, favorable International Prognostic Index, localized disease, and, among stage II patients, cervical lymphadenopathy that is unilateral and nonbulky.[65-67]

Differential Diagnosis

Reactive lymphoid hyperplasia often causes enlargement of one or more of the components of Waldeyer's ring, sometimes forming mass lesions mimicking a neoplasm. Preservation of reactive follicles and crypts favors a reactive process. Infectious mononucleosis due to acute EBV infection can mimic DLBCL or classical Hodgkin's lymphoma, but some architectural preservation, polymorphic composition, positive in situ hybridization for EBER, and clinical features (particularly age) can be helpful in the differential diagnosis. Before making a diagnosis of DLBCL or classical Hodgkin's lymphoma in Waldeyer's ring in a child or adolescent, evalutation for evidence of acute EBV infection is essential. Infiltration of crypt epithelium by lymphoid cells is normal and does not suggest mucosa-associated lympohid tissue (MALT) lymphoma. Reactive hyperplasia with monotypic immunoglobulin light-chain expression in plasma cells that are polyclonal by molecular genetic analysis has been reported in Waldeyer's ring in children, representing a pitfall in the diagnosis of MALT lymphoma in this site.[73] The pleomorphic variant of mantle cell lymphoma may mimic DLBCL, and assessment for CD5 and cyclin D1 expression should be considered in cases of what appear to be DLBCL in this area. Undifferentiated nasopharyngeal carcinoma and large B-cell lymphoma may be difficult to distinguish on routine sections, but immunophenotyping readily establishes a diagnosis.

NASAL CAVITY AND PARANASAL SINUSES

Among malignancies arising in the sinonasal area, lymphomas are second in frequency only to squamous cell carcinoma.[74] Sinonasal lymphomas account for 0.2% to 2% of all lymphomas[75] and less than 5% of extranodal lymphomas.[70] The incidence of lymphomas in this anatomic site is higher in Asia and South America.[76,77] Two main types of lymphoma are found in the sinonasal tract: DLBCL and extranodal NK/T-cell lymphoma. Lymphomas that arise in paranasal sinuses are almost always DLBCL, and the majority of lymphomas arising in the nasal cavity are extranodal NK/T-cell lymphomas.[77-80] Extranodal NK/T-cell lymphoma is discussed in Chapter 28. Other types of sinonasal lymphoma are discussed here.

Clinical Features

Paranasal sinus lymphomas affect men more often than women (male-to-female ratio 1.5:1 to 2:1). They affect predominantly middle-aged to older adults[75,78] and occasionally children.[81] A few patients have been HIV$^+$ or iatrogenically immunosuppressed.[78,82,83] Symptoms include nasal obstruction or discharge, facial swelling, pain or numbness, epistaxis, sinus pressure, toothache, or headache. The lymphoma may invade adjacent structures such as the orbit, base of the skull, CNS, pterygopalatine fossa, nasopharnyx, and palate.[81,82,84] Such patients may present with neurologic abnormalities, proptosis, diplopia, decreased visual acuity, and even blindness.[75,76,78,81,82,85-87] Patients occasionally have fever and night sweats.[78,82] Among the paranasal sinuses, the maxillary sinus is the most common site of involvement, followed by the ethmoid sinus, sphenoid sinus, and frontal sinus. Frequently, multiple sinuses are involved concurrently.[75,78,81,82,88] These lymphomas are often associated with destruction of adjacent bone.

Pathologic Features

In Western countries the most common lymphoma is DLBCL, followed by extranodal NK/T-cell lymphoma. Other types are infrequent or rare, but Burkitt's lymphoma, follicular lymphoma,[76,81,82,86,88] marginal zone lymphoma,[78] peripheral T-cell lymphoma, not otherwise specified, and adult T-cell leukemia/lymphoma[78,87] presenting with sinus involvement have been described. The lymphomas in HIV$^+$ patients are DLBCL and Burkitt's lymphoma.[82] Those in children are most often Burkitt's lymphoma, followed by DLBCL.[78,89] Immunophenotypic features are similar to those seen in other sites. The proportion of sinonasal B-cell lymphomas containing EBV varies among different series[77,86,90]; in a study performed at Massachusetts General Hospital, EBV was encountered only in DLBCLs in patients with underlying immunodeficiencies.[78]

Staging, Treatment, and Outcome

The majority of cases are localized at presentation. In one series, 71% of lymphomas of all types were stage I, 8% stage II, 2% stage III, and 18% stage IV.[78] Patients with stage IV disease may have involvement of CNS, lung, bone, kidney, or gastrointestinal tract.[81,82] Most patients receive radiation and chemotherapy. Some authorities recommend prophylactic treatment of the CNS to achieve long-term disease-free survival.[91] When the lymphomas relapse or progress, they frequently involve lymph nodes and may also involve a variety of extranodal sites, including the CNS, lung, bone, ovary, testis, marrow, liver, spleen, and skin.[75,79,84,86] Results of follow-up vary widely, with 5-year survival ranging from 29%[86] to 80%[88] in different series of paranasal lymphoma patients treated with combined-modality therapy.

Differential Diagnosis

DLBCL and extranodal NK/T-cell lymphoma may be difficult to distinguish on routine sections. Angioinvasion and angiocentric localization, prominent necrosis, epitheliotropism, and pseudoepitheliomatous hyperplasia favor NK/T-cell lymphoma. DLBCL more commonly arises in paranasal sinuses, whereas nasal localization and midfacial destructive disease favor the NK/T-cell type.[78,88,92] Most DLBCLs are composed of a diffuse proliferation of large cells; therefore, any other cellular composition with a diffuse pattern, especially a mixture of small and large cells or medium-sized cells, should raise the question of NK/T-cell lymphoma.[92] B-cell and NK/T-cell lymphomas can be distinguished easily with immunophenotyping. Absence of EBV tends to exclude NK/T-cell lymphoma.

SALIVARY GLAND

Clinical Features

Lymphomas account for 2% to 5% of salivary gland malignancies.[21,93] The lymphomas arise in the parotid in at least 70% of cases, in the submaxillary gland in 15% to 25% of cases, and in the sublingual and minor salivary glands in less than 10% of cases. Almost all patients are older than 50 years, with a slight female preponderance. Patients present with an enlarging mass that is usually painless but is occasionally accompanied by facial nerve paralysis or cervical lymphadenopathy. Underlying Sjögren's syndrome, lymphoepithelial sialadenitis, or rheumatoid arthritis is common.[21,93,94]

Pathologic Features

Extranodal marginal zone B-cell lymphoma of MALT (see Chapter 18) and DLBCL account for nearly all lymphomas arising in the salivary glands and occur in roughly equal numbers. MALT lymphoma is the most common type that arises in salivary gland parenchyma. The lymphomas in patients with Sjögren's syndrome are mostly MALT type. MALT lymphoma affects predominantly females, in accordance with the greater incidence of Sjögren's syndrome in women. MALT lymphoma often arises in a background of lymphoepithelial sialadenitis with lymphoepithelial lesions. In contrast to lymphoepithelial sialadenitis without lymphoma, the lymphoepithelial lesions in MALT lymphoma are surrounded by large halos and broad, intersecting strands and sheets of monocytoid B cells, distorting and obliterating the salivary gland parenchyma. Also present are scattered reactive follicles and plasma cells, sometimes in large aggregates. In salivary glands other than the parotid, lymphoepithelial lesions may be less conspicuous, but the histologic features are otherwise similar. Follicular lymphoma may also arise in the salivary gland region but usually involves lymph nodes in the vicinity rather than salivary gland parenchyma. The pathologic features are similar to those of other nodal follicular lymphomas (see Chapter 17). At least some cases of DLBCL most likely represent large cell transformation of an underlying marginal zone lymphoma or follicular lymphoma.[21,93,94] Rare cases of Burkitt's lymphoma,[93] peripheral T-cell lymphoma, unspecified type, anaplastic large cell lymphoma, and extranodal NK/T-cell lymphoma have also been reported.[95]

Staging, Treatment, and Outcome

The majority of patients with salivary gland lymphoma present with localized disease. Patients with marginal zone lymphoma can develop extrasalivary disease in lymph nodes or in other

MALT sites. In a minority of cases the lymphoma undergoes cell transformation to DLBCL, which may behave in an aggressive manner.[21,93,94]

Differential Diagnosis

In the differential diagnosis of marginal zone lymphoma and lymphoepithelial sialadenitis, extensive monocytoid B-cell proliferation outside lymphoepithelial lesions and extensive glandular obliteration favor lymphoma. Monocytoid B cells confined to lymphoepithelial lesions and even discrete halos around such lesions can be seen in lymphoepithelial sialadenitis, but broad, intersecting bands of monocytoid B cells support a diagnosis of lymphoma. Demonstration of monotypic immunoglobulin in lymphoid cells or plasma cells supports lymphoma. Molecular genetic studies are usually not helpful because B-cell clones are found in more than 50% of cases of lymphoepithelial sialadenitis.[96] HIV-associated cystic lymphoid hyperplasia involves lymph nodes, is often bilateral, and typically consists of multiple dilated ducts surrounded by floridly hyperplastic follicles with attenuated mantles. Lymphoepithelial lesions are not conspicuous, although large numbers of lymphoid cells may be found within the epithelium of dilated ducts. The differential diagnosis may also include chronic sclerosing sialadenitis (Kuttner's tumor), which typically involves submandibular glands. These patients may have dry mouth and may carry a clinical diagnosis of Sjögren's syndrome. Chronic sclerosing sialadenitis may have prominent follicular hyperplasia and a dense lymphoid infiltrate with numerous plasma cells, but lymphoepithelial lesions are not seen, and there is typically band-like sclerosis. In a proportion of the cases, there is an excess of IgG4-containing plasma cells, suggesting a relationship to other IgG4-mediated diseases such as autoimmune pancreatitis.[97]

ORAL CAVITY

Clinical Features

Approximately 2% of all extranodal lymphomas arise in the oral cavity (palate, gingiva, tongue, buccal mucosa, floor of the mouth, lips).[46,98] Lymphoma arising in the bones of the jaw may invade adjacent soft tissues and present as an oral cavity lesion.[99] Most patients are immunocompetent, middle-aged to older adults, with a median age in the sixth or seventh decade; there is a slight male preponderance.[98-102] In recent years there has been an increase in lymphomas of the oral cavity because of the tendency for patients with HIV infection to develop lymphoma in this site.[100,101,103] Almost all HIV-infected patients are younger males, with an approximate median age of 40 years.[100,103,104] Oral lymphomas have also been rarely reported in transplant recipients.[101]

Patients present with soft tissue swelling, pain, mucosal ulceration or discoloration, paresthesias, anesthesia, and loosening of teeth.[99,101,103,105,106] The sites most often affected, in both HIV$^+$ and HIV$^-$ patients, are the palate, maxilla, and gingiva, with the tongue, buccal mucosa, floor of the mouth, and lips affected less often.[98-100,103,104] Physical examination reveals an exophytic, often polypoid mass in the majority of cases. In a minority of cases the lymphoma is an infiltrative, ulcerated lesion with raised margins.[98]

Pathologic Features

A wide variety of lymphomas arise in the oral cavity. Among nonimmunosuppressed patients, approximately half are DLBCL. The next most common type is follicular lymphoma (Fig. 62-5), followed by marginal zone (MALT) lymphoma, mantle cell lymphoma, peripheral T-cell lymphoma, not otherwise specified, extranodal NK/T-cell lymphoma, Burkitt's lymphoma, and others.[99,100,102] MALT lymphomas may arise in minor salivary glands. Follicular lymphoma has a predilection to involve the palate.[101] Mycosis fungoides occasionally involves the oral cavity; the majority of these cases are found in the setting of long-standing, advanced disease, but in exceptional cases the first manifestation of mycosis fungoides is in the oral cavity. It has been suggested that the uncommon aggressive epidermotropic CD8$^+$ cutaneous T-cell lymphoma is more likely to involve the oral cavity than the more common mycosis fungoides type.[107,108]

Oral lymphomas in HIV-infected individuals are less heterogeneous than those found in the general population; they are almost all high-grade lymphomas. Most are DLBCL, with occasional peripheral T-cell lymphoma, unspecified, and

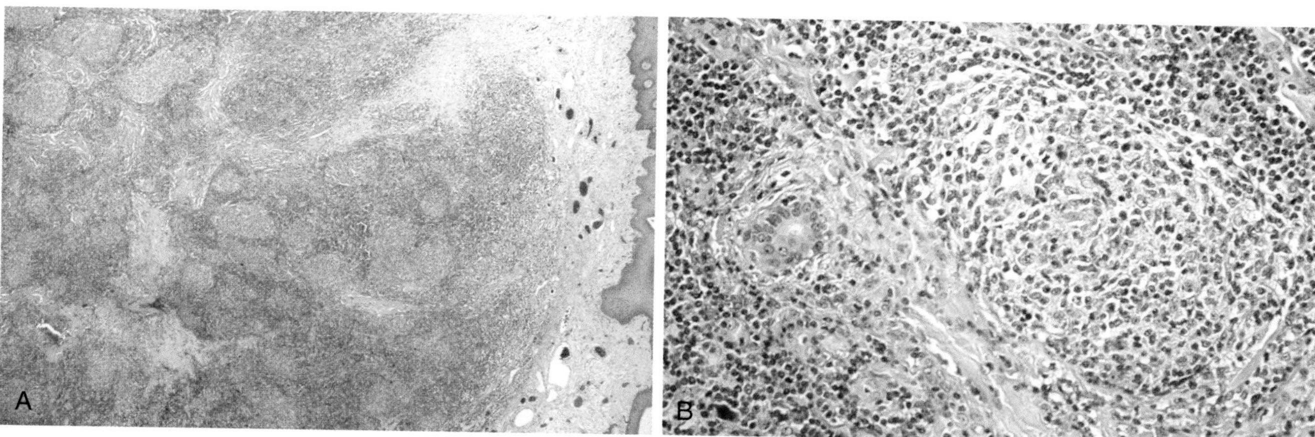

Figure 62-5. Follicular lymphoma in the oral cavity. This lymphoma was a relapse from an orbital primary tumor. **A,** Low power shows crowded follicles within soft tissue beneath squamous epithelium. **B,** Poorly circumscribed neoplastic follicles contain predominantly centrocytes and are seen adjacent to small acini of minor salivary gland.

a few cases of Burkitt's lymphoma and anaplastic large cell lymphoma.[21,100,101,103,104] Plasmablastic lymphoma is a distinctive subset of HIV-associated DLBCL that often occurs in the oral cavity; it is composed of cells with the appearance of immunoblasts or plasmablasts with vesicular nuclei, prominent nucleoli, abundant eccentrically placed cytoplasm with a paranuclear hof, high mitotic rate, frequent single-cell necrosis, and scattered tingible body macrophages. The immunophenotype is distinctive: neoplastic cells usually lack both leukocyte common antigen (CD45) and CD20, although they are usually CD138$^+$, IRF4/MUM-1$^+$, and CD79a$^+$; often contain cytoplasmic immunoglobulin; and show clonal immunoglobulin heavy-chain gene rearrangement, confirming their B lineage.[104,109]

The majority of HIV-associated oral lymphomas, both B- and T-cell types, including plasmablastic lymphoma, contain EBV.[100,101,103,104] In contrast, only about 9% of oral lymphomas in nonimmunosuppressed patients are EBER$^+$.[100,101] EBV may play a role in the pathogenesis of the majority of HIV-associated lymphomas, but it is not a major factor in the pathogenesis of oral lymphoma in the general population.

Staging, Treatment, and Outcome

Staging reveals localized disease in approximately 70% of cases.[99,104] The proportion with localized and disseminated disease is similar in HIV$^+$ and HIV$^-$ patients. Outcome depends on stage, type of lymphoma, and HIV status. Patients with localized, histologically low-grade lymphomas have an excellent outcome, whereas patients with high-grade lymphoma or disseminated disease have significantly worse survival rates.[21,99,106] AIDS patients have a very poor prognosis; 75% of patients die within 18 months of the diagnosis of lymphoma, although other HIV-associated illnesses may contribute to their deaths.[99,104]

Differential Diagnosis

The most important diagnostic pitfall is failing to consider lymphoma during the physical examination. Oral lymphomas can mimic dental conditions such as periodontal disease, acute necrotizing gingivitis, and dental infections.[103,105] The appearance of some lesions suggests carcinoma.[99] In HIV$^+$ patients, Kaposi's sarcoma, deep fungal infections, and HIV-associated periodontal disease also enter the differential diagnosis.[103]

THYROID

Clinical Features

Primary lymphomas of the thyroid are uncommon and have distinctive clinical and pathologic features. They account for 1% to 5% of all thyroid malignancies and 1% to 2.5% of all lymphomas.[110] Patients have a wide age range, but most are older adults with a median age between 60 and 70 years. There is a striking female preponderance.[110-113] Almost all patients have evidence of Hashimoto's thyroiditis. Patients with Hashimoto's thyroiditis have an estimated 40- to 80-fold increased risk for lymphomas compared with individuals without this disorder.[111] Patients complain of the presence of a mass, sometimes described as rapidly enlarging. They may also have dysphagia, cough, dyspnea, and hoarseness.The lesion may result in tracheal compression.[110-113]

Pathologic Features

On gross examination the tumors range from 0.5 to 19 cm (mean, 7 cm) and form multinodular or diffuse, firm or soft masses with smooth, pale tan or white-gray surfaces on sectioning.[111] DLBCL is the most common type, accounting for 50% to more than 90% of cases. Extranodal marginal zone (MALT) lymphoma is the next most common type, accounting for 10% to 28% of cases. In approximately half of the cases of DLBCL there is a component of MALT lymphoma, consistent with transformation of an underlying low-grade lymphoma. All other types of lymphoma are quite uncommon; among those reported are Burkitt's lymphoma, follicular lymphoma, and rare peripheral T-cell lymphomas, including anaplastic large cell lymphoma.[110-113]

The histologic features of these lymphomas are similar to those seen in other sites, although thyroidal MALT lymphoma has some distinctive characteristics. Tumors often contain a characteristic type of lymphoepithelial lesion consisting of round aggregates of marginal zone cells filling and expanding the lumens of thyroid follicles—so-called MALT-ball lymphoepithelial lesions.[111] Follicular colonization tends to be prominent, in some cases resulting in a follicular architecture so striking that it mimics follicular lymphoma. Blast transformation of neoplastic cells within colonized follicles is more common in the thyroid than elsewhere.[114] Changes of Hashimoto's thyroiditis are often seen adjacent to the lymphoma (Fig. 62-6).[111] The immunophenotypic features are similar to those seen in other sites. Recently, three of six marginal zone lymphomas of the thyroid were found to have a previously undescribed translocation involving the genes for FOXP1 and IGH ([3;14][p14.1;q32]) that results in upregulation of FOXP1 and could play a role in the pathogenesis of marginal zone lymphoma.[115]

Staging, Treatment, and Outcome

The majority of patients have localized disease at presentation; 50% to 70% of patients have stage I disease, and most of the remainder have stage II disease, usually with cervical or perithyroidal lymph node involvement. A minority of patients have more widespread nodal and extranodal involvement. Extranodal sites that may be involved include the bone marrow, gastrointestinal tract, lung, liver, and bladder.[111-113] MALT lymphomas are almost always localized (stage I or II). Stage III and IV lymphomas are usually DLBCL.[110-113]

Treatment has not been uniform. Some patients with marginal zone lymphoma have been treated with surgery alone; others have also received radiation or chemotherapy, or both.[110,111] The 5-year disease-specific survival of thyroid lymphoma patients ranges from 46% to 79%. Patients with marginal zone lymphoma and patients with stage I disease, regardless of histologic type, have an excellent prognosis. The outcome is less favorable for those with higher-stage disease or large B-cell lymphoma.[110,111,113]

Differential Diagnosis

Both Hashimoto's thyroiditis and MALT lymphoma have reactive lymphoid follicles and lymphoepithelial lesions, but obliteration of thyroid parenchyma by a diffuse infiltrate of marginal zone B cells and lymphoid or plasma cells expressing monotypic immunoglobulin favor marginal zone lymphoma. Lymphoepithelial lesions are larger and much

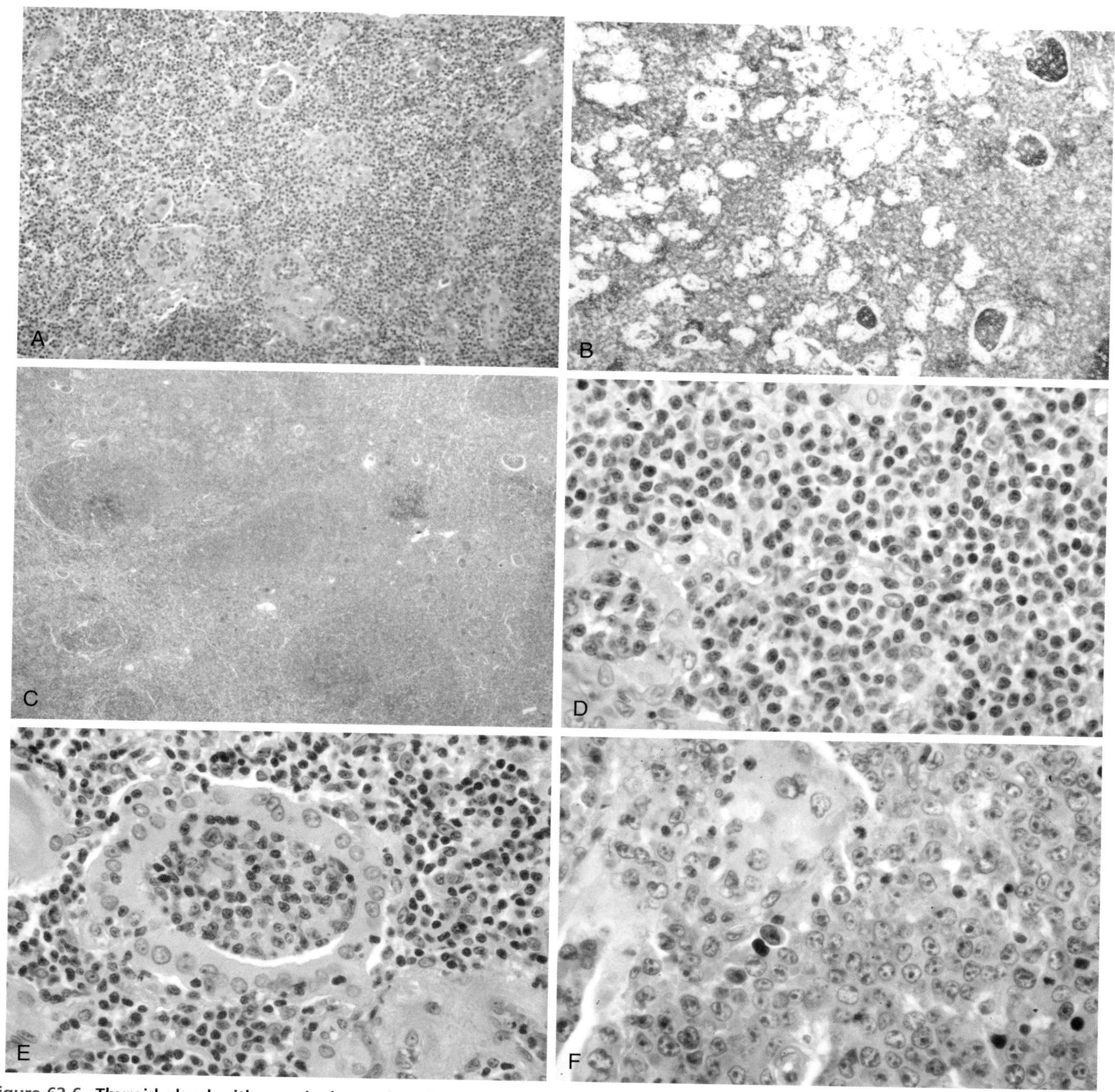

Figure 62-6. Thyroid gland with marginal zone lymphoma (A to E) with large cell transformation (F). Other areas showed Hashimoto's thyroiditis. **A**, Low power shows obliteration of the normal parenchyma. **B**, CD20 stain highlights the diffuse infiltrate of B cells; several rounded lymphoepithelial lesions are seen (immunoperoxidase technique on paraffin section). **C**, In some areas there is vague nodularity, consistent with colonization of reactive follicles by neoplastic marginal zone cells. **D**, The marginal zone cells are small, with oval to slightly irregular nuclei and a moderate amount of pale cytoplasm. **E**, MALT-ball lymphoepithelial lesion. The epithelium of the thyroid follicle shows oxyphil change. **F**, An area of large cell transformation. Many of the neoplastic cells are immunoblasts.

more numerous in MALT lymphoma. A number of cases of extramedullary plasmacytoma arising in the thyroid have been described; it is likely that at least some of these represent MALT lymphomas with marked plasmacytic differentiation. Reactive follicles; an extrafollicular component of B cells, particularly if they have the morphology of marginal zone cells; and lymphoepithelial lesions make plasmacytoma unlikely.[111,113] It may be difficult to distinguish undifferentiated carcinoma from DLBCL on routine sections, but a diagnosis can be established using immunohistochemical studies.

LARYNX

Clinical Features

Primary laryngeal lymphomas are rare, accounting for less than 1% of laryngeal neoplasms.[116] Patients are mostly middle-aged to older adults, with a few young adults and children also affected. There is a slight male preponderance.[21,116-120] Several patients have had concurrent laryngeal squamous cell carcinoma or other malignancies.[118,119] Rare patients are HIV⁺ or have another underlying immunodeficiency.[21,120,121]

Patients present with hoarseness, dyspnea, progressive or acute laryngeal obstruction, sore throat, foreign body sensation, or dysphagia.[21,116,118,119] The tumors are usually smooth-surfaced, submucosal, raised, often polypoid lesions.[118,120,122] Pedunculated tumors may prolapse into the airway.[119,120] Laryngeal lymphomas may arise from the lymphoid tissue found in the larynx, mainly in the epiglottis and supraglottic larynx, correlating with the distribution of lymphomas at this site.[122]

Pathologic Features

The two main types of laryngeal lymphomas are DLBCL and extranodal marginal zone (MALT) lymphoma, together accounting for approximately 80% of cases. Their pathologic features are similar to those found in other sites.[116-119,122,123] Rare cases of follicular lymphoma[116] and peripheral T-cell lymphoma,[118,124] several cases of extranodal NK/T-cell lymphoma,[120,124,125] and an EBV⁺ B-cell lymphoma in a boy with Wiskott-Aldrich syndrome[121] have been described.

Staging, Treatment, and Outcome

Information on staging is limited, but in approximately three quarters of cases there is Ann Arbor stage I disease; most of the remainder are stage II.[21,116,118-120,125] In a few cases of MALT lymphoma the larynx has been involved simultaneously with other extranodal sites in the head and neck.[21,126] Most patients with MALT lymphoma and DLBCL can be treated successfully with a combination of surgery and radiation or chemotherapy,[21,127] although laryngeal lymphoma sometimes results in sudden death due to acute airway obstruction.[122] When patients with MALT lymphoma develop relapses, they tend to be isolated extranodal tumors in the upper respiratory tract, stomach, orbit, or skin; even when relapses occur, there may be long disease-free intervals. This behavior is similar to that of MALT lymphoma in other sites.[21,118]

TRACHEA

Primary tracheal lymphomas are rare. Patients are mainly older adults, both men and women. Patients present with dyspnea, wheezing, stridor, or cough.[128,129] Rare patients are HIV⁺.[130] Examination reveals a nodular or polypoid tumor with a smooth or friable surface that narrows the tracheal lumen. Most of the few cases that have been characterized using newer lymphoma classifications were extranodal marginal zone MALT lymphoma. High-grade lymphomas have also been described. Patients usually respond well to treatment, and most are well on follow-up.[123,128,129,131]

LUNGS

Primary pulmonary lymphomas are traditionally defined as lymphomas presenting as pulmonary lesions with no clinical, pathologic, or radiographic evidence of lymphoma elsewhere in the past, at present, or for 3 months after presentation.[132,133] Some pathologists include cases in which staging reveals disease outside the lung, as long as pulmonary disease predominates.[134]

Clinical Features

Primary pulmonary lymphomas account for 0.3% of primary lung neoplasms,[133] less than 1% of all lymphomas,[135,136] and 3.6% of extranodal lymphomas.[133] Patients are typically adults, with a median age of about 60 years. It is very uncommon before age 30,[132,134-138] although rare cases in younger patients have been reported.[139,140] Most studies show a slight male predominance.[134-136] One third or more of patients are asymptomatic when the lymphoma is discovered. The remainder have pulmonary (cough, dyspnea, hemoptysis, chest pain) or constitutional symptoms. Virtually all asymptomatic patients have low-grade lymphomas.[132,134,137-139,141,142] Up to 29% of patients have an associated autoimmune disease,[138] most commonly Sjögren's syndrome.[134,135,138] A small number of patients are HIV⁺ men.[143] Lung allograft recipients may develop posttransplant lymphoproliferative disorders involving the lung.[135]

Radiologic Features and Patterns of Involvement

Patients have single or multiple, unilateral or bilateral lesions that take the form of nodules, masses, or infiltrates that may resemble consolidated lung. Air bronchograms are common.[132,134-138,141,142] Pulmonary lymphomas rarely show endobronchial or diffuse submucosal involvement.[135] Less than 10% of cases are associated with a pleural effusion.[132,134]

Pathologic Features

Approximately 70% of cases are extranodal marginal zone (MALT) lymphoma,[132,134,135,139] with features similar to those seen in other anatomic sites. In the lung the lymphoma spreads in a diffuse and interstitial pattern. Most cases have interspersed intact or disrupted reactive lymphoid follicles, and nearly all cases have lymphoepithelial lesions formed with bronchial or bronchiolar epithelium (Fig. 62-7). Infiltration of the pleura is frequent.[134,138,144] Occasional cases are associated with amyloid deposition[137,138,144]; this seems to be more frequent in the lung than in other sites. Monoclonal paraproteins are relatively common,[132,134] being found in up to 43% of cases.[138] A translocation described only in MALT lymphomas, t(11;18)(q21;q21), results in *API2-MALT1* gene fusion; it is more common in pulmonary MALT lymphoma than at other sites.[57,145,146]

DLBCL is the next most common type of primary pulmonary lymphoma, accounting for approximately 20% of cases; however, many of them have a component of MALT lymphoma, consistent with large cell transformation of the low-grade lymphoma.[132,134,138,139,141] Other types of lymphoma are distinctly uncommon; those reported include follicular lymphoma,[134,137,139] Burkitt's lymphoma,[134] lymphomatoid granulomatosis[139] (see Chapter 23), peripheral T-cell lymphoma, unspecified,[134,139] anaplastic large cell lymphoma,[133] and rare cases of classical Hodgkin's lymphoma.[135] Among HIV⁺ patients, nearly all cases have been diffuse, high-grade, EBV⁺ B-cell lymphomas.[143,147]

Staging, Treatment, and Outcome

Staging may reveal lymphoma confined to the lungs or disease involving lymph nodes or other extranodal sites,

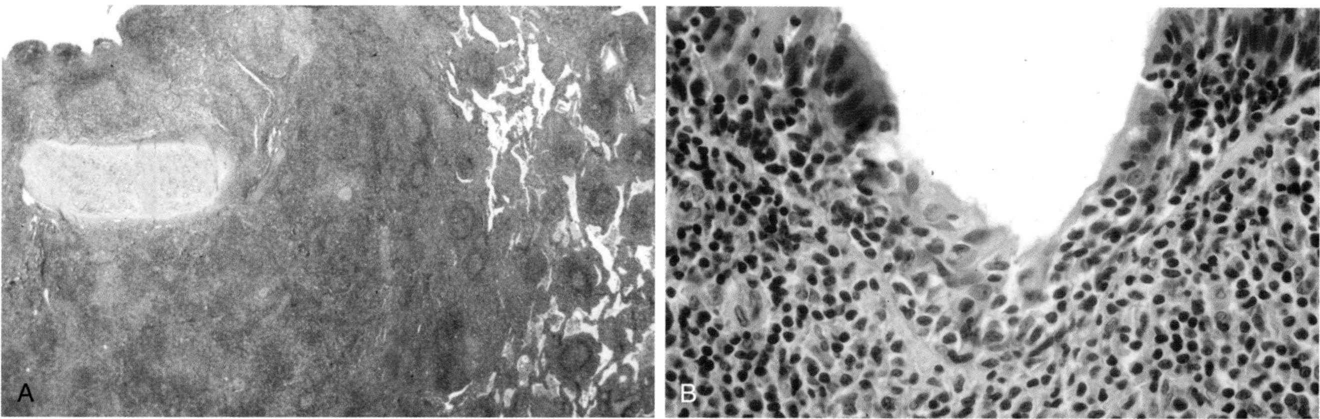

Figure 62-7. Marginal zone B-cell lymphoma in the lung. A, A dense, diffuse lymphoid infiltrate extends from the bronchial lumen (*upper left*), past the bronchial cartilage, into the surrounding lung. At the periphery there is an interstitial pattern. Reactive follicles are scattered evenly throughout the lymphoid infiltrate. **B,** Higher power shows bronchial epithelium with lymphoepithelial lesions.

especially those known to give rise to marginal zone lymphoma.[136,142] Patients with MALT lymphoma may develop relapses in the lung and at other MALT sites, especially the stomach and salivary glands, as well as in lymph nodes; some may undergo transformation to DLBCL. Overall, however, patients do well, and survival is good regardless of the therapy given.[132,134,135,138,139,142,144] The prognosis of pulmonary DLBCL is similar to[138,139] or somewhat worse than[132,134] that of pulmonary MALT lymphoma. The more aggressive therapy usually given to patients with these lymphomas could account for the lack of difference in outcome that some have observed.

Differential Diagnosis

The main problem is distinguishing MALT lymphoma from chronic inflammatory processes with lymphoid hyperplasia. In favor of lymphoma is a predominance of B cells with the morphology of marginal zone cells in a diffuse pattern outside follicles, CD43 coexpression by B cells, and monotypic immunoglobulin expression by lymphocytes or plasma cells. In favor of a reactive process is a mixture of B and T cells. Lymphoepithelial lesions occur frequently in lymphoid hyperplasia but less frequently than in marginal zone lymphoma, and the intraepithelial lymphocytes can be B or T cells, in contrast to the predominance of B cells seen in marginal zone lymphoma.[137]

PLEURA AND PLEURAL CAVITY

Lymphomas rarely arise primarily in the pleural cavity. Two distinctive types have been described: primary effusion lymphoma (see Chapter 55) and pyothorax-associated lymphoma (see Chapter 22).

THYMUS

Three types of non-Hodgkin's lymphomas arise in the thymus: mediastinal (primary thymic) large B-cell lymphoma (see Chapter 22), precursor T-lymphoblastic leukemia/lymphoma (see Chapter 41), and extranodal marginal zone B-cell MALT lymphoma (see Chapter 18). Thymic MALT lymphoma is a rare but distinctive subtype, which forms lymphoepithelial lesions with Hassall's corpuscles and usually expresses IgA (Fig. 62-8).[148]

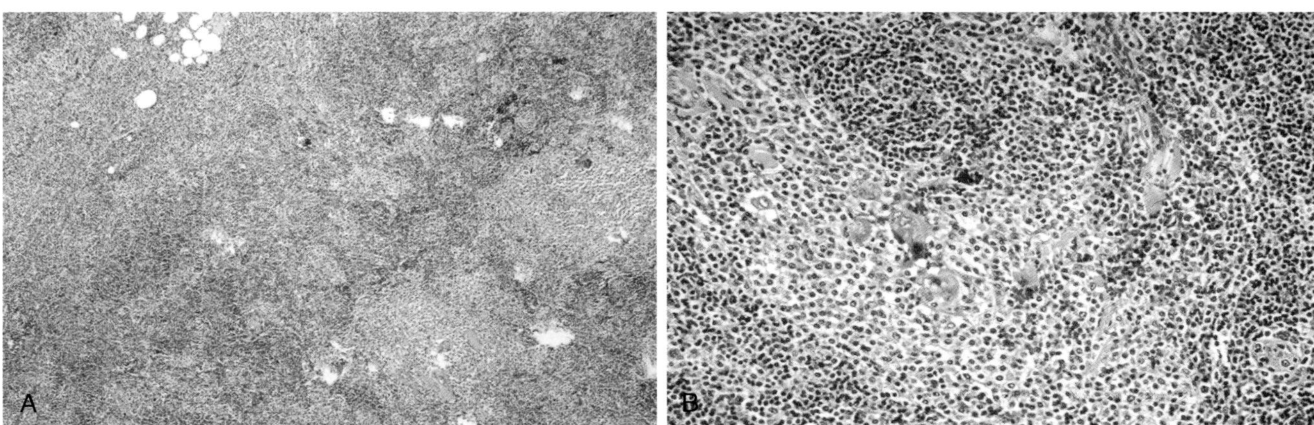

Figure 62-8. Marginal zone B-cell lymphoma in the thymus. A, The normal thymic tissue is obliterated by a mottled pale and dark lymphoid infiltrate. **B,** Pale areas correspond to aggregates of marginal zone cells, shown here surrounding and invading a Hassall's corpuscle.

HEART

Clinical Features

Primary cardiac lymphomas are defined as lymphomas predominantly or exclusively involving the heart.[149,150] Cardiac lymphomas are very rare. The heart only occasionally gives rise to tumors, and lymphomas account for only 1% to 2% of primary cardiac neoplasms.[149,151] A number of cardiac lymphomas have been reported in HIV⁺ patients, and a few cases have been described in renal or cardiac transplant recipients (Figs. 62-9 and 62-10).[152,153] Cardiac lymphomas occurring sporadically affect mainly older adults, with a slight male preponderance.[150-152,154,155] Those arising in HIV⁺ individuals affect a younger population with a more striking male preponderance.[152] Children rarely develop primary cardiac lymphoma.[156,157] Patients may present with chest pain, dyspnea, congestive heart failure, syncope, or arrhythmias.[150,152] Pericardial effusion, sometimes with tamponade, and pleural effusion are common. Complete atrioventricular block has been described.[158]

Lymphomas most often involve the myocardium; extension to valves is rare.[149] Lymphomas usually involve the right side of the heart. The left ventricle is occasionally involved, but involvement of the left atrium, the most common site of myxoma, is quite uncommon.[152] The tumor can be localized by echocardiogram, computed tomography scan, or magnetic resonance imaging. Transesophageal echocardiography is an especially sensitive technique for identifying these lesions.[159] Diagnosis may be based on an examination of biopsy specimens (open biopsy, endomyocardial biopsy, or percutaneous

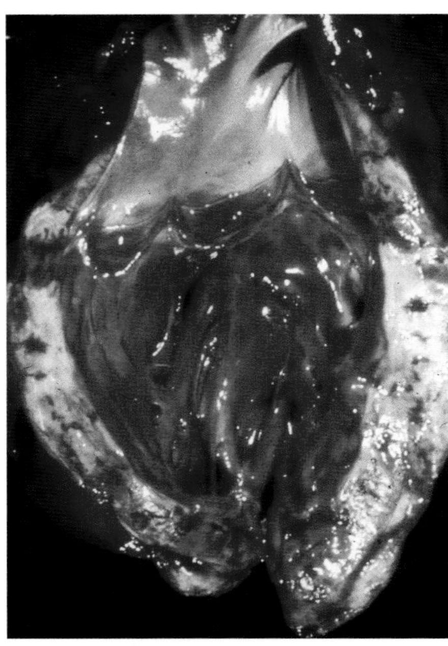

Figure 62-9. Cardiac lymphoma in a renal transplant recipient. Yellow tumor can be seen on cross section, replacing normal myocardium. (From Monaco AP, Harris NL. Case record of the Massachusetts General Hospital. Weekly clinicopathological exercises. Case 4-1985. A 36-year-old man with a cardiac mass three years after renal transplantation. *N Engl J Med*. 1985;312:226-237. Reprinted with permission. Copyright 1985 Massachusetts Medical Society. All rights reserved.)

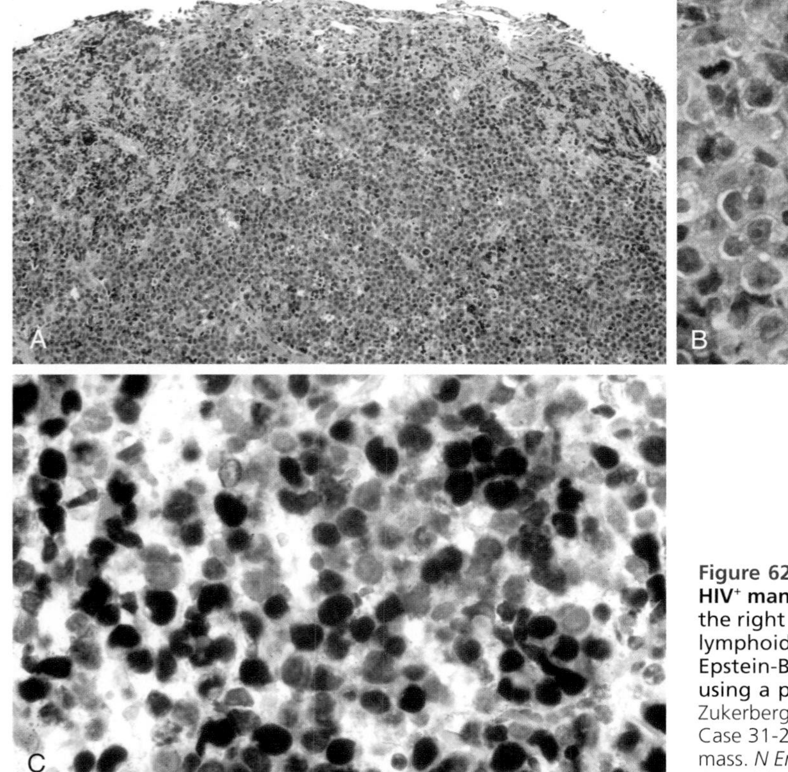

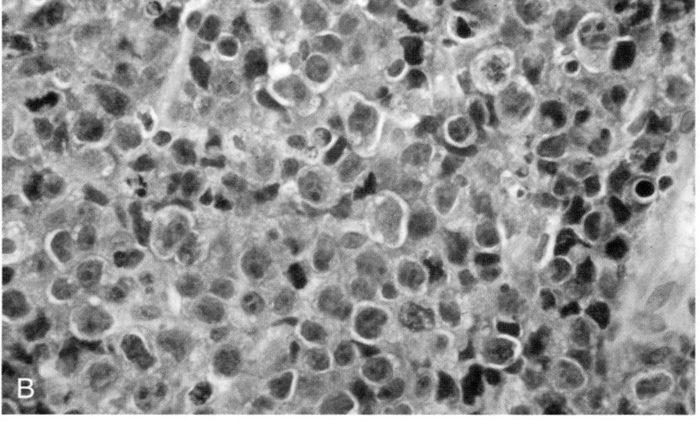

Figure 62-10. Diffuse large B-cell lymphoma in the heart of an HIV⁺ man. A, A dense lymphoid infiltrate forms a mass involving the right side of the heart. **B,** Higher power shows large atypical lymphoid cells with frequent mitoses. **C,** Neoplastic cells contain Epstein-Barr virus (in situ hybridization on a paraffin section using a probe for EBER). (From Kaplan LD, Afridi NA, Homvang G, Zukerberg LR. Case records of the Massachusetts General Hospital. Case 31-2003. A 44-year-old man with HIV infection and a right atrial mass. *N Engl J Med*. 2003;349:1369-1377. Reprinted with permission. Copyright 2003 Massachusetts Medical Society. All right reserved.)

biopsy with transesophageal echocardiographic imaging) or of pericardial fluid.[152,155,159,160] The prognosis has been poor because the diagnosis was often delayed (or made postmortem) and because chemotherapy could be accompanied by fatal arrhythmias.[150] Among cases reported more recently, however, the prognosis appears to be better because of earlier diagnosis and improvements in imaging and therapy, including careful monitoring of cardiac function at the beginning of therapy. Patients treated expeditiously with chemotherapy, with or without radiation therapy, may attain a sustained complete remission.[149,151,161]

Pathologic Features

The lymphomas are nearly exclusively DLBCL (see Fig. 62-10); their immunophenotypic features are similar to those seen in other sites.[150,152,158,160,161] B-lymphoblastic lymphoma and Burkitt's lymphoma have been described in children.[156,157] Genetic features have not been well studied.

Differential Diagnosis

Because of the rarity of cardiac lymphomas, the diagnosis is rarely suspected before biopsy (or, in some cases, autopsy). Clinically, it can mimic much more common nonneoplastic causes of cardiac dysfunction. Once a mass is identified radiographically, the combination of right-sided tumor and high lactate dehydrogenase levels, particularly in an immunocompromised patient, is suspicious for lymphoma.

BREAST

Clinical Features

Primary lymphomas of the breast are usually defined as lymphomas confined to one or both breasts, with or without ipsilateral axillary lymph node involvement but without evidence of disease elsewhere at presentation, in a patient without a prior history of lymphoma.[162] The lymphoma should be seen in close proximity to mammary tissue.[163,164] The breast is among the least common sites to give rise to lymphomas, possibly correlating with the very sparse endogenous lymphoid tissue at this site.[162] At most, only about 0.5% of primary malignancies of the breast are lymphomas.[164] Most patients are middle-aged to elderly women, although occasionally young women and, rarely, adolescents are affected.[162-167] Occasionally lymphomas in the breast arise in pregnant or lactating women.[164,168] Almost all patients present with a palpable breast mass.[169] In a few asymptomatic patients, the lymphoma has been detected by mammography.[166,167,170] Constitutional symptoms are uncommon.[163] In 0% to 25% of cases in different series, patients present with bilateral disease.[162-164] On physical examination, patients usually have discrete, mobile masses, without fixation to either superficial or deep structures. Involvement of the overlying skin has been described,[171] and it may be inflamed,[172] mimicking inflammatory carcinoma. The proportion of cases with ipsilateral axillary lymphadenopathy varies widely among series, from 11%[166] to about 50%.[163]

Pathologic Features

On gross examination the tumors vary greatly in size, from approximately 1 to 12 cm. They are usually discrete but nonencapsulated, with a fleshy or soft consistency and a whitish gray or whitish pink color. In some cases there is more than one discrete mass.[162,164,166,172] In most series DLBCL is most common, constituting approximately 70% of cases (Fig. 62-11).[165,169,170,173] The remainder are mainly low-grade lymphomas of either follicular or marginal zone (MALT) type (Fig. 62-12). However, some recent data suggest that low-grade B-cell lymphomas are more prevalent, with MALT lymphoma being more common, followed by follicular lymphoma.[167] It is possible that a greater number of low-grade lymphomas are being detected owing to the identification of asymptomatic lesions by mammography.[167] Burkitt's lymphoma is uncommon, but dramatic presentations with bilateral breast involvement have been reported in pregnant or lactating women.[166,168,173] T-cell lymphomas are very rare.[167,172]

DLBCL affects women over a wide age range. Follicular and MALT lymphomas appear to affect middle-aged and older women. Burkitt's lymphoma is found mainly in young pregnant or postpartum women and may be associated with synchronous bilateral disease; a minority of DLBCLs are also found in this clinical setting.[162,164,166,168,172-174] Burkitt's lymphoma patients are often from Africa.[175]

Although breast lymphomas appear circumscribed, they often exhibit some invasion into surrounding tissues at the periphery of the mass.[166] The neoplastic cells infiltrate around

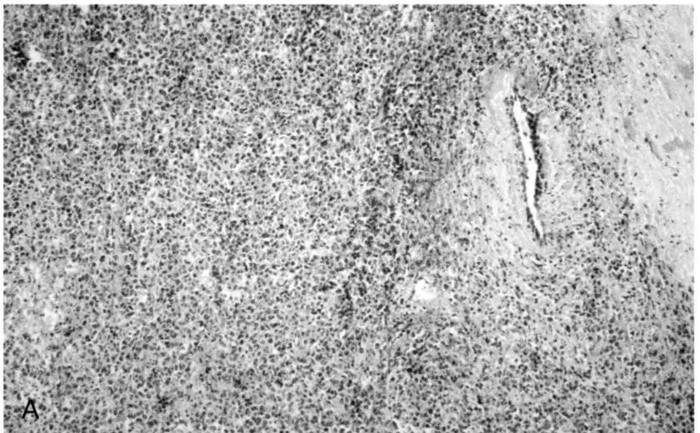

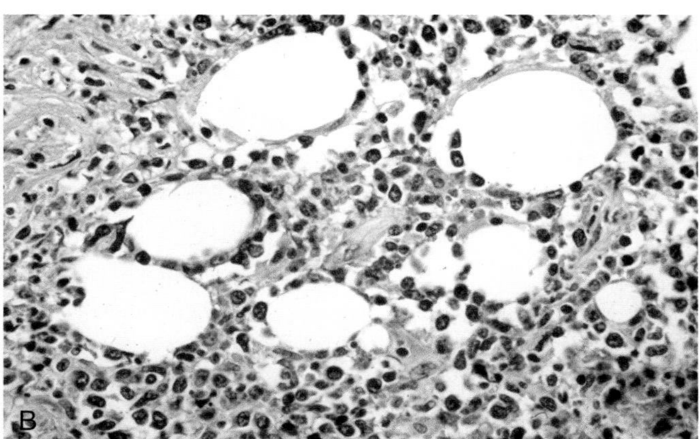

Figure 62-11. Diffuse large B-cell lymphoma in the breast. A, Low power shows a dense, diffuse lymphoid infiltrate surrounding a ductule and replacing normal tissue. **B,** Large atyical lymphoid cells with irregular nuclei infiltrate fat.

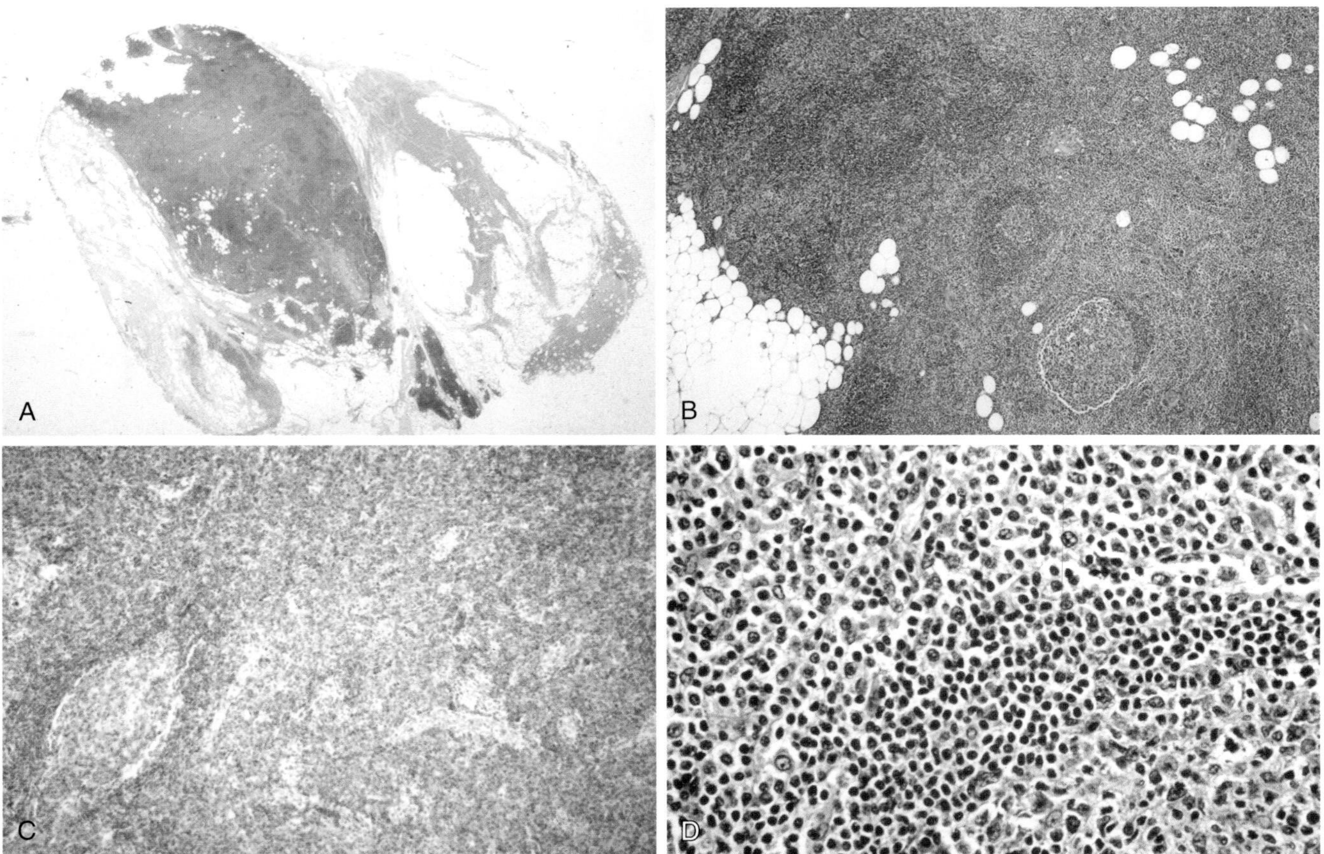

Figure 62-12. Marginal zone B-cell lymphoma in the breast. A, Whole mount of the excisional biopsy specimen shows a well-delineated nodule of lymphoid tissue. **B,** Medium power shows a diffuse lymphoid infiltrate with scattered reactive follicles. **C,** CD20 stain shows staining of the follicle and of most of the extrafollicular lymphoid cells (immunoperoxidase technique on paraffin section). **D,** The lower right corner contains a portion of a reactive follicle with a mantle of small lymphocytes. The rest of the field is occupied by marginal zone cells.

and within mammary ducts and lobules, sometimes with obliteration of these structures. Follicular lymphomas of all grades (1 to 3) have been reported. Marginal zone lymphoma has an appearance similar to that in other sites, except that lymphoepithelial lesions are usually absent.[166,167,172] Rare cases of lymphoma arising adjacent to saline or silicone breast implants have been described; surprisingly, the majority have been anaplastic lymphoma kinase (ALK)–negative anaplastic large cell lymphomas.[176] Immunophenotypic and genetic features are similar to those of the same types of lymphoma arising at other sites.[166,172,177]

Treatment and Outcome

The outcome of patients with lymphomas of the breast has improved over time. DLBCL can spread to lymph nodes and a wide variety of extranodal sites, including the CNS, contralateral breast, liver, spleen, and gastrointestinal tract.[164,165,173] MALT lymphoma patients typically remain well after treatment or develop relapses that are extranodal (subcutis, larynx, chest wall, parotid, orbit); lymph nodes are occasionally involved, but usually without generalized disease. Large cell transformation has been reported. Thus, mammary MALT lymphoma behaves in a manner similar to MALT lymphoma elsewhere.[166,168,173] Follicular lymphoma may be associated with the development of generalized disease, similar to nodal follicular lymphoma.[166] Burkitt's lymphoma and the subset of DLBCL occurring in young women are aggressive lymphomas with a high risk of spread to the ovaries, gastrointestinal tract, and CNS.[168,172] This group of patients has a poor prognosis, but with aggressive therapy, long-term survival may be possible.[174]

Differential Diagnosis

Because of the rarity of lymphomas of the breast, the diagnosis is almost never suspected preoperatively. The clinical impression is usually carcinoma.[172] On pathologic grounds, the differential diagnosis includes carcinoma in cases of high-grade lymphoma and a reactive lymphoid infiltrate in cases of low-grade lymphoma. Lymphomas (and other breast lesions) may be sampled via incisional or excisional biopsy, Tru-cut needle biopsy, or fine-needle aspiration (Fig. 62-13). The tissue may be submitted for permanent or frozen section. The greatest number of misdiagnoses have occurred when breast lymphoma is submitted for frozen section. Large B-cell lymphoma is frequently misdiagnosed as medullary carcinoma or undifferentiated carcinoma in this setting.[172] The same problem can occur with permanent sections, especially when small, artifactually distorted tissue is submitted. Careful

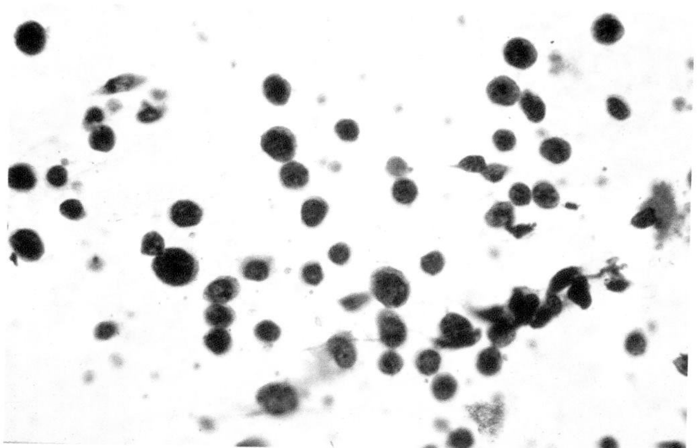

Figure 62-13. B-cell lymphoma in the breast, sampled by fine-needle aspiration. Atypical lymphoid cells in a range of sizes are present. Flow cytometric analysis revealed a population of CD10$^+$, CD5$^-$, CD23$^-$, CD43$^-$ B cells expressing monotypic kappa light chain, confirming the diagnosis of lymphoma.

attention to cytologic detail and to the discohesive nature of the lymphoid cells should lead to a consideration of lymphoma. The diagnosis can then be confirmed by immunophenotyping. In the differential diagnosis of low-grade lymphoma and chronic inflammatory processes, the presence of large numbers of B cells outside follicles favors a diagnosis of MALT lymphoma, especially if the cells have the morphology of marginal zone cells and express monotypic immunoglobulin. In distinguishing follicular hyperplasia from follicular lymphoma, criteria similar to those used in lymph nodes can be applied.

The uncommon reactive process known as lymphocytic mastopathy, diabetic mastopathy, or autoimmune mastopathy may be seen in patients with diabetes mellitus or immunologic disorders or in women who are otherwise well. It usually presents as a palpable breast mass in young or middle-aged women.[175,178] Microscopic examination reveals a lobulocentric, sometimes perivascular lymphocytic infiltrate composed predominantly of B cells, sometimes with germinal center formation. Some cases also show lobular atrophy and sclerosis.[175,178] The tight perilobular distribution, lack of cytologic atypia, and lack of monotypic immunoglobulin help distinguish this disorder from lymphoma.

GASTROINTESTINAL TRACT

The gastrointestinal tract is the most common extranodal site for the development of lymphomas; between 4% and 20% of all non-Hodgkin's lymphomas arise in this site. The stomach is most often involved, followed by the small intestine, colon, and esophagus.[179-181] Predisposing factors include infection, in particular by *Helicobacter pylori*; celiac disease; and possibly inflammatory bowel disease. The gastrointestinal tract is one of the most common sites for lymphoma in patients with congenital immunodeficiency syndromes (see Chapter 54), HIV infection (see Chapter 56), and iatrogenic immunosuppression (see Chapter 55).

The clinical findings associated with gastrointestinal lymphomas are pain, anorexia, weight loss, bleeding, obstruction, palpable mass, diarrhea, nausea or vomiting, fever, and perforation. Intussusception may be seen with bulky lymphomas in the ileocecal region.[182-187]

Stomach

The stomach is the primary site in 55% to 75% of cases of gastrointestinal lymphomas. Between 1% and 7% of gastric malignancies are lymphomas.[179,188] DLBCL is the most common type, followed by extranodal marginal zone (MALT) lymphoma (see Chapter 18). Other lymphomas, including Burkitt's lymphoma and peripheral T-cell lymphoma, are uncommon.

Gastric Diffuse Large B-Cell Lymphoma

Clinical Features

This is mainly a disease of older adults, with a median age in the seventh decade; younger adults are occasionally affected. There is a slight male preponderance.[189-191]

Pathologic Features

Gross examination reveals single or occasionally multiple large ulcerated or exophytic lesions that are usually transmurally invasive and sometimes associated with invasion of adjacent structures.[192] Microscopic examination reveals a diffuse proliferation of large cells with round or oval, irregular or lobated nuclei, distinct nucleoli, and scant cytoplasm. An estimated one third of cases have a concomitant component of low-grade marginal zone lymphoma, consistent with large cell transformation.[188]

Immunophenotypic features are similar to those of DLBCL at other sites.[193] A subset of large B-cell lymphomas are CD10$^+$ and BCL6$^+$, suggesting germinal center B-cell origin.[190]

Rearrangement of the *BCL6* gene is more common, and *BCL2* gene rearrangement is less common, in gastric than in nodal DLBCL.[194] Frequent loss of heterozygosity on chromosome 6q in sites of putative tumor suppressor genes and occasional cases with loss of heterozygosity of other tumor suppressor genes, including *TP53* and *APC*, have been reported.[195] *MYC* translocation and homozygous deletion of p16 have been described in some high-grade lymphomas. Despite the high frequency of t(11;18) and trisomy 3 in MALT lymphomas, they are uncommon in DLBCLs, implying that MALT lymphomas with these cytogenetic abnormalities are unlikely to undergo large cell transformation.[196,197] Other trisomies (most often of chromosomes 12 and 18) are more common in DLBCLs that have arisen through transformation of MALT lymphoma than in de novo large B-cell lymphomas.[196]

Staging, Treatment, and Outcome

In most cases (78% to 95%) patients present with stage I or II disease.[188-190,193] A few have more distant spread to marrow, liver, or other sites.[188] Patients have been treated with surgery, radiation, chemotherapy, or a combination of these modalities. The estimated 5-year survival is 65%.[192] In some series the subtype of large B-cell lymphoma did not significantly impact prognosis[193]; in others, certain subsets had a significantly better or worse outcome. In one study DLBCL associated with MALT lymphoma had a 5-year survival of 92%,

CD10⁺ large B-cell lymphoma had a 5-year survival of 89%, and CD10⁻ large B-cell lymphoma without a low-grade component had a 5-year survival of only 30%.[190] In another study DLBCL associated with a component of MALT lymphoma had a 5-year cause-specific survival of 84%, compared with 64% for de novo DLBCL.[189] Stage is also prognostically important: patients with stage Ie or IIe1 disease have a better outcome than those with stage IIe2 or higher.[190,193]

Differential Diagnosis

Poorly differentiated carcinomas may be composed of discohesive-appearing cells with little or no gland formation, mimicking DLBCL. Lymphoid cells may show artifactual vacuolar change and mimic signet ring cells. Stains for mucin and immunohistochemical studies are helpful in establishing a diagnosis.

Small and Large Intestinal Lymphoma

The small intestine is the primary site in 15% to 35% of cases of gastrointestinal lymphomas.[179,182,183,188,198] Lymphomas account for approximately 25% of small intestinal neoplasms.[179] The most common type is DLBCL, followed by MALT lymphoma (including the distinctive subtype known as immunoproliferative small intestinal disease; see Chapter 18), Burkitt's lymphoma, enteropathy-type intestinal T-cell lymphoma (see Chapter 37), mantle cell lymphoma (see Chapter 21), and follicular lymphoma (see Chapter 17).[179,182,184,192,198] The ileum is more commonly affected than the duodenum or jejunum.

Seven percent to 20% of gastrointestinal lymphomas arise in the large intestine.[183,198] Lymphomas account for only 0.5% of malignancies in the colon.[179,199] The most common type of lymphoma is DLBCL, followed by MALT lymphoma, mantle cell lymphoma, and rare cases of follicular lymphoma, Burkitt's lymphoma, and peripheral T-cell lymphoma. Large intestinal lymphomas most often involve the cecum, followed by the rectum; other portions of the colon are only rarely affected.[179] Anal lymphomas are very rare; they are usually DLBCL.[200] Plasmablastic lymphoma of the type that most commonly arises in the oral cavity may be primary in the large or small intestine, particularly the anal region.[201]

Intestinal Diffuse Large B-Cell Lymphoma

Clinical Features

Most patients are older adults, with a few cases occurring in younger adults or children. There is a slight male preponderance among adults, whereas affected children are almost exclusively boys. DLBCL in children is found virtually only in the ileocecal area.[184,187,199] Less than 1% of gastrointestinal lymphomas arise in the setting of ulcerative colitis.[185] Ulcerative colitis–associated lymphomas, which are mostly DLBCL, are often distally located in the colon, almost always in sites of active inflammation. Compared with DLBCL of the colon in the general population, DLBCL in patients with ulcerative colitis is more often multiple (38% versus 10%).[202,203] DLBCL generally appears in patients with long-standing ulcerative colitis,[202] although recent evidence indicates that the incidence may be increasing, with a shorter interval to the development of lymphoma in patients treated with immunosuppressive therapy.[204] The findings suggest that immunosuppression may accelerate lymphomagenesis in this susceptible population.

Pathologic Features

The gross and microscopic appearance is similar to that of gastric DLBCL (Fig. 62-14).[182,184,186-188] In a subset of cases a component of MALT lymphoma is found,[188] consistent with transformation of the low-grade lymphoma. The reported proportion of cases with an associated MALT lymphoma varies widely, from 10%[188] to more than 50%.[182,184,186] The immunophenotypic and genotypic features are similar to those of gastric DLBCL.

Staging, Treatment, and Outcome

In the majority of cases disease is confined to the intestine, with or without regional lymph node involvement.[188] Treatment is usually surgical resection followed by chemotherapy. The estimated 5-year survival ranges from 25% to 67%.[192,197] DLBCL arising in association with MALT lymphoma may have a better prognosis than de novo large B-cell lymphoma.[186]

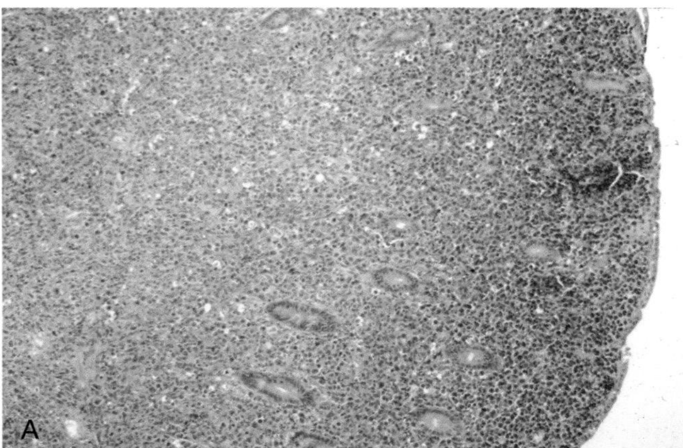

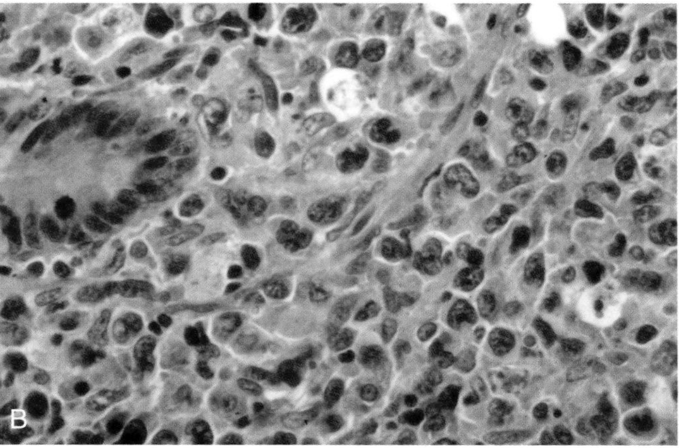

Figure 62-14. Diffuse large B-cell lymphoma in the colon. A, Lymphoma invades deep into the wall of the bowel. **B,** The large atypical neoplastic cells are highly irregular and often multilobated.

Mantle Cell Lymphoma

The gastrointestinal manifestations of mantle cell lymphoma (see Chapter 21) include lymphomatous polyposis involving long segments of bowel,[186,197] usually with mesenteric lymph nodal involvement[197] and widespread disease away from the gastrointestinal tract. The prognosis is similar to that of other cases of mantle cell lymphoma.

Follicular Lymphoma

Follicular lymphoma occasionally arises in the gastrointestinal tract; any portion may be involved,[205] but the duodenum is the most common site, particularly the area of the ampulla of Vater.[198,206-208] Patients are adults, with women affected more often than men; they present with abdominal pain or are asymptomatic.[205] Endoscopy reveals mucosal nodularity or small polypoid masses.[198,205] Larger, deeply invasive lesions cause biliary obstruction, mimicking pancreatic or duodenal carcinoma.[208] The histologic, immunohistologic, and genetic features are similar to those of nodal follicular lymphoma (see Chapter 17), except that frequent expression of IgA and the mucosal homing receptor $\alpha 4\beta 7$ has been described.[206] In most cases the follicular lymphoma is low grade (grade 1 or 2). Some patients have regional lymph node involvement,[198,205-208] but widespread disease is usually absent.[198,207,208] Nonduodenal gastrointestinal follicular lymphoma tends to be more widespread than duodenal disease.[207] Duodenal follicular lymphoma has a favorable prognosis.[198,205,208] The reason for the preferential duodenal localization is uncertain, but clinical and pathologic findings suggest that follicular lymphoma of the duodenum may originate from local antigen-responsive B cells.[206]

Burkitt's Lymphoma

Clinical Features

In the World Health Organization (WHO) classification of tumors of the hematopoietic and lymphoid tissues,[209] three clinical variants of Burkitt's lymphoma are described: endemic, sporadic, and immunodeficiency associated. Involvement of the ileocecal region is the most common manifestation of sporadic Burkitt's lymphoma. Ileocecal disease may also be seen in a minority of endemic and immunodeficiency-associated Burkitt's lymphomas. Burkitt's lymphoma rarely affects other portions of the gastrointestinal tract, such as the stomach[188] and more distal portions of the colon. Burkitt's lymphoma most often affects children and young adults, with a marked male preponderance.[182] In some cases staging reveals disease beyond the gastrointestinal tract.

Pathologic Features

The tumors are usually bulky exophytic lesions that may be associated with intussusception when they occur in the ileocecal area.[186] Histologic, immunophenotypic, and genetic features are similar to those seen in other sites. Burkitt's lymphoma is discussed in detail in Chapter 24.

Appendix

Clinical Features

The appendix is a rare primary site for lymphomas, accounting for only 2% to 3% of all gastrointestinal lymphomas.[185] This could be an underestimate, because some large ileocecal lymphomas might arise from the appendix without the primary site being identifiable. Appendiceal lymphomas affect mainly children and young adults,[210-212] with a slight male preponderance and a mean age of 26 years—substantially younger than the mean age for lymphomas in other parts of the gastrointestinal tract.[212] Patients present with right lower quadrant abdominal pain, mimicking acute appendicitis.[212] Some have a palpable mass.

Pathologic Features

Gross examination shows nodular, fleshy, whitish gray masses confined to the distal appendix or involving the appendix more extensively and protruding into the cecum.[210-212] The most common type appears to be DLBCL, followed by Burkitt's lymphoma.[184,211] MALT lymphoma and periperal T-cell lymphoma have also been reported.[210,211]

Staging, Treatment, and Outcome

Most reported cases have been Ann Arbor stage I disease.[211,212] Low-grade lymphomas are often treated with resection alone, and higher grade tumors are usually treated with resection combined with radiation or chemotherapy, with almost all patients free of disease at follow-up.[210-212] The favorable prognosis may be related to the limited nature of the disease in most cases.

Hodgkin's Lymphoma

Clinical Features

Primary gastrointestinal Hodgkin's lymphoma is very rare, with less than 0.5% of cases of Hodgkin's disease arising in this site.[213] The disease affects adults, with a male preponderance. Some have inflammatory bowel disease, especially Crohn's disease, or other immunologic abnormalities. In the general population the stomach is most often involved, followed by the small intestine and the colon. In patients with inflammatory bowel disease, the inflamed area is most likely to be involved.[213,214] Patients have a favorable prognosis, with a good response to therapy in many cases.[213-216]

Pathologic Features

There is usually transmural invasion of the bowel wall, which is often multifocal.[213,215] Reported cases have been of the mixed cellularity and nodular sclerosis subtypes, with immunophenotypic features of classical Hodgkin's disease (see Chapter 27).[213-215] Neoplastic cells are typically positive for EBV.[213,215] The occurrence of Hodgkin's disease in areas of Crohn's disease, the history of azathioprine or prednisone use in many cases, and the presence of EBV suggest that chronic inflammation and immunosuppression combine to play a role in the genesis of some cases of gastrointestinal Hodgkin's disease.[213]

LIVER

Clinical Features

Primary hepatic lymphomas are uncommon. A recent increase in frequency has been suggested,[217,218] although it is possible that these lymphomas are just being identified, biopsied, and diagnosed more frequently.[218] Most patients are middle-aged and older adults with a wide age range (median age, 50 years; range, 7 to 87 years) and a male-to-female ratio of approximately 2:1. Patients present with right upper quadrant or epigastric pain, nausea, vomiting, anorexia, or weakness. About half of them have fever, night sweats, or weight loss, but jaundice is uncommon. On physical examination, hepatomegaly is often found.[219,220] In a few cases of MALT lymphoma, the lymphoma was an incidental finding during abdominal surgery performed for other reasons.[221] Lactate dehydrogenase is frequently elevated, and hepatic transaminases may also be elevated; however, alpha fetoprotein and carcinoembryonic antigen levels are typically normal or only slightly elevated.[219,220,222,223]

In up to 40% of cases patients have another disorder, such as immunodeficiency, chronic infection, or autoimmune disease.[218,222] These include hepatitis A, B, or C virus infection; HIV infection; prior organ transplantation; systemic lupus erythematosus; Felty's syndrome; autoimmune cytopenias; primary biliary cirrhosis; prior Hodgkin's disease; and active tuberculosis, among others.[217,218,220,222,224-228] HIV-infected patients are younger and almost exclusively male.[227]

Pathologic Features

In approximately half the cases, the lymphomas form a large solitary mass. In most of the remainder, there are multiple nodules that may tend to be confluent. In about 5% of cases, there is diffuse hepatic enlargement without a discrete mass.[218-220,222] Most lymphomas are DLBCL. The remainder are Burkitt's lymphoma, MALT lymphoma, lymphoplasmacytic lymphoma, follicular lymphoma, and peripheral T-cell lymphomas.[217,219,220,223-226] Almost all lymphomas in HIV+ patients have been DLBCL or Burkitt's lymphoma.[227] Necrosis is common; sclerosis is infrequent. Lymphomas with diffuse hepatic enlargement may show prominent sinusoidal involvement.[219] Some of these are DLBCL; some are hepatosplenic T-cell lymphoma (see Chapter 33). MALT lymphoma has histologic features similar to those seen in other sites. The marginal zone B cells markedly expand the portal tracts; form intersecting, broad, serpiginous bands that entrap nodules of hepatocytes; and, in some areas, produce a diffuse, confluent infiltrate. Neoplastic cells form lymphoepithelial lesions with bile duct epithelium.[221,228,229] Immunohistochemical features are similar to those seen in the same types of lymphoma at other anatomic sites.[221]

Outcome

In the small number of patients with low-grade primary hepatic lymphomas for whom follow-up information is available, some have survived free of disease following resection alone, and others have died of unrelated causes.[221,228,229] Among patients with DLBCL, the prognosis is relatively good.[222] In one study the 5-year cause-specific survival was 87%.[220] Among HIV+ patients the outcome is worse, with mortality greater than 60%.[217,227]

Differential Diagnosis

The finding of one or more hepatic lesions can suggest hepatocellular carcinoma or metastatic carcinoma. The combination of high lactate dehydrogenase and normal carcinoembryonic antigen and alpha fetoprotein, particularly in a patient with an underlying immunologic abnormality, can suggest lymphoma.[222]

GALLBLADDER

Rare cases of primary lymphomas in the gallbladder have been reported.[230-234] Most patients have been older adults. One patient had a history of HIV infection,[235] and a few have had gallstones.[231] Patients present with symptoms that often mimic cholecystitis, cholelithiasis, or choledocholithiasis, such as right upper quadrant pain,[233] nausea, vomiting, or, rarely, jaundice.[230] Follow-up information is limited. Gross inspection shows mural thickening or one or more discrete tumor nodules.[231,232,234] Almost all these lymphomas have been diffuse large cell type (B lineage when immunophenotyped)[232] or MALT lymphoma.[230,231,234] The few cases of MALT lymphoma reported have mainly arisen in women.[234]

EXTRAHEPATIC BILIARY TREE

Lymphomas occasionally involve porta hepatis lymph nodes and compresses the extrahepatic biliary tree, resulting in jaundice. Lymphomas arising primarily from the extrahepatic biliary tree is very rare, with 13 cases reported in the last 20 years. Patients present with obstructive jaundice. The clinical and radiographic features often suggest carcinoma or sclerosing cholangitis. The walls of the bile ducts appear thickened. These lymphomas have often been characterized using older classifications, making analysis difficult; however, DLBCL appears to be more common than any other type.[236,237]

PANCREAS

Clinical Features

Primary pancreatic lymphomas are rare, accounting for less than 0.2% of pancreatic malignancies[238] and less than 0.7% of non-Hodgkin's lymphomas.[46] Patients are adults, with ages ranging from the third to ninth decades (mean age, 60 years) and a male-to-female ratio of approximately 2:1.[239-242] Other than rare HIV+ patients,[240] affected individuals have no conditions predisposing to lymphoma. Patients complain of abdominal pain, anorexia, weight loss, nausea, or vomiting.[239,241] They are often jaundiced and may have a palpable mass.[239] The preoperative clinical diagnosis is often pancreatic adenocarcinoma. The prognosis is difficult to assess because this tumor is rare and patients have not been treated uniformly. However, more than 50% of patients die of lymphoma.[241]

Pathologic Features

Tumors form large masses (generally >6 cm) most often involving the pancreatic head, although the lymphoma may involve the body or tail or the entire pancreas.[239,241,242] These lymphomas have been characterized using a variety of classification systems, and immunophenotyping is not always reported, but most appear to be DLBCL.[241,243] Rare cases of MALT lymphoma[242] and peripheral T-cell lymphomas have also been reported.[241]

Differential Diagnosis

The main entity in the clinical differential diagnosis is pancreatic adenocarcinoma. Lymphomas are larger than most carcinomas.[243] On endoscopic retrograde cholangiopancreatography, lymphoma may compress or distort ductal structures but generally does not invade their walls, in contrast to carcinoma.[239] Establishing a diagnosis requires obtaining tissue for pathologic examination.

ADRENAL

Clinical Features

Lymphomas arising in the adrenal gland are rare, with only approximately 100 cases reported.[244,245] Patients are adults, with a median age of 60 years and a male-to-female ratio of 2:1 to 3:1.[244,246] Rare patients are HIV+,[247] and several have had autoimmune disorders,[245,248] but there are no known specific predisposing factors. Patients present with abdominal pain, fever, night sweats, or weight loss.[245-248] Nearly half have manifestations of adrenal insufficiency, and all such patients have bilateral adrenal involvement.[248,249] A variety of radiographic techniques, including ultrasonography, computed tomography, and magnetic resonance imaging, can be used to detect the characteristically bulky tumors. In approximately 75% of cases both adrenals are involved, often with no detectable disease outside the adrenals.[246-248]

Pathologic Features

Almost all well-documented cases have been DLBCL, with rare cases of peripheral T-cell lymphomas and other types, including cases diagnosed as lower-grade lymphomas.[244,246-249] In one study 45% of cases were positive for EBV by in situ hybridization. Mutations of the *TP53* and *c-KIT* genes are frequent.[244]

Staging, Treatment, and Outcome

The prognosis is poor, and many cases are diagnosed only at autopsy.[248] However, improved diagnostic techniques leading to earlier diagnosis have resuted in improved outcomes following complete surgical excision and combination chemotherapy.[245,246,249]

KIDNEY

Clinical Features

Most cases reported as primary renal lymphomas are lymphomas presenting with renal involvement but not necessarily confined to the kidney. An estimated 0.7% of extranodal lymphomas present in the kidney.[46] Nearly all patients are middle-aged or older adults, with a mean age in the sixth decade and a slight male preponderance.[250-259] A few cases have been described in children,[253] HIV+ patients,[253] or iatrogenically immunosuppressed allograft recipients. Patients with other malignancies, autoimmune diseases, or other disorders have been reported,[250,251,253,254,260] but no risk factors specific for renal lymphomas have been identified. Patients present with flank pain, loss of appetite, nausea, hematuria, weight loss, fever, renal insufficiency, or fatigue.[252-254,256,261] Rarely, the lymphoma is an incidental finding.[254]

Pathologic Features

Renal lymphomas are unilateral in approximately three quarters of cases; the remainder have bilateral involvement. Bilateral disease is much more often associated with renal insufficiency.[250,252-254,256] The lesions range from less than 5 cm to massive, with obliteration of the kidney. Frequently the tumors invade adjacent tissues, including perinephric fat, psoas muscle, and even pancreas and duodenum. There may be vascular or ureteral encasement by the lymphoma. Occasional cases show extension into the renal vein and inferior vena cava, analogous to renal cell carcinoma.[252-254] The most common renal lymphoma is DLBCL, accounting for slightly more than half the cases. The remainder are a variety of low- and high-grade types, nearly always of B lineage, including extranodal marginal zone (MALT) lymphoma,[256,261] lymphoplasmacytic lymphoma, follicular lymphoma, lymphoblastic lymphoma, Burkitt's lymphoma,[250,252-254,257,259] and anaplastic large cell lymphoma.[258] Lymphomas in HIV+ patients are usually DLBCL or Burkitt's lymphoma.[253] Renal lymphomas in children are usually Burkitt's lymphoma or, less often, lymphoblastic lymphoma.[253]

Staging, Treatment, and Outcome

Only about 25% of patients presenting with renal lymphomas have Ann Arbor stage I disease.[252-256] In one review, 42% of patients were alive and free of disease at last follow-up, 4% were alive with disease, and 54% had died, usually of lymphoma and less often of complications of surgery or chemotherapy or of unrelated causes. Survival is slightly better in the subset of patients treated with combination chemotherapy.[254] However, renal lymphomas often present with features that correlate with a poor prognosis, especially the high frequency of disseminated disease.[252] Patients with renal lymphomas most likely have an outcome similar to that of other lymphoma patients with similar prognostic factors.[262] The renal insufficiency found in some cases of bilateral renal lymphomas usually responds promptly to chemotherapy, but many of these patients eventually die of lymphoma.[263] Patients with bilateral disease tend to have a worse prognosis than those with unilateral disease.[253,255,262]

Differential Diagnosis

Renal lymphomas, particularly when unilateral, may be mistaken clinically and radiographically for renal cell carcinomas.[251,253,260,261] Less often, they may mimic polycystic kidney disease,[253] soft tissue tumors,[264] inflammatory lesions,[264] or Wilms' tumor.[253] Bilateral lymphoma is much more common than bilateral renal cell carcinoma, so bilateral disease may suggest lymphoma preoperatively.[254] Lymphomas can generally be readily distinguished from other entities in the clinical differential diagnosis on microscopic examination.

URETER

Lymphomas occasionally involve the ureters. Manifestations include abdominal pain, nausea and vomiting, dysuria, hematuria, fever, renal insufficiency, hydronephrosis, and hydroureter.[253,265,266] Lymphomas confined to the ureters at presentation are exceedingly unusual but have been described.[266,267] In most cases lymphoma is widespread at presentation, or the ureters are secondarily involved via extension from retroperitoneal disease. The majority are DLBCLs. The differential diagnosis includes idiopathic retroperitoneal fibrosis.[267,268] Idiopathic retroperitoneal fibrosis can be associated with ureteral obstruction and a chronic inflammatory cell infiltrate, and retroperitoneal lymphomas can be associated with marked sclerosis and crush artifact, so differentiating the two may be difficult. Cytologic atypia of lymphoid cells and a diffuse infiltrate composed predominantly of B cells support a diagnosis of lymphoma.

URINARY BLADDER AND URETHRA

Clinical Features

Primary lymphomas of the urinary bladder are rare, and even less common are lymphomas arising in the urethra. Lymphomas arising in these sites share a number of clinical and pathologic features..[253,269] They affect predominantly older adults, with a female preponderance.[253,269-275] Patients present with hematuria, urinary frequency, dysuria, or obstructive symptoms. Analogous to the pathogenesis of marginal zone B-cell lymphomas at other sites, marginal zone lymphomas in the bladder may be related to prior inflammatory disease, with a number of patients having a history of chronic cystitis or bacteriuria.[253,269,270,276]

Pathologic Features

Cystoscopic or gross pathologic examination reveals single or occasionally multiple submucosal, exophytic, sessile nodules ranging from less than 1 to 15 cm. Sectioning usually reveals pale, firm tissue, although some tumors are soft and of variable color.[253,269] Lymphoma does not usually invade beyond the bladder.[253,277] In women with urethral lymphomas, a mass may protrude from the urethral meatus, mimicking a caruncle.[253,273,277] Most cases are extranodal marginal zone (MALT) lymphoma.[253,269,275,276,278] Histologic features are similar to those seen in other sites. Lymphoepithelial lesions may form in association with cystitis cystica,[279] cystitis glandularis,[269,270,275] or transitional surface epithelium.[271] Associated follicular cystitis is sometimes seen. A minority of cases are DLBCL; some may represent large cell transformation of an underlying marginal zone lymphoma.[271,277,278] The most common urethral lymphoma is DLBCL.[272,280,281] Many of the remainder have been characterized based on older classification systems, but descriptions suggest that some are marginal zone lymphomas.[253,273,274]

Staging, Treatment, and Outcome

Nearly all patients have localized disease at presentation.[253,269,275,279] The prognosis is favorable because the lymphomas tend to be localized and are frequently low grade and responsive to therapy.[253,269,271,275] DLBCL may behave in a more aggressive manner. The outlook for patients with marginal zone lymphoma is very good.

Differential Diagnosis

The main entity in the differential diagnosis of DLBCL is poorly differentiated carcinoma,[253] but other high-grade malignancies, including rhabdomyosarcoma, can also be considered.[267] Low-grade lymphomas may be mistaken for chronic inflammatory disorders.[253,275] Urothelial carcinoma may have a dense inflammatory infiltrate or undifferentiated neoplastic cells and may mimic either low- or high-grade lymphomas or Hodgkin's lymphoma.[282]

MALE GENITAL TRACT

Testis and Epididymis

Clinical Features

Lymphomas account for about 5% of testicular tumors. Lymphomas are the most frequent testicular neoplasms in men older than 50 years.[283] Children are only rarely affected.[253,284-287] The mean age is in the late 50s or 60s in most large series.[253,283,285,286,288] Lymphomas are the most common bilateral tumors of the testis.[253,285] A few patients have been HIV$^+$,[289] but there is no known predisposing factor specific for testicular lymphoma. Patients typically present with a hard, painless scrotal mass. In a minority of cases patients present with constitutional symptoms[253,289] or with symptoms related to extratesticular disease, such as abnormal neurologic findings.[285] Lymphomas arising in the epididymis are much less common than testicular lymphomas, and lymphomas arising in the spermatic cord are extremely rare; the clinical and pathologic features of lymphomas in these sites appear to be similar to those of testicular lymphomas.[285,290-295]

Pathologic Features

Gross examination of orchiectomy specimens reveals a circumscribed, fleshy or firm, tan, gray, or white tumor ranging from a few millimeters to 16 cm in greatest dimension.[285] In half the cases lymphoma penetrates the tunica albuginea. The epididymis is involved in the majority of cases. In nearly 40% of cases, the spermatic cord is involved.[285]

On microscopic examination, the lymphoma typically obliterates the seminiferous tubules in at least some areas, with peripheral areas that may show intertubular tumor spread. In most cases neoplastic cells invade the seminiferous tubules, occupying the periphery of the tubules, displacing germ cells and Sertoli cells centrally, or filling the tubules completely. In one third of cases the tumor is associated with sclerosis.[285] Nearly all primary testicular lymphomas are DLBCL.[283,285,286,289] Most are composed of centroblasts (large noncleaved cells), but some cases of DLBCL show a predominance of immunoblasts or multilobated lymphoid cells. In a few cases there may be minor foci with neoplastic follicle formation.[285] Immunohistochemical analysis reveals features similar to those of DLBCL at other sites.[253,285,286] BCL2 protein expression is frequent, but the *BCL2* translocation is usually absent.[296]

Among patients aged 21 years and younger, the small number of reported cases have not shown the striking predominance of DLBCL seen in the adult population. Primary testicular lymphomas in childhood are rare, but most cases are localized follicular lymphoma, grade 3 of 3. They express pan–B-cell antigens and usually BCL6, but unlike most other follicular lymphomas, they are typically BCL2 protein negative, with no *BCL2* gene rearrangement.[287,297]

Only a few cases of T-lineage lymphomas, including peripheral T-cell lymphoma, unspecified type, anaplastic large cell lymphoma, and precursor T-lymphoblastic lymphoma, have been described.[298,299] Extranodal NK/T-cell lymphoma of the nasal type may involve the testis. These are aggressive, CD56+, EBV+ lymphomas associated with a poor prognosis (see Chapter 28). Because CD56 is expressed in normal testis and has the capacity for homophilic binding, CD56 expression could play a role in the testicular presentation of these lymphomas.[300,301]

Staging, Treatment, and Outcome

Approximately 70% to 80% of patients who present with testicular involvement by lymphoma have limited-stage disease (Ann Arbor stage I or II),[253,283,286,288] and more than half have stage I disease.[285] Testicular DLBCL was traditionally considered to have a poor prognosis, and although advances in therapy have improved the prognosis somewhat, median survival for patients presenting with stage I or II disease is only about 60 months, so there is room for improvement.[283,286,288,289,302] When relapse occurs it often involves extranodal sites, most commonly the CNS[283,286,302,303] but also the opposite testis, bone, lung, skin, Waldeyer's ring, liver, kidney, and other sites; relapse may also involve the lymph nodes.[283,285,286,289] The best outcomes are associated with orchiectomy combined with doxorubicin (Adriamycin)–based combination chemotherapy. Because of the high risk of relapse in the CNS and opposite testis, some investigators suggest that intrathecal chemotherapy, cranial irradiation, and irradiation of the opposite testis should be considered in cases of testicular lymphoma.[283,289,304]

A number of clinical and pathologic features affect the prognosis of patients with DLBCL. Patients presenting with localized disease have a better outcome than those with widespread disease.[283,285,288,302,304] Sclerosis and follicle formation are associated with a favorable prognosis. In one study, lymphomas with sclerosis had a much better outcome than those without sclerosis (72% versus 16% 5-year disease-free survival for all patients; 90% versus 34% 5-year disease-free survival for stage I patients).[285] Patients presenting with bilateral testicular involvement have a worse prognosis, possibly because they are more likely to have disease outside the testis.[285]

Differential Diagnosis

The most important entity in the differential diagnosis of testicular lymphoma is seminoma.[285] Compared with seminoma, lymphoma affects older patients, is more often bilateral, is more likely to involve the epididymis and spermatic cord, and is more likely to metastasize to sites such as bone or CNS.[285] Seminomas are composed of nests of neoplastic cells with abundant glycogen-rich cytoplasm and uniform oval, euchromatic nuclei with prominent nucleoli delineated by fibrous septa that contain small lymphocytes and, sometimes, granulomas. Seminomas express placental alkaline phosphatase and Oct-4. Testicular DLBCLs, particularly those with prominent sclerosis and large numbers of admixed non-neoplastic lymphocytes, may suggest a diagnosis of orchitis, including bacterial, viral, or granulomatous orchitis. Acute inflammation with abscess formation and granulomas strongly favors an inflammatory process. Other unusual entities, including plasmacytoma[305] and rhabdomyosarcoma, can occasionally enter the differential diagnosis, but clinical and histologic features, augmented by immunophenotyping, establish the diagnosis.

Prostate

Clinical Features

Primary lymphomas of the prostate account for 0.1% of all non-Hodgkin's lymphomas and 0.09% of prostatic neoplasms.[306] In a large series of prostate biospies, transurethral resection specimens, and prostatectomies, 0.17% of cases harbored primary prostatic lymphomas.[307] Patients' ages range from 18 to 86 years, with a mean of approximately 60 years.[253,306,308-310] Most patients present with symptoms of bladder outlet obstruction, sometimes with hematuria.[307,308,310,311] In a few cases there has been hydronephrosis,[310] sometimes with renal failure.[306] On physical examination the prostate is usually diffusely enlarged and firm, but not as hard as in cases of carcinoma.[309] Patients are often thought to have benign prostatic hyperplasia,[253] and lymphoma is only rarely suspected.

Pathologic Features

The lymphomas are of various types, but the most common appears to be DLBCL. Others are almost always B-cell lymphomas, with reported cases including follicular lymphoma,[308,309] Burkitt's lymphoma,[306] and several cases of marginal zone (MALT) lymphoma (Fig. 62-15).[311,312] Microscopic examination reveals an atypical lymphoid infiltrate that is usually patchy but may be unifocal, extensive and obliterative, or perivascular. The lymphoma infiltrates among fibromuscular bundles and occasionally infiltrates glandular epithelium.[309]

Staging, Treatment, and Outcome

Staging has shown the disease to be Ann Arbor stage I in the majority of cases, although involvement of abdominal lymph nodes and of extranodal sites is not uncommon. The prognosis has been considered poor, although patients treated in recent years with optimal therapy have had a better outcome.[306]

Differential Diagnosis

The differential diagnosis of prostatic lymphomas includes poorly differentiated carcinoma and prostatitis. However, even in poorly differentiated carcinoma, neoplastic cells at least focally form cords, cohesive sheets, and sometimes glandular spaces. When considering prostatitis, the presence of a dense, monomorphic, cytologically atypical lymphoid infiltrate favors lymphoma.

FEMALE GENITAL TRACT

Lymphomas only rarely present with involvement of the female genital tract. The ovaries are most commonly affected, followed by the uterine cervix, uterine corpus, vagina, vulva, and fallopian tube. Nearly all cases are non-Hodgkin's lymphomas of B lineage, with DLBCL being the most common type throughout the female genital tract. T-cell lymphoma and Hodgkin's lymphoma are vanishingly rare.[253,313] Except in rare cases of lymphoma arising in the setting of HIV infection or iatrogenic immunosuppression[314,315] or in the case of endemic Burkitt's lymphoma, there are no known predisposing factors for the development of female genital tract lymphoma.

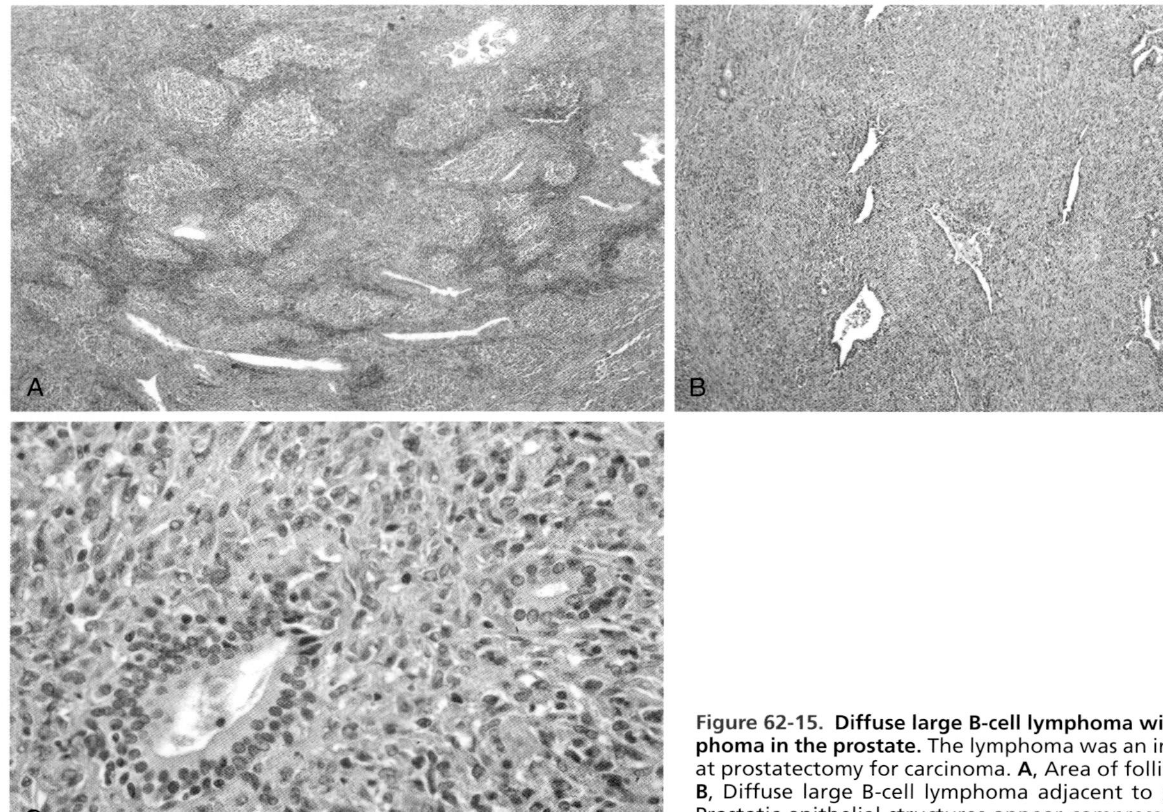

Figure 62-15. Diffuse large B-cell lymphoma with follicular lymphoma in the prostate. The lymphoma was an incidental finding at prostatectomy for carcinoma. **A,** Area of follicular lymphoma. **B,** Diffuse large B-cell lymphoma adjacent to prostatic glands. Prostatic epithelial structures appear compressed and atrophic. **C,** Area of diffuse large B-cell lymphoma.

Ovary

Clinical Features

Most series of ovarian lymphomas consist of cases in which patients presented with ovarian involvement but also had extraovarian disease.[316] Less than 1% of lymphomas present with ovarian involvement.[46,253,317] In countries where Burkitt's lymphoma is endemic, however, approximately 50% of malignant ovarian tumors in childhood are Burkitt's lymphoma.[318] Patients range in age from 18 months to 74 years,[253,319] with a peak incidence in the fourth or fifth decade.[253,317,320] Cases have been discovered during pregnancy.[253] The most common presenting complaints are abdominal pain and increasing abdominal girth.[317,320,321] A minority of patients have weight loss, fatigue, fever, or abnormal vaginal bleeding.[317,319]

Pathologic Features

On gross examination, ovarian lymphomas range from microscopic (incidental findings)[320] to 25 cm in diameter, with an average diameter of 11 to 14 cm.[253,320] They typically have an intact external surface that may be smooth or nodular. The consistency ranges from soft and fleshy to firm and rubbery, depending on the degree of associated sclerosis. On sectioning, the tumors are usually white, tan, or gray-pink. A minority have cystic degeneration, hemorrhage, or necrosis.[253,319,322] Very rare cases of lymphoma involving the ovary in association with, or possibly arising from, a teratoma have been described.[323]

The most common lymphoma is DLBCL, followed by Burkitt's lymphoma and follicular lymphoma.[317] Rare cases of anaplastic large cell lymphoma and B- and T-lymphoblastic lymphoma have been reported.[313,320] Among children and adolescents, Burkitt's lymphoma appears to be most common.[313,319] In contrast to adults, who develop lymphomas of a variety of types, younger patients almost always have aggressive lymphomas.

The histologic appearance of lymphomas in the ovary is similar to that seen in extraovarian sites, although there is often associated sclerosis. In addition, tumor cells may appear to grow in cords and nests, simulating carcinoma,[318] or to have an elongated shape and grow in a storiform pattern, mimicking spindle cell sarcoma. Ovarian lymphomas may preferentially spare a peripheral rim of cortical tissue, corpus luteum, corpus albicans,[253] and follicles,[319] but otherwise they typically obliterate normal ovarian parenchyma. Lymphomas are rarely associated with hyperplasia and luteinization of the adjacent stroma, with menstrual disturbances.[253] Ovarian lymphomas have immunophenotypic features similar to those of the same kinds of lymphomas at other sites. The genetic features have been studied in few cases.[253,320]

Staging, Treatment, and Outcome

Laparotomy shows involvement of one or both ovaries with approximately equal frequency.[319,322] Extraovarian spread is found in most cases, most commonly to pelvic or para-aortic lymph nodes and occasionally to the peritoneum, other portions of the female genital tract, or more distant

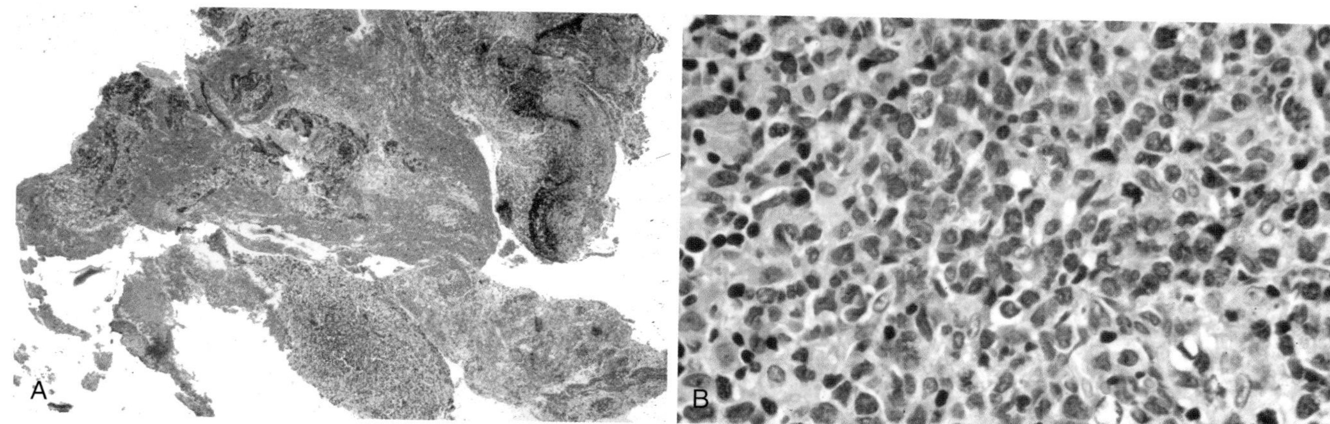

Figure 62-16. Diffuse large B-cell lymphoma in the uterine cervix. A, Curetted fragments of lymphoma admixed with blood. **B**, Higher power shows large atypical lymphoid cells with irregular nuclei.

sites.[253,317] Ovarian lymphomas have been considered aggressive tumors with a poor outcome, although with aggressive combination chemotherapy, the prognosis appears to be similar to that of nodal lymphomas of comparable stage and histologic type.[316,317,320]

Differential Diagnosis

The differential diagnosis of ovarian lymphomas includes dysgerminoma, undifferentiated carcinoma, metastatic carcinoma (particularly from the breast),[319] primary small cell carcinoma, adult granulosa cell tumor,[321] spindle cell sarcoma, and myeloid sarcoma.[253] Attention to cytologic detail and familiarity with the spectrum of histologic features of ovarian lymphomas are helpful in establishing a diagnosis. Immunohistochemical studies are of assistance in difficult cases.

Fallopian Tube

Primary malignant lymphomas of the fallopian tube are vanishingly rare, with one possible case of primary tubal follicular lymphoma reported.[253] Among patients with lymphomas of the ovaries, secondary tubal involvement is found in more than 25%. DLBCL and Burkitt's lymphoma are most common.[319,324]

Uterus

Clinical Features

Malignant lymphomas arising in the uterus are rare; less than 1% of extranodal lymphomas arise in this site.[46] Lymphomas arise much more often in the cervix than in the corpus, with a ratio as high as 10:1 in one series.[325] Ages range from 20 to 80 years,[326] with a median in the fifth decade.[326-328] The most common presenting symptom is abnormal vaginal bleeding.[253,324,326,327] Less common complaints are dyspareunia or perineal, pelvic, or abdominal pain. Constitutional symptoms are unusual.[253,328] Only a minority of cervical lymphomas yields a positive cervical smear, presumably because lymphomas are usually not ulcerated.[329]

Pathologic Features

On gross examination, cervical lymphomas usually produce bulky lesions that are readily identifiable on pelvic examination. The classic appearance is diffuse, circumferential enlargement of the cervix ("barrel-shaped" cervix). The lymphoma may also form a discrete submucosal tumor,[326] a polypoid or multinodular lesion,[326,330,331] or a fungating, exophytic mass; ulceration is unusual.[326] The tumors have been variously described as fleshy, rubbery, or firm. They are usually homogeneous in color and white-tan to yellow.[326] Extensive local spread to sites such as the vagina, parametria, or even pelvic side walls is common.[326,330] Ureteral obstruction with hydronephrosis is common.[253,326] Lymphomas of the uterine corpus are usually fleshy or soft and pale gray, yellow, or cream colored. They may form a polypoid mass or diffusely coat the endometrium, sometimes with deep invasion of the myometrium.[253,326]

The majority of lymphomas are DLBCL (Fig. 62-16).[324,325,331] Follicular lymphoma is next most common (Fig. 62-17). A few cases of Burkitt's lymphoma[313] and several cases of extranodal marginal zone (MALT) lymphoma[253,313,324,325,332,333] have been reported. Also described are rare cases of B-lymphoblastic lymphoma,[313] peripheral T-cell lymphomas,[334,335] and extranodal NK/T-cell lymphoma.[324]

The microscopic appearance of the lymphomas are similar to that seen in nodal and other extranodal sites. In the cervix there is often a band of uninvolved normal tissue just beneath

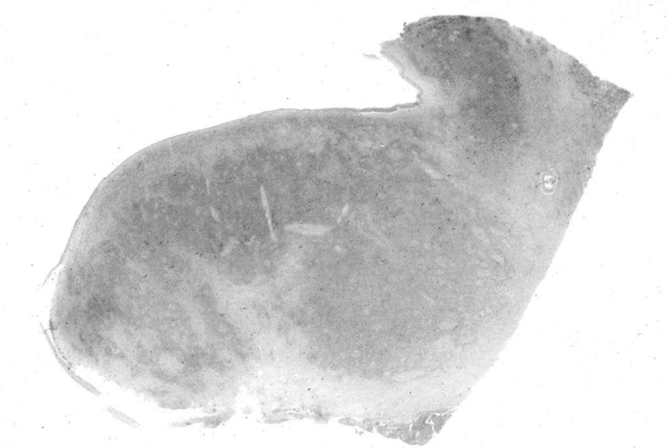

Figure 62-17. Follicular lymphoma in the uterine cervix, whole mount. Neoplastic follicles invade deep into the wall of the cervix.

the mucosa, and the overlying mucosa is usually intact. In a large biopsy or hysterectomy specimen, deep invasion of the cervical wall is usually seen. In cases of follicular lymphoma, perivascular spread of tumor is often a feature.[329] Cervical lymphomas are frequently associated with prominent sclerosis,[331] which may be associated with a cord-like arrangement or spindle-shaped tumor cells.[326] In small biopsies, squeeze artifact is often prominent and may restrict the pathologist's ability to render a diagnosis. Immunohistochemical studies have documented a B lineage in nearly all cases.[253,313,326,331]

Staging, Treatment, and Outcome

Although most uterine lymphomas are bulky and locally invasive, the majority are stage I and have a relatively good prognosis.[253,324] The optimal therapy has not been determined, but a combination of chemotherapy and radiation appears to offer the best chance of a cure.[336] In a few cases young women have been successfully treated using combination chemotherapy,[331] and some of them have maintained fertility.[253] The 5-year survival for cervical lymphomas is approximately 80%.[327] There is not enough information to draw definite conclusions about the prognosis of the rare endometrial lymphomas. However, patients with localized disease tend to do well, and those with advanced disease presenting with endometrial involvement tend to fare poorly.[326,333]

Vagina and Vulva

Lymphomas rarely arise in the vagina[253,328,337] and even less often in the vulva.[253,314,338,339] Patients are affected over a wide age range. They present with vaginal bleeding, discharge, pain or discomfort, dyspareunia, urinary frequency, or a mass. Surface epithelium is usually intact. Papanicolaou smears are generally negative.[340] Nearly all the lymphomas are DLBCL,[253,313,337,339,341] but rare cases of follicular lymphoma,[313,326] Burkitt's lymphoma, lymphoplasmacytic lymphoma,[313] and T-cell lymphomas[253,340] have been reported. Vaginal lymphomas are often associated with marked sclerosis and tend to present with localized disease. Treatment has not been uniform, and follow-up information is limited, but vaginal lymphoma appears to have a favorable prognosis.[328,337,340] Vulvar lymphomas are relatively aggressive, but occasional patients have achieved long disease-free survival.

Secondary involvement of the vagina by lymphoma is much more common than primary vaginal lymphomas.[253] In cases with widespread lymphoma presenting with vaginal involvement, the prognosis is not as favorable as for primary vaginal lymphoma of the same histologic type.[337,340] Secondary involvement of the vulva by lymphoma is rare.[342]

Differential Diagnosis of Lower Female Genital Tract Lymphomas

The most common entities in the differential diagnosis are poorly differentiated carcinomas (especially lymphoepithelioma-like carcinoma and small cell carcinoma) and a reactive lymphoid infiltrate.[253,326] Unlike carcinomas, which tend to invade and obliterate normal structures, lymphomas tend to infiltrate around them, with relative preservation of endometrial and endocervical glands and sparing of the most superficial subepithelial stroma.[253] Adjacent in situ squamous carcinoma or adenocarcinoma favors carcinoma.

Marked chronic inflammation is common in the uterus, particularly the cervix, and less often in the vagina and vulva. It is occasionally so dense and extensive that it raises the question of lymphoma. In favor of an inflammatory process are the absence of a grossly recognizable mass, a superficial location, association with erosion or ulceration of the overlying epithelium, and a polymorphic composition consisting of follicle center cells, immunoblasts, small lymphocytes, plasma cells, and neutrophils. Marked chronic inflammatory processes involving the endometrium are generally associated with areas of more typical-appearing chronic endometritis. Rarely, these lesions are associated with EBV infection.[343] In contrast, lymphomas usually produce a grossly recognizable mass with extension into adjacent structures. On microscopic examination, lymphomas tend to invade deeply, spare a narrow subepithelial zone, be composed of a monomorphic population of lymphoid cells (often with sclerosis), and spread in proximity to blood vessels.[343]

A rare entity that may raise the question of uterine lymphomas is leiomyoma with lymphoid infiltration. This designation is used for uterine leiomyomas with a moderate to dense infiltrate of small lymphocytes with scattered larger lymphoid cells, occasional germinal centers, numerous plasma cells, and, rarely, eosinophils. The inflammatory cells are largely confined to the leiomyoma. The polymorphic nature of the infiltrate and its confinement to the leiomyoma help distinguish it from lymphoma. In all reported cases of leiomyoma with lymphoid infiltration, follow-up has been uneventful.[344]

BONE

Clinical Features

Primary lymphomas of bone are defined as lymphomas arising in bone, with or without extension into adjacent soft tissue, without lymphoma elsewhere on staging. Some authorities include cases with regional lymph node involvement.[345,346] Primary lymphomas of bone have a slight male preponderance. Patients may be of any age, from young children to the elderly; however, most are adults, with a median age in the 40s or 50s.[345,347-355] Primary lymphomas of bone account for 3% of primary neoplasms of bone,[355,356] less than 1% of all lymphomas,[345,350] and approximately 5% of extranodal non-Hodgkin's lymphomas.[46] Among children, primary lymphomas of bone account for a higher proportion of non-Hodgkin's lymphomas, estimated to be 2.8% to 4.2%.[357] The cause is unknown, and there are no known risk factors.

Patients present with pain localized to the involved bone.[345,346,350,355,357] A minority also have swelling or a palpable mass, fracture, or loss of neurologic function.[350,356] Patients rarely present with constitutional symptoms.[350,357] The bones most commonly affected are the long bones of the extremities, with the femur involved most often, followed by the tibia and the humerus. Next most commonly affected are the flat bones of the shoulder and pelvis, followed by the remainder of the axial skeleton and the cranial and jaw bones.[349-351,355] Small bones of the hands and feet are only rarely involved.[349,358] In most cases the disease is monostotic; in a minority of cases it is polyostotic.[345,346,351,353,357,359] The radiographic features are not specific. Radiographic examination most often shows a destructive, lytic lesion with ill-defined margins; however, in a minority of cases the appearance is blastic or mixed blastic and lytic. Radiographs may also show soft tissue extension associated with a periosteal reaction or a pathologic fracture.[345,348,353,355,356]

Pathologic Features

In adults, nearly all primary lymphomas of bone are DLBCL. Most are composed of cells with large irregular or multilobated nuclei; a minority are composed of centroblasts with oval nuclei, immunoblasts, or bizarre pleomorphic cells.[347-349,351,352,355,360] Large cleaved cells may become elongated and resemble spindle cells.[355] Occasional cases of Burkitt's lymphoma as well as rare cases of other types of lymphoma have been reported, including T-cell and null cell anaplastic large cell lymphomas (ALK$^+$ and ALK$^-$) (Fig. 62-18),[360] B-lymphoblastic lymphoma,[361] low-grade lymphomas, peripheral T-cell lymphoma, not otherwise specified,[345] and adult T-cell lymphoma/leukemia (human T-lymphotropic virus 1 positive).[362,363]

Rare cases of classical Hodgkin's lymphoma presenting in bone have been reported,[356,364,365] and although workup reveals lymph node involvement in most cases,[365] some appear to represent primary osseous Hodgkin's lymphoma.[364] Unifocal and multifocal Hodgkin's lymphomas primary in bone have been described.[364]

In children, approximately 40% of bone lymphomas are lymphoblastic lymphoma, 10% are Burkitt's lymphoma, and 50% are DLBCL. Lymphoblastic lymphoma is more likely to be associated with high-stage disease than is DLBCL, which is more often localized.[357,361,366]

Primary DLBCL of bone expresses IgG more often than IgM,[355] in contrast to most lymphomas, which usually express IgM. Immunophenotypic features of the various lymphomas that arise in bone are otherwise similar to those seen in other sites. In one study approximately half the cases had a germinal center immunophenotype (CD10$^+$, BCL6$^+$); the remainder had an indeterminate (CD10$^-$, BCL6$^+$) or post–germinal center (CD10$^-$, BCL6$^-$) phenotype.[359] Like other extranodal DLBCLs,

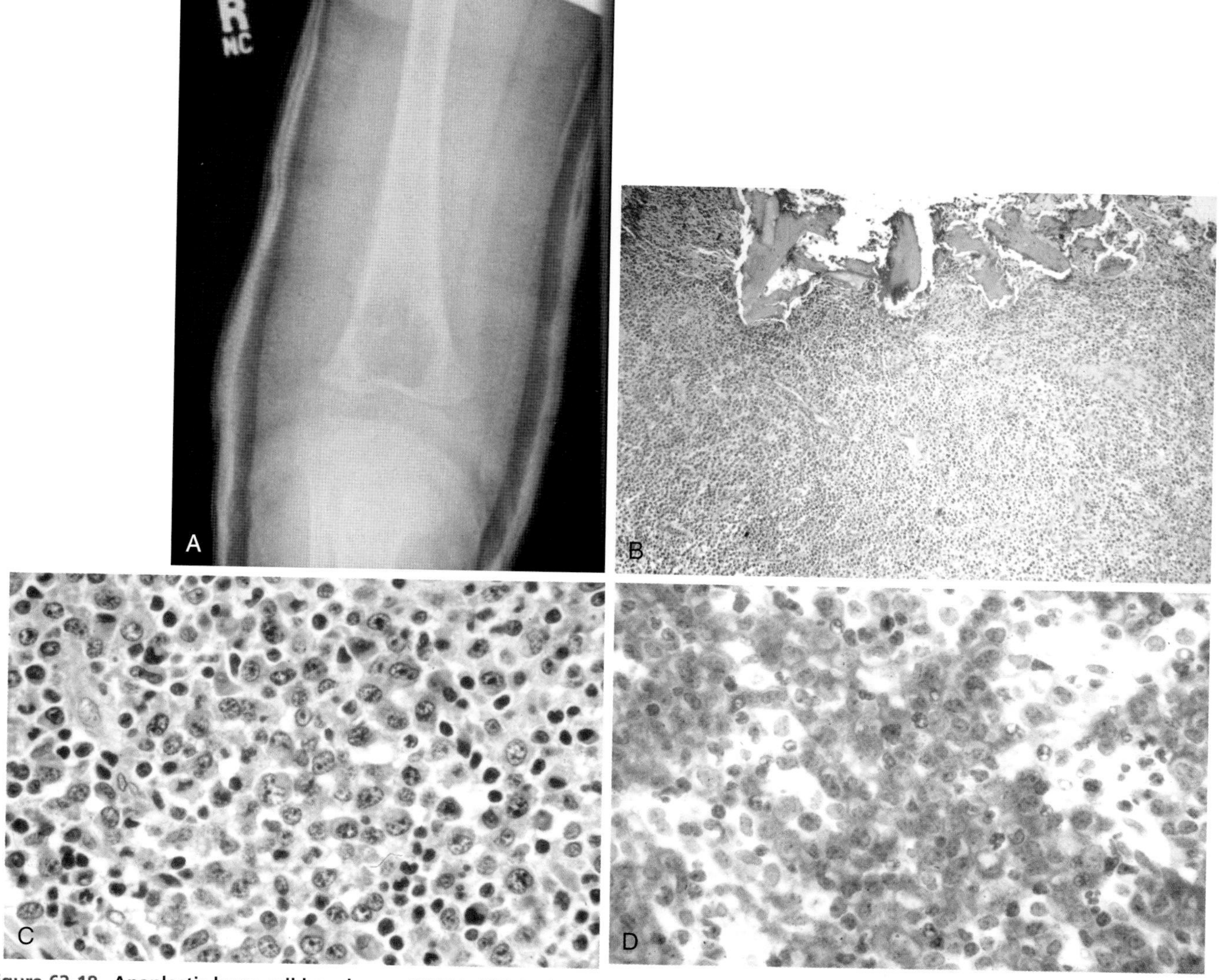

Figure 62-18. Anaplastic large cell lymphoma, CD30$^+$, ALK-1$^+$, in a child. A, A destructive lytic lesion involves the metaphysis of the distal femur. **B,** The lymphoma is associated with bony destruction. **C,** The lymphoma is composed of large atypical cells with oval or indented nuclei and pink cytoplasm. **D,** Neoplastic cells are intensely positive for CD30 (immunoperoxidase technique on a paraffin section).

and in contrast to nodal large B-cell lymphomas, the *BCL2* translocation is very uncommon.[351,359]

Staging, Treatment, and Outcome

Staging in patients presenting with apparently localized disease may reveal more widespread disease, most often involving regional lymph nodes or other bones.[347,353,359] Primary lymphoma of bone has a better prognosis than other bony malignancies.[367] Patients receiving local treatment alone (surgery, radiation) have a distant relapse rate of about 50%.[346,357,367] A combination of chemotherapy and radiation is usually recommended to increase the chance of cure.[347,350,368] Chemotherapy alone is currently the preferred treatment for children because it achieves a good outcome and may avoid complications, such as secondary sarcomas in radiated bone.[366] In patients with localized disease who are optimally staged and treated, 5-year disease-free survival may be as high as 90%.[350,366] A variety of factors can affect the prognosis. Prognosis is worse with higher-stage polyostotic disease, extension into soft tissue, primary tumor in the pelvis or spine, and older age. Lymphomas arising in a long bone have a better prognosis.[347,348,350,354,357] Among DLBCLs, a better outcome has been associated with cases composed of large irregular (cleaved) cells or multilobated cells[348,349,352,360] and a germinal center–like phenotype,[359] with a worse outcome associated with noncleaved, immunoblastic, or pleomorphic cells.[348,349]

The most common sites of relapse are other bones and lymph nodes.[345,346,351,353,355,360,366] Other sites include adjacent soft tissue, lung, bone marrow, and CNS.[355,360] Patients with lymphoblastic lymphoma may relapse in the form of acute lymphoblastic leukemia.[357,366] The strong tendency of primary bone lymphoma to spread to other bones suggests that it has homing properties that distinguish it from primary nodal lymphoma.[346]

Differential Diagnosis

Rendering the correct diagnosis may be difficult because of associated fibrosis, crush artifact, overdecalcification, small sample size, and an admixture of many reactive cells.[355,357] The differential diagnosis of bone lymphomas is broad, and in many series, lymphomas were initially misdiagnosed as other types of neoplasms or as reactive, inflammatory processes.[348,349,354,356,357] Bone lymphomas can be misdiagnosed as a reactive process such as chronic osteomyelitis[354,356,357] or as a simple fracture[356] if there is a large reactive component and neoplastic cells are present in small numbers or are not well preserved. In some cases, particularly those with associated sclerosis, neoplastic cells are elongated and resemble spindle cells, causing spindle cell sarcoma to enter the differential diagnosis.[354,355] Tumor cells may also grow in an Indian file pattern or a nested pattern, often in association with sclerosis. Some have cytoplasmic clearing and resemble signet ring cells,[354] so a diagnosis of metastatic carcinoma may be considered. Because bone lymphomas (and other neoplasms involving bone) can be associated with reactive woven bone formation, it can be misinterpreted as osteosarcoma. Eosinophilic granuloma and poorly differentiated plasmacytoma may be considered in the differential diagnosis, but cytologic features and immunophenotyping help establish a diagnosis. Myeloid sarcoma can mimic lymphomas, especially lymphoblastic lymphoma. If the myeloid sarcoma has a component of monocytes with irregular nuclei, the appearance can resemble DLBCL with large cleaved or multilobated cells. Lymphomas may also raise the consideration of a small round cell tumor, but Ewing's sarcoma has cytoplasmic glycogen and a more cohesive growth pattern and less pleomorphic nuclei than lymphoma. Neuroblastoma may present with bony metastases. The tumor cells may form rosettes; they are pear-shaped or carrot-shaped cells, with denser chromatin than lymphoma. For the rare patient with Hodgkin's lymphoma involving bone, the differential diagnosis includes acute or chronic osteomyelitis, depending on the composition of the reactive population, particularly if large neoplastic cells are present in small numbers.[364]

Pearls and Pitfalls

- The types of lymphomas encountered in extranodal sites differ to some extent from those encountered in lymph nodes. These lymphomas vary by the specific extranodal site. Familiarity with the types of lymphomas arising in different extranodal sites facilitates diagnosis.
- Carcinomas are much more common than lymphomas in many extranodal sites, and this may lead to failure to consider a diagnosis of lymphoma. Lymphoma should be considered when the specimen shows an undifferentiated-appearing malignant neoplasm.
- In certain extranodal sites, such as bone and the lower female genital tract, crush artifact may be a significant barrier to establishing a diagnosis. In such cases pathologists should request more tissue until an adequate specimen is obtained.
- Certain types of extranodal lymphomas tend to occur in certain age groups or ethnic groups or in association with underlying immunodeficiency or autoimmune disorders. Clinical correlation is important in establishing the correct diagnosis.
- Infectious mononucleosis can mimic both classical Hodgkin's lymphoma and diffuse large B-cell lymphoma; infectious mononucleosis should be considered in the differential diagnosis of atypical lymphoid proliferations in Waldeyer's ring, especially in young patients.
- Certain extranodal diffuse large B-cell lymphomas, such as primary effusion lymphoma and plasmablastic lymphoma, are characteristically $CD20^-$. If morphology suggests lymphoma and CD20 is negative, the possibility of lymphoma should not be excluded until immunostaining with a broader panel of markers is performed.

References can be found on Expert Consult @ www.expertconsult.com

Appendix

Staining Techniques

Phuong L. Nguyen

SETUP

Preparation of Buffy Coat Smears

Aspirate 1 mL of fluid marrow into a syringe *without* anticoagulant. Then, as quickly as possible, transfer most of it into a paraffin-coated vial to which disodium EDTA powder has been added (1 mg EDTA for 1 to 2 mL marrow; 0.5 mg EDTA for <1 mL marrow). (Save a few drops of the remaining un-anticoagulated marrow aspirate in the syringe for preparing direct smears.) Invert the vial several times to mix. Pour this mixture of EDTA-anticoagulated marrow into a Petri dish. Using a Pasteur pipette, transfer the fluid component to a 1-mL Wintrobe hematocrit tube. When the tube is filled, cap it with parafilm and centrifuge it at 2800 revolutions per minute for 8 to 10 minutes. This results in the separation of the marrow aspirate into four layers, from top to bottom:

1. Fat and perivascular layer. Using a pipette, transfer this white, cloudy top layer onto a slide and crush it with another slide. Because of the relatively increased number of macrophages associated with perivascular tissue, the crush preparation of this layer is excellent for assessing storage iron.
2. Plasma layer. Remove this clear layer and set it aside.
3. Buffy coat layer. This layer, also known as the myeloid-erythroid layer, is rich in nucleated cells. Transfer it onto a clean, paraffin-lined Petri dish, and mix gently and thoroughly with two volumes of plasma. Place individual drops of this mixture on 6 to 10 glass slides, and prepare push smears using a spreader device. These smears should be dried quickly before being used for routine Wright-Giemsa staining, Dacie staining, or other special cytochemical staining. This buffy coat layer can also be used for ultrastructural studies by electron microscopy when needed (see later).
4. Erythrocyte layer. Discard.

Preparation of Marrow Samples for Electron Microscopic Examination

To collect a marrow sample for ultrastructural studies by electron microscopy, aspirate 1 mL of fluid marrow and transfer it to a paraffin-coated vial into which powdered disodium EDTA has already been added (1 mg EDTA for 1 to 2 mL marrow aspirate). Process the EDTA-anticoagulated marrow mixture to obtain the buffy coat layer (described earlier). Then follow these steps:

1. Discard the fat and perivascular and plasma layers.
2. Layer a few drops of cold 4% glutaraldehyde on top of the buffy coat and allow to stand for 15 to 20 minutes.
3. To fix the lower layer, score the Wintrobe tube at the lower reading where the buffy coat layer meets the erythrocyte layer, crack the tube cleanly, and place the cracked end of the tube with the exposed lower layer into cold 4% glutaraldehyde for 15 to 20 minutes while retaining the top portion of the Wintrobe tube that contains the buffy coat.
4. To remove the now partially fixed buffy coat layer, push it out and into another vial of fresh, cold 4% glutaraldehyde for an additional 15 to 20 minutes, then cut the layer cleanly into 1-mm cubes while still in glutaraldehyde to optimize fixation.

The specimen can remain as such, or it can be transferred to fresh glutaraldehyde, where it can stay for up to 2 weeks at 4°C before processing. To demonstrate platelet peroxidase by electron microscopy, tannic acid is used as a fixative instead of glutaraldehyde, and other specific modifications to the processing procedure are required before electron microscopic examination.[1,2]

STAINING PROCEDURES

Hematoxylin-Eosin Staining of Sections

Harris hematoxylin is a regressive stain in which sections are overstained in a neutral solution of hematoxylin. The excess stain is removed by acid alcohol and then neutralized by an alkaline solution.

Reagents

Reagent	Mixture
Harris hematoxylin; eosin Y	
Stock acid alcohol	9.5 mL concentrated hydrochloric acid (37%) in 950 mL 70% ethanol
Working acid alcohol	70% ethanol in stock acid alcohol in 1:1 volume
Bluing reagent	3 to 4 drops of 28% ammonium hydroxide (NH_4OH) in 250 mL deionized or distilled water
5% sodium thiosulfate ($Na_2S_2O_3 \bullet 5H_2O$)	Dissolve in distilled or deionized water
Stock iodine solution	Iodine crystals in 70% ethanol to saturate
Working iodine solution	Stock iodine solution in 70% ethanol to make an amber-colored solution

Fixatives

Zenker's, B5 fixative, or formalin (omit steps 5 and 6 with formalin fixation).

Procedure

Heat-fix mounted sections in a 60°C to 70°C oven for 45 minutes.

Step	Task	Solution	Repetition/Duration
1	Immerse slides	Xylol	2 changes for 5 minutes each
2	Immerse slides	100% ethanol	2 changes for 3 minutes each
3	Immerse slides	95% ethanol	2 changes for 3 minutes each
4	Immerse slides	70% ethanol	3 minutes
5	Immerse slides	Working iodine solution	6 minutes
6	Rinse to remove excess iodine	Deionized water	
7	Immerse slides	5% sodium thiosulfate	6 minutes
8	Wash	Running tap water	5 minutes
9	Rinse slides	Deionized water	10 dips
10	Immerse slides	Bluing solution	1 minute
11	Rinse	Deionized water	10 dips
12	Immerse slides	Hematoxylin	5 minutes for particle clot sections 20-40 minutes for Zenker's-fixed bone cores 5-10 minutes for Formalin-fixed bone cores 5-10 minutes for B5-fixed bone cores
13	Rinse to remove excess hematoxylin	Running tap water	
14	Dip	Acid alcohol	1 dip (may vary according to tissue)
15	Rinse to remove excess acid alcohol	Running tap water	
16	Rinse	Deionized water	
17	Dip slides	Bluing solution	10 slow dips
18	Wash	Running tap water	5 minutes
19	Check hematoxylin staining		If too light, repeat steps 10-18 If too dark, repeat steps 14-18
20	Immerse slides	70% ethanol	3 minutes
21	Dip	Eosin	2-5 dips (formalin- and B5-fixed tissue may require more time)
22	Dip slides	70% ethanol	4 changes, 3 dips each
23	Immerse slides	95% ethanol	2 changes, 10 dips each
24	Immerse slides	100% ethanol	2 changes, 3 minutes each
25	Immerse slides	100% ethanol/ xylol	3 minutes
26	Immerse slides Check eosin in first change of xylol	Xylol	3 changes, 3 minutes each If too light, process back through solutions to 70% ethanol, and repeat steps 21-26 If too dark, process back through solutions to 95% ethanol (or 70% ethanol if very dark), and repeat steps 23-26
27	Cover slip	Micromount, Permount, or other organic solvent mounting medium	

STAINS

Wilder's Reticulin Stain

Sections are treated with phosphomolybdic acid, which acts as an oxidizer to enhance the impregnation of fibers; this step is followed by a uranyl nitrate solution, which acts as a sensitizer. This procedure initiates deposits of silver when the sections are exposed to silver hydroxide. The reducing solution (uranium nitrate plus formaldehyde) reduces silver to develop the color on the fibers; toning is with gold chloride, an oxide. Unreduced silver is then removed by sodium thiosulfate.

Reagents

Reagent	Mixture
10% phosphomolybdic acid ($P_2O_5 \bullet 24MoO_3 \times H_2O$) solution	
1% uranium nitrate ($UO_2[NO_3]_2 \bullet 6H_2O$) solution	
28% ammonium hydroxide (NH_4OH)	
3.1% sodium hydroxide (NaOH)	
10.2% silver nitrate ($AgNO_3$)	
Neutral formaldehyde	5 g calcium carbonate ($CaCO_3$) powder in 50 mL 37% formaldehyde
Reducing solution	0.5 mL 37% neutral formaldehyde and 1.5 mL 1% uranium nitrate in 50 mL deionized water (make the solution fresh, just before use)
1% gold chloride solution ($HAuCl_4 \bullet 3H_2O$)	
Working gold chloride solution	5 mL 1% gold chloride solution in 45 mL deionized water
5% sodium thiosulfate ($Na_2S_2O_3 \bullet 5H_2O$) solution	
Counterstain (optional)	1% safranin O
Working ammoniacal silver solution	To 5 mL 10.2% silver nitrate, add 28% ammonium hydroxide, drop by drop, until the precipitate that forms is almost dissolved; then add 5 mL 3.1% sodium hydroxide, followed by 28% ammonium hydroxide, drop by drop, until the resulting precipitate is just dissolved (approximately 20-25 drops); back-titrate with 10.2% silver nitrate until a faint turbidity remains (approximately 20-25 drops); dilute resulting ammoniacal silver solution with deionized water, up to 50 mL; *use at once*

Fixatives

Formalin, Zenker's, or B5 fixative.

Procedure

Note: If beginning with hematoxylin-eosin-stained sections, can decolorize with acid alcohol, then perform reticulin stain.

Step	Task	Solution	Repetition/ Duration
1	Deparaffinize sections	Deionized water; if necessary, remove mercury deposits with iodine solution and 5% sodium thiosulfate	
2	Wash	Deionized water	3 changes
3	Immerse slides	10% phosphomolybdic acid (to oxidize)	2 minutes
4	Wash	Running tap water	1 minute
5	Rinse	Deionized water	10-15 dips
6	Immerse slides	1% aqueous uranium nitrate (to sensitize)	2 minutes
7	Rinse	Deionized water	10-15 dips
8	Immerse slides	Working ammoniacal silver solution	2 minutes
9	Dip quickly	50% ethanol	1 quick dip
10	Immerse slides	Reducing solution	2 minutes
11	Rinse well	Deionized water	
12	Dip slides	Working gold chloride solution	Until sections lose yellow background color
	Dip slides (in working gold chloride solution) and rinse (in deionized water)	Gold chloride solution	Check toning under microscope, until completed
	Rinse	Deionized water	
13	Rinse well	Deionized water	
14	Dip slides to remove excess silver	5% sodium thiosulfate	2-3 dips
15	Wash	Running tap water	5 minutes
16	Counterstain (optional)	0.1% safranin O	3-5 dips
17	Rinse	Deionized water	15-16 dips
18	Dehydrate	70%, 95%, and 100% ethanol through xylene or xylene substitute	
19	Cover slip	Micromount or Permount	

Results: reticulin fibers should be black; collagen should be rose colored

Wright-Giemsa Stain for Smears

The Wright polychrome stain is a Romanowsky stain composed of methylene blue, oxidative products of methylene blue (azures), and eosin dyes. Giemsa, which contains azures, is added to the stain to intensify nuclear features and azurophilic and toxic granulation.

Reagents

Stock Wright-Giemsa Stain Solution	Combine as Follows
• 13 g Wright stain dry powder (Richard Allen. Kalamazoo, MI) • 3 g Wright stain dry powder (Fisher Scientific. Houston, TX) • 0.4 g Giemsa stain dry powder in 4 L absolute methyl alcohol (CH_3OH); methyl alcohol must be free of acetone	• Rinse reagent bottle twice with methanol • Pour 2 L methanol into prerinsed reagent bottle • Add magnetic stirrer and mix • Add weighted amount of Wright stain powders and Giemsa stain powder • Add remaining 2 L of methanol • Cover top and mix for 2-3 hours; incubate overnight at 37.5°C • Next day, mix again for 2-3 hours • Filter with doubled filter paper before using

Other Reagents	Mixture
Methanol	
Giemsa stain solution (Richard Allen Scientific—# 89002)	
Phosphate buffer (pH 6.4 ± 0.05)	26.52 g potassium monobasic phosphate (KH_2PO_4) and 10.24 g sodium dibasic phosphate (Na_2HPO_4) in 4 L deionized water
Working Wright-Giemsa buffer solution	25 mL stock Wright-Giemsa stain solution and 25 mL Giemsa stain solution in 200 mL stock phosphate buffer (expires in 1 hour)

Dip Procedure for Wright-Giemsa Stain with Slide Holders

Procedure

1. Place slides in the slide holder, feather edge up.
2. Fix in staining dish of methyl alcohol (acetone free) for 2 minutes.
3. Move to stock Wright-Giemsa stain for 4 minutes; agitate a few times.
4. Move to working Wright-Giemsa buffer solution for 20-25 minutes; agitate a few times. Staining time may vary with each batch of Wright stain.
5. Rinse stain off in staining dish of approximately 5 mL methanol/200 mL deionized water.
6. Rinse in three consecutive staining dishes of deionized water—6 to 8 dips each. The deionized water should be changed after each batch.
7. Optional: Wipe dye from back of slide if present (this step is usually not necessary).
8. Place in a slide rack in a vertical position to air-dry under a fan.

Notes

- Be sure the slide holder is dry before placing slides in it; the slide holder can be rinsed in a separate boat of methyl alcohol to clean it and remove water.
- Change methyl alcohol and stock Wright-Giemsa stain each day.
- Change Wright-Giemsa buffer solution after 2 batches of slides or after 1 hour, even if used less than twice.
- If stain is too light, reprocess stained slides in stock Wright-Giemsa stain and Wright-Giemsa buffer solution.
- Because of the difficulty of controlling staining quality, my laboratory no longer uses a flat-rack staining procedure.

Results

- Erythrocytes: salmon pink
- Leukocyte and megakaryocyte nuclei: purple-blue
- Platelets: purple-blue to lilac cytoplasm containing red-purple granules

Iron Stains

The Prussian blue stain detects the presence of nonhemoglobin iron (Fe^{+++}) in the form of a blue-green insoluble compound that is seen mainly in erythrocytes (siderocytes), normoblasts (sideroblasts), and reticuloendothelial cells. The reaction must take place in an acidic environment to free iron from binding proteins.

Dacie Method for Unstained Aspirate Smears

Reagent	Mixture
Stock Iron Reagents	
2% potassium ferrocyanide ($K_4Fe[CN]_6 \bullet 3H_2O$)	Solution is pale to moderate yellow, is stored in the dark, and expires in 1 week
0.2N hydrochloric acid	16.7 mL 37% hydrochloric acid in 983.3 mL deionized water
Other Reagents	
Working Dacie iron reagent	2% ($K_4Fe[CN]_6 \bullet 3H_2O$) in 0.2N hydrochloric acid in 1:1 volume (solution is pale yellow) Note: The solution should be made just before use (it expires in 1 hour) and can be used *once*
0.1% aqueous safranin O	

Procedure. Specimens consist of air-dried films of peripheral blood; bone marrow aspirate, including buffy coat smears; cellular fluids; or cytospins of urine sediment. Crush preparations are not satisfactory because fat is dissolved by the methanol.

Procedure

1. Fix in absolute methanol—15 minutes.
2. Air-dry under a fan—do not wash.
3. Incubate slides in working Dacie iron solution in a 50°C to 56°C oven for 10 minutes. (Note: excessive heat or prolonged incubation can alter the reaction.)
4. Rinse with deionized water.
5. Wash in running tap water—20 minutes.
6. Rinse with deionized water. Do not dry (drying before counterstaining may cause artifact).
7. Counterstain with 0.1% safranin O—10-20 seconds (may use 0.1% eosin).
8. Rinse with deionized water, and air-dry under a fan.

Results

- Diffuse and particulate iron: vivid blue to blue-green
- Nuclei: bright pink
- Cytoplasm: pale pink

Prussian Blue Reaction on Crush Preparations of Fat-Perivascular Layer

Reagent	Mixture
Fixative	10% formalin fumes Place a piece of filter paper in the lid of a Coplin jar, and place 2 small drops of 10% formalin (10 mL 37% formaldyhyde in 90 mL deonizied water) on the filter paper for each use
Stock iron reagent	2% potassium cyanide ($K_4Fe[CN]_6 \bullet 3H_2O$) Solution is pale to moderate yellow, is stored in the dark, and expires in 1 week
Working iron reagent	15 mL 2% potassium ferro cyanide ($K_4Fe[CN]_6 \bullet 3H_2O$) in 45 mL 0.5% hydrochloric acid
0.5% hydrochloric acid	Solution is filtered into a Coplin jar, is pale yellow, and should be made just before use

Procedure. Note that crush preparations are from the fat and perivascular layer, which results from preparation of the marrow's buffy coat. If no layer is present, a particle crush preparation can be used.

Procedure

1. Fix dried film in a Coplin jar with weak formalin vapors (10% formalin)—10 minutes. (Excess formalin causes a black granular precipitate.)
2. Do not wash.
3. Immerse in working iron reagent—10 minutes.
4. Wash thoroughly with deionized water.
5. Wash under running tap water—2 minutes.
6. Air-dry under a fan.
7. Coverslip with a solvent-soluble mounting medium, if desired.

Results

- Diffuse and particulate iron: vivid blue or blue-green

References can be found on Expert Consult @ www.expertconsult.com

Index

A

Note: Page numbers followed by b, f, and t indicate boxes, figures and tables, respectively.

D

E

F

G

H

J

K

L

M

O

P

Q

R

S

T